Gastrointestinal Disease

Volume 1

Pathophysiology
Diagnosis
Management

FOURTH EDITION

MARVIN H. SLEISENGER, M.D.

Professor of Medicine
Vice Chairman for Academic Affairs
Department of Medicine
Director, Clinical Training Program in Gastroenterology
University of California, San Francisco
Attending Physician, Moffitt-Long Hospital
San Francisco, California

JOHN S. FORDTRAN, M.D.

Professor of Medicine,
Chief, Department of Internal Medicine,
Baylor University Medical Center,
Dallas, Texas

with a foreword by

THOMAS P. ALMY, M.D.

1989

W.B. SAUNDERS COMPANY
Harcourt Brace Jovanovich, Inc.
Philadelphia London Toronto Montreal Sydney Tokyo

Gastrointestinal Disease

Volume 1

Pathophysiology
Diagnosis
Management

FOURTH EDITION

W. B. SAUNDERS COMPANY
Harcourt Brace Jovanovich, Inc.

The Curtis Center
Independence Square West
Philadelphia, PA 19106

Library of Congress Cataloging-in-Publication Data

Gastrointestinal disease: pathophysiology, diagnosis,
  management/ [edited by] Marvin Sleisenger, John S.
  Fordtran; with a foreword by Thomas P. Almy.—4th ed.
    p. cm.

Includes bibliographical references and index.

ISBN 0–7216–2298–4 (set)

1. Gastrointestinal system—Diseases. I. Sleisenger,
  Marvin H. II. Fordtran, John S.

RC801.G384 1989

616.3'3—dc19   88–15668

Listed here is the latest translated edition of this book together
with the language of the translation and the publisher.

Italian *(3rd Edition)*—Piccin Nuova Libraria S.P.A., Padova, Italy.
Spanish *(3rd Edition)*—Panamericana, Buenos Aires, Argentina.
Portuguese *(2nd Edition)*—Editora Guanabara Koogan S.A., Rio de Janeiro, Brazil.

Editor: Edward Wickland
Developmental Editor: David Kilmer
Designer: W. B. Saunders Staff
Production Manager: Bob Butler
Manuscript Editor: Mark Coyle
Illustration Coordinator: Peg Shaw
Indexer: Helene Taylor

Single Volume	ISBN	0–7216–2078–7
Volume I	ISBN	0–7216–2079–5
Volume II	ISBN	0–7216–2080–9
Set	ISBN	0–7216–2298–4

Gastrointestinal Disease

Last digit is the print number: 9   8   7   6   5   4   3

CONTRIBUTORS

THOMAS P. ALMY, M.D.
Professor of Medicine and Community and Family Medicine, Emeritus, Dartmouth Medical School; Staff Member, Mary Hitchcock Memorial Hospital, Hanover, New Hampshire, and Veterans Administration Hospital, White River Junction, Vermont
Diverticular Disease of the Colon

DAVID H. ALPERS, M.D.
Professor of Medicine and Chief, Gastroenterology Division, Washington University School of Medicine; Physician, Barnes Hospital, St. Louis, Missouri
Absorption of Vitamins and Divalent Minerals; Eating Behavior and Nutrient Requirements; Nutritional Deficiency in Gastrointestinal Disease; Dietary Management and Vitamin-Mineral Replacement Therapy

DAVID F. ALTMAN, M.D.
Associate Dean of Student and Curricular Affairs, University of California, San Francisco, School of Medicine; Director, Gastroenterology Clinic, University of California Medical Center, San Francisco, California
The Effect of Age on Gastrointestinal Function; Neoplasms of the Gallbladder and Bile Ducts

MARVIN E. AMENT, M.D.
Professor of Pediatrics, University of California, Los Angeles, School of Medicine; Chief, Division of Pediatric Gastroenterology and Nutrition, and Chief, Hospital Parenteral and Enteral Nutritional Support Service, UCLA Medical Center, Los Angeles, California
The Stomach and Duodenum: Anatomy, Embryology, and Developmental Anomalies

JAMES L. AUSTIN, M.D.
Assistant Professor of Surgery, University of Missouri School of Medicine; Staff Surgeon, Truman Veterans Administration Hospital, Columbia, Missouri
Abdominal Abscesses and Gastrointestinal Fistulas

JOHN G. BARTLETT, M.D.
Professor of Medicine, Johns Hopkins University School of Medicine; Chief of Infectious Diseases Division, Johns Hopkins Hospital, Baltimore, Maryland
The Pseudomembranous Enterocolitides

THEODORE M. BAYLESS, M.D.
Professor of Medicine, Johns Hopkins University School of Medicine; Medical Director, Meyerhoff Digestive Disease–Inflammatory Bowel Disease Center, Johns Hopkins Hospital, Baltimore, Maryland
Small Intestinal Ulcers and Strictures: Isolated and Diffuse

MICHAEL D. BENDER, M.D.
Associate Clinical Professor of Medicine and Family and Community Medicine, University of California, San Francisco, School of Medicine, San Francisco, California; Chief of Medicine and Director of Medical Education, Peninsula Hospital, Burlingame, California
Ascites; Diseases of the Peritoneum, Mesentery, and Diaphragm

JEFFREY A. BILLER, M.D.
Assistant Clinical Professor of Pediatrics, Tufts University School of Medicine; Pediatric Gastroenterologist, Division of Pediatric Gas-

troenterology and Nutrition, The Floating Hospital, New England Medical Center, Boston, Massachusetts
Pancreatic Disorders in Childhood

HENRY J. BINDER, M.D.
Professor of Medicine and Director, Gastrointestinal Research Training Program, Yale University School of Medicine; Director, General Clinical Research Center, Yale–New Haven Medical Center, New Haven, Connecticut
Absorption and Secretion of Water and Electrolytes by Small and Large Intestine

C. RICHARD BOLAND, M.D.
Associate Professor of Medicine, University of Michigan Medical School; Chief of Gastroenterology, Ann Arbor Veterans Administration Medical Center, Ann Arbor, Michigan
Colonic Polyps and the Gastrointestinal Polyposis Syndromes

GEORGE W. BO-LINN, M.D.
St. John's Mercy Medical Center, St. Louis, Missouri
Obesity, Anorexia Nervosa, Bulimia, and Other Eating Disorders

JOHN H. BOND, M.D.
Professor of Medicine, University of Minnesota; Chief, Gastroenterology Section, Veterans Administration Medical Center, Minneapolis, Minnesota
Intestinal Gas

H. WORTH BOYCE, JR., M.S., M.D.
Professor of Medicine; Director, Division of Digestive Diseases and Nutrition; Director, The Center for Swallowing Disorders, University of South Florida College of Medicine, Tampa, Florida
Tumors of the Esophagus

ROBERT S. BRESALIER, M.D.
Assistant Professor of Medicine, University of California, San Francisco, School of Medicine; Attending Physician, Veterans Administration Medical Center, San Francisco, California
Malignant Neoplasms of the Large and Small Intestine

JOHN P. CELLO, M.D.
Associate Professor of Medicine, University of California, San Francisco, School of Medicine; Chief of Gastroenterology, San Francisco General Hospital, San Francisco, California
Ulcerative Colitis; Chronic Pancreatitis; Carcinoma of the Pancreas

RAY E. CLOUSE, M.D.
Assistant Professor of Medicine, Washington University School of Medicine; Assistant Physician, Barnes Hospital, St. Louis, Missouri
Motor Disorders of the Esophagus; Intensive Nutritional Support

SIDNEY COHEN, M.D.
Professor, Temple University School of Medicine; Chairman, Department of Medicine, Temple University Hospital, Philadelphia, Pennsylvania
Movement of the Small and Large Intestine

JEFFREY CONKLIN, M.D.
Assistant Professor, Division of Gastroenterology, Department of Internal Medicine, University of Iowa Hospitals and Clinics, Iowa City, Iowa
Gastrointestinal Smooth Muscle

JEFFREY R. CRIST, M.D.

Instructor in Medicine, Harvard Medical School; Assistant in Medicine, Gastroenterology Division, Beth Israel Hospital, Boston, Massachusetts
Neurology of the Gut

GLENN R. DAVIS, M.D.

Assistant Clinical Professor, University of Arkansas for Medical Science; Staff Physician, St. Vincent Infirmary, Little Rock, Arkansas
Neoplasms of the Stomach

JOHN DELVALLE, M.D.

Instructor of Internal Medicine, Division of Gastroenterology, University of Michigan Medical School, Ann Arbor, Michigan
Secretory Tumors of the Pancreas

GHISLAIN DEVROEDE, M.D.

Professor of Surgery and Physiology, Université de Sherbrooke; Attending Physician, Centre Hospitalier Universitaire, Sherbrooke, Québec, Canada
Constipation

NICHOLAS E. DIAMANT, M.D., F.R.C.P.(C)

Professor of Medicine and Physiology, University of Toronto; Head, Division of Gastroenterology, Toronto Western Hospital, Toronto, Ontario, Canada
Physiology of the Esophagus

WYLIE J. DODDS, M.D.

Professor of Radiology and Medicine, Medical College of Wisconsin; Staff Radiologist, Milwaukee County Medical Center and Froedtert Memorial Lutheran Hospital, Milwaukee, Wisconsin
Gastroesophageal Reflux Disease (Reflux Esophagitis)

ROBERT M. DONALDSON, JR., M.D.

David Paige Smith Professor of Medicine, Yale University School of Medicine; Attending Physician, Yale–New Haven Hospital, New Haven, Connecticut
The Relation of Enteric Bacterial Populations to Gastrointestinal Function and Disease; The Blind Loop Syndrome; Crohn's Disease

DOUGLAS A. DROSSMAN, M.D.

Associate Professor of Medicine and Psychiatry, Division of Digestive Diseases, University of North Carolina School of Medicine; Associate Attending, North Carolina Memorial Hospital, Chapel Hill, North Carolina
The Physician and the Patient: Review of the Psychosocial Gastrointestinal Literature with an Integrated Approach to the Patient

DAVID L. EARNEST, M.D.

Professor of Medicine, University of Arizona College of Medicine; Attending Physician, Gastroenterology Section, University of Arizona Health Sciences Center, Tucson, Arizona
Radiation Enteritis and Colitis; Other Diseases of the Colon and Rectum

ABRAM M. EISENSTEIN, M.D.

Clinical Professor of Medicine, University of Texas Southwestern Medical School at Dallas; Chief of Gastroenterology, Presbyterian Hospital of Dallas; Attending Physician, Parkland Memorial Hospital, Dallas, Texas
Caustic Injury to the Upper Gastrointestinal Tract

THOMAS H. ERMAK, Ph.D.

Assistant Research Cell Biologist, Department of Medicine, University of California, San Francisco, School of Medicine; Attending Staff, Cell Biology and Aging Section, Veterans Administration Medical Center, San Francisco, California
The Pancreas: Anatomy, Histology, Embryology, and Developmental Anomalies

ANTHONY S. FAUCI, M.D.

Director, National Institute of Allergy and Infectious Diseases, National Institutes of Health, Bethesda, Maryland
Acquired Immunodeficiency Syndrome (AIDS)

MARK FELDMAN, M.D.

Professor of Internal Medicine, University of Texas Southwestern Medical School at Dallas; Associate Chief of Staff for Research and Development, Dallas Veterans Administration Medical Center, Dallas, Texas
Nausea and Vomiting; Gastric Secretion in Health and Disease

KENNETH D. FINE, M.D.

Resident in Internal Medicine, Baylor University Medical Center, Dallas, Texas
Diarrhea

JOHN S. FORDTRAN, M.D.

Professor of Medicine and Chief, Department of Internal Medicine, Baylor University Medical Center, Dallas, Texas
Diarrhea

SCOTT L. FRIEDMAN, M.D.

Assistant Professor of Medicine, University of California, San Francisco, School of Medicine; Attending Physician, San Francisco General Hospital, San Francisco, California
Gastrointestinal Manifestations of AIDS and Other Sexually Transmissible Diseases

SHERWOOD L. GORBACH, M.D.

Professor of Community Health and Medicine, Tufts University School of Medicine, Boston, Massachusetts
Infectious Diarrhea

RAJ K. GOYAL, M.D.

Charlotte F. and Irving W. Rabb Professor of Medicine, Harvard Medical School; Chief, Gastroenterology Division, Beth Israel Hospital, Boston, Massachusetts
Neurology of the Gut; Gastrointestinal Smooth Muscle

DAVID Y. GRAHAM, M.D.

Professor of Medicine and Virology, Baylor College of Medicine; Chief of Digestive Disease Division, Veterans Administration Medical Center, Houston, Texas
Complications of Peptic Ulcer Disease and Indications for Surgery

RICHARD J. GRAND, M.D.

Professor of Pediatrics, Tufts University School of Medicine; Chief, Division of Pediatric Gastroenterology and Nutrition, The Floating Hospital, New England Medical Center, Boston, Massachusetts
Pancreatic Disorders in Childhood

JAMES H. GRENDELL, M.D.

Assistant Professor of Medicine and Physiology, University of California, San Francisco, School of Medicine; Attending Physician, San Francisco General Hospital, San Francisco, California
The Pancreas: Anatomy, Histology, and Developmental Anomalies; Chronic Pancreatitis; Vascular Diseases of the Bowel

J. KENT HAMILTON, M.D.

Clinical Instructor of Medicine, University of Texas Southwestern Medical School at Dallas; Attending Physician, Baylor University Medical Center, Dallas, Texas
Foreign Bodies in the Gut

MELVIN B. HEYMAN, M.D., M.P.H.

Assistant Professor, Department of Pediatrics, University of California, San Francisco, School of Medicine; Associate Director, Division of Pediatric Gastroenterology and Nutrition, University of California Children's Medical Center, San Francisco, California
Food Sensitivity and Eosinophilic Gastroenteropathies

MARTIN F. HEYWORTH, M.D., M.R.C.P.

Associate Professor of Medicine, University of California, San Francisco, School of Medicine; Staff Physician, Veterans Administration Medical Center, San Francisco, California
Maldigestion and Malabsorption

ALAN F. HOFMANN, M.D., Ph.D.

Professor of Medicine in Gastroenterology, University of California, San Diego, School of Medicine; Professor of Medicine, University of California, San Diego, Medical Center
The Enterohepatic Circulation of Bile Acids in Health and Disease

WALTER J. HOGAN, M.D.

Professor of Medicine, Medical College of Wisconsin; Chief, Gastrointestinal Diagnostic Laboratory, Froedtert Memorial Lutheran Hospital, Milwaukee, Wisconsin
Gastroesophageal Reflux Disease (Reflux Esophagitis)

R. THOMAS HOLZBACH, M.D.

Head, Gastrointestinal Research Unit, Research Institute, and Department of Gastroenterology, Cleveland Clinic Foundation, Cleveland, Ohio
Pathogenesis and Medical Treatment of Gallstones

STEVEN H. ITZKOWITZ, M.D.

Assistant Professor of Medicine, University of California, San Francisco, School of Medicine; Research Associate, Veterans Administration Medical Center, San Francisco, California
Chronic Polyps and the Gastrointestinal Polyposis Syndromes

GRAHAM H. JEFFRIES, M.S., Ch.B. (N.Z.), D. Phil. (Oxon), F.A.C.P.

Professor and Chairman, Department of Medicine, Pennsylvania State University College of Medicine, Hershey, Pennsylvania
Protein-Losing Gastroenteropathy

R. SCOTT JONES, M.D.

Stephen H. Watts Professor and Chairman, Department of Surgery, University of Virginia; Surgeon-in-Chief, University of Virginia Medical Center, Charlottesville, Virginia
Intestinal Obstruction, Pseudo-Obstruction, and Ileus

PAUL H. JORDAN, JR., M.D.

Professor of Surgery, Baylor College of Medicine; Senior Attending Surgeon, The Methodist Hospital, Houston, Texas
Operations for Peptic Ulcer Disease and Early Postoperative Complications

MARTIN F. KAGNOFF, M.D.

Professor of Medicine, University of California, San Diego, School of Medicine; Attending Physician, University of California, San Diego, Medical Center, San Diego, California
Immunology and Disease of the Gastrointestinal Tract

GORDON L. KAUFFMAN, JR., M.D.

Professor of Surgery and Physiology, and Chief, Division of General Surgery, The Milton S. Hershey Medical Center, Pennsylvania State University, Hershey, Pennsylvania
Stress Ulcers, Erosions, and Gastric Mucosal Injury

YOUNG S. KIM, M.D.

Professor of Medicine and Pathology, University of California, San Francisco, School of Medicine; Director, Gastrointestinal Research Laboratory, Veterans Administration Medical Center, San Francisco, California
Colonic Polyps and the Gastrointestinal Polyposis Syndromes; Malignant Neoplasms of the Large and Small Intestine

FREDERICK A. KLIPSTEIN, M.D.

Professor of Medicine, University of Rochester; Attending Physician, Strong Memorial Hospital, Rochester, New York
Tropical Sprue

O. DHODANAND KOWLESSAR, M.D.

Professor of Medicine and Associate Chairman, Department of Medicine, Jefferson Medical College of Thomas Jefferson University, Philadelphia, Pennsylvania
The Carcinoid Syndrome

GUENTER J. KREJS, M.D.

Professor and Chairman, Department of Internal Medicine, Karl Franzens University, Graz, Austria
Diarrhea

MICHAEL D. LEVITT, M.D.

Professor of Medicine, University of Minnesota; Associate Chief of Staff for Research, Veterans Administration Medical Center, Minneapolis, Minnesota
Intestinal Gas

MARVIN LIPSKY, M.D.

Research Fellow in Medicine, Harvard Medical School; Research/ Clinical Fellow in Medicine, Brigham and Women's Hospital, Boston, Massachusetts
The Short Bowel Syndrome

PETER M. LOEB, M.D.

Clinical Professor of Medicine, University of Texas Southwestern Medical School at Dallas; Gastroenterologist, Presbyterian Hospital; Attending Gastroenterologist, Parkland Memorial Hospital and Veterans Administration Medical Center, Dallas, Texas
Caustic Injury to the Upper Gastrointestinal Tract

TIMOTHY P. MARONEY, M.D.

Assistant Professor of Radiology, University of California, San Francisco, School of Medicine; Attending Physician, University of California Medical Center, San Francisco, California
Endoscopic/Radiologic Treatment of Biliary Tract Diseases

HENRY MASUR, M.D.

Deputy Chief, Critical Care Medicine Department, Clinical Center, National Institutes of Health, Bethesda, Maryland; Clinical Professor of Medicine, George Washington University School of Medicine, Washington, D.C.
Acquired Immunodeficiency Syndrome (AIDS)

RICHARD W. McCALLUM, M.D., F.A.C.P., F.R.A.C.P. (Aust.), F.A.C.S.

Paul Janssen Professor of Medicine, University of Virginia School of Medicine; Chief, Division of Gastroenterology, University of Virginia Medical Center, Charlottesville, Virginia; Director of Gastrointestinal Fellowship Program at University of Virginia and Salem Veterans Administration Center, Salem, Virginia
Motor Function of the Stomach in Health and Disease

GEORGE B. McDONALD, M.D.

Professor of Medicine, University of Washington School of Medicine; Attending Physician, Veterans Administration Medical Center, Fred Hutchinson Cancer Research Center, University Hospital, Harborview Medical Center, and Pacific Medical Center, Seattle, Washington
Esophageal Diseases Caused by Infection, Systemic Illness, and Trauma

JAMES E. McGUIGAN, M.D.

Professor and Chairman, Department of Medicine, University of Florida College of Medicine; Physician-in-Chief, Shands Hospital, Gainesville, Florida
Anatomy, Embryology, and Developmental Anomalies; The Zollinger-Ellison Syndrome

JAMES H. MEYER, M.D.

Chief of Gastroenterology, Veterans Administration Medical Center, Sepulveda, California
Chronic Morbidity after Ulcer Surgery; Pancreatic Physiology

ARTHUR NAITOVE, M.D.

Professor of Surgery, Dartmouth Medical School; Attending Physician, Mary Hitchcock Memorial Hospital, Hanover, New Hampshire; Attending Physician, Veterans Administration Medical Center, White River Junction, Vermont
Diverticular Disease of the Colon

THOMAS F. O'BRIEN, JR., M.D.

Professor of Medicine, East Carolina University School of Medicine, Greenville, North Carolina
Benign Neoplasms and Vascular Malformations of the Large and Small Intestine

ROBERT K. OCKNER, M.D.

Professor of Medicine, University of California, San Francisco, School of Medicine; Chief, Division of Gastroenterology, Moffitt-Long Hospitals; Attending Physician, San Francisco General Hospital and Veterans Administration Medical Center; Consultant, Letterman Army Medical Center, San Francisco, California
Ascites; Vascular Diseases of the Bowel

ROBERT L. OWEN, M.D.

Professor of Medicine, Epidemiology, and International Health, University of California, San Francisco, School of Medicine; Staff Physician, Veterans Administration Medical Center, San Francisco, California
Parasitic Diseases; Gastrointestinal Manifestations of AIDS and Other Sexually Transmissible Diseases

WALTER L. PETERSON, M.D.

Associate Professor of Internal Medicine, University of Texas Southwestern Medical School at Dallas; Chief, Gastroenterology Section, Dallas Veterans Administration Medical Center, Dallas, Texas
Gastrointestinal Bleeding

SIDNEY F. PHILLIPS, M.D.

Professor of Medicine, Mayo Medical School; Director, Gastroenterology Unit, Mayo Clinic, Rochester, Minnesota
Megacolon: Congenital and Acquired; Conventional and Alternative Ileostomies

DANIEL E. POLTER, M.D.

Clinical Professor of Medicine, University of Texas Southwestern Medical School at Dallas; Attending Staff, Baylor University Medical Center, Dallas, Texas
Foreign Bodies in the Gut

CHARLES E. POPE, II, M.D.

Professor of Medicine, University of Washington School of Medicine; Chief, Gastroenterology, Veterans Administration Medical Center, Seattle, Washington
Heartburn, Dysphagia, and Other Esophageal Symptoms; The Esophagus: Anatomy and Developmental Anomalies; Rings and Webs; Diverticula

STEVEN B. RAFFIN, M.D., F.A.C.P.

Associate Clinical Professor of Medicine, University of California, San Francisco, School of Medicine, San Francisco, California; Attending Physician, Peninsula Hospital and Medical Center, Burlingame, California
The Stomach and Duodenum: Diverticula, Rupture, and Volvulus; Bezoars

HOWARD A. REBER, M.D.

Professor of Surgery and Vice Chairman, Department of Surgery, University of California, Los Angeles, School of Medicine, Los Angeles, California; Chief, Surgical Service, Sepulveda Veterans Administration Hospital, Sepulveda, California
Abdominal Abscesses and Gastrointestinal Fistulas

CHARLES T. RICHARDSON, M.D.

Patterson Professor of Medicine, University of Texas Southwestern Medical Center at Dallas; Chief of Staff, Dallas Veterans Administration Medical Center, Dallas, Texas
Gastric Ulcer

ERNEST J. RING, M.D.

Professor of Radiology and Chief of Interventional Radiology, University of California, San Francisco, School of Medicine
Endoscopic/Radiologic Treatment of Biliary Tract Diseases

ANDRÉ ROBERT, M.D., Ph.D.

Senior Scientist, Drug Metabolism Research, The Upjohn Company, Kalamazoo, Michigan
Stress Ulcers, Erosions, and Gastric Mucosal Injury

IRWIN H. ROSENBERG, M.D.

Professor of Medicine and Nutrition, and Director of USDA Human Nutrition Research Center on Aging, Tufts University; Attending Physician, New England Medical Center, Boston, Massachusetts
Eating Behavior and Nutrient Requirements; Nutritional Deficiency in Gastrointestinal Disease; Intensive Nutritional Support

TODD L. SACK, M.D.

Assistant Professor of Medicine in Residence, University of California, San Francisco, School of Medicine; Attending Physician, University of California Medical Center and Veterans Administration Medical Center, San Francisco, California
Effects of Systemic and Extraintestinal Disease on the Gut; Oral Diseases and Cutaneous Manifestations of Gastrointestinal Disease

BRUCE F. SCHARSCHMIDT, M.D.

Professor of Medicine, University of California, San Francisco, School of Medicine; Attending Physician, University of California, San Francisco, Affiliated Hospitals, San Francisco, California
Jaundice; Bile Formation and Gallbladder and Bile Duct Function

LAWRENCE R. SCHILLER, M.D.

Clinical Assistant Professor of Internal Medicine, University of Texas Southwestern Medical School at Dallas; Associate Attending Physician and Director, Gastroenterology Physiology Laboratory, Baylor University Medical Center, Dallas, Texas
Fecal Incontinence

BRUCE D. SCHIRMER, M.D.

Assistant Professor of Surgery, University of Virginia Medical Center, Charlottesville, Virginia
Intestinal Obstruction, Pseudo-Obstruction, and Ileus

DAVID J. SCHNEIDERMAN, M.D.

Assistant Professor of Medicine, University of Arizona School of Medicine; Director, Gastrointestinal Endoscopy Unit, Arizona Health Sciences Center, Tucson, Arizona
Ulcerative Colitis; Other Diseases of the Colon and Rectum

THEODORE SCHROCK, M.D.

Professor of Surgery, University of California, San Francisco, School of Medicine, San Francisco, California
Complications of Gastrointestinal Endoscopy; Acute Appendicitis; Examination of the Anorectum, Rigid Sigmoidoscopy, Flexible Sigmoidoscopy, and Diseases of the Anorectum

MARVIN M. SCHUSTER, M.D., F.A.C.P., F.A.P.A.

Professor of Medicine with Joint Appointment in Psychiatry, Johns Hopkins University School of Medicine; Director, Division of Digestive Diseases, Francis Scott Key Medical Center, Baltimore, Maryland
Irritable Bowel Syndrome

HOWARD A. SHAPIRO, M.D.

Clinical Professor of Medicine, University of California, San Francisco, School of Medicine; Attending Physician, University of California, Medical Center, San Francisco, California
Endoscopic/Radiologic Treatment of Biliary Tract Diseases

JAMES SHOREY, M.D.

Chief, Hepatology Section, Medical Service, Dallas Veterans Administration Medical Center, Dallas, Texas
Evaluation of Mass Lesions in the Liver

SOL SILVERMAN, JR., M.A., D.D.S.

Professor and Chairman, Division of Oral Medicine, University of California, San Francisco, School of Dentistry; Attending Dentist, Moffitt-Long Hospital, San Francisco, California
Oral Diseases and Cutaneous Manifestations of Gastrointestinal Disease

DENNIS R. SINAR, M.D.

Associate Professor of Medicine, East Carolina University School of Medicine; Chairman, Laser Committee, Pitt County Memorial Hospital, Greenville, North Carolina
Benign Neoplasms and Vascular Malformations of the Large and Small Intestine

MARVIN H. SLEISENGER, M.D.

Professor of Medicine and Vice Chairman for Academic Affairs, Department of Medicine; Director, Clinical Training Program in Gastroenterology, University of California, San Francisco, School of Medicine; Attending Physician, Moffitt-Long Hospital, San Francisco, California
Effects of Systemic and Extraintestinal Disease on the Gut; Cholelithiasis; Chronic and Acute Cholecystitis; Biliary Obstruction, Cholangitis, and Choledocholithiasis; Postoperative Syndromes

WILLIAM J. SNAPE, JR.

Professor of Medicine, University of California, Los Angeles, School of Medicine; Chief of Gastroenterology, Harbor-UCLA Medical Center, Los Angeles, California
Movement of the Small and Large Intestine

KONRAD H. SOERGEL, M.D.

Professor of Medicine and Chief, Division of Gastroenterology, Medical College of Wisconsin; Chief, Gastroenterology Service, Froedtert Memorial Lutheran Hospital and Milwaukee County Medical Complex, Milwaukee, Wisconsin
Acute Pancreatitis

ANDREW H. SOLL, M.D.

Professor of Medicine, University of California, Los Angeles, School of Medicine; Key Investigator, Center for Ulcer Research and Education, Wadsworth Veterans Administration Medical Center, Los Angeles, California
Duodenal Ulcer and Drug Therapy

M. MICHAEL THALER, M.D.

Professor of Pediatrics and Director, Pediatric Gastroenterology and Nutrition, University of California, San Francisco, School of Medicine; Attending Physician, University of California Medical Center, San Francisco, California
The Biliary Tract: Embryology and Anatomy; Biliary Disease in Infancy and Childhood

RICHARD C. THIRLBY, M.D.

Staff Surgeon, The Virginia Mason Clinic, Seattle, Washington
Postoperative Recurrent Ulcer

PHILLIP P. TOSKES, M.D.

Professor of Medicine and Director, Division of Gastroenterology, Hepatology and Nutrition, University of Florida College of Medicine and Gainesville Veterans Administration Medical Center; Attending Physician, Shands Hospital of the University of Florida, Gainesville, Florida
The Relation of Enteric Bacterial Populations to Gastrointestinal Function and Disease; The Blind Loop Syndrome

ROGER B. TRAYCOFF, M.D.

Associate Professor of Medicine and Anesthesiology, Department of Medicine, Section of Algology, Southern Illinois University School of Medicine, Springfield, Illinois
The Management of Abdominal Pain

JERRY S. TRIER, M.D.

Professor of Medicine, Harvard Medical School; Co-Director, Gastroenterology Division, and Senior Physician, Brigham and Women's Hospital, Boston, Massachusetts
Anatomy, Embryology, and Developmental Abnormalities of the Small and Large Intestine and Colon; The Short Bowel Syndrome; Celiac Sprue; Whipple's Disease; Radiation Enteritis and Colitis

REBECCA W. VAN DYKE, M.D.

Assistant Professor of Medicine, University of California, San Francisco, School of Medicine; Attending Physician, Moffitt-Long Hospital, University of California Medical Center, San Francisco, California
Mechanisms of Digestion and Absorption of Food

JOHN H. WALSH, M.D.

Professor of Medicine, Division of Gastroenterology, University of California, Los Angeles, School of Medicine; Director, Center for Ulcer Research and Education, Wadsworth Veterans Administration Medical Center, Los Angeles, California
Gastrointestinal Peptide Hormones

LAWRENCE W. WAY, M.D.

Professor of Surgery, University of California, San Francisco, School of Medicine; Attending Surgeon, University of California Medical Center; Chief, Surgical Service, Veterans Administration Medical Center, San Francisco, California
Abdominal Pain; Cholelithiasis; Chronic and Acute Cholecystitis; Biliary Obstruction, Cholangitis, and Choledocholithiasis; Postoperative Syndromes; Neoplasms of the Gallbladder and Bile Ducts

WILFRED M. WEINSTEIN, M.D.

Professor of Medicine, Division of Gastroenterology, University of California, Los Angeles, School of Medicine; Attending Physician, UCLA Medical Center, Los Angeles, California
Gastritis

HARLAND S. WINTER, M.D.

Assistant Professor of Pediatrics, Harvard Medical School; Associate in Gastroenterology, The Children's Hospital; Associate Pediatrician, Massachusetts General Hospital, Boston, Massachusetts
Anatomy, Embryology, and Developmental Abnormalities of the Small Intestine and Colon

TERESA L. WRIGHT, B.M., B.S., M.D.

Assistant Professor of Medicine, University of California, San Francisco, School of Medicine; Attending Staff, Veterans Administration Medical Center, San Francisco, California
Maldigestion and Malabsorption

TADATAKA YAMADA, M.D.

Professor of Internal Medicine and Chief of Division of Gastroenterology, University of Michigan Medical School, Ann Arbor, Michigan
Secretory Tumors of the Pancreas

FOREWORD

Since its first publication in 1973, the appearance of a new edition of this widely acclaimed text has served as a milestone in the progress of our knowledge of digestive disease. For twenty years the Editors, themselves deeply involved in the logarithmic growth of fundamental research and in the rising standards of clinical training and education, have enlisted more than one hundred of the major North American participants in that progress as contributors to this trusted resource for learning and for patient care.

Like its predecessors, the Fourth Edition affords the reader a sound orientation to current concepts of biology, human behavior, pathophysiology, pharmacology, and nutrition essential for understanding the broad spectrum of manifestations of digestive illness; yet its chief emphasis is on the rational and effective management of the principal gastrointestinal diseases and disorders encountered in developed Western countries. As before, the Editors have excluded from the scope of the book only the diseases of the liver, some conditions common in children, and most specific infections of the gut, in view of excellent coverage of those fields by other texts.

The veteran reader of this work will find extensive revisions, incorporating new advances in the basic and clinical aspects of our field and bringing into play the insights of thirteen new authors or coauthors. Eight wholly new chapters present important fresh perspectives on, among other things, the acquired immunodeficiency syndrome (AIDS), the gastrointestinal effects of aging, the management of intrahepatic masses disclosed by modern methods of imaging, and the endoscopic treatment of biliary tract disease. The material on cytoprotection of the gut mucosa, on the pathogenesis of gallstones, on premalignant conditions in the digestive tract, and on psychological interactions between physician and patient has been thoroughly updated. The section on nutritional management has been revised to reflect recent advances in basic nutritional concepts and to provide authoritative guidance on the benefits and limitations of enteral and parenteral feedings for functionally impaired patients. The coverage of new diagnostic procedures is no less extensive than in the previous edition but will be found, suitably indexed, in the chapters that describe their most important clinical applications. This change should facilitate the most appropriate, timely, and cost-effective use of these rapidly evolving and expensive resources.

The Editors are to be congratulated on their conspicuous success in keeping their far-flung readership abreast of the current rapid advances in digestive disease. Their Fourth Edition is a volume of large but still manageable proportions, whose weight will be measured not in pounds but by its continuing impact on the modern practice of gastroenterology.

THOMAS P. ALMY

ACKNOWLEDGMENTS

The Editors are grateful to the many authors of this book who have written wisely and well. Numerous colleagues have aided us by their constant encouragment and support; among them we would like especially to thank Dick Root, Holly Smith, Bob Ockner, John Cello, Bruce Scharschmidt, and Young Kim; and Boone Powell, Jr., Don Seldin, Dan Foster, Floyd Rector, Carol Santa Ana, and Lawrence Schiller. The Editors have also benefited from the continuing advice and support of the veteran contributors who helped to plan the First Edition: Bob Donaldson, Chuck Pope, Jerry Trier, and Larry Way, and Dave Alpers and Irv Rosenberg for their efforts in behalf of the section on Nutrition. For excellent secretarial assistance we thank Eva Fruit, Connie Van, Janie Francis, Marcia Horvitz, and Sharon Michael. We also happily acknowledge the fine efforts of the professionals at the W. B. Saunders Company: Lew Reines, Ed Wickland, Bob Butler, Dave Kilmer, Mark Coyle, Peg Shaw, and Helene Taylor.

We are especially proud to acknowledge the encouragement of our wives, Lenore Sleisenger and Jewel Fordtran; and of our children and grandchildren, Tom Sleisenger; Bill, Micki, Joey, and Amy Fordtran; and Bess, Bryan, Emily and Sarah Stone.

Again, we cannot fail to mention the influence of the late Mort Grossman and the late Franz Ingelfinger, and the continuing encouragement of Tom Almy. Directly and indirectly they all influenced this work. We hope we have justified their efforts and confidence.

PREFACE

In the five years since the Third Edition, the avalanche of information has been greater than during the intervals between preceding editions. Once again we have found it impossible to eliminate enough of the older material in making way for the newer to maintain constant the size of the work. So, the Fourth Edition is a bit bigger. Fortunately, availability of thinner and lighter paper has allowed this to be done with little increase in the book's weight. The bibliography remains rather complete, reflecting our belief that all important statements require documentation.

Many chapters have been completely rewritten, and all the others were thoroughly updated. In Part I, Some Psychologic and Biologic Aspects of Gastrointestinal Disease, we have a new chapter, The Effect of Age on Gastrointestinal Function. New additions to Part II, Major Symptoms and Syndromes, include chapters on Complications of Gastrointestinal Endoscopy, Fecal Incontinence, and Evaluation of Mass Lesions in the Liver. We have also given greater emphasis to the oral and cutaneous manifestations of gastrointestinal disease by discussing these important clinical findings in a separate chapter. In Part V, The Small and Large Intestine, there is a new chapter on Acquired Immunodeficiency Syndrome, and several chapters have been expanded considerably (including those on Colon Cancer and Food Sensitivity and Eosinophilic Gastroenteropathies. Part VI, The Biliary Tract: Anatomy, Physiology, and Disease, contains a new chapter on Endoscopic and Radiologic Treatment. Finally, much new information on nutrition will be found in Part IX, particularly on the biomedical effects of alcohol, on vitamin and mineral deficiencies, and on enteral nutrition therapy.

We have deleted the section in the Third Edition entitled Special Diagnostic Procedures. Indications for endoscopy of the upper intestinal tract, biliary tract, pancreas, and colon and for the various scanning techniques will be found in the chapters devoted to the diseases of the various organ systems.

Although we have tried our best to control it, we are still guilty of some repetition. We hope it will be looked upon as educational reinforcement rather than poor editing. We hope this Fourth Edition will be found both helpful and stimulating for all who are interested in the theory and practice of gastroenterology.

CONTENTS

PART I

SOME PSYCHOLOGIC AND BIOLOGIC ASPECTS OF GASTROINTESTINAL FUNCTIONS AND DISEASES

PART II

MAJOR SYMPTOMS AND SYNDROMES: PATHOPHYSIOLOGY, DIAGNOSIS, AND MANAGEMENT

PART III

THE ESOPHAGUS: ANATOMY, PHYSIOLOGY, AND DISEASE

PART IV

THE STOMACH AND DUODENUM:
ANATOMY, PHYSIOLOGY, AND DISEASE

PART V
THE SMALL AND LARGE INTESTINE: ANATOMY, PHYSIOLOGY, AND DISEASE

PART VI

THE BILIARY TRACT: ANATOMY, PHYSIOLOGY, AND DISEASE

PART VII

THE PANCREAS: ANATOMY, PHYSIOLOGY, AND DISEASE

PART VIII

DISEASES OF THE INTRA-ABDOMINAL VASCULATURE AND SUPPORTIVE STRUCTURES

PART IX

NUTRITIONAL MANAGEMENT

COLOR PLATES

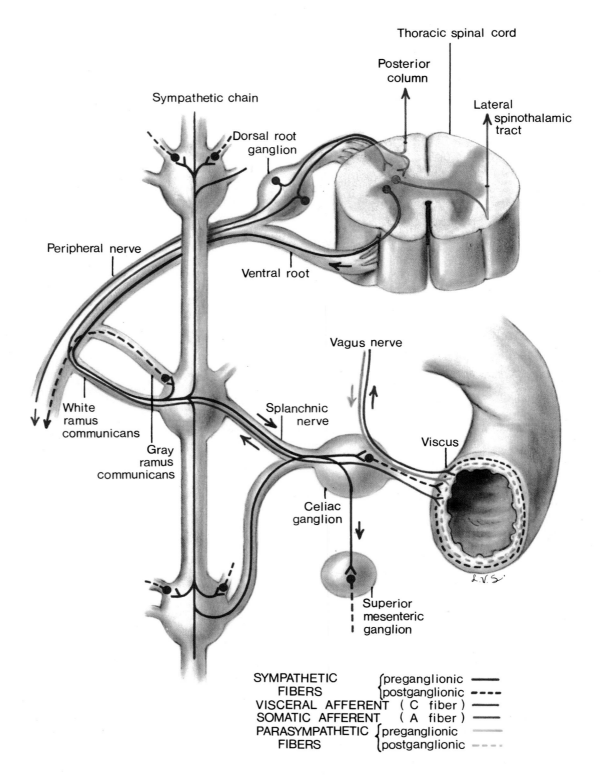

Thoracic spinal cord

Posterior column

Lateral spinothalamic tract

Sympathetic chain

Dorsal root ganglion

Peripheral nerve

Ventral root

Vagus nerve

White ramus communicans

Splanchnic nerve

Viscus

Gray ramus communicans

Celiac ganglion

Superior mesenteric ganglion

| SYMPATHETIC FIBERS | { preganglionic ——— |
| | postganglionic - - - - |
| VISCERAL AFFERENT (C fiber) —— |
| SOMATIC AFFERENT (A fiber) —— |
| PARASYMPATHETIC FIBERS | { preganglionic |
| | postganglionic - - - - |

Figure 15–2. Relationship of visceral afferent fibers that transmit pain impulses to autonomic and somatic afferent fibers. The visceral afferents for pain pass through the splanchnic ganglia, reach the sympathetic chain in the splanchnic nerves, and enter the dorsal root via the white ramus communicans. They synapse with cell bodies in the dorsal horn that send impulses toward the brain in the lateral spinothalamic tract. These relays may be inhibited by sensory impulses that enter in large afferents from the periphery (A fibers). The connections undoubtedly are much more complex than shown here. (Adapted from Netter.)

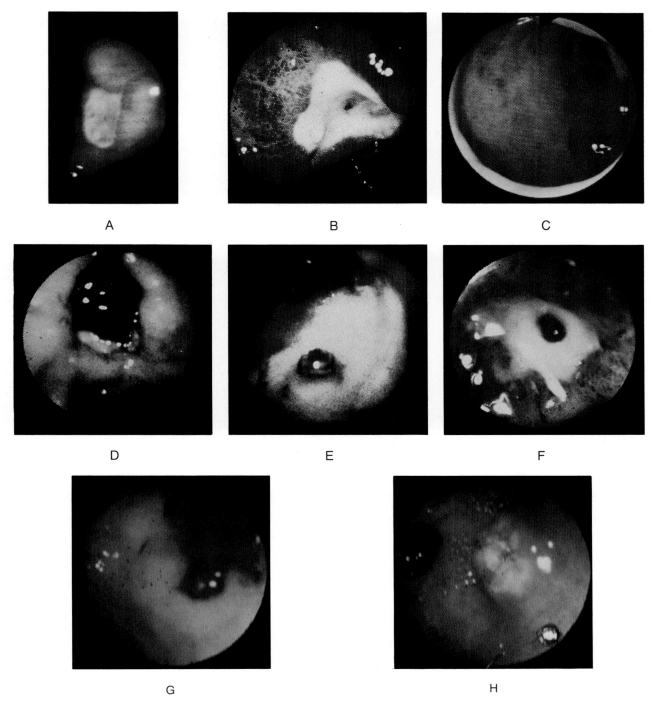

A   B   C

D   E   F

G   H

Figure 25–4. Bleeding peptic ulcers. *A*, Clean base. *B*, Central spot. *C*, Fresh clot. *D*, Black clot. *E* and *F*, Visible vessels (sentinel clots). *G*, Active bleeding. *H*, After electrocoagulation. (Photos courtesy of D. Fleischer, M.D. [C]; H. Parker, M.D. [D and E]; and J. Morrissey, M.D. [G, H].)

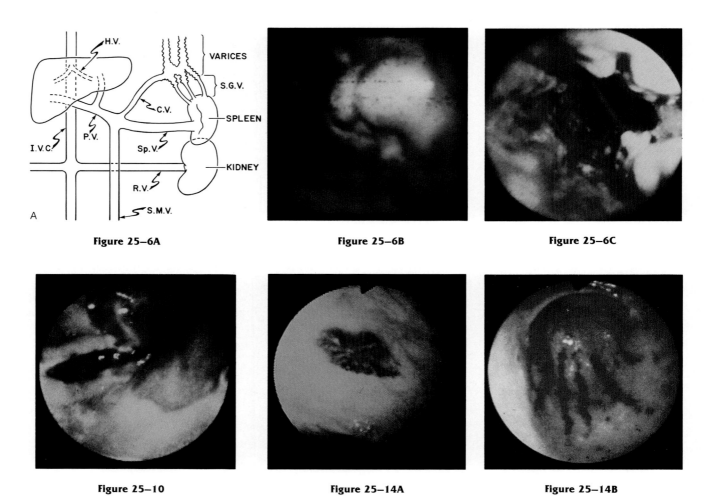

Figure 25–6A   Figure 25–6B   Figure 25–6C

Figure 25–10   Figure 25–14A   Figure 25–14B

Figure 25–6. *A*, Diagrammatic representation of the portal circulation showing esophagogastric varices. H.V., hepatic vein; I.V.C., inferior vena cava; P.V., portal vein; C.V., coronary vein; Sp.V., splenic vein; R.V., renal vein; S.M.V., superior mesenteric vein; S.G.V., short gastric veins. *B,* Large, nonbleeding varices. *C,* Actively bleeding esophageal varix. (Courtesy of J. Morrissey, M.D.)

Figure 25–10. Mallory-Weiss tear at gastroesophageal junction. (Courtesy of J. Noble, M.D.)

Figure 25–14. *A,* Cecal vascular ectasia. (Courtesy of H. Parker, M.D.). *B,* Antral vascular ectasia. (Reprinted with permission from: Gastric antral vascular ectasia: The watermelon stomach, by Jabbari, M., Cherry, R., Lough, J. O., et al. Gastroenterology 87:1165. Copyright 1984 by The American Gastroenterological Association.)

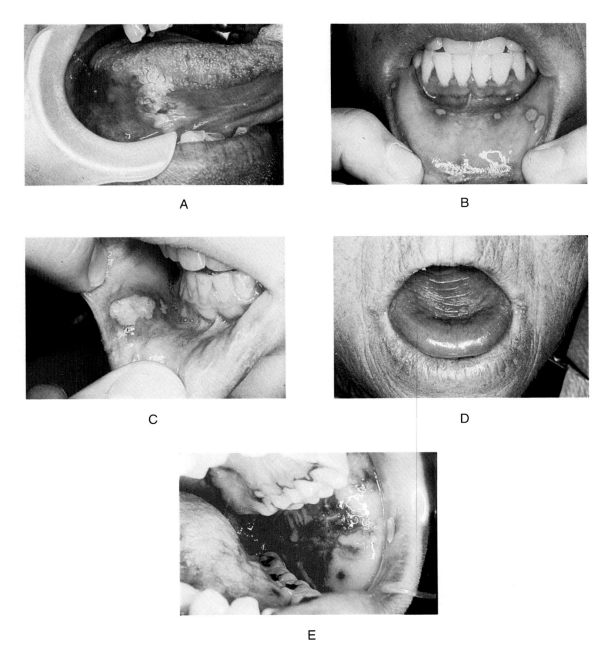

Figure 30–2. Oral lesions associated with gastrointestinal disorders. *A,* Oral leukoplakia and associated squamous carcinoma. *B,* Multiple minor aphthous ulcers. *C,* Major aphthous ulcer. *D,* Glossitis in a patient with diabetes and malabsorption. The tongue is smooth (depapillation) and red; angular cheilitis is present. *E,* Marked erythema and ulceration associated with erythema multiforme. This patient had Stevens-Johnson syndrome.

Illustration continued on following page

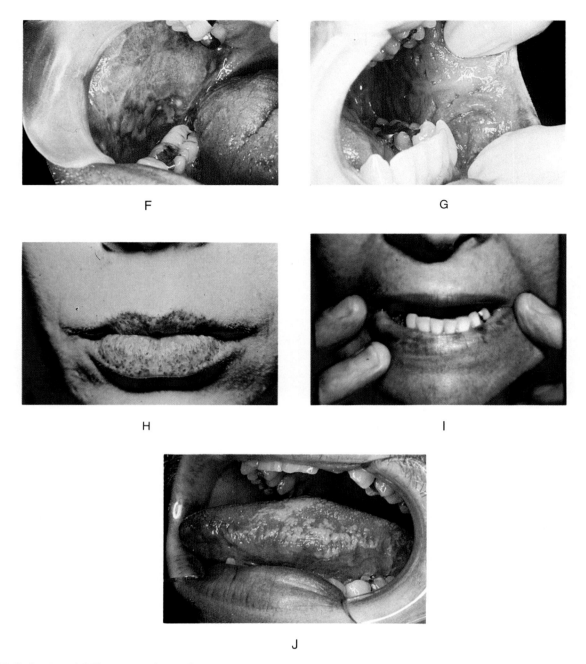

Figure 30–2 *Continued F,* The erosive form of oral lichen planus involving the buccal mucosa. Note lace-like keratoses, erythema, and ulceration. *G,* Pyostomatitis vegetans in a patient with ulcerative colitis. Biopsy revealed micro-abscesses. *H,* Hereditary hemorrhagic telangiectasia (Osler-Weber-Rendu disease). *I,* Mucocutaneous pigmentation of Peutz-Jeghers syndrome. *J,* Hairy leukoplakia in a patient with AIDS. (Courtesy of Sol Silverman Jr., D.D.S., and Victor Newcomer, M.D.)

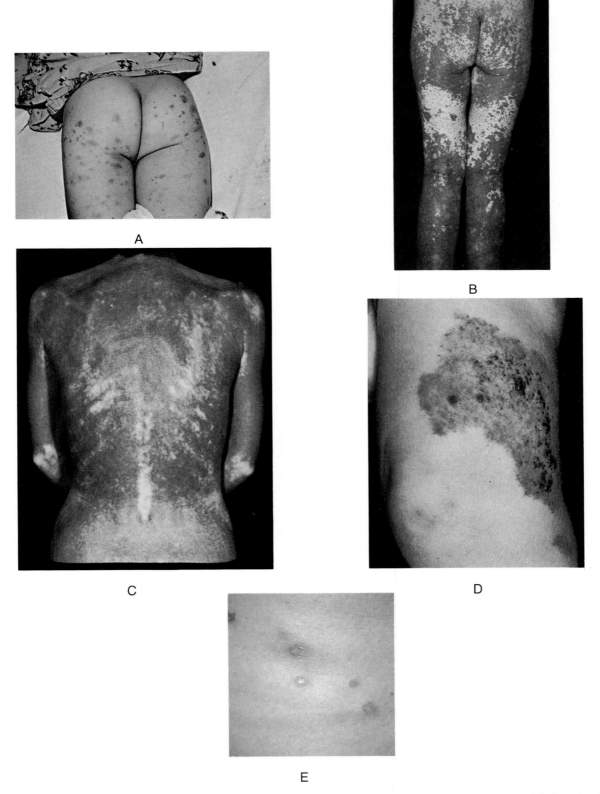

Figure 30–3. Cutaneous lesions associated with gastrointestinal disorders. *A*, Henoch-Schönlein purpura. *B*, Cryoglobulinemia with drug eruption. *C*, Urticaria pigmentosa in a patient with systemic mastocytosis. *D*, Cutaneous vascular hemangioma associated with intestinal hemorrhage. *E*, Degos' disease, with vasculitic lesions of different stages.

Illustration continued on following page

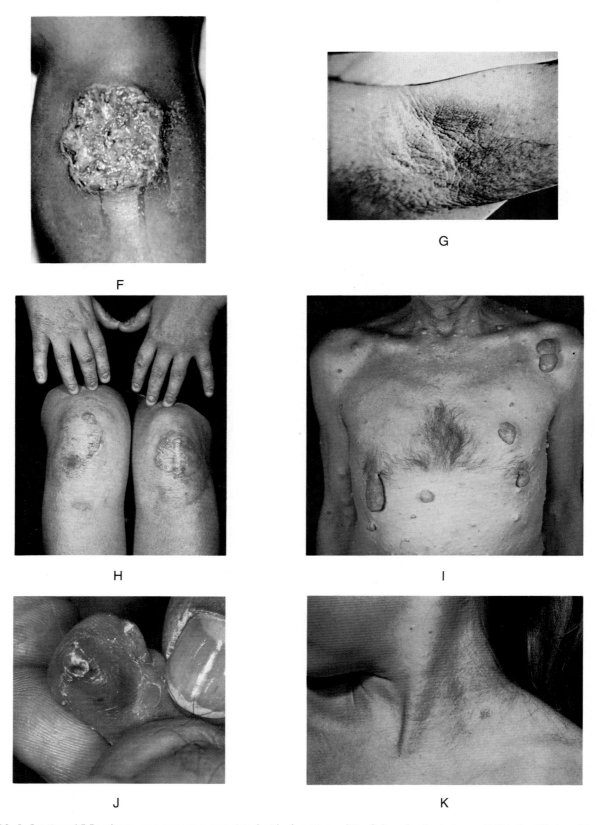

F

G

H

I

J

K

Figure 30–3 *Continued F,* Pyoderma gangrenosum associated with ulcerative colitis. *G,* Acanthosis nigricans. *H,* Skin fragility in epidermolysis bullosa dystrophica. *I,* Neurofibromatosis. *J,* Finger tip lesion in blue rubber bleb nevus syndrome. *K,* Pseudoxanthoma elasticum. (Courtesy of Victor Newcomer, M.D.)

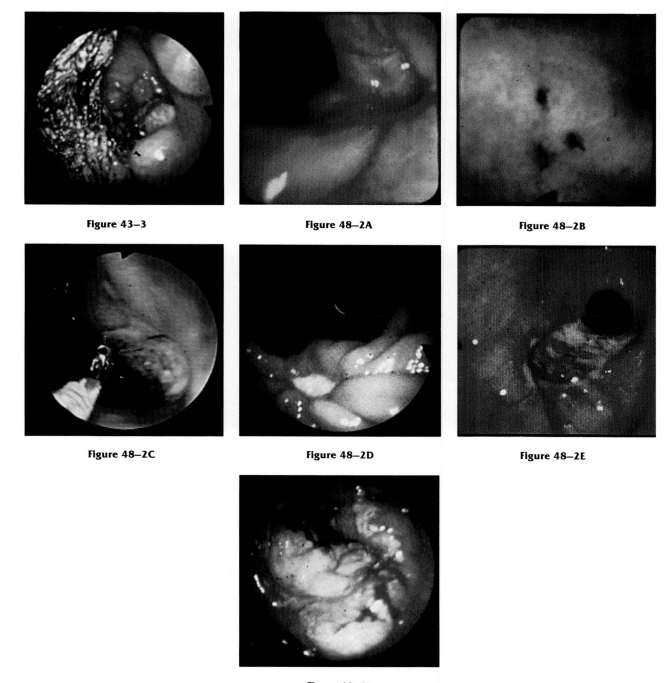

Figure 43–3

Figure 48–2A

Figure 48–2B

Figure 48–2C

Figure 48–2D

Figure 48–2E

Figure 48–2F

Figure 43–3. Endoscopic view of trichobezoar adjacent to an area of nodular gastritis. (Courtesy of Emmet B. Keefe, M.D.)

Figure 48–2. *A*, Endoscopic picture of a relatively deep, benign-appearing gastric ulcer. Folds radiate to the ulcer margin. *B*, Endoscopic picture illustrating blood-tinged, superficial erosions. In this patient the erosions resulted from therapy with indomethacin. (Courtesy of Frank Lanza, M.D.) *C*, Endoscopic picture illustrating gastric ulcer. Biopsy forceps can be seen obtaining tissue from edge of the ulcer crater. (Courtesy of Doug Thurman, M.D.) *D*, Endoscopic picture demonstrating folds radiating to a benign-appearing gastric ulcer. The edges of the crater are regular but slightly indurated. *E*, Oval or somewhat linear gastric ulcer. The pylorus is seen in the background. *F*, Malignant-appearing gastric ulcer.

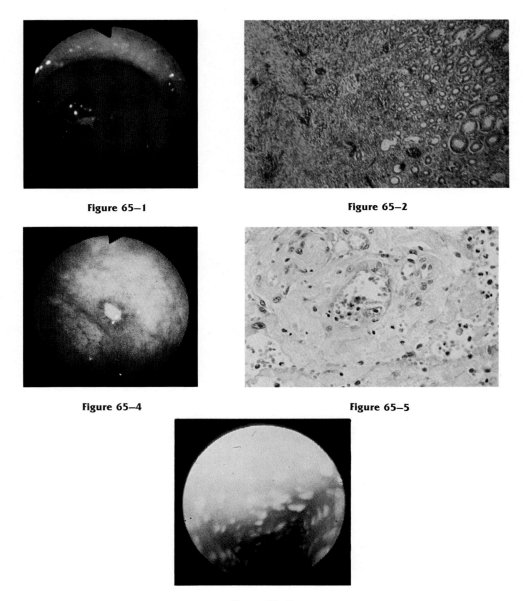

Figure 65—1

Figure 65—2

Figure 65—4

Figure 65—5

Figure 65—6

Figure 65—1. Endoscopic view of Kaposi's sarcoma involving the gastric antrum. There is a nodular lesion along the incisura angularis, as well as submucosal hemorrhage in the prepyloric region. (Courtesy of D. F. Altman, M.D.)

Figure 65—2. Endoscopic biopsy specimen of Kaposi's sarcoma of the sigmoid colon. There is hemorrhage and infiltration of the submucosa and lamina propria by numerous spindle-shaped cells. Hematoxylin and eosin stain, ×50. (Reprinted with permission from: Gastrointestinal Kaposi's sarcoma in patients with acquired immunodeficiency syndrome: endoscopic and autopsy findings, by Freidman, S. L., Wright, T. L., and Altman, D. F. Gastroenterology 89:102—108. Copyright 1985 by The American Gastroenterological Association.)

Figure 65—4. Endoscopic view of a focal colonic mucosal ulcer due to cytomegalovirus. (Courtesy of J. P. Cello, M.D.)

Figure 65—5. Endoscopic biopsy specimen of cytomegalovirus infection of the colon, demonstrating characteristic CMV inclusion in a capillary endothelial cell. Hematoxylin and eosin stain, ×50. (Courtesy of D. F. Altman, M.D.)

Figure 65—6. Endoscopic appearance of *Candida* eosphagitis, demonstrating focal mucosal exudates and erythema. (From Blackstone, M. O. Endoscopic Interpretation: Normal and Pathologic Appearances of the Gastrointestinal Tract, 1984. Used by permission of Raven Press, New York).

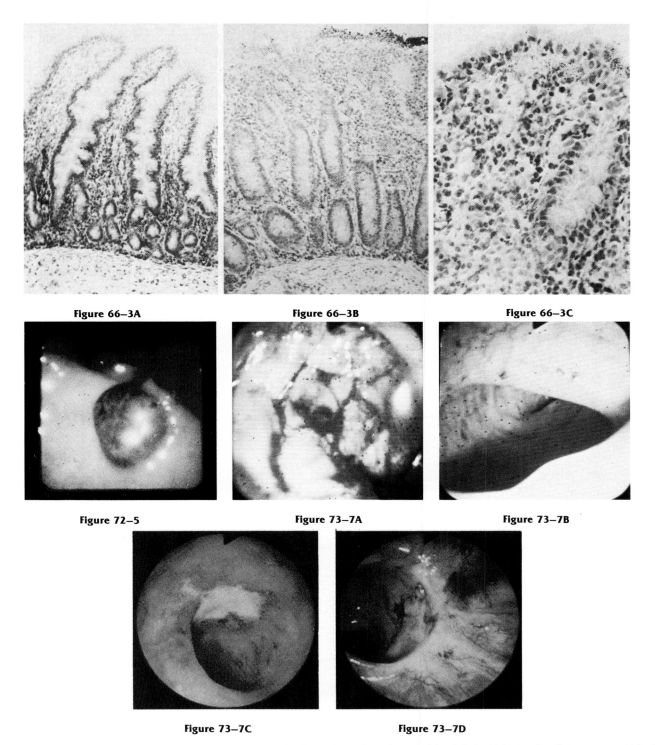

Figure 66–3A   Figure 66–3B   Figure 66–3C

Figure 72–5   Figure 73–7A   Figure 73–7B

Figure 73–7C   Figure 73–7D

Figure 66–3. Lipid distribution in jejunal biopsies stained with oil-red-O. *A,* Normal control (× 84). Lipid (stained red) is present within the basal portion of the lamina propria. *B,* Celiac disease (× 84). Lipid is present within the surface epithelium. *C,* Tropical sprue (× 210). Lipid is located principally subjacent to the surface epithelium.

Figure 72–5. Kaposi's sarcoma of the sigmoid colon. Although malignant histologically, such tumors of gut behave biologically in a benign fashion. (Courtesy of Dr. M. H. Sleisenger.)

Figure 73–7. Endoscopic changes in colorectal mucosa induced by radiation therapy. *A,* Acute radiation proctitis with mucosal hemorrhage may appear much the same as acute idiopathic inflammatory bowel disease. *B,* Small telangiectatic vessels on pale, opaque mucosa may be all that is seen in a later stage. (*A* and *B* courtesy of Jerome D. Waye, M.D.) *C,* Radiation-induced ulceration with surrounding telangiectasia located at rectosigmoid junction. *D,* Healing of an indolent radiation-induced rectal ulcer may lead to scar formation, retraction, and ultimately a stricture. (*C* and *D* from Silverstein, F. E., and Tytgat, G. N. J. Atlas of Gastrointestinal Endoscopy. London, Gower Medical Publishing, and Philadelphia, W. B. Saunders Co., 1987. Used by permission.)

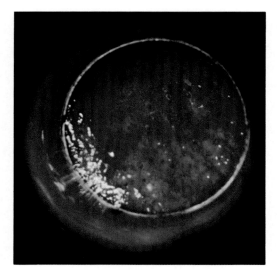

Figure 78–3A

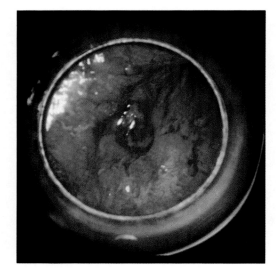

Figure 78–3B

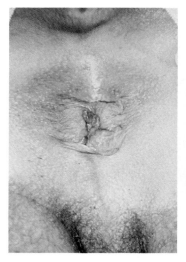

Figure 83–6

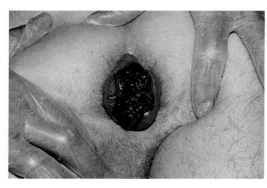

Figure 83–7

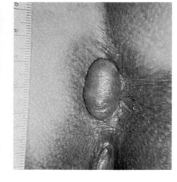

Figure 83–8

Figure 78–3. Proctoscopic views of colonic mucosa in two patients with ulcerative colitis. *A,* Granularity and minute bleeding mucosal ulcerations. *B,* Minimal granularity, but mucosa is friable and a pseudopolyp can be seen. (Courtesy of M. H. Sleisenger, M.D.)

Figure 83–6. Typical prolapsing mixed internal and external hemorrhoids. The patient is prone. Note hemorrhoidal masses in the three primary locations: left lateral, right posterior, and right anterior. Radial grooves are prominent between adjacent hemorrhoids.

Figure 83–7. Acute prolapsed, thrombosed internal hemorrhoids. Note congestion and edema of the external components below the pectinate line. Mucosal ulceration has developed.

Figure 83–8. Thrombosed external hemorrhoid. The mass is entirely covered by skin.

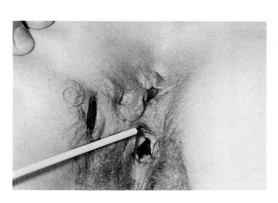

Figure 83–12

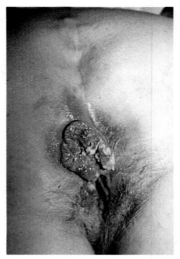

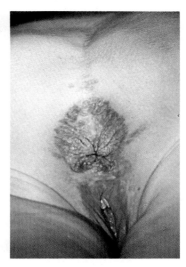

Figure 83–13   Figure 83–14

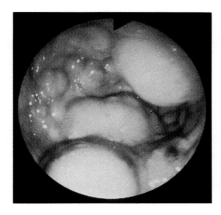

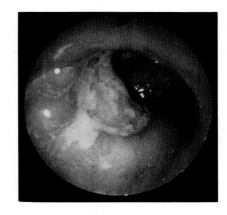

Figure 84–5   Figure 84–9

Figure 83–12. Complex anorectal fistulas due to Crohn's disease in a young woman. Pointer indicates rectovaginal fistula. The anus is edematous and deformed. A large secondary fistula orifice gapes open on the left.

Figure 83–13. Large epidermoid carcinoma involving much of the circumference at the anal verge.

Figure 83–14. Perianal Bowen's disease.

Figure 84–5. Pneumatosis coli as seen by fiberoptic colonoscopy. The tense air cysts are often mistaken for sessile polyps but collapse with a popping sound when biopsy samples are taken. (From Silverstein, F. E., and Tytgat, G. N. J. Atlas of Gastrointestinal Endoscopy. London, Gower Medical Publishing, and Philadelphia, W. B. Saunders Co., 1987. Used by permission.)

Figure 84–9. Solitary rectal ulcer. Sharply demarcated ulceration is present in the anterior wall of the rectum. The ulcer size can vary from several millimeters to 5 centimeters and may have an irregular outline or be linear in shape. The ulcer edge is often flat but clearly demarcated from normal mucosa by a thin line of hyperemia. The surrounding mucosa may have a nodular appearance. (From Silverstein, F. E., and Tytgat, G. N. J: Atlas of Gastrointestinal Endoscopy. London, Gower Medical Publishing, and Philadelphia, W. B. Saunders Co., 1987. Used by permission.)

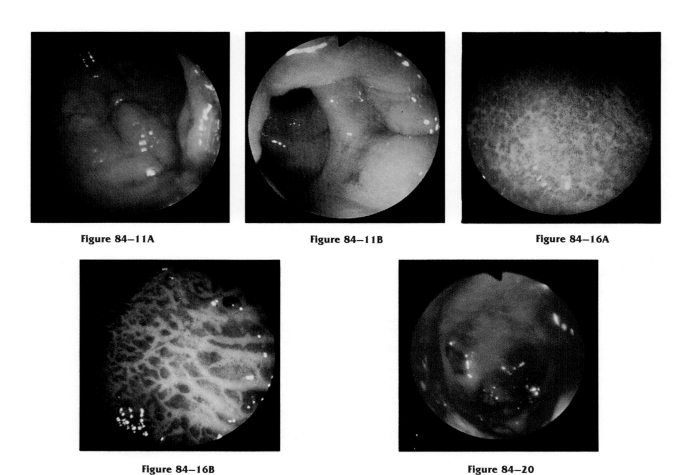

Figure 84–11A

Figure 84–11B

Figure 84–16A

Figure 84–16B

Figure 84–20

Figure 84–11. Two endoscopic photographs of colitis cystica profunda in the rectum. The cysts are covered by normal-appearing mucosa and appear as submucosal wounds or plaques. In some cases, the mucosa may be edematous, hyperemic or even ulcerated similar to that shown in Figure 84–9. (From Silverstein, F. E., and Tytgat, G. N. J. Atlas of Gastrointestinal Endoscopy. London, Gower Medical Publishing, and Philadelphia, W. B. Saunders Co., 1987. Used by permission.)

Figure 84–16. A, Endoscopic photograph of rectal mucosa showing melanosis coli. B, Close-up view showing that darker areas are divided in a polyhedral design by lighter areas of less pigmentation. The gross appearance of the mucosa may vary from light brown to black coloration.

Figure 84–20. Endoscopic photograph of rectal mucosa in an elderly woman with acute colitis following a hydrogen peroxide enema. There is marked mucosal hyperemia, areas of bullous-like edema and necrotic ulceration. (Courtesy of P. Bryan Hudson, Ph.D., M.D.)

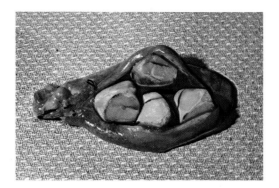

Figure 89–1

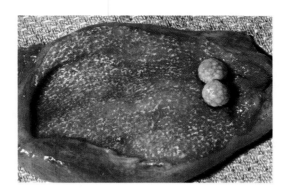

Figure 89–2

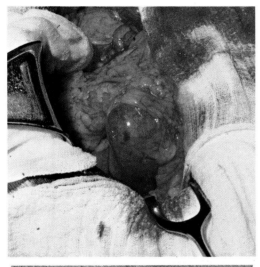

Figure 89–3

Figure 97–14

Figure 89–1. Gallbladder removed for episodic biliary colic. There is moderate thickening of the gallbladder wall from chronic inflammation and collagen deposition. The stones are typical faceted mixed-cholesterol gallstones.

Figure 89–2. Gallbladder showing prominent cholesterolosis of the mucosal surface. Operation was performed for episodic colic. The gallbladder had opacified on the preoperative oral cholecystogram. The gallstones are "mulberry stones," which are almost pure cholesterol.

Figure 89–3. The gallbladder as seen at laparotomy in a case of early acute cholecystitis. Onset of the attack was less than 48 hours before operation. The gallbladder is inflamed and edematous and surrounded by adherent omentum. The open specimen *(inset)* shows two bilirubin pigment stones as well as mucosal inflammation and minor submucosal hemorrhages. At the start of the operation, one stone had been lodged in the infundibulum, obstructing the gallbladder.

Figure 97–14. Endoscopic appearance of a *choledochocele*. An enlarged, hemispherical structure is seen protruding into the duodenal lumen after injection of contrast material into the common bile duct. The duodenoscope and cannulation catheter have been withdrawn. The orifice of the papilla of Vater is not visible; it is eccentrically placed, behind and slightly inferior to the protruding choledochocele. Same patient as in Figure 97–15, page 1837.

I

SOME PSYCHOLOGIC AND BIOLOGIC ASPECTS OF GASTROINTESTINAL FUNCTIONS AND DISEASES

The Physician and the Patient

DOUGLAS A. DROSSMAN

Review of the Psychosocial Gastrointestinal Literature with an Integrated Approach to the Patient

Physicians are aware of the major role that psychosocial factors play in the illnesses of many of their patients.* For example, the most frequent clinical diagnosis made by gastroenterologists is that of a "functional disorder."[2] They relate such patients' complaints to "stress." Another large proportion of the gastroenterologist's patients have chronic or debilitating disease. These patients frequently exhibit anxiety and depression and are encumbered with a variety of social difficulties. Traditionally, physicians have separated psychologically mediated conditions from disease (i.e., a condition is either organic or functional) or, in the context of an existing disease, have labeled emotional and social factors as secondary. The purposes of this chapter are to discuss the limitations of this perspective and to describe an integrative approach to the diagnosis and treatment of all patients. Consider the case of Mrs. R.

A 42-year-old woman is admitted for abdominal discomfort and constipation, and plain film of the abdomen shows increased air in the small bowel and a colon filled with stool. She gives a history of chronic constipation beginning in early childhood. Her father died before her birth, and the mother gave her to foster parents for the first six years of life in order to pursue other interests. The foster mother was seen by Mrs. R. as being dominant and controlling. The patient remembers receiving enemas when she missed bowel movements. As a teenager, she began using laxatives. Upon entering college, she became depressed and had a brief psychiatric hospitalization. At that time she became aware of her sensitivity to loss and rejection as a result of earlier life experiences (which she attempted to manage by maintaining control over herself, her environment, and those close to her). Being away from home and in a new setting was thus an overwhelming experience. She had a successful clinical response to psychotherapy, married, raised a family, and maintained an active career.

Five years before admission, the patient had a hysterectomy and postoperatively developed clinical evidence of bowel obstruction. Barium contrast studies did not reveal an anatomic source, and she responded to nasogastric suction and discontinuation of the postoperative narcotic analgesic. Two and one-half years before the present admission, she separated from her husband after learning that he was seeing other women. She continued her responsibilities at work and home, claiming to "need no one to be the good mother I should be." Six months later she became aware of arthralgias and cold-related discoloration of the digits. A diagnosis of scleroderma with Raynaud's syndrome was made. Because of her chronic constipation, a gastroenterologist was consulted. Results of esophageal and rectal manometry and colonoscopy to the terminal ileum were normal except for melanosis coli. The patient admitted to frequent use of anthracine-type laxatives for symptoms of abdominal swelling and constipation (defined by her as the inability to pass a stool within 48 hours), and she was strongly advised to take a bulk laxative instead of a bowel stimulant.

Two months before the current admission, she was hospitalized elsewhere with the same gastrointestinal complaints. An abdominal film showed air-fluid levels in the small bowel and air in the colon, but no bowel dilatation. Esophageal manometry was again normal. Her serum potassium was 1.8 mEq per liter. Barium contrast studies of the intestine were again nondiagnostic. No renal or metabolic cause for the hypokalemia could be determined, and drug ingestion was suspected, although the patient denied diarrhea or use of laxatives or diuretics. With a presumed diagnosis of pseudo-obstruction, she was treated with metoclopramide and potassium chloride replacement. One week after discharge she discontinued the metoclopramide because of an unfavorable clinical response and the development of dizziness.

The current admission was prompted by complaints of worsening constipation. She volunteered that many doctors had been unable to solve her problem and referred to herself as an "orphan patient." She denied heartburn, dysphagia, vomiting, fever, or weight loss. She had been informed recently of her natural mother's diagnosis of cancer and had begun taking an anticholinergic medicine for worsening of the abdominal discomfort. Serum potassium was 2.8 mEq per liter.

I will return to this patient at the end of the chapter. At this point it is enough to say that this is a complex case involving the *interaction* of biologic, psychologic, and sociocultural processes. The following pertinent questions raised by Mrs. R's case history will be discussed in the context of a review of epidemiologic, psychosomatic, and biomedical literature.

1. What is "stress"?
2. How do environmental stimuli affect intestinal function?

---

*A semantic distinction is made here. *Disease* relates to abnormalities in structure and function of organs and tissues, whereas *illness* involves the individual's personal experience of ill health or bodily dysfunction.[1] Although this distinction is used herein for clarity of presentation, it is my intention to show that these terms cannot be conceptualized independently.

3. What are the possible effects of early life experiences on later bowel function and patient behavior?

4. What is the association of psychosocial variables with illness and susceptibility to disease?

5. What are the possible mechanisms that might lead us to understand these associations?

6. How do psychosocial factors influence the patient's experience and response to illness?

7. How should the physician evaluate the patient and effect optimal care?

REVIEW OF THE LITERATURE

Special Problems in Behavioral Research and Its Application to Clinical Care

Before reviewing the pertinent literature, it is necessary to emphasize certain methodologic limitations. First, there is the problem of integrating the research among the biomedical and behavioral disciplines. Investigators from different disciplines often do not agree on conceptualization, terminology, selection criteria, identification of the variables for study, and the conclusions that are drawn from the data. Second, our ability to study the human organism in its natural environment is extremely limited. Much psychophysiologic research has involved recording data from subjects placed in hospital and laboratory environments where they are removed from the relevant psychosocial variables. Subjects are fasted, even purged, and tubes or electrodes are placed, all of which further limit the relevance to everyday living. Third, human behavior is multidetermined, less predictable, and difficult to measure. With the enormous growth of the neocortex relative to that of other animals, the complexity and range of psychologic and environmental influences on both the visceral components of the gut and the individual's behavior make the design of completely controlled studies in man beyond present capability. Extrapolation from animal models is of limited clinical use. For example, in laboratory rats avoidance activity and defecation in response to an acute noxious stimulus such as pain is expected, but a similar stimulus in humans results in far more variable effects owing to the ability of man to modulate such stimuli through cortical processes. Furthermore, the effects of a *symbolic* stimulus (a fantasy or fear) are hard to quantify and may produce profound physiologic effects owing to early experiences or cultural attitudes (e.g., hex, phobias). Fourth, even the best behavioral research is usually retrospective or cross-sectional in design. Therefore, significant associations between psychosocial factors and physiologic disturbances or medical disease do not necessarily indicate causation.

Ultimately, we must depend upon experienced clinicians to elicit the subtle and complex biopsychosocial data and to provide a framework for clinical care; such observations cannot easily be verified by experimental techniques and are subject to bias. For example, most of the early psychosomatic concepts were based on case studies, often by single observers. Some of these concepts have been appropriately criticized, while others have been misunderstood. The research scientist is often left with more questions than answers, and yet it is the clinician's responsibility to evaluate the total context of patients' illnesses whether or not the validity of clinically obtained data has been clearly established. Despite methodologic limitations, psychosomatic, psychophysiologic, and behavioral research are discussed to give a historical perspective and to provide plausible concepts that explain clinical experience. Future confirmation of these concepts will require the use of well-designed multidisciplinary studies in the behavioral and biomedical sciences.

The Concept of "Stress"

Stress is difficult to understand and even harder to study; no definition is entirely satisfactory.[3] The human organism functions in a constantly changing environment. Any influence on the person's steady state that requires adjustment or adaptation can, in its broadest sense, be considered stress. The term is completely nonspecific and has traditionally encompassed both the stimulus and its effects. The stimulus can be a biologic event such as infection, a social event such as a change of residence, or merely a disturbing thought. Despite its traditional connotation, stress can be desirable as well as undesirable. Some stimuli, such as pain, sex, or threat of injury, will often elicit a predictable response in animals and man. In contrast, life events or other psychologic processes have more varied influences on the individual. For example, loss of a job may be of little concern to one person, yet seem fraught with crisis to another who views the event as a personal failure. A stimulus may produce a variety of responses among individuals or within the same individual at different times. There may be no observable effect, a psychologic response (anxiety, depression), physiologic changes (diarrhea, diaphoresis), disease onset (asthma, colitis), or any combination of these reactions. Both a person's interpretation of events as stressful or not and his or her response depend on prior experience, attitudes, coping mechanisms, personality, cultural influences, and biologic factors, including susceptibility to disease. The nonspecific nature of the term *stress* precludes its use as a distinct variable for research. Therefore, in the literature review that follows, the psychosocial variables studied will be identified as specifically as possible.

Effects of Environmental Stimuli on Intestinal Function

The correlation of gastrointestinal system disturbance with various environmental stimuli has been a part of the writings of poets and philosophers for centuries.[4] Healthy subjects commonly report abdominal distress or change in bowel function when they are upset or distressed,[5] and clinicians usually take this association into account when evaluating and treating their patients. Clinical reports and psychophysiologic studies in animals and man have supported these empirically derived observations. Cannon, at the turn of the century, noted a cessation in bowel activity among cats reacting to a growling dog.[6] Beaumont observed changes in gastric mucosal appearance and activity in response to psychologic and physical stimuli in his patient with a traumatic fistula.[7] Later investigation by Pavlov[8] and others studying surgically produced fistulas in dogs led eventually to our understanding of how psychic factors affect acid secretion via the vagus nerve. Studies of Tom and Monica, two people with gastric fistulas,[9, 10] demonstrated that different emotional configurations produce distinct changes in gastric function. Gastric hyperemia and increased motility and secretion occurred with feelings of anger, intense pleasure, or aggressive behavior patterns related to the subject's active engagement with the environment. Conversely, mucosal pallor and decreased secretion and motor activity occurred with fear or depression—states of withdrawal ("giving-up behavior") or disengagement from others.

Similar observations have been made for esophageal and colonic activity. Esophageal spasm in response to strong emotion was reported over 60 years ago.[11] More recent use of manometric recording devices indicates that experimental noise and complicated cognitive tasks produce high-amplitude, high-velocity peristaltic contractions.[12] Grace and coworkers[13] studied four colostomy patients with prolapsed segments of bowel and observed decreased motility when patients expressed feelings of depression and increased motility when they expressed anger and resentment. Among pediatric patients with colostomies, pain or the threat of pain produced blanching of the mucosa, while the sight of appetizing food caused vascular engorgement.[14] Almy and colleagues reported increased rectal motility and vascular engorgement among subjects in response to a variety of noxious physical and psychologic stimuli.[15] Almy also correlated increased motility with concurrent states of aggression or coping behavior during his interviews with irritable bowel syndrome patients who had clinical histories of pain and constipation. Similarly, the irritable bowel syndrome patients who had histories of diarrhea expressed helplessness, defeat, and withdrawal concurrent with laboratory observations of decreased colonic motility.[16] These patterns were not consistent over time but varied as the attendant mood changed. These data suggest that changes in bowel appearance or function are bodily concomitants of emotion.

The relationship of these psychophysiological responses to symptoms or to specific gastrointestinal disorders (e.g., irritable bowel syndrome, "nutcracker esophagus," functional abdominal pain) has not been determined and requires further investigation. However, from these and other studies, we are left with the conclusion that the gut responds to psychologic stimuli and that, although visceral reactions to such stimuli may vary, this effect is a normal part of daily living.

Early Life Experience, Patient Behavior, and Bowel Function

Having accepted that the bowel is responsive to environmental stimuli, we can consider whether early experiences can contribute to bowel dysfunction later in life.

Psychoanalytic Concepts

Psychoanalytic theory states that situations of conflict arise in early life that confront the child's innate impulses with external environmental constraints, and that normal personality development involves successful resolution of these conflicts. The processes of feeding and elimination are two such examples. These complex behaviors, sources of intense gratification to the infant, must gradually be controlled by the growing child according to the prevailing mores of family and society. To varying degrees during development and later in life, these adopted constraints remain in conflict with desires for immediate gratification. With increased motor development, the child can either defy or comply with environmental constraints by choosing to eat, resist eating, bite, defecate, or withhold stool. When and how these behaviors are displayed will depend upon the child's needs and the quality and intensity of the environmental controls. Behaviors learned during this period are considered pivotal in the child's personality and development and later interaction with the environment: the development of autonomy, of distinguishing right from wrong, and of disciplining impulses in a socially acceptable manner. Conversely, failure to resolve these early conflicts may make the adult vulnerable in situations that tax these character traits. Thus the obstinate (sic "obstipation") person withholds or resists when feeling controlled.

These early derivatives of personality development still play a role in adult behavior as expressed in folklore, dreams, and language development.[17] Terms such as "I could eat you up" or "She's as sweet as honey" reflect personal endearment derived in part from early associations with feeding and the primitive wish to incorporate the desired object. Other associations include "biting sarcasm" (oral aggression), being "fed up" (to take no more), and "you (that) make(s) me want to vomit" (oral rejection of undesirables). The patients with certain gastroenterologic disorders who have also undergone psychoanalysis report the association of highly emotionally charged and/or repressive interactions with parents over the processes of feeding and elimination. Examples include functional constipation,[18] psychogenic vomiting,[19] adult rumination or merycism,[20] and anorexia nervosa.[21] It also follows that patients who develop a variety of gastrointestinal diseases may have irrational beliefs or unwarranted fears that are derived from these early periods of life.

Behavioral Concepts

Early life experiences may also influence later bowel function through learning. The field of behavioral psychology provides plausible explanations as to how established patterns of visceral dysfunction may evolve and offers the potential for treating some of the psychophysiologic* and somatic gastrointestinal disorders. Two types of learning systems have been extensively studied in animals; both mechanisms may affect human gastrointestinal system function.[22] *Classical conditioning*, as originally described by Pavlov, involves linking a neutral food or unconditioned stimulus (sound of a bell) with a conditioned stimulus (food) that elicits a conditioned response (salivation). After several trials, the unconditioned stimulus is able to produce the conditioned response. Other visceral functions, such as the secretion of digestive juices and motility of the gallbladder, stomach, and intestine, can be classically conditioned.[23] The stimulus can be enteroceptive as well as exteroceptive. For example, the *thought* of sucking on a lemon can cause increased salivation.[24] *Operant conditioning* or *instrumental learning* involves the development of a desired response through motivation and reinforcement. Playing basketball is one example. Accuracy improves through practice; the correct behavior is reinforced by scoring a basket. The same reward can condition a number of responses, and any response may be conditioned by a variety of rewards. Negative feedback (punishment) can also produce learned responses, an example being training a rat to avoid shock by learning to push a lever. In humans, abstract rewards such as gaining approval or accomplishing a task can serve as reinforcers. Visceral responses to operant conditioning have been shown in dogs. Using water as a reward, Miller and Carmona trained one group of thirty dogs to increase salivation (as measured by parotid duct secretion) and another to decrease salivation.[25]

Conditioned learning may be the basis for gastrointestinal system dysfunction, symptoms, and patient behavior. Miller[26] cites the example of a child who might develop abdominal distress to avoid unpleasant situations. A child may wake up on the day of a dreaded examination at school and develop several nonspecific autonomically mediated symptoms. If the parent singles out a symptom, such as abdominal distress or diarrhea, as the particular reason for keeping the child home and subsequently repeats this pattern, the child's relief in avoiding the feared situation might reinforce the development of such symptoms in future distressing circumstances. Recent data suggest that some clinical disorders, such as the irritable bowel syndrome, may result in part from behavioral reinforcement of bowel complaints either by toys and other extra rewards[27] or by frequent school absences due to illness[28] beginning early in life. Similarly, patients with hypochondriacal complaints may have learned their behavior in an environment where love and attention were more often reserved for the sick.

Changing established patterns of visceral function or dysfunction can be achieved through biofeedback, a clinical application of operant conditioning. Special instrumentation is used so the patient can monitor and change autonomic function that is not usually under conscious control. The subject can be instructed to increase or decrease pressures or electrical activity (e.g., EMG), the reward being accomplishment of the task. Subjects can alter esophageal sphincter pressures[29] and intestinal motility.[30] Currently, one clinical use of biofeedback is in the treatment of patients with anal sphincter dysfunction and fecal incontinence.[31]

Relationship of Psychosocial Factors to Disease Susceptibility

There is increasing evidence that psychosocial processes act as "conditional stressors"; i.e., they alter physiologic, endocrine, or immune function so as to make the organism more or less susceptible to medical disorders. Thus, it is more appropriate to speak of determinants of or influences on, rather than causes of disease. Support for this hypothesis is derived from animal research, epidemiologic studies, and psychiatric or psychologic assessment.

Animal Research

Alteration in the social environment of animals can affect infant mortality rates and the incidence of arteriosclerosis, neoplasia, and infection. Animal research affords the opportunity to restrict the variety of social factors that contribute to susceptibility to these and other diseases and helps develop hypotheses for further human investigation.

A traditional model for "stress" research is the induction of acute gastric erosions in rats. Selye first observed gastric erosions in rats exposed to a variety of noxious stimuli.[32] Later, more refined studies showed that these erosions developed in rats restrained during periods of peak activity[33] or in those prematurely separated from their mothers.[34] Fewer erosions developed when the rats could exhibit some control over their environment by pressing a lever to make the timing of shocks predictable.[35]

Chronic gastrointestinal lesions were reported in 11 of 19 rhesus monkeys in response to restraint and conditioned anxiety.[36] More recently, the cotton-topped tamarin[37] has been found to develop human-like colitis and also to have a high frequency of colon carcinoma. There is preliminary evidence that the incidence of these diseases may increase after the animal is captured, and behavioral factors such as readjustment to a new social environment may be contributory.[38]

Psychophysiologic reactions involve psychologically induced alterations in function of target organs without structural change. They are often viewed as physiologic concomitants of an affect such as anger or fear, although the person is not always aware of the affect. The persistence of an altered physiologic state or the enhanced physiologic response to psychologic stimuli is considered by some as a *psychophysiologic disorder*.

The relationship of these pathologic states to chronic ulcers and inflammatory bowel disease in humans is not established. What is important to remember from these studies is that social alteration, in a reproducible fashion, may lead to acute or chronic end-organ damage. Interestingly, the nature of these social alterations in animal life is not unlike certain situations in human experience that are generally perceived as distressing and, as will be shown, can precede the onset of illness.

Epidemiologic Studies

Cassel had emphasized the importance of social structure as a factor in human susceptibility to disease.[39] Persons with a marginal status in society (oppressed ethnic minority groups, socially isolated individuals) and those who experience disorganization (broken homes) are more susceptible to a variety of disorders, including tuberculosis, schizophrenia, stroke, and alcoholism.

The idea that highly pressured jobs might have an increased association with certain diseases (hypertension, peptic ulcer disease, diabetes) was supported in a study by Cobb and Rose.[40] They found a severalfold higher prevalence and incidence of hypertension and double the prevalence of peptic ulcer disease among air traffic controllers as compared with second-class airmen. The relationship was more significant for those working at the busiest towers.

In studying the effects of life change on illness, Holmes and colleagues developed a 43-item questionnaire of life events, weighted for degree of social change and coping needed.[41] On the basis of both retrospective and prospective study designs[42] they reported that major changes in a person's lifestyle correlated with the subsequent incidence of illness or injury. The greater the cumulative score, the greater the likelihood of a significant change in health status. When this type of questionnaire is applied to patients with gastrointestinal disorders, the patients' scores are significantly different from those of normals or other medical groups. Those with peptic ulcer disease report negative life events as more severe.[43] However, patients with irritable bowel syndrome *minimize* the impact of negative life events, possibly reflecting the tendency of these patients to deny relevant psychosocial experiences.[44] These findings suggest that the group differences relate to the way these items are experienced and reported; they highlight the need in this type of research to determine the personal meaning of life events.

The work of Schmale,[45] using interviews with patients hospitalized for various medical diseases, complements the previous studies in his attempt to evaluate the personal experience of psychosocial events on feeling states. Eighty per cent of the patients interviewed reported a state of "giving up"; feelings of "helplessness" and "hopelessness" characterized by decreased abilities to cope with losses and a sense of futility in resolving difficulties. To determine if such feeling states relate to disease susceptibility, he studied women with atypical Pap smears, and reported that those previously identified as feeling "hopeless" by predefined criteria were more likely to have carcinoma in situ (as diagnosed by cervical conization) than those who felt they had some control over their environent.[46] These data suggest that environmental situations, psychologic states, or patient attitudes and behaviors may influence susceptibility to disease or the timing of its onset.

Psychiatric and Psychological Assessment

Psychiatric Reports. A major area of research during the psychoanalytically dominated era of psychosomatic medicine (1920 to 1955) was psychosomatic specificity, that is, whether specific psychologic features were associated with and necessary for the development of a particular disease. Alexander[47] and his associates at the Chicago Psychoanalytic Institute emphasized the role for psychodynamic conflict as a necessary factor in the development of specific personality characteristics for several medical diseases. Based on their evaluation of medical patients, they identified several diseases (asthma, rheumatoid arthritis, ulcerative colitis, essential hypertension, neurodermatitis, thyrotoxicity, and duodenal ulcer) as being psychosomatic.* The diseases were not caused solely by psychologic conflict but also required a biologic predisposition (X factor) for the diseases to develop later, if given the proper environmental setting.

One example of application of this theory is in peptic ulcer disease. Patients with this disorder were defined as having a conflict between a desire for independent accomplishment and a wish to be dependent and cared for by others. This conflict was believed to lead to certain compensatory and predictable personality traits (the "ulcer-prone personality"). The concept was further refined by Mirsky,[48] who stated that the genetic or early-acquired biologic factor was the *primary* defect that led to the specific psychologic characteristics. For example, the presence of acid hypersecretion in the infant might lead to a greater requirement for feeding in order to neutralize the excess secretion and relieve some internal tension state. If this need were not met by a gratifying environment (mother), then a chronic or repetitive state of tension would develop. The child might generalize this experience and later have difficulty gaining confidence in the environment as a source of support. A psychodynamic pattern (oral-dependent) for securing gratification would develop to satisfy the increased needs.

Thus, a person with this personality pattern would be more likely to view the real or threatened loss of a

---

Psychosomatic is an overused term considered by some as synonymous with *psychogenic* (i.e., caused by a psychologic mechanism in the absence of functional or structural organ change) and by others as reflective of all disorders in which psychologic variables contribute to the illness state. The classical definition is used in the context of this historical review. Thus, a psychosomatic disorder was considered a condition with morphologic end-organ change believed to result from both pre-existent biologic susceptibility and specific psychologic characteristics.

source of support as distressing. Examples would be the death of a loved one or moving away from home. Later, others theorized that in such situations the individual might develop a lowered gastric mucosal resistance to acid or might increase acid secretion, thus enhancing the susceptibility to ulcer formation. Increased acid secretion was reported to occur in ulcer patients when they experience tension, anxiety, anger, or other dysphoric states.[49]

The hypothesis that the pre-existing biologic tendency to gastric hypersecretion (as measured by elevated serum pepsinogen values) in combination with "ulcer-prone" personality characteristics may predispose such people to react to the typical conflict situation by developing a duodenal ulcer was tested in a prospective study of 2073 Army recruits in basic training.[50] It was presumed that leaving home and entering basic training would be an appropriate stressful environment to activate the specific dependent-independent conflict. A group of 63 acid hypersecretors and 57 hyposecretors were selected for psychologic testing and gastroenterologic X-ray examination. Ten men (8 per cent of the total sample of 120 men) were selected by psychiatrists blinded to the medical findings as most likely to have or to develop a duodenal ulcer. By the end of the study, 9 of the 120 men were found to have an ulcer initially or on subsequent X-ray examination. They were all hypersecretors. Most interestingly, seven of these nine ulcer patients were among the sample of ten selected by the psychiatrists. Thus, recognition of the characteristic psychologic pattern predicted the occurrence of ulcer disease among members of a larger group with similar capacity for hypersecretion. The hypothesis was supported.

This study can be criticized since the population of young males is not representative of the general ulcer population, the psychologic findings were never validated on another patient sample, and the proteolytic bioassay used for pepsinogen was crude and subject to daily variation. Nevertheless, the results must be considered compelling, unless and until a study using more sophisticated techniques produces contrasting findings.

The onset or exacerbation of disease symptoms at the time of personally distressing events has frequently been observed when these data are sought. Using ulcerative colitis as an example, Karush[51] reviewed case reports by psychiatrists and analysts of hundreds of patients with this disorder. The common thread reported for symptom exacerbation was activation of a conflict relating to an intensely dependent relationship with a controlling and dominating mother or other key figure.[52–56] This conflict was believed to explain the observations that ulcerative colitis patients are overly sensitive to rejecting attitudes. As a result they seem reluctant to develop trusting relationships with some people, but may also become very dependent on certain key persons and place unrealistic demands upon them.[56] A real or threatened disruption of this key relationship, such as marriage, the death of the dominant person, his or her disapproval of the patient, or the assumption of increased responsibility by the patient (thereby fostering a greater sense of independence) was associated with symptom flare-ups. Bleeding and diarrhea were sometimes reported to occur within 24 hours of the stressful event.[53, 56] For these reasons Engel has stressed the importance of a predictable and consistent physician-patient relationship as the keystone of treatment of ulcerative colitis patients. He warns that a flare of symptoms may occur if the patient is unprepared for any disruption in this relationship.[57] To validate this hypothesis prospective studies are needed that involve a less selected group of patients (i.e., not just those in psychoanalysis) in comparison with other medical patients and healthy subjects.

Standardized Psychologic Assessment. The use of standardized psychologic tests offers the advantages of reliability, consistency, and reproducibility of results, and allows for the control of the effects of the medical illness on the patient. Yet, when such tests are applied to patients with gastrointestinal disorders, either there is a lack of consistency in the results or there is great variation (psychologic heterogeneity)[58, 59] which would tend to refute the previous psychosomatic specificity hypothesis. However, standardized methods of psychologic assessment cannot evaluate the personal meaning of events and cannot always account for distortion of answers by patients due to defensiveness or a desire to give socially acceptable responses. Therefore standardized tests must be viewed as complementary to clinically elicited data.[59] For example, if the psychiatric observations just discussed are correct, then these patients, either unable or unwilling to disclose personal information before a trusting relationship is established, will not give the needed data in questionnaires or structured interviews. Indeed, some psychologic data suggest that patients with ulcerative colitis are not emotionally expressive[53] and fail to see the connection between their symptoms and any feelings of distress.[60] These clinical observations have led to the concept of "alexithymia," an affective and cognitive defect in certain patients' abilities to experience and report thoughts, fantasies, and feeling states.[61–63]

Our concepts of illness are changing with the results of new research. One point seems likely: The interaction of psychosocial variables is much more complex than the one formulated by the early psychosomatic theories of disease specificity. Nevertheless, the psychoanalytic work has provided a foundation for future study in understanding the role of early environmental influences in disease onset and patient experience of illness. Furthermore, it underscores the need to carry out multidisciplinary collaborative work in the behavioral and biologic sciences.

Current Research: Mechanisms

Just *how* psychologic and environmental factors influence susceptibility to illness and disease remains speculative, but recent data from multidisciplinary research in behavioral medicine and the basic sciences offer hypotheses for future clinical study.

Effects on Immune Function

Like many other physiologic systems, the immune system is sensitive to environmental influences via the central nervous system.[64] The capacity of rats to cope with their environment can influence tumor growth and mortality or their susceptibility to a host of infections.[65, 66] Clinical observations, case reports, and early epidemiologic studies in humans provide evidence for an association of stressful life events, such as bereavement or divorce, and higher rates of morbidity and mortality, and this relationship may be mediated through the immune system.[67] In one prospective study,[68] 15 men whose wives had advanced breast cancer showed a poorer blastogenic response to mitogens after their wives' deaths than before bereavement. In a cross-sectional study,[69] women recently separated from their husbands had significantly poorer responsiveness to mitogens and lower percentages of helper T lymphocytes than married women. Furthermore, poorer immune function and greater depression was associated with shorter separation periods and greater continued attachment to the former husband, suggesting that psychosocial adaptation to the experience may lead to recovery in immune function. These effects are also observed with more commonplace events such as stressful examinations. Among medical students significant declines in natural killer (NK) cell activity[70] and interferon production by stimulated lymphocytes[71] developed during final examinations. These effects were associated with higher subjective levels of distress and could not be explained by differences in personality, nutritional status, or sleep. Finally, a possible role for subjective distress in carcinogenesis has been implicated. In one study,[72] distressed (as measured by a depression scale) psychiatric inpatients had significantly poorer DNA repair of their irradiated leukocytes than their nondistressed patient counterparts. The authors propose that altered psychosocial states may have effects on carcinogenesis through alterations in DNA repair, in addition to the previously reported indirect effects through impaired immune surveillance of mutant cells.

Of possible clinical interest is that immune response may be directly modified through behavioral interventions. Ader and Cohen[73] have developed a model for altering immune function through classical conditioning. They have shown that a neutral stimulus (a flavored drink) paired with the immunosuppressive effects of a pharmacologic drug (cyclophosphamide) can produce a conditioned response such that the rat's antibody response to a later antigenic stimulus is attenuated in the conditioned rat when exposed to the drinking solution alone. In other words, the rat is conditioned to become immunosuppressed by the neutral stimulus when the active drug is no longer present. Using this model, the authors have also been able to significantly delay the development of murine lupus erythematosus in NZB-NZW hybrid mice.[74] In a human study of geriatric residents who were randomly assigned to relaxation training, social contact, or no intervention, immune response was possibly enhanced in the relaxation training group as evidenced by greater NK cell activity and lower antibody titers to a herpes simplex type I antigen, and this was concomitant with decreases in distress-related symptoms.[75]

These immune changes may be mediated through the hypothalamus and perhaps the limbic system. The hypothalamus is at the interface between environmental input to the brain and peripheral regulatory systems that include immunity, endocrine release, autonomic control, and behavior.[76] Ablation of portions of the hypothalamus in the guinea pig prevents lethal anaphylaxis (as a model for humoral response)[77] and suppresses the cell-mediated cutaneous response to tuberculin.[78] In vitro measures of lymphocyte stimulation by phytohemagglutinin and the antigen tuberculin PPD in guinea pigs following anterior hypothalamic ablation showed significant blunting of responses compared with control and sham-operated animals.[79] Hypothalamic modulation of immune response may also occur through its control over endocrine and neurotransmitter release. Corticosteroids, growth hormone, thyroid hormone, and beta-adrenergic stimulation, all of which are regulated by the hypothalamus, can alter immune reactivity to antigenic stimuli.[76]

These studies indicate a relationship between transient altered psychosocial states, in vitro evidence of immune function, and possible modification of immune response through behavioral conditioning. While further work is needed to determine the clinical relevance of these findings in relation to disease susceptibility in humans, the implications are significant. They may explain the previously discussed clinical observations that relate psychosocial changes with onset or exacerbation of disease, and empiric reports that strong belief systems (e.g., via faith healers and cults) attenuate disease or prolong life in patients with terminal illnesses. From a practical standpoint, behavioral interventions such as supportive interpersonal care or formalized psychologic interventions may influence the way individuals respond to stressful events, and by ameliorating distress, may have an impact on associated changes in immune function, and ultimately on health.

Brain-Gut Peptides

The immunohistochemical mapping of brain-gut peptides may establish linkages between psychologic states and other CNS phenomena and physiologic responses in the intestine. The opiate peptides, enkephalin and endorphins, and their receptors, isolated in the brain, play a major role in pain perception. In one study, administration of naloxone, an opiate receptor antagonist, reduced the probability of a placebo response and caused a significantly greater increase in pain ratings among placebo responders than among nonresponders.[80] These substances may also be involved in human behavior and certain disorders such as schizophrenia.[81] The pronounced effects of opiates on intestinal motility have long been recognized; the opiate receptors in the gut are similar to those identified for endogenous opiates in the brain. In addition, intestinal peptides such as vasoactive intestinal peptide, bombesin, secretin, cholecystokinin (CCK), and substance P, to name a few, are also present in the brain.[82] Their effects depend upon their location, and the roles of these peptides in brain function and psychologic behavior are only beginning to be studied. For example, it is known that the exogenous administration of cholecystokinin and bombesin inhibits feeding activity and elicits postprandial satiety in several animals.[83] Determination of the role that food-stimulated endogenous release of CCK plays in human eating patterns and the disorders of eating (anorexia nervosa and morbid obesity) must await the development of methods for measuring these peptides in the circulation. Certain properties of these peptides highlight the complexity and variety of possible interactions between the central nervous system and gut function. They can be released locally *or* systemically (neurocrine, paracrine, endocrine), are found as neurotransmitters in the brain *and* gut ("peptidergic" system), and have extremely varied effects depending upon the target organ.

Neurophysiology of the Gut

A final area of promising research is in the study of the intestinal smooth muscle response to various stimuli and its implications for understanding the functional gastrointestinal disorders. It is possible that the hyperactive gut response to endocrine and neuropsychologic stimuli can be affected by differences in myoelectrial activity. Using the irritable bowel syndrome (IBS) as a model, Snape[84] and Taylor[85] have reported a higher prevalence of a 3 cycle per minute slow-wave electrical activity in the rectosigmoid in IBS patients than in normal individuals and propose this to be the biologic basis for the disorder. In the resting state, colonic motor activity is the same for both groups; however, when CCK or pentagastrin was given, increased motor activity occurred in the IBS patients, at the same frequency of 3 cycles per minute. The authors propose that when the intestine is stimulated, this abnormality in *electrical* activity predisposes to an abnormal pattern of colonic *motor* activity that is manifested as symptoms.[86] In another series of studies, Bueno and coworkers[87] suggest that IBS type symptoms are mediated by differences in electrical spike-burst (action potential) activity rather than slow-wave activity. When using a long intracolonic electromyographic recording probe, they report that among IBS patients constipation is associated with an increased incidence of short spike bursts and diarrhea is associated with a decreased incidence of spike bursts. Furthermore, symptoms of abdominal pain were seen to correlate with increased spike-bursts and nonperistaltic muscle contraction waves. More recently, Kumar and Wingate[88] have reported specific motor abnormalities to exist in the small intestine of IBS patients. When compared with normal people or patients with inflammatory bowel disease, IBS patients have spontaneous and stress-induced abolition of the migrating motor complex

(MMC "housekeeper") and abnormal irregular contractile activity.

There remains a great deal of variation among laboratories as to how these patterns are measured and interpreted, and the prevalence of these findings and their specificity for gastrointestinal disorders have yet to be confirmed.[89] Nevertheless, the data provide preliminary evidence as to *how* psychosocial factors produce their physiologic effects.

Psychosocial Influences on the Patient's Experience of and Response to Illness

Effects on the Experience of Illness

As a practical matter, clinicians must often be more concerned with how environmental events, personality, and behavior contribute to a patient's illness than with their effects on the development of disease. Gastroenterology practices include patients who are genuinely incapacitated with symptoms that are probably of psychologic origin and patients who must adapt psychologically to a chronic disease. Throughout life, personality, family, and society shape the individual's attitudes, expectations, and behaviors about illness. This learning influences how the person experiences disease and how he or she copes, uses medical facilities, and complies with treatment. For example, one person who awakens with abdominal pain may go to work if he or she recognizes the pain to be minor, believes that complaining is a "weakness," or is worried about losing a day's pay. Another individual with the same experience but who recently lost a loved one to intestinal cancer, who is conditioned by early family memories to expect excessive attention when ill, or who is employed at a place with liberal sick leave policies would be more likely to stay at home or to see a physician. The varying patterns of how symptoms are perceived, evaluated, and acted upon are designated as *illness behavior*.[90] In order to allow optimal patient care to be provided, the factors mediating this behavior must be sought among patients with chronic gastrointestinal disease or those in whom psychologic factors are the major determinants for the illness.

Societal norms will influence how symptoms are experienced and reported. In China, mental illness is highly stigmatized, and patients with minor psychiatric problems will present with physical symptoms.[91] Ethnic differences regarding pain behavior among patients in a New York City hospital were reported by Zborowski.[92] First- and second-generation Jews and Italians were observed to be more dramatic in their response to pain, whereas the Irish tended to deny their symptoms and the "Old Americans" remained more stoic. Attitudes about pain relief also differed. While Italians were satisfied with relief of pain, the Jewish patients continued to be preoccupied with their symptoms, concerned with the meaning of the pain and the future consequences. Although this information may not apply as well to later-generation ethnic groups, the concept of cultural influences on patient experience of illness and response to it is important.

Effects on Health Care Seeking. Although nearly all patients with acute severe illness will eventually seek medical care, social and psychologic factors play a major role in *whether* or *when* patients with chronic disease or mildly discomforting symptoms go to the doctor. Between 70 and 90 per cent of all self-recognized illnesses are managed outside traditional medical facilities, often with self-help groups or religious/cult practitioners providing a substantial portion of the care.[93] Although these practitioners are not trained to diagnose and treat disease, several studies show them to be more effective than traditional medicine in restoring a sense of well-being in their clients, even without objective evidence of improvement.[93] Studies of irritable bowel syndrome patients support the idea that patterns of seeking health care are culturally and psychologically determined. The female:male sex ratio of IBS in Western nations is 2:1,[94] but in India, where women are not expected to see physicians unless seriously ill, the sex ratio is reversed.[95] Furthermore, in a multivariate analysis of IBS patients and IBS nonpatients who had never been to physicians, when controlling for symptom severity, the primary determinants of patient status were personality factors, illness behaviors, and reaction to stressful life events.[44]

The Role of Personality Characteristics. Just as patients with occult disease may have no symptoms, so patients may have bodily complaints without evident disease or may display symptom behaviors that are out of proportion to the clinical findings. Such patients see themselves as ill and, wittingly or unwittingly, derive certain benefits from the "sick role." Parsons lists such benefits as exemption from work or family obligations, avoidance of stressful situations, and gratification of needs through a dependent relationship with a physician.[96] The mechanisms of this abnormal illness behavior[97] vary among individuals but are usually understood on the basis of underlying personality patterns, psychiatric disorders, or social influence.

For example, *hypochondriacal patients* are preoccupied with bodily functions and have numerous seemingly innocuous complaints that are magnified into worries about serious illness. Many of these patients have limited social relationships outside the health care system. Their persistent complaints serve to maintain self-esteem and provide a means of social communication.[98] The physician must accept their illness without challenge and at the same time avoid compulsion or patient pressure to undertake unneeded studies or treatments.

People with *histrionic personality* features (somatization disorder, "hysteria") are also likely to develop bodily complaints in situations that might produce mental distress and tend to dramatize their symptoms. They have a strong need to depend on others for gratification and support, and all these characteristics readily influence them to seek the care of physicians. Diagnostic evaluation will involve basing clinical decisions on data from the history, physical examination, and laboratory that suggest other medical disorders rather than relying solely on the intensity of the patients' complaints or their behavior. Care of such patients involves maintaining a consistent and supportive, but not overly involved, relationship.[99]

Patients with *depression* (major or atypical affective disorder) may have symptoms that simulate occult or organic disease. Some of these patients relate feelings of discouragement, loss of interest, and sadness about being physically ill and report their concerns in terms of bodily complaints such as anorexia, weight loss, and a variety of pain symptoms, including persistent severe abdominal pain. The diagnosis may be missed if the observed signs of depression are accepted as secondary to some overlooked disease. Often an exploration of the setting and circumstances preceding the onset of illness and an awareness of the behavioral characteristics of depression are helpful in making the diagnosis. These patients may benefit from treatment with antidepressant medication.

Once any disease becomes manifest to the patient as an illness, he or she will respond psychologically to the experience. For example, when health-related quality of life is evaluated by a standardized test (Sickness Impact Profile) in patients with inflammatory bowel disease, there is greater impairment of psychosocial (work, sleep and rest, recreation, social interaction, emotional behavior) than physical function.[100] Therefore it becomes an unnecessary exercise to determine whether the psychosocial or physical effects are the main problems. Usually both are major factors, and treatment will be based on the determination of which aspects of the illness are remediable.

The psychologic adaptations required of patients with chronic disease are considerable. The meaning of illness in relation to the organ system involved, its severity, the perceived alterations in body image (e.g., colostomy), social acceptability, implications in terms of future function at work and at home, and the likelihood of surgery or untimely death must all be dealt with by the patient. How the physician assists in these adaptations can be crucial to the patient's psychologic well-being and clinical course. It is not surprising that the chronically ill patient will regress and often behave in a dependent manner. The continued complaints about symptoms and the increased caretaking needs that the patients display may tax family, friends, and physician, all of whom may feel helpless to give enough emotional or medical assistance. Conversely, other patients will resist the help of others to avoid acknowledging their imposed dependence. The family must deal with feelings of guilt and anger, the expressions of which, though unavoidable, are not usually socially permitted. It is often the physician who not only bears the brunt of such feelings in the patient and family but must also reconcile these difficulties among the various parties. In most instances, the problems are worked out and the patient establishes a pattern of coping. However, if the patient has limited capacity to cope psychologically with the illness, if the disorder is particularly incapacitating, or if the interpersonal family relationships are unstable, more physician and ancillary effort (social service, psychologic counseling, peer support groups such as the National Foundation for Ileitis and Colitis) will be required to achieve a satisfactory adjustment.

CLINICAL APPLICATIONS

A Comprehensive Approach to Patient Evaluation and Care

There are two messages from our analysis of the psychosocial literature. The first is that a close association among the environment, the mind, and the digestive tract in function and disease exists, but that methodologic difficulties in studying these variables preclude full clarification of the relationship. The second message is that future multidisciplinary collaborative research is needed to confirm and establish the mechanisms underlying these associations. However, the clinicians who must address daily all the biologic, psychologic, and sociocultural variables that contribute to the illnesses among their patients are not in a position to wait.

The limitations of a nonintegrated approach (i.e., psychologic *or* physical) to both diagnosis and patient care are evident. To diagnose a patient's physical complaint as "functional" can be done only with the recognition that serious disease might present with nonspecific or atypical symptoms. Furthermore, since disease may occur or be exacerbated at times of life events requiring psychosocial adaptation,[42] the attribution of illness to psychosocial factors apart from disease has no specificity in explaining the true basis of patient complaints. Similarly, it is frequently assumed that directed treatment of a patient's disease is sufficient; any secondary psychologic difficulties will resolve. Yet patients do not always have anticipated clinical responses to even the most reliable treatment. A patient with a duodenal ulcer may continue to have pain despite endoscopically proved healing, while another will become asymptomatic before healing occurs.[101] With the same diagnosis, one patient might minimize the symptoms and be noncompliant to treatment, while another might focus on the symptoms and request that the physician certify a claim for disability insurance.

What the clinician needs is a framework that embraces interaction among, rather than separation of, biologic and behavioral dimensions. One, proposed by Engel,[102, 103] is based on observations in biology.[104, 105] This biopsychosocial model of illness describes a hierarchy of related subsystems extending from the molecule to the organ, the person, the family, and the society within which he or she lives (Fig. 1–1). Thus, our biomedical knowledge of disease is framed within a more comprehensive system. Each level in the hierarchy is composed of less complex subsystems and is itself a component of a larger system (Fig. 1–2). For example, the human being is the highest level of the organismic hierarchy and at the same time the lowest unit of the social hierarchy. All the subsystems are

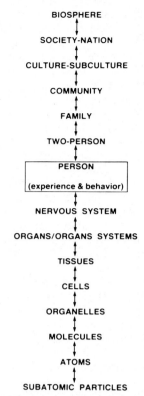

Figure 1–1. Hierarchy of related subsystems. (From Engel, G. Am. J. Psychiatr. *137*:535, 1980. Used by permission.)

interrelated so that a change, for example, at the cellular level (e.g., development of AIDS) has the potential of affecting organ systems, the person, the family, and society. In a clinical setting, information is first obtained from the person via the interview and physical examination. Further evaluation may include gathering data at any other level (testing for immune competency, assessment of organ damage, cultures, biopsies, identification of contacts, public health assessment within the community, and so forth).

Consider the use of this model in the evaluation of a recently widowed male alcoholic with chronic pancreatitis who is brought to the hospital in acute abdominal pain hours after an automobile accident. Several interrelated factors are evident. His pain can be explained by the pre-existent pancreatic disease and/or a new episode of acute pancreatitis due to increased alcohol intake or trauma. From a psychologic standpoint unresolved conflicts relating to the loss of the spouse can produce pain in some individuals on a psychogenic basis.[106] Finally, the patient may have drunk to ease the pain of his chronic disease, to console himself during his acute grief, or to gather the courage to kill himself (via drunk driving) and join his wife. Few, if any, of these contributing, or possibly primary, factors will be recognized if the physician ends the evaluation with confirmation of acute pancreatitis. Long-term success in this patient's care will depend on intervention at several levels.

A model such as this does not have to increase the

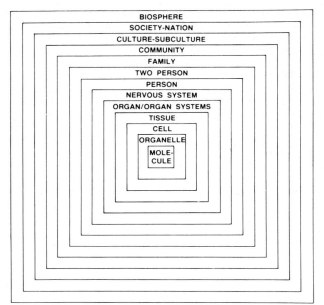

Figure 1–2. Continuum of systems. Each level is composed of less complex subsystems.

demands on clinicians; rather, it reorients them so that what is already known to constitute optimal evaluation and care of patients becomes operational. Furthermore, its use avoids the pitfall of trying to decide whether a problem is functional or organic[107] or of assuming that *if* the behavioral influences are considered, less attention will be paid to the proper treatment of the disease.

The following suggestions serve only as guidelines to what is an *individualized* approach to patient evaluation and care. They can be applied to all patients but are of particular value for those suspected to have mainly psychosocial determinants for their illnesses[108] or those with chronic disorders whose behavior or clinical response does not fit patterns expected from the clinical findings.

Obtaining the Data—The History

The physician's interview technique is his most important asset in making a diagnosis and planning treatment, yet this clinical skill is often underutilized. Consider the information obtained in this office interview:

Dr.: "How can I help you?"
Pt.: "I developed a flare-up of my Crohn's . . . the pain, nausea and vomiting, when I came back from vacation . . . (pause) . . . I . . ."
Dr.: "Was the pain like what you had before?"
Pt.: "Yes . . . well almost . . . I think."
Dr.: "Was it made worse by food?"
Pt.: "Yes."
Dr.: "Did you have fever? or diarrhea?"
Pt.: "Well yes, I think, but I didn't take my temperature."

Dr.: "So you had fever and diarrhea?"
Pt.: "Uh no, well, they were a little loose . . . I guess."

In this case, the physician eventually diagnosed partial small bowel obstruction secondary to Crohn's disease. However, some relevant information was not elicited in this interview, and because of the interruptions and use of leading questions, the accuracy of the information after the first question is uncertain.

The medical history is obtained by encouraging the patient to tell the story in his own way so that the events contributing to the illness unfold naturally;[109] this is called the patient-centered, nondirective interview. Open-ended questions produce the most accurate data. Additional information is obtained with facilitating expressions: "Yes?", "Can you tell me more?", repeating the patient's previous statements, head nodding, or even silence with an expectant look. Avoid closed-ended (yes-no) questions at first, though they may be used later in the interview to further characterize the symptoms. Never use multiple choice or leading questions because the patient's desire to comply may bias his responses.

The traditional "medical" and "social" histories should not be separated but elicited together, so the medical problem is described in the context of the psychosocial events surrounding the illness. The setting of symptom onset or exacerbation should always be obtained. At all times, the questions should communicate the physician's willingness to address both biologic and psychologic aspects of the illness.

Dr.: "How can I help you?"
Pt.: "I developed a flare-up of my Crohn's . . . the pain, nausea and vomiting, when I came back from vacation . . . (pause) . . ."
Dr.: "Yes? . . ."
Pt.: "I was about to start my new position as floor supervisor, and thought I'd take vacation to get prepared . . . and then all this happened."
Dr.: "Oh, I see . . . (pause) . . . so then you got sick."
Pt.: "Yes. I started getting that crampy feeling right here . . . and then it got worse after eating. So I knew I'd be obstructed again if I didn't get in to see you."
Dr.: "Any other symptoms?"
Pt.: "Well, I felt warm, but didn't take my temperature."
Dr.: "What about your bowel pattern?"
Pt.: "They started getting loose when I was on vacation. Now they're slowing down. I haven't gone today."

Note that the number of verbal exchanges is the same, yet the patient says more. The clinical features are clearer and additional knowledge of the symptoms associated with beginning a new job situation is obtained. This interview method also encourages patient self-awareness and provides for possible behavioral treatment intervention (stress-reduction techniques, job change, counseling) that may ameliorate future symptom flare-ups.

The historical information should be obtained from the perspective of the patient's understanding of the illness. Personal beliefs and family and cultural mores will influence whether and how the symptoms are reported. Important questions to ask include, "What do you think is causing this problem?", Why did it happen now?", "What kind of treatment do you think you should receive?", and "What do you fear most about your illness?"[93, 110]

A 29-year-old black woman continued to have severe abdominal pain after hospital evaluation failed to yield a diagnosis and despite use of analgesic medication. When asked what she thought could be causing the pain, after some hesitation she reported that she believed that "roots" (a hex) were put on her by the friend of a woman who was seeing her husband. She was later treated by her own "root doctor" with amelioration of the symptoms within days.

This case illustrates the need to understand the problem from the patient's perspective and highlights the power of cultural belief systems in influencing the illness.[111]

Evaluating the Data

In planning the diagnostic and treatment approach the physician should assess the relative influences of the biologic, psychologic, and social dimensions on the illness. Both medical and psychologic hypotheses should be considered. It is just as inappropriate (and possibly harmful) to subject a patient with "functional" illness to unneeded diagnostic studies while failing to explore psychologic determinants as it is to obtain a psychiatric consultation in a patient presenting with fulminant colitis and toxic megacolon. A negative medical evaluation is insufficient data for making the diagnosis of a psychosocial disorder. Therefore, psychiatric consultation should be considered when the psychological data could clarify the illness or improve patient care. Examples include psychiatric diagnoses that would benefit from specific treatment (e.g., psychopharmacologic agents, electroconvulsive therapy), situations in which the patient's level of psychosocial functioning is seriously impaired in the absence of significant physical abnormalities (e.g., inability to work), or when invasive diagnostic or therapeutic strategies are being considered on the basis of patient complaints without clear indications from medical data.

As with medical diagnoses, the certainty of a psychologic diagnosis depends on obtaining valid data:[112]

A 27-year-old married childless legal secretary developed symptoms of nausea, vomiting, and painful "swelling" of her abdomen, which she perceived as due to constipation. After two years of taking laxatives to relieve her abdominal swelling, she developed weakness and muscle cramps. She was hospitalized and found to have hypokalemia, metabolic alkalosis, and mild renal insufficiency. Medical evaluation was otherwise nondiagnostic.

The patient came from a large family and had planned, in accordance with her family's wishes, to have several children. There was some difficulty conceiving, but after four years she succeeded, only to hemorrhage two weeks before the

due date and deliver a stillborn child. A funeral was held without her knowledge prior to her discharge from the hospital; subsequently, any desire of hers to talk about the events or to cry was discouraged by her overprotective family. The vomiting and abdominal "swelling" began at this time. Over the next few months, she was discouraged from talking about the event, lost interest in visiting the grave, and stopped going to church. The hospitalization for the metabolic disturbance occurred on the second anniversary of the childbirth.

After discharge from the hospital, she was seen regularly as an outpatient and with gradual encouragement became aware of her mixed feelings about having children. *Though strongly encouraged by her husband and parents to be a mother, at times she saw this role as an impediment to her freedom.* These thoughts were shameful to her and led to feelings of guilt over possibly contributing to the child's death. In addition, she harbored resentment toward the family for not allowing her to grieve.

This patient's successful clinical response began during outpatient visits with her reliving of the traumatic event and with further discussion of her ambivalence toward being a mother. Active grieving of the stillborn child ensued. She became clinically depressed and recognized that her nausea, abdominal swelling, and pain, which she attempted to treat by taking laxatives, occurred when thinking about the baby.

After several months, the laxative use ended and the symptoms resolved. The patient became pregnant a second time but lost the fetus in the fourth month. This time she experienced active grieving without recurrence of symptoms or use of laxatives. One year later she delivered a healthy girl and continues without symptoms.

In this confirmed case of psychogenic pain and vomiting complicated by laxative abuse and metabolic disturbances, the underlying conflict was between the desire to be working and childless and the social and family expectations for her to be a mother and homemaker. Pregnancy was accompanied by unconscious angry feelings toward the child, who would eventually limit her freedom. Thus, for her, the stillbirth was a very distressing event. The underlying negative feelings about the unborn child made her feel responsible for its death. The nausea, vomiting, and abdominal swelling, modeled after the symptoms of pregnancy, served symbolically to deny the death of the fetus, thus freeing her from feeling guilty. The resolution of the symptoms after discussion of the conflicts and mourning were permitted offers further evidence for the diagnosis.[113]

In accepting the multidetermined nature of illness, it follows that medical diagnoses are not made to the exclusion of psychologic diagnoses, and vice versa.

A 25-year-old white single woman was hospitalized with a two and one-half year history of abdominal, back, and neck pain, anorexia, and weight loss. Worsening pain and profound weight loss up to 50 pounds had developed in the six months prior to hospitalization. After numerous negative diagnostic studies over the years, her recent deterioration prompted referral by her family physician for further evaluation. Initial work-up was again unrevealing except for evidence of malnutrition, some midabdominal tenderness, and the finding of a 2-cm left supraclavicular node, on which a biopsy was performed. Laboratory studies revealed a mildly elevated serum alkaline phosphatase and low serum albumin, both of which were attributed to malnutrition.

Without a certain diagnosis, psychiatric consultation was obtained before the laboratory report on the node was returned. The psychiatrist uncovered a pathologic grief reaction with depression and on this basis reported that psychologic factors were contributing to her symptoms. Her father had died in a plane accident when she was eight years old, but she continued to talk as if he were still alive. Many of the feelings about her father were displaced onto a younger brother who "looked and acted just like him." The symptoms began when her brother left for Okinawa after joining the army. She maintained feelings of loneliness and sadness, with frequent crying spells, anorexia, lack of motivation, constipation, and sleep disturbance with nocturnal awakening.

A diagnosis of metastatic squamous cell carcinoma was made. The patient died four months later.

The presence of carcinoma does not minimize the significance of the psychologic data obtained or its long-standing contribution to the patient's prior illness. The pitfall to the physician would be to assume (prior to the node biopsy) that her problem was psychologic without adequate exploration of possible somatic causes, or conversely (after the node biopsy), that the entire two and one-half year illness was fully explained by the cancer. A point worth considering from the previously discussed studies is whether her profound and prolonged state of depression had increased her susceptibility to cancer at such an early age.

Decision-Making in Diagnosis

To establish a diagnosis, further studies may be needed. Deciding which tests to order requires considering their usefulness within the clinical context. It it safe? Is it cost-effective? Will the results make a difference in treatment? Patients who are persistent in their complaints or who challenge their physician's competence may tempt the physician to schedule unneeded studies or surgery out of uncertainty, or just to "do something." This behavior has been called "furor medicus"[114] and can be avoided by basing decisions on careful and objective evaluation of data (e.g., blood in the stool, fever, abnormal serum chemistries) rather than solely on the patient's illness behavior.

The patient with persistent and unexplained abdominal pain is one example familiar to the gastroenterologist.[113, 115] In a review of 64 patients hospitalized for diagnosis of this problem and followed up to seven years, 85 per cent had no diagnosis made, and only four of the ten patients with a diagnosis eventually required surgical intervention (adhesive small bowel obstruction in two, common duct stones, and carcinoma of the pancreas).[116] The interesting finding for the purposes of this discussion is that 36 per cent of the group had exploratory laparotomy performed at some time over that seven-year period. A diagnosis was made in only one patient (duodenal ulcer), suggesting that the likelihood of laparotomy establishing an explanation for pain in a patient with an otherwise negative evaluation is small. Since the study was performed prior to the routine use of modern imaging techniques (e.g., ultrasound, CT and MRI scanning),

it is now likely that the diagnostic yield of laparotomy for referred patients with chronic pain would be even lower. In prospective series of similar medical and surgical patients who were also studied psychologically, many patients had psychiatric diagnoses established.[113, 117, 118]

Decisions must often be made with incomplete or nonspecific information. When studies are unrevealing and the patient is clinically stable, it is wiser to tolerate the uncertainty in diagnosis and observe the patient for new developments over a period of time ("Don't just do something—stand there!").

A 59-year-old black woman with diabetes for two years presented with severe abdominal pain and a 40-pound weight loss due to anorexia, nausea, and postprandial vomiting over a six-month period. She was hospitalized and found to have an unexplained anemia of chronic disease, a gastric motility disorder secondary to her diabetes, and an elevated sedimentation rate. She described her pain as constant, severe, and associated with sleep loss and frequent crying spells. Psychiatric consultation disclosed that she seemed mildly depressed, which was presumed secondary to her medical illness, and that symptoms began several weeks after the death of an aunt who had raised her as a child. There were insufficient psychologic data to make any specific diagnosis. It was observed that her family and friends paid a great deal of attention to her during the period of her illness. She stated that they cared for her "like my aunt did." The social support from her family (secondary gain) was thought to possibly contribute to the maintenance of her illness state, possibly explaining the dramatization of her symptoms and increased helplessness she displayed when the family was present in the room.

There was no evidence of occult bleeding, and X-ray and endoscopic study of the upper gastrointestinal tract, small bowel, and colon showed only delayed gastric emptying. CT scan of the abdomen was negative. ERCP showed a normal biliary sytem, but the pancreatic duct could not be cannulated. Secretin-stimulated cytologies were negative. Bone marrow biopsies produced no specific diagnosis. Immunologic studies and rheumatologic consultation disclosed no evidence for vasculitis or an immune disorder.

A diagnostic laparotomy was actively considered, but it was decided to follow the patient clinically for several weeks with a trial of metoclopramide and tricyclic antidepressants. Six months later she regained some weight, vomiting resolved, and the pain, though still present, became less distressing. The anemia and elevated sedimentation rate have persisted.

With this patient, medical, psychologic, and social factors could be identified as contributing to her illness, yet many features of her condition remained unexplained. The possibility of an occult neoplasm was of concern, yet the risk of surgery and the low likelihood of affecting the patient's course favorably if cancer were found led to the decision to tolerate the uncertainty in diagnosis rather than attempt further invasive procedures.

Treatment

Establish a Therapeutic Relationship

The behavioral treatment strategy must be individualized since patients vary in the degree of negotiation and participation they require. The physician should nonjudgmentally show interest in the patient's well-being regardless of cause. It is often the fear of disapproval and lack of trust that prevent the patient from sharing the intimate thoughts and feelings that may be important in understanding the illness or planning treatment. When the patient is unwilling or unable to accept the role of psychosocial factors in the illness, the physician should not attempt to provide such "insight." If asked whether the problem is "in my head," the physician can explain that illness is rarely one or the other, and that it is important to understand the role of all factors, including the patient's feelings. The physician may cite examples of how many chronic conditions can be associated with depression or unrealistic fears. When appropriate, the patient should be reassured that his or her fears are unwarranted. However, premature or inappropriate reassurance may be perceived by the patient as a lack of thoroughness on the part of the physician. The physician must respond to the patient's needs empathically and nonjudgmentally, although this does not mean "going along" with the patient when it would not be in his or her best interest. For example, disability can be a disincentive for the patient to reestablish "wellness" and return to gainful employment. If the physician thinks the patient does not qualify, this should be stated clearly and firmly.

Recognize Patient Adaptations to Chronic Illness

With chronic illness patients develop adaptations that interfere with the motivation to improve. From the patient's perspective, more may initially be lost by giving up the illness (loss of family attention, stopping of narcotic medication, increased responsibility at home or at work) than is gained by relief of the discomfort.

A 28-year-old single male machinist with a long-standing history of Crohn's colitis was receiving disability compensation because of symptoms of chronic diarrhea, perianal disease, and weight loss from a colonic fistula eroding into his jejunum. Because of his chronic disease, he moved in with his parents to be cared for by them. He did not want to have surgery, but after several years of poor control with medical management, he agreed and had a proctocolectomy and ileostomy. This led to objective improvement with weight gain and healing of the perianal disease. Nevertheless, for the next 18 months he continued to complain of lethargy and weakness, increased his alcohol intake, and felt unable to return to work, requesting continuation of his disability benefits.

The physician must accept that clinical improvement in these situations may take a long time but may be advanced if he or she attends to helping the patient to return to more normal psychosocial function as well as to cope with the illness.

Help the Patient Develop Independence to Grow Out of the "Sick Role"

The obvious reinforcers for illness behavior include increased attention from others and social and financial compensation. However, many of the physician's behaviors, though appropriate with certain patients having acute illness, will actually maintain sick role behavior among patients with chronic illness. Such behaviors include paying a great deal of attention to patient complaints to the exclusion of other issues, acting on each complaint by ordering diagnostic studies or giving prescriptive medication, or maintaining a dominant position in the interaction by assuming total responsibility for the patient's well-being. The patient learns that the physician's interest is contingent on continued illness behavior rather than on clinical improvement and that he or she should maintain a passive and compliant manner. The physician's role with chronically ill patients is to modify their behavior by encouraging them to take more responsibility in their care. An example would be to give the patient the option of choosing among several indicated medications (e.g., high-fiber diet and/or psyllium seed preparation for constipation). Thus, the physician gives up some control in the treatment plan in an effort to encourage patient responsibility. In addition, the physician should pay more attention to other aspects of the patient's life, while limiting discussion about the patient's symptoms (the "organ recital") to no more than is needed to satisfy any medical considerations. This technique of differential attention is a form of operant conditioning that reinforces a more adaptive form of social communication.

Use of Psychopharmacologic Medications

Psychopharmacologic medications, while often overprescribed, can be a treatment adjunct for selected patients with chronic gastrointestinal complaints. Their indications should be based not on the severity of the symptoms but on the patient's emotional and behavioral condition. The acutely anxious patient (evidenced by observing speech and nonverbal behavior) with impairment of daily function can be treated briefly with a benzodiazepine agent. These drugs are not indicated for mild self-limited anxiety or for the treatment of chronic anxiety states. Tricyclic antidepressants are most helpful in the patient with so-called organic signs of depression—sleep disturbance, weight loss, constipation, loss of libido, psychomotor retardation, and loss of interest in activities.[119] Evidence for these signs in the patient with unexplained gastrointestinal complaints would warrant a therapeutic trial, even when the patient denies feeling sad (masked depression). Some data suggest that tricyclic antidepressants, monoamine oxidase inhibitors, or combinations of antidepressants and phenothiazines[119-121] can be helpful in patients with unexplained pain syndromes. Their effectiveness may relate to treatment of an underlying depression or to an effect on pain perception via endogenous endorphin release or facilitation of CNS descending inhibitory pain pathways.[122]

A 64-year-old auto mechanic was referred for evaluation of a nine-month history of mid-abdominal pain and 15-lb weight loss. Extensive diagnostic evaluation by his referring physician was unrevealing. The patient reported that the pain kept him from eating, sleeping, and working and from assuming his usual interests. He angrily requested that "something be done" or he will "go to the Mayo Clinic." While he denied symptoms of depression, his sister volunteered that he had actually lost interest in all activities since his wife died of uterine cancer one year earlier. A trial of a tricyclic antidepressant was begun with the explanation that the medication is used for control of chronic pain.

Three months later the patient still complained of the pain, but acknowledged being able to sleep better and resume part-time work. He had gained back 10 lb.

In this case history, behavioral signs of depression were present even with the patient's denial of sadness. A treatment trial led to clinical improvement despite the persistence of pain symptoms.

Patients with psychotic delusions may present to the gastroenterologist with bodily complaints. These patients, who may respond to phenothiazine or other antipsychotic agents, are often identified by their bizarre beliefs about the symptoms. For example, a patient complaining of abdominal pain might, when asked, state that it is due to insects devouring the stomach. The description is not reported metaphorically; the patient truly believes it. These patients require psychiatric referral.

Psychiatric Treatment

The indications for psychiatric consultation have been discussed. Psychiatric treatment should be based on an assessment of the extent to which the illness produces a personal, social, and economic hardship. It is not necessarily dependent on a psychiatric diagnosis but rather on the likelihood that the patient will respond to some therapeutic intervention (e.g., with lithium, psychotherapy, and so forth). The patient must see psychiatric care as relevant to personal needs. The patient who agrees to see the psychiatrist "to prove I'm not crazy" is not likely to be helped.

The type of treatment must be individualized. For the psychologically minded and motivated patient, insight-oriented psychotherapy can be recommended. The patient with limited finances who is not intimidated by sharing personal thoughts with others might benefit from group therapy. Crisis intervention (i.e., four or five sessions designed to get the individual over a particularly difficult period) can help the patient with chronic illness who experiences identifiable causes for recent deterioration in function. Family or marital counseling is indicated when difficulties in the family interaction contribute to the illness state or to the patient's maladaptive behavior. Some patients do well with brief visits to a psychopharmacology clinic. Finally, behavioral modification, relaxation training, biofeedback, and other operant techniques can be used in the patient with a psychophysiologic disorder who is motivated toward taking personal responsibility in the treatment.

Physician Considerations

Patients with unexplained complaints or chronic gastrointestinal disease can be taxing on physicians who want all their patients to become symptom-free and compliant within a short period. It is no wonder that patients who abuse themselves (e.g., chronic alcoholics) or who derive traditionally unacceptable benefits from the health care system (e.g., hypochondriacs) are called "crocks," "turkeys," or "gomers." These inexcusable terms seem to allay the frustration that develops when physicians feel helpless to benefit them.[123] Medicine is not an exact science, and physicians must learn to tolerate uncertainty; however, recognition of the psychosocial dimensions of illness will often put the patient's problems into better perspective. Finally, the physician must set realistic goals in treatment of patients with chronic or unexplained illness. Often the goal is not total relief but improvement in psychosocial function *despite* the symptoms.

CONCLUSION AND EPILOGUE

The physician is confronted daily with patients whose illnesses need to be understood within a psychosocial context. The purposes of this chapter have been to explore the possible associations among biologic, psychologic, and sociocultural variables in illness and disease and to present a patient-centered rather than disease-oriented approach to diagnosis and care.

We can now return to Mrs. R., the subject of the first case study presented in this chapter. Given a comprehensive framework, such questions as "Is there obstruction *or* is the problem functional?" need to be reframed: for example, "Given this patient's long and complicated history, what types of treatments and interventions (surgery, bowel training, bran, psychotherapy, metoclopramide, and so forth) are likely in combination to effect a clinical response?" Although more data are needed before her illness can be fully clarified and treatment plans instituted, several points with relevance to many such cases can be made.

The patient's long-standing history of constipation should be judged carefully. Her working definition of constipation (within 48 hours) is well within the limits of normal function.[5] Rather than being constipated by standards of stool consistency or frequency, this patient may simply pay more attention to bowel function than most persons do. Her foster mother's use of enemas when she was young may have some bearing on this preoccupation, a possibility that is supported by the patient's early and continued use of laxatives. Their relationship early in her life may in itself, through operant conditioning, have altered her bowel pattern over the years. As a means of resisting her dominating foster mother, the child may have withheld stool. The psychic reward she gained (controlling her body and thwarting her mother) may have reinforced the inhibition of the defecation reflex, and this gradually contributed to later constipation.[124]

Later in life, Mrs. R. experienced episodes of pseudo-obstruction that coincided with a number of possible biologic determinants—possible scleroderma bowel disease, habit constipation, use of drugs that impair intestinal motility (narcotic analgesics and anticholinergics), and hypokalemia. In addition, three events related to real or threatened loss (hysterectomy, separation from her husband, and serious illness in her natural mother) preceded the onset of bowel dysfunction, of disease (possible scleroderma), and of behaviors that worsened her clinical condition (increased use of laxatives and anticholinergics). That such events would be more significant to her than to others is supported by her hospitalization for depression shortly after leaving home for college and her observations from psychotherapy. The more-than-coincidental association of these events and the inability to attribute a specific biologic or psychologic cause to her illness have been the basis for this discussion.

Whatever treatments are ultimately chosen for this "orphan" patient, the management of issues of *control*, as evidenced by her noncompliance to treatment recommendations, and *perceived rejection* will influence their efficacy. In the treatment plan, the physician should probably include a promise to Mrs. R. that he or she is committed to caring for her medically for an extended time. Furthermore, she should be invited to participate in the decisions made about specific treatment; for example, she may choose between a high-fiber diet and a bulk laxative.

The balance between psychosocial and biological influences will vary considerably among patients in a medical practice. For Mrs. R., the psychosocial influences on her illness may prove to outweigh the biologic ones. It is good clinical practice to consider all the variables in diagnosis and to attend to both the emotional and the medical needs of patients. Research in recent years has provided some scientific basis for the clinical observations presented. This chapter has been an attempt to synthesize our new knowledge and place it within a clinical framework. Much is yet to be learned about mechanisms and interactions. Because of our developing scientific understanding, however, we now know that the common practice of separating the psychologic state of the patient from the physiologic state can no longer be justified.

References

1. Reading, A. Illness and disease. Med. Clin. North Am. *61*:703, 1977.
2. Mitchell, C. M., and Drossman, D. A. Survey of the AGA membership relating to patients with functional GI disorders. Gastroenterology *92*:1282, 1987.
3. Hinkle, L. E., Jr. The concept of "stress" in the biological and social sciences. *In* Lipowski, Z. J., et al. (eds.). Psychosomatic Medicine. Current Trends and Clinical Applications. New York, Oxford University Press, 1977, pp. 27–49.
4. Wolf, S. The psyche and the stomach. Gastroenterology *80*:605, 1981.
5. Drossman, D. A., Sandler, R. S., McKee, D. C., and Lovitz, A. J. Bowel patterns among subjects not seeking health care: Use of a questionnaire to identify a population with bowel dysfunction. Gastroenterology *83*:529, 1982.
6. Cannon, W. B. The movements of the intestine studied by means of roentgen rays. Am. J. Physiol. *6*:251, 1902.
7. Beaumont, W. *In* Experiments and Observations on the Gastric Juice and the Physiology of Digestion. Plattsburg, F. P. Allen, 1883.
8. Pavlov, I. *In* The Work of the Digestive Glands. English translation from the Russian by W. H. Thompson. London, C. Griffin and Company, 1910.
9. Wolf, S., and Wolff, H. G. Human Gastric Function. 1st ed. New York, Oxford University Press, 1943.
10. Engel, G. L., Reichsman, F., and Segal, H. L. A study of an infant with gastric fistula. I. Behavior and the rate of total hydrochloric acid secretion. Psychosom. Med. *18*:374, 1956.
11. Jacobson, E. Spastic esophagus and mucous colitis. Arch. Intern. Med. *37*:443, 1927.
12. Young, L. D., Richter J. E., Anderson K. O., Bradley, L. A., Katz, P. O., McElveen, L., Obrecht, W. F., Dalton C., and Snyder, R. M. The effects of psychological and environmental stressors on peristaltic esophageal contractions in healthy volunteers. Psychophysiology *24*(2):132, 1987.
13. Grace, W. J., Wolf, S., and Wolff, H. G. The Human Colon. New York, Paul B. Hoeber, 1951.
14. Friedman, M. H. F., and Snape, W. J. Color changes in the mucosa as affected by food and psychic stimuli. Fed. Proc. *5*:30, 1946.
15. Almy, T. P., Kern, F., Jr., and Tulin, M. Alteration in colonic function in man under stress: II. Experimental production of sigmoid spasm in healthy persons. Gastroenterology *12*:425, 1949.
16. Almy, T. P. Experimental studies on the irritable colon. Am J. Med. *10*:60, 1951.
17. Glaser, J. P., and Engel, G. L. Psychodynamics, psychophysiology, and gastrointestinal symptomatology. Clin. Gastroenterol. *6*:507, 1977.
18. Buxbaum, E., and Sodergren, S. S. A disturbance of elimination and motor development. The mother's role in the development of the infant. Psychoanal. Study Child *32*:195, 1977.
19. Hill, O. W. Psychogenic vomiting. Gut *9*:348, 1968.
20. Philippopoulos, G. S. The analysis of a case of merycism: Psychopathology-psychodynamics. Psychother. Psychosom. *22*:364, 1973.
21. Drossman, D. A., Ontjes, D. A., and Heizer, W. D. Anorexia nervosa. Gastroenterology *77*:1115, 1979.
22. Miller, N. E. Effect of learning on gastrointestinal functions. Clin. Gastroenterology *6*:533, 1977.
23. Bykov, K. M. The Cerebral Cortex and the Internal Organs. Translation by W. H. Gantt. New York, Chemical Publishing, 1957.
24. Razran, G. The observable unconscious and the inferable conscious in current Soviet psychophysiology: Interceptive conditioning, semantic conditioning and the orienting reflex. Psychol. Rev. *68*:81, 1961.
25. Miller, N. E., and Carmona, A. Modification of a visceral response: Salivation in thirsty dogs by instrumental training with water reward. J. Comp. Physiol. *63*:1, 1967.
26. Miller, N. E. Learning of visceral and glandular responses. Science *163*:434, 1969.
27. Whitehead, W. E., Winget, C., Fedoravicius, A. S., Wooley, S., and Blackwell, B. Learned illness behavior in patients with irritable bowel syndrome and peptic ulcer. Dig. Dis. Sci. *27*:202, 1982.
28. Lowman, B. C., Drossman, D. A., Cramer, E. M., and McKee, D. C. Recollection of childhood events in adults with irritable bowel syndrome. J. Clin. Gastroenterol. *9*:324, 1987.
29. Schuster, M. M., Nikoomanesh, P., and Welles, D. Biofeedback control of lower esophageal sphincter contraction. Clin. Res. *21*:521, 1973.
30. Furman, S. Intestinal biofeedback in functional diarrhea: A preliminary report. J. Behav. Therap. Exp. Psychiatr. *4*:317, 1973.
31. Wald, A. Biofeedback therapy for fecal incontinence. Ann. Intern. Med. *95*:146, 1981.
32. Selye, H. The general adaptation syndrome and the diseases of adaptation. J. Clin. Endocrinol. Metab. *6*:117, 1946.
33. Ader, R. Gastric erosions in the rat: Effects of immobilization at different points in the activity cycle. Science *145*:406, 1964.
34. Ackerman, S. H., Hofer, M. A., and Weiner, H. Age at maternal separation and gastric erosion susceptibility in the rat. Psychosom. Med. *37*:180, 1975.
35. Weiss, J. M. Somatic effects of predictable and unpredictable shock. Psychosom. Med. *32*:397, 1970.

36. Porter R. W., Brady, J. V., Conrad, D., Mason, J. W., Galambos, R., and Rioch, D. M. Some experimental observations on gastrointestinal lesions in behaviorally conditioned monkeys. Psychosom. Med. *20*:379, 1958.

37. Chalifoux, L. V., and Bronson, R. T. Colonic adenocarcinoma associated with chronic colitis in cotton top marmosets, *Saguinus oedipus*. Gastroenterology *80*:942, 1981.

38. Drossman, D. A. Is the cotton-topped tamarin a model for behavioral research? Dig. Dis. Sci. *30*:24s, 1985.

39. Cassel, J. The contribution of the social environment to host resistance. Am. J. Epidemiol. *104*:107, 1976.

40. Cobb, S., and Rose, R. M. Hypertension, peptic ulcer and diabetes in air traffic controllers. JAMA *224*:489, 1973.

41. Holmes, T. H., and Rahe, R. H. The social readjustment scale. J. Psychosom. Res. *11*:213, 1967.

42. Holmes, T., and Masuda, M. Life changes and illness susceptibility. *In* Dohrenwend, B. S., and Dohrenwend, B. P. (eds.). Stressful Life Events. New York, John Wiley & Sons, Inc., 1974.

43. Feldman, M., Walker, P., Green J. L., and Weingarden, K. Life events stress and psychosocial factors in men with peptic ulcer disease. Gastroenterology *91*:1370, 1986.

44. Drossman, D. A., McKee, D. C., Sandler, R. S., Mitchell, C. M., Lowman, B. C., Burger, A. L., and Cramer, E. M. Psychosocial factors in the irritable bowel syndrome: A multivariate study of patients and nonpatients with IBS. Gastroenterology *92*:1374, 1987.

45. Schmale, A. H. Giving up as a final common pathway to changes in health. Adv. Psychosom. Med. *8*:20, 1972.

46. Schmale, A. H., and Iker, H. Hopelessness as a predictor of cervical cancer. Soc. Sci. Med. *5*:95, 1971.

47. Alexander, F. Psychosomatic Medicine: Its Principles and Applications. New York, W. W. Norton, 1950.

48. Mirsky, I. A. Physiologic, psychologic and social determinants in the etiology of duodenal ulcer. Am. J. Dig. Dis. *3*:285, 1958.

49. Mittellman, B., Wolff, H. G., and Scharf, M. P. Emotions and gastroduodenal function: Experimental studies on patients with gastritis, duodenitis and peptic ulcer. Psychosom. Med. *4*:5, 1942.

50. Weiner, H., Thaler, M., Reiser, F., and Mirsky, I. A. Etiology of duodenal ulcer. I. Relation of specific psychological characteristics to rate of gastric secretion. Psychosom. Med. *19*:1, 1957.

51. Karush, A. A review of the psychosomatic literature on chronic ulcerative colitis. *In* Karush, A. (ed.). Psychotherapy in Chronic Ulcerative Colitis. Philadelphia, W. B. Saunders Company, 1977, pp. 39–58.

52. Murray, C. D. Psychogenic factors in the etiology of ulcerative colitis and bloody diarrhea. Am. J. Med. Sci. *180*:239, 1930.

53. Sullivan, A. J. Psychogenic factors in ulcerative colitis. Am. J. Dig. Dis. Nutr. *2*:651, 1935.

54. Daniels, G. E. Psychiatric aspects of ulcerative colitis. N. Engl. J. Med. *226*:178, 1942.

55. Lindemann, E. Modifications in the course of ulcerative colitis in relationship to changes in life situations and reaction patterns. Proc. Assoc. Res. Nerv. Ment. Dis. *29*:706, 1949.

56. Engel, G. L. Studies of ulcerative colitis. III. The nature of the psychologic processes. Am. J. Med. *19*:231, 1955.

57. Engel, G. L. Studies of ulcerative colitis. V. Psychological aspects and their implications for treatment. Am. J. Dig. Dis. *3*:315, 1958.

58. Magni, G., Di Mario, F., Rizzardo, R., Pulin, S., and Naccarato, R. Personality profiles of patients with duodenal ulcer. Am. J. Psychiatry *143*:1297, 1986.

59. Drossman, D. A., Psychosocial aspects of ulcerative colitis and Crohn's disease. *In* Kirsner, J. B., and Shorter, R. G. (eds.). Inflammatory Bowel Disease. Philadelphia, Lea & Febiger, in press.

60. Groen, J., and Bastiaans, J. Studies on ulcerative colitis: Personality structure, emotional conflict, situations and effects of psychotherapy. *In* Modern Trends in Psychosomatic Medicine. London, Butterworth and Company, 1955, p. 242.

61. Sifneos, P. E. The prevalence of "alexithymic" characteristics in psychosomatic patients. Psychother. Psychosom. *22*:255, 1973.

62. Nakagawa, T., Sugita, M., Nakai, Y., and Ikemi, Y. Alexithymic features in digestive diseases. Psychother. Psychosom. *32*:191, 1979.

63. Keltikangas-Jarvinen, L. Concept of alexithymia: I. The prevalence of alexithymia in psychosomatic patients. Psychother. Psychosom. *44*:132, 1985.

64. Rogers, M. P., Dubey, D., and Reich, P. The influence of the psyche and the brain on immunity and disease susceptibility. A critical review. Psychosom. Med. *41*:147, 1979.

65. Sklar, L. S., and Anisman, H. Stress and coping factors influence tumor growth. Science *205*:513, 1979.

66. Ader, R. Psychosomatic and psychoimmunologic research. Psychosom. Med. *42*:307, 1980.

67. Kiecolt-Glaser, J. K., and Glaser, R. Psychological influences on immunity. Psychosomatics *27*:621, 1986.

68. Schleifer, S. J., Keller, S. E., Camerino, M., Thornton, J. C., and Stein, M. Suppression of lymphocyte stimulation following bereavement. JAMA *250*:374, 1984.

69. Kiecolt-Glaser, J. K., Fisher, L. D., Ogrocki, P., et al. Marital quality, marital disruption and immune function. Psychosom. Med. *49*(1):13, 1987.

70. Kiecolt-Glaser, J. K., Garner, W., Speicher, C. E., Penn, G. M., Holliday, J., and Glaser, R. Psychosocial modifiers of immunocompetence in medical students. Psychosom. Med. *46*:7, 1984.

71. Kiecolt-Glaser, J. K., Glaser, R., Strain, E. C., Stout, J. C., Tarr, K. L., Holliday, J. E., and Speicher, C. E. Modulation of cellular immunity in medical students. J. Behav. Med. *9*:5, 1986.

72. Kiecolt-Glaser, J. K., Stephens, R. E., Lipetz, P. D., Speicher, C. E., and Glaser, R. Distress and DNA repair in human lymphocytes. J. Behav. Med. *8*:311, 1985.

73. Ader, R., and Cohen, N. Behaviorally conditioned immunosuppression. Psychosom. Med. *37*:333, 1975.

74. Ader, R., and Cohen, N. Behaviorally conditioned immunosuppression and murine systemic lupus erythematosus. Science *215*:1534, 1982.

75. Kiecolt-Glaser, J. K., Glaser, R., Williger, D., Stout, J., Messick, G., Sheppard, S., et al. Psychosocial enhancement of immunocompetence in a geriatric population. Health Psychol. *4*:25, 1985.

76. Stein, M., Keller, S., and Schleifer, S. The hypothalamus and the immune response. *In* Weiner, H., Hofer, M. A., and Stunkard, A. J. (eds.) Brain, Behavior, and Bodily Disease, Vol. 59. New York, Raven Press, 1981, pp. 45–65.

77. Szentivanyi, A., and Filipp, G. Anaphylaxis and the nervous system, Part II. Ann. Allergy *16*:143, 1958.

78. Macris, N. T., Schiavi, R. C., Camerino, M. S., and Stein, M. Effect of hypothalamic lesions on immune processes in the guinea pig. Am. J. Physiol. *219*:1205, 1970.

79. Keller, S. E., Stein, M., Camerino, M. S., Schleifer, S. J., and Sherman, J. Suppression of lymphocyte stimulation by anterior hypothalamic lesions in the guinea pig. Cell. Immunol. *52*:334, 1980.

80. Levine, J. D., Gordon, N. C., and Fields, H. L. The mechanism of placebo analgesia. Lancet *2*:654, 1978.

81. Guillemin, R. Beta-lipotropin and endorphins: Implications of current knowledge. Hosp. Pract. 53, Nov., 1978.

82. Dockray, G. J. Brain-gut peptides. Viewpoints Dig. Dis. *13*:5, 1981.

83. Smith, G. P. Satiety effect of gastrointestinal hormones. *In* Beers, R. F., Jr., and Bassett, E. G. (eds.). Polypeptide Hormones. New York, Raven Press, 1980, pp. 413–420.

84. Snape, W. J., Carlson, G. M., and Cohen, S. Colonic myoelectric activity in the irritable bowel syndrome. Gastroenterology *70*:326, 1978.

85. Taylor, I., Darby, C., Hammond, P., and Basu, P. Is there a myoelectrical abnormality in the irritable colon syndrome? Gut *19*:391, 1978.

86. Snape, W. J., Carlson, G. M., Matarazzo, S. A., and Cohen, S. Evidence that abnormal myoelectrical activity produces colonic motor dysfunction in the irritable bowel syndrome. Gastroenterology *72*:383, 1977.

87. Bueno, L., Fioramonti, J., Ruckebusch, Y., Frexinos, J., and

Coulom, P. Evaluation of colonic myoelectrical activity in health and functional disorders. Gut 21:480, 1980.

88. Kumar, D., and Wingate, D. L. The irritable bowel syndrome: a paroxysmal motor disorder. Lancet 2:973, 1985.

89. Whitehead, W. E., and Schuster, M. M. (eds.). Irritable bowel syndrome. In Gastrointestinal Disorders: Behavioral and Physiological Basis for Treatment. New York, Academic Press, 1985.

90. Mechanic, D. The concept of illness behavior. J. Chron. Dis. 15:189, 1962.

91. Tseng, W. S. The nature of somatic complaints among psychiatric patients: The Chinese case. Compr. Psychiatry 16:237, 1975.

92. Zborowski, M. Cultural response to pain. J. Social Issues 8(4):16, 1952.

93. Kleinman, A., Eisenberg, L., and Good, B. Culture, illness and care. Clinical lessons from anthropologic and cross-cultural research. Ann. Intern. Med. 88:251, 1978.

94. Drossman, D. A., Powell, D. P., and Sessions, J. T., Jr. The irritable bowel syndrome. Gastroenterology 73:811, 1977.

95. Pimbarker, B. D. Irritable colon syndrome. J. Indian Med. Assoc. 54:95, 1970.

96. Parsons, T. The Social System. New York, Fress Press of Glencoe, 1951.

97. Pilowski, I. Abnormal illness behavior. Br. J. Med. Psychol. 42:347, 1969.

98. Altman, N. Hypochondriasis in psychological care of the medically ill. In Strain, J. T., and Grossman, S. (eds.). A Primer in Liaison Psychiatry. New York, Appleton-Century-Crofts, 1975, pp. 76–92.

99. Kahana, R. J., and Bibring, G. L. Personality types in medical management. In Psychiatry and Medical Practice in a General Hospital, 1964.

100. Drossman, D. A., Patrick, D. L., Mitchell, C. M., and Zagami, E. Health related quality of life in IBD: Functional status. Gastroenterology 92:1375, 1987.

101. Peterson, W. L., Sturdevant, A. L., Frankl, H. D., Richardson, C. A., Isenberg, J. I., Elashoff, J. D., Sones, J. Q., Gross, R. A., McCallum, R. W., and Fordtran, J. S. Healing of duodenal ulcer with an antacid regimen. N. Engl. J. Med. 297:341, 1977.

102. Engel, G. L. The need for a new medical model: A challenge for biomedicine. Science 196:129, 1977.

103. Engel, G. L. The clinical application of the biopsychosocial model. Am. J. Psychiatr. 137:535, 1980.

104. Von Bertalanffy, L. General System Theory. New York, Braziller, 1968.

105. Weiss, P. The living system: Determinism stratified. In Koestler, A., and Smythies, J. R. (eds.). Beyond Reductionism. New York, Macmillan Publishing Company, 1969, pp. 3–55.

106. Pilowsky, I. Psychodynamic aspects of the pain experience. In Sternbach, R. A. (ed.). The Psychology of Pain. 2nd ed. New York, Raven Press, 1986, pp. 181–195.

107. Lipkin, M. Functional or organic? A pointless question. Ann. Intern. Med. 71:1013, 1969.

108. Drossman, D. A. The problem patient. Evaluation and care of medical patients with psychosocial disturbances. Ann. Intern. Med. 88:366, 1978.

109. Morgan, J., and Engel, G. The Clinical Approach to the Patient. Philadelphia, W. B. Saunders Company, 1969, pp. 26–79.

110. Barsky, A. J. Hidden reasons some patients visit doctors. Ann. Intern. Med. 94:492, 1981.

111. Snow, L. F. Sorcerers, saints, charlatans: Black folk healers in urban America. Culture Med. Psychiatr. 2:69, 1978.

112. Drossman, D. A. Can the primary care physician be better trained in the psychosocial dimensions of patient care? Int. J. Psychiatr. Med. 8:169, 1977–1978.

113. Drossman, D. A. Patients with psychogenic abdominal pain: Six years' observation in the medical setting. Am. J. Psychiatr. 139:1549, 1982.

114. DeVaul, R. A., and Faillace, L. A. Persistent pain and illness insistence. A medical profile of proneness to surgery. Am J. Surg. 135:828, 1978.

115. Drossman, D. A. The patient with chronic undiagnosed abdominal pain. Hosp. Pract. 21(11A):22, 1986.

116. Sarfeh, I. J. Abdominal pain of unknown etiology. Am. J. Surg. 131:22, 1976.

117. Gomez, J., and Dally, P. Psychologically mediated abdominal pain in surgical and medical outpatient clinics. Br. Med. J. 1:1451, 1977.

118. Woodhouse, C. R. J., and Bockner, S. Chronic abdominal pain: A surgical or psychiatric symptom? Br. J. Surg. 66:348, 1979.

119. Hollister, L. E. Tricyclic antidepressants. N. Engl. J. Med. 299:1106, 1978.

120. Merskey, H., and Hester, R. A. The treatment of chronic pain with psychotropic drugs. Postgrad. Med. J. 48:594, 1972.

121. Walsh, T. C. Antidepressants in chronic pain. Clin. Neuropharm. 6:271, 1983.

122. Hendler, N. The anatomy and psychopharmacology of chronic pain. J. Clin. Psych. 43(Suppl):15, 1982.

123. Anon. Gomers. JAMA 243:2333, 1980.

124. Cooke, W. T. Laxative abuse. Clin. Gastroenterol. 6:659, 1977.

Neurology of the Gut

RAJ K. GOYAL
JEFFREY R. CRIST

2

The nervous system exerts a major influence on the control of all aspects of gastrointestinal function, including motor, secretory, and absorptive activities. This influence is largely dependent upon three component levels of organization: (1) the afferent or sensory neurons gather a variety of sensory information and relay it to a large array of interneurons; (2) the interneurons serve as central computers to integrate a variety of sensory information and formulate various commands, which are then passed on to efferent or motor neurons; and (3) the motor neurons then exert their influence directly on target cells such as smooth muscle, secretory cells, or absorptive cells in the gut. The nervous system also provides for interaction between the gastrointestinal tract and other organs of the body.

The purpose of this chapter is to summarize the general principles of neurobiology and salient features of the organization and function of nerves involved in the physiology and pathophysiology of digestive organs and digestive diseases described in various chapters throughout this book.

GENERAL NEUROBIOLOGY

Anatomy of Neurons

The neuron (Fig. 2–1) is the fundamental anatomic and functional unit of the nervous system. All neural circuits or reflex pathways are composed of individual neurons arranged in a simple or complex sequence. The most remarkable feature of all neurons is the presence of one or more protoplasmic processes that arise from the cell body (perikaryon or soma).[1] These protoplasmic neural processes are divided into dendrites and axons. Dendrites are extensions of the nerve cell surface that function as a zone serving to transduce chemical signals into electrical signals. Axons are signal-conducting structures that carry electrical impulses along the nerve fibers to axonal endings. Axonal endings are specialized membrane and cytoplasmic endings of axons responsible for neurosecretory activity and synaptic transmission.

Cell Body (Perikaryon or Soma)

The cell body is responsible for generation, maintenance, and repair of its processes, as well as the production of neurotransmitters or enzymes responsible for the synthesis of neurotransmitters. The plasma membrane of the cell body also serves as a transducer of chemical influences into electrical signals.

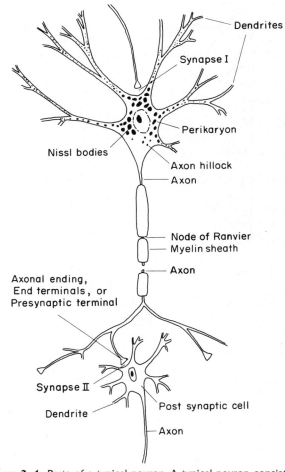

Figure 2–1. Parts of a typical neuron. A typical neuron consists of a single cell body (perikaryon or soma), many dendrites, and an axon, which arises from the perikaryon at the axon hillock. The axon can be myelinated, i.e., possess a myelin sheath, which is interrupted at intervals by regions known as nodes of Ranvier. The terminal part of the axon branches into specialized axonal endings or end terminals. These axonal endings make close contacts or synapses with other cells called postsynaptic cells. The axonal endings are also called presynaptic endings and contain neurotransmitter substances that exert their effect on the postsynaptic cell. Note that presynaptic and postsynaptic configuration of neurons is made in reference to a given synapse. Thus the typical neuron shown here is a presynaptic cell in reference to Synapse II and a postsynaptic cell in reference to Synapse I.

Based upon the number of processes arising from the cell body, neurons are classified anatomically as unipolar, bipolar, or multipolar neurons (Fig. 2–2). In the so-called T-shaped unipolar neuron, the single process emanating from the cell body or stem divides into a peripheral and a central process at a variable distance from its origin from the soma. These neurons are sensory neurons and are characteristically present in dorsal root ganglia. Their peripheral axonal process is connected with specialized sensory receptors and conducts the electrical impulses generated by them. The electrical spike carried by this peripheral axonal process is often conducted along the central axonal process to its axonal endings. The bipolar neurons also possess a peripheral and a central axon. They also serve as sensory neurons and are typically present in the nodose ganglion. The multipolar neurons possess many dendritic processes and a single axon. They serve as sensory neurons, motor neurons, or interneurons and provide for complex integration of activity. They are typically present in brain, spinal cord, and peripheral autonomic and enteric ganglia.

Dendrites

Dendrites are usually defined as extensions of the nerve cell body that serve to transduce the effects of chemical neurotransmitters released by other neurons into electrical signals. According to this functional definition, a neuron may be more appropriately considered to possess a "dendritic zone," which in most neurons may include not only the dendritic extensions but also the neural cell body itself; both the cell body and the dendrites participate in the receptive or trans-

ducer function of the neuron.[1] In unipolar or bipolar sensory neurons the dendrite zone is reduced to a small area of the sensory ending and, as described below, no dendrites arising from the nerve cell body are present.

Nerve Fiber (Axon)

The nerve fiber or axon is usually a long process defined functionally by its ability to conduct electrical impulses. It includes both peripheral and central processes of unipolar neurons and bipolar neurons. The origin of the axon from the nerve cell body is frequently identified as the axon hillock. This specialized mass of conical protoplasm is characterized by the absence of Nissl bodies (ribosomes). The axon hillock is usually not well developed in enteric neurons.[2] Peripheral to this initial hillock segment the axon contains mitochondria, neurofilaments, microtubules, smooth endoplasmic reticulum, and neurosecretory vesicles.

The diameter of individual nerve fibers may vary from 0.5 to 20 μ. Those less than 2 μ are typically unmyelinated, whereas those larger than 2 μ are almost always myelinated. In the central nervous system oligodendrocytes form and maintain the myelin sheath, whereas in the peripheral nervous system the myelin sheath is formed and maintained by Schwann cells.

Sensory Nerve Endings and Sensory Organs (Fig. 2–3)

Afferent nerve endings of sensory neurons serve as specialized transducers that transduce mechanical or chemical activity into electrical signals, which are then

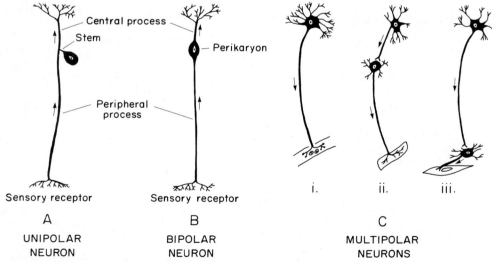

Figure 2–2. Types of neurons associated with the gastrointestinal tract. Based upon the number of processes arising from the cell body, neurons are classified as unipolar, bipolar, or multipolar neurons. A, A T-shaped unipolar neuron. A single stem process arises from the cell body and then divides into a peripheral process that is connected with sensory receptors. The central process extends to make contact with second order neurons. Arrows indicate the direction of electrical spike conduction. Such cells are typically present in dorsal root ganglia. B, A bipolar neuron. In these neurons the peripheral process is connected with sensory receptors and conducts spike potentials to the perikaryon. The central process also arises from the cell and extends to second order neurons. They are present in the nodose ganglion of the vagus. C, Multipolar neurons. Multipolar neurons may be sensory neurons, interneurons, or motor neurons. (i) A typical alpha motor neuron, (ii) pre- and postganglionic neurons of sympathetic pathways, and (iii) pre- and postganglionic neurons of parasympathetic pathways. The majority of enteric neurons are also multipolar.

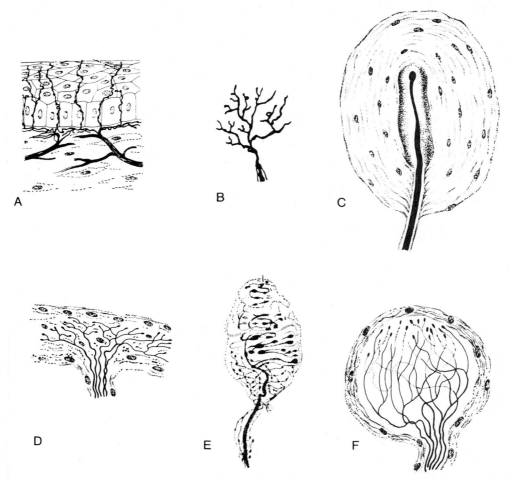

Figure 2–3. Various types of sensory endings or sensory receptors in the gut. *A* and *B*, Free nerve endings are the only type of endings in the mucosal and muscle layers of the gut. They sense a variety of mechanical, chemical, and pain stimuli. *C*, Pacinian corpuscles are present in the mesentery and sense pressure. *D*, Ruffini organs sense tactile sensation. *E*, Meissner's corpuscles sense light touch. *F*, Krause end organs sense special tactile sensations. The specialized sensory receptors in *D, E,* and *F* are present in anal canal mucosa. (From Junqueira, L. C., and Carneiro, J. Basic Histology. 4th ed. Los Altos, CA, Lange Medical Publications, 1983. Used by permission.)

conducted along the sensory nerves. The sensory endings are also known as sensory receptors. Many sensory endings that serve as transducers for a variety of mechanical, thermal, chemical, or painful stimuli do not typically show morphologic specialization and are therefore known as free nerve endings. However, in certain circumstances the sensory endings are recognized as distinctive encapsulated structures on light microscopy and are called sensory organs. Examples of sensory organs include pacinian corpuscles (for pressure sensations), Meissner's corpuscles (for touch sensations), end organs of Krause (for special tactile sensations), and Ruffini's corpuscles (also for tactile sensations).

Axonal End Terminals or Axonal Endings

Axons make contact with target cells by means of specialized cytoplasmic and membrane endings (Fig. 2–4). These axonal endings are called presynaptic axonal end terminals or simply axonal endings. The target cell is called the postsynaptic cell and the contact area is called a synapse. The endings of axons of somatic efferents which innervate striated muscle are highly specialized and are known as motor endplates.[1] The motor endplate is an axonal end terminal which sits within a trough on the muscle cell surface. The ending is covered only by a thin cytoplasmic layer of Schwann sheath and contains numerous mitochondria and acetylcholine-containing synaptic vesicles. The synaptic cleft is a 20- to 30-nm space between the endplate and the muscle cell membrane which is thrown into numerous deep junctional folds. A motor axon may innervate a single muscle fiber, or more commonly branch to innervate over a hundred muscle fibers.

The endings of visceral efferent axons to smooth muscle, blood vessels, and glands are usually called varicosities.[3] These axons often end in a simple arborization pattern, branching initially into an extensive intramuscular plexus and then into fine terminals. The branches form bulbous expansions or varicosities. These varicosities are 0.5 to 2 μ in diameter and contain numerous mitochondria and neurosecretory granules

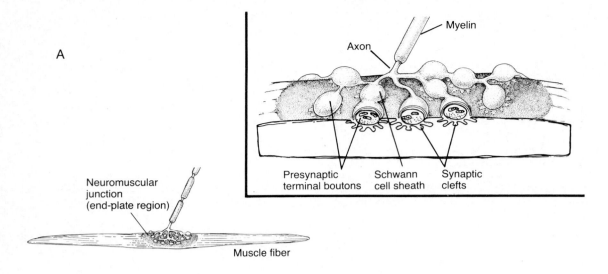

A

Myelin

Axon

Neuromuscular
junction
(end-plate region)

Muscle fiber

Presynaptic
terminal boutons

Schwann
cell sheath

Synaptic
clefts

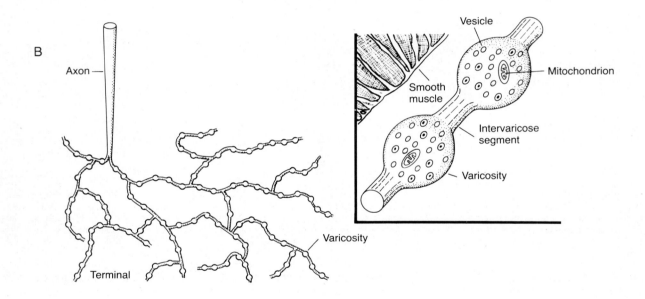

B

Axon

Terminal

Varicosity

Vesicle

Smooth
muscle

Mitochondrion

Intervaricose
segment

Varicosity

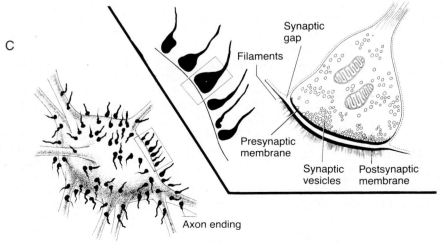

C

Synaptic
gap

Filaments

Presynaptic
membrane

Synaptic
vesicles

Postsynaptic
membrane

Axon ending

Figure 2—4. *Legend on opposite page.*

The Schwann sheath covering is absent or markedly attenuated over the area of the varicosity, thereby allowing release of neurotransmitter. The postsynaptic membrane of these synapses shows no specialization, and the distance between the varicosity and the target cell membrane is much larger than the width of the neural synaptic or motor endplate cleft.

When the target cell is a neuron, the axonal ending is usually called a presynaptic terminal.[3] The axons that synapse with other neurons may form bulbous expansions, basket-like structures, or club-shaped terminations. Frequently an axon branch along its course has many presynaptic terminals that synapse with other neural structures. In these synapses the plasma membrane of the presynaptic axon and the postsynaptic neurons are thickened and in some instances bound together by means of dense filaments. The synaptic gap is usually about 20 nm. The synapses are between axon endings of one cell and the dendrite (axodendritic), soma (axosomatic), or even axons (axoaxonic) of another cell.[4]

Functions of Neurons

The two fundamental functions of neurons are (1) generation and propagation of electrical action potentials to the axonal ending, and (2) synthesis and transport of neurotransmitters or their synthetic enzymes to the axonal endings for neurotransmitter release.

Electrical Events in Neurons

Membrane Potential. The resting membrane potential in the neuron is negative inside as compared to outside the cell by about 65 millivolts.[4] This negativity is due to multiple factors such as the large number of negatively charged ions which cannot diffuse out of the cell membrane, the constant tendency of K^+ to leak out of the cell via the K^+ channels in the plasma membrane, and the disproportionate extrusion of positively charged sodium ions outside as compared to the intrusion of positively charged potassium ions by the Na^+/K^+ pump present in the plasma membrane. This net outward movement of positive charges is a result of the sodium-potassium pump, which moves three sodium ions to the exterior for every two potassium ions to the interior of the neuron.[5]

Changes in membrane potential of the neuron can be produced by application of active chemicals or by neurotransmitter released onto its surface due to stimulation of presynaptic axonal terminals. These manip-

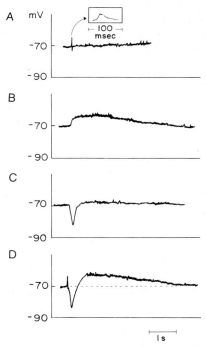

Figure 2–5. Types of postsynaptic potentials recorded from enteric neurons. *A,* A fast excitatory postsynaptic potential (fast EPSP), which is a transient depolarization lasting only milliseconds. *B,* A slow EPSP, which is a slow depolarization lasting several seconds. *C,* An inhibitory postsynaptic potential, which is a state of hyperpolarization lasting less than 1 second in this example. *D,* Fast EPSP, IPSP, and slow EPSP in the same neuron. When depolarization exceeds a certain threshold, spikes are produced.

ulations can cause either excitation (depolarization, i.e., decrease in the negativity of the potential) or inhibition (hyperpolarization, i.e., increase in the negativity of the potential) of the resting cell membrane.[6] Excitation and inhibition caused by presynaptic nerve stimulation are called excitatory postsynaptic potentials (EPSPs) and inhibitory postsynaptic potentials (IPSPs), respectively. The EPSP that develops rapidly and lasts briefly (less than 50 msec) is called the fast EPSP. In contrast, the EPSP that develops slowly and lasts for several seconds to minutes is called the slow EPSP. Depending upon the nature of presynaptic stimulation and the postsynaptic neuron one or more of these postsynaptic potentials can be observed in the same neuron (Fig. 2–5).[5] The fast EPSP is seen in the majority of myenteric and submucous neurons, as well as postganglionic adrenergic and alpha-motor neurons. It is due to a nonselective increase in permeability of all cations leading to Na^+ and Ca^{2+} movement

Figure 2–4. Types of axonal endings in the gut. Axonal endings come in close contact with effector cells at certain areas which are called synapses. *A,* The nerve striated muscle synapse (motor endplate). This synapse is between specialized axonal endings of alpha motor neurons and the specialized area on the striated muscle membrane. *B,* Nerve–smooth muscle contacts in which axonal endings are represented by multiple varicosities on the fine branches of the axon. The contact space between the varicosities and smooth muscle cell is wider than the synaptic cleft of the motor endplate. *C,* Nerve–nerve synapses. The axonal endings may be represented either by multiple swellings along the course of an axonal branch (varicosity) or a terminal swelling on an axon branch (shown here). The axonal endings are also called presynaptic terminals (*A* and *B* modified from Kandel, E. R., and Schwartz, J. H. Principles of Neural Science. 2nd ed. New York, Elsevier, 1985; and Junqueira, L. C. *C* modified from Carneiro, J. Basic Histology. 4th ed. Los Altos, CA, Lange Medical Publications, 1983.)

inside and K$^+$ movement outside the cell. However, owing to a greater electrochemical gradient for sodium to enter the cell than for potassium to leave, there is a net cation movement inside the cell causing depolarization. The fast EPSP is most commonly due to nicotinic actions of acetylcholine.[5, 6]

The slow EPSP is characterized by its more leisurely time course and is due to a receptor-mediated decrease in potassium conductance resulting in depolarization of the cell membrane. The slow EPSP in many neurons is due to muscarinic actions of acetylcholine.[5]

The IPSP is associated with membrane hyperpolarization. This is usually due to a receptor-mediated opening of K$^+$ channels. Movement of K$^+$ outside the cell causes hyperpolarization of the cell membrane.[4] In submucosal neurons, noradrenaline usually mediates inhibitory postsynaptic potentials.[7]

Action (Spike) Potential. When the neural cell body depolarizes it causes an opening of voltage-gated Na$^+$ channels. Because the axon hillock of the neuron has the highest concentration of voltage-gated sodium channels, an action potential is generated at this site when the cell membrane depolarizes beyond a certain critical "threshold for excitation" (usually +15 to +20 millivolts).[8] The action potential is defined as a sudden and transient depolarization of the cell membrane (Fig. 2–6). The spike potential is usually only 1 to 2 msec in duration, because opening of voltage-dependent sodium channels occurs only momentarily. The action potential is produced in an all-or-none fashion, and, once produced, it travels peripherally along the axon and centrally to the soma and dendrites. The spike portion of the action potential is followed by a state of hyperpolarization which lasts many milliseconds (up to 50 msec) called the "afterhyperpolarization."[4, 6] It is particularly prominent in some enteric neurons called Type 2 (AH) neurons. The afterhyperpolarization is due to opening of potassium channels, which persists for several milliseconds after the membrane repolarization process is complete.

Membrane potential changes similar to those described for neurons also occur in sensory receptors.[9]

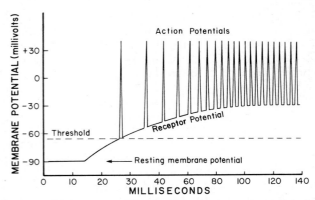

Figure 2–7. Action potential generation at a sensory receptor site. Deformation of a mechanoreceptor generates a state of depolarization or receptor potential. When the receptor potential crosses a certain threshold, action potentials are generated. The action potentials are then propagated along the axons of sensory neurons. (From Guyton, A. C. Textbook of Medical Physiology. 7th ed. Philadelphia, W. B. Saunders Co., 1986.)

Mechanical deformity (mechanoreceptors), application of specific chemicals (chemoreceptors) or changes in temperature (thermoreceptors) lead to changes in ionic permeability and depolarization. This depolarization is called a receptor potential (Fig. 2–7). When the receptor potential rises above a certain threshold value, a spike potential is generated by activation of voltage-gated sodium channels. Generation of action potentials at the sensory receptors is, thus, very similar to that in a neuron.

When the excitatory state of a neuron or a sensory receptor remains above the threshold of excitation, the axon hillock of the soma or regenerative region of the sensory receptor continues to generate action potentials, which are repetitive as long as the excitatory state of the neuron remains above the threshold level.[9] The rate of these repetitive action potentials is dependent upon how much the excitatory state is above threshold. The firing rate at a certain excitatory state in a neuron is dependent upon the magnitude and duration of the afterhyperpolarization. Different nerve cells have different thresholds for spike generation and firing rates.

Once generated, the spike potential propagates along the axon. The propagation of the action potential (called the nerve impulse) occurs as a spreading wave of increased Na$^+$ permeability.[8] In the unmyelinated axon, as this wave moves along the axon, the axon membrane behind the wave returns to its resting stage because the active ion-transporting system redistributes sodium and potassium ions to the resting level of the axon membrane. In myelinated axons local increased sodium conductance occurs only at the nodes of Ranvier. Therefore the conduction occurs by jumping of the impulse from one node to another. This type of spike conduction is called saltatory conduction and is significantly faster than continuous conduction.[5] The nerve impulse conduction can be blocked by the puffer fish poison, tetrodotoxin, which acts on the outside of cell membrane to block voltage dependent Na$^+$ channels.[10] Tetrodotoxin has served as an important tool

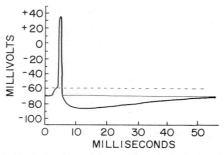

Figure 2–6. Typical action potential. Action (spike) potential is a transient depolarization lasting milliseconds. Action potential is generated when the excitatory postsynaptic potential reaches a certain threshold value called the threshold for excitation (−60 mV in this example). Action potential is followed by a prolonged state of hyperpolarization called afterhyperpolarization. (Modified from Guyton, A. C. Textook of Medical Physiology. 7th ed. Philadelphia, W. B. Saunders Co., 1986.)

in the investigation of neural control in the gastrointestinal tract. Cooling, pressure, and local anesthetics also block axonal conduction.[5]

The conduction velocity is dependent upon the diameter of the fiber and the presence of myelination.[1, 11] Conduction velocity increases from 1 meter/sec in a 1 μ diameter unmyelinated fiber to 120 meters/sec in a 20 μ diameter myelinated fiber. Different groups of nerve fibers are characterized by their conduction velocities (or size). However, classification of the fibers by different investigators using different terminologies has led to unnecessary confusion.[1, 12] In general, all fibers are divided into A and C types. C fibers are unmyelinated, are about 1 μ in diameter, and usually conduct at velocities of less than 2 meters/sec. A fibers are myelinated, 1 to 20 μ in diameter and conduct from 6 to 120 meters/sec. Based upon their diameter and conduction velocities, A fibers are further classified into large (A alpha), medium (A beta), small (A gamma), and very small (A delta) fibers.

Neurosecretory Events of Neurons

Neurotransmitter Candidates. A wide variety of chemical substances may serve as neurotransmitters in the gastrointestinal tract (Table 2–1). In general, they can be classified into two groups: Group I consists of low-molecular-weight substances, including acetylcholine, biogenic amines, and products of general metabolism. The biogenic amines include dopamine, norepinephrine, and 5-hydroxytryptamine (5HT). The products of general metabolism in Group I include gamma-aminobutyric acid (GABA), adenosine triphosphate (ATP), and adenosine. Group II consists of peptides, which include generally accepted neurotransmitters such as substance P, vasoactive intestinal peptide, opioid peptides, and somatostatin as well as many other potential candidates such as bombesin-like peptide, calcitonin gene–related peptide, cholecystokinin, galanin, neuropeptide Y, and peptide-histamine-isoleucine. The list of potential neuropeptides is rapidly increasing.

Synthesis, Transport, and Release of Neurotransmitters. Low-molecular-weight substances such as acetylcholine, norepinephrine, dopamine, and 5HT are synthesized in the presynaptic terminals.[13] The enzymes responsible for synthesis of these compounds are synthesized on free ribosomes in the cell body[14] and subsequently released into the neuronal cytoplasm for transportation along the axon by slow axoplasmic flow at a rate of less than 0.5 mm/hr.[15] These enzymes are distributed throughout the neuron but are more prevalent at the axon terminal where neurotransmitter is synthesized for local release. In general, these low-molecular weight compounds are utilized by neurons which have long axons, where local synthesis of neurotransmitters is most desirable. Synthesized transmitter is packaged into vesicles which are derived from: (1) smooth endoplasmic reticulum along the axon, (2) internalization of coated pits of presynaptic terminals, and (3) recycling of previously released vesicles.[16–18] Figures 2–8 and 2–9 summarize synthesis and release of acetylcholine and norepinephrine at cholinergic and adrenergic synapses, respectively.

Neuroactive peptides are formed in ribosomes attached to rough endoplasmic reticulum and subsequently packaged into vesicles within the Golgi apparatus.[13] The neuropeptide vesicles then move along the axons in microtubules at a rate of about 1.7 cm/hr. Neuropeptides are generally contained in neurons that have shorter axons. The storage and release of neurotransmitters involves the packaging of neurotransmitter substances into synaptic vesicles. The synaptic vesicles vary greatly depending upon the type of neuron.[19] They are typically spherical or ovoid and range in diameter from 20 to 120 nm and are most concentrated at nerve terminals.[2, 20] The storage of neurotransmitter in vesicles prevents their degradation by cytosolic enzymes. Neurotransmitter release is initiated by the arrival of an action potential at the axonal ending. The axonal endings are characterized by the presence of a large number of voltage-gated calcium channels. When the action potential depolarizes the ending, large numbers of Ca^{2+} ions along with Na^+ ions flow into the axon terminal. It is believed that elevated free Ca^{2+} activates proteins in dense bars attached to the internal surface of the presynaptic membrane. The activated proteins cause binding of dense bars with transmitter vesicles. This complex of dense bars and vesicles extrudes neurotransmitter from the ending by the process of exocytosis.[21, 22]

Each vesicle contains a quantum of neurotransmitter which is released in an all-or-none fashion into the

Table 2–1. NEUROTRANSMITTER CANDIDATES

Low-Molecular-Weight Substances
  Acetylcholine
  Biogenic amines
    Catecholamines
      Dopamine
      Norepinephrine (NE)
      Epinephrine
      Tyramine
      Octopamine
    5-Hydroxytryptamine (5HT)
  Products of general metabolism
    Amino acids
      Glycine
      Gamma-aminobutyric acid (GABA)
      Glutamate, aspartate
    Purines
      Adenosine triphosphate (ATP)
      Adenosine

Neuropeptides
  Bombesin-like
  Cholecystokinin (CCK)
  Calcitonin gene–related peptide (CGRP)
  Galanin
  Neuropeptide Y (NPY)
  Dynorphin
  Enkephalin (Leu, Met)
  Beta-endorphin
  Somatostatin
  Substance P (SP)
  Vasoactive intestinal peptide (VIP)

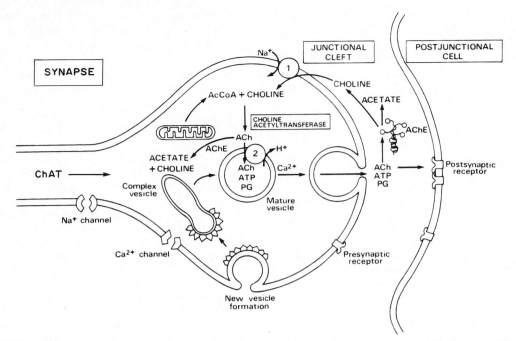

Figure 2–8. Schematic illustration of a generalized cholinergic junction. Two cellular structures, the cholinergic nerve terminal (left) and the postjunctional cell (right) are separated by the junctional (synaptic) cleft. Choline is transported into the nerve terminal by a carrier (1). Inside the nerve terminal, choline combines with activated acetate (AcCoA) in a reaction catalyzed by choline acetyltransferase to form acetylcholine (ACh). Choline acetyltransferase is synthesized in the cell body and is transported along the axons to the nerve terminals. Formation of storage vesicles is initiated by the deposition of clathrin molecules on the inner surface of the terminal membrane (shown as the fencelike structure on the new vesicle). Upon pinching off from the surface, a "complex vesicle" is formed that eventually gives rise to a mature storage vesicle. ACh is transported into the storage vesicle by the action of a carrier (2) that utilizes the outward flux of protons as its source of energy. ATP and proteoglycan (PG) are also stored in the vesicle. Release of transmitter occurs when an action potential, carried down the axon by the action of voltage-sensitive sodium channels, invades the nerve terminals. Voltage-sensitive calcium channels in the terminal membrane are opened, allowing an influx of calcium. The increase in intracellular calcium causes fusion of vesicles with the surface membrane, resulting in exocytotic expulsion of ACh, ATP, and proteoglycan into the junctional cleft. ACh reaching postjunctional (and possibly prejunctional) receptors modifies the function of the corresponding cell. ACh also diffuses into contact with the enzyme acetylcholinesterase (AChE), a polymeric enzyme that splits ACh into choline and acetate. (From Junqueira, L. C., and Carneiro, J. Basic Histology. 4th ed. Los Altos, CA, Lange Medical Publications, 1983. Used by permission.)

synaptic cleft. The number of vesicles that discharge their contents is directly related to the level of cytosolic Ca^{2+}.

Neurotransmitter release can be facilitated or inhibited by a variety of influences on the axonal endings.[23] For example, inhibition of neurotransmitter release may occur due to (1) an inability of the action potential to pass along the axon and arrive at the axon terminal, for example, after tetrodotoxin treatment or application of local anesthetic; (2) marked reduction in extracellular Ca^{2+}; (3) axoaxonal synapses which may act by inhibiting influx of Ca^{2+}; and (4) presynaptic inhibitory autoreceptors whose activation by the released transmitter leads to feedback inhibition of further transmitter release. Prominent examples of presynaptic autoreceptors are presynaptic alpha-2-adrenoreceptors and presynaptic muscarinic receptors.[5]

Fate of Released Neurotransmitters. The released neurotransmitters bind with respective receptors on the postsynaptic and presynaptic cell surface and induce a variety of ionic and biochemical changes in the target cell.[5, 24, 25] The width of the synaptic cleft influences the rate of diffusion and concentration of neurotransmitter at the receptor sites. At motor end-

plates and neural synapses the synaptic cleft is narrow and receptors are localized specifically to the postsynaptic membrane. These are called highly directed synapses, as a high concentration of neurotransmitter is achieved locally at the cleft and there is little diffusion of the transmitter. On the other hand, neurotransmitter release from nerve varicosities at visceral neuromuscular and neuroglandular sites is diffused over wide areas because of the large distance between varicosities and effector sites. These are called nondirected synapses. Appropriately, the neurotransmitter receptors on smooth muscles and glands are diffusely present on the cell surface, in contrast to their localized presence at the motor end plate.

After the released transmitter has exerted its effect, it must be disposed of. Three mechanisms exist for disposal of neurotransmitter from the synaptic cleft. They are (1) reuptake, (2) diffusion, and (3) enzymatic degradation.[26] Reuptake of neurotransmitter from the synaptic cleft by the presynaptic cell is a common mechanism of neurotransmitter inactivation at the synapse. Uptake mechanisms have been shown to exist for choline, GABA, and other biogenic amines.[26] Diffusion of neurotransmitter from the synaptic cleft

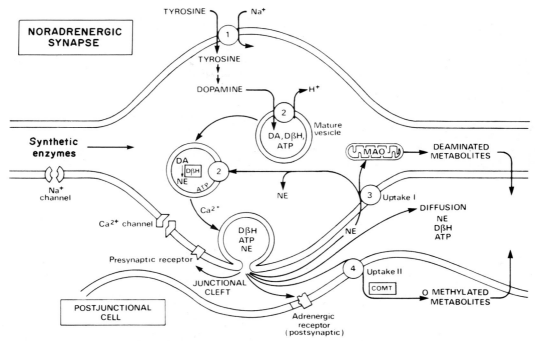

Figure 2–9. Schematic diagram of the neuroeffector junction of the peripheral sympathetic nervous system. The nerves terminate in complex networks with varicosities or enlargements that form synaptic junctions with effector cells. Some of the processes occurring in the noradrenergic varicosity (e.g., new vesicle formation) are analogous to those in cholinergic terminals. Tyrosine is decarboxylated to dopa and then hydroxylated to form dopamine (1) in the cytoplasm. Dopamine is transported into the vesicle by a carrier mechanism (2). The same carrier transports norepinephrine (NE) and several other amines into these granules. Dopamine is converted to norepinephrine through the catalytic action of dopamine beta-hydroxylase (DβH). ATP is also present in high concentration in the vesicle. Release of transmitter occurs when an action potential is conducted to the varicosity by the action of voltage-sensitive sodium channels. Depolarization of the varicosity membrane opens voltage-sensitive calcium channels and results in an increase in intracellular calcium. The elevated calcium facilitates exocytotic fusion of vesicles with the surface membrane and expulsion of norepinephrine, ATP, and some of the dopamine beta-hydroxylase. Norepinephrine reaching either pre- or postsynaptic receptors modifies the function of the corresponding cells. Norepinephrine also diffuses out of the cleft, or it may be transported into the cytoplasm of the varicosity (uptake I) or into the postjunctional cell (uptake II). (From Junqueira, L. C., and Carneiro, J. Basic Histology. 4th ed. Los Altos, CA, Lange Medical Publications, 1983. Used by permission.)

probably plays some role in the inactivation of all neurotransmitters. This role may be particularly important in the removal of neuroactive peptides from the synaptic site. Enzymatic degradation of neurotransmitter is particularly important in the cholinergic synapses.[27]

Actions of Neurotransmitters on the Postsynaptic Cell. Neurotransmitters act on receptors on the postsynaptic cell to produce (1) changes in membrane potential associated with changes in ionic channels; (2) biochemical changes in adenylate or guanylate cyclases and phosphatidylinositol turnover; and (3) changes in intracellular Ca^{2+}. These three groups of events may be interrelated.[28, 29]

Neurotransmitters may cause either depolarization leading to increased excitability or hyperpolarization leading to decreased excitability of neurons.[4–6] Depolarization may be mediated by several different ionic channels in the plasma membrane, including (1) opening of nonselective cation channels, (2) opening of Na^+ channels, (3) opening of Ca^{2+} and Na^+ channels (also called slow channels), and (4) closing of K^+ channels. On the other hand, neurotransmitters cause hyperpolarization almost solely by opening of K^+ channels. In many neurons brief depolarization associated with a spike potential is associated with subsequent hyperpolarization. In these instances, depolarization of the cell activates voltage dependent Na^+ and K^+ channels. However, Na^+ channels open and close abruptly and are responsible for spike potentials, whereas K^+ channels are relatively slow to open and close. This slow opening and closing of K^+ channels is responsible for the afterhyperpolarization that follows the spike potential.

Biochemical changes associated with neurotransmitter action may include a wide variety of effects, including elevations or reductions in cyclic AMP or cyclic GMP, diacylglycerol, and inositol triphosphate.[30–32] These changes in intracellular messengers can in turn cause changes in ionic fluxes, membrane potentials, and intracellular calcium levels. In many instances neurotransmitter actions on the target cells lead to directly or indirectly mediated changes in intracellular calcium that may serve as a final mediator of secretory, absorptive, or mechanical events in secretory, absorptive, or muscle cells, respectively.

Coexistence of Neurotransmitters in a Neuron. In the past, it was thought that one neuron contained only a single neurotransmitter. Recently, however, it has become clear that the presence of multiple neuro-

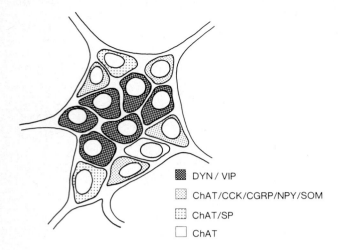

DYN / VIP
ChAT/CCK/CGRP/NPY/SOM
ChAT/SP
ChAT

Figure 2–10. Co-localization of transmitters in neurons in the submucous ganglia of guinea pig small intestine. Note that the majority of neurons have more than one neurotransmitter. About half (45 per cent) of the neurons contain dynorphin and vasoactive intestinal peptide (VIP). The other half contain choline acetyltransferase along with cholecystokinin (CCK), calcitonin gene-related peptide (CGRP), neuropeptide Y (NPY), and somatostatin (about 30 per cent); choline acetyltransferase along with substance P (about 10 per cent); or choline acetyltransferase alone (about 15 per cent). Also note the topography of different neuron types within the ganglion. (From Costa, M., Furness, J. B., and Llewellyn-Smith, I. J. *In* Johnson, L. R. [ed.]. Physiology of the Gastrointestinal Tract. New York, Raven Press, 1987. Used by permission.)

transmitters in a neuron is more of a rule than an exception.[33] Figure 2–10 summarizes coexistence of neurotransmitters in submucous neurons.

It has also been shown that some neurons in culture can produce different transmitters based upon alterations in culture conditions.[34]

GENERAL ORGANIZATION OF NERVES OF THE GUT

Although most of the gastrointestinal tract is insensitive to common cutaneous sensations, it is richly innervated by sensory nerves which carry a variety of mechanical and chemical information directly to the CNS or through synaptic pathways involving sympathetic or intramural ganglia.[35] At each of these sites sensory information is processed and appropriate secretomotor responses are formulated and executed by activation of various efferent pathways (Fig. 2–11). Examples of these efferent pathways include (1) motor neurons and sympathetic and parasympathetic preganglionic neurons in the CNS, (2) sympathetic postganglionic neurons in the sympathetic ganglia, and (3) parasympathetic postganglionic neurons and other intramural neurons in the enteric nervous system. Apart from mediating reflex control of gastrointestinal function, the sensory information from the gut can also modify neurally mediated functions of other organs in the body or can proceed to cortical levels in the brain.

Sensory Receptors

Gastrointestinal sensory receptors can be classified based upon their location, function, specificity, and adaptability (Table 2–2). Based on location, sensory nerves can be classified into mucosal, muscle, and serosal sensory receptors.

Mucosal Sensory Receptors

At least five types of mucosal sensory receptors are present in gastrointestinal mucosa. These respond to

mechanical, chemical, osmotic, thermal, or painful stimuli.[36–40]

Mechanoreceptors that respond selectively to mucosal pinching or stroking are present throughout the gastrointestinal tract. Many mechanoreceptors are multimodal, responding to mechanical as well as thermal and chemical stimuli. They discharge only upon initiation and termination of the stimulus, and therefore are referred to as rapidly adapting mechanoreceptors.[35, 41–43] Mechanoreceptors that respond to light touch are present in the pharynx and the anal canal. These receptors are slowly adapting in nature in that they continue to fire during prolonged activation.

Chemoreceptors sensitive to alkali, acid, glucose, and amino acids have been demonstrated in the gut and the liver. In general, chemoreceptors are connected to small-diameter unmyelinated fibers. They do not fire spontaneously and are specific in that they are activated only by certain chemical substances. Alkali and acid receptors have been described in the stomach and small intestine. They respond to either strong acids or strong alkalis, but not to both.[35] Multimodal neu-

Table 2–2. CLASSIFICATION OF GASTROINTESTINAL SENSORY RECEPTORS

Based on location and function
  Mucosal Sensory Receptors
    Mechanoreceptors (touch, pressure, stretch)
    Chemoreceptors (alkali, acid, glucose, amino acids)
    Osmoreceptors
    Thermoreceptors (cooling, warming, or both)
    Nociceptors
  Muscle Sensory Receptors
    Tension receptors
    Nociceptors
  Serosal and mesenteric sensory receptors
    Pressure sensitive (pacinian corpuscles)
    Nociceptors
Based on specificity
  Unimodal (i.e., activated selectively by a specific sensory stimulus)
  Multimodal (i.e., activated by multiple stimuli; most nociceptors are multimodal)
Based on adaptability
  Rapidly adapting (responding only to dynamic events or changes in stimulus)
  Slowly adapting (responding continuously to a sensory stimulus)

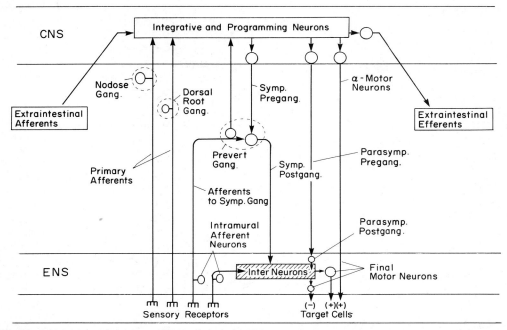

Figure 2–11. General organization of the innervation of the gut. The sensory fibers connected to sensory receptors in the gut can be classified into three groups: (1) Primary afferents are carried directly to CNS. They accompany either the vagus and have their cell bodies in the nodose ganglia or the sympathetic nerves and have their cell bodies in the dorsal root ganglia. (2) Afferents to prevertebral sympathetic ganglia, where they connect with postganglionic sympathetic neurons and with other afferent neurons that are connected to the CNS. (3) Intramural afferents, which remain within the gut wall and are connected to intramural neurons.

The efferent neurons can also be classified into 3 groups: (1) Those located in the CNS are alpha motor neurons, preganglionic parasympathetic neurons, and preganglionic sympathetic neurons. The alpha motor neurons directly innervate gastrointestinal striated muscle, the preganglionic parasympathetic fibers innervate postganglionic neurons in the enteric nervous system, and the preganglionic sympathetic fibers innervate postganglionic sympathetic nerves in the prevertebral ganglia. (2) Those located in the prevertebral sympathetic ganglia are postganglionic sympathetic neurons that project to enteric neurons. (3) Final motor neurons are all located in the enteric nervous system (except alpha motor neurons). Thus integration of intestinal reflexes occurs in the central nervous system (CNS), prevertebral ganglia, and enteric nervous system (ENS). The CNS also integrates extraintestinal afferent activity with gastrointestinal motor activity and integrates gastrointestinal afferent influences with extraintestinal motor activity.

ronal chemoreceptors responding to either acids or alkalis have also been described.[35] Glucoreceptors are present in the antrum of the stomach, duodenum, jejunum, ileum, and liver.[35, 36, 39, 44, 45] Their afferents are carried in vagus and splanchnic nerves.[45] Amino acid receptors have been demonstrated in the small intestine of cats. Like other chemoreceptors, they are quite specific and activated only by mucosal contact with amino acids. These receptors have been shown to exhibit differential sensitivity to the various amino acids.[46]

Specific osmoreceptors are present in the liver. These liver osmoreceptors discharge at a rate proportional to the osmotic pressure of the solution, independent of the chemical nature of the osmotic agent.[47] The presence of osmoreceptors in duodenal mucosa was first suggested in studies showing that gastric emptying was slowed by highly osmotic duodenal contents.[48] However, specific osmoreceptors that are connected to primary afferent fibers have not been demonstrated in the gut. Single fiber recordings show that receptors that are activated by osmotic activity are multimodal in that they are also stimulated by mechanical, thermal, and other chemical stimuli.[35, 45]

Thermoreceptors are sensitive to visceral cooling or warming, or in some instances to both. Such receptors have been demonstrated in the esophagus, stomach, and small intestine. Thermoreceptors are slow-adapting and do not show basal activity at normal body temperatures.[49] Thermoreceptors located in esophageal mucosa and submucosa are connected to unmyelinated afferent fibers in the vagus, whereas those in the parietal peritoneum are connected to splanchnic unmyelinated fibers.[35]

Mucosal nociceptors have not been investigated in any detail because defining pain receptors in the gastrointestinal mucosa is difficult. According to one view they represent a distinct receptor population. The polymodal receptors described above may also serve as nociceptors.[50, 51] The nature of receptors that mediate heartburn or peptic ulcer pain is unknown. Except for specialized tactile sensory receptors in the anal canal, all mucosal mechanoreceptors, thermoreceptors, and nociceptors are represented by free nerve endings. The identity of chemoreceptors is not clear. It has been suggested that at least some of them may be represented by specialized mucosal cells (like the taste cells in the tongue) that may activate a sensory ending by release of a chemical transmitter. All these receptors are connected to unmyelinated or thin myelinated fibers. The identity of sensory neurons mediating mucosal sensations involved in local reflexes within the intestinal wall is unknown.

Muscle Sensory Receptors

Most of the gastrointestinal tract has been shown to contain slowly adapting tension receptors in its muscle layers. These receptors are often spontaneously active and have a low threshold for stretch or contractile stimulation. The anatomic nature and location of these receptors are not known. Recently subcapsular ganglionic endings connected to sensory neurons have been described, and these may serve as tension receptors.[4] Muscle nociceptive receptors may be represented by free nerve endings and are connected to unmyelinated fibers. These receptors generally act as high-threshold tension receptors and show no evidence of adaptation. They also discharge vigorously and continuously in response to vascular ischemia and administration of algesic agents such as bradykinin, 5HT, and capsaicin.[39, 40]

Serosal and Mesenteric Sensory Receptors

Pacinian corpuscles are located in the serosa and mesentery, particularly around blood vessels. These receptors are sensitive to pressure and may monitor local changes in blood flow. They are rapidly adapting and are connected to myelinated fibers that are carried in splanchnic afferents.[43] The serosa and mesentery also contain polymodal nociceptive receptors that are connected to unmyelinated fibers and are carried in splanchnic afferents.

Afferent Projections

Sensory receptors are connected to afferent neurons, which carry sensory information to other neurons in the CNS, the prevertebral ganglia, and the enteric plexuses (Fig. 2–11). The neurons that carry sensory information to the CNS are called primary afferents and, depending upon the pathway taken, are described as vagal or splanchnic primary afferents.

Vagal Primary Afferents

Vagal primary afferent neurons are bipolar or pseudobipolar and have their cell bodies located in the inferior (nodose) ganglion of the vagus.[35] This ganglion is 2.5 cm in length and appears as a fusiform enlargement of the vagus nerve just as it passes caudally through the jugular foramen at the base of the skull. The peripheral processes of these neurons are predominantly unmyelinated fibers or small-diameter myelinated fibers that lose their myelin sheath as they extend from the nodose ganglion.[52] These peripheral processes run in the vagus nerves in close association with parasympathetic preganglionic fibers, which they outnumber by as much as 9 to 1. These fibers are distributed to a large variety of mucosal and muscle sensory receptors throughout the gut, including the esophagus, stomach, small intestine, gallbladder, liver, pancreas, and large bowel as far as the mid transverse colon. They do not carry impulses from mesenteric sensory receptors and probably do not carry impulses

from any nociceptive receptors. The central processes of these neurons ascend rostrally from the nodose ganglion through the jugular foramen into the medulla oblongata as the solitary fasciculus.[47, 53–59] These neurons contain substance P and calcitonin gene–related peptide, both of which may serve as sensory neurotransmitters.[60]

Splanchnic Primary Afferents

Splanchnic primary afferent neurons are T-shaped unipolar cells whose cell bodies are located segmentally in dorsal root ganglia of the spinal cord from T2 through S3.[61] The peripheral processes of these cells carry impulses from sensory endings in the gut and travel along blood vessels in association with sympathetic postganglionic efferent fibers. They pass uninterrupted through paravertebral sympathetic ganglia to eventually enter the gray ramus and dorsal root ganglia.[44] The splanchnic afferents have both unmyelinated and myelinated fibers. Unmyelinated fibers outnumber myelinated fibers by 10 to 1.[62] In contrast with the vagus nerve, in which approximately 80 per cent of the fibers are afferent, only 20 per cent of the fibers in the greater splanchnic nerve are afferent.[63, 64] The splanchnic afferents carry pain sensations as well as a wide variety of sensory information from various portions of the gut.[35, 45, 65] Sectioning of these nerves is sometimes used in the treatment of intractable pain, for example that of pancreatic carcinoma.

The dorsal root ganglia contain the cell bodies of the primary splanchnic afferent fibers and appear as ovoid swellings on dorsal nerve roots of the spinal cord just before their junction with the corresponding ventral root.[12] Dorsal root ganglia also contain cell bodies of neurons that provide segmental innervation to somatic structures such as skin and skeletal muscle. Two types of cells have been identified in these ganglia.[12] Type A are large cells with myelinated processes. They may be connected to pacinian corpuscles from the serosa and mesentery. The neurotransmitter content of these cells is not known. Type B cells are smaller and have small-diameter myelinated or unmyelinated processes. These cells can be further divided into two subpopulations based upon their neuropeptide content. Substance P and cholecystokinin (CCK) exist in one population of these cells, whereas somatostatin exists in a separate population.[66] Both these populations of type B cells innervate viscera as well as somatic sensory structures. Substance P–containing neurons may be involved in nociceptive sensations.[67, 68] The central processes of the T-shaped unipolar sensory neurons arise from the dorsal root ganglia and enter the spinal cord in their respective segments.[61, 62, 69–71]

Sensory Neurons in Enteric Ganglia

Some sensory neurons whose cell bodies are located in the enteric plexuses send processes that exit the gut wall and travel along the blood vessels to prevertebral ganglia, where they make synaptic contact with postganglionic sympathetic neurons.[72–75] They are activated by stimulation of tension receptors (bowel distention) and may exert their influence on postganglionic sympathetic neurons by releasing acetylcholine, bombesin-like peptide, CCK, enkephalin, substance P, and vasoactive intestinal peptide.[76-78]

Other sensory neurons whose cell bodies are located in the enteric ganglia carry information solely to other enteric ganglia along the gut. These sensory nerves are connected to mechanoreceptors that play an important role in local intramural reflexes along the gut such as secondary esophageal peristalsis and the intestinal peristaltic reflex. Electrophysiologic studies have revealed both slowly adapting and rapidly adapting mechano-sensitive neurons in the myenteric ganglia.[4] Although little is known about these intramural sensory neurons, it is probable that they are also connected to chemo-receptors, osmoreceptors, and thermoreceptors.

Efferent Projections (Fig. 2–12)

The central nervous system influences the function of the gastrointestinal tract through motor neurons whose axons exit the CNS to innervate the gastrointestinal tract either directly or indirectly via other neurons. These motor neurons include alpha motor neurons and preganglionic sympathetic and parasympathetic neurons. The alpha motor neurons belong to the group of general somatic and special visceral efferent systems. The preganglionic sympathetic and parasympathetic neurons belong to the group of general visceral efferents of the spinal cord and brainstem.

Special Visceral Outflow: Striated Muscle Innervation

Striated muscle is present at the proximal (pharynx and cervical esophagus) and distal (external anal sphincter) ends of the gastrointestinal tract. These striated muscles are innervated by alpha motor neurons, which are large multipolar neurons having myelinated axons 10 to 13 μ in diameter. The axons travel uninterrupted to the striated muscle, where they terminate at the motor end plate. The neurotransmitter of these alpha motor neurons is acetylcholine. These nerves provide excitatory but no inhibitory innervation to the muscles they innervate. The somas of alpha motor neurons that innervate the striated muscles of the pharynx and the upper part of the esophagus are located in the nucleus ambiguus, and their axons are carried in the glossopharyngeal, vagus, and spinal accessory nerves. The somas of alpha motor neurons innervating the external anal sphincter are located in the anterior horn cells of spinal segments S2 through S4 and their axons are carried in the pudendal nerve and eventually the inferior rectal nerve. Lesions of alpha motor neurons or defects in neuromuscular transmission at the motor end plate (e.g., myasthenia gravis) lead to paralysis of muscles supplied by these neurons. Clinically such lesions lead to pharyngeal and esophageal paralysis resulting in oropharyngeal dysphagia (see pp. 563–567) and paralysis of the external anal sphincter resulting in fecal incontinence (see pp. 317–331).

General Visceral Outflow: Sympathetic Projections

The soma of preganglionic sympathetic neurons to the gut are located in the intermediolateral column of spinal cord segments T2 through L2. The preganglionic fibers innervating the gut emerge from the spinal cord and travel in the ventral roots through the white ramus and the paravertebral ganglion to enter the prevertebral ganglia.[79] The preganglionic fibers are approximately 3 μ in diameter, thinly myelinated and have conduction velocities of 3 to 15 meters/sec. They synapse with one or more postganglionic neurons in the prevertebral ganglia. The postganglionic axons are very small (less than 2 μ in diameter), unmyelinated, and slowly conducting (less than 2 meters/sec) fibers. They extend to the effector organ and enter it in the company of blood vessels.[79] The main axon gives rise to many preterminal axons that branch and become continuous with terminal axons. The terminal axons ramify and form a meshwork called the ground plexus in the effector organ.

The postganglionic sympathetic axons provide rich innervation to the myenteric plexus (both the ganglia and the interganglionic strands) and the submucous plexus[80] (Fig. 2–13). In humans, there is very sparse adrenergic innervation of the longitudinal and circular muscle coats and muscularis mucosae.[81] In certain species, some sphincters of the gut may be more densely innervated.[80, 82, 83] A few adrenergic fibers extend into the villi, and a small number of axons form an open network around the mucosal glands. In contrast, the vasculature of the gut is densely innervated by adrenergic terminals. The preganglionic fibers from the upper thoracic segments provide segmental innervation to the upper esophagus.[84] The preganglionic fibers from segments T5 through T9 typically run along the greater splanchnic nerve and synapse with postganglionic sympathetic neurons in the celiac ganglion. The postganglionic sympathetic neurons from the celiac ganglion are distributed to the lower part of the esophagus, stomach, duodenum, pancreas, and biliary tract.[84] The preganglionic fibers from segments T10 and T11 are carried in lesser splanchnic nerves to the superior mesenteric ganglion, where they synapse with postganglionic neurons. The postganglionic sympathetic fibers accompany the superior mesenteric artery to innervate most of the small intestine and the right half of the colon.[79] The preganglionic fibers from segments T12, L1, and L2 are carried in the smallest splanchnic nerve to the inferior mesenteric and pelvic ganglia, where they synapse with postganglionic neurons.[85, 86] The postganglionic processes of neurons in the inferior mesenteric ganglion run along the inferior mesenteric artery and innervate the left half of the transverse colon, the descending colon, and the sigmoid colon. The postganglionic processes of the pelvic ganglia innervate the rectum and anal canal.[87]

Sympathetic Ganglia and Synaptic Transmission. Prevertebral sympathetic ganglia contain postganglionic multipolar neurons, small interneurons, glial cells, and presynaptic endings of preganglionic and

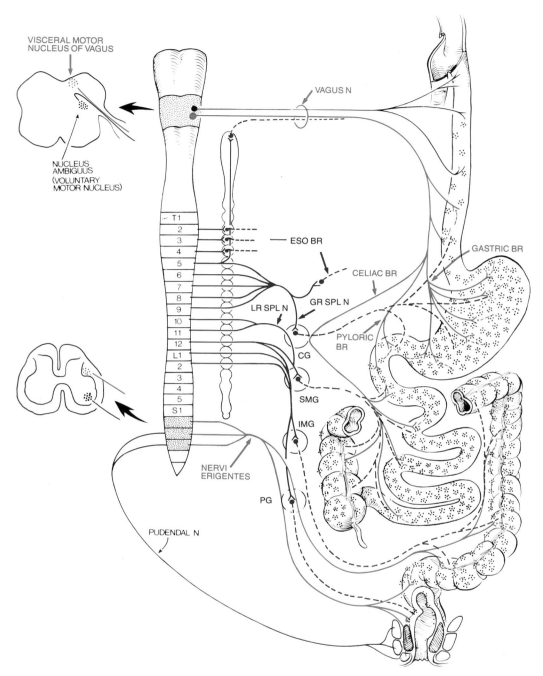

Figure 2–12. Efferent innervation of the gastrointestinal tract. Alpha motor neurons are shown in black. They innervate skeletal muscle at either end of the gut. The alpha motor neurons to the pharynx and upper esophagus are present in the nucleus ambiguus and their axons are carried in the vagus nerve. The alpha motor neurons to the external anal sphincter are present in Onuf's nucleus and their axons are carried in the pudendal nerve. The sympathetic pathway, shown in blue, consists of cell bodies of preganglionic neurons located in spinal cord segments T2 through L2. The preganglionic fibers, shown in solid blue lines, are carried in the greater splanchnic nerve (GR SPL N), lesser splanchnic nerve (LR SPL N), and smallest splanchnic nerve (not labeled) to terminate in the celiac ganglion (CG), superior mesenteric ganglion (SMG), inferior mesenteric ganglion (IMG), and pelvic ganglion (PG). The postganglionic sympathetic neurons, shown in broken blue lines, are distributed in a segmental fashion to the gastrointestinal tract. The parasympathetic pathway, shown in green, consists of vagal and sacral outflows. The vagal pathway, shown in solid green lines, consists of preganglionic parasympathetic axons whose cell bodies are present in the dorsal motor nucleus of vagus. The vagal parasympathetics supply the gastrointestinal tract up to the right half of the colon. Sacral preganglionic parasympathetic fibers arising from neurons in spinal cord segments S2 to S4 (nervi erigentes) supply the left half of the colon, including the rectum and the internal anal sphincter. The postganglionic parasympathetic nerves and fibers, shown in green broken lines, are present intramurally in the gut wall. The enteric nervous system is shown in red. Sympathetic and parasympathetic nerves make extensive contacts with neurons in the enteric nervous system.

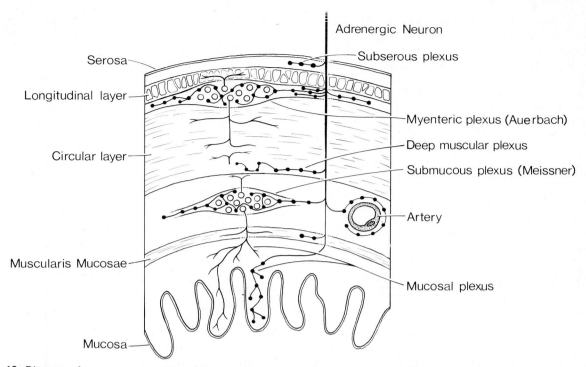

Figure 2–13. Diagram of a transverse section of the gut showing enteric plexuses and the distribution of adrenergic neurons. Note the ganglionic plexuses of Auerbach and Meissner. The deep muscular plexus contains a few, the subserosal contains an occasional, and the mucosal plexus contains no ganglia. The processes of enteric neurons have varicosities, which are not shown. The adrenergic fibers are all extrinsic and arise from adrenergic neurons in the prevertebral sympathetic ganglia. The adrenergic fibers (shown here with varicosities) are distributed largely to the myenteric, submucous, and mucosal plexuses and to blood vessels.

sensory neurons whose cell bodies are located in enteric ganglia.[79] Ultrastructural studies of sympathetic ganglia show extensive dendrodendritic contacts between postganglionic neurons. These contacts provide a means for extensive interaction among neurons within the ganglia.[79] In addition, axoaxonal synapses between preganglionic fibers have been demonstrated that may provide a means of presynaptic inhibition or facilitation among preganglionic nerves.[88] The sympathetic preganglionic neurons are primarily cholinergic, but some also contain enkephalin.[89, 90] It has been suggested that enkephalins may act as presynaptic inhibitors of acetylcholine release from presynaptic terminals.[91] These ganglia also contain nerve terminals that contain bombesin-like peptide, cholecystokinin, calcitonin gene–related peptide, enkephalin, substance P, and vasoactive intestinal peptide (VIP).[92–94] These peptides may represent the neurotransmitters of the axons of sensory nerves arising from the gut.[73]

Preganglionic sympathetic stimulation causes three recognizable membrane potential changes in sympathetic ganglia.[79, 95, 96] These include fast excitatory postsynaptic potentials (EPSPs) (mediated by nicotonic receptors), inhibitory postsynaptic potential (IPSPs) (mediated by M2 muscarinic and adrenergic receptors), and slow EPSPs (mediated in part by M1 muscarinic receptors). M2 cholinergic autoreceptors on the presynaptic terminal also inhibit the release of acetylcholine, providing feedback control of acetylcholine release.[7, 35] Many noncholinergic fibers arising in the gut and terminating in sympathetic ganglia cause slow

EPSPs in postganglionic neurons (presumably due to substance P and bombesin-like peptides).[97–99]

The prevertebral sympathetic ganglia contain mainly adrenergic neurons. However, peptidergic neurons containing neuropeptide Y (NPY), somatostatin, substance P (SP), enkephalin, and VIP have also been demonstrated which may project to distinct structures within the gut.[100–102] In one study it was found that there are four distinct groups of postganglionic neurons. One group contain only norepinephrine (NE) and project to myenteric neurons. A second group contain NE and NPY and project to mucosal blood vessels. A third group contain NE and somatostatin and project to submucous ganglia. A final group of cells contain only VIP and are the only cells not containing NE.

General Functions of Sympathetic Nerves. Sympathetic efferent stimulation generally causes inhibition of gastrointestinal motor and secretory activity, and contraction of gastrointestinal sphincters and blood vessels.[75, 103, 104] The generalized inhibitory effects of sympathetic stimulation on motility and secretion are more prominent in the stomach, small bowel, and large bowel than in the esophagus and rectum. Clinically, sympathetic stimulation generally leads to gastric stasis, adynamic or paralytic ileus, or colonic ileus[2,105] (see pp. 379–380). Stimulation of sympathetic or parasympathetic afferents can mediate stimulation of sympathetic efferents, and these reflexes are called sympathosympathetic and parasympathosympathetic reflexes, respectively. Reflex mediated generalized sympathetic stimulation may involve all parts of the gut. However, in many reflexes only one segment of the gut may be involved. For example, stimulation of sympathetic fibers to the stomach by small bowel chemoreceptor activation may be responsible for control of gastric emptying by means of the chemical composition of food entering the duodenum.[48] On the other hand, the major clinical manifestation of surgical sympathectomy or visceral neuropathy involving sympathetic nerves (e.g., diabetes mellitus) is usually diarrhea due to the loss of tonic inhibitory effects of sympathetic nerves on small intestinal motility and intestinal secretion[106, 107] (see pp. 296–298). Because surgical sympathectomy involves visceral afferent fibers as well as adrenergic motor fibers, sympathectomy is also associated with deranged mediation of many visceral sensations including visceral pain.

General Visceral Outflow: Parasympathetic Projection

The parasympathetic efferent projections to the gut consist of cranial (vagus) and sacral (pelvic splanchnic) outflow tracts. The vagal parasympathetic preganglionic fibers arise from the dorsal motor nucleus of the vagus, which provides parasympathetic innervation to practically all thoracic and abdominal viscera except the pelvic region.[108] The dorsal motor nucleus is 10 to 11 mm in length and is located in the floor of the fourth ventricle in the medulla oblongata.[84] The parasympathetic preganglionic fibers arising from this nucleus are contained in the vagi as they descend in the thorax. The vagi branch to form an esophageal plexus that innervates the esophagus, heart, and other thoracic structures.[109] At a variable distance above the esophageal hiatus in the diaphragm, the fibers of the plexus merge into anterior and posterior vagal trunks.

The anterior trunk gives off gastric, hepatic, and celiac branches. The gastric branches run along the lesser curvature and supply the anterior surface of the stomach almost as far as the pylorus.[109] The pyloric branches run to the right between the layers of lesser omentum close to the hepatic plexus, and then downward to reach the pyloric antrum, the pylorus, and the proximal part of the duodenum. Small celiac branches run alongside the left gastric artery to reach the celiac ganglion.

The posterior vagal trunk gives off gastric and celiac branches. The gastric branches radiate to the posterior surface of the stomach and supply it from the fundus to the pyloric antrum.[109] The celiac branch is large and reaches the celiac plexus alongside the left gastric artery. Sometimes it joins a similar branch from the anterior vagal trunk before entering the celiac plexus. The celiac branch is distributed to the pylorus, duodenum, pancreas, small bowel, and large bowel up to the mid-transverse colon.

The gross anatomic description of the distribution of the vagus nerves does not give true information regarding the distribution of the parasympathetic efferent fibers. This is due to the fact that the vagus is predominantly a sensory nerve with afferent fibers constituting over 80 per cent of all fibers.[52]

The sacral outflow provides parasympathetic innervation to the hindgut, namely, the anorectal area, descending colon, and left half of the transverse colon.[84] Sacral parasympathetic preganglionic neurons are located along the lateral aspect of the anterior gray horn in spinal cord segments S2 to S4. Axons from these cells accompany the roots of segments S2 to S4 and depart from them soon after emerging from the anterior sacral foramina. These nerves join to form the nervi erigentes. After a short course, these nerves join the hypogastric nerves, which are the paired continuations of the superior hypogastric plexus, to form the pelvic plexuses. The pelvic plexus contains sympathetic, parasympathetic, and afferent fibers and many autonomic ganglia. The sacral preganglionic fibers synapse with ganglia on the serosal surface of the colon and rectum.[77, 110] The postganglionic neurons send axons that ascend between longitudinal and circular muscles as far as the mid-colon. These bundles, which have been called intramural nerves of the colon, make contact with intramural enteric neurons.[111, 112] The preganglionic neurons in the parasympathetic pathway are generally believed to be cholinergic. However, some vagal parasympathetic neurons contain catecholamines[113–115] and enkephalin.[101, 116–119]

The second order neuron (postganglionic neuron) in the parasympathetic pathway to the gut may be a final motor neuron or an interneuron located between the preganglionic and final motor neuron. The precise nature of the final motor neuron in the parasympathetic pathway to the gut is not currently known. There is strong evidence demonstrating that it consists of both cholinergic and noncholinergic nerves. The cholinergic nerves are always excitatory and the noncholinergic nerves are both excitatory and inhibitory in nature.[120] Pharmacologic studies of the lower esophageal sphincter suggest that synaptic transmission between vagal preganglionic fibers and postganglionic noncholinergic inhibitory neurons involves both muscarinic and nicotinic receptors of acetylcholine.[121, 122] In some instances a 5HT interneuron may also be involved.[123]

General Functions of Parasympathetic Nerves. Vagal efferent fibers exert discrete effects on the gastrointestinal tract. For example, activation of the deglutition reflex activates certain fibers that innervate the esophagus and proximal stomach.[124, 125] Moreover, sham feeding causes selective activation of vagal preganglionic fibers that mediate secretomotor activity of the stomach and pancreas (see p. 957). There is also evidence to suggest that separate groups of vagal preganglionic fibers separately innervate inhibitory or excitatory neurons in the same organ.[124] For example, sensory stimuli that are subthreshold for the full deglutition reflex activate only those vagal fibers that innervate inhibitory neurons in the esophagus and lower esophageal sphincter, leading to inappropriate relaxation of the lower esophageal sphincter[126] (see p. 586). Moreover, deglutition causes activation of those vagal fibers that innervate inhibitory postganglionic neurons followed by activation of those vagal fibers that innervate excitatory intramural neurons. This sequential activation of vagal fibers leads to deglutitive inhibition, which precedes esophageal peristaltic contractions.[126, 127] Innervation of inhibitory and excitatory postganglionic neurons by separate preganglionic fibers also allows for more efficient inhibitory or excitatory effects of vagus neurons. For example, excitation of the vagal fibers that synapse with inhibitory neurons with simultaneous inhibition of vagal fibers that synapse with postganglionic excitatory neurons leads to more efficient vagal inhibition of the lower esophageal sphincter or the stomach.[125]

Electrical stimulation of vagal efferents produces indiscriminate and simultaneous activation of all preganglionic vagal parasympathetic fibers. Therefore such studies do not always closely mimic the physiologic influences of the vagus observed in certain well-defined reflexes in which only a selected population of fibers may be activated at one time. In general, electrical vagal efferent stimulation produces excitatory as well as inhibitory effects.[128] After blockade of cholinergic (muscarinic) excitatory influences, vagal stimulation usually produces inhibition or inhibition followed by excitation. Both of these responses (i.e., inhibition or inhibition followed by excitation) are mediated by noncholinergic transmitters.[120, 129]

Vagal influences are more prominent in the more proximal (esophagus, stomach, and duodenum) than distal (small bowel and proximal colon) portions of the gastrointestinal tract. Bilateral vagotomy at the cervical region involving preganglionic vagal fibers leads to major motor and secretory dysfunctions of the esophagus, stomach, duodenum, and pancreas and only minor derangement of function of the gallbladder, small bowel, and right side of the colon.[125] Cervical vagotomy causes loss of primary esophageal peristalsis associated with swallowing, but secondary esophageal peristalsis is largely unaffected.[122] Bilateral truncal vagotomy at the level of the lower esophagus is clinically used for treatment of peptic ulcer. Bilateral truncal vagotomy leads to reduction in gastric acid secretion but is accompanied by serious gastric motility disorders leading to gastric stasis.[125, 130] To obviate the complications of gastric stasis, truncal vagotomy is always combined with some sort of gastric drainage procedure (see p. 941). Gastric stasis associated with vagotomy can also be obviated by performing selective vagotomy in which vagal fibers that innervate the gastric body are sectioned but vagal fibers that supply the antrum and pylorus are preserved (see p. 943). Selective vagotomy also avoids other deleterious effects of truncal vagotomy, such as post-vagotomy diarrhea, by preserving normal vagal control of gallbladder, small bowel, and pancreatic function.[125]

The sacral parasympathetic nerves exert important effects on colorectal motility and the internal anal sphincter.[87, 131–134] Sacral parasympathetic damage leads to impaired defecation reflex and constipation.

CENTRAL NERVOUS SYSTEM CONNECTIONS OF GASTROINTESTINAL NERVES

Projections of Afferent Nerves in the CNS

The central projections of sensory cells in the nodose ganglia extend to the nucleus tractus solitarius, area postrema, and dorsal motor nucleus of the vagus.[84] Neurons whose cell bodies are located in these nuclei in turn make extensive synaptic contacts with other brainstem and hypothalamic nuclei.

The sensory unmyelinated (C) fibers of dorsal root ganglia cells terminate on neurons in lamina II and III of the dorsal horn (substantia gelatinosa Rolandi). These neurons serve as interneurons, which then terminate on neurons in lamina V of the spinal cord.[84] By means of the anterior spinothalamic tract, neurons from this lamina send ipsilateral and some contralateral projections to thalamic nuclei and other nuclei in the reticular formation.[61, 71] The thalamus is in turn connected with many cortical and other brain areas. These pathways are thought to carry visceral pain.[68] In the spinal cord visceral pain fibers are intermixed with fibers containing somatic segmental pain, which explains the referral of visceral pain to somatic segments.[56] This pain pathway is also connected with central algesic pathways, which include opioid-containing neurons.[68] These neurons reduce pain by inhibiting sensory input of the pain-carrying fibers.

The sensory small myelinated fibers of dorsal root ganglia cells terminate on neurons located in lamina I and V of the spinal cord.[113] Axons of these neurons pass along the lateral spinothalamic tract projecting directly to neurons in the reticular formation.

CNS Connection with Motor Neurons of the Gut and Centrally Mediated Reflexes

The motor efferent neurons to the gastrointestinal tract (alpha motor neurons, vagal and sacral parasympathetic neurons, and thoracolumbar sympathetic neurons) receive projections from neurons in cortical and subcortical areas, including the limbic system, the hypothalamus, and various brainstem centers, and also directly from gastrointestinal afferent neurons. The afferent fibers make direct contacts with motor neurons and thus mediate monosynaptic reflexes. The polysynaptic pathways are involved in a variety of gastrointestinal reflexes as well as integration of activities involving behavior, viscerosomatic reflexes, and pain perception.

The sympathetic and parasympathetic afferents and efferents and their connections in the CNS are involved in a large variety of specific reflex activities. These activities can be grouped as:

1. Reflexes in which both afferents and efferents belong to the gastrointestinal tract. These may be sympathoparasympathetic, sympathosympathetic, par-

asympathosympathetic or parasympathoparasympathetic depending on the sympathetic or parasympathetic nature of afferents and efferents.[75, 135, 136]

2. Reflexes in which gastrointestinal afferents mediate visceral pain, or other visceral, somatic or behavioral changes. Some examples of these reflexes include deglutition tachycardia, deglutition bradycardia, nausea and vomiting, deglutition reflex, defecation reflex, hunger, and satiety.[48, 87, 135, 137] There are also many behavior-related disorders of the gastrointestinal tract, such as irritable bowel syndrome and bulimia (see pp. 185–194).

3. Reflexes in which afferents arising from extraintestinal sites induce gastrointestinal changes.[138] An example of an extraintestinal intestinal reflex includes the cephalic phases of acid and pancreatic secretion, in which increased secretion occurs in response to the sight or smell of food.[9, 139]

ENTERIC NERVOUS SYSTEM

The most remarkable feature of the innervation of the gut is its own intramural nervous system, called the enteric nervous system. The enteric nervous system has a functional and structural organization which is similar to that of CNS. Interestingly, there are more neurons in the enteric nervous system than there are in the spinal cord. The enteric nervous system is capable of functioning independently of any extrinsic innervation or central nervous system control. The enteric nervous system receives sensory input through its sensory neurons, integrates this information through intramural interneurons, and generates appropriate motor responses that are mediated to the effector tissue by means of intramural motor neurons. This enteric pathway can, however, be modulated by the central nervous system by means of sympathetic and parasympathetic efferent nerves that are connected to enteric nerves. Although it is not known with certainty, some of the final motor neurons in the enteric nervous system may also be the second order (postganglionic) neurons in the parasympathetic pathway.

General Anatomy of Enteric Plexus (Fig. 2–14)

The enteric nervous system consists of two major and three minor networks or plexuses of neurons and their processes. The two main ganglionated plexuses are the myenteric (Auerbach's) plexus, and the submucous (Meissner's) plexus. They contain collections of neuronal cell bodies, also called ganglion cells. The myenteric plexus lies between the circular and longitudinal muscle layers and extends from the esophagus to the internal anal sphincter, including the biliary tract.[2] The features of the myenteric plexus vary considerably along the length of the gut and there are many species differences.[140–142] In the esophagus, the myenteric plexus is an irregular network with sparse small-sized ganglia. Interestingly, the neuronal count

decreases distally along the esophagus and increases again in the lower esophageal sphincter. The myenteric plexus is more prominent in the stomach than in the esophagus. The proximal stomach also contains thick nerve bundles that extend in a straight course from the proximal portion of the lesser curvature to the greater curvature of the stomach. These so-called shunt fascicles may represent the intramural course of bundles of extrinsic nerves. In the small bowel the myenteric plexus is very highly developed and consists of a regular network of interconnecting nerve bundles with ganglia located at bundle intersections. The density of ganglia is greater in the duodenum and jejunum than in the ileum. In the ascending and transverse colon the myenteric plexus is also well developed and located mainly under the teniae coli. The myenteric ganglia become irregular and less densely populated distally along the colon. In the lower part of the anal canal myenteric ganglia are virtually absent. The distal colon, like the stomach, has many prominent intramural fascicles.

The submucous or Meissner's plexus is located in the submucosa of the gut wall between the muscularis mucosa and circular muscle layers. The submucous plexus, like the myenteric plexus, varies in meshwork density and nerve cell content along the length of the gut.[143] In the esophagus the submucous plexus is sparsely populated and essentially nonexistent in some mammals. The submucous ganglia are better developed in the stomach than in the esophagus. They are most developed in the small bowel. The neuronal density in the submucous ganglia in the colon gradually decreases caudally, so that neurons are also virtually absent in the anal canal distal to the pectinate line. Submucosal ganglia are smaller than those in the myenteric plexus and contain fewer cells. For instance, in the guinea pig ileum there are approximately 8 neurons per ganglion in the submucosal plexus as compared with 43 neurons per ganglion in the myenteric plexus.[144]

In addition to the two major plexuses, there are three variably developed plexuses:

1. The subserous plexus is situated between the serosa and consists of bundles of nerve fibers with few or no ganglia.

2. A deep muscular plexus is situated within the circular muscle. Fibers within this plexus are continuous with fine branches from the myenteric plexus and the adjacent submucous plexus. This deep muscular plexus may have occasional nerve cell bodies.

3. Mucosal plexuses are named according to their position in the mucosa, namely, subglandular, intraglandular, and intravillous mucosal plexuses. These mucosal plexuses are best developed in the small intestine. They do not contain ganglion cells and consist of fine branches from neurons in the submucous ganglia, adrenergic postganglionic neurons, and sensory endings of primary afferent fibers.

Ultrastructural studies of enteric plexuses demonstrate a degree of structural organization that in many ways resembles the complexity of the central nervous system.[145–148] The ganglia are composed of glial cells and tightly packed aggregations of neurons and their

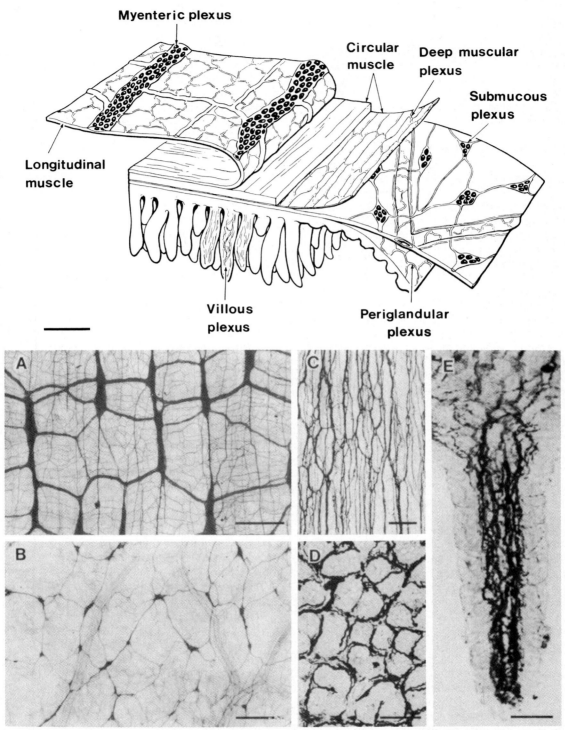

Figure 2–14. Anatomy of enteric plexuses. The diagram at the top shows the myenteric plexus present between longitudinal and circular muscle layers and the submucous plexus in the submucosa. It also shows between circular and muscularis mucosa the deep muscular plexus near the innermost layers of the circular muscle and the periglandular and villous plexuses in and around the mucosal glands and villi, respectively. The micrographs in A, B, and C are whole mounts stained with Z10 technique to show myenteric (A) and submucous (B) plexuses and nerve fibers in circular muscle layers (C). The micrographs in D and E are stained for cholinesterase to show periglandular (D) and villous plexuses (E). Calibration: diagram 200 μm; A and B 500 μm; C, D, and E 50 μm. (From Costa, M., Furness, J. B., and Llewellyn-Smith I. J. *In* Johnson, L. R. [ed.]. Physiology of the Gastrointestinal Tract. New York, Raven Press, 1987. Used by permission.)

processes which form the neuropil and glial cells. The ganglia characteristically contain very little intercellular space and their outer surfaces are covered with a continuous sheet of basal lamina of variable thickness. Connective tissue elements and blood vessels never enter the ganglia themselves.[2, 144] The size and shape of neurons vary considerably within the ganglia. A particularly distinct feature of enteric ganglia is the finding that large portions of neuronal cytoplasm come in close contact with the surrounding basal lamina. This close contact of large portions of neuronal cytoplasm with the basal lamina, along with the absence of blood vessels extending within the ganglia, suggest that neurons rely upon diffusion of nutrients through the basal lamina from the extraganglionic interstitial fluid.

Axodendritic and axosomatic synapses are commonly observed in enteric ganglia, but axoaxonic (or presynaptic) synapses are rarely seen. The synapses within the enteric ganglia are morphologically asymmetrical, with the postsynaptic density usually being more prominent and thicker than the presynaptic density.[20, 147, 149] There is great variability in the size and shape of the active zone and degree of accumulation of vesicles in the enteric ganglia. Presynaptic terminals in the enteric ganglia demonstrate small granular (10 to 50 nm) vesicles, small agranular (10 to 50 nm) vesicles, granular vesicles of heterogenous size and nature, large opaque (50 to 200 nm) vesicles, and large granular vesicles. Different vesicle types may contain different neurotransmitters, and a number of attempts have been made to classify nerve profiles within the ganglia according to the types of vesicles they contain. However, most nerve profiles contain more than one type of vesicle.

Glial cells throughout the nervous system are believed to play a supportive role for neurons. In the CNS glial cells are most prominent and outnumber neurons by 10 to 50 times. In enteric ganglia, glial cells generally outnumber neurons by two to one and are smaller and lack the large cytoplasmic expanses of neurons.[145] The enteric glial cells contain large numbers of gliofilaments gathered in bundles than run primarily along the long axis of the cell. These glial cells are distinctly different from the satellite cells of the autonomic ganglia and the Schwann cells of the peripheral nerves and in many ways are more similar to the astrocytes of the central nervous system.[150, 151] Moreover, recent studies have shown that enteric glial cells contain a protein called glial fibrillary acidic protein that had previously been thought to be specific to astrocytes of the central nervous system.

Enteric Neurons

Enteric neurons are either sensory neurons (which carry information from sensory receptors), final motor neurons (which make contact with muscle, secretory, or other target cells), or interneurons (which integrate information they receive from sensory neurons and provide motor programs to the motor neurons). The interneurons and final motor neurons can be either excitatory or inhibitory in nature. The functional nature of enteric neurons cannot be defined by their morphology. For example, recognition of argyrophilic or argyrophobic neurons does not provide any useful information.[152]

Most enteric neurons are multipolar. These multipolar neurons may be sensory neurons, motor neurons, or interneurons. Unipolar neurons are less commonly seen in enteric ganglia and probably function as sensory neurons. Based upon electron microscopic features nine types of nerves in enteric ganglia have been identified.[2] The functional significance of this classification is not known.

A wide variety of pharmacologic and electrophysiologic studies involving the motor or secretory responses to nerve stimulation have provided important information concerning the possible role of various enteric neurons in the regulation of gastrointestinal activity. This task, however, has been complicated by the fact that enteric neurons may utilize many neurotransmitter substances (over 14 potential candidates so far) to produce their actions on the gut. Although recent studies have provided a great deal of information concerning the electrical properties and neurotransmitter content of enteric neurons, the physiologic role of these many different neurons is not yet fully defined. Most of the currently available information on enteric neurons comes from studies of the guinea pig ileum.

Electrical Properties of Enteric Neurons

Using intracellular recording techniques, two basic types of neurons can be distinguished in enteric ganglia.[4, 6] Type 1 neurons are also called S type ("S" for synaptic input) because stimulation of the nerves which synapse on them evokes prominent fast EPSPs. Their action potential is due to the opening of Na^+ channels and is blocked by tetrodotoxin. These neurons discharge spikes continuously during long-lasting depolarizing current pulses (Fig. 2–15). These features of type 1 neurons are in many ways similar to those of other autonomic neurons. Type 2 neurons are also called AH neurons ("AH") for afterhyperpolarization). They are characterized by the prolonged afterhyperpolarization that follows an action potential. They have a prominent calcium component to their action potential that is not blocked by tetrodotoxin. These neurons do not exhibit prominent fast EPSPs in response to fiber tract stimulation, and they typically discharge only a single spike at the onset of a long depolarizing current (Fig. 2–15). Type 2 (AH) neurons have characteristics unique to that of enteric nerves. Although a small number of enteric neurons in the guinea pig ileum cannot be easily classified according to this system, myenteric ganglia contain approximately 50 per cent type 1 (S) and 50 per cent type 2 (AH) neurons and submucosal ganglia contain approximately 90 per cent type 1 (S) and 10 per cent type 2 (AH) neurons.

Using extracellular recording techniques, various types of enteric neurons have been classified based

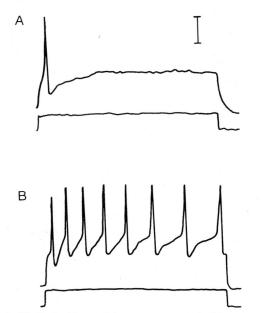

Figure 2–15. Comparison of the responses evoked by intracellular injection of depolarizing current in an AH/type 2 neuron and an S/type 1 neuron in the myenteric plexus of guinea pig small intestine. *A,* Injection of a 200-msec duration depolarizing pulse evoked a single spike only at the onset of the current pulse in the AH/type 2 neuron. *B,* Injection of a 200-msec duration depolarizing pulse evoked multiple spike discharges throughout the current pulse in the S/type 1 neuron. Upper trace is transmembrane voltage; lower trace is current. Vertical calibration 20 mV; 1 nA. (From Wood, J. D. *In* Johnson, L. R. [ed.]. Physiology of the Gastrointestinal Tract. New York, Raven Press, 1987. Used by permission.)

upon their response to mechanical distortion and the pattern of their spike discharge[4] (Fig. 2–16). Extracellular recordings are suitable only for recording spike activity, but have an advantage over intracellular recording techniques in that they can record from a localized area of the cell membrane.

Mechanosensitive sensory neurons are those that respond to mechanical distortion. Three types of mechanosensitive neurons have been identified in enteric ganglia: (1) slowly adapting mechanoreceptor types maintain a discharge throughout the stimulus; (2) rapidly adapting mechanoreceptor types discharge upon initiation and termination of the stimulus; and (3) "tonic type" mechanoreceptive neurons discharge in a set pattern for long periods extending far beyond termination of the stimulus (up to 40 sec).

The discharge rate is independent of intensity of mechanical stimulation. There are two major types of neurons that do not seem to respond to mechanical distortion of the ganglion. They are known as single spike–type and burst-type neurons. The single spike neurons discharge continuously at low frequencies and without a consistent pattern of activity. These neurons exhibit fast EPSPs with nerve tract stimulation and their overall behavior is similar to type 1 (S) neurons demonstrated using intracellular studies. The burst-type neurons discharge spikes in bursts that occur with regular or irregular interspike intervals.

Chemical Nature of Enteric Neurons

In the past, all enteric neurons were thought to be postganglionic neurons in the parasympathetic pathway and were considered to be cholinergic in nature. Subsequently, pharmacologic studies suggested that many nerves in the enteric nervous system were neither cholinergic nor adrenergic and suggested that noncholinergic, nonadrenergic nerves were purinergic in nature. However, it is now obvious that there are many noncholinergic, nonadrenergic neurotransmitters that include a large number of regulatory peptides.These peptides have largely been identified by their immunohistochemical localization to enteric neurons. There is a remarkable similarity in noncholinergic, nonadrenergic transmitters that are involved in the CNS and those involved in the enteric nervous system.

Cholinergic Neurons. A large number of neurons in the myenteric and submucous plexuses are cholinergic. Apart from pharmacologic studies, cholinergic nerves can be identified by staining for choline acetyltransfer-

MECHANOSENSITIVE NEURONS

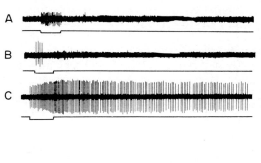

SINGLE SPIKE NEURON

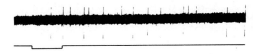

BURST TYPE NEURON

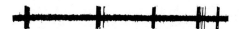

Figure 2–16. Patterns of spike discharges from myenteric neurons as recorded by extracellular recordings. The top panel shows mechanosensitive neurons. These neurons discharge in response to deformation of the ganglia. *A* shows slowly adapting neurons that continue to discharge throughout the period of deformation. *B* shows a rapidly adapting mechanosensitive neuron that fires only upon initiation of the deformation. *C* shows a tonic type mechanosensitive neuron that discharges in response to mechanical stimulation and continues for a long time even after the removal of the deformation. The middle panel shows the discharge pattern of a single spike neuron. These neurons are not mechanosensitive and discharge single spikes continuously. The bottom panel shows the discharge pattern of a burst type neuron. Note that the spikes occur in bursts that may be regular or irregular. (From Wood, J. D. *In* Johnson, L. R. [ed.]. Physiology of the Gastrointestinal Tract. New York, Raven Press, 1987. Used by permission.)

ase, the enzyme that synthesizes acetylcholine.[27, 153] Because of technical reasons, distribution of cholinergic nerves and their projections in the gut is not yet fully known. Cholinergic fibers from the myenteric plexus are generally distributed to the longitudinal and circular muscle layers as well as to other myenteric nerves, whereas those from the submucous plexus are distributed to other submucosal ganglia, mucosal glands, and blood vessels. Many cholinergic enteric neurons serve as final motor neurons. Stimulation of enteric cholinergic nerves causes contraction of smooth muscle, increase in intestinal secretion, release of intestinal hormones, and dilation of blood vessels. Many of these effects on target tissue are mediated by M2 muscarinic receptors.[120, 154]

Cholinergic preganglionic parasympathetic neurons and many intramural cholinergic interneurons make synaptic contacts with other myenteric and submucous neurons. Activation of cholinergic presynaptic terminals cause fast EPSPs in neurons of both the plexuses. The fast EPSP is mediated by nicotinic receptors for acetylcholine.[7] Activation of cholinergic nerves also causes a slow EPSP in some neurons. This slow-rising, long-lasting postsynaptic potential (lasting up to 90 sec after termination of stimulus) provides for prolonged excitation of postsynaptic neurons and is observed in submucosal and myenteric neurons. It is mediated by M1 muscarinic receptors.[6] The cholinergic excitatory input may impinge on either excitatory motor neurons

(which may be cholinergic or noncholinergic) or noncholinergic inhibitory motor neurons, resulting in the end effect on the target cell being either excitatory or inhibitory in nature. Cholinergic nerves in the enteric plexus have also been shown to possess presynaptic M2 muscarinic receptors, which serve to provide inhibitory modulation of acetylcholine release.[7, 155]

Many cholinergic neurons also contain neuropeptides. Some have been shown to contain SP or enkephalin, while others contain CCK, NPY, and somatostatin.[156, 157] The physiologic importance of such combinations of transmitters in these nerves is not yet known.

Adrenergic Neurons (Fig. 2–17). All adrenergic innervation to myenteric and submucous plexuses, mucosa, and blood vessels is derived from extrinsic sympathetic nerves. Intrinsic adrenergic neurons in the gut have not been identified.[81, 158]

5-Hydroxytryptamine Neurons (Fig. 2–17). A small number of 5HT-containing neurons have been identified in the myenteric plexus.[159–161] Axons from these neurons usually descend aborally and are distributed to the myenteric and submucous plexuses. There are no projections to the muscle layers or the mucosa. There are no 5HT-containing neurons in the submucous plexus of the guinea pig small intestine. These observations suggest that 5HT neurons serve primarily as interneurons in the enteric plexuses.[158] 5HT interneurons appear to mediate a prolonged excitatory state

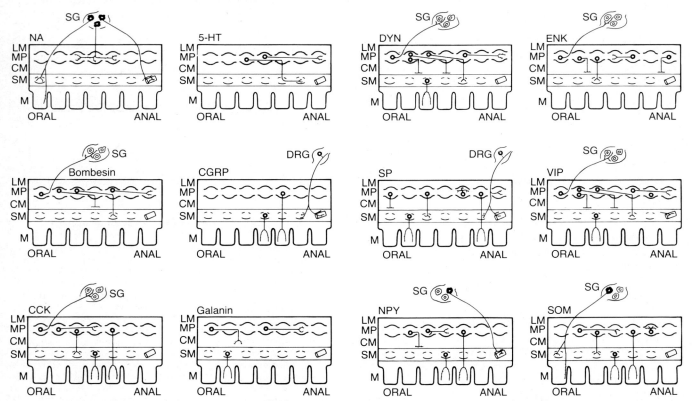

Figure 2–17. Diagrammatic representation of the projections of different types of neurons in the gut. Please refer to the text for details. 5-HT, 5-hydroxytryptamine. See Figure 2–18 legend for other abbreviations. (From Costa, M., Furness, J. B., and Llewellyn-Smith, I. J. *In* Johnson, L. R. [ed.]. Physiology of the Gastrointestinal Tract. New York, Raven Press, 1987. Used by permission.)

in cholinergic nerves containing substance P and VIP that are responsible for muscle excitation, intestinal secretion, and sphincter relaxation.

ATP (Purinergic) Neurons. There is some evidence to suggest that adenosine triphosphate (ATP) is a neurotransmitter in noncholinergic, nonadrenergic nerves.[162-164] ATP is present in neuronal vesicles containing other transmitters, suggesting that it may serve as a cotransmitter.[120] ATP has been shown to cause excitation and inhibition in gut smooth muscle, and to increase intestinal secretion by acting directly on the enterocyte.[154] Adenosine, which may be produced by breakdown of ATP, produces prominent effects by acting on adenosine receptors, which are different from ATP receptors. Antagonism of ATP or adenosine receptors does not antagonize vagally mediated relaxation of the lower esophageal sphincter.[165] Hence, the role of these purines as noncholinergic, nonadrenergic transmitters remains uncertain. Location and distribution of purinergic nerves in the gut is not known.

GABA Neurons. GABA is an inhibitory transmitter in interneurons of the spinal cord, cerebellum, dorsal ganglia, and several areas of the cortex. Several recent studies suggest that GABA may also act as a neurotransmitter in certain enteric neurons.[166-170]

Bombesin-like Peptide Neurons (Fig. 2–17). Bombesin is a 14 amino acid peptide that has a C-terminal amino acid sequence common to that of the 27 amino acid peptide known as gastrin releasing peptide (GRP). Bombesin-like peptide–containing nerve cell bodies have been localized in both myenteric and submucosal ganglia in the stomach and the small and large intestines.[171-176] Fibers from these neurons are widely distributed to longitudinal and circular muscle layers, to other aborally located myenteric and submucous ganglia, and perhaps to the mucosa of stomach and intestines. Bombesin-like peptide nerves send long (up to 2 cm) projections aborally along the gut. They may serve as excitatory interneurons mediating the peristaltic reflex. Bombesin-like peptides cause release of many gastrointestinal peptides, particularly gastrin. They also stimulate acid secretion and secretion by enterocytes and cause contraction of longitudinal and circular muscles.[154] The excitatory effect on smooth muscle is mediated directly as well as indirectly via other excitatory neurons.[177, 178] Bombesin-like peptide neurons may also play an important physiologic role in gastrin release.[179] Some of these neurons send fibers to prevertebral sympathetic ganglia and may serve as sensory neurons.[158]

Calcitonin Gene–Related Peptide Neurons (Fig. 2–17). Calcitonin gene–related peptide (CGRP) is a recently discovered 37 amino acid peptide whose existence was predicted on the basis of the analysis of calcitonin gene expression.[180] Nerve cell bodies of CGRP neurons are present in both myenteric and submucosal ganglia of the rat large and small intestine.[181] In the intestine immunoreactive cell bodies are more prevalent in the submucosal than in the myenteric ganglia and are more prevalent in small bowel than in the more proximal portions of the GI tract. CGRP-containing nerve fibers project to the circular, longi-

tudinal, and muscularis mucosae muscle layers, to blood vessels, and to the mucosa throughout the rat gut. In the esophagus, a marked reduction in immunoreactivity following ablation of the nodose ganglion suggests that a large number of these CGRP-containing nerves are sensory in nature.[182] Studies in the central nervous system have shown that CGRP often coexists with substance P or acetylcholine.[60] Whether this is true in the gastrointestinal tract has yet to be shown.

CGRP causes dilatation of blood vessels, resulting in increased intestinal blood flow. It also causes contraction of ileal and colonic longitudinal muscle, relaxation of the lower esophageal sphincter, inhibition of esophageal body contractions, relaxation of strips of aorta, and inhibition of gastric acid secretion.[183-186] The inhibitory action of CGRP on the lower esophageal sphincter is mediated directly and also indirectly through stimulation of inhibitory neurons. CGRP-containing nerves may serve as inhibitory neurons in the gut and also as afferent nerves in the vagal afferent pathway.

Cholecystokinin Neurons (Fig. 2–17). Cholecystokinin (CCK) is a 33 amino acid peptide with its biologic activity in the terminal 8 amino acids (CCK8). It is related to the family of gastrin-like peptides. A variety of enteric neurons show immunoreactivity for CCK-like peptides.[157, 176] These neurons generally also contain other potential transmitters such as acetylcholine, CGRP, NPY, and somatostatin. CCK can stimulate cholinergic and noncholinergic excitatory neurons as well as noncholinergic inhibitory neurons. CCK neurons may mediate vagal inhibition of acid secretion and gastrin release by stimulating somatostatin cells, which provide inhibitory input to parietal and gastrin cells.[187] CCK stimulates pancreatic secretion and causes contraction of the gallbladder and relaxation of the sphincter of Oddi. It increases small bowel transit and increases frequency of electrical spike activity in the colon. CCK has been shown to be a neuropeptide in sensory pathways between the stomach and the hypothalamus involved in mediating satiety.[188] CCK also stimulates gastric tension receptors, which may be involved in mediating satiety. Many of these effects of CCK are due to its hormonal rather than its neurotransmitter actions.

Galanin Neurons (Fig. 2–17). Galanin is a 29 amino acid peptide that has been localized to neurons in myenteric and submucous plexuses throughout the gut in rodents.[189-191] The cells from the myenteric plexus send projections to circular and longitudinal muscle layers and to other myenteric neurons. Fibers from neurons in the submucous plexus project to the mucosa. Galanin causes contraction of jejunal longitudinal muscle and circular muscle of the opossum lower esophageal sphincter. However, it causes inhibition of jejunal circular muscle. Excitatory or inhibitory effects of galanin are exerted directly on these muscles.[192] Galanin also causes inhibition of myenteric neurons,[193] and, because galanin fibers project anally for long distances (up to 2 cm), galanin may serve as an inhibitory transmitter of interneurons involved in the peristaltic reflex. The effect of galanin on mucosal function is not known. The role of galanin-containing nerves in intestinal physiology is not yet known.

Dynorphin and Enkephalin Neurons (Fig. 2–17). Three opioid peptides have been demonstrated in mammalian enteric nerves. These include dynorphin, Met enkephalin, and Leu enkephalin. Dynorphin is a 17 amino acid peptide and enkephalins are pentapeptides. Met and Leu enkephalins have the same amino acid sequences except the presence of Methionine or Leucine, respectively, at the carboxyl terminals. Dynorphine neurons are present in myenteric and submucous plexuses. The project caudally to other myenteric neurons and to circular and longitudinal muscle layers. Some fibers of neurons in the myenteric plexus also project to prevertebral sympathetic ganglia. These neurons serve as sensory neurons. Fibers from dynorphin neurons in the submucous plexus project to the mucosa. Enkephalin neurons are present in myenteric but not submucous ganglia in a number of mammalian species.[194–197] Axons of the enkephalin neurons project to circular muscle and the submucous plexus. Some also project orally to other myenteric neurons, while others project to sympathetic ganglia and serve as sensory neurons. Many enkephalin-containing neurons also contain dynorphin as well as VIP. Both enkephalin and dynorphin cause presynaptic inhibition of transmitter release as well as direct inhibition of postsynaptic neurons.[7, 198] Their major antisecretory effect is via inhibition of submucous plexus neurons.[154] The role of opioid projections to circular muscle is not clear. Enkephalins may cause direct excitation of certain circular muscle, while dynorphin inhibits others.[199] Opioids may also act to inhibit transmission at the neuromuscular site. The overall effect of exogenous opioids is to inhibit gastrointestinal transit through inhibition of tonic inhibitory neurons, resulting in enhancement of myogenic segmental contractions.[196] This, along with their antisecretory effects, results in constipation.

Neuropeptide Y (NPY) Neurons (Fig. 2–17). NPY is a 36 amino acid peptide structurally related to pancreatic polypeptide. NPY is present in some neurons in myenteric ganglia but more frequently in submucous neurons.[157, 200–204] Myenteric NPY-containing neurons send projections to other myenteric ganglia, to circular muscle, and directly to the base of the intestinal mucosa. NPY neurons in the submucosal plexus send projections to the intestinal mucosa exclusively. NPY is contained in enteric cholinergic neurons to the mucosa, whereas the NPY neurons that project from the myenteric ganglia to the mucosa also contain acetylcholine, CCK, CGRP, and somatostatin. NPY neurons that project to the mucosa from submucosal ganglia contain acetylcholine, CCK, and somatostatin. Neuropeptide Y is also contained in adrenergic neurons that have their cell bodies in the prevertebral sympathetic ganglia and supply the mucosal blood vessels.[100, 102, 205] Interestingly, NPY is present in VIP-containing nerves in the esophagus. Neuropeptide Y has been shown to cause vasoconstriction and decreased intestinal absorption of electrolytes.[206] The physiologic role

of neuropeptide Y in cholinergic, adrenergic, or VIP nerves is not known.

Somatostatin Neurons (Fig. 2–17). Somatostatin is a 28 amino acid peptide that has been localized in myenteric and submucosal neurons throughout the gut.[197, 207, 208] Somatostatin neurons in the myenteric plexus project aborally to other myenteric ganglia but not to any muscle layers, suggesting that they act exclusively as interneurons. In the submucous plexus somatostatin is contained in cholinergic neurons, which also contain CCK and NPY.[157] These neurons project to other submucous ganglia and the mucosal plexus. Somatostatin is also contained in extrinsic adrenergic neurons that project to the submucous plexus and mucosa.[209] Somatostatin inhibits cholinergic excitatory neurons and stimulates noncholinergic inhibitory neurons to the circular smooth muscle of the small bowel. It may therefore play a role in descending inhibition in the peristaltic reflex.[210] Somatostatin appears to inhibit intestinal secretion via its inhibitory effect on submucous neurons and by a direct action on secretory cells.[7, 154] In the stomach somatostatin cells make intimate contact with parietal and gastrin cells. Activation of these somatostatin-containing cells by cholinergic or CCK-containing nerves causes inhibition of acid secretion and gastrin release.[187] Overall, somatostatin appears to play an important inhibitory role in secretory processes in the gut.

Substance P Neurons (Fig. 2–17). Substance P is an 11 amino acid peptide belonging to a family of related tachykinins including substance K. Substance P–containing neurons are located in both myenteric and submucosal ganglia.[200, 211, 212] Substance P neurons in the myenteric plexus send projections to adjacent myenteric ganglia, submucous ganglia, circular and longitudinal muscle layers, and muscularis mucosae. Some substance P–containing neurons send projections that exit from the gut and proceed to prevertebral sympathetic ganglia. They may serve as sensory neurons. In the submucous plexus substance P is contained in cholinergic neurons that project primarily to the mucosa.[158]

Substance P causes contraction of longitudinal muscle, circular muscle, and muscularis mucosae by a direct action and also via stimulation of cholinergic neurons.[213] Substance P appears to serve as a noncholinergic excitatory neurotransmitter involved in peristalsis of the gut.[214–220] Substance P also causes vasodilation (particularly of bowel and coronary vessels), stimulation of salivary and intestinal secretion, and inhibition of acid secretion.[154, 214] The role of substance P as a neurotransmitter of sensory nerves, particularly those carrying nociceptive stimuli, is well established.[66, 221] Substance P–containing sensory fibers have their cell bodies in the dorsal root ganglia and are selectively stimulated and then destroyed by capsaicin.

Vasoactive Intestinal Peptide (VIP) Neurons (Fig. 2–17). VIP is a 28 amino acid peptide related to secretin. VIP is present in large numbers of submucous neurons and less frequently in myenteric neurons.[118, 176, 222–224] VIP neurons in the submucous plexus supply

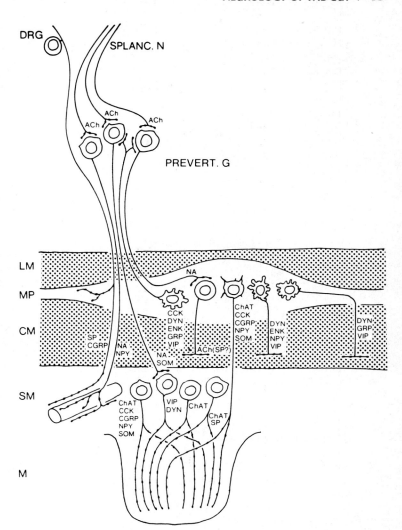

Figure 2–18. Diagram of projections of neurons with different neurochemical codes in the small intestine of the guinea pig. The text should be consulted for further details. ACh, acetylcholine; CCK, cholecystokinin; CGRP, calcitonin gene-related protein; ChAT, choline acetyltransferase; CM, circular muscle; DRG, dorsal root ganglion; DYN, dynorphin; ENK, enkephalin; GRP, gastrin-releasing peptide; LM, longitudinal muscle; M, mucosa; MP, myenteric plexus; NA, norepinephrine; NPY, neuropeptide Y; PREVERT. G, prevertebral ganglion; SM, submucosa; SOM, somatostatin; SP, substance P; SPLANC. N, splanchnic nerve; VIP, vasoactive intestinal peptide. (From Costa, M., Furness, J. B., and Llewellyn-Smith, I. J. *In* Johnson, L. R. [ed.]. Physiology of the Gastrointestinal Tract. New York, Raven Press, 1987. Used by permission.)

the mucosa and blood vessels, whereas those in myenteric ganglia send axons to circular muscle, submucous ganglia, and other myenteric ganglia. Some VIP fibers also project to sympathetic ganglia. VIP relaxes smooth muscle of the blood vessels, lower esophageal sphincter, pylorus, and internal anal sphincter. However, it produces contractions in the esophageal body and duodenum.[225–229] VIP stimulates small bowel and pancreatic secretion but inhibits acid secretion.[154, 230] VIP may serve as an inhibitory or excitatory neurotransmitter in the gut.

Summary of Enteric Neurons and Their Fiber Projections (Fig. 2–18)

The most detailed study of the nature of the neurons and their projections has been done in the guinea pig small bowel. In the guinea pig ileum myenteric neurons contain acetylcholine, 5-hydroxytryptamine, bombesin-like peptide, CCK, CGRP, galanin, dynorphin, enkephalin, NPY, somatostatin, substance P, and VIP. Myenteric neurons containing acetylcholine, bombesin-like peptide, CCK, CGRP, galanin, dynorphin, enkephalin, NPY, SP, and VIP (but not 5HT or somato-

statin) send projections to the circular muscle layer and are therefore candidates as transmitters at the neuromuscular junctions. Acetylcholine, bombesin-like peptide, and substance P cause excitation of smooth muscle and are candidates as excitatory neurotransmitters, whereas ATP, CGRP, galanin, and VIP cause either excitation or inhibition, depending upon the tissue involved, and are candidates as inhibitory or excitatory neurotransmitters.

All of the various peptide-containing myenteric neurons send projections to other myenteric neurons. These projections are usually aborally directed, but enkephalin, somatostatin, and SP neurons also send projections orally in the myenteric plexus. Because of their oral projections, it appears that some neurons containing enkephalin, somatostatin, and substance P may mediate proximal contraction in the peristaltic reflex. Myenteric neurons containing 5HT, bombesin-like peptide, CCK, galanin, dynorphin, enkephalin, somatostatin, substance P, and VIP also send projections to submucosal ganglia. Myenteric neurons containing acetylcholine, bombesin-like peptide, CCK, CGRP, NPY, and somatostatin also send projections directly to the intestinal mucosa.

The submucous ganglia contain primarily acetylcholine- and VIP-containing neurons (Fig. 2–18). They also contain CCK, CGRP, galanin, NPY, somatostatin, and substance P. Neurons containing 5HT, bombesin-like peptide, and enkephalin are not present in submucosal ganglia. Many submucous neurons appear to contain more than a single neurotransmitter candidate. For example, some cholinergic neurons contain substance P, whereas others contain bombesin-like peptide, CCK, NPY, and somatostatin. Cholinergic as well as VIP-containing neurons send dense projections to the subepithelial plexus. VIP-containing neurons also innervate the submucous arterioles.

The subepithelial plexus is believed to contain primarily nerve fibers that are involved in the innervation of the mucosa. This plexus contains fibers that originate in the submucous plexus, myenteric plexus, and sympathetic ganglia (Fig. 2–18). Among the agents present in the subepithelial plexus, acetylcholine, VIP, and substance P exert prominent secretory effects directly on enterocytes, and NPY and somatostatin exert prominent antisecretory effects on enterocytes. Adrenergic terminals are also antisecretory and enhance absorption via alpha receptors. Submucosal blood vessels receive rich innervation from extrinsic adrenergic fibers and intrinsic fibers containing substance P, CGRP, and VIP.

Synaptic Transmission in Enteric Ganglia

The enteric neurons have a wide variety of chemicals that are potential candidates for synaptic transmission from one neuron to another. A single stimulus applied to interganglionic nerves elicits a fast EPSP in the majority of neurons in both the myenteric and submucous plexuses. These fast EPSPs are mediated largely by nicotinic receptors for acetylcholine. This suggests that cholinergic terminals make synaptic contacts with the vast majority of neurons in the enteric plexuses. Stimulation of interganglionic nerve bundles also produces a slow EPSP in the majority of myenteric and submucous neurons. There are several neurotransmitter candidates that might be involved in this response, including acetylcholine (muscarinic M1 receptor), 5HT, ATP, bombesin-like peptide, CCK, GABA, somatostatin, substance P, and VIP. All these candidate transmitters produce depolarization in neurons of both enteric plexuses.

Inhibitory postsynaptic potentials (IPSPs) in response to single or repetitive nerve stimulation are very prominent in submucous neurons but occur rarely in myenteric neurons. IPSPs in submucous neurons in the guinea pig are mediated by adrenergic nerves (alpha-2 receptors). Neurotransmitter candidates for producing IPSPs in myenteric neurons include noradrenaline, 5HT, CCK, enkephalin, dynorphin, and somatostatin.

Some substances also act presynaptically to depress synaptic transmission in the enteric ganglia. These substances include acetylcholine, noradrenaline, opiate peptides, and 5HT. Such presynaptic inhibition occurs through axoaxonic ("presynaptic") synapses or inhibitory "autoreceptors" located on the presynaptic terminal. The latter instance provides a means by which neurons can control their own release of transmitter.

The Final Motor Neuron and Neuroeffector Transmission

There are several different final motor neurons that exert their effect directly on such effector cells as smooth muscle, secretory (e.g., chief cells, parietal cells, enterocytes, mucosal cells, exocrine and pancreatic cells), endocrine cells (e.g., gastrin cells), or paracrine cells (e.g., somatostatin cells in the stomach) in the gut. Their effect can be either excitatory or inhibitory. In order to establish the probable identity of a neurotransmitter at a neuroeffector site, it is necessary to show that (1) the candidate substance exists in the axon ending that makes contact with target cells, (2) the potential neurotransmitter candidate acts directly on the effector cells to produce changes that mimic those of presynaptic nerve stimulation (endogenously released transmitters), and (3) a selective antagonist of the neurotransmitter antagonizes the effect of presynaptic nerve stimulation. Transmural stimulation of enteric nerves in circular muscle usually shows a cholinergic excitatory response, which is antagonized by atropine. After blockade of this cholinergic response, an inhibitory response followed by an excitatory response is usually seen. The postinhibition excitatory response may represent a postinhibitory rebound contraction or a response to the release of an excitatory neurotransmitter. There is convincing evidence that acetylcholine is an important excitatory neurotransmitter at neuromuscular, neurosecretory cell, and neuroendocrine cell sites. However, the functional identity of noncholinergic inhibitory and noncholinergic excitatory transmitters remains uncertain. Candidate inhibitory transmitters include ATP, CGRP, galanin, and NPY. VIP is a probable inhibitory neurotransmitter at the neuromuscular site in the lower esophageal sphincter, pylorus, and internal anal sphincter.[122, 226] The candidate noncholinergic excitatory neurotransmitter is bombesin-like peptide and the probable excitatory neurotransmitter is substance P. The wide distribution of multiple various neurotransmitters and their co-localization in the same nerves, along with the heterogeneity of their distribution in different organs in the same species and in different species, suggest the following general principles: (1) one neurotransmitter can serve many different functions, (2) multiple transmitters may be involved in initiating the same response, (3) similar responses in different organs may be due to different transmitters, and (4) there are many species differences. Therefore, generalizations regarding neurotransmitter involvement should be made with great caution and reservation.

Functions of Enteric Nerves

The function of enteric nerves is to convert the uncontrolled and purposeless motor and secretory activity of the gut into purposeful and coordinated intestinal activity. The enteric nerves serve in generating propulsive activities such as peristalsis and other propagated motor complexes including the migrating motor complex. They also generate reverse peristalsis, modulate segmental contractions, and coordinate activities of the gastrointestinal sphincters.

The role of enteric nerves in the control of gastrointestinal function can be appreciated by considering the consequences of ablation of all enteric nervous activity. Enteric nerve activity can be experimentally blocked by administration of tetrodotoxin (a neurotoxin that blocks conduction of all spike activity in nerves). Clinically, near complete loss of enteric neurons can occur in achalasia (in the esophagus),[122] Hirschsprung's disease (in the colon),[231, 232] and some cases of intestinal pseudo-obstruction syndrome that may involve enteric neurons (particularly in the small bowel).[233] In the absence of any neural input, the only motor activity that remains is that controlled by hormonal influences or intrinsic activity of muscle or secretory cells. In such an instance, the esophageal body is quiescent and the lower esophageal sphincter is tonically contracted. Neither primary nor secondary peristalsis occurs and the sphincter fails to relax with swallows, resembling a clinical picture of achalasia. The gastric fundus is quiescent and the body and antrum show action potentials with or without associated contraction. Whatever contraction occurs may lack orderly propagation. The pylorus is tonically contracted. The small bowel shows continuous slow waves with or without superimposed irregular segmental contractions. The net effect of enteric nerves on the circular muscle layer is inhibitory in nature. Hence, in the total absence of enteric nerves, myogenic contractions of the small bowel increase in frequency. The sphincter of Oddi shows phasic and tonic contractions. The colon is usually contracted. The rectum has tonic and phasic contractions, and the internal anal sphincter is tonically contracted. It should be obvious from the above description that the gastrointestinal tract is quite active in the absence of intrinsic or extrinsic innervation. In fact, one of the major effects of nerves in the small and large intestine and sphincters is to provide an inhibitory influence on gastrointestinal activity.

The enteric plexuses contain neurons that serve different functions such as sensory, integrating, motor programming, and final motor effect on target cells. Currently, little is known about the precise connections and chemical nature of these component neurons.

Specific clinical disorders of the gut associated with loss of one or the other type of enteric neurons are not currently well characterized. There is evidence to suggest that simultaneously released transmitters may determine the final response of the target cell. For example, acetylcholine released along with noncholinergic transmitter has been shown to affect the latency and amplitude of esophageal circular muscle contraction. And it has been suggested that regional gradients of cholinergic and noncholinergic transmitters in the esophagus may be involved in the genesis of esophageal peristalsis.[234] The disorders of the enteric nerves of the gut involving selective loss of one or another type of enteric neuron lead to a variety of functional disturbances of the gut. For example, with selective loss of excitatory influence (e.g., with atropine treatment) the contractile activity is markedly inhibited. Selective loss of inhibitory influences, on the other hand, leads to excessive myogenic contractions. With selective loss of excitatory nerves, the excitatory activity of the gut shows even greater inhibition than with total loss of all intramural nerves, because the action of inhibitory nerves is unopposed after selective loss of excitatory nerves. The net result of either total or selective loss of inhibitory or excitatory influence of enteric nerves is to impair intestinal transit. Vigorous nonperistaltic contractions occur, for example, in diffuse esophageal spasm, in certain types of intestinal pseudo-obstruction syndromes, and in Hirschsprung's disease. Minimal propulsion continues, associated with myogenic progression of contraction waves and decreasing rates of contractions distally along the small bowel. In patients in whom there is extensive damage of enteric nerves (such as in those with intestinal pseudo-obstruction syndrome), propulsion of food residues through the gut nearly ceases.[233] Continued intestinal secretion along with continued oral intake eventually leads to dilation of the gut (see pp. 377–379).

The enteric nerves also control the activity of secretory cells even though spontaneous and hormonally mediated secretory processes continue in the absence of enteric nerves. Overall, cholinergic, VIP, and possibly purinergic intrinsic nerves directly enhance intestinal secretion. Other intrinsic nerves, such as enkephalin and somatostatin nerves, inhibit secretion largely by inhibiting excitatory nerves. The sympathetic nerves play a particularly important role in this regard as they inhibit intestinal secretion indirectly by inhibiting excitatory nerves but also directly by stimulating absorption by the villous cells.[154]

References

1. Stevens, C. F. The neuron. Sci. Am. *241*:54, 1979.
2. Gabella, G. Structure of muscle and nerves in the gastrointestinal tract. *In* Johnson, L. R. (ed.): Physiology of the Gastrointestinal Tract. New York, Raven Press, 1987, pp. 335–381.
3. Heuser, J. E., and Reese, T. S. Structure of the synapse. *In* Kandel, E. R. (ed.). Handbook of Physiology. Section 1: The Nervous System, Vol. 1. Bethesda, American Physiological Society, 1977, pp. 261–294.
4. Wood, J. D. Physiology of the enteric nervous system. *In* Johnson, L. R. (ed.). Physiology of the Gastrointestinal Tract. New York, Raven Press, 1987, pp. 67–109.
5. Hille, B. Ionic Channels of Excitable Membranes. Sunderland, MA, Sinauer, 1984.
6. North, R. A. Electrophysiology of enteric ganglia. Neuroscience 7:315, 1982.
7. Surprenant, A. Transmitter mechanisms in the enteric nervous system: An electrophysiological vantage point. Trends in Autonomic Pharmacology *3*:71, 1985.

8. Koester, J. Voltage-gated channels and the generation of the action potential. *In* Kandel, E. R., and Schwartz, J. H. (eds.). Principles of Neural Science. New York, Elsevier, 1985, pp. 75–86.

9. Guyton, A. C. Textbook of Medical Physiology. Philadelphia, W. B. Saunders Company, 1985.

10. Narahashi, T., Haas, H. G., and Therrien, E. F. Saxitoxin and tetrodotoxin: Comparison of nerve blocking mechanism. Science *157*:1441, 1967.

11. Boyd, I. A., and Davey, M. R. Compositions of Peripheral Nerves. Edinburgh, E. and S. Livingstone Ltd., 1968.

12. Schmidt, R. F. (ed.). Fundamentals of Sensory Physiology. New York, Springer-Verlag, 1982.

13. Holtzman, E. The origin and fate of secretory packages, especially synaptic vesicles. Neuroscience *2*:327, 1977.

14. Burnstock, G., Hokfelt, T., Gershon, M. D., Iversen, L. L., Kosterlitz, H. W., and Szurszewski, J. H. Non-adrenergic, non-cholinergic autonomic neurotransmission mechanisms. Neurosci. Res. Program Bull. *17*:377, 1979.

15. Schwartz, J. H. The transport of substances in nerve cells. Sci. Am. *249*:152, 1980.

16. Grafstein, B., Forman, D. S. Intracellular transport in neurons. Physiol. Rev. *60*:1167, 1980.

17. Loh, Y. P., Brownstein, M. J., and Gainer, H. Proteolysis in neuropeptide processing and other neural functions. Annu. Rev. Neurosci. *7*:189, 1984.

18. Tucek, S. Acetylcholine synthesis in neurons. London, Chapman and Hall, 1978.

19. Campbell, G., and Gibbins, I. L. Nonadrenergic, noncholinergic transmission in the autonomic nervous system: Purinergic nerves. *In* Kalsner, S. (ed.). Trends in Autonomic Pharmacology, Vol. 1. Baltimore, Urban and Schwarzenburg, 1979, pp. 103–144.

20. Burnstock, G. Ultrastructural identification of neurotransmitters. Scand. J. Gastroenterol. (Suppl.) *70*:1, 1981.

21. Fawcett, D. W. Purinergic nerves. *In* The Cell. Philadelphia, W. B. Saunders Company, 1981.

22. Heuser, J. E., Reese, T. S., Dennis, M. J., Jan, Y., Jan, L., and Evans, L. Synaptic vesicle exocytosis captured by quick freezing and correlated with quantal transmitter release. J. Biol. *81*:275, 1979.

23. Kelly, R. B., Deutsch, J. W., Carlson, S. S., Wagner, J. A. Biochemistry of neurotransmitter release. Annu. Rev. Neurosci. *2*:399, 1979.

24. Cohen, P. The role of protein phosphorylation in neural and hormonal control of cellular activity. Nature *296*:613, 1982.

25. Hartzell, H. C. Mechanisms of slow postsynaptic potentials. Nature *291*:539, 1981.

26. Schwartz, J. H. Molecular steps in synaptic transmission. *In* Kandel, E. R., Schwartz, J. H. (eds.). Principles of Neural Science. New York, Elsevier, 1985, pp. 169–175.

27. Blusztajn, J. K., and Wurtman, R. J. Choline and cholinergic neurons. Science *221*:614, 1983.

28. Cooper, J. R., Bloom, F. E., and Roth, R. H. The Biochemical Basis of Neuropharmacology. New York, Oxford University, 1982.

29. Nicoll, R. A. Neurotransmitters can say more than just "yes" or "no." Trends Neurosci. *5*:369, 1982.

30. Berridge, M. J., and Irvine, R. F. Inositol trisphosphate, a novel second messenger in cellular signal transduction. Nature *312*:315, 1984.

31. Rodbell, M. The role of hormone receptors and GTP-regulatory proteins in membrane transduction. Nature *284*:17, 1980.

32. Schwartz, J. H. Molecular aspects of postsynaptic receptors. *In* Kandel, E. R., Schwartz, J. H. (eds.). Principles of Neural Science. New York, Elsevier, 1985, pp. 159–168.

33. Chan-Palay, V., and Palay, S. L. Purinergic nerves. *In* Coexistence of Neuroactive Substances in Neurons. New York, Wiley, 1984.

34. Willard, A. L., and Nishi, R. Neurons dissociated from rat myenteric plexus retain differentiated properties when grown in cell culture. III. Synaptic interactions and modulatory effects of neurotransmitter candidates. Neuroscience *16*:213, 1985.

35. Mei, N. Intestinal chemosensitivity. Physiol. Rev. *65*:211, 1985.

36. Clarke, G. D., and Davison, J. S. Mucosal receptors in the gastric antrum and small intestine of the rat with afferent fibres in the cervical vagus. J. Physiol. (Lond.) *284*:55–67, 1978.

37. Clerc, N., and Mei, N. [Demonstration of mucous mechanoreceptors in the lower esophageal sphincter. Comparison with muscle mechanoreceptors.] C. R. Soc. Biol. (Paris) *175*:352, 1981.

38. Cottrell, D. F., and Iggo, A. Tension receptors with vagal afferent fibres in the proximal duodenum and pyloric sphincter of sheep. J. Physiol. (Lond.) *354*:457, 1984.

39. Cottrell, D. F., and Iggo, A. Mucosal enteroceptors with vagal afferent fibres in the proximal duodenum of sheep. J. Physiol. (Lond.) *354*:497, 1984.

40. Cottrell, D. F., Iggo, A. The responses of duodenal tension receptors in sheep to pentagastrin, cholecystokinin and some other drugs. J. Physiol. (Lond.) *354*:477, 1984.

41. Clerc, N., and Mei, N. Vagal mechanoreceptors located in the lower oesophageal sphincter of the cat. J. Physiol. (Lond.) *336*:487, 1983.

42. Clerc, N., and Mei, N. Thoracic esophageal mechanoreceptors connected with fibers following sympathetic pathways. Brain Res. Bull. *10*:1, 1983.

43. Floyd, K., Hick, V. E., and Morrison, J. F. Mechanosensitive afferent units in the hypogastric nerve of the cat. J. Physiol (Lond.) *259*:457, 1976.

44. Mei, N., Perrin, J., Crousillat, J., and Boyer, A. Comparison between the properties of the vagal and splanchnic glucoreceptors of the small intestine. Involvement in insulin release. J. Auton. Nerv. Syst. *10*:275, 1984.

45. Perrin, J., Crousillat, J., and Mei, N. Assessment of true splanchnic glucoreceptors in the jejuno-ileum of the cat. Brain Res. Bull. *7*:625, 1981.

46. Jeanningros, R. Vagal unitary responses to intestinal amino acid infusions in the anesthetized cat: A putative signal for protein induced satiety. Physiol. Behav. *28*:9, 1982.

47. Adachi, A. Projection of the hepatic vagal nerve in the medulla oblongata. J. Auton. Nerv. Syst. *10*:287, 1984.

48. Hunt, J. N. Mechanisms and disorders of gastric emptying. Annu. Rev. Med. *34*:219, 1983.

49. El Ouazzani, T., and Mei, N. Electrophysiologic properties and role of the vagal thermoreceptors of lower esophagus and stomach of cat. Gastroenterology *83*:995, 1982.

50. Blumberg, H., Haupt, P., Janig, W., and Kohler, W. Encoding of visceral noxious stimuli in the discharge patterns of visceral afferent fibres from the colon. Pflugers Arch. *398*:33, 1983.

51. Haupt, P., Janig, W., and Kohler, W. Response pattern of visceral afferent fibres, supplying the colon, upon chemical and mechanical stimuli. Pflugers Arch. *398*:41, 1983.

52. Mei, N., Condamin, M., and Boyer, A. The composition of the vagus nerve of the cat. Cell Tissue Res. *209*:423, 1980.

53. Chernicky, C. L., Barnes, K. L., Ferrario, C. M., and Conomy, J. P. Afferent projections of the cervical vagus and nodose ganglion in the dog. Brain Res. Bull. *13*:401, 1984.

54. Cooke, H. J. Neurobiology of the intestinal mucosa. Gastroenterology *90*:1057, 1986.

55. Hermann, G. E., and Rogers, R. C. Convergence of vagal and gustatory afferent input within the parabrachial nucleus of the rat. J. Auton. Nerv. Syst. *13*:1, 1985.

56. Knyihar, E., Csillik, G. Regional distribution of acid phosphatase–positive axonal systems in the rat spinal cord and medulla, representing central terminals of cutaneous and visceral nociceptive neurons. J. Neural Transm. *40*:227, 1977.

57. Sawchenko, P. E. Central connections of the sensory and motor nuclei of the vagus nerve. J. Auton. Nerv. Syst. *9*:13, 1983.

58. Scharoun, S. L., Barone, F. C., Wayner, M. J., and Jones, S. M. Vagal and gastric connections to the central nervous system determined by the transport of horseradish peroxidase. Brain Res. Bull. *13*:573,1984.

59. Stansfeld, C. E., and Wallis, D. I. Properties of visceral primary afferent neurons in the nodose ganglion of the rabbit. J. Neurophysiol. *54*:245, 1985.

60. Gibbins, I. L., Furness, J. B., Costa, M., MacIntyre, I., Hillyard, C. J., and Girgis, S. Co-localization of calcitonin gene–related peptide–like immunoreactivity with substance P

in cutaneous, vascular and visceral sensory neurons of guinea pigs. Neurosci. Lett. *57*:125, 1985.

61. Neuhuber, W. The central projections of visceral primary afferent neurons of the inferior mesenteric plexus and hypogastric nerve and the location of the related sensory and preganglionic sympathetic cell bodies in the rat. Anat. Embryol. (Berl.) *164*:413, 1982.

62. Cervero, F., Connell, L. A., Lawson, S. N. Somatic and visceral primary afferents in the lower thoracic dorsal root ganglia of the cat. J. Comp. Neurol. *228*:422, 1984.

63. Kuo, D. C., Krauthamer, G. M., and Yamasaki, D. S. The organization of visceral sensory neurons in thoracic dorsal root ganglia (DRG) of the cat studied by horseradish peroxidase (HRP) reaction using the cryostat. Brain Res. *208*:187, 1981.

64. Kuo, D. C., Yang, G. C., Yamasaki, D. S., and Krauthamer, G. M. A wide field electron microscopic analysis of the fiber constituents of the major splanchnic nerve in cat. J. Comp. Neurol. *210*:49, 1982.

65. Ranieri, F., Mei, N., and Crousillat. J. Splanchnic afferents arising from gastro-intestinal and peritoneal mechanoreceptors. Exp. Brain Res. *16*:276, 1973.

66. Hokfelt, T., Elde, R., Johansson, O., Luft R., Nilsson, G., and Arimura, A. Immunohistochemical evidence for separate populations of somatostatin-containing and substance P–containing primary afferent neurons in the rat. Neuroscience *1*:131, 1976.

67. Hokfelt, T., Kellerth, J. O., Nilsson, G., and Pernow, B. Experimental immunohistochemical studies on the localization and distribution of substance P in cat primary sensory neurons. Brain Res. *100*:235, 1975.

68. Hokfelt, T., Ljungdahl, A., Terenius, L., Elde, R., and Nilsson, G. Immunohistochemical analysis of peptide pathways possibly related to pain and analgesia: Enkephalin and substance P. Proc. Natl. Acad. Sci. USA *74*:3081, 1977.

69. Cervero, F., and Connell, L. A. Fine afferent fibers from viscera do not terminate in the substantia gelatinosa of the thoracic spinal cord. Brain Res. *294*:370, 1984.

70. Matsushita, M., and Tanami, T. Contralateral termination of primary afferent axons in the sacral and caudal segments of the cat, as studied by anterograde transport of horseradish peroxidase. J. Comp. Neurol. *220*:206, 1983.

71. Neuhuber, W. L., Sandoz, P. A., and Fryscak, T. The central projections of primary afferent neurons of greater splanchnic and intercostal nerves in the rat. A horseradish peroxidase study. Anat. Embryol. (Berl.) *174*:123, 1986.

72. Feher, E., and Vajda, J. Evidence of sensory neurons in the wall of the small intestine revealed by horseradish peroxidase technique. Z. Mikrosk. Anat. Forsch. *96*:2, 1982.

73. King, B. F., and Szurszewski, J. H. Mechanoreceptor pathways from the distal colon to the autonomic nervous system in the guinea-pig. J. Physiol. (Lond.) *350*:93, 1984.

74. Kreulen, D. L., Szurszewski, J. H. Nerve pathways in celiac plexus of the guinea pig. Am. J. Physiol. *237*:E90, 1979.

75. Szursezewski, J. H. Physiology of mammalian prevertebral ganglia. Annu. Rev. Physiol. *43*:53, 1981.

76. Kreulen, D. L., and Peters, S. Non-cholinergic transmission in a sympathetic ganglion of the guinea-pig elicited by colon distension. J. Physiol. (Lond.) *374*:315, 1986.

77. Krier, J., and Hartman, D. A. Electrical properties and synaptic connections to neurons in parasympathetic colonic ganglia of the cat. Am. J. Physiol. *247*:G52, 1984.

78. Peters, S., and Kreulen, D. L. Fast and slow synaptic potentials produced in a mammalian sympathetic ganglion by colon distension. Proc. Natl. Acad. Sci. USA *83*:1941, 1986.

79. Simmons, M. A. The complexity and diversity of synaptic transmission in the prevertebral sympathetic ganglia. Prog. Neurobiol. *24*:43, 1985.

80. Furness, J. B., and Costa, M. The adrenergic innervation of the gastrointestinal tract. Ergeb. Physiol. *69*:2, 1974.

81. Llewellyn-Smith, I. J., Furness, J. B., O'Brien, P. E., and Costa, M. Noradrenergic nerves in human small intestine. Distribution and ultrastructure. Gastroenterology *87*:513, 1984.

82. Baumgarten, H. G., and Lange, W. Adrenergic innervation of the oesophagus in the cat (*Felis domestica*) and Rhesus monkey (*Macacus rhesus*). Z. Zellforsch. Mikrosk. Anat. *95*:529, 1969.

83. Furness, J. B., and Costa, M. The ramifications of adrenergic nerve terminals in the rectum, anal sphincter and anal accessory muscles of the guinea-pig. Z. Anat. Entwicklungsgesch. *140*:109, 1973.

84. Carpenter, M. B. Human Neuroanatomy. Baltimore, Williams and Wilkins, 1983.

85. Bahr, R., Bartel, B., Blumberg, H., and Janig, W. Functional characterization of preganglionic neurons projecting in the lumbar splanchnic nerves: Vasoconstrictor neurons. J. Auton. Nerv. Syst. *15*:131, 1986.

86. Kuo, D. C., Hisamitsu, T., de Groat W. C. A sympathetic projection from sacral paravertebral ganglia to the pelvic nerve and to postganglionic nerves on the surface of the urinary bladder and large intestine of the cat. J. Comp. Neurol. *226*:76, 1984.

87. Bouvier, M., and Gonella, J. Nervous control of the internal anal sphincter of the cat. J. Physiol. (Lond.) *310*:457, 1981.

88. Elfvin, L. G. Ultrastructural studies on the synaptology of the inferior mesenteric ganglion of the cat. 3. The structure and distribution of the axodendritic and dendrodendritic contacts. J. Ultrastruct. Res. *37*:432, 1971.

89. Falsgaard, C. J., Hokfelt, T., Elfvin, L. G., Terenius, L. Enkephalin-containing sympathetic preganglionic neurons projecting to the inferior mesenteric ganglion: Evidence from combined retrograde tracing and immunohistochemistry. Neuroscience *7*:2039, 1982.

90. Krier, J., Schmalz, P. F., and Szurszewski, J. H. Central innervation of neurones in the inferior mesenteric ganglion and of the large intestine of the cat. J. Physiol. (Lond.) *332*:125, 1982.

91. Konishi, S., Tsunoo, A., and Otsuka, M. Enkephalins presynaptically inhibit cholinergic transmission in sympathetic ganglia. Nature *282*:515, 1979.

92. Dalsgaard, C. J., Hokfelt, T., Schultzberg, M., Lundberg, J. M., Terenius, L., Dockray, G. J., Goldstein, M. Origin of peptide-containing fibers in the inferior mesenteric ganglion of the guinea-pig: Immunohistochemical studies with antisera to substance P, enkephalin, vasoactive intestinal polypeptide, cholecystokinin and bombesin. Neuroscience *9*:191, 1983.

93. Hokfelt, T., Elfvin, L. G., Schultzberg, M., Goldstein, M., and Nilsson, G. On the occurrence of substance P–containing fibers in sympathetic ganglia: Immunohistochemical evidence. Brain Res. *132*:29, 1977.

94. Schultzberg, M., Hokfelt, T., Terenius, L., Elfvin, L. G., Lundberg, J. M., Brandt, J., Elde, R. P., and Godstein, M. Enkephalin immunoreactive nerve fibres and cell bodies in sympathetic ganglia of the guinea-pig and rat. Neuroscience *4*:249, 1979.

95. Crowcroft, P. J., and Szurszewski, J. H. A study of the inferior mesenteric and pelvic ganglia of guinea-pigs with intracellular electrodes. J. Physiol. (Lond.) *219*:421, 1971.

96. Hartman, D. A., and Krier, J. Synaptic and antidromic potentials of visceral neurones in ganglia of the lumbar sympathetic chain of the cat. J. Physiol. (Lond.) *350*:413, 1984.

97. Dun, N. J., and Jiang, Z. G. Non-cholinergic excitatory transmission in inferior mesenteric ganglia of the guinea-pig: Possible mediation by substance P. J. Physiol. (Lond.) *325*:145, 1982.

98. Dun, N. J., Karczmar, A. G. Actions of substance P on sympathetic neurons. Neuropharmacology *18*:215, 1979.

99. Dun, N. J., and Ma, R. C. Slow non-cholinergic excitatory potentials in neurones of the guinea-pig coeliac ganglia. J. Physiol. (Lond.) *351*:47, 1984.

100. Lundberg, J. M., Hokfelt, T., Anggard, A., Terenius, L., Elde R., Markey, K., Goldstein, M., and Kimmel, J. Organizational principles in the peripheral sympathetic nervous system: Subdivision by coexisting peptides (somatostatin–, avian pancreatic polypeptide–, and vasoactive intestinal polypeptide–like immunoreactive material). Proc. Natl. Acad. Sci. USA *79*:1303. 1982.

101. Lundberg, J. M., Hokfelt, T., Nilsson, G., Terenius, L., Rehfeld, J., Elde, R., and Said, S. Peptide neurons in the vagus, splanchnic and sciatic nerves. Acta Physiol. Scand. *104*:499, 1978.

102. Macrae, I. M., Furness, J. B., and Costa, M. Distribution of subgroups of noradrenaline neurons in the coeliac ganglion of the guinea-pig. Cell Tissue Res. *224*:173, 1986.

103. Reed, J. D., Sanders, D. J., and Thorpe, V. The effect of

splanchnic nerve stimulation on gastric acid secretion and mucosal blood flow in the anaesthetized cat. J. Physiol. (Lond.) *241*:1, 1971.

104. Sjovall, H., Redfors, S., Hallback, D. A., Eklund, S., Jodal, M., and Lundgren, O. The effect of splanchnic nerve stimulation on blood flow distribution, villous tissue osmolality and fluid and electrolyte transport in the small intestine of the cat. Acta Physiol. Scand. *117*:359, 1983.

105. Hulten, L. Extrinsic nervous control of colonic motility and blood flow. An experimental study in the cat. Acta Physiol. Scand. (Suppl.)*335*:1, 1969.

106. Chang, E. B., Fedorak, R. N., and Field, M. Experimental diabetic diarrhea in rats. Intestinal mucosal denervation hypersensitivity and treatment with clonidine. Gastroenterology *91*:564, 1986.

107. Graffner, H., Ekelund, M., Hakanson, R., Oscarson, J., Rosengren, E., and Sundler, F. Effects of upper abdominal sympathectomy on gastric acid, serum gastrin, and catecholamines in the rat gut. Scand. J. Gastroenterol. *19*:711, 1984.

108. Fox, E. A., and Powley, T. L. Longitudinal columnar organization within the dorsal motor nucleus represents separate branches of the abdominal vagus. Brain Res. *341*:269, 1985.

109. Zhu, T. L., Tan, J. S., Zhang, Z. X., Zang, B. K., and Ma, Y. P. Vagus nerve anatomy at the lower esophagus and stomach. A study of 100 cadavers. Chin. Med. J. [Engl.] *93*:629, 1980.

110. de Groat, W. C., and Krier, J. An electrophysiological study of the sacral parasympathetic pathway to the colon of the cat. J. Physiol. (Lond.) *260*:425, 1976.

111. Fukai, K., Fukuda, H. The intramural pelvic nerves in the colon of dogs. J. Physiol. (Lond.) *354*:89, 1984.

112. Fukai, K., and Fukuda, H. Three serial neurones in the innervation of the colon by the sacral parasympathetic nerve of the dog. J. Physiol. (Lond.) *362*:69, 1985.

113. Gwyn, D. G., Ritchie, T. C., and Coulter, J. D. The central distribution of vagal catecholaminergic neurons which project into the abdomen in the rat. Brain Res. *328*:139, 1985.

114. Kalia, M., Fuxe, K., Goldstein, M., Harfstrand, A., Agnati, L. F., Coyle, J. T. Evidence for the existence of putative dopamine-, adrenaline- and noradrenaline-containing vagal motor neurons in the brainstem of the rat. Neurosci. Lett. *50*:57, 1984.

115. Ritchie, T. C., Westlund, K. N., Bowker, R. M., Coulter, J. D., and Leonard, R. B. The relationship of the medullary catecholamine containing neurones to the vagal motor nuclei. Neuroscience 7:1471, 1982.

116. Edin, R., Lundberg, J., Terenius, L., Dahlstrom, A., Hokfelt, T., Kewenter, J., and Ahlman, H. Evidence for vagal enkephalinergic neural control of the feline pylorus and stomach. Gastroenterology *78*:492, 1980.

117. Glazer, E. J., Bashbaum, A. I. Leucine enkephalin: Localization in and axoplasmic transport by sacral parasympathetic preganglionic neurons. Science *208*:1479, 1980.

118. Lundberg, J. M., Hokfelt, T., Kewenter, J., Pettersson, G., Ahlman, H., Edin, R., Dahlstrom, A., Nilsson, G., Terenius, L., Uvnas-Wallensten, K., and Said, S. Substance P–, VIP–, and enkephalin–like immunoreactivity in the human vagus nerve. Gastroenterology *77*:468, 1979.

119. Vincent, S. R., Dalsgaard, C. J., Schultzberg, M., Hokfelt, T., Christensson, I., and Terenius, L. Dynorphin-immunoreactive neurons in the autonomic nervous system. Neuroscience *11*:973, 1984.

120. Goyal, R. K., and Rattan, S. Neurohumoral, hormonal, and drug receptors for the lower esophageal sphincter. Gastroenterology *74*:598, 1978.

121. Gilbert, R., Rattan, S., Goyal, R. K. Pharmacologic identification, activation and antagonism of two muscarine receptor subtypes in the lower esophageal sphincter. J. Pharmacol. Exp. Ther. *230*:284, 1984.

122. Goyal, R. K., and Cobb, B. W. Motility of the pharynx, esophagus, and esophageal sphincters. *In* Johnson, L. R. (ed.): Physiology of the Gastrointestinal Tract. New York, Raven Press, 1981, pp. 359–391.

123. Rattan, S., and Goyal, R. K. Evidence of 5-HT participation in vagal inhibitory pathway to opossum LES. Am. J. Physiol. *234*:E273, 1978.

124. Gidda, J. S., Goyal, R. K. Swallow-evoked action potentials in vagal preganglionic efferents. J. Neurophysiol. *52*:1169, 1984.

125. Roman, C., and Gonella, J. Extrinsic control of digestive tract motility. *In* Johnson, L. R. (eds.). Physiology of the Gastrointestinal Tract. New York, Raven Press, 1987, pp. 507–553.

126. Paterson, W. G., Rattan, S., Goyal, R. K. Experimental induction of isolated lower esophageal sphincter relaxation in anesthetized opossums. J. Clin Invest. *77*:1187, 1986.

127. Gidda, J. S., Goyal, R. K. Regional gradient of initial inhibition and refractoriness in esophageal smooth muscle. Gastroenterology *89*:843, 1985.

128. Rattan, S., and Goyal, R. K. Neural control of the lower esophageal sphincter: Influence of the vagus nerves. J. Clin. Invest. *54*:899, 1974.

129. Goyal, R. K., and Rattan, S. Nature of the vagal inhibitory innervation to the lower esophageal sphincter. J. Clin. Invest. *55*:1119, 1975.

130. Cooke, A. R. Control of gastric emptying and motility. Gastroenterology *68*:804, 1975.

131. Burleigh, D. E., and D'Mello, A. Neural and pharmacologic factors affecting motility of the internal anal sphincter. Gastroenterology *84*:409, 1983.

132. de Groat, W. C., and Krier, J. The sacral parasympathetic reflex pathway regulating colonic motility and defaecation in the cat. J. Physiol. (Lond.) *276*:481, 1978.

133. Frenckner, B. Function of the anal sphincters in spinal man. Gut *16*:638, 1975.

134. Frenckner, B., Ihre, T. Influence of autonomic nerves on the internal anal sphincter in man. Gut *17*:306, 1976.

135. Devroede, G., and Lamarche, J. Functional importance of extrinsic parasympathetic innervation to the distal colon and rectum in man. Gastroenterology *66*:273, 1974.

136. Kreulen, D. L., and Szurszewski, J. H. Reflex pathways in the abdominal prevertebral ganglia: Evidence for a colo-colonic inhibitory reflex. J. Physiol. (Lond.) *295*:21, 1979.

137. Bajaj, S. C., Ragaza, E. P., Silva, H., and Goyal, R. K. Deglutition tachycardia. Gastroenterology *62*:632, 1972.

138. Bouvier, M., Grimaud, J. C., Salducci, J., and Gonella, J. Role of vesical afferent nerve fibres involved in the control of internal anal sphincter motility. J. Auton. Nerv. Syst. *10*:243, 1984.

139. Read, N. W., Cooper, K., and Fordtran, J. S. Effect of modified sham feeding on jejunal transport and pancreatic and biliary secretion in man. Am. J. Physiol. *234*:E417, 1978.

140. Christensen, J., Rick, G. A. Shunt fascicles in the gastric myenteric plexus in five species. Gastroenterology *88*:1020, 1985.

141. Christensen, J., Rick, G. A., Robison, B. A., Stiles, M. J., and Wix, M. A. Arrangement of the myenteric plexus throughout the gastrointestinal tract of the opossum. Gastroenterology *85*:890, 1983.

142. Christensen, J., Stiles, M. J., Rick, G. A., and Sutherland, J. Comparative anatomy of the myenteric plexus of the distal colon in eight mammals. Gastroenterology *86*:706, 1984.

143. Christensen, J., Rick, G. A. Nerve cell density in submucous plexus throughout the gut of cat and opossum. Gastroenterology *89*:1064, 1985.

144. Wilson, A. J., Furness, J. B., and Costa, M. The fine structure of the submucous plexus of the guinea-pig ileum. II. Description and analysis of vesiculated nerve profiles. J. Neurocytol. *10*:785, 1981.

145. Gabella, G. Ultrastructure of the nerve plexuses of the mammalian intestine: The enteric glial cells. Neuroscience *6*:425, 1981.

146. Gabella, G. On the ultrastructure of the enteric nerve ganglia. Scand. J. Gastroenterol. [Suppl.] *71*:15, 1982.

147. Komuro, T., Baluk, P., and Burnstock, G. An ultrastructural study of nerve profiles in the myenteric plexus of the rabbit colon. Neuroscience 7:295, 1982.

148. Komuro, T., Baluk, P., and Burnstock, G. An ultrastructural study of neurons and non-neuronal cells in the myenteric plexus of the rabbit colon. Neuroscience 7:1797, 1982.

149. Hoyes, A. D., Barber, P. Axonal terminal ultrastructure in the myenteric ganglia of the guinea-pig stomach. Cell Tissue Res. *209*:329, 1980.

150. Bjorklung, H., Dahl, D., and Seiger, A. Neurofilament and glial fibrillary acid protein-related immunoreactivity in rodent enteric nervous system. Neuroscience *12*:277, 1984.
151. Jessen, K. R., and Mirsky, R. Glial cells in the enteric nervous system contain glial fibrillary acidic protein (GFAP). Nature *286*:736, 1980.
152. Richardson, K. C. Studies on the structure of autonomic nerves in the small intestine correlating the silver impregnated image in light microscopy with permanganate fixed ultrastructure in electromicroscopy. J. Anat. *94*:457, 1960.
153. Lolova, I. Histochemical study of the cholinesterase activity in cat myenteric ganglia during postnatal development. J. Neural Transm. *50*:297, 1981.
154. Gwyn, D. G., Leslie, R. A., and Hopkins, D. A. Gastric afferents to the nucleus of the solitary tract in the cat. Neurosci. Lett. *14*:13, 1979.
155. Kilbinger, H., and Nafziger, M. Two types of neuronal muscarine receptors modulating acetylcholine release from guinea-pig myenteric plexus. Naunyn Schmiedebergs Arch. Pharmacol. *328*:304, 1985.
156. Furness, J. B., Costa, M., and Eckenstein, F. Neurones localized with antibodies against choline acetyltransferase in the enteric nervous system. Neurosci. Lett. *40*:105, 1983.
157. Furness, J. B., Costa, M., Keast, J. R. Choline acetyltransferase and peptide immunoreactivity of submucous neurons in the small intestine of the guinea-pig. Cell Tissue Res. *237*:329, 1984.
158. Costa, M., Furness, J. B., and Llewellyn-Smith, I. J. Histochemistry of the Enteric Nervous System. In Johnson L. R. (ed.): Physiology of the Gastrointestinal Tract. New York, Raven Press, 1987, pp. 1–40.
159. Furness, J. B., and Costa, M. Neurons with 5-hydroxytryptamine–like immunoreactivity in the enteric nervous system: Their projections in the guinea-pig small intestine. Neuroscience *7*:341, 1982.
160. Griffith, S. G., and Burnstock, G. Serotoninergic neurons in human fetal intestine: An immunohistochemical study. Gastroenterology *85*:929, 1983.
161. Kurian, S. S., Ferri, G. L., De Mey, J., and Polak, J. M. Immunocytochemistry of serotonin-containing nerves in the human gut. Histochemistry *78*:523, 1983.
162. Burnstock, G. Purinergic nerves. Pharmacol. Rev. *24*:509, 1972.
163. White, T. D. Characteristics of neuronal release of ATP. Prog. Neuropsychopharmacol. Biol. Psychiatry *8*:487, 1984.
164. White, T. D., Leslie, R. A. Depolarization-induced release of adenosine 5′-triphosphate from isolated varicosities derived from the myenteric plexus of the guinea pig small intestine. J. Neurosci. *2*:206, 1982.
165. Rattan, S., and Goyal, R. K. Evidence against purinergic inhibitory nerves in the vagal pathway to the opossum lower esophageal sphincter. Gastroenterology *78*:898, 1980.
166. Kaplita, P. V., Waters, D. H., Triggle, D. J. Gamma-aminobutyric acid action in guinea-pig ileal myenteric plexus. Eur. J. Pharmacol. *79*:43, 1982.
167. Krantis, A., Costa, M., Furness, J. B., and Orbach, J. Gamma-aminobutyric acid stimulates intrinsic inhibitory and excitatory nerves in the guinea-pig intestine. Eur. J. Pharmacol. *67*:461, 1980.
168. Krantis, A., and Kerr, D. I. The effect of GABA antagonism on propulsive activity of the guinea-pig large intestine. Eur. J. Pharmacol. *76*:111, 1981.
169. Krantis, A., Kerr, D. I., and Dennis, B. J. Autoradiographic study of the distribution of [3H]gamma-aminobutyrate–accumulating neural elements in guinea-pig intestine: Evidence for a transmitter function of gamma-aminobutyrate. Neuroscience *17*:1243, 1986.
170. Ong, J., and Kerr, D. I. Evidence for a physiological role of GABA in the control of guinea-pig intestinal motility. Neurosci. Lett. *50*:339, 1984.
171. Buffa, R., Solovieva, I., Fiocca, R., Giorgino, S., Rindi, G., Solcia, E., Mochizuchi, T., Yanaihara, C., and Yanaihara, N. Localization of bombesin and GRP (gastrin releasing peptide) sequences in gut nerves or endocrine cells. Histochemistry *76*:457, 1982.
172. Costa, M., Furness, J. B., Yanaihara, N., Yanaihara, C., and
Moody, T. W. Distribution and projections of neurons with immunoreactivity for both gastrin-releasing peptide and bombesin in the guinea-pig small intestine. Cell Tissue Res. *235*:285, 1984.
173. Daniel, E. E., Costa, M., Furness, J. B., and Keast, J. R. Peptide neurons in the canine small intestine. J. Comp. Neurol. *237*:227, 1985.
174. Dockray, G. J., Vaillant, C., Walsh, J. H. The neuronal origin of bombesin-like immunoreactivity in the rat gastrointestinal tract. Neuroscience *4*:1561, 1979.
175. Ekblad, E., Ekman, R., Hakanson, R., and Sundler, F. GRP neurones in the rat small intestine issue long anal projections. Regul. Pept. *9*:279, 1984.
176. Hutchison, J. B., Dimaline, R., and Dockray, G. J. Neuropeptides in the gut: Quantification and characterization of cholecystokinin octapeptide–, bombesin– and vasoactive intestinal polypeptide–like immunoreactivities in the myenteric plexus of the guinea-pig small intestine. Peptides *2*:23, 1981.
177. Erspamer, V., Erspamer, G. F., Inselvini, M., and Negri, L. Occurrence of bombesin and alytesin in extracts of the skin of three European discoglossid frogs and pharmacological actions of bombesin on extravascular smooth muscle. Br. J. Pharmacol. *45*:333, 1972.
178. Zetler, G. Antagonism of the gut-contracting effects of bombesin and neurotensin by opioid peptides, morphine, atropine or tetrodotoxin. Pharmacology *21*:348, 1980.
179. Dockray, G. J. Physiology of enteric neuropeptides. In Johnson L. R. (ed.). Physiology of the Gastrointestinal Tract. New York, Raven Press, 1987, pp. 41–66.
180. Rosenfeld, M. G., Mermod, J. J., Amara, S. G., Swanson, L. W., Sawchenko, P. E., Rivier, J., Vale, W. W., and Evans, R. M. Production of a novel neuropeptide encoded by the calcitonin gene via tissue-specific RNA processing. Nature *304*:129, 1983.
181. Clague, J. R., Sternini, C., and Brecha, N. C. Localization of calcitonin gene–related peptide–like immunoreactivity in neurons of the rat gastrointestinal tract. Neurosci. Lett. *56*:63, 1985.
182. Rodrigo, J., Polak, J. M., Fernandez, L., Ghatei, M. A., Mulderry, P., and Bloom, S. R. Calcitonin gene–related peptide immunoreactive sensory and motor nerves of the rat, cat, and monkey esophagus. Gastroenterology *88*:444, 1985.
183. Aggestrup, S. Effect of regulatory polypeptides on the substance P stimulated lower esophageal sphincter pressure in pigs. Regul. Pept. *12*:1, 1985.
184. Brain, S. D., Williams, T. J., Tippins, J. R., Morris, H. R., and MacIntyre, I. Calcitonin gene–related peptide is a potent vasodilator. Nature *313*:54, 1985.
185. Goodman, E. C., and Iversen, I. L. Calcitonin gene–related peptide: Novel neuropeptide. Life Sci. *38*:2169, 1986.
186. Lenz, H. J., Rivier, J. E., and Brown, M. R. Biological actions of human and rat calcitonin and calcitonin gene–related peptide. Regul. Pept. *12*:81, 1985.
187. Soll, A. H., Amirian, D. A., Park, J., Elashoff, J. D., and Yamada, T. Cholecystokinin potently releases somatostatin from canine fundic mucosal cells in short-term culture. Am. J. Physiol. *248*:G569, 1985.
188. Walsh, J. Gastrointestinal hormones. In Johnson, L. R. (ed.): Physiology of the Gastrointestinal Tract. New York, Raven Press, 1987, pp. 181–253.
189. Ekblad, E., Ekman, R., Hakanson, R., and Sundler, F. GRP neurones in the rat small intestine issue long anal projections. Regul. Pept. *9*:279, 1984.
190. Melander, T., Hokfelt, T., Rokaeus, A., Fahrenkrug, J., Tatemoto, K., and Mutt, V. Distribution of galanin-like immunoreactivity in the gastrointestinal tract of several mammalian species. Cell Tissue Res. *239*:253, 1985.
191. Tatemoto, K., Rokaeus, A., Jornvall, H., McDonald, T. J., and Mutt, V. Galanin—a novel biologically active peptide from porcine intestine. Febs. Lett. *164*:124, 1983.
192. Fox, J. E., McDonald, T. J., Kostolanska, F., and Tatemoto, K: Galanin: An inhibitory neural peptide of the canine small intestine. Life Sci. *39*:103, 1986.
193. Ekblad, E., Hakanson, R., Sundler, F., and Wahlestedt, C. Galanin: Neuromodulatory and direct contractile effects on smooth muscle preparations. Br. J. Pharmacol. *86*:241, 1985.

194. Costa M., Furness, J. B., and Cuello, A. C. Separate populations of opioid containing neurons in the guinea-pig intestine. Neuropeptides 5:445, 1985.

195. Furness, J. B., Costa, M., Miller, R. J. Distribution and projections of nerves with enkephalin-like immunoreactivity in the guinea-pig small intestine. Neuroscience 8:653, 1983.

196. North, R. A., and Egan, T. M. Actions and distributions of opioid peptides in peripheral tissues. Br. Med. Bull. 39:71, 1983.

197. Schultzberg, M., Hokfelt, T., Nilsson, G., Terenius, L., Rehfeld, J. F., Brown, M., Elde, R., Goldstein, M., and Said, S. Distribution of peptide- and catecholamine-containing neurons in the gastrointestinal tract of rat and guinea-pig: Immunohistochemical studies with antisera to substance P, vasoactive intestinal polypeptide, enkephalins, somatostatin, gastrin/cholecystokinin, neurotensin and dopamine beta-hydroxylase. Neuroscience 5:689, 1980.

198. Yau, W. M., Dorsett, J. A., and Youther, M. L. Inhibitory peptidergic neurons: Functional difference between somatostatin and enkephalin in myenteric plexus. Am. J. Physiol. 250:G60, 1986.

199. Daniel, E. E. Pharmacology of adrenergic, cholinergic and drugs acting on other receptors in gastrointestinal muscle. In Bertaccini, G. (ed.). Mediators and Drugs in Gastrointestinal Motility. New York, Springer-Verlag, 1982, pp. 249–322.

200. Ekblad, E., Ekelund, M., Graffner, H., Hakanson, R., and Sundler, F. Peptide-containing nerve fibers in the stomach wall of rat and mouse. Gastroenterology 89:73, 1985.

201. Feher, E., and Burnstock, G. Electron microscopic study of neuropeptide Y–containing nerve elements of the guinea pig small intestine. Gastroenterology 91:956, 1986.

202. Furness, J. B., Costa, M., Emson, P. C., Hakanson, R., Moghimzadeh, E., Sundler, F., Taylor, I. L., and Chance, R. E: Distribution, pathways and reactions to drug treatment of nerves with neuropeptide Y–and pancreatic polypeptide–like immunoreactivity in the guinea-pig digestive tract. Cell Tissue Res. 234:71, 1983.

203. Furness, J. B., Costa, M., Gibbins, I. L., Llewellyn-Smith, I. J., and Oliver, J. R. Neurochemically similar myenteric and submucous neurons directly traced to the mucosa of the small intestine. Cell Tissue Res. 241:155, 1985.

204. Sundler, F., Moghimzadeh, E., Hakanson, R., Ekelund, M., and Emson, P. Nerve fibers in the gut and pancreas of the rat displaying neuropeptide-Y immunoreactivity. Intrinsic and extrinsic origin. Cell Tissue Res. 230:487, 1983.

205. Lindh, B., Dalsgaard, C. J., Elfvin, I. G., Hokfelt, T., and Cuello, A. C. Evidence of substance P immunoreactive neurons in dorsal root ganglia and vagal ganglia projecting to the guinea pig pylorus. Brain Res. 269:365, 1983.

206. Friel, D. D., Miller, R. J., and Walker, M. W. Neuropeptide Y: A powerful modulator of epithelial ion transport. Br. J. Pharmacol. 88:425, 1986.

207. Costa M., Furness, J. B., Smith, I. J., Davies, B., and Oliver, J. An immunohistochemical study of the projections of somatostatin-containing neurons in the guinea-pig intestine. Neuroscience 5:841, 1980.

208. Keast, J. R., Furness, J. B., and Costa, M. Somatostatin in human enteric nerves. Distribution and characterization. Cell Tissue Res. 237:299, 1984.

209. Costa, M., Furness, J. B. Somatostatin is present in a subpopulation of noradrenergic nerve fibres supplying the intestine. Neuroscience 13:911, 1984.

210. Furness, J. B., and Costa, M. Actions of somatostatin on excitatory and inhibitory nerves in the intestine. Eur. J. Pharmacol. 56:69, 1979.

211. Costa, M., Furness, J. B., Llewellyn-Smith, I. J., and Cuello, A. C. Projections of substance P–containing neurons within the guinea-pig small intestine. Neuroscience 6:411, 1981.

212. Leander, S., Brodin, E., Hakanson, R., Sundler, F., and Uddman, R. Neuronal substance P in the esophagus. Distribution and effects on motor activity. Acta Physiol. Scand. 115:427, 1982.

213. Yau, W. M., Dorsett, J. A., and Youther, M. L. Calcium-dependent stimulation of acetylcholine release by substance P and vasoactive intestinal polypeptide. Eur. J. Pharmacol. 120:241, 1986.

214. Bartho, L., and Holzer, P. Search for a physiological role of substance P in gastrointestinal motility. Neuroscience 16:1, 1985.

215. Costa, M., Furness, J. B., Pullin, C. O., and Bornstein, J. Substance P enteric neurons mediate non-cholinergic transmission to the circular muscle of the guinea-pig intestine. Naunyn Schmiedebergs Arch. Pharmacol. 328:446, 1985.

216. Crist, J. R., Gidda, J., Goyal, R. K. Role of substance P nerves in longitudinal smooth muscle contractions of the esophagus. Am. J. Physiol. 250:G336, 1986.

217. Donnerer, J., Bartho, L., Holzer, P., and Lembeck, F. Intestinal peristalsis associated with release of immunoreactive substance P. Neuroscience 11:913, 1984.

218. Franco, R., Costa, M., and Furness, J. B. Evidence for the release of endogenous substance P from intestinal nerves. Naunyn Schmiedebergs Arch. Pharmacol. 306:195, 1979.

219. Fujisawa, K., and Ito, Y. The effects of substance P on smooth muscle cells and on neuro-effector transmission in the guinea-pig ileum. Br. J. Pharmacol. 76:279, 1982.

220. Holzer, P., and Petsche, U. On the mechanism of contraction and desensitization induced by substance P in the intestinal muscle of the guinea-pig. J. Physiol. (Lond.) 342:549, 1983.

221. Dalsgaard, C. J., Vincent, S. R., Hokfelt, T., Lundberg, J. M., Dahlstrom, A., Schultzberg, M., Cokray, G. J., Cuello, A. C. Coexistence of cholecystokinin and substance P–like peptides in neurons of the dorsal root ganglia of the rat. Neurosci. Lett. 33:159, 1982.

222. Costa, M., and Furness, J. B. The origins, pathways and terminations of neurons with VIP-like immunoreactivity in the guinea-pig small intestine. Neuroscience 8:665, 1983.

223. Edin, R. Lundberg, J. M., Ahlman, H, Dahlstrom, A., Fahrenkrug, J., Hokfelt, T., Kewenter, J. On the VIP-ergic innervation of the feline pylorus. Acta Physiol. Scand. 107:185, 1979.

224. Ferri, G. L., Botti, P., Biliotti, G., Rebecchi, L., Bloom, S. R., Tonelli, L., Labo, G., and Polak J. M. VIP–, substance P– and met-enkephalin–immunoreactive innervation of the human gastroduodenal mucosa and Brunner's glands. Gut 25:948, 1984.

225. Aggestrup, S., Uddman, R., Jensen, S. L., Sundler, F., Schaffalitzky de Muckadell, O., Holst, J. J., Hakanson, R., Ekman, R., and Sorensen, H. R. Regulatory peptides in the lower esophageal sphincter of man. Regul. Pept. 10:167, 1985.

226. Biancani, P., Walsh, J., and Behar, J. Vasoactive intestinal peptide: A neurotransmitter for relaxation of the rabbit internal anal sphincter. Gastroenterology 89:867, 1985.

227. Fahrenkrug, J., and Emson, P. C. Vasoactive intestinal polypeptide: Functional aspects. Br. Med. Bull. 38:265, 1982.

228. Goyal, R. K., Rattan, S., and Said, S. I. VIP as a possible neurotransmitter of non-cholinergic non-adrenergic inhibitory neurones. Nature 288:378, 1980.

229. Grider, J. R., Cable, M. B., Said, S. I., and Makhlouf, G. M. Vasoactive intestinal peptide as a neural mediator of gastric relaxation. Am. J. Physiol. 248:G73, 1985.

230. Dharmsathaphorn, K., Mandel, K. G., Masui, H., and McRoberts, J. A. Vasoactive intestinal polypeptide–induced chloride secretion by a colonic epithelial cell line. Direct participation of a basolaterally localized Na^+, K^+, Cl^- cotransport system. J. Clin. Invest. 75:462, 1985.

231. Rothman, T. P., and Gershon, M. D. Regionally defective colonization of the terminal bowel by the precursors of enteric neurons in lethal spotted mutant mice. Neuroscience 12:1293, 1984.

232. Ziegler, H. W., Heitz, P. U., Kasper, M., Spichtin, H. P., and Ulrich, J. Aganglionosis of the colon. Morphologic investigations in 524 patients. Pathol. Res. Pract. 178:543, 1984.

233. Schuffler, M. D., and Jonak, Z. Chronic idiopathic intestinal pseudo-obstruction caused by a degenerative disorder of the myenteric plexus: The use of Smith's method to define the neuropathology. Gastroenterology 82:476, 1982.

234. Crist, J. R., Gidda, J. S., Goyal, R. K. Intramural mechanism of esophageal peristalsis: Roles of cholinergic and noncholinergic nerves. Proc. Natl. Acad. Sci. USA 81:3595, 1984.

3

Gastrointestinal Smooth Muscle

JEFFREY CONKLIN
RAJ K. GOYAL

In humans, the smooth muscle portion of the gut extends as a continuous structure from midesophagus to the anal canal, making smooth muscle a major constituent of the hollow viscera that compose the gut. In addition to being a prominent structural component of the gut wall, smooth muscle contractile properties such as the abilities to contract rhythmically or maintain tone over long periods enable gastrointestinal organs to perform a wide variety of specialized tasks. These tasks include (1) the transport, storage, and mixing of luminal contents with gastrointestinal secretions so that efficient digestion may take place; (2) the propulsion of luminal contents through various segments of the gut so that the absorption of nutrients and fluid may occur efficiently; and (3) the expulsion of food residues from the gastrointestinal tract. This chapter describes the general features of smooth muscle with particular reference to gastrointestinal smooth muscles. Its purpose is to provide an understanding of smooth muscles so that the cellular physiology and pathophysiology of smooth muscle disorders described in various chapters of this book may be better understood.

ORGANIZATION OF SMOOTH MUSCLE IN THE GUT

In general, the smooth muscle portion of the gastrointestinal tract consists of a continuous outer longitudinal and a much thicker inner circular muscle layer. Muscle layers are named according to the orientation of the long axes of their constituent cells.[1] In humans, there are two major deviations from this general pattern: the proximal stomach is invested by a third muscle layer, the oblique layer, and the longitudinal muscle of the colon is condensed into three longitudinal bands, the teniae coli. The longitudinal and circular muscle layers are usually distinct and are separated by a connective tissue space that contains the myenteric plexus. However, there are many interconnections between the muscle cells within each muscle layer. In the regions of the sphincters, the orientation of muscle fibers becomes somewhat haphazard and the clear cleavage between longitudinal and circular muscle layers disappears. Both the longitudinal and circular muscle layers play important roles in the digestion and movement of luminal contents.[2-5] In general, longitudinal muscle contraction shortens the distance over which peristaltic contraction must move luminal contents. Alternating contractions and relaxations of the longitudinal muscle also help mix luminal contents. The circular muscle layer usually produces ringlike contractions that help in the mixing or propulsion of luminal contents, depending upon whether these contractions are segmental or propagated along the gut wall.

The alimentary tract consists of serially joined segments: the esophagus, stomach, and small and large bowel. Each has a distinct function. These segments are separated from one another by gastrointestinal sphincters. Sphincters are specialized circular muscles that obstruct the gut lumen by remaining contracted under basal conditions. They relax in response to appropriate stimuli so that luminal contents may pass from one gut segment to the next. Thus, they insure the timely delivery of luminal contents from one visceral organ to the next, so that each may perform its task efficiently. For example, the pyloric sphincter serves as a unique controller for the delivery of gastric contents into the duodenum.[3] Sphincters also block the retrograde flow of contents from one organ to the other. For example, the lower esophageal sphincter provides an important barrier to reflux of gastric contents into the esophagus.[2]

There is also a continuous thin sheet of muscle lying between the submucosa and the lamina propria. This is the muscularis mucosae. Many muscle fibers arising from the muscularis mucosae extend into lamina propria to make muscular baskets around glandular structures and to provide attachment of the muscularis mucosae to the mucosa.

Characteristically, each muscle layer within the smooth muscle tissue is subdivided into bundles by intramuscular septa made up predominantly of collagen fibrils. Septa extend across the entire thickness of the muscle layer and run parallel to the long axes of muscle cells constituting the muscle layer. Individual septa run only a few hundred microns along the length of tissue before giving way to other septa. This arrangement allows groups of muscle cells bounded by septa to function as individual force generating units. The forces produced by these multicellular units are propagated throughout the rest of the muscle by the septa enclosing them.

The smooth muscle of gut does not have elaborate

neuromuscular junctions like the motor end plates of the striated muscle. Instead, autonomic nerve axons make fine arborizations within the muscle tissue. Along their courses, axonal branches have multiple dilations called varicosities (see p. 23). These varicosities contain neurotransmitters which are released upon stimulation. The distance between varicosities and the smooth muscle cell surfaces varies from 10 nm to more than 100 nm. In the latter case, the neurotransmitter released from the varicosities diffuses for long distances through intervening connective tissues to produce its effect on the smooth muscle cell.

Within the gut wall there is also a population of nonneural and nonmuscle cells called interstitial cells of Cajal.[6, 7] These cells have large nuclei, an abundance of large mitochondria, many caveolae, considerable rough endoplasmic reticulum, and long processes. In the small bowel, interstitial cells make up an extensive two-dimensional plexus between the longitudinal and circular muscle layers that penetrates the circular layer for a short distance. They form gap junctions with other interstitial cells as well as with muscle cells from circular and longitudinal layers. Neurons from the myenteric plexus make synaptic connections with interstitial cells. A similar plexus of interstitial cells is found at the junction between the muscularis propria and submucosa of the colon. These histologic characteristics make interstitial cells ideal candidates for pacemaker cells, which generate and propagate slow waves into the muscularis propria.

In the absence of any neurohormonal stimulation, some gastrointestinal smooth muscles remain inactive, for example, smooth muscle of the esophageal body. However, most smooth muscles generate spontaneous, phasic contractions, as is the case with gastric, colonic, and small intestinal smooth muscle. The smooth muscles of the gastrointestinal sphincter produce sustained tonic contractions. When stimulated by neurohormonal agents most gastrointestinal smooth muscles generate phasic contractions. The frequency of phasic contractions produced by stimulation is a unique property of each gastrointestinal muscle. For example, the distal stomach contracts at a maximum rate of 5 contractions per minute, while the duodenum contracts to a rate of 12 contractions per minute.[3, 4]

SMOOTH MUSCLE CELLS

Individual smooth muscle cells are small, spindle-shaped cells that measure 200 to 300 μ in length and 10 to 20 μ in diameter. The smooth muscle plasma membrane consists of an 8 to 10 nm thick lipid bilayer similar to that of other animal cells. Embedded within the bilayer are various specialized protein molecules. These include proteins anchoring the contractile apparatus (e.g., dense bands), sites of contact between adjacent cells (e.g., gap junction, intermediate junctions), ion pumps, ion channels, and receptors for neurohumoral substances.[8]

The surfaces of individual cells are organized into alternating regions of structural specialization composed primarily of caveolae and dense bands (Fig. 3–1). *Caveolae* are small flask-shaped involutions of the plasma membrane that extend about 120 nm into the cell and communicate with the extracellular space through a narrow neck. Although they may occur as isolated structural features of the plasma membrane, they are most often arranged in rows one to several caveolae wide, oriented parallel to the long axis of the cell.[9, 12] Because caveolae are so numerous, occurring at a density of 20 to 30 per square micron, they add as much as 50 per cent to the cell surface. The functional significance of smooth muscle caveolae remains unclear. Similar structures from cardiac and endothelial cells are responsible for endocytosis; that is, they selectively transport extracellular molecules into the cell via specific plasma membrane acceptor proteins. Smooth muscle caveolae do not appear to be involved in the endocytic process.[9] Smooth muscle caveolae are often found overlying cisternae of the sarcoplasmic reticulum. Action potentials propagating along the plasma membrane are conducted into the caveolae, bringing them into close proximity to the sarcoplasmic reticulum. Changes in the sarcoplasmic reticulum membrane brought about by action potentials trigger calcium release, initiating contraction. Thus, smooth muscle caveolae may be functional analogues of striated muscle T tubules.[10]

Dense bands are small fusiform patches of amorphous electron-dense material attached to the cytoplasmic side of the plasma membrane (Fig. 3–1). They are distributed along the length of the cell between rows of caveolae and occupy most of the remaining cell surface. Dense bands are composed of at least two proteins: alpha-actinin, which is also a structural component of the Z line in striated muscle, and vinculin.[13, 14] Thin (actin) filaments emerge from dense bands to run into the cytoplasmic compartment, where they interact with other components of the contractile apparatus. Dense bands serve as sites where the contractile machinery is anchored to the plasma membrane. Because they are distributed over as much as 50 per cent of the plasma membrane, forces generated by the contractile proteins are transmitted to many discrete patches of plasma membrane over the cell surface. This results in the plasma membrane being retracted at many distinct points and bulging out between dense bands during contraction[15, 16] (Fig. 3–2).

The major intracellular organelles, other than contractile proteins, include the nucleus, sarcoplasmic reticulum, and mitochondria. The *sarcoplasmic reticulum* is a closed system of membranous tubules scattered throughout the cell. Some components of the reticulum are located near the nucleus, where they are responsible for the synthesis of cellular proteins. The majority of the reticulum is situated at the periphery of the cell, where it is located directly beneath and parallel to plasma membrane structures. The peripheral sarcoplasmic reticulum, although it makes up less than 2 per cent of the cell volume, is the major intracellular storage site from which calcium is released to initiate

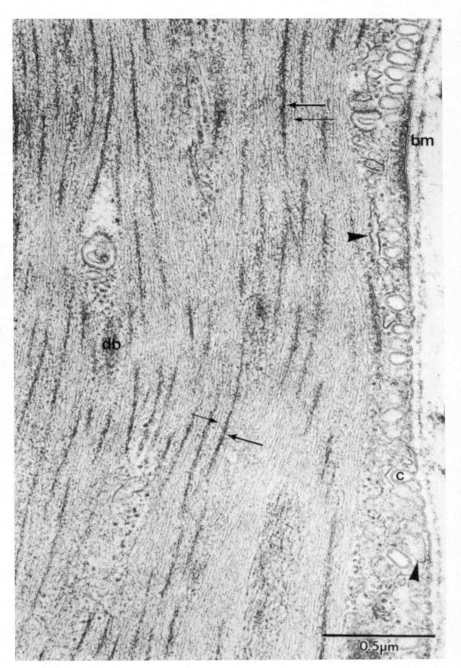

Figure 3–1. Transmission electron micrograph showing longitudinal section of a smooth muscle cell. The plasma membrane is cut tangentially so the caveolae (c) appear as vesicles or pits. Tubules of the sarcoplasmic reticulum *(arrowheads)* form a network in association with caveolae. Between rows of caveolae, there is a dense band (bm). Large arrows point to thick filaments which are surrounded by adjacent parallel thin filaments *(small arrows)*. Cytoplasmic dense body (db) is also seen. (Photograph by A. V. Somlyo. From Hartshorne, D. J. *In* Johnson, L. R. [ed.]. Physiology of the Gastrointestinal Tract. 2nd ed. New York, Raven Press, 1987. Used by permission.)

contraction. It is also the major storage site into which cytoplasm Ca^{2+} is sequestered during relaxation. Beneath regions of the plasma membrane occupied by caveolae, the sarcoplasmic reticulum exists either as tubules running between rows of caveolae or as an extensively branching network surrounding caveolae.[17] The extensive branching of the sarcoplasmic reticulum around caveolae greatly increases the amount of plasma membrane in close contact with the reticulum. This relationship increases the amount of sarcoplasmic reticulum releasing Ca^{2+} in response to an action potential. In other areas, where the plasma membrane is not occupied by caveolae, cisternae of the sarco-plasmic reticulum are situated 12 to 20 nm from the plasma membrane.[17, 18] Although this close relationship ensures that action potentials will influence these elements of the sarcoplasmic reticulum, it also ensures that second messenger molecules produced in response to receptor-hormone interactions must diffuse only a short distance before interacting with the sarcoplasmic reticulum. Such short diffusion distances make for a rapid and efficient release of the calcium required for the initiation of contraction in response to neurohumoral agents. *Mitochondria* are located primarily at the poles of the nucleus and at the periphery of the cell, in locations where energy utilization is high. Near

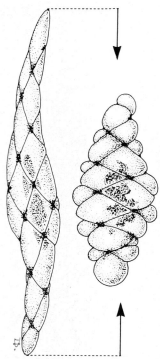

Figure 3–2. An interpretive diagram of contraction in the smooth muscle fiber. Bundles of intermediate filaments from cable-like systems stretch from one dense body to another and to dense bands on the plasma membrane. Intermediate filaments harness the force generated by the sliding of thin filaments past thick filaments. Contractile proteins (thick and thin filaments) also stretch from one dense body to another and to dense bands on the plasma membrane. The force pull generated by the sliding of thin filaments past thick filaments shortens the distance between dense bodies and retracts the dense bands. As the dense bands of the cell membrane are pulled inward, the long axis of the muscle shortens and the regions of plasma membrane between the dense bands balloon out. (From Cormack, D. H. Introduction to Histology. Philadelphia, J. B. Lippincott Company, 1984. Used by permission.)

the nucleus protein synthesis occurs, and near the plasma membrane many active ion pumps and energy-requiring enzymes are present.

Adjacent individual smooth muscle cells contact one another by two types of junctions, intermediate junctions and nexuses. *Intermediate junctions* are sites of tight mechanical coupling between neighboring smooth muscle cells (Fig. 3–3). This junction appears morphologically as an area of plasma membrane occupied by a dense band on one smooth muscle cell juxtaposed to a similar structure on an adjacent smooth muscle cell. At these junctions, the intercellular space between abutting membranes is narrowed to 30 to 40 nm and is filled by a focal condensation of intercellular matrix.[19] Since intermediate junctions are made up of juxtaposed dense bands, they are sites where the contractile machinery of adjacent cells is mechanically coupled. This mechanical coupling allows forces developed by the contractile apparatus of one cell to be transmitted to the contractile apparatus of its neighbor. The *nexus* or *gap junction,* another well-defined junction, couples plasma membranes of contiguous smooth muscle cells

in a different way[20–24] (Fig. 3–4). This structure consists of a small round or oval patch of plasma membrane juxtaposed to a similar structure on an adjacent smooth muscle cell. The intercellular space at the nexus is narrowed to 2 to 3 nm and is traversed by closely packed intramembranous particles which also span the thickness of adjacent plasma membranes. These intra-membranous particles represent intercellular channels that form tunnels from one cell to the other. These channels allow the free movement of ions and small molecules between neighboring cells.[21, 22, 25] The number of gap junctions per cell varies depending on the muscle studied. Gap junctions, because they provide direct communication between the cytoplasmic compartments of adjacent cells, serve as low-resistance electrical pathways[26] between neighboring cells. Functionally, this means that electrical, chemical, or ionic changes in one cell can easily spread to its neighbor. Thus, gap junctions are responsible for the syncytial nature of smooth muscle.

There is a stroma between cells that consists of collagen fibers, elastic fibers, and ground substance. Collagen and elastic fibers are linked by microfilaments to the plasma membrane over areas occupied by dense bands.[9, 19] This mechanical coupling of connective tissue elements to plasma membrane sites where the contractile apparatus is anchored allows the direct transmission of forces generated by a smooth muscle cell contraction throughout the tissue. Since individual smooth muscle cells generate little if any passive force over a wide range of stretch,[27] the make-up and orientation of connective tissue elements within the extracellular stroma plays a major role in determining the passive mechanical properties of smooth muscle tissues.

CONTRACTILE APPARATUS: CONTRACTILE PROTEINS

Eighty to 90 per cent of the volume of a smooth muscle cell is made up of filamentous contractile proteins and dense bodies. The filamentous proteins include thin (actin) filaments, thick (myosin) filaments, and intermediate (desmin) filaments.[19, 28, 29] Although these smooth muscle contractile filaments do not exist in the highly ordered repeating arrays characteristic of striated muscle (sarcomeres), there is considerable order to their arrangement[30, 31] (Fig. 3–5).

Thin (actin) filaments (5- to 7-nm filaments) in smooth muscle are made up of globular polypeptides called globular actin or G-actin. In physiological salt solution G-actin molecules polymerize to form filamentous actin or F-actin, which consists of two strands of actin molecules twisted into a double helix. Actin molecules are organized into bundles that can be thought of as cables running nearly parallel to the long axis of the cell[17, 18, 21] (Fig. 3–5*A*). Another protein, tropomyosin, is present in the groove between twists of the actin helix. The function of tropomyosin in smooth muscle is not known. Bundles of actin filaments are anchored to the plasma membrane by dense bands,

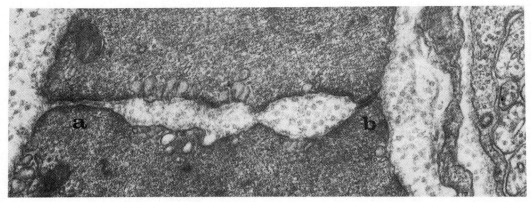

Figure 3–3. Transverse section of intestinal muscle showing two intermediate junctions joining adjacent smooth muscle cells. The intermediate junctions are identified as a narrowing of the intracellular space between segments of adjacent smooth muscle cell membrane occupied by dense bands. The intermediate junction on the left (a) is broader than that on the right (b). At each junction the intercellular space is narrowed and occupied by electron-dense material. The intercellular space at junction (a) is 30 nM, while that at junction (b) is 15 nm. Intermediate junctions serve as sites of mechanical coupling between adjacent smooth muscles. The laminar process of an interstitial cell and a nerve are present at far right. (From Gabella, G. *In* Johnson, L. R. [ed.]. Physiology of the Gastrointestinal Tract. 2nd ed. New York, Raven Press, 1987. Used by permission.)

Figure 3–4. *A,* Transverse section of intestinal muscle to show a gap junction *(arrows)* between adjacent smooth muscles. × 25,000. *B,* Surface view of gap junctions, demonstrated by using freeze fracture technique. (*A* and *B* from Gabella, G. *In* Johnson, L. R. [ed.]. Physiology of the Gastrointestinal Tract. 2nd ed. New York, Raven Press, 1987. Used by permission.) *C,* Diagram of a gap junction. The gap junction consists of a number of intramembranous proteins called connexons, which make tunnels connecting the cytoplasmic compartments of adjacent cells. (Reprinted by permission of the publisher from: Principles underlying electrical and chemical synaptic transmission, by Kandel, E. R., and Siegelbaum, S. *In* Kandel, E. R., and Schwartz, J. H. [eds.]. Principles of Neural Science. 2nd ed. Copyright 1985 by Elsevier Science Publishing Co., Inc.)

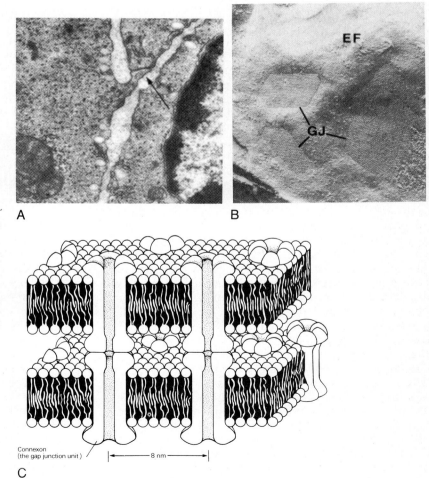

Connexon
(the gap junction unit)

8 nm

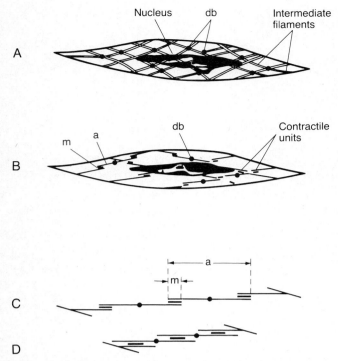

Figure 3–5. A diagrammatic presentation of components of contractile units in smooth muscle. *A,* Structural network formed by bundles of intermediate filaments and dense bodies. *B,* Contractile units which generate the contraction. The contractile unit consists of dense bodies (db), actin filaments (a) arising from the dense bodies, and myosin filaments (m). *C,* In the relaxed state thick filaments are just overlapped by thin filaments. *D,* During contraction actin filaments slide past the myosin filaments. Sliding is limited mechanically because myosin filaments cannot slide past the dense body to which the actin filaments are attached. (Modified from Squire, J. M. The Structural Basis of Muscular Contraction. New York, Plenum Press, 1981. Used by permission.)

and to one another within the cytoplasmic compartment by dense bodies. Dense bodies are composed of two isoforms of actinin, alpha actinin and gamma actinin. They are oriented so their long axes are parallel to the long axis of the cell, and they have actin filaments attached at each pole (Figs. 3–5B and 3–6). Thus, dense bodies are smooth muscle analogues of the Z lines in striated muscle that anchor actin filaments converging from opposite directions. Actin filaments emerging from opposite ends of the dense body run nearly parallel to the long axis of the cell for an unknown distance before encountering the thick filaments (Figs. 3–5B and C and 3–6). This organizational schema for the smooth muscle contractile apparatus, that is, actin filaments of opposite polarity being anchored to dense bodies and extending to interdigitate with myosin filaments, is analogous to the sarcomere of striated muscle. The smooth muscle sarcomere analogue is the interval between dense bodies, instead of Z lines. Many such sarcomere-like units one after the other make up what is termed a "contractile unit."[30, 31] The contractile unit spans relatively long distances along the cell length, anchoring to plasma membrane–associated dense bands at both of its ends[15, 33] (Fig. 3–5B and C).

Thick (myosin) filaments (about 15-nm filaments) interdigitate with actin filaments. They are made up of multiple myosin molecules, each having a molecular weight of about 480,000. Myosin is an asymmetrical molecule consisting of a long tail region and a globular head region.[34] The tail is composed of two identical subunits that are coiled around one another to form a long, rodlike alpha-helix. At one end of the myosin molecule, the coiled structure changes into a globular formation with each subunit giving rise to a globular head. Each head region contains an actin binding site and an actin-activated Mg^{2+}-ATPase. Each myosin head is also associated with two regulatory proteins called myosin light chains, one of which must be phosphorylated for actin to interact with myosin. There are three regions along the myosin molecule that have hingelike properties (Fig. 3–7). One of these regions, located near the myosin head, allows the head region to rotate about the tail[35] (Fig. 3–7). Thick filaments are aggregates of many myosin molecules packed together so that their tail regions make up a filamentous core with the globular heads projecting radially from the core. Many radial projections from myosin filaments can be seen interacting with adjacent actin filaments during contraction.[18] These structures are the same as the myosin crossbridges described in striated muscle.

Intermediate filaments (10-nm filaments) are composed of the protein desmin. They link plasma membrane–bound dense bands and cytoplasmic dense bodies, forming a cytoskeletal network that extends throughout the cytoplasm. The association of intermediate filaments with dense bodies suggests that they serve as a framework on which the myofilaments are organized and that they are a cellular mechanism for the distribution of contractile forces throughout the cell[1, 36] (Figs. 3–5A and 3–6).

MECHANISM OF CONTRACTION IN SMOOTH MUSCLE

As is the case with striated muscle, smooth muscle contraction is described by the sliding filament model.[31, 37] According to this model, repeated interactions of the myosin heads with adjacent actin filaments produce the sliding of thick and thin filaments past one another in much the same way as repeated oar strokes move a boat through water. As the oarsmen must use energy to move their boat relative to the water, energy in the form of ATP hydrolysis is used to produce the sliding of thick and thin filaments past one another.

The sliding of thick and thin filaments past one another decreases the distance between dense bodies making up individual contractile units,[38, 39] shortening the contractile unit and generating force. This force is transmitted to the plasma membrane via the dense bands to which the contractile unit is anchored (Figs. 3–5 and 3–6). When many contractile units shorten, the result is contraction of the smooth muscle cell.[38, 39]

The molecular mechanism by which actin and myosin interact to produce contraction is called *crossbridge*

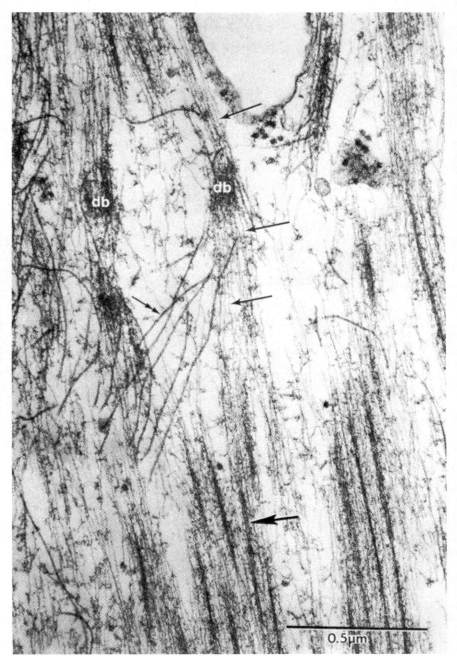

Figure 3–6. Longitudinal section of a smooth muscle showing the relationship of dense bodies (db) to intermediate (10-nm) filaments *(double arrow)*. Note that intermediate filaments form a network connecting neighboring dense bodies. A number of thin actin filaments *(small arorws)* are attached to the dense bodies. Some can be traced from dense bodies to thick myosin filaments *(large arrows)*. Special tissue fixation was used to wash out many soluble cytoplasmic proteins, thereby allowing better visualization of the contractile apparatus of the cell. (Photograph by A. V. Somlyo. From Hartshorne, D. J. *In* Johnson, L. R. [ed.]. Physiology of the Gastrointestinal Tract. 2nd ed. New York, Raven Press, 1987. Used by permission.)

cycling.[37, 40–42] A model of crossbridge cycling in smooth muscle has been described by Eisenberg and Hill[42] (Fig. 3–8). The essential concept of this model is that the myosin head alternates between two structural conformations that have differing affinities for actin. In one of its conformations, the 90° conformation, the myosin head is oriented with its long axis perpendicular to the bodies of the thick filament and adjacent thin filament. In this conformation, the binding of the myosin head to actin is weak. In its other conformation, the myosin head makes a 45° angle to its adjacent actin filament, and is bound tightly to actin.

The crossbridge cycle is initiated when the 20,000-dalton light chains associated with the myosin heads of a myosin molecule are phosphorylated. Phosphoryla-

tion of the myosin light chains activates the myosin-Mg^{2+}-ATPase and increases crossbridge cycling by as much as 1000 fold.[37] This initiates contraction. An abbreviated version of the crossbridge cycle in smooth

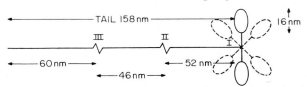

Figure 3–7. Diagrammatic representation of the myosin molecule to show two hingelike regions (II and III) in the tail and at the junction of the head and the neck (I). (From Hartshorne, D. J. *In* Johnson, L. R. [ed.]. Physiology of the Gastrointestinal Tract. 2nd ed. New York, Raven Press, 1987. Used by permission. Data from Onishi and Wakabayashi.[34])

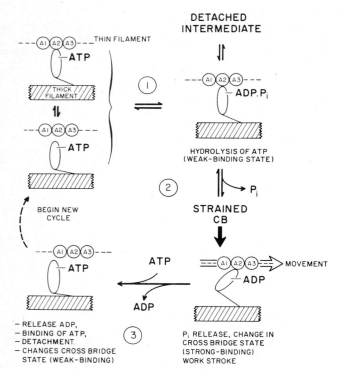

Figure 3–8. Representation of the crossbridge cycle. Only one of the two myosin heads is shown. A1, A2, and A3 represent actin monomers in the thin filament. Refer to the text for the explanation of the kinetic scheme. (From Hartshorne, D. J. *In* Johnson, L. R. [ed.]. Physiology of the Gastrointestinal Tract. 2nd ed. New York, Raven Press, 1987. Used by permission.)

muscle[37] is shown (Fig. 3–8). At the beginning of a crossbridge cycle, ATP is bound to the myosin head in its 90° conformation and the myosin head is only weakly bound to an adjacent actin molecule. Since the interaction between actin and myosin is weak, crossbridges exist in the attached and detached states. The first step in the crossbridge cycle is the hydrolysis of ATP to $ADP + P_i$ by the myosin-Mg^{2+}-ATPase. Hydrolysis of ATP occurs whether the actin and myosin are associated or dissociated. At the end of this step ADP and P_i remain bound to the myosin head, and the attached and detached crossbridges remain in equilibrium. The next step (step 2), in which P_i dissociates from the myosin head, is the force-generating step. It is during this step that the myosin head binds tightly to its adjacent actin molecule and tilts into its 45° state. When the myosin head tilts it becomes strained, much like the spring component of a catapult is strained prior to releasing its load. When the springlike component of the myosin head unloads, it produces the sliding of actin and myosin molecules past one another. During the next step, ADP dissociates from the attached myosin head and ATP binds in its place. The rebinding of ATP returns the myosin head to its 90° position, and its weak binding state. Since the myosin head assumes its 90° position while bound to actin, the crossbridge is strained once again. However, the strain is opposite that which produced filament sliding when the crossbridge went from the 90° conformation to the

45° conformation. Negative work is not produced because the myosin head returns to its weak binding state and dissociates from actin simultaneously.

During muscle contraction, hundreds of myosin heads on each thick filament are repeatedly undergoing similar changes in conformation, and pulling against the actin molecule. The force developed by this process is proportional to the number of crossbridges acting in parallel.[43] Not all of the myosin crossbridges are cycling synchronously, so that at any point in time during contraction, myosin heads on a thick filament can be found at all stages in the crossbridge cycle. This asynchronous cycling of literally millions of myosin crossbridges allows the cell to contract in a continuous fashion rather than like a ratchet.

When compared with striated muscle, two of the most striking features of smooth muscle contraction are its economy of energy utilization and slowness. These features are explained by a slower cycling of crossbridges in smooth muscle. This slowing occurs at step 3 in the crossbridge cycle, when ADP on the myosin head is replaced by ATP and the myosin head undergoes its conformational change from the strong to the weak binding state (Fig. 3–8).[40] Specifically, detachment of ADP from the actomyosin complex occurs 100 times more slowly in the smooth muscle than in striated muscle. For this reason, the smooth muscle myosin molecule remains bound to actin and generating force for a much greater percentage of time than does the striated muscle myosin molecule.[44, 45] Since the crossbridge remains in its force-generating state for a longer period of time, less ATP is hydrolyzed per unit of time to maintain an equivalent level of force production. Functionally, this translates into a contraction that is much slower than striated muscle contraction, but is much more efficient. Since normal gastrointestinal function does not require rapid contractile changes, and often depends upon sustained contraction, these properties of the smooth muscle crossbridge cycle are appropriate to the tasks of the gastrointestinal smooth muscle.

Role of Intracellular Calcium and Myosin Light Chain Kinase in Smooth Muscle Contraction

As with striated muscles, changes in intracellular ionized calcium ($[Ca^{2+}]_i$) result in changes in the contractile state of smooth muscle—contraction occurring at higher concentrations and relaxation at lower concentrations. However, the mechanisms by which changes in $[Ca^{2+}]_i$ regulate the contractile apparatus are different in the two muscle types. In striated muscle, the proteins troponin and tropomyosin, both of which are located on the actin molecule, are responsible for regulating the actin-myosin interaction. When no contraction is occurring, tropomyosin shields the site on the actin filament that can bind with the myosin head. A rise in $[Ca^{2+}]_i$ produces a shift in the troponin and tropomyosin molecules, allowing the myosin head to interact with its binding site on the actin molecule.[46] This type of regulation has been termed "thin filament–linked regulation." Since no troponin or troponin-like molecules exist in smooth muscle, this regulatory system does not function in smooth muscle. Instead, it is a modification of the myosin molecule brought about by its interaction with a Ca^{2+}-calmodulin-myosin light chain kinase complex that allows the crossbridge cycle to proceed.[37, 47, 48] Therefore, the regulation of the smooth muscle crossbridge cycle is termed "myosin-linked regulation."

The modification of the myosin head that allows crossbridge cycling to occur is the phosphorylation of a 20,000-dalton constituent of the myosin molecule called myosin light chain.[49, 50] Myosin light chain phosphorylation is brought about by the interaction of (1) Ca^{2+}, (2) a specific enzyme responsible for phosphorylating the myosin light chains called myosin light chain kinase (MLCK), and (3) a calcium-activated protein called calmodulin (Fig. 3–9).

When the smooth muscle cell is at rest, free intracellular calcium concentrations ($[Ca^{2+}]_i$) are low (0.1 to 0.2 μM). Therefore, little Ca^{2+} is bound to calmodulin, and calmodulin is not associated with MLCK. Excitation of the cell leads to a rise of $[Ca^{2+}]_i$ (1.0 to 4.0 μM). When this occurs, Ca^{2+} binds to calmodulin. Each calmodulin molecule contains four Ca^{2+} binding sites, which are sequentially filled as the $[Ca^{2+}]_i$ rises. Filling of the first two binding sites produces a large conformational change in the calmodulin molecule, but the molecule is unable to interact with and activate MLCK until the third and fourth sites are occupied.[51] The Ca^{2+}-calmodulin-MLCK complex then brings about the hydrolysis of ATP to generate the P_i with which myosin light chains are phosphorylated. Phosphorylation of the 20,000-dalton myosin light chain on each myosin head brings about a conformational change in the myosin head. This conformational change allows filamentous actin to activate the myosin-Mg^{2+}-ATPase, and the crossbridge cycle proceeds.

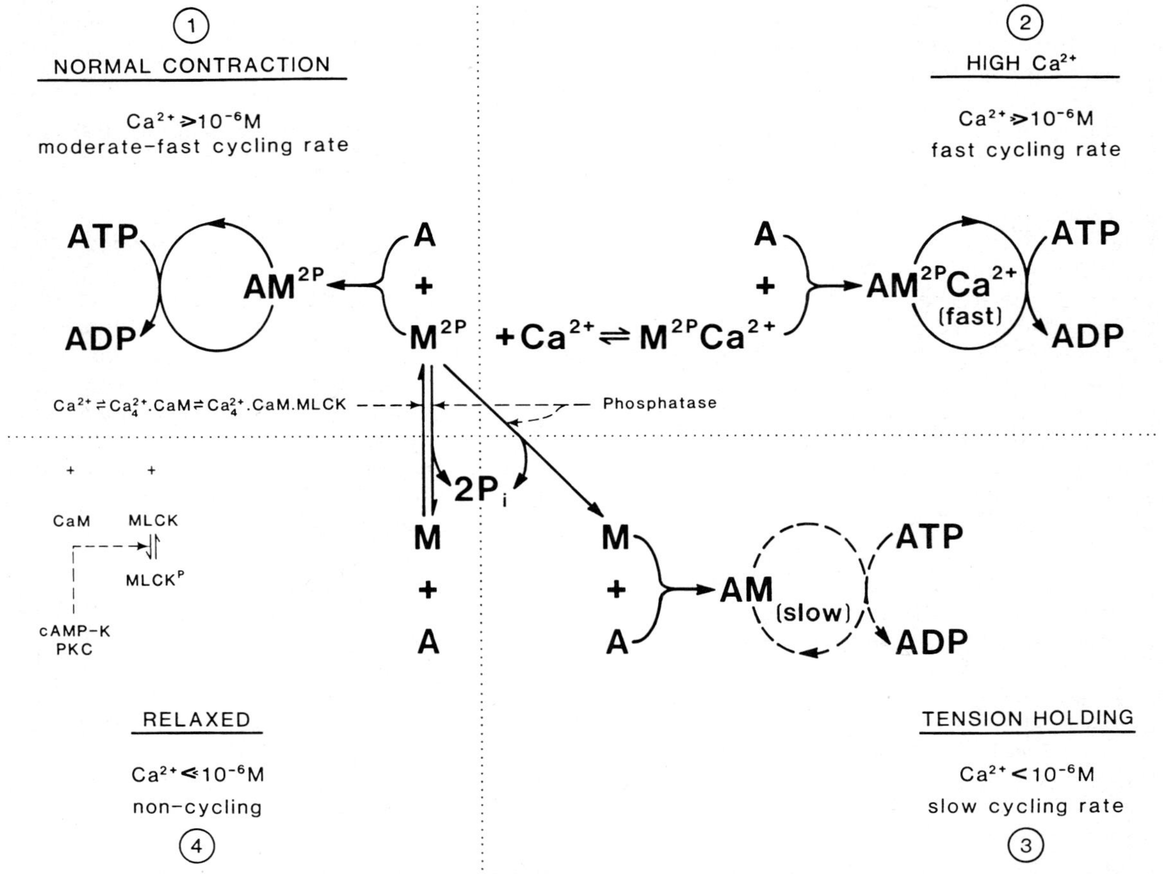

Figure 3–9. Diagrammatic representation of events involved in contraction-relaxation cycle in smooth muscle. Sections 1 and 2 represent events during tension development. The initial contractile response is associated with a moderate crossbridge cycling rate associated with phosphorylation of myosin light chains. The cycling rate becomes faster, presumably owing to binding of Ca^{2+} to phosphorylated myosin. The cycling rate corresponds to the velocity of shortening. Section 3 depicts events in tension holding or stress maintenance. It usually follows an initial contraction and may continue for prolonged periods in certain muscles. With stress maintenance, crossbridge cycling continues at a slower rate. The crossbridge cycle slows because actin and myosin spend a greater time in the bound state. This is also called the *latch state.* It is associated with low rates of myosin phosphorylation, and it requires some calcium. Section 4 depicts events during relaxation. Here there is very little crossbridge cycling occurring. It results from a fall in $[Ca^{2+}]_i$ or inactivation of myosin light chain kinase by its phosphorylation. See text for details. M, myosin; A, actin; CaM, calmodulin; MLCK, myosin light-chain kinase. (From Hartshorne, D. J. *In* Johnson, L. R. [ed.]. Physiology of the Gastrointestinal Tract. 2nd ed. New York, Raven Press, 1987. Used by permission.)

Inactivation of MLCK occurs when $[Ca^{2+}]_i$ drops to resting levels. As the $[Ca^{2+}]_i$ drops, Ca^{2+} dissociates from calmodulin and the calmodulin-MLCK interaction is disrupted. Smooth muscle cells also possess several myosin light chain phosphatases capable of dephosphorylating the myosin light chain, thus interrupting cycling of crossbridges and returning muscle cells to the relaxed state.

Contraction-Relaxation Cycles in Gastrointestinal Smooth Muscle

Some gastrointestinal smooth muscles contract and then relax soon after reaching their maximal contraction, producing a monophasic contraction wave. This is called a phasic contraction, and the muscles sharing this behavior are called phasic muscles. Circular muscles of nonsphincter parts of the gut are examples of phasic muscles. Other smooth muscles maintain their contracted states following activation. The period of maintained stress is called tonic contraction. In the case of gastrointestinal sphincters, tonic contraction occurs in the absence of any neurohumoral stimulation and is due to a unique property intrinsic to the sphincter muscles. This allows the maintenance of tone under basal conditions. Muscles able to maintain prolonged stress are called tonic muscles.[52]

Many smooth muscles show both phasic and tonic contractile properties. The cellular mechanisms underlying phasic and tonic behaviors of different muscles are not fully understood but, as will be discussed later, may be due to differences in their electrical properties, differences in the ways cells maintain intracellular Ca^{2+} concentrations, and subtle differences in the properties of their contractile proteins. The final effect of these differing properties is a difference in crossbridge cycling rate, which is the ultimate determinant of the phasic and tonic behavior of muscles. Figure 3–9 summarizes four of the crossbridge cycling states in phasic and tonic contraction and relaxation of smooth muscles.[37] Active contraction and the velocity of muscle shortening correlate with the rate of the crossbridge cycling. The rate of crossbridge cycling is, in turn, dependent upon the intracellular Ca^{2+} ion concentration and the activity of myosin light-chain kinase. These relationships are such that cycling increases at higher Ca^{2+} concentration and with greater kinase activity.[53]

On the other hand, the maintenance of tonic contraction occurs at lower Ca^{2+} concentrations and is characterized by much slower rates of crossbridge cycling, resulting in actin and myosin remaining bound for a greater percentage of time during the crossbridge cycle. This phenomenon has been called the latch state.[55, 56] This process requires calcium but in smaller concentrations than active shortening, and is associated with very low rates of myosin light chain phosphorylation. The latch state allows tonic contraction of sphincter muscles with very low levels of energy expenditure.

Stress maintenance in phasic muscles requires much more energy. Relaxation of smooth muscle occurs when $[Ca^{2+}]_i$ drops below levels capable of activating the contractile proteins as described above. This drop in $[Ca^{2+}]_i$ may occur by several mechanisms. First, hyperpolarization of the plasma membrane by neurohumoral agents closes voltage-gated Ca^{2+} channels, thereby decreasing entry of Ca^{2+} into the cell. It also decreases cell excitability by requiring a greater excitatory stimulus for the plasma membrane to reach threshold for action potential production. The interactions of inhibitory neurohumoral agents with their receptors also lower $[Ca^{2+}]_i$ through other mechanisms that are not dependent on membrane potential. These mechanisms include (1) increasing the activity of the plasma membrane and sarcoplasmic membrane Ca^{2+} pumps, (2) increasing the activity of a plasma membrane bound Na^+-Ca^{2+} exchanger, and (3) the phosphorylation of myosin light chain kinase so it cannot be activated and the crossbridge cycle cannot be stimulated. Specific phosphatases can dephosphorylate myosin light chains, leading to relaxation. However, their importance in the normal relaxation process is unclear.[57, 58] These processes will be discussed in detail below.

Regulation of Intracellular Calcium Concentration

Since the major mechanism by which activation of contractile proteins takes place is an increase in $[Ca^{2+}]_i$ from 0.1 to 0.2 μM in relaxed cells to only 1.0 to 4.0 μM in maximally contracted cells,[59-64] close regulation of $[Ca^{2+}]_i$ is required for normal muscle function. Because the extracellular free calcium ion concentration is 2.0 μM, the cell must be able to maintain a 10,000-fold lower $[Ca^{2+}]_i$ when relaxed. The maintenance of this Ca^{2+} gradient is one of the major tasks of smooth muscle cells. The two structures most responsible for maintaining and modulating $[Ca^{2+}]_i$ are the plasma membrane and sarcoplasmic reticulum (Fig. 3–10).

By virtue of its function as a barrier between intracellular and extracellular Ca^{2+} pools, the plasma membrane is the major cellular organelle responsible for maintaining cellular Ca^{2+} homeostasis (Fig. 3–10). In relaxed cells, the plasma membrane maintains a large inwardly directed electrochemical gradient to Ca^{2+}. This gradient is due to a 50 to 60 mV transmembrane potential difference and a 10,000-fold concentration difference between the extracellular space and the cytoplasmic compartment, both of which favor Ca^{2+} movement into the cell. This large electrochemical gradient and a low $[Ca^{2+}]_i$ are maintained because the plasma membrane has a very low permeability to Ca^{2+} and possesses a very efficient mechanism for transporting from the cell any Ca^{2+} that may enter, either by a passive leak or during the excitation process.

In smooth muscle, Ca^{2+} is transported out of the cell primarily by a plasma membrane–associated and calmodulin-stimulated $(Ca^{2+}$-$Mg^{2+})$-ATPase[65-68] (Fig.

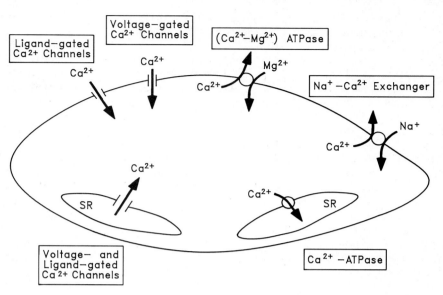

Figure 3–10. Schematic representation of $[Ca^{2+}]_i$ homeostasis in smooth muscle cell. In relaxed smooth muscles the intracellular calcium concentration is 0.1–0.2 μM, as compared with 2 mM in the extracellular fluid. The low $[Ca^{2+}]_i$ is maintained by a Ca^{2+}–Na^+ exchanger in the plasma membrane and Ca^{2+} pumps in the plasma membrane and sarcoplasmic reticulum. Increases in $[Ca^{2+}]_i$ that initiate smooth muscle contraction result from the opening of ligand-gated and/or voltage-gated channels in the plasma membrane and endoplasmic reticulum. $[Ca^{2+}]_i$ values of 1 to 4 μM are associated with maximal contraction. These values are substantially below extracellular Ca^{2+} concentrations.

3–10). When the smooth muscle is stimulated to contract, $[Ca^{2+}]_i$ rises to around 1 μM. As the Ca^{2+} concentration increases, Ca^{2+} begins to bind with a regulatory calcium-binding protein called calmodulin. The binding of four Ca^{2+} ions to a calmodulin molecule induces a conformational change that allows calmodulin to bind with and activate the $(Ca^{2+}\text{-}Mg^{2+})$-ATPase. As the Ca^{2+} pump lowers $[Ca^{2+}]_i$, Ca^{2+} dissociates from calmodulin, the calmodulin–$(Ca^{2+}\text{-}Mg^{2+})$-ATPase complex dissociates, and Ca^{2+} pump activity decreases to basal levels. Since the pump moves Ca^{2+} out of the cell against its electrochemical gradient, it requires energy in the form of ATP hydrolysis. It transports Ca^{2+} at a half-maximal rate when $[Ca^{2+}]_i$ is 0.25 μM and is maximally active at 1 μM. This means that the pump is active over the range of $[Ca^{2+}]_i$ encountered in resting smooth muscle cells, and is maximally activated at $[Ca^{2+}]_i$ levels that are associated with maximal contraction. These kinetic characteristics make this $(Ca^{2+}\text{-}Mg^{2+})$-ATPase a key regulator of $[Ca^{2+}]_i$ in resting and activated cells. Whether this mechanism plays a role in relaxation caused by neurohumoral agents is not known. Smooth muscle plasma membranes also possess a Na^+-Ca^{2+} exchanger that is able to transport Ca^{2+} out of the cell in exchange for transporting Na^+ into the cell. The energy required to transport Ca^{2+} against its electrochemical gradient is obtained from Na^+ moving down its electrochemical gradient. This exchange mechanism may play a role in ligand-induced relaxation.

The sarcoplasmic reticulum serves as the major intracellular Ca^{2+} storage pool[69-71] and is able to remove Ca^{2+} from the cytoplasm by means of an ATP-dependent Ca^{2+} uptake mechanism (Ca^{2+} pump)[65, 72, 73] (Fig. 3–10). Although this Ca^{2+} pump is like the pump found in plasma membrane, in that it utilizes ATP to transport Ca^{2+} against a concentration gradient, it is structurally different from its plasma membrane counterpart, and does not transport Mg^{2+}.[74, 75] The interaction of inhibitory neurohormonal agents with plasma

membrane receptors results in the activation of the sarcoplasmic reticulum Ca^{2+}-ATPase, thereby lowering $[Ca^{2+}]_i$ and producing relaxation. This Ca^{2+} pump also allows the sarcoplasmic reticulum to rapidly reaccumulate Ca^{2+} released during activation of contraction. This insures the intracellular Ca^{2+} supply needed during repetitive contractions in response to repeated neurohumoral or electrical stimulation.

Excitation-Contraction Coupling

During excitation $[Ca^{2+}]_i$ is increased as a result of Ca^{2+} release from the sarcoplasmic reticulum and from the opening of plasma membrane Ca^{2+} channels.[62-64] Excitation-contraction coupling refers to the mechanism by which excitation of the smooth muscle cell produces an increase in $[Ca^{2+}]_i$ and contraction.[76] There are two general mechanisms by which smooth muscle excitation elevates $[Ca^{2+}]_i$. One of these mechanisms involves cell membrane depolarization, while the other one is not associated with any membrane potential change.[77] It is important to point out that both of these mechanisms can occur simultaneously in the same cell, and that one neurohumoral agent may utilize one or both of these mechanisms.

The term *electromechanical coupling* is used to describe the phenomenon by which depolarization of plasma membrane leads to an increase in $[Ca^{2+}]_i$ and contraction. There are three mechanisms by which plasma membrane depolarization may lead to an increased $[Ca^{2+}]_i$: (1) by the diffusion of Ca^{2+} through voltage-gated Ca^{2+} channels during action potentials;[78-80] (2) by Ca^{2+} release from the sarcoplasmic reticulum in response to plasma membrane depolarization;[77, 81] and (3) by Ca^{2+} release from the sarcoplasmic reticulum in response to elevations in $[Ca^{2+}]_i$ brought about by action potentials (Ca^{2+}-induced Ca^{2+} release).[82] The mechanism by which smooth muscle spike potentials raise $[Ca^{2+}]_i$ is described later on in this chapter. The mechanisms for voltage-gated and Ca^{2+}-dependent release from sarcoplasmic reticulum remain unknown.

Although Ca^{2+} influx accompanying action potentials elevates $[Ca^{2+}]_i$ sufficiently to produce maximal contraction in some cells, this is not universally true.[77, 83] Therefore, voltage-dependent and Ca^{2+}-dependent Ca^{2+} release from the sarcoplasmic reticulum in response to action potentials must contribute to the $[Ca^{2+}]_i$ required for maximal contraction. The contribution of each mechanism to stimulated increases in $[Ca^{2+}]_i$ probably varies with different muscles and different stimuli.

Pharmacomechanical coupling refers to muscle contraction in response to drugs or neurohormonal agents without depolarizing the plasma membrane. It is normally due to a rise in $[Ca^{2+}]_i$ caused by release of calcium from sarcoplasmic reticulum. Inositol 1,4,5-trisphosphate appears to be the second messenger responsible for initiating this Ca^{2+} release (see Fig. 3–15).

ELECTRICAL ACTIVITY OF SMOOTH MUSCLES

All smooth muscle cells exhibit voltage differences between the cell interior and exterior that are brought about by the asymmetric distribution and movement of small inorganic ions across the plasma membrane.[59–61] This voltage difference is called the transmembrane potential difference. The important charge carrying ions responsible for generating potential differences include Na^+, Cl^-, K^+ and Ca^{2+}. The distribution and movement of ions across the plasma membrane are determined by specific plasma membrane properties and constituents. The plasma membrane is a lipid bilayer. It is practically impermeable to ions, because they are charged and surrounded by a large halo of H_2O in an aqueous environment such as the extracellular fluid. Therefore, all transmembrane ionic movements must occur by some process other than diffusion through the matrix of the lipid bilayer. Embedded within and spanning the plasma membrane are two classes of proteins responsible for transmembrane ion movements, ion pumps and ion channels (Table 3–1).

Ion pumps are proteins able to translocate ions across the plasma membrane. When pumps move ions against their electrochemical gradients, energy is required. Three important ion pumps are involved in regulation of ionic distribution across the smooth muscle cell. The pump most important for maintaining resting membrane potential is the *Na^+-K^+ pump ($[Na^+$-$K^+]$-ATPase)*[43] (see Fig. 3–12). It actively pumps Na^+ out of the cell and K^+ into the cell, thereby maintaining a greater K^+ concentration inside the cell than outside, and a greater Na^+ concentration outside than inside.[84, 85] Because the stoichiometry for transport is 3 Na^+ ions out for every 2 K^+ ions moved into the cell, Na^+ pump activity results in a net movement of

positive charge out of the cell, generating a more negative transmembrane potential difference. The Na^+-K^+ pump is able to control intracellular Na^+ concentration ($[Na^+]_i$) over a narrow range because its activity is very dependent upon $[Na^+]_i$. When $[Na^+]_i$ is increased, pump activity is stimulated, and Na^+ efflux is increased. The pump remains activated until $[Na^+]_i$ returns to resting levels. Pump activity is also stimulated when extracellular K^+ concentrations are increased. Because the Na^+-K^+ pump must transport both Na^+ and K^+ against their concentration gradients, energy is required. The energy to drive the pump is supplied by the hydrolysis of one ATP molecule for every 3 Na^+ and 2 K^+ ions translocated. *Calcium pumps* located in the plasma membrane and the sarcoplasmic reticulum have been described above. The *chloride pump,* which is present as a constituent of the plasma membrane, actively transports Cl^- into the cell against its electrochemical gradient to maintain resting intracellular Cl^- concentrations.[86, 87] Little is known about this transport mechanism.

Ion-selective channels are proteins that form aqueous tunnels spanning the plasma membrane. Thus, they provide hydrophilic pathways allowing the passive diffusion of charged ions through the lipid bilayer. Channel proteins exist in two interconvertible structural conformations, open and closed. In their open conformation, channels allow the free diffusion of ions across the plasma membrane, and in their closed conformation ion movement is blocked. Many different types of ion channels have been described. Most of the channels are ion selective. That is, they act as selectivity filters, allowing the passage of only one ionic species. In smooth muscle K^+-selective and Ca^{2+}-selective channels have been identified. Some channels are selective for cations but do not distinguish between different species of cations. It should also be remembered that there may be several species of channels that are selective for a particular ion. For example, one type of K^+ channel is controlled by changes in membrane potential, while another is controlled by hormones.

Ion selective channels can be either nongated or gated. The nongated ion channels are also called passive or leak channels, as they always remain open.[88] Although there are some questions regarding the existence of the passive ion channels, passive K^+ channels are considered to be primarily responsible for the resting membrane potential. Gated ion channels, also called active channels, can be opened and closed by changes in membrane potential difference, or by neurohormonal agents.[78, 79] Accordingly, gated ion channels are classified as voltage- or ligand-gated ion channels, respectively[43] (see Fig. 3–12).

Voltage-gated ion channels are defined as channels that open and close in response to changes in transmembrane potential difference (Fig. 3–11). Some voltage-gated ion channels are also ion-selective, allowing the passage of one particular ionic species. For example, there are voltage-gated Ca^{2+} and voltage-gated K^+ channels. Different types of voltage-gated channels also have different voltage sensitivities,[80] so at a partic-

Table 3–1. CHARACTERISTICS AND FUNCTIONS OF ION PUMPS AND CHANNELS IN SMOOTH MUSCLE

Transport System	Characteristics	Function
Ion Pumps		
Na$^+$-K$^+$ pump (Na$^+$-K$^+$-ATPase)	Constituent of cell membrane Transports 3 Na out for 2 K into the cell Activity increased by [Na$^+$]$_i$; [K$^+$]$_e$	Maintains large K$^+$ and Na$^+$ concentration gradients across plasma membrane Contributes to resting membrane potential Responsible for repolarization phase of slow waves
Ca^{2+} pump (Ca^{2+}-Mg^{2+}-ATPase)	Present in plasma membrane	Pumps Ca^{2+} outside of the cell and maintains 1000-fold lower Ca^{2+} concentration intracellularly
Ca^{2+} pump (Ca^{2+}-ATPase)	Present on endoplasmic reticulum	Pumps Ca^{2+} into sarcoplasmic reticulum
Cl$^-$ pump (Not known)	Present in plasma membrane Transports Cl$^-$ into the cells against electrochemical gradient	Maintains Cl$^-$ concentration gradient Contributes to resting membrane potential
Ion Exchangers		
Na$^+$-Ca^{2+} exchanger	Transports Ca^{2+} out of and Na$^+$ into the cell Does not require ATP hydrolysis for energy	Plays a role in neurotransmitter-induced relaxation
Ion-Selective Channels		
PASSIVE CHANNELS		
Na$^+$-K$^+$ leak channels	They always remain open Their presence not well documented	Thought to contribute to resting membrane potential
VOLTAGE-GATED CHANNELS		
K$^+$ channels (Ca^{2+}-activated K$^+$ channel)	Depolarization and ↑[Ca^{2+}]$_i$ increase probability of channel being open	Increases K$^+$ efflux Responsible for repolarizing phase of AP
Ca^{2+} channels	Majority closed at RMP Probability of being open increases with depolarization	Responsible for (1) rising phase of AP and (2) plateau of slow waves in cat intestine
LIGAND-GATED CHANNELS		
K$^+$ channels	Inhibitory agents, e.g., β-adrenergics or VIP, increase probability of channel being open Excitatory agents, e.g., substance P or muscarinic agonists, decrease probability of channel being open	Increases K$^+$ efflux, resulting in hyperpolarization Decreases K$^+$ efflux, resulting in depolarization
Cation selective	Most are closed at RMP Opened by excitatory agents (muscarinic agonists or substance P)	Opening increases transmembrane cation fluxes, resulting in depolarization
Cl$^-$ channels	Not clearly demonstrated in smooth muscle	Changing Cl$^-$ conductance may depolarize or hyperpolarize the cell, depending on membrane potential

RMP, resting membrane potential; AP, action potential.
It is not known whether excitatory and inhibitory agents modulate the same channel.

(A) LIGAND-GATED CHANNEL

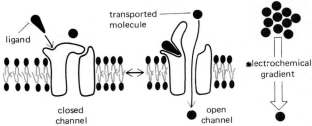

Figure 3–11. Schematic diagram of gated ion channels. Ion channels allow ions to pass down their electrochemical gradient only when the channel proteins are in their open configuration. The channel in *A* is ligand-gated. It is opened either when a neurohormonal agent binds to it or when a second messenger generated at a separate receptor site interacts with the channel. Voltage-gated channels *(B)* are open by changes in membrane potential. Depending upon the channel, depolarization or hyperpolarization may be the stimulus for opening. *B* depicts a voltage-gated channel that opens during depolarization of the membrane. (From Alberts, B., Bray, D., Lewis, J., et al. Molecular Biology of the Cell. New York, Garland Publishing, 1983. Used by permission.)

(B) VOLTAGE-GATED CHANNEL

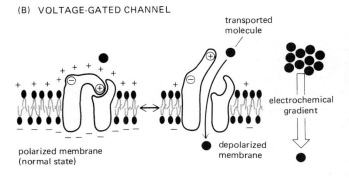

ular membrane potential some ion-selective voltage-gated channels will be open, while others will be closed. For example, at resting potential almost all the Ca^{2+}-selective voltage-gated channels are closed, while a significant proportion of the K^+-selective voltage-regulated channels are open.

The mechanism by which membrane potential controls voltage-gated channels is best understood by considering the behavior of channels as charged proteins in a large electrical field.[89, 90] When such a molecule is placed in a strong electrical field, such as that generated by membrane potential differences, the field interacts with charged surface groups on the protein. Changes in the electrical field brought about by changes in membrane potential distort the spatial configuration of voltage-gated channels. Depending on the membrane potential difference, this allows voltage-gated channels to adopt any of three relatively stable conformations. These include: (1) a closed conformation that does not allow the diffusion of ions through the channel, but that can be opened by a change in membrane potential; (2) an active and open conformation that allows free diffusion of one ionic species across the channel; and (3) in some voltage-gated channels an inactivated state that does not allow ions to pass whether the channel is in the open or closed conformation. Voltage-gated channels are able to make almost instantaneous transitions between open and closed states, while the transition from the active to the inactive conformation is slower, and occurs after a change in membrane potential has transformed a channel to its open state.

Ligand-gated channels are transmembrane ion channels that are opened or closed in response to the direct interaction of hormones or neurotransmitters with their plasma membrane receptors (Fig. 3–11). When a stimulatory agent binds to and activates its receptor, a signal is produced that changes the conformation of the ion channel—either opening or closing the channel, depending on the receptor occupied. This alters ion movement across the plasma membrane, thereby changing membrane potential and smooth muscle cell excitability. It is likely that some ligand-gated channels contain receptors as part of their structure, while other ligand-gated channels and their receptors are separate proteins that communicate via intracellular second messengers such as inositol-1,4,5-trisphosphate or cAMP.

Resting Membrane Potential

Resting membrane potential is the voltage difference across the plasma membrane when the cell is under no excitatory or inhibitory influences. It is defined in electrical terms as a steady state; that is, the membrane potential at which net ionic flow across the plasma membrane is 0. Depending on the gastrointestinal smooth muscles studied, this potential ranges from -40 mV to -75 mV (Table 3–2, Fig. 3–12), with the interior of the cell being negative relative to its exterior. The resting membrane potential is generated by the diffusion of ions through ion-selective channels (Fig. 3–12).

Most of the resting potential is due to K^+ diffusing out of the cell through K^+-selective channels, a certain proportion of which remain open at rest. This diffusion of K^+ out of the cell, down its concentration gradient, makes the cell interior negative relative to its exterior. Because the equilibrium potential for K^+, that is, the potential difference at which there would be no net movement of K^+, is -89 mV, the outward movement of K^+ continues at the resting membrane potential. The diffusion of other inorganic ions across the plasma membrane contributes little to resting membrane potential, because the resting membrane is much less

Table 3–2. RESTING MEMBRANE POTENTIAL, SPONTANEOUS CHANGES IN MEMBRANE POTENTIAL, AND SPONTANEOUS CONTRACTIONS IN SOME GASTROINTESTINAL SMOOTH MUSCLES

	Resting Membrane Potential	Spontaneous Membrane Depolarizations	Spontaneous Contractions
Esophagus			
Esophageal body	-48 mV	None	None
Lower esophageal sphincter	-40 mV	Spikes	Tonic
Stomach			
Fundus	-48 mV	None	Tonic
Midcorpus	-60 mV	Slow waves 5/min (with prepotentials)	5/min
Caudad corpus	-63 mV	Slow waves (3.5/min)	3.5/min
Antrum	-70 mV	Slow waves (0.5/min) ($\pm$ spikes)	0.5/min
Pyloric ring	-75 mV	Slow waves (0.5/min) + oscil. pot. + spikes	0.5/min
Small Intestine			
Duodenum	-68 mV	Slow waves 12/min ($\pm$ spikes)	12/min
Jejunum		Slow waves 8/min ($\pm$ spikes)	8/min
Ileum		Slow waves 5/min ($\pm$ spikes)	5/min
Large Intestine			
Colon—taenia 1/1–5 min (human, dog)	-50 mV	Oscil. pot. (17–36/min) $\pm$ spike burst 1–5 min	
Colon—circular (human) 6/min		Oscil. pot. (14–58/min) $\pm$ spikes	
Colon—circular (dog)		Slow waves (6–8/min)	
Internal anal sphincter		Oscil. pot. ($\sim$ 20/min) Tonic	

Oscil. pot., oscillation potential.

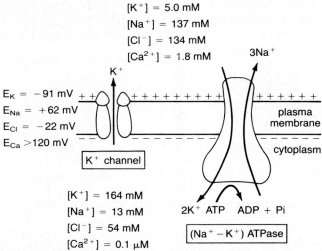

$[K^+] = 5.0$ mM
$[Na^+] = 137$ mM
$[Cl^-] = 134$ mM
$[Ca^{2+}] = 1.8$ mM

$E_K = -91$ mV
$E_{Na} = +62$ mV
$E_{Cl} = -22$ mV
$E_{Ca} > 120$ mV

plasma membrane
cytoplasm

K$^+$ channel

$[K^+] = 164$ mM
$[Na^+] = 13$ mM
$[Cl^-] = 54$ mM
$[Ca^{2+}] = 0.1$ μM

2K$^+$ ATP   ADP + Pi
(Na$^+$–K$^+$) ATPase

Figure 3–12. The origin of smooth muscle resting membrane potential, transmembrane ion distributions in the resting cell, and equilibrium potentials (E_x) for ionic species contributing to resting potential. The (Na$^+$-K$^+$)-ATPase generates the Na$^+$ and K$^+$ concentration gradients depicted. Open K$^+$ channels make the membrane much more permeable to K$^+$ than any other ionic species, and allow K$^+$ diffusion out of the cell, down its concentration gradient. The result is a resting transmembrane potential difference, with the interior of the cell being negative relative to its exterior.

permeable to ions other than K$^+$. However, at resting potential there is some inward Na$^+$ diffusion and outward Cl$^-$ diffusion, making resting potential somewhat less negative than would be the case for a membrane permeable only to K$^+$.

The Na$^+$-K$^+$ pump and Cl$^-$ pump are responsible for maintaining the transmembrane concentration gradients for Na$^+$, K$^+$, and Cl$^-$. Without these pumps the diffusion of ions occurring at rest would run down the transmembrane concentration gradients and the resting membrane potential would be lost. In addition, since the Na$^+$-K$^+$ pump translocates 3 Na$^+$ out of the cell for every 2 K$^+$ into the cell, there is a net movement of positive charge out of the cell. This charge movement contributes about -5 mV to resting membrane potential. Moreover, a Cl$^-$ pump, which transports Cl$^-$ into the cell, appears to contribute from -5 to -15 mV to resting membrane potential.[59]

The resting membrane potential is important in determining how easily a muscle cell may be excited. For example, the resting potential of muscle cells from the gastric fundus is less negative than the resting potential of cells from the antrum. This results in muscle from the fundus being more easily excited than muscle from the antrum.

Spontaneous and Repetitive Membrane Depolarization

The membrane potential difference in most smooth muscle is not a steady value. Instead, it exhibits spontaneous and repetitive depolarizations and repolarizations[91] (Fig. 3–13). There are several patterns of

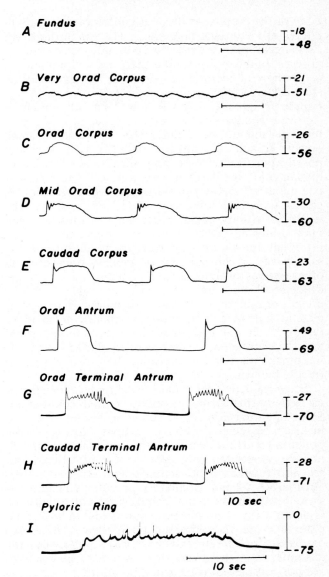

Figure 3–13. Spectrum of intracellular resting membrane potentials and spontaneous and repetitive depolarizations in smooth muscle. This illustration demonstrates the heterogeneity of electrical behavior of different smooth muscles. (From Szurszewski, J. H. *In* Johnson, L. R. [ed.]. Physiology of the Gastrointestinal Tract. 2nd ed. New York, Raven Press, 1987. Used by permission.)

spontaneous and repetitive membrane depolarization in gastrointestinal smooth muscle. For the sake of description they can be classified into: (1) slow, short-duration oscillations of membrane potential occurring at frequencies of 20 to 50 per minute, *oscillatory potentials;* (2) slower and longer duration oscillations of membrane potential occurring at frequencies of 1 to 18 per minute, *slow waves;* (3) very slow, long-duration depolarizations of the plasma membrane lasting over a minute; and (4) brief spike-like membrane depolarizations, *spike potentials.*

The patterns of spontaneous and repetitive membrane depolarizations are different in different gastrointestinal muscles (Table 3–2). For example, in the body of the esophagus there are no spontaneous oscillations of membrane potential,[92] whereas in the lower esophageal sphincter there is continuous spike activity at rest.[93] In the gastric fundus there are no spontaneous oscillations of membrane potential, but in the distal stomach slow waves recur at a rate of 3 to 5 per minute[3] (Fig. 3–13). Small bowel smooth muscle is characterized by slow waves that occur at a rate of 5 to 12 per minute, depending upon the site in the small bowel.[4] In addition, spike potentials may be superimposed upon slow waves. The membrane potential of human colon oscillates at a fast rate of 14 to 58 cycles per minute.[94] Apart from organ-to-organ variation in electrical activity observed within one species, the electrical activity of the same smooth muscle organ may vary from species to species. For example, guinea pig small intestine is characterized by absence of any slow waves, in contrast to very stable slow waves in all other species of animals.[4] The circular muscle of the dog colon[95] generates slow waves at a rate of 6 to 8 cycles per minute, whereas the membrane potential of circular human colonic muscle oscillates much more rapidly.[94] The patterns of resting membrane potential and the spontaneous membrane depolarization in different smooth muscles determine their distinctive contractile behavior.[3]

The term action potential is used to describe electrical activity that results in smooth muscle contraction. Spike potentials are action potentials because they are invariably associated with contractions. Slow wave-like potentials with a wide plateau that occur in the stomach are also associated with prominent contractions, and are also referred to as action potentials (Fig. 3–13). On the other hand, oscillatory potential changes and slow membrane potential changes are not usually associated with a prominent contraction unless spike potentials are superimposed upon them. Therefore, oscillatory potentials and slow wave potentials—for example, those occurring in small and large bowel—are not considered to be action potentials.

Slow Waves

Slow waves are slow, low-amplitude oscillations of muscle membrane potential.[96] Individual slow waves consist of a rapid depolarizing phase, a partial repolarization, a prolonged plateau potential lasting from one to several seconds, and a slow repolarization to resting membrane potential. Slow wave amplitude ranges from 15 to 30 mV. The frequency of their recurrence, while relatively constant for any organ, varies from 3 cycles per minute in the stomach to 12 cycles per minute in the duodenum. Slow waves propagate over varying lengths of bowel from their site of origin. When the plasma membrane of a smooth muscle generating slow waves is depolarized by neurohumoral stimulation, the plateau phase of a slow wave becomes more positive, reaching a membrane potential more positive than the threshold for spike potential production, and a burst of spike potentials is triggered on the plateau of

depolarized phase. This results in contraction. Since the slow waves set the pace for spike burst generation and hence contractions, the slow waves are also called pacesetter potentials.

Slow waves are generated by interstitial cells present at the boundary between the longitudinal and circular muscle layers of the small bowel[6, 7, 97] and at the junctional zone between the submucosa and circular muscle layer of the colon.[98]

The ionic basis of slow waves is not the same in all gastrointestinal viscera.[96] Slow waves of cat intestine result from the cyclical turning on and off of a plasma membrane–bound electrogenic sodium pump, the (Na^+-K^+)-ATPase. The model of slow wave generation in the cat intestine proposes that there is a continuous leak of Na^+ into the cell through Na^+ channels. When the Na^+ pump is turned off, this Na^+ conductance results in depolarization of the plasma membrane, accounting for the rising phase of the slow waves. Turning the pump on during the plateau phase repolarizes the cell to resting membrane potential by generating an outward Na^+ current that is greater than the passive Na^+ leak current. There is considerable experimental evidence to support this hypothesis. First, when the plasma membrane is experimentally held at resting potential and transmembrane current flow is measured, rhythmic inward currents recurring at the slow wave frequency are seen. These inward currents occur without a change in membrane resistance, indicating that they arise by a mechanism other than changes in membrane permeability. Second, the addition of ouabain to or the removal of K^+ from the experimental bathing solution—both maneuvers that inhibit (Na^+-K^+)-ATPase activity—abolishes slow wave activity. Third, the intracellular injection of Na^+—a maneuver that increases (Na^+-K^+)-ATPase activity—increases slow wave amplitude. Fourth, Na^+ efflux from cat smooth muscle tissues is maximal during the early repolarizing phase of the slow wave, as would be expected if increased Na^+ pump activity is responsible for the repolarizing phase of the slow wave. The plateau phase (plateau potential) of the slow wave is produced by an increase in membrane permeability to Ca^{2+} that results from the opening of voltage-gated Ca^{2+} channels as the membrane depolarizes. The evidence supporting an increased Ca^{2+} conductance as the mechanism for plateau potentials comes from studies in which cat intestinal muscle was incubated either in Ca^{2+}-deficient or Mg^{2+}-containing solutions. Both of these interventions, which are known to inhibit transmembrane Ca^{2+} flux, diminish the amplitude and duration of plateau potentials without influencing slow wave frequency.

In the rabbit small intestine, the rising phase of each slow wave is generated by a transient increase in membrane permeability to Na^+ and the plateau potential is the result of an increase in Cl^- movement down its electrochemical gradient out of the cell. The increased Cl^- conductance results from the opening of certain ill-defined Cl^- channels by membrane depolarization. The evidence in favor of this hypothesis includes: (1) a decreased membrane resistance at the peak of slow wave depolarization, indicating the opening of ion channels; (2) the loss of slow wave activity when tissues are bathed in Na^+-deficient solutions; and (3) the reduction of the amplitudes and durations of plateau potentials when Cl^- is replaced by less permeant ions.

After originating in the interstitial cell of Cajal, slow waves follow a complex propagation path into the muscularis propria. Connor and coworkers have hypothesized that low-amplitude slow waves of the small intestine first passively spread from their generator sites into the circular layer, where they initiate an active response that amplifies the slow wave enough to generate spike potentials.[99] The amplified current then spreads back to the longitudinal muscle, where it reinforces the slow wave in the longitudinal muscle. Alternatively, Bortoff and Sachs have proposed that slow waves are conducted along the small intestine primarily by local currents in the longitudinal muscle, and spread passively into the circular muscle.[100]

The slow waves spread at a rate of approximately 10 cm/sec; they spread 5 to 10 times faster circumferentially than longitudinally.[96, 101] Exact rates vary from organ to organ. This difference appears to be due to the fact that smooth muscle cells in the circular layer are coupled by many low-resistance gap junctions, while muscle cells in the longitudinal muscle have few if any gap junctions.

When electrical recordings are made from an intact length of small bowel, slow waves arise in the proximal portion and propagate aborally. However, when the bowel is cut circumferentially into 1- to 2-cm lengths, slow wave generators in each segment are unmasked.[3, 96, 102] Each segment generates slow waves at a different frequency, with each more aboral segment generating slow waves at an intrinsic frequency that is lower than the preceding segment. Thus, the propagated slow wave is replaced by numerous autonomous slow wave generators that describe a gradient in slow wave frequency, with the highest frequency at the orad end. This production of propagated slow waves by the interaction of a series of slow wave generators or "pacemakers" is best modeled as a chain of relaxation oscillators coupled to one another through a resistance.[102] The oscillator with the highest frequency occupies the most proximal site, and the oscillator with the lowest frequency the most distal site. When coupled in a chain, the oscillator with the highest frequency controls the frequency of the others over a considerable length of the chain. In smooth muscle tissues, slow waves from the fastest pacemaker site passively spread to the next slower pacemaker. Upon its arrival the slow wave stimulates the generation of a slow wave by the slower generator, at a time when it normally would not produce a slow wave. In this way, the faster pacemaker "entrains" its neighbor to a more rapid frequency. The process of slow wave propagation and regeneration by spread from pacemaker to pacemaker continues until the frequency of a distant pacemaker cannot be entrained by the faster pacemaker. When oscillators are uncoupled from the chain, each oscillates at its own intrinsic frequency.[4] Because the slow wave frequency and propagation velocity determine the frequency and velocity of propagation of smooth muscle contractions, disorders of slow waves are associated with several motor disorders of the gut such as tachygastria, gastric arrhythmia,[103] and intestinal motor disorders.[4, 5]

Spike Potentials

Spike potentials in smooth muscle are single, rapid voltage transients lasting 100 to 200 msec. Each consists of a rapid depolarizing phase that peaks in 10 to 25 msec and a slower repolarizing phase that brings the membrane back to resting potential. Under physiologic conditions the peak potential is seldom more positive than 0 mV.

Spikes may occur spontaneously in smooth muscle cells that have resting membrane potentials above the threshold value for generation of spike potential, as is the case at the lower esophageal sphincter. Alternatively, spikes occur when membrane potential is depolarized above a certain threshold voltage (-25 to -35 mV) by slow waves or stimulatory neurohumoral agents. Smooth muscle spikes are due to rapid movement of Ca^{2+} into the cell. The cellular mechanism underlying spike potentials is as follows. When the muscle membrane depolarizes, some voltage-gated Ca^{2+} channels make a rapid transition to their open state. The subsequent influx of positively charged Ca^{2+} ions depolarizes the membrane more, thereby opening more channels and producing more depolarization.[104-106] This positive feedback loop is responsible for the rapid depolarizing phase of the action potential. It will continue to drive plasma membrane toward the equilibrium potential for Ca^{2+} (> 120 mV), if other mechanisms do not intervene. Since action potentials seldom overshoot 0 mV, the cell must possess mechanisms for breaking this positive feedback loop, and subsequently repolarizing the cell. One way the positive feedback mechanism is interrupted is by the transition of open Ca^{2+} channels to their inactive conformation.[107] This decreases Ca^{2+} conductance and arrests the rising phase of the action potential. The other mechanism tending to restore resting membrane potential is the initiation of an outward K^+ current during the depolarizing phase of the action potential.[80] This increased K^+ conductance drives the membrane potential to more negative values. The increased K^+ conductance occurs through Ca^{2+}-activated K^+ channels[80, 108-110] that open in response to increases in $[Ca^{2+}]_i$. These K^+ channels are also voltage-gated, so that they are opened by membrane depolarization. Thus, increasing $[Ca^{2+}]_i$ and membrane depolarization, both of which occur during action potentials, increase K^+ conductance. With the lowering of $[Ca^{2+}]_i$ and increasing membrane potential to their resting values, Ca^{2+}-activated K^+ channels close and the steady state is once again attained.

Smooth muscle cells in which spike potentials originate can be recognized by occurrence of prepotential or initial depolarization, which drives the membrane potential to its threshold for spike production. Once generated, the spike potential is propagated to other electrically coupled cells. The muscle cells that conduct action potentials do not have prepotentials.

Induced Changes in Membrane Potential

Excitatory stimuli, such as electrical currents spreading from neighboring smooth muscle cells, or stretch or excitatory neurohumoral agents interacting with their smooth muscle receptors, make the membrane potential more positive. That is, they depolarize the cell.[111, 112] On the other hand, inhibitory neurohumoral agents make the membrane potential more negative, that is, they hyperpolarize the cell.[113] These changes in membrane potential are brought about either by changes in plasma membrane permeability to specific ions (opening or closing ion-selective channels), or by changing (Na^+-K^+)-ATPase activity. If the smooth muscle is spontaneously active—that is, if its membrane potential spontaneously oscillates, as is the case with slow waves—the effects of external stimuli will be superimposed upon spontaneous electrical activity. Thus, excitatory stimuli depolarize the muscle and accentuate spontaneous oscillations. Hyperpolarizing stimuli attenuate spontaneous depolarizations.

Ligand-induced changes in membrane potential are exemplified by the action of acetylcholine or VIP. In many smooth muscles, the interaction of acetylcholine with muscarinic cholinergic receptors closes a population of K^+ channels that are open at rest.[111] The accompanying decrease in K^+ conductance results in membrane depolarization. In other smooth muscles, muscarinic receptor stimulation causes depolarization by opening a population of channels that are not selective for any one ionic species, but allow the passage of several cationic species, including K^+, Na^+, and Ca^{2+}.[112] The net effect of such a simultaneous increase in membrane permeability to several cations is depolarization. These mechanisms of depolarization may allow the membrane potential to exceed the threshold for generation of spike potentials. In most smooth muscle, threshold is from -25 to -35 mV. The interaction of VIP with its smooth muscle receptors increases the proportion of open K^+ channels, thereby increasing the plasma membrane permeability to K^+. The resultant increase in K^+ efflux produces membrane hyperpolarization. Plasma membrane hyperpolarization reduces smooth muscle cell excitability, inhibiting contractions.

SECOND MESSENGERS MEDIATING EFFECTS OF NEUROHORMONAL AGENTS

The interactions of neurotransmitters, hormones, or drugs with specific plasma membrane receptor proteins can produce contraction or relaxation of smooth muscle cells. Such receptors exert their effect either by modulating ion channels directly, or by stimulating the production of intracellular mediators, called second messengers, which may modify the activity of ion channels, membrane pumps, or the contractile proteins themselves. Two major second messengers are inositol 1,4,5-triphosphate (Fig. 3–14) and cyclic nucleotides (Fig. 3–15).

A group of lipids known as the inositol lipids are present on the inner leaflet of the plasma membrane (Fig. 3–14). Binding of an excitatory neurohumoral agent, like acetylcholine, to its receptor activates a specific phosphodiesterase (phospholipase C),[114–116] which hydrolyzes one of the inositol lipids, phosphatidylinositol 4,5-biphosphate (PIP$_2$), to inositol 1,4,5-triphosphate and diacylglycerol. Both of these com-

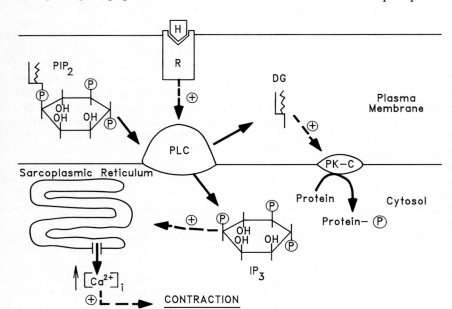

Figure 3–14. The role of inositol 1,4,5-triphosphate as the excitatory second messenger responsible for pharmacomechanical coupling in smooth muscle. Hormone (H) binds to its receptor (R). Receptor activation turns on a specific phosphodiesterase, phospholipase C (PLC), which hydrolyzes phosphatidylinositol 4,5-biphosphate (PIP$_2$) to inositol 1,4,5-triphosphate (IP$_3$) and diacylglycerol (DG). IP$_3$ becomes a second messenger, releasing Ca^{2+} from the sarcoplasmic reticulum, and DG activates protein kinase C.

Figure 3–15. Cyclic AMP as a second messenger responsible for smooth muscle relaxation. Plasma membrane–bound adenylate cyclase is a complex of five components: a stimulatory receptor (R_s); an inhibitory receptor (R_i); a stimulatory guanine nucleotide–binding protein (G_s); an inhibitory guanine nucleotide–binding protein (G_i); and a catalytic subunit (C). Binding of hormone to R_s leads to an increase in cAMP production, as described in the text. Cyclic AMP activates cAMP-dependent protein kinase, which is able to phosphorylate many target proteins, including (1) a portion of the plasma membrane (Na^+-K^+)-ATPase; (2) myosin light chain kinase (MLCK); (3) a sarcoplasmic reticulum Ca^{2+}-ATPase; and (4) plasma membrane channel proteins, particularly the K^+ channel. Phosphorylation of each target protein can result in inhibition of contraction. Binding of hormone to R_i leads to a decrease in cAMP production, as described in the text.

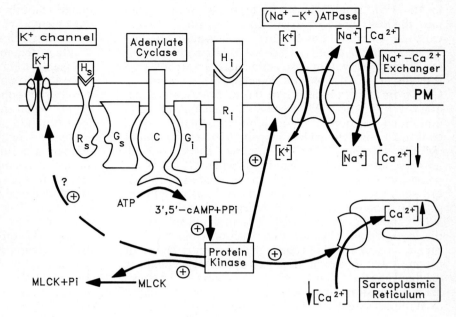

pounds serve as second messengers. Inositol 1,4,5-triphosphate diffuses through the cytoplasm to the endoplasmic reticulum, where it initiates Ca^{2+} release. Although the mechanism by which this Ca^{2+} release occurs is not known, recent work on striated muscle indicates that the sarcoplasmic reticulum contains Ca^{2+} channels that can be opened by second messenger molecules.[117] Once inositol 1,4,5-triphosphate has dissociated from its binding site, the sarcoplasmic reticulum sequesters free cytoplasmic calcium and inositol 1,4,5-triphosphate is recycled to phosphatidylinositol 4,5-biphosphate via a number of enzymatic reactions. It is not known whether inositol 1,4,5-triphosphate or some other signal modulates the ligand-gated channels responsible for membrane depolarization in response to muscarinic receptor stimulation. Diacylglycerol activates a Ca^{2+}-dependent and phospholipid-dependent protein kinase (protein kinase C). Protein kinase C phosphorylates a number of cellular proteins. Although activation of protein kinase C can alter the contractile state of smooth muscle, results to date are conflicting and its physiologic role remains unclear.

The activation of adenylate cyclase is a major pathway by which inhibitory neurohumoral agents inhibit smooth muscle contraction. The adenylate cyclase complex consists of five separate plasma membrane–bound components (Fig. 3–15).[118, 119] There are two types of receptors: stimulatory receptors (R_s), like VIP and beta-adrenergic receptors, that stimulate adenylate cyclase when activated, and inhibitory receptors (R_i), like muscarinic acetylcholine receptors, that inhibit adenylate cyclase when activated. There are also two different guanine nucleotide–binding proteins. One is inhibitory (G_i) and inhibits adenylate cyclase when activated by R_i, while the other is stimulatory (G_s) and stimulates adenylate cyclase when activated by R_s. Finally, there is a catalytic subunit (C) that converts ATP to cAMP. When neither receptor type is activated

by agonist, G_s and G_i bind GDP and are inactive. The result is a slow basal conversion of ATP to cAMP. Activation of stimulatory receptors (e.g., by beta-adrenergic agonists or VIP) increases the affinity of stimulatory guanine nucleotide–binding protein for GTP. Binding GTP allows the interaction of guanine nucleotide–binding protein with the catalytic unit, and results in stimulation of adenylate cyclase activity. The activated state is short-lived, however, because guanine nucleotide–binding protein has intrinsic GTPase activity that hydrolyzes GTP to GDP. GTP hydrolysis results in the uncoupling of guanine nucleotide–binding protein from the catalytic unit, and a fall in cyclase activity to basal levels. Activation of inhibitory receptors by agonists, like acetylcholine, initiates an almost identical series of events, except that inhibitory guanine nucleotide–binding protein is activated, thereby decreasing adenylate cyclase activity. Thus, muscarinic receptor activation initiates contraction by simultaneously turning on excitatory mechanisms (inositol 1,4,5-triphosphate and ligand-gated channels) and turning off inhibitory effector systems (adenylate cyclase).

Cyclic AMP generated by hormone-stimulated adenylate cyclase becomes a second messenger and exerts its effects on smooth muscle by activating specific cellular enzymes—cAMP-dependent protein kinases.[120, 121] Activated protein kinases then phosphorylate target proteins throughout the cell, thereby regulating their activities. Many of these target proteins play crucial roles in the control of contractile function. Cyclic AMP–dependent mechanisms inhibit smooth muscle contraction by decreasing $[Ca^{2+}]_i$ in two ways. First, cAMP-dependent phosphorylation of the plasma membrane (Na^+-K^+)-ATPase increases Na^+-K^+ pump activity. Increased Na^+ export brought about by activation of the pump accelerates a Na^+-Ca^{2+} exchanger that lowers $[Ca^{2+}]_i$ by exchanging extracellular Na^+ for intracellular Ca^{2+}. In addition, since the pump translocates 3 Na^+ out of the cell for each 2 K^+ translocated into the cell, there is a net loss of positive charge, which results in membrane hyperpolarization and decreased cell excitability. Cyclic AMP–dependent protein kinase activation also stimulates a sarcoplasmic reticulum Ca^{2+}-ATPase that lowers $[Ca^{2+}]_i$ by pumping Ca^{2+} from the cytoplasm into the sarcoplasmic reticulum.[123, 124] Cyclic AMP-dependent mechanisms also inhibit contraction by modulating the activity of a contractile protein called myosin light chain kinase (MLCK) (see Fig. 3–9).[125] As discussed earlier, smooth muscle contraction is initiated only when MLCK phosphorylates a particular protein associated with the myosin head—the myosin light chain. Phosphorylation of MLCK occurs by a cAMP-dependent mechanism.[126] When phosphorylated, MLCK cannot phosphorylate the myosin light chain and contraction cannot occur. Finally, in many cell types, the phosphorylation of plasma membrane ion channels by cAMP-dependent mechanisms may increase K^+ permeability.[127] This also leads to membrane hyperpolarization and decreased excitability. Although such a mechanism is very likely in smooth muscle, its existence has not been firmly proved.

Stimulation of guanylate cyclase by activation of certain receptors leads to elevation of intracellular guanosine 3′,5′-monophosphate cGMP. Elevation of cyclic GMP levels may also cause phosphorylation of myosin light chain kinase, leading to relaxation of smooth muscle.[128] Lower esophageal sphincter relaxation has been shown to be mediated by either cAMP or cGMP.[129]

SMOOTH MUSCLE ENERGY METABOLISM

Smooth muscle cells depend upon a steady and continuous supply of energy to carry out their cellular functions. These functions include: (1) the maintenance of transmembrane ion gradients and resting membrane potential by the (Na^+-K^+)-ATPase; (2) force generation resulting from the cyclical activity of actin-activated myosin ATPase (the crossbridge cycle); and (3) the regulation of $[Ca^{2+}]_i$ by sarcoplasmic reticulum and plasma membrane–bound Ca^{2+}-ATPases. The immediate sources of energy used to carry out these functions are ATP and high-energy compounds like phosphocreatine that readily give up their phosphates to ADP when ATP turnover is rapid. In smooth muscle, the reservoirs of ATP and phosphocreatine are so small that they can sustain contractile or other metabolic activity for only a few minutes in the absence of continuous and well-regulated ATP synthesis.[130]

The biochemical pathways for ATP synthesis in smooth muscle include enzyme systems for glycogenolysis, glycolysis (the Embden-Meyerhof pathway), the Krebs cycle, and the respiratory chain. These pathways utilize glycogen, glucose, free fatty acids, and free amino acids as substrates for ATP synthesis. Oxidative phosphorylation is the major pathway by which unstimulated smooth muscles support their basal energy requirements. The preferred substrate for oxidation in the resting cell is free fatty acids.[131]

When the smooth muscle is stimulated to contract, ATP utilization increases linearly with active isometric force.[132] The amount of isometric force generated can be altered either by changing the concentration of agonist when the tissue is held at a constant length, or by maintaining a constant stimulus and changing overall tissue length. In each case, the increase in ATP utilization occurring with active isometric force generation can be divided into two components: the ATP utilized by the contractile machinery, and ATP utilized by other energy-requiring processes stimulated during activation. This second group includes such things as ion pumps.

The ATP utilized by myosin ATPase during crossbridge cycling is almost exclusively provided through oxidative phosphorylation.[133] Glycogen is the substrate for oxidation (Fig. 3–16). The intracellular signal that appears to couple glycogen breakdown (glycogenolysis) with contraction is Ca^{2+}. The steps by which this occurs are as follows. When the cell is stimulated to contract, $[Ca^{2+}]_i$ increases. In addition to initiating Ca^{2+}-calmodulin-MLCK activation, the increased $[Ca^{2+}]_i$ also activates phosphorylase kinase.[134] Activated kinase phosphorylates glycogen phosphorylase b, converting it to the activated phosphorylase a. Phosphorylase a breaks down glycogen. Glycogenolysis and contraction are closely coupled because phosphorylase kinase and contraction are activated over the same range of $[Ca^{2+}]_i$. Once glycogen is broken down to glycose 1-phosphate, it can be metabolized to pyruvate through the glycolytic pathway and then utilized by the Krebs cycle and the respiratory chain to produce ATP. Glucose is not directly utilized as a substrate for oxidative phosphorylation.

The plasma membrane–bound (Na^+-K^+)-ATPase uses ATP supplied by aerobic glycolysis, not oxidative phosphorylation, as its energy supply.[114, 116] Glucose is the sole substrate for aerobic glycolysis in both stimulated and unstimulated smooth muscle (Fig. 3–16). Stimulation of the (Na^+-K^+)-ATPase is accompanied by an increase in cellular glucose uptake.[135] The intracellular signal that stimulates this glucose transport is not known. After being taken up, glucose is metabolized to lactate through aerobic glycolysis to produce ATP. Since aerobic glycolysis produces lactate and not pyruvate in smooth muscle, glucose is not used for oxidative phosphorylation.

The discussion above indicates that aerobic glycolysis and oxidative phosphorylation are compartmentalized within the cell, and that they are coupled independently to different energy-requiring processes. Thus, energy production can be closely regulated according to the needs of specific cellular processes. Glycogenolysis and oxidative phosphorylation are able to produce the large quantities of ATP needed during contractions, and the coupling of aerobic glycolysis to (Na^+-K^+)-ATPase activity provides an efficient and sensitive way to coordinate energy production with ion transport.

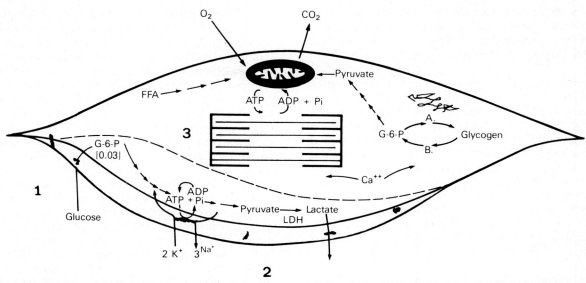

Figure 3–16. Schematic representation of energy utilization in a smooth muscle cell. (1) Glucose is the substrate for aerobic glycolysis. Its rate of transport is determined by glucose utilization. (2) Aerobic glycolysis is the sole source for the ATP used by the Na^+ pump. This means that glucose utilization and transport are coupled to $(Na^+\text{-}K^+)$-ATPase activity. (3) The ATP utilized by contractile proteins during contraction comes from the breakdown of glycogen and oxidative phosphorylation. (From Lynch, R. M., and Paul, R. J. Experientia *41*:970, 1985. Used by permission.)

MECHANICS OF SMOOTH MUSCLE

Depending upon the physiologic function demanded of a gastrointestinal smooth muscle, its activation may result in the production of force with little or no change in overall muscle length (isometric contraction), or it may result in significant shortening against a relatively constant load (isotonic contraction). Moreover, the amount of force generated by a muscle when activated depends upon the length to which the muscle is stretched prior to activation. The mechanical properties of the smooth muscle layer are defined by a model that includes passive elastic elements and active contractile elements (Fig. 3–17).

The force generated by smooth muscle when it is contracting against a fixed load is called *isotonic contraction*. When the load is less than the maximal force a muscle is able to produce, shortening occurs. The velocity of shortening is determined by the load on the muscle, as illustrated by the hyperbolic force-velocity curve[136] in Fig. 3–17*B2*. This force-velocity relationship comes about because the velocity of shortening is determined by the crossbridge cycling rate. Greater loads decrease cycling rate and the velocity of shortening. Heavier loads decrease crossbridge cycling rate by increasing the average time myosin spends in its attached (force-generating) conformation. Conceptually, this is most easily thought of as the myosin head

Figure 3–17. A model for mechanical properties of smooth muscle. The schematic *(A)* shows the mechanical analogue of mechanical characteristics of smooth muscle. It is represented by two passive elastic elements, one of which is in series and the other of which is in parallel with the contractile elements. The parallel component represents connective tissue elements, while the series component arises from the crossbridge. *B1* shows force-length relationships due to activation of the contractile element (active tension). Note that the maximal force generated gradually increases, reaches a maximum, and then decreases as the length of the contractile element is increased. *B2* shows the force-velocity relationship of contractile elements. Note that as the force (load) is decreased, the velocity of shortening increases. *B3* shows the force-length relationship passive elastic elements. Note that passive elements generate no force until a certain length is reached and then, with increasing lengths, the force increases exponentially. P, force; L, length; V, velocity of shortening. (From Paul, R. J. *In* Johnson, L. R. [ed.]. Physiology of the Gastrointestinal Tract. 2nd ed. New York, Raven Press, 1987. Used by permission.)

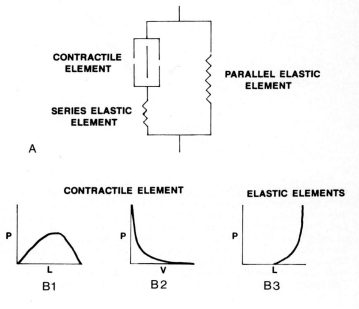

requiring more time to pull the actin filament a set distance in the presence of an external load. Shortening velocity and crossbridge cycling rate both correlate with the degree of myosin light chain phosphorylation.[137]

Isometric force is the force measured when a muscle is fixed at a constant overall length and allowed to contract maximally. The amount of isometric force a muscle can generate depends upon its length, as depicted in Figure 3–17*B1*. Stretching a relaxed smooth muscle results in a passive force-length relationship (Fig. 3–17*B3*). At small degrees of stretch, muscles generate little passive force. As more stretch is applied, the amount of passive force rapidly increases. Since single smooth muscle cells generate almost no passive force as their length is increased, the passive force-length curve for tissues reflects elastic properties of extracellular connective tissues, primarily collagen and elastin.[27, 138]

When measurement of the isometric force-length relationship is repeated under conditions ensuring maximal and constant contraction, a total force-length curve is generated (Fig. 3–18). The difference between total and passive force-length relationships is the active

force-length relationship. Active force-length curves reflect the ability of actin and myosin to generate force at any fixed overall tissue length. The active force-length curve is typically a bell-shaped curve. At short lengths, the muscle strip is unable to develop active tension. Active tension develops and then increases progressively as the length is increased until at a certain length (L_o or optimal length) maximal tension development occurs. At lengths greater than L_o, the tension falls until no active tension is developed. Correlative structural and mechanical studies done on striated muscles reveal that active isometric force is proportional to the overlap between thick and thin filaments in the sarcomere.[139] At smooth muscle lengths less than that for maximal force generation, smooth muscle cells and their contractile filaments are misaligned so maximal activation does not produce maximal contraction.[140] Although other ultrastructural and biochemical reasons for less than maximal force generation probably exist, they have not been identified. As the muscle is stretched, muscle cells and contractile filaments become better aligned, and force generation increases. When the muscle is stretched beyond its optimal length (L_o), some myosin molecules are no longer able to

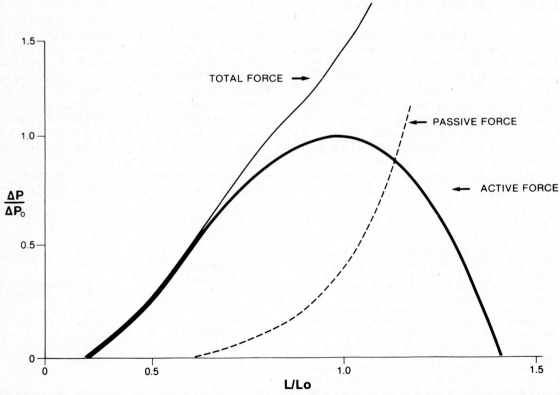

Figure 3–18. The relationship between isometric force and muscle length in smooth muscle. The passive force-length curve represents the force generated by a relaxed muscle when it is stretched passively. This curve represents the force generated by the elastic component of the connective tissues making up the stroma. The total force curve represents the force generated when the stretched muscle is stimulated to contract maximally. The active force curve is the total force curve minus the passive force curve. The active force curve represents the maximal force generated by the contractile proteins making up the smooth muscle. The maximum active tension and the length at which the maximal tension develops are assigned a value of 1. L/L_o represents tissue length/tissue length at maximal tension development (L_o) and $\Delta P/\Delta P_o$ represents the force developed at a particular length/maximal force (P_o). Sphincter smooth muscle, which is tonically contracted even in the unstimulated state, generates steeper resting force length curves. (From Paul, R. J. *In* Johnson, L. R. [ed.]. Physiology of the Gastrointestinal Tract. 2nd ed. New York, Raven Press, 1987. Used by permission.)

interact with adjacent thin filaments. At and beyond this length, isometric force falls linearly with the decrease in overlap between thick and thin filaments. In part, this explains why massively dilated segments of bowel are unable to generate contractile force.

Different gastrointestinal smooth muscles are characterized by different force-length relationships in the unstimulated state. For example, sphincteric muscles generate a much steeper force-length curve than circular muscles from adjacent organs.[141, 142] The steeper force-length curves of unstimulated sphincteric muscle occur because the contractile machinery of the sphincter muscle is partially and continuously activated through some intrinsic myogenic system.[141, 142] That is, the sphincter is tonically contracted as a result of some property of the muscle and not as a result of neural or hormonal stimulation.[143]

References

1. Cormack, D. H. Introduction to Histology. Philadelphia, J. B. Lippincott Company, 1984, p. 240.
2. Goyal, R. K., and Paterson, W. G. Esophageal motility. *In* Wood, J. D. (section ed.). Handbook of Physiology: Motility. Baltimore, Williams & Wilkins, 1987, in press.
3. Szurszewski, J. H. Electrical basis for gastrointestinal motility. *In* Johnson, L. R. (ed.). Physiology of the Gastrointestinal Tract. 2nd ed. New York, Raven Press, 1987, pp. 383–422.
4. Weisbrodt, N. W. Motility of the small intestine. *In* Johnson, L. R. (ed.). Physiology of the Gastrointestinal Tract. 2nd ed. New York, Raven Press, 1987, pp. 631–663.
5. Christensen, J. Motility of the colon. *In* Johnson, L. R. (ed.). Physiology of the Gastrointestinal Tract. 2nd ed. New York, Raven Press, 1987, pp. 665–693.
6. Thunenberg, L. Interstitial cells of Cajal: Intestinal pacemaker cells. Adv. Anat. Embryol. Cell Biol. *71*:1, 1982.
7. Suzuki, N., Prosser, C. L., and Dahms, V. Boundary cells between longitudinal and circular layers: Essential for electrical slow waves in cat intestine. Am. J. Physiol. *250*:G287, 1986.
8. Brading, A. F., and Casteels, R. The physiology of the smooth muscle: An interdisciplinary review. Parts I and II. Experientia *41*:837–1088, 1985.
9. Somlyo, A. V. Ultrastructure of vascular smooth muscle. *In* Bohr, D. F., Somlyo, A. P., and Sparks, H. V. (eds.). Handbook of Physiology: Section 2, The Cardiovascular System, Vol. 2. Vascular Smooth Muscle. Baltimore, Williams & Wilkins, 1980, pp. 33–67.
10. Somlyo, A. P. Excitation contraction coupling and the ultrastructure of smooth muscle. Circ. Res. *57*:497, 1985.
11. Prosser, C. L., Burnstock, G., and Kahn, J. Conduction in smooth muscle: Comparative structural properties. Am. J. Physiol. *199*:545, 1960.
12. Wells, G. S., and Wolowyk, M. K. Freeze-etch observations on membrane structure in smooth muscle of guinea-pig taenia coli. J. Physiol. (Lond.) *218*:11, 1971.
13. Geiger, B., Dutton, A. H., Tokayasu, T., and Singer, S. J. Immunoelectron microscope studies of membrane-microfilament interaction: Distributions of alpha-actinin, tropomyosin, and vinculin in intestinal epithelial brush border and chicken gizzard smooth muscle cells. J. Cell. Biol. *91*:614, 1981.
14. Schollmeyer, J. E., Furcht, L. T., Goll, D. E., Robinson, R. M., and Stromer, M. H. Localization of contractile proteins in smooth muscle cells and in normal and transformed fibroblasts. *In* Goldman, R., Pollard, T., and Rosenbaum, J. (eds.). Cell Motility, Vol. 3a. Cold Spring Harbor, Cold Spring Harbor Laboratories, 1976, pp. 361–388.
15. Fay, F. S., Fogarty, K., Fujiwara, K., and Tuft, R. Contractile mechanism of single isolated smooth muscle cells. *In* Twarog, B. M., Levine, R. J. C., and Dewey, M. M. (eds.). Basic Biology of Muscles: A Comparative Approach. New York, Raven Press, 1982, pp. 143–157.
16. Fay, F. S., and Delise, C. M. Contraction of isolated smooth muscle cells—structural changes. Proc. Natl. Acad. Sci. USA *70*:641, 1973.
17. Gabella, G. Structure of muscles and nerves in the gastrointestinal tract. *In* Johnson, L. R. (ed.). Physiology of the Gastrointestinal Tract. 2nd ed. New York, Raven Press, 1987, pp. 335–381.
18. Somlyo, A. V., and Franzini-Armstrong, C. New views of smooth muscle structure using freezing, deep-etching and rotary shadowing. Experientia *41*:841, 1985.
19. Gabella, G. Structural apparatus for force transmission in smooth muscle. Physiol. Rev. *64*:455, 1984.
20. Dewey, M. M., and Barr, L. A study of the structure and distribution of the nexus. J. Cell. Biol. *23*:553, 1964.
21. Perachia, C. Structural correlates of gap junction permeation. Int. Rev. Cytol. *66*:81, 1980.
22. Staehelin, L. A. Structure and function of intercellular junctions. Int. Rev. Cytol. *39*:199, 1974.
23. Gabella, G., and Blundell, D. Nexus between the smooth muscle cells of the guinea-pig ileum. J. Cell. Biol. *82*:239, 1979.
24. Fry, G. N., Devine, C. E., and Burnstock, G. Freeze-fracture studies of nexuses between smooth muscles. J. Cell. Biol. *72*:26, 1977.
25. Kandel, E. R., and Siegelbaum, S. Principles underlying electrical and chemical synaptic transmission. *In* Kandel, E. R., and Schwartz, J. H. (eds.). Principles of Neural Science. 2nd ed. New York, Elsevier, 1985, pp. 89–107.
26. Barr, L., Berger, W., and Dewey, N. M. Electrical transmission of the nexus between smooth muscle cells. J. Gen. Physiol. *51*:347, 1968.
27. Fay, F. S. Mechanical properties of single isolated smooth muscle cells. *In* Smooth Muscle Physiology and Pharmacology, Vol. 50. Paris, INSERM Colloquia, 1975, pp. 327–342.
28. Cooke, P. Organization of contractile fibers in smooth muscle. *In* Dowben, R. M., and Shay, J. W. (eds.). Cell and Muscle Motility, Vol. 3. New York, Plenum Press, 1983, pp. 57–77.
29. Shoenberg, C. F., and Haselgrove, J. C. Filaments and ribbons in vertebrate smooth muscle. Nature (Lond.) *249*:152, 1974.
30. Small, J. V., and Squire, J. M. Structural basis of contraction in vertebrate smooth muscle. J. Mol. Biol. *67*:117, 1972.
31. Squire, J. M. Vertebral smooth muscle. *In* The Structural Basis of Muscular Contraction. New York, Plenum Press, 1981, p. 459.
32. Heumann, H. G. Smooth muscle: Contraction hypothesis based on the arrangement of actin and myosin filaments in different states of contraction. Philos. Trans. R. Soc. Lond. [Biol.] *265*:213, 1973.
33. Small, J. V. Studies of isolated smooth muscle cells: The contractile apparatus. J. Cell Sci. *24*:327, 1977.
34. Onishi, H., and Wakabayashi, T. Electron microscopic studies of myosin molecules from chicken gizzard muscle. 1: The formation of the intramolecular loop in the myosin tail. J. Biochem. (Tokyo) *92*:871, 1982.
35. Elliott, A., and Offer, G. Shape and flexibility of the myosin molecule. J. Mol. Biol. *123*:505, 1978.
36. Lazarides, E. Intermediate filaments as mechanical integrators of cellular space. Nature *283*:249, 1980.
37. Hartshorne, D. J. Biochemistry of the contractile process in smooth muscle. *In* Johnson, L. R. (ed.). Physiology of the Gastrointestinal Tract. 2nd ed. New York, Raven Press, 1987, pp. 423–482.
38. Murphy, R. A. Filament organization and contractile function in vertebrate smooth muscle. Annu. Rev. Physiol. *41*:737, 1979.
39. Fay, F. S., Rees, D. D., and Warshaw, D. M. The contractile mechanism of smooth muscle. *In* Bittar, E. E. (ed.). Membrane Structure and Function, Vol. 4. New York, John Wiley and Sons, 1981, pp. 79–130.
40. Marston, S. B. Myosin and actomyosin ATPase kinetics. *In* Stephens, N. L. (ed.). Biochemistry of Smooth Muscle, Vol. 1. Boca Raton, FL, CRC Press, 1983, pp. 167–191.
41. Marston, S. B., and Taylor, E. W. Mechanics of myosin and actomyosin ATPase in chicken gizzard smooth muscle. FEBS Letters *86*:167, 1978.
42. Eisenberg, E., and Hill, T. L. Muscle contraction and free

energy transduction in biological systems. *Science* 227:999, 1985.

43. Alberts, B., Bray, D., Lewis, J., et al. Molecular Biology of the Cell. New York, Garland Publishing, Inc., 1983, pp. 292, 549–609.

44. Warshaw, D. M., Fay, F. S. Crossbridge elasticity in single smooth muscle cells. J. Gen. Physiol. 82:157, 1983.

45. Warshaw, D. M., Fay, F. S. Tension transients in single isolated smooth muscle cells. Science 216:1438, 1983.

46. Huxley, A. F. Muscle structure and theories of contraction. Prog. Biophys. Mol. Biol. 7:257, 1957.

47. Hartshorne, D. J., and Gorecka, A. The biochemistry of the contractile proteins of smooth muscle. *In* Bohr, D. F., Somlyo, A. P., and Sparks, H. V. (eds.). Handbook of Physiology: Section 2, The Cardiovascular System, Vol. 2. Vascular Smooth Muscle. Baltimore, Williams & Wilkins, 1980, pp. 93–120.

48. Small, J. V., and Sobreszek, A. The contractile apparatus of smooth muscle. Int. Rev. Cytol. 64:241, 1980.

49. Ikebe, M., and Hartshorne, D. The role of myosin phosphorylation in the contraction-relaxation cycle of smooth muscle. Experientia 41:1006, 1985.

50. Ballin, G. Structure and function of calmodulin-dependent smooth muscle myosin light chain kinase. Experientia 40:1185, 1984.

51. Burger, D., Cox, J. A., Comte, M., and Stein, E. A. Sequential conformational changes in calmodulin upon binding of calcium. Biochemistry 23:1966, 1984.

52. Rüegg, J. C. Smooth muscle tone. Physiol. Rev. 51:201, 1971.

53. Kuriyama, H., Ito, Y., Suzuki, H., Kitamure, K., and Itoh, T. Factors modifying contraction-relaxation cycle in vascular smooth muscles. Am. J. Physiol. 243:H641, 1982.

54. Guth, K., and Junge, J. Low Ca^{2+} impedes cross-bridge detachment in chemically skinned taenia coli. Nature 300:775, 1982.

55. Chatterjee, M., and Murphy, R. A. Calcium-dependent stress maintenance without myosin phosphorylation in skinned smooth muscle. Science 221:464, 1983.

56. Weisbrodt, N. W., and Murphy, R. A. Myosin phosphorylation and contraction of feline esophageal smooth muscle. Am. J. Physiol. 249:C9, 1985.

57. Pato, M. D., and Adelstein, R. S. Dephosphorylation of the 20,000-dalton light chain of myosin by two different phosphatases from smooth muscle. J. Biol. Chem. 255:6535, 1980.

58. Pato, M. D., and Kerc, E. Purification and characterization of a smooth muscle myosin phosphatase from turkey gizzards. J. Biol. Chem. 260:12359, 1985.

59. Casteels, R. Membrane potential in smooth muscle cells. *In* Bülbring, E., Brading, A. F., Jones, A. W., and Tomita, T. (eds.). Smooth Muscle: An Assessment of Current Knowledge. Austin, University of Texas Press, 1981, pp. 105–126.

60. Bortoff, A. Smooth muscle of the gastrointestinal tract. *In* Christensen, J., and Wingate, D. L. (eds.). A Guide to Gastrointestinal Motility. Bristol, England, John Wright and Sons Ltd., 1983, pp. 48–74.

61. Jones, A. W. Content and fluxes of electrolytes. *In* Bohr, D. F., Somlyo, A. P., and Sparks, H. V. (eds.). Handbook of Physiology: Section 2, The Cardiovascular System. Baltimore, Williams & Wilkins, 1980, pp. 253–299.

62. Morgan, K. G., Morgan, J. P., and DeFeo, T. T. Determination of absolute ionized calcium concentrations in vascular smooth muscle cells using aequorin. Fed. Proc. 43:767, 1984.

63. Williams, D. A., Fogarty, K. E., Tesin, R. Y., and Fay, F. S. Calcium gradients in single smooth muscle cells revealed by the digital imaging microscope using Fura-2. Nature. 318:558, 1985.

64. Williams, D., and Fay, F. S. Calcium transients and resting levels in isolated smooth muscle cells monitored with quin 2. Am. J. Physiol. 250:C779, 1986.

65. Grover, A. K. Ca-pumps in smooth muscle: One in plasma membrane and another in the endoplasmic reticulum. Cell Calcium 6:227, 1985.

66. Wuytack, F., Raeymaekers, L., and Casteels, R. Ca^{2+}-transport ATPases in smooth muscle. Experientia 41:900, 1985.

67. Daniel, E. E. The use of subcellular membrane fractions in analysis of control of smooth muscle function. Experientia 41:905, 1985.

68. Popescu, L. M., and Ingnat, P. Calmodulin-dependent Ca^{2+} pump ATPase of human smooth muscle sarcolemma. Cell Calcium 4:219, 1983.

69. Sugi, H., and Daimon, T. Translocation of intracellularly stored calcium during contraction-relaxation cycle in guinea pig taenia coli. Nature 269:436, 1977.

70. Heumann, H. G., The subcellular localization of calcium in invertebrate smooth muscle: Calcium-containing and calcium-accumulating structures in muscle cells of mouse intestine. Cell Tissue Res. 169:221, 1976.

71. Bond, M., Kitazawa, T., Somlyo, A. P., and Somlyo, A. V. Release and recycling of calcium by the sarcoplasmic reticulum in guinea-pig vein smooth muscle. J. Physiol. (Lond.) 357:185, 1984.

72. Endo, M., Yagi, S., and Lino, M. Tension-pCa relation and sarcoplasmic reticulum responses in chemically skinned smooth muscle fibers. Fed. Proc. 41:2245, 1982.

73. Raeymaekers, L. The sarcoplasmic reticulum of smooth muscle fibers. Z. Naturforsch. 37c:481, 1982.

74. Wuytack, F. L., Raeymaekers, L., Verbist, J., DeSmedt, H, and Casteels, R. Evidence for the presence in smooth muscle of two types of Ca^{2+}-transport ATPase. Biochem. J. 224:445, 1984.

75. Raeymaekers, L., Wuytack, F., and Casteels, R. Subcellular fractionation of pig stomach smooth muscle. A study of the distribution of the $(Ca^{2+}-Mg^{2+})$-ATPase activity in plasmalemma and endoplasmic reticulum. Biochim. Biophys. Acta 815:441, 1985.

76. Morgan, J. P., and Morgan, K. G. Stimulus-specific patterns of intracellular calcium levels in smooth muscle of ferret portal vein. J. Physiol. (Lond.) 351:155, 1984.

77. Johansson, B., and Somlyo, A. P. Electrophysiology and excitation contraction coupling. *In* Bohr, P. F., Somlyo, A. P., Sparks, H. V. (eds.). Handbook of Physiology: Section 2, The Cardiovascular System, Vol. 2. Vascular Smooth Muscle. Baltimore, Williams & Wilkins, 1980, pp. 301–323.

78. Hurwitz, L. Pharmacology of calcium channels and smooth muscle. Ann. Rev. Pharmacol. Toxicol. 26:225, 1986.

79. Bolton, T. B. Mechanisms of action of transmitters and other substances on smooth muscle. Physiol. Rev. 59:606, 1979.

80. Walsh, J. V., and Singer, J. J. Voltage clamp of single freshly dissociated smooth muscle cells: Current-voltage relationships for 3 currents. Pflügers Arch. 390:207, 1981.

81. Rasmussen, H., and Barrett, P. Q. Calcium messenger system: An integrated view. Physiol. Rev. 64:938, 1984.

82. Itoh, T., Ueno, H., and Kuriyama, H. Calcium-induced calcium release in vascular smooth muscles—assessments based on contractions evoked by intact saponin-treated skinned muscles. Experientia 41:989, 1985.

83. Itoh, T., Kuriyama, H., and Suzuki, H. Excitation-contraction coupling in smooth muscle cells of the guinea-pig mesenteric artery. J. Physiol. (Lond.) 321:513, 1981.

84. Widdicombe, J. H. The ionic properties of the sodium pump in smooth muscle. *In* Bülbring, E., Brading, A. F., Jones, A. W., and Tomita, T. (eds.). Smooth Muscle: An Assessment of Current Knowledge. Austin, University of Texas Press, 1981, pp. 93–104.

85. Fleming, W. W. The electrogenic Na^+, K^+ pump in smooth muscle: Physiologic and pharmacologic significance. Ann. Rev. Pharmacol. Toxicol. 20:129, 1980.

86. Brading, A. F. Ionic distribution and mechanisms of transmembrane ion movements in smooth muscle. *In* Bülbring, E., Brading, A. F., Jones, A. W., and Tomita, T. (eds.). Smooth Muscle: An Assessment of Current Knowledge. Austin, University of Texas Press, 1981, pp. 65–92.

87. Aickin, C. C., and Brading, A. F. Intracellular chloride activity of guinea-pig vas deferens. J. Physiol. (Lond.) 308:56P, 1986.

88. Koester, J. Nongated channels and passive membrane properties of the neuron. *In* Kandel, E. R., and Schwartz, J. H. (eds.). Principles of Neural Science. 2nd ed. New York, Elsevier, 1985, pp. 58–65.

89. Stevens, C. F. Interactions between intrinsic membrane protein and electric field: An approach to studying nerve excitability. Biophys. J. 22:295, 1978.

90. Hille, B. Ionic channels in excitable membranes: Current problems and biophysical approaches. Biophys. J. 22:283, 1978.

91. Prosser, C. L., and Mangel, A. W. Mechanisms of spike and slow wave pacemaker activity in smooth muscle cells. *In* Carpenter, D. O. (ed.). Cellular Pacemakers. New York, Wiley-Interscience, 1982, pp. 273–301.

92. Goyal, R. K., and Gidda, J. S. Relationship between electrical and mechanical activity in the opossum esophagus. Am. J. Physiol. *240*:G305, 1981.

93. Asoh, R., and Goyal, R. K. Manometry and electromyography of the upper esophageal sphincter in the opossum. Gastroenterology *74*:835, 1978.

94. Chambers, M. M., Bowes, K. L., Kingma, Y. J., Bannister, C., and Cole, K. R. In vitro electrical activity in human colon. Gastroenterology *81*:502, 1981.

95. Chambers, M. M., Kingma, Y. J., and Bowes, K. L. Intracellular electrical activity in circular muscle of canine colon. Gut *25*:1268, 1984.

96. Tomita, T. Electrical activity (spikes and slow waves) in gastrointestinal smooth muscles. *In* Bülbring, E., Brading, A., Jones, A. W., and Tomita, T. (eds.). Smooth Muscle: An Assessment of Current Knowledge. Austin, University of Texas Press, 1981, pp. 127–156.

97. Hara, Y., Kuboto, M., Szurszewski, J. H. Electrophysiology of smooth muscle of the small intestine of small mammals. J. Physiol. (Lond.) *372*:501, 1986.

98. Durdle, N. G., Kingma, Y. J., Bowes, K. L., and Chambers, M. M. Origin of slow waves in the canine colon. Gastroenterology *84*:374, 1983.

99. Conner, J. A., Kreulin, D., Prosser, C. L., and Weigel, R. Interaction between longitudinal and circular muscle in intestine of cat. J. Physiol. (Lond.) *273*:665, 1977.

100. Bortoff, A., and Sachs, F. Electrotonic spread of slow waves in circular muscle of small intestine. Am. J. Physiol. *218*:576, 1970.

101. Publicover, N. G., and Sanders, K. M. Myogenic regulation of propagation in gastric smooth muscle. Am. J. Physiol. *248*:G512, 1985.

102. Sarna, S, K., Daniel, E. E., Kingma, Y. J. Simulation of slow-wave electrical activity of small intestine. Am. J. Physiol. *221*:166, 1971.

103. You, C. H., Chey, W. Y., Lee, K. Y., Menguy, R., and Bortoff, A. Gastric and small intestine dysrhythmia associated with chronic intractable nausea and vomiting. Ann. Intern. Med. *95*:449, 1981.

104. Walsh, J. V., and Singer, J. J. Calcium action potentials in single freshly isolated smooth muscle cells. Am. J. Physiol. *239*:C162, 1980.

105. Ganikevich, V. Y., Shuba, M. F., and Smirnov, S. V. Potential-dependent calcium inward current in a single isolated smooth muscle cell of the guinea-pig taenia caeci. J. Physiol. (Lond.) *380*:1, 1986.

106. Benham, C. D., Bolton, T. B., and Lang, R. J. Membrane potential and voltage clamp recording from single smooth muscle cells of rabbit jejunum. J. Physiol. (Lond.) *353*:67P, 1984.

107. Jmari, K., Mironneau, C., and Mironneau, J. Inactivation of calcium current in rat uterine smooth muscle: Evidence for calcium- and voltage-mediated mechanisms. J. Physiol. (Lond.) *380*:111, 1986.

108. Benham, S. D., Bolton, T. B., Lang, R. J., and Takewaki, T. Calcium-activated potassium channels in single smooth muscle cells of rabbit jejunum and guinea-pig mesenteric artery. J. Physiol. (Lond.) *371*:45, 1986.

109. Weigel, R. J., Conner, J. A., and Prosser, C. L. Two roles of calcium during the spike in circular muscle of small intestine in cat. Am. J. Physiol. *237*:C247, 1979.

110. Mitra, R., and Morad, M. Ca^{2+} and Ca^{2+}-activated K^+ currents in mammalian gastric smooth muscle cells. Science *229*:269, 1985.

111. Sims, S. M., Singer, J. J., Walsh, J. V. Cholinergic agonists suppress a potassium current in freshly dissociated smooth muscle cells of the toad. J. Physiol. (Lond.) *367*:503, 1985.

112. Benham, C. D., Bolton, T. B., and Lang, R. J. Acetylcholine activates an inward current in single mammalian smooth muscle cells. Nature *316*:345, 1985.

113. Morgan, K. G., Schmalz, P. F., and Szurszewski, J. H. The inhibitory effects of vasoactive intestinal polypeptide on the mechanical and electrical activity of canine antral smooth muscle. J. Physiol. (Lond.) *282*:437, 1978.

114. Berridge, J., and Irvine, R. F. Inositol trisphosphate, a novel second messenger in cellular signal transduction. Nature *312*:315, 1985.

115. Somlyo, A. V., Bond, M., Somlyo, A. P., and Scarpa, A. Inositol triphosphate–induced calcium release and contraction in vascular smooth muscle. Proc. Natl. Acad. Sci. USA *82*:5231, 1985.

116. Baron, C. A., Cunningham, M., Strauss, J. F., and Coburn, R. F. Pharmacomechanical coupling in smooth muscle may involve phosphatidylinositol metabolism. Proc. Natl. Acad. Sci. USA *81*:6899, 1984.

117. Smith, J. S., Coronado, R., and Meissner, G. Sarcoplasmic reticulum contains adenosine nucleotide–activated calcium channels. Nature *316*:446, 1985.

118. Birnbaumer, L., Codina, J., Mattera, R., Cerione, R. A., Hildebrandt, J. D., Sunyer, T., Rojas, F. J., Caron, M. G., Lefkowitz, R. J., and Iyengar, R. Regulation of hormone receptors and adenylate cyclases by guanine nucleotide binding N proteins. Rec. Prog. Horm. Res. *41*:41, 1985.

119. Tomlinson, S., MacNeil, S., and Brown, B. L. Calcium, cyclic AMP and hormone action. Clin. Endocrinol. *23*:595, 1985.

120. Hardman, J. G. Cyclic nucleotides and smooth muscle contraction: Some conceptual and experimental considerations. *In* Bülbring, E., Brading, A., Jones, A. W., and Tomita, T. (eds.). Smooth Muscle: An Assessment of Current Knowledge. Austin, University of Texas Press, 1981, pp. 249–262.

121. Cohen, R. The role of protein phosphorylation in neural and hormonal control of cellular activity. Nature *296*:613, 1982.

122. Scheid, C. R., Honeyman, T. W., and Fay, F. S. Mechanisms of β-adrenergic relaxation of smooth muscle. Nature *227*:32, 1979.

123. Bhalla, R. C., Webb, R. C., Sigh, D., and Brock, T. Role of cyclic AMP in rat aortic microsomal phosphorylation and calcium uptake. Am. J. Physiol. *234*:H508, 1978.

124. Nichikori, K., and Maeno, H. Close relationship between adenosine 3':5'-monophosphate–dependent endogenous phosphorylation of a specific protein and stimulation of calcium uptake in rat uterine microsomes. J. Biol. Chem. *254*:6099, 1979.

125. deLanerolle, P., Nishikawa, M., Yost, D. A., and Adelstein, R. S. Increased phosphorylation of myosin light chain kinase after an increase in cyclic AMP in intact smooth muscle. Science *223*:1415, 1984.

126. Adelstein, R. S., Conti, M. A., Hathaway, D. R., and Klee, C. B. Phosphorylation of smooth muscle myosin light chain kinase by the catalytic subunit of adenosine 3':5'-monophosphate–dependent protein kinase. J. Biol. Chem. *253*:8347, 1978.

127. Levitan, I. B. Phosphorylation of ion channels. J. Memb. Biol. *87*:177, 1985.

128. Nishikawa, M., deLanerolle, P., Lincoln, T. M., and Adelstein, R. S. Phosphorylation of mammalian myosin light chain kinases by the catalytic subunit of cyclic AMP–dependent protein kinase and by cyclic GMP–dependent protein kinase. J. Biol. Chem. *259*:8429, 1984.

129. Miller, C. A., Barnette, M. S., Ormsbee, H. S., and Trophy, T. J. Cyclic nucleotide–dependent protein kinases in the lower esophageal sphincter. Am. J. Physiol. *251*:G794, 1986.

130. Paul, R. J. Smooth muscle mechanochemical energy conversion: Relationship between metabolism and contractility. *In* Johnson, L. R. (ed.). Physiology of the Gastrointestinal Tract. 2nd ed. New York, Raven Press, 1987, pp. 483–506.

131. Chace, K. U., and Odessey, R. The utilization by rabbit aorta of carbohydrates, fatty acids, ketone bodies and amino acids as substrates for energy production. Cir. Res. *48*:850, 1981.

132. Lynch, R. M., and Paul, R. J. Energy metabolism and transduction in smooth muscle. Experientia *41*:970, 1985.

133. Davidheiser, S., Joseph, J., Davies, R. E. Separation of aerobic glycolysis from oxidative metabolism and contractility in rat anococcygeus muscle. Am. J. Physiol. *247*:C335, 1984.

134. Namm, D. H. The activation of glycogen phosphorylase in arterial smooth muscle. J. Pharmacol. Exp. Ther. *178*:299, 1971.

135. Lynch, R. M., and Paul, R. J. Glucose uptake in porcine carotid artery: Relation to alteration in Na-K transport. Am. J. Physiol. *247*:C433, 1984.

136. Gordon, A. R., and Siegman, M. J. Mechanical properties of smooth muscle. I. Length-tension and force-velocity relations. Am. J. Physiol. *221*:1243, 1971.

137. Murphy, R. A., Aksoy, M. O., Dillon, P. F., Gerthoffer, W. T., and Kamm, K. E. The role of myosin light chain phosphorylation in regulation of the crossbridge cycle. Fed. Proc. *42*:51, 1983.

138. Van Dijk, A. M., Wiering, P. A., van der Meer, M., and Laird, J. D. Mechanics of resting isolated single vascular smooth muscle cells from bovine carotid artery. Am. J. Physiol. *246*:C277, 1984.

139. Gordon, A. M., Huxley, A. F., and Julian, F. J. The variation in isometric tension with sarcomere length in vertebrate muscle fibers. J. Physiol. (Lond.) *184*:170, 1966.

140. Siegman, M. J., Davidheiser, S., Butler, T. M., and Mooers, S. U. What is the length-tension relation in smooth muscle? Fed. Proc. *44*:457, 1985.

141. Christensen, J., Conklin, J. L., Freeman, B. W. Physiologic specialization of the esophagogastric junction in three species. Am. J. Physiol. *225*:1265, 1973.

142. Christensen, J., Conklin, J. L. Studies on the origin of distinctive mechanisms of smooth muscle of the esophagogastric junction. *In* Daniel, E. E. (ed.). Proceedings of the Fourth International Symposium on Gastrointestinal Motility. Vancouver, Canada, Mitchell Press, 1973, pp. 63–71.

143. Goyal, R. K., and Rattan, S. Genesis of basal sphincter pressure: Effect of tetrodotoxin on lower esophageal sphincter pressure in opossum in vivo. Gastroenterology, *71*:62, 1976.

4

Gastrointestinal Peptide Hormones

JOHN H. WALSH

Since the last edition of this book was published, many new developments have occurred in the field of gastrointestinal regulatory peptides. It is apparent that the name "gastrointestinal hormones" is not sufficient to designate regulatory peptides delivered to their targets by pathways not involving the blood. For example, neuropeptides act in the area of the nerve terminals where they are released. Paracrine peptides also influence their neighbors by local diffusion. The new family of peptides classified as "growth factors" undoubtedly are important regulators of gut development in the fetus and newborn and of other functions in the adult, but little is known about their physiologic roles and delivery mechanisms. Finally, the concept of autocrine regulation has been applied to tumors that produce their own growth factors. The major pathways by which regulatory peptides are delivered to their target cells are shown in Figure 4–1. Although "hormone" traditionally refers to circulating regulators, "hormone" will be used in this chapter to indicate any peptide regulatory substance regardless of its method of delivery.

As more knowledge is acquired, clinical relevance is becoming more well defined for hormones and neuropeptides of the gut. This chapter emphasizes the knowledge about gastrointestinal peptides most likely to be relevant to diseases of the human gut. A vast literature has accumulated about the physiology and biochemistry of gastrointestinal peptides and brain-gut peptides. Those readers who wish to learn more about the physiology of these peptides are referred to recent reviews of gastrointestinal hormones,[1] neuropeptides,[2] and paracrine agents.[3]

LOCALIZATION OF GUT HORMONES

Hormones

Gastrointestinal peptides are found in endocrine cells and in nerves. Most of the endocrine peptides are localized in cells restricted to a defined region of the gut: stomach, pancreas, upper small intestine, or lower small intestine and colon.[4] Somatostatin is the exception, being found in all these locations (Table 4–1). Gastrin is the major peptide of the stomach. Insulin, glucagon, and pancreatic polypeptide are found in the pancreas. Secretin, cholecystokinin, gastric inhibitory peptide, motilin, and substance P are found in the upper small intestine. Enteroglucagon, neurotensin, peptide YY, and substance P are found in the lower small intestine and colon.[5] The cells that produce these peptides have been named either for their electron microscopic appearance or because they can be identified by antibodies against their peptide product.

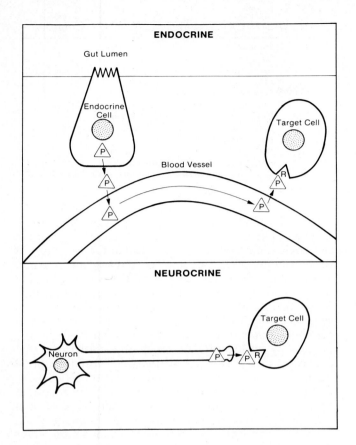

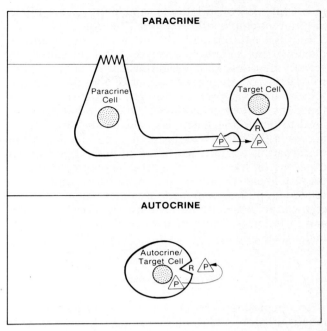

Figure 4–1. Pathways for delivery of regulatory peptides (P) to their specific receptors (R).

Neuropeptides

Neuropeptides also are distributed in distinctive patterns in the gut.[6] The previous chapter has indicated that gut nerves are either extrinsic or intrinsic. Extrinsic parasympathetic preganglionic innervation is provided by the vagus nerve and by pelvic nerves. Sympathetic innervation is provided by postganglionic nerves arising in the sympathetic ganglia. Most of the gut neuropeptides are produced by the intrinsic nervous system of the gut. Therefore extrinsic innervation by vagotomy and/or sympathectomy does not significantly alter gut neuropeptides.

Neuropeptides found in the gut wall are listed in Table 4–2. Some neuropeptides, including somatostatin, cholecystokinin, and substance P, also are classic hormones. Several others are found in the gut only in nerves.[7] Most of these peptides also are produced in the brain. They constitute the so-called gut-brain peptide axis.

One confusing aspect of gut neuropeptides is that several peptides often are found in the same neuron. Furthermore, peptides also are found in nerves that contain acetylcholine or norepinephrine. Neuropeptides can be classified partially by their concurrence in cholinergic or sympathetic nerves. However, this classification does not completely describe the complex pattern in which as many as six peptides can be found

Table 4–1. GASTROINTESTINAL ENDOCRINE CELLS

Location	Endocrine Product	Cell Type
Stomach	Gastrin	G
	Somatostatin	D
Pancreas	Insulin	B
	Glucagon	A
	Pancreatic polypeptide	PP (F/D$_1$)
	Somatostatin	D
Duodenum/jejunum	Secretin	S
	Cholecystokinin	CCK
	Motilin	M
	GIP	GIP
	Somatostatin	D
Ileum/colon	Enteroglucagon	L
	Peptide YY	L
	Neurotensin	N
	Somatostatin	D

Table 4–2. NEUROPEPTIDES OF THE GUT

Calcitonin gene–related peptide (CGRP)
Dynorphin (DYN)
Enkephalins (Leu ENK, Met ENK)
Galanin
Gastrin releasing peptide (GRP)
Neuropeptide Y (NPY)
Peptide HI (PHI or PHM)
Somatostatin
Substance K (neurokinin A)
Substance P
Vasoactive intestinal peptide (VIP)

in a single neuron, while the same peptides are found in different combinations in other neurons.

Intrinsic neurons with cell bodies in the myenteric plexus or the submucous plexus of the gut can act as sensory neurons, as interneurons, or as efferent neurons acting on a variety of target cells in the gut. The sensory nervous system of the gut is extensive, but its functions are largely unknown. One tool that has been used to define the function of the small-fiber sensory nerves is their selective destruction by administration of capsaicin, a substance found in hot peppers. Such experiments have shown that a large proportion of sensory fibers contain substance P or calcitonin gene–related peptide.[8] Capsaicin treatment markedly decreases the concentration of these peptides in the gut and in the dorsal horn of the spinal cord, where they make their primary synapses.

Growth Factors

The peptide growth factors of the gut include hormones, neuropeptides, and locally produced peptides. Gastrin acts as a trophic hormone for the stomach. Cholecystokinin is trophic for the pancreas. Gastrin releasing peptide is trophic for antral gastrin cells.

Epidermal growth factor, or urogastrone, is the best-characterized growth factor in the gut that does not act as a hormone or neuropeptide.[9] Instead it is produced in the salivary glands, in Brunner's glands of the duodenum, and in other sites including the kidney and breast.[10, 11] Urogastrone/epidermal growth factor is secreted into the saliva and into the duodenal lumen;[12] in the blood it is bound to platelets.[13] In newborns, epidermal growth factor from breast milk may serve as a regulator of gut development, either by acting locally on the mucosa or after being absorbed.[14] Less is known about the fate of this peptide in adults. Insulin-like growth factor I, also known as somatomedin C, is the growth-stimulating factor that is secreted by several tissues, including liver, under stimulation by growth hormone.[15] It, rather than growth hormone itself, appears to account for trophic responses to growth hormone. Another form of this peptide, known as insulin-like growth factor II, is secreted in the fetus and regulates fetal tissue development.[16] Other growth factors are produced by macrophages, fibroblasts, and platelets.[17, 18] Some of these factors are listed in Table 4–3. The conditions under which these factors are produced and secreted in gut tissues have not yet been identified clearly.

HORMONE CHEMISTRY

Transcription, Translation, and Posttranslational Processing

All of the hormones and neuropeptides considered in this chapter, with the exception of insulin, are composed of a single peptide chain. All are formed in

Table 4–3. GROWTH FACTORS OF THE GUT

Hormones
    Gastrin
    Cholecystokinin
Neuropeptides
    Gastrin releasing peptide
Local cell products
    Epidermal growth factor/urogastrone
    Insulin-like growth factor I (somatomedin C)
    Insulin-like growth factor II
    Platelet-derived growth factor
    Fibroblast-derived growth factor

their cells of origin by a similar process (Fig. 4–2) Sequences of genetic DNA, known as exons, contain the nucleotide triplets that determine the structure of the hormone precursor, known as the prepropeptide. These exon sequences of genomic DNA are separated by intervening DNA sequences known as introns. Messenger RNA (mRNA) is complementary to exon sequences of DNA. The process by which mRNA is formed is known as transcription. Translation is the process by which mRNA directs the synthesis of the prepropeptide. Newly synthesized prepropeptide undergoes removal of an amino terminal portion, known as the signal peptide, to form a propeptide. Propeptides are processed further by cleavage of peptide bonds to lead to smaller fragments, some of which become hormones. In addition to cleavage of larger precursors into smaller fragments, various modifications can occur to individual amino acids. Some of these modifications make the peptide more resistant to degradation, and some alter the interaction of peptide with its receptor.

Multiple Active Peptides from Single Prohormones

As soon as it became possible to determine the sequence of mRNA by production and sequence analysis of the complementary DNA (cDNA), it became apparent that the propeptides predicted from the gene sequence often contained more than one potentially active peptide sequence. The best-known example is the proopiomelanocortin gene that contains the sequence of β-endorphin, ACTH, and MSH.[19] The proenkephalin gene was found to contain five copies of Met enkephalin and one copy of Leu enkephalin.[20, 21] Inspection of other cDNA sequences has led to the discovery of additional active peptides encoded by the same mRNA as a known active peptide. Examples include peptide HI (PHI), found as a second product of the VIP gene,[22] and substance K (neuromedin A), found as a second product of the substance P gene.[23] If posttranslational processing proceeds normally, each time one gene product is produced the other biologically active peptides encoded by the same mRNA also are produced.

The same genetic information can be used to produce

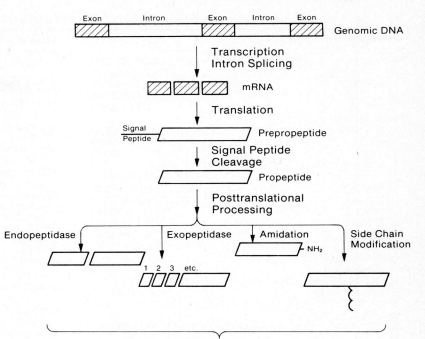

Figure 4–2. General biochemical process by which genes direct the synthesis of biologically active peptides.

different hormones by a process known as alternate mRNA splicing. This process was discovered when mRNA was found that had regions identical to the mRNA encoding calcitonin but also had a unique region. The portion of the calcitonin mRNA that was translated into calcitonin was missing and was replaced by a new portion that was translated into a completely new peptide, known as calcitonin gene–related peptide.[24] The basis for this change in mRNA was found to be substitution of the coding sequence from one exon on the calcitonin gene by an adjacent exon that contained the sequence information for the calcitonin gene–related peptide. Several other examples of alternate mRNA splicing now have been discovered, including alternate splicing of the substance P gene.[25] This process provides a method for tissue-specific gene expression in which one type of endocrine cell or neuron can produce one biologically active peptide and another tissue can produce a second peptide by utilizing all but a small part of the same genetic machinery.

Another type of posttranslational modification leading to multiple hormonal forms is selective cleavage of a large prohormone into smaller fragments that are biologically active because they all contain the critical amino acid sequence that determines bioactivity. Examples include gastrin, cholecystokinin, and somatostatin.[1] Each of these hormones is found in at least two naturally occurring forms that differ only in the length of the peptide chain amino terminal to an active carboxyl terminal sequence.

Other Posttranslational Modifications

The most common amino acid modification that leads to biologic activity is amidation of the carboxyl terminal amino acid residue. Amidated peptides comprise about half of the biologically active gut hormones and neuropeptides. Amidation is not a random process, but depends on a specific sequence of amino acids at the carboxy terminal end of the prohormone. Enzymes cause a sequence of events leading to production of an amide group from a glycine residue by a specific amidating enzyme.[26, 27] In most cases amidation is necessary for biologic activity.

Side chain modifications also may alter biologic activity greatly. Sulfation of the tyrosine residue near the carboxyl terminus of cholecystokinin increases the potency for interaction with specific CCK receptors by about 1000-fold.[28] On the other hand, sulfation of an equivalent tyrosine residue in gastrin has little effect on acid-stimulating activity.

Families of Related Hormones

Examination of the amino acid sequences of the gastrointestinal hormones and neuropeptides reveals that many of them have much greater similarity than can be explained by chance alone. The best explanation for the similarities is that gene duplication during evolution has led to the development of peptides derived from the same primative precursor that perform new specialized functions by activation of newly specialized receptors on target tissues. The structures shown in Table 4–4 are arranged according to potential gene families.

Gastrin-Cholecystokinin Family. All members of this family contain the same biologically active region, the carboxyl terminal sequence Gly-Trp-Met-Asp-Phe-amide.[29] The mRNAs from which these peptides are translated are even more similar because their prohor-

Table 4–4. STRUCTURES OF GASTROINTESTINAL PEPTIDES

Gastrin-Cholecystokinin Family
Gastrin
34 MW 3849	pQLGP QGPPH LVADP SKKQG PWLEE
	EEEAY GWMDF*
17 MW 2098	pQG PWLEE EEEAY GWMDF*
14 MW 1833	WLEE EEEAY GWMDF*
6 MW 817	Y GWMDF*

Cholecystokinin
58 MW 6706	VSQ RTDGE SRAHL GALLA-RYIQQ
	ARKAP SGRMS IVKNL QNLDP SHRIS
	DRDŶM GWMDF*
39 MW 4687	YIQQ ARKAP SGRMS IVKNL QNLDP SHRIS
	DRDŶM GWMDF*
33 MW 3927	KAP SGRMS IVKNL QNLDP SHRIS
	DRDŶM GWMDF*
8 MW 1125	DŶM GWMDF*
7 MW 1010	ŶM GWMDF*
5 MW 654	GWMDF*

Secretin/Glucagon/VIP Family
Secretin MW 3054
    HSDGT FTSEL SRLRE GARLQ RLLQG LL*
Glucagon MW 3483
    HSQGT FTSDY SKYLD SRRAQ DVFQW LMNT
Oxyntomodulin MW 4422
    HSQGT FTSDY SKYLD SRRAQ DVFQW LMNTK RNKNN
    IA
Glicentin MW 8236
    RSLQN TEEKS RSFPA PQTDP LDDPD QMTED KR-
    HSQGT FTSDY SKYLD SRRAQ DVFQW LMNTK RNKNN
    IA
Gastric inhibitory peptide (GIP) MW 4975
    YAEGT FISDY SIAMD KIRQQ DFVNW LLAQK GKKSD
    WHKNI TQ
Growth hormone releasing factor (GRF) MW 5040
    YADAI FTNSY RKVLG QLSAR KLLQD IHSRQ QGESN
    QERGA RARL*
Vasoactive intestinal peptide (VIP) ME 3326
    HSDAV FTDNY TRLRK QMAVK KYLNS ILN*
Peptide HI/HM (PHI/PHM) MW 2985
    HADGV FTSDF SKLLG QLSAK KYLES LM*
Glucagon-like peptide 1 MW 4111
    HDEFE RHAEG TFTSD VSSYL EGQAA KEFIA WLVKG
    R*
Glucagon-like peptide 2 MW 3922
    HADGS FSDEM NTILD NLAAR DFINW LIQTK ITDR

Pancreatic Polypeptide Family
Pancreatic polypeptide (PP) MW 4162
    APLEP VDPGD QATPE QMAQY AAELR RYINM LTRPR
    Y*
Peptide YY (PYY) MW 4241
    YPAKP EAPGE DASPE ELSRY YASLR HYLNL VTRQR
    Y*
Neuropeptide Y (NPY) MW 4368
    YPSKP DNNPGE DAPAE DLARY YSALR HYINL ITRQR
    Y*

Tachykinin/Bombesin Family
Substance P MW 1348
    R PKPQQ FFGLM*
Substance K (neurokinin A) MW 1133
    HKTDS FVGLM*
Neuromedin K (neurokinin B) MW 1216
    DHHDF FVGLM*
Gastrin releasing peptide (GRP) MW 2859
    VP LPAGG GTVLT KMYPR GNHWA VGHLM*
GRP decapeptide MW 1120
    GNHWA VGHLM*

Tachykinin/Bombesin Family *Continued*
Neuromedin B MW 1155
    GHLWA TGHFM*

Opioid Peptides
Proenkephalin Gene Products
Met enkephalin MW 574
    YGGFM
Leu enkephalin MW 556
    YGGFL
Met enkephalin Arg-Phe MW 877
    YGGFMRF
Met enkephalin Arg-Gly-Leu MW 900
    YGGFMRGL
Proopiomelanocortin Gene Products
β endorphin MW 3465
    YGGFM TSEKS QTPLV TLFKN AIIKN AYKKG E
ACTH MW 4541
    SYSME HFRWG KPVGK KRRPV KVYPN GAEDE SAEAF
    PLEF
α MSH MW 1665
    Ac-SYSME HFRWG KPV*
β MSH MW 2176
    DEGPY KMEHF RWGSP PKD
α MSH MW 1464
    GVMGH FRWDR FG
Predynorphin Gene Products
Dynorphin MW 2263
    YGGFL RRIRP KLKWD DNQ
Leu enkephalin MW 556
    YGGFL
β neoendorphin MW 1100
    YGGFL RKYP
Leumorphin MW 3352
    YGGFL RRQFK VVTRS QEDPN AYSGE LFDA

Insulin Family
Insulin MW 5795
    GIVEQ CCTSI CSLYQ LENYC NFVNQ HLCGS B-chain
    HLVEA LYLVC GERGF FYTPK T A-chain
Insulin-like growth factor I MW 7654
    GPETL CGAEL VDALQ FVCGD RGFYF NKPTG YGSSS-
    RRAPQ TGIVD ECCFR SCDLR RLEMY CAPLK PAKSA

Epidermal Growth Factor Family
Epidermal growth factor/urogastrone MW 6222
    NSDSE CPLSH DGYCL HDGVC MYIEA LDKYA CNCVV
    GYIGE RCQYR DLKWW ELR

Somatostatin Family
Somatostatin 28 MW 3150
    SANSN PAMAP RERKA GCKNF FWKTF TSC
Somatostatin 14 MW 1640
    A GCKNF FWKTF TSC

Calcitonin Family
Calcitonin MW 3420
    CGNLS TCMLG TYTQD FNKFH TFPQT AIGVG AP*
Calcitonin gene–related peptide MW 3791
    ACDTA TCVTH RLAGL LSRSG GVVKN NFVPT NVGSK
    AF*

Other Gastrointestinal Peptides
Motilin MW 2699
    FVPIF TYGEL QRMQE KERNK GQ
Neurotensin MW 1696
    pQLYEH KPRRP YIL
Galanin MW 3210
    GWTLN SAGYL LGPHA IDNHR SFHDK YGLA*
Thyrotropin releasing hormone (TRH) MW 362
    pQHP*

---

pQ, pyroglutamyl; *, C-terminal amide; Ŷ, tyrosine sulfate.

mones have a common amino acid sequence that is removed to form the carboxyl terminal amide group.[30, 31] Gastrin and cholecystokinin are characterized by multiple proteolytic processing sites, leading to great variation in the size of biologically active peptides that can be isolated from tissues and blood.[32] Posttranslational processing of cholecystokinin also includes sulfation of the tryosine residue seven amino acids from the carboxyl terminus. This sulfation is necessary for full biologic potency of cholecystokinin, but a similar sulfation in gastrin, found in about half the gastrin molecules, has little effect on gastrin biologic activity.

Secretin/Glucagon/VIP Family. This group of peptides includes the largest number of members. The mRNAs from at least two members encode for more than one biologically active peptide. Peptides in this group are distributed almost equally between hormones and neuropeptides. The oldest known member of this family is secretin.[33] The cDNA sequence for secretin has not been reported. Other members include glucagon, glucagon-related peptides, gastric inhibitory polypeptide (GIP), vasoactive inhibitory polypeptide (VIP), peptide histidine isoleucine (PHI), and growth hormone releasing factor (GRF).[1] VIP and PHI are encoded by the same mRNA,[22] as are glucagon and glucagon-related peptides.[34] PHI was isolated originally from the pig and was named for its first and last amino acids. In man the last amino acid is methionine rather than isoleucine, so some prefer to call the human peptide PHM instead of PHI.

Pancreatic Polypeptide Family. The three peptides in this family all contain the same number of amino acids and have other structural similarities including a carboxyl terminal tyrosine amide.[35] Pancreatic polypeptide and peptide tyrosine tyrosine (PYY) are hormones, while neuropeptide Y (NPY) is a neuropeptide.[36–38]

Opioid Peptide Family. Members of this family are products of three different genes: proenkephalin gene, proopiomelanocortin gene, and prodynorphin gene.[39] The proenkephalin gene product is subjected to posttranslational processing that yields four copies of Met enkephalin, one of Leu enkephalin, and one each of Met enkephalin Arg-Phe and Met enkephalin Arg-Gly-Leu. The proopiomelanocortin gene produces β-endorphin, ACTH, α-MSH, β-MSH, and γ-MSH. The prodynorphin gene produces dynorphin, Leu enkephalin, and β-neoendorphin.

Tachykinin-Bombesin Family. Substance P is the prototype of mammalian tachykinins. One of two genes that encodes substance P also encodes another biologically active neuropeptide known as substance K or neurokinin A or neuromedin L. Another gene produces neuromedin K, also known as neurokinin B.[39] The bombesin-like peptides are structurally related to the tachykinins. All members of this family have a carboxyl terminal methionine amide residue that is necessary for biologic activity. The major product of the bombesin-type gene is gastrin releasing peptide (GRP), a 27 amino acid neuropeptide. The decapeptide of GRP also is produced by posttranslational processing of this gene product.[40] Another gene encodes for a related peptide known as neuromedin B.

Insulin Family. Insulin and two other peptides, insulin-like growth factor I (IGF-I) and insulin-like growth factor II (IGF-II), all are produced from different genes.[15, 16] Each reacts at lower affinity with the receptors for the other two peptides.

Epidermal Growth Factor Family. Urogastrone is the human equivalent of epidermal growth factor (EGF) isolated from mice.[9] Transforming growth factor A (TGF-A) reacts with epidermal growth factor receptors but is produced by a different gene.[41]

Calcitonin Family. Calcitonin and calcitonin gene–related peptide (CGRP) are produced by differential gene splicing of the same gene.[42] CGRP is expressed in the gut as a neuropeptide, while calcitonin is not expressed by gut tissues.

Somatostatin Family. The only members of the somatostatin family that definitely are present in mammals are two products that represent cleavage of the same precursor at different sites, somatostatin-14 and somatostatin-28.[43] Other somatostatin-like peptides that have been found in lower species have not been found in mammals.

Peptides without Families. The list of peptides that do not fit into known families is small. Motilin and neurotensin are two such hormones. Several amphibian peptides are structurally related to neurotensin. The newly discovered neuropeptide galanin does not appear to have any relatives. Pancreostatin is a very new pancreatic peptide that has structural similarity to a portion of chromogranin, a peptide found in the granule membranes of endocrine and neuropeptide cells. Thyrotropin releasing hormone also belongs on this list, although its gene encodes several copies of this tripeptide amide neuropeptide.

GUT PEPTIDE HORMONE RECEPTORS

All biologic actions of peptide hormones and neuropeptides depend on interactions between these peptides and specific receptor proteins located on the surface of target cells. Receptors must have high affinity and specificity to recognize individual peptides, and they must possess mechanisms to relay signals generated by hormone-receptor coupling to the interior of the target cell. Interactions of peptides with their receptors lead to cellular responses that are proportional to the number of receptors occupied, although not necessarily on a one-to-one basis. Cellular responses to one peptide may be enhanced or suppressed by the action of other peptides on separate sets of receptors on the same cell.

Bioassays relating peptide concentration to cellular response measure receptor function indirectly. Only in homogeneous cell preparation can the cells possessing specific receptors be identified with certainty. In complex tissues, hormones and neuropeptides may influence target cells indirectly by altering release of other transmitters from nerves or paracrine cells.

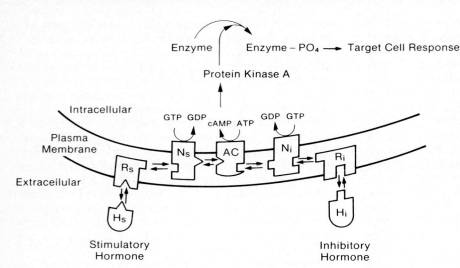

Figure 4–3. Stimulatory and inhibitory pathways involving adenylate cyclase modulation by peptide-receptor interactions. Occupation of a stimulatory (Rs) or inhibitory (Ri) receptor sends a stimulatory or inhibitory signal to adenylate cyclase (AC). These signals are transmitted by GTP binding regulatory proteins (Ns and Ni). The activity of adenylate cyclase determines the rate of formation of cAMP, which in turn regulates the activity of protein kinase A. This enzyme activates certain intracellular enzymes and other regulatory intracellular proteins by causing phosphorylation of specific amino acid side chains.

Receptor-mediated cell activation involves recognition and binding of the peptide to a specific receptor followed by transduction of the signal produced by receptor occupation to produce a cellular response. Usually receptors activate one of two major pathways. One pathway involves stimulation or inhibition of adenylate cyclase in the cell membrane, leading to changes in intracellular cyclic AMP (Fig. 4–3). Stimulation or inhibition of adenylate cyclase activity is

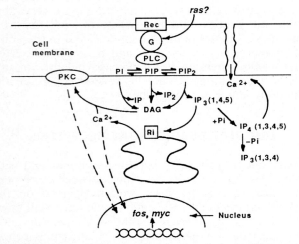

Figure 4–4. Pathways by which receptor occupation causes cell activation by calcium, inositol phosphates, and protein kinase C (PKC). An agent that works through the PI system first binds to a specific receptor (Rec) on the cell surface. This signal is transmitted through a G protein (G), which may be the cellular ras gene product, to the enzyme phospholipase C (PLC). This enzyme splits PIP_2 to diacylglycerol (DAG) and inositol trisphosphate [IP_3 (1,4,5)], and may also split the other phosphatidylinositide lipids (PI and PIP). The DAG and the calcium ions that are released by inositol trisphosphate from the cell's internal stores activate the enzyme protein kinase C. The inositol trisphosphate is also converted to inositol-1,3,4,5-tetrakisphosphate (IP_4), which apparently stimulates calcium ion entry from the cell exterior. The IP_4 is broken down to the 1,3,4-isomer of inositol trisphosphate. The effects of protein kinase C activity and elevated calcium ion concentrations include the activation of the fos and myc oncogenes. (From Marx, J. L. Science 235:974, 1987. Copyright 1987 by the American Association for the Advancement of Science. Used by permission.)

coupled to occupation of stimulatory or inhibitory receptors by guanylate binding proteins. The protein that activates cAMP production is known as the stimulatory subunit, N_s, and the protein that inhibits cAMP production is known as the inhibitory subunit, N_i. Stimulation of the cAMP pathway leads to activation of a protein kinase known as protein kinase A.

Another pathway is more complex and has received great attention in the past few years. It originally was called the calcium pathway. Now it is recognized that messengers in this pathway include inositol trisphosphate, diacylglycerol, and protein kinase C as well as calcium. Changes in intracellular calcium may be transient despite prolonged responses. Both the cAMP and the calcium/inositol/protein kinase C pathways lead to activation of specific protein kinases. Kinases are enzymes that phosphorylate proteins in the cell that are responsible for further cell activation. A schematic illustration of the major pathways for receptor activation of cell function through this pathway is given in Figure 4–4.

Studies of receptor function include radioligand analysis of binding affinity and receptor number; measurement of cellular cAMP, calcium, inositol phosphates, diacylglycerol, and protein kinase C; and measurement of cell responses to stimulation. Receptor binding studies also are quite useful for evaluating receptor antagonists. The most satisfactory system for performing such studies is a preparation of purified, healthy whole cells. However, useful information also can be obtained from plasma membrane preparations and from more complex tissues.

Great progress is being made in analysis of receptor structure-function relationships because of success in cloning the cDNA and determining complete amino acid sequences of several receptors. Among the receptors that have been completely analyzed are those for insulin and for epidermal growth factor. Precise information now can be obtained about peptide binding sites. In addition, the intracellular activities of the receptor can be studied. The intracellular portions of both the insulin and the epidermal growth factor receptors have tyrosine kinase activity, meaning that they cause phosphorylation of tyrosine groups in specific intracellular proteins.

The most complete information about gastrointestinal receptors has been obtained in pancreatic acinar cells. Other cells that have been studied in some detail are the gastric oxyntic (parietal) cell, smooth muscle cells, and enterocytes. Considerable information has been deduced about receptors on endocrine cells. The following is a brief synopsis about some of the receptor studies done on these cell systems.

Pancreatic Acinar Cell Receptors. The two classes of receptors are well defined on pancreatic acinar cells (Table 4–5). Secretin, VIP, and PHI are the natural ligands for two classes of acinar receptor. One is called secretin-preferring and the other is VIP-preferring. The secretin-preferring receptors probably are the most important for stimulation of pancreatic bicarbonate secretion in man. The calcium/inositol/protein kinase C pathways can be activated by occupation of at least four different acinar receptors: cholecystokinin, cholinergic, bombesin/GRP, and substance P. Occupation of any of these receptors produces an equivalent intracellular response. Activation of one of these receptors plus one that increases cAMP causes potentiation of enzyme secretion. Progress has been made in the purification and chemical characterization of the CCK receptor, and the complete amino acid sequence soon may be determined.

Gastric Oxyntic (Parietal) Cell Receptors. Studies with isolated parietal cells have revealed biologic evidence for the presence of separate receptors for gastrin, histamine, and acetylcholine. Whereas the CCK receptor in the pancreas is highly specific for CCK, and gastrin has 1000-fold lower potency, the gastric receptor has almost equal affinity for gastrin and CCK. This probably means that CCK inhibits acid secretion *in vivo* by acting on some other cell type that inhibits the parietal cell. It is possible that the inhibitory agent is somatostatin, but specific receptors for somatostatin have been difficult to identify on the parietal cell. Both gastrin and acetylcholine activate the calcium/inositol/protein kinase C pathways, while histamine activates cAMP production. Histamine H_2 receptor antagonists prevent cAMP stimulation by histamine by direct in-

Table 4–5. PATHWAYS FOR ACINAR CELL ACTIVATION

Receptor activation pathways
Activators of adenylate cyclase/protein kinase A pathway
Secretin
VIP
PHI/PHM
Cholera toxin
Activators of Ca^+/inositol/protein kinase C pathway
Acetylcholine
Cholecystokinin
GRP/bombesin
Substance P

Activation of both pathways produces potentiated enzyme secretion

teraction with the histamine receptor. Prostaglandins of the E series inhibit histamine activation of adenylate cyclase indirectly. The combination of histamine receptor activation with either gastrin or acetylcholine receptor activation results in potentiation of acid secretion. This interaction probably explains why histamine receptor antagonism is highly effective *in vivo* to inhibit all forms of gastric acid stimulation.

Smooth Muscle Receptors. Preparations of dispersed smooth muscle cells have simplified the distinction between muscle cell receptors and nerve receptors in smooth muscle tissues. Isolated muscle cells have revealed very high sensitivity to several hormones and neuropeptides, with good correlations between contractile responses and direct studies of receptor binding. The best direct receptor binding results have utilized radiolabeled substance P, substance K, or VIP. Functional responses to CCK8 and to acetylcholine also have been analyzed. Receptors on smooth muscle from specific tissues often demonstrate high-affinity receptors for certain peptides predicted from biologic responses to those peptides *in vivo,* for example, high-affinity receptors for CCK in the gallbladder.

Endocrine Cell Receptors. Although many studies with isolated gut endocrine cells are preliminary, it is clear that they have receptors that explain *in vivo* endocrine responses to peptides. Thus gastrin cells have high-affinity receptors for bombesin and GRP that lead to gastrin release and receptors for somatostatin that inhibit gastrin release. Somatostatin cells are stimulated to release somatostatin by activation of a high-affinity CCK receptor and a somewhat lower-affinity gastrin receptor. Neurotensin cells have responses that resemble those of gastrin cells. Acetylcholine causes hormone release from most endocrine cells but inhibits release from somatostatin cells.

Enterocyte Receptors. Although intestinal mucosal cells respond to a number of hormones and neuropeptides, the only peptide receptor that has been characterized by direct binding studies is the VIP receptor. Activation of this receptor, located on the basolateral membrane, causes an increase in cellular cAMP in the enterocyte.

Peptic (Chief) Cell Receptors. No peptide receptors have been demonstrated on chief cells, although they are suspected from physiologic studies. Chief cells contain stimulatory cholinergic receptors and stimulatory beta-adrenergic receptors.

HORMONE MEASUREMENT: RADIOIMMUNOASSAY

Most published information concerning concentrations of hormones in the blood has been based on radioimmunoassay measurements performed on plasma or serum specimens. The general principles of radioimmunoassay are well known and are based on specific inhibition of the reaction between a labeled ligand and an antibody specific for that ligand by unlabeled material. The principles of radioimmunoassay have been applied very successfully to studies of gastrointestinal physiology and disease.[44] Almost all known gastrointestinal peptides can be measured by radioimmunoassay. Several of these peptides also can be measured successfully by bioassay. One peptide for which bioassay may offer some advantage is cholecystokinin. The multiplicity of biologically active forms and the chemical similarity of the biologically active region to gastrin, coupled with the exquisite sensitivity of the pancreatic acinus to CCK but not to gastrin, have led to the development of a very satisfactory bioassay for CCK. However, suitable radioimmunoassays also have been developed for CCK. For all other gut hormones and neuropeptides, radioimmunoassay offers the best method for specific measurement.

Potential Pitfalls

Several pitfalls may lead to invalid radioimmunoassay measurement of peptides. Most hormones are destroyed by plasma enzymes, although at rates that vary greatly. Rapid cooling and centrifugation of blood samples followed by immediate freezing of plasma will minimize the initial degradation. Appropriate enzyme inhibitors also can be used successfully. Unfortunately, trypsin is not a major cause of peptide inactivation by plasma, so the most commonly used inhibitor, aprotinin (Trasylol), often is not protective. Calcium chelation with EDTA or 1,10-phenanthroline will inhibit the action of metalloenzymes. Phosphoramidon inhibits the action of another common endopeptidase, EC 3.4.24.11 ("enkephalinase").[45] Acidification of plasma or immediate extraction into organic solvents also can be used in some cases. The appropriate method for collection of samples should be established for each hormone before embarking on studies that involve its measurement. Similar studies must be performed in the radioimmunoassay laboratory to determine assay conditions that do not lead to losses by enzymatic degradation or by absorption to glass and plastic surfaces during the assay procedure. It is quite helpful to obtain a known amount of standard peptide and use this to develop internal standards to monitor recovery of the peptide when it is added to blood or plasma.

A second problem that arises in radioimmunoassay measurement of peptides is falsely increased values due to interference in binding of labeled peptide to the antibody by substances other than the peptide being measured. Nonspecific interference can be produced by a variety of plasma proteins, including albumin. Anticoagulants such as heparin can produce falsely high or low values. Degradation of labeled peptide by plasma enzymes can lead to misleading values unless the plasma is treated to remove or inactivate enzymes. Hormone concentrations are measured by comparing the inhibition produced by an unknown sample with the inhibition produced by known amounts of standard peptide. If the peptide standard has lost activity during storage, the values obtained for unknown peptide

concentrations will be falsely elevated. Finally, related peptides and biologically inactive degradation products can inhibit antibody-label binding and cause misleading values. A good example is neurotensin, for which values obtained with amino terminal antibodies are much higher than those obtained with carboxyl terminal antibodies because of the presence of large amounts of biologically active amino terminal degradation product in the blood.[46] An example of potential interference between related peptides is cholecystokinin, which has the same active carboxyl terminal pentapeptide sequence as gastrin. Some antibodies specific for this region recognize both peptides equally, while others preferentially recognize one peptide, usually gastrin, but retain some reactivity with the other.

Extraction of tissues to determine hormone concentration presents other problems. Tissue enzymes rapidly degrade peptides, and homogenization of tissue at neutral pH greatly speeds up the process. Basic peptides, including most of the hormones and neuropeptides except gastrin, are extracted poorly in neutral or basic conditions. They remain bound to tissue proteins, even after these proteins are denatured by boiling, unless the solution is acidified. Many peptides will adhere to surfaces of containers unless appropriate carriers are included. Therefore extractions are best done in laboratories experienced in this type of work and should include addition of an internal standard to monitor purification.[47] Usually it is safe to freeze tissue samples immediately on dry ice, or preferably in liquid nitrogen, and to store them at temperatures of $-45°C$ or lower before they are analyzed. Long-term storage of plasma or tissue at common freezer temperatures of $-20°C$ can lead to marked losses of peptide activity. If no other freezer is available, some method of inactivation, such as boiling in water and saving the tissue and the water, should be considered.

Clinical Applications

For practical use in clinical situations, the major role of hormone measurement is to detect hypersecretion of hormones by tumors or due to endocrine cell hyperplasia or hyperactivity. The gastrointestinal hormones and neuropeptides that are produced by tumors include gastrin, VIP, somatostatin, pancreatic polypeptide, neurotensin, substance P, substance K, and other tachykinins. Insulin and glucagon also are produced by islet cell tumors. When these hormones are analyzed for clinical purposes it is important to assure that the sample has been collected under conditions that prevent degradation by plasma enzymes. The blood samples should be obtained under conditions that do not produce physiologic increases in hormone concentration that can be confused with pathologic concentrations in the fasting patient. For example, gastrin and pancreatic polypeptide are increased markedly after a meal, while VIP and other neuropeptides are relatively unchanged.

Units of Measurement

The other major consideration is the upper limit of normal and the range obtained for each hormone in normal and abnormal clinical conditions in the laboratory performing the test. It is not satisfactory to refer to published normal values because there is too much variation between laboratories. Each laboratory may obtain internally consistent results, but differences in standards, antibodies, nonspecific interference by plasma proteins, and assay conditions may lead to wide differences in normal values. For example, the upper limit of normal plasma gastrin concentrations varies between 100 and 300 pg/ml among laboratories that produce internally consistent results. A value of 300 is consistent with gastrinoma in one laboratory but is normal in another.

It should be kept in mind that hormone concentrations are reported in different units. The designation pg/ml, meaning picograms per milliliter, is based on the weight of the peptide without regard to its molecular weight. It is more correct chemically to express results in molar terms. The term pM means picomolar, or picomoles per liter. The designation "pico," abbreviated p, refers to a unit of 10^{-12}, while "femto," abbreviated f, refers to 10^{-15}, and "nano," abbreviated n, refers to 10^{-9}. The use of a capital M refers to moles per liter. Thus a value of 50 pM, or 50 pmoles per liter, is the same as 50 fmol/ml. To convert pg/ml to pM or fmol/ml, look up the molecular weight of the standard peptide, divide that number by 1000, then divide the pg/ml value by the result. For example, the molecular weight of gastrin is 2100. A plasma gastrin value of 63 pg/ml is divided by 2.1 to give the equivalent molar value, 30 pM or 30 fmol/ml. Some assays retain the archaic designation of "units" or "clinical units." These originally were determined by arbitrary bioassay testing when no other chemical or immunologic measurements were available. One microgram of secretin is equal roughly to 4 clinical units. One microgram of cholecystokinin is roughly equal to 3 clinical units. A clinical unit of secretin thus is equal roughly to 80 nanomoles, and a clinical unit of CCK to 100 nanomoles. One microunit/ml thus would be equivalent to 80 pM or 80 fmol/ml for secretin and 100 pM or 100 fmol/ml for CCK. All other peptides except insulin now are expressed in terms of weight or molar concentration rather than units.

HORMONE RELEASE AND POSTSECRETORY PROCESSING

Peptide hormones are released by endocytosis, similar to the mechanism for release of pancreatic enzymes from acinar cells. Once released, peptides either diffuse locally to interact with receptors on nearby cells, characteristic for neuropeptides and paracrine agents, or they enter the blood stream and become true circulating hormones. Peptides produced by cells or nerves in the gastrointestinal mucosa also frequently can be detected in the gut lumen. Each endocrine cell responds in a characteristic way to the presence of specific nutrients in the gut lumen. Endocrine cells also are influenced by parasympathetic and sympathetic neurotransmitters. Most endocrine and neural peptide release is inhibited by somatostatin, and most gut endocrine cells are stimulated by gastrin releasing peptide/bombesin. The factors regulating neuropeptide release are less well defined but may be similar to factors regulating release of classical neurotransmitters. Release or inhibition of release is the effect usually described, but alteration of synthesis by regulation of mRNA transcription frequently parallels the changes in peptide release.

Regulation of Hormone Release by Gut Luminal Contents

A brief synopsis of the known regulators of the more important gastrointestinal hormones[1] includes:

Gastrin. Digested proteins and amino acids, especially phenylalanine and tryptophan, stimulate gastrin release. Release is inhibited by luminal acidification and by somatostatin. Other unidentified components in coffee, wine, and beer are good gastrin releasers *in vivo*. Calcium in the lumen of the stomach is a good gastrin releaser, while intravenous calcium is relatively ineffective. Beta-sympathetic stimulation and GABA can increase gastrin release. Vagal parasympathetic release is complicated. Sham feeding and gastric distention both cause gastrin release, but this stimulation is enhanced by atropine. Bombesin and GRP are especially effective gastrin releasers.

Cholecystokinin. The same types of protein and amino acids that release gastrin also release cholecystokinin, but digestible fat and fatty acids also are strong releasers. Glucose may have a moderate stimulatory activity in man. Acid in the upper intestine does not inhibit, and may enhance, cholecystokinin release. Divalent cations including calcium, magnesium, and zinc also act as luminal stimulants. Bombesin/GRP peptides are effective releasers.

The most complex regulation of cholecystokinin release involves the action of pancreatobiliary juice, particularly trypsin. In the rat diversion of pancreatic juice from the intestinal lumen leads to cholecystokinin release, and administration of trypsin reverses the stimulation. Trypsin inhibitors also cause cholecystokinin release in rats. Similar effects in man are more difficult to demonstrate, possibly because it is necessary to inhibit both trypsin and chymotrypsin to produce good stimulation.

Secretin. Secretin release is stimulated by acidification of the duodenal mucosa to a pH of 3 to 4 or lower. Fatty acids may be modest secretin releasing agents, while certain components of spicy foods such as 1-phenylpentanol are highly effective. Bile appears to enhance secretin release. Unlike most other gut hormones, secretin is not responsive to exogenous bombesin or GRP.

Gastric Inhibitory Polypeptide. GIP is an upper intestinal hormone that is released by all major classes of nutrients, carbohydrates, proteins, and fats. It also is released in response to bombesin and to beta-adrenergic stimulation.

Motilin. Motilin is unusual in that its release is maximal during fasting. Peak plasma concentrations of motilin occur approximately every 90 to 100 minutes during fasting. This cyclical release pattern is abolished by ingestion of a meal. However, fat may cause an increase in motilin. Pancreatobiliary juice may also be stimulatory. Certain antibiotics such as erythromycin appear to cause motilin release.

Somatostatin. The factors regulating somatostatin release are poorly understood and are complicated by the potential for this peptide to act as a paracrine agent or as a neuropeptide, in addition to its activity as a hormone.[48] Various food components have been found to cause an increase in plasma somatostatin, but the results have not been consistent. Fat appears to be the best candidate as a nutrient releaser of somatostatin. In isolated systems somatostatin in the stomach appears to be released by luminal acid. Cholinergic agents inhibit somatostatin release *in vitro*, but the effect of vagal and cholinergic stimulation *in vivo* is more difficult to determine. *In vitro* somatostatin also can be released by beta-adrenergic stimulants and in isolated stomach by a wide variety of peptides that inhibit gastrin release and acid secretion, including secretin, GIP, VIP, glucagon, and cholecystokinin. Bombesin may release somatostatin by an indirect mechanism.

Neurotensin. The major neurotensin releasing factor in food is fat. Bombesin also is an effective releaser.

Enteroglucagon. Enteroglucagon release is stimulated strongly by fat and probably to a lesser degree by carbohydrates. It too is released by bombesin.

Pancreatic Polypeptide. This peptide is released strongly by the same peptides and amino acids that release gastrin. Other nutrients also may cause pancreatic polypeptide release, but their effects may be secondary to gastric distention rather than to a specific nutrient effect. Pancreatobiliary juice has been reported to release pancreatic polypeptide. Release of pancreatic polypeptide is highly sensitive to anticholinergic medications and is virtually abolished by moderate doses of atropine. Release can be stimulated by cephalic stimulation, sham feeding, or gastric distention. Stimulation by these reflex mechanisms and by protein meals is virtually abolished by atropine and by vagotomy. Release may return gradually months or years after vagotomy. Since the pancreatic polypeptide cells in the pancreas are not in direct contact with the bowel lumen, some secondary mechanism must be involved. One possibility is cholecystokinin, which is a moderate releasing agent for this peptide. However, the patterns of release of pancreatic polypeptide and of cholecystokinin are different, since fat is a strong CCK releaser but a poor pancreatic polypeptide releaser. A reflex involving gastrin releasing peptide could be involved, since GRP and bombesin are strong

pancreatic polypeptide releasers and their effects are markedly inhibited by atropine.

Peptide YY. This peptide is released strongly by the presence of fat in the intestinal lumen, as are the other distal intestinal hormones. Bombesin also is effective in releasing PYY.

Regulation of Neuropeptide Release

Neuropeptides are released from granules located in nerve terminals. These peptides are destroyed by enzymes in the tissues where they are released. Some fraction of the released peptide may enter the circulation or the gut lumen and provide a possibility of monitoring its release in the tissues, but the concentrations found in these fluids cannot be translated directly into concentrations of peptide present at target sites.

The factors regulating neuropeptide release also are more difficult to study than those regulating hormone release. Most of the data obtained have utilized *in vitro* animal experiments that may not be applicable to intact humans.[39] Occasionally, as in the case of VIP, it has been possible to release enough peptide into the blood to permit measurement in plasma.

Release of neuropeptides can be demonstrated by the same general types of stimulation that are used to produce release of other neurotransmitters. The most commonly used stimulants are high concentrations of potassium in the presence of adequate concentrations of calcium, electrical depolarization, and nicotinic cholinergic ganglionic stimulants. Electrical stimulation of the vagus or sympathetic nerves can be performed *in vivo* in animals. So far, these approaches have not produced a picture of specific release mechanisms for specific neuropeptides.

Use of specific blocking agents can reveal that a substance is released in physiologically relevant amounts but does not indicate whether the substance is released constantly or in pulses. Thus, the inhibition of gastric secretion by naloxone indicates that some opioid mechanism in the stomach stimulates gastric acid secretion but does not reveal the location or nature of the substance. Few other blocking agents are available. An alternate method for blocking receptors is desensitization. Use of desensitization to substance P has revealed that bombesin probably acts in the esophageal sphincter and cholecystokinin probably acts in the ileum through substance P release. Other substances that can release substance P from nerves include serotonin and neurotensin, while opiate withdrawal also causes substance P release.

Some physiologic models in animals have shown the release of two peptides, substance P and VIP, by physiologic reflexes. Substance P is released by increases in small intestinal luminal pressure, and the pressure generated during a peristaltic wave is sufficient to cause this effect. Vasoactive intestinal polypeptide is released in the stomach by esophageal distention and in the intestine by intestinal distention. VIP also can be released by electrical vagal stimulation, by intraduodenal fat or acid, by serotonin, by oxytocin, and by intestinal ischemia. Experimental evidence also has been obtained for physiologically relevant release of GRP/bombesin peptides in rats. Passive immunization with bombesin antibody prevents release of gastrin in some experimental systems, implying that these peptides mediate gastrin release *in vivo.*

Inhibitors of Neuropeptide Release

Proof of neural regulation of a response often includes the demonstration that nerve blockade prevents the response. This type of antagonism is difficult to produce for specific neuropeptides, but general inhibition of nerve transmission in experimental systems can be produced with the sodium channel blocker tetrodotoxin. Tetrodotoxon-sensitive responses usually are caused by release of neurotransmitters. One of the major clues for the involvement of neuropeptides in physiologic processes is demonstration that the response is not inhibited by usual cholinergic and adrenergic antagonists but is inhibited by treatment with tetrodotoxon. Unfortunately this agent is highly poisonous and cannot be used in conscious animals. Other evidence for neuropeptide action is provided when ganglionic blocking agents prevent a response but adrenergic and cholinergic agents do not. Low calcium can be used to prevent neurotransmitter release *in vitro,* but this approach cannot be used *in vivo.*

A few physiologic and pharmacologic factors have been identified that inhibit local neuropeptide release. Met enkephalin release is inhibited by intestinal distention. Substance P release is inhibited by opiates, hexamethonium, and alpha-adrenergic stimulants. Since intestinal distention is known to release substance P, it is possible that this release is mediated in part by inhibition of enkephalin release. VIP release also is inhibited by alpha-adrenergic activity induced by splanchnic nerve stimulation and can be inhibited by serotonin antagonists.

Regulation of Growth Factor Release

The stimulants for release of the hormonal growth factors gastrin and cholecystokinin are the same as for their release as hormonal regulators of gastric and pancreatic secretion. End-organ failure often causes compensatory hormone release. This is the case for gastrin in patients with atrophic gastritis and chronic achlorhydria. Increased release of cholecystokinin in patients with pancreatic insufficiency also has been reported. Conditions leading to increased release of gastrin releasing peptide have not been established, but this peptide is secreted as a growth factor by many small cell lung carcinomas.[49]

Some growth factors, including EGF/urogastrone and a peptide resembling bombesin, are present in milk.[50] Since the fetal and neonatal intestine absorbs many proteins intact, it is likely that such peptides regulate growth and development of the intestine and of other organs in fetal and neonatal life.

Release of EGF/urogastrone and of other local growth factors such as platelet-derived growth factors has not been studied in detail. Both of these peptides are contained in platelets and are likely to be released during the early phases of platelet adhesion following vascular damage.[13, 51] EGF/urogastrone also is secreted into the saliva and duodenal juice.[12] Factors regulating this secretion are unknown.

Postsecretory Processing, Clearance, and Degradation

After hormones and neuropeptides are released they have a relatively brief half-life in the body as active peptides before they are degraded. In some cases the initial degradation steps produce peptides that retain biologic activity. Such breakdown from larger to smaller active forms is known as postsecretory processing. The best-known examples are for gastrin and cholecystokinin; initial enzymatic processing at the amino terminal end of these molecules produces smaller peptides with full biologic activity. It is possible that some peptides might actually increase in activity as a result of such processing in the blood, but no good examples are available.

Most active peptides in blood have circulating half-lives between 2 and 30 minutes. Any peptide with a half-life less than 15 minutes must be degraded at multiple sites, because the blood flow to any single organ such as the kidney is not sufficient to permit complete removal in such a short time. Various studies have revealed that there are arteriovenous gradients for biologically active peptides across numerous capillary beds. The presence of a gradient means that the tissue is taking up some of the peptide. When a gradient exists under steady state conditions the tissue also must be degrading the peptide. Several enzyme systems that are capable of degrading multiple hormones and neuropeptides have been described. The best characterized are angiotensin converting enzyme, "enkephalinase" (EC 3.4.24.11), and several aminopeptidases. The major activity of these enzymes seems to be in tissues rather than in blood, but their exact location and relative importance have not been determined. It is possible that inhibition of the degrading systems could lead to prolonged activity of both circulating and locally released transmitters. For example, the elevated concentrations of many peptides found in uremia cannot be explained simply by loss of renal clearance, and some general defect in hormone metabolism may occur in the uremic syndrome.

Differential clearance rates account for the relative amounts of molecular forms of peptides found in the blood. For example, gastrin 34 clearance is about six to eight times slower than gastrin 17 clearance, so gastrin 34 is the most abundant form of gastrin in blood although more gastrin 17 is released from the antrum.[52] Large forms of cholecystokinin also seem to predominate in blood compared with the octapeptide, also possibly for the same reason.[32] Somatostatin 14 is cleared much faster than somatostatin 28, and somatostatin 28 has been the major form found in the human circulation although the largest tissue stores of somatostatin contain a preponderance of somatostatin 14.

Metabolites of hormones may have longer half-lives than the biologically active hormone and accumulate at higher concentrations in blood. The principal example among gastrointestinal hormones is neurotensin. Peptidases in blood cleave the 13 amino acid parent molecule into two fragments that have little or no biologic activity. The amino terminal 1–8 fragment has a much longer half-life than the parent and accumulates in blood. Failure to recognize this phenomenon has led to misleading estimates of the concentrations of circulating hormone. For example, measurement of neurotensin with an antibody specific for the amino terminal portion reveals mainly the inactive fragment.

Although the pathways for tissue degradation are not known for all hormones or neuropeptides, they have been studied *in vivo* for a few. Hollow fibers implanted in tissues have been used as artificial lymphatics to study degradation of labeled neuropeptides. Such studies revealed that neurotensin, GRP decapeptide, and substance P are broken down by a system having the characteristics of "enkephalinase."[53] This enzyme has been purified from kidney and from stomach.

PHYSIOLOGIC ACTIONS OF GUT HORMONES

Criteria for Physiologic Activity

In order to qualify completely as a physiologically important hormone, a peptide must meet several criteria. The peptide must be released into blood during the time that a biologic response in a target organ is being stimulated or inhibited. Infusion of the pure natural peptide intravenously must reproduce the effect on the target organ. The chemistry of the peptide should be known completely so that synthetic peptide can be prepared and shown to reproduce the effects found with the natural peptide. The circulating concentrations of the peptide that cause artificial stimulation of the target should be the same as those producing a similar degree of stimulation under physiologic conditions of release. When more than one form of the same peptide is produced, it must be shown that the activities of the sum of active peptides in the circulation accounts for biologic responses. Furthermore, it must be shown that the radioimmunoassay used for detection of peptide in the circulation is not measuring biologically inactive degradation products. It is extremely useful to have a bioassay of plasma that has high enough sensitivity to confirm the results obtained by radioimmunoassay. This goal has been achieved for cholecystokinin by development of a highly sensitive and specific pancreatic acinar cell bioassay.[54]

Finally, in order to confirm the biologic significance of a circulating peptide as a hormone, it should be possible to prevent the physiologic response to a stimulant by removing the peptide from the blood or by specific antagonism at its receptor. Resection or destruction of one gut endocrine cell without disturbing other physiologic systems has been quite difficult. However, it has been possible to use antibodies for specific immunoneutralization of several peptides. Such studies have added greatly to establishing the hormonal role of secretin, gastrin, and motilin and to establishing a possible role for GIP but have made an important role for pancreatic polypeptide appear less likely. Use of receptor antagonists has been useful for establishing the physiologic roles of gastrin and cholecystokinin.

The most likely physiologic roles for gastrointestinal hormones are described below. Only a few of these have been proved by all the criteria described in the preceding paragraphs. In fact, gastrin, secretin, cholecystokinin, and motilin are the only ones for which all results, including blockage of action by antibody and/or receptor inhibition, have revealed clear-cut hormonal status. Somatostatin recently has been found to be involved in the inhibition of acid secretion by fat, but it is not known if the inhibition of this effect was due to neutralization of somatostatin as a circulating hormone or to local neutralization of its paracrine activity in the stomach. GIP is an example of a peptide for which the only antibody study appears to indicate a role as a circulating hormone, but peptide infusion studies do not agree. Specific hormonal roles have not yet been proved for any of the distal intestinal hormones.

Physiologic Activities of Specific Hormones

Insulin and Glucagon. The physiologic importance of these two peptides in glucose homeostasis is well known. No other specific roles in gut physiology have been proved.

Gastrin. Gastrin has been shown by all criteria to be a major hormonal stimulant of gastric acid secretion caused by the presence in the stomach of food and other substances contained in coffee and wine.[55] It also may mediate the acid response to gastric distention, but probably plays only a minor role in the acid response to sham feeding. Gastrin also has a significant trophic action on the acid-secreting gastric mucosa that is physiologic in rats and possibly also in man.

Cholecystokinin. Cholecystokinin has the widest range of actions likely to be physiologic of any gastrointestinal hormone, with the possible exception of somatostatin. Use of receptor blockade with proglumide and newer CCK-specific blockers, combined with radioimmunoassay and bioassay of plasma cholecystokinin, indicates that this hormone is important in the stimulation of pancreatic enzyme secretion and of gallbladder contraction caused by fat in the intestine.[56] Other physiologic actions of CCK that are very likely include relaxation of the sphincter of Oddi and stimulation of pancreatic growth.[57] There is reasonable evidence that physiologic concentrations of CCK inhibit gastric emptying[58] and enhance insulin release. The possible role of CCK as a hormonal inhibitor of acid secretion remains questionable. Cholecystokinin may produce reduction in food intake when given peripherally or in the central nervous system, but there is little evidence for a physiologic satiety effect caused by circulating CCK.[59]

Secretin. It is now well established that duodenal acidification causes physiologically important release of secretin for stimulation of pancreatic bicarbonate secretion.[60] Physiologic concentrations of secretin also may inhibit gastric emptying in man. The role of secretin in inhibition of acid secretion caused by gastric and duodenal acidification has not been established completely. In animals, secretin appears to be important in inhibition of acid caused by duodenal acidification.[61] In man, inhibition of acid secretion caused by acidification of a liquid peptide meal appeared to be due to inhibition of gastrin release and independent of secretin release.[62]

Motilin. Motilin is involved in the initiation of the intestinal interdigestive myoelectric complex. Whether the increase in motilin observed at the onset of this gastric and upper intestinal activity was cause or effect was in doubt until recently. However, two antibody neutralization studies indicate that motilin has an important role in initiating these complexes.[63, 64]

Gastric Inhibitory Polypeptide. There is little doubt that GIP has an important role in enhancing insulin release in the presence of hyperglycemia. One study also indicated that antibodies to GIP decreased the inhibition of gastric acid secretion in dogs caused by fat. However, intravenous infusion studies do not suggest an important role for GIP as an enterogastrone in man.

Somatostatin. Somatostatin could act physiologically in three ways: as a hormone, as a paracrine agent, and as a neuropeptide. The specific physiologic role of somatostatin therefore has been more difficult to assess than that of other hormones. There are no good receptor blockers and useful blocking antibodies have been developed only recently. There is *in vivo* evidence that somatostatin acts as an inhibitor of insulin release, as an inhibitor of intestinal absorption, and as an inhibitor of acid secretion when fat enters the intestine. The hormonal or paracrine nature of these actions has been difficult to resolve. Somatostatin also appears to have an important paracrine action to inhibit gastrin release in isolated gastric preparations. Similar physiologic paracrine inhibition of release of gastrin and possibly of several intestinal hormones is likely but remains to be proved convincingly.

Pancreatic Polypeptide. Infusion studies in dogs appeared to produce good evidence that pancreatic polypeptide acts as a physiologic inhibitor of pancreatic exocrine secretion. However, recent antibody neutralization studies failed to show any alteration in pancreatic secretion and have cast doubt on a physiologic role for pancreatic polypeptide as a pancreatic exocrine inhibitor.[65]

Enteroglucagon. Enteroglucagon consists of two peptides: a 69 amino acid peptide known as glicentin and a 37 amino acid peptide C-terminal fragment of glicentin known as oxyntomodulin. Few physiologic studies have been done with these peptides because of poor availability. The two most likely physiologic roles are stimulation of intestinal mucosal growth and inhibition of gastric acid secretion, but neither has been proved.

Neurotensin. The potential role for neurotensin as an inhibitor of acid secretion has not been well established. This peptide also could have a role in regulation of fat absorption or in intestinal vasodilation.

Peptide YY. PYY is a new peptide and studies are incomplete, but it is a reasonable candidate as a hormonal inhibitor of pancreatic secretion and a weaker candidate as a physiologic inhibitor of acid secretion.

Physiologic Actions of Gut Neuropeptides

Physiologic roles are much more difficult to establish for neuropeptides than for hormones. Because local release and concentrations of these peptides are hard to measure, much more reliance must be put on receptor antagonism and other methods for blockage such as desensitization or immunoneutralization. The latter method presents greater difficulty for neuropeptides than for hormones because it is difficult to determine whether or not antibody has entered the appropriate tissue spaces to neutralize a locally released neuropeptide. Most of the results obtained to date have resulted from experiments carried out *in vitro* in isolated organ and tissue systems that contained nerves but did not reproduce the normal physiologic condition.

Endogenous Opioids. Naloxone provides the best pharmacologic tool for antagonism of a family of neuropeptides *in vivo*. There are a number of different endogenous opioids, and they react with at least three classes of receptors.[66] Naloxone preferentially blocks the mu receptor but has enough inhibitory activity on the other two to be useful as a general antagonist *in vivo*. The two most widely predicted physiologic effects of endogenous opioids, based on comparison with the effects of exogenous morphine, were inhibition of intestinal motility and inhibition of pain. Unfortunately, naloxone has not provided clear-cut evidence for the importance of opioids in these effects; treatment with opioids does not prevent ileus or cause greatly exaggerated visceral pain. On the other hand, naloxone decreases gastric acid secretion under several conditions of stimulation, pointing to a significant stimulatory role for endogenous opioids as stimulants of gastric secretion.[67] Opioids also may have significant roles in regulating pyloric sphincter contraction and in modulating intestinal salt and water absorption. They also may regulate colonic contraction.[68] The most obvious *in vitro* effect of opioids on gut nerves is presynaptic inhibition of acetylcholine release from the myenteric plexus. The enkephalins therefore could serve as important inhibitory interneuron messengers.

Substance P and Other Tachykinins. There is reasonably good evidence that substance P is a stimulatory neuropeptide involved in propagation of esophageal and intestinal peristaltic contractions.[69] It also seems to mediate contraction of the lower esophageal sphincter caused by acidification of the esophagus.[70] It may have an important role in splanchnic vasodilation. Since substance P is a major component of the sensory nervous system of the gut, it may participate in the afferent limb of various reflexes. It also may have a role in the transmission of pain impulses. The other major tachykinin, substance K (neurokinin A), has a different distribution of receptors on smooth muscle of the gut and may also be a physiologic regulator of motility.

Vasoactive Intestinal Polypeptide. The three major types of effects of VIP that may be physiologic in the gut are relaxation of smooth muscle, vasodilatation, and stimulation of pancreatic and intestinal secretion. VIP appears to be an important mediator of lower esophageal sphincter relaxation and of internal anal sphincter relaxation.[71, 72] Receptive relaxation of the upper stomach induced by distention of the esophagus also appears to be mediated by VIP. All of these actions have been blocked by VIP antibodies under various experimental conditions. There is also evidence that reflex vasodilatation in the small intestine caused by stroking of the mucosa is mediated by VIP.[73] VIP also participates in descending relaxation in the peristaltic reflex.[74] Physiologic secretory effects of VIP are less well documented. There is reasonably good evidence that pancreatic VIP nerves mediate neural stimulation of bicarbonate secretion in pigs,[75] but VIP has little effect on human pancreatic bicarbonate secretion. Recent attempts to demonstrate a physiologic role for VIP in neurally stimulated intestinal secretion, which seems very reasonable because of the presence of many VIP nerves in the intestinal mucosa and the dramatic secretory effects of circulating VIP in the VIPoma syndrome, were unsuccessful.[76] VIP antibody had no inhibitory effect on intestinal secretion caused by electrical field stimulation of the intestine.

Gastrin Releasing Peptide/Bombesin. This neuropeptide seems likely to mediate neural release of antral gastrin. Antibodies to bombesin prevent gastrin release in the isolated rat stomach during neural stimulation.[77] GRP nerves in the pancreas may mediate neural stimulation of pancreatic enzyme secretion.[78] Bombesin is known to release substance P in the colonic muscularis mucosae and from the lower esophageal sphincter, and these may be physiologic effects of GRP. Finally, GRP is a potential excitatory neurotransmitter of enteric interneurons.

Cholecystokinin. CCK is known to release acetylcholine from the myenteric plexus, where it could act as an interneuron transmitter. It also releases substance P in the ileum, and this could be important in generation of the peristaltic wave as an excitatory transmitter. There is good evidence that CCK activates peripheral sensory nerve endings in the upper gut that transmit messages to the brainstem, for example after gastric distention.[79] CCK also may be involved in splanchnic vasodilatation.

Somatostatin. The most likely role for neural somatostatin is to inhibit acetylcholine release from the myenteric plexus of the intestine. It is known to inhibit acetylcholine release stimulated by CCK and by neurotensin but not by substance P. Thus somatostatin may function as an inhibitory transmitter in the peristaltic reflex.

Neuropeptide Y. NPY is co-localized in sympathetic postganglionic nerve fibers that contain norepinephrine and augments the vasoconstrictor effects of norepinephrine. These two transmitters may act together to regulate blood flow. Also NPY decreases acetylcholine release caused by electrical stimulation, probably by a preganglionic action similar to the inhibitory action of norepinephrine.

Calcitonin Gene–Related Peptide. CGRP is heavily concentrated in small sensory nerve fibers and is markedly depleted by treatment with the sensory neurotoxin capsaicin. Thus it is likely to have a role in the sensory transmission of gut reflexes, possibly sharing this role with substance P. Other peptides that could be involved in sensory transmission include CCK, VIP, somatostatin, and the opioids.

HORMONES IN GASTROINTESTINAL DISEASES

Hormone-Secreting Tumors of the Pancreas

The most clinically obvious consequences of gut hormone secretion are the syndromes produced by gut endocrine tumors.[80] Most of these tumors arise in the pancreas. They are known as islet cell tumors, although the variety of hormones secreted by these tumors is greater than the normal islet cell endocrine products: insulin, glucagon, somatostatin, and pancreatic polypeptide. Gastrin is produced in the fetal pancreas but not in the adult pancreas. Vasoactive intestinal polypeptide is a pancreatic neuropeptide. The cellular origin of rarer tumor products such as ACTH and growth hormone releasing factor is unknown. The histologic characteristics of these tumors have led pathologists to describe them as carcinoid tumors of the pancreas. This is a histologically descriptive term rather than a biochemical description of these tumors, because pancreatic "carcinoid tumors" rarely contain serotonin.

Pancreatic endocrine tumors usually become clinically apparent because of their secretory products. Clinical syndromes associated with pancreatic endocrine tumors are summarized in Table 4–6. More complete discussions of the major gastrointestinal syndromes produced by gastrinomas and by VIPomas are presented in later chapters of this book.

Table 4–6. CLINICAL SYNDROMES ASSOCIATED
WITH ISLET TUMORS

Tumor Product	Clinical Manifestation
Gastrin	Peptic ulcer, diarrhea
VIP	Secretory diarrhea
Insulin	Fasting hypoglycemia
Glucagon	Skin disease, hyperglycemia
Pancreatic polypeptide	None
Somatostatin	Malabsorption, gallstones
ACTH	Cushing's syndrome
GFR	Acromegaly

Flushing in the Carcinoid Syndrome: Role of Tachykinins

The carcinoid syndrome is characterized clinically by diarrhea and flushing. These tumors secrete serotonin in amounts that could account for the diarrhea but not for the flushing.[81] Although flushing may occasionally be caused by secretion of another bioactive amine by the tumors, such as histamine, the active agent or agents have been a mystery for many years. Recent evidence suggests that substance P and related gene products, known collectively as the tachykinins, may account for the flushing found in the carcinoid syndrome (see pp. 1560–1570).

Flushing often is brought on by eating and also can be provoked pharmacologically by pentagastrin, epinephrine, isoproterenol, ethanol, or calcium. In most cases the flush can be prevented by concurrent administration of somatostatin.[82, 83] No changes in plasma concentrations of several hormones produced by islet cell tumors, including gastrin, VIP, and neurotensin, have been found during these provoked episodes of flushing. Intravenous pentagastrin also can induce the carcinoid flush without any change in plasma serotonin.[84]

Substance P is now well established to be present in gut carcinoid tumors. Tumor extracts contain other peptides derived from the beta-preprotachykinin gene, including substance K (neurokinin A) and neuropeptide K.[85] Biologically active substance P fragments also have been isolated from metastatic carcinoids.[86]

Infusion of low doses of substance P intravenously causes lacrimation and flushing.[87] Plasma concentrations required to produce transient flushing fall within the normal range, while supranormal concentrations lead to prolonged flushing. Substance P–induced flushing is not accompanied by diarrhea. Plasma concentrations of substance K (neurokinin A) and neuropeptide K were increased in patients with flushing attacks induced by pentagastrin, food, or alcohol, while concentrations of substance P were less consistently elevated.[88] The greater increases measured for the other tachykinins compared with substance P may reflect the very short half-life of substance P in the circulation.[87] Presently nothing is known about the effects of substance K and neurokinin K infusions in man, but it is reasonable to suppose that they could produce flushing similar to substance P.

Treatments that diminish flushing also decrease plasma tachykinin concentrations. Patients who responded to interferon with a decrease in flushing episodes and diarrhea also had a decrease in plasma tachykinins. On the other hand, decreased urinary excretion of 5-HIAA, indicating decreased serotonin production, correlates with lessened diarrhea in patients treated with a long-acting somatostatin analogue.[89] The relationship between plasma tachykinins and improvement in flushing attacks during somatostatin analogue treatment is not yet well documented. It is not known if tachykinins can cause the hypotension and bronchoconstriction that sometimes are provoked during operations in patients with carcinoid syndrome, but it is likely that these episodes can be prevented or reversed by somatostatin.[81]

In summary, substance P and other tachykinins are found in the tumors of patients with the carcinoid syndrome, intravenous substance P mimics carcinoid flushing, tachykinins are released by agents that provoke carcinoid flushing, and tumor treatments that diminish tachykinin release appear to diminish the incidence and severity of flushing. Tachykinins therefore are very likely to account for carcinoid flushing in many patients with the carcinoid syndrome. On the other hand, diarrhea appears to be more highly correlated with serotonin secretion by the tumors, and flushing may also be caused by other tumor products such as histamine.

Hormones in Renal Failure

The overall role of the kidneys in clearance of hormones from the blood is not great for those with very short half-lives, including most gut hormones. Only those with half-lives of 30 minutes or more, such as gastrin 34, could theoretically be cleared by the kidney alone. Enzymes in the kidney degrade most of the hormones filtered by the glomerulus, so that only small fractions of the cleared hormones appear in the urine.

Increased circulating concentrations of hormones are common in patients with renal failure. It is suspected that reduced renal clearance explains the high hormone levels only partially. For unexplained reasons, catabolism of hormones by other organs may be impaired in renal failure.[90]

Responsiveness to hormones may be impaired in their target organs and increased hormone release may occur as a compensatory mechanism. For example, about 20 to 25 per cent of patients with renal failure have low or absent gastric acid secretion. These patients usually have hypergastrinemia, but uremic patients with normal or increased rates of acid secretion usually have normal plasma gastrin.[91] Chronic hypochlorhydria in patients with renal failure is associated with antral gastrin cell hyperplasia, just as it is in patients with chronic hypochlorhydria due to atrophic gastritis. Gastrin 34 is the predominant molecular form of gastrin elevated in the blood of renal failure patients.

It has been determined that total body clearance rates of gastrin 17 are not altered in hypergastrinemic patients with renal failure.[92] However, the kidney probably plays a more important role in the clearance of gastrin 34 than of gastrin 17.[92] Patients with renal failure appear to have higher proportions of gastrin 34 in the blood than patients with equivalent hypergastrinemia due to atrophic gastritis. Thus the hypergastrinemia of renal failure is likely to reflect two factors: increased gastrin production due to gastric hypoacidity, and decreased renal clearance of gastrin 34.

Other gastrointestinal hormones are elevated to variable extents in renal failure. Pancreatic polypeptide is increased but somatostatin is slightly decreased in patients with renal failure and hypergastrinemia.[91] Other peptides reported to be elevated include gastric inhibitory polypeptide and neurotensin. On the other hand, no increase in plasma secretin has been found.

Increased plasma motilin is common in patients with renal failure. The increase is due mainly to a plasma component larger than motilin. By analogy with gastrin, this may be a large molecular form of motilin that normally is cleared efficiently by the kidneys, while true motilin may be cleared in other parts of the body as well as the kidney.[93] Other peptides that are elevated in blood, neurotensin and GIP, also exist in multiple molecular forms. It is possible that it is mainly the large forms that are increased in the plasma in renal failure. This finding would be predicted if the kidney generally plays a more important role in clearance of prohormones and other forms larger than the most common biologically active form from the circulation.

Hormones in Gastric and Duodenal Diseases

Hypergastrinemia with Acid Hypersecretion

Gastrinoma: The Zollinger-Ellison Syndrome. Gastrinoma is one of the most dramatic examples of gastrointestinal hormone overproduction. The association of gastric acid secretion and severe peptic ulcer disease with a gastrin-producing non-beta islet cell tumor constitutes the Zollinger-Ellison syndrome. The manifestations of this disease, including peptic ulcer disease and diarrhea, can be explained entirely by overstimulation of the stomach by circulating gastrin. This disease is discussed in detail on pages 909 to 925.

Gastrinoma is by far the most common cause of marked hypergastrinemia (over 500 pg/ml) in patients with peptic ulcer disease. The diagnosis is supported strongly if basal acid hypersecretion is confirmed and if the plasma gastrin concentration increases by more than 200 pg/ml after intravenous administration of secretin, 2 units/kg.[94, 95] Calcium infusion produces equivalent stimulation but takes longer.[96, 97] The presence of hypercalcemia due to hyperparathyroidism in a patient with hypergastrinemia and peptic ulcer is a strong indication for multiple endocrine neoplasia, type I.[94] Occasionally plasma gastrin may be normal in gastrinoma patients.[98] This happens most often after successful resection of parathyroid adenoma leads to correction of hypercalcemia. Gastrinoma patients typically have minimal gastrin responses to food, but large increases are not uncommon in patients with previous gastric surgery.

Antral Gastrin Cell Hyperfunction or Hyperplasia. Although antral gastrin cells become hyperplastic and hypersecrete gastrin under several conditions in which gastric acid secretion is suppressed, primary hypersecretion of antral gastrin associated with gastric acid hypersecretion is rare. A few well-documented cases have been reported.[99, 100] The primary distinguishing feature of this disorder is exaggerated food-stimulated gastrin response combined with moderately elevated fasting gastrin and moderate to marked basal acid hypersecretion. Patients with this condition tend to have duodenal ulcers resistant to treatment. There is evidence for familial distribution in some cases, and autosomal dominant inheritance has been suspected.[101]

Whether or not antral gastrin cell hyperfunction usually is associated with hyperplasia of antral gastrin cells is unclear. In isolated cases no hyperplasia was found.[102] However, in two studies increased antral gastrin cell density was found in hypergastrinemia patients compared with other patients with peptic ulcer disease.[99, 100] There is no evidence that these patients have decreased antral somatostatin cells or decreases in somatostatin cell numbers. Also, they appear to have normal pH inhibitory mechanisms and demonstrate normal suppression of food-stimulated gastrin responses at low pH.[103]

Antral gastrin cell hyperfunction and hyperplasia also may occur after chronic treatment with potent acid-inhibiting drugs and is very common after vagotomy. These changes are due to hypoacidity with an appropriate antral gastrin response. It is not known whether or not chronic antisecretory drug treatment that fails to heal an ulcer can lead to gastrin cell hyperfunction.

The most specific treatment for antral gastrin cell hyperfunction associated with peptic ulcer is antrectomy. This operation has led to normalization of fasting and food-stimulated gastrins in several patients, proving that their hypergastrinemia originated in the antrum.[102] Although some of these patients respond poorly to H₂ blockers, it is possible that antrectomy could be avoided if stronger antisecretory agents such as omeprazole were used. It is possible that the hypergastrinemia could be reversed by use of one of the prostaglandin compounds that decrease gastrin responses to meals. Also the therapeutic responses to vagotomy have not been established. Until larger numbers of patients with this condition can be identified, the optimal therapeutic approach will remain unknown.

Isolated Retained Antrum. The failure to resect the distal antrum during Billroth II gastrectomy, leaving antrum at the proximal margin of a blind duodenal pouch, sets the stage for possible isolated retained antrum syndrome. For this syndrome to be complete, the antral pouch must secrete enough gastrin to cause gastric acid hypersecretion leading to recurrent ulcer. Despite frequent histologic evidence for retained antrum, the syndrome is extremely rare. One explanation is that antrectomy usually is combined with vagotomy, so that the remaining stomach is relatively insensitive to gastrin. Also it appears that gastrin release from a retained antrum may remain low unless the pouch is extremely large or the distal end of the pouch becomes obstructed.

The diagnostic findings that lead to suspicion of isolated retained antrum in a patient with previous antrectomy and gastrojejunostomy include recurrent ulcer, increased basal gastrin, abnormally high acid secretion, negative responses to provocative testing for gastrinoma with secretin and/or calcium, and little or no gastrin response to food.[104] Bombesin, which releases antral gastrin, may cause a positive response in these patients.[105, 106] Technetium scanning also may reveal an area of high uptake in the region of the retained antrum due to the normal antral property of secreting technetium into the gastric lumen.[107]

Hypergastrinemia Not Associated with High Acid Secretion

Decreased gastric acidity in patients with functionally normal antral mucosa leads to gastrin cell hyperplasia and hypergastrinemia. This increase in gastrin is physiologically appropriate. The mechanism may involve decreased release of antral somatostatin in the absence of luminal acid. An increase in plasma gastrin does not occur immediately after the gastric contents are neutralized, but begins within 8 to 12 hours.[108] Neutralization of the gastric lumen also increases gastrin responses to food by preventing the normal pH feedback inhibition of gastrin release. Peak gastrin responses to food may not be increased by H_2 blockers or antacids, but the gastrin response is prolonged if gastric contents remain above pH 3 beyond the time when food buffering normally is overcome by gastric acid.

Atrophic Gastritis and Pernicious Anemia. Atrophic gastritis is very common in the elderly. It is the leading cause of increased plasma gastrin values in the population.[109, 110] Although plasma gastrin values can be as high as 1000 to 10,000 pg/ml, there should be no confusion of these patients with gastrinoma patients. However, mistakes can arise if gastric secretion is not measured before antisecretory drugs are begun. Low gastric secretion can be determined indirectly by blood tests. Very low plasma group I pepsinogen is a reliable indicator of low acid secretory capacity.[111] Decreased plasma secretin response after pentagastrin stimulation is another indication of low acid secretion. These tests are not widely available, so direct aspiration of gastric contents and measurement of volume output and acidity after pentagastrin stimulation remains the best method for quickly excluding achlorhydria.

The combination of high basal gastrin and a negative secretin stimulation test is characteristic of atrophic gastritis. False positive secretin tests occur occasionally. Feeding tests typically produce exaggerated responses. Gastric acidification by instillation of 0.1 M HCl often lowers plasma gastrin in these patients.[112] The decrease is measured best between 30 minutes and one hour after acidification and does not occur in all patients.

Although the majority of patients with severe atrophic gastritis have hypergastrinemia, including the rare subpopulation with pernicious anemia, about 20 per cent do not. These patients usually have antral gastritis severe enough to destroy a major portion of the gastrin cell mass. Patients with hypogammaglobulinemia and atrophic gastritis also often have antral gastritis and normal plasma gastrin.[113] Any other disease associated with atrophic gastritis, such as rheumatoid arthritis, usually has a secondary hypergastrinemia.[114]

Vagotomy. All types of vagotomy, truncal and highly selective, lead to basal hypergastrinemia if the antrum remains intact.[115] There is a corresponding increase in antral gastrin cells.[116] Vagotomy leads to decreased gastric acid secretion and decreased sensitivity to gastrin.[117] This is one explanation for the hypergastrinemia. Vagotomy also removes an inhibitory factor that suppresses gastrin release and gastrin cell proliferation. The nature of this factor is unknown. It is important to recognize that considerable elevations of gastrin can occur after vagotomy and that hypergastrinemia does not indicate gastrinoma. Gastrinoma in the vagotomized patient can be detected by the usual methods—demonstration of increased acid secretion and an increase in gastrin after intravenous secretin.

Uremia. About 25 per cent of uremic patients have hypergastrinemia. Almost all of them have very low acid secretion. The pathogenesis of this type of hypergastrinemia is discussed in the section on renal failure.

Antisecretory Drugs. Ordinary doses of histamine H_2 receptor blockers lead to very mild increases in serum gastrin.[116] It is not necessary to stop giving these drugs for more than 12 hours when screening patients for gastrinoma.

Omeprazole produces more prolonged acid inhibition than H_2 blockers and can lead to much higher gastrin values.[118, 119] If this drug becomes approved for clinical use in peptic ulcer disease, hypergastrinemia may be a major side effect. The hypergastrinemia is dose-related and may not be a problem at ordinary therapeutic doses.

Certain prostaglandin compounds such as enprostil can decrease gastrin release stimulated by food.[120, 121] Whether or not this property will have any therapeutic advantage remains to be determined.

When Should Plasma Gastrin Be Measured?

There is no completely satisfactory answer to this question. Gastrin should be measured when there is suspicion of gastrinoma or other pathologic hypergastrinemia. The most obvious circumstance occurs when a patient has peptic symptoms and/or diarrhea associated with evidence for hyperparathyroidism or a pituitary tumor. A similar circumstance would be peptic ulcer in a patient with a family history of multiple endocrine neoplasia. Any patient with evidence of marked gastric hypersecretion, either by acid secretory studies, endoscopy, or radiographic findings, is a candidate for gastrin measurement. Any patient with ulcer disease severe enough to lead to possible ulcer surgery should have gastrin measurement. Duodenal ulcer associated with unexplained diarrhea is another indication. Beyond these indications there is a gray zone in which patients with peptic ulcer disease resistant to treatment with ordinary drug regimens and patients with frequent symptomatic recurrences may have gastrin measurements.

Interpretation of gastrin values requires some additional information. The most common cause of borderline elevated values is recent ingestion of food. A borderline value always should be repeated with careful attention to fasting. Antisecretory drugs should be withheld for at least 12 hours. In the case of moderate elevations it is important to establish the presence of acid secretion. Duodenal ulcer is evidence enough that acid is present, but gastric ulcer may be malignant and may be associated with atrophic gastritis in a patient with gastric cancer. Since atrophic gastritis is *by far* the most common cause of hypergastrinemia, gastrinoma treatment never should be instituted on the basis of elevated plasma gastrin alone. If borderline gastrin values are found in a patient with acid hypersecretion, provocative testing with secretin and feeding usually will establish the cause of gastrinoma or antral gastrin cell hyperfunction.

Hormones and Pathophysiology of Peptic Ulcer

The role of gastrin in peptic ulcer disease associated with gastrinoma and with antral gastrin cell hyperfunction is clear. These diseases illustrate the effects of excessive stimulation to secrete acid and the trophic effects of gastrin on the acid-secreting gastric mucosa. Hormones, especially gastrin and somatostatin, also could play an important part in the pathogenesis of ordinary duodenal ulcer disease. The pathophysiology of duodenal ulcer disease is discussed on pages 823 to 831. Common findings in duodenal ulcer that could be explained either by increased gastrin activity or by decreased somatostatin activity include increased maximal acid output due to hyperplasia of parietal cells, increased acid responses to physiologic stimulants, and decreased inhibition of acid secretion by gastric acidification or by fat. In gastric ulcer there is less evidence for excessive gastric acid secretion and the pathogenesis appears to be related to damage of the gastric mucosa (see pp. 880–887). The alterations in gastric hormones found in gastric ulcer are likely to be secondary to the gastritis associated with the disease rather than primary. It will be apparent from the following sections that no single hormonal factor has reached common acceptance as being important in the pathogenesis of duodenal ulcer. Some findings appear to be reprodu-

cible in certain countries but absent in others. The possibility of genetically determined population differences should not be discarded.

Exaggerated Gastrin Release

Most studies of gastrin release in duodenal ulcer patients have found normal basal gastrin concentrations in plasma, but one recent study showed a modest increase in ulcer patients.[122] Some groups have found increased postprandial gastrin release in duodenal ulcer patients, while the majority of studies have not.[123] Postprandial hypergastrinemia appears to be especially common in duodenal ulcer patients in Germany and some other parts of Europe.[124] Our own studies and those of several other groups in the United States have not revealed postprandial hypergastrinemia, especially when intragastric pH is controlled. Amino terminal gastrin fragments in blood may be increased in duodenal ulcer patients even when carboxyl terminal biologically active fragments are not. The few patients with antral gastrin cell hyperfunction appear to fall into a second population.

Hypergastrinemia Secondary to Antisecretory Drugs

With the widespread use of potent antisecretory drugs it is possible that hypergastrinemia secondary to prolonged acid suppression will become more common. This type of hypergastrinemia would not contribute to pathogenesis of the original ulcer but could play a role in continuation of acid hypersecretion. Ordinary single nocturnal doses of H_2 blockers produce minor changes in gastrin release, but larger doses may lead to secondary increases in gastrin production and release. Long-acting agents such as omeprazole produce more dramatic increases in gastrin stores and gastrin release.

Alterations in Antral Gastrin and Somatostatin Cell Ratios

Some groups have found increased antral gastrin stores and/or decreased antral somatostatin stores, while others have not.[125] Similar findings have been reported for density of antral gastrin and somatostatin cells.[126] At the present time there is no clear evidence for a primary change in gastrin or somatostatin number or hormone production in ordinary duodenal ulcer disease.[127] Gastrin cells may be increased without a change in somatostatin cells in antral gastrin cell hyperfunction. Secondary changes in antral endocrine cells are common.[125] Chronic gastric hypersecretion in the Zollinger-Ellison syndrome leads to decreased antral gastrin cells and increased somatostatin cells. Vagotomy leads to gastrin cell hyperplasia.

Decreased pH Inhibition of Gastrin Release

There is some evidence that the mechanism by which low gastric pH inhibits gastrin release is defective in duodenal ulcer patients. The most positive results have been obtained when inhibition was produced at an intragastric pH of 2.5.[128] When the intragastric pH is further lowered to 1.0, there is no evidence for a defect in ulcer patients.[129]

Increased Parietal Cell Sensitivity to Gastrin

Whether or not duodenal ulcer patients are hypersensitive to gastrin is a difficult question to answer. Comparisons of sensitivity are difficult when basal and maximal acid secretion differ between the groups being compared. When duodenal ulcer patients are matched with control patients for maximal acid secretion, some studies have found that duodenal ulcer patients are hypersensitive to gastrin.[130] The dose of pentagastrin or of gastrin required to produce half maximal acid responses was lower in the ulcer patients than in the controls.[131] Other studies have found no evidence for gastrin hypersensitivity in matched groups or after mathematical correction for differences in acid secretion.[132, 133] A third finding was that duodenal ulcer patients were more sensitive to exogenous gastrin but that they had decreased clearance of gastrin in the blood so that they were not more sensitive than control subjects when comparisons were based on circulating gastrin concentrations.[117] It is possible that all findings are correct and that the populations being studied had different characteristics. Until further studies are performed, no general conclusion about gastrin receptors on the parietal cells of duodenal ulcer patients is possible.

Increased Gastrin Cell Responsiveness to Bombesin/GRP

Although many groups have failed to find increased gastrin release in response to luminal stimulants, there are reports that duodenal ulcer patients are hypersensitive to bombesin.[132] As this peptide is the amphibian equivalent to gastrin releasing peptide found in nerves in the antral glands, it could indicate gastrin hyperresponsiveness to neural rather than luminal stimulants in duodenal ulcer. However, increased gastrin responses to the best-known neural stimulants, sham feeding and gastric distention, have not been shown convincingly in duodenal ulcer patients.[134]

Increased Growth Stimulation by Gastrin or Other Trophic Hormones

Increased parietal cell mass is the best-established abnormality in duodenal ulcer. The age at which parietal cell hyperplasia is established in ulcer patients has not been determined. Gastrin and epidermal growth factor (urogastrone) are two peptides that produce hyperplasia of the gastric acid–secreting mucosa and parietal cell hyperplasia. Overproduction or hypersensitivity of the proliferative cells in the gastric mucosa to either of these peptides could explain the parietal cell hyperplasia of peptic ulcer disease. Unfortunately there are no good data that examine these hypotheses.

Hormones in Pancreatic Diseases

Chronic Pancreatitis: Pancreatic Polypeptide

Chronic pancreatitis that destroys most of the gland leads to malabsorption due to enzyme deficiency and to diabetes mellitus secondary to insulin deficiency. A blood test that would permit diagnosis of pancreatic insufficiency without direct measurement of pancreatic function and prior to the onset of diabetes would be useful. Pancreatic polypeptide (PP) is produced almost exclusively in the pancreas and is released into the blood by meals. It is easily measured by radioimmunoassay. Several studies have explored the usefulness of PP in the diagnosis and monitoring of chronic pancreatic disease associated with pancreatic insufficiency.[135, 136] The conclusion has been that serious pancreatic insufficiency usually is accompanied by depressed PP responses. The diagnostic usefulness of this finding is limited, however, because a significant number of normal people have low PP responses to food. Similar conclusions pertain to PP released by cholecystokinin, secretin, or bombesin.[137, 138] The same conclusion can be made about PP release in cystic fibrosis.[139] However, serial measurements of PP might be useful to monitor the development of pancreatic insufficiency in patients with known chronic pancreatitis or cystic fibrosis.

Gastic inhibitory polypeptide release is increased in patients with mild chronic pancreatitis but is less abnormal in patients with severe pancreatic insufficiency.[140]

Pancreatic Endocrine Tumors: Pancreatic Polypeptide

Pancreatic polypeptide often is increased in plasma of patients with pancreatic endocrine tumors producing other hormones.[141] This finding is especially common in VIPoma. About three quarters of patients with this tumor have increased plasma PP. The proportion with elevated PP varies with other endocrine tumors. It is lowest, about one quarter, in gastrinoma. Increased pancreatic polypeptide also is common in multiple endocrine neoplasia. Since pancreatic polypeptide concentrations in blood tend to increase with age, it would be desirable to have a simple test that would distinguish between the benign PP hypersecretion associated with aging and malignant elevations of PP. The release of this hormone is normally greatly depressed by atropine. An atropine suppression test has been advocated to distinguish benign from malignant elevations in PP.[141] However, the results have been mixed. Some groups have reported that administration of atropine provided useful information, while others have found that atropine inhibited PP release in patients with or without tumors.[142, 143] It is possible that atropine does not inhibit PP release from tumors but that the test is of limited usefulness because patients with pancreatic endocrine tumors often have benign hyperplasia of PP cells in the remaining normal pancreas. This hyperplasia may lead to increased PP blood levels and normal inhibitory responses to atropine.

Experimental Pancreatitis: Cholecystokinin

Large doses of cholecystokinin produce acute pancreatitis when given to animals. Cholecystokinin antagonists lessen the severity of experimental pancreatitis in animals.[144] There is no evidence that excessive secretion of cholecystokinin produces pancreatitis in man. However, a therapeutic trial of cholecystokinin antagonists has not yet been reported in man.

Hormones in Intestinal Diseases

Celiac Disease

See also pages 1134 to 1152.

Celiac disease causes extensive damage to the duodenal and jejunal mucosa associated with malabsorption. Although loss of absorptive surface is a major cause of steatorrhea in these patients, poor pancreatic secretory responses to test meals have also been found. Impaired pancreatic responses can be explained by decreased release of two hormones that are concentrated in the proximal small intestinal mucosa, secretin and cholecystokinin. Patients with celiac disease responded to duodenal acidification with markedly diminished secretin responses, despite more pronounced duodenal acidification due to poor acid neutralization by the diseased duodenum.[145] Treatment with a gluten-free diet caused partial recovery of the secretin response.

Impaired pancreatic function in celiac disease also may be due to decreased release of cholecystokinin. Decreased immunoreactive CCK has been found in small bowel mucosal biopsies and in postprandial plasma from patients with untreated celiac disease.[146] Poor gallbladder emptying in untreated celiac patients also was related to markedly diminished CCK release, and both gallbladder and CCK responses to meals recovered in parallel during successful treatment with a gluten-free diet.[147] Another upper gastrointestinal peptide with diminished release in celiac disease is GIP.[148]

It might be supposed that gut hormones that are primarily located in the proximal small intestine would all be diminished in celiac disease patients but that those found in the unaffected distal portions of the small intestine would be released in excess by meals that were poorly digested in the upper intestine. This prediction has been supported to a significant extent by the study of Besterman and colleagues.[149] Secretin and GIP release were markedly diminished in untreated patients and returned toward normal after treatment. Markedly exaggerated enteroglucagon responses were found in the same patients, while neurotensin responses were only modestly increased. Peptide YY responses are markedly increased in patients with tropical sprue.[141] Exaggerated enteroglucagon responses were reversed by treatment. Measurement of enteroglucagon responses to meals may be a useful way to monitor treatment of celiac patients, since the high levels found in patients with active disease are easy to measure.[150] This approach has been used successfully in management of children with celiac disease and also to select patients for diagnostic small bowel biopsy.[150]

Dumping Syndrome

See also pages 939 to 952.

Dumping syndrome results from abnormally rapid gastric emptying of nutrients, especially of hyperosmolar carbohydrates. As expected, the gastrointestinal hormones normally released by carbohydrates demonstrate an exaggerated release when exposed to a large carbohydrate load. Gastric inhibitory peptide and enteroglucagon are especially raised during dumping. Exaggerated neurotensin and VIP responses also have been reported when the meal contains fat.[151] It has not been established whether or not rapid increases in GIP or enteroglucagon contribute to reactive hypoglycemia found in this syndrome.[152] Somatostatin was found to lessen the reactive hypoglycemia, implying that hormones might play a significant role in the pathogenesis.[153] However, somatostatin also decreases the rate of carbohydrate absorption from the intestine. Neurotensin release also is increased in patients with dumping syndrome, but this peptide does not reproduce symptoms of the syndrome.[154] Peptide YY release also is increased in this syndrome.[155]

Diarrhea

See also pages 290 to 316.

The only types of diarrhea that have undisputed hormonal etiology are those produced by endocrine tumors. VIPoma causes secretory diarrhea, carcinoid syndrome causes diarrhea because of both increased motility and intestinal secretion, and gastrinoma causes diarrhea because of increased gastric acid secretion. Other idiopathic secretory diarrhea syndromes may have a hormonal etiology, as indicated by the fact that somatostatin sometimes causes marked improvement. However, no peptide hormone other than VIP has been shown to cause clinically significant diarrhea. Motilin and other hormones sometimes are abnormal in patients with acute bacterial or functional diarrhea, but it has not been possible to distinguish causal roles from secondary responses.[156, 157]

Varied abnormalities in hormone release were found in patients with Crohn's disease. No specific abnormalities in neuropeptides were found in these patients.[158]

Regulation of Tumors by Hormones

Responsiveness of Tumors to Gastrin and Cholecystokinin

Several cell lines established from carcinomas of the colon, pancreas, or stomach contain specific binding sites for gastrin or for cholecystokinin. Similar binding sites have been found in tumor lines established from gastrointestinal smooth muscle tumors. In some cases these binding sites appear to be true receptors that modulate increased cell proliferation when stimulated by gastrin or cholecystokinin. Gastrin and cholecystokinin also have trophic actions in the normal stomach, colon, and pancreas. The significance of receptors for gastrin and cholecystokinin in the regulation of tumor growth *in vivo* has not been established. There is no good evidence that patients with chronic hypergastrinemia, due either to gastrinoma or to atrophic gastritis, have increased colon cancer. Gastric cancer is increased somewhat in patients with atrophic gastritis, but a relationship with hypergastrinemia has not been established.

Autocrine Regulation of Tumors

Certain tumors are known to produce growth factors that enhance their own growth. A peptide that is secreted by a tumor cell is considered to be an autocrine peptide if the cell line contains receptors for that peptide and occupation of those receptors increases cell proliferation.[159] Binding of the peptide or inhibition of the receptor should decrease cell growth. There is good evidence that certain tumors secrete peptides that meet these criteria. One of the best-established examples is secretion of gastrin releasing peptide by small cell lung cancers.[49] Bombesin and gastrin releasing peptide are growth factors for small cell tumor lines *in vitro,* and cell growth is inhibited by antibodies to bombesin/GRP. Growth of tumors in nude mice also is inhibited by these antibodies. The effects of similar treatment in man have not been established.

Gastrointestinal tumors may produce growth factors. Rat hepatocyte cell lines produce a substance that reacts with epidermal growth factor receptors and causes proliferation of normal rat hepatocytes.[160] It will be interesting to determine what additional growth factors are produced by other gastrointestinal tumors.

Role of Peptide Products of Oncogenes

Oncogenes are normal constituents of the human genome that frequently are expressed abnormally in malignancy. They are activated either by increased gene expression, by gene amplification, or by mutation to form a product with increased tumor-promoting activity. The origins and mechanisms of action of these genes are only partially understood.[161] More than 30 human oncogenes have been identified. They can be subclassified, according to the location of their gene products, as either nuclear or cytoplasmic. The cytoplasmic oncogenes cause formation of proteins that either are secreted from the cell, are inserted into the cell membrane, or act in the cytoplasm. These cytoplasmic oncogene products appear to correspond to known normal proteins that regulate cell function. Some resemble hormones, others resemble hormone receptors, and others resemble guanosyl triphosphate–binding proteins or intracellular protein kinases.[162]

Those oncogene products that are secreted from cells might act as autocrine growth factors. One product, produced by the sis oncogene, resembles one of the two peptide chains of platelet derived growth factor and is known to induce cell proliferation. Many of the

growth factors are regulated by oncogenes that do not directly encode the growth factors but somehow regulate their expression. Another way that oncogenes can cause cell activation is by altering normal growth factor receptors or by expressing new receptors that activate intracellular pathways in the absence of normal growth factors. There is still no proof that activation of human proto-oncogenes is sufficient or necessary to cause cancer.[163]

The significance of oncogenes in gastrointestinal malignancies is being learned along with knowledge about oncogenes in other types of malignancy. A few studies have indicated that measurement of oncogene products may give useful information about the malignant potential of gut cells. For example, the expression of the ras oncogene appears to be different in benign and malignant colonic diseases.[164] This is an area that is producing a great deal of new knowledge at a rapid rate.

Neuropeptides in Disease

Achalasia

See also pages 567 to 580.

Achalasia is a neuromuscular disorder involving the lower esophagus and lower esophageal sphincter. A prominent feature is failure of the lower esophageal sphincter to relax during swallowing. Vasoactive intestinal peptide has been identified as a neuropeptide in the esophagus that is likely to be a major mediator of relaxation during swallowing. Normal lower esophageal sphincter muscle contains a rich innervation with VIP-containing neurons. The number of these fibers is markedly diminished in patients with achalasia.[165] The loss of VIP fibers may contribute directly to impaired sphincter relaxation found in these patients.

Other neural abnormalities have been found in achalasia patients. In idiopathic achalasia, and in Chagas' disease, which is an infectious disease counterpart of this disorder, there is extensive destruction of the myenteric plexus in the esophagus and often in the stomach.[166] Some patients with these diseases exhibit decreased gastric secretory responses to sham feeding and decreased neural release of pancreatic polypeptide.

Eating Disorders

See also pages 173 to 199.

Possible involvement of hormones and neuropeptides in eating disorders presently is only conjectural. Cholecystokinin and gastrin releasing peptide are neuropeptides that have peripheral and central actions to decrease food intake.[167, 168] Neuropeptide Y has a potent central nervous action to increase food intake.[169] Disorders of central or peripheral release or activity of these peptides could be important in syndromes of obesity or anorexia but have not been demonstrated.

The Prader-Willi syndrome is a childhood disease characterized by obesity associated with infantile hypotonia, abnormal pubertal development, central nervous system dysfunction, and abnormal appearance.

Children with this disease have defective release of pancreatic polypeptide without any abnormality in release of other pancreatic hormones.[170] Whether this pancreatic polypeptide deficiency contributes to overeating in this disease has not been established.

Receptor Disorders in Gut Disease

Atrophic Gastritis: Gastrin Receptor Antibodies

Atrophic gastritis is one of the diseases often associated with tissue-specific antibodies. Patients with this disorder commonly have circulating antibodies directed at antigens on the parietal cell. Some of these antibodies are directed at antigens on the parietal cell surface and appear to be cytotoxic. Recent evidence suggests that at least a proportion of these antibodies react with the gastrin receptor and prevent binding of gastrin to this receptor.[171] Interference with the parietal cell gastrin receptor could be a cause for decreased acid secretion. In atrophic gastritis the number of parietal cells is markedly diminished along with the number of chief cells. Both of these cells are derived from a proliferative stem cell that appears to be stimulated by activation of a gastrin receptor. Gastrin receptor antibodies therefore could cause gastric atrophy by blocking the activity of the trophic gastrin receptors on these cells.

Insulin Receptor Antibodies: Hyperglycemia and Hypoglycemia

Antibodies directed against insulin receptors have been identified in patients with hyperglycemia or with hypoglycemia.[172] In hyperglycemia these antibodies block the normal action of insulin, while other antibodies directly activate the insulin receptor and cause hypoglycemia. Some of these antibodies appear to develop spontaneously. Others develop in patients who have been treated with insulin and have developed anti-insulin antibodies. Antibodies that react with insulin receptors represent anti-idiotypic antibodies in these patients. The receptor antibodies are directed against the insulin binding site of anti-insulin antibodies and react with receptors because insulin receptors are structurally similar to the insulin binding site on the insulin antibody. This anti-idiotype phenomenon can occur as an endogenous response to any antibody directed against the biologically active portion of a hormone. They are most commonly identified as reacting with the insulin receptor because so many people are treated with insulin and develop antibodies to this peptide.

Other Potential Receptor Disorders

Antibodies against the muscarinic cholinergic receptor on skeletal muscle appear to be responsible for causing myasthenia gravis.[173] A similar phenomenon in the gut causing motility disturbances is possible but has not been described.

Some of the manifestations of hyperthyroidism are caused by long-acting thyroid stimulator. This immunoglobulin reacts with receptors for thyroid stimulating hormone. Similar phenomena in the gut could cause hyperplasia or hypoplasia if antibodies were developed against gastrointestinal growth factor receptors.

Diagnostic Uses of Gastrointestinal Peptides

Gastrointestinal peptides have been used to evaluate gastric and pancreatic secretory function, to stimulate gallbladder contraction, as adjuncts in radiologic and endoscopic examinations of the tubular gut, and as provocative tests for endocrine tumors.

Pentagastrin Gastric Secretory Testing

Pentagastrin is a synthetic analogue of gastrin, t-Boc-β-Ala-Trp-Met-Asp-Phe-NH$_2$ (MW 768), that has the biologic activity of gastrin. It has largely replaced histamine as a stimulant of gastric acid secretion.[174] The standard dose is 6 μg/kg given subcutaneously. Gastric acid stimulation occurs within 10 minutes, peaks at 20 to 30 minutes, and lasts an hour or more. Peak acid stimulation produced by pentagastrin is equivalent to that produced by histamine, but the side effects with pentagastrin are much less. This test is primarily useful to exclude achlorhydria in patients with gastric ulcer. It also may be used in the preoperative evaluation of patients undergoing vagotomy for peptic ulcer disease.

Pentagastrin Provocative Tests for Carcinoid and Medullary Carcinoma

Pentagastrin has been used to provoke episodes of carcinoid flushing to reproduce the clinical symptoms found after eating and to permit blood sampling to measure substance P and other suspected mediators of flushing.[175] Pentagastrin also regularly releases calcitonin from medullary tumors of the thyroid.[174] Often it is superior to calcium infusion, but either test may be superior in an individual patient.

Secretin Pancreatic Secretory Testing

Purified natural porcine secretin is available for clinical use.[176] The structure of human secretin has been determined partially, but synthetic human secretin is not yet available. Secretin is supplied in vials containing 75 units, equivalent to about 25 μg. It is available from Pharmacia.

For pancreatic secretory testing, the usual dose is 1 unit/kg intravenously.[174] Duodenal contents are aspirated continuously and divided into aliquots, usually at 20-minute intervals. Volume and bicarbonate are measured in each aliquot. The earliest change in chronic pancreatitis is said to be a decrease in bicarbonate concentration to less than 90 mM. This finding often is combined with a decrease in volume to less than 2 ml/kg/80 min. Low volume and normal bicarbonate concentration may be found in patients with pancreatic carcinoma. The secretin test also may be used to aid collection of samples for pancreatic cytology. Secretin sometimes is given in combination with cholesystokinin for evaluation of pancreatic enzyme secretion.[177]

Secretin Provocative Testing for Gastrinoma

Secretin suppresses postprandial gastrin release and has little effect on basal gastrin in normal subjects and patients with ordinary duodenal ulcer disease. It decreases basal gastrin in patients with pernicious anemia or other forms of atrophic gastritis, but this decrease is seen best at 30 minutes or later.

In patients with gastrinoma, secretin usually produces a rapid increase in plasma gastrin concentration. Rapid intravenous infusion of secretin, 2 units/kg, leads to an increase over basal of more than 100 pg/ml in more than 90 per cent of gastrinoma patients.[95, 178] The size of the response is related to the basal gastrin level, but the test is most useful in patients with gastrin concentrations less than 1000 pg/ml. Peak responses occur between 2 and 10 minutes after injection and may disappear by 30 minutes. False positives are rare but have been reported in occasional patients with atrophic gastritis and after vagotomy.[179] Therefore a positive test alone should not be used to diagnose gastrinoma without also measurement of gastric acid secretion. Use of impure secretin preparations, such as Boots, can cause false positives if the radioimmunoassay used to measure gastrin also measures cholecystokinin that contaminates such preparations.

Secretin in Pancreatic Radiology

Secretin has been used to increase pancreatic blood flow in angiography of the pancreas. This has been useful in visualizing small blood vessels and small vascular tumors such as endocrine tumors of the pancreas.[180]

Cholecystokinin in Biliary Imaging

Cholecystokinin and cholecystokinin octapeptide both produce gallbladder contraction similar to that produced by a fatty meal. They have been used widely in radiographic and ultrasonic studies of gallbladder emptying. There seems to be no particular advantage over the fatty meal in the results obtained.[181] Cholecystokinin also can provoke symptoms resembling biliary colic in some patients with repeated episodes of right upper quadrant pain. Symptoms produced by cholecystokinin do not predict success of cholecystectomy in relief of the clinical symptoms in these patients, however.[182]

Bombesin in Retained Antrum

Bombesin is an experimental drug. Intravenous infusion of bombesin causes release of gastrin from normal gastrin cells.[183] Intravenous bombesin causes exaggerated release of gastrin in patients with antral gastrin cell hyperfunction, either due to atrophic gastritis or associated with duodenal ulcer.[184] However, bombesin seems to offer no advantage over a protein meal in these patients. Theoretically bombesin should be useful in diagnosis of isolated retained antrum. A few case reports support this use. This is a very rare condition. Response to bombesin is not a reliable indication of retained antrum after partial gastrectomy and gastroduodenostomy, because some gastrinomas are responsive to bombesin.

Glucagon in Gastrointestinal Radiography and Endoscopy

Glucagon has a general relaxing effect on smooth muscle in the tubular gut.[185] It has been used widely and successfully to reduce spasm during various gastrointestinal procedures including colonoscopy, barium enema, duodenoscopy, ERCP, and hypotonic duodenography.

Therapeutic Uses of Gastrointestinal Hormones

Peptides are not widely used as chronic therapeutic agents except for replacement therapy of essential hormones such as insulin and vasopressin. Destruction by the gut prevents orally administered peptides from having systemic activity in most cases. Rapid catabolism produces a short half-life for potential therapeutic activity. These drawbacks can be circumvented to some extent by chemical modifications of the peptides that decrease breakdown without decreasing biologic activity. Improved delivery systems that are being developed for insulin probably could be applied to other gut peptides. These include long-acting implanted minipumps, nasal sprays, and agents that increase absorption through the skin. However, new uses for gut hormones will need to be devised before widespread administration is common. The peptide that has demonstrated some definite promise as a therapeutic agent is somatostatin.

Somatostatin in Treatment of Endocrine Tumor Syndromes

Somatostatin has the advantage of suppressing both hormone release and hormone action for several peptides produced by endocrine tumors. It has been used to treat the secretory diarrhea caused by VIPoma, the diarrhea and flushing of carcinoid syndrome, the gastric hypersecretion of gastrinoma, and several other endocrine tumor syndromes. A cyclic somatostatin derivative that has a smaller ring and contains D-amino acids to decrease the rate of degradation[186, 187] (Sandostatin) has been used in numerous endocrine tumor patients. It has a long enough half-life to be given subcutaneously only one to three times a day.

Early results with long-acting somatostatin indicate good clinical improvement in diarrhea and flushing episodes in the majority of patients with carcinoid syndrome. Good results also have been obtained in several patients with secretory diarrhea due to VIP-oma.[188] Less dramatic improvements have been found in patients with gastrinoma. The beneficial effects of somatostatin in these patients often appear to be due to peripheral antagonism of the endocrine tumor products rather than to decreased release of tumor peptides. Rarely do the tumors shrink. Somatostatin is known to antagonize the secretory effects of gastrin in the stomach and of VIP in the small intestine. These appear to be the most important effects when the somatostatin analogue is used therapeutically in patients with tumors that secrete these hormones. Decreased hormone release from the tumors is not a regular effect of the somatostatin analogue. Somatostatin improves the skin lesions found in the glucagonoma syndrome.[189] The mechanism for this effect is unknown. In carcinoid syndrome, suppressed release of serotonin and of the tachykinins may be more important in relief of diarrhea and flushing. There is no evidence that somatostatin or its analogues has a useful role in halting progression of tumor growth in most patients, although there are a few exceptional patients in whom tumor size has decreased.

Other Therapeutic Uses of Somatostatin

Somatostatin has been tested in several conditions in which inhibition of peptide release could have a therapeutic advantage. It has been used successfully in patients with idiopathic secretory diarrhea or diarrhea due to mucosal disease of the intestine, but was ineffective in treatment of Asiatic cholera.[190] Somatostatin also may improve healing of gastrointestinal fistulas by decreasing gastrointestinal secretions. It produced some amelioration of symptoms of dumping.[153] At least one study reported a beneficial effect of somatostatin in acute pancreatitis.[191] There were preliminary reports that somatostatin was beneficial in severe upper gastrointestinal bleeding, but more recent studies have failed to show benefit in bleeding ulcers or esophageal varices.

Potential Therapeutic Uses of Cholecystokinin

Because of its wide range of actions, cholecystokinin has several potential uses and several potential side effects. One use that may soon become established is the intermittent administration of cholecystokinin to patients undergoing hyperalimentation to prevent biliary stasis. These patients are known to have a high rate of gallstone development. Preliminary data suggest that this cholelithiasis can be prevented if the gallbladder is emptied periodically by administration of cholecystokinin.

Cholecystokinin induces gastrointestinal motility and increases peristalsis in the normal gut. It was hoped that this peptide would be useful in treatment of postoperative ileus. Unfortunately, most patients with postoperative ileus appear to be unresponsive to cholecystokinin.[192]

Another potential use for cholecystokinin is in treatment of obesity. Intravenous or subcutaneous administration of this peptide causes acute decreases in food intake. Unfortunately, chronic administration does not appear to lead to sustained decrease in food intake.

Because of its trophic effects on the pancreas, cholecystokinin could be considered as a potential agent to restore pancreatic exocrine function in patients with pancreatic atrophy. This use has not been reported. It probably would succeed if the pancreatic tissue was normal but understimulated, as in patients with celiac disease and impaired cholecystokinin release, but would not likely succeed in patients with pancreatic destruction due to chronic pancreatitis.

References

1. Walsh, J. H. Gastrointestinal hormones. *In* Johnson, L. R. (ed.). Physiology of the Gastrointestinal Tract. 2nd ed. New York, Raven Press, 1987, p. 181.
2. Dockray, G. J. Physiology of enteric neuropeptides. *In* Johnson, L. R. (ed.). Physiology of the Gastrointestinal Tract. 2nd ed. New York, Raven Press, 1978, p. 41.
3. Yamada, T. Local regulatory actions of gastrointestinal peptides. *In* Johnson, L. R. (ed.). Physiology of the Gastrointestinal Tract. 2nd ed. New York, Raven Press, 1987, p. 131.
4. Solcia, E., Capella, C., Buffa, R., Usellini, L., Fiocca, R., and Sessa, F. Endocrine cells of the digestive system. *In* Johnson, L. R. (ed.). Physiology of the Gastrointestinal Tract. 2nd ed. New York, Raven Press, 1987, p. 111.
5. Sjolund, K., Sanden, G., Hakanson, R., and Sundler, F. Endocrine cells in human intestine: An immunocytochemical study. Gastroenterology 85:1120, 1983.
6. Costa, M., Furness, J. B., and Llewellyn-Smith, I. J. Histochemistry of the enteric nervous system. *In* Johnson, L. R. (ed.). Physiology of the Gastrointestinal Tract. 2nd ed. New York, Raven Press, 1987, p. 1.
7. Keast, J. R., Furness, J. B., and Costa, M. Distribution of certain peptide-containing nerve fibres and endocrine cells in the gastrointestinal mucosa in five mammalian species. J. Comp. Neurol. 236:403, 1985.
8. Gibbins, I. L., Furness, J. B., Costa, M., MacIntyre, I., Hillyard, C. J., and Girgis, S. Co-localization of calcitonin gene–related peptide-like immunoreactivity with substance P in cutaneous, vascular and visceral sensory neurons of guinea pigs. Neurosci. Lett. 57:125, 1985.
9. Gregory, H., and Preston, B. M. The primary structure of human urogastrone. Int. J. Pept. Protein. Res. 9:107, 1977.
10. Heitz, P. U., Kasper, M., van Noorden, S., Polak, J. M., Gregory, H., and Pearse, A. G. Immunohistochemical localisation of urogastrone to human duodenal and submandibular glands. Gut 19:408, 1978.
11. Hirata, Y., and Orth, D. N. Epidermal growth factor (urogastrone) in human tissues. J. Clin. Endocrinol. Metab. 48:667, 1979.
12. Gregory, H., Walsh, S., and Hopkins, C. R. The identification of urogastrone in serum, saliva, and gastric juice. Gastroenterology 77:313, 1979.
13. Oka, Y., and Orth, D. N. Human plasma epidermal growth factor/beta-urogastrone is associated with blood platelets. J. Clin. Invest. 72:249, 1983.
14. Okamoto, S., and Oka, T. Evidence for physiological function of epidermal growth factor: Pregestational sialoadenectomy of mice decreases milk production and increases offspring mortality during lactation period. Proc. Natl. Acad. Sci. USA 81:6059, 1984.
15. Jansen, M., van-Schaik, F. M., Ricker, A. T., Bullock, B., Woods, D. E., Gabbay, K. H., Nussbaum, A. L., Sussenbach,

J. S., and Van-den-Brande, J. L. Sequence of cDNA encoding human insulin-like growth factor I precursor. Nature *306*:609, 1983.

16. Bell, G. I., Merryweather, J. P., Sanchez-Pescador, R., Stempien, M. M., Priestley, L., Scott, J., and Rall, L. B. Sequence of cDNA clone encoding human preproinsulin-like growth factor II. Nature *310*:775, 1984.

17. Herschman, H. R., Lusis, A. J., and Groopman, J. E. Growth factors. Ann. Intern. Med. *92*:650, 1980.

18. Sporn, M. B., and Roberts, A. B. Peptide growth factors and inflammation, tissue repair, and cancer. J. Clin. Invest. *78*:329, 1986.

19. Nakanishi, S., Inoue, A., Kita, T., Nakamura, M., Chang, A. C. Y., and Numa, S. Nucleotide sequence of cloned cDNA for bovine corticotropin-β-lipotropin precursor. Nature *278*:423, 1979.

20. Gubler, U., Seeburg, P., Hoffman, B. J., Gage, L. P., and Udenfriend, S. Molecular cloning establishes proenkephalin as precursor of enkephalin-containing peptides. Nature *295*:206, 1982.

21. Noda, M., Furutani, Y., Takahahi, H., Toyasato, M., Hirose, T., Inayama, S., Nakanishi, S., and Numa, S. Cloning and sequence analysis of cDNA for bovine adrenal proenkephalini. Nature *295*:202, 1982.

22. Itoh, N., Obata, K., Yanaihara, N., and Okamoto, H. Human pre-provasoactive intestinal polypeptide contains a novel PHI-27–like peptide, PHI-27. Nature *304*:547, 1983.

23. Nawa, H., Hirose, T., Takashima, H., Inayama, S., and Nakanishi, S. Nucleotide sequences of cloned cDNAs for two types of bovine brain substance P precursor. Nature *306*:32, 1983.

24. Rosenfeld, M. G., Mermod, J.-J., Amara, S. G., Swanson, L. W., Sawchenko, P. E., Rivier, J., Vale, W. W., and Evans, R. M. Production of a novel neuropeptide encoded by the calcitonin gene via tissue-specific RNA processing. Nature *304*:129, 1983.

25. Nawa, H., Kotani, H., and Nakanishi, S. Tissue-specific generation of two preprotachykinin mRNA's from one gene by alternative RNA splicing. Nature *312*:729, 1984.

26. Bradbury, A. F., Finnie, M. D. A., and Smyth, D. G. Mechanism of C-terminal amide formation by pituitary enzymes. Nature *298*:686, 1982.

27. Mains, R. E., Myers, A. C., and Eipper, B. A. Hormonal, drug, and dietary factors affecting peptidyl glycine alpha-amidating monooxygenase activity in various tissues of the adult male rat. Endocrinology *116*:2505, 1985.

28. Jensen, R. T., Lemp, G. F., and Gardner, J. D. Interaction of cholecystokinin with specific membrane receptors on pancreatic acinar cells. Proc. Natl. Acad. Sci. USA *77*:2079, 1980.

29. Gregory, R. A. A review of some recent developments in the chemistry of the gastrins. Bioorg. Chem. *8*:497, 1979.

30. Wiborg, O., Berglund, L., Boel, E., Norris, K., Rehfeld, J. F., Marcker, K. A., and Vuust, J. Structure of a human gastrin gene. Proc. Natl. Acad. Sci. USA *81*:1067, 1984.

31. Takahashi, Y., Kato, K., Hayashizaki, Y., Wakabayashi, T., Ohtsuka, E., Matsuki, S., Ikehara, M., and Matsubara, K. Molecular cloning of the human cholecystokinin gene by use of a synthetic probe containing deoxyinosine. Proc. Natl. Acad. Sci. USA *82*:1931, 1985.

32. Reeve, J. R., Jr., Eysselein, V., Walsh, J. H., Ben-Avram, C. M., and Shively, J. E. New molecular forms of cholecystokinin. Microsequence analysis of forms previously characterized by chromatographic methods. J. Biol. Chem. *261*:16392, 1986.

33. Mutt, V., Jorpes, J. E., and Magnusson, S. Structure of porcine secretin: The amino acid sequence. Eur. J. Biochem. *15*:513, 1970.

34. Bell, G. I., Sanchez-Pescador, R., Laybourn, P. J., and Najarian, R. C. Exon duplication and divergence in the human preproglucagon gene. Nature *304*:368, 1983.

35. Chance, R. E., Moon, N. E., and Johnson, M. G. Human pancreatic polypeptide (HPP) and bovine pancreatic polypeptide (BPP). *In* Jaffe, B. M., and Behrman, H. R. (eds.). Methods of Hormone Radioimmunoassay. New York, Academic Press, 1979, 'p. 657.

36. Leiter, A. B., Keutmann, H. T., and Goodman, R. H. Struc-

ture of a precursor to human pancreatic polypeptide. Am. J. Biol. Chem. *259*:14702, 1984.

37. Tatemoto, K. Isolation and characterization of peptide YY (PYY), a candidate gut hormone that inhibits pancreatic exocrine secretion. Proc. Natl. Acad. Sci. USA *79*:2514, 1982.

38. Tatemoto, K. Neuropeptide Y: Complete amino acid sequence of the brain peptide. Proc. Natl. Acad. Sci. USA *79*:5485, 1982.

39. Dockray, G. J. Physiology of enteric neuropeptides. *In* Johnson, L. R. (ed.). Physiology of the Gastrointestinal Tract. 2nd ed. New York, Raven Press, 1987, p. 41.

40. Reeve, J. R., Jr., Walsh, J. H., Chew, P., Clark, B., Hawke, D., and Shively, J. E. Amino acid sequences of three bombesin-like peptides from canine intestine extracts. J. Biol. Chem. *258*:5582, 1983.

41. Marquardt, H., Hunkapiller, M. W., Hood, L. E., and Todaro, G. J. Rat transforming growth factor type 1: Structure and relation to epidermal growth factor. Science *223*:1079, 1984.

42. Rosenfeld, M. G., Amara, S. G., and Evans, R. M. Alternative RNA processing: Determining neuronal phenotype. Science *225*:1315, 1984.

43. Shen, L.-P., and Rutter, W. J. Sequence of the human somatostatin I Gene. Science *224*:168, 1984.

44. Geokas, M. C., Yalow, R. S., Straus, E. W., and Gold, E. M. Peptide radioimmunoassays in clinical medicine. Ann. Intern. Med. *97*:389, 1982.

45. Kenny, A. J. Endopeptidase-24.11: An ectoenzyme capable of hydrolysing regulatory peptides at the surfaces of many different cell types. *In* Kreutzberg, G. W., Reddington, M., and Zimmermann, N. (eds.). Cellular Biology of Ectoenzymes. Berlin, Heidelberg, Springer-Verlag, 1986, p. 257.

46. Lee, Y. C., Allen, J. M., Utterthal, L. O., Walker, M. C., Shemilt, J., Gill, S. S., and Bloom, S. R. The metabolism of intravenously infused neurotensin in man and its chromatographic characterization in human plasma. J. Clin. Endocrinol. Metab. *59*:45, 1984.

47. Walsh, J. H. Radioimmunoassay methodology for articles published in Gastroenterology [editorial]. Gastroenterology *75*:523, 1978.

48. Yamada, T. Local regulatory actions of gastrointestinal peptides. *In* Johnson, L. R. (ed.). Physiology of the Gastrointestinal Tract. 2nd ed. New York, Raven Press, 1987, p. 131.

49. Cuttita, F., Carney, D. N., Mushine, J., Moody, T. W., Fedorko, J., Fischler, A., and Minna, J. D. Bombesin-like peptides can function as autocrine growth factors in human small-cell lung cancer. Nature *316*:823, 1985.

50. Carpenter, G. Epidermal growth factor is a major growth-promoting agent in human milk. Science *210*:198, 1980.

51. Savage, A. P., Chatterjee, V. K., Gregory, H., and Bloom, S. R. Epidermal growth factor in blood. Regul. Pept. *16*:199, 1986.

52. Eysselein, V. E., Maxwell, V., Reedy, T., Wunsch, E., and Walsh, J. H. Similar acid stimulatory potencies of synthetic human big and little gastrins in man. J. Clin. Invest. *73*:1284, 1984.

53. Bunnett, N. W., Kobayashi, R., Orloff, M. S., Reeve, J. R., Turner, A. J., and Walsh, J. H. Catabolism of gastrin releasing peptide and substance P by gastric membrane-bound peptidases. Peptides *6*:277, 1985.

54. Liddle, R. A., Green, G. M., Conrad, C. K., and Williams, J. A. Proteins but not amino acids, carbohydrates, or fats stimulate cholecystokinin secretion in the rat. Am. J. Physiol. *251*:G243, 1986.

55. Peterson, W. L., Barnett, C., and Walsh, J. H. Effect of intragastric infusions of ethanol and wine on serum gastrin concentration and gastric acid secretion. Gastroenterology *91*:1390, 1986.

56. Loewe, C. J., Grider, J. R., Gardiner, J., and Vlahcevic, Z. R. Selective inhibition of pentagastrin- and cholecystokinin-stimulated exocrine secretion by proglumide. Gastroenterology *89*:746, 1985.

57. Yamaguchi, T., Tabata, K., and Johnson, L. R. Effect of proglumide on rat pancreatic growth. Am. J. Physiol. *249*:G294, 1985.

58. Liddle, R. A., Morita, E. T., Conrad, C. K., and Williams, J.

A. Regulation of gastric emptying in humans by cholecystokinin. J. Clin. Invest. 77:992, 1986.

59. Pappas, T. N., Melendez, R., Strah, K. M., and Debas, H. T. Cholecystokinin is not a peripheral satiety signal in the dog. Am. J. Physiol. 249:G733, 1985.

60. Chey, W. Y., Kim, M. S., Lee, K. Y., and Chang, T.-M. Effect of rabbit antisecretin on postprandial pancreatic secretion in dogs. Gastroenterology 77:1268, 1979.

61. Chey, W. Y., Kim, M. E., Lee, K. Y., and Chang, T.-M. Secretin is an enterogastrone in the dog. Am. J. Physiol. 240:G239, 1981.

62. Kleibeuker, J. H., Eysselein, V. E., Maxwell, V. E., and Walsh, J. H. Role of endogenous secretin in acid-induced inhibition of human gastric function. J. Clin. Invest. 73:526, 1984.

63. Lee, K. Y., Chang, T.-M., and Chey, W. Y. Effect of rabbit antimotilin serum on myoelectric activity and plasma motilin concentration in fasting dog. Am. J. Physiol. 245:G547, 1983.

64. Poitras, P. Motilin is a digestive hormone in the dog. Gastroenterology 87:909, 1984.

65. de Jong, A. J., Singer, M. V., and Lamers, C. B. Effect of rabbit anti-pancreatic polypeptide serum on postprandial pancreatic exocrine secretion in dogs. Gastroenterology 90:1926, 1986.

66. Olson, G. A., Olson, R. D., and Kastin, A. J. Endogenous opiates: 1985. Peptides 7:907, 1986.

67. Feldman, M., Walsh, J. H., and Taylor, I. Effect of naloxone and morphine on gastric acid secretion and on serum gastrin and pancreatic polypeptide concentrations in man. Gastroenterology 79:294, 1980.

68. Sjoqvist, A., Hellstrom, P. M., Jodal, M., and Lundgren, O. Neurotransmitters involved in the colonic contraction and vasodilatation elicited by activation of the pelvic nerves in the cat. Gastroenterology 86:1481, 1984.

69. Crist, J., Gidda, J., and Goyal, R. K. Role of substance P nerves in longitudinal smooth muscle contractions of the esophagus. Am. J. Physiol. 250:G336, 1986.

70. Reynolds, J. C., Ouyang, A., and Cohen, S. A lower esophageal sphincter reflex involving substance P. Am. J. Physiol. 246:G346, 1984.

71. Biancani, P., Walsh, J. H., and Behar, J. Vasoactive intestinal polypeptide. A neurotransmitter for lower esophageal sphincter relaxation. J. Clin. Invest. 73:963, 1984.

72. Biancani, P., Walsh, J. H., and Behar, J. Vasoactive intestinal polypeptide. A neurotransmitter for relaxation of the rabbit internal anal sphincter. Gastroenterology 89:867, 1985

73. Grider, J. R., Cable, M. B., Said, S. I., and Makhlouf, G. M. Vasoactive intestinal peptide as a neural mediator of gastric relaxation. Am. J. Physiol. 248:G73, 1985.

74. Grider, J. R., and Makhlouf, G. M. Clonic peristaltic reflex: Identification of vasoactive intestinal peptide as mediator of descending relaxation. Am. J. Physiol. 251:G40, 1986.

75. Holst, J. J., Fahrenkrug, J., Knuhtsen, S., Jensen, S. L., Poulsen, S. S., and Nielsen, O. V. Vasoactive intestinal polypeptide (VIP) in the pig pancreas: Role of VIPergic nerves in control of fluid and bicarbonate secretion. Regul. Pept. 8:245, 1984.

76. Cooke, H. J., Zafirova, M., Carey, H. V., Walsh, J. H., and Grider, J. Vasoactive intestinal polypeptide actions on the guinea pig intestinal mucosa during neural stimulation. Gastroenterology 92:361, 1987.

77. Schubert, M. L., Saffouri, B., Walsh, J. H., and Makhlouf, G. M.: Inhibition of neurally mediated gastrin secretion by bombesin antiserum. Am. J. Physiol. 248:G456, 1985.

78. Knuhtsen, S., Holst, J. J., Jensen, S. L., Knigge, U., and Nielsen, O. V. Gastrin-releasing peptide: Effect on exocrine secretion and release from isolated perfused procine pancreas. Am. J. Physiol. 248:G281, 1985.

79. Raybould, H., and Tache, Y. Cholecystokinin-8 inhibits gastric motility and emptying by capsaicin sensitive vagal afferent pathways in the rat. Gastroenterology, in press, 1987.

80. Lips, C. J., Vasen, H. F., and Lamers, C. B.: Multiple endocrine neoplasia syndromes. CRC Crit Rev Oncol. Hematol. 2:117, 1984.

81. Oates, J. A. The carcinoid syndrome [editorial]. N. Engl. J. Med. 315:702, 1986.

82. Frolich, J. C., Bloomgarden, Z. T., Oates, J. A., McGuigan, J. E., and Rabinowitz, D. The carcinoid flush. Provocation by pentagastrin and inhibition by somatostatin. N. Engl. J. Med. 299:1055, 1978.

83. Long, R. G., Peters, J. R., Bloom, S. R., Brown, M. R., Vale, W., Rivier, J. E., and Grahame-Smith, D. G.: Somatostatin, gastrointestinal peptides, and the carcinoid syndrome. Gut 22:549, 1981.

84. Richter, G., Stockmann, F., Conlon, J. M., and Creutzfeldt, W. Serotonin release into blood after food and pentagastrin. Studies in healthy subjects and in patients with metastatic carcinoid tumors. Gastroenterology 91:612, 1986.

85. Conlon, J. M., Deacon, C. F., Richter, G., Schmidt, W. E., Stockmann, F., and Creutzfeldt, W. Measurement and partial characterization of the multiple forms of neurokinin A–like immunoreactivity in carcinoid tumours. Regul. Pept. 13:183, 1986.

86. Roth, K. A., Makk, G., Beck, O., Faull, K., Tatemoto, K., Evans, C. J., and Barchas, J. D. Isolation and characterization of substance P, substance P 5–11, and substance K from two metastatic ileal carcinoids. Regul. Pept. 12:185, 1985.

87. Schaffalitzky de Muckadell, O. B., Aggestrup, S., and Stentoft, P. Flushing and plasma substance P concentration during infusion of synthetic substance P in normal man. Scand. J. Gastroenterol. 21:498, 1986.

88. Norheim, I., Theodorsson-Norheim, E., Brodin, E., and Oberg, K. Tachykinins in carcinoid tumors: Their use as a tumor marker and possible role in the carcinoid flush. J. Clin. Endocrinol. Metab. 63:605, 1986.

89. Kvols, L. K., Moertel, C. G., O'Connell, M. J., Schutt, A. J., Rubin, J., and Hahn, R. G. Treatment of the malignant carcinoid syndrome. Evaluation of a long-acting somatostatin analogue. N. Engl. J. Med. 315:663, 1986.

90. Loly, J., Depresseu, J. C., Brassinne, A., and Nizet, A.: Renal control of the peripheral uptake of exogenous gastrin in the dog. Eur. J. Physiol. 395:171, 1982.

91. Hallgren, R., Landelius, J., Fjellstrom, K. E., and Lundqvist, G. Gastric acid secretion in uraemia and circulating levels of gastrin, somatostatin, and pancreatic polypeptide. Gut 20:763, 1979.

92. Taylor, I. L., Sells, R. A., McConnell, R. B., and Dockray, G. J. Serum gastrin in patients with chronic renal failure. Gut 21:1062, 1980.

93. Shima, K., Shin, S., Tanaka, A., Hashimura, E., Nishino, T., Imagawa, K., Kumahara, Y., and Yanaihara, N. Heterogeneity of plasma motilin in patients with chronic renal failure. Horm. Metab. Res. 12:328, 1980.

94. Lamers, C. B., Buis, J. T., and van Tongeren, J. Secretin-stimulated serum gastrin levels in hyperparathyroid patients from families with multiple endocrine adenomatosis type I. Ann. Intern. Med. 86:719, 1977.

95. Mignon, M., Rigaud, D., Cambray, S., Chayvialle, J. A., Accary, J. P., Rene, E., Vatier, J., and Bonfils, S. A comparative evaluation of secretin bolus and secretin infusion as secretin provocation tests in the Zollinger-Ellison sydnrome. Scand. J. Gastroenterol. 20:791, 1985.

96. Thompson, J. C., Reeder, D. D., Villar, H. V., and Fender, H. R. Natural history and experience with diagnosis and treatment of the Zollinger-Ellison syndrome. Surg. Gynecol. Obstet. 140:721, 1975.

97. Deveney, C. W., Deveney, K. S., Jaffe, B. M., Jones, R. S., and Way, L. W. Use of calcium and secretin in the diagnosis of gastrinoma (Zollinger-Ellison syndrome). Ann. Intern. Med. 87:680, 1977.

98. Wolfe, M. M., Jain, D. K., and Edgerton, J. R. Zollinger-Ellison syndrome associated with persistently normal fasting serum gastrin concentrations. Ann. Intern. Med. 103:215, 1985.

99. Lewin, K. J., Yang, K., Ulrich, T., Elashoff, J. D., and Walsh, J. H. Primary gastrin cell hyperplasia: Report of five cases and a review of the literature. Am. J. Surg. Pathol. 8:821, 1984.

100. Keuppens, F., Willems, G., De Graef, J., and Woussen-Colle, M. C. Antral gastrin cell hyperplasia in patients with peptic ulcer. Ann. Surg. 191:276, 1980.

101. Rotter, J. I., Petersen, G., Samloff, I. M., McConnell, R. B., Ellis, A., Spence, M. A., and Rimoin, D. L. Genetic hetero-

geneity of hyperpepsinogenemic I and normopepsinogenemic I duodenal ulcer disease. Ann. Intern. Med. *91*:372, 1979.

102. Lamers, C. B., Ruland, C. M., Joosten, H. J., Verkooyen, H. C., Van Tongeren, J. H., and Rehfeld, J. F. Hypergastrinemia of antral origin in duodenal ulcer. Am. J. Dig. Dis. *23*:998, 1978.

103. Cooper, R. G., Dockray, G. J., Calam, J., and Walker, R. Acid and gastrin responses during intragastric titration in normal subjects and duodenal ulcer patients with G-cell hyperfunction. Gut *26*:232, 1985.

104. Webster, M. W., Barnes, E. L., and Stremple, J. F. Serum gastrin levels in the differential diagnosis of recurrent peptic ulceration due to retained gastric antrum. Am. J. Surg. *135*:248, 1978.

105. Basso, N., Lezoche, E., Giri, S., Percoco, M., and Speranza, V. Acid and gastrin levels after bombesin and calcium infusion in patients with incomplete antrectomy. Am. J. Dig. Dis. *22*:125, 1977.

106. Jansen, J. B., and Lamers, C. B. Serum gastrin responses to bombesin and food in patients with hypergastrinemia. Dig. Dis. Sci. *27*:303, 1982.

107. Cortot, A., Fleming, C. R., Brown, M. L., Go, V. L., and Malagelada, J. R. Isolated retained antrum diagnosis by gastrin challenge tests and radioscintillation scanning. Dig. Dis. Sci. *26*:748, 1981.

108. Peters, M. N., Feldman, M., Walsh, J. H., and Richardson, C. T. Effect of gastric alkalinization on serum gastrin concentrations in humans. Gastroenterology *85*:35, 1983.

109. McGuigan, J. E., and Trudeau, W. L.: Serum gastrin concentrations in pernicious anemia. N. Engl. J. Med. *282*:358, 1970.

110. Strickland, R. G., Bhathal, P. S., Korman, M. G., and Hansky, J. Serum gastrin and the antral mucosa in atrophic gastritis. Br. Med. J. *4*:451, 1971.

111. Varis, K., Samloff, I. M., Ihamaki, T., and Siurala, M. An appraisal of tests for severe atrophic gastritis in relatives of patients with pernicious anemia. Dig. Dis. Sci. *24*:187, 1979.

112. Fahrenkrug, J., Schaffalitzky de Muckadell, O. B., Hornum, I., and Rehfeld, J. F. The mechanism of hypergastrinemia in achlorhydria. Effect of food, acid, and calcitonin on serum gastrin concentrations and component pattern in pernicious anemia, with correlation to endogenous secretin concentrations in plasma. Gastroenterology *71*:33, 1976.

113. Hughes, W. S., Brooks, F. P., and Conn, H. O. Serum gastrin levels in primary hypogammaglobulinemia and pernicious anemia. Studies in adults. Ann. Intern. Med. *77*:746, 1972.

114. de Witte, T. J., Geerdink, P. J., Lamers, C. B., Boerbooms, A. M., and van der Korst, J. K. Hypochlorhydria and hypergastrinaemia in rheumatoid arthritis. Ann. Rheum. Dis. *38*:14, 1979.

115. Becker, H. D., Reeder, D. D., and Thompson, J. C. Effect of truncal vagotomy with pyloroplasty or with antrectomy on food-stimulated gastrin values in patients with duodenal ulcer. Surgery *74*:580, 1973.

116. Gehling, N., Lawson, M. J., Alp, M. H., Rofe, S. B., and Butler, R. N. Antral gastrin concentrations in duodenal ulcer patients after cimetidine and highly selective vagotomy. Aust. N.Z. J. Surg. *56*:793, 1986.

117. Blair, A. J., Richardson, C. T., Walsh, J. H., Chew, P., and Feldman, M. Effect of parietal cell vagotomy on acid secretory responsiveness to circulating gastrin in humans. Relationship to postprandial serum gastrin concentration. Gastroenterology. *90*:1001, 1986.

118. Festen, H. P., Thijs, J. C., Lamers, C. B., Jansen, J. M., Pals, G., Frants, R. R., Defize, J., and Meuwissen, S. G. Effect of oral omeprazole on serum gastrin and serum pepsinogen I levels. Gastroenterology. *87*:1030, 1984.

119. Pappas, T., Hamel, D., and Debas, H., Walsh, J., and Tache, Y. Spantide: Failure to antagonize bombesin-induced stimulation of gastrin secretion in dogs. Peptides *6*:1001, 1985.

120. Mahachai, V., Walker, K., Sevelius, H., and Thomson, A. B. Antisecretory and serum gastrin lowering effect of enprostil in patients with duodenal ulcer disease. Gastroenterology *89*:555, 1985.

121. Thomas, F. J., Koss, M. A., Hogan, D. L., and Isenberg, J. I. Enprostil, a synthetic prostaglandin E2 analogue, inhibits meal-stimulated gastric acid secretion and gastrin release in patients with duodenal ulcer. Am. J. Med. *81*:44, 1986.

122. Blair, J. A., III, Feldman, M., Barnett, C., Walsh, J. H., and Richardson, C. T. Detailed comparison of basal and food-stimulated acid secretion rates and serum gastrin concentrations in duodenal ulcer patients and normal subjects. J. Clin. Invest. *79*:582, 1987.

123. Taylor, I. L., Dockray, G. J., Calam, J., and Walker, R. J. Big and little gastrin responses to food in normal and ulcer subjects. Gut *20*:957, 1979.

124. Mayer, G., Arnold, R., Feurle, G., Fuchs, K., Ketterer, H., Track, N. S., and Creutzfeldt, W. Influence of feeding and sham feeding upon serum gastrin and gastric acid secretion in control subjects and duodenal ulcer patients. Scand. J. Gastroenterol. *9*:703, 1974.

125. Arnold, R., Creutzfeldt, W., Ebert, R., Becker, H. D., Borger, H. W., and Schafmayer, A. Serum gastric inhibitory polypeptide (GIP) in duodenal ulcer disease: Relationship to glucose tolerance, insulin, and gastric release. Scand. J. Gastroenterol. *13*:41, 1978.

126. Gutierrez, O., Rene, E., Accary, J. P., Lehy, T., Laigneau, J. P., Chayvialle, J. A., and Bonfils, S. Antral gastrin- and somatostatin-producing cells and intraluminal peptide secretion in normal subjects and duodenal ulcer patients with and without vagotomy. Regul. Pept. *14*:133, 1986.

127. Colturi, T. J., Unger, R. H., and Feldman, M. Role of circulating somatostatin in regulation of gastric acid secretion, gastrin release, and islet cell function. Studies in healthy subjects and duodenal ulcer patients. J. Clin. Invest. *74*:417, 1984.

128. Walsh, J. H., Maxwell, V., Ferrari, J., and Varner, A. A. Bombesin stimulates human gastric function by gastrin-dependent and independent mechanisms. Peptides *2*:193, 1981.

129. Thompson, J. C., and Swierczek, J. S. Acid and endocrine responses to meals varying in pH in normal and duodenal ulcer subjects. Ann. Surg. *186*:541, 1977.

130. Lam, S. K., Isenberg, J. I., Grossman, M. I., Lane, W. H., and Walsh, J. H. Gastric acid secretion is abnormally sensitive to endogenous gastrin release after peptone test meals in duodenal ulcer patients. J. Clin. Invest. *65*:555, 1980.

131. Halter, F., Bangerter, U., Hacki, W. H., Schlup, M., Varga, L., Wyder, S., Rotzer, A., and Galeazzi, R. Sensitivity of the parietal cell to pentagastrin in health and duodenal ulcer disease: A reappraisal. Scand. J. Gastroenterol. *17*:539, 1982.

132. Hirschowitz, B. I., Tim, L. O., Helman, C. A., and Molina, E. Bombesin and G-17 dose responses in duodenal ulcer and controls. Dig. Dis. Sci. *30*:1092, 1985.

133. Aly, A., and Emas, S. Sensitivity of the oxyntic and peptic cells to pentagastrin in duodenal ulcer patients and healthy subjects with similar secretory capacity. Digestion *25*:88, 1982.

134. Knutson, U., Bergegardh, S., and Olbe, L. The effect of intragastric pH variations on the gastric acid response to sham feeding in duodenal ulcer patients. Scand. J. Gastroenterol. *9*:357, 1974.

135. Adrian, T. E., Besterman, H. S., Mallinson, C. N., Garalotis, C., and Bloom, S. R. Impaired pancreatic polypeptide release in chronic pancreatitis with steatorrhea. Gut *20*:98, 1979.

136. Valenzuela, J. E., Taylor, I. L., and Walsh, J. H. Pancreatic polypeptide response in patients with chronic pancreatitis. Dig. Dis. Sci. *24*:862, 1979.

137. Owyang, C., Scarpello, J. H., and Vinik, A. I. Correlation between pancreatic enzyme secretion and plasma concentration of human pancreatic polypeptide in health and in chronic pancreatitis. Gastroenterology *83*:55, 1982.

138. Lamers, C. B., Diemel, C. M., and Jansen, J. B. Comparative study of plasma pancreatic polypeptide responses to food, secretin, and bombesin in normal subjects and in patients with chronic pancreatitis. Dig. Dis. Sci. *29*:102, 1984.

139. Stern, A., Davidson, G. P., Kirubakaran, C. P., Deutsch, J., Smith, A., and Hansky, J. Pancreatic polypeptide secretion. A marker for disturbed pancreatic function in cystic fibrosis. Dig. Dis. Sci. *28*:870, 1983.

140. Ebert, R., Creutzfeldt, W., Brown, J. C., Frerichs, H., and Arnold, R. Response of gastric inhibitory polypeptide (GIP) to test meal in chronic pancreatitis—relationship to endocrine and exocrine insufficiency. Diabetologia *12*:609, 1976.

141. Adrian, T. E., Uttenthal, L. O., Williams, S. J., and Bloom, S. R. Secretion of pancreatic polypeptide in patients with pancreatic endocrine tumors. N. Engl. J. Med. *315*:287, 1986.

142. Lamers, C. B., and Diemel, C. M. Basal and postatropine serum pancreatic polypeptide concentrations in familial multiple endocrine neoplasia type I. J. Clin. Endocrinol. Metab. *55*:774, 1982.

143. Oberg, K., and Lundqvist, G. Meal-stimulated and atropine-inhibited secretion of pancreatic polypeptide in healthy subjects, members of MEA I families and patients with malignant endocrine tumours of the gastrointestinal tract. Regul. Pept. *5*:273, 1983.

144. Niederau, C. Liddle, R. A., Ferrell, L. D., and Grendell, J. H. Beneficial effects of cholecystokinin-receptor blockade and inhibition of proteolytic enzyme activity in experimental acute hemorrhagic pancreatitis in mice. Evidence for cholecystokinin as a major factor in the development of acute pancreatitis. J.Clin. Invest. *78*:1056, 1986.

145. Rhodes, R. A., Tai, H. H., and Chey, W. Y. Impairment of secretion release in celiac sprue. Am. J. Dig. Dis. *23*:833, 1978.

146. Calam, J., Ellis, A., and Dockray, G. J. Identification and measurement of molecular variants of cholecystokinin in duodenal mucosa and plasma. Diminished concentrations in patients with celiac disease. J. Clin. Invest. *69*:218, 1982.

147. Maton, P. N., Selden, A. C., Fitzpatrick, M. L., and Chadwick, V. S. Defective gallbladder emptying and cholecystokinin release in celiac disease. Reversal by gluten-free diet. Gastroenterology *88*:391, 1985.

148. Creutzfeldt, W., Ebert, R., Arnold, R., Freichs, H., and Brown, J. C. Gastric inhibitory polypeptide (GIP), gastrin and insulin: Response to test meal in coeliac disease and after duodeno-pancreatectomy. Diabetologia *12*:279, 1976.

149. Besterman, H. S., Bloom, S. R., Sarson, D. L., Blackburn, A. M., Johnston, D. I., Patel, H. R., Stewart, J. S., Modigliani, R., Guerin, S., and Mallinson, C. N. Gut-hormone profile in coeliac disease. Lancet *1*:785, 1978.

150. Kilander, A. F., Dotevall, G., Lindstedt, G., and Lundberg, P. A. Plasma enteroglucagon related to malabsorption in coeliac disease. Gut *25*:629, 1984.

151. Lawaetz, O., Blackburn, A. M., Bloom, S. R., Aritas, Y., and Ralphs, D. N. Gut hormone profile and gastric emptying in the dumping syndrome. A hypothesis concerning the pathogenesis. Scand. J. Gastroenterol. *18*:73, 1983.

152. Jorde, R., Schulz, T. B., Burhol, P. G., and Schulz, L. B. The response of plasma gastric-inhibitory polypeptide (GIP) to slow and fast glucose ingestion in Billroth II resected patients and normal controls. Regul. Pept. *2*:391, 1981.

153. Long, R. G., Adrian, T. E., and Bloom, S. R. Somatostatin and the dumping syndrome. Br. Med. J. [Clin. Res.] *209*:886, 1985.

154. Pedersen, J. H., Beck, H., Shokouh-Amiri, M., and Fischer, A. Effect of neurotensin in the dumping syndrome. Scand. J. Gastroenterol. *21*:478, 1986.

155. Adrian, T. E., Long, R. G., Fuessl, H. S., and Bloom, S. R. Plasma peptide YY (PYY) in dumping syndrome. Dig. Dis. Sci. *30*:1145, 1985.

156. Besterman, H. S., Christofides, N. D., Welsby, P. D., Adrian, T. E., Sarson, D. L., and Bloom, S. R. Gut hormones in acute diarrhoea. Gut *24*:665, 1983.

157. Besterman, H. S., Mallinson, C. N., Modigliani, R., Christofides, N. D., Pera, A., Ponti, V., Sarson, D.L., and Bloom, S. R. Gut hormones in inflammatory bowel disease. Scand. J. Gastroenterol. *18*:845, 1983.

158. Sjolund, K., Schaffalitzky de Muckadell, O. B., Fahrenkrug, J., Hakanson, R., Peterson, B. G., and Sundler, F. Peptide-containing nerve fibres in the gut wall in Crohn's disease. Gut *24*:724, 1983.

159. Sporn, M. B., and Roberts, A. B. Autocrine growth factors and cancer. Nature *313*:745, 1985.

160. Luetteke, N. C., and Michalopoulos, G. K. Partial purification and characterization of a hepatocyte growth factor produced by rat hepatocellular carcinoma cells. Cancer Res. *45*:6331, 1985.

161. Bishop, J. M. Viral oncogenes. Cell *42*:23, 1985.

162. Weinberg, R. A. The action of oncogenes in the cytoplasm and nucleus. Science *230*:770, 1985.

163. Duesberg, P. H. Activated proto-onc genes: Sufficient or necessary for cancer? Science *228*:669, 1985.

164. Thor, A., Horan Hand. P., Wunderlich, D., Caruso, A., Muraro, R., and Schlom, J. Monoclonal antibodies define differential ras gene expression in malignant and benign colonic diseases. Nature *311*:562, 1984.

165. Aggestrup, S., Uddman, R., Sundler, F., Fahrenkrug, J., Hakanson, R., Srensen, H., and Hambraeus, G. Lack of vasoactive intestinal polypeptide nerves in esophageal achalasia. Gastroenterology *84*:924, 1983.

166. Dooley, C. P., Taylor, I. L., and Valenzuela, J. E. Impaired acid secretion and pancreatic polypeptide release in some patients with achalasia. Gastroenterology *84*:809, 1983.

167. Kissileff, H. R., Pi-Sunyer, F. X., Thornton, J., and Smith, G. P. C-terminal octapeptide of cholecystokinin decreases food intake in man. Am. J. Clin. Nutr. *34*:154, 1981.

168. Smith, G. P., and Gibbs, J. Gut peptides and postprandial satiety. Fed. Proc. *43*:2889, 1984.

169. Levine, A. S., and Morley, J. E. Neuropeptide Y: A potent inducer of consummatory behavior in rats. Peptides *5*:1025, 1984.

170. Zipf, W. B., O'Dorisio, T. M., Cataland, S., and Dixon, K. Pancreatic polypeptide responses to protein meal challenges in obese but otherwise normal children and obese children with Prader-Willi syndrome. J. Clin. Endocrinol. Metab. *57*:1074, 1983.

171. de Aizpurua, H. J., Ungar, B., and Toh, B. H. Autoantibody to the gastrin receptor in pernicious anemia. N. Engl. J. Med. *313*:479, 1985.

172. Dons, R. F., Havlik, R., Taylor, S. I., Baird, K. L., Chernick, S. S., and Gorden, P. Clinical disorders associated with autoantibodies to the insulin receptor. Simulation by passive transfer of immunoglobulins to rats. J. Clin. Invest. *72*:1072, 1983.

173. Drachman, D. B. Immunopathology of myasthenia gravis. Fed. Proc. *38*:2613, 1979.

174. Walsh, J. H., and Taylor, I. L. Pharmacology of gastrointestinal hormones. *In* Thompson, J. H., and Bevin, J. A. (eds.). Essentials of Pharmacology. Philadelphia, Harper and Row, 1983, p. 530.

175. Ahlman, H., Dahlstrom, A., Gronstad, K., Tisell, L. E., Oberg, K., Zinner, M. J., and Jaffe, B. M. The pentagastrin test in the diagnosis of the carcinoid syndrome. Blockade of gastrointestinal symptoms by ketanserin. Ann. Surg. *201*:81, 1985.

176. Grossman, M. I. Food and Drug Administration status of secretin and cholecystokinin for use in human subjects [editorial]. Gastroenterology *75*:324, 1978.

177. Heij, H. A., Obertop, H., Schmitz, P. I., von Blankenstein, M., and Westbroek, D. L. Evaluation of the secretin-cholecystokinin test for chronic pancreatitis by discriminant analysis. Scand. J. Gastroenterol. *21*:35, 1986.

178. Lamers, C. G., and Van Tongeren, J. H. Comparative study of the value of the calcium, secretin, and meal stimulated increase in serum gastrin to the diagnosis of the Zollinger-Ellison syndrome. Gut *18*:128, 1977.

179. Feldman, M., Schiller, L. R., Walsh, J. H., Fordtran, J. S., and Richardson, C. T. Positive intravenous secretin test in patients with achlorhydria-related hypergastrinemia. Gastroenterology, in press, 1987.

180. Debas, H. T., Soon-Shiong, P., McKenzie, A. D., Bogoch, A., Greig, J. H., Dunn, W. L., and Magill, A. B. Use of secretin in the roentgenologic and biochemical diagnosis of duodenal gastrinoma. Am. J. Surg. *145*:408, 1983.

181. Hopman, W. P., Rosenbusch, G., Jansen, J. B., de Jong, A. J., and Lamers, C. B. Gallbladder contraction: Effects of fatty meals and cholecystokinin. Radiology *157*:37, 1985.

182. Byrne, P., Hunter, G. J., and Vallon, A. Cholecystokinin cholecystography: A three year prospective trial. Clin. Radiol. *36*:499, 1985.

183. Varner, A. A., Modlin, I. M., and Walsh, J. H. High potency of bombesin for stimulation of human gastrin release and gastric acid secretion. Regul. Pept. *1*:289, 1981.

184. Hirschowitz, B. I., and Molina, E. Relation of gastric acid and pepsin secretion to serum gastrin levels in dogs given bombesin and gastrin-17. Am. J. Physiol. *244*:G546, 1983.

185. Miller, R. E., Chernish, S. M., Rosenak, B. D., and Rodda, B. E. Hypotonic duodenography with glucagon. Radiology *108*:35, 1973.

186. Kraenzlin, M. E., Ch'ng, J. L., Wood, S. M., Carr, D. H., and Bloom, S. R. Long-term treatment of a VIPoma with somatostatin analogue resulting in remission of symptoms and possible shrinkage of metastases. Gastroenterology *88*:185, 1985.

187. Wood, S. M., Kraenzlin, M. E., Adrian, T. E., and Bloom, S. R. Treatment of patients with pancreatic endocrine tumours using a new long-acting somatostatin analogue: Symptomatic and peptide responses. Gut *26*:438, 1985.

188. Santangelo, W. C., O'Dorisio, T. M., Kim, J. G., Severino, G., and Krejs, G. J. Pancreatic cholera syndrome: Effect of a synthetic somatostatin analog on intestinal water and ion transport. Ann. Intern. Med. *103*:363, 1985.

189. Boden, G., Ryan, I. G., Eisenschmid, B. L., Shelmet, J. J., and Owen, O. E. Treatment of inoperable glucagonoma with the long-acting somatostatin analogue SMS 201-995. N. Engl. J. Med. *314*:1686, 1986.

190. Molla, A. M., Gyr, K., Bardhan, P. K., and Molla, A. Effect of intravenous somatostatin on stool output in diarrhea due to *Vibrio cholerae*. Gastroenterology *87*:845, 1984.

191. Usadel, K. H., Leuschner, U., and Uberla, K. K. Treatment of acute pancreatitis with somatostatin: A multicenter double blind study [letter]. N. Engl. J. Med. *303*:999, 1980.

192. Frisell, J., Magnusson, I., Leijonmarck, C. E., and Ihre, T. The effect of cholecystokinin on postoperative bowel function. Acta Chir. Scand. *151*:557, 1985.

The Relation of Enteric Bacterial Populations to Gastrointestinal Function and Disease

5

ROBERT M. DONALDSON, JR.
PHILLIP P. TOSKES

The importance of enteric microorganisms is clearly documented by their effects on germ-free or pathogen-free host animals,[1, 2] on the structure and function of small bowel mucosa,[3] on the intraluminal metabolism of sterols, including cholesterol, bile salts, and steroidal hormones,[4] and on the metabolism of drugs[5] and a variety of nutrients.[6] Also clear is the involvement of the intestinal flora in diverse human diseases ranging from hepatic coma to tropical sprue. This chapter summarizes the nature of the bacterial populations of the human alimentary tract, the host factors that affect those populations, the effects of indigenous microorganisms on intestinal morphology and function, and the role of the enteric flora in certain disease states. Detailed reviews of these subjects are available.[6–10]

NATURE AND DEVELOPMENT OF ENTERIC BACTERIAL POPULATIONS

Information about the nature of intestinal flora depends greatly upon how microorganisms are collected, cultured, isolated, identified, and enumerated.[9, 10] Particularly important is rigorous attention to anaerobic techniques, including the use of media preserved in the oxygen-free state and provision of an anaerobic environment for inoculation and transfer of material.

Although proposed many years ago as a promising approach to the identification and quantification of intestinal microbial populations,[11] biochemical analyses are now widely used, and investigators still rely largely on classic microbiologic techniques.[12] Using peroral intubation to collect samples, workers have developed over the years a reasonably complete picture of the enteric microflora. Table 5–1 provides a general indication of the kinds and numbers of microorganisms that normally populate the various portions of the alimentary canal. This table also shows the pH in the intestinal lumen and the corresponding redox potential (i.e., the potential difference generated by the relative state of oxidation or reduction). In an increasingly anaerobic environment the redox potential becomes increasingly negative.

In healthy individuals the stomach and small bowel contain relatively small numbers of bacteria. In fact, jejunal cultures fail to identify any bacterial growth in about one third of healthy volunteers. When organisms are present, they are usually gram-positive aerobes or facultative anaerobes such as lactobacilli and enterococci, which are usually present in concentrations of up to 10^4 viable organisms per gram of jejunal contents. Coliforms may be transiently present in healthy jejunum, but rarely exceed 10^3 organisms per gram and probably represent ingested "contaminants" en route

Table 5–1. NORMAL MICROBIAL POPULATIONS OF THE ALIMENTARY TRACT

	Stomach	Jejunum	Ileum	Cecum
Total bacterial counts*	$0–10^3$	$0–10^4$	$10^5–10^8$	$10^{10}–10^{12}$
Aerobes and facultative anaerobes				
Streptococci	$0–10^3$	$0–10^4$	$10^2–10^5$	$10^4–10^9$
Lactobacilli	$0–10^3$	$0–10^4$	$10^2–10^5$	$10^6–10^{10}$
Staphylococci	$0–10^2$	$0–10^2$	$10^2–10^5$	$10^2–10^5$
Enterobacteria	$0–10^2$	$0–10^3$	$10^3–10^8$	$10^5–10^8$
Fungi	$0–10^2$	$0–10^2$	$10^2–10^4$	$10^4–10^6$
Anaerobes				
Bacteroides	0	0	$10^3–10^7$	$10^9–10^{12}$
Bifidobacteria	0	0	$10^3–10^6$	$10^8–10^{10}$
Clostridia	0	0	$10^2–10^4$	$10^8–10^9$
Eubacteria	0	0	0	$10^9–10^{12}$
Redox potential (mV)	+150	−50	−150	−200
pH	3.0	6.0–7.0	7.5	6.8–7.3

Data compiled from Donaldson,[10] Savage,[6] and Simon and Gorbach.[9]

*Viable microorganisms per gram of contents.

to the colon. Normally, anerobic bacteroides are not found in proximal small bowel. In patients who are otherwise healthy but do not secrete gastric acid, the numbers of bacteria present in the stomach and jejunum may be somewhat higher than those described in Table 5–1.

As many as 10^4 to 10^8 microorganisms per ml of contents can be recovered from the stomach and jejunum of achlorhydric subjects who may otherwise be quite well.[13] Production of symptoms usually requires higher bacterial concentrations; also important are *total* numbers of microorganisms and the rate at which they pass along the intestine.

In the distal small intestine the pH is maintained above 7.0 and the redox potential is markedly reduced. Although the ileum may harbor a relatively sparse flora in about one third of healthy subjects, the majority of volunteers show a distinct change in bacterial populations when the distal small bowel is cultured. Microbiologically, the ileum appears to represent a zone of transition from the sparse populations of aerobic flora found in the stomach and proximal bowel and the very dense bacterial populations of anaerobic microorganisms found in the colon. In the ileum the concentrations of microorganisms increase to levels of 10^5 to 10^9 organisms per gram of contents. Enterobacteria, including coliforms, occur only transiently and in small numbers in the proximal bowel but are regularly found in substantial numbers in the ileum. Strict anaerobes, which normally cannot survive in the jejunum, frequently colonize the ileum, where the redox potential is markedly reduced.

The most dramatic change in the enteric flora occurs across the ileocecal valve. The total number of microorganisms increases up to one million fold and approximates 10^9 to 10^{12} microorganisms per gram of colonic contents. The large bowel flora is dominated by fastidious anaerobic organisms such as bacteroides, anaerobic lactobacilli, and clostridia. These microorganisms, although difficult to culture, actually outnumber aero-

bic and facultative organisms by as much as 10,000:1 within the lumen of the colon. The complexity of the colonic flora is illustrated by the fact that comprehensive bacterial analyses have demonstrated more than 400 different species in the colon of a single individual.[14]

The alimentary canal of the host is sterile at birth, and animals raised in a germ-free environment harbor no microorganisms in the gut lumen. Thus the enteric flora is derived exclusively from the environment, and enteric bacteria colonize the human infant in an oral-to-anal direction.[15] In a wide variety of animal species, including man, coliforms and streptococci colonize the alimentary canal within a few hours of birth. Anaerobic lactobacilli and enterococci become established at 24 hours and slowly increase in numbers during the next 10 to 21 days, a period when the number of coliforms decreases dramatically. Bacteroides, destined to become the dominant constituent of the colonic flora, first make their appearance at ten days and rapidly proliferate during the next two weeks. Approximately three to four weeks after birth, the flora characteristic for the host is fairly well established and, except under unusual circumstances, does not change significantly thereafter.

FACTORS THAT INFLUENCE THE ENTERIC FLORA

Bacterial populations of the gut vary considerably from one individual to another, but the enteric flora in a given individual remains remarkably stable.[9] The remarkable capacity of intestinal bacteria to proliferate under optimal culture conditions means that mechanisms must exist to prevent the host from being overwhelmed by its own intestinal flora and to prevent the bowel from being colonized by a single dominant microorganism.

Host factors that are crucial for limiting microbial growth include gastric acid and intestinal motility. Achlorhydria resulting from gastric mucosal atrophy or gastric surgery permits increased numbers of viable microorganisms to pass into the small bowel.[16] The major factor responsible for limiting bacterial proliferation in the small bowel is undoubtedly the cleansing action of normal propulsive motility of the intestinal canal. In the relatively stagnant contents of the large bowel, bacterial growth is luxuriant, whereas microorganisms are rapidly cleared from the small intestine. Quantitative investigations have demonstrated that although microorganisms are destroyed in the acid contents of the stomach, those bacteria that survive and pass into the small bowel remain viable as they are swept into the colon at a relatively rapid rate. Of particular importance in this regard is the interdigestive migrating motor complex responsible for sweeping the bowel clean (see pp. 1090–1091). Mucus may aid in this mechanical process for removing bacteria, a possibility that is supported by the fact that microorganisms tend to concentrate in the mucous layer that lines the gastrointestinal mucosa. The crucial importance of normal small bowel peristalsis is emphasized by the fact that whenever normal motility is slowed or interrupted, bacterial overgrowth (more than 10^7 microorganisms per ml of jejunal contents) rapidly ensues.

In addition to host factors, the *environment* undoubtedly influences the nature of enteric flora. When animals are rigorously raised in strict germ-free or pathogen-free environments there occur predictable effects on intestinal bacterial populations.[17] However, there is little evidence for a profound impact of environmental factors on the intestinal flora of healthy humans. For example, the biomedical literature is replete with the effects of diet on intestinal microbial populations, but most of the findings are conflicting. Probably only extreme unphysiologic alterations in diet influence the kinds and numbers of microorganisms in the intestinal canal.[9] Since not only food but also desquamated intestinal cells and various gastrointestinal secretions serve to nourish the microbial populations of the gut, and since most of the diet is absorbed before ingested nutrients reach the bacteria-rich colon, it is not surprising that extreme changes in diet have only slight effects on colonic microorganisms.

Bacterial interactions within the gut lumen undoubtedly represent an important, if still poorly understood, determinant of the bacterial populations inhabiting the alimentary canal.[8] Such interactions are numerous and complex and include (1) mutual competition for available nutrients, (2) alteration of intraluminal pH or redox potential, (3) production of toxic metabolites, (4) bowel synthesis of growth factors, (5) enzyme-sharing, and (6) transfer of antibiotic resistance. It is important to recognize, for example, that without the oxygen-utilizing aerobes such as coliforms and enterococci, the colon would not be sufficiently anaerobic to maintain the large populations of fastidious anaerobes such as the bacteroides.

Microbial interactions probably have considerable clinical relevance. It is clear, for example, that enteric bacteria impair colonization of the bowel by *Candida albicans*.[18] Moreover, patients who are carriers of *Salmonella typhosa* or *Vibrio cholerae* may harbor these organisms in the gallbladder or small bowel at a time when fecal cultures are consistently negative. These organisms survive passage through the proximal small bowel only to be destroyed within the colon by bacterially produced antibiotics such as the "colicines" and certain short-chain fatty acids. In a variety of nonspecific or viral diarrheal disorders, diarrhea itself appears to alter the enteric flora. During severe diarrhea, time for microbial interactions to occur is inadequate, and coliforms tend to increase while the numbers of strict anaerobes may diminish.[9]

The effects of antibiotics on enteric bacteria are complex and depend upon the intraluminal and antimicrobial properties of the agents used and the secondary effects resulting from altered bacterial interactions. Nevertheless, a few generalizations are possible. Nonabsorbable, broad-spectrum antibiotics transiently reduce enteric coliforms and other aerobes without greatly altering anaerobic organisms.[9] Antibiotics that decrease the number of gram-negative aerobes effectively decrease infections in patients undergoing colon surgery[19] or those afflicted with granulocytopenia.[20] Because they persist during broad-spectrum antibiotic prophylaxis, anaerobes continue to stabilize the enteric flora and thus prevent overgrowth with pathogens.[21]

EFFECTS OF ENTERIC FLORA ON THE INTESTINE

Morphology

The bowel of the germ-free animal differs considerably from that of conventionally reared animals. The villi of small bowel mucosa are thin and remarkably regular, while the depth of crypts is diminished.[3] Leukocytic infiltration of the lamina propria, the size and number of Peyer's patches, the number of mitotic figures in crypt epithelium, and the rate of mucosal regeneration are all dramatically reduced. When the germ-free animal is monocontaminated by cultures of one or another microorganism, the intestinal mucosa rapidly assumes the "normal" appearance of "physiologic inflammation" observed in conventionally reared animals.

Intestinal Absorption

Compared with their effects on intestinal morphology, the influence of normal enteric bacterial populations on intestinal absorption is much less dramatic. Although small bowel transit is slowed and activity of microvillus membrane peptidases and disaccharidases appears to be increased in germ-free animals[6, 22] there is little evidence that these changes lead to a substantial increase in nutrient absorption. When intestinal bacterial populations are diminished, quantitative measurements show that laboratory animals absorb xylose, amino acids, and calcium more effectively, but differences are not quantitatively impressive.[10]

Intraluminal Metabolism

Of obvious importance is the effect of intestinal bacteria on the metabolism of various sterols and steroids, including cholesterol and bile acids.[4] Of increasing interest is the fact that the capacity of enteric bacteria to metabolize cholesterol and bile salts is increased in patients who ingest large amounts of cholesterol and in those with colon cancer.[23] Enteric bacteria generate cholesterol dehydrogenase, which oxidizes this important sterol. Intestinal microorganisms are also capable of hydrolyzing the primary conjugated bile acids secreted by the liver. In addition, bacterial 7-dehydroxylase removes the hydroxyl group at the 7 position of the primary bile acids, converting cholic to deoxycholic acid and chenodeoxycholic acid to lithocholic acid. Although quantitatively less important, a wide variety of other bacterial metabolites are also formed. Of these metabolites lithocholate appears to be the most toxic, although it should be pointed out that the minor bacterial derivatives have not been extensively studied.

Intestinal bacteria also alter other biologically active sterols such as androgens and estrogens. Bacterial beta-glucuronidase and sulfatase hydrolyze the conjugated forms of these hormones, which are excreted in bile. This deconjugation is necessary for intestinal reabsorption and consequent enterohepatic circulation of estrogens and androgens. Considerable evidence[9] now indicates that antibiotic suppression of the enteric flora diminishes the enterohepatic circulation of estriol, progesterone, and androgens, thus reducing the levels of these hormones in plasma and urine.

As previously reviewed,[10] it has long been known that lipids, proteins, and carbohydrates that reach the large bowel are rapidly metabolized by enteric microorganisms (Table 5-2). They hydrolyze glycerides and synthesize lipids from simpler organic compounds such as acetate. Fecal fatty acids differ from dietary fatty acids because the branched and hydroxylated fatty acids recovered from feces result from bacterial synthesis. It is possible *in vitro* to demonstrate conversion of long-chain fatty acids to hydroxy fatty acids with pure cultures of a variety of microorganisms.

Enteric bacteria degrade protein and urea within the intestinal lumen to produce ammonia. Ammonia production in antibiotic-treated or germ-free animals is markedly reduced. Although the implications of this ammonia production in health are not entirely understood, bacterial production becomes important when the body is unable to handle ammonia properly because of hepatic insufficiency or a primary metabolic defect in the urea cycle. Serum and spinal fluid levels of ammonia are decreased and hepatic encephalopathy improves when enteric bacterial populations are substantially diminished by the administration of poorly absorbed, broad-spectrum antibiotics together with enemas and cathartics.

Colonic bacterial disaccharidases split any unab-

sorbed dietary sugars and ferment them to form acetic, propionic, and butyric acids, which can be absorbed through the colonic mucosa. By converting unabsorbed carbohydrate to organic acids that can be absorbed by passive diffusion through the intestine, colonic bacteria aid the host in conserving energy.[24] Indeed the ability of some patients to maintain their weight despite substantial intestinal malabsorption may be explained in part by this capacity of colonic microorganisms to degrade unabsorbed carbohydrates with resulting energy conservation. Some bacterially produced organic acids, however, can be deleterious. In patients with malabsorption, including those with intestinal bypass surgery, bacterial production of D-lactate can lead to episodes resembling ethanol intoxication as a result of accumulation of D-lactic acid in the blood.[25]

METABOLISM OF DRUGS AND OTHER COMPOUNDS BY ENTERIC BACTERIA

Intraluminal microbial metabolism continues to attract interest.[5, 26, 27] Bacterial actions on drugs include: (1) the conversion of sulfasalazine to sulfapyridine and 5-aminosalicylic acid, the agent responsible for suppressing intestinal inflammation; (2) deconjugation of biliary-secreted conjugates of chloramphenicol and digoxin with subsequent absorption and enterohepatic cycling of the metabolites; (3) degradation of digoxin to inactive metabolites; and (4) metabolism of L-dopa to dopamine (which cannot cross the blood-brain barrier), leading to ineffective therapy of Parkinson's disease.

Also of potential importance to the host is bacterial metabolism of various nitrogenous substances. Bacterial decarboxylases are capable of converting aromatic amino acids to various biologically active amines. Whether enteric production and subsequent accumulation of potentially "toxic" amines play a meaningful role in the clinical manifestations of disorders such as hepatic failure or uremia has long been a subject of speculation and investigation. Although diminished protein intake and suppression of the enteric flora improves hepatic and, to a lesser extent, uremic encephalopathy, no specific microbially produced agents have yet been identified as responsible.

Bacterial glucoronidases, sulfatases, reductases, and decarboxylases are capable of profoundly affecting the transport properties and consequent toxicity of a wide variety of nitrogenous compounds consumed in modern diets. Examples include the formation of a carcinogen, cyclohexylamine, from dietary cyclamates and bacterial conversion of nitrates used as food preservatives to potentially carcinogenic nitrosamines. Rats fed cycasin provide an experimental model of bacterially induced colon cancer. Microbial beta-glucosidase converts inert cycasin to methylazomethanol, an active mutagen that regularly produces tumors. A recent review[9] considers in detail these and other actions of enteric bacteria that may be relevant to colon cancer.

Table 5-2. BACTERIAL ALTERATION OF UNABSORBED NUTRIENTS

Substrate	Products	Importance to Host
Carbohydrates	Organic acids	Colonic absorption conserves calories Osmotic diarrhea
	Hydrogen	Breath tests for malabsorption
	Methane	Cause of explosions during colonoscopy
	D-Lactate	Impaired cerebral function
Triglycerides	Fatty acids	Diarrhea
	Hydrolylated fatty acids	Diarrhea
Proteins	Ammonia, amines	Metabolic encephalopathy
	Indoles, skatoles	Questionable

ROLE OF INDIGENOUS FLORA IN INTESTINAL DISEASE

Small Bowel Bacterial Overgrowth

As might be expected, malabsorption due to bacterial proliferation within the small bowel lumen occurs when, for whatever reason, there is stasis of small bowel contents, particularly when such stasis is combined with impaired or absent gastric acid secretion.[28] The specific disorders known to be associated with small bowel bacterial overgrowth are discussed on pages 1289 to 1297. Here we need only state that any small abnormality conducive to local stasis or recirculation of small bowel contents is likely to be accompanied by marked intraluminal proliferation of microorganisms. Gastric atrophy and gastric surgery also increase the number of microorganisms residing in the small bowel lumen, and the so-called *blind loop* or *stagnant loop syndrome* occurs most frequently among elderly hypochlorhydric patients. Moreover, gastric surgery with or without readily demonstrable concomitant small bowel stasis may be followed by clinically significant bacterial overgrowth.

Within the small bowel of patients or experimental animals with small bowel bacterial overgrowth, bacterial populations are extremely complex and closely resemble those of normal colonic contents. Bacterial counts can be truly impressive and often reach 10^8 to 10^{10} viable microorganisms per gram of small bowel content. *Bacteroides* and *anaerobic lactobacilli* usually predominate, but *enterobacteria, enterococci, clostridia,* and *diphtheroids* may also be present in high concentrations.

Cobalamin (vitamin B_{12}) malabsorption that is not corrected by intrinsic factor is a characteristic feature of clinically significant small bowel bacterial overgrowth. The mechanism for cobalamin malabsorption was clarified 25 years ago by experiments that showed in rats with surgically induced bacterial overgrowth that bacterial uptake of cobalamin prevents the vitamin from being absorbed by enterocytes.[29] This mechanism has subsequently been confirmed repeatedly in a wide variety of experimental and clinical settings, and alternative explanations have consistently been found wanting.[6, 9, 28] Competitive uptake of the vitamin is particularly characteristic of gram-negative aerobes and various anaerobes. Intrinsic factor effectively inhibits aerobic microbial uptake of cobalamin but has no effect on uptake of cobalamin by gram-negative anaerobes (bacteroides). Thus anaerobes can bind cobalamin even when the vitamin is "protected" by its attachment to intrinsic factor.[30]

Enteric microorganisms also synthesize cobalamin and thus ought to be a rich source of this vitamin. Because viable bacteria retain the vitamin, however, it never becomes available to the host. Thus in treating patients with small bowel bacterial overgrowth, one is faced with a paradoxical situation: cobalamin deficiency develops even though large quantities of the vitamin are present in the small bowel lumen.

Enteric bacteria also synthesize folic acid but, in contrast to vitamin B_{12}, folate is released by the microorganism. Folate generated by colonic bacteria is not available to the host, however, because this nutrient is not transported across colonic mucosa. On the other hand, species such as the rat derive considerable folate from coprophagy and can be made folate-deficient only when treated with antibiotics.[31] In the blind loop syndrome small bowel bacteria produce and release folate that can be absorbed, and patients with the blind loop syndrome rarely, if ever, become folate-deficient. In fact, serum folate levels tend to be high rather than low.[32]

For more than two decades, investigators have recognized the importance of bacterial alteration of bile salts in the pathogenesis of fat malabsorption.[33] At the pH of intestinal contents conjugated bile salts normally exist as fully ionized, water-soluble bile salts capable of forming mixed micelles with the products of fat digestion. These ionized bile salts are not readily reabsorbed from the proximal intestine and thus remain in the lumen, where they are needed to "solubilize" lipids. To be absorbed, conjugated bile salts require a specific transport mechanism present only in the ileum (see pp. 144–161). When bacteria proliferate in the small bowel, however, they hydrolyze conjugated bile salts to form free bile acids. The latter are present at the pH of small bowel contents as protonated bile acids, which are readily reabsorbed from the jejunum and do not attain concentrations sufficient to form micelles. Thus, if bacterial hydrolysis of conjugated bile salts is sufficiently rapid, bile salt micelle formation is impaired. By labeling the glycine moiety of primary bile acids, one can estimate *in vivo* the rate of bile salt hydrolysis as determined by the appearance of $^{14}CO_2$ in the breath or specific activity of labeled bile salt secreted in bile.

Deficiency of bile salt unquestionably limits intestinal transport of monoglyceride and fatty acids, but deficiency is probably not the only factor responsible for steatorrhea. Feeding bile salts does not correct fat malabsorption,[33] and rats with experimentally produced bacterial overgrowth have more severe lipid malabsorption than rats with complete bile duct ligation.[34] Accumulation of "toxic" concentrations of free bile acids may also contribute to steatorrhea, since intestinal transport of lipids is decreased by free bile acid metabolites that have been generated by enteric bacteria.[35] As discussed below, the patchy intestinal mucosal lesion seen regularly in the blind loop syndrome almost certainly plays an additional role.

Although it has been difficult to document carbohydrate malabsorption, xylose tolerance tests are abnormal in the clinical as well as in the experimental blind loop syndrome. When rats with blind loops are fed ^{14}C-xylose, urinary excretion of xylose is diminished to about the same extent as breath $^{14}CO_2$ excretion is increased.[36] This observation emphasizes the importance of intraluminal bacterial degradation of carbohydrates in the blind loop syndrome and serves as the basis for the ^{14}C-xylose breath test in the clinical diagnosis of small bowel bacterial overgrowth (see p. 1295). Further evidence for bacterial fermentation of carbohydrates comes from increased intraluminal levels of organic acids in the setting of bacterial overgrowth.[37] In addition, however, intestinal levels of disaccharidases are reduced, and absorption of monosaccharides by the jejunum is diminished. Thus, impaired assimilation of carbohydrate in the setting of small bowel bacterial overgrowth involves both intraluminal bacterial metabolism of carbohydrates and decreased digestion and transport of sugars by enterocytes.

Protein depletion occurs frequently in cases of bacterial overgrowth and probably results from a combination of decreased mucosal uptake of amino acids,[38] intraluminal degradation of protein precursors by bacteria,[39] and antibiotic-reversible protein-losing enteropathy.[40] In the experimental blind loop syndrome both fecal and urinary nitrogen are increased.[34]

In general, malabsorption can be attributed to intraluminal effects of proliferating bacteria combined with damage to the enterocyte itself. Although patchy and variable in severity, a small bowel mucosal lesion can be readily identified both in experimental animals and in patients with overgrowth.[28, 38, 41] Moderate blunting of villi occurs, along with loss of structural integrity of some of the surface epithelial cells and increased cellular infiltration of the lamina propria. Other manifestations of cellular damage include diminished disaccharidase activity; decreased transport of monosaccharides, amino acids, and fatty acids; and protein-losing enteropathy. The cause of mucosal damage is unknown but has been attributed to bacterial proteases, lectins, mucus degradation, bile acids, hydroxylated fatty acids, organic acids, alcohols, and acetaldehyde.[28, 35, 37, 42–45]

Three additional factors may contribute to the clinical features of the blind loop syndrome (see pp. 1290–1293). First, bacterial production of organic acids increases osmolarity of small bowel contents and decreases intraluminal pH.[6] Second, bacterial metabolites such as free bile acids, hydroxylated fatty acids, and organic acids stimulate intestinal secretion of water and electrolytes.[6, 23, 45] Finally, experimental bacterial overgrowth in rats leads to small bowel motility disturbances, which are reversible with antibiotics.[45]

Specific Enteric Infections

See also pages 1191 to 1232.

During acute diarrhea, the enteric flora may be markedly altered.[9] When active diarrhea is caused by *Vibrio cholerae, Shigella, Salmonella,* or pathogenic *Escherichia coli*, the concentration of specific pathogen in feces is on the order of 10^7 to 10^9 viable organisms per milliliter. On the other hand, the concentration of anaerobes usually diminishes. Since similar decreases in the number of anaerobes can be demonstrated with saline-induced catharsis, it seems likely that rapid passage of contents through the bowel creates an unfavorable environment for maintaining fastidious anaerobes. On the other hand, changes in the indige-

nous microflora can influence the course of specific enteric infections by (1) altering the susceptibility of the bowel to colonization by pathogens, (2) generating enteropathogenic strains of "normal" species, and (3) changing the sensitivity of pathogens to antibiotics.

In several experimental situations the indigenous microflora appears to suppress proliferation of enteropathogenic bacteria.[47] Salmonellae, for example, do not ordinarily colonize mouse intestine, but certain strains of *S. enteritidis* proliferate readily when mice are pretreated with streptomycin. Furthermore, germ-free mice and guinea pigs show an increased susceptibility to infection with *Salmonella* and *Shigella*. The normal microorganisms specifically responsible for resistance to invasion by pathogens have not been clearly delineated, but there is some evidence that *Bacteroides* and nonpathogenic *E. coli* play an important role.

Many instances of so-called nonspecific diarrhea occur in situations in which one might expect alterations in the enteric flora. This is certainly the case in traveler's diarrhea, in which an individual is exposed to a completely different environment and climate; in weanling diarrhea, which occurs when the infant is exposed to large numbers of new microorganisms for the first time; and in the diarrhea that occurs following the administration of antibiotics. Whether diarrhea in these situations always results from microorganisms that at that particular time become pathogenic for that particular host is an important question that remains to be settled. Certainly most cases of traveler's diarrhea result from enteropathogenic strains of *E. coli*.[9, 47] Many, but not all, cases of antibiotic-induced diarrhea (see pp. 1307–1320) are due to a toxin-producing strain of *Clostridium difficile*. This bacillus multiplies because other anaerobes that normally act as competitive inhibitors of this organism have been decreased or eliminated by antibiotic therapy.

E. coli is part of the normal fecal flora, but different strains cause diarrhea by different mechanisms. Classic enteropathogenic strains of *E. coli* are invasive. Other strains elaborate heat-labile (LT) or heat-stable (ST) enterotoxins. LT is similar to cholera toxin and produces secretion through the adenyl cyclase mechanism, whereas ST induces secretion through the guanyl cyclase mechanism. For diarrhea to ensue, *E. coli* must adhere to the mucosa of the small intestine, a process that depends upon specific binding of bacterial structures called pili to receptors on the enterocytes of some hosts but not others. Receptors for *E. coli* enterotoxins are also under genetic control, and absence of such receptors may explain why some individuals do not develop diarrhea when exposed to an enterotoxin.

Normal bacteria can also influence infectious diarrhea by inducing resistance of the pathogen to antibiotics. Resistance to one or several antibiotics can be transferred from one enteric microorganism to another by means of self-replicating extrachromosomal genetic elements that resemble episomes and are called R factors.[48] The transfer of drug resistance from one bacterial cell to another is mediated by a portion of the R factor known as the resistance transfer factor.

Transferable resistance to penicillin, ampicillin, streptomycin, tetracycline, various sulfonamides, furazolidone, kanamycin, and neomycin or to any combination of these drugs has been demonstrated. How often transfer of antibiotic resistance from one strain to another is important in acute diarrheal disorders remains questionable, but it is clear that indigenous Enterobacteriaceae resistant to one or several antibiotics can transfer this resistance to pathogenic microorganisms.

Tropical Sprue

Several observations suggest that either some change in the indigenous flora or actual infection by a pathogen causes tropical sprue.[49] The disease often begins as an episode of acute gastroenteritis, which then progresses to the more typical chronic malabsorption (see pp. 1281–1289). Epidemics of tropical sprue have been described in prisoner of war camps and in villages in south India. The inflammatory changes present in the small bowel mucosa are consistent with a bacterial effect. Finally, impressive and lasting remissions consistently follow treatment with broad-spectrum antibiotics.

Although alterations in the host's flora may well be important in the pathogenesis of tropical sprue, the disease does not simply result from proliferation of bacteria within the small bowel lumen. There are distinct differences between tropical sprue and the blind loop syndrome.[9] Small bowel biopsies from patients with tropical sprue consistently show distortion of villus architecture, in contrast to the blind loop syndrome, in which morphologic abnormalities are patchy and of variable severity. Steatorrhea and cobalamin malabsorption in patients with the blind loop syndrome can be corrected within a few days by appropriate administration of antibiotics, whereas meaningful response to antibiotics usually requires several weeks in tropical sprue. Although coliforms may be modestly increased in the small bowel of some patients with tropical sprue, one certainly does not see the massive overgrowth of anaerobes that is found in the blind loop syndrome.

Since deficiencies of folate, cobalamin, or protein all favor the development of intestinal mucosal abnormalities, it is possible that even mild deficiencies of one or more of these nutrients might increase the mucosal susceptibility to injury by a microorganism that in the healthy host would be nonpathogenic. Certainly, administration of folic acid produces at least partial remission in patients with tropical sprue. Acute diarrhea, particularly when it occurs in the tropics, can be associated with transient but definite inflammatory changes in the small bowel, cobalamin malabsorption, and steatorrhea. Thus, although far from proved, the disorder known as tropical sprue may result from a combination of factors, including invasion by microorganisms that tend to flourish in the tropics, subclinical deficiency of critical nutrients, and pathophysiologic alterations resulting from diarrhea.[50]

References

1. Coates, M. E., and Fuller, B. The gnotobiotic animal in the study of gut microbiology. *In* Clarke, R. T. J., and Bauchop, T. (eds.). Microbial Ecology of the Gut. New York, Academic Press, 1977, pp. 311–346.
2. Gordon, H. A., and Pesti, L. The gnotobiotic animal as a tool in the study of host microbial relationships. Bacteriol. Rev. *35*:390, 1971.
3. Abrams, G. D. Microbial effects on mucosal structure and function. Am. J. Clin. Nutr. *30*:1880, 1977.
4. Hylemon, P. B., and Glass, T.L. Biotransformation of bile acids and cholesterol by the intestinal microflora. *In* Hentges, D. J. (ed.). Human Intestinal Microflora in Health and Disease. New York, Academic Press, 1983, pp. 189–214.
5. Boxenbaum, H. G., Bejersky, I., Jack, M. L., and Kaplan, S. A. Influence of gut microflora on bioavailability. Drug Metab. Rev. *9*:259, 1979.
6. Savage, D. C. Gastrointestinal microflora in mammalian nutrition. Ann. Rev. Nutr. *6*:155, 1986.
7. Hill, M. J. Diet and the human intestinal bacterial flora. Cancer Res. *41*:3778, 1981.
8. Rolfe, R. D. Interactions among microorganisms of the indigenous intestinal flora and their influence on the host. Rev. Inf. Dis. *67*:S73, 1984.
9. Simon, G. L., and Gorbach, S. L. The human intestinal microflora. Dig. Dis. Sci. *31*(Suppl.):1475, 1986.
10. Donaldson, R. M. Role of indigenous enteric bacteria in intestinal function and disease. *In* Code C. F. (ed.). Handbook of Physiology. Baltimore, Williams & Wilkins Company, 1968.
11. Moore, W. E. C., and Holdeman, L. V. Identification of anaerobic bacteria. Am. J. Clin. Nutr. *25*:1306, 1972.
12. Hentges, D. J. (ed.). Human Intestinal Microflora in Health and Disease. New York, Academic Press, 1983, p. 568.
13. Drasar, B. S., Shiner, M., and McLeod, G. M. Studies on the intestinal flora. I. The bacterial flora of the gastrointestinal tract in healthy and achlorhydric persons. Gastroenterology *56*:71, 1969.
14. Moore, W. E. C., and Holdeman, L. V. Discussion of current bacteriologic investigations of the relationships between intestinal flora, diet, and colon cancer. Cancer Res. *35*:3418, 1975.
15. Rotimi, V. O., and Duerden, B. I. The bacterial flora in normal neonates. J. Med. Micr. *14*:51, 1981.
16. Bjorneklett, A., Fausa, O., and Midtveldt T. Small bowel bacterial overgrowth in the post gastrectomy syndrome. Scand. J. Gastroenterol. *18*:277, 1983.
17. Coates, M. E., Gustafsson, B. E. (eds.). The Germ-Free Animal in Biomedical Research. London, Laboratory Animals, 1984, p. 442.
18. Kennedy, M. J., and Voz, P. A. Ecology of *Candida albicans* gut colonization. Infect. Immun. *49*:654, 1985.
19. Clarke, J. S., Condon, R. E., Bartlett, J. G., Gorbach, S. L., Nichols, R. L., and Ochi, S. Preoperative oral antibiotics reduce septic complications of colon operations. Ann. Surg. *181*:251, 1977.
20. Guiot, H. F. Selective antimicrobial modulation of the intestinal microbial flora for infection prevention in patients with hematologic malignancies. Scand. J. Infect. Dis. *18*:53, 1986.
21. Guiot, H. F., van der Meer, J. W. M., and van Furth, R. Selective antimicrobial modulation of human microbial flora: Infection prevention in patients with decreased host defense mechanisms by selective elimination of potentially pathogenic bacteria. J. Infect. Dis. *143*:644, 1981.
22. Wostman, B. S. The germ-free animal in nutritional studies. Ann. Rev. Nutr. *2*:257, 1981.
23. Hill, M. J. Bile, bacteria and bowel cancer. Gut *24*:871, 1983.
24. Bond, J. H., Currier, B. E., Buchwald, H., and Levitt, M. Colonic conservation of malabsorbed carbohydrate. Gastroenterology *78*:444, 1980.
25. Halverson, J., Gale, A., Lazarus, C., and Avioli, L. V. D-Lactic acidosis and other complications of intestinal bypass surgery. Arch. Intern. Med. *144*:357, 1984.
26. Pradham, A. Metabolism of some drugs by intestinal lactobacilli and their toxicological considerations. Acta Pharmacol. Toxicol. *58*:11, 1986.

27. Midtvedt, T., Carlstedt-Duke, B., Høverstad, T., Lingaas, E., Norin, E., Saxerholt, H., and Steinbakk, M. Influence of peroral antibiotics upon the biotransformatory activity of the intestinal microflora in healthy subjects. Eur. J. Clin. Invest. *16*:11, 1986.
28. Gracey, M. The contaminated small bowel syndrome. *In* Hentges, D. J. (ed.). Human Intestinal Microflora in Health and Disease. New York, Academic Press, 1983, pp. 495–516.
29. Donaldson, R. M., Jr. Malabsorption of ⁶⁰Co-labelled cyanocobalamin in rats with intestinal diverticula. I. Evaluation of possible mechanisms. Gastroenterology *43*:271, 1962.
30. Welkos, S. A., Toskes, P. P., Baer, H., and Smith, G. W. Importance of anaerobic bacteria in the cobalamin malabsorption of experimental rat blind loop syndrome. Gastroenterology *80*:313, 1981.
31. Barnes, R. H. Nutritional implications of coprophagy. Nutr. Rev. *20*:289, 1962.
32. Hoffbrand, A. V., Tabaqchali, S., and Mollin, D. L. High serum folate levels in intestinal blind loop syndrome. Lancet *1*:1339, 1966.
33. Kim, Y. S., Spritz, N., Blum, M., Terz, J., and Sherlock, P. The role of altered bile acid metabolism in the steatorrhea of experimental blind loop. J. Clin. Invest. *45*:956, 1966.
34. Donaldson, R. M., Jr. Role of enteric microorganisms in malabsorption. Fed. Proc. *26*:1426, 1967.
35. Wanitschke, R., and Ammon, H. V. Effects of dihydroxy bile acids and hydroxy fatty acids in the absorption of oleic acid in the human jejunum. J. Clin. Invest. *61*:178, 1978.
36. Toskes, P. P., King, C. E., Spivey, J. C., and Lorenz, E. Xylose catabolism in experimental rat blind loop syndrome: Studies including newly developed d-(¹⁴C) xylose breath test. Gastroenterology *74*:691, 1978.
37. Prizont, R., Whitehead, J. S., and Kim, Y. S. Short chain fatty acids in rats with jejunal blind loops. I. Analysis of SCFA in small intestine, cecum feces, and plasma. Gastroenterology *69*:1254, 1975.
38. Sherman, P., Wesley, A., and Forstner, G. Sequential disaccharidase loss in rat intestinal blind loops. Impact of malnutrition. Am. J. Physiol. *248*:626, 1985.
39. Varcoe, R., Holliday, D., and Tavill, A. Utilization of urea nitrogen for albumin synthesis in the stagnant loop syndrome. Gut *15*:898, 1974.
40. King, C. E., and Toskes, P. P. Protein-losing enteropathy in the human experimental rat blind loop syndrome. Gastroenterology *80*:504, 1981.
41. Toskes, P. P., Giannella, R. A., Jervis, H. R., Rout, W. R., and Takeuchi, A. Small intestinal mucosal injury in the experimental blind loop syndrome. Gastroenterology *68*:1193, 1975.
42. Riepe, S. P., Goldstein, J. G., and Alpers, D. H. Effect of secreted bacteroides proteases on human intestinal brush border hydrolases. J. Clin. Invest. *66*:314, 1980.
43. Baraona, E., Julkunen, R., Tannenbaum, L., and Lieber, C. S. Role of intestinal bacterial overgrowth in ethanol production and metabolism in rats. Gastroenterology *90*:103, 1986.
44. Banwell, J. G., Boldt, D. H., Meyers, J., and Weber, F. L., Jr. Phytohemagglutinin derived from red kidney bean (*Phaseolus vulgaris*): A cause for intestinal malabsorption associated with bacterial overgrowth in the rat. Gastroenterology *84*:506, 1984.
45. Cline, W. S., Lorenzsonn, V., Benz, L., Bass, P., and Olsen, W. A. The effects of sodium ricinoleate on small intestinal function and structure. J. Clin. Invest. *58*:380, 1976.
46. Justus, P. G., Fernandez, A., Martin, J. L., King, C. E., Toskes, P. P., and Mathias, J. R. Altered myoelectric activity in the experimental blind loop syndrome. J. Clin. Invest. *72*:1064, 1983.
47. Giannella, R. A. Pathogenesis of acute bacterial diarrheal disorders. Ann. Rev. Med. *32*:341, 1981.
48. Watanabe, T. Infectious drug resistance in enteric bacteria. N. Engl. J. Med. *275*:888, 1981.
49. Cook, G. C. Aetiology and pathogenesis of post infective tropical malabsorption (tropical sprue). Lancet *1*:721, 1984.
50. Tomkins, A. Tropical malabsorption: Recent concepts on pathogenesis and nutritional significance. Clin. Sci. *60*:131, 1981.

6 Immunology and Disease of the Gastrointestinal Tract

MARTIN F. KAGNOFF

This chapter focuses on aspects of the immune system that are important to the function of the gastrointestinal tract and to normal host-environment interactions that take place in the gut. It also highlights how the immune system may be relevant to the etiology and pathogenesis of several intestinal diseases and disorders.

New knowledge of the function and regulation of the immune response is substantially increasing our understanding of disease processes. Thus, it is now recognized that abnormalities in the genetic regulation of lymphoid cell functions have important implications for human disease. In the technical arena, monoclonal antibodies and methods in molecular immunology are being applied to disease diagnosis and treatment. The eventual ability to manipulate the intestinal immune response promises an exciting future.

The first section outlines the normal physiology of the immune system in the digestive tract. The second section examines the role of the immune system in the pathogenesis of specific diseases that affect the gastrointestinal tract.

GENERAL CHARACTERISTICS AND DEVELOPMENT OF THE IMMUNE SYSTEM

The immune system is composed of lymphocytes that recognize and interact with antigen using specific receptors on their cell surface. Less mature lymphocytes respond to antigen by proliferating and/or differentiating into mature effector lymphoid cells that can mediate a spectrum of different immune effector functions.

There are two well-described lineages of lymphocytes—the thymus-derived or T lymphocyte lineage and the bone marrow–derived or B lymphocyte lineage. As shown schematically in Figure 6–1, T lymphocytes develop from stem cells under the influence of the thymus, whereas B lymphocytes develop from stem cells in the fetal liver and bone marrow. Because of their role in lymphocyte ontogeny, the thymus, fetal liver, and bone marrow are termed central lymphoid organs. B and T lymphocytes leave the central lymphoid organs during development and populate the peripheral lymphoid organs. Peripheral lymphoid organs include lymphoid tissue in the gastrointestinal tract (termed gut-associated lymphoid tissue or GALT), the spleen, and the peripheral and mesenteric lymph nodes.

Mature T lymphocytes have regulatory activities (i.e., helper function or suppressor function) or cytotoxic properties (i.e., cytotoxic T lymphocyte). In contrast, mature B lymphocytes (plasma cells) produce and secrete antibody belonging to one of several immunoglobulin classes (e.g., IgM, IgA, IgG, or IgE).

Antigenic materials that stimulate the intestinal immune system include those derived from gut bacteria, viruses, parasites, ingested foods, drugs, or chemicals.

Characteristics of T Cells

T lymphocytes undergo development in the thymus. T lymphocytes as well as other mononuclear cells frequently are categorized into subsets based on the presence of varying arrays of markers on their cell surface. Such markers are termed clusters of differentiation (CD) and are detected usually by monoclonal antibodies. CD2 is an early marker on the cell surface of thymocytes.[1] Later, thymocytes coexpress the two additional surface markers, CD4 (detected by the OKT4 or Leu 3 monoclonal antibodies) and CD8 (detected by OKT8 or Leu 2 monoclonal antibodies). Minor subpopulations of thymocytes lack CD4 and CD8 or express one but not the other marker. Before migrating to the periphery, T cells in the thymus subsequently acquire CD3 and the T cell antigen receptor.[2, 3] In the periphery T cells generally are divided into subsets based on whether or not they have the CD4 or CD8 markers and based on differences in their functional activities (e.g., helper or suppressor activity, cytotoxic activity).

T cells do not respond to soluble antigens. Rather, the T cell receptor (TcR) for antigen recognizes antigen on the surface of cells in association with major histocompatibility complex (MHC) molecules[4] (Fig. 6–2). The MHC in humans is termed HLA. Regulatory T

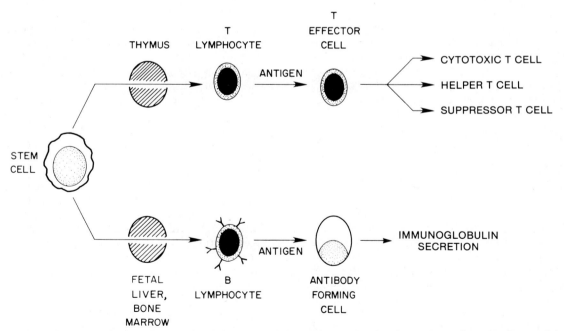

Figure 6–1. Development of the immune system. Thymus-derived (T) lymphocytes develop from stem cells in the thymus. B lymphocytes develop from stem cells in the fetal liver and bone marrow. After stimulation, T lymphocytes proliferate and mature into T effector cells (e.g., helper T cells, suppressor T cells, cytotoxic T cells), whereas B lymphocytes proliferate and mature into antibody-forming cells (i.e., plasma cells) that synthesize and secrete immunoglobulin. (From Kagnoff, M. F. *In* Johnson, L. R. [ed.]. Physiology of the Gastrointestinal Tract. New York, Raven Press, 1987. Used by permission.)

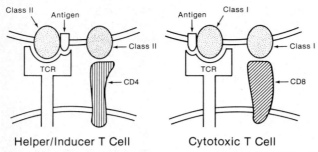

Figure 6–2. The T cell receptor for antigen (TCR) recognizes antigen in association with HLA molecules. T cells bearing the CD4 marker recognize antigen in association with class II HLA antigens and generally function as helper/inducer T cells. T cells bearing the CD8 marker recognize antigen in association with class I HLA antigens and generally function as cytotoxic T cells (or suppressor T cells). As illustrated, CD4 and CD8 also function as accessory binding molecules in cellular interactions between T cells and cells bearing class II or class I HLA molecules respectively. Not shown, the TCR is closely associated also with the CD3 complex on the cell membrane.

cells that help in the induction of immune responses (e.g., B cell responses, cytotoxic T cell responses) are termed helper/inducer T cells. Such T cells generally recognize antigen in association with class II HLA molecules. T cells that suppress the immune response and cytotoxic T cells generally recognize a combination of antigen and class I HLA molecules (i.e., such T cells can be termed class I or class II restricted T cells). The HLA locus on chromosome 6 is divided into several regions and subregions.[5] Molecules coded for by the HLA-A, -B and -C region genes are termed class I molecules and are present on all nucleated cells. In contrast, molecules coded for by HLA-D region genes (includes the HLA-DP, -DQ and -DR subregions) are termed class II molecules and are present mainly on B cells, macrophages and dendritic reticular cells, activated T cells, and, under some conditions, on intestinal epithelial cells and other cell types.

The receptor on the T cell that recognizes antigen in conjunction with MHC molecules is a disulfide-linked glycoprotein dimer that consists of an alpha chain and a beta chain.[6] The alpha and beta chains of the T cell antigen receptor (TcR) are coded for by linked variable and constant region gene segments on chromosomes 14 and 7, respectively.[7, 8] During the formation of a complete gene for the TcR, these linked gene segments undergo DNA rearrangements, the net result of which is to amplify greatly the number of different antigens that can be recognized by different T cells (i.e., the T cell repertoire). On the cell surface, the TcR for antigen is noncovalently associated with a set of 3 membrane molecules termed the CD3 complex (also referred to as T3).[9] The CD3 complex appears to be involved in transferring a signal from the T cell receptor to the inside of the cell. A second receptor for antigen consisting of a gamma chain and a proposed delta chain may also exist on a subset of T cells.

T cells can be categorized phenotypically by the presence or absence of different arrays of cell surface molecules that generally are detected by monoclonal antibodies. The CD3 marker (i.e., marker of the CD3 complex associated with the T cell antigen receptor) is present on most mature T cells.[9] CD8 is present on T cells that interact with class I MHC molecules, whereas CD4 is present on T cells that interact with class II MHC molecules[10, 11] (Fig. 6–2). CD4 and CD8 function as accessory binding molecules in interactions between T cells and antigen-presenting cells or target cells that express class II and class I HLA molecules respectively. The CD2 complex appears to function in triggering T cell activation.[12] CD2 also contains a binding site for sheep erythrocytes that is used, in the laboratory, to purify T cells through the formation of sheep erythrocyte (E)–T cell rosettes (i.e., E-rosettes).[12] Lymphocyte function–associated antigen-1 (LFA-1) on T cells appears to function as an adhesion molecule in cytotoxic reactions.[13] Further, subpopulations of T cells have receptors for the Fc portion of immunoglobulin on their surface. These latter T cells may help or suppress B cells in the production of specific immunoglobulin classes and subclasses.[14, 15]

T cells secrete soluble factors termed lymphokines that influence T and B cell activation, growth, and differentiation.[16] Many of these lymphokines have been well characterized by biochemical analysis or gene cloning (e.g., interleukin-2 [IL-2], interleukin-3 [IL-3], interleukin-4 [IL-4], interleukin-5 [IL-5], and gamma interferon [γ-IFN]), and have multiple effects on the growth and differentiation of more than one cell type. Interleukin-2 is a 15-kilodalton glycoprotein that binds to specific membrane receptors for IL-2 and stimulates activated T cells to proliferate. IL-2 also has effects on B cell growth and differentiation. IL-4 (BSF-1) and IL-5 (BCGF II) affect B cell growth and differentiation, including immunoglobulin class expression, and together with IL-3 (multi-CSF) variably influence the growth and differentiation of other cells of the hematopoietic system (e.g., mast cells, eosinophils). Gamma interferon affects the expression of class II HLA molecules on antigen-presenting cells, whereas IL-4 affects the expression of such markers on B cells.[17, 18]

Characteristics of B Cells

B cells that are stimulated by antigen develop, in the presence of helper T cells and/or T cell lymphokines, into mature plasma cells that produce antibody (immunoglobulin) directed against the stimulating antigen. Unlike T cells, B cells can recognize soluble antigens. The receptors for antigen on B cells are membrane-associated immunoglobulin molecules that have the same recognition structure for antigen as the antibody that is subsequently produced and secreted by the B cell. These receptors recognize determinants on the antigen itself rather than antigenic determinants in association with MHC molecules. Further, the three-dimensional conformation of the antigen is very important in the formation of many of the antigenic determinants. Thus, antigenic determinants often do

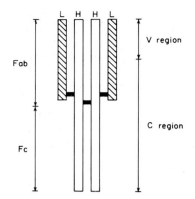

Figure 6–3. Diagram of an immunoglobulin molecule. Each monomer is composed of four polypeptide chains—two heavy chains (H) and two light chains (L). Disulfide bonds bridging the light and heavy chains are indicated by solid bars. The immunoglobulin molecule consists of two regions, each coded for by distinct exons in the genome. The variable (V) region determines antigen recognition, and the constant (C) region determines the effector functions of the molecule. By enzymatic (pepsin) cleavage, the immunoglobulin molecule can be split into Fab and Fc fragments. These fragments correlate respectively with an antigen-binding fragment (Fab) and a fragment that mediates biologic effector function (Fc).

cell-mediated cytotoxicity) are mediated by the Fc fragment that includes a major part of the constant region, whereas antigen recognition and binding are mediated by the Fab fragment that includes the variable region and a smaller part of the constant region (Fig. 6–3).

Immunoglobulin classes or subclasses (isotype) are determined by the heavy chain constant region. In humans there are five immunoglobulin classes: IgM, IgG, IgA, IgE, and IgD. The IgG class is composed of four subclasses (IgG1, IgG2, IgG3, and IgG4), and the IgA class has two subclasses (IgA1 and IgA2). IgA in human serum is mostly monomer, but IgA in secretions is mostly dimer (i.e., two monomer units). IgG is a monomer, whereas IgM is a pentamer (i.e., five monomer units).

The heavy chain of each immunoglobulin molecule is coded for by several coding regions (exons) in the genome. The sequence order of these exons on human chromosome 14 is depicted schematically in Fig. 6–4. Not all immunoglobulin isotypes are capable of mediating the same effector functions. Of note, some isotypes (e.g., IgG2, IgG4, IgA2, and IgE) are present in low amounts in serum. Quantitative measurements of total IgG or IgA levels may not reveal deficiencies within those minor isotypes, although they may be important in certain host defenses and in disease.

The variable region of the immunoglobulin molecule mediates antigen recognition. The variable region of the heavy chain is coded for by three different coding regions (V, D, and J region exons) (Fig. 6–4), whereas the variable region of the light chain is coded by two coding regions (V and J). Both the heavy-chain and light-chain variable regions contribute to the antigen-combining site of the antibody molecule. Because of their uniqueness, portions of the variable region of the antibody molecule can themselves act as antigenic determinants. Variable region antigenic determinants are termed idiotypic determinants. Such idiotypic determinants and antibodies to idiotypic determinants are being used in attempts to deliberately manipulate the regulation of the immune response and in experimental approaches to develop new vaccines.

The gene segments that code for immunoglobulin and the T cell antigen receptor have a characteristic property of undergoing DNA rearrangements to form

not consist of continuous amino acid sequences, but arise by virtue of amino acid sequences that are juxtaposed to each other on the surface of the protein through protein folding (i.e., conformational determinants).[19] In addition to receptors for antigen, B cells variably have receptors for complement components, the Fc region of immunoglobulin, and mitogen or hormone receptors.

Immunoglobulin molecules have four polypeptide chains; two light chains (either kappa or lambda) and two heavy chains (Fig. 6–3). This structural unit is termed a monomer. Heavy chains are coded for by genes on chromosome 14, whereas the kappa and lambda light chains are coded for by genes on chromosomes 2 and 22, respectively.[20] Each heavy and light chain has a variable (V) region that determines antigen recognition and a constant (C) region that determines the effector function of the immunoglobulin molecule. Immunoglobulin can be cleaved enzymatically into Fc and Fab fragments. Most effector functions (e.g., complement fixation, opsonization, antibody-dependent

Figure 6–4. The genetic region on human chromosome 14 encoding the heavy chain of immunoglobulin. This region consists of four linked families of gene segments: variable (V) region, diversity (D) region, joining (J) region, and constant (C) region gene segments. C region gene segments determine the class or subclass (isotype) of the heavy chain. There are five classes of the H chain (μ, δ, γ, ϵ, and α), four subclasses of the γ-chain (γ_1, γ_2, γ_3, and γ_4), and two subclasses of the α-chain (α_1, α_2). Each isotype is coded for by separate gene segments (exons). As shown, gene

HUMAN HEAVY CHAIN IMMUNOGLOBULIN GENES

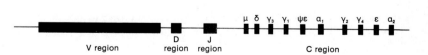

Chromosome 14

segments coding for γ, ϵ, and α are interspersed with each other, and there is a nonexpressed pseudo ϵ gene (ψ ϵ) closely linked to the α_1 gene. When an active heavy chain gene is formed by a VDJ segment joining, the μ gene is the first to be expressed. Other C genes such as the γ or α genes are subsequently expressed by heavy chain switching mechanisms, which likely involve deletion of the C genes located between the expressed V gene and the newly expressed γ or α gene. (From Kagnoff, M. F. *In* Johnson, L. R. [ed.]. Physiology of the Gastrointestinal Tract. New York, Raven Press, 1987. Used by permission.)

a complete coding gene.[21] This mechanism substantially increases the diversity of the antigen recognition repertoire of immunoglobulin molecules and T cell receptors. It also enables the immunoglobulin variable region to associate with one of several different constant regions, thereby diversifying the effector functions that can be mediated by a single antigen recognition unit.

Antigen-Presenting Cells

Several different cell types (e.g., macrophages, dendritic reticular cells, Langerhans cells, Kupffer cells) can function as "antigen-presenting cells." Some antigens require intracellular processing by antigen-presenting cells before being presented to T cells. This involves the uptake of antigen into the antigen-presenting cells and internal lysosomal processing or other mechanisms of internal cellular processing. The processed antigen subsequently is transported to and displayed on the cell surface in association with HLA class I or class II molecules,[22] in which form it is presented to the T cell. Dendritic reticular cells appear to be involved mainly in the presentation and not the processing of antigen. B lymphocytes and perhaps intestinal epithelial cells with class II molecules on their surface also appear to function as antigen-presenting cells.[23] In addition, antigen-presenting cells may produce soluble factors such as interleukin-1 that have an important role in T cell activation.

Other Cells

Mast cells, eosinophils, and basophils are important in immune effector mechanisms. The function of mast cells in the intestinal mucosa of humans is now an area of active study. Some mast cells in the intestinal mucosa contain biochemical mediators that may differ from those found in mast cells in extraintestinal sites.[24] Mast cell mediators (e.g., histamine, prostaglandins, leukotrienes) can interact with lymphoid cells and other cell types and thus participate in a broad spectrum of allergic, cytotoxic, and inflammatory reactions. In addition, mast cell mediators can directly alter smooth muscle function and vascular permeability.

Subpopulations of lymphocytes (i.e., natural killer [NK] cells and killer [K] cells) have receptors for the Fc region of immunoglobulin, but may lack other cell-surface markers typical of B or T cells. Such lymphocytes can be shown to have cytotoxic properties. Thus, lymphocytes termed "natural killer" cells are cytotoxic for certain tumor cells in *in vitro* assays, whereas "killer" cells are cytotoxic *in vitro* for target cells coated with antibody (i.e., antibody-dependent cell-mediated cytotoxic reactions).

THE INTESTINE AS A LYMPHOID ORGAN

Lymphoid tissue in the gut is an important part of the immune system. In fact, the human gastrointestinal

tract contains as much lymphoid tissue as the spleen. The gastrointestinal-associated lymphoid tissue (GALT) can be divided on anatomic, morphologic, and functional grounds into three major populations; the Peyer's patches, lamina propria lymphoid cells, and intraepithelial lymphocytes.[25] Peyer's patches are organized collections of small lymphoid follicles in the small intestine. They are a sampling site for intestinal antigens, play a major role in the initiation of the intestinal immune response, and contain many of the precursor lymphocytes that subsequently migrate to and populate the two other major GALT populations. The lamina propria lymphoid population is made up of B and T lymphocytes and plasma cells situated in the lamina propria region of the intestinal mucosa. The majority of B cells in the lamina propria are committed to produce immunoglobulin of the IgA class, and most lamina propria T cells have the CD4 phenotype (i.e., class II restricted and associated with helper/inducer function). The intraepithelial lymphocyte (IEL) population consists of lymphocytes located between intestinal epithelial cells. IEL are heterogeneous morphologically and phenotypically. Their functional properties are only now being defined. In addition to GALT, lymphocytes in the mesenteric lymph nodes (MLN) and reticuloendothelial cells in the liver (Kupffer cells) function as an important part of the intestinal immune system.

The intestinal immune system is one of several protective mechanisms that shield the host's internal milieu from the external environment. Lymphocytes in the three subdivisions of the GALT come into close proximity with gut antigens. Intraepithelial lymphocytes are separated from direct exposure to gut antigens only by the tight junctions between enterocytes. Peyer's patch lymphocytes are separated from gut luminal contents by specialized cells, termed membranous cells (M cells), that are involved in the uptake of antigen into Peyer's patches.[26] Lymphocytes and plasma cells in the lamina propria exist in the environment of a rich lymphatic and blood supply and are separated from contact with the luminal contents by mucosal epithelial cells and the basement membrane. The mechanical barrier formed by intestinal epithelial cells, their glycocalyx and the mucous coat, and intestinal motility are important also in protecting the host from bacteria and other toxic materials. Of note, these barriers are not totally efficient under normal conditions, and they are particularly inefficient when intestinal inflammatory processes disrupt the normal mucosa. Thus, the need for a multifaceted system for host protection is readily apparent.

Lymphoid Cell Populations of the Intestinal Tract
Peyer's Patches

Peyer's patches play an important role in the initiation and expression of the mucosal immune response.[25] These lymphoid aggregates extend through the mucosa and into the submucosa of the small intestine. Peyer's

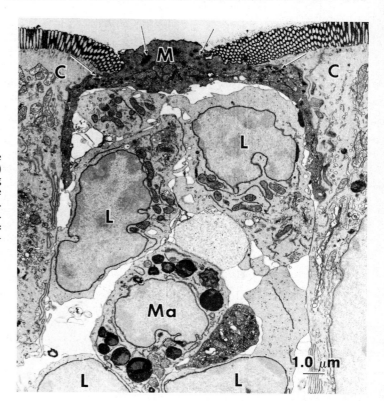

Figure 6–5. Peyer's patch M cell (M), stretched membrane-like between columnar cells (C), encloses four lymphoid cells (L) and a macrophage (Ma). Arrows mark vesicles transporting exogenously administered horseradish peroxidase from the intestinal lumen to the space surrounding the lymphoid cells. Lead citrate stain, ×8450. (From Owen, R. L., and Nemanic, P. Antigen processing structures of the mammalian intestinal tract: An SEM study of lymphoepithelial organs. Scan. Electron Microsc. *2*:367, 1978. Used by permission.)

patches first appear in the human fetus at 24 weeks' gestation and are most prominent in the ileum. They increase in number and size until 12 to 14 years of age and decrease thereafter. Nonetheless, they still can be detected in individuals who are in their nineties.

Antigens enter Peyer's patch lymphoid follicles through the specialized follicle-associated epithelium (FAE) that overlies these structures. FAE differs from the epithelium associated with the surrounding villi in two respects: (1) it contains M cells between columnar enterocytes,[26] and (2) it has a paucity of mucus-producing goblet cells. M cells lack fully developed microvilli on their luminal surface, consist of many folds, are pinocytotic, contain numerous vesicles, and form cytoplasmic bridges that separate adjacent lymphocytes from the intestinal lumen (Fig. 6–5). In humans, M cells transport macromolecules and particulate material from the lumen of the gut into Peyer's patch. Similar specialized epithelium overlies tonsillar and appendiceal lymphoid tissue.

The entry of lymphocytes into Peyer's patches is selective and takes place through the endothelial cells that line the postcapillary high endothelial venules.[27, 28] Molecules on the cell surface of lymphocytes appear to govern the preferential homing of populations of B and T lymphocytes to sites such as Peyer's patches rather than to peripheral lymph nodes, and vice versa.[29] Within Peyer's patches, lymphocytes are compartmentalized into two distinct regions—lymphoid follicles that contain mostly B cells and the interfollicular area that contains mostly class II restricted (CD4) T cells (Fig. 6–6). Follicles contain a dense outer rim of lymphocytes and a central germinal center that contains dividing B cells.

Many of the dividing B cells (i.e., B blast cells) in the germinal centers become committed to the IgA class. Seventy per cent of surface immunoglobulin–positive B cells in Peyer's patches stain for IgA. T cells within Peyer's patches have a special role in providing help for the development of IgA-committed B cells.[15, 30, 31] Although B cells are primed by exposure to gut antigens in Peyer's patches and become committed to the IgA class in that site, it is important to note that they do not mature into antibody-secreting plasma cells in Peyer's patches.[32–34] Rather, IgA B cells in Peyer's patches leave that organ and undergo a migratory pathway before ultimately populating the lamina propria region of the intestine. In the lamina propria many of the IgA-committed B cells ultimately differentiate into IgA-secreting plasma cells.[35, 36]

T cells in Peyer's patches also can be primed by exposure to intestinal antigens. Thus, in animal studies, exposure to enteric viruses and tumor cells has been shown to expand precursor T cell populations within Peyer's patches. After further maturation, such T cells could mediate regulatory or cytotoxic functions.[37–40]

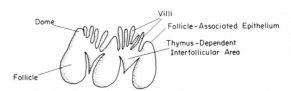

Figure 6–6. Schematic representation of a Peyer's patch depicting the follicle, dome, thymus-dependent interfollicular area, and specialized follicle-associated epithelium. (From Kagnoff, M. F. *In* Johnson, L. R. [ed.]. Physiology of the Gastrointestinal Tract. New York, Raven Press, 1987. Used by permission.)

However, precursor cytotoxic T lymphocytes (CTL) do not develop into mature effector CTL within the Peyer's patch. Rather, primed T cells appear to migrate from the Peyer's patch to other intestinal lymphoid compartments where they mediate their effector function. T cells predominate in Peyer's patches at birth (65 to 80 per cent T cells). In contrast, B cells predominate in the Peyer's patches of adults.[25]

In summary, Peyer's patches hold the key to the expression of the mucosal immune response and are an important source of B and T cells that ultimately populate other regions of the gut mucosa. Studies to develop more effective oral immunization protocols will require an in-depth understanding of the contribution of Peyer's patches to the generation of mucosal immunity.

Lamina Propria Lymphoid Cells

B lymphocytes and plasma cells, T lymphocytes, macrophages, eosinophils, and mast cells are scattered throughout the connective tissue of the lamina propria (Fig. 6–6). Seventy to 90 per cent of B lymphocytes and plasma cells in the lamina propria stain for IgA by immunofluorescence or immunoperoxidase techniques, whereas 15 to 20 per cent produce IgM and approximately 2 per cent produce IgE.[25] The striking lack of IgG-producing cells in the normal lamina propria contrasts markedly with the situation in extraintestinal sites like the peripheral lymph nodes and spleen, which are rich in IgG-producing cells.

Approximately 25 to 40 per cent of lymphocytes in the lamina propria are T cells. The majority of these T cells have the CD4 marker and other markers characteristic of T helper/inducer cells (i.e., class II restricted T cells).[41, 42] These T cells are presumed to be important in the activation, growth, and differentiation of B cells in the lamina propria. A small population of lamina propria T cells have CD8 and additional markers (e.g., 9.3) that are associated usually with class I restricted cytotoxic T lymphocytes.[42] However, few CD8 T cells with markers generally associated with suppressor T cells (e.g., CD11) are found in the lamina propria.

The lamina propria also contains macrophages, mast cells, and eosinophils. The macrophages are presumed to process and present antigen to T lymphocytes in the intestinal mucosa and to produce soluble factors (e.g., interleukin-1) that are important for T lymphocyte activation. Such macrophages likely play a role also in bacterial phagocytosis, as illustrated in diseases like Whipple's disease and disseminated *Mycobacterium avium intracellulare* infection in which lamina propria macrophages contain large quantities of bacteria in varying states of digestion.[43, 44] Mast cells are abundant in the lamina propria relative to other mucosal and nonmucosal sites, and can be identified readily in appropriately fixed tissue specimens.[45] In rodents, mast cells in the mucosa are heterogeneous, based on biochemical and functional studies. Currently, the degree of heterogeneity of lamina propria mast cells in humans is less clear. Mast cells can be stimulated to degranulate by immunologic and nonimmunologic stimuli. They release mediators that alter vascular permeability, muscle contraction, mucous production, and the recruitment of inflammatory cells. The degree to which such mast cell mediators contribute to diarrheal syndromes associated with idiopathic inflammatory disease and allergic disorders in the gut is an area of active study. Finally, eosinophils are abundant in the lamina propria. Although the role of eosinophils in the normal mucosa is not yet well defined, abnormalities associated with striking increases in such cells are seen in diseases like the eosinophilic enteritis syndromes as described on pages 1123 to 1131.

Lymphoid cells that do not belong to the T or B cells lineage also have been variably noted in the intestinal mucosa. Studies of natural killer cells which frequently appear as large granular lymphocytes bearing the Leu 7 and CD16 markers and lacking CD3, CD4, and CD8 have yielded varying results. Thus, based on phenotypic markers, different studies have noted either a paucity[46, 47] or significant numbers of such cells[48, 49] in the lamina propria of the small intestine.

Intraepithelial Lymphocytes

The lymphocytes located between the columnar epithelial cells that line the villous surface are termed intraepithelial lymphocytes (IEL). These cells lie between the enterocytes in close proximity to the base of the epithelial cells and the basement membrane. Normally, there is approximately one IEL per five to eight epithelial cells in adult small intestine and approximately one IEL per 20 epithelial cells in the colon[46, 50] (Fig. 6–7). IEL vary in morphology from typical small

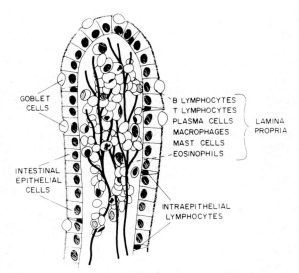

Figure 6–7. Schematic representation of an intestinal villus. B lymphocytes, T lymphocytes, plasma cells, macrophages, mast cells, and eosinophils are interspersed in the vascular and lymphatic-rich connective tissue of the lamina propria. Intraepithelial lymphocytes are situated near the basement membrane between intestinal epithelial cells. (From Kagnoff, M. F. *In* Johnson, L. R. [ed.]. Physiology of the Gastrointestinal Tract. New York, Raven Press, 1987. Used by permission.)

lymphocytes (20 per cent of IEL) to medium-sized or large lymphocytes (approximately 80 per cent of IEL).

Most human IEL appear to be T cells as characterized by phenotypic markers.[46, 47, 51, 52] The majority of such cells express Leu-1, a pan T cell marker, CD3, and/or CD2. Eighty to 90 per cent of IEL express CD8, whereas 10 to 20 per cent express CD4. This distribution contrasts strikingly with the T cell distribution in the lamina propria in which CD4-positive T cells predominate. B cells and plasma cells are not present in the IEL (< 1 per cent),[51, 52] and IEL rarely express antigens characteristic of natural killer cells (Leu-7, CD16).[46, 50, 51] There are apparent differences between IEL in humans and in mice. Approximately 80 to 90 per cent of murine IEL have the class I T cell–associated marker Lyt2 (i.e., analogous to CD8). However, in contrast to IEL in humans, a major fraction of these murine IEL do not have other known thymic markers.[53, 54]

Approximately 20 per cent of isolated IEL are medium to large lymphocytes that contain metachromatic granules, a feature that is characteristic also of NK cells, and some CTL in sites outside the gut. In rodents, IEL have been shown to mediate a broad array of cytotoxic activities including those characteristic of CTL, natural killer cells, spontaneous cytotoxic cells, and natural cytotoxic cells.[55] Further, culture studies of murine IEL have indicated a relationship between IEL that function as classic cytotoxic T lymphocytes and those with natural killer cell activity.[55-57] In contrast, human IEL have not been demonstrated, thus far, to mediate NK activity in cell culture assays or the broad array of cytotoxic functions that are mediated by murine IEL.[50, 51, 55, 58]

IEL can develop in the intestine independent of direct environmental antigen exposure.[59] Nonetheless, their numbers are increased considerably by the presence of food and bacterial antigens in the intestine. It has been suggested that once exposed to luminal antigens, IEL re-enter the lamina propria and recirculate in the host. However, there currently are insufficient data to prove or disprove this notion. Studies in mice suggest that a fraction of Peyer's patch T cells can migrate to the IEL region.[60]

IEL are prominent in the small intestinal mucosa of patients with active celiac disease, tropical sprue, and *Giardia lamblia* infestation. They have been reported to be increased also in the small intestine, but not in the colon, of patients with the acquired immunodeficiency syndrome (AIDS).[47, 50, 61] Nonetheless, their role in the production of mucosal damage in these diseases, either via direct cytotoxic activity or by the release of mediators, has not been defined. However, morphologic studies suggest an interaction between IEL and the parasite *Microsporidium* in AIDS patients.[62] Recent studies have developed long-term cloned cell lines of IEL[56, 57] as well as monoclonal antibodies that recognize surface antigens on IEL in rodent systems.[63] Such approaches may lead to better understanding of the regulation of IEL and their role in immune defense and disease.

Other Intestinal Lymphoid Tissue

Isolated lymphoid follicles, sometimes containing germinal centers, are abundant in the intestinal mucosa. These lymphoid follicles have been postulated to have functions analogous to those of Peyer's patches.[64] In addition, the appendix contains large lymphoid follicles that structurally resemble Peyer's patches. Mesenteric lymph nodes (MLN) receive the lymphatic drainage from the small and large intestine. Although they share structural features with peripheral lymph nodes, immunochemical and cell migration studies indicate that MLN also are part of the mucosal immune system. For example, dividing MLN B cells express a high degree of commitment to the ultimate production of IgA.[65]

Migration of Intestinal Lymphocytes and the Common Mucosal Immune System

Lymphocytes migrate from Peyer's patches to the lamina propria and intraepithelial region of the small intestine. B cells in Peyer's patches are the precursors of the more mature B cells that produce IgA in the intestinal lamina propria.[66] T cells from Peyer's patches populate both the intestinal lamina propria and the intraepithelial region.[60] Thus, there is a close relationship between the different populations of intestinal lymphocytes that compose the GALT.

There also is a close relationship between gut lymphocyte populations and those in the lung, mammary gland, and female genital tract. The migration of lymphocytes between these sites appears to be selective. This has led to the notion of a common mucosal immune system that involves the lymphoid cells in those sites.[67] The migration of lymphocytes from the gut to other mucosal sites is important to host defense. For example, gut lymphocytes migrate to the breast mostly in the late stages of pregnancy and during lactation, and the antigen specificity of colostral IgA and IgA-producing B cells reflects the antigenic exposure that those B cells previously had in the gut.[68] This mechanism is important for the protection of the suckling newborn against enteric microorganisms.

The model of lymphocyte migration in Figure 6–8 is based on data from animal studies. After stimulation by antigen, B and T lymphocytes in Peyer's patches leave that site and migrate to the mesenteric lymph node, the superior mesenteric duct, and the thoracic duct before entering the systemic circulation and returning to the intestinal lamina propria and intraepithelial regions. A proportion of Peyer's patch B cells also localize in the bronchus-associated lymphoid tissue, the mammary glands, and the female genital tract.

The Secretory IgA Immune System

IgA is the major immunoglobulin in human intestinal secretions, whereas it constitutes only 10 to 15 per cent

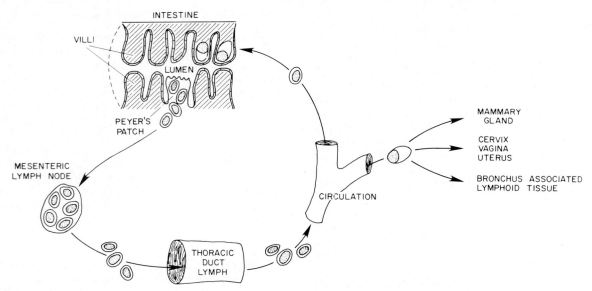

Figure 6–8. Migration pathway of Peyer's patch cells. Lymphocytes from Peyer's patches enter the mesenteric lymph node and thoracic duct lymph before entering the circulation. These cells then disseminate to the lamina propria of the intestine and to extraintestinal sites such as the bronchus-associated lymphoid tissue. Cells from the mesenteric lymph nodes can disseminate also to extraintestinal sites such as the mammary gland, female genital tract, or bronchus-associated lymphoid tissue. (From Kagnoff, M. F. *In* Johnson, L. R. [ed.]. Physiology of the Gastrointestinal Tract. New York, Raven Press, 1987. Used by permission.)

of serum immunoglobulin. Antibody responses at intestinal mucosal surfaces are mediated by IgA that is produced by plasma cells in the lamina propria and secreted into the intestinal lumen.[69, 70] The intestinal IgA system is fully developed by two years of age, whereas the quantity of IgA in serum gradually increases until puberty.

Most IgA in the intestinal secretions exists as secretory IgA (sIgA), a molecule that differs structurally from serum IgA[25] (Fig. 6–9). Whereas 85 to 90 per cent of human IgA is a monomer that is produced in the bone marrow and in other nonmucosal sites, sIgA is produced in the intestinal mucosa as a dimer and contains two additional polypeptide chains—secretory component (mol. wt. 70,000 daltons) and J chain (mol. wt. 15,000 daltons). Secretory component and J chain confer distinct structural and antigenic properties on the sIgA molecule. Only small amounts of sIgA normally are present in serum, but increased quantities can be found in patients with inflammatory disorders affecting the intestinal mucosa.

Secretory component (SC) is also known as the polyimmunoglobulin receptor. SC is a glycoprotein produced by intestinal epithelial cells and is present as an integral membrane protein on the basal and lateral membranes of those cells.[71] SC acts as the epithelial cell surface receptor for (IgA)$_2$J. After dimeric (IgA)$_2$J binds to SC, the (IgA)$_2$J-SC complex is endocytosed and transported across the intestinal epithelial cell to the apical plasma membrane. The membrane-anchoring domain of SC is proteolytically cleaved from this complex, and the (IgA)$_2$J dimer, covalently bound to the remainder of the SC molecule, is released into the intestinal secretions.[72] In addition to its transport function, SC appears to stabilize IgA in the intestine against degradation by proteolytic enzymes. SC also transports polymeric IgM into intestinal secretions—hence the term "polyimmunoglobulin receptor."

J chain is a polypeptide produced by plasma cells and is a component of the polymeric immunoglobulins (i.e., IgM, polymeric IgA). This molecule appears to govern the initiation and extent of immunoglobulin polymerization.[73] The size and structural differences between monomeric serum and polymeric secretory IgA require consideration when conducting and interpreting laboratory tests to quantify IgA levels in intestinal secretions.

There are two subclasses of IgA in humans: IgA1 and IgA2. These subclasses are coded for by different genes in the immunoglobulin heavy chain constant region, and have some differences in their primary amino acid structure.[74] A major difference involves a

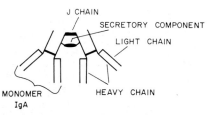

Figure 6–9. Schematic representation of a secretory IgA (sIgA) molecule. sIgA is a dimer that contains two monomer IgA subunits as well as two extra polypeptide chains, secretory component, and J chain. (From Kagnoff, M. F. *In* Johnson, L. R. [ed.]. Physiology of the Gastrointestinal Tract. New York, Raven Press, 1987. Used by permission.)

13 amino acid sequence that is present in the IgA1, but not in the IgA2 heavy chain. These molecules also differ in their carbohydrate composition, antigenic determinants (allotype markers), and susceptibility to microbial IgA proteases. For example, several pathogenic microorganisms produce IgA proteases with substrate specificity for IgA1, and these appear to correlate with bacterial pathogenicity.[75] Serum contains 80 to 90 per cent IgA1 and 10 to 20 per cent IgA2, whereas the intestinal mucosa contains approximately 50 per cent IgA2-producing cells.[76] The IgA2 subclass can be further categorized into two allelic forms on the basis of allotypic markers that reflect inherited amino acid substitutions between individuals in the IgA2 heavy chain; A2m(1) and A2m(2).[77] A2m(1) is more common in Caucasians and differs from A2m(2) at 6 amino acid positions. In IgA2 having the A2m(1) allotype, light chains are not joined to heavy chains by disulfide bonds.

IgA produced by intestinal lamina propria plasma cells is transported, mainly in the crypt area, into the intestinal lumen. As illustrated in Figure 6–9, dimer IgA (IgA1 or IgA2) containing J chain couples with SC on the surface of the epithelial cell membrane. The IgA–J chain–SC complex then is taken up and transported through the cell, and released into the intestinal lumen. As shown in Figure 6–10, dimer IgA also can enter the draining lymphatics, and, subsequently, the thoracic duct lymph and circulation.

· Human hepatic bile contains IgA, most of which is polymeric and contains SC.[78] Dimer IgA appears to be transported into human bile through the intrahepatic and extrahepatic biliary epithelium via a SC-dependent mechanism.[78] This mechanism may function to remove immune complexes that contain macromolecules bound to IgA from the circulation.[79, 80] Transport of IgA into bile is quantitatively more important in rodents than in humans, and in those species takes place mostly through hepatocytes, which, unlike human hepatocytes, have SC on their sinusoidal surface.[81]

IgA production is a terminal step in a differentiation process that begins with pre-B cells. Pre-B cells express IgM heavy chain in their cytoplasm, but have no detectable immunoglobulin on their surface. As pre-B cells mature, they begin to express cytoplasmic light chain. Later, complete IgM molecules and, subsequently, IgM and IgD molecules are expressed on the B cell surface. IgA develops still later in the differentiation of such B cells into antibody-forming cells. Production and secretion of the IgA class is highly dependent on helper function provided by class II restricted helper/inducer T cells, including lymphokines produced by those cells.[15, 31] For example, interleukin 5 in mice is now known to be a key IgA enhancing factor.[81a]

The accumulation and subsequent expansion in the lamina propria of B cells destined to produce IgA involves mechanisms that are independent as well as those that are dependent on antigen stimulation. Antigen stimulation is not required for the entry of B lymphocytes into the lamina propria. Antigen stimulation does, however, significantly influence the location, magnitude, and persistence of the mucosal IgA response.[82] For example, in experimental systems, IgA

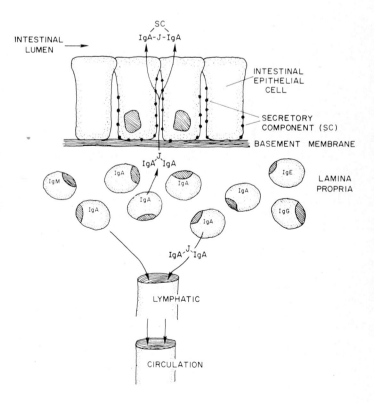

Figure 6–10. Transport of IgA into intestinal secretions. Dimer IgA containing J chain is secreted by plasma cells in the lamina propria. This molecule may couple with secretory component (SC) on the basal or lateral surface of the epithelial cell. The sIgA molecule then is transported through the cell and into the intestinal lumen. As indicated, IgA produced in the lamina propria also can enter the draining lymphatics and circulation before being provided to distant secretions. In addition, cells producing IgA can disseminate to extraintestinal secretory sites such as the mammary gland and bronchus-associated lymphoid tissue. (Adapted from Kagnoff, M. F. *In* Johnson, L. R. [ed.]. Physiology of the Gastrointestinal Tract. New York, Raven Press, 1987. Used by permission.)

antibody against a stimulating antigen is confined largely to the area of the intestine stimulated by that antigen.

The biologic activities of sIgA differ substantially from those of other immunoglobulin classes and reflect, in large measure, the antigen-binding properties of sIgA. sIgA can bind dietary antigens in the intestine and limit their absorption.[83] As discussed later, many IgA deficient individuals have increased titers of serum antibodies against food antigens. Further, sIgA binds bacteria (e.g., *Escherichia coli* and *Vibrio cholerae*) and prevents their adherence to and colonization of intestinal epithelial cell surfaces.[84] Studies with cholera toxin and human polio vaccine have shown that sIgA can neutralize bacterial toxins and can limit the replication and mucosal penetration of viruses.[85] Serum antibody is recognized to prevent viral dissemination from the mucosa. On the other hand, the presence of serum antiviral antibody with a concurrent lack of mucosal antiviral antibody might favor the development of a viral carrier state in the gut.

IgA does not participate in several inflammatory responses or reactions that are initiated by interactions between the Fc region of other immunoglobulin classes and lymphoid cells or components of the complement system. Thus, unlike IgM or IgG, IgA does not lead to complete activation of the complement cascade, does not significantly participate in antibody-dependent cell-mediated cytotoxic reactions, and is not an opsonizing antibody.[25, 86] Since the intestinal mucosa is continually exposed to a broad array of antigenic material with the potential for activating mucosal inflammatory reactions, it seems logical that IgA, an isotype that normally does not participate in inflammatory responses, would predominate in that site.

Other Antibody Classes and Subclasses

IgM is produced in the intestinal mucosa by lamina propria plasma cells and is transported across epithelial cells and into intestinal secretions bound to SC.[87] In addition, a small portion of the IgM in intestinal secretions may derive from serum. The concentration of IgM in intestinal secretions is 20-fold lower than that of IgA. IgM can activate the complement system. However, unique functions for secreted IgM have not been described. In patients with selective IgA deficiency, there often is an increase in intestinal lamina propria IgM-producing plasma cells. In these patients, IgM may compensate functionally for the lack of IgA.[88]

IgE is the crucial antibody class involved in allergic disorders. IgE binds to specific receptors on mast cells. When IgE on the mast cell surface is cross-linked by antigen, mast cells release biologically active products and allergic-type reactions ensue. The intestinal mucosa, relative to other lymphoid sites, is rich in IgE-producing cells and mast cells.[25] The prevalence of such cells in the gut suggests that IgE responses likely are important in intestinal inflammatory responses and immediate-type hypersensitivity reactions. Sensitiza-

tion by the intestinal route also may be a key factor in the development of a variety of host-systemic allergic disorders. In addition, IgE in the gut has a recognized role in helminth infections. Local IgE responses need not be accompanied by elevated serum IgE levels. Nonetheless, much remains to be learned about mucosal and mesenteric lymph node IgE production and about the interactions between eosinophils, IgE-producing B cells, and mast cells in the gut.

The lack of IgG-producing cells in the normal intestinal lamina propria is striking. IgG is the major immunoglobulin class produced in response to parenteral immunization, but generally is only a minor constituent of the intestinal immune response. Increases in IgG-producing cells are seen in the intestinal lamina propria in inflammatory diseases of the intestine, and IgG response may be important in the pathogenesis of such diseases. In this respect, most IgG subclasses fix complement and can participate in target cell damage by directing the specificity of antibody-dependent cell-mediated cytotoxic reactions. IgD antibodies function almost exclusively as membrane receptors for antigen.

INTESTINAL CELL-MEDIATED CYTOTOXIC RESPONSES

Lymphoid cells from GALT participate in cytotoxic responses that are important to host defense and under some circumstances may participate in the pathogenesis of disease. A number of different cell-mediated cytotoxic activities have been described based largely on morphologic and phenotypic characteristics of the "killer" cell, the type of target cell killed *in vitro,* the requirements for killer cell activation, and the mechanism of target cell recognition and damage.

Cytotoxic T cells (CTL) play a major role in host defense to many viruses, fungi and intracellular bacteria. Most CTL are class I restricted. CTL recognize and kill target cells having foreign antigens (e.g., viral antigens) on their surface in association with the host's self class I MHC determinants (i.e., HLA-A, -B, and -C molecules), or alternatively target cells having foreign (allogeneic) class I MHC molecules on their surface. Class II T cells also can function as CTL under some circumstances. In mice, it has been shown that CTL in the IEL population can be activated by antigen stimulation and that precursor CTL populations in Peyer's patches can be expanded by enteric stimulation with alloantigens or viral antigens[38, 40, 55–57] In addition to their role in defense against certain types of infectious agents, CTL appear to contribute to intestinal injury in graft-versus-host disease and perhaps also to mucosal damage in other intestinal diseases.

Natural killer (NK) cells also mediate cytotoxic reactions. NK cells are defined functionally by their ability to kill tumor cells (e.g., K562) in *in vitro* cytotoxicity assays, in the absence of stimulation by antigen. They are thought to be important in host tumor cell surveillance and perhaps also to mediate some regulatory functions. The activation and killing properties of NK cells are not MHC restricted.[89] In the periphery, NK cells often appear as large granular lymphocytes (LGL) that contain azurophilic cytoplasmic granules. They carry variable arrays of phenotypic markers including DC16, Leu-7, HNK1, and NKH1 (Leu-19).[90] The human intestine appears to have relatively few NK cells as assessed in functional assays,[51, 58] although lymphocytess bearing markers often associated with NK cells (i.e., NKH1, Leu-7) have been detected in mucosal lymphocyte populations in some studies.[46, 47, 49, 58, 91]

K cells kill target cells that are coated with antibody directed to intrinsic target cell surface antigens or extrinsic antigens associated with the target cell surface. Their mechanism of killing is termed antibody-dependent cell-mediated cytotoxicity (ADCC). The killer cell (K cell) appears to be a normal lymphocyte that has Fc receptors for IgG (CD16) but lacks other known T and B cell markers, although some K cells also have CD3.[92] Antibody of the IgG class is usually required for killing, although in some experimental systems, IgM or IgA has been reported to mediate low-level ADCC reactions. ADCC assay systems have been used as a readout system to assess the cytotoxic properties of serum factors and lyymphocytes in inflammatory bowel disease (IBD). ADCC assays have been used also as a readout in attempts to identify IBD specific antigens.[93, 94] Of note, granulocytes and macrophages also can kill target cells by an ADCC mechanism. Whether or not the human intestinal mucosa contains K cells capable of mediating ADCC reactions has been disputed.[58, 95, 96]

The intestinal lamina propria appears to contain lymphocytes that can be activated to be cytotoxic and kill tumor cells following incubation with the lymphokine IL-2.[97] Whether or not these mucosal lymphocytes are the same as the populations of "lymphokine activated killer cells" (LAK cells) obtained from peripheral blood is not known.[98] Understanding the function and regulation of mucosal cytotoxic cell types in normal host defense and in inflammatory diseases of the bowel will be of considerable importance.

Genetic Control and Regulation of the Immune Response

Studies in genetics and molecular immunology have provided new insights into how immune responses are

regulated and the structural basis of immune response genes. Genetically determined abnormalities in the regulation of the immune response can contribute to the development of human disease. MHC (HLA) genes code for the class I and II gene products that ultimately govern T cell recognition of antigen, antigen presentation, and interactions between lymphoid cell subsets.

HLA is located on the short arm of chromosome 6 and contains three major gene families: the class I, II, and III genes[5] (Fig. 6–11). Class I and class II genes code for cell surface proteins, whereas class III genes code for complement components. Proteins coded for by class I genes are present on the surface of all nucleated cells. There are three polymorphic class I loci in humans; HLA-A, -B, and -C (Fig. 6–11). Class I HLA genes code for a polymorphic 45,000-dalton class I heavy chain that is noncovalently associated on the cell surface with beta-2 microglobulin, a nonpolymorphic 12,000-dalton protein (Fig. 6–12). Cytotoxic and suppressor T lymphocytes recognize foreign antigens in conjunction with class I molecules (HLA-A, -B, or -C molecules) on the cell surface. Such interactions are said to be class I restricted.[10, 11]

Class II genes are located in the HLA-D region, which contains subregions termed -DP, -DQ, and -DR (Fig. 6–11).[99] Genes in this region commonly are referred to as immune response genes because the class II molecules they code for mediate immune response gene function.[100] Class II molecules are found on the surface of B lymphocytes, macropohages, dendritic reticular cells, and activated T lymphoycytes. Class II DR molecules have been detected also on intestinal epithelial cells[23, 101] and several other cell types. Further, the T cell lymphokine gamma-interferon can increase the expression of certain class II molecules on some of those cell types.[46]

Class II molecules exist on the cell surface as heterodimers, each containing an alpha chain of approximately 34,000 daltons and a beta chain of approximately 29,000 daltons (Fig. 6–12). The T cell receptor for antigen on CD4 T cells (i.e., mainly helper/inducer T cells) recognizes antigen in conjunction with class II molecules (Fig. 6–12). Such interactions are said to be class II restricted.

Polymorphism is an important characteristic of class I and class II MHC genes and their gene products. Thus, serologic testing in humans has revealed more than 47 allelic specificities at the HLA-B locus and at least 14 allelic specificities at the HLA-DR locus, 3 at HLA-DQ, and 6 at HLA-DP.[5]

Figure 6–11. Schematic map of the HLA region on the short arm of human chromosome 6. Genes mapping to the HLA-DP, -DQ, and -DR region code for the HLA class II molecules on B cells, macrophages, other antigen presenting cells, and activated T cells. Genes mapping to the HLA-B, -C, and -A locus code for the HLA class I molecules present on all nucleated cells. Class III genes code for components of the complement system. The two genes encoding steroid 21-hydroxylase are closely linked to the genes encoding C4A and C4B.

MAP OF THE HLA REGION

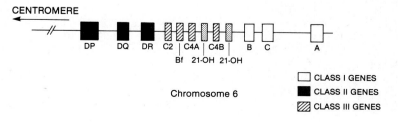

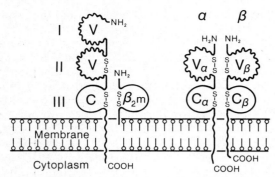

Figure 6–12. Schematic figure of human MHC (HLA) class I and II molecules. Class I molecules consist of a polymorphic heavy chain with three domains that is noncovalently associated on the cell surface with the nonpolymorphic 2 microglobulin (β2m). Class II molecules exist on the cell surface as heterodimers each containing an alpha and a beta chain. Class I and II molecules have variable (V) and constant (C) domains as indicated. Domain structure is maintained by intrachain disulfide (S—S) bonds.

Expression of class II HLA-DR molecules on colon epithelial cells in humans has been observed in association with active inflammatory disease of the colon, and increased expression of class II HLA-DR has been noted on small intestinal epithelial cells in celiac disease.[46, 102] Such molecules are expressed on the basolateral membrane and in the apical part of the cytoplasm of the enterocyte. They do not appear on the microvilli or the enterocyte surface in direct contact with the gut lumen. It may be that class II molecules on intestinal epithelial cells play a role in antigen presentation within the intestinal mucosa.

HLA class II genes code for complement components (i.e., C2, C4A, C4B, Bf). The currently proposed gene order of the HLA complex on chromosome 6 is depicted in Figure 6–11.

Susceptibilty to more than 40 diseases has been variably associated with particular HLA-A, -B, or -D region serologic markers. For example, susceptibility to rheumatic diseases in which sacroiliitis and spondylitis are prominent features, to reactive arthritis, and to Reiter's syndrome is associated with HLA-B27. A majority of patients with inflammatory bowel disease accompanied by sacroiliitis have the HLA-B27 antigen.[103] Celiac disease and chronic active hepatitis[104, 105] are among the best examples of diseases associated with HLA-D region markers, and in particular with specific serologic markers of the HLA-DR and -DQ subregions. Nonetheless, these diseases develop in only a minority of persons having those serologic markers. Further, not all persons with those diseases have the serologically defined "HLA susceptibility" marker. This suggests that, in addition to putative immune response genes in the HLA region, other environmental or genetic factors may be required in the pathogenesis of those diseases. Using direct biochemical analysis of class II HLA molecules and methods in molecular biology, it is now clear that many individuals that appear to have the same HLA class II molecules by serologic tests, in fact, differ at the genetic and protein level. Such methods have, in some cases, identified

even more striking associations between specific HLA class II genes and molecules and disease.[106, 106a]

Stimulation and Suppression of the Mucosal Immune Response

A mucosal antibody response to enteric antigens may occur in the absence of a detectable systemic antibody respose, or may be accompanied by a systemic immune response.[25] Further, routes of immunization markedly influence the isotype of immunoglobulin that is produced. Induction of the local secretory IgA immune response depends upon many factors, including the chemical nature of the antigen and the dose and frequencey of antigen exposure. Most enterically administered proteins are not effective at stimulating a local mucosal IgA response. In contrast, antigens that persist in the intestinal tract and antigens that selectively bind to the mucosal surface (e.g., cholera toxin) are particularly effective in stimulating mucosal IgA responses.[25]

Compartmentalization of the mucosal antibody response has been well demonstrated in immunization studies with polio virus in humans having "double-barreled" colostomies. Application of virus to the distal colostomy segment stimulated the production of IgA antibody confined largely to the distal colostomy segment. When poliovirus was given orally after reanastomosis of the distal and proximal colonic segments, viral replication was inhibited in the distal immunized segment, but not in the proximal nonimmunized segment.[107]

In rodents, studies suggest taht parenteral immunization can suppress the subsequent production of an enterically stimulated mucosal immune response.[108] However, the effect of prior parenteral immunization on the subsequent abilty to stimulate mucosal IgA resposes in humans is not well understood. This may be of some importance since parenteral vaccines are used in immunization programs to prevent enteric infections. Hypothetically it is possible that transient mucosal protection due to a high level of serum antibody after parenteral immunization may be followed by suppression of the mucosal immune response, and perhaps an intestinal carrier state when serum antibody levels decline.

Suppression and Stimulation of Systemic Immune Responses by Enteric Antigens

"Oral tolerance" has followed enteric immunization with several different types of antigens including soluble proteins, particulate antigens, reactive chemicals, bacteria, and inactivated viruses.[109-114] It has been studied mostly in animals, and is characterized by a diminished or absent immune response when the antigen-fed host is challenged parenterally with the same antigen used for feeding. The impaired ability to stimulate systemic IgM, IgG, IgA, and IgE antibody responses and delayed-type hypersensitivity reactions[115, 116] after antigen feeding can last for several months after intestinal antigen exposure is stopped. The decreased systemic immune response is highly specific for the enterically administered antigen. Oral tolerance has been shown to be mediated by suppressor T cells, antibody (possibly including anti-idiotypic antibody), and/or antigen-antibody complexes.[109, 117] Conversely, enteric immunization also can result in the priming and stimulation of immune responses in extraintestinal sites.[109] In addition to the nature of the stimulatory antigen, several other factors influence whether or not oral tolerance or systemic priming follows enteric antigen exposure. These include the age and genetic background of the immunized host, prior antigen exposure history, and the nature of the intestinal microflora.

Antigens in the intestine can, under some circumstances, activate a dual process characterized by the production of an IgA mucosal antibody response and the concurrent suppression of sytemic immune responses (i.e., oral tolerance) to the same antigen in animal models.[112, 117] The former mechanism appears to limit antigen absorption. The latter mechanism seems advantageous to the host since small quantities of otherwise harmless nonpathogenic antigens absorbed across the normal or inflamed intestine might stimulate systemic allergic reactions or cross-react with self components and lead to autoimmune responses.[109] The regulatory mechanisms that permit coexistence of mucosal immunity and concurrent decreased systemic immunity to the same antigen are currently being studied.[118] In contrast to nonreplicating, noninvasive microorganisms and protein antigens, invasive pathogenic viruses, bacteria, and certain bacterial products in the gut do not result in oral tolerance. Instead such antigens activate pathways that result in the production of protective systemic immune responses. This likely reflects the direct invasion by these organisms through the bastrointestinal tract and/or their site of interaction with the GALT.

IMMUNODEFICIENCIES

Selective IgA Deficiency and IgA-Associated Disorders

Selective IgA deficiency is one of the most common forms of immunodeficiency. As assessed by blood donor screening, it occurs with a prevalence of approximately 1 in 700 in the general population.[119] Patients with selective IgA deficiency have low levels of serum IgA (less than 5 mg/dl) accompanied by normal to increased concentrations of other serum immunoglobulins and normal cell-mediated immunity.[88] The majority have low levels of secretory IgA at intestinal and other mucosal surfaces. However, individuals with low levels of serum IgA and normal levels of secretory IgA, or normal levels of serum IgA but low levels of secretory IgA[120] can be encountered.

The etiology of selective IgA deficiency is unknown in most cases. However, its increased occurrence in family members of index cases suggests that genetic factors play a role. Studies have reported an association between IgA deficiency and HLA haplotypes, and indicated that a gene in the C4 or 21-hydroxylase locus may affect IgA production.[121] Rarely, IgA deficiency is the result of a deletion of IgA genes.[122] The number of B cells with cell-surface IgA can be normal or, less often, decreased. The majority of patients have a primary defect in the maturation of B cells that involves the terminal differentiation of IgA B cells into IgA plasma cells. However, as many as one fifth of patients with this disorder appear to have a defect in immune regulation wherein suppressor T cells selectively inhibit IgA production.[123] Selective IgA deficiency should be differentiated from IgA deficiency secondary to the administration of drugs (e.g., sulfasalazine, gold salts, D-pencillamine, phenytoin, and fenclofenac).[124–128]

The clinical picture in selective IgA deficiency is quite variable. Thus, some individuals may reach the sixth or seventh decade without symptoms. Others experience chronic or recurrent sinopulmonary infections, autoimmune disorders, collagen vascular disease, or allergic disorders.

Gastrointestinal disease is not prominent in most patients. This may be because the IgA deficiency can be compensated for by increased numbers of IgM-producing cells in the gut. Further, the IgA deficiency tends to affect the IgA1 more than the IgA2 subclass. Since IgA2 is more prevalaent in the gastrointestinal tract than in serum,[129] the production of small amounts of IgA2 in the gut may play a protective role in patients with IgA deficiency. Infections, when they occur, tend to be sinopulmonary. *Giardia lamblia* infestations and intestinal lymphoid nodular hyperplasia are not common; these diseases are far more striking in the common variable immunodeficiency syndromes, discussed later, than in selective IgA deficiency.

IgA deficiency has been reported in association with several intestinal diseases. For example, 2 per cent of celiac disease patients have IgA deficiency, an approximately tenfold increase over that expected in the general population.[130] However, no cause-and-effect relationship has been established, and such patients respond to treatment with a gluten-free diet. Except for an increase in lamina propria IgM plasma cells, the intestinal biopsy is similar to that seen in others with celiac disease. One patient with malabsorption, villous atrophy, and IgA deficiency was reported to have serum IgG antibody reactive with intestinal epithelial cells and responded to treatment with cyclophosphamide.[131] Patients with both Crohn's disease and selective IgA deficiency have been reported,[132] and anti-IgA antibodies may be present in more than 80 per cent of these individuals.[133] Finally, a patient with secretory component deficiency, mucocutaneous candidiasis, and severe malabsorption has been described. This patient's serum IgA level was normal, but, as would be expected, IgA was absent from the intestinal secretions.[119]

Autoimmune and connective tissue disease (e.g., rheumatoid arthritis, systemic lupus erythematosus, thyroiditis, pernicious anemia, dermatomyositis, Sjögren's syndrome, chronic active hepatitis), autoantibodies in the absence of apparent disease, allergic disorders, and malignancy are reported to be increased in the population with selective IgA deficiency.[134] Such individuals often have circulating antibodies to food proteins (more than one third have antibody to cow's milk proteins) and circulating immune complexes.[135] This suggests that local IgA responses normally limit the absorption of antigenic material from the gut or that there is an abnormality in immunoregulation in patients with selective IgA deficiency. It can be postulated that antibodies to certain antigens absorbed from the intestinal tract might cross-react with host self components (i.e., autoantibodies). In some instances, such antibodies might result in autoimmune disease. Other antibodies could result in allergic disorders.

A group of patients having IgA deficiency and IgG2 and/or IgG4 deficiency with accompanying pulmonary infections has been described.[136, 137] This syndrome should be differentiated from selective IgA deficiency. IgG2 is important in the systemic immune response to bacterial polysaccharide antigens. Since IgG2 and IgG4 represent only a small portion of serum IgG, deficiencies in these minor IgG subclasses may not be detected by standard measurements of total serum IgG. Further, IgA deficiency may be accompanied by IgE deficiency.[138] In those cases, IgA deficiency may reflect a more generalized abnormality in B cell differentiation. Finally, 70 per cent or more of patients with ataxia telangiectasia, an autosomal recessive disease characterized by telangiectasia, progressive ataxia, and sinopulmonary infections beginning in childhood, exhibit IgA deficiency. Frequently, these individuals also have accompanying low levels of IgE and abnormalities in cell-mediated immunity.

Evaluation of the symptomatic IgA deficient patient should include assessment of the possible coexistence of other immunoglobulin class or subclass defects, determination of IgA in secretions, assessment for the presence or absence of secretory component, studies of B and T cell function, and quantitative determination of the patient's ability to develop an antibody response to protein and polysaccharide antigens.[88]

There is no specific treatment for IgA deficiency. Diseases associated with this disorder are treated as they are in non-IgA-deficient individuals. Prophylaxis or routine treatment with immune serum globulin is not advised, as approximately 25 to 40 per cent of such patients have IgG anti-IgA antibodies and severe anaphylactic reactions can occur.[133, 139] Such antibodies can be directed to subclass-specific or allotype-specific antigens on IgA.[133] When blood products must be administered, the risk of severe transfusion reactions can be diminished by the use of autologous blood, frozen-thawed-washed cells, or IgA-deficient products.[140, 141] Patients with concomitant IgG defects are candidates for gamma globulin replacement therapy.

It is of note that IgA derived from the intestinal mucosa has been postulated to play a role in several diseases. In Berger's disease (IgA mesangial nephropathy), Henoch-Schönlein purpura, and alcoholic cirrhosis, elevated serum polymeric IgA and IgA immune complexes, often containing C3, have been reported.[142–144] Various studies indicate that both IgA1 and IgA2 are present in the immune complexes, which suggests a possible derivation from the gut mucosa, or alternatively that the complexes have predominantly IgA1, which suggests a nonmucosal origin.[145, 146] High-molecular-weight rheumatoid factor with anti-IgG activity has been noted in the serum of Berger's disease patients,[144, 147] and it has been proposed that these individuals have an underlying abnormaltiy in T cell regulation of the IgA response.[148] Patients with IgA nephropathy may have circulating IgA anti-basement membrane antibodies that react with determinants on collagen. These patients also may have elevated serum antibody titers to respiratory pathogens and dietary antigens.[150, 151]

Common Variable Immunodeficiency

The term common variable immunodeficiency (CVI) refers to a collection of immune deficiency disorders, and not a single disease. Patients with CVI have decreased serum immunoglobulins, impaired antibody responses, and, in some cases, abnormalities in T cell function. The onset of disease is after infancy, and most commonly in the second or third decade. Serum immunoglobulin levels vary, but IgG levels generally are less than 300 mg/dl and may be accompanied by diminished IgM and/or IgA levels.

CVI can be classified into B cell abnormalities that reflect various B cell maturation defects, or less frequently abnormalities in T cell regulation.[152–154] Some patients have very few circulating B cells, or pre-B cells that do not differentiate into early B cells. In others, the number of circulating B cells is normal but B cells may exhibit abnormalities in growth and differentiation. For example, B cells may not differentiate into plasma cells on stimulation with mitogens or antigens. In some, B cells can synthesize but do not secrete immunoglobulin. In others, B cells secrete IgM but little or no IgG and IgA. A subset of patients with CVI have normal B cells that do not function *in vivo* because of an abnormality in immunoregulatory T cells. These individuals may have a lack of sufficient T cell help for the B cell response or suppressor T cells that inhibit B cell function.[152, 154] The specific nature of these various defects is of interest because of the future possibility of using defined T cell products or pharmacologic reagents to influence B cell growth and differentiation. Plasma cells usually are absent or markedly deficient in peripheral lymphoid sites, including the intestinal lamina propria.

Chronic gastrointestinal disorders, often including diarrhea, occur in as many as 60 per cent of patients. Twenty to 30 per cent of patients have mild to moderate malabsorption, frequently associated also with small intestinal infestation with *Gardia lamblia*.[155] The enteropathy in CVI may be accompanied also by a deficiency in jejunal brush border enzymes.[156] Villous architecture can be normal or abnormal with partial villous atrophy. Treatment of *Giardia lamblia* infestation usually reverses the malabsorption and villous abnormalities. In patients whose malabsorption persists after therapy for giardiasis, improvement occasionally is noted in response to gluten withdrawal, treatment with corticosteroids, or gamma globulin therapy. In others, bacterial infection of the gut with pathogens like *Campylobacter* sp.[157] or more generalized bacterial overgrowth of the small intestine may contribute to the diarrhea and malabsorption, warranting a trial of antibiotics. In rare cases, persistent infection with other parasites (e.g., stronglyloidiasis) has been reported.[158]

Nodular lymphoid hyperplasia (NLH) of the small intestine, and occasionally of the stomach, colon, and rectum, can be detected by X-ray or biopsy in as many as 60 per cent of patients with CVI.[155] The finding of NLH does not correlate directly with the presence of diarrhea or malabsorption, and treatment of giardiasis in those with NLH does not eliminate the NLH. Germinal centers of the lymphoid nodules lack plasma cells, but have been reported to contain B lymphocytes with surface IgM.[159] The cause of the lymphoid nodules is not known, but they may result from chronic antigenic stimulation coupled with an abnormality in negative feedback regulation.

Achlorhydria is present in one third to one half of CVI patients.[155] In addition, a pernicious anemia-like syndrome with intrinsic factor deficiency, gastric atrophy, loss of parietal cells, and low serum levels of vitamin B_{12} may develop. Unlike classic pernicious anemia, this disease usually develops at an earlier age, the gastric mucosa lacks a plasma cell infiltrate, and there is no increase in antibodies to parietal cells or intrinsic factor. Patients with adult onset CVI also appear to be at increased risk to develop gastric carcinoma[160] and carcinoma or lymphoma of the small intestine and/or colon.[161]

Other gastrointestinal disorders reported in CVI include an increased occurrence of cholelithiasis and disorders of both exocrine and endocrine pancreatic function.[155] Crohn's disease, ulcerative colitis, and ulcerative proctitis with a variable response to steroids have been noted also in CVI patients. Autoimmune disorders, including chronic active hepatitis,[162] may dominate the clinical course. Autoantibodies are more frequent than in the normal population. In addition, there may be a family history of immunologic aberrations including thyroid and gastric parietal cell autoantibodies, autoimmune hemolytic anemia, and thrombocytopenia.

The major treatment modality in CVI is parenteral gamma globulin therapy, although adverse reactions to IgA in such preparations may occur.[163–165] In some patients, steroids have partially reversed the immunoglobulin abnormalities.[166] In certain cases cimetidine has been reported to decrease suppressor cell activity and allow endogenous immunoglobulin production.[167] With greater understanding of B cell growth and dif-ferentiation, some individuals with CVI may be treatable ultimately with defined B cell growth and/or differentiation factors.[168]

Infantile and Childhood Immunodeficiency Syndromes

Several immunodeficiency disorders in infants and children that affect B cells, T cells, or other mononuclear cell types can be associated with gastrointestinal manifestations.

X-Linked Infantile Agammaglobulinemia (Bruton's Type)

This B cell disease affects antibody production in males. It becomes apparent with the decline of maternally acquired immunoglobulin around six months of age. All classes of immunoglobulin are virtually absent and circulating B cells are lacking, although pre-B cells are present. There is an inability to make antibody after stimulation with antigen, and the gut lamina propria and other lymphoid sites lack plasma cells. T cells are normal in number and function. Recurrent pyogenic infections pose a major problem. Intestinal manifestations occur less often than in common variable immunodeficiency. Malabsorption associated frequently with *Giardia lamblia* infestation can be seen, and chronic diarrhea with persistent rotavirus[169] has been reported. Recommended treatment is with parenteral gamma globulin.

Thymic Hypoplasia (DiGeorge's Syndrome)

T cells have a direct role in the elimination of viral and fungal infections and an indirect role in the control of bacterial infections. Severe defects in T cell function predictably result in increased susceptibility to viral, fungal, protozoal, and bacterial infections.

Thymic hypoplasia results from a failure of formation of the third and fourth pharyngeal pouches with consequent absence or hypoplasia of the thymus and parathyroid glands.[170] The T cell deficiency can be partial or complete. Gastrointestinal manifestations are usually limited to diarrhea, malabsorption, and chronic *Candida albicans* infection. Some patients have esophageal atresia.

Combined Immunodeficiency Diseases

Severe combined immunodeficiency (SCID) is inherited in either an X-linked or autosomal recessive mode. One half of patients exhibiting the autosomal recessive mode of inheritance have adenosine deaminase deficiency.[171] The clinical syndrome in infants is characterized by a lack of T and B cell immunity, and consequent viral, fungal, protozoal, and bacterial infections. Individuals with SCID can have serious gastrointestinal manifestations. Chronic diarrhea, malabsorption, and *Candida albicans* infection are common.

On proctoscopy, the rectal mucosa may be edematous and friable. Crypt abscesses are noted on biopsy. The intestinal lamina propria is depleted of lymphocytes and plasma cells, the villi are blunted, and large vacuolated macrophages can be seen. Unless treated successfully, children with SCID often die within the first few years of life from bacterial, viral, and fungal infections. In those treated with bone marrow transplants, graft-versus-host disease may develop.

Combined B and T cell defects also occur in the Wiskott-Aldrich syndrome, an X-linked recessive immunodeficiency. This disease is characterized by eczema, thrombocytopenia, and recurrent infections. Defects in the membrane glycoproteins of both T cells and platelets have been demonstrated. Melena and hematemesis may result in severe blood loss. An inability to form antibody to polysaccharide antigens and an immunoglobulin pattern showing a low IgM but a high IgA and IgE are characteristic. Wiskott-Aldrich syndrome can be successfully treated by bone marrow transplantation.[172]

Chronic Granulomatous Disease of Childhood

Chronic granulomatous disease of childhood occurs predominantly in males and may have an X-linked inheritance pattern. Patients have a defect in the ability of polymorphonuclear leukocytes and monocytes to kill catalase-positive microorganisms following phagocytosis, secondary to a presumed enzyme deficiency. However, T and B cell function is normal. Ulcerative stomatitis and partial or complete gastric outlet obstruction secondary to antral deformity can be seen. A colonic disease resembling Crohn's disease as well as rectal fistula and perianal abscesses also can be part of the clinical picture. The bowel wall may be thickened and contain granulomas.[173] Other intestinal manifestations include diarrhea, steatorrhea, and vitamin B_{12} malabsorption. Rectal biopsies and biopsies of the lamina propria may reveal characteristic lipid-filled pigmented histiocytes, giant cells, and granulomas. The Crohn's disease–like picture may show an initial response to treatment with corticosteroids.[173]

Protein-Losing Enteropathy and Immunodeficiency

Protein-losing enteropathies are associated with the gastrointestinal loss of serum proteins, including albumin and immunoglobulins. Extensive immunoglobulin loss can result in hypogammaglobulinemia that affects all antibody classes. Cell-mediated immune defects can occur in patients whose protein loss also is accompanied by the intestinal loss of lymphocytes and lymphocytopenia. Extensive protein loss with or without low lymphocyte counts can be seen in congenital or acquired intestinal lymphangiectasia, constrictive pericarditis, Whipple's disease, regional enteritis, alpha heavy chain disease, and acute graft-versus-host disease.

Gastrointestinal immunoglobulin losses may also occur in patients with celiac sprue, ulcerative colitis, Menetrier's disease (giant hypertrophy of the gastric mucosa), and allergic gastroenteropathy. In these patients, immunoglobulin synthesis is normal or increased, antibody responses to exogenous antigens usually are normal, and increased susceptibility to infection is not common. Prognosis and treatment of this disorder depends on the underlying disease.

Iatrogenic Immunodeficiency Syndromes

The host that is immunocompromised by chemotherapy or radiation therapy (e.g., in preparation for bone marrow transplant) is susceptible to bacterial, viral, parasitic, and fungal infections. Such immunosuppressed individuals may have severe lymphocyte depletion in Peyer's patches and lymph node tissues, depressed T cell function, and abnormally low immunoglobulin levels. Clinically, they may present with esophagitis secondary to *Candida albicans*, herpes simplex virus, or cytomegalovirus (CMV) infection. Gastric and duodenal infections with CMV and herpes simplex may also occur. If there is accompanying granulocytopenia, invasive infections with gram-negative bacteria can be seen. Such individuals may develop intestinal ulcerations with complicating septicemia, perforation, or bleeding. Individuals maintained on antibiotic therapy may develop pseudomembranous colitis due to *Clostridium difficile* toxin. CMV may cause deep ulcerating small intestine and colon lesions. Parasitic infections include infestation with *Giardia lamblia, Isospora belli,* and coccidial parasites such as *Cryptosporidium* sp. and *Microsporidium.* In the case of *Cryptosporidium,* successful elimination of the parasite depends on the reversibility of the immunodeficiency state. Finally, in severely immunosuppressed individuals, malignant B cell lymphoproliferative syndromes may develop and reflect Epstein-Barr virus infection. Such B cell proliferation sometimes may be reversible after withdrawal of immunosuppressive drugs or treatment with antivirals (e.g., acyclovir).

Acquired Immunodeficiency Syndrome

In the acquired immunodeficiency syndrome (AIDS), infections similar to those described in the iatrogenic immunodeficiency syndromes have been noted. The primary immune abnormality in AIDS is impaired function and depletion of class II restricted CD4-bearing T cells (ile., mostly helper/inducer T cells) that are infected, via the CD4 determinant, with the human immunodeficiency virus (HIV). Since CD4 T cells are a major immunoregulatory cell population in the induction of many B and T cell resposes, depletion of those T cells results in wide-ranging abnormalities of immune responses mediated by both T and B cells.

The abnormal representation of T lymphocyte subsets in the circulation of AIDS patients results in a reversal of the normal CD4/CD8 T cell ratio. A similar abnormality can be seen in the peripheral blood in homosexual men with the lymphadenopathy syndrome (LAS) and in some apparently healthy homosexual men.[49]

There is a significant decrease in T cells in the intestinal mucosa of male homosexual subjects with LAS and AIDS. This decrease most markedly affects CD4 T cells. Concurrently, the proportion of CD8 T cells in the intestinal mucosa of AIDS subjects (i.e., class I restricted T cells) is significantly increased.[49]

Differences in the distribution of T cell subsets in the circulation compared with the intestinal mucosa have been noted in healthy homosexual men.[49] Thus, reversed CD4/CD8 T cell ratios frequently noted in the peripheral blood of healthy homosexual men are not paralleled in the intestinal mucosa of the same individuals. In contrast, the CD4/CD8 T cell ratio is reversed in both the circulation and intestinal mucosa of AIDS and LAS subjects (Fig. 6–13). T cell abnormalities in the intestinal mucosa may render AIDS and LAS subjects more susceptible to opportunistic infections.

ALPHA HEAVY CHAIN DISEASE AND INTESTINAL LYMPHOMA

Alpha heavy chain disease is characterized by plasma cell infiltration of the small intestinal lamina propria and malabsorption, which sometimes evolves to malignant lymphoma.[174, 175] The majority of patients are between the ages of 10 and 30. This disease was initially observed in the Mediterranean area and Middle East among populations exposed to poor hygiene, but now

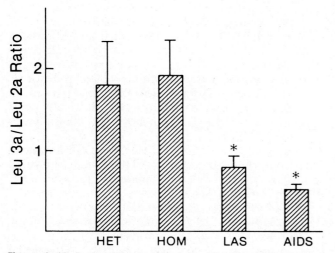

Figure 6–13. Ratio of T cells having the CD4 (Leu 3a) phenotype associated with helper/inducer T cells or the CD8 (Leu 2a) phenotype associated with suppressor/cytotoxic T cells in the intestinal mucosa of healthy heterosexual males (HET), healthy homosexual males (HOM), and males with lymphadenopathy syndrome (LAS) or AIDS. There is a reversal in the normal "helper/suppressor" T cell ratio in the intestinal mucosa of subjects with LAS or AIDS (p<0.05). (From Rodgers, V. D., Fassett, R., and Kagnoff, M. F. Gastroenterology 90:552–558, 1986. Used by permission.)

has been noted in other areas. Alpha chain disease appears to be an immunoproliferative B cell disorder of the secretory IgA system. It is the most common of the heavy chain disease. Fragments of incomplete IgA heavy chains, devoid of light chains, are found in the serum and/or secretions of these patients. Studies of alpha heavy chain disease protein have revealed a structural defect characterized by an internal deletion in the normal amino acid sequence of the alpha heavy chain. In intestinal fluids and urine, the alpha heavy chain disease protein may be associated with J chain and secretory component.

Alpha heavy chain disease usually involves primarily the small intestine and mesenteric lymph nodes, but disease limited to the stomach or involving the colon also has been reported.[176, 177] Early, there is diffuse infiltration of the small intestinal lamina propria, but not the submucosa, with mature plasma cells and, in some cases, small lymphocytes. The mesenteric lymph nodes are similarly infiltrated in the follicles, but nodal architecture is preserved. Alpha heavy chain protein can be detected in the serum or intestinal fluid. This early stage disease appears benign, although patients may experience malabsorption and weight loss. Clinically, there have been instances in which the disease, treated with antibiotics at this point, has remitted.[174, 178] Later, there is infiltration of the submucosa and muscularis propria with dysplastic and atypical plasma cells and immunoblasts, and obliteration of lymph node architecture. Late-stage disease is characterized by an immunoblastic malignant lymphoma. Cells at that stage do not secrete alpha heavy chain protein, but may have alpha chains incorporated into their plasma membrane. The large cells of the immunoblastic lymphoma appear to arise from the same B cell clone that gave rise to the initial plasma cell proliferation.[179] Detection of transition from a benign to a malignant stage can be achieved by ultrastructural studies of plasma cells in biopsy specimens.[180]

Clinically, patients often present with malabsorption, weight loss, and colicky abdominal pain. Protein-losing enteropathy, bacterial overgrowth, and parasitic infestation with *Giardia lamblia* are common. Elevated serum alkaline phosphatase reflects the intestinal isoenzyme. The small bowel is usually involved to a greater extent proximally than distally. Small bowel biopsy may reveal a patchy or a more generalized partial or total villous atrophy with intact surface epithelium. Oral antibiotics often result in improvement in the malabsorption, suggesting a contribution of the enteric bacterial flora and/or parasitic infestation to the malabsorption syndrome.

Diagnosis depends on athe laboratory detection of alpha heavy chain protein in the serum or intestinal fluid. In some cases this can be difficult. Serum protein electrophoresis patterns may exhibit an abnormal broad band extending from the alpha-2 to the gamma region in approximately 50 per cent of patients; however, in many cases the only electrophoretic abnormality may be a mild increase in alpha-2 globulin.[174] Immunoelectrophoretic analyses may reveal an abnormal protein component that reacts with monospecific antisera to IgA heavy chains but not to kappa or lambda light chains. Serum IgM and IgG levels are often low. Definite diagnosis can be made by demonstrating the lack of conformational IgA Fab determinants using highly selected precipitating antisera or, alternatively, by demonstrating the absence of light chain determinants using specialized sera to kappa and lambda chains or Fab alpha chain fragments combined with immunoelectrophoresis.[181, 182]

GRAFT-VERSUS-HOST DISEASE

In graft-versus-host disease (GVHD), donor lymphoid cells damage host tissue. This ocurs when there is (1) an immunodeficient host, (2) an immunocompetent graft, and (3) histoincompatibility between the graft and the host. Lymphocytes in the graft recognize the host as foreign. GVHD is seen most often after attempts to reconstitute the immune system of an immunodeficient patient with bone marrow, fetal liver, or thymus. However, infusion of blood components containing viable lymphocytes into an immunodeficient host can be sufficient to initiate GVHD. The major factor determining the severity of the GVHD is the degree of disparity in histocompatibility. GVHD occurs in cases of HLA-A, -B and -D region incompatibility, but HLA-D region disparity is the most important in determining the magnitude of the GVHD. Transfers between HLA-A and -B nonidentical, but HLA-D identical donors often result in milder disease. Diagnostic confirmation of GVHD can be obtained by demonstrating cell chimerism by sex chromosome analysis or HLA typing.

GVHD is classified as acute or chronic.[183, 184] In acute GVHD, any region of the intestinal tract can be affected, but disease is often most severe in the distal small intestine, cecum, and ascending colon.[183] Typically, acute disease occurs within two weeks to two months of the transfer of allogeneic (i.e., histoincompatible) lymphoid cells. Patients may experience large-volume watery diarrhea (i.e., up to 10 to 15 liters/day) and lower abdominal pain with or without upper gastrointestinal symptoms. Stool exam usually reveals fecal leukocytes, occult blood, and considerable cellular debris. Evidence of the presence of *Cryptosporidium* sp. should be sought.[185] When more severe bleeding is noted, it may result from accompanying herpes virus or fungal infections, causing esophagitis and gastric or duodenal erosions. Severe protein loss through the intestinal tract is common. Involvement of the stomach and proximal small intestine by GVHD or accompanying CMV infection may lead to symptoms of nausea, vomiting and upper abdominal pain.

Small intestinal X-rays in acute GVHD may reveal mucosal or submucosal edema, most common in the distal small intestine, whereas barium enema studies document mucosal ulceration and thickening of the colon wall. Such changes are not pathognomonic, however, as they occur also in CMV enteritis, which may accompany GVHD. Endoscopic findings vary from mild or patchy erythema to mucosal sluffing. Of note, the gastric and rectal mucosa can appear grossly normal despite extensive changes in the proximal colon and distal small intestine. Nonetheless, biopsy specimens from the stomach or rectum of these patients may reveal microscopic changes.[186]

The intestinal lesion in the small bowel in acute GVHD is characterized by villous atrophy and an inflammatory infiltrate of lymphocytes, plasma cells, and occasional eosinophils. Early findings on colonic biopsy simply may reveal necrosis of individual crypt epithelial cells and sparing of enterochromaffin cells.[187] Such lesions may progress to frank crypt necrosis, crypt abscess formation, and ultimately epithelial denudation. The early lesion may be caused by cytotoxic T lymphocyte–mediated crypt epithelial cell lysis.[183]

Other early manifestations of acute GVHD can include skin and liver disease.[183] A maculopapular rash may involve the trunk, palms, soles, and ears and can progress to become confluent and desquamative.[188] Liver disease varies from being subclinical, with abnormalities of a biochemical nature, to more severe. Hepatic involvement usually is manifested as cholestatic jaundice accompanied by a marked increase in serum alkaline phosphatase. Subsequently, hyperbilirubinemia, mild hepatomegaly, and clinical jaundice may ensue. The bile duct epithelium appears to be a major site of immune injury.[189] Like intestinal epithelium, bile duct epithelium in acute GVHD may express class II MHC antigens. Distinguishing between liver involvement secondary to GVHD and other causes of liver disease (e.g., acute or chronic hepatitis, primary biliary cirrhosis) often is difficult. In the clinical setting of GVHD, liver biopsies usually are not warranted. However, when looked for, histologic changes include abnormalities in the intralobular bile ducts, destruction of small bile ducts, and ductular proliferation.[190] Of note, some patients may experience mainly intestinal symptoms without skin or hepatic manifestations.

Chronic GVHD develops between 3 and 12 months after the receipt of allogeneic lymphoid cells, and affects as many as 30 per cent of long-term survivors of bone marrow transplantation.[184] Most individuals with chronic GVHD have previously experienced an acute reaction, although up to one third of individuals with chronic GVHD may not have had clinically apparent acute GVHD.

Intestinal symptoms in chronic GVHD differ markedly from those in acute GVHD. Small intestinal symptoms are not a major component of the syndrome, although some individuals develop fibrotic strictures of the small intestine after several months of acute GVHD. More than 10 per cent of patients with chronic GVHD have esophageal involvement.[191] Symptoms may include dysphagia, odynophagia, retrosternal pain, or mainly insidious weight loss. Pathologically, desquamation of the epithelium of the upper esophagus and midesophagus, upper esophageal webs, ringlike narrowings, and tapering strictures can be seen. Biopsy findings include infiltration of the esophageal mucosa with lymphocytes, neutrophils, and eosinophils, necrosis of individual squamous cells in the basal layer, and desquamation of the superficial epithelium. Submucosal fibrosis also can occur. Treatment of the esophageal manifestations includes symptomatic therapy and periodic dilatations as required for strictures and esophageal rings.

Chronic liver disease is seen in the vast majority of patients with chronic GVHD and usually parallels disease in other organ systems.[189, 192] Striking elevations of alkaline phosphatase are common, but hepatic failure, portal hypertension, and cirrhosis are unusual. Biopsy in patients with prolonged chronic GVHD may reveal reduced numbers or an absence of small bile ducts, cholestasis, and portal area plasma cell infiltrates.[193] Chronic GVHD affecting the liver must be differentiated from other liver disease (e.g., hepatitis B; non-A, non-B hepatitis; primary biliary cirrhosis; CMV hepatitis) and hepatotoxic reactions including cholestasis caused by drugs used in the treatment of chronic GVHD (e.g., azothioprine and cyclosporine).

Skin changes are a prominent component of chronic GVHD. Common changes include increased pigmentation, contractures, and a scleroderma-like syndrome. Polyserositis and ocular manifestations may also accompany chronic GVHD.

Prognosis following acute GVHD is variable. With sustained engraftment of donor cells, disease can be severe with a 10 to 30 per cent mortality. In general, treatment has included corticosteroids, cyclosporine, methotrexate, and antithymocyte globulin.[183, 184] Techniques that have been used in attempting to prevent acute GVHD after bone marrow transplantation include better patient selection for histocompatibility, the use of the immunosuppressive agents cyclosporine and methotrexate, the use of protected environments (e.g., laminar air flow rooms, oral nonabsorbable antibiotics, and sterile food), and the treatment of bone marrow *in vitro* to delete T cells prior to cell transfer.[194] Of note, the latter may decrease the incidence and severity of GVHD, but also can be associated with an increased prevalence of graft failure. Resolution of the liver disease of acute GVHD often takes weeks to months, and more than 50 per cent of patients with severe acute GVHD who become long-term survivors develop chronic liver involvement.[193] Attempts to treat chronic GVHD often are effective and include the use of corticosteroids and immunosuppressant drugs (e.g., cyclosporine) after transplantation.[195] Hepatic abnormalities in chronic GVHD may respond to treatment with immunosuppressive drugs.[184] Although treatment may need to be prolonged, a significant number of individuals remain free of chronic GVHD after immunosuppressive drugs are discontinued.[188, 195]

INFLAMMATORY BOWEL DISEASE

Evidence that immune mechanisms are important in the pathogenesis of tissue injury in inflammatory bowel disease (IBD) derives from the histologic and clinical features of these diseases, and from laboratory studies of humoral and cell-mediated immunity in IBD patients.[196] Increased numbers of mononuclear cells including lymphocytes, plasma cells, and/or mast cells often are seen in the intestine of these patients, and granulomas are a prominent feature of Crohn's disease. Clinically, IBD can occur in association with other diseases in which immune mechanisms play an important role (i.e., autoimmune hemolytic anemia, thrombocytopenic purpura). The current mainstay of therapy in IBD involves drugs that are known to alter the immune response such as corticosteroids, immunosuppressants, and sulfasalazine.[197, 198] Further, the extraintestinal manifestations of IBD (i.e., pericholangitis, chronic active hepatitis, erythema nodosum, pyoderma gangrenosum, ankylosing spondylitis, erythema multiforme) suggest that immune mechanisms may be important. Nonetheless, there currently is insufficient evidence to classify IBD as a primary immunologic disease.

Key questions regarding the role of the immune system in IBD remain unanswered. Currently, the exact relationship between ulcerative colitis and Crohn's disease is not known, and it is possible that each of these clinical entities encompasses more than a single disease in terms of etiology and pathogenesis. It is not known whether antibody or T cell–mediated immune responses are more important in disease pathogenesis. Further, the cells and cell-associated molecules that represent the major targets of immune injury in these diseases are not known. Immune responses leading to tissue injury in IBD might reflect a host response to exogenous antigens (e.g., bacteria, viruses). Alternatively, a specific or more generalized abnormality, acquired or inherited, in the regulation of humoral and/or cell-mediated immune responses, an autoimmune reaction directed against self or altered self components, or a combination of these or other mechanisms may be important in disease pathogenesis. Definition of the major genetic factors that play a role in IBD, including genetic factors that govern the induction and expression of immune responses, remain to be elucidated. It is not likely that unraveling the role of immune, genetic, and environmental factors in IBD will be a simple task. As outlined briefly below, substantial effort has gone into addressing these and other important questions in IBD.

Humoral Immune Responses

Many ulcerative colitis patients, but not healthy controls, have serum antibodies to cytoplasmic colon epithelial cell mucopolysaccharide determinants. Such antibody reacts with antigens extracted from sterile fetal and adult colon and is not directed to ABO blood group substances. Serum antibodies to *E. coli* 014 polysaccharide also are frequently seen in the serum of ulcerative colitis patients. Since the bacterial and colon antigens are serologically cross-reactive, bacterial antigens have been suspected of stimulating an "autoimmune" response. However, the presence of these serum antibodies does not correlate with the extent or severity of ulcerative colitis, and similiar antibodies can be found in Crohn's disease as well as in healthy relatives of IBD patients,[199] and occasionally in other gastrointestinal diseases. Consequently, such antibodies have been regarded as of little significance in the etiopathogenesis of IBD. However, closer examination of these antibodies in terms of their antigen specificities and their ability to mediate specific effector functions might yield new insights.[200]

Ulcerative colitis patients were noted to have a serum IgG antibody that specifically reacted with their colon tissue, but not with normal colon or other tested tissues.[201] The same group of investigators also described a correlation between the clinical activity of ulcerative colitis and the presence of a serum antibody that could kill a long-term cultured human colon cancer cell line by an antibody-dependent cell-mediated cytotoxic mechanism,[202] but the relationship to each other, if any, of these serum antibodies is not known. In different studies, this same group reported an IgG antibody bound to colon tissue in ulcerative colitis patients.[203] Further examination of the tissue-bound antibody indicated that it reacted with a 40,000 molecular weight protein present in either normal or diseased colon tissue but not in the other tissues tested (i.e., a possible colon-specific antigen).[204] However, recent data with a monoclonal antibody to the 40,000 molecular weight protein indicated it reacted also with determinants in skin and biliary epithelium. Additional studies variably have suggested that Crohn's disease tissue has several major proteins of > 100,000 kd that specifically react with serum from subjects with Crohn's disease.[205, 206] Currently, there is not sufficient evidence to conclude that such serum or tissue-bound antibodies or tissue antigens play a role in the etiopathogenesis of IBD.

An abnormality in the ability to stimulate antigen-specific antibody responses in Crohn's disease has been proposed. Thus, Crohn's disease patients were reported to have impaired IgG antibody responses to tetanus toxoid.[198, 207] On the other hand, increased serum antibody titers to milk proteins (i.e., casein, beta-lactoglobulin, and alpha-lactalbumin) and to bovine serum albumin often are found in IBD patients. The latter findings may reflect stimulation of the immune system by antigens that pass through an inflamed intestine, whereas the former may point to a more fundamental abnormality in the regulation of humoral antibody production.

Antibodies to synthetic double-stranded RNA in approximately one fourth of Crohn's disease patients and antibodies cytotoxic for T and B cells (i.e., lymphocytotoxic antibodies) in more than 40 per cent of IBD patients and their families[208] have been interpreted to suggest a role for viral infection in the pathogenesis of IBD. More recently, Crohn's disease patients also were reported to have serum antibody to Z-DNA.[209] Finally, sera from Crohn's disease patients and their first-degree relatives and spouses who were household members was shown to react with lymphoid tissues

from athymic (nude) mice that were injected previously with Crohn's disease tissue filtrates.[210–212] Those studies were interpreted to suggest that a common environmental factor may be important in the pathogenesis of Crohn's disease.[210–212]

An increase in IgG B cells has been noted in the colonic mucosa of patients with ulcerative colitis and in Crohn's disease. Variable increases in mucosal IgA- and IgM-producing cells also can be seen in ulcerative colitis. In contrast, the numbers of mucosal T cells and the distribution of mucosal T cell subsets in patients with Crohn's disease and ulcerative colitis has not differed from normal controls.[42, 213] Recent technical advances have enabled investigators to obtain lymphoid cells directly from the normal or diseased intestinal mucosa and to study these cells in tissue culture systems. In such studies, B cells from IBD patients spontaneously secreted less IgA than B cells from controls.[214] However, compared with controls, IBD B cells secreted more monomer IgA, and particularly IgA1. The mechanism responsible for this phenomenon and its importance in the pathogenesis of IBD is not yet known.

Cell-Mediated Immune Responses

Investigations of cell-mediated immune responses in IBD have led to a number of striking observations but, thus far, have not revealed a unifying picture. Measurements of the numbers of B and T cells in the circulation and the response of such cells to mitogenic stimuli frequently have yielded conflicting results, either for technical reasons or because different subpopulations of patients have been examined.[215, 216] It is assumed that immune reactions important in the pathogenesis of IBD likely are mediated by lymphoid cells localized at or near the site of disease in the intestine. For this reason, human small intestinal and colonic lymphoid populations from IBD patients have been isolated and studied.[217, 218] Investigations comparing normal and IBD patients have assessed the numbers of T cells and proportions of T cell subsets in the intestinal mucosa, the responses of those cells to mitogens, and the cytotoxic properties of such cells in *in vitro* assay systems.[42, 58, 95, 96, 213, 219, 220]

Peripheral blood lymphocytes (PBL) from most ulcerative colitis and Crohn's disease patients, but not from those with other diseases, were noted to be cytotoxic for isolated colonic epithelial cells. Cytotoxicity was specific for colon epithelial cells (i.e., it was not seen when cells from other tissues or epithelial cells from other gastrointestinal sites such as the small bowel were used as targets).[221, 222] Further, the cytotoxic lymphocytes had Fc receptors but did not appear to be B or T cells (i.e., a characteristic of K and NK cells).[223, 224] PBL from normal individuals were cytotoxic also to colon epithelial cells if they were first incubated in serum from IBD patients. More recently, the same investigators demonstrated a similar phenomenon using colon mononuclear cells from IBD patients and autologous colon epithelial cells as targets.[225] These data were interpreted to represent a form of antibody-dependent cell-mediated cytotoxicity in which the lymphocytes that mediated cytotoxicity became "armed" with an immune complex or a serum antibody present in IBD serum and directed against antigens present on colon epithelial cells. Although mononuclear cells from the mucosa of colon cancer patients were similarly cytotoxic for their own colon epithelial cells, the mechanism of cell damage appeared to differ.[225] Others have used different assay systems to demonstrate that mesenteric lymph nodes from areas of affected and unaffected tissue of Crohn's disease patients contain increased numbers of K cells capable of mediating antibody-dependent cell-mediated cytotoxic reactions.[226] There does not appear to be a striking difference between IBD patients and controls in the representation of T cell subsets in the intestinal mucosa.[42, 213]

Other approaches have assessed possible abnormalities in cell-mediated immunity in IBD by measuring *in vitro* parameters of cell-mediated immunity. This strategy assumes that changes in those parameters parallel *in vivo* changes in function. Evidence suggests that lymphocytes from IBD patients may be sensitized to bacterial and/or colon antigens,[227] but whether this reflects a primary event or is secondary to tissue damage is not known. Studies of delayed-type hypersensitivity (DTH) reactions have utilized recall antigens to test immunologic memory (e.g., PPD, mumps, fungal antigens) as well as 2,4-dinitrochlorobenzene to test the ability to contact sensitize for a DTH reaction *de novo*.[228] Generally such studies have revealed depressed DTH in Crohn's disease and ulcerative colitis. However, results have varied considerably, possibly reflecting the heterogeneity of the patient populations, their treatment with different therapeutic regimens, and the variable nutritional status of the patients.[229, 230] Studies of the response of PBL to T cell mitogens have demonstrated decreased responsiveness in some patients, but here too results have varied markedly. Lymphocytes isolated from the lamina propria of ulcerative colitis patients, compared with controls, have shown decreased stimulation by mitogens such as phytohemagglutinin, concanavalin A, and pokeweed mitogen.[231] It is not known whether this reflects the presence in the IBD mucosa of an already highly activated population of lymphocytes that is difficult to stimulate further, or whether other factors render these lymphocytes relatively unresponsive.

A further approach has asked whether there are abnormalities in regulation of the immune system in IBD. Using the T cell mitogen concanavalin A to activate suppressor cells, PBL from patients with moderately severe to severe IBD were reported to have a decreased ability to be stimulated *in vitro* to suppressor activity.[232] In a totally different system, others reported an increase in peripheral blood suppressor cells capable of inhibiting IgM synthesis in some patients with mild Crohn's disease.[233] Such suppressor cell activity could not be demonstrated using lamina propria mononuclear cells from Crohn's disease patients.[234] Thus far, studies

of suppressor cell activity in the circulation or the mucosa have yielded disparate results, in part owing to the use of different methods to assess suppressor cell activity, and in part due to the differences in patient populations studied (i.e., disease activity, use of medications).[235, 236] As greater fundamental understanding of immune regulatory mechanisms and antigen-specific and nonspecific T cell–mediated suppressor mechanisms become available, key questions about immunoregulation that relate to IBD, including approaches to understanding whether or not T cell lymphokines that affect lymphocyte growth and differentiation are important in these diseases, may lead to a clearer disease model that is testable by experimental approaches.

An alternative approach to define the role of cell-mediated immune responses in the pathogenesis of IBD has involved attempts to identify antigens on epithelial cells that might serve as the targets of cell-mediated immune attack. Peripheral blood and intestinal lamina propria mononuclear cells from IBD subjects, but not controls, were reported to damage chicken red blood cells coated with biochemically purified components from rodent intestinal epithelial cells. Peripheral blood mononuclear cells were weakly cytotoxic for these antigen-coated cells in the presence of patient serum, and the mechanism of killing appeared to be an antibody-dependent cell-mediated cytotoxic reaction.[93] In contrast, the T cell fraction of lamina propria mononuclear cells mediated low levels of cytotoxicity and cell damage did not require the addition of antibody, indicating involvement of a different type of cytotoxic mechanism.[94] It appears that greater definition of the importance of cell-mediated immune responses and/or autoimmunity in the pathogenesis of IBD will require further experimentation to test proposed models of these diseases.

Genetic Factors

Genetically controlled regulatory mechanisms govern the processes by which B and T lymphocytes interact with each other and with antigen-presenting cells. Such mechanisms also govern the interaction between cytotoxic, helper, and suppressor T cells and their targets. In addition, the repertoires of receptors for antigen on B and T cells are genetically encoded and differ between individuals.

One approach to investigation of the possible abnormalities of the immune response in IBD has been to examine genes and gene products that are related to the regulation of the immune response (e.g., HLA and immunoglobulin allotype genes) in IBD patients and compare them with those of control subjects. Studies have tested for differences in the distribution of HLA antigens, as determined by serologic assays, between ulcerative colitis or Crohn's disease patients and control groups; thus far, however, such studies have not demonstrated consistent differences. An exception is in patients with IBD and ankylosing spondylitis, who have a high prevalence of the class I antigen HLA-B27.[103] One group suggested that patients with HLA-B27 and reactive arthritis may have subclinical ileal inflammation (i.e., Crohn's disease)[237] and reported that the joint disease in such subjects responds to therapy with sulfasalazine.[238] Studies of the distribution of immunoglobulin allotype markers using serologic methods have indicated that Northern European Caucasians with the Gm(a,x,g) haplotype may be at increased risk for the development of Crohn's disease.[239] Newer approaches to examine genes that regulate the immune response using molecular probes are in progress in IBD patients. Finally, it is noteworthy that class II HLA-DR antigens are expressed on intestinal epithelial cells, particularly during inflammatory reactions such as those noted in IBD.[102] Whether such antigens simply are a consequence of an ongoing immune reaction or whether they contribute to disease pathogenesis through their involvement in the processing and presentation of antigen to lymphocytes in IBD patients is not known.

Immune Complexes and Complement

A further area of controversy about IBD surrounds studies of immune complexes. Circulating immune complexes have been noted by some, but not other, investigators in IBD patients.[240-245] Such immune complexes do not appear to correlate with disease activity or extraintestinal manifestations of IBD.[245] Whether or not these circulating immune complexes deposit in the tissues and cause tissue damage is not known. Alterations in serum complement and complement consumption and depressions in serum properdin and properdin convertase, both components of the alternative pathway of complement activation, also have been noted in IBD.[246-248] The relevance of these observations to the pathogenesis of IBD is not known.

Summary

A reasonable interpretation of data available thus far is that humoral and/or cell-mediated immune reactions may play a role in producing tissue injury in IBD. Often, during ongoing tissue injury, more than one effector mechanism and several lymphoid cell types are involved concurrently. Although the function of the immune response normally is to protect the host, environmental factors may activate potentially damaging immune responses in the IBD population. Tissue damage might be secondary to an immune reaction to an environmental antigen, or the immune attack could be autoimmune (i.e., directed to self components associated with, or that cross-react with, the environmental antigen). Once initiated, similar antigens or different factors might perpetuate tissue injury. Further studies on the immune system and genetic factors in IBD may help to elucidate its pathogenesis as well as provide useful clinical tests to detect disease, and to

predict prognosis. Ultimately, the ability to specifically manipulate components of the immune system may provide exciting new therapeutic modalities for the patient with IBD.

CELIAC DISEASE

See also pages 1134 to 1152.

Celiac disease (gluten-sensitive enteropathy) in children and adults is characterized by small intestinal mucosal damage and the malabsorption of most nutrients.[104] Disease is precipitated by the ingestion of dietary wheat gluten and similar alcohol-soluble proteins (prolamins) in rye, barley, and oats. In genetically susceptible individuals, ingestion of such proteins can result in epithelial cell damage and a loss of the normal intestinal villous architecture. The latter is characterized by villous atrophy and crypt hyperplasia, most striking in the proximal small bowel.

The role of wheat gluten in this disease has been studied extensively. Gluten is composed of gliadin and glutenin. The gliadin fraction of wheat gluten contains the proteins responsible for activating disease.[104] However, gliadin from a single wheat variety contains at least 40 components. These components can be assigned on the basis of electrophoretic mobilities into four major groups (alpha-, beta-, gamma- and omega-gliadins), all of which are rich in the amino acids glutamine and proline.[249] Based on limited studies in patients, there is some debate as to whether all gliadin fractions or only alpha-gliadins can activate disease.[250-252]

How gliadin results in epithelial cell damage and villous atrophy is not known. Current evidence favors the importance of immune mechanisms, and not a direct toxicity of gliadin or its peptides for the mucosa. Thus, a striking feature of celiac disease is the infiltration of the lamina propria with plasma cells and the relative increase in IEL.[253] Increased mucosal anti-gluten antibody synthesis, increased serum antibody titers to gluten and gliadin, as well as to reticulin and some dietary proteins (i.e., milk and egg proteins), have been reported in these patients.[254-257] Among different celiac disease patients, anti-gliadin antibodies appear to be directed to different gliadin components and determinants.[258] Thus, the peptides of the gliadin molecule that stimulate humoral antibody production appear to vary from individual to individual. Little is known with regard to determinants on gliadin that interact with T cells.[259] As with other immunologically mediated diseases, the intestinal lesion in celiac disease may reflect tissue damage caused by both cell-mediated and antibody-mediated immune effector mechanisms.

The discovery that specific MHC class II antigens (i.e., HLA-DR3 and -DQw2), as detected by serology, occur in up to 90 per cent or more of European Caucasians with celiac disease compared with 20 to 30 per cent of the normal population added strong support to the notion that immune mechanisms are important in the pathogenesis of this disease.[104, 260] Thus, genes that code for the class II cell surface molecules on B cells, antigen-presenting cells, activated T cells, and some intestinal epithelial cells. These cell surface molecules govern the host's ability to respond to soluble protein antigens and to mediate a variety of immune functions. They ultimately determine the magnitude and quality of the immune response. Although the serologic markers HLA-DR3 and -DQw2 are highly associated with celiac disease, less than 1 per cent of the general population with those markers develop celiac disease.[104] Recent studies using molecular probes and Southern blot analysis to assess genomic DNA restriction fragment length polymorphisms indicate that a subset of individuals with both the serologic HLA-DR3 DQw2 markers and a 4.0 kilobase genomic DNA fragment that includes a DPβ chain gene are at least 40-fold more likely to develop celiac disease than those with the HLA-DR3 DQw2 haplotype that lack the 4.0 Kb fragment.[106, 260a] In mice, the magnitude of the anti-gliadin antibody response has been shown to be regulated both by genes mapping to the MHC and by genes mapping to the immunoglobulin heavy chain locus.[261] In some celiac disease patients, persistence of the antibody response to gliadin has correlated also with immunoglobulin heavy chain markers.[262]

Celiac disease appears to be concordant in only 70 per cent of monozygotic twins and in about 30 per cent of serologically HLA-identical siblings.[104] This led to the suggestion that genes other than those in HLA and environmental factors other than gliadin or other grain proteins might be important in the pathogenesis of celiac disease. In this regard, genes in or linked to the immunoglobulin heavy chain constant region have been proposed as a second genetic locus important in celiac disease.[262, 263] Other studies have reported a region of amino acid sequence homology between alpha-gliadins and a protein coded for by a human intestinal adenovirus.[264] The latter observation led to the suggestion that molecular mimicry, likely involving T cell recognition of a gliadin protein and a viral protein, may be important in the initiation of celiac disease.[265]

Serologic HLA markers similar to those found in celiac disease (i.e., HLA-DR3, -DQw2) are present also in as many as 90 per cent of patients with dermatitis herpetiformis.[266] The latter is a skin disease associated with cutaneous deposits of IgA and small bowel changes histologically similar to those seen in celiac disease.[267] Further, during treatment with a gluten-free diet, both the intestinal and skin disease improve.[268] The genetic and immunologic relationship between these diseases is currently being studied.

WHIPPLE'S DISEASE

Whipple's disease is a rare multisystem, male-predominant disease with a major involvement of the gastrointestinal tract. The disease is characterized by malabsorption, polyarthritis, hyperpigmentation, and variable involvement of other organs, particularly the central nervous system and heart, as discussed on pages

1297 to 1306. The lamina propria contains abundant PAS-positive macrophages. However, the latter finding is not pathognomonic for Whipple's disease and can be seen also in individuals with disseminated *Mycobacterium avium intracellulare* infection (e.g., in AIDS).[43, 44] Rod-shaped microorganisms in the lamina propria suggest a bacterial etiology,[269, 270] but definitive identification of the bacteria has been elusive. Factors that predispose to Whipple's disease and what proportion of individuals exposed to the bacteria develop the disease also are not known.

Several studies have sought abnormalities in the immune response in Whipple's disease patients. Thus far, these studies have not demonstrated a consistent abnormality in the humoral immune system or complement system. Serum antibodies to material within the macrophages, possibly bacterial carbohydrate determinants, have been noted, and abnormalities in cell-mediated immunity have been reported.[271, 272] Decreased numbers of peripheral blood T lymphocytes, depressed delayed-type cutaneous hypersensitivity reactions to skin test antigens, and decreased responses to T cell mitogens can be seen, but are not a consistent finding in all patients. Following treatment, delayed-type cutaneous hypersensitivity reactions and responses to mitogens may return to normal, but in some patients they remain abnormal.[273, 274] Whether these putative immune defects in Whipple's disease are primary or secondary to the disease process is unknown. There is no experimental evidence to support a primary functional abnormality in the macrophage-monocytic series. However, morphologic observations suggest a failure of complete macrophage destruction of bacteria after phagocytosis.

References

1. IVIS-WHO Nomenclature Subcommittee Announcement. J. Immunol. *134*:659, 1985.
2. Reinherz, E. L., and Schlossman, S. F. The differentiation and function of human T lymphocytes. Cell *19*:821, 1980.
3. Reinherz, E. L., Kung, P. C., Goldstein, G., Levey, R. H., and Schlossman, S. F. Discrete stages of intrathymic differentiation: Analysis of normal thymocytes and leukemic lymphoblasts of T-cell lineage. Proc. Natl. Acad. Sci. USA *77*:1588, 1980.
4. Benacerraf, B., and McDevitt, H. O. Histocompatibility linked immune response genes. Science *175*:273, 1972.
5. Bodmer, J., and Bodmer, W. Histocompatibility. Immunology Today *5*:251, 1984.
6. Acuto, O., and Reinherz, E. L. The human T-cell receptor. Structure and function. N. Engl. J. Med. *312*:1100, 1985.
7. Toyonaga, B., Yanagi, Y., Suciu-Foca, N., Minden, M., and Mak, T. W. Rearrangements of T-cell receptor gene YT35 in human DNA from thymic leukemia T-cell lines and functional T-cell clones. Nature *311*:385, 1984.
8. Yoshikai, Y., Kimura, N., Toyonaga, B., and Mak, T. W. Sequences and repertoire of human T cell receptor chain variable region genes in mature T lymphocytes. J. Exp. Med. *164*:90, 1986.
9. Reinherz, E. L., Meuer, S. C., Fitzgerald, K. A., Levine, H., and Schlossman, S. F. Antigen recognition by human T lymphocyte is linked to surface expression of the T3 molecular complex. Cell *30*:735, 1982.
10. Engleman, E. G., Benike, C. J., Grumet, F. C., and Evans, R. L. Activation of human T lymphocyte subsets: Helper and

suppressor/cytotoxic T cells recognize and respond to distinct histocompatibility antigens. J. Immunol. *127*:2124, 1981.

11. Meuer, S. C., Schlossman, S. F., and Reinherz, E. L. Clonal analysis of human cytotoxic T lymphocytes: T4+ and T8+ effector cells recognize products of different major histocompatibility complex regions. Proc. Natl. Acad. Sci. USA *79*:4395, 1982.

12. Meuer, S. C., Hussey, R. E., Fabbi, M., Fox, D., Acuto, O., Fitzgerald, K. A., Hodgdon, J. C., Protentis, J. P., Schlossman, S. F., and Reinherz, E. L. An alternative pathway of T-cell activation: A functional role for the 50 kd T11 sheep erythrocyte receptor protein. Cell *36*:897, 1984.

13. Golde, W. T., Kappler, J. W., Greenstein, J., Malissen, B., Hood, L., and Marrack, P. Major histocompatibility complex–restricted antigen receptor on T cells. VIII. Role of the LFA-1 molecule. J. Exp. Med. *161*:635, 1985.

14. Hoover, R. G., and Lynch, R. G. Isotype-specific suppression of IgA:suppression of IgA responses in BALB/c mice by T cells. J. Immunol. *130*:521, 1983.

15. Kiyono, H., Mosteller-Barnum, L. M., Pitts, A. M., Williamson, S. I., Michalek, S. M., and McGhee, J. R. Isotype-specific immunoregulation, IgA-binding factors produced by Fc receptor–positive T cell hybridomas regulate IgA responses. J. Exp. Med. *161*:731, 1985.

16. Howard, M., and Paul, W. E. Regulation of B cell growth and differentiation by soluble factors. Ann. Rev. Immunol. *1*:307, 1983.

17. King, D. P., and Jones, P. P. Induction of Ia and H-2 antigens on a macrophage cell line by immune interferon. J. Immunol. *131*:315, 1983.

18. Noma, Y., Sideras, P., Naito, T., Bergstedt-Lindquist, S., Azuma, C., Severinson, E., Tanabe, T., Kinashi, T., Matsuda, F., Yaoita, Y., and Honjo, T. Cloning of cDNA encoding the murine IgG1 induction factor by a novel strategy using SP6 promoter. Nature *319*:640, 1986.

19. Barlow, D. J., Edwards, M. S., and Thornton, J. M. Continuous and discontinuous protein antigenic determinants. Nature *322*:747, 1986.

20. McBridge, O. W., Hieter, P. A., Hollis, P. A., Swan, D., Otey, M. C., and Leder, P. Chromosomal location of human kappa and lambda immunoglobulin light chain constant region genes. J. Exp. Med. *155*:1480, 1982.

21. Maki, R., Traunecker, A., Sakano, H., Roeder, W., and Tonegawa, S. Exon shuffling generates an immunoglobulin heavy chain gene. Proc. Natl. Acad. Sci. USA *77*:2138, 1980.

22. Germain, R. N. The ins and outs of antigen processing and presentation. Nature *322*:687, 1986.

23. Scott, H., Solheim, B. G., Brandtzaeg, P., and Thorsby, E. HLA-DR–like antigens in the epithelium of the human small intestine. Scand. J. Immunol. *12*:77, 1980.

24. Befus, A. D., Goodacre, R., Dyck, N., and Bienenstock, J. Isolation and characterization of human intestinal mast cells. Fed. Proc. *43*:1973, 1984.

25. Kagnoff, M. F. Immunology of the digestive system. *In* Johnson, L. R. (ed.). Physiology of the Gastrointestinal Tract. New York, Raven Press, 1987.

26. Owen, R. L., and Nemanic, P. Antigen processing structures of the mammalian intestinal tract: An SEM study of lymphoepithelial organs. Scan. Electron Microsc. *2*:367, 1978.

27. Butcher, E. C., Scollay, R. G., and Weissman, I. L. Organ specificity of lymphocyte migration mediation by highly selective lymphocyte interaction with organ-specific determinants on high endothelial venules. Eur. J. Immunol. *10*:556, 1980.

28. Kraal, G., Weissman, I. L., and Butcher, E. C. Differences in *in vivo* distribution and homing of T cell subsets to mucosal vs non-mucosal lymphoid organs. J. Immunol. *130*:1097, 1983.

29. Gallatin, W. M., Weissman, I. L., and Butcher, E. C. A cell-surface molecule involved in organ-specific homing of lymphocytes. Nature *304*:30, 1983.

30. Kawanishi, H., Saltzman, L., and Strober, W. Mechanisms regulating IgA class-specific immunoglobulin production in gut-associated lymphoid tissues. I. T cells derived from Peyer's patches that switch sIgM B cells in vitro. J. Exp. Med. *157*:433, 1983.

31. Murray, P. D., and Kagnoff, M. F. Regulation of the anti-α(1,3) dextran response: Two populations of dextran-reactive B cells that differ in their T cell requirements for induction to antibody synthesis. J. Immunol. *138*:2439, 1987.

32. Kagnoff, M. F., and Campbell, S. Functional characteristics of Peyer's patch lymphoid cells. I. Induction of humoral antibody and cell-mediated allograft reactions. J. Exp. Med. *139*:398, 1974.

33. Kagnoff, M. F. Functional characteristics of Peyer's patch cells. IV. Effect of antigen feeding on the frequency of antigen-specific B cells. J. Immunol. *118*:992, 1977.

34. Kagnoff, M. F. Immunological unresponsiveness after enteric antigen administration. *In* Strober, W., and Hanson, L. A. (eds.). Recent Advances in Mucosal Immunity. New York, Raven Press, 1982, pp. 95–111.

35. Cebra, J. J., Crandall, C. A., Gearhart, P. J., Robertson, S. M., Tseng, J., and Watson, P. M. Cellular events concerned with the initiation, expression and control of the mucosal immune response. *In* Ogra, P. L., and Dayton, D. (eds.). Immunology of Breast Milk. New York, Raven Press, 1979, pp. 1–18.

36. Craig, S. W., and Cebra, J. J. Peyer's patches. An enriched source of precursors for IgA-producing immunocytes in the rabbit. J. Exp. Med. *134*:188, 1971.

37. Kagnoff, M. F. Functional characteristics of Peyer's patch cells. III. Carrier priming of T cells by antigen feeding. J. Exp. Med. *142*:1425, 1975.

38. Kagnoff, M. F. Effects of antigen-feeding on intestinal and systematic immune responses. I. Priming of precursor cytotoxic T cells by antigen feeding. J. Immunol. *120*:395, 1978.

39. Ngan, J., and Kind, L. S. Suppressor T-cells for IgE and IgG in Peyer's patches of mice made tolerant by the oral administration of ovalbumin. J. Immunol. *120*:861, 1978.

40. London, S. D., Rubin, D. H., and Cebra, J. J. Cytotoxic potential of murine Peyer's patch lymphocytes. (Abstract) 6th Int. Cong. Immunol. 1986, p. 56.

41. Janossy, G., Tidman, N., Selby, W. S., Thomas, J. A., and Granger, S. Human T-lymphocytes of inducer and suppressor type occupy different microenvironments. Nature *288*:81, 1980.

42. James, S. P., Fiocchi, C., Graeff, A. S., and Strober, W. Phenotypic analysis of lamina propria lymphocytes. Predominance of helper-inducer and cytolytic T cell phenotypes and deficiency of suppressor-inducer phenotypes in Crohn's disease and control patients. Gastroenterology *91*:1483, 1986.

43. Roth, R. I., Owen, R. L., Keren, D. F., and Volberding, P. A. Intestinal infection with *Mycobacterium avium* in acquired immune deficiency syndrome (AIDS). Histological and clinical comparison with Whipple's disease. Dig. Dis. Sci. *30*:497, 1985.

44. Strom, R. L., and Groninger, R. P. AIDS with *Mycobacterium avium intracellulare* lesions resembling those of Whipple's disease. N. Engl. J. Med. *309*:1323, 1983.

45. Barret, K. E., and Metcalfe, D. D. Mast cell heterogeneity: Evidence and implications. J. Clin. Immunol. *4*:253, 1984.

46. Cerf-Bensussan, N., Schneeberger, E. E., and Bhan, A. K. Immunohistologic and immunoelectron microscopic characterization of the mucosal lymphocytes of human small intestine by the use of monoclonal antibodies. J. Immunol. *130*:2615, 1983.

47. Selby, W. S., Janossy, G., Bofill, M., and Jewell, D. P. Lymphocyte subpopulations in the human small intestine. The findings in normal mucosa and in the mucosa of patients with adult coeliac disease. Clin. Exp. Immunol. *52*:219, 1983.

48. Chiba, M., Hiromasa, O. H. T. A., Nagasaki, A., Arakawa, H., and Masamune, O. Lymphoid cell subsets in normal human small intestine. Gastroenterol. Jpn. *21*:336, 1986.

49. Rodgers, V. D., Fassett, R., and Kagnoff, M. F. Abnormalities in intestinal mucosal T cells in homosexual populations including those with the lymphadenopathy syndrome and acquired immunodeficiency syndrome. Gastroenterology *90*:552, 1986.

49a. Rodgers, V. D., and Kagnoff, M. F. Gastrointestinal manifestations of the acquired immunodeficiency syndrome. Western J. Med. *146*:57, 1987.

50. Dobbins, W. O. Human intestinal intraepithelial lymphocytes. Gut *27*:972, 1986.

51. Cerf-Bensussan, N., Guy-Grand, D., and Griscelli, C. Intra-epithelial lymphocytes of human gut: Isolation, characterization and study of natural killer activity. Gut *26*:81, 1985.

52. Selby, W. S., Janossy, G., and Jewell, D. P. Immunohistolog-ical characterization of intraepithelial lymphocytes of the hu-man gastrointestinal tract. Gut *22*:169, 1981.

53. Ernst, P. B., Befus, A. D., and Bienenstock, J. Leukocytes in the intestinal epithelium: An unusual immunological compart-ment. Immunology Today *6*:50, 1985.

54. Klein, J. R. Ontogeny of the Thy-1⁻, Lyt-2⁺ murine intestinal intraepithelial lymphocyte. Characterization of a unique pop-ulation of thymus-independent cytotoxic effector cells in the intestinal mucosa. J. Exp. Med. *164*:309, 1986.

55. Klein, J. R., and Kagnoff, M. F. Nonspecific recruitment of cytotoxic effector cells in the intestinal mucosa of antigen-primed mice. J. Exp. Med. *160*:1931, 1984.

56. Klein, J. R., Lefrancois, L., and Kagnoff, M. F. A murine cytotoxic T lymphocyte clone from the intestinal mucosa that is antigen specific for proliferation and displays broadly reactive inducible cytotoxic activity. J. Immunol. *135*:3697, 1985.

57. Kagnoff, M. F., and Klein, J. P. Spontaneous *in vitro* evolution of lytic specificity of cytotoxic T lymphocyte clones isolated from murine intestinal epithelium. J. Immunol., *138*:58, 1987.

58. Chiba, M., Bartnik, W., ReMine, S. G., Thayer, W. R., and Shorter, R. G. Human colonic intraepithelial and lamina pro-prial lymphocytes: Cytotoxicity *in vitro* and the potential effects of the isolation method on their functional properties. Gut *22*:177, 1981.

59. Ropke, C., and Everett, N. B. Kinetics of intraepithelial lymphocytes in the small intestine of thymus-deprived mice and antigen-deprived mice. Anat. Rec. *185*:101, 1976.

60. Guy-Grand, D., Griscelli, C., and Vassalli, P. The mouse gut T lymphocytes, a novel type of T cell. Nature, origin and traffic in mice in normal and graft-versus-host conditions. J. Exp. Med. *148*:1661, 1978.

61. Kotler, D. P., Gaetzh, P., Lang, M., Klein, E. B., Hott, P. R. Enteropathy associated with acquired immunodeficiency syndrome. Ann. Int. Med. *101*:421, 1984.

62. Dobbins, W. I., and Weinstein, W. M. Electron microscopy of the intestine and rectum in acquired immuno-deficiency syn-drome. Gastroenterology *88*:738, 1985.

63. Cerf-Bensussan, N., Guy-Grand, D., Lisowska-Grospierre, B., Griscelli, C., and Bhan, A. K. A monoclonal antibody specific for rat intestinal lymphocytes. J. Immunol. *136*:76, 1986.

64. Keren, D. F., Holt, P. S., Collins, H. H., Gembski, P., and Formal, S. B. The role of Peyer's patches in the local immune response of rabbit ileum to live bacteria. J. Immunol. *120*:1892, 1978.

65. McWilliams, M., Phillips-Quagliata, J. A., and Lamm, M. E. Mesenteric lymph node B lymphoblasts which home to the small intestine are precommitted to IgA synthesis. J. Exp. Med. *145*:866, 1977.

66. Craig, S. W., and Cebra, J. J. Peyer's patches: An enriched source of precursors for IgA-producing immunocytes in the rabbit. J. Exp. Med. *134*:188, 1971.

67. McDermott, M. R., and Bienenstock, J. Evidence for a com-mon mucosal immunologic system. I. Migration of B immu-noblasts into intestinal, respiratory, and genital tissues. J. Immunol. *122*:1892, 1979.

68. Lamm, M. E., Weisz-Carrington, P., Roux, M. E., Mc-Williams, M., and Phillips-Quagliata, J. M. Mode of induction of an IgA response in the breast and other secretory sites by oral antigen. *In* Ogra, P. L., and Dayton, D. (eds.). Immu-nology of Breast Milk. New York, Raven Press, 1979, pp. 105–114.

69. Kagnoff, M. F., Donaldson, R. M., Jr., and Trier, J. S. Organ culture of rabbit small intestine: Prolonged *in vitro* steady-state protein synthesis and secretion and secretory IgA secretion. Gastroenterology *63*:541, 1972.

70. Kagnoff, M. F., Serfilippi, D., and Donaldson, R. M., Jr. *In vitro* kinetics of intestinal secretory IgA secretion. J. Immunol. *110*:297, 1973.

71. Mostov, K. E., Friedlander, M., and Blobel, G. The receptor of transepithelial transport of IgA and IgM contains multiple immunoglobulin-like domains. Nature *308*:37, 1984.

72. Kuhn, L. C., and Kraehenbuhl, J. P. Role of secretory com-ponent, a secreted glycoprotein, in the specific uptake of IgA dimer by epithelial cells. J. Biol. Chem. *254*:11072, 1979.

73. Koshland, M. E. Structure and function of the J chain. Adv. Immunol. *20*:41, 1975.

74. Flanagan, J. G., Lefranc, M. P., and Rabbitts, T. H. Mecha-nisms of divergence and convergence of the human immuno-globulin 1 and 2 constant gene sequences. Cell *36*:681, 1984.

75. Kornfeld, S. J., and Plaut, A. G. Secretory immunity and the bacterial IgA proteases. Rev. Infect. Dis. *3*:521, 1981.

76. Andre, C., Andre, F., and Fargier, M. C. Distribution of IgA1 and IgA2 plasma cells in various normal human tissues and in the jejunum of plasma IgA-deficient patients. Clin. Exp. Im-munol. *33*:327, 1978.

77. van Loghem, E., and Biewenga, J. Allotypic and isotypic aspects of human immunoglobulin A. Mol. Immunol. *20*:1001, 1983.

78. Nagura, H., Smith, P. D., Nakane, P. K., and Brown, W. R. IgA in human bile and liver. J. Immunol. *126*:587, 1981.

79. Peppard, J., Orlans, E., Payne, A. W. R., and Andrew, E. The elimination of circulating complexes containing polymeric IgA by excretion in the bile. Immunology *42*:83, 1981.

80. Russess, M. W., Brown, T. A., and Mestecky, J. Role of serum IgA. Hepatobiliary transport of circulating antigen. J. Exp. Med. *153*:968, 1981.

81. Socken, D. J., Jeejeebhoy, K. N., Bazin, H., and Underdown, B. J. Identification of secretory component as an IgA receptor on rat hepatocytes. J. Exp. Med. *150*:1538, 1979.

81a. Murray, P. D., McKenzie, D. T., Swain, S. L., and Kagnoff, M. F. Interleukin 5 and interleukin 4 produced by Peyer's patch T cells selectively enhance immunoglobulin A expression. J. Immunol. *139*:2669, 1987.

82. Husband, A. J., and Gowans, J. L. The origin and antigen-dependent distribution of IgA-containing cells in the intestine. J. Exp. Med. *148*:1146, 1978.

83. Walker, W. A., Isselbacher, K. J., and Bloch, K. J. Intestinal uptake of macromolecules: Effect of oral immunization. Sci-ence *177*:608, 1972.

84. Williams, R. C., and Gibbons, R. J. Inhibition of bacterial adherence by secretory immunoglobulin A: A mechanism of antigen disposal. Science *177*:697, 1972.

85. Ogra, P. L., Karzon, D. T., Righthand, F., and MacGillivray, M. Immunoglobulin response in serum and secretions after immunization with live and inactivated poliovaccine and natural infection. N. Engl. J. Med. *279*:893, 1968.

86. Kagnoff, M. F., and Campbell, S. Antibody-dependent cell-mediated cytotoxicity; comparative ability of murine Peyer's patch and spleen cells to lyse lipopolysaccharide-coated and uncoated erythrocytes. Gastroenterology *70*:341, 1976.

87. Brown, W. R. Relationships between immunoglobulins and the intestinal epithelium. Gastroenterology *75*:129, 1978.

88. Fassett, R. T., and Kagnoff, M. F. Clinical significance of se-lective IgA deficiency. Int. Med. for the Specialist, *8*:90, 1987.

89. Trinchieri, G., and Perussia, B. Human natural killer cells: Biologic and pathogenic aspects. Lab. Invest. *50*:489, 1984.

90. Lanier, L. L., Le, A. M., Civin, C. I., Loken, M. R., and Phillips, J. H. The relationship of CD16 (Leu-11) and Leu-19 (NKH-1) antigen expression on human peripheral blood NK cells and cytotoxic T lymphocytes. J. Immunol. *136*:4480, 1986.

91. Shanahan, F., Brogan, M., Naversina, R., and Targan, S. Spontaneous and lymphokine activated killer cells exist in the human intestine as phenotypically distinct subpopulations (ab-stract). Gastroenterology *90*:1629, 1986.

92. Lanier, L. L., Kipps, T. J., and Phillips, J. H. Functional properties of a unique subset of cytotoxic CD3 + T lymphocytes that express Fc receptors for IgG (CD16/Leu-11 antigen). J. Exp. Med. *162*:2089, 1985.

93. Aronson, R. A., Cook, S. L., and Roche, J. K. Sensitization to epithelial antigens in chronic mucosal inflammatory disease. I. Purification, characterization, and immune reactivity of mu-

rine epithelial cell-associated components (ECAC). J. Immunol. *131*:2796, 1983.

94. Roche, J. K., Fiocchi, C., and Youngman, K. Sensitization to epithelial antigens in chronic mucosal inflammatory disease. Characterization of human intestinal mucosa–derived mononuclear cells reactive with purified epithelial cell–associated components *in vitro*. J. Clin. Invest. 75:522, 1985.

95. MacDermott, R. P., Franklin, G. O., Jenkins, K. M., Kodner, I. J., Nash, G. S., and Weinrieb, I. J. Human intestinal mononuclear cells. I. Investigation of antibody-dependent, lectin-induced and spontaneous cell-mediated cytotoxic capabilities. Gastroenterology 78:47, 1980.

96. Falchuk, Z. M., Barnhard, E., and Machado, I. Human colonic mononuclear cells: Studies of cytotoxic function. Gut 22:290, 1981.

97. Fiocchi, C., Tubbs, R. R., Youngman, K. R. Human intestinal mucosa mononuclear cells exhibit lymphokine-activated killer cell activity. Gastroenterology 88:625, 1985.

98. Grimm, E. A., Mazumder, A., Zhang, H. Z., Rosenberg, S. A. Lymphokine-activated killer cell phenomenon. Lysis of natural killer–resistant fresh solid tumor cells by interleukin 2–activated autologous human peripheral blood lymphocytes. J. Exp. Med. *155*:1823, 1982.

99. Giles, R. C., and Capra, J. D. Biochemistry of MHC class II molecules. Tissue Antigens 25:57, 1985.

100. Elson, C. O., Kagnoff, M. F., Fiocchi, C., Befus, A. D., and Targan, S. Intestinal immunity and inflammation: Recent progress. Gastroenterology *91*:746, 1986.

101. Barclay, A. N., and Mason, D. W. Induction of Ia antigen in rat epidermal cells and gut epithelium by immunological stimuli. J. Exp. Med. 15:1665, 1982.

102. Poulsen, L. O., Elling, P., Sørensen, F. B., and Hedt-Rasmussen, K. HLA-DR expression and disease activity in ulcerative colitis. Scand. J. Gastroenterol. 24:364, 1986.

103. Mallas, E. G., Mackintosh, P., Asquith, P., and Cooke, W. T. Histocompatibility antigens in inflammatory bowel disease. Their clinical significance and their association with arthropathy with special reference to HLAB27 (W27). Gut 17:906, 1976.

104. Cole, S. G., and Kagnoff, M. F. Celiac disease. Annu. Rev. Nutr. 5:241, 1985.

105. Mackay, I. R., and Tait, B. D. HLA association with autoimmune-type chronic active hepatitis: Identification of B8-DRw3 haplotype by family studies. Gastroenterology 79:95, 1980.

106. Howell, M. D., Austin, R. K., Kelleher, D., Nepom, G., and Kagnoff, M. F. An HLA-D region restriction fragment length polymorphism associated with celiac disease. J. Exp. Med. *164*:333, 1986.

106a. Howell, M. D., Smith, J. R., Austin, R. K., Kelleher, D., Nepom, G. T., Volk, B., and Kagnoff, M. F. An extended HLA-D region haplotype associated with celiac disease. Proc. Natl. Acad. Sci., in press, 1987.

107. Ogra, P. L., and Karzon, D. T. Distribution of poliovirus antibody in serum, nasopharynx and alimentary tract following segmental immunization of lower alimentary tract with poliovaccine. J. Immunol. *102*:1423, 1969.

108. Pierce, N. F., and Koster, F. T. Priming and suppression of the intestinal immune response to cholera toxoid/toxin by parenteral toxoid in rats. J. Immunol. *124*:307, 1980.

109. Kagnoff, M. F. Oral tolerance. Ann. N.Y. Acad. Sci. 392:248, 1982.

110. Kagnoff, M. F. Effects of antigen-feeding on intestinal and systematic immune responses. III. Antigen-specific serum-mediated suppression of humoral antibody responses after antigen feeding. Cell. Immunol. 40:186, 1978.

111. Rubin, D., Weiner, H. L., Fields, B. N., and Greene, M. I. Immunologic tolerance after oral administration of reovirus: Requirement for two viral gene products for tolerance induction. J. Immunol. *127*:1697, 1981.

112. Challacombe, S. J., and Tomasi, T. B., Jr. Systemic tolerance and secretory immunity after oral immunization. J. Exp. Med. *152*:1459, 1980.

113. Richman, L. K., Chiller, J. M., Brown, W. R., Hanson, D. G., and Vaz, N. M. Enterically induced immunologic tolerance. I. Induction of suppressor T lymphocytes by intragastric administration of soluble proteins. J. Immunol. *121*:2429, 1978.

114. Asherson, G. L., Zembala, M., Perera, M. A. C. C., Mayhew, B., and Thomas, W. R. Production of immunity and unresponsiveness in the mouse by feeding contact sensitizing agents and the role of suppressor cells in the Peyer's patches, mesenteric lymph nodes and other lymphoid tissues. Cell. Immunol. 33:145, 1977.

115. Kagnoff, M. F. Effects of antigen-feeding on intestinal and systemic immune responses. II. Suppression of delayed-type hypersensitivity responses. J. Immunol. *120*:1509, 1978.

116. Miller, S. D., and Hanson, D. G. Inhibition of specific immune responses by feeding protein antigens. IV. Evidence of tolerance and specific active suppression of cell-mediated immune responses to ovalbumin. J. Immunol. *123*:2344, 1979.

117. Kagnoff, M. F. Oral tolerance, enteric immunity and autoimmunity. *In* Spondyloarthropathies: Involvement of the Gut. Proceedings of the First Conference on Spondyloarthropathies: Involvement of the Gut, Ghent, 10–13 September 1986. H. Mielants and E. M. Veys, editors. Elsevier Science Publishers B. V. (Biomedical Division), Excerpta Medica, Amsterdam, 1987, pp. 187–198.

118. Suzuki, I., Kitamura, K., Kiyono, H., Kurita, T., Green, D. R., and McGhee, J. R. Isotype-specific immunoregulation. Evidence for a distinct subset of T contrasuppressor cells for IgA responses in murine Peyer's patches. J. Exp. Med. *164*:501, 1986.

119. Rupars, C., Muller, A., Paint, N., Beige, D., and Avenard, G. Large scale detection of IgA deficient blood donors. J. Immunol. Meth. 54:183, 1982.

120. Strober, W., Krakauer, R., Klaeveman, H. L., Reynolds, H. Y., and Nelson, D. L. Secretory component deficiency. A disorder of the IgA immune system. N. Engl. J. Med. 294:351, 1976.

121. Wilton, A. N., Cobain, T. J., and Dawkins, R. L. Family studies of IgA deficiency. Immunogenetics 21:333, 1985.

122. van Loghem, E., Zegers, B. J. M., Bast, E. J. E. G., and Kater, L. Selective deficiency of immunoglobulin A2. J. Clin. Invest. 72:1918, 1983.

123. Schwartz, S. A. Heavy chain–specific suppression of immunoglobulin synthesis and secretion by lymphocytes from patients with selective IgA deficiency. J. Immunol. *124*:2034, 1980.

124. Leickly, F. E., and Buckley, R. H. Development of IgA and IgG2 subclass deficiency after sulfasalazine. J. Pediatr. *108*:481, 1986.

125. van Riel, P. L., van de Putte, L. B., Gribnau, F. W., and de Waal, R. M. IgA deficiency during aurothioglucose treatment. A case report. Scand. J. Rheumatol. *13*:334, 1984.

126. Webster, A. D. B. Laboratory investigation of primary deficiency of the lymphoid system. Clin. Immunol. Allergy 5:447, 1985.

127. Savilahti, E. Sulphasalazine induced immunodeficiency. Br. Med. J. 287:759, 1983.

128. Farr, M., Struthers, G. R., Scott, D. G., and Bacon, P. A. Fenclofenac-induced selective IgA deficiency in rheumatoid arthritis. Br. J. Rheumatol. 24:367, 1985.

129. Andre, C., Andre, F., and Fargier, M. C. Distribution of IgA1 and IgA2 plasma cells in various normal human tissues and in the jejunum of plasma IgA-deficient patients. Clin. Exp. Immunol. 33:327, 1978.

130. Crabbe, P. A., and Heremans, J. F. Selective IgA deficiency with steatorrhea. A new syndrome. Am. J. Med. 42:319, 1967.

131. McCarthy, D. M., Katz, S. I., Gazze, L., Waldmann, T. A., Nelson, D. L., and Strober, W. Selective IgA deficiency associated with total villous atrophy of the small intestine and an organ-specific antiepithelial cell antibody. J. Immunol. *120*:932, 1978.

132. Hodgson, H. J., and Jewell, D. P. Selective IgA deficiency and Crohn's disease: Report of two cases. Gut 18:644, 1977.

133. Petty, R. E., Sherry, D. D., and Johannson, J. M. IgG anti-IgA1 and anti-IgA2 antibodies: Their measurement by an enzyme-linked immunosorbent assay and their relationship to disease. Int. Arch. Allergy Appl. Immunol. 80:337, 1986.

134. Ammann, A. J., and Hong, R. Disorders of the IgA system. *In* Stiehm, E. R., and Fulginiti, V. A. (eds.). Immunologic Disorders in Infants and Children. Philadelphia, W. B. Saunders Company, 1980, pp. 260–273.

135. Cunningham-Rundles, C., Brandeis, W. R., Good, R. A., and Day, N. K. Milk precipitins, circulating immune complexes and IgA deficiency. Proc. Natl. Acad. Sci. USA 75:3387, 1978.

136. Oxelius, V.-A., Laurell, A.-B., Lindquist, B., Golebiowska, H., Axelson, U., Bjorkander, J., and Hanson, L. IgG subclasses in selective IgA deficiency. N. Engl. J. Med. 304:1476, 1981.

137. Ugazio, A. G., Out, T. A., Plebani, A., Duse, M., Monafo, V., Nespoli, L., and Burgio, G. R. Recurrent infections in children with selective IgA deficiency: Association with IgG2 and IgG4 deficiency. Birth Defects 19:169, 1983.

138. Polmar, S. H., Waldmann, T. A., Balestra, S. T., Jost, M. C., and Terry, W. D. Immunoglobulin E in immunologic deficiency diseases. I. Relation of IgE and IgA to respiratory tract disease in isolated IgE deficiency, IgA deficiency, and ataxia telangiectasia. J. Clin. Invest. 51:326, 1972.

139. Buckley, R. H. Immunodeficiency. J. Allergy Clin. Immunol. 72:627, 1983.

140. Cunningham-Rundles, C., Wong, S., Bjordkander, J., and Hanson, L. A. Use of an IgA-depleted intravenous immunoglobulin in a patient with an anti-IgA antibody. Clin. Immunol. Immunopathol. 38:141, 1986.

141. Clark, J. A., Callicoat, P. A., Brenner, N. A., Bradley, C. A., and Smith, D. M. Selective IgA deficiency in blood donors. Am. J. Clin. Pathol. 80:210, 1983.

142. Andre, C., Berthoux, F. C., Andre, F., Gillon, J., Genin, C., and Sabatier, J.-C. Prevalence of IgA2 deposits in IgA nephropathies. A clue to their pathogenesis. N. Engl. J. Med. 303:1343, 1980.

143. Montoliu, J., Darnell, A., Torras, A., and Revert, L. Glomerular disease in cirrhosis of the liver: Low frequency of IgA deposits. Am. J. Nephrol. 6:199, 1986.

144. Czerkinsky, C., Koopman, W. J., Jackson, S., Collins, J. E., Crago, S. S., Schrohenloher, R. E., Julian, B. A., Galla, J. H., and Mestecky, J. Circulating immune complexes and immunoglobulin A rheumatoid factor in patients with mesangial immunoglobulin A nephropathies. J. Clin. Invest. 77:1931, 1986.

145. Coppo, R., Basolo, B., Piccoli, G., Mazzucco, G., Bulzomi, M. R., Roccatello, D., DeMarchi, M., Carbonara, A. O., and DiBelgiojoso, G. B. IgA1 and IgA2 immune complexes in primary IgA nephropathy and Henoch-Schönlein nephritis. Clin. Exp. Immunol. 57:583, 1984.

146. Conley, M. E., and Cooper, M. D., and Michael,, A. F. Selective deposition of immunoglobulin A₁ in immunoglobulin A nephropathy, anaphylactoid purpura nephritis, and systemic lupus erythematosus. J. Clin. Invest. 66:1432, 1980.

147. Sinico, R. A., Fornasier, A., Oreni, N., Benuzzi, S., and D'Amico, G. Polymeric IgA rheumatoid factor in idiopathic IgA mesangial nephropathy (Berger's disease). J. Immunol. 137:536, 1986.

148. Sakai, H., Nomoto, Y., and Arimori, S. Decrease of IgA specific suppressor T cells activity in patients with IgA nephropathy. Clin. Exp. Immunol. 50:77, 1979.

149. Cederholm, B., Wieslander, J., Bygren, P., and Heinegard, D. Patients with IgA nephropathy have circulating anti–basement membrane antibodies reacting with structures common to collagen I, II, and IV. Proc. Natl. Acad. Sci. 83:6151, 1986.

150. Sancho, J., Egido, J., Rivera, F., and Hernando, L. Immune complexes in IgA nephropathy: Presence of antibodies against diet antigens and delayed clearance of specific polymeric IgA immune complexes. Clin. Exp. Immunol. 54:194, 1983.

151. Galla, J. H., Russell, M. W., Hammond, D., Spotswood, M., and Mestecky, J. Environmental antigens (E Ag) in IgA nephropathy (IgAN). Kidney Int. 27:210, 1985.

152. Siegal, F. P., Siegal, M., and Good, R. A. Role of helper, suppressor, and B cell defects in the pathogenesis of the hypogammaglobulinemias. N. Engl. J. Med. 229:172, 1978.

153. Waldmann, T. A., Blaese, R. M., Broder, S., and Krakauer, R. S. Disorder of suppressor immunoregulatory cells in the pathogenesis of immunodeficiency and autoimmunity. Ann. Intern. Med. 88:226, 1978.

154. Reinherz, E. L., Cooper, M. D., Schlossman, S. F., and Rosen, F. S. Abnormalities of T cell maturation and regulation in human beings with immunodeficiency disorders. J. Clin. Invest. 68:699, 1981.

155. Hermans, P. E., Diaz-Buxo, J. A., and Stobo, J. D. Idiopathic late-onset immunoglobulin deficiencies. Am. J. Med. 61:221, 1976.

156. Dawson, J., Bryant, M. G., Bloom, S. R., and Peters, T. J. Jejunal mucosal enzyme activities, regulatory peptides and organelle pathology of the enteropathy of common variable immunodeficiency. Gut 27:273, 1986.

157. Henochowicz, S. Chronic diarrhea and weight loss in a patient with common variable immunodeficiency. Ann. Allergy 56:382, 1986.

158. Shelhamer, J. H., Neva, F. A., and Finn, D. R. Persistent strongyloidiasis in an immunodeficient patient. Am. J. Trop. Med. Hyg. 31:746, 1982.

159. Nagura, H., Kohler, P. F., and Brown, W. R. Immunocytochemical characterization of the lymphocytes in nodular lymphoid hyperplasia of the bowel. Lab. Invest. 40:66, 1979.

160. Hermans, P. E., and Huizenga, K. A. Association of gastric cancer with idiopathic late immunoglobulin deficiency. Ann. Intern. Med. 76:605, 1972.

161. Ament, M. E. Immunodeficiency syndromes and the gut. Scand. J. Gastroenterol. 20(Suppl. 114):127, 1985.

162. Conley, M. E., Park, C. L., and Douglas, S. D. Childhood common variable immunodeficiency with autoimmune disease. J. Pediatr. 108:915, 1986.

163. Wahn, V., Good, R. A., Gupta, S., Pahwa, S., and Day, N. K. Evidence of persistent IgA/IgG circulating immune complexes associated with activation of the complement system in serum of a patient with common variable immune deficiency: Anaphylactic reactions to intravenous gammaglobulin. Acta Pathol. Microbiol. Immunol. Scand. [Suppl.]284:49, 1984.

164. Bjorkander, J., Wadsworth, C., and Hanson, L. A. 1040 prophylactic infusions with an unmodified intravenous immunoglobulin product causing few side-effects in patients with antibody deficiency syndromes. Infection 13:102, 1985.

165. Frankel, S. J., Polmar, S. H., Grumet, F. C., and Wedner, H. J. Anti-IgA antibody associated reactions to intravenous gammaglobulin in a patient who tolerated intramuscular gammaglobulin. Ann. Allergy 56:436, 1986.

166. Wahn, V., Grosse-Wilde, H., Rosin, H., Carls, C., and Gobel, U. Partial in vivo response to corticosteroid treatment in common variable immune deficiency. Infection 13:15, 1985.

167. White, W. B., Ballow, M. Modulation of suppressor-cell activity by cimetidine in patients with common variable hypogammaglobulinemia. N. Engl. J. Med. 312:198, 1985.

168. Mayer, L., Fu, S. M., Cunningham-Rundles, C., and Kunkel, H. G. Polyclonal immunoglobulin secretion in patients with common variable immunodeficiency using monoclonal B cell differentiation factors. J. Clin. Invest. 74:2115, 1984.

169. Saulsbury, F. T., Winkelstein, J. A., and Yolken, R. H. Chronic rotavirus infection in immunodeficiency. J. Pediatr. 97:61, 1980.

170. DiGeorge, A. M. Congenital absence of the thymus and its immunologic consequences: Concurrence with congenital hypoparathyroidism. Birth Defects 4:116, 1968.

171. Thompson, L. F., and Seegmiller, J. E. Adenosine deaminase deficiency and severe combined immunodeficiency disease. Adv. Enzymol. 51:167, 1980.

172. Parkman, R., Rappeport, J., Geha, R., Belli, J., Cassady, R., Levy, R., Nathan, D. G., and Rosen, F. S. Complete correction of the Wiskott-Aldrich syndrome by allogeneic bone marrow transplantation. N. Engl. J. Med. 298:921, 1978.

173. Werling, S. L., Chusid, M. J., Caya, J., and Oechler, H. W. Colitis in chronic granulomatous disease. Gastroenterology 82:328, 1982.

174. Seligmann, M., Mihaesco, E., Preud'Homme, J.-L., Danon, F., and Brouet, J.-C. Heavy chain diseases: Current findings and concepts. Immunol. Rev. 48:145, 1979.

175. Seligmann, M., and Rambuad, J. C. Alpha-chain disease: An immunoproliferative disease of the secretory immune system. Ann. N.Y. Acad. Sci. 409:478, 1983.

176. Coulbois, J., Galian, P., Galian, A., and Couteaux, B. Gastric form of alpha chain disease. Gut 27:719, 1986.

177. Cho, C., Linscheer, W. G., Bell, R., and Smith, R. Colonic lymphoma producing alpha-chain disease protein. Gastroenterology 83:121, 1982.

178. Rambaud, J.-C., Piel, J.-L., Galian, A., Leclerc, J.-P., Danon,

F., Girard-Pipeau, F., Modigliani, R., and Illoul, G. Complete clinical, histological and immunological remission in a patient with alpha-chain disease treated by oral antibiotics. Gastroenterol. Clin. Biol. 2:49, 1978.

179. Brouet, J. C., Mason, D. Y., Danon, F., Preud'Homme, J. L., Seligmann, M., Reyes, F., Navab, F., Galian, A., Rene, E., and Rambaud, J. C. Alpha chain disease: Evidence for a common clonal-origin of intestinal immunoblastic lymphoma and plasmacytic proliferation. Lancet 1:861, 1977.

180. Veloso, F. T., Saleiro, J. V., Oliveira, A. O., and de Freitas, A. F. Atypical plasma cells in alpha-chain disease. Cancer 52:79, 1983.

181. Doe, W. F., and Spiegelberg, H. L. Characterization of an antiserum specific for the Fab alpha fragment. Its use for detection of alpha-heavy chain disease protein by immunoselection. J. Immunol. 122:19, 1979.

182. Doe, W. F., Danon, F., and Seligmann, M. Immunodiagnosis of alpha chain disease. Clin. Exp. Immunol. 36:189, 1979.

183. McDonald, G. B., Shulman, H. M., Sullivan, K. M., and Spencer, G. D. Intestinal and hepatic complications of human bone marrow transplantation. Part I. Gastroenterology 90:460, 1986.

184. McDonald, G. B., Shulman, H. M., Sullivan, K. M., and Spencer, G. D. Intestinal and hepatic complications of human bone marrow transplantation. Part II. Gastroenterology 90:770, 1986.

185. Manivel, C., Filipovich, A., and Snover, D. C. Cryptosporidiosis as a cause of diarrhea following bone marrow transplantation. Dis. Colon Rectum 28:741, 1985.

186. Snover, D. C., Weisdorf, S. A., Vercellotti, G. M., Rank, B., Hutton, S., and McGlave, P. A histopathologic study of gastric and small intestinal graft-versus-host disease following allogeneic bone marrow transplantation. Hum. Pathol. 16:387, 1985.

187. Lampert, I. A., Thorpe, P., van Noorden, S., Marsh, J., Goldman, J. M., Gordon-Smith, E. C., and Evans, D. J. Selective sparing of enterochromaffin cells in graft versus host disease affecting the colonic mucosa. Histopathology 9:875, 1985.

188. Sullivan, K. M. Graft-versus-host disease. In Blume, K. G., and Petz, L. D. (eds.). Clinical Bone Marrow Transplantation. New York, Churchill Livingstone, 1983, p. 91.

189. Shulman, H. M., McDonald, G. B. Liver disease after marrow transplantation. In Sale, G. E., Shulman, H. M. (eds.). The pathology of bone marrow transplantation. New York, Masson, p. 104, 1984.

190. Snover, D. C., Weisdorf, S. A., Ramsay, N. K., McGlave, P., and Kersey, J. H. Hepatic graft versus host disease: A study of the predictive value of liver biopsy in diagnosis. Hepatology 4:123, 1984.

191. McDonald, G. B., Sullivan, K. M., Schuffler, M. D., Shulman, H. M., and Thomas, E. D. Esophageal abnormalities in chronic graft-versus-host disease in humans. Gastroenterology 80:914, 1981.

192. Storb, R., Prentice, R. L., Sullivan, K. M., Shulman, H. M., Deeg, H. J., Doney, K. C., Buckner, C. D., Clift, R. A., Witherspoon, R. P., Appelbaum, F. A., Sanders, J. E., Stewart, P. S., and Thomas, E. D. Predictive factors in chronic graft-versus-host disease in patients with aplastic anemia treated by marrow transplantation from HLA-identical siblings. Ann. Intern. Med. 98:461, 1983.

193. Shulman, H. M., Sullivan, K. M., Weiden, P. L., McDonald, G. B., Striker, G. E., Sale, G. E., Hackman, R., Tsoi, M. S., Storb, R., and Thomas, E. D. Chronic graft-versus-host syndrome in man. A long-term clinicopathologic study of 20 Seattle patients. Am. J. Med. 69:204, 1980.

194. Storb, R., Deeg, H. J., Whitehead, J., Appelbaum, F., Beatty, P., Bensinger, W., Buckner, D., Clift, R., Doney, K., Farewell, V., Hansen, J., Hill, R., Lum, L., Martin, P., McGuffin, R., Sanders, J., Stewart, P., Sullivan, K., Witherspoon, R., Yee, G., and Thomas, E. D. Methotrexate and cyclosporine compared with cyclosporine alone for prophylaxis of acute graft versus host disease after marrow transplantation for leukemia. N. Engl. J. Med. 314:729, 1986.

195. Sullivan, K. M., Storb, R., Witherspoon, R., et al. Biology

and treatment of chronic graft-versus-host disease. In Gale, R. P. (ed.). Recent Advances in Bone Marrow Transplantation. New York, Alan R. Liss, 1983, p. 331.

196. Jewell, D. P., and Patel, C. Immunology of inflammatory bowel disease. Scand. J. Gastroenterol. [Suppl.] 114:119, 1985.

197. MacDermott, R. P., Kane, M. G., Steele, L. L., and Stenson, W. F. Inhibition of cytotoxicity by sulfasalazine. I. Sulfasalazine inhibits spontaneous cell-mediated cytotoxicity by peripheral blood and intestinal mononuclear cells from control and inflammatory bowel disease. Immunopharmacology 11:101, 1986.

198. Brogan, M., Hiserodt, J., Oliver, M., and Stevens, R. The effect of 6-mercaptopurine on natural killer–cell activities in Crohn's disease. J. Clin. Immunol. 5:204, 1985.

199. Lagercrantz, R., Perlmann, P., and Hammarstrom, S. Immunological studies in ulcerative colitis. V. Family studies. Gastroenterology 60:381, 1971.

200. Chapman, R. W., Cottone, M., Selby, W. S., and Shepherd, H. A. Serum autoantibodies, ulcerative colitis and primary sclerosing cholangitis. Gut 27:86, 1986.

201. Nagai, T., and Das, K. M. Demonstration of an assay for specific cytolytic antibody in sera from patients with ulcerative colitis. Gastroenterology 80:1507, 1981.

202. Das, K. M., Kadono, Y., and Fleischner, G. M. Antibody-dependent cell-mediated cytotoxicity in serum samples from patients with ulcerative colitis. Relationship to disease activity and response to total colectomy. Am. J. Med. 77:791, 1984.

203. Das, K. M., Dubin, R., and Nagai, T. Isolation and characterization of colonic tissue-bond antibodies from patients with idiopathic ulcerative colitis. Proc. Natl. Acad. Sci. USA 75:4528, 1978.

204. Takahashi, F., and Das, K. M. Isolation and characterization of a colonic autoantigen specifically recognized by colon tissue-bound immunoglobulin G from idiopathic ulcerative colitis. J. Clin. Invest. 76:311, 1985.

205. Bagchi, S., and Das, K. M. Detection and partial characterization of Crohn's disease tissue specific proteins recognized by Crohn's disease sera. Clin. Exp. Immunol. 55:41, 1984.

206. Bagchi, S., Baral, B., and Das, K. M. Isolation and characterization of Crohn's disease tissue-specific glycoproteins. Gastroenterology 91:326, 1986.

207. Stevens, R., Oliver, M., Brogan, M., Heiserodt, J., and Targan, D. Defective generation of tetanus-specific antibody–producing B cells after in vivo immunization of Crohn's disease and ulcerative colitis patients. Gastroenterology 88:1860, 1985.

208. Korsmeyer, S. J., Williams, R. C., Jr., Wilson, I. D., and Strickland, R. G. Lymphocytotoxic and RNA antibodies in inflammatory bowel disease: A comparative study in patients with their families. Ann. N.Y. Acad. Sci. 278:574, 1976.

209. Allinquant, B., Malfoy, B., Schuller, E., and Leng, M. Presence of Z-DNA specific antibodies in Crohn's disease, polyradiculoneuritis and amyotrophic lateral sclerosis. Clin. Exp. Immunol. 58:29, 1984.

210. Zuckerman, M. J., Valenzuela, I., Williams, S. E., Kadish, A. S., Das, K. M. Persistence of an antigen recognized by Crohn's disease sera during in vivo passage of a Crohn's disease–induced lymphoma in athymic nude mice. J. Lab. Clin. Med. 104:69, 1984.

211. Das, K. M., Simon, M. R., Valenzuela, I., Weinstock, J. V., and Marcuard, S. M. Serum antibodies from patients with Crohn's disease and from their household members react with murine lymphomas induced by Crohn's disease tissue filtrates. J. Lab. Clin. Med. 107:95, 1986.

212. Manzione, N. C., Das, K. M. Immunofluorescence assay using Crohn's disease tissue–injected athymic nude mouse lymph nodes in the diagnosis of inflammatory bowel diseases. Am. J. Med. 80:1060, 1986.

213. Selby, W. S., Janossy, G., Befill, M., and Jewell, D. P. Intestinal lymphocyte subpopulations in inflammatory bowel disease: An analysis by immunohistological and cell isolation techniques. Gut 25:32, 1984.

214. MacDermott, R. P., Nash, G. S., Bertovich, M. J., and Mohrman, R. F. Altered patterns of secretion and monomeric IgA and IgA subclass 1 by intestinal mononuclear cells in inflammatory bowel disease. Gastroenterology 91:379, 1986.

215. Thayer, W. R., Jr., Charland, C., and Field, C. E. The subpopulations of circulating white blood cells in inflammatory bowel disease. Gastroenterology 71:379, 1976.
216. Auer, I. O., Gotz, S., Ziemer, E., Malchow, H., and Elms, H. Immune status in Crohn's disease. 3. Peripheral blood B lymphocytes, enumerated by means of F(ab)₂ antibody fragments, null and T lymphocytes. Gut 20:261, 1979.
217. Bartnik, W., Remine, S. G., Chiba, M., Thayer, W. R., and Shorter, R. G. Isolation and characterization of human colonic intraepithelial and lamina propria lymphocytes. Gastroenterology 78:976, 1980.
218. MacDermott, R. P. Cell-mediated immunity in gastrointestinal disease. Hum. Pathol. 17:219, 1986.
219. Fiocchi, C., Battisto, J. R., and Farmer, R. G. Gut mucosal lymphocytes in inflammatory bowel disease. Isolation and preliminary functional characterization. Dig. Dis. Sci. 24:705, 1979.
220. Bookman, M. A., and Bull, D. M. Characteristics of isolated mucosal lymphoid cells in inflammatory bowel disease. Gastroenterology 77:503, 1979.
221. Shorter, R. G., Cardoza, M., Spencer, R. J., and Huizenga, K. A. Further studies of in vitro cytotoxicity of lymphocytes from patients with ulcerative and granulomatous colitis for allogeneic colonic epithelial cells including the effects of colectomy. Gastroenterology 56:304, 1969.
222. Shorter, R. G., Cardoza, M., Huizanga, K. A., Remine, S. G., and Spencer, R. J. Further studies of in vitro cytotoxicity of lymphocytes for colonic epithelial cells. Gastroenterology 57:30, 1969.
223. Stobo, J. D., Tomasi, T. B., Huizenga, K. A., Spencer, R. J., and Shorter, R. G. In vitro studies of inflammatory bowel disease: Surface receptors of the mononuclear cell required to lyse allogeneic colonic epithelial cells. Gastroenterology 70:171, 1976.
224. Kemler, B. J., and Alpert, E. Inflammatory bowel disease: Study of cell mediated cytotoxicity for isolated human colonic epithelial cells. Gut 21:353, 1980.
225. Shorter, R. G., McGill, D. B., and Bahn, R. C. Cytotoxicity of mononuclear cells for autologous colonic epithelial cells in colonic diseases. Gastroenterology 86:13, 1984.
226. Britton, S., Ecklund, A. E., and Bird, A. G. Appearance of killer (K) cells in the mesenteric lymph nodes in Crohn's disease. Gastroenterology 75:218, 1978.
227. Bull, D. M., and Ignaczak, T. F. Enterobacterial common antigen–induced lymphocyte reactivity in inflammatory bowel disease. Gastroenterology 64:43, 1973.
228. Meyers, S., Sachar, D. B., Taub, R. N., and Janowitz, H. D. Significance of anergy to dinitrochlorobenzene (DNCB) in inflammatory bowel disease: Family and postoperative studies. Gut 19:249, 1978.
229. Fujita, K., Okabe, N., and Yao, T. Immunological studies on Crohn's disease. II. Lack of evidence for humoral and cellular dysfunctions. J. Clin. Lab. Immunol. 16:155, 1985.
230. Harries, A. D., Danis, V. A., and Heatley, R. V. Influence of nutritional status on immune functions in patients with Crohn's disease. Gut 25:465, 1984.
231. MacDermott, R. P., Bragdon, M. J., Jenkins, K. M., Franklin, G. O., Shedlofsky, S., and Kodner, I. J. Investigation of T cell function by isolated human intestinal mononuclear cells. Gastroenterology 78:1213, 1980.
232. Hodgson, H. J. F., Wands, J. R., and Isselbacher, K. J. Decreased suppressor cell activity in inflammatory bowel disease. Clin. Exp. Immunol. 32:451, 1978.
233. Elson, C. O., Graeff, A. S., James, S. P., and Strober, W. Covert suppressor T cells in Crohn's disease. Gastroenterology 80:1513, 1981.
234. Elson, C. O., Machelski, E., and Weiserbs, D. B. T cell–B cell regulation in the intestinal lamina propria in Crohn's disease. Gastroenterology 89:321, 1985.
235. James, S. P., Neckers, L. M., Graeff, A. S., Cossman, J., Balch, C. M., and Strober, W. Suppression of immunoglobulin synthesis by lymphocyte subpopulations in patients with Crohn's disease. Gastroenterology 86:1510, 1984.
236. Elson, C. O., James, S. P., Graeff, A. S., Berensdon, R. A.,

and Strober, W. Hypogammaglobulin due to abnormal suppressor T cell activity in Crohn's disease. Gastroenterology 86:569, 1984.
237. Mielants, H., Veys, E. M., Cuvelier, C., De Vos, M., and Botelberghe, L. HLA-B27 related arthritis and bowel inflammation. Part 2. Ileocolonoscope and bowel histology in patients with HLA-B27 related arthritis. J. Rheumatol. 12:294, 1985.
238. Mielants, H., and Veys, E. M. HLA-B27 related arthritis and bowel inflammation. Part 1. Sulfasalazine (salazopyrin) in HLA-B27 related reactive arthritis. J. Rheumatol. 12:287, 1985.
239. Kagnoff, M. F. Association between Crohn's disease and immunoglobulin heavy chain (Gm) allotypes. Gastroenterology 85:1044, 1983.
240. Hodgson, H. J. F., Porter, B. J., and Jewell, D. P. Immune complexes in inflammatory bowel disease. Clin. Exp. Immunol. 29:187, 1977.
241. Nielson, H., Binder, V., Daugharty, H., and Svehag, S. E. Circulating immune complexes in ulcerative colitis. I. Correlation to disease activity. Clin. Exp. Immunol. 31:72, 1978.
242. Elmgreen, J., Wiik, A., Nielsen, H., and Nielsen, O. H. Demonstration of circulating immune complexes by the indirect leukocyte phagocytosis test in chronic inflammatory bowel disease. Relation to results of a standard complement consumption assay. Acta Med. Scand. 218:73, 1985.
243. Soltis, R. D., Hasz, D., Morris, M. J., and Wilson, J. D. Evidence against the presence of circulating immune complexes in chronic inflammatory bowel disease. Gastroenterology 76:1380, 1979.
244. Kemler, B. J., and Alpert, E. Inflammatory bowel disease associated circulating immune complexes. Gut 21:195, 1980.
245. Knoflach, P., Vladutiu, A. O., Swierczynska, Z., Weiser, M. M., and Albini, B. Lack of circulating immune complexes in inflammatory bowel disease. Int. Arch. Allergy Appl. Immunol. 80:9, 1986.
246. Hodgson, H. J. F., Potter, B. J., and Jewell, D. P. Humoral immune system in inflammatory bowel disease. I. Complement levels. Gut 18:749, 1977.
247. Ross, I. N., Thompson, R. A., Montgomery, R. D., and Asquith, P. Significance of serum complement levels in patients with gastrointestinal disease. J. Clin. Pathol. 32:798, 1979.
248. Lake, A. M., Stitzel, A. E., Urmson, J. R., Walker, W. A., and Spitzer, R. E. Complement alterations in inflammatory bowel disease. Gastroenterology 76:1374, 1979.
249. Kasarda, D. D., Bernardin, J. E., and Nimmo, C. C. In Pomeranz, Y. (ed.). Advances in Cereal Science and Technology, Vol. I. St. Paul, MN, American Association of Cereal Chemists, 1976, p. 158.
250. Jos, J., Charbonnier, L., Mougenot, J. F., Mosse, J., and Rey, J. Isolation and characterization of the toxic fraction of wheat gliadin in coeliac disease. In McNicholl, B., McCarthy, C. F., and Fottrell, P. F. (eds.). Perspectives in Coeliac Disease: Proceedings of the 3rd Symposium on Coeliac Disease. Baltimore, University Park Press, 1977, pp. 75–89.
251. Kumar, P. J., Sinclair, T. S., Farthing, M. J. G., Ohannesian, A. D., Jones, D., Emmett, S., Waldron, N., Clark, M. L., and Dawson, A. M. Clinical toxicity testing of pure gliadins in coeliac disease. Gastroenterology 86:1147, 1986.
252. Ciclitira, P. J., Evans, D. J., Fragg, N. L., Lennox, E. S., and Dowling, R. H. Clinical testing of gliadin fractions in coeliac patients. Clin. Sci. 66:357, 1984.
253. Holmes, G. K. T., Asquith, P., Stokes, P. L., and Cooke, W. T. Cellular infiltrate of jejunal biopsies in adult coeliac disease in relation to gluten withdrawal. Gut 15:278, 1974.
254. Falchuk, Z. M., and Strober, W. Gluten-sensitive enteropathy: Synthesis of antigliadin antibody in vitro. Gut 15:947, 1974.
255. Brandtzaeg, P., and Baklien, D. Immunohistochemical studies of the formation and epithelial transport of immunoglobulins in normal and diseased human intestinal mucosa. Scand. J. Gastroenterol. 11(Suppl. 36):1, 1976.
256. Kenrick, K. G., and Walker, K. J. Immunoglobulins and dietary protein antibodies in childhood coeliac disease. Gut 11:635, 1970.
257. Maury, C. P., Teppo, A. M., Vuoristo, M., Turunen, U., and

Virtanen, I. Autoantibodies to gliadin-binding 90 kDa glyco-protein in coeliac disease. Gut 27:147, 1986.

258. Levenson, S. D., Austin, R. K., Dietler, M. D., Kasarda, D. D., and Kagnoff, M. F. Specificity of anti-gliadin antibody in celiac disease. Gastroenterology 89:1, 1985.
259. Kagnoff, M. F., Austin, R. K., Johnson, H. C. L., Bernardin, J. E., Dietler, M. D., and Kasarda, D. D. Celiac sprue: Correlation with murine T cell responses to wheat gliadin components. J. Immunol. 129:2693, 1982.
260. Tosi, R., Vismara, D., Tanigaki, N., Ferrara, G. B., Cicimarra, F., Baffolano, W., Follow, D., and Aurichhio, S. Evidence that coeliac disease is primarily associated with a DC locus allelic specificity. Clin. Immunol. Immunopathol. 28:395, 1983.
260a. Howell, M. D., Resner, J., Austin, R. K., and Kagnoff, M. F. Rapid identification of hybridization probes for chromosomal walking. Gene 55:41, 1987.
261. Kagnoff, M. F. Two genetic loci control the murine immune response to A-gliadin, a wheat protein that activates coeliac sprue. Nature 296:158, 1982.
262. Weiss, J. B., Austin, R. K., Schanfield, M. S., and Kagnoff, M. F. Gluten-sensitive enteropathy. IgG heavy-chain (Gm) allotypes and the immune response to wheat gliadin. J. Clin. Invest. 72:96, 1983.
263. Kagnoff, M. F., Weiss, J. B., Brown, R. J., Lee, T., and Schanfield, M. S. Immunoglobulin allotype markers in gluten-sensitive enteropathy. Lancet 1:952, 1983.
264. Kagnoff, M. F., Austin, R, K., Hubert, J. J., and Kasarda, D. D. Possible role for a human adenovirus in the pathogenesis of celiac disease. J. Exp. Med. 160:1544, 1984.
265. Kagnoff, M. F., Paterson, Y. J., Kumar, P. J., Kasarda, D. D., Carbone, F. R., Unsworth, D. J., and Austin, R. K. Evidence for the role of a human intestinal adenovirus in the pathogenesis of celiac disease. Gut 28:995, 1987.

266. Sachs, J. A., Awad, J., McCloskey, D., Navarrete, C., Festenstein, H., Elliot, E., Walker-Smith, J. A., Griffiths, C. E. M., Leonard, J. N., and Fry, L. Different HLA associated gene combinations contribute to susceptibility for coeliac disease and dermatitis herpetiformis. Gut 27:515, 1986.
267. Seah, P. P., and Fry, L. Immunoglobulins in the skin of dermatitis herpetiformis and their relevance in diagnosis. Br. J. Dermatol. 92:157, 1975.
268. Leonard, J., Haffenden, G., Tucker, W., Unsworth, J., Swain, F., McMinn, R., Holborow, J., and Fry, L. Gluten challenge in dermatitis herpetiformis. N. Engl. J. Med. 308:816, 1983.
269. Kent, S. P., and Kirkpatrick, P. M. Whipple's disease. Immunological and histochemical studies of eight cases. Arch. Pathol. Lab. Med. 104:544, 1980.
270. Keren, D. F., Weisburger, W. R., Yardley, J. H., Salyer, W. R., Arthur, R. R., and Charache, P. Whipple's disease: Demonstration by immunofluorescence of similar bacterial antigens in macrophages from three cases. Johns Hopkins Med. J. 139:51, 1976.
271. Gupta, S., Pinching, A. J., Onwubalili, J., Vince, A., Evans, D. J., and Hodgson, H. J. F. Whipple's disease with unusual clinical, bacteriologic, and immunologic findings. Gastroenterology 90:1286, 1986.
272. Evans, D. J., and Ali, M. H. Immunocytochemistry in the diagnosis of Whipple's disease. J. Clin. Pathol. 38:372, 1985.
273. Barbier, P., Balasse-Ketelbant, P., Kennes, B., Menu, R., Platteborse, R., and Parmentier, R. Whipple's disease. An immunologic and electron-microscopy study. Arch. Fr. Mal. Appar. Dig. 64:659, 1975.
274. Haeney, M. R., and Ross, I. N. Whipple's disease in a female with impaired cell-mediated immunity unresponsiveness to cotrimoxazole and levamisole therapy. Postgrad. Med. J. 54:45, 1978.

7 | The Enterohepatic Circulation of Bile Acids in Health and Disease

ALAN F. HOFMANN

When food enters the small intestine, cholecystokinin-pancreozymin and secretin are released, causing secretion of bile acid pancreatic juice. Together, these secretions mediate the chemical hydrolysis and physical dispersion of nutrients—the process known as digestion. The active constituents of bile are the bile acids, which disperse, in the form of mixed micelles, the fatty acid and 2-monoglyceride formed by the action of pancreatic lipase on dietary triglyceride. Micellar solubilization of fatty acid and monoglyceride greatly increases their diffusion through the unstirred layer to the membrane of the enterocyte (see pp. 1068–1075). Bile acids are only slightly absorbed in the proximal small intestine, where the majority of nutrients are

absorbed, and are mostly absorbed by an active process in the terminal ileum. After absorption, bile acids are efficiently removed by the liver and promptly secreted into bile.

If the sole function of the bile acids were to facilitate fat absorption, their metabolism and enterohepatic cycling would be of nutritional significance only. But the importance of bile acids to clinical gastroenterology is far greater. First, bile acids induce bile flow and biliary lipid secretion; in man, their active secretion into the canaliculus is the major determinant of biliary flow and biliary cholesterol secretion. Second, bile acids are the water-soluble excretory products of cholesterol; in addition, by forming mixed micelles in bile, they permit the elimination of cholesterol as such in bile. Thus bile acids are lipid transporters, and their metabolism is intimately connected to cholesterol metabolism. Third, as noted, bile acids facilitate fat absorption, and indeed are essential for adequate absorption of fat-soluble vitamins. Thus, a bile acid deficiency has serious metabolic consequences, especially in growing children. Fourth, bile acids bind calcium ions, not only when present as micelles, but even when present in monomeric form. Bile acids thus decrease Ca^{2+} activity in bile, which prevents the formation of calcium-containing gallstones and solubilizes Ca^{2+} in small intestinal content; this may enhance absorption of calcium and also prevent calcium soap formation. Fifth, the major two dihydroxy bile acids present in bile induce colonic secretion of water when present in the colonic lumen in pathologically high concentrations; bile acid malabsorption causes bile acid diarrhea. Sixth, chenodeoxycholic acid (CDCA) and its 7β-hydroxy epimer, ursodeoxycholic acid (UDCA), when administered, induce the secretion of bile that is unsaturated in cholesterol; chronic administration of these agents induces gradual dissolution of cholesterol gallstones. Finally, bile acids are being explored as diagnostic agents, since their serum level provides information on intestinal and hepatic function, and increased fecal loss is a sign of bile acid malabsorption. Thus, bile acids are endobiotics with essential physiologic functions; they are causal agents in some intestinal diseases; they may be used to dissolve gallstones; and their concentration in body fluids may give useful information on hepatic and intestinal function.

The purpose of this chapter is to summarize their circulation in health and disease, to indicate how this circulation is impaired in disease, and to describe the consequences of this impairment. Other chapters deal with specific aspects of bile acid physiology: the role of bile acids in bile secretion (pp. 1656–1668), the use of bile acids to dissolve gallstones (pp. 1668–1691), the role of bile acid malabsorption in the short bowel syndrome (pp. 1106–1112), and the significance of bile acid deconjugation in the blind loop syndrome (pp. 1289–1297). For more complete coverage of the topics discussed here, the reader is referred to specialized texts[1, 2] on bile acids as well as a symposium on the physical chemistry of bile.[3] Biennial symposia on bile acids are held, and their proceedings are published.[4-7]

OVERALL PHYSIOLOGY

The *enterohepatic circulation* of bile acids should be viewed as a continuous stream of transport molecules, which carries nutrient lipids to the intestinal mucosa and transports cholesterol from the liver into bile, permitting its elimination from the body in feces. This movement of molecules accelerates with meals and slows during fasting, but its motion never stops (Fig. 7–1). As a consequence, the biliary tract and small intestine are continuously cleansed by a stream of surfactant molecules and mixed micelles.

Anatomically, in health, the majority of the bile acids are in the gallbladder during fasting and in the small intestinal lumen during digestion. The driving forces of the enterohepatic circulation are (1) convective flow (gastrointestinal propulsion and blood circulation), which is responsible for interorgan flow, and (2) cellular transport (by enterocytes and hepatocytes), which is responsible for transorgan flow.

During fasting, the majority of the bile acids are in the gallbladder. Some bile acids bypass the gallbladder and enter the duodenum, but these move only slowly along the small intestine, and the amount of bile acids entering portal blood is low. When a meal is eaten, the gallbladder contracts and the bile acid pool is discharged into the small intestine. Intestinal propulsion moves the bile acids along the intestine. Some passive absorption of the more lipophilic conjugated bile acids occurs throughout the intestine, but the majority of bile acids reach the terminal ileum, where an active transport process efficiently extracts the bile acids from the luminal contents; more than 90 per cent of the bile acids secreted with a meal are reabsorbed by the small intestine. After reabsorption, the bile acids are carried in the portal venous system to the liver, where they are efficiently extracted and promptly secreted once again into bile. A small fraction (10 to 50 per cent, depending on the bile acid) spills over

Figure 7–1. Schematic depiction of the enterohepatic circulation of bile acids in man. Gallbladder filling is determined by contraction of the sphincter of Oddi (not shown) and emptying by gallbladder contraction, which delivers stored bile acids to the intestine. The movement of the enterohepatic circulation is largely mediated by intestinal motility and the circulation of the blood. The serum level of bile acids is determined by spillover into the circulation of the fraction of bile acids returning from the intestine that is not removed by the liver. In healthy man, individual bile acids are eliminated from the body only in feces. The composition of the circulating bile acids is determined by (1) input of primary bile acids by synthesis from cholesterol, (2) input from the intestine of secondary bile acids formed by bacterial enzymes (not shown), (3) further hepatic biotransformation of secondary bile acids, and (4) the efficiency of intestinal conservation of primary and secondary bile acids.

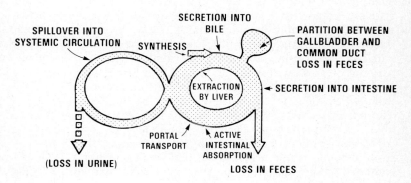

into the general circulation. However, these molecules are quickly returned to the liver in the hepatic arterial and mesenteric circulation, and are thus once again exposed to the efficient extraction process of the liver. The half-life of any bile acid molecule in the systemic circulation is only a few minutes.[8]

The enterohepatic circulation is composed of chemical pumps, mechanical pumps, valves, and storage chambers. The mechanical pumps comprise the canaliculi, the biliary tract, and the small intestine, which propel bile and small intestinal content, respectively, as well as the heart, which propels the circulation. The chemical pumps comprise active transport systems of the hepatocyte, ileal enterocytes, and renal tubular cells; the canalicular pump is noteworthy since it actually secretes bile acids with a measurable secretory pressure. There are two valves. The first is the sphincter of Oddi, which regulates gallbladder filling and discharge of bile into the duodenum. During overnight fasting, its contraction continuously diverts about half of the secreted bile acids into the gallbladder. The second is the ileocecal valve, which acts to retard passage of ileal contents into the cecum and thus promotes the absorption of bile acids from the terminal ileum before they are degraded by the enzymes of the anaerobic bacterial flora of the cecum. The major storage chamber is the gallbladder; the proximal small intestine is a minor storage area. During overnight fasting, gallbladder concentration permits storage of an increasing mass of bile acids without a proportional increase in gallbladder volume. The proximal small intestine also acts as a storage area during overnight fasting, although before breakfast, the majority of bile acids are stored in the gallbladder.

The anatomic localization of the enterohepatic circulation is determined by the anatomy of the hepatic circulation, by the activity of its pumps, by the extensive binding of bile acids by plasma proteins, and by the impermeability to bile acids of the epithelium of the storage chambers. Efficient ileal extraction is responsible for the passage of only small amounts of bile acids into the colon; efficient hepatic extraction from portal blood is responsible for the extremely low concentration of bile acids in the systemic circulation. All bile acids are protein-bound, the proportion varying from 80 per cent for the most hydrophilic bile acids to above 99 per cent for the most lipophilic bile acids.[9] Such protein binding decreases the movement of bile acids into other tissues and greatly decreases the passage of bile acids into the glomerular filtrate. The small fraction of plasma bile acids that are filtered are efficiently reabsorbed by the renal tubules, thus explaining the virtual absence of bile acids in urine. The absorbed bile acids return to the systemic circulation, from which they are efficiently extracted by the liver. The impermeability of the biliary and proximal small intestinal epithelium to bile acids maintains the concentration gradient established in the canaliculus: the concentration of bile acids in bile and small intestinal content is more than 1000 times greater than that in the surrounding cells.

The chemical pumps of the enterohepatic circulation are not regulated. What regulates the movement of bile acids in the enterohepatic circulation is the degree of sequestration of bile acids in the storage chambers and small intestinal motility. Storage in the gallbladder is mediated by contraction of the sphincter of Oddi, and in the proximal small intestine by the slowing of propulsive motility during overnight fasting. With ingestion of a meal, gallbladder contraction delivers the stored bile acids to the small intestine, and the bile acids present in the proximal small intestine are delivered to the distal intestine.

Of the organic constituents of bile, only the bile acids participate in a true enterohepatic circulation. Biliary phospholipid is hydrolyzed to lysolecithin and fatty acid by pancreatic phospholipase; the hydrolysis products are re-esterified in the intestinal mucosa and absorbed mostly as surface lipids of chylomicrons. These exchange with phospholipids of circulating lipoproteins and tissue membranes. The minority (20 to 40 per cent) of cholesterol is absorbed from the small intestine, the majority being excreted. Glucuronide and sulfate conjugates of drugs and steroids are poorly reabsorbed from the small intestine. Thus, the glycine or taurine of unconjugated bile acids serve as "signals" permitting active absorption by the specific transport system located in the terminal ileum.

Bile acids are always present in the systemic circulation because hepatic clearance of bile acids returning from the intestine is not complete. It now seems likely from much animal and human investigation that the fraction of bile acids cleared by the liver remains relatively constant and independent of the load delivered to the liver.[10] Accordingly, the concentration of bile acids in peripheral plasma is directly proportional to the load of bile acids presented to the liver from the intestine. As would be anticipated, the level of bile acids rises during meals when bile acid absorption increases, and falls between meals and during overnight fasting, when bile acid absorption decreases.

Bile acids differ from bilirubin, whose concentration in peripheral plasma remains constant. The hepatic extraction of bilirubin is much less efficient than that of bile acids—about 15 per cent for bilirubin, compared with 50 to 90 per cent for bile acids. The amount of bilirubin entering the plasma each day from the reticuloendothelial system is about 500 μM—the daily production rate; in contrast, about 30,000 μM of bile acids enters the plasma from the intestine each day. Nonetheless, the concentration of bilirubin in peripheral blood is 10 to 20 μM/L, whereas that of bile acids, even during digestion, is less than 8 μM/L.

CHEMICAL CONSTITUENTS: STEADY-STATE DESCRIPTION

Steroid Moiety

The bile acids participating in the enterohepatic circulation are primary bile acids formed in the liver and secondary bile acids formed from primary bile acids by the action of intestinal bacteria.

In man, two primary bile acids are formed in the liver from cholesterol. *Cholic acid* (CA), a trihydroxy acid, is $3\alpha,7\alpha,12\alpha$-trihydroxy-5β-cholanoic acid (Fig. 7–2). The other primary bile acid is *chenodeoxycholic acid* (CDCA), which is $3\alpha,7\alpha$-dihydroxy-5β-cholanoic acid. The synthesis rate of CA is about twice that of CDCA.[11] After formation, the bile acids are amidated with glycine or taurine as *N*-acyl conjugates to form the four conjugated bile acids, cholylglycine, cholyltaurine, chenodeoxycholyl(chenyl)glycine, and chenyltaurine. Conjugation is virtually complete in the hepatocyte, so that almost all bile acids leaving the hepatocyte are conjugated. Conjugation also has functional significance, in that conjugated bile acids are far stronger bile acids than their respective precursors. The pK_a of unconjugated bile acids is 5.0, that of glycine conjugates about 3.8, and that of taurine conjugates less than 1.0.[12] Since the conjugated bile acids are strong acids, they resist precipitation in the presence of acid or calcium ions and are much more slowly absorbed by passive, nonionic diffusion in the biliary tract and proximal small intestine.

The cholyl and chenyl conjugated bile acids are excreted in bile, and then into the small intestine where they promote fat digestion and absorption. The amide bond is completely resistant to pancreatic enzymes, and most are reabsorbed in the small intestine without deconjugation. Nonetheless, about one-fourth of the primary bile acid conjugates are deconjugated by bacterial enzymes in the ileum, liberating an unconjugated

steroid moiety. The majority of these bile acids are reabsorbed to return to the liver, where they are reconjugated with glycine or taurine (Fig. 7–3). Thus, for the primary bile acids there is synthesis and conjugation in the liver, followed by partial deconjugation in the intestine, with complete reconjugation in the liver (Fig. 7–3).[13]

Each day, one third to one fourth of the primary bile acid pool is lost and then converted by anaerobic bacteria to secondary bile acids. The most important change is 7-dehydroxylation, which converts CA to *deoxycholic acid* (DCA) ($3\alpha,12\alpha$-dihydroxy-5β-cholanoic acid) and CDCA into *lithocholic acid* (LCA) (3α-hydroxy-5β-cholanoic acid). The fates of these two secondary bile acids differ. About one third to one half of the DCA that is formed is reabsorbed; the absorbed, unconjugated DCA passes to the liver, where it is conjugated with glycine or taurine to form deoxycholylglycine or deoxycholyltaurine. The deoxycholyl conjugates are secreted in bile and reabsorbed with an efficiency similar to that of the dihydroxy primary bile acid conjugates, chenylglycine and chenyltaurine. Again, a fraction of the deoxycholylglycine and deoxycholyltaurine is deconjugated, and again, most of the liberated, unconjugated moiety is reabsorbed to return to the liver to be reconjugated with glycine or taurine. Thus, DCA, after its absorption, resembles a primary bile acid in its subsequent metabolism (Fig. 7–4).

LCA is insoluble at body temperature, and probably adsorbs strongly to colonic bacteria. About one fifth of the newly formed LCA is reabsorbed. It passes to

THE BILE ACIDS OF MAN

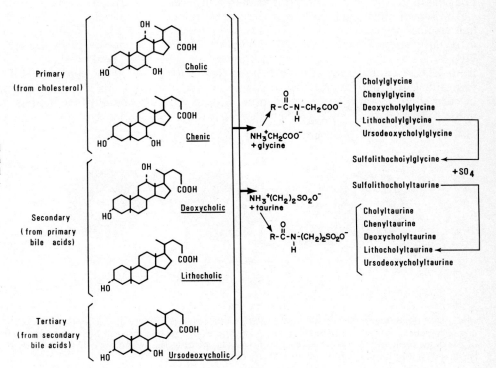

Figure 7–2. Chemical structures and trivial names of major biliary bile acids in human bile. The sulfate group is added at the 3 position of lithocholic. For average composition, see Figure 7–5.

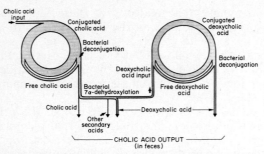

Figure 7–3. Enterohepatic circulation of cholic acid (left) and deoxycholic acid (right) in man. Only a fraction of the deoxycholic acid that is formed in the intestine is absorbed; this passes to the liver, where it is conjugated. The deoxycholyl conjugates then recycle in a manner similar to that of the primary bile acid conjugates. This figure also shows the two requirements for hepatic conjugation: unconjugated bile acid synthesized in the liver from cholesterol, and unconjugated bile acid formed in the small intestine.

the liver, where it is amidated with glycine or taurine. In addition, the majority of the LCA conjugates are then sulfated at the 3 position to form two new lithocholyl conjugates (Fig. 7–2), sulfolithocholylglycine and sulfolithocholyltaurine.

The subsequent fate of individual species of lithocholyl conjugates has not been well defined. In all probability, the unsulfated lithocholylglycine and lithocholyltaurine, which compose less than one third of biliary lithocholates, are efficiently reabsorbed from the small intestine and returned to the liver, where they are mostly sulfated. Thus, each lithocholate molecule is eventually sulfated and amidated. The sulfated conjugates, sulfolithocholylglycine and sulfolithocholyltaurine, are poorly absorbed from the small intestine, pass into the colon, and are eliminated in feces.

The fourth most common bile acid in many individuals is *ursodeoxycholic acid* (UDCA) (3α,7β-dihydroxy-5β-cholanoic acid), the 7β epimer of CDCA. UDCA is probably formed in the intestine by bacteria from CDCA. Some may also be formed in the liver from the 7-oxo (keto) derivative of CDCA, which can be formed in the intestine by the action of bacterial 7-dehydrogenases on CDCA. When the 3-hydroxy, 7-

oxo compound reaches the liver, it is reduced in part to UDCA, although the majority is converted to CDCA. These two bile acids are conjugated and secreted in the intestine, where they may be dehydrogenated to the 7-oxo derivative. This again may be absorbed and once again reduced to UDCA and CDCA during hepatic passage. Thus, CDCA undergoes reversible oxidation and reduction at the 7 position, so that CDCA and UDCA are both precursor and product of each other. However, the overall direction of these interconversions is markedly in favor of CDCA.

Bile also contains trace constituents of other secondary bile acids, which are mostly 3-oxo (keto) or 12-oxo acids.[14] Both the 3-oxo group and the 12-oxo group are reduced to their respective α-hydroxy groups during hepatic passage, so that the presence of these oxo bile acids in small amounts indicates incomplete reduction of presumably a larger fraction. At present, their physiologic significance is dubious, and their presence merely indicates uncommon bacterial biotransformations and the failure of the liver to reduce the oxo groups completely.

It is likely that trace amounts of many other secondary bile acids are absorbed from the large intestine and secreted in urine, where they can be identified by mass spectrometry.[15] The absence of these uncommon bile acids in bile probably has several explanations. Some, for example 23-carbon (C_{23} or "nor") bile acids, are poorly amidated in the hepatocyte and as a consequence reflux into the sinusoidal plasma. Others are glucuronidated or sulfated rather than amidated in the hepatocyte, and these conjugates are poorly secreted by the canalicular enzymes.

Bile acids are the only steroids in the body that are excreted solely by the fecal route and that are completely transformed by bacteria before elimination (Fig. 7–5). In most individuals, the predominant fecal bile acids are the secondary bile acids, DCA and LCA. The daily fecal loss is equal to hepatic synthesis of bile acids, since the bile acid molecule is considered to remain intact during intestinal passage. Thus, in healthy individuals, daily fecal bile acid loss is about 0.2 g of DCA and 0.1 g of LCA, reflecting hepatic

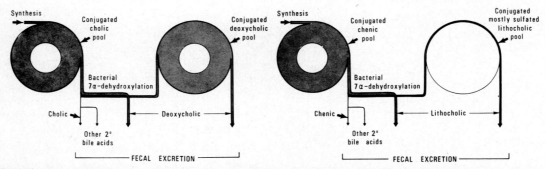

Figure 7–4. Enterohepatic circulation of steroid moiety of major primary and secondary bile acids. Ursodeoxycholic acid is not shown. The ring represents the right half of the loop shown in Figure 7–1, so that for each bile acid there is a loop, the left half representing the fraction of bile acids returning to the liver, which spill over into plasma. The proportion of lithocholic acid in biliary bile acids is least, as its input is least, and its loss is more rapid than that of any other bile acid.

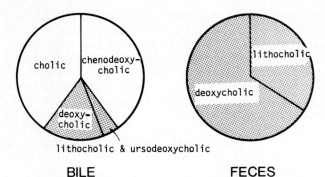

BILE   FECES

Figure 7–5. Average bile acid composition of bile (left) and feces (right) in healthy man. Cholic acid, chenic (chenodeoxycholic) acid, and deoxycholic acid together constitute usually more than 95 per cent of the biliary bile acids. The proportion of ursodeoxycholic and lithocholic acids is highly variable, but rarely above 5 per cent. The majority of lithocholic acids in bile is present in sulfated form, i.e., as sulfolithocholylglycine and sulfolithocholyltaurine. Trace bile acids that are present not only in bile and feces, but also in urine, are not shown.

synthesis of that amount of CA and CDCA, respectively. The CA and CDCA "families" are considered to maintain their individuality—there is no bacterial 12-dehydroxylation or hepatic 12-hydroxylation of bile acids. Thus, all LCA in the fecal bile acids is derived from CDCA and all DCA in bile originates from CA.[16]

The mass of any bile acid that is present in the enterohepatic circulation and exchanges with an injected tracer dose of that bile acid is defined as the bile acid pool. The steady-state size of the bile acid pool of any given bile acid is determined by the relative rates of input (synthesis or oral administration or both) and loss (from the intestine). The relative size of the individual bile acid pools determines biliary bile acid composition. In man, about twice as much CA as CDCA is synthesized; however, the conjugates of CDCA are more efficiently absorbed from the small intestine than those of CA; and as a consequence, the turnover rate of CDCA is slower, and its proportion in biliary bile acids is equal to or greater than that of CA. About one third to one half of the DCA formed in the colon is absorbed; its turnover rate is identical to that of CDCA; and as a consequence, its proportion in bile, which averages 15 to 20 per cent, may exceed that of the primary bile acids in some individuals. LCA has the lowest proportion in bile, since its input (from the colon) is least and its turnover rate is highest, since its sulfated amidates are poorly conserved by the small intestine.[11, 13, 17]

When bile acids are administered, the administered bile acids accumulate in the enterohepatic circulation. The overall effect of bile acid administration depends on a number of factors. The administered bile acid will accumulate in the enterohepatic circulation until its input (equal to ingestion if it is fully absorbed) is balanced by loss of its conjugates. This in turn is determined by the capacity of the intestine to actively (and passively) absorb the conjugates of the administered bile acid. The administered bile acid may be dehydroxylated in the large intestine, and these dehy-

droxylated derivatives may also accumulate. Finally, the administered bile acid may suppress the synthesis of primary bile acids in the liver.[17] Lastly, one bile acid (hyodeoxycholic acid, $3\alpha,6\alpha$-dihydroxy-5β-cholanoic acid) is glucuronidated, and the glucuronide conjugates are not reabsorbed from the small intestine and are excreted in part in urine.[18] Thus, when this bile acid is administered chronically, it does not accumulate in the enterohepatic circulation.

Conjugation Moieties

Bile acids are nearly completely conjugated in hepatic bile in man. Conjugation occurs exclusively in the liver, via a bile acid–coenzyme A intermediate. In health, bile acids are conjugated predominantly (60 to 80 per cent) with glycine. The remainder are conjugated with taurine, and no other conjugating groups have as yet been identified other than sulfate and glucuronidate. The only non-amidate present in bile in appreciable proportions are the sulfates of the lithocholyl amidates. Conjugation with glycine or taurine is strongly influenced by side chain structure. C_{23} nor-bile acids with a side chain containing one less methylene group are not amidated with glycine or taurine, but instead form a C_{23} ester, glucuronide.

The conjugating system prefers taurine for conjugation. The availability of taurine for conjugation depends on its rate of active uptake from plasma by the hepatocyte in relation to its rate of usage for bile acid conjugation.[19] Plasma taurine, and consequently hepatocyte taurine (and in turn bile acid amidation with taurine), are increased by diets rich in taurine-containing foodstuffs (for example, meat) or by ingestion of exogenous taurine. When taurine is administered, the majority of bile acids become conjugated with taurine. This has little effect on overall bile acid metabolism. (There is some decrease in the pool of chenyl amidates, which is likely to be explained by less efficient intestinal conservation of dihydroxy bile acids amidated with taurine, since these cannot undergo passive absorption in the proximal small intestine because of their being such strong acids.)

The proportion of bile acids amidated with glycine or taurine reflects the relative rates of deconjugation and reconjugation. In most individuals, hepatic conjugation is largely with glycine, and the glycine conjugates are more rapidly deconjugated during transit in the distal small intestine than the corresponding taurine conjugates. Thus, the glycine moiety of bile acids turns over more rapidly than the steroid moiety. For taurine conjugated bile acids, the two moieties of the molecule have similar turnover rates.

As was discussed, most bile acids are absorbed from the small intestine without deconjugation. The majority of the unconjugated bile acids formed in the distal small intestine are reabsorbed. The remainder pass into the large intestine.

Bacterial deconjugation occurs rapidly and completely in the cecum. There is probably little reabsorption of the intact glycine or taurine molecule. Glycine is metabolized to ammonia and carbon dioxide; taurine is metabolized to ammonia, carbon dioxide, and sulfate. All of these substances are partly absorbed to enter their respective metabolic pools and partly incorporated into bacterial metabolites.

In health, the only bile acids that undergo appreciable sulfation are the glycine and taurine amidates of LCA. LCA sulfates are excreted solely in bile; there is no urinary elimination. Probably a majority of LCA sulfates are hydrolyzed by bacterial sulfatases during passage of these bile acids through the colon, as careful fecal analyses have shown that most of the LCA in feces is not sulfated. Some of the sulfate is absorbed from the colon to enter the body's sulfate pools.

DYNAMICS OF ENTEROHEPATIC CIRCULATION

When a meal is ingested, the gallbladder contracts and bile acids are secreted into the intestine. Some passive absorption of dihydroxy glycine amidates occurs in the proximal small intestine, but the majority of bile acids pass to the terminal ileum, where they are actively absorbed. Bile acid secretion can be measured by duodenal perfusion techniques and is 30 to 60 mM (12 to 24 gm) per day, depending on the dietary intake.[20] The pool is 5 to 10 mM (2 to 4 gm), so it cycles about 3 to 12 times daily on the average. Bile acid secretion is unrelated to bile acid pool size, at least in many studies. Patients with small bile acid pools have a secretion rate similar to that of patients with large pools, because the small pool cycles more frequently. The size of the bile acid pool can be expanded by agents that slow transit and can be diminished by agents that accelerate transit.[21] If bile acids are administered, the pool expands until intestinal transport is "saturated." Thus, the limit for transport of bile acids in the enterohepatic circulation is the absorptive capacity of the small intestine.

Bile acids are absorbed solely in portal blood; there is no lymphatic absorption. Bile acids are efficiently extracted by the liver and promptly secreted into the biliary canaliculus. Uptake of polar conjugated bile acids involves a saturable, sodium-dependent process; uptake of lipophilic, unconjugated bile acids is passive and sodium-independent. Cellular transport does not involve ligandin, and other binding proteins are being sought and identified. The concentration of bile acids in the hepatocyte is considered to remain very low at all times, since canalicular transport, which is an active process, is extremely efficient. Cellular transport of bile acids is under active investigation in many laboratories at present.[22, 23]

Gallbladder bile has a bile acid concentration of 50 to 200 mM, and dilution in the small intestine lowers this concentration to 5 to 10 mM. Portal blood has a concentration of 0.01 to 0.02 ml, and peripheral blood has a concentration of 0.002 to 0.006 mM. The concentration in the canaliculus is unknown, but based on animal studies it is likely to be 5 to 100 mM.

Although it is tempting to consider the bile acid pool as a single entity, it is in fact composed of the individual bile acid pools, each with its own enterohepatic cycling pattern. Conjugates of CDCA and DCA undergo more passive jejunal absorption and therefore return to the liver more rapidly than conjugates of CA. When they reach the liver, they are extracted less efficiently than cholyl conjugates, so that a greater fraction spills into the peripheral plasma compartment. As a consequence, plasma bile acids are always enriched in CDCA and DCA.[24] For a given steroid moiety, the unconjugated fraction which is always being absorbed from the intestine is also extracted less efficiently than the corresponding conjugated fraction. Thus, plasma bile acids are always enriched in unconjugated bile acids.

The rhythm of the enterohepatic circulation—its acceleration during eating and deceleration during fasting—is determined by the pattern of dietary intake. Most individuals eat three meals a day and sleep at night. Accordingly, the enterohepatic circulation has three postprandial bursts of activity during the day (Fig. 7–6). The greater the intake, the greater the duration of the postprandial increase in plasma bile

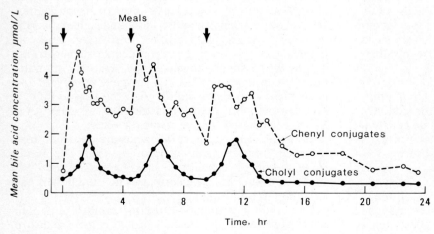

Figure 7–6. Profile of serum bile acid levels over a 24-hour period in healthy individuals ingesting three equicaloric meals. For each bile acid, there is a postprandial rise caused by spillover into the plasma compartment of bile acids returning to the liver. The spillover represents a rather constant spillover of an increased load. The serum level of chenodeoxycholyl conjugates is higher than that of cholyl conjugates, as the first-pass clearance of chenyl conjugates is less than that of cholyl conjugates.

acids. During overnight fasting, the enterohepatic circulation of bile acids slows but does not cease. Each cycle of the interdigestive migrating motility complex is associated with a weak contraction of the gallbladder and relaxation of the sphincter of Oddi, so that a small bolus of bile acids moves down the small intestine to the ileum.

The level of bile acids in peripheral blood always represents the instantaneous balance between intestinal absorption and hepatic uptake. Since the fractional clearance of each bile acid remains relatively constant, the diurnal variation in the level of bile acids in peripheral blood actually mirrors the movements of the enterohepatic circulation.

A physiologic pharmacokinetic model has been developed that describes in broad outline the input, interorgan flow, biotransformation, and liver and intestinal transport and loss of the bile acids during their enterohepatic cycling. The model has been used to simulate satisfactorily the enterohepatic circulation of CA,[25] CDCA,[24] and DCA[26] over a 24-hour period in man.

Bile Acid Structure and Function

Bile acids have a number of functions, and it is helpful whenever possible to relate these functions to the chemical structure and physicochemical properties of bile acids. The functions may be summarized: (1) generation of bile acid–dependent bile flow, (2) stimulation of bile acid–dependent biliary lipid secretion, (3) transport of lipids in bile and small intestinal content, (4) transport and buffering of metal ions such as calcium and iron, (5) regulation of bile acid and cholesterol metabolism, and (6) modulation of colonic desiccation, that is, cathartic activity.

Bile Acid–Dependent Flow. Conjugated bile acids are actively secreted into the canaliculus and induce bile acid–dependent flow by their osmotic properties which induce the movement of water and filtrable solute from plasma in the space of Disse (across the paracellular junctional complexes).[24] The bile acid molecules are too large to back-diffuse across these junctional complexes. Conjugated bile acids are strong acids and fully ionized at the pH of hepatic bile; their size and charge also prevent passive absorption in the biliary tree and thus maintain their osmotic effect in the lumen.

Stimulation of Bile Acid–Dependent Biliary Lipid Secretion. Bile acids induce the secretion of phospholipid and cholesterol into the canaliculus, presumably in the form of lipid vesicles. The mechanism of this effect is not known, and indeed the effect is not present in all species. In general, the more lipophilic the bile acid, the greater the stimulation of phospholipid and cholesterol. However, there are species differences in this stimulatory effect. In man, but not most other animals, CDCA and UDCA dissociate the secretion of phospholipid and cholesterol, so that the ratio of

cholesterol to phospholipid falls.[27] This effect is the rationale for the treatment of cholesterol cholelithiasis with these bile acids (see below).

Transport of Lipids in Bile and Small Intestinal Content. Bile acids form mixed micelles with polar lipids such as lecithin (phosphatidylcholine) and the mixture of fatty acids and monoglycerides formed by the action of lipases on dietary triglycerides. These mixed micelles can in turn solubilize other lipids such as cholesterol and fat-soluble vitamins in their hydrocarbon interiors. The ability of bile acids to form mixed micelles with such lipids is related to their amphipathic structure. The natural bile acids have a hydrophobic side and a hydrophilic side; they are mildly surface-active and aggregate to form micelles over a narrow concentration range (2 to 10 mM), often termed the critical micellar concentration (CMC).[12] Amidation with glycine or taurine, although lowering the pK_a of the bile acid, has little effect on the CMC value. The natural bile acids can be modified chemically (by altering the arrangement of the nuclear hydroxy groups) such that the hydrophobic side of the molecule becomes hydrophilic; such nonamphipathic bile acids have extremely high CMC values. The CMC is also influenced by the length of the side chain; as the side chain is shortened, the CMC rises exponentially. In general, the more "amphipathic" a bile acid is, the greater is its ability to form mixed micelles with polar lipids such as lecithin. In animals, replacement of the bile acid pool by nonamphipathic bile acids results in decreased efficiency of fat-soluble vitamins.[28]

Transport and Buffering of Metal Cations. Bile acids complex metal cations such as Ca^{2+}. Such complexation decreases Ca^{2+} activity in hepatic bile, thus decreasing the degree of supersaturation with insoluble calcium salts such as calcium carbonate. Complexation of Fe^{2+} in the duodenum may inhibit its precipitation and enhance its absorption. In the gallbladder, Ca^{2+} moves freely through the paracellular junctions. The activity of Ca^{2+} in bile is predicted by the rules of Donnan's equilibrium, since the gallbladder epithelium is impermeable to bile acid ions.[29]

Regulation of Bile Acid, Cholesterol, and Lipoprotein Metabolism. Bile acids induce biliary secretion of about 1 gm of cholesterol daily, and their daily synthesis is about one third to one fourth of this value. Most of the bile acids transported by the hepatocyte are "old" bile acids, that is, bile acids that have made multiple trips through the enterohepatic circulation. Normally, of the bile acids secreted into bile, less than 5 per cent are "new" bile acids, that is, bile acids just synthesized from cholesterol.

Nonetheless, the capacity of the liver for bile acid synthesis is immense. Normally bile acid synthesis is "down-regulated" or suppressed, since it is one fifth to one twentieth of its maximal rate. When the enterohepatic circulation is interrupted surgically (by bile fistula or ileal resection), pharmacologically (by ingestion of bile acid binding agents such as cholestyramine) or pathologically (by ileal disease), bile acid synthesis increases. The increase is proportional to the degree of interruption until the maximal rate of synthesis (4 to 6 gm/day) is achieved.[30]

The converse is also true, as was noted. The administration of most of the natural bile acids suppresses bile acid biosynthesis.

The mechanism(s) responsible for this apparent negative feedback inhibition has not been elucidated at a biochemical level. The simplest view is that bile acid biosynthesis is regulated indirectly by the concentration of bile acids in the hepatocyte. When this concentration falls, bile acid synthesis increases; when it increases, bile acid synthesis falls. The rate limiting enzyme has long been believed to be cholesterol 7-hydroxylase; however, the role of 26-hydroxylation is under active investigation as a rate limiting step in bile acid biosynthesis.[31]

Bile acid synthesis is equivalent to cholesterol degradation to an end product; in man, most cholesterol is eliminated as cholesterol rather than as bile acids (Fig. 7–7). Bile acid synthesis and cholesterol synthesis are intimately linked: any increase in bile acid biosynthesis must be followed by an increase in cholesterol synthesis. Increased synthesis of cholesterol by the hepatocye is generally accompanied by an up-regulation of LDL receptors, which increases the hepatic uptake of LDL, thus lowering the serum level of LDL cholesterol. The most potent up-regulation of LDL receptors is achieved by the simultaneous administration of inhibitors of HMG CoA reductase (the rate-limiting enzyme for cholesterol biosynthesis) and bile acid sequestrants. Under these circumstances, the hepatocyte appears to seek plasma cholesterol avidly; the marked increase in LDL receptors causes a dramatic fall in the serum LDL cholesterol levels.[32] The converse appears to be true. If bile acids and cholesterol are administered simultaneously, there is increased input into the hepatocyte cholesterol pool, and at the same time, inhibition of bile acid biosynthesis. As a consequence, LDL receptors are down-regulated; serum LDL cholesterol levels increase; and accelerated atherosclerosis occurs, at least in some species.

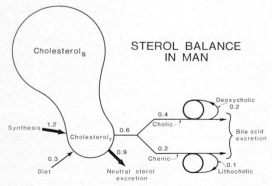

Figure 7–7. Schematic depiction of cholesterol metabolism in the healthy adult. The subscripts indicate the rapidly exchanging (r) and slowly exchanging (s) cholesterol pools. In man, in contrast to many other vertebrates, the majority of cholesterol is lost from the body as cholesterol. In many other vertebrates, most cholesterol is eliminated in the chemical form of bile acids.

To date, the structure-activity relationships for this regulatory effect of bile acids have had little investigation. CDCA increases serum cholesterol levels in man and, as noted, shares with CA and DCA (but not UDCA) the ability to suppress primary bile acid biosynthesis.[33, 34]

Inhibition of Colonic Desiccation: Cathartic Properties. At least 1 L of water enters the colon daily and about 80 to 90 per cent of this is absorbed. If colonic absorption of water is deficient, diarrhea results; if it is overly efficient, feces may become extremely hard, causing obstipation. Whether bile acids modulate colonic water absorption is not known, but there are a number of observations suggesting that bile acids may be important in normal colonic desiccation and stool formation:

1. When the aqueous concentration of bile acids is decreased in the colonic lumen by the administration of bile acid sequestrants, constipation is often noted.

2. When bile acids are present in elevated concentrations in the colon, diarrhea is observed.[35]

3. In a patient with defective bile acid biosynthesis, constipation was a severe clinical problem.[36]

4. In perfusion studies, dihydroxy bile acids induce colonic secretion of water and electrolytes as well as increase colonic motility.

The mechanism by which bile acids influence colonic electrolyte transport is not known. The current view is that conjugated bile acids pass paracellularly and act at the basolateral membrane level, possibly to increase cytosolic Ca^{2+}. Unconjugated bile acids can be absorbed passively and may reach the basolateral membrane by a transcellular route.[37] Much work is needed to clarify the significance and mechanisms of these effects.

DISTURBANCES IN THE ENTEROHEPATIC CIRCULATION OF BILE ACIDS

Disturbances in the enterohepatic circulation may be categorized as follows: (1) defective input, that is, defective biosynthesis from cholesterol, (2) defective transport (by the liver or intestine), (3) defective biotransformation (by hepatic or bacterial enzymes), (4) defective interorgan flow (cholecystectomy or portal-systemic venous shunting), and (5) combinations of any of the preceding.[17]

Defective Bile Acid Biosynthesis

Defective bile acid biosynthesis lies in the realm of inborn errors of metabolism. At least 12 enzymatic steps are involved in the conversion of cholesterol to conjugated bile acids, and to date, defects in at least four of these steps have been identified. No patient has been reported with a total absence of bile acid biosynthesis; presumably such a defect is fatal.

Cerebrotendinous xanthomatosis is a classic garrodian defect which presents clinically with tendinous xanthomas, normal blood cholesterol but elevated blood cholestanol, and neurologic disturbances. The defect (autosomal recessive) is attributable to defective mitochondrial 26-hydroxylation, so that normal side chain oxidation of cholesterol does not occur.[31] Bile acid synthesis, especially that of CDCA, is defective. Exuberant hydroxylation of the side chain occurs at positions other than the 26 carbon, and these bile alcohols are excreted as glucuronides in bile and urine in massive amounts, thus providing an alternative route for cholesterol elimination. The deficiency of bile acids leads to loss of feedback inhibition of cholesterol biosynthesis. Large amounts of 7-hydroxy cholesterol are formed; this is 7-dehydroxylated and hydrogenated in the liver to form cholestanol; the accumulation of this saturated sterol in myelin may be responsible for the neurologic manifestations of this rare genetic disease. Treatment with CDCA suppresses cholesterol synthesis, decreases cholestanol production, and results in a biochemical cure, sometimes with neurologic improvement. Treatment with UDCA is ineffective.[38]

Other defects of bile acid biosynthesis have been reported but are exceptionally rare. These include a deficiency in the 3-oxo-Δ^4-dehydrogenase-reductase, as well as deficient 24-hydroxylation.[39] The latter is one of many biochemical defects present in Zellweger's syndrome, a generalized defect in peroxisome formation. One case of defective 12-hydroxylase activity has been reported, associated with defective CA synthesis. The case presented clinically as severe constipation.[36]

Defective Transport

Cholestasis, whether caused by defective canalicular transport, increased ductular permeability, or obstruction to bile flow, causes bile acid retention. Secondary bile acids cannot form, since bile acids are not exposed to bacterial enzymes. The primary bile acids accumulate in the hepatocyte and undergo sulfation and glucuronidation after amidation. These sulfates and glucuronides reflux from the hepatocyte and are excreted in urine.[40] Bile acid synthesis is greatly reduced, as is cholesterol biosynthesis. Biliary phospholipid and cholesterol accumulate in blood as liquid crystalline aggregates, which associate with other lipoproteins and albumin to form "lipoprotein X." In this new steady state, cholesterol metabolism is characterized by absent secretion into and absorption from the intestine, by greatly decreased hepatic synthesis of cholesterol and bile acids, and by urinary loss of bile acids, mostly as sulfates, although some unsulfated bile acids as well as glucuronidated bile acids are also present in urine.

The second type of defective transport is defective intestinal transport causing bile acid malabsorption. Such defects are caused by ileal disease or loss of the ileum; several cases of an apparent acquired defect of ileal bile acid transport have been reported.

Several syndromes of bile acid malabsorption can be distinguished.

Bile Acid Excess in the Colon Causing Bile Acid Diarrhea. When there is a loss of ileal absorptive function because of a small resection or inflammatory

disease, the increased synthesis leads to a new steady state with increased amounts of bile acids passing into the colon. As noted, bile acid synthesis increases five to twenty fold. Provided bile acid malabsorption is not too great, bile acid secretion is probably normal in the morning, but declines gradually during the day. The bile acid pool is restored during overnight fasting because of the greatly increased synthetic rate. Fat digestion is relatively unimpaired, especially during the early part of the day. Even if there is some deficient micellar solubilization of lipolytic products during digestion of the evening meal, fat can be absorbed because there is an ample anatomic reserve.[35, 41]

The important abnormality of the enterohepatic circulation in these individuals is the greatly increased amount of bile acids passing into the colon (Fig. 7–8). The clinical consequences of this colonic excess of bile acids appear to depend on the interaction between the bile acids and the resident bacteria. The problem is complex because the bile acids influence the biotransforming activity of the bacteria, and the bacterial biotransformations influence the cathartic activity of the bile acids. In some patients, the increased concentration of bile acids passing into the colon appears to overwhelm the anaerobic species mediating 7-dehydroxylation, and primary bile acids persist in solution, since both CA and CDCA are soluble when the pH of colonic content is above about pH 6.8. The concentration of CDCA remains above its secretory concentration, and normal colonic desiccation does not occur. The result is a watery diarrhea caused by CDCA. If stool is ultracentrifuged, CDCA is present at a concentration of 2 to 6 mM in the supernatant solution.

In other patients, bacterial dehydroxylation continues to be complete, despite the increased load of bile

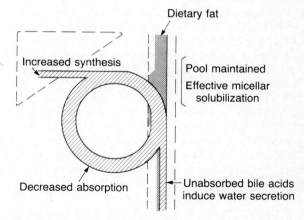

Figure 7–8. Mechanism of diarrhea in patients with bile acid malabsorption consequent to small ileal resection. In such patients, bile acid secretion is relatively unimpaired, at least during the first and second meals of the day. The relatively normal micellar solubilization, together with little loss of anatomic reserve, results in only mild fat absorption. The high concentration of bile acids entering the colon inhibits sodium and water absorption, causing diarrhea. Cholestyramine binds bile acids throughout the small intestine and reduces the concentration of bile acids in the colon, allowing normal sodium and water absorption; diarrhea is improved. In some patients, colonic pH is sufficiently acid that bile acids precipitate from solution, and diarrhea is not present.

acids passing into the colon. When dehydroxylation occurs, DCA is formed. If colonic pH is sufficiently high (pH >7.0), it remains in solution and causes diarrhea. On the other hand, if colonic pH is below 7, DCA is insoluble and diarrhea is minimal.[35]

Some patients with ileal resections have intermittent diarrhea. Possible explanations are changes in the dehydroxylating activity of the colonic flora or changes in intraluminal pH that influence bile acid solubility; however, the extent to which the colon adapts to a high intraluminal concentration of bile acids has not been clarified.

In individuals with diarrhea and elevated concentrations of dihydroxy bile acids in the colon, whether primary or secondary, cholestyramine administration causes immediate improvement of the diarrhea; indeed, the dose must be titrated, since obstipation may be induced.[41]

Bile Acid Deficiency in the Small Intestine Causing Fat Maldigestion, Fat Malabsorption, and Fatty Acid Diarrhea. In patients with large ileal resections, the increased bile acid synthesis cannot compensate for the increased loss, and bile acid secretion into the duodenum falls. In some patients, the compensatory increase in bile acid biosynthesis may be less than in patients with small resections. In such patients, bile acid secretion is decreased during breakfast and falls still further throughout the day. In addition, the secreted bile acid precipitate in part is insoluble calcium salts. The end result is that the concentration of bile acids is too low to solubilize in micellar form the products of fat digestion. As a consequence, dietary fat is absorbed far more slowly and throughout the length of the small intestine. Because of the loss of the anatomic reserve, the unabsorbed fatty acid passes into the colon, where, like bile acids, it induces water secretion, contributing to diarrhea (Fig. 7–9).[42] In the colon, bacterial dehydroxylation is efficient, and the secondary bile acids also rapidly precipitate from solution. Stringent reduction of dietary fat may improve the diarrhea, but the symptomatic benefit must be weighed against the inconvenience and unpalatability of a fat-free diet.

Bile acid deficiency in the small intestine also occurs in cholestasis or in patients with biliary drainage. In such instances, as in patients with large ileal resections, triglyceride lipolysis occurs normally, and fatty acids are absorbed by diffusion of fatty acid monomers. Fat absorption is greatly slowed and occurs throughout the length of the small intestine. Considerable fat absorption does occur (often about 50 per cent). The extent of absorption may depend on the nature of dietary fatty acids, since animal studies suggest that unsaturated fatty acids are absorbed more efficiently than saturated fatty acids when bile acids are deficient. Medium-chain fatty acids are efficiently absorbed, because of their high aqueous solubility. There is profound malabsorption of fat-soluble vitamins, and vitamin supplementation is necessary.

Bile acid replacement cannot be used in most pa-

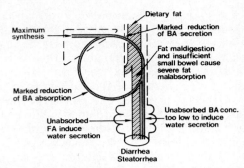

Figure 7–9. Mechanism of steatorrhea and diarrhea in patients with severe bile acid malabsorption induced by an extensive resection of the ileum. Hepatic synthesis of bile acids increases, but secretion of bile acids into the intestine falls progressively during the day. Micellar solubilization of digestion products of dietary fat is impaired and, together with the loss of anatomic reserve, becomes the major reason for severe malabsorption of fat. Unabsorbed fatty acids entering the colon inhibit the normal absorption of sodium and water. This "fatty acid diarrhea" is improved by removing fat from the diet. Bile acids appear to play little role in the diarrhea of such patients, because their concentration is too low to influence sodium and water absorption. The low concentration of bile acids in the small intestine is explained not only by decreased secretion but also by precipitation, perhaps as insoluble calcium salts. In the large intestine, primary bile acids are 7α-dehydroxylated to secondary bile acids, and this also contributes to their remaining in an insoluble physical state. (Based on published and unpublished data of Hofmann, A. F., and Poley, J. R. Gastroenterology 62:918, 1972.)

tients with bile acid deficiency in the small intestine. The administered bile acids may improve fat digestion and absorption, but very large quantities are required to simulate the normal hepatic secretion of bile acids during digestion—about 4 to 6 gm per meal. If this amount of bile acids is given, the diarrhea of such patients usually worsens because of the induction of colonic secretion.[43] There is one report of an ileostomy patient with steatorrhea and severe bile acid malabsorption secondary to ileal resection. Bile acid replacement caused a clinically useful improvement in steatorrhea and little worsening of diarrhea in this patient.[44] There is a need for an inexpensive bile acid replacement that does not induce diarrhea. An additional requirement for patients with cholestasis is that such a hypothetical agent not be absorbed.

Other Consequences of Severe Bile Acid Malabsorption. Steatorrhea caused by severe bile acid malabsorption can also cause hyperabsorption of dietary oxalate,[45] the mechanism of which is discussed on page 1863. Oxalate is a metabolic end-product, so that absorbed oxalate is promptly excreted in urine, causing hyperoxaluria. Hyperoxaluria, in turn, may cause oxalate nephrolithiasis if the solubility product of calcium oxalate is exceeded and crystal nucleation occurs.

Gallstones also occur more frequently in patients with severe bile acid malabsorption. Their pathogenesis is likely to involve a deficiency of bile acids in the biliary tree. This in turn leads to defective solubilization of cholesterol, causing cholesterol gallstones, or defective complexation of calcium, causing calcium carbonate gallstones.[46]

Defective Biotransformation

Defective bile acid conjugation has not been identified. Increased bile acid deconjugation occurs in the stagnant loop syndrome and may contribute to fat malabsorption since the liberated unconjugated bile acids are passively absorbed throughout the small intestine and also precipitate from solution at small intestinal pH.

Increased bile acid deconjugation is evidenced by high concentrations of unconjugated bile acids in the plasma. If cholyl-1-^{14}C-glycine is administered, $^{14}CO_2$ rapidly appears in breath.[47] However, not all patients with bacterial overgrowth have increased bile acid deconjugation.

Altered Interorgan Flow

In sprue patients, decreased cholecystokinin release causes defective gallbladder contraction evidenced by a large gallbladder and an expanded exchangeable bile acid pool.[48] Whether the intraluminal bile acid deficiency which occurs in such patients contributes to their fat malabsorption has not been clarified.

Cholecystectomy removes the major storage chamber for bile acids, and bile acids must be stored in the small intestine between meals. Astonishingly, the effect of cholecystectomy on the enterohepatic circulation is rather small: there is a tendency for the fasting-state bile acid level to increase and the postprandial increase to be "blunted," but these changes are minor.[49] Postprandial bile acid concentrations in the jejunal lumen during digestion are normal. Some patients develop diarrhea following cholecystectomy, but it is claimed that bile acid malabsorption does not play a major causal role in these patients, who are extremely heterogeneous; nonetheless, a brief therapeutic trial of cholestyramine is always warranted.[50] It is possible that the propulsion of bile acids in the distal small intestine is malregulated so that bile acids are absorbed less efficiently by the ileum and a greater fraction of bile acids spills into the colon. Post-cholecystectomy diarrhea appears to encompass a variety of clinical conditions, some of which may present as the irritable bowel syndrome. A therapeutic trial of cholestyramine should always be performed.

In portal-systemic shunting of bile acids, the bile acid load delivered by the intestine is shunted directly into the systemic circulation. The effect of such shunting on plasma bile acid levels is considerable and its magnitude depends on (1) the first-pass fractional extraction of the compound in question, (2) the degree of shunting, (3) whether or not there is a compensating increase in hepatic arterial blood flow, and (4) whether defective hepatic uptake is also present. The effect of portal-systemic shunting on plasma bile acid levels has been modeled using computer simulation, and it has been concluded that the effect of total portal-systemic shunting (for a compound with a fractional extraction of about 90 per cent) is to increase plasma levels by a factor of four, if blood flow is maintained by increasing arterial blood flow. If arterial blood flow is not increased, the level increases 16-fold. Thus, an increase in plasma bile acid levels that is greater than 16-fold is likely to indicate a defect in hepatic uptake in addition to shunting.

In liver disease, there are often multiple defects, such as shunting together with defective hepatic uptake. In cirrhosis, capillarization of the sinusoids may occur. In this defect, the fenestrations of the sinusoidal endothelial cells become smaller, causing a restriction to the diffusion of albumin-bound molecules into the space of Disse.[51] Such a defect should impair the hepatic extraction of extensively albumin-bound bile acid classes (for example, CDCA conjugates) to a greater extent than it impairs that of bile acid classes that are not so strongly bound to albumin (conjugates of CA). As predicted, the plasma level of CDCA conjugates increases to a greater extent than those of CA conjugates in patients with cirrhosis.[52]

BILE ACIDS IN THERAPY

The potential uses of bile acids in therapy follow from their functions.

Choleretic Agents

Bile acids induce bile flow, and it is logical to use bile acids as choleretic agents. At present, bile acids are not used in the Western world for this purpose

Figure 7–10. Bile acid composition of serum and urine (percentages, normalized to 100 per cent) from 23 patients with cholestasis, shown using circular coordinates. Only cholic and chenodeoxycholic acids are shown, as other bile acids constituted less than 5 per cent of the total bile acids in any sample. Urinary excretion of bile acids averaged 32 mg per day in these patients, compared with less than 0.5 mg per day in healthy controls. Bile acid glucuronides are also formed and excreted in urine in patients with cholestasis. (From van Berge Henegouwen, G. P., Brandt, K. H., Eyssen, H., et al. Gut 17:861, 1976. Used by permission.)

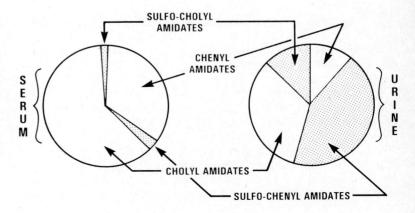

since there are no controlled studies showing that the induction of bile flow is of therapeutic benefit; moreover, there are probably a number of agents whose ability to induce bile flow is as great as that of bile acids. Dehydrocholate, a derivative of CA in which each hydroxy group has been oxidized to an oxo group, has been used as a choleretic for nearly 60 years. It induces bile flow osmotically, and the choleresis is greater than that induced by the natural bile acids, since dehydrocholate does not form micelles (it forms dimers above 40 mM). One gram of dehydrocholate induces about 25 ml of bile flow. However, the compound is completely metabolized to CA during a single passage through the liver. New bile acids have been synthesized with greater choleretic activity, but their clinical utility has not been tested. CDCA and UDCA, which are widely used for gallstone dissolution, also have considerable choleretic activity.[53]

Induction of Biliary Lipid Secretion

As noted above, CDCA and UDCA induce the formation of bile that is unsaturated in cholesterol. Chronic administration leads to enrichment of the bile with the administered bile acid, which in turn induces the formation of unsaturated bile in most patients.[54, 55] Radiolucent gallstones will dissolve in about half of the patients who ingest optimal doses of CDCA or UDCA (or the combination). Gallstones that are resistant to such therapy are likely to contain calcium salts on the surface.[56]

Complexation of Metal Ions

The ability of bile acid monomers and micelles to complex metals such as Ca^{2+} or Fe^{2+} has not been exploited in therapy.

Transport of Lipolysis Products of Dietary Fat

Bile acid replacement is not successful in cases of bile acid deficiency (cholestasis or interruption of the enterohepatic circulation because of biliary fistula or bile acid malabsorption), as was discussed earlier.

Regulators of Cholesterol Metabolism

In cerebrotendinous xanthomatosis, a disease of defective CDCA biosynthesis, therapy with CDCA is curative.[38]

In healthy individuals or in gallstone patients, the chronic administration of CDCA causes decreased cholesterol biosynthesis and down-regulation of LDL receptors, causing increased serum LDL cholesterol.[33] Accordingly, a major pharmacologic effort has been made to increase cholesterol and bile acid biosynthesis by the administration of ion exchange resins that bind bile acids in the intestinal lumen, decreasing their

intestinal absorption. A large, well-designed multicenter study showed that cholestyramine administration reduced serum cholesterol levels and coronary events in patients with hypercholesterolemia.[57]

Bile Acid Sequestration in the Intestine Induced by Administration of Binding Resins

Binding resins (cholestyramine, colestipol) are ion exchange resins and consist of a polymeric skeleton containing multiple positively charged sites. The agents are usually administered with the binding site occupied by a chloride counterion; in the intestine, the chloride ion is exchanged for another molecule. In the small intestine, such agents bind all anionic substances to some extent, but they have a special affinity for anionic substances that contain large hydrophobic regions, such as bile acids, fatty acids, and anionic drugs, since binding may involve both ionic and "hydrophobic" binding.

When cholestyramine is administered, bile acids are bound throughout the small intestine, inducing maldigestion.[58] The degree of maldigestion depends on the ratio of the amount of bile acid secreted to the amount of cholestyramine discharged from the stomach. Maldigestion is probably least at breakfast and greatest toward evening. As a consequence of fat maldigestion, fat is absorbed throughout the length of the small intestine; indeed, mild steatorrhea is frequent. The absorption of biliary and dietary cholesterol is impaired, and this decrease in cholesterol input also contributes to the known hypocholesterolemic action of these agents. Diarrhea is not present in such patients, since the concentration of bile acids and fatty acids in the aqueous phase of colonic contents is quite low. What is present is bloating and distention, which may arise from the involvement of the distal small intestine in the absorptive process. The increased bile acid synthesis appears to compensate for the increased loss, and steatorrhea increases only modestly. Bile acid binding is rather inefficient, probably because anions such as phosphate or sulfate compete with bile acid anions for binding. Synthesis, unlike postsurgical interruption of the enterohepatic circulation, is less than maximal.

In patients with mild bile acid malabsorption and bile acid–induced diarrhea, cholestyramine administration may cause striking symptomatic improvement with complete elimination of diarrhea. In some of these patients, diarrhea does not return when cholestyramine therapy is stopped.

DIAGNOSTIC VALUE OF SERUM BILE ACID MEASUREMENTS

Overview and Chemical Methodology

The level of serum bile acids represents the instantaneous balance between absorption from the intestine (input) and hepatic uptake (removal) and therefore reflects enterohepatic integrity.[8, 59] The value of serum bile acid measurements in the detection and management of hepatic or intestinal disease is limited, not because serum bile acid measurement is not a specific test, but largely because it does not represent a substantial benefit over existing tests.

Serum bile acids may be determined enzymatically with the use of a hydroxy steroid dehydrogenase from *Pseudomonas testosteroni*, which oxidizes the 3-hydroxy group to a 3-oxo group. The reaction requires DPN, and the reaction is quantitated by coupling DPN reduction to oxidation of a fluorescent indicator or a tetrazolium dye.[60] This method is simple, is moderately sensitive, and measures all bile acids—whether free or conjugated—that have a free 3-hydroxy group. Sensitivity can be increased greatly by coupling the DPN reduction to luciferase in a recently described bioluminescence procedure.[61] Serum bile acids may also be measured by radioimmunoassay; usually a class of conjugates—conjugates of cholic acid[62] or conjugates of CDCA[63]—is measured. Radioimmunoassay and bioluminescence have similar sensitivities.[64] Serum bile acids may also be quantitated by gas-liquid chromatography,[52, 65] and this in turn may be coupled with mass spectrometry.[66] This method is extremely sensitive but difficult technically, and can be performed only in research laboratories. It is the only method that provides complete chemical information on the composition of the steroid moieties of the bile acids present in the serum sample.

Plasma Bile Acid Measurements in the Detection of Liver Disease

Recent work suggests that the fasting-state serum bile acid level is a moderately sensitive but highly specific indicator of acute or chronic parenchymal liver disease; that is, bile acid levels are increased in patients who have liver disease as shown by biopsy yet have normal serum bilirubin levels.[67–69] For the detection of viral hepatitis type B, bile acids and transaminase appear to be of about equal sensitivity.[70] Bile acid measurement does not appear to be useful as a screening test to detect early liver injury caused by excess alcohol consumption[71] and is not as sensitive as the transaminase level for detecting carriers of non-A, non-B viral hepatitis.[72] Serum bile acid levels provide little or no information on the type of liver disease,[73] and early claims that postprandial measurements of bile acids provided greater sensitivity than fasting-state levels have not stood the test of time.

Whether fasting-state serum bile acid measurements actually provide clinically useful information remains unestablished. An elevated unconjugated bilirubin level coexisting with a normal serum bile acid level suggests Gilbert's syndrome.[74] Some, but not all, studies have suggested that the level of serum bile acids is helpful in distinguishing chronic persistent from chronic active hepatitis, probably because patients with chronic active hepatitis have some degree of portal-systemic shunting, as well as impaired hepatic uptake.[75] The sensitivity of serum bile acid levels appears to be superior to that of most other conventional liver tests for detecting early cirrhosis because probably no other plasma measurement is as sensitive as serum bile acid levels for detecting portal-systemic shunting (Fig. 7–11).[76] It has been claimed that in cirrhotic patients, the level of plasma bile acids is the best liver test for predicting survival.[77]

The fasting-state level of bile acids is much higher in the neonate and falls during the first year.[78] This decline is considered to indicate maturation of the hepatic transport mechanism. Interpretation of the serum bile acid level in infants is more difficult than in adults because of the greater difficulty in defining accurate confidence limits for normal values.

As noted earlier, in healthy individuals the fasting-state serum bile acid level is determined by the instantaneous balance between intestinal absorption and hepatic uptake. Intestinal absorption in the fasting state is determined by the amount of bile acids released into the intestine by the sphincter of Oddi and by intestinal transport, which in the fasting state is controlled by the interdigestive complex.

Because of this inherent ambiguity in fasting-state levels, several groups have explored the use of an oral tolerance test in which an unconjugated bile acid, such as UDCA, is administered orally and the increase in its level in serum is monitored.[79] Such tests are inconvenient but appear to have excellent specificity and some sensitivity. Definition of their clinical utility is

Figure 7–11. Schematic depiction of mechanism for elevated serum bile acid levels in patients with cirrhosis. In such patients, both portal-systemic shunting and decreased hepatic uptake occur (in part because of intrahepatic shunting as well as decreased permeability of the endothelial cells). The major factor likely to be responsible for increased serum bile acid levels is portal-systemic shunting.

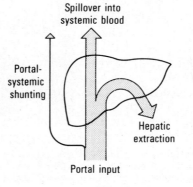
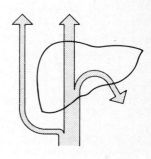

Spillover into systemic blood

Portal-systemic shunting

Hepatic extraction

Portal input

HEALTH

CIRRHOSIS

under study. At best, however, such tests can never distinguish blood flow defects (shunting or capillarization) from uptake defects.

Bile acid patterns may be obtained by gas-liquid chromatography, but at the moment these appear to be of little diagnostic value. The sole value of gas-liquid chromatography is its ability to signal the presence of novel bile acids in children with inborn errors of bile acid metabolism.[39]

Plasma Bile Acid Measurements in the Detection of Bile Acid Malabsorption

The significance of mild bile acid malabsorption is that it may cause diarrhea, the symptoms of which can be ameliorated by cholestyramine administration. In principle, the presence of bile acid malabsorption also has diagnostic significance, since the literature suggests that bile acid malabsorption is present more commonly than vitamin B_{12} malabsorption in patients with ileitis. However, many ileitis patients have no evidence of bile acid or vitamin B_{12} malabsorption,[80, 81] no specific therapy is available for ileitis, and it is not known whether prognosis or management of ileitis will be improved by the availability of a more sensitive test for assessing ileal transport function.

The postprandial increase in cholyl conjugates occurs because of active ileal transport of an increased load of bile acids and constant fractional hepatic uptake. Several patients have been reported to have a syndrome of primary bile acid malabsorption, which, by definition, is documented bile acid malabsorption occurring without evidence of anatomic abnormalities. In these patients and in the far more common condition of dysfunction because of ileal pathology or ileal resection, the fasting-state level is lower, and the postprandial elevation of cholyl conjugates is much lower than in healthy individuals.[4, 55] Further, the postprandial increase declines progressively during the day, so

that the increase following the evening meal is barely detectable (Fig. 7–12).

Since chenyl conjugates have considerably more passive absorption in the proximal small intestine, their postprandial increases are not as severely disturbed as those of the cholyl conjugates.

Administration of cholylglycine-1-^{14}C indicates bile acid malabsorption,[47, 82] so that both deconjugation (by breath $^{14}CO_2$ analysis) and bile acid conservation may be measured with this radiochemical. Bile acid absorption can also be assessed by measuring the serum level of bile acids after a meal, as noted,[49, 83] or after oral administration of a bile acid.[79]

A ^{75}Se (gamma emitting) derivative (SeHCAT) of cholyltaurine has recently become available and may be used to detect bile acid malabsorption by following retention in the body (using the gamma camera and counting over the gallbladder area) or by measuring the rate of fecal excretion.[84] The technique appears to be accurate, and its utility is being explored by departments of nuclear medicine. Chemical measurements of fecal bile acids also can be used to detect bile acid malabsorption, but the measurement is not useful as a screening procedure because bile acid loss may increase secondarily in other diarrheal conditions. Nonetheless, such measurements may be of value in the individual patient to define the degree of compensatory increase in bile acid biosynthesis that occurs in bile acid malabsorption.

METHODS FOR QUANTIFYING INDIVIDUAL COMPONENTS OF THE ENTEROHEPATIC CIRCULATION OF BILE ACIDS

For characterizing individual components of the enterohepatic circulation of bile acids in man, one requires accurate analytic techniques or radioactivity measurements or both; for interpretation of data, one

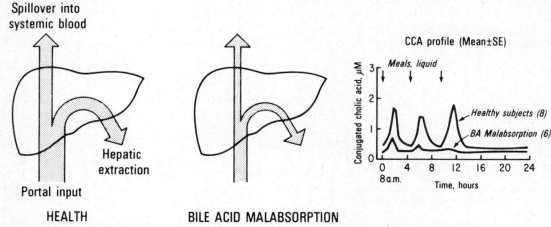

Figure 7–12. Schematic depiction of mechanism for decreased postprandial elevation of cholyl conjugates in patients with bile acid malabsorption. The amount of bile acids returning to the liver is less, and the hepatic first-pass clearance is similar to that in healthy individuals. Consequently, the postprandial elevation in the level of serum bile acids in these patients is less than that in healthy persons.

requires an understanding of the physiology of the normal and perturbed enterohepatic circulation. Available methods have been tabulated.[13]

Bile acid secretion is a flux of molecules and can be measured only in its accessible part, the small intestine, by perfusion techniques.[85] Bile acid synthesis can be measured by quantitating fecal bile acid output or by isotope dilution techniques.[11, 56, 57] The exchangeable bile acid pool may be measured by isotope dilution using either a single sample[58] or multiple samples[11, 57] of bile. Methods for measuring bile acid absorption have already been discussed.

The uptake of bile acids by the liver is probably best determined by direct measurements, that is, portal vein and hepatic vein concentrations.[86, 87] Hepatic uptake of bile acids may be determined indirectly by measuring the spillover into peripheral plasma of a bile acid administered by mouth and comparing the area under the curve (AUC) with the AUC after intravenous administration.[88] In principle, measurement of bile acid clearance after intravenous injection is the best way of characterizing hepatic uptake of bile acids. In practice, however, mixing and distribution problems complicate the problem of deconvoluting the plasma disappearance curve to obtain an accurate estimate of hepatic uptake kinetics; thus, intravenous bile acid clearance tests are likely to have little clinical utility.[89]

For determination of the composition of the bile acid pool, chromatography is necessary; gas-liquid chromatography[64, 65] is being replaced by reversed-phase high-pressure liquid chromatography.[90] Chromatography of fecal bile acids[91] gives information on the extent of bacterial biotransformation of bile acids lost from the enterohepatic circulation, but the input of secondary bile acids into the enterohepatic circulation can be quantitated only by the isotope dilution technique.[11] As noted, the composition of urinary bile acids reflects the balance between intestinal input and hepatic excretion. Urinary bile acids are extremely complex, as many minor bile acids appear to be absorbed from the intestine and excreted in urine rather than bile. Analytic methods capable of separating individual bile acids have been developed by Sjoevall and coworkers and applied to the analysis of urinary bile acids[15] and fecal bile acids[92] in health and disease. Thorough investigation of perturbed bile acid metabolism in gastrointestinal or hepatobiliary disease generally requires the collaboration of a chemically oriented clinician and a clinically oriented chemist.

References

1. Nair, P. P., and Kritchevsky, D. The Bile Acids. 3 vols. Vol. 1, Chemistry, 1971. Vol. 2, Physiology and Metabolism, 1973. Vol. 3. Pathophysiology, 1976. New York, Plenum Press.
2. Danielsson, H., and Sjoevall, J. Sterols and Bile Acids. Elsevier, New York, 1985.
3. Hofmann, A. F. The Physical Chemistry of Bile in Health and Disease. Hepatology (Suppl.) 4:1S, 1984.
4. Paumgartner, G., Stiehl, A., and Gerok, W. Enterohepatic Circulation of Bile Acids and Sterol Metabolism. Lancaster, MTP Press, 1985.
5. Paumgartner, G., Stiehl, A., and Gerok, W. Bile Acids and the Liver. Lancaster, MTP Press, 1987, in press.
6. Barbara, L., Dowling, R. H., Hofmann, A. F., and Roda, E. Bile Acids in Gastroenterology. Lancaster, MTP Press, 1983.
7. Barbara, L., Dowling, R. H., Hofmann, A. F., and Roda, E. Recent Advances in Bile Acid Research. New York, Raven Press, 1985.
8. van Berge Henegouwen, G. P., and Hofmann, A. F. Systemic spill-over of bile acids. Eur. J. Clin. Med. 13:433, 1983.
9. Aldini, R., Roda, A., Morselli Labate, A. M., Capelleri, G., Roda, E., and Barbara, L. Hepatic bile acid uptake: effect of conjugation hydroxyl and keto groups, and albumin binding. J. Lipid Res. 23:1167, 1982.
10. Angelin, B., Bjorkhem, I., Einarsson, K., and Ewerth, S. Hepatic uptake of bile acids in man. Fasting and postprandial concentrations of individual bile acids in portal venous and systemic blood serum. J. Clin. Invest. 70:724, 1982.
11. Hofmann, A. F., and Cummings, S. A. Measurement of bile acid and cholesterol kinetics in man by isotope dilution: principles and applications. In Barbara, L., Dowling, R. H., Hofmann, A. F., and Roda, E. (eds.). Bile Acids in Gastroenterology. Lancaster, MTP Press, 1983, pp. 75–117.
12. Hofmann, A. F., and Roda, A. Physicochemical properties of bile acids and their relationship to biological properties: an overview of the problem. J. Lipid Res. 25:1477, 1984.
13. Hofmann, A. F. The enterohepatic circulation of bile acids in man. Clin. Gastroenterol. 6:3, 1977.
14. Stellaard, F., Klein, P. D., Hofmann, A. F., and Lachin, J. M. Mass spectrometry identification of biliary bile acids in bile from gallstone patients before and during treatment with chenodeoxycholic acid. An ancillary study of the National Cooperative Gallstone Study (NCGS). J. Lab. Clin. Med. 105:504, 1985.
15. Alme, B., Bremmelgaard, A., Sjoevall, J., and Thomassen, P. Analysis of metabolic profiles of bile acids in urine using a lipophilic anion exchanger and computerized gas–liquid chromatography–mass spectrometry. J. Lipid Res. 18:339, 1977.
16. Danielsson, H., Eneroth, P., Hellstrom, K., Lindstedt, S., and Sjoevall, J. On the turnover and excretory products of cholic and chenodeoxycholic acid in man. J. Biol. Chem. 238:2299, 1963.
17. Hofmann, A. F. The enterohepatic circulation of bile acids. In Handbook of Physiology. Section on the Gastrointestinal System. In press.
18. Sacquet, E., Parquet, M., Riotto, M., Raizman, A., Jarrig, P., Huguet, C., and Infante, R. Intestinal absorption, excretion, and biotransformation of hyodeoxycholic acid in man. J. Lipid Res. 24:604, 1983.
19. Hardison, W. G. Relation of hepatic taurine pool size to bile-acid conjugation in man and animals. In Sulfur Amino Acids: Biochemical and Clinical Aspects. New York, Alan R. Liss, 1983, pp. 407–418.
20. Northfield, T. C., and Hofmann, A. F. Biliary lipid output during three meals and an overnight fast. I. Relationship to bile acid pool size and cholesterol saturation of bile in gallstone and control subjects. Gut 16:1, 1975.
21. Hardison, W. G. M., Tomaszewski, N., and Grundy, S. M. Effect of acute alterations in small bowel transit time upon the biliary excretion rate of bile acids. Gastroenterology 76:568, 1979.
22. Berk, P. D., and Stremmel, W. Hepatocellular uptake of organic anions. Prog. Liver Dis. 8:125, 1986.
23. Boyer, J. L. Mechanisms of bile secretion and hepatic transport. In Andreoli, T. E., Hoffman, J. F., Fanestil, D. D., and Schultz, S. G. (eds.). Physiology of Membrane Disorders. New York, Plenum Medical, 1986, pp. 609–636.
24. Molino, G., Hofmann, A. F., Cravetto, C., Belforte, G., and Bona, B. Simulation of the metabolism and enterohepatic circulation of endogenous chenodeoxycholic acid in man using a physiological pharmacokinetic model. Eur. J. Clin. Invest. 16:397, 1986.
25. Hofmann, A. F., Molino, G., Milanese, M., and Belforte, G. Description and simulation of a physiological pharmacokinetic model for the metabolism and enterohepatic circulation of bile acids in man. Cholic acid in healthy man. J. Clin. Invest. 71:1003, 1983.

26. Hofmann, A. F., Cravetto, C., Molino, G., Belforte, G., and Bona, B. Simulation of the metabolism and enterohepatic circulation of endogenous deoxycholic acid in man using a physiological pharmacokinetic model for bile acid metabolism. Gastroenterology 93:693, 1987.

27. Carulli, N., Loria, P., Bertolotti, M., Ponz de Leon, M., Menozzi, D., Medici, G., and Piccagli, I. Effects of acute changes of bile acid pool composition on biliary lipid secretion. J. Clin. Invest. 74:614, 1984.

28. Borgstrom, B., Krabische, L., Lindstrom, M., Lillienau, J., Midtvedt, T., and Corrie, M. Effects of feeding ursocholic acid to germfree rats. Scand. J. Clin. Lab. Invest. 46:183, 1986.

29. Moore, E. W. The role of calcium in the pathogenesis of gallstones: Ca^{++} electrode studies of model bile salt solutions and other biologic systems (with a hypothesis on structural requirements for Ca^{++} binding to proteins and bile acids). Hepatology (Suppl.) 4:228S, 1984.

30. Dowling, R. H., Mack, E., and Small, D. M. Effects of controlled interruption of the enterohepatic circulation of bile salts by biliary diversion and by ileal resection on bile salt secretion, synthesis, and pool size in the rhesus monkey. J. Clin. Invest. 49:232, 1970.

31. Bjorkhem, I. Mechanism of bile acid biosynthesis in mammalian liver. In Danielsson, H., and Sjoevall, J. (eds.): Sterols and Bile Acids. Amsterdam, Elsevier, 1985, pp. 231–278.

32. Brown, M. S., and Goldstein, J. L. A receptor-mediated pathway for cholesterol homeostasis. Science 232:34, 1986.

33. Albers, J. J., Grundy, S. M., Cleary, P. A., Small, D. M., Lachin, J. M., Schoenfield, L. J., and the National Cooperative Gallstone Study Group. National Cooperative Gallstone Study. The effects of chenodeoxycholic acid on lipoproteins and apolipoproteins. Gastroenterology 82:638, 1982.

34. Nilsell, K., Angelin, B., Leijd, B., and Einarsson, K. Comparative effects of ursodeoxycholic acid and chenodeoxycholic acid on bile acid kinetics and biliary lipid secretion in humans. Evidence for different modes of action on bile acid synthesis. Gastroenterology 85:1248, 1983.

35. Fromm, H., and Malavolti, M. Bile acid–induced diarrhoea. Clin. Gastroenterol. 15:567, 1986.

36. Dowling, R. H. Bile acids in constipation and diarrhoea. In Barbara, L., Dowling, R. H., Hofmann, A. F., and Roda, E. (eds.): Bile Acids in Gastroenterology. Lancaster, MTP Press, 1983, pp. 157–171.

37. Dharmsathaphorn, K., Pandol, S. J. Jr., and Ammon, H. V. Cl^- secretion induced by bile salts: a study of the mechanism of action based on a cultured colonic epithelial cell line. J. Clin. Invest., in press.

38. Beringer, V. M., Salen, G., and Shefer, S. Long-term treatment of cerebrotendinous xanthomatosis with chenodeoxycholic acid. N. Engl. J. Med. 311:1649, 1984.

39. Setchell, K. D. R., and Street, J. M. Inborn errors of bile acid synthesis. Semin. Liver Dis. 7:85, 1987.

40. Stiehl, A. Disturbances of bile acid metabolism in cholestasis. Clin. Gastroenterol. 6:45, 1977.

41. Hofmann, A. F., and Poley, J. R. Role of bile acid malabsorption in pathogenesis of diarrhea and steatorrhea in patients with ileal resection. I. Response to cholestyramine or replacement of dietary long chain triglyceride by medium chain triglyceride. Gastroenterology 62:918, 1972.

42. Ammon, H., and Phillips, S. F. Inhibition of colonic water and electrolyte absorption by fatty acids in man. Gastroenterology 65:744, 1973.

43. Hardison, W. G. M., and Rosenberg, I. H. Bile salt deficiency in the steatorrhea following resection of the ileum and proximal colon. N. Engl. J. Med. 277:337, 1967.

44. Fordtran, J. S., Bunch, F., and Davis, G. R. Ox bile treatment of severe steatorrhea in an ileectomy-ileostomy patient. Gastroenterology 82:564, 1982.

45. Chadwick, V. S., Modha, K., and Dowling, R. H. Mechanism for hyperoxaluria in patients with ileal dysfunction. N. Engl. J. Med. 298:172, 1973.

46. Heaton, K. W., and Read, A. E. Gallstones in patients with disorders of the terminal ileum and disturbed bile salt metabolism. Br. Med. J. 3:494, 1969.

47. Hess Thaysen, E. Diagnostic value of the ^{14}C-cholylglycine breath test. Clin. Gastroenterol. 6:227, 1977.

48. Low-Beer, T. S., Heaton, K. W., Pomare, E. W., and Read, A. E. The effect of coeliac disease upon bile salts. Gut 14:204, 1973.

49. LaRusso, N. F., Korman, M. G., Hoffman, N. E., and Hofmann, A. F. Dynamics of the enterohepatic circulation of bile acids. Postprandial serum concentrations of conjugates of cholic acid in health, cholecystectomized patients, and patients with bile acid malabsorption. N. Engl. J. Med. 291:689, 1974.

50. Fromm, H., Tunuguntla, A. K., Malavolti, M., Sherman, C., and Ceryak, S. Absence of significant role of bile acids in diarrhea of the heterogenous group of post-cholecystectomy patients. Dig. Dis. Sci. 32:33, 1987.

51. Huet, P-M., Goresky, C. A., Villeneuve, J-P., Marleau, D., and Lough, J. D. Assessment of liver microcirculation in human cirrhosis. J. Clin. Invest. 70:1234, 1982.

52. van Berge Henegouwen, G. P., Brandt, K-H., Eyssen, H., and Parmentier, G. Sulfated and unsulfated bile acids in serum, bile and urine of patients with cholestasis. Gut 17:861, 1976.

53. Okolicsanyi, L., Lirussi, F., Strazzabosco, M., Jemmolo, R. M., Orlando, R., Nassuato, G., Muraca, M., and Crepaldi, G. The effect of drugs on bile flow and composition. An overview. Drugs 31:430, 1986.

54. Bachrach, B. H., and Hofmann, A. F. Ursodeoxycholic acid in the treatment of cholesterol cholelithiasis: a review. Dig. Dis. Sci. 27:737 and 833, 1982.

55. Maton, P. N., Iser, J. H., Reuben, A., Saxton, H. M., Murphy, G. M., and Dowling, R. H. The final outcome of CDCA-treatment in 125 patients with radiolucent gallstones: factors influencing efficacy, withdrawal, symptoms, and side effects and post-dissolution recurrence. Medicine 61:86, 1982.

56. Freilich, H. S., Malet, P. F., Schwartz, J. S., and Soloway, R. D. Chemical and morphologic characteristics of cholesterol gallstones that failed to dissolve on chenodiol. The National Cooperative Gallstone Study. Gastroenterology 91:713, 1986.

57. Lipid Research Clinics Program. The lipid research clinics coronary primary trial results. I. Reduction in incidence of coronary heart disease. II. The relationship of reduction incidents of coronary heart disease to cholesterol lowering. JAMA 251:351, 1984.

58. Poley, J. R., and Hofmann, A. F. Role of fat maldigestion in pathogenesis of steatorrhea in ileal resection. Fat digestion after two sequential test meals with and without cholestyramine. Gastroenterology 71:38, 1976.

59. Paumgartner, G. Serum bile acids. Physiological determinants and results in liver disease. J. Hepatol. 2:291, 1986.

60. Dworsky, E., Corneliussen, L., Wold, K., and Krutnes, M-B. Determination of 3β-hydroxy bile acids in serum: a direct enzymatic colorimetric method. In Proceedings of the First International Symposium on Bile Acids in Hepatobiliary and Gastrointestinal Diseases. Oxford, IRL Press, 1984, pp. 25–36.

61. Roda, A., Kricka, L. J., DeLuca, M., and Hofmann, A. F. Bioluminescent measurement of primary bile acids using immobilized 7β-hydroxysteroid dehydrogenase: application to serum bile acids. J. Lipid Res. 23:1354, 1982.

62. Simmonds, W. J., Korman, M. G., Go, V. L. W., and Hofmann, A. F. Radioimmunoassay of conjugated cholyl bile acids in serum. Gastroenterology 65:705, 1973.

63. Schalm, S. W., LaRusso, N. F., Hofmann, A. F., Hoffman, N. E., van Berge Henegouwen, G. P., and Korman, M. G. Diurnal serum levels of primary conjugated bile acids. Assessment by specific radioimmunoassays for conjugates of cholic and chenodeoxycholic acid. Gut 19:1006, 1978.

64. Roda, A. Sensitive methods for serum bile acid analysis. In Barbara, L., Dowling, R. H., Hofmann, A. F., and Roda, E. (eds.): Bile Acids in Gastroenterology. Lancaster, MTP Press, 1983, pp. 57–68.

65. Setchell, K. D. R., and Matsui, A. Serum bile acid analysis. Clin. Chim. Acta 127:1, 1983.

66. Bjorkhem, I., and Falk, O. Assay of the major bile acids in serum by isotope dilution—mass spectrometry. Scand. J. Clin. Lab. Invest. 43:163, 1983.

67. Cravetto, C., Molino, G., Biondi, A. M., Cavanna, A., Avag-

nina, P., and Frediani, S. Evaluation of the diagnostic value of serum bile acids in the detection and functional assessment of liver diseases. Ann. Clin. Biochem. 22:596, 1985.

68. Ferraris, R., Colombatti, G., Fiorentini, M. T., Carosso, R., Arossa, W., and De la Pierre, M. Diagnostic value of serum bile acids and routine liver function tests in hepatobiliary diseases. Dig. Dis. Sci. 28:129, 1983.

69. Festi, D., Morselli Labate, A. M., Roda, A., Bassoli, F., Frabboni, R., Rucci, P., Taroni, F., Aldini, R., Roda, E., and Barbara, L. Diagnostic effectiveness of serum bile acids in liver diseases as evaluated by multivariate statistical methods. Hepatology 3:707, 1983.

70. Gitnick, G. L., Brezina, M. L., and Mullen, R. L. Application of alanine aminotransferase, carcinoembryonic antigen, and cholyl glycine levels to the prevention and evaluation of acute and chronic hepatitis. In Vyas, G. N., Cohen, S. N., and Schmid, R. (eds.). Viral Hepatitis: A Contemporary Assessment of Etiology, Epidemiology, Pathogenesis, and Prevention. Philadelphia, Franklin Institute Press, 1978, pp. 431–438.

71. Tobiasson, P., and Boeryd, B. Serum bile acids in alcoholic liver disease. In Proceedings of the First International Symposium on Bile Acids in Hepatobiliary and Gastrointestinal Diseases. Oxford, IRL Press, 1984, pp. 111–120.

72. Mishler, J. M. IV., Barbosa, L., Mihalko, L. J., and McCarter, H. Serum bile acids and alanine aminotransferase concentrations. JAMA 246:2340, 1981.

73. Linnet, K., and Andersen, J. R. Differential diagnostic value in hepatobiliary disease of serum conjugated bile acid concentrations and some routine liver tests assessed by discriminant analysis. Clin. Chim. Acta 127:217, 1983.

74. Vierling, J. M., Berk, P. D., Hofmann, A. F., Martin, J. F., Wolkoff, A. W., and Scharschmidt, B. F. Normal fasting-state levels of serum cholyl-conjugated bile acids in Gilbert's syndrome: an aid to the diagnosis. Hepatology 2:340, 1982.

75. Monroe, P. S., Baker, A. L., Schneider, J. F., Krager, S., Klein, P. D., and Schoeller, D. The aminopyrine breath test and serum bile acids reflect histologic severity in chronic hepatitis. Hepatology 2:317, 1982.

76. Mannes, G. A., Stellaard, F., and Paumgartner, G. Increased serum bile acids in cirrhosis with normal transaminases. Digestion 25:217, 1982.

77. Mannes, G. A., Thieme, C., Stellaard, F., Wang, T., Sauerbruch, T., and Paumgartner, G. Prognostic significance of serum bile acids in cirrhosis. Hepatology 6:50, 1986.

78. Balistreri, W. F. Immaturity of hepatic excretory function and the ontogeny of bile acid metabolism. J. Pediatr. Gastroenterol. Nutr. 2(Suppl. 1):S207, 1983.

79. Miescher, G., Paumgartner, G., and Preisig, R. Portal-systemic spill-over of bile acids: a study of mechanisms using ursodeoxycholic aids. Eur. J. Clin. Invest. 13:439, 1983.

80. Lenz, K. An evaluation of the "breath test" in Crohn's disease. Scand. J. Gastroenterol. 10:665, 1975.

81. Sarva, R. P., Farivar, S., Fromm, H., Bazzoli, F., Wald, A., and Amin, P. M. Comparative sensitivity of eight- and 24-hour bile acid breath tests and Schilling test in ileopathies. Am. J. Gastroenterol. 76:432, 1981.

82. Fromm, H., Thomas, P. J., and Hofmann, A. F. Sensitivity and specificity in tests of distal ileal function: prospective comparison of bile acid and vitamin B_{12} absorption in ileal resection patients. Gastroenterology 64:1077, 1973.

83. Aldini, R., Roda, A., Festi, D., Mazzella, G., Morselli, A. M., Sama, C., Roda, E., Scopinaro, N., and Barbara, L. Diagnostic value of serum primary bile acids in detecting bile acid malabsorption. Gut 23:829, 1982.

84. Sciarretta, G., Vicini, G., Fagioli, G., Verri, A., Ginevra, A., and Malaguti, P. Use of 23-selena-25-homocholyltaurine to detect bile acid malabsorption in patients with ileal dysfunction or diarrhea. Gastroenterology 91:1, 1986.

85. Reuben, A., Maton, P. N., Murphy, G. M., and Dowling, R. H. Bile lipid secretion in obese and non-obese individuals with and without gallstones. Clin. Sci. 69:71, 1985.

86. Marigold, J. K., Gilmore, I. T., and Thompson, R. P. H. Effects of a meal on plasma clearance of [^{14}C]-glycocholic acid and indocyanine green in man. Clin. Sci. 61:325, 1981.

87. Ewerth, S., Angelin, B., Einarsson, K., Nilsell, K., and Bjorkhem, I. Serum concentrations of ursodeoxycholic acid in portal venous and systemic venous blood of fasting humans as determined by isotope dilution–mass spectrometry. Gastroenterology 88:126, 1985.

88. van Berge Henegouwen, G. P., and Hofmann, A. F. Pharmacology of chenodeoxycholic acid. II. Absorption and metabolism. Gastroenterology 73:300, 1977.

89. Thjodleifsson, B., Barnes, S., Chitranukroh, A., Billing, B. H., and Sherlock, S. Cholyl-^{14}C-glycine clearance and serum bile acid concentration for the detection of liver disease. (Abstract.) Digestion 14:553, 1976.

90. Rossi, S. S., Converse, J. L., and Hofmann, A. F. High pressure liquid chromatographic analysis of conjugated bile acids in human bile: simultaneous resolution of sulfated and unsulfated lithocholyl amidates and the common conjugated bile acids. J. Lipid Res. 28:589, 1987.

91. Setchell, K. D. R., Street, J. M., and Sjoevall, J. Fecal bile acids. In Kritchevsky, D., Nair, P. P., and Setchell, K. D. R. (eds.): The Bile Acids. Volume 4. New York, Plenum Press, in press.

92. Setchell, K. D. R., Lawson, A. M., Tanida, N., and Sjoevall, J. General methods for the analysis of metabolic profiles of bile acids and related compounds in feces. J. Lipid Res. 24:1085, 1983.

8 The Effect of Age on Gastrointestinal Function

DAVID F. ALTMAN

I grow old . . . I grow old . . .
I shall wear the bottoms of my trousers rolled.
Shall I part my hair behind? Do I dare to eat a peach?

"The Love Song of J. Alfred Prufrock"
T. S. Eliot

The population of the United States is rapidly aging. In 1900, 4.1 per cent of Americans were over 65 years old; by the year 2000, it is expected that 11.3 per cent will be over that age.[1] With this change of our population we are becoming more aware of the special medical needs of the elderly.

Gastrointestinal complaints comprise a large portion of the reasons for elderly individuals to seek health care. The gastrointestinal tract is certainly subject to the influence of aging, both with respect to normal changes in function and with altered manifestations of diseases in older patients. There are also a number of important diseases of the gut that are seen almost exclusively in the elderly.

CHANGES IN GUT FUNCTION WITH AGING
(Table 8–1)

Esophagus

Pharyngoesophageal function appears to change with age, but the clinical significance of these changes remains unclear. Piaget and Fouillet, in radiographic

Table 8–1. THE EFFECTS OF AGING ON THE GASTROINTESTINAL TRACT

Esophagus	Motility	Hypopharyngeal dysfunction
		Diminished lower esophageal sphincter
Stomach	Morphology	None
	Motility	Slowed gastric emptying of liquids and solids
	Secretion	Diminished secretion of acid and pepsin
Small intestine	Morphology	Minor increase in crypt length
	Motility	None
	Absorption	Decreased disaccharidase activity
Colon	Motility	Uncertain
	Anorectal function	Decreased rectal capacitance
Pancreas	Morphology	Ductal dilatation
		Fibrosis
Biliary tree	Motility	Unchanged
	Bile composition	Increased lithogenicity

examinations of 100 asymptomatic subjects over 65 years old, showed abnormal hypopharyngeal function in 22, with pharyngeal hypotonicity, incomplete opening of the cricopharyngeus muscle, pooling of barium in the pyriform sinuses, or aspiration of barium.[2] In addition, studies of motility in the body of the esophagus and lower esophageal sphincter have shown diminished amplitude of peristaltic contractions, frequent tertiary contractions, delayed esophageal emptying, incomplete sphincter relaxation, and esophageal dilation. This complex had been termed presbyesophagus, but carefully conducted studies by Hollis and Castell in elderly men without diabetes or neurologic diseases showed only diminished amplitude of contraction, a change of little if any clinical significance.[3] Thus presbyesophagus may be a reflection of the increased frequency of conditions such as stroke and diabetes in the elderly, rather than a reflection of diminished esophageal function per se.

Stomach

Morphologic Changes

The incidence of chronic gastritis and gastric atrophy increase with age, and the juncture of fundic and pyloric mucosae also migrates proximally.[4] However, these changes do not appear to be normal concomitants of aging, as studies by Bird and colleagues have shown normal gastric mucosa in a third of patients over age 80 and over half of those over age 90.[5]

Gastric Motility

Gastric motility and gastric emptying appear to diminish progressively with age. Studies using radiolabeled solid and liquid phases of meals have shown that it is primarily the vagally mediated liquid emptying that is slowed; the antrally determined emptying of solids is the same in the elderly as in the young.[6] These observations are confounded, however, by the influence of acid on gastric emptying: the emptying of solids is slowed by the presence of acid, but with achlorhydria relatively common in the elderly it is not yet possible to know the contribution of the decreased acid secretion or of any underlying disease of the gastric wall on emptying. In one study of achlorhydric patients with pernicious anemia or atrophic gastritis, gastric emptying of solids was accelerated by the intragastric instillation of acid and pepsin, although not into the range

162

observed in healthy controls.[7] The addition of metoclopramide did improve emptying to normal. These results suggest that although intragastric pH may have some role in determining the rate of emptying, diminished capacity of the antral musculature might be more important.

Gastric Secretory Function

Acid. It is generally accepted that gastric acid secretion diminishes with age. In classic studies reported by Grossman and co-workers in 1963 using betazole (Histalog) stimulation, basal and stimulated acid production diminished after age 50, particularly in men.[8] In addition, the frequency of basal achlorhydria increased with age. Thus, in those over age 60, 43 per cent of the men and 36 per cent of the women had basal achlorhydria, and stimulated acid was absent in 21 per cent of the men and 10 per cent of the women. It is intriguing to note that in 1932 Vanzant and colleagues reported a decrease in achlorhydria after age 65, and suggested that those with retained gastric acid secretion were more biologically "fit."[9] This remains unconfirmed.

Pepsin. The pattern of change of pepsin secretion with age is less well defined than that of acid. This is in part related to methodologic difficulties of testing. Using serum pepsinogen I as a marker of pepsin secretion, Samloff and associates found that 40 per cent of individuals over age 70 had levels less than 50 ng/dl, compared with only 5 per cent of those under age 40.[10] However, the relationship of these changes to age, independent of conditions such as atrophic gastritis, has not been clarified.

Small Intestine

Cellular Morphology and Absorptive Function

Although most of the information about small intestinal changes with age comes from animal studies, general nutritional surveys would indicate that, in at least some of the elderly, poor nutrition is not related solely to diminished intake but rather to altered intestinal function. So-called covert malabsorption in the elderly has not yet been clinically documented, yet some subtle alterations in intestinal morphology and nutrient absorption have been described.

Numerous studies have suggested a change in the architecture of the small bowel mucosa, with villi becoming leaf-shaped, disorganized, or atrophic. However, Holt and co-workers have shown that in carefully controlled studies of aging rats in which variables such as nutritional status are eliminated, no major morphologic changes occur, although crypts are longer and there are more crypt cells.[11] Cell turnover appears to be unchanged.

Despite the apparent lack of change of morphology with aging, there are changes in nutrient absorption. Carbohydrate malabsorption has been documented using both xylose, which is absorbed by passive diffusion,

and more complex carbohydrates. Some diminution in brush border disaccharidases may account for the latter, but whether other factors are critical in these changes is not known. The changes do seem to progress with advancing age.[12] Fat absorption has not been well studied in human subjects, owing at least in part to the difficulties in performing adequate fat balance studies, particularly 72-hour stool collections, in other than institutionalized individuals. Some decrease in fat absorption has been documented, but the contribution of altered pancreatic, biliary, or intestinal function to this has not been adequately studied. Protein absorption, in the few studies that have been done, appears to remain intact with aging.

The absorption of vitamins and minerals has also been difficult to assess. Water-soluble vitamins are probably absorbed normally, and the handling of vitamin B_{12} in those without gastric atrophy is also maintained with aging. A defect in the intestinal handling of vitamin D seems to develop commonly, although the exact nature of this defect has not been clarified. Whatever the mechanism, the active transport of calcium is impaired in the elderly and may be an important contributing factor in the development of osteoporosis and osteomalacia.[13]

Motility

Small intestinal motility seems to remain intact with aging. Careful studies have shown preservation of all phases of the migrating motor complex and only minor changes in the motility index and amplitude of contraction.[14] No clinical consequences of these latter changes have been described. Certainly, pronounced changes in intestinal motility can accompany many of the systemic diseases frequent in the elderly, such as amyloidosis and diabetes mellitus, and can be induced by a number of medications.

Colon

Motility

Constipation is possibly the most frequent digestive complaint of the elderly. Yet the contribution of altered colonic motility to this remains unclear. Both segmental contraction of the colon and mass movements increase after meals in all age groups, but this is associated with propulsive activity only in those who are physically active.[15] In addition, numerous medications, such as anticholinergics and narcotic analgesics, are known to affect colonic motility. These factors may thus be of greater importance than aging in causing constipation.

Anorectal Function

Defecation and continence are intimately related to normal anorectal function. Several distinct anatomic and physiologic phenomena contribute, particularly the anorectal angle as maintained by the puborectalis muscle, and the internal and external anal sphincters. Ihre demonstrated decreased rectal elasticity with advancing age in studies of healthy elderly subjects.[16] With this decreased capacitance the rectal volume at which external sphincter tonic activity is lost also decreases. However, subjective sensations of rectal volume are maintained. None of these changes would serve to explain the altered bowel habits that so frequently concern the elderly.

Pancreas

The pancreas undergoes both anatomic and physiologic changes with aging. The main pancreatic duct becomes ectatic, and this is associated histologically with ductal epithelial hyperplasia and intralobular fibrosis. Rarely this fibrosis may lead to pancreatic atrophy.[17] These senescent pathologic changes are not uniformly reflected in altered pancreatic function, although there is a decline in the volume of stimulated pancreatic secretion after the fourth decade, and enzyme output diminishes progressively with advancing age.[18] The importance of these changes in causing any clinical dysfunction or nutritional impairment has not been fully elucidated, although one study demonstrating impaired absorption of radiolabeled lipids in elderly subjects showed improvement with the administration of exogenous pancreatic enzymes.[19]

Biliary Tree

Biliary morphology and motility appear not to change with aging. The composition of bile itself has been shown to be increasingly lithogenic in some populations, and this lithogenicity has been related to an increase in biliary cholesterol.[20] Total bile salt pool and cholic acid turnover are maintained, suggesting no change in the enterohepatic circulation of bile salts with aging. These changes in bile composition are similar to those seen in obesity.

NUTRITIONAL REQUIREMENTS OF THE ELDERLY

Understanding the nutritional requirements of the elderly has been confounded by the complex interaction of multiple, poorly understood variables, some of which have been mentioned in the preceding sections. Certainly physical activity will affect caloric needs, and common conditions of aging such as degenerative arthritis can profoundly affect limb mobility and thus general activity. Changes in gut absorptive function that may occur with age must also be taken into account in making nutritional recommendations. Finally, and perhaps of most profound importance, sociologic conditions of loneliness and isolation may play the largest role in the malnutrition frequently seen in the elderly.

Schneider and colleagues recently reviewed the difficulties in the development of recommended daily allowances (RDAs) for the elderly.[21] They concluded that the RDAs should be aimed at the maintenance of optimal physiologic function and the prevention of age-dependent diseases, keeping in mind the substantial heterogeneity of the elderly population with respect to underlying diseases, use of medications, and other individual factors. Also, nutrient-nutrient interactions (e.g., fiber and trace element absorption) and medication-nutrient interactions need to be more fully explained.

Role of Energy Expenditure

It may be fairly stated that for most individuals the quantity of food eaten is a more important determinant of nutritional status than is the composition of the diet. Most nutrients will be supplied in adequate quantity if the total amount eaten is reasonable. Thus a balance of energy intake and energy expenditure is critical. A deviation either way could result in considerable differences in body mass and composition.

Body mass generally declines with age. This has been attributed to a decrease in height, muscle mass, and skeletal mass, all of which are accompanied by an increase in total fat mass.[22] A reduction of basal metabolic rate of about 10 per cent occurs by age 60, with another 10 per cent reduction by age 75.[23]

Physical activity is a highly variable and obviously important factor. The influences of occupation, leisure, and illness on activity need to be assessed in each individual. Thus it is apparent that generalizations about total caloric requirements for the elderly are inadequate. Published data need to be viewed in light of these important variables.

Recommended Intake

Protein

Although conflicting data with respect to nitrogen balance in the elderly exist in the literature, true protein deficiency is unusual in this group. A protein requirement of 0.6 gm/kg per day, or something less than 40 gm of protein daily, has been calculated.[24] A decreased whole-body turnover of protein and the reduced skeletal muscle mass may account for this lower requirement.

Calcium

As noted earlier, the incidence of osteoporosis and osteomalacia in the elderly may be related in part to alterations in the handling of vitamin D and calcium by the intestinal tract. It has been recommended that the current RDA of 800 mg of calcium be increased to 1000 mg in women over the age of 50 and men over 60.[25] The role of vitamin D intake and sunlight exposure in the elderly on net calcium balance remains to be clarified.

Vitamins and Minerals

There exists a paucity of data on vitamin deficiencies in the elderly. Vitamin absorption, of both water-soluble and fat-soluble vitamins, seems to be generally preserved. Even so, some experts have recommended multivitamin supplementation, given the difficulty of clinical assessment of vitamin deficiencies and the relatively low cost of such preparations.

Dietary trace elements are essential to the maintenance of health, yet here too data are scarce. Zinc has been studied most often. Attempts made to establish a link between zinc deficiency and the impaired olfactory sensation of the elderly have not been successful. Zinc deficiency does occur as part of some diseases to which the elderly are subject, such as cirrhosis, chronic renal failure, and malabsorption. Still, there seems little justification for routine zinc supplementation. Similar conclusions can be drawn with regard to iron and copper supplementation, despite the claims of enthusiasts.

Fiber

The role of fiber in the diet is also controversial. The potential benefit of increased stool bulk in light of the prevalance of constipation needs to be balanced against the risk of impaired nutrient absorption that moderate amounts of dietary fiber can induce.[26] Generally, diets containing fresh fruits and vegetables and whole-meal grains seem beneficial for most individuals.

GASTROINTESTINAL DISEASES OF THE ELDERLY

Functional Diseases

Elderly patients, like patients of all ages, may manifest major psychosocial stress in somatic complaints related to the gastrointestinal tract. In a study of patients over 65 years old followed in an urban clinic for over one year, complaints in 58 per cent were believed to have a psychosomatic basis.[27] Given the major life changes encountered by aging individuals, with retirement, changes in living situations, loss of agility, and so forth, it is not surprising that health would be affected.

The primary symptoms of functional gastrointestinal disease may be dyspepsia, intermittent diarrhea, and, most commonly, constipation. Weight loss should alert the physician to a possible "organic" cause of symptoms, although this might also be an important indication of depression or of poor nutrition, the latter caused by the social problems mentioned previously or subtle changes in smell or taste that may impair eating.

Management is generally supportive. This is an area where a primary care physician is essential. Family and community supports must be mustered insofar as they are available. Tricyclic antidepressants must be used with caution and reserved for the more severely depressed patients.

Malignancies

Malignancies of the esophagus, stomach, and colon are all highly age-related. Generally, the course and prognosis are similar in all age groups. Certain distinctions are worth noting. Carcinoma of the stomach may present with obscure symptoms such as weight loss, anorexia, or vague abdominal pains. Meticulous evaluation of these complaints may be necessary, including carefully done double-contrast barium studies and endoscopy with biopsy. Carcinoma of the colon may be the most common malignancy in individuals over the age of 70 in some parts of the world. Screening procedures for colon cancer should be continued in the elderly.

Kaposi's sarcoma, now most often recognized as a manifestation of the acquired immunodeficiency syndrome, has long been known as a neoplasm affecting the elderly, particularly men of Eastern European or Italian descent. Involvement of the viscera occurs in the majority of patients, but only 10 per cent have clinical manifestations of this involvement, with intestinal obstruction, hemorrhage, or perforation being most common.[28] Kaposi's sarcoma is significantly associated with other lymphoreticular malignancies.

Atrophic Gastritis

There is an increased frequency of atrophic changes of the gastric mucosa with advancing age. The relationship of atrophy to frank gastritis and the incidence of these lesions is controversial (see pp. 792–813). Certainly, factors other than age may play a role in the development of gastritis, such as genetic and endocrine factors, systemic diseases, and exogenous toxins such as alcohol, nicotine, and medications. Most patients are asymptomatic, but clinical presentations with anemia or gastric ulcer are common. Perhaps the greatest clinical importance is the recognized potential for malignancy in these conditions. Although surveillance has been recommended, the optimal timing and means of such surveillance have not been determined.

Peptic Ulcer

See also pages 814 to 909.

The incidence of peptic ulcer disease is very nearly the same in the young and the old, although probably because of the decline in gastric acid secretion associated with aging the ratio of duodenal to gastric ulcer does fall. However, in several large series of hospitalized patients with duodenal ulcer, elderly patients make up nearly a third of the population. It is also of interest that the proportion of women with peptic ulcer increases with age.

The clinical presentation of peptic ulcer may be different in the elderly. Abdominal pain is often absent, and even in the presence of perforation, which can be the first manifestation of the ulcer, fever, leukocytosis, and expected physical signs may not be present.

The course of peptic ulcer in the elderly may be more severe, particularly in patients with complicating medical illnesses such as atherosclerotic cardiovascular disease or chronic obstructive pulmonary disease. Patients with bleeding complications fare worse, with a greater requirement for blood transfusion and a higher incidence of rebleeding.[29] Although this has been attributed to impaired contraction of blood vessels causing poor hemostasis, this has not been confirmed by pathologic studies. It is not surprising that mortality from peptic ulcer in the elderly is higher, with reports of up to 65 per cent mortality for octogenarians with bleeding gastric ulcers.

Management of elderly patients with peptic ulcer requires familiarity with drugs and their side effects. Cimetidine can cause confusion in elderly patients, and sucralfate can exacerbate constipation.[30] Surgical mortality is also greater in the elderly, as would be expected. Complications of surgical therapy, particularly partial gastrectomy, in the elderly can include gastric pouch cancer, bezoar formation, and nutritional deficiencies.

Cholelithiasis

See also pages 1691 to 1714.

Gallstone prevalence rises with age, and cholecystectomy may be the most common abdominal operation performed in those over age 60.[31] Disease presentation in the elderly may be nonspecific and vague. Cobden and associates reported patients with vague mental and physical disabilities that improved after cholecystectomy.[32] Empyema of the gallbladder, septic cholangitis, or gallstone ileus may be the initial manifestation of gallstone disease in the elderly.

Surgery remains the primary means of management of cholelithiasis. Gallstone dissolution with oral bile salts or with the use of methyl tert-butyl ether (MTBE) may be preferred in selected patients at high risk. Although carcinoma of the gallbladder is associated with the presence of gallstones, the low incidence of this complication would not warrant prophylactic cholecystectomy (see pp. 1734–1740).

Celiac Disease

See also pages 1134 to 1152.

Gluten-sensitive enteropathy is often thought of as a disease of childhood, yet in one study 7 per cent of newly diagnosed cases were in patients over 60 years old, and in another study celiac disease was the most common cause of steatorrhea in those over age 50.[33] Only a quarter of elderly patients in one study presented with classic symptoms of malabsorption, and in over half of these patients the diagnosis was first suspected because of abnormal blood counts.[34] In elderly patients sprue must be kept in mind when there is evidence of metabolic bone disease, unexplained cachexia, anemia, bleeding diathesis, or neurologic signs.

Malignancy, especially lymphoma and carcinoma, is a well-recognized complication of celiac disease. When patients are refractory to gluten withdrawal, or when an exacerbation of malabsorption occurs in those who were previously stable, or especially in those with abdominal pain as a symptom of their disease, one must strongly suspect the development of a malignancy.

Vascular Ectasias

See also pages 1363 to 1368.

Vascular ectasias or arteriovenous malformations of the bowel may be the cause of recurrent episodes of bleeding in the elderly.[35] The bleeding may be chronic and low grade or it may be intermittent and massive. The cause of the lesions is not known, but their prominence in the cecum and ascending colon has led to speculation that in areas of high wall tension, chronic venous obstruction causes tortuosity of the venules and capillaries of the mucosa and loss of competency of the precapillary sphincter.[36] The true incidence of the condition is unknown, owing in part to the absence of a simple, reliable diagnostic test for this condition. An interesting association of the lesion with valvular aortic stenosis has been suggested but not confirmed.

The diagnosis is often not confirmed until surgical partial colectomy. Recently, endoscopic laser photocoagulation has become a practical tool in treatment of these lesions, but its effect on the natural history of this condition is uncertain.[37]

Intestinal Ischemia

See also pages 1903 to 1932.

The extensive overlapping of blood supply to the intestinal tract effectively protects it from the effects of the atherosclerotic changes so prevalent in the elderly. However, when these changes are sufficiently extensive both acute and chronic ischemic changes can be observed and can affect either the small or large intestine.

Acute mesenteric vascular occlusion is often embolic in origin, either from atherosclerotic plaques or from a cardiac mural thrombus. Other causes of acute occlusion include atherosclerotic blockage of two mesenteric vessels and aortic dissection. The severity of the clinical condition is related to the size of the embolus (when that is the precipitating cause), the extent of vascular occlusion, and the adequacy of collaterals. For example, when collaterals are extensive, mild ischemic injury can resolve spontaneously and completely.

Nonocclusive intestinal infarction can occur in the setting of congestive heart failure, anoxia, or shock. In these patients surgical intervention can be of great risk, particularly in light of the multiple medical complications frequently present, but it also can be lifesaving.

Chronic mesenteric vascular occlusion is less common and may present as so-called intestinal angina. This syndrome is marked by the onset of cramping or dull abdominal pain 15 to 30 minutes after a meal, which lasts for up to a few hours. Patients lose weight because of a fear of eating. Physical findings are nonspecific and the diagnosis depends heavily on clinical suspicion and the presence of occlusion of at least two major vessels on angiography. Surgical therapy has yielded short-term benefit, but long-term outcomes are uncertain. The role of balloon catheter dilation of these vessels is under investigation.

Ischemic colitis most often occurs in patients over age 50 with extensive atherosclerotic vascular disease. The clinical manifestations may be highly variable, depending in part upon the degree of disruption of the blood supply. In patients presenting with an acute, fulminant picture the diagnosis may be made only at surgery. In others with a chronic, indolent course a colonic stricture may be the first clinical manifestation of colitis. The differentiation of ischemic colitis, especially with rectosigmoid involvement, from inflammatory bowel disease may be difficult. Ischemia as a cause of colitis must be kept in mind when an older patient presents with symptoms and signs of colitis. Angiography can be helpful but may not detect occlusion localized to smaller blood vessels.

Diverticular Disease

See also pages 1419 to 1434.

The incidence of diverticular disease of the colon is strikingly related to age, with postmortem examinations revealing diverticula in more than 50 per cent of persons in the eighth or ninth decades of life.[38] The absence of fiber in Western diets has been cited as an important factor in the pathogenesis of diverticula. Studies of colonic motility have shown a relationship of abnormal motility with symptomatic diverticulosis. They have also demonstrated that high-fiber diets improve motility and reduce pain. However, most diverticulosis is asymptomatic, and the correlations with motility in asymptomatic individuals is less clear.

Complications of diverticulosis—diverticulitis and hemorrhage—are more common with longer duration of disease. Thus these problems may become more prominent in elderly patients, who with their other medical conditions might be greater risks for significant morbidity and mortality. In addition, at the time of presentation, diverticulitis can be difficult to differentiate from other important conditions, including inflammatory bowel disease, ischemia, and malignancy.

Inflammatory Bowel Disease

See also pages 1327 to 1358 and 1435 to 1477.

Chronic ulcerative colitis and Crohn's disease are usually thought of as diseases of the young; their incidence, however, is nearly the same in those over age 50 as in younger patients. The symptoms, clinical course, and response to treatment of these diseases is similar to that seen in younger patients.[39, 40] However, as many physicians are unaware of the incidence of these diseases in the elderly, diagnosis can be delayed and symptoms and signs confused with those of diverticulitis or malignancy. Differentiation from the former can be especially difficult, with barium enema often not helpful. If sigmoidoscopy or colonoscopy shows mucosal inflammation, this should be interpreted as indicating the presence of inflammatory bowel disease, as such changes are distinctly unusual in diverticulitis. Management of inflammatory bowel disease in the elderly can be complicated by the high incidence of associated diseases such as diabetes, hypertension, atherosclerosis, and osteoporosis. Systemic corticosteroids and sulfasalazine are well tolerated, however. The results of surgical therapy are also generally gratifying, depending, of course, on any other medical conditions present. Surgery should not be withheld solely on the basis of a patient's age. Patients mistakenly operated upon for diverticulitis who have inflammatory bowel disease fare poorly when subjected to a simple colostomy or partial colectomy without ileostomy.[41]

Constipation and Fecal Impaction

As noted previously, constipation is certainly a most common complaint among the elderly. Studies by Lanfranchi and co-workers have divided patients with constipation into two types: those with painful constipation are regarded as having an irritable or spastic bowel, while painless constipation is thought to be consistent with an atonic colon possibly with reduced colonic sensitivity.[42] The latter appears to be the most common in older people, and has been called by Brocklehurst the "terminal reservoir syndrome."[15] Immobility seems to be the critical factor in predisposing the elderly to constipation. There may be a lack of stimulus to cause mass contraction in immobile people; alternately, the need for help in being able to defecate may cause an elderly person not to respond to the urge to defecate, and later the patient may not be able to defecate at will. With distention, the rectal stretch receptors could lose their sensitivity, leading to decreased urge, thus beginning a classic vicious circle.

Other causes of constipation are listed in Table 8–2. It is critical to keep in mind iatrogenic causes, as many drugs, especially anticholinergic, anti-parkinsonian, and tricyclic antidepressant drugs, can cause severe constipation in the elderly (see p. 336).

Table 8–2. CAUSES OF CONSTIPATION

Obstruction
  Neoplasm
  Stricture
Painful anal lesions
Neurologic diseases
Endocrine and metabolic disorders
  Myxedema
  Hypercalcemia
  Hypokalemia
Psychologic
  Depression
  Dementia
Drugs

The important complications of constipation in the elderly are fecal impaction, idiopathic megacolon, sigmoid volvulus, and fecal incontinence. The presentation of impaction may be difficult to distinguish from that of intestinal obstruction of other causes. The plain abdominal radiograph may be most helpful, especially when it shows feces throughout the colon. Digital rectal examination can be misleading in patients with an impaction high in the rectum or in the sigmoid colon. Impaction itself can lead to complications of stercoral ulceration and rectal prolapse. Studies in patients with previous impaction have shown a decrease in both rectal pressure and response to rectal distention compared with aged-matched controls.[43] The findings are similar to those described in patients with low spinal cord injuries.

Idiopathic megacolon in the elderly has been thought to be due to long-standing constipation, with use of laxatives being a possible contributing factor. This form of megacolon appears to predispose to the development of sigmoid volvulus. This can be an abdominal catastrophe, with a mortality rate of 35 per cent per episode. Although nonsurgical reduction of the volvulus is possible, evidence from recent trials suggests that elective surgical resection should follow.[44]

Fecal Incontinence (Table 8–3)

As noted earlier, the maintenance of continence involves the complex interaction of the rectal reservoir, the anorectal angle as determined by the puborectalis muscle, and the internal and external anal sphincters. It is perhaps paradoxical that the most important cause of incontinence in the elderly may be constipation; fecal impaction can lead to so-called overflow diarrhea and incontinence. An obstructing rectal neoplasm can have the same effect. Another important form of incontinence is neurogenic, with either global cerebral disease such as dementia or spinal cord lesions causing a decreased awareness of impending defecation, or with diminished power of pelvic musculature, particularly the puborectalis and external anal sphincter muscles as can be seen in patients with diabetes. Finally, surgical or radiotherapeutic trauma to the anorectum can be occasional causes.

Treatment of these conditions can be a challenge. The routine use of laxatives to prevent impaction can itself lead to difficulties, as noted. The use of routine twice-weekly enemas in institutionalized patients has been recommended.[45] The neurogenic form of incontinence may be best managed simply by arranging for the patient to be sitting on a commode at the times before the gastrocolic reflex is to occur. The use of

Table 8–3. CAUSES OF FECAL INCONTINENCE

Impaction with overflow diarrhea
Previous anal surgery
Neuropathic (e.g., diabetes, dementia)
Idiopathic

opiates during the day and senna at night to stimulate morning evacuation has also been recommended.

References

1. Schneider, E. L., and Williams, T. F. Geriatrics and gerontology: imperatives in education and training. (Editorial.) Ann. Intern. Med. *104*:432, 1986.
2. Piaget, F., and Fouillet, J. Le pharynx et l'oesophage senile: etude clinique, radiologique et radio-cinematographique. J. Med. Lyon *40*:961, 1959.
3. Hollis, J. B., Castell, D. O. Esophageal function in elderly men: a new look at "presbyesophagus." Ann. Intern. Med. *80*:371, 1974.
4. Kimura, K. Chronological transition of the fundic pyloric border determined by stepwise biopsy of the lesser and greater curvatures of the stomach. Gastroenterology *63*:584, 1972.
5. Bird, T., Hall, M. R. P., and Schade, R. O. K. Gastric histology and its relation to anemia in the elderly. Gerontology *23*:309, 1977.
6. Moore, J. G., Tweedy, C., Christian, P. E., and Datz, F. L. Effect of age on gastric emptying of liquid and solid meals in man. Dig. Dis. Sci. *28*:340, 1983.
7. McCallum, R. W., Frank, E. B., and Lange, R. Abnormal gastric emptying in patients with atrophic gastritis with or without pernicious anemia. (Abstract.) Gastroenterology *80*:1151, 1981.
8. Grossman, M. I., Kirsner, J. B., and Gillespie, I. E. Basal and Histalog-stimulated gastric secretion in control subjects and in patients with peptic ulcer or gastric ulcer. Gastroenterology *45*:14, 1963.
9. Vanzant FR, et al.: The normal range of gastric acidity from youth to old age. Arch. Intern. Med. *49*:345, 1932.
10. Samloff, I. M., Liebman, W. M., and Panitch, N. M. Serum group I pepsinogens by radioimmunoassay in control subjects and patients with peptic ulcer. Gastroenterology *69*:83, 1975.
11. Holt, P. R., Pascal, R. R., and Kotler, D. P. Effect of aging upon small intestinal structure in the Fischer rat. J. Gerontol. *39*:642, 1984.
12. Feibusch, J., and Holt, P. R. Impaired absorptive capacity for carbohydrates in the elderly. Am. J. Clin. Nutr. *32*:942, 1979.
13. Holt, P. R. Intestinal absorption and malabsorption. *In* Texter, E. C., Jr. (ed.). The Aging Gut. New York, Masson, 1983, pp. 33–36.
14. Anuras, S., and Sutherland, J. Jejunal manometry in healthy elderly subjects. Gastroenterology *86*:1016, 1984.
15. Brocklehurst, J. C., Kirkland, J. L., Martin, J., and Ashford, J. Constipation in long-stay elderly patients. Gerontology *29*:181, 1983.
16. Ihre, T. Studies on anal function in continent and incontinent patients. Scand. J. Gastroenterol. *9*:5, 1974.
17. Kreel, L., and Sandin, B. Changes in pancreatic morphology associated with aging. Gut *14*:962, 1973.
18. Langier, R., and Sarles, H. Gastrointestinal disorders of the elderly: the pancreas. Clin. Gastroenterol. *14*:749, 1985.
19. Citi, S., and Salvani, L. The intestinal absorption of ^{131}I labelled olein triolein, of ^{58}Co vitamin B_{12} and ^{59}Fe in the aged subjects. G. Gerontol. *12*:123, 1964.
20. Valdivieso, V., Palma, R., Wünkhaus, R., Antezana, C., Severin, C., and Contreras, A. Effect of aging on biliary lipid composition and bile acid metabolism in normal Chilean women. Gastroenterology *74*:871, 1978.
21. Schneider, E. L., Vining, E. M., Hadley, E. C., and Farnham, S. A. Recommended daily allowances and the health of the elderly. N. Engl. J. Med. *314*:157, 1986.
22. Tzamnoff, S. P., and Norris, A. H. Effect of muscle mass decrease on age related BMR changes. J. Appl. Physiol. *43*:1001, 1977.
23. Magnus-Levy, A. Basal metabolism in the same person after an interval of fifty years. JAMA *118*:1369, 1942.
24. Zanni, E., Calloway, D. H., and Zezulka, A. Y. Protein requirements of elderly men. J. Nutr. *109*:513, 1979.

25. Nordin, B. E. C. Calcium, Phosphate, and Magnesium Metabolism, Clinical Physiology and Diagnostic Procedures. Edinburgh, Churchill Livingstone, 1976.
26. Southgate, D. A. T., and Durnin, J. V. G. A. Calorie conversion factors: an experimental reassessment of the factors used in the calculation of the energy value of human diets. Br. J. Nutr. 24:517, 1970.
27. Schuster, M. M. Disorders of the aging GI system. In Reichal, W. (ed.). The Geriatric Patient. New York, HP Publishing Co., 1978, pp. 73–81.
28. Safai, B., and Good, R. A. Kaposi's sarcoma: a review and recent developments. CA 31:2, 1981.
29. Permutt, R. P., and Cello, J. P. Duodenal ulcer disease in the hospitalized elderly patient. Dig. Dis. Sci. 27:1, 1982.
30. Sucralfate for peptic ulcer—a reappraisal. Med. Lett. Drugs Ther. 26:43, 1984.
31. Stroll, E. L., Diffenbaugh, W. G., and Anderson, R. E. Biliary tract surgery in the aged patient. Geriatrics 19:275, 1964.
32. Cobden I, Lendrum, R., Venables, C. W., and James, O. F. W. Gallstones presenting as mental and physical debility in the elderly. Lancet 1:1062, 1984.
33. Price, H. L., Gazzard, B. G., and Dawson, A. M. Steatorrhoea in the elderly. Br. Med. J. 1:1582, 1977.
34. Swinson, C. M., and Levi, A. J. Is coeliac disease underdiagnosed? Br. Med. J. 281:1258, 1980.
35. Meyer, C. T., Troncale, F. J., Galloway, S., and Sheahan, D. G. Arteriovenous malformations of the bowel: an analysis of 22 cases and a review of the literature. Medicine 60:36, 1981.
36. Boley, S. J., Sammartino, R., Adams, A., DiBiase, A., Kleinhaus, S., and Sprayregen, S. On the nature and etiology of vascular ectasias of the colon. Gastroenterology 72:650, 1977.
37. Cello, J. P., and Grendell, J. H. Endoscopic laser treatment for gastrointestinal vascular ectasias. Ann. Intern. Med. 104:352, 1986.
38. Almy, T. P., and Howell, D. A. Diverticular disease of the colon. N. Engl. J. Med. 302:324, 1980.
39. Law, D. H., Steinberg, H., and Sleisenger, M. H. Ulcerative colitis with onset after the age of 50. Gastroenterology 41:457, 1961.
40. Harper, P. C., McAuliffe, T. L., and Beeken, W. L. Crohn's disease in the elderly. Arch. Intern. Med. 146:753, 1986.
41. Schmidt, G. T., Lennard-Jones, J. E., Morson, B. C., and Young, A. C. Crohn's disease of the colon and its distinction from diverticulitis. Gut 9:7, 1968.
42. Lanfranchi, G. A., Bazzocchi, G., Brignola, C., Campieri, M., and Labo, G. Different patterns of intestinal transit time and anorectal motility in painful and painless chronic constipation. Gut 25:1352, 1984.
43. Read, N. W., Abourezky, L., Read, M. G., Howell, P., Ottewell, D., and Donnelly, T. C. Anorectal function in elderly patients with fecal impaction. Gastroenterology 89:959, 1985.
44. Bak, M. P., and Boley, S. J. Sigmoid volvulus in elderly patients. Am. J. Surg. 151:71, 1986.
45. Brocklehurst, J. C. Colonic disease in the elderly. Clin. Gastroenterol. 14:725, 1985.

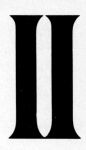

MAJOR SYMPTOMS AND SYNDROMES: PATHOPHYSIOLOGY, DIAGNOSIS, AND MANAGEMENT

Obesity, Anorexia Nervosa, Bulimia, and Other Eating Disorders

GEORGE W. BO-LINN

9

OBESITY

If one uses the criteria for obesity of the National Center for Health Statistics (body mass index of 27.8 determined by weight in kilograms divided by surface area in meters squared), about 34 million adult Americans were overweight between 1976 and 1980.[1] This group represents over a quarter of all Americans aged 20 to 75 years, of whom 12.4 million were severely overweight. The recently completed National Health and Nutrition Examination Survey (NHANES II) shows that increasing age is associated with increasing overweight, particularly among black women.[2] A consensus development conference sponsored by the National Institutes of Health (NIH) recently addressed aspects of this problem.[3] Nonetheless, despite an annual commitment of $24 million by the NIH to obesity research, and untold millions of dollars spent in treating obesity and the major health problems associated with it, obesity remains one of the most serious public health problems in the United States.

Definition. Any definition of obesity must begin with the distinction from overweight, which refers to a body weight greater than arbitrarily set standards whether the excessive weight is due to fat, muscle, or bone. Conceptually, obesity is simply excessive body fat. However, problems arise not only in determining what is "excessive," but also as regards which method one uses to measure fat. Whereas body weight is easily quantified, body fat has been variously measured by densitometry, tritiated water dilution, skinfold measurements, whole-body potassium, uptake of lipid-soluble inert gases, total-body electrical conductivity, and, most recently, computerized tomography.[4, 5] Furthermore, measuring body fat as a fraction of body weight alone may be insufficient since regional patterns of fat distribution have important health implications; for example, abdominal obesity is an independent risk factor for ischemic heart disease, strokes, and death.[6]

Therefore, it is understandable albeit unfortunate that obesity has been used interchangeably with overweight. By defining obesity as being a weight greater than 20 per cent more than that desirable for a person of a given height, one assumes a correlation between weight and adiposity that is often misleading in individual cases. Problems with the widespread use of height-weight tables include variation in skeletal mass, bone density, and selection of relative weight indices. Operationally, however, the disadvantages of height-weight tables are outweighed, so to speak, by its widespread acceptance, ease of measurement, and conceptual simplicity. Variations of traditional height-weight tables are being used. The NHANES II used the body mass index (weight/height ratio known as Quetelet's index), which correlates fairly well with other estimates of body fat. Figure 9–1 shows a nomogram for converting height and weight measurements to body mass index. Replacement of relative weight tables must await development of methods permitting easy and accurate measurement of total and regional body adiposity, and numbers and size of adipose cells.

Classification. Because the etiology of obesity remains unclear, classifications of obesity have been based on a variety of schema, such as anatomic distribution of body fat (generalized, gynoid [fat distribution characteristic of women], or android [fat distribution characteristic of men]), psychologic (developmental, reactive), period of onset (juvenile, mature, or pregnancy-related), or morphology of adipose tissue (hyperplastic or hyperplastic-hypertrophic). The latter two methods of classification are particularly interesting.

Juvenile-onset obesity has been studied because many obese children grow up to become obese adults, and this type of obesity is especially difficult to treat.[7] However, available data suggest that an obese infant or child has only a slightly increased tendency to remain obese with maturity.[8] This predictive relationship appears established by age 1 year, and the longer the child remains obese, the higher is the probability that adult obesity will become a problem.[7] Theories of adipose tissue morphology find support in this trend, holding that childhood-onset obesity is characterized by hyperplasia and hypertrophy, that is, excess numbers and enlarged size of fat cells.[9] Lewis and colleagues recently demonstrated that overfeeding during infancy in baboons increased fat depot mass later in life primarily by fat cell hypertrophy rather than by hyperplasia.[10] Adult-onset obesity is generally considered to be characterized by hypertrophy without hyperplasia. However, small increases in adipocyte cell number even in patients with adult-onset obesity have been reported.[11] These concepts for classification of obesity obviously remain controversial. Since obesity is a clinical manifestation and multifactorial in etiology, any one classification will be inadequate. Obese patients constitute a heterogeneous population with only their evident adiposity serving as the common link. Hence, the various classification schemes serve to underscore the lack of understanding regarding the underlying cause of obesity.

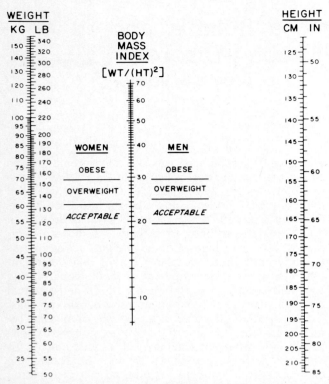

Figure 9–1. Nomogram for determining body mass index (BMI). A straight edge is attached from the individual's weight on the left side to the point on the right-hand line corresponding to the person's height. The BMI (weight/height²) is the point at which this line connecting height and weight crosses the central vertical line. By the NHANES II criteria, a man is considered "overweight" when his BMI equals or exceeds 27.8, and "severely overweight" when his BMI equals or exceeds 31.1. For a woman, these cutoff points are 27.3 and 32.3, respectively. Please see text. (From Bray, G. A. Int. J. Obesity *2*:99, 1978. Used by permission.)

Physiology of Appetite

By a reductionistic viewpoint, obesity results from calorie intake excessive to calorie needs. Hence, to study obesity one should understand factors regulating hunger, appetite, satiety, and metabolism. *Hunger* is generally a clear signal by the body that energy needs are not being met and is accompanied by unpleasant sensations ("hunger pangs") to motivate food acquisition. *Appetite* is a desire to eat, often unrelated to physiologic need, and easily influenced by external stimuli. *Satiety* is the loss of this desire. The regulation of food intake is therefore a complex process involving "true" and "perceived" needs, as terminated by the satiety response to a meal.

Central Control of Appetite. The control of appetite lies in a central system and a peripheral system. The central system classically involves the hypothalamus, which includes the so-called feeding center (lateral hypothalamus) and satiety center (ventromedial hypothalamus). Evidence for the existence of such centers comes from animal experiments wherein destroying the lateral hypothalamus causes aphagia and, likewise, placing bilateral lesions in the ventromedial nucleus causes hyperphagia.[12, 13] Whether these concepts are applicable to humans is still unclear. Certainly some hypothalamic lesions in humans have been associated with hyperphagia and obesity. Furthermore, the paraventricular nucleus, ventral tegmental area, amygdala, globus pallidus, and area postrema also appear to be involved in the central control of appetite.[14] Hence, rather than a specific "center" *per se* in the hypothalamus, one should conceptualize neuroendocrine tracts that in concert regulate appetite. One model of the central control of appetite is shown in Figure 9–2. Thus, satiety is mediated by activity of the

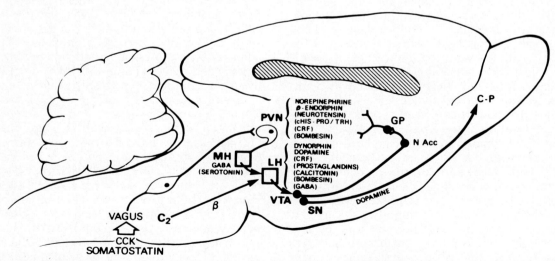

Figure 9–2. The neuroanatomic and neurotransmitter substrates of the central control of appetite. Substrates are shown in their anatomic location of activity. Substrates in parentheses have less firmly established anatomic localization. PVN, paraventricular nucleus; MH, medial hypothalamus; GABA, gamma-aminobutyric acid; LH, lateral hypothalamus; VTA, ventral tegmental area; SN, substantia nigra; N Acc, nucleus accumbens; C-P, caudate putamen; GP, globus pallidus; C_2, rostral area of medulla oblongata; CCK, cholecystokinin; cHis-Pro, cyclo-histidylproline diketopiperazine; TRH, thyrotropin-releasing hormone; CRF, corticotropin-releasing factor; and β, beta-adrenergic input. (From Morley, J. E., and Levine, A. S. Lancet *1*:398, 1983. Used by permission.)

raphe nuclei (serotonergic) tract and the ventral adrenergic bundle, which pass through the piriform area near the ventromedial hypothalamus. The lateral hypothalamus is associated with the dopaminergic nigrostriatal tracts.

Therefore, appetite regulation is more appropriately considered as neuropharmacologic interactions rather than as anatomic centers in the hypothalamus. Release of neurotransmitters may be stimulated by "appetostats," nutrients that induce feeding or satiety behavior. The glucostatic theory was first proposed by Carlson in 1916, and modified later by Mayer.[15] This theory holds that cells exist in the brain that control appetite by monitoring arteriovenous differences in glucose concentration. Glucoreceptors have been found in the ventromedial hypothalamus and appear to respond to iontophoretic application of glucose.[16]

The lipostatic theory similarly proposes that fatty acids released during lipolysis stimulate appetite.[17] An aminostatic theory has also been proposed and has support in the known activity of gamma-aminobutyric acid in inhibiting satiety-inducing substances such as prostaglandins, calcitonin, corticotropin-releasing factor, and phenylethylamine.[18]

Incorporating the concept of nutrients acting to regulate appetite is Brobeck's classical thermostatic theory, which proposes that body temperature as adjusted by the heat of the metabolized nutrients ultimately regulates appetite.[19] The search for appetostats is stimulated by the known ability of animals to regulate the proper mix and total intake of nutrients for their energy needs.[20] The implication for obesity in humans is whether obese people have lost this ability because of a deranged or absent appetostat system.

The list of specific neurotransmitters that may stimulate or inhibit feeding behavior is growing. Opiates, both exogenous and endogenous, stimulate feeding, most likely via the kappa receptors in the brain.[21] Dynorphin (1–17), a potent endogenous opioid peptide and ligand of the kappa receptor, induces feeding in rats when injected in their central nervous systems, and abnormal levels of dynorphin are found in brains of rats with feeding disorders.[22, 23] Exogenous kappa receptor agonists such as cyclazocine compounds induce feeding. Furthermore, the opiate antagonist naloxone inhibits feeding; the kappa antagonist MR-2266 is even more potent.[24, 25] The role of opioids in obesity is unclear, but it is intriguing that stress-induced eating in rats seems to be mediated through activation of endogenous opioids.[26]

Interaction of endogenous opioid peptides with the monoamines has been postulated. The dopaminergic nigrostriatal tracts associated with the lateral hypothalamus also contain opiate binding sites.[27] Stimulation of dopamine synthesis and release can be initiated by activation of these opiate receptors.[28] Another monamine, serotonin, appears to be involved in satiety, since serotonin agonists produce anorexia.[29] The adrenergic system also affects feeding. The alpha-adrenergic agonists stimulate appetite, perhaps by stimulating gamma-aminobutyric acid (GABA) release, which

in turn inhibits the serotonergic tract associated with the ventromedial hypothalamus.[30] The beta-adrenergic agonists cause satiety by inhibiting the lateral hypothalamic feeding center, perhaps also via GABA, since GABA inhibits dopaminergic transmission from the nigrostriatal tracts associated with the lateral hypothalamus.[31]

The list of neuropeptides believed to influence appetite includes calcitonin, 41-aminoacid corticotropin-releasing factor (CRF), bombesin, thyrotropin-releasing hormone and its active metabolite histidylproline diketopiperazine, and neurotensin. Unlike the opioid peptides, however, these neuropeptides inhibit rather than stimulate feeding. Calcitonin is particularly potent when administered centrally where calcitonin receptors have been found in the brain of rats.[32] Appetite is presumably suppressed via calcitonin's inhibition of calcium uptake into hypothalamic neurons.

Peripheral Control of Appetite. The regulation of food intake also depends on the peripheral control of appetite. A feedback system to signal satiety or hunger must involve the intestinal tract. Initiation of these signals is complex, and the signals probably reach the hypothalamus via the nervous system or via the blood stream as gastrointestinal peptide hormones. Factors that may induce satiety are shown in Table 9–1.

Attention has naturally centered on the stomach, the first recipient of ingested food. A gastromechanical theory of hunger, first proposed by Cannon in 1912, postulated that glucoprivation stimulated gastric "hunger" contractions that in turn caused afferent signals to the hypothalamus to initiate food-seeking behavior.[33] While this theory has since been disproved, the physiologic mechanism to explain "hunger" has not been found.

Satiety, however, has been extensively studied and a number of explanations for postprandial satiety have been proposed. The gastric distention theory derives from evidence that distention receptors exist in the wall of the stomach and that bulky meals cause more satiety than meals consisting of refined carbohydrates of equal caloric value.[34, 35] The signal of gastric distention may be vagally mediated. However, vagotomy does not abolish the satiety associated with food distention of the stomach, which suggests a hormonal mechanism independent of the vagus nerve.[36] Gastrin, somatostatin, and bombesin have all been proposed since they are released from the stomach by food. Bombesin is the most likely candidate since it, unlike

Table 9–1. FACTORS THAT MAY INDUCE SATIETY

Site	Factor That Signals Satiety
Oral	Chemical (taste, smell)
Gastric	Mechanical distention
	Hormones (gastrin, somatostatin, bombesin)
Intestinal	Nutrient "appetostats" (glucose, fatty acids, amino acids)
	Hormones (cholecystokinin, secretin, neurotensin, gastric inhibitory peptide)
Pancreatic	Hormones (pancreatic polypeptide, glucagon)

the other two, retains its satiety effect despite complete denervation of the stomach.[37]

Beyond the stomach, satiety can be induced by placement of food in the small intestine.[38] In 1967, a purified extract of small intestine with enterogastrone activity was found to stimulate satiety in mice. Smith reported that cholecystokinin (CCK) produced a dose-related inhibition of food intake in rats, but secretin did not.[39] Subsequent work with CCK-8 demonstrated molecular and behavioral specificity for this satiating effect. The molecular specificity depends on the presence of a sulfate group on the tryosine moiety in the seventh position from the carboxyl-terminal end. Behavioral specificity exists because doses of CCK-8 inhibit food intake in food-deprived rats but not water intake in water-deprived rats and produce satiety *per se* without causing toxic side effects.[39, 40] This satiating effect of CCK-8 is synergistic with the satiety effect of oral food stimuli and of gastric distention.[41]

Because abdominal vagotomy abolishes the satiety effect of CCK-8 and because of the blood-brain barrier, the site of action must be in the periphery and must be carried to the brain via visceral afferent pathways. The relative importance of vagal efferent and afferent fibers is unanswered by experiments involving total abdominal vagotomy. But pharmacologic inhibition of peripheral postganglionic muscarinic receptors with atropine methylnitrate to simulate loss of vagal efferent fibers did not change the satiety effects of CCK-8.[42] Hence, the gastric vagal afferent limb probably is critical for the central effect of CCK-8. Exactly how CCK-8 interacts with these vagal afferent fibers to produce satiety is still unknown despite several hypotheses.[43]

Other "satiety hormones" have been postulated, including somatostatin and pancreatic glucagon. They, like CCK-8, have behavioral specificity and their satiety effects are abolished by abdominal vagotomy. Interestingly, selective hepatic vagotomy reportedly blocks the effects of glucagon, suggesting some connection with glucagon's known glycogenolytic action in the liver.[44]

Despite interest in these "satiety" hormones, it is still not proven that these hormones have a physiologic role in satiety following endogenous release by ingested food. Stimulation of feeding in rats has been found following intraperitoneal injection of antibodies to glucagon, but this evidence is not compelling.[45]

Energy Expenditure in Obesity

While obesity obviously is the end result of energy intake chronically exceeding energy consumption, it remains unclear whether obese persons ingest too much or metabolize too little energy. Many dietary surveys indicate that hyperphagia is not the primary cause of obesity.[46, 47] Although methodologic problems exist in dietary surveys, such as inaccurate measurement of food intake, change in eating behavior during the survey, and unreliable calculation of food caloric con-

tent, interest nonetheless has shifted to studies of energy expenditure in the obese.[48, 49]

Energy expenditure consists of three components: physical activity, basal metabolic rate, and thermogenesis. As regards physical activity, studies comparing obese individuals with lean persons in this regard are inconclusive.[50] Basal metabolic rate (BMR) represents the energy necessary for the basic maintenance of the body and is primarily dependent on the lean body mass, thyroid hormones, and protein turnover. In general, BMR of the obese is greater than that of lean subjects.[51] This finding is not particularly surprising since obese persons have a greater lean body mass, necessary to maintain their extra fat. Therefore, in terms of caloric intake, physical activity, and basal metabolic rate, there are no strong data to support the generally accepted opinion that obese persons are fat because of gluttony and sloth. The concept, then, has developed that obese persons are inherently very efficient in energy metabolism, being "energy thrifty" as compared with lean persons.[52]

Part of this concept involves the "set-point" hypothesis, wherein each person's energy regulatory system attempts to maintain body weight at a constant level, even when challenged by increased or decreased energy (dietary) intakes. This hypothesis is very appealing because it would explain why some people remain lean on high levels of calorie ingestion, while others remain obese despite their seemingly best efforts at dieting. Two classic single-subject studies seem to support the set-point hypothesis. Neumann in 1902 and Gulick in 1922 published the results of systematically altering their energy intakes over a period of months while monitoring their respective body weights.[53, 54] Despite wide variations in their calorie consumptions, their body weights appeared to remain constant, giving rise to the term "luxus consumption." Neumann postulated that when he overate, his body automatically compensated by wasting the excess calories as heat. Recently, however, these studies have been closely re-examined by Garrow, who instead found that changes in energy intake were indeed reflected in changes in body weight.[55] Although the set-point hypothesis remains conjecture, it has stimulated tremendous interest in metabolic (thermogenic) responses by the body to overfeeding.

Thermogenesis, or more precisely facultative thermogenesis, is defined as the energy expenditure above that required to maintain the basal state, or BMR. Thermogenesis is highly variable and is affected by external factors such as effects of food intake, thermogenic agents, and cold exposure. Components of facultative thermogenesis include exercise by muscles, cold-induced shivering, and diet-induced thermogenesis. The latter component is the subject of intense study in hopes of understanding the metabolic control of body weight.

Diet-induced thermogenesis, also known as specific dynamic action of food, postprandial thermogenesis, and thermic effect of food, consists of obligatory and facultative components. The obligatory component represents the energy expended to digest, absorb, process, and store nutrients, and varies according to the metabolic fate of the nutrient, be it carbohydrate, fat, or protein. About 10 per cent of the metabolizable energy ingested as a mixed diet is lost as heat. The facultative component of diet-induced thermogenesis represents energy lost in excess of the obligatory component and is the most controversial area of obesity research.[56, 57]

Animal models provide the most convincing support for diet-induced thermogenesis. While methodologic problems exist, young animals (from weaning up to sexual maturity) will overeat when presented with a "cafeteria diet," otherwise known as a "snack diet" or "trash-feeding diet" consisting of cakes, cookies, candy bars, and so forth. Despite increasing their food intake by up to 100 per cent, these animals remain lean and deposit very little weight or fat, while older animals eating the same diet become obese.[58] This phenomenon in young animals has been attributed to diet-induced thermogenesis, which causes a compensatory increase in metabolic rate.

The mechanism of diet-induced thermogenesis is similar to if not the same as that for nonshivering thermogenesis, a form of heat production during cold exposure. Nonshivering thermogenesis is derived from brown adipose tissue. Activation of the sympathetic nervous system releases norepinephrine, which in turn leads to depolarization of brown adipocytes and release of free fatty acids. These fatty acids are utilized by the mitochondria in generating ATP from ADP, thus consuming energy.[59] However, in humans, the role of diet-induced thermogenesis and brown adipose tissue in obesity remains unclear. While infants have abundant amounts of brown adipose tissue, this amount diminishes with age. Whether it functions as an energy outlet is unproven.

Another concept of how energy can be dissipated and leanness preserved is via "substrate" or futile cycling in glycolytic-gluconeogenic pathways.[60] This concept proposes that excess energy is "burned off" in independent (nonequilibrium) forward and reverse reactions that result in ATP consumption and heat production. Rates of cycling are reportedly increased in brown adipose tissue and white adipose tissue in response to cold stress, nonadrenergic stimulation, and feeding. Hence, a defect in futile cycles results in increased energy efficiency and thus could contribute to the development of obesity.

The ubiquitous sodium-potassium pump maintains appropriate intracellular sodium and potassium concentrations and consequently requires large amounts of energy, estimated to be as much as 20 to 50 per cent of total energy expenditure. Hence, decreased Na-K ATPase activity could result in diminished energy consumption and conceivably lead to obesity. For example, the genetically obese (ob/ob) mouse has reduced levels of Na-K ATPase in muscles and in liver. Similarly reduced levels have been found in the diabetic obese (db/db) mouse. De Luise and colleagues reported decreased Na-K ATPase activity in red blood cells of obese persons which did not increase with weight reduction.[61] However, other investigators have demonstrated increased erythrocyte Na-K ATPase activity in obese individuals when compared with that in lean persons.[62, 63] Increased activity has also been found in liver homogenates from obese subjects.[64] Furthermore, recent studies suggest that Na-K ATPase activity may be influenced more by ethnic origin than by obesity.[65] These findings cast considerable doubt on the significance of Na-K ATPase pump activity in the pathogenesis of human obesity.

In summary, the pathophysiology of obesity is unknown. The relative roles of excessive calorie intake and defective ("too thrifty") energy metabolism in the development and maintenance of obesity remain to be defined. Most of the studies involving humans that have addressed this area have serious methodologic shortcomings. The problems include difficulties in performing accurate calorimetric studies in humans, determining whether and by how much energy metabolism differs in preobese persons who become obese from that in obese persons who stay obese, and identifying homogeneous subgroups of obese patients to study. Sims and Danforth[65a] recently provided a fascinating perspective on energy balance in man.

Heredity and Obesity

A question of philosophic and physiologic importance is whether obesity is genetically predetermined. Certainly, human obesity is highly heritable. Obese parents generally beget obese children. For example, two obese parents are estimated to have a 73 per cent chance of having an obese child, while two lean parents have only a 9 per cent chance of doing so.[66] However, whether these children are predestined to corpulence or simply eat their way to that state is highly controversial. Cultural, social, and behavioral factors play a tremendous role in food intake, particularly during the early years of childhood and adolescence, when eating habits are developed. When bombarded by advertising and television commercials for calorie-dense "junk" foods, children (and adults) will consume more.[67] Other factors such as child-rearing practices, socioeconomic stratum, and urban lifestyle are associated with obesity.[68] Schacter's externality theory proposes that obese persons are more susceptible to external cues than are lean persons and, as a consequence, eat more and more frequently.[69] This susceptibility presumably develops during the formative years of infancy and childhood.

Separating the relative importance of environmental influences as noted above from genetic ones has been difficult. Studies of twins raised by adoptive parents have been conflicting in their results.[70-73] A recent study by Stunkard and colleagues examined 540 adult Danish adoptees.[74] They concluded that genetic influences have an important role in determining obesity, while environmental factors do not. Another study of over 4000 twins found that human fatness is under substantial genetic control.[75] Also noteworthy is the familial dependence of the resting metabolic rate, which suggests a possible genetic link among family members.[76] These conclusions, however, do not demonstrate that environmental factors are unimportant in prevention and treatment of obesity. Certainly, a genetic predisposition to obesity should not dissuade one from adopting prudent dietary habits.

Medical Problems of Obesity

The morbidity and mortality of obesity will not be discussed here in detail. The reader is referred to several recent reviews of the health hazards associated with obesity.[77] The impact of obesity of premature mortality may be even more pronounced than previously thought, since a recent study suggests that excessive mortality occurs at relative weights at least 10 per cent lower than U.S. average "desirable" weights.[78] However, medical problems of obese individuals that are of particular interest to the gastroenterologist will be discussed.

Life insurance statistics demonstrate that excess weight is associated with higher mortality rate. Digestive diseases, primarily gallbladder disease, are a prominent manifestation of this health risk. The association of gallbladder disease and obesity is well known.[79] Increased cholesterol production and secretion, with greater saturation of bile with cholesterol, have been documented in obese subjects.[80] Furthermore, obesity also increases the risk of dying from gallbladder disease.[81]

As regards esophageal disease, effects of obesity on esophageal function are not clear-cut. O'Brien measured lower esophageal sphincter pressures in 25 morbidly obese women and found them to be in the normal range in 22 subjects, with reflux demonstrated in only 4 of 21 patients studied with pH electrodes.[82] Similar findings have been noted in patients studied prior to undergoing gastric bypass surgery.[83] However, there is almost universal agreement that obesity predisposes to gastroesophageal reflux. An elevated gastroesophageal pressure gradient has been demonstrated in obese patients.[84] This increased gradient, presumably reflecting increased intra-abdominal pressure due to large panniculi, has been postulated to decrease the velocity of the esophageal peristaltic wave. Prolonged esophageal transit times have been measured with radionuclide scintigraphy and may predispose to reflux esophagitis if injurious agents such as refluxed acid and bile are allowed greater mucosal contact time.[85]

Abnormalities of gastric emptying in obese patients were documented by Horowitz and associates using double isotope techniques with a mixed solid-liquid meal.[86] Obese patients (all were at least 50 per cent in excess of ideal body weight) had delayed gastric emptying of solids that correlated positively with increasing body weight. Liquid emptying in obese patients was not different from that in normal subjects. Other

studies have shown variable and sometimes conflicting results, a reflection of both methodologic problems and selection of definition criteria for obesity.[87, 88] For example, Wright and associates measured rates of fluid/solid gastric emptying in 46 obese subjects (averaging 77 per cent over ideal body weight). They found that obese subjects, especially men, had much more rapid gastric emptying of solids than that of nonobese controls. Liquid emptying rates did not differ between obese and nonobese subjects. No correlation between body surface area and gastric emptying rates of solids or liquids were found.[89] Obese persons appear to have greater tolerance to distention of the stomach when compared with normal subjects.[90] A significant increase in gastric volume may explain the sometimes observed delayed gastric emptying. Whether these abnormalities improve after weight reduction is unknown.

Liver abnormalities occur frequently in obese individuals. Steatosis is found in up to 94 per cent of obese patients and is usually the only abnormality noted in most studies.[91] Minimal or slight portal fibrosis and/or inflammation occurs in 30 to 50 per cent of cases, pericellular fibrosis in 10 to 25 per cent of cases, and "early" cirrhosis in 3 to 5 per cent of cases.[92] Recently, steatonecrosis has been described, mainly in obese women, which simulates the steatonecrosis seen in alcoholic liver disease.[93] However, Braillon and coworkers studied 50 obese individuals and found no evidence that obesity *per se* caused severe liver disease, suggesting instead the existence of concurrent hepatotoxic agents such as alcohol and certain drugs.[94] Whether a consistent relationship exists between severity of histologic liver abnormalities and the severity or duration of obesity is unclear.[95] Furthermore, there is a poor relationship between histologic abnormalities and abnormalities of commonly used "liver function" tests.[96]

Pharmacokinetics of drugs in obesity are generally unknown.[97] Obesity has been reported as a predictor of poor antibody response to hepatitis B plasma vaccine irrespective of injection site.[98] Possible explanations include poor mobilization of the antigen in obese persons and poor immune response.[99] Cimetidine disposition and clearance in obesity appears to be normal when the drug is administered intravenously.[100] Since cimetidine is rapidly and almost completely absorbed after oral administration and drug absorption is normal in obesity, one would predict similar unaltered pharmacokinetics of oral cimetidine.

The risks of surgery in obesity are considerable and are generally due to impaired cardiopulmonary function, thromboembolic disease, wound complications, and technical difficulties of operating in the obese patient.[101] In one study, duodenal ulcer surgery in patients weighing at least 15.9 kg over ideal body weight for height had more wound infections, and a trend toward more atelectasis, thrombophlebitis, and mortality when compared with nonobese patients.[102] In obese patients undergoing cholecystectomy, wound infections and pneumonitis occurred more frequently than in nonobese patients.[103]

Evaluation of Obesity

Causes of obesity other than idiopathic are very uncommon and, in general, quite apparent. The differential diagnosis of obesity is shown in Table 9–2. Despite the many protestations of a "glandular problem" causing their morbid obesity, these patients rarely have primary endocrine disease. Serum thyroid hormone concentration is normal. A few patients with idiopathic obesity may have an elevated triiodothyronine (T_3), presumably secondary to carbohydrate overfeeding.[104] Cushing's syndrome or disease has a characteristic fat distribution and accompanying laboratory abnormalities. Hypothalamic obesity is well established. It usually develops before the fourth decade and rarely results in morbid obesity.[105] Craniopharyngiomas are the most common lesions; trauma and infections are other causes. Stein-Leventhal syndrome is associated with obesity in women and has physical features distinguishing it from idiopathic obesity.

The rare genetic disorders associated with obesity include Laurence-Moon-Bardet-Biedl syndrome, Alström-Hallgren syndrome, Prader-Willi syndrome, Cohen's syndrome, Carpenter's syndrome, and Blount's disease. These disorders present in childhood and are generally made clinically evident by the associated congenital abnormalities.

In summary, an extensive evaluation for secondary obesity is unnecessary. In adults, hypothyroidism and Cushing's syndrome can be eliminated from consideration by measuring serum thyroid hormone levels and by performing a dexamethasone suppression test, respectively. If the obese patient has headaches, visual disturbances, growth disorder, or endocrine dysfunction, computerized tomography of the head should be performed.

Treatment of Obesity

To lose weight, one needs to either decrease calorie intake or to increase energy expenditure. Despite the simplicity of this concept, no one has yet found a satisfactory way to achieve long-term weight reduction. Many techniques work for weeks to months, some with dramatic weight loss, but almost all have failed in the long run. Furthermore, few objective data are available to judge the success of these programs, much less their risks and comparative efficacy. Some guidelines are available, but for the most part deciding which modality to propose to one's patient must be based on common sense.[106]

Diets

Dieting remains the simplest, least complicated way to lose weight. In general, one must have an energy deficit of 7500 kilocalories to lose a kilogram of weight. To achieve this energy deficit, one can try to increase poorly absorbable foods in the diet ("high-fiber diet"), decrease absorption of normal foods ("starch block-

Table 9–2. DIFFERENTIAL DIAGNOSIS OF OBESITY

Hypothalamic Disorders
Tumors
   Solid tumors: most common is craniopharyngioma
   Leukemia
Trauma
Infection/inflammation
   Tuberculosis
   Sarcoidosis
   Arachnoiditis
   Encephalitis
Adipsia/hypernatremia syndrome
Basal encephalocele
Pseudotumor cerebri (?)

Endocrine Disorders
Hypothyroidism
Hyperadrenocorticism
Hypogonadism (Fröhlich's syndrome)
Polycystic ovaries (Stein-Leventhal syndrome)
Pseudohypoparathyroidism

Congenital Syndromes
Laurence-Moon-Bardet-Biedl syndrome
Alström-Hallgren syndrome
Prader-Willi syndrome
Cohen's syndrome
Carpenter's syndrome
Blount's disease
Morgagni-Stuart-Morel syndrome

Drug-Induced (Increased Food Intake)
Cyproheptadine
Phenothiazine

ers," bile acid binders), or even use nonabsorbable food substitutes (sucrose polyester). These methods either simply do not work, as is the case with "starch blockers," or they hold theoretical interest of doubtful clinical usefulness. Hence, the most direct approach is to reduce calorie intake. A multitude of weight-loss diets have been proposed. Table 9–3 lists some of the most popular diets.

Low-Calorie Diets. To achieve greater and faster weight loss, low-calorie (800 kcal), very-low-calorie diets (240 to 330 kcal), and even total fasts have been proposed. When very-low-calorie diets were first popularized, they consisted of hydrolyzed collagen as the only calorie source. By 1977, at least 60 deaths in obese persons on liquid protein diets had been reported.[107] Most of these deaths were attributed to cardiac arrhythmias.[108] These and other complications appear to be less frequent when the protein source is of high biologic value, such as egg albumin or milk soya. Furthermore, when formulated as a nutritionally complete diet albeit containing only 400 kcal, these very-low-calorie diets have been shown to be relatively safe and effective when used under experienced medical supervision.[109] Problems may arise when these diets are available commercially and sold to consumers by "diet counselors."[110, 111] Currently, these regimens are to be considered for only the morbidly obese under direct physician supervision with periodic biochemical and electrocardiographic monitoring. Certainly, patients with severe chronic disease, children, pregnant women, or mildly obese persons should be excluded.

Table 9–3. CATEGORIES OF WEIGHT-LOSS DIETS

Type of Diet	Examples
Nutritionally Balanced	
Restricted calories	Weight Watchers, TOPS (Take Off Pounds Sensibly), Dr. Rechtschaffen's Diet (1980), Redbook's Wise Woman's Diet (1981), Prudent Diet (1972), Rotation Diet (when supplemented with minerals, vitamins) (1986)
Nutritionally Unbalanced	
High-carbohydrate	Pritikin Diet (1979), F-plan Diet (1983), Dr. Cooper's Fabulous Fructose Diet (1979), Rice Diet Report (1985)
Low-carbohydrate	Dr. Atkins Superenergy Diet (1976), Doctor's Quick Weight-loss Diet (1968), Complete Scarsdale Diet (1978)
High-protein	I Love New York Diet (1982), Richard Simmon's Never-Say-Diet Book (1980), Slendernow Diet (1982), Southampton Diet (1982)
High-fat	Dr. Herman Taller's Calories Don't Count Diet (1961), Dr. Atkins Diet Revolution (1972)
Fad Diets	Beverly Hills Diet (1981), Dolly Parton Diet, Krebs Cycle K-28 Diet (1978), Fit for Life (1985), Herbalife, Grapefruit Diet, Enzyme Catalyst Diet (1976), Zen macrobiotic
Very-Low-Calorie Diets	
Protein-sparing modified Fasts	Medical supervision required
Formula diets	
Liquid protein diets	Last Chance Diet (1976)
Chemically defined	Cambridge Diet (1980), Fasting: The Ultimate Diet (1975)

The diet should be terminated when the patient becomes less than 20 per cent above ideal body weight, since at that weight the patient is no longer considered to be at increased risk for complications of obesity. One should remember that once the very-low-calorie diet is stopped, weight reduction is rarely maintained. The same can be said for total fasting and semistarvation-ketogenic regimens (such as the protein-sparing modified fast).[112]

Novelty (Fad) Diets. Food faddism and cultism are key components of popular diets that propose a unique, undiscovered, or "natural" approach to weight loss. Most of these diets severely limit food choices or even eliminate any choice, resulting in a grossly unbalanced diet.[113, 114] Despite very strong condemnations from the medical community, these diets continue to be frustratingly popular.[115]

In summary a hypocaloric (about 1000 kcal/day) diet should include (1) 100 per cent of the recommended dietary allowances for vitamins and minerals, (2) a minimum of 100 gm of carbohydrate, representing about 50 per cent of total calories and consisting mostly of complex carbohydrates, (3) a minimum of 15 gm of essential fatty acids, and (4) a minimum of 0.8 gm of protein per kilogram of ideal body weight, representing about 15 per cent of total calories. This diet would be recommended for persons wishing to lose 9 kg or less over a two-month period.[116] Despite the seeming simplicity of this goal and regimen, most patients will fail. Protests to the contrary, the vast majority of patients will underestimate their intake.[117] Some investigators have reported that a hypocaloric diet induces a metabolic adaptation, such that obese patients may develop lower energy requirements. However, this adaptation, if it exists, is probably of insufficient magnitude to jeopardize the diet regimen.[118]

Exercise

Exercise should always be included in a weight-reduction program. Potential benefits of increased exercise and physical conditioning in the treatment of obesity include (1) increased caloric expenditure, (2) increased ratio of lean body mass to fat, (3) cardiovascular conditioning, and (4) improved psychologic well-being.[119] Data regarding the effects of exercise on food intake are conflicting.[120] In one study of obese women, Woo and colleagues did not demonstrate a compensatory rise in food intake with increased caloric expenditure from an exercise program.[121] However, one should recall that extensive exercise is needed to increase caloric expenditure significantly. The caloric equivalent of 1 pound of adipose tissue is approximately 3500 kcal, or the energy expenditure of a 100-kg person walking at 1 mile per hour for 35 miles. It is quite easy to "reward" oneself with a calorie-dense snack following an invigorating but calorically insignificant jog.

Since few obese people have the dedication to adhere to strict, repetitive exercise regimens, the drop-out rate from exercise programs is quite high, as it is from diet programs. As such, one should consider exercise as a *pattern* of behavior, amenable to modification.[122] Furthermore, physical activity can be categorized as (1) a programmed regimen of concentrated exercise, for example, running, swimming, cycling, and (2) general activity as part of one's lifestyle. Since the latter can be incorporated or "modified" into one's day-to-day patterns of living, it is easier for patients to begin and *adhere to* exercise by asking them to park their car some distance from the store and walking the remaining distance or to use the stairs and not the elevator, than for patients to swim three times a week.[123] While these "lifestyle" activities have little metabolic consequence, they do boost patient morale, which improves adherence to an *overall* weight-loss program.

Behavioral Modification

Because of the high dropout rate associated with balanced-deficit dieting, behavioral modification has been added with some success. When combined with very-low-calorie diets, behavior modification has improved the otherwise dismal long-term results of either program alone.[122, 124] The major elements of a behavioral weight-control program should include (1) self-monitoring by patients of food types, meal times, circumstances, and so forth to characterize their eating behavior fully, (2) control of the stimuli that precede eating, (3) development of techniques to control eating behavior, such as counting each mouthful of food and each swallow, (4) reinforcement, usually positive, of dieting behavior, (5) cognitive behavior modification to eliminate negative thoughts and to set realistic goals, (6) nutrition education, and (7) exercise.[125]

Because such a behavioral weight-control program is beyond the expertise and patience of most physicians, paramedical and lay staff are usually recruited. Self-help and commercially run organizations, such as Weight Watchers, Overeaters Anonymous, and Take Off Pounds Sensibly, probably provide the safest, most accessible, and most successful treatment modality available for weight reduction and maintenance.

Pharmacologic Treatment

In 1985, Americans spent over $200 million on diet drugs.[126] The hope is to reduce appetite (and thus energy intake) or to increase energy expenditure.

Anorectic drugs include the amphetamines (diethylproprion, fenfluramine, mazindol, and phentermine resin), related compounds, and phenylpropanolamine. Recent reviews describe their clinical pharmacology and central mode of action.[127, 128] Since these drugs do nothing to modify basic eating behavior, they should not be used except within an overall weight-reduction program. Short-term weight loss has been repeatedly documented, but not long-term efficacy.[129, 130]

So-called peripherally acting drugs for treatment of obesity include bulk fillers to cause stomach distention and satiety, and agents to decrease nutrient absorption (cholestyramine, amylase inhibitors popularly known as "starch blockers"). These agents are of no benefit in treating obesity.[131]

Hormonal preparations to increase energy expenditure have also been tried without benefit. Thyroidal hormones have produced short-term weight loss, but this loss is mostly from the lean body mass rather than from fat stores.[132] Other hormones include human growth hormone, progesterone, and human chorionic gonadotropin.[133] Because of the role of alpha-adrenergic receptors in adipocyte metabolism, blocking agents that promote lypolysis are being studied.[134] Unfortunately, these agents also enhance insulin release.

Miscellaneous Treatment

In the quest for losing weight, Americans spent about $5 billion in 1985.[126] One can easily seen how this fact is not lost on the entrepreneurial mind. In 1982, starch blockers were the rage before they were shown to be ineffective.[135] Other methods ranging from ear acupuncture to constricting belts have been proposed.[136] One of the latest entries is gastric balloon implantation. These "artificial bezoars" allegedly stimulate satiety by reducing gastric capacity. A variety of balloons have been used including "dime-store" balloons and mammary implants.[137] A commercially available, aggressively marketed balloon has achieved popularity among the public and some gastroenterologists. The Garren-Edwards Gastric Bubble is a cylindrically shaped elastomeric bubble introduced into the stomach via a modified orogastric feeding tube after endoscopic "screening" of the stomach. Inflated to 200 ml, the bubble is left in place after a second endoscopy confirms proper inflation and correct position. The patient is then supposed to enter a program of low-calorie diet (800 to 1000 kcal/day) and behavior modification. After four months, a third endoscopy is performed to puncture and remove or replace the bubble. The FDA has approved this bubble for use in persons who are 20 per cent or more above their ideal weight, a potential market of at least 30 million customers. Training seminars for endoscopists are being conducted throughout the country by the manufacturer.

Reported complications of balloon or bubble therapy include gastrointestinal ulceration and hemorrhage, acute pancreatitis, obstruction requiring laparotomy, and fatal peritonitis.[138, 139] Spontaneous deflation occurs in about 9 per cent of inserted balloons.[140] Following reports of more complications, the FDA approved labeling changes for the gastric bubble wherein the manufacturer calls for bubble removal after 12 weeks (instead of 16 weeks) and recommends the insertion of the bubble only in morbidly obese patients (generally considered to be patients being 100 per cent or 100 pounds over ideal weight).

Weight loss has been reported with balloon therapy. Whether the balloon contributes to the weight reduction as a "satiety-inducing" agent or the weight loss is caused by the low-calorie diet and behavioral modification alone is unknown. A panel of physicians asked by the American Medical Association to address the safety and efficacy of the Garren gastric bubble recently judged it to be investigational and called for controlled clinical trials.[141] At least three such studies are under way. A preliminary report from one study concluded that the gastric bubble does not increase weight loss when compared with diet and behavior modification alone (personal communication, R. Hogan, M.D., Jackson, MS).

Jaw wiring has had limited success.[142] It can be performed in an outpatient setting and has little morbidity.[143] Its major risk is that of aspiration pneumonia. Long-term success has not been reported and is unlikely.

Surgical Therapy of Obesity

Because of the dismal long-term results with medical therapy of obesity, a variety of surgical procedures have been devised to cause malabsorption of nutrients or to decrease food intake.

Patient Selection. Guidelines for surgery for morbid obesity have been proposed by the Task Force of the American Society for Clinical Nutrition.[144] Before being considered for bariatric surgery, the patient

Table 9–4. ELIGIBILITY CRITERIA FOR SURGICAL TREATMENT OF OBESITY

1. Body weight exceeds average desirable weight by 100 pounds or 100% for at least 3 years
2. Presence of serious medical complication(s) of obesity
3. Repeated failure of acceptable nonsurgical methods of treating obesity
4. Well-informed, cooperative patient aged 18 to 50 years
5. Optimal preoperative cardiopulmonary status
6. Absence of correctable metabolic or endocrine disease that could cause obesity
7. Absence of disqualifying conditions such as stroke, recently treated malignancy, or serious organ dysfunction
8. Stable adult life pattern without significant psychopathology or substance abuse
9. Commitment by surgeon, hospital, and patient to life-long follow-up.

should be at least 45.5 kg or 100 per cent over average desirable weight or have at least one serious medical complication of morbid obesity. Furthermore, the patient should have a history of having failed nonsurgical means of weight reduction and of having been morbidly obese for at least 3 years, and should be considered able to tolerate the anesthesia and surgery. Table 9–4 shows a summary of eligibility criteria. Preoperative evaluations, preferably made separately by an internist, a surgeon, and a psychiatrist, are recommended to judge probable postoperative success.[145] Preoperative studies should also include a nutritional assessment. Radiographic evaluation of the gastrointestinal tract is probably advisable particularly in patients undergoing gastric reduction surgery, although only an oral cholecystogram has been reported to be of sufficient yield to warrant use as a preoperative screening test (unless the patient has symptoms to suggest disease elsewhere or has had previous gastrointestinal surgery).[146]

Intestinal Bypass Operations. These operations are based on the concept of iatrogenic malabsorption. Ironically, the mechanism of weight loss after these bypass operations is believed to be decreased food intake (due to decreased appetite) while the pathophysiology of its many complications stem from the malabsorption.[147] Intestinal bypass operations have fallen into disfavor and are rarely performed nowadays.[148] However, since over 10,000 patients have had these operations, they remain of more than historical interest.

In 1969, Payne and DeWind described a bypass wherein 36 cm of jejunum is anastomosed end-to-side to the ileum 10 cm proximal to the ileocecal valve (Fig. 9–3).[149] Because this technique was associated with unpredictable weight loss (presumably due to nutrient reflux into the bypassed ileum) and a high rate of bypass enteritis, Scott and associates proposed a modification in 1970.[150] This technique has the 30 cm of jejunum anastomosed end-to-end to the ileum 20 cm proximal to the ileocecal valve with the distal end of the defunctionalized small intestine anastomosed to the colon (Fig. 9–4). Other malabsorption-producing procedures, such as Scopinaro's pancreaticobiliary bypass and Hallberg's biliointestinal bypass, have been tried but have not achieved the popularity of the Payne-DeWind and Scott procedures.

Judgment about these procedures must weigh the benefits against the complications.[151] The beneficial effects of these intestinal bypass operations include predictable weight loss that generally stabilizes within the first postoperative year, improved glucose tolerance, decreased serum levels of cholesterol and tri-

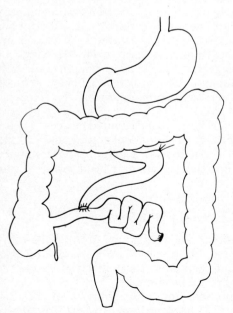

Figure 9–3. The jejunoileal bypass by Payne and DeWind. This procedure consists of 36 cm of jejunum anastomosed end-to-side to the ileum 10 cm proximal to the ileocecal valve.

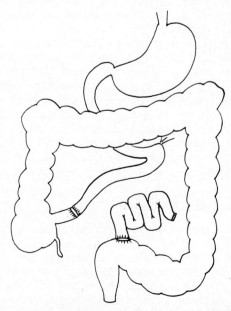

Figure 9–4. The jejunoileal bypass by Scott. This procedure consists of 30 cm of jejunum anastomosed end-to-end to the ileum 20 cm proximal to the ileocecal valve. The distal end of the defunctionalized bowel is anastomosed end-to-side to the sigmoid colon.

glyceride, improved cardiovascular function, and enhanced psychosocial interactions (improved body image, sex life, interpersonal relations, self-esteem, and job effectiveness).[152] The complications of jejunoileal bypass operations are many and have been extensively reviewed.[153] Table 9–5 lists the reported complications and proposed mechanisms. Among the most serious complications are liver disease and malnutrition.

The incidence of liver disease following jejunoileal bypass varies according to the parameter examined. Fatty steatosis is found most often, but one should remember that 60 to 100 per cent of morbidly obese patients had this abnormality preoperatively. However, lipid concentrations in the liver do increase after bypass, presumably owing mostly to a rise in triglyceride concentration.[154] The mechanism of liver injury is not known, although many explanations have been proposed.[155] The most worrisome hepatic complication is hepatic failure, which occurs to some degree in 5 per cent of patients, with 1 per cent progressing to cirrhosis.[155, 156] Death from liver failure or cirrhosis occurs in 0.5 to 2 per cent of patients. Liver changes are most pronounced within the first postoperative year (during the period of maximum weight loss) and generally reverse and stabilize as the weight stabilizes.[156] Liver biopsies may show disorders ranging from minimal to marked steatosis to central sclerosis and central fibrosis with an inflammatory reaction resembling alcoholic hepatitis (including hyalin and Mallory's bodies) and to frank cirrhosis.[157]

In general, neither liver function tests nor imaging correlate with liver histologic findings in bypass patients. Hence, sequential liver biopsies should be performed postoperatively (at least at the end of the first postoperative year) to identify those patients with severe histologic changes before irreversible cirrhosis develops. This surveillance is worthwhile since liver failure is often reversible after intestinal continuity is re-established.

Malnutrition develops because of malabsorption from markedly diminished intestinal surface area. Increased fecal excretion of fat, nitrogen, electrolytes, calcium, magnesium, zinc, copper, and minerals has been reported.[158] Symptoms due to depletion of these nutrients include weakness, muscle cramps, and disturbances in acid-base balance. Malabsorption of fat-soluble vitamins is particularly significant, with bone disease developing in 17 to 48 per cent of patients with low plasma levels of 25-OH vitamin D_3 and high plasma parathyroid hormone.[159]

In view of the many complications associated with jejunoileal bypass operations, the question arises as to whether a patient who has had this procedure should have prophylactic restoration of intestinal continuity, since reanastomosis corrects most of the metabolic problems.[160] As it is, up to 40 per cent of patients have already suffered complications serious enough to require reanastomosis or revision. Usually, however, the patient is resistant to such a recommendation, even if much of the initial postoperative weight loss has been

Table 9–5. COMPLICATIONS OF INTESTINAL BYPASS PROCEDURES

Complication	Proposed Mechanism

Liver disease
  Fatty metamorphosis
  Hepatitis
  Centrolobular fibrosis
  Cirrhosis
  Liver failure
	Rapid mobilization of lipid, nutritional deficiencies (protein, choline, methionine, essential fatty acids), toxic insult (toxins from anaerobic bacterial overgrowth, bile salts, production of endogenous alcohol)

Gallstones	Bile acid loss, mobilization of cholesterol
Nutritional deficiencies Vitamins	Malabsorption
Vitamin B_{12}	Ileum bypassed
Vitamin K	Steatorrhea
Vitamin D	Steatorrhea
Vitamin A	Steatorrhea
Vitamin E	Steatorrhea
Electrolytes/minerals (potassium, calcium, magnesium, copper, zinc)	Malabsorption
Diarrhea, enteropathy	Decreased absorptive surface, decreased transit time, disaccharidase deficiency, excessive colonic bile and fatty acids, steatorrhea, bacterial overgrowth
Intestinal problems Intussusception, herniation, pneumatosis cystoides intestinalis, pseudo-obstruction, transmural ileocolitis	Postsurgical, multifactorial

Renal disease
  Urolithiasis
  Oxaluria
	Excess oxalate absorption (undigested fat binds intraluminal calcium, allowing increased absorption of oxalate)

Tubular acidosis	Secondary to hypokalemia
Arthropathy	Bacterial toxins
Dermatitis (maculopapular, vesicular or pustular)	Bacterial toxins
Encephalopathy	D-Lactic acidemia from colonic fermentation of carbohydrates
Tuberculosis (especially reactivation)	Protein malnutrition, immunoreactive changes
Bone disease (osteomalacia)	Alterations in vitamin D metabolism due to malabsorption, liver disease, bacterial overgrowth
Alopecia (temporary)	Protein deficiency

regained. Hence, one must generally combine small intestinal reanastomosis with gastroplasty or gastric partition in an effort to maintain some weight loss.[161, 162]

Gastric Operations (Gastric Partition, Gastroplasty)

Techniques. Gastric operations for weight loss are designed to restrict oral intake by reducing the amount of food that can comfortably be accommodated by the small gastric reservoir created. First developed by Mason and Ito in 1967, the gastric bypass subsequently was modified.[163] Originally (1966 to 1970), the procedure involved totally dividing the stomach and creating a 100-ml pouch with a 20-mm loop gastroenterostomy. From 1970 to 1977, modifications proposed reducing

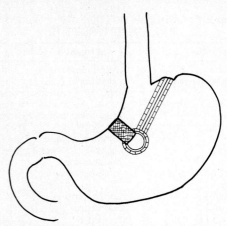

Figure 9–5. Mason's vertical gastroplasty. The procedure consists of a 50-ml gastric reservoir and a 12-mm channel located on the lesser curvature. A complete through-and-through stapled opening is made on the lesser curvature, and a double line of staples beginning at the angle of His to this opening creates the upper pouch. The stoma is reinforced with a collar of polypropylene mesh around the lesser curvature channel.

the pouch size (to 60 ml) and narrowing the stoma (to 8 mm). These procedures were technically difficult to perform in obese patients and had attendant unacceptably high morbidity and mortality. In 1971, Mason developed gastroplasty, wherein a partial transection of the stomach was performed along the lesser curvature, leaving a channel along the greater curvature.[164] Other modifications of gastric bypass were reported (Alden's loop gastric bypass with stapled partition and antecolic gastrojejunostomy in 1977 and Griffen's Roux-en-Y bypass in 1979). However, bypass operations became less frequently performed after 1982 as autostapling devices made gastroplasty easier. Different techniques of gastroplasty (Mason's vertical gastroplasty [Fig. 9–5], Gomez's horizontal gastroplasty with reinforced stoma [Fig. 9–6], O'Leary's lesser curvature gastroplasty, Laws' gastroplasty with silastic collar reinforced stoma) each try to achieve a small (30 to 55 ml) pouch, small outlet stoma (10 to 12 mm), and reinforced partition to prevent enlargement of either pouch or stoma.[165]

Physiologic Changes. Most of the weight loss occurs in the first six weeks.[165] After gastroplasty, a dramatic fall in the intake of energy and nutrients is responsible for the weight loss.[166] Although no metabolic measurement—respiratory oxygen consumption, urine urea nitrogen, or basal metabolic rate—is predictive of degree of weight loss, a metabolic shift to fat utilization with sparing of lean body mass has been reported.[167] Patients eat less presumably because of the earlier satiety that occurs owing to gastric pouch distention. However, the mechanism of action is unclear. Prolonged retention of food and liquids in the pouch does not occur.[168, 169] However, since gastric emptying in obese patients in general is not well defined, methodologic questions of emptying from gastric pouches remain.

Various changes in postprandial gastrointestinal hormones occur after gastric bypass surgery. Basal serum pancreatic polypeptide concentration is reduced, but meal-stimulated secretion is increased.[170, 171] Meal-stimulated serum gastrin levels are similarly increased.[172] Among the serum lipid changes that occur after gastroplasty is an increase in high-density lipoprotein that has been proposed as another advantage of gastroplasty over jejunoileal bypass operations.[173] Postoperatively, glucose tolerance and insulin sensitivity improve.[174]

Complications. The short- and long-term morbidity and mortality of gastric bariatric surgery are less than that of intestinal bypass procedures.[175, 176] The operative mortality has decreased to 1 per cent in experienced hands depending on the particular technique used. Early deaths are generally due to anastomotic leaks and peritonitis (which in the obese patient is not always obvious), gastric ischemia, and perforation. Late operative complications occur in up to 17 per cent of patients and include stomal obstruction (usually in the first postoperative month), stomal ulcers, incisional hernias, persistent nausea and vomiting, cholelithiasis, and cholecystitis.[177] A number of radiologic techniques have been described to assess patients with stomal complications following gastroplasty and gastric bypass surgery.[178, 179] However, to detect and evaluate stomal disruption in addition to the integrity of the partitioned stomach, endoscopy is superior to radiography.[180] Furthermore, endoscopic pneumatic balloon catheter dilation has been used successfully to treat stomal stenosis.[181]

Hepatic. Initially, there were no reports of liver disease developing after gastric operations. Indeed, improvement in liver histology was found. However, a clinical picture similar to alcoholic hepatitis has been described in a patient whose liver biopsy showed alcoholic-like hyalin.[182]

Hematologic. Similar to reports of anemia developing in patients after partial gastrectomy, anemia is a frequent complication after gastric exclusion surgery.

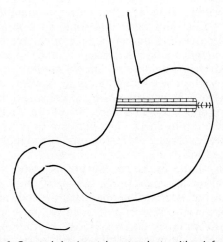

Figure 9–6. Gomez's horizontal gastroplasty with reinforced stoma. The procedure consists of a 60-ml fundic reservoir and a 12-mm channel located on the greater curvature of the stomach. A seromuscular ring of nonabsorbable suture reinforces the stoma and is supposed to prevent expansion of the channel. Unfortunately, this reinforcement has not been as successful as hoped.

Iron-deficiency anemia, which is easily treated with oral supplementation, occurs in almost half of patients.[183] Folate deficiency and vitamin B_{12} deficiency occur in 18 per cent and 40 per cent of patients, respectively.[183] Megaloblastic anemia due to vitamin B_{12} deficiency has been reported, although neurologic disease was not found.[184, 185] Consequently, all patients following gastric exclusion surgery should receive supplemental iron and multivitamins during the first postoperative year of maximum weight loss and thereafter, should periodic follow-up examinations reveal deficiencies developing.

Neurologic. Syndromes of ataxia, weakness, peripheral neuropathy, postural hypotension, diplopia, confusion, and agitation have been described.[177, 186] The etiologies are multifactorial, but in some cases have responded to parenteral thiamine.[186] Wernicke-Korsakoff syndrome and Guillain-Barré syndrome can also occur.[187] At autopsy in one patient who developed ataxia, chorea, and polyneuropathy, investigators found extensive demyelination, presumably due to starvation-induced neuronal and Schwann cell lipidoses.[188]

Miscellaneous. Because of the malnutrition that can follow gastric surgery, a variety of complications can occur including immunologic impairment, protein and zinc deficiency (with sometimes profound but reversible hair loss during the first postoperative year), renal stones, and osteomalacia.[189, 190]

Effectiveness. While it remains unclear whether decreased food intake in patients following gastric exclusion surgery is due to early adverse conditioning from epigastric pain when eating too much, the net result is generally substantial weight loss. Griffen and Ward reported a mean weight loss of 47.6 kg in a study of nearly 1600 patients.[191] The greater the initial weight of the patient, the greater is the weight loss, although some of these patients will gain weight after two to three years because of increased food intake from accommodation to gastric distention, stomal dilation, and circumvention of the small stoma (by consuming calorie-dense liquids).[192]

Few studies have compared gastric surgery with other modalities of weight reduction. Andersen and colleagues found in one randomized controlled trial that gastroplasty produced as much initial weight loss as diet alone.[193] Alden analyzed 200 patients in a nonrandomized manner, noting similar weight loss but considerably more frequent and severe complications following jejunoileal bypass as compared with gastric bypass.[194] Griffen and associates and Buckwalter, in two prospective randomized studies, also favored gastric bypass because of fewer complications and similar degrees of weight loss.[175, 176] However, it must be remembered that all of these studies suffer from a high drop-out rate and lack of sufficient long-term follow-up of their patients.

EATING DISORDERS

An eating disorder can be defined as a disturbance in eating behavior that results in injury to a person's physical or psychologic health. Eating disorders recognized by the American Psychiatric Association include anorexia nervosa, bulimia, pica, and rumination disorder of infancy. While the latter problems are also important, I shall restrict my discussion to anorexia nervosa and bulimia.

History and Prevalence

Anorexia nervosa was first described three hundred years ago by Richard Morton when he described a 17-year-old girl who was "like a skeleton only clad with skin."[195] Although Sir William Gull and Charles Lasegue, a French contemporary, each described additional patients in more clinical detail, Gull coined the term "anorexia nervosa."[196]

Actually, the term "anorexia nervosa" is a misnomer since such patients have no loss of appetite, but rather are morbidly preoccupied with food and the fear of becoming fat. Similarly, bulimia, which means "ox hunger," is a misnomer as regards the patient. While these patients binge-eat enormous numbers of calories, they are not driven by hunger and instead carefully plan their binges and subsequent purging. Patients with bulimia nervosa have, as the name implies, characteristics of both anorexia nervosa and bulimia. The majority of these patients have a prior history of true or cryptic anorexia nervosa and use self-induced vomiting and purging to counteract the effects of eating.

The prevalence of eating disorders is unknown. The incidence of anorexia nervosa has doubled over the last 20 years according to some studies.[197, 198] Bulimia also appears to be increasing in incidence and prevalence, particularly among young people in the higher socioeconomic strata in developed countries. Estimates of prevalence range from 1 to 50 per cent of adolescent women and 10 per cent of college-age men.[199, 200] Purging behavior—self-induced vomiting and laxative and diuretic use—among teenagers is as high as 13 per cent, with women purgers outnumbering men purgers 2 to 1.[201] However, the apparent increasing incidence of eating disorders is based for the most part on questionnaire studies. Whether there truly is an epidemic of anorexia nervosa and related disorders has recently been questioned.[202] Exact estimates of incidence and prevalence are difficult because of varying definitions, the covert nature of patients not wishing to arouse suspicion of their eating behavior, and the subclinical forms of the disorders.

Natural History

Anorexia Nervosa. While the clinical picture of anorexia nervosa has been well reviewed recently, certain characteristic features are worth emphasizing.[203, 204]

Anorexia nervosa usually begins in the teenager, primarily in women, most often 4 to 5 years after menarche. The patient is usually from an affluent white family and of at least normal intelligence. Having dieted sporadically, she is slightly overweight initially or perceives herself as overweight, and her reactive mechanism results in severe restriction of food intake ("restricters") or in binge-purge behavior alternating with periods of self-starvation ("bulimia nervosa"). Anorectic patients are intensely fearful of becoming obese, and consequently are preoccupied with food and meal preparation. Since a disturbance of body image underlies anorexia nervosa, actual food intake is pathologically reduced to induce starvation and thus to achieve the desired, albeit distorted, appearance. Excessive exercise is also used to achieve weight loss and may even be a clue to incipient anorexia nervosa.

Bulimia. Bulimia begins at a later age than anorexia nervosa, usually between 17 and 25 years.[205] However, presentation to medical attention may not occur until the patient is in her third or fourth decade of life. The typical bulimic patient is also preoccupied with food and eating, but, unlike the anorectic, she utilizes self-induced emesis or laxatives rather than starvation to control her weight. The critical sensation during binge-eating episodes is a distressing loss of control with feelings of guilt and shame.[206] Hence, she is more willing to seek professional help than the anorectic.

The eating pattern of a bulimic is typically one of binge-eating often precipitated by anxiety and tension, frustration, or depression.[206, 207] "Forbidden foods" high in carbohydrates and fat content, such as doughnuts, cakes, and ice cream, are consumed rapidly and usually in secrecy, and therefore often at night while alone. Up to 20,000 kcal may be ingested during one binge.[208] Binges stop with abdominal discomfort or social interruption, followed by self-induced emesis, laxatives, or diuretics in hopes of undoing the binge eating. The binge-purge episodes are almost automatic, and the bulimics feel driven and depersonalized. Other impulsive behavior may be found, such as alcohol and drug abuse, sexual promiscuity, and stealing, sometimes to support the expenses of the food binges.[209]

Psychologic Features

The frequent association of depression with eating disorders is striking; up to 50 per cent of anorectics and 20 per cent of bulimics are depressive.[210] In some cases, the affective symptoms precede the onset of the disease.[211] Similarities between patients with depression and those with eating disorders include an increased frequency of the HLA-BW16 antigen, failure to suppress cortisol in response to dexamethasone, decreased urinary excretion of 3-methoxy-4-hydroxyl phenyl glycol, and decreased levels of platelet monoamine oxidase.[203]

Psychometric studies of anorectics indicate high levels of depression. However, one also needs to consider the confounding effect of prolonged fasting *per se* that results in "semistarvation neurosis," a constellation of behavioral and psychologic changes that resemble those found in anorectics. When compared with control subjects (with personality disorders only) and patients with diagnosed depression, anorectic patients tend to

fall between the two groups, and generally exhibit depression of mild to moderate severity. However, the patients with bulimia nervosa are more depressed than anorectics and tend to have a poorer psychologic (and medical) prognosis. Impaired psychologic development as described by Bruch[212] may explain the high prevalence of psychologic dysfunction. Psychometric studies of bulimic subjects are scant but generally reveal fewer depressive symptoms. Once again, however, bulimia nervosa subjects had high scores on the psychopathic deviate and depression scale.

Family studies have found a very high prevalence of depressive symptoms and affective disorders among relatives of anorectic and bulimic patients.[213] However, no convincing evidence of genetic or sociofamilial transmission has been found. Rather, the patient may be the product of a family whose pathologic interactions predispose or contribute to these diseases.

Behaviorally, the patient with anorexia nervosa may be noteworthy for her "good behavior." Often an overachiever in school, she is generally compliant and perfectionistic. However, when the physiologic impact of her calorie restriction becomes marked with weakness and fatigue, she exhibits apathy, passivity and withdrawal, and regression ("semi-starvation neurosis"). The bulimic, in contrast, may appear completely normal, both in behavior and physical appearance. Since the binge-purge episodes are surreptitious, the only outward signs of dysfunction, other than the metabolic complications of purging, may be antisocial behavior and mild depression.

Symptoms and Physical Features

. . . . all the conditions in this case were negative, and may be explained by the anorexia which led to starvation, and a depression of all the vital functions.

W. W. Gull, M.D., 1874

The medical complications of anorexia nervosa are generally those of starvation. The symptoms and physical findings bring to mind the cachectic survivors of prisoner-of-war camps. While patients with anorexia nervosa tend to minimize their symptoms, they will usually have amenorrhea, sleep disturbances, cold intolerance (often accompanied by cyanosis and numbness of the extremities), and skin changes, such as hairiness, scaliness, and desquamation.[214, 215]

The physical examination in patients with classic anorexia nervosa is notable for inanition. As with symptoms, the patients tend to mask the severity of their illness. By wearing long sleeves, slacks, or long skirts, they can hide their severe weight loss. The bradycardia and mild hypotension of cachexia is present, as is some degree of peripheral edema, usually due to failure to mobilize fluid from the legs rather than to hypoalbuminemia. Of some diagnostic usefulness is the faintly yellow cast to the skin due to carotenemia, not present in patients with other forms of semi-starvation.

Despite the similarities between starved patients (such as prisoners of war and famine victims) and patients with anorexia nervosa, there are notable differences. Since anorectic patients have self-induced starvation, they usually "select" certain food categories to avoid, and take vitamin supplements, thus avoiding frank vitamin deficiency.[216] Muscle strength and breast tissue are also generally maintained, for reasons not entirely clear.

There is no diagnostic complex of physical signs and laboratory findings in patients with eating disorders. Hence, once must rely on diagnostic criteria that include both psychologic and physical changes. However, the laboratory profile is helpful in that findings that are not generally associated with eating disorders, such as an elevated erythrocyte sedimentation rate or white blood cell count, should make the physician suspicious that another diagnosis needs to be considered.

In contrast to patients with classic anorexia nervosa, bulimic patients are usually distressed by their eating disorder, and are less apt to hide or deny their problems and symptoms. Furthermore, the bulimic is usually of normal weight. Hence, the complications of bulimia more often result from binge eating followed by purging with laxatives and diuretics, rather than from self-imposed starvation. Symptoms of bulimia are then less common as compared with those of anorexia nervosa. For example, normal menses are usually present, probably a reflection of the patient's normal weight. Depression is often a complaint, as are episodes of impulsive behavior, such as alcohol and drug abuse. Symptoms of substance abuse in a female adolescent should trigger one's suspicion of bulimia.

As for the physical examination, bulimics are usually not cachectic and do not exhibit the physical findings described in anorectic patients. However, there may be stigmata of drug abuse or episodes of self-mutilation.

Laboratory Findings

Just as the physical findings reflect the degree of inanition (anorexia nervosa) or binge-purge behavior (bulimia), so do the laboratory findings. Hence, neither anorectic nor bulimic patients have "diagnostic" laboratory abnormalities. Severe malnutrition, whatever the cause, can result in anemia, low white cell and platelet numbers, and relative lymphocytosis. Two laboratory abnormalities of interest are elevated beta-carotene levels and high cholesterol levels in the blood.[217, 218] There is no ready explanation for either finding.

Complications

The medical complications of anorexia nervosa are generally those of starvation, while those of bulimia result from the physical and metabolic derangements of binge eating and purging (Table 9–6).[219]

Dental and Oral. Patients with anorexia nervosa or bulimia can present with the following: perimylolysis, dental caries, periodontal disease, and damage to oral mucous membranes.[220] Perimylolysis is a loss of enamel and dentin on the lingual surfaces of the teeth caused by the chemical effects of regurgitated gastric acid and

Table 9–6. MEDICAL COMPLICATIONS OF ANOREXIA NERVOSA AND BULIMIA

Organ System	Anorexia Nervosa	Bulimia
Oral		Gum disease, perimylolysis, caries, parotid enlargement, pharyngitis (hoarseness)
Gastrointestinal		
Esophageal		Esophagitis, Mallory-Weiss tear, rupture, rumination
Gastric	Delayed gastric emptying, decreased acid secretion	Acute gastric dilation, rupture
Intestinal	Constipation, superior mesenteric artery syndrome	Cathartic colon, ileus, rectal prolapse, hemorrhoids
Hepatic, pancreatic	Elevated hepatic enzymes	Pancreatitis, elevated serum amylase
Cardiovascular	Hypotension, bradycardia, arrhythmias (sometimes lethal), pericardial effusion	Ipecac-induced cardiotoxicity, pneumopericardium
Pulmonary		Aspiration pneumonia, pneumomediastinum
Endocrine/metabolic	Amenorrhea, decreased estrogen, euthyroid sick syndrome, increased growth hormone, decreased somatomedin C, decreased or erratic vasopressin secretion, increased etiocholanolone, decreased norepinephrine, hypercarotenemia, hypothermia, decreased gonadotropin, abnormal dexamethasone suppression	Menstrual irregularities
Renal	Dehydration, azotemia, decreased glomerular filtration rate, calculi, edema	Edema, hypokalemia, hypochloremic metabolic alkalosis, hypophosphatemia
Hematologic	Anemia, leukopenia, thrombocytopenia	
Musculoskeletal	Osteoporosis	Ipecac-induced myopathy
Neurologic	Caffeine-induced psychosis, compression peripheral neuropathy	Electroencephalographic abnormalities
Dermatologic	Lanugo hair, dry skin, yellow cast to skin	Bruises and lacerations of fingers (self-induced emesis), phenolphthalein fixed drug reaction, ecchymoses on face and neck (forceful emesis), conjunctival hemorrhages, self-mutilation

the mechanical trauma of the tongue against the surface of the teeth.[221] Bruxism, teeth clenching, and abnormal swallowing habits may contribute to the damage. Excessive carbohydrate intake and poor oral hygiene result in an increase in dental caries.

Parotid gland enlargement occurs in patients with eating disorders, particularly those with bulimia.[222] The enlargement may be painful or painless. The parotid enlargement in patients with malnutrition is due to an increase in acinar size.[223] However, once the malnutrition has been corrected, the parotid gland may remain enlarged. Hence, a mechanism other than malnutrition *per se* may be present, such as the effects of binge eating with resultant abrupt and sustained parotid gland stimulation.

Gastrointestinal. *Esophageal*. Esophageal complications in patients with eating disorders include esophagitis, esophageal erosions and ulcers, Mallory-Weiss tears, and rupture. These complications occur because of the mechanical and chemical injury to the esophagus from repeated vomiting. Dysphagia, esophageal stricture, and Barrett's esophagus reportedly occur more frequently in bulimic patients who vomit chronically.[219] Retching places tremendous stress on the esophagus, with rapid rises in esophageal pressures as high as 300 mm Hg, and can cause Mallory-Weiss tears. Perforation can result from vigorous vomiting.

Rumination in patients with eating disorders has been described.[224–226] Previously thought to occur predominantly in infants and mentally retarded children and adults, rumination in adults of normal intelligence with bulimia or anorexia nervosa suggests underlying neuromotility disturbances of the esophagus.[227]

***Gastric and Intestinal*.** Gastric complications of eating disorders include gastritis, decreased acid secretion, delayed gastric emptying, acute gastric dilatation, and rupture. Basal and stimulated acid output have been described as significantly less in patients with anorexia nervosa than that in normal subjects. This decrease persists even after patients gain weight.[228] McCallum and colleagues, however, noted no decrease in basal maximal acid output in patients with anorexia.[229] Delayed gastric emptying also occurs and may contribute to postprandial discomfort, fullness, and abdominal pain noted by some anorectic patients.[229–231] The mechanism of the impaired emptying is unknown, although bethanechol, a parasympathomimetic agent, temporarily increases gastric emptying in these patients. Improvement has also been reported with domperidone, metoclopramide, and cisapride.[232–235] Acute gastric dilatation is an uncommon but well-described complication.[236, 237] A combination of factors play a role, but dilatation may be due in part to rapid ingestion of large meals, exacerbated by delayed gastric emptying. Should dilatation be so severe that intragastric pressure exceeds gastric venous pressure, then ischemia and infarction can occur. Gastric rupture, another life-threatening complication, can then result.[238, 239]

Intestinal complications include the superior mesenteric artery syndrome (SMAS) wherein the artery compresses the transverse duodenum, causing intestinal obstruction. A chronic and an acute form of this syndrome exist. Chronic SMAS presents as severe postprandial pain and bloating, often accompanied by bilious vomiting. Acute SMAS presents with classic symptoms of acute small-bowel obstruction. This form of the syndrome occurs most commonly in anorectic patients following rapid and marked weight loss.[240, 241] The diagnosis is suggested by the history and confirmed radiographically. Medical management includes correcting the malnutrition and restoring normal weight and habitus. Rarely, surgery is necessary.

Colonic complications generally occur from laxative abuse. Although ineffective in significantly reducing calorie absorption, laxatives are often used in enormous quantities.[242] The electrolyte and water depletion can be life-threatening. Other consequences of laxative abuse include "cathartic colon," which is dilated, hypomotile, and neurologically damaged.[243] Rectal prolapse, hemorrhoids, and bleeding also plague laxative abusers, probably related to excessive straining of stool.[244] Laxative abuse can rarely cause steatorrhea and protein-losing enteropathy.

***Pancreatic*.** Acute pancreatitis with its attendant severe abdominal pain and severe complications has been reported in patients with eating disorders.[245, 246] Most of the patients have been markedly malnourished young women who developed pancreatitis when refeeding was initiated. One proposed mechanism for pancreatitis in anorectic patients is obstruction of the duodenum and subsequent duodenopancreatic reflux secondary to the superior mesenteric artery syndrome (see above).[219] Another mechanism may be excessive stimulation of pancreatic secretions coupled with outflow obstruction.

Hyperamylasemia without clinical evidence for pancreatitis occurs in nearly one third of patients with eating disorders.[247] Salivary rather than pancreatic isoenzyme elevation is usually the explanation for the hyperamylasemia.[248] Hence, measurement of serum lipase or pancreatic isoamylase activity should be the initial step in evaluating hyperamylasemia in these patients.

Cardiovascular. Patients with eating disorders may have impaired cardiovascular function with decreased blood pressure and reduced cardiac output and heart rate. The heart is abnormal with thinning of the left ventricle and reduction of cardiac chamber size.[249] Presumably these changes are in response to malnutrition. Many electrocardiographic changes have been reported. Electrolyte abnormalities cause many of the cardiac arrhythmias. However, intrinsic conduction defects have been found, and sudden deaths tragically occur. In addition, ipecac abuse has been linked to several deaths of patients with eating disorders.[250] Alkaloid emetine, an ingredient of ipecac syrup, has marked cardiotoxicity.

Pulmonary. Because of self-induced vomiting, the anorectic or bulimic patient risks aspiration pneumonia and pneumomediastinum. Bulimic patients may also be abusing drugs and alcohol. Vomiting when under the influence of these substances can result in vomitus being aspirated into the lungs. Furthermore, vigorous emesis can rupture lung tissue, and air can dissect into the mediastinum and pericardial sac.[251]

Endocrine/Metabolic. It appears that the endocrine abnormalities that have been described in eating disorders are secondary to starvation, since there is no evidence for primary pituitary, gonadal, thyroid, or adrenal dysfunction. The abnormalities are more severe as weight loss becomes more pronounced.

The most common endocrine abnormality is amenorrhea and estrogen deficiency.[204] Approximately 20 per cent of patients develop amenorrhea prior to the onset of overt anorexia nervosa; about half cease menses at the onset of calorie restriction, and the rest cease menses as cachexia develops. The primary defect resides in the hypothalamus as release of gonadotropin releasing hormone is impaired, resembling a prepubertal pattern.[252] With weight gain, some restoration of the normal pattern generally occurs, but in at least 25 per cent of patients the amenorrhea persists. The reason for impaired release of gonadotropin releasing hormone in anorexia nervosa is unknown, although psychologic stress has been proposed as one cause.

Low estrogen levels are due to gonadotropin deficiency. Similarly in male patients with anorexia nervosa, serum testosterone levels are low, which may explain the impotence and low libido in these patients.[253]

Other pituitary hormones have been found to be at abnormal levels in anorexia nervosa. Growth hormone levels are often elevated, probably owing to decreased somatomedin C levels.[254] Without somatomedin C, the normal feedback inhibition on growth hormone secretion is missing. Decreased plasma somatomedin C is probably a consequence of both decreased synthesis and impaired bioactivity, a finding in most patients with severe weight loss for any reason.[255]

Vasopressin secretion is depressed or erratic in patients with anorexia nervosa, as it is also in patients who have been starved.[256] While the defect appears to be in the hypothalamus, there may be relative renal insensitivity to vasopressin because of damage to the kidney from chronic potassium deficiency.[256] Consequently, these patients may have polyuria or frank diabetes insipidus.

Thyroid. Although anorectic patients have signs and symptoms suggestive of hypothyroidism, such as slow pulse rate, constipation, cold intolerance, dry skin, and low basal metabolic rate, they do not have a true low thyroid state. Under the stress of malnutrition, the peripheral conversion of thyroxine to triiodothyronine is decreased, a condition of any "euthyroid sick" patient.[257] Hence, they have low normal serum T_4, low T_3, and high reverse T_3 levels. Interestingly, lethargy is not a usual finding in patients with anorexia nervosa, as it is in other patients with malnutrition. Elevated T_4 and reverse T_3 levels are sometimes found in these patients. This pattern represents another form of the "euthyroid sick" syndrome. Therefore, clinically significant hypothyroidism or hyperthyroidism is not a feature of anorexia nervosa, and treatment is not indicated.

Adrenal. Malnourished anorectic patients may have a shift of adrenal metabolism that results in altered levels of active androgen. An elevated etiocholanolone level is, in fact, characteristic of anorexia nervosa.[258]

Mean plasma cortisol levels are normal or elevated in anorexia nervosa. Elevated levels may be secondary to decreased metabolism of cortisol or to increased cortisol production.[259, 260] In addition, dexamethasone suppression tests are abnormal. Whether this is because of concomitant depression or of anorexia nervosa *per se* is unclear. Norepinephrine levels are low, as they are in any starved patients.[260] The levels return to normal once weight gain is achieved.

Renal. Because of fluid and electrolyte depletion from vomiting and purging, the bulimic patient is particularly at risk for life-threatening complications.[261] Chronically dehydrated, often hypokalemic, the bulimic patient can develop urolithiasis, renal insufficiency, and even renal failure. The typical hypochloremic, hypokalemic metabolic alkalosis of chronic vomiting requires immediate identification and treatment.

Furthermore, these patients develop edema, which becomes particularly severe when the patient attempts to discontinue diuretic or cathartic abuse. The very high aldosterone level stimulated by chronic volume contraction causes increased sodium retention. It may take months before normal renal equilibrium is reestablished. Hence, the patient must be repeatedly persuaded not to resume her purging habits during this temporary period of worsening peripheral edema.

Hematologic. Leukopenia, decreased white blood cell function, thrombocytopenia, and mild anemia may occur in anorexia nervosa. The bone marrow is often hypocellular with decreased fat content.[262] The degree of these abnormalities does not correlate with the amount or duration of weight loss. However, the abnormalities may resolve as the patient gains weight. Even if they do not resolve, anorectic patients are not more prone to infections.[263] Immunocompetency is preserved in anorexia nervosa until weight loss is extremely severe.

Musculoskeletal. Osteoporosis is an increasingly recognized complication of anorexia nervosa.[264] Low calcium intake and estrogen deficiency probably account for the reduced bone mass. Since anorectic patients often exercise frequently and vigorously, some protection to the bone is attained. Nevertheless, complications occur, such as rib fractures that can result from self-induced, forceful vomiting.

Muscle abnormalities may be secondary to electrolyte depletion such as hypocalcemia and hypophosphatemia. Chronic ipecac syrup ingestion can cause a toxic peripheral myopathy and cardiomyopathy.[265]

Neurologic. Few neurologic complications have been described. Hypoglycemic and hyperglycemic comas are probably the most serious. Although the occurrence of an eating disorder in a patient with diabetes mellitus is relatively uncommon, inability to control the blood glucose should alert the physician to this possibility.[266]

Shaul and colleagues described a patient with anorexia nervosa who developed acute psychosis as a result of caffeine toxicity.[267] Patients with eating disorders may ingest tremendous amounts of caffeine in diet pills, diuretics, and cola soft drinks.

Peripheral nerve palsies can occur secondary to nerve compression from marked cachexia and loss of cushioning subcutaneous tissue.[268] The peroneal nerve is particularly vulnerable. However, recovery usually follows restoration of normal body habitus.

Dermatologic. Patients with eating disorders, particularly those who self-induce vomiting and purging, may exhibit several dermatologic complications. Bruises and lacerations over the knuckles occur from inserting the fingers into the mouth to induce retching. Ecchymoses and conjunctival hemorrhages may also result from excessive and forceful vomiting. Furthermore, vitamin K deficiency, a rare complication of bulimia nervosa, will exacerbate the bruising.[269]

Phenolphthalein, an ingredient in most over-the-counter laxatives, can cause a fixed drug reaction.[270] These inflammatory skin lesions recur at the same site upon repeated exposure to phenolphthalein and may develop brownish-gray hyperpigmentation over time.

Pathogenesis

Five major eras in the study of anorexia nervosa have been defined, namely, descriptive era, pituitary era, rediscovery era, psychoanalytic era, and the current modern era.[273] The prevalent view is that anorexia nervosa, and eating disorders in general, result from complex interactions of physiologic, psychologic, and sociocultural dysfunction.

Sociocultural pressures peculiar to women involve concepts of sexuality and attractiveness. The physical ideal for affluent women in Western society is thinness, as emphasized continually by fashion, entertainment media, and peer pressure. The physical changes of puberty in young women signal both a new appearance and sexual maturity. Bruch, emphasizing perceptual and conceptual disturbances in anorexia nervosa, suggests that "anorectics to be" are unable to differentiate between external and visceral cues during childhood.[212] As adolescence ensues, the girl is unable to respond to visceral cues but rather acts only in response to external demands coming from other people and situations. Inevitably, emerging physical and sexual maturity with its many pressures and challenges then reinforces insecurity, and the anorectic begins to perceive her adult body as alien and threatening.[271] In order to regain control, then, she resorts to dieting, which serves to reassure her of mastery of her own body and, further, to effectively reverse the pubertal process.

Specific etiologic factors to explain why certain persons develop eating disorders have been sought in both the psychologic and physiologic spheres. That family psychopathology exists is evidenced by the increased incidence of depression and alcoholism in first-degree and second-degree relatives of anorectic and bulimic patients.[272] Bruch states that early disturbances in the mother-child relationship establish an overall sense of ineffectiveness that is central to the psychopathology.[212] In the physiologic sphere, numerous studies report hormonal and neuroendocrine disturbances in patients with eating disorders. The hypothalamus has been suggested as the mediator of the pathophysiologic mechanism of the disease. However, whether these physiologic abnormalities are primary or whether the alterations are secondary to starvation remains unknown.

Conceptualizing eating disorders as bio-psychosocial diseases most accurately represents the current thinking on its pathogenesis (Fig. 9–7).[273] Pathologic vulnerability, psychologic predisposition, and social pressures interact upon the individual in whom the disease will develop. The challenges and conflicts of pubertal changes may initiate the disorder. The cumulative effect leads to dieting and other means of weight loss. This in turn results in malnutrition and "starvation

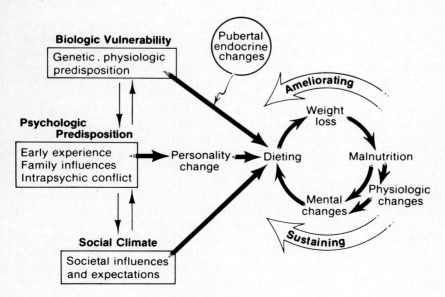

Figure 9–7. Biopsychosocial model for anorexia nervosa. (From Lucas, A. R. Mayo Clin. Proc. 56:254, 1981. Used by permission.)

neurosis." The vicious circle of psychologic dysfunction fostering further dieting and psychologic denial becomes established and may lead relentlessly to death.

Diagnosis

There is no single physiologic and psychologic characteristic to identify patients with an eating disorder. The first and most important diagnostic tool is taking an appropriate history and being aware that these patients often present with a complication of the disorder while denying its existence. The diagnosis depends on identifying the underlying but intense fear of becoming fat as a result of "losing control over eating." Bruch described several characteristic disturbances of psychologic function in anorectics: (1) a disturbance in body image, (2) a disturbance in the accuracy of perception or cognitive interpretation of enteroceptive stimuli, with failure to recognize hunger, fatigue, or anger, and (3) a paralyzing sense of ineffectiveness, which is central and pervasive in their thinking and activities.

As regards the bulimic patient, the physician's skill at history-taking is even more important since, unlike anorectics, the bulimic is usually near normal weight and typically practices binge-purge activities in secrecy. A series of open-ended questions has been suggested for the initial interview, for example, "How has your weight been recently? Are you happy with your weight and appearance? How has your mood been recently? Does eating cause your moods or feelings to change?" before moving on to direct questions, such as "Do you eat when you are not hungry? Does overeating make you feel guilty or depressed? Do you try to control your weight by vomiting or taking laxatives or diuretics?"[274]

The American Psychiatric Association has recently revised its diagnostic criteria for both anorexia nervosa and bulimia (Table 9–7). The criteria of Feighner and colleagues[274a] have been most widely used in research studies, and are more specific as regards anorexia nervosa since they include the presence of at least two of the following: amenorrhea, lanugo, bradycardia, periods of overactivity, and episodes of bulimia or emesis. The clinical usefulness of these criteria is to exclude diseases other than eating disorders and to lend confidence to the diagnosis as treatment is contemplated.

As regards bulimia, the former DSM-III diagnostic criteria (1980) of the American Psychiatric Association have been criticized for the following: (1) using the term bulimia to denote both a symptom (gross overeating) and a syndrome (a constellation of psychologic features); (2) defining bulimia basically as recurrent acts of binge-purge behavior; and (3) failing to clarify the relationship between anorexia nervosa and bulimia. The last criticism bears upon the disorder bulimia nervosa, best described by Russell in 1979.[275] These distinctions are worthwhile since interpretations of treatment studies suffer from both overly broad and

Table 9–7. DSM-III-R DIAGNOSTIC CRITERIA FOR ANOREXIA NERVOSA AND BULIMIA NERVOSA

Anorexia Nervosa
A. Refusal to maintain body weight over a minimal normal weight for age and height, e.g., weight loss leading to maintenance of body weight 15% below that expected; or failure to make expected weight gain during period of growth, leading to body weight 15% below that expected.
B. Intense fear of gaining weight or becoming fat, even though underweight.
C. Disturbance in the way in which one's body weight, size, or shape is experienced, e.g., the person claims to "feel fat" even when emaciated, believes that one area of the body is "too fat" even when obviously underweight.
D. In females, absence of at least three consecutive menstrual cycles when otherwise expected to occur (primary or secondary amenorrhea). (A woman is considered to have amenorrhea if her periods occur only following hormone, e.g., estrogen, administration.)

Bulimia Nervosa
A. Recurrent episodes of binge eating (rapid consumption of a large amount of food in a discrete period of time).
B. A feeling of lack of control over eating behavior during the eating binges.
C. The person regularly engages in either self-induced vomiting, use of laxatives or diuretics, strict dieting or fasting, or vigorous exercise in order to prevent weight gain.
D. A minimum average of two binge eating episodes a week for at least three months.
E. Persistent overconcern with body shape and weight.

Reprinted with permission from the Diagnostic and Statistical Manual of Mental Disorders, Third Edition, Revised. Copyright 1987, American Psychiatric Association.

unduly strict diagnostic criteria. The DSM-III-R of the American Psychiatric Association no longer includes bulimia, *per se,* as an eating disorder. Rather, it provides diagnostic criteria for bulimia nervosa, thus addressing some but not all of the concerns discussed above.

Differential Diagnosis

The differential diagnosis of eating disorders includes both physical and psychologic diseases. For anorexia nervosa, the major differential includes gastrointestinal diseases that cause malabsorption, malignancies, and depression. For bulimia, wherein the patient is often normal weight, the primary concern is whether the patient has schizophrenia or other psychiatric disorders. In general, a careful history and review of systems and routine laboratory studies eliminate the diseases that mimic anorexia nervosa or bulimia (Table 9–8).

Physical Diseases. The diseases to consider in a patient with gastrointestinal symptoms, amenorrhea, and weight loss with concomitant biochemical abnormalities include malignancy, diseases of the central nervous system, metabolic disorders, and gastrointestinal diseases. Malignancy is the fourth leading cause of death in the adolescent age group, with the most common cancers being leukemia and lymphoma.[276] However, it would be the unusual case that was not readily distinguished from anorexia nervosa following

Table 9–8. TESTS FOR EVALUATION OF PATIENTS WITH EATING DISORDERS

1. Careful history to include eating attitudes
2. General physical examination
3. Nutritional assessment
4. Laboratory: complete blood count, serum electrolytes, blood urea nitrogen, creatinine, liver enzymes, amylase, albumin, erythrocyte sedimentation rate, urinalysis, thyroid function tests, fasting plasma cortisol level
5. Electrocardiogram
6. If clinically indicated: chest roentgenogram; stool examination for blood, fat, parasites; flexible sigmoidoscopy and mucosal biopsy; upper GI series with small bowel follow-through, air-contrast barium enema; head CT scan with contrast medium

physical examination and evaluation of routine laboratory studies. In the elderly, malignancy is much more likely to explain progressive weight loss than is anorexia nervosa. However, cases of anorexia nervosa have been reported in women up to the age of 94.

Diseases of the central nervous system can cause anorexia, particularly tumors of the hypothalamus.[277] A history of headaches or visual problems suggestive of increased intracranial pressure and localized findings of papilledema and cranial nerve involvement do not occur in anorexia nervosa. The rare concomitant occurrence of anorexia nervosa and a hypothalamic tumor should nonetheless be kept in mind.[278]

Endocrine disorders to consider include hyperthyroidism, hypothyroidism, adrenal insufficiency, diabetes, hyperparathyroidism, and hypercalcemia. While these diseases are often associated with weight loss, they are also easily distinguished by the history, physical examination, and routine laboratory studies.

Gastrointestinal diseases that can be mistaken for an eating disorder are primarily those associated with malabsorption syndromes, for example, celiac sprue, pancreatic insufficiency, parasitosis, and inflammatory bowel disease. Symptoms of abdominal pain, bloating, nausea, vomiting, diarrhea, and weight loss can occur in patients with eating disorders due either to presumed motility disturbances or to laxatives used to control weight. Patients with eating disorders alone do not have steatorrhea, fever, leukocytosis, anemia, hypoalbuminemia, or the elevated erythrocyte sedimentation rate found with organic disease. More importantly, the patient with an eating disorder can be distinguished by her intense, morbid preoccupation with food, an attitude toward eating that is absent with organic disease.

Psychiatric Disorders. In addition to eliminating physical disease as the cause for the patient's problem, the physician must also differentiate eating disorders from psychiatric conditions such as conversion reactions, schizophrenia, depression, anxiety reactions, and adjustment disorders of adolescence. Furthermore, one should consider whether substance abuse may explain the patient's weight loss and behavioral problems. A mental health professional may be necessary to determine whether a patient has schizophrenia or depression as the cause for anorexia or bizarre eating behavior. A variety of psychometric tests are available to uncover the patient's underlying attitude toward food, including the Goldberg Anorectic Attitude Scale, the Eating Attitudes Test, and techniques to investigate body self-image.[279] As regards the latter, some question remains whether there is a body image disturbance in eating disorders and, if so, whether it is specific enough to be clinically useful.[280]

Treatment

Treatment of patients with eating disorders has several goals: nutritional restitution with alleviation of symptoms, increased self-esteem, and progress toward personal and social development.[212] Therefore, a team approach to treatment is optimal, with the internist managing the medical care while serving as a liaison among psychiatric/psychologic and nutritional professionals. Both the physician and patient may find assistance and valuable information by contacting such organizations as the American Anorexia/Bulimia Association, 133 Cedar Lane, Teaneck, NJ 17666 (201–836–1800), or the National Association of Anorexia Nervosa and Associated Disorders, Box 271, Highland Park, IL 60035 (312–831–3438).

Medical Management. All anorectics and some bulimics require some nutritional management. An accurate assessment of the degree of malnutrition is necessary to determine those patients in need of aggressive nutritional support (Table 9–9). Those patients with a Prognostic Nutritional Index (PNI) less than 30 per cent can receive nutritional counseling and be managed on an outpatient basis; those with PNI scores between 30 and 59 per cent need nutritional supplementation that can be oral and generally without hospitalization (250 to 500 kcal/day); however, those patients with PNI scores greater than 60 per cent (or weight loss greater than 40 per cent of ideal weight or greater than 25 per cent loss within 3 months) should be hospitalized and receive 400 to 600 kcal/day supplementation. Other compelling reasons for hospitalization include severe metabolic derangements (markedly abnormal vital signs, hypokalemia, azotemia, etc.), severe depression or suicide risk, severe binge-purge activity, psychosis, or family crisis (Table 9–10).[281] While the oral route is always preferable, enteral alimentation or, rarely, parenteral alimentation may

Table 9–9. DEFINITION OF THE PROGNOSTIC NUTRITIONAL INDEX (PNI)

PNI (%) = $158 - 16.6$ (ALB) $- 0.78$ (TSF) $- 0.20$ (TFN) $- 5.8$ (DH), where ALB = serum albumin (gm/dl); TSF = triceps skin fold (mm); TFN = serum transferrin (mg/dl); and DH = delayed hypersensitivity reactivity to *Candida* (0 = nonreactive, 1 = <5 mm, 2 = ≥5 mm reactivity.

PNI <30%, low risk
PNI 30%–59%, intermediate risk
PNI ≥60%, high risk

From Drossman, D. A. Anorexia nervosa: a comprehensive approach. Adv. Intern. Med. *28*:339, 1983. Copyright 1983, Year Book Medical Publishers. Reproduced with permission.

Table 9–10. INDICATIONS FOR HOSPITALIZATION·
OF PATIENTS WITH EATING DISORDERS

Medical Complications
1. Severe malnutrition: e.g., weight loss greater than 40% of ideal body weight or greater than 25% weight loss within last 3 months
2. Severe metabolic derangements: e.g., serum potassium less than 2.5 mEq/L, blood urea nitrogen greater than 25 mg/dl, hypotension, cardiac arrhythmia

Psychologic Problems
1. Severe depression, psychosis, or suicide risk
2. Severe binge-purge activity
3. Intercurrent condition such as substance abuse, alcoholism, family dysfunction, failure of support systems
4. Failure to respond to previous treatment

be necessary if the patient refuses to eat or has several medical complications of malnutrition. Some caution is indicated during refeeding to avoid congestive heart failure, acute gastric dilation, or pancreatitis.[282] Serum electrolytes, chemistries, and hepatic and renal functions need careful observation in severely malnourished patients and bulimics with chronic laxative/diuretic abuse or self-induced emesis. Initial weight gain will consist mostly of water, and peripheral edema may be severe and very discouraging for the patient. Calorie intake should be gradually increased over a two-week period until a daily intake of 3000 to 5000 calories is achieved. The patient should never eat alone. A behavioral approach (positive reinforcement) to gain weight may be possible. Only after restoration of normal body weight can pharmacotherapy and psychotherapy be effective.[283]

Psychotherapy. A variety of therapies for anorexia nervosa have been tried, including individual psychotherapy (insight-oriented therapy), behavioral modification, group therapy (dynamic, psychoeducational, or self-help), and family therapy (structural, systemic, or strategic). None has been shown to be consistently effective or, if effective, long-lasting. In fact, in patients without an underlying psychiatric disorder, no form of psychotherapy may be effective.

Since patients with bulimia usually realize that their behavior is maladaptive and are receptive to treatment, the treatment of bulimia focuses on the control of eating as the primary problem. Treatment is accomplished in three stages: (1) self-monitoring of eating behavior (two to three visits per week for four to six weeks) with positive reinforcement by the physician; (2) recognition of stress-binge association and development of coping strategies; and (3) maintenance (semimonthly for two months) wherein the physician reinforces adaptive coping mechanisms.[283]

Pharmacotherapy. A wide range of psychotropic drugs have been tried. None has an established place in the treatment of eating disorders. Antidepressants, most often monoamine oxidase inhibitors and the tricyclics, have been used, but if the patient does not have an underlying depressive disorder, these drugs are unlikely to be helpful, although there is some evidence that antidepressant drug therapy for bulimia

may be of benefit.[90] Cyproheptadine, a serotonin and histamine antagonist, has been reported to be helpful in treating certain patients with anorexia nervosa, although initial studies were conflicting.[284, 285] By inhibiting serotonergic tracts associated with the ventrolateral hypothalamus (satiety center), one hopes to induce weight gain.

Because patients with eating disorders often display an addictive behavior to dieting similar to the behavior of addicts to drugs, some investigators believe that while anorexia may begin as a psychologic disorder, anorectics become "addicted" to endogenous opioid peptides released during prolonged starvation. The opioid peptides stimulate feeding behavior in rats. The anorectic, however, consciously does not eat, and becomes "addicted" to the presumed euphoria of the increased levels of opioids. Hence, opioid blockade reportedly assists treatment of the anorectic by breaking the addiction to dieting.[286, 287] The role of endogenous opioid peptides in bulimics is equally speculative, although a recent report suggests that naltrexone, a long-acting opioid antagonist, significantly reduced binge-purge activity.[288]

Outcome and Prognosis

Very few long-term studies have examined the natural history and treatment response of anorexia nervosa, and fewer still have looked at bulimia. Two recent reviews of anorexia nervosa, both with at least a two-year follow-up period, found that the average mortality rate was 6 per cent, with three fourths of the patients improved overall despite the fact that only one third were eating normally.[289, 290] Even in patients who are successfully treated in the hospital, about 50 per cent relapse within a year.[291]

A poor prognosis for recovery from anorexia nervosa is suggested by early onset, chronicity, premorbid obesity particularly when associated with binge-purge behavior ("bulimia nervosa"), inability to develop and maintain secure peer relationships, and disturbed parental relationship.

Since bulimia is a relatively newly described disorder, much less is known about outcome and prognosis. Heterogeneity of severity and chronicity of bulimia among patients makes interpretation of the literature difficult. Lowenkopf has identified three groups of patients with possibly different psychopathology and prognoses.[292] The mildest forms of bulimia occur among college women who respond to brief group therapy and behavioral techniques. The second group, mostly college students, consume more food and vomit more frequently each day than the first group, and require more intensive treatment, often in the hospital. The third group consists of older patients, sometimes in their late thirties and forties, who have chronic and stable bulimia that generally occurs daily, remains surreptitious, and does not disrupt their daily activities. These patients have "come to terms with their disorder." In the absence of more data, the physician should individualize treatment of the patient with an eating disorder. It is worth remembering that it may not be *what* treatment is given that determines outcome, but rather *how* it is offered. A solid, interactive physician-patient relationship based on trust is critical for successful treatment.

References

1. Van Itallie, T. B. Health implications of overweight and obesity in the United States. Ann. Intern. Med. *103*:983, 1985.
2. National Center for Health Statistics. Plan and operation of the National Health and Nutrition Examination Survey, 1976–80. Washington, U.S. Public Health Service. DHHS Publ. No. (PHS) 81–1317, 1981.
3. Foster, W. R., and Burton, B. T. Health implications of obesity. National Institutes of Health Consensus Development Conference. Ann. Intern. Med. *103*:997, 1985.
4. Cunningham, J. J. New approaches to the noninvasive assessment of body composition: bio-electrical impedance analysis and total body electrical conductance. Nutr. Int. *3*:6, 1987.
5. Ashwell, M., Cole, T. J., and Dixon, A. K. Obesity: new insight into the anthropometric classification of fat distribution shown by computerized tomography. Br. Med. J. *290*:1692, 1985.
6. Bjorntorp, P. Regional patterns of fat distribution. Ann. Intern. Med. *103*:994, 1985.
7. Heald, F. P., and Hollander, R. J. The relationship between obesity in adolescence and early growth. J. Pediatr. *67*:35, 1965.
8. Rimm, I. J., and Rimm, A. A. Association between juvenile onset obesity and severe adult obesity in 73,532 women. Am. J. Publ. Health *66*:479, 1976.
9. Knittle, J. L., Timmers, K., Ginsberg-Fellner, F., Brown, R. E., and Katz, D. P. The growth of adipose tissue in children and adolescents: cross-sectional and longitudinal studies of adipose cell number and size. J. Clin. Invest. *63*:239, 1979.
10. Lewis, D. S., Bertrand, H. A., McMahan, C. A., McGill, H. C., Jr., Carey, K. D., and Masoro, E. J. Preweaning food intake influences the adiposity of young adult baboons. J. Clin. Invest. *78*:899, 1986.
11. Salans, L. B., Cushman, S. W., and Weismann, R. E. Studies of human adipose tissue. Adipose cell size and number in nonobese and obese patients. J. Clin. Invest. *52*:929, 1973.
12. Powley, T. L., McFarlane, B. A., Markell, M. S., and Opsahl, C. A. Different effects of vagotomy and atropine on hypothalamic stimulation of feeding. Behav. Biol. *23*:306, 1978.
13. Anand, B. K., and Brobeck, J. R. Hypothalamic control of food intake in rats and cats. Yale J. Biol. Med. *24*:123, 1951.
14. Morley, J. E., and Levine, A. A. Neuropeptides and appetite regulation. Med. J. Aust. *142*:S11, 1985.
15. Mayer, J. Regulation of energy intake and the body weight: the glucostatic theory and lipostatic hypothesis. Ann. N.Y. Acad. Sci. *63*:15, 1955.
16. Oomura, Y. Significance of glucose, insulin, and free fatty acid in the hypothalamic feeding and satiety neurons. *In* Noxin, D., Wyrwicka, W., and Bray, G. (eds.). Hunger: Basic Mechanisms and Clinical Implications. New York, Raven Press, 1976, p. 145.
17. Lemagnon, J., Devos, M., Gaudilliere, J. P., Louis-Sylvestre, J., and Tallon, S. Role of a lipostatic mechanism in regulation by feeding of energy balance in rats. J. Comp. Physiol. Psychol. *84*:1, 1973.
18. Mellinkoff, S. M., Frankland, M., Boyle, D., and Greipel, M. Relationship between serum amino acid concentrations and fluctuations in appetite. J. Appl. Physiol. *8*:535, 1956.
19. Brobeck, J. R. Food intake as a mechanism of temperature regulation. Yale J. Biol. Med. *20*:545, 1948.
20. Kissileff, H. R., and Van Itallie, T. B. Physiology of the control of food intake. Ann. Rev. Nutr. *2*:371, 1982.
21. Morley, J. E., and Levine, A. S. The role of endogenous opiates as regulators of appetite. Am. J. Clin. Nutr. *35*:757, 1982.
22. Morley, J. E., Levine, A. S., Grace, M., and Kneip, J. Dynorphin (1–13), dopamine and feeding in rats. Pharmacol. Biochem. Behav. *16*:701, 1982.
23. Reid, L. D., Konecka, A. M., Przewlocki, R., Millan, M. H., Millan, M. J., and Herz, A. Endogenous opioids, circadian rhythms, nutrient deprivation, eating and drinking. Life Sci. *31*:1829, 1982.
24. Morley, J. E., Levine, A. S., Grace, M., and Kneip, J. An investigation of the role of kappa opiate receptor agonists in the initiation of feeding. Life Sci. *31*:2617, 1982.
25. Ferguson-Segall, M., Flynn, J. J., Walker, J., and Margules, D. L. Increased immunoreactive dynorphin and leu-enkephalin in posterior pituitary of obese mice (ob/ob) and supersensitivity to drugs that act at kappa receptors. Life Sci. *31*:2233, 1982.
26. Morley, J. E., and Levine, A. S. Stress induced eating is mediated through endogenous opiates. Science *209*:1259, 1980.
27. Pollard, H., Llorens, C., Schwartz, J. C., Gros, C., and Dray, F. Localization of opiate receptors and enkephalins in the rat striatum in relationship with the nigrostriatal dopaminergic system. Brain Res. *151*:392, 1978.
28. Urwyler, S., and Tabakoff, B. Stimulation of dopamine synthesis and release by morphine and D-ala-d-leu-enkephalin in the mouse striatum in vivo. Life Sci. *28*:2277, 1981.
29. Blundell, J. E. Serotonin and feeding. *In* Esmon, W. B. (ed.). Serotonin in Health and Disease. Vol. 5, Clinical Applications. New York, Spectrum, 1979, pp. 403–450.
30. Morley, J. E. The neuroendocrine control of appetite: the role of the endogenous opiates, cholecystokinin, TRH, gamma-amino butyric acid and the diazepam receptor. Life Sci. *27*:355, 1980.
31. Liebowitz, S. F. Neurochemical systems of the hypothalamus in control of feeding and drinking and water electrolyte excretion. *In* Morgane, P., and Panksepp, J. (eds.). Handbook of the Hypothalamus. Vol. 3. New York, Marcel Dekker, 1980. pp. 299–437.
32. Levine, A. S., and Morley, J. E. Reduction of feeding in rats by calcitonin. Brain Res. *222*:187, 1981.
33. Cannon, W. B., and Washburn, A. L. An explanation of hunger. Am. J. Physiol. *29*:441, 1912.
34. Paintal, A. S. A study of gastric stretch receptors. Their role in the peripheral mechanism of satiation of hunger and thirst. J. Physiol. (Lond.) *126*:255, 1954.
35. Harvey, R. F. Gut peptides and the control of food intake. Br. Med. J. *287*:1572, 1983.
36. Kraly, F. S., and Gibbs, J. Vagotomy fails to block the satiating effect of food in the stomach. Physiol. Behav. *24*:1007, 1980.
37. Smith, G. P., Jerome, C., and Gibbs, J. Abdominal vagotomy does not block the satiety effect of bombesin in the rat. Peptides *2*:409, 1981.
38. Gibbs, J., Maddison, S. P., and Rolls, E. T. Satiety role of the small intestine examined in sham-feeding rhesus monkeys. J. Comp. Physiol. Psychol. *95*:1003, 1981.
39. Gibbs, J., Young, R. C., and Smith, G. P. Cholecystokinin decreases food intake in rats. J. Comp. Physiol. Psychol. *84*:488, 1973.
40. Pi-Sunyer, F. X., Kissileff, H. F., Thornton, J., and Smith, G. P. C-terminal octapeptide of cholecystokinin decreases food intake in obese men. Physiol. Behav. *29*:627, 1982.
41. Moran, T. H., and McHugh, P. R. Cholecystokinin suppresses food intake by inhibiting gastric emptying. Am. J. Physiol. *242*:R491, 1982.
42. Smith, G. P., Jerome, C., Cushin, B. J., Eterno, R., and Simansky, K. J. Abdominal vagotomy blocks the satiety effect of cholecystokinin in the rat. Science *213*:1036, 1981.
43. Smith, G. P. The peripheral control of appetite. Lancet *1*:88, 1983.
44. VanderWeele, D. A., Haraczkiewicz, E., and DiConte, M. Pancreatic glucagon administration, feeding, glycemia, and liver glycogen in rats. Brain Res. Bull. *5*(Suppl. 4):17, 1980.
45. Langhans, W., Ziegler, V., Scharrer, E., and Geary, N. Stimulation of feeding in rats by intraperitoneal injection of antibodies to glucagon. Science *218*:894, 1982.
46. Thomason, A. M., Billewicz, N. Z., and Passmore, R. The relationship between caloric intake and body weight in man. Lancet *1*:1027, 1961.

47. Vasselli, J. R., Cleary, M. P., and Van Itallie, T. B. Modern concepts of obesity. Nutr. Rev. *41*:361, 1983.

48. Spıtzer, L., Rodin, J. Human eating behavior: a critical review of studies in normal weight and overweight individuals. Appetite 2:293, 1981.

49. Jéquier, E. Energy expenditure in obesity. Clin. Endocrinol. Metab. *13*:563, 1984.

50. Porikos, K., Pi-Sunyer, F. X. Regulation of food intake in human obesity: studies with caloric dilution and exercise. Clin. Endocrinol. Metab. *13*:547, 1984.

51. Ravussin, E., Burnard, B., Schutz, Y., and Jéquier, E. Twenty-four hour energy expenditure and resting metabolic rate in obese, moderately obese, and control subjects. Am. J. Clin. Nutr. *35*:566, 1982.

52. Garrow, J. S., and Webster, J. Are pre-obese people energy thrifty? Lancet *1*:670, 1985.

53. Neumann, R. O. Experimentelle Beiträge zur Lehre von dem täglichen Nahrungsbedarf des Menschen unter bosonderer Berücksichtigung der notwendigen Eiweissmenge. Arch. Hyg. *45*:1, 1902.

54. Gulick, A. A study of weight regulation in the adult human body during overnutrition. Am. J. Physiol. *60*:371, 1922.

55. Garrow, G. B. Energy intake and body weight: a reexamination of two "classic" studies. Am. J. Clin. Nutr. *39*:349, 1984.

56. Rothwell, N. J., and Stock, M. J. Diet-induced thermogenesis. Nutr. Int. 2:95, 1986.

57. Pi-Sunyer, F. X. Thermogenesis in human obesity. Curr. Concepts Nutr. *13*:87, 1984.

58. Rothwell, N. J., and Stock, M. J. Energy expenditure of "cafeteria-fed" rats determined from measurements of energy balance and indirect calorimetry. J. Physiol. *328*:371, 1982.

59. Levin, B. E., and Sullivan, A. C. Regulation of thermogenesis in obesity. Int. J. Obes. *8*(Suppl. 1):159, 1984.

60. Newsholme, E. A. A possible metabolic basis for the control of body weight. N. Engl. J. Med. *302*:399, 1980.

61. De Luise, M., Blackburn, G. L., and Flier, J. S. Reduced activity of the red-cell sodium-potassium pump in human obesity. N. Engl. J. Med. *303*:1017, 1980.

62. Mir, M. A., Charalambous, B. M., Morgan, K., and Evans, P. J. Erythrocyte sodium-potassium-ATPase and sodium transport in obesity. N. Engl. J. Med. *305*:1264, 1981.

63. Simat, B. M., Mayrand, R. R., From AHL, Morley, J. E., Billington, C., Fullerton, D. S., and Ahmed, K. Is the erythrocyte sodium pump altered in human obesity? J. Clin. Endocrinol. Metab. *56*:925, 1983.

64. Bray, G. A., Kral, J. G., and Bjorntorp, P. Hepatic sodium-potassium-dependent ATPase in obesity. N. Engl. J. Med. *304*:1580, 1981.

65. Beutler, E., Kuhl, W., and Sacks, P. Sodium-potassium-ATPase activity is influenced by ethnic origin and not by obesity. N. Engl. J. Med. *309*:756, 1983.

65a. Sims, E. A. H., and Danforth, E., Jr. Expenditure and storage of energy in man. J. Clin. Invest. *79*:1019, 1987.

66. Gurnay, R. Hereditary factors in obesity. Arch. Intern. Med. *57*:557, 1936.

67. Dietz, W. H., Jr., and Gortmaker, S. L. Do we fatten our children at the television set? Obesity and television viewing in children and adolescents. Pediatrics *75*:807, 1985.

68. Goldblatt, P. B., Moore, M. E., and Stunkard, A. J. Social factors in obesity. JAMA *192*:1039, 1965.

69. Stunkard, A. J., and Penul, S. B. Behavior modification in the treatment of obesity. The problem of maintaining weight loss. Arch. Gen. Psychiatry *36*:801, 1979.

70. Hartz, A., Giefer, E., and Rimm, A. A. Relative importance of the effect of family, environment, and heredity on obesity. Ann. Human Genet. *41*:185, 1977.

71. Garn, S. M., Cole, P. E., and Bailey, S. M. Effect of parental fatness levels on the fatness of biological and adoptive children. Ecol. Food Nutr. *7*:91, 1977.

72. Withers, R. F. J. Problems in the genetics of human obesity. Eugen. Rev. *56*:81, 1964.

73. Annest, J. L., Sing, C. F., Biron, P., and Mongeau, J. G. Family aggregation of blood pressure and weight in adoptive families. III. Analysis of the role of shared genes and shared household environment in explaining family resemblance for height, weight and selected height/weight indices. Am. J. Epidemiol. *117*:492, 1983.

74. Stunkard, A. J., Sorensen, T. I. A., Hanis, C., Teasdale, T. W., Chakraborty, R., Schull, W. J., and Schulsinger, F. An adoption study of human obesity. N. Engl. J. Med. *314*:193, 1986.

75. Stunkard, A. J., Foch, T. T., and Hrubec, Z. A twin study of human obesity. JAMA *256*:51, 1986.

76. Bogardus, C., Lillioja, S., Ravussin, E., Abbot, W., Zawadski, J. K., Young, A. Y., Kowler, W. C., Jacobowitz, R., and Moll, P. P. Familial dependence of the resting metabolic rate. N. Engl. J. Med. *315*:96, 1986.

77. Cohen, J. Obesity: a review. J. Roy. Coll. Gen. Pract. *35*:435, 1985.

78. Manson, J. E., Stampfer, M. J., Hennekens, C. H., and Willett, W. C. Body weight and longevity. A reassessment. JAMA *257*:353, 1987.

79. Leijd, B. Cholesterol and bile acid metabolism in obesity. Clin. Sci. *59*:203, 1980.

80. Nestel, P. J., Schreibman, P. H., and Ahrens, E. H., Jr. Cholesterol metabolism in human obesity. J. Clin. Invest. *52*:2389, 1973.

81. Build Study, 1979. Chicago, Society of Actuaries and Association of Life Insurance Medical Directors of America, 1980.

82. O'Brien, T. F., Jr. Lower esophageal sphincter pressure (LESP) and esophageal function in obese humans. J. Clin. Gastroenterol. 2:145, 1980.

83. Backman, L., Granstrom, L., Lindahl, J., and Melcher, A. Manometric studies of lower esophageal sphincter in extreme obesity. Acta Chir. Scand. *149*:193, 1983.

84. Mercer, C. D., Wren, S. F., and DaCosta, L. R. Gastroesophageal pressure gradients and lower esophageal sphincter pressures in severely obese patients. Gastroenterology *82*:1129, 1982.

85. Mercer, C. D., Rue, C., and Hanelin, L. Effect of obesity on esophageal transit. Am. J. Surg. *149*:177, 1985.

86. Horowitz, M., Collins, P. J., and Cook, D. J. Abnormalities of gastric emptying in obese patients. Int. J. Obesity 7:415, 1983.

87. Lavigne, M. E., Wiley, Z. D., Meyer, J. H., and MacGregor, I. L. Gastric emptying as a function of body size. Gastroenterology *74*:1258, 1978.

88. Moore, J. G., Christian, P. E., and Coleman, R. E. Gastric emptying of varying meal weight and composition in man. Evaluation by dual liquid and solid-phase isotopic method. Am. J. Dig. Dis. *26*:16, 1981.

89. Wright, R. A., Krinsky, S., Fleeman, C., Trujillo, J., and Teague, E. Gastric emptying and obesity. Gastroenterology *84*:747, 1983.

90. Granstrom, L., and Backman, L. Stomach distention in extremely obese and in normal subjects. Acta Chir. Scand. *151*:367, 1985.

91. Nasrallah, S. M., Wills, C. E., Jr., and Galambos, J. T. Hepatic morphology in obesity. Dig. Dis. Sci. *26*:325, 1981.

92. Andersen, T., and Gluud, C. Liver morphology in morbid obesity: a literature review. Int. J. Obesity *8*:97, 1984.

93. Itoh, S., Matsuo, S., Ichinoe, A., Yamaba, Y., and Miyazawa, M. Nonalcoholic steatohepatitis and cirrhosis with Mallory's hyalin with ultrastructural study of one case. Dig. Dis. Sci. *27*:341, 1982.

94. Braillon, A., Capron, J. P., Herve, M. A., Degott, C., and Quenum, C. Liver in obesity. Gut *26*:133, 1985.

95. Andersen, T., Christoffersen, P., and Gluud, C. The liver in consecutive patients with morbid obesity: a clinical morphological and biochemical study. Int. J. Obes. *8*:107, 1984.

96. Galambos, J. T., and Wills, C. E. Relationship between 505 paired liver tests and biopsies in 242 obese patients. Gastroenterology *74*:1191, 1978.

97. Abernethy, D. R., and Greenblatt, D. J. Pharmacokinetics of drugs in obesity. Clin. Pharmacokinet. *7*:108, 1982.

98. Weber, D. J., Rutala, W. A., Samsa, G. P., Santimaw, J. E., and Lemon, S. M. Obesity is a predictor of poor antibody response to hepatitis B plasma vaccine. JAMA *254*:3187, 1985.

99. Weber, D. J., Rutala, W. A., Samsa, G. P., Bradshaw, S. E., and Lemon, S. M. Impaired immunogenicity of hepatitis B vaccine in obese persons. N. Engl. J. Med. *314*:1393, 1986.

100. Abernethy, D. R., Greenblatt, D. J., Matlis, R., Gugler, R. Cimetidine disposition in obesity. Am. J. Gastroenterol. *79*:91, 1984.

101. Pasulka, P. S., Bistrian, B. R., Benotti, P. N., and Blackburn, G. L. The risks of surgery in obese patients. Ann. Intern. Med. *104*:540, 1986.

102. Postlethwait, R. W., and Johnson, W. D. Complications following surgery for duodenal ulcer in obese patients. Arch. Surg. *105*:438, 1972.

103. Pemberton, L. B., and Manax, W. G. Relationship of obesity to postoperative complications after cholecystectomy. Am. J. Surg. *121*:87, 1971.

104. Danforth, E., Jr., Horton, E. S., O'Connell, M., Sims, E. A. H., Burger, A. G., Ingbar, S. H., Braverman, L., and Vagenakis, A. G. Dietary-induced alterations in thyroid hormone metabolism during overnutrition. J. Clin. Invest. *64*:1336, 1979.

105. Bray, G. A., and Gallagher, T. F., Jr. Manifestations of hypothalamic obesity in man: a comprehensive investigation of eight patients and a review of the literature. Medicine *54*:301, 1975.

106. Weinsier, R. L., Wadden, T. A., Ritenbaugh, C., Harrison, G. G., Johnson, F. S., Willmore, J. H. Recommended therapeutic guidelines for professional weight control programs. Am. J. Clin. Nutr. *40*:865, 1984.

107. Felig, P. Very-low-calorie protein diets. N. Engl. J. Med. *310*:589, 1984.

108. Lantigua, R. A., Amatruda, J. M., Biddle, T. L., Forbes, G. B., and Lockwood, D. H. Cardiac arrythmias associated with a liquid protein diet for the treatment of obesity. N. Engl. J. Med. *303*:735, 1980.

109. Wadden, T. A., Stunkard, A. J., and Brownell, K. D. Very low calorie diets: their efficacy, safety, and future. Ann. Intern. Med. *99*:675, 1983.

110. Wadden, T. A., Stunkard, A. J., Brownell, K. D., and Van Itallie, T. B. The Cambridge Diet. More mayhem? JAMA *250*:2833, 1983.

111. Gotto, A. M., and Goodrick, G. K. Evaluating commercial weight-loss clinics. Arch. Intern. Med. *142*:682, 1982.

112. Wadden, T. A., Stunkard, A. J., Brownell, K. D., and Day, S. C. A comparison between two very-low-calorie diets: protein-sparing modified fast versus protein-formula liquid diet. Am. J. Clin. Nutr. *41*:533, 1985.

113. Dazzi, A., and Dwyer, J. Nutritional analyses of popular weight reduction diets in books and magazines. Int. J. Eating Disorders *3*:61, 1984.

114. Schroeder, L. A. Weight control—fad, fact, or fiction? Popular approaches to weight control. Nutr. Int. *2*:281, 1986.

115. Newmark, S. R., and Williamson, B. Survey of very-low-calorie weight reduction diets. I. Novelty diets. Arch. Intern. Med. *143*:1195, 1983.

116. Newmark, S. R., and Williamson, B. Survey of very-low-calorie weight reduction diets. II. Total fasting, protein-sparing modified fasts, chemically defined diets. Arch. Intern. Med. *143*:1423, 1983.

117. Southgate, D. A. T. Obese deceivers? Br. Med. J. *292*:1692, 1986.

118. James, W. P. T. Dietary aspects of obesity. Postgrad. Med. J. (Lond.). *60*(Suppl. 3):50, 1984.

119. Horton, E. S. The role of exercise in the prevention and treatment of obesity. *In* Bray, G. H. (ed.). Obesity in Perspective. DHEW Publication No. (NIH) 75–708, 1973, p. 62.

120. Blair, S. N., Ellsworth, N. M., and Haskell, W. L. Comparison of nutrient intake in middle-aged men and women runners and controls. Medical Science and Sports Exercise *13*:310, 1981.

121. Woo, R., Garrow, J. S., and Pi-Sunyer, F. X. Voluntary food intake during prolonged exercise in obese women. Am. J. Clin. Nutr. *36*:478, 1982.

122. Stunkard, A. J. Behavioral management of obesity. Med. J. Aust. *142*(Suppl.):S13, 1985.

123. Blundell, J. E. Behavior modification and exercise in the treatment of obesity. Postgrad. Med. J. *60*(Suppl. 3):37, 1984.

124. Stunkard, A. J., Penick, S. B. Behavior modification in the treatment of obesity: the problem of maintaining weight loss. Arch. Gen. Psychiatry *36*:801, 1979.

125. Stunkard, A. J., Berthold, H. C. What is behavior therapy? A very short description of behavioral weight control. Am. J. Clin. Nutr. *41*:821, 1985.

126. Sheraton, M., Harbison, G., and Wurmstedt, R. C. Dieting: the losing game. Time, January 20, 1986.

127. Douglas, J. G., and Munro, J. F. Drug treatment and obesity. Pharmacol. Ther. *18*:351, 1982.

128. Silverstone, T., and Goodall, E. The clinical pharmacology of appetite suppressant drugs. Int. J. Obes. *8*(Suppl. 1):23, 1984.

129. Silverstone, T. Clinical use of appetite suppressants. Drug and Alcohol Depend. *17*:151, 1986.

130. Weintraub, M., Hasday, J. D., Mushlin, A. L., and Lockwood, D. H. A double-blind clinical trial in weight control. Use of fenfluramine and phentermine alone and in combination. Arch. Intern. Med. *144*:1143, 1984.

131. Cawthorne, M. A., and Arch, J. R. S. The search for peripherally acting drugs for the treatment of obesity—a review. Int. J. Obes. *6*:1, 1982.

132. Koppeschaar, H. P. F., Meinders, A. E., and Schwarz, F. Metabolic responses in grossly obese subjects treated with a very-low-calorie diet with and without triiodothyronine treatment. Int. J. Obes. *7*:133, 1983.

133. Rivlin, R. S. Therapy of obesity with hormones. N. Engl. J. Med. *292*:26, 1975.

134. Curtis-Prior, P. B., and Tan, S. Application of agents active at the alpha-2 adrenoceptor of fat cells to the treatment of obesity—a critical appraisal. Int. J. Obes. *8*(Suppl. 1):201, 1984.

135. Bo-Linn, G. W., Santa Ana, C. A., Morawski, S. G., and Fordtran, J. S. Starch blockers: their effect on calorie absorption from a high-starch meal. N. Engl. J. Med. *307*:1413, 1982.

136. Bin, X., and Jiuzhi, F. Clinical observation of the weight-reducing effects of ear acupuncture in 350 cases of obesity. J. Trad. Chin. Med. *5*:87, 1985.

137. Percival, W. L. "The balloon diet": a noninvasive treatment for morbid obesity. Preliminary report of 108 patients. Can. J. Surg. *27*:135, 1984.

138. Holland, S., Bach, D., and Duff, J. Balloon therapy for obesity—when the balloon bursts. J. Can. Assoc. Radiol. *36*:347, 1985.

139. Boyle, T. M., Agus, S. G., and Bauer, J. J. Small intestinal obstruction secondary to obturation by a Garren gastric bubble. Am. J. Gastroenterol. *82*:51, 1987.

140. Garren, L., Garren, M., Garren, R., and Giordano, F. Gastric balloon implantation for weight loss in the morbidly obese (abstract). Am. J. Gastroenterol. *80*:860, 1985.

141. Cole, H. M. (ed.). Diagnostic and therapeutic technology assessment. Garren gastric bubble. JAMA *256*:3282, 1986.

142. Ramsey-Stewart, G., and Martin, L. Jaw wiring in the treatment of morbid obesity. Aust. N.Z. J. Surg. *55*:163, 1985.

143. Wood, G. D. The early results of treatment of the obese by a diet regime enforced by maxillo-mandibular fixation. J. Oral Surg. *35*:461, 1977.

144. Van Itallie, T. B., Bray, G. A. Connor, W. E., Faloon, W. W., Kral, J. G., Mason, E. E., and Stunkard, A. J. Guidelines for surgery for morbid obesity. Am. J. Clin. Nutr. *42*:904, 1985.

145. Ramsey, Stewart, G. The perioperative management of morbidly obese patients (a surgeon's perspective). Anaesth. Intern. Care *13*:399, 1985.

146. Griffin, W. O., Jr. Preoperative evaluation before surgery for morbid obesity. Am. J. Surg. *147*:427, 1984.

147. Bray, G. A., Barry, R. E., and Benfield, J. Intestinal bypass surgery for obesity decreases food intake and taste preferences. Am. J. Clin. Nutr. *29*:779, 1976.

148. Baddeley, R. M. An epilogue to jejunoileal bypass. World J. Surg. *9*:842, 1985.

149. Payne, J. H., and DeWind, L. T. Surgical treatment of obesity. Am. J. Surg. *118*:141, 1969.

150. Scott, H. W., Dean, R., and Shull, H. J. New considerations in use of the jejunoileal bypass in patients with morbid obesity. Ann. Surg. *177*:723, 1973.

151. Alpers, D. H. Surgical treatment for obesity. N. Engl. J. Med. *308*:1026, 1983.

152. Stunkard, A. J., Foster, G. D., and Grossman, R. F. Surgical treatment of obesity. Adv. Psychosom. Med. *15*:140, 1986.

153. Carey, L. C., Martin, E. W., Jr., and Mojzisik, C. The surgical treatment of morbid obesity. Curr. Probl. Surg. *21*:1, 1984.

154. Holzbach, R. T., Wieland, R. G., Lieber, C. S., DeCarli, L. M., Koepke, K. R., and Green, S. G. Hepatic lipids in morbid obesity. Assessment at the subsequent to jejunoileal bypass. N. Engl. J. Med. *290*:296, 1974.

155. O'Leary, J. P. Hepatic complications of jejunoileal bypass. Semin. Liver Dis. *3*:203, 1983.

156. Marubbio, A. T., Rucker, R. D., Jr., Schneider, P. D., Horstmann, J. P., Varco, R. L., and Buchwald, H. The liver in morbid obesity and following bypass surgery for obesity. Surg. Clin. North Am. *59*:1079, 1979.

157. Peters, R. L. Patterns of hepatic morphology in jejunoileal bypass patients. Am. J. Clin. Nutr. *30*:53, 1977.

158. Faloon, W. W., Flood, M. S., Aroesty, S., and Sherman, C. D. Assessment of jejunoileostomy for morbid obesity—some observations since 1976. Am. J. Clin. Nutr. *33*:431, 1980.

159. Adibi, S. A., and Stanko, R. T. Perspectives on gastrointestinal surgery for treatment of morbid obesity: the lesson learned. Gastroenterology *87*:1381, 1984.

160. Hocking, M. P., Duerson, M. C., O'Leary, J. P., and Woodward, E. R. Jejunoileal bypass for morbid obesity. Late followup in 100 cases. N. Engl. J. Med. *308*:995, 1983.

161. Yale, C. E. Gastric bypass combined with reversal of intestinal bypass for morbid obesity. World J. Surg. *4*:4723, 1980.

162. Hanni, C. L., Pool, L. R., Dean, R. E., and Cronquist, J. C. Treatment of jejunoileal bypass failure by reanastomosis and gastroplasty in a single-stage procedure. Am. Surg. *50*:354, 1984.

163. Mason, E. E., and Ito, C. Gastric bypass in obesity. Surg. Clin. North Am. *47*:1345, 1967.

164. Mason, E. E., Printen, K. J., Blommers, T. J., Lewis, J. W., and Scott, D. H. Gastric bypass in morbid obesity. Am. J. Clin. Nutr. *33*:395, 1980.

165. Mason, E. E., Printen, K. J., and Bloomers, T. J. Gastric bypass for obesity after ten years experience. Int. J. Obes. *2*:197, 1978.

166. Miskowiak, J., Honoré, K., Larsen, L., and Andersen, B. Food intake before and after gastroplasty for morbid obesity. Scand. J. Gastroenterol. *20*:925, 1985.

167. Tsoi, C. M., Westenskow, D. R., and Moody, F. G. Weight loss and metabolic changes of morbidly obese patients after gastric partitioning operation. Surgery *96*:545, 1984.

168. Horowitz, M., Collins, P. J., Chatterton, B. E., Harding, P. E., Watts, J., and Shearman, D. J. C. Gastric emptying after gastroplasty for morbid obesity. Br. J. Surg. *71*:435, 1984.

169. Arnstein, N. B., Shapiro, B., Eckhauser, F. E., Dmuchowski, C. F., Knol, J. A., Strodel, W. E., Nakajo, M., and Swanson, D. P. Morbid obesity treated by gastroplasty: radionuclide gastric emptying studies. Radiology *156*:501, 1985.

170. Schrumpf, E., Linnestad, P., Nygaard, K., Giercksky, K. E., and Fausa, O. Pancreatic polypeptide secretion before and after gastric bypass surgery for morbid obesity. Scand. J. Gastroenterol. *16*:1009, 1981.

171. Amland, F. F., Jorde, R., Kildebo, S., Burhol, P. G., and Giercksky, K. E. Effects of a gastric partitioning operation for morbid obesity on the secretion of gastric inhibitory polypeptide and pancreatic polypeptide. Scand. J. Gastroenterol. *19*:857, 1984.

172. Miskowiak, J., Andersen, B., Stadil, F., and Pedersen, J. H. Serum gastrin and blood glucose levels in gastroplasty for morbid obesity. Scand. J. Gastroenterol. *19*:669, 1984.

173. Ranlov, R. J. Serum lipid changes after gastroplasty for morbid obesity. Acta Med. Scand. *216*:503, 1984.

174. Schrumpf, E., Bergan, A., Djoseland, O., Fausa, O., Flaten, O., Skagen, D. W., and Tronier, B. The effect of gastric bypass operation on glucose tolerance in obesity. Scand. J. Gastroenterol. *20*(Suppl. 107):24, 1985.

175. Buckwalter, J. A. A prospective comparison of the jejunoileal and gastric bypass operations for morbid obesity. World J. Surg. *1*:757, 1977.

176. Griffen, W. O., Young, V. L., and Stevenson, C. C. A prospective comparison of gastric and jejunoileal bypass operations for morbid obesity. Ann. Surg. *186*:500, 1977.

177. Bass, J., and Freeman, J. B. Complications of gastric partitioning for morbid obesity. Adv. Surg. *18*:223, 1984.

178. Grundy, A., McFarland, R. J., Gazet, J. C., and Pilkington, T. R. E. Radiological appearances following vertical banded gastroplasty. Clin. Radiol. *36*:395, 1985.

179. Cope, J. R., Moseley, H. S., Haynid, C. C., Kingsley, J. R., and Gustavson, R. The radiology of gastric reduction surgery for obesity. Clin. Radiol. *34*:279, 1983.

180. Messmer, J. M., Wolper, J. C., and Sugerman, H. J. Stomal disruption in gastric partition in morbid obesity (comparison of radiographic and endoscopic diagnosis). Am. J. Gastroenterol. *79*:603, 1984.

181. Wolper, J. C., Messmer, J. M., Turner, M. A., and Sugerman, H. J. Endoscopic dilation of late stomal stenosis. Its use following gastric surgery for morbid obesity. Arch. Surg. *119*:836, 1984.

182. Hamilton, D. L., Vest, T. K., Brown, B. S., Shah, A. N., Menguy, R. B., and Chey, W. Y. Liver injury with alcoholiclike hyalin after gastroplasty for morbid obesity. Gastroenterology *85*:722, 1983.

183. Amaral, J. F., Thompson, W. R., Caldwell, M. D., Martin, H. F., and Randall, H. T. Prospective hematologic evaluation of gastric exclusion surgery for morbid obesity. Ann. Surg. *201*:186, 1985.

184. Crowley, L. V., and Olson, R. W. Megaloblastic anemia after gastric bypass for obesity. Am. J. Gastroenterol. *78*:406, 1983.

185. Schilling, R. F., Gohdes, P. N., and Hardie, G. H. Vitamin B$_{12}$ deficiency after gastric bypass surgery for obesity. Ann. Intern. Med. *101*:501, 1984.

186. Maryniak, O. Severe peripheral neuropathy following gastric bypass surgery for morbid obesity. Can. Med. Assoc. J. *131*:119, 1984.

187. Fawcett, S., Young, G. B., and Holliday, R. L. Wernicke's encephalopathy after gastric partitioning for morbid obesity. Can. J. Surg. *27*:169, 1984.

188. Feit, H., Glasberg, M., Ireton, C., Rosenberg, R. N., and Thal, E. Peripheral neuropathy and starvation after gastric partitioning for morbid obesity. Ann. Intern. Med. *96*:453, 1982.

189. MacLean, L. D., Rhode, B. M., and Shizgal, H. M. Nutrition following gastric operations for morbid surgery. Ann. Surg. *198*:347, 1983.

190. Crowley, L. V., Seay, J., and Mullin, G. Late effects of gastric bypass for obesity. Am. J. Gastroenterol. *79*:850, 1984.

191. Griffen, J. R., and Ward, O. Gastric bypass for morbid obesity. Surg. Clin. North Am. *59*:1103, 1979.

192. Halverson, J. D., and Koehler, R. E. Gastric bypass: analysis of weight loss and factors determining success. Surgery *90*:446, 1981.

193. Andersen, T., Backer, O. G., Stokholm, K. H., and Quaade, F. Randomized trial of diet and gastroplasty compared with diet alone in morbid obesity. N. Engl. J. Med. *310*:352, 1984.

194. Alden, J. F. Gastric and jejunoileal bypass. Arch. Surg. *112*:799, 1977.

195. Morton, R. Phthisiologia: sue exercitationes de phthisi. London, S. Smith, 1689.

196. Gull, W. W. Address in medicine. Lancet *2*:171, 1868.

197. Jones, D. J., Fox, M. M., Babigian, H. M., and Hutton, H. E. Epidemiology of anorexia nervosa in Monroe County, New York: 1960–1976. Psychosom. Med. *42*:551, 1980.

198. Willi, J., and Grossmann, S. Epidemiology of anorexia nervosa in a defined region of Switzerland. Am. J. Psychiatry *140*:564, 1983.

199. Crisp, A. H., Palmer, R. L., and Kalucy, R. S. How common is anorexia nervosa? A prevalence study. Br. J. Psychiatry *128*:549, 1976.

200. Harris, R. T. Bulimarexia and related serious eating disorders with medical complications. Ann. Intern. Med. *99*:800, 1983.

201. Killen, J. D., Taylor, C. B., Telch, M. J., Saylor, K. E., Maron, D. J., and Robinson, T. N. Self-induced vomiting and laxative and diuretic use among teenagers. Precursors of the binge-purge syndrome? JAMA *255*:1447, 1986.

202. Williams, P., and King, M. The "epidemic" of anorexia nervosa: another medical myth? Lancet 1:205, 1987.

203. Herzog, D. B., and Copeland, P. M. Eating disorders. N. Engl. J. Med. 313:295, 1985.

204. Balaa, M. A., and Drossman, D. A. Anorexia nervosa and bulimia: the eating disorders. DM. 31:9, 1985.

205. Halmi, K. A., Casper, R. C., and Eckert, E. D. Unique features associated with the age of onset of anorexia nervosa. Psychiatry Res. 1:209, 1979.

206. Abraham, S. F., and Beumont, P. J. Y. How patients describe bulimia or binge eating. Psychol. Med. 12:625, 1982.

207. Casper, R. C., Eckert, E. D., Halmi, K. A., Goldberg, S. C., and Davis, J. M. Bulimia—its incidence and clinical importance in patients with anorexia nervosa. Arch. Gen. Psychiatry 37:1030, 1980.

208. Mitchell, J. E., Pyle, R. L., and Eckert, E. D. Frequency and duration of binge-eating episodes in patients with bulimia. Am. J. Psychiatry 138:835, 1981.

209. Casper, R. C. The pathophysiology of anorexia nervosa and bulimia nervosa. Ann. Rev. Nutr. 6:299, 1986.

210. Swift, W. J., Andrews, D., Barklage, N. E. The relationship between affective disorder and eating disorders: a review of the literature. Am. J. Psychiatry 143:290, 1986.

211. Cantwell, D. P., Sturzenberger, S., Burroughs, J., Salkin, B., and Green, J. K. Anorexia nervosa: an affective disorder? Arch. Gen. Psychiatry 34:1087, 1977.

212. Bruch, H. Eating Disorders: Obesity, Anorexia Nervosa, and the Person Within. New York, Basic Books, 1973.

213. Hatsukami, D. K., Mitchell, J. E., Eckert, E. D. Eating disorders: a variant of mood disorders? Psychiatr. Clin. North Am. 7:349, 1984.

214. Warren, M. P., VandeWeile, R. L. Clinical and metabolic features of anorexia nervosa. Am. J. Obstet. Gynecol. 117:435, 1975.

215. Crisp, A. H., Hsu, L. K. G., Harding, B., and Hartshorn, J. Clinical features of anorexia nervosa. A study of a consecutive series of 102 female patients. J. Psychosom. Res. 24:179, 1980.

216. Casper, R. C., Kirschner, B., and Sandstead, H. An evaluation of trace metals, vitamins, and taste function in anorexia nervosa. Am. J. Clin. Nutr. 33:1801, 1980.

217. Schwabe, A. D., Lippe, B. M., Chang, R. J., Pops, M. A., and Yager, J. Anorexia nervosa. Ann. Intern. Med. 94:371, 1981.

218. Mordasini, R., Klose, G., and Greten, H. Secondary type II hyperlipoproteinemia in patients with anorexia nervosa. Metabolism 27:71, 1978.

219. Cuellar, R. E., and VanThiel, D. H. Gastrointestinal complications of the eating disorders: anorexia nervosa and bulimia. Am. J. Gastroenterol. 81:1113, 1986.

220. Abrams, R. A., and Ruff, J. C. Oral signs and symptoms in the diagnosis of bulimia. J. Am. Dent. Assoc. 113:761, 1986.

221. Hellström, I. Oral complications in anorexia nervosa. Scand. J. Dent. Res. 85:71, 1977.

222. Levin, P. A., Falco, J. M., Dixon, K., Gallup, E. M., and Saunders, W. Benign parotid enlargement in bulimia. Ann. Intern. Med. 93:827, 1980.

223. DuPlessis, D. J. Parotid enlargement in malnutrition. S. Afr. Med. J. 302:700, 1956.

224. LaRocca, F. E. F., and Della-Fera, M. A. Rumination: its significance in adults with anorexia nervosa. Psychosomatics 27:209, 1986.

225. Blinder, B. J. Rumination: a benign disorder? Int. J. Eating Disorders 5:385, 1986.

226. Fairburn, C. G., and Cooper, P. J. Rumination in bulimia nervosa. Br. Med. J. 288:826, 1984.

227. Shay, S. S., Johnson, L. F., Wong, R. K. H., Curtis, D. J., Rosenthal, R., Lanott, J. R., and Owensby, L. C. Rumination, heartburn, and daytime gastroesophageal reflux. A case study with mechanisms defined and successfully treated with biofeedback therapy. Am. J. Gastroenterol. 8:115, 1986.

228. DuBois, A., Gross, H. A., Ebert, M. H., and Castell, D. O. Altered gastric emptying and secretion in primary anorexia nervosa. Gastroenterology 77:319, 1979.

229. McCallum, R. W., Grill, B. B., Lange, R., Planky, M., Glass, E. E., and Greenfield, D. G. Definition of a gastric emptying

230. Holt, S., Ford, M. J., Grant, S., and Heading, R. C. Abnormal gastric emptying in primary anorexia nervosa. Br. J. Psychiatry 139:550, 1981.

231. DuBois, A., Gross, H. A., Richter, J. E., and Ebert, M. H. Effect of bethanechol on gastric functions in primary anorexia nervosa. Dig. Dis. Sci. 26:598, 1981.

232. Russell, D. M., Freedman, M. L., Feiglin, D. H. I., Jeejeebhoy, K. N., Swinson, R. P., and Garfinkel, P. E. Delayed gastric emptying and improvement with domperidone in a patient with anorexia nervosa. Am. J. Psychiatry 140:1235, 1983.

233. Saleh, J. W., and Lebwohl, P. Gastric emptying studies in patients with anorexia nervosa: effect of metoclopramide. Gastroenterology 76:1233, 1979.

234. Stacher, G., Bergmann, H., Weisnagrotzki, S., Kiss, A., Höbarth, J., and Mittelbach, G. Delayed gastric emptying in patients with anorexia nervosa and bulimia: effects of cisapride. Dig. Dis. Sci. 30:796, 1985.

235. Stacher, G., Kiss, A., Weisnagrotzki, S., Bergmann, H., Höbarth, J., and Schneider, C. Oesphageal and gastric motility disorders in patients categorised as having primary anorexia nervosa. Gut 27:1120, 1986,.

236. Brook, G. K. Acute gastric dilatation in anorexia nervosa. Br. Med. J. 2:499, 1977.

237. Mitchell, J. E., Pyle, R. L., and Miner, R. A. Gastric dilatation as a complication of bulimia. Psychosomatics 23:96, 1982.

238. Saul, S. H., Dekker, A., and Watson, C. G. Acute gastric dilatation with infarction and perforation. Report of fatal outcome in patient with anorexia nervosa. Gut 22:978, 1981.

239. Breslow, M., Yates, A., and Shisslak, C. Spontaneous rupture of the stomach: a complication of bulimia. Int. J. Eating Disorders 5:137, 1986.

240. Sours, J. A., Vorhaus, L. J. Superior mesenteric artery syndrome in anorexia nervosa: a case report. Am. J. Psychiatry 138:519, 1981.

241. Pentlow, B. D., and Dent, R. G. Acute vascular compression of the duodenum in anorexia nervosa. Br. J. Surg. 68:665, 1981.

242. Bo-Linn, G. W., Santa Ana, C. A., Morawski, S. G., and Fordtran, J. S. Purging and calorie absorption in bulimic patients and normal women. Ann. Intern. Med. 99:14, 1983.

243. Mitchell, J. E., and Boutacoff, L. I. Laxative abuse complicating bulimia: medical and treatment implications. Int. J. Eating Disorders 5:325, 1986.

244. Crisp, A. H. Gastrointestinal disturbance in anorexia nervosa. Postgrad. Med. J. 61:3, 1985.

245. Rampling, D. Acute pancreatitis in anorexia nervosa. Med. J. Aust. 2:194, 1982.

246. Backett, S. A. Acute pancreatitis and gastric dilatation in a patient with anorexia nervosa. Postgrad. Med. J. 61:39, 1985.

247. Mitchell, J. E., Pyle, R. L., Eckert, E. D., Hatsukami, D., and Lentz, R. Electrolyte and other physiologic abnormalities in patients with bulimia. Psychol. Med. 13:273, 1983.

248. Humphries, L. L., Adams, L. J., Eckfeldt, J. H., Levitt, M. D., and McClain, C. J. Hyperamylasemia in patients with eating disorders. Ann. Intern. Med. 106:50, 1987.

249. Fohlin, L. Body composition, cardiovascular and renal function in adolescent patients with anorexia nervosa. Acta Paediatr. Scand. (Suppl.) 268:1, 1977.

250. Palmer, E. P., and Guay, A. T. Reversible myopathy secondary to abuse of ipecac in patients with eating disorders. N. Engl. J. Med. 313:1457, 1985.

251. Donley, A. J., and Kemple, T. J. Spontaneous pneumomediastinum complicating anorexia nervosa. Br. Med. J. 1:1604, 1978.

252. Boyar, R. M., Katz, J., Finkelstein, J. W., Kapen, S., Weiner, H., Weinzman, E. D., and Hellman, L. Anorexia nervosa: immaturity of the 24-hour luteinizing hormone secretory pattern. N. Engl. J. Med. 291:861, 1974.

253. McNab, D., and Hawton, K. Disturbance of sex hormones in anorexia nervosa in the male. Postgrad. Med. J. 57:254, 1981.

254. Frankel, R. J., Jenkins, J. S. Hypothalamic-pituitary function in anorexia nervosa. Acta Endocrinol. (Copenh.) 78:209, 1975.

255. Clemmons, D. R., Libanski, A., and Underwood, L. E. Reduction of plasma innumo-reactive somatomedin C during fasting in humans. J. Clin. Endocrinol. Metab. *53*:1247, 1981.

256. Gold, P. W., Kaye, W., Robertson, G. L., and Ebert, M. Abnormalities in plasma and cerebrospinal-fluid arginine vasopressin in patients with anorexia nervosa. N. Engl. J. Med. *308*:1117, 1983.

257. Moshang, T., Jr., and Utiger, R. D. Low triiodothyronine euthyroidism in anorexia nervosa. *In* Vigersky, R. A. (ed.). Anorexia Nervosa. New York, Raven Press, 1977, pp. 263–270.

258. Boyar, R. M., Hellman, L. D., Roffwarg, H., and Katz, J. Cortisol secretion and metabolism and anorexia nervosa. N. Engl. J. Med. *296*:190, 1977.

259. Walsh, B. T., Katz, J. L., Levin, J., Kream, J., Fukushima, D. K., Weiner, H., and Zumoff, B. The production rate of cortisol declines during recovery from anorexia nervosa. J. Clin. Endocrinol. Metab. *53*:203, 1981.

260. Young, J. B., and Landsberg, L. Suppression of sympathetic nervous system during fasting. Science *196*:1473, 1977.

261. Oster, J. R. The binge-purge syndrome: a common albeit unappreciated cause of acid-base and fluid-electrolyte disturbances. South. Med. J. *80*:58, 1987.

262. Myers, T. J., Perkerson, M. D., Witter, B. A., and Granville, N. B. Hematologic findings in anorexia nervosa. Conn. Med. *45*:14, 1981.

263. Bowers, T. K., and Eckert, E. Leukopenia in anorexia nervosa. Lack of increased risk of infection. Arch. Intern. Med. *138*:1520, 1978.

264. Rigotti, N. A., Nussbaun, S. R., Herzog, D. B., and Neer, R. M. Osteoporosis in women with anorexia nervosa. N. Engl. J. Med. *311*:1601, 1984.

265. Brotman, M. C., Forbath, N., and Garfinkel, P. E. Myopathy due to ipecac syrup poisoning in a patient with anorexia nervosa. Can. Med. Assoc. J. *125*:453, 1981.

266. Hillard, J. R., and Hillard, P. J. A. Bulimia, anorexia nervosa, and diabetes. Deadly combinations. Psychiatr. Clin. North Am. *7*:367, 1984.

267. Shaul, P. W., Farrell, M. K., and Maloney, M. J. Caffeine toxicity as a cause of acute psychosis in anorexia nervosa. J. Pediatr. *105*:493, 1984.

268. Schott, G. D. Anorexia nervosa presenting as foot drop. Postgrad. Med. J. *55*:58, 1979.

269. Niiya, K., Kitagawa, T., Fujishita, M., Yoshimoto, S., Kobayashi, M., Kubonishi, I., Taguchi, H., and Miyoshi, I. Bulimia nervosa complicated by deficiency of vitamin K–dependent coagulation factors. JAMA *250*:792, 1983.

270. Wyatt, E., Greaves, M., Sondergaard, J. Fixed drug eruption (phenolphthalein). Evidence for a blood-borne mediator. Arch. Dermatol. *106*:671, 1972.

271. Crisp, A. H. Anorexia Nervosa: Let Me Be. London Academic Press, 1980.

272. Hudson, J. I., Pope, H. G., Jr., Jonas, J. M., and Yurgelun-Todd, D. Family history study of anorexia nervosa and bulimia. Br. J. Psychiatry *142*:133, 1983.

273. Lucas, A. Toward the understanding of anorexia nervosa as a disease. Mayo Clin. Proc. *56*:254, 1981.

274. Harris, R. T. Eating disorders: diagnosis and management by the internist. South. Med. J. *79*:871, 1986.

274a. Feighner, J. P., Robins, E., Guze, S., Woodruff, R. A., Winokur, G., and Munoz, R. Diagnostic criteria for use in psychiatric research. Arch. Gen. Psychiatry *26*:57, 1972.

275. Fairburn, C. G., and Garner, D. M. The diagnosis of bulimia nervosa. Int. J. Eating Disorders *5*:403, 1986.

276. Nussbaum, M. P., Shenker, I. R., Shaw, H., and Frank, S. Differential diagnosis and pathogenesis of anorexia nervosa. Pediatrician *12*:110, 1985.

277. Udvarhelyi, G. B., Adamkiewicz, J. I., and Cook, R. E. "Anorexia nervosa" caused by a fourth ventricle tumor. Neurology *16*:565, 1966.

278. White, J. H., Kelly, P., and Dorman, K. Clinical picture of atypical anorexia nervosa associated with hypothalamic tumor. Am. J. Psychiatry *134*:323, 1977.

279. Chiodo, J. The assessment of anorexia nervosa and bulimia. Prog. Behav. Modif. *19*:255, 1985.

280. Slade, P. A review of body-image studies in anorexia nervosa and bulimia nervosa. J. Psychiatr. Res. *19*:255, 1985.

281. Crisp, A. H. Anorexia nervosa. Br. Med. J. *287*:855, 1983.

282. Brotman, A. W., Rigotti, N. A., and Herzog, D. B. Medical complications of eating disorders. Compr. Psychiatry *26*:258, 1985.

283. Fairburn, C. G. The place of cognitive behavioral approach in the management of bulimia. *In* Darby, P. L., Garfinkel, P. E., and Garner, D. M. (eds.). Anorexia Nervosa: Recent Developments in Research. New York, Alan R. Liss, 1983.

284. Pope, H. G., Jr., and Hudson, J. I. Antidepressant drug therapy for bulimia: current status. J. Clin. Psychiatry *47*:339, 1986.

285. Halmi, K. A., Eckert, E., and Falk, J. R. Cyproheptadine for anorexia nervosa (letter). Lancet *1*:1357, 1982.

286. Opioid blockage for anorexia? Medical World News, October 13, 1986.

287. Kaye, W. H., Pickar, D., Naber, D., and Ebert, M. H. Cerebrospinal fluid opioid activity in anorexia nervosa. Am. J. Psychiatry *139*:643, 1982.

288. Jonas, J. M., and Gold, M. S. Naltrexone reverses bulimic symptoms (letter). Lancet *1*:807, 1986.

289. Hsu, L. K. G. Outcome of anorexia nervosa. A review of the literature (1954 to 1978). Arch. Gen. Psychiatry *37*:1041, 1980.

290. Schwartz, D. M., and Thompson, M. G. Do anorectics get well? Current and future needs. Am. J. Psychiatry *138*:319, 1981.

291. Collins, M., Hodas, G. R., and Liebman, R. Interdisciplinary model for the inpatient treatment of adolescents with anorexia nervosa. J. Adolesc. Health Care *4*:3, 1983.

292. Lowenkopf, E. L. Bulimia: concepts and therapy. Compr. Psychiatry *24*:546, 1983.

10

Heartburn, Dysphagia, and Other Esophageal Symptoms

CHARLES E. POPE, II

Three symptoms—heartburn, dysphagia, and pain on swallowing (odynophagia)—should immediately suggest an esophageal cause to the clinician. Other symptoms which may be of esophageal origin but are not specific include chest pain, gastrointestinal bleeding, and respiratory symptoms such as coughing and wheezing. A complete medical history can be one of the most useful tools in the investigation of these esophageal symptoms, and it should suggest the esophageal etiology of the symptoms in most cases.

DYSPHAGIA

Dysphagia is one of the most specific symptoms produced by gastrointestinal disease and always indicates malfunction of some type in the esophagus. Some studies suggest that the prevalence of psychiatric disorders is high in patients with motor disorders of the esophagus.[1] Individual patients with achalasia (a condition with structural esophageal abnormalities) will note increased dysphagia during periods of emotional stress. In these situations, the esophagus may be the target of mind-gut interactions. Nevertheless, it is necessary to investigate the structure and function of the esophagus when dysphagia is present and not to dismiss dysphagia as a psychiatric abnormality.

Normally, the act of swallowing proceeds without producing any symptoms at all. Dysphagia is present when the patient is aware that something has gone wrong soon after swallowing. Patients say that the food "sticks," "hangs up," or "stops," or they feel that the food "just won't go down right." Dysphagia is experienced immediately after the act of deglutition. A sensation of something always "stuck in the throat" may be due to a foreign body or to globus histericus, but it should not be interpreted as dysphagia.

A specific type of dysphagia is pharyngeal or transfer dysphagia, which is inability to initiate deglutition successfully. Food or fluid is often propelled around in the mouth, but the patient is not successful in passing the bolus into the esophagus. "I just can't seem to get it started down" is the usual complaint. Patients with transfer dysphagia will cough and sputter with a liquid bolus as their attempts to swallow propel some of the fluid into the larynx. This symptom may be caused by pharyngeal muscular weakness or by failure in the neural coordination of swallowing. In the former case, there may be a nasal quality to the voice and regurgitation of fluid into the nasopharynx during swallowing.

Esophageal dysphagia is produced by two different processes (Table 10–1). Mechanical narrowing of the lumen either from intrinsic causes (carcinoma, peptic stricture, or web) or from extrinsic causes (mediastinal tumors) is one main category. The other category is a motor disorder (failure of the muscular pump) such as achalasia or scleroderma.

Differentiation between mechanical obstruction and a motor disorder can be made by establishment of the type of bolus which is arrested, the time course of the progression of dysphagia, and the mechanisms used by the patient to relieve obstruction. Arrest of liquids as well as solids points more to a motor disorder unless there is very high grade mechanical obstruction or unless a previously swallowed solid bolus has impacted in the esophagus and produced obstruction. If the time course of the dysphagia shows rapid progression of dysphagia for solids, then a carcinoma should be suspected. Very intermittent dysphagia for solids might be produced by an esophageal web (see pp. 632–635). Constant low-grade dysphagia for solids, especially when associated with heartburn and regurgitation, might point either to a peptic stricture or just to the presence of significant gastroesophageal reflux disease (see pp. 594–619). Relief of the obstruction by vomiting or regurgitation of the bolus usually points to an organic narrowing; if the impacted bolus is dislodged by repeated swallowing, by performing a Valsalva maneuver, or by drinking water, then a motor disorder is usually the underlying cause of the dysphagia.

The patient's localization of the site of bolus impaction is of limited help in determining the area of difficulty. Subxiphoid or high epigastric localization is usually more accurate than when the site of obstruction is felt in the substernal notch. In the latter case, the

Table 10–1. ESOPHAGEAL DYSPHAGIA

	Mechanical Narrowing (Tumors, Strictures)	Motor Disorder (Achalasia, Scleroderma)
Onset	Gradual or sudden	Usually gradual
Progression	Often	Usually not
Type of bolus	Solids (unless high-grade obstruction)	Solids and/or liquids
Temperature-dependent	No	Worse with cold liquids; may improve with warm liquids
Response to bolus impaction	Often must be regurgitated	Can usually be passed by repeated swallowing or by washing it down with fluids

Table 10–2. CHARACTERISTICS OF DYSPHAGIA IN CERTAIN ILLNESSES

1. Cancer	Progressive nature, halitosis, dysphagia for solids and then liquids; must regurgitate bolus
2. Stricture	History of heartburn; long time course
3. Lower esophageal ring	Intermittent obstruction of solid bolus; total obstruction; no heartburn or weight loss
4. CNS diseases	Transfer dysphagia, aspiration of fluids, nasal voice
5. Achalasia	Dysphagia for solids and liquids; regurgitation of food eaten 24 hours earlier; pulmonary symptoms
6. Diffuse spasm	Dysphagia during pain attacks
7. Scleroderma	Postural effects on dysphagia

bolus may well be lodged in the distal esophagus, yet may be felt in the lower neck. The unwary radiologist may be misled by this disparity and may spend time taking many spot films of the cervical area when attention should be directed further down. Many of these factors have been organized into a diagnostic algorithm, which can have a diagnostic accuracy as high as 80 per cent when 39 questions are answered sequentially.[2] Certain esophageal conditions tend to have characteristic groups of symptoms, as listed in Table 10–2.

Patients with reflux disease will sometimes complain of "bolus awareness." Although the bolus will not actually stop and produce the sensation of dysphagia, the patient will be able to track the progress of the bolus down the esophagus until it reaches the stomach. Administering a barium-soaked bolus and watching by X-ray as a bony finger tracks the bolus will confirm this ability.

HEARTBURN (PYROSIS)

Heartburn is a term that the interviewer should use with caution, as the lay perception of the meaning of heartburn is so variable. After asking the patient whether heartburn is present, the next response to a positive reply is to ask the patient to define the meaning of the term. True heartburn, a manifestation of gastroesophageal reflux disease, is usually described as a "hot, burning" sensation; "It feels as if fire will come out my mouth." The term "burning" rather than "pain" is usually used by the patient unless the sensation of heartburn becomes so intense that "pain" is an appropriate term. Heartburn often comes in waves and is located substernally. An internationally common gesture often accompanies the patient's description of heartburn—the open hand moves from epigastrium to neck and back again. Contrast this with the stationary clenched fist gesture of the patient suffering from the discomfort of coronary insufficiency.

There is another aspect of heartburn due to reflux which is so characteristic that it should always be sought. This is the relief of the sensation of burning by the ingestion of antacids, albeit only transiently. If a burning sensation in the chest is not at all affected

by antacid ingestion, then it may well be of esophageal origin, but it is not heartburn.

Heartburn is often intensified by bending over or lifting heavy objects. Many patients will notice the sensation after retiring, especially if a bedtime snack has preceded retirement. Patients will often report that heartburn is more pronounced when lying on the right side in bed. Production or intensification of heartburn by taking citrus fruit juices is another feature of most patients' symptom complex. Other dietary features often mentioned include worsening of the substernal burning after meals high in fat, sugars, or alcohol. Wine drinkers usually report that a good robust red wine is more likely to produce symptoms than is a delicate white. Intermittent cigarette smokers may notice heartburn soon after lighting up; constant smokers usually do not associate their habit with heartburn symptoms.

Heartburn may be accompanied by the appearance of fluid in the mouth, either a salty fluid (water brash) or regurgitated gastric contents. Water brash is fluid secreted by the salivary glands. The fluid refluxed from the stomach is often described as "bitter" rather than "sour," and may be yellow or green, suggesting the presence of bile in the regurgitated fluid. Belching may precede regurgitation of fluid or the occurrence of heartburn.

The presence of heartburn does not allow prediction of the macroscopic or microscopic appearance of the esophageal mucosa. Many patients with severe prolonged heartburn will have a normal-appearing esophageal lining on endoscopy. Some of these normal-appearing linings will show polymorphonuclear leukocytes on biopsy; other normal-appearing mucosa will show an increase in the thickness of the basal cell layer on histologic examination, and still other linings will appear microscopically normal (see pp. 603–605).

PAIN ON SWALLOWING (ODYNOPHAGIA)

The third symptom specific for esophageal involvement is pain on swallowing. This symptom usually indicates that an inflammatory process is involving the esophageal mucosa or, rarely, the esophageal muscle. Odynophagia can occur after caustic ingestion, peptic digestion of the esophageal mucosa, mucosal infection by fungal or viral agents, or a chemical burn caused by retention of a pill or capsule. Rarely, a nonobstructing esophageal carcinoma can produce odynophagia. Odynophagia is temporally related to the ingestion of either a solid or liquid bolus. Odynophagia can be so intense as to preclude the ingestion of any material whatsoever, including the patient's own saliva.

CHEST PAIN

The esophagus is only one of many structures that can produce chest pain. Chest pain of esophageal origin can be intense and mimic the pain of coronary insufficiency almost exactly. The pain can arise either from motor disorders or from a sensitive mucosa. Chest pain of esophageal origin (esophageal colic) is usually substernal and classically radiates directly through to the back. It can also radiate to the neck, jaw, shoulders, or down one or both arms. Chest pain of esophageal origin can be fleeting, or can persist for as long as four to six hours. A few unfortunates can suffer almost constantly from chest pain of esophageal origin. In approximately half of the patients suffering from esophageal colic, the discomfort can be precipitated by exercise, although the relationship between the amount of exercise and the production of pain is less strict than in chest pain of coronary insufficiency. Esophageal colic can be triggered by drinking very cold or very warm liquids. Solid bolus ingestion is less likely to provoke an attack. Emotional stress can also precipitate attacks, and it sometimes misdirects investigation into purely psychologic channels.

Ingestion of antacids will occasionally but not reliably relieve esophageal colic which has been produced by acid sensitivity of the esophageal mucosa. Antacids, of course, will be of no benefit when the colic is produced by motor disorders of the esophagus (see pp. 559–593). These in turn can occasionally be relieved by sublingual nitroglycerin, which can further confound differentiation between esophageal colic and coronary insufficiency.

RESPIRATORY SYMPTOMS

The production of respiratory symptoms by esophageal reflux has been receiving increasing attention in both the pediatric and adult populations. The pulmonary manifestations of reflux can range from life-threatening aspiration of gastric contents during emergency anesthesia to recurrent wheezing, which is less clearly related to esophageal reflux. The mechanism of such wheezing may be direct irritation of the bronchial mucosa by aspirated fluid or by reflexes stimulated by chemical irritation of the esophageal or laryngeal epithelium. Some of the characteristics of reflux-induced pulmonary symptoms are listed in Table 10–3.

Occasionally, the patient will awake from sleep with respiratory stridor and a mouthful of gastric contents. Most commonly, the patient will not be aware of regurgitation of fluid, and in fact, regurgitation or heartburn may not be a prominent part of the history but must be obtained by careful questioning. Because reflux can follow bouts of coughing and intense respiratory efforts, it is sometimes difficult to determine

Table 10–3. CHARACTERISTICS OF PULMONARY SYMPTOMS OF ESOPHAGEAL ORIGIN

Late onset in life
No family history of allergy
Nocturnal wheezing
Hoarseness
Sensation of laryngeal foreign body
Need to clear throat repeatedly

whether reflux is the cause or the result of pulmonary problems. Recognition of reflux in infants is even more difficult; sometimes recurrent bouts of pneumonia, anemia, or failure to thrive are the only clues to the presence of pathologic reflux.

BELCHING

Belching can be considered an esophageal symptom although it usually does not denote the presence of esophageal disease. Air is normally ingested during "dry" swallows or along with solid or liquid material. Gas may be ingested in carbonated beverages or, rarely, may be produced by fermentation in the stomach. Some individuals have trained themselves to belch voluntarily, either to signal extreme gastronomic appreciation or else to disrupt the classroom. The extreme example of this feat is esophageal speech. Under the fluoroscope, the esophageal speaker can be shown to fill the esophagus with air and then expel the air in controlled bursts, while forming words with the lips.

Belching has been studied experimentally.[3] Infusion of air into the stomach results in the unappreciated reflux of gas into the esophagus. Secondary peristalsis returns the gas to the stomach, only to have the sequence repeated. Occasionally, an increase in intra-abdominal pressure is associated with escape of air not only from the stomach but also from the esophagus, and an audible belch is produced. Experimentally, belching consists therefore of both an "internal" and an "external" belch. It would seem logical to presume that the same dichotomy is present in the well-fed individual after a meal.

RUMINATION

An uncommon symptom, but one that has attracted medical attention since the seventeenth century, is that of rumination.[4] Patients who ruminate notice that 10 to 15 minutes after eating, the mouth suddenly fills with portions of the meal recently eaten. This material is either expectorated, or chewed and reswallowed, only to reappear again in a relentless cycling. The food that unexpectedly returns in this fashion usually does not taste acid to the ruminator; in fact, the rumination usually ceases after 30 or 40 minutes when the food begins to taste acid. This act is involuntary and is often a cause of chronic social embarrassment to the patient, who is often reluctant to mention this process to the physician. If the act is brought to medical attention, it is usually referred to as "vomiting," from which it can usually easily be differentiated by the absence of accompanying nausea. Ruminators, when questioned, are often aware of an involuntary twitch of the abdominal muscles that immediately precedes the appearance of material into the mouth. This can be documented manometrically by showing a simultaneous spike in gastric and esophageal pressure just before the bolus appears.[5] Recognition of this sequence of events can even be helpful in arranging for treatment of this condition by biofeedback.[6]

References

1. Clouse, R. E., and Lustman, P. J. Psychiatric illness and contraction abnormalities of the esophagus. N. Engl. J. Med. *309*:1337, 1983.
2. Edwards, D. A. W. Discriminative information in the diagnosis of dysphagia. J. R. Coll. Physicians Lond. *9*:257, 1975.
3. McNally, E. F., Kelly, J. E., Jr., and Ingelfinger, F. J. Mechanism of belching: Effects of gastric distension with air. Gastroenterology *46*:254, 1964.
4. Fabricius ab Aquapendente. Tractatus de gula, ventriculo et intestinis. Padua, 1618.
5. Amarnath, R. P., Abell, T. L., and Malagelada, J.-R. The rumination syndrome in adults. Ann. Intern. Med. *105*:513, 1986.
6. Shay, S. S., Johnson, L. F., Wong, R. K. H., Curtis, D. J., Rosenthal, R., Lamott, J. R., and Owensby, L. C. Rumination, heartburn, and daytime gastroesophageal reflux. J. Clin. Gastroenterol. *8*:115, 1986.

Caustic Injury to the Upper Gastrointestinal Tract

11

PETER M. LOEB
ABRAM M. EISENSTEIN

The ingestion of caustic agents can initiate a progressive and devastating injury to the esophagus and stomach.[1-4] Since the introduction of concentrated liquid alkaline cleansers in the 1960s, the incidence of severe injury has increased.[1, 5, 6] If the patient survives the acute effects of caustic ingestion, the reparative response can result in esophageal and gastric stenosis and an increased incidence of esophageal cancer. Management of these problems is complicated further because the individuals most susceptible to injury are the psychotic, the suicidal, the alcoholic, and the very young.[1] About 80 per cent of caustic ingestions occur as accidents in children under five years of age who have access to strong household cleansers. These substances are often stored in food or drink containers, and unfortunately, liquid lye has an appearance similar to milk.

CAUSTIC AGENTS

Caustic injury is usually produced by strong alkaline or acidic agents. Lye is a broad term for strong alkali used in cleansing agents.[7] Sodium and potassium hydroxides in granular, paste, and liquid forms are used for drain cleaners, washing powders, Clinitest tablets, and soaps. Concentrations of these alkali vary from 9.5 to 32 per cent in the liquid form to 100 per cent in the solid form.[1, 4, 6, 8] Sodium carbonate, introduced as a substitute for the noncaustic phosphate detergents, can be equally corrosive.[9] Milder injuries are usually caused by ammonium hydroxide and bleaches (sodium and calcium hypochloride, and hydrogen peroxide), although severe damage can also result from these agents.[10]

Acids are commonly available as toilet bowl cleaners (sulfuric, hydrochloric, phosphoric), soldering fluxes (hydrochloric), antirust compounds (hydrochloric, oxalic), battery fluids (sulfuric), and swimming pool and slate cleaners (hydrochloric).[10] There are innumerable other agents that cause caustic injury, but such injuries usually occur as isolated events.[4]

PATHOGENESIS AND PATHOLOGY

The extent of injury to the gastrointestinal tract depends upon the type of agent; its concentration, quantity, and physical state; and the duration of exposure.[11-13] Accidental ingestions are sometimes halted by the odor of the agent or by oropharyngeal irritation.[13] Acidic solutions usually cause immediate pain, and unless ingestion is intentional, the agent is rapidly expelled. Caustic agents in solid form adhere to mucous membranes and are more difficult to swallow. The alkali liquid solutions are often tasteless and odorless and thus are swallowed before protective reflexes can be invoked. Patients with abnormal esophageal emptying will have prolonged exposure and more severe esophageal injury, whereas caustic agents entering the stomach in the postprandial state will be diluted and partially neutralized.[14]

The primary difference between alkaline and acidic injury is the rapid penetration into tissue by alkali.[1, 15] Experimental studies in cats reveal that 1 ml of 30.5 per cent sodium hydroxide solution exposed for one second can penetrate the full thickness of the cat's esophagus.[1] Alkali has a potent solvent action on the lipoprotein lining, producing a liquefaction necrosis with intense inflammation and saponification of the mucous membranes, submucosa, and muscularis of the esophagus and stomach.[1, 14, 16–21] Thrombosis of adjacent vessels results in further necrosis, followed by bacterial colonization. Sloughing of the superficial necrotic layer occurs two to four days after injury and is followed by increased fibroblastic activity.[13] Ulceration may persist for months, even as collagen formation occurs in adjacent tissue. Whereas granular agents often produce limited focal injury to the oropharyngeal and proximal esophageal mucosa, liquid alkaline solutions can cause extensive contiguous damage to the entire esophagus and stomach.[2, 11, 22–24] Severe injury frequently occurs with liquid agents, whereas only 10 to 25 per cent of patients ingesting granular agents have serious injury.[23, 24] Animal studies have shown that, after ingestion of liquid alkali, violent regurgitation occurs in the esophagus, followed by propulsion of the alkali back into the stomach. This to-and-fro action lasts for several minutes, with eventual passage of the alkali into the duodenum.[25] The extent of injury is then limited only by the quantity and concentration of the compound ingested. Certainly, the stomach is not resistant to alkali ingestion, and the neutralizing effect of gastric acidity is insignificant compared with the total alkalinity of small volumes of strong alkali.[26]

Acid agents produce a coagulation necrosis, resulting in a firm protective eschar that delays injury and limits penetration.[27] The alkaline environment and the rapid transit time limit injury of the oropharynx and esophagus by the more hydrophilic acid compounds.[14, 16, 27] Acidic agents were thought to spare the esophagus and injure the stomach. However, ingestion of highly concentrated sulfuric or hydrochloric acid penetrates the esophageal mucosa and produces severe esophageal injury in about one of two patients.[10, 26, 27] In one study, there was no difference in the percentage of patients who developed esophageal injury after alkali and acid exposure.[28] In the fasting patient, caustic acids will diffusely sear the gastric mucosa along the magenstrasse to the antrum, often sparing the fundus.[14, 29] When the stomach is full, the hydrophilic acidic agents mix with gastric contents and cause diffuse injury. Although pylorospasm usually occurs, in some cases the solutions pass into the duodenum.

Caustic injuries to the gastrointestinal mucosa are classified pathologically in the same manner as skin burns.[13, 30]

First-degree is superficial injury producing edema and erythema of only the mucosa. The mucosa subsequently sloughs without scar or stricture formation.

Second-degree is penetration through the submucosa into the muscular layers. In one to two weeks, the layers slough, producing deep ulcerations followed by granulation tissue. A fibroblastic reaction ensues during the second and third weeks, and over a period of weeks to months the collagen undergoes contraction. With contiguous involvement, a narrowing of the lumen of the esophagus or stomach can result.[1, 19] Scar formation appears to be complete within eight weeks in about 80 per cent of patients but can take as long as eight months.[5, 31] Infection and additional trauma may result in increased injury and progressive damage.[19] Esophageal strictures tend to occur where the caustic agents pool at the cricopharyngeus, at the level of the aortic arch and tracheal bifurcation, and at the lower esophageal sphincter.[12] Likewise, most gastric strictures occur in the antrum of persons who are injured when fasting, as opposed to the midbody in those who have previously ingested food.

Third-degree is penetration of the caustic agent through the wall of the esophagus or stomach, with the development of mediastinitis and peritonitis or involvement of contiguous organs. Most perforations occur within 48 hours of ingestion and are usually the result of alkali in the esophagus and liquid alkali or acid in the stomach.

CLINICAL FEATURES

The patient with a history of caustic ingestion may present with a wide spectrum of clinical findings.[11, 13, 14, 32, 33] The diagnosis is usually not difficult if an accurate history is obtained and a physical examination is performed. Family and friends should be sent to retrieve the agent or container if the type of substance has not been clearly identified.

Acute Manifestations. In many cases, the patient may have no complaints, and examination of the mouth and pharynx may be normal. However, one cannot predict the extent of esophageal or gastric involvement from the findings in the oropharynx or larynx.[4, 30, 34, 35] The patient may have persistent salivation or even the inability to swallow. Oropharyngeal lesions occur more frequently after solid lye ingestion. Edema, ulceration, or a white membrane may be present over the palate, uvula, and pharynx. The lesions bleed easily and are painful.[16, 36] Hoarseness and stridor indicate laryngeal, epiglottal, and even hypopharyngeal involvement.[35] With esophageal damage, many patients complain of dysphagia and odynophagia. These esophageal and respiratory symptoms may develop rapidly or may be delayed for several hours.[36] Severe gastric injury may present as epigastric pain, retching or emesis of tissue, blood, or only coffee-ground material.

With third-degree injury of the esophagus, tachypnea, dyspnea, stridor, and shock may develop rapidly. Physical findings of mediastinitis may be present. Likewise, gastric perforation may result in acute peritonitis. Progressive necrosis with perforation of the stomach or esophagus may not develop for 48 hours.[36]

Late Manifestations. Although the patient's symptoms are usually progressive, they may disappear with recovery from the acute injury, only to recur over the next three to eight weeks when the development of obstructive features such as scar formation occurs. Dysphagia heralds the onset of an esophageal stricture and develops in 15 to 25 per cent of caustic exposures.[36, 39] Early satiety, weight loss, and progressive emesis are symptoms suggestive of gastric outlet obstruction. Stenosis may become apparent as late as one year after injury.[7, 34]

Mortality. The mortality rate after caustic ingestion is high but in the last 20 to 30 years has been reduced from 20 per cent to 1 to 3 per cent.[12, 18, 36–38] Most deaths result from mediastinitis and peritonitis acutely and malnutrition and aspiration chronically.

DIAGNOSTIC STUDIES

The poor correlation between symptoms, physical findings, and esophageal and gastric lesions; the inability to predict the presence or extent of injury; and the current medical and surgical management of caustic injuries make it imperative that careful diagnostic studies be performed.[28]

Esophagogastroduodenoscopy. Many experts have recommended endotracheal intubation with general anesthesia for endoscopy and limitation of endoscopic advancement to the site of severe injury.[4, 13, 30, 33, 34, 38, 40, 41] Most endoscopic perforations occur with the use of the rigid instrument in children and in uncooperative patients.[42, 43] With the use of smaller flexible endoscopes, general anesthesia is usually unnecessary, and endotracheal intubation is indicated only in patients with respiratory distress. A complete examination of esophageal and gastric mucosae usually can be performed, unless there is evidence of perforation or severe injury that prevents gentle passage of the endoscope.[7, 11, 20, 23, 33, 42] Endoscopic examination should be performed as soon as the patient's cardiovascular and respiratory status is stable. Patients who are not seen until 48 hours after injury should also undergo endoscopy, for there is no evidence to support the earlier-held concept that perforation would be more likely.

Perhaps the most reliable finding by endoscopy is the absence of esophageal and gastric lesions. Over 50 per cent of patients with a history of caustic ingestion are found to have no evidence of injury.[4, 24, 28, 36] Classification of the depth of injury is not so precise as pathologic classification. The extent of involvement is more easily defined. First-degree burns (superficial burns), manifested by scattered foci of edema, erythema, or hemorrhage, usually can be delineated without difficulty.[4] With diffuse contiguous involvement, it is difficult to determine the depth of injury.[13] Membranous exudate and blisters suggest that second-degree burns are present. Deep ulcerations with black discoloration indicate that full-thickness necrosis of third-degree injury has occurred and perforation is impending or present.[41, 42] Isolated areas of ulceration and necrosis may also be present, without circumferential involvement. Although no controlled studies are available, the results of retrospective studies indicate some correlation between the degree of injury assessed endoscopically and the clinical course.[38] About 30 per cent of second-degree injuries and over 90 per cent of third-degree injuries develop strictures.[24, 39] However, Estrera et al. discovered that three of eight patients diagnosed endoscopically as having second-degree burns were found at surgery to have full-thickness necrosis.[44] Some investigators classify injury as mild or severe, depending on the presence of circumferential lesions. Certainly, circumferential ulcerations of the esophagus are more likely to result in stricture formation.[4, 24]

Radiologic Studies. In the acute phase of caustic injury, chest roentgenograms may reveal evidence of esophageal perforation, such as air in the mediastinum, mediastinal thickening, or pneumothorax.[7] The esophagus may be dilated after severe injury. Upright chest films and abdominal plain roentgenograms may confirm a gastric perforation by the presence of free air or an extragastric mass.

In the acute stages of the illness, barium contrast films of the esophagus and stomach are usually not adequately sensitive to delineate the severity and extent of injury.[7, 31, 34, 45, 46] Furthermore, barium ingestion may interfere with endoscopic evaluation and is usually deferred. If barium studies are performed acutely, it appears that the effects of alkaline and acidic injury to the esophagus are similar.[29] There may be mucosal and submucosal edema manifested by blurred, irregular, and scalloped margins. Plaque-like linear defects represent irregular ulceration and sloughing of the mucosa.[47] The esophagus often appears atonic and dilated. The changes persist for up to three weeks. Strictures can be short or long, with smooth or irregular margins (Fig. 11–1).

Barium studies of the stomach in the severely injured patient may demonstrate thick, irregular folds, ulcers, atony, and rigidity, which are found most prominently in the body and antrum of the stomach.[48] Gastric dilatation may occur, and the pylorus becomes rigid and dilated, although acutely there is intense pylorospasm. Effects of acid caustic injury are often seen in the duodenum. Edema, ulceration, and dilatation of the bulb and even of the second and third portions of the duodenum may be present. After about two weeks, the edema and dilatation resolve and stenosis of the antrum may develop. This stenotic lesion may have an appearance similar to an infiltrative gastric carcinoma (Fig. 11–2).[49]

TREATMENT OF CAUSTIC INJURIES

Emergency Treatment

Neutralization of Caustics. The manufacturers of many home alkali products recommend that acid neutralizers be given immediately after caustic ingestion. However, most studies suggest that the heat produced in the neutralization reaction of alkali or acidic sub-

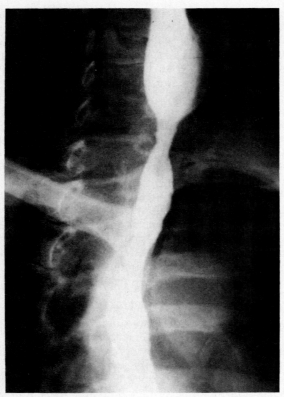

Figure 11–1. Stricture in the upper esophagus with narrowing of the midesophagus several weeks after caustic ingestion. (Courtesy of R. N. Berk, M.D., University of California, San Diego.)

stances may increase tissue injury.[20, 26, 41, 50] Attempts to dilute alkaline substances may also result in increased heat release through the exothermic properties of dilution and neutralization. Furthermore, alkali injuries occur so rapidly that even immediate attempts to neutralize them probably would be unsuccessful. Any maneuver that might induce emesis could produce aspiration or re-exposure of the esophagus and even

the larynx to the caustic agent.[7, 26, 41, 50, 51] With acid injury, the immediate use of large volumes of water or milk may dilute and neutralize the acid substance without producing further injury from the heat of reaction.[17, 20]

Resuscitation. Once the patient has been brought to the hospital, he or she should be allowed nothing by mouth.[13] If there is clinical evidence of laryngeal involvement or respiratory difficulties, rapid establishment of an airway by means of oral endotracheal intubation under direct visualization or tracheostomy is critical. Blind endotracheal intubation should not be performed. In any case, direct evaluation of the oropharynx and laryngoscopic examination are recommended.[7] Laryngeal edema may not develop until 24 hours after ingestion.[13, 25] Hypotension should be immediately corrected with isotonic fluid and blood products.

Endoscopic examination with a flexible, small-caliber endoscope should be performed when the patient's condition is stable. If esophageal or gastric perforation is suggested by clinical evaluation or plain films of the chest and abdomen, thoracotomy or laparotomy is indicated as soon as resuscitation is complete.[13, 37]

Specific Therapeutic Measures

A number of treatment modalities are available. The goals are to prevent perforation and to avoid progressive fibrosis and stenosis of the esophagus and stomach. Only emergency surgery can prevent or treat perforation, whereas corticosteroids, collagen synthesis inhibitors, antibiotics, intraesophageal stents, esophageal dilatation or surgery could be used to prevent or treat stenosis. The problems with choosing among these approaches are as follows:

1. The degree of injury is difficult to assess with endoscopy because the depth of injury cannot be determined accurately.

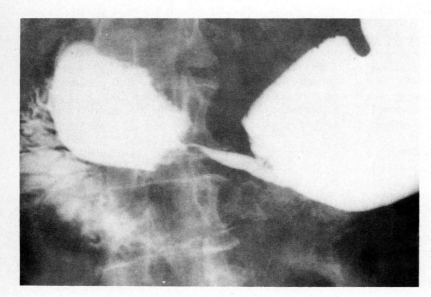

Figure 11–2. Chronic antral stricture. (Courtesy of R. N. Berk, M.D., University of California, San Diego.)

2. The spectrum of injury varies greatly, depending upon the type, concentration, and amount of agent ingested.

3. There are no clinical controlled trials that assess the efficacy of any of these modalities.

Perforation. Although emergency surgery is clearly indicated in cases of esophageal or gastric perforation, it is difficult to predict which patients will develop perforation in the first 24 to 48 hours. With the emergence of liquid caustics as a major cause of injury, several investigators have recommended immediate surgery after either liquid alkali or acid ingestion in patients with severe, contiguous, second-degree burns.[13, 37, 44, 53, 54] Surgical exploration allows more definitive diagnosis, and gastrectomy or esophagectomy can be performed if perforation or transmural injury is found. The absence of acid in the stomach with nasogastric aspiration is considered by some surgeons as a sign of severe gastric injury and is an additional factor in favor of surgery.[13, 44, 50] Unfortunately, no study evaluating the significance or predictive value of achlorhydria after gastric injury has been performed.[37] However, early surgery and gastric resection have been condemned by some authors because the extent of the injury often cannot be delineated, and leaks at anastomotic sites can occur when injured tissue is anastomosed.[14, 16, 55, 56] Most investigators admit that in selected cases early surgery would be prudent, but the criteria to select these cases are not known.[26] Estrera et al. argue that the reduced mortality rate achieved by early detection of impending or actual perforation outweighs the morbidity and mortality rate associated with surgical exploration in patients with endoscopically diagnosed second-degree burns.[44]

Prevention of Stricture

Corticosteroids. A number of studies in animals have shown that corticosteroids inhibit granulation and fibroblastic tissue reaction if given within 24 hours after alkali injury.[5, 31, 34, 57, 58] Additional animal studies indicate that the use of corticosteroids after alkali injury markedly decreases the incidence of esophageal strictures.[34, 59] There are a number of anecdotal clinical reports claiming that corticosteroids reduce the incidence of strictures.[15, 24, 34, 58, 59] However, other investigators feel that corticosteroids may obscure evidence of peritonitis and mediastinitis and that they fail to reduce the incidence of stricture formation.[1, 13, 24, 27, 33, 60] No clinical or experimental studies relating to acid injury are reported.

Collagen Synthesis Inhibitors. In experimental animals, beta-aminopropionitrile, penicillamine, and N-acetylcysteine have been shown to prevent alkali-induced esophageal strictures.[61-63] These lathyrogenic compounds impair synthesis and weaken collagen by interfering with covalent crosslinks. To date, no clinical studies have been performed with these agents.

Antibiotics. Controlled animal studies reveal that if steroids are used after alkali ingestion, there is a marked increased incidence of local infection that can be prevented by administration of broad-spectrum antibiotics.[5, 37, 57] Local infections may increase granulation response, with resultant increase in tissue fibrosis and stricture formation. No human studies are available, although most investigators recommend the use of antibiotics.[4, 15, 24, 27, 35, 41, 59] Other authors assert that antibiotics should be withheld until specific indications develop.[7]

Total Parenteral Nutrition (TPN). Intravenous hyperalimentation has been recommended in patients with severe caustic injury to the esophagus or stomach,[35] since further injury to the esophagus may occur if the patient is fed.[19] Di Costanzo et al. proposed that patients be fasted after severe caustic injury and that nutrition be maintained by intravenous TPN.[35] Adequate nutrition certainly plays a role in the healing process in the severely injured patient, but there are no data to support the notion that fasting and hyperalimentation will prevent stricture formation.

Esophageal Dilatation. Some physicians have recommended esophageal dilatation starting immediately after injury.[12, 53, 64-66] In this case, dilatation is performed at frequent intervals until healing occurs. Early dilatation has been criticized by some who suggest that perforation or increased damage and accelerated fibrosis and stricture formation may occur.[13, 24] These groups recommend that dilatation be performed only when stricture formation develops.[13, 40] Others pass a string or nasogastric tube as part of the initial therapy to maintain the esophageal lumen.[4, 13, 40, 67] With careful clinical evaluation and the use of frequent radiographic or endoscopic studies, the development of an esophageal stricture can be anticipated or detected early.

Esophageal Stents. A number of investigators have placed intraluminal Silastic stents under endoscopic guidance in patients with deep circumferential burns.[44, 54, 68-70] Estrera et al. have combined aggressive early exploration to assess the degree of injury and placement of esophageal stents to prevent stenosis.[44] This allows resection of the esophagus and/or stomach in patients with transmural injury and endoscopic stenting of patients with second-degree injury. The stent is removed about three weeks after surgery. Unfortunately, a majority of these patients required later esophageal dilatation.

Recommended Approach[15, 36, 38]

Patients who have first-degree injury to the esophagus or stomach will require no further therapy.

Patients with circumferential and contiguous injury are at risk for development of esophageal stricture. Generally, the results of the experimental animal data indicate that steroids are of value and therefore should be administered. Methylprednisolone, 40 to 60 mg per day intravenously, is usually recommended.[11, 65] Broad-spectrum antibiotics should be administered. Penicillin, tetracycline, and ampicillin have been used, but new cephalosporins and aminoglycosides would best cover the oropharyngeal flora. Antibiotics and corticosteroids should probably be continued for at least three weeks. Patients with contiguous burns who do not undergo surgery should be followed closely for evidence of mediastinitis or peritonitis. The use of intravenous nutrition and fasting appears to be the most rational means of providing nutrition and avoiding additional injury. Reducing gastric secretion with intravenous H_2 blockers also seems reasonable. Esophageal dilatation should probably be delayed until it appears that a stricture will develop. However, one must observe the patient carefully, with barium swallows administered every two to four months for the first year. Patients who have suspected perforation of either the esophagus or stomach should undergo exploration by experienced surgeons. If perforation is present or appears imminent, resection should be performed. Although liquid caustic ingestions are associated with a high incidence of perforations and strictures in some series, in other reports the mortality rate is low and complete healing can occur without immediate surgical intervention in patients with severe panesophagogastric involvement.[1, 11, 50, 71] The use of prophylactic esophageal stents remains to be proved clinically effective.

Since none of these therapeutic modalities has yet been proved to be of benefit, it is likely that experience with early surgery or early esophageal dilatation by one group of interested physicians may weigh in favor of use of these approaches at any given institution. It is to be hoped that carefully controlled clinical studies evaluating corticosteroids, collagen inhibitors, antibiotics, early dilatation, and emergency surgery will be forthcoming.

LATE COMPLICATIONS

Stricture. Once a stricture has developed, peroral dilatation should be instituted.[13] The frequency is determined by the clinical response. Efforts should be made to dilate the lumen to greater than No. 40 or No. 42 French bougie so that solids can be swallowed without difficulty. Antacids, H_2 blockers, and a regimen for preventing gastroesophageal reflux should theoretically be useful.

Surgery is indicated if the stricture cannot be dilated, if the patient cannot tolerate repeated dilatation, or if nutrition cannot be adequately maintained.[72] Esophageal resection or bypass can be performed, with esophagogastric anastomosis or colon or jejunal interposition.

Antral Stenosis. Antral stenosis may develop progressively after the injury or in five to six weeks but may not appear for several years.[73] Pyloroplasty and gastroenterostomy have been applied successfully to a few patients, but gastric resection is usually recommended. Although many patients are initially achlorhydric, vagotomy is usually performed, since acid production may return. With extensive injury, subtotal or total gastrectomy or partial esophagectomy may be necessary. More recently, endoscopic balloon dilata-

tion has been used successfully and should be considered as an initial maneuver in patients with antral stenosis.[74]

Carcinoma of the Esophagus. There is a strong association between caustic injury and squamous cell carcinoma of the esophagus.[75, 76] Between 1 and 7 per cent of patients with carcinoma of the esophagus have a history of caustic ingestion. It has been estimated that there is a 1000- to 3000-fold increase in the expected incidence of esophageal carcinoma after caustic ingestion.[77] Such a relationship is supported by the location of the cancer at the site of the stricture (scar carcinoma) and the younger ages of patients with caustic ingestion-related carcinomas. The interval between injury and the development of squamous cell carcinoma averages 40 years. Prognosis in these carcinomas appears to be somewhat better than that for other squamous cell carcinomas with combined surgical and radiation therapy. This is probably because the patients are younger and have symptoms earlier, since the carcinoma develops in an already compromised lumen. Furthermore, the scar tissue may limit the spread of the cancer.[77]

Carcinoma of the Stomach. Carcinoma of the stomach has been reported after caustic injury, and squamous metaplasia may occur in the gastric mucosa.[78] These reports are isolated, and there is no evidence of increased risk of development of gastric carcinoma in patients with previous caustic injury.

References

1. Leape, L. L., Ashcraft, K. W., Scarpelli, D. G., and Holden, T. M. Hazard to health—liquid lye. N. Engl. J. Med. 284:578, 1971.
2. Messersmith, J. K., Oglesby, J. E., Mahoney, W. D., and Baugh, J. H. Gastric erosion from alkali ingestion. Am. J. Surg. 119:740, 1970.
3. Ray, J. F., Myers, W. O., Lawton, B. R., Lee, F. Y., Wenzel, F. J., and Sautter, R. D. The natural history of liquid lye ingestion. Arch. Surg. 109:436, 1974.
4. Hawkins, D. B., Demeter, M. J., and Barrett, T. E. Caustic ingestion: Controversies in management. A review of 214 cases. Laryngoscope 90:98, 1980.
5. Rosenberg, N., Kunderman, P. J., Vroman, L., and Moolten, S. E. Prevention of experimental lye strictures of the esophagus by cortisone. Arch. Surg. 63:147, 1951.
6. Muhlendahl, K. E., Oberdisse, U., and Krienke, E. G. Local injuries by accidental ingestion of corrosive substances by children. Arch. Toxicol. 39:299, 1978.
7. Buttross, S., and Brouhard, B. H. Acute management of alkali ingestion in children: A review. Texas Med. 77:57, 1981.
8. Lowe, J. E., Graham, D. Y., Boisaubin, E. V., and Lanza, F. L. Corrosive injury to the stomach: The natural history and role of fiberoptic endoscopy. Am. J. Surg. 137:803, 1979.
9. Lee, J. R., Simonowitz, D., and Block, G. E. Corrosive injury of the stomach and esophagus by non-phosphate detergents. Am. J. Surg. 123:652, 1972.
10. Scher, L. A., and Maull, K. I. Emergency management and sequelae of acid ingestion. JACEP 7:206, 1978.
11. Cello, J. P., Fogel, R. P., and Boland, R. Liquid caustic ingestion spectrum of injury. Arch. Intern. Med. 140:501, 1980.
12. Tucker, J. A., and Yarington, C. T. The treatment of caustic ingestion. Otolaryngol. Clin. North Am. 12:343, 1979.
13. Kirsh, M. M., and Ritter, F. Caustic ingestion and subsequent damage to the oropharyngeal and digestive passages. Ann. Thorac. Surg. 21:74, 1976.

14. Steigmann, F., and Dolehide, R. Corrosive (acid) gastritis. Management of early and late cases. N. Engl. J. Med. *254*:981, 1956.
15. Haller, J. A., and Backman, K. The comparative effects of current therapy on experimental caustic burns of the esophagus. Pediatrics *34*:236, 1964.
16. Citron, B. P., Pincus, I. J., Geokac, M. C., and Haverback, B. J. Chemical trauma of esophagus and stomach. Surg. Clin. North Am. *48*:1303, 1968.
17. Poteshman, N. Corrosive gastritis due to hydrochloric acid ingestion. Am. J. Roentgenol. *99*:182, 1967.
18. Ritter, F. N., Gago, O., Kirsh, M. M., Komom, R. M., and Orvald, T. O. The rationale of emergency esophagogastrectomy in the treatment of liquid caustic burns of the esophagus and stomach. Ann. Otol. Rhinol. Laryngol. *80*:513, 1971.
19. Krey, H. Treatment of corrosive lesion in the esophagus. Acta Otolaryngol. (Suppl.) *102*:1, 1952.
20. Rumack B. H., and Burrington, J. D. Caustic ingestion: A rationale look at diluents. Clin. Toxicol. *11*:27, 1977.
21. Allen, R., Thoshinsky, M., Stallone, R. J., and Hunt, T. K. Corrosive injuries of stomach. Arch. Surg. *100*:409, 1970.
22. Leon, H. R., Stanley, R., and Wise, L. Gastric bullae—an early roentgen finding in corrosive gastritis following alkali ingestion. Radiology *115*:597, 1975.
23. Bikhazi, B., Thompson, E. R., and Shumrick, D. A. Caustic ingestion: Current status. Arch. Otolaryngol. *89*:770, 1969.
24. Middlekamp, J. N., Ferguson, T. B., Roper, C. L., and Hoffman, F. D. The management and problem of caustic burns in children. J. Thorac. Cardiovasc. Surg. *57*:341, 1969.
25. Ritter, F., Newman, M. H., and Newman, D. E. A clinical and experimental study of corrosive burns of the stomach. Ann. Otol. Rhinol. Laryngol. *78*:830, 1968.
26. Penner, G. E. Acid ingestion: Toxicity and treatment. Ann. Emerg. Med. *9*:374, 1980.
27. Ashcraft, K. W., and Padula, R. The effect of dilute corrosives on the esophagus. Pediatrics *53*:226, 1974.
28. Gaudreault, P., Parent, M., McGuigan, M. A., Chicoine, L., and Lovejoy, F. H. Predictability of esophageal injury from signs and symptoms: A study of caustic ingestion in 378 children. Pediatrics *71*:767, 1983.
29. Muhletaler, C. A., Gerlock, A. J., DeSoto, L., and Halter, S. A. Acid corrosive esophagitis: Radiologic findings. Am. J. Roentgenol. *134*:1137, 1980.
30. Hollinger, P. H. Management of esophageal lesions caused by chemical burns. Ann. Otol. Rhinol. Laryngol. *77*:819, 1968.
31. Webb, W. R., Koutras, P., Ecker, R. R., and Sugg, W. L. An evaluation of steroids and antibiotics in caustic burns of the esophagus. Ann. Thorac. Surg. *9*:95, 1970.
32. Bosch del Marco, L. Contribucion al estudio de la gastritis corrisiva: Estudio cinico y experimental. An. Fac. Med. Montevideo *34*:891, 1949.
33. Nicosia, J. F., Thornton, J. P., Folk, F. A., and Saletta, J. D. Surgical management of corrosive gastric injuries. Ann. Surg. *180*:139, 1974.
34. Haller, J. A., Andrews, H. G., White, J. J., Tamer, M. A., and Cleveland, W. W. Pathophysiology and management of acute corrosive burns of the esophagus: Results of treatment in 285 children. J. Pediatr. Surg. *6*:578, 1971.
35. Di Costanzo, J., Noirclerc, M., Jouglard, J., Escoffier, J. M., Cano, N., Martin, J., and Gauthier, A. New therapeutic approach to corrosive burns of the upper gastrointestinal tract. Gut *21*:370, 1982.
36. Postlethwait, R. W. Chemical burns of the esophagus. Surg. Clin. North Am. *63*:915, 1983.
37. Gago, O., Ritter, F. N., Martel, W., Orvald, T. O., Delavan, J. W., Dieterle, R. V. A., Kirsh, M. M., Kahn, D. R., and Sloan, H. Aggressive surgical treatment for caustic injury of the esophagus and stomach. Ann. Thorac. Surg. *13*:243, 1972.
38. Cardona, J. C., and Daly, J. F. Current management of corrosive esophagitis. Ann. Otol. *80*:521, 1971.
39. Symbas, P. N., Vlasis, S. E., and Hatcher, C. R. Esophagitis secondary to ingestion of caustic material. Ann. Thorac. Surg. *36*:73, 1983.
40. Daly, J. F. Corrosive esophagitis. Otolaryngol. Clin. North Am. *1*:119, 1968.
41. Feldman, M., Iben, A., and Hurley, E. J. Corrosive injury to oropharynx and esophagus. Calif. Med. *118*:6, 1973.
42. Chung, R., and DenBesten, L. Fiberoptic endoscopy in treatment of corrosive injury of stomach. Arch. Surg. *110*:725, 1971.
43. Welsh, J. J., and Welsh, L. W. Endoscopic examination of corrosive injuries of the upper gastrointestinal tract. Laryngoscope *88*:1300, 1978.
44. Estrera, A., Taylor, W., Mills, L. J., and Platt, M. R. Corrosive burns of the esophagus and stomach: A recommendation for an aggressive surgical approach. Ann. Thorac. Surg. *41*:276, 1986.
45. Marchand, P. Caustic strictures of esophagus. Thorax *10*:171, 1956.
46. Stannard, M. W. Corrosive esophagitis in children. Am. J. Dis. Child. *132*:596, 1978.
47. Martel, W. Radiologic features of esophagogastritis secondary to extremely caustic agents. Radiology *103*:31, 1972.
48. Muhletaler, C. A., Gerlock, A. J., DeSoto, L., and Halter, S. A. Gastroduodenal lesion of ingested acids: Radiologic findings. Am. J. Roentgenol. *135*:1247, 1980.
49. Holzbach, R. Corrosive gastritis resembling carcinoma due to ingestion of acid. JAMA *205*:883, 1967.
50. Kirsh, M. M., Peterson, A., Brown, J.W., Orringer, M. B., Ritter, F., and Sloan, H. Treatment of caustic injuries of the esophagus. Ann. Surg. *188*:675, 1978.
51. Ray, J. F. Liquid caustic ingestion. A flag of caution. Arch. Intern. Med. *140*:471, 1980.
52. Knopp, R. Caustic ingestions. *In* Tintinalli, J. E., Rothstein, R. J., and Krome, R. L. (eds.). Emergency Medicine: A Comprehensive Study Guide. Dallas American College of Emergency Physicians, 1985, pp. 229–234.
53. Kiviranta, U. K. Corrosion carcinoma of the esophagus: 381 cases of corrosion and nine cases of corrosion carcinoma. Acta Otolaryngol. *42*:89, 1952.
54. Fell, S. C., Denize, A., Becker, N. H., and Hurwitt, E. S. The effect of intraluminal splinting in the prevention of caustic stricture of the esophagus. J. Thorac. Cardiovas. Surg. *52*:675, 1966.
55. Marks, I. N., Bank, S., Werbeloff, L., Farman, J., and Louw, J. H. The natural history of corrosive gastritis. Am. J. Dig. Dis. *8*:509, 1963.
56. Chong, G., Beahrs, O., and Payne, W. Management of corrosive gastritis due to ingested acid. Mayo Clin. Proc. *49*:861, 1974.
57. Spain, D. M., Molomut, N., and Habert, A. The effect of cortisone on the formation of granulation tissue in mice. Am. J. Pathol. *26*:710, 1950.
58. Weiskoff, A. Effects of cortisone on experimental lye burns of the esophagus. Ann. Otol. *61*:681, 1952.
59. Knox, W. G., Scott, J. R., Zintel, H. A., Guthrie, R., and McCabe, R. E. Bouginage and steroids used singly or in combination in experimental corrosive esophagitis. Ann. Surg. *166*:930, 1967.
60. Aceto, T., Terplan, K., Fiore, R. R., and Muschauer, R. W. Chemical burns of the esophagus in children on a glucocorticoid therapy. J. Med. (Basel) *10*:1, 1970.
61. Butler, C., Madden, J. W., and Peacock, E. E. Morphologic aspects of experimental esophageal lye strictures. II. Effect of steroid hormones, bougienage, and induced lathyrism of acute lye burns. Surgery *81*:431, 1977.
62. Gehanno, P., and Guedon, C. Inhibition of experimental esophageal lye strictures by penicillamine. Arch. Otolaryngol. *107*:145, 1981.
63. Liu, A. J., and Richardson, M. A. Effects of N-acetylcysteine on experimentally induced esophageal lye injury. Ann. Otol. Rhinol. Laryngol. *94*:477, 1985.
64. Salzer, H. Fruhbehandlung des Speisehrenversatzung. Wien Clin. Wochenschr. *33*:307, 1920.
65. Boyce, H. W., and Palmer, E. O. Techniques of Clinical Gastroenterology. Springfield, Illinois, Charles C Thomas, Publisher, 1975, p. 264.
66. Marshall, F. Caustic burns of the esophagus: Ten year results of aggressive care. South. Med. J. *72*:1236, 1979.
67. Beukers, M. M., Bartelsman, T. F., Heymans, H. S., and Jager, E. C. D. Nasogastric intubation as sole treatment of caustic esophageal lesions. Ann. Otol. Rhinol. Laryngol. *94*:337, 1985.
68. Coln, D., and Chang, J. H. T. Experience with esophageal

stenting for caustic burns in children. J. Pediatr. Surg. *21*:591, 1986.

69. Mills, L. J., Estrera, A. S., and Platt, M. R. Avoidance of esophageal stricture following severe caustic burns by the use of an intraluminal stent. Ann. Thorac. Surg. *28*:60, 1979.
70. Reyes, H. M., and Hill, J. L. Modification of the experimental stent technique for esophageal burns. J. Surg. Res. *20*:65, 1976.
71. Balasegaram, M. Early management of corrosive burns of the esophagus. Br. J. Surg. *62*:444, 1975.
72. Campbell, G. S., Burnett, H. F., Ransom, J. M., and Williams, D. Treatment of corrosive burns of the esophagus. Arch. Surg. *112*:495, 1977.
73. Maull, K. I., Scher, L. A., and Greenfield, L. J. Surgical implications of acid ingestion. Surg. Gynecol. Obstet. *148*:895, 1925.

74. Hogan, R. B., and Polter, D. E., Nonsurgical management of lye-induced antral stricture with hydrostatic balloon dilation. Gastrointest. Endosc. *32*:228, 1986.
75. Appelqvist, P., and Salmo, M. Lye corrosion carcinoma of the esophagus. Cancer *45*:2655, 1980.
76. Hopkins, R. A., and Postlethwait, R. W. Caustic burn and carcinoma of the esophagus. Ann. Surg. *194*:146, 1981.
77. Csíkos, M., Horvath, O., Petri, A., Petri, I., and Imre, J. Late malignant transformation of chronic corrosive oesophageal strictures. Langenbecks Arch. Chir. *365*:231, 1985.
78. Eaton, H., and Tennekoon, G. E. Squamous carcinoma of the stomach following corrosive acid burns. Br. J. Surg. *59*:382, 1972.

12

Foreign Bodies in the Gut

J. KENT HAMILTON
DANIEL E. POLTER

Foreign bodies in the gut represent a common problem facing gastroenterologists and surgeons. The challenge is to determine the appropriate application of endoscopy, surgery, and expectant management. The ready availability of fiberoptic endoscopy has changed expectant management, especially in regard to intragastric and colonic foreign bodies.

The management of foreign bodies is based on collected experience, not upon controlled clinical research. In each situation, one must evaluate the type of object, the organ involved, the patient's condition, and the type of symptoms in deciding when and how to intervene. The concept that most foreign objects will pass safely through the intestinal tract has been validated by the literature from the pre-endoscopic era.[1, 2] In Carp's report of 31 patients studied before the advent of endoscopy, over 80 per cent of ingested foreign objects passed within one month, the average time being one week. The remaining five patients required operations, with two deaths resulting.[2] Flexible endoscopes now allow retrieval of objects formerly accessible only by surgical intervention. Some, but not all, objects should be retrieved, depending on size, shape, location, risk of perforation, or obstruction or for relief of symptoms.[3]

Reviews of foreign body perforation of the gastrointestinal tract indicate that some objects, such as bones, pins, and toothpicks, carry a significant risk of perforation.[4, 5] Perforation may occur at any level but is more likely at anatomic sites where a foreign object may arrest because of angulation or narrowing of the bowel lumen (Fig. 12–1). The ileocecal area is most frequently the site of perforation. In one series of patients with perforations the majority were edentulous and unaware of swallowing the offending object. These patients presented with peritonitis, hemorrhage, abdominal mass, obstruction, or abscess. One of 12 patients with foreign body perforation of the gut died.[4]

THE HYPOPHARYNX

The upper airway at the level of the hypopharynx is a frequent site of arrest of food and foreign bodies. This situation usually does not present itself to the gastroenterologist for management. This "café coronary" syndrome must be managed immediately at the moment of occurrence by measures such as the Heimlich maneuver. Obstruction above the level of the upper esophageal sphincter with airway compromise is best treated by the ENT physician or surgeon who can manage acute airway obstruction with tracheostomy if necessary. It should be remembered that airway obstruction may occur by losing a foreign body as it is withdrawn. Kelly or McGill forceps and a laryngoscope must always be immediately available.[6]

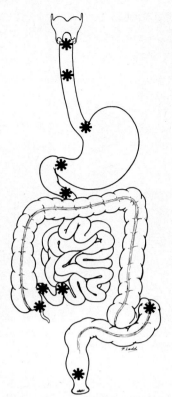

Figure 12–1. Anatomic areas in the alimentary canal where foreign objects may arrest after ingestion.

THE ESOPHAGUS

The esophagus is the most common site of acute foreign body obstruction, usually by a food bolus above a mechanically obstructing lesion.[6, 7] In adults, this typically is a stricture or lower esophageal ring but occasionally may be a tumor or diverticulum. A more dangerous situation is encountered when a bone or other sharp object impales the esophagus. Sharp objects, such as bones, toothpicks, and pins may perforate the esophagus with fatal septic or hemorrhagic consequences. Individuals with penetrating esophageal injuries due to foreign objects should be investigated urgently and seen with surgical consultation.[7, 8] Esophageal perforation is discussed on page 647. Foreign bodies may lodge at the level of the cervical esophagus, aortic arch, gastroesophageal junction, or any site of pathologic constriction.

Special mention should be made of ingestion of small alkaline batteries found in electronic equipment. Toddlers are especially attracted to these thin, round objects. Fatal esophageal perforations due to the prompt local corrosive effects of these batteries have been reported. Such batteries usually contain a 45 per cent solution of potassium hydrochloride and are not water tight. Alkaline batteries in the esophagus should be retrieved on an emergent basis and any sign of perforation should be treated surgically.[9, 10]

Controversy exists as to management of batteries which pass the esophagus. Recent evidence indicates that those smaller than 20 mm in diameter will pass uneventfully under radiographic observation.[9] Heavy metal intoxication (manganese, mercury, silver) does not seem to be a problem in most circumstances. If radiographic follow-up demonstrates fragmentation of the battery, urine and blood screening for mercury intoxication should be done. Induced vomiting was ineffective in one large report. The National Button Battery Ingestion Study has a 24-hour emergency line at (202) 625–3333.

Clinical Manifestations. The patient who presents with acute esophageal obstruction may be in mild to severe distress. He may relate a history of choking while eating, with obstruction perceived at the level of obstruction or referred to the sternal notch. The location of perceived discomfort may not correlate with anatomic location. There may be substernal pain that at times can be severe, mimicking myocardial infarction. The patient will usually gag and try to regurgitate the bolus. Many patients will relate antecedent dysphagia or prior bouts of obstruction, but some will not. Excessive salivation usually will be present.

Patients may also present with a history of odynophagia while eating. The food is usually thought to contain a chicken or fish bone. There may be a continued sensation of something being lodged in the throat or esophagus. At this point the question is whether or not the object is still present in the esophagus. Physical examination is usually normal, but crepitation should always be sought.

Diagnosis. Radiographic films are helpful in elucidating the type and location of foreign bodies. Plain films of the neck, with soft tissue technique, are indicated when there is pain or the sensation of a foreign body in the throat. Lateral films of the neck, chest films, and occasionally xeroradiography are especially useful in visualizing small bones in the neck and cervical esophagus (Figs. 12–2 and 12–3). Some objects such as aluminum pull tabs, small fish bones, and wood are radiolucent, or nearly so. Failure to visualize an object on X-ray does not preclude its presence. If pain or foreign body sensation persists, then endoscopy with intubation under direct vision is appropriate because of the dire consequences of esophageal perforation. The administration of thin barium and cotton pledgets makes subsequent examination difficult and adds another foreign body. Barium examination may be useful if symptoms have abated or partial distal obstruction by a food bolus is suspected.

Occasionally difficulty arises in determining whether an object is in the esophagus or trachea. Esophageal foreign bodies align themselves in the frontal plane and are best seen on AP projections (Fig. 12–4). In contrast, tracheal foreign bodies align themselves saggitally and are best seen on lateral projections.

Management. Medical therapy with glucagon (0.5 to 1.0 mg given intravenously) and mild sedation may allow spontaneous passage of impacted food boluses.[11] Tube decompression of the esophagus, especially if a contrast medium examination has been performed,

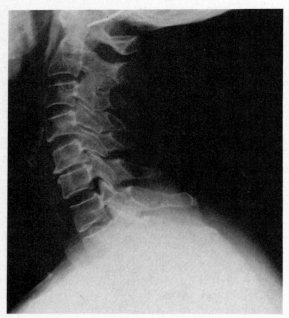

Figure 12–2. A lateral neck view demonstrating a chicken bone lodged in the cervical esophagus. Contrast this with Figure 12–3.

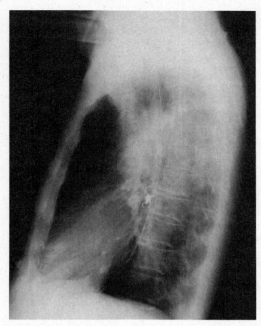

Figure 12–4. A swallowed dental bridge. In this case the nasogastric tube denotes esophageal location.

facilitates endoscopy and reduces the risk of aspiration. The patient should be given intravenous fluids, and the head of the bed is elevated. Instillation of papain has been used for enzymatic dissolution of an impacted meat bolus in the distal esophagus. However, it is not recommended because of reports of fatal esophageal perforation and aspiration of this agent. In addition papain may not effectively digest meat.[12] The use of magnets and Foley catheters to remove foreign bodies has been reported. Their worth is unknown. The

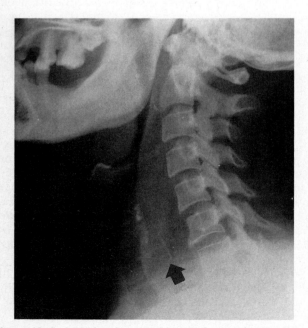

Figure 12–3. A chicken bone that has perforated the esophagus, causing an abscess. Note the prevertebral bulging.

offending object may be lost easily in the pharynx or upper airway during retrieval.

Endoscopic techniques for the removal of food boluses and foreign bodies require a variety of accessory equipment (Fig. 12–5). Most obstructing boluses are best retrieved with a snare or basket. Insufflation of air to distend the esophagus, parenteral glucagon for esophageal relaxation, and orientation of flat objects in the frontal plane are useful maneuvers to bring objects through the esophagus. Before attempting to remove any object, a "dry run" with a similar object, using the available accessories, is advisable to determine which device will grasp the object securely. A useful device for retrieval of sharp objects is an overtube (Fig. 12–6) of approximately 60 cm in length and 15 mm in internal diameter. This can be made from large-bore Tygon tubing. If the tube is homemade, beveling of the end is recommended. The object is drawn into the tube, and both are withdrawn with the endoscope. It is also useful for piecemeal removal of a food bolus, avoiding repetitive intubations.[13]

An additional technique has been described recently. A latex hood is fitted just above the bending portion of an endoscope. When the endoscope is retracted up the esophagus, the hood everts to cover the foreign body. Experience is limited, but small objects within the diameter of the endoscope may be removed safely. Larger, rigid objects may cut through the latex and cause injury.

The Garren balloon or gastric bubble is a foreign body that may deflate, causing obstruction. Prior to removal, these devices should be deflated thoroughly by multiple holes made by a thermal cautery device. Grasping the balloon with two rat tooth forceps via a two-channel endoscope will give enough traction to allow balloon retrieval.

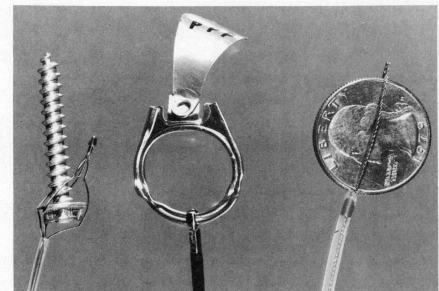

Figure 12–5. Three commonly available endoscopic forceps used to retrieve foreign bodies: the spiral basket, the rat-tooth forceps, and the polypectomy snare.

General anesthesia may be needed in uncooperative patients or to obtain adequate relaxation for removal of large objects. The large-bore rigid esophagoscope is useful for removing embedded or large objects using forceps that can crush and divide material such as bone. Objects with multiple sharp protrusions, such as dental bridges, may have to be removed surgically if they become embedded in the esophageal wall.[7]

Several additional points deserve mention. First, perforation rates as high as 12 per cent have been reported during removal of esophageal foreign bodies with rigid esophagoscopes. Perforations with flexible endoscopes may also occur during removal of esophageal foreign bodies.[14] Second, if mucosal disruption or bleeding is observed or if the patient reports pain, it may be wise to defer dilation of a stricture or ring until a later date. Third, some patients will continue to have pain after dislodgement owing to mucosal laceration. Such pain suggests the possibility of perforation and should be investigated with oral contrast studies.

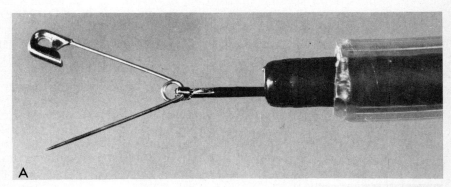

Figure 12–6. A homemade overtube demonstrating the capture (A) and retraction (B) of an open safety pin into an overtube for safe passage through the esophagus.

A

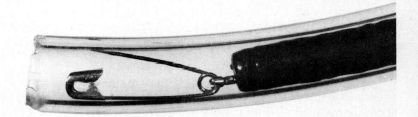

B

THE STOMACH

In contrast to the esophagus, where symptoms of obstruction and the danger of perforation demand expedient action, foreign objects in the stomach usually cause few, if any, symptoms. The question then becomes whether or not the object will safely traverse the intestine. The most frequent victims are prisoners, young children, persons with dentures, or intoxicated or mentally disturbed individuals.[3] Accidental ingestion may also occur as a result of using the mouth as a third hand.

Clinical Manifestations. Many patients will be asymptomatic or will be brought in by their parents with the history of having swallowed something. The presence of pain, fever, bleeding, or vomiting should suggest pyloric obstruction, mucosal disruption, or penetration by the object. Objects may be multiple and may have been present for a long period of time. Multiple ingestions are common among mentally deranged individuals.

Diagnosis. Plain films of the abdomen serve to determine the nature of the object and help monitor its transit through the intestine. At times, the question of penetration and location will arise. Contrast studies will be valuable in this regard. An abdominal X-ray should be obtained prior to endoscopy to determine if the object remains in the stomach.

Management. It is well established that the majority of ingested foreign objects will pass through the intestinal tract. This is based on observations made in mental hospitals in the pre-endoscopic era, and has been confirmed more recently.[15, 16] Certain objects such as bones, toothpicks, pins, needles, denture fragments, razor blades, and long, thin objects such as pieces of wire should be removed if endoscopically accessible because of the risk of bleeding, obstruction, or perforation.[17] The nature of the object, its size, presence of sharp or pointed ends, arrested progress under observation, or the onset of symptoms will determine whether or not to intervene endoscopically or surgically.

Swallowed coins are common in children. Smaller coins such as nickels will generally pass. A quarter will pass in most cases but may not in smaller children. A frequent question is how long to wait for an object to pass the pylorus. In general, objects 20 mm in diameter or 5 cm in length are less likely to pass. Observation of a coin in the stomach for a period of three days or longer has been recommended.[18, 19] If an object remains in the stomach several days, it may become embedded in the gastric wall, making endoscopic removal difficult or impossible. Therefore, it is advisable to remove the object if no progress is made after three to seven days. During the waiting period, all stools should be inspected to document passage of the object. If an object passes through the pylorus, passage through the remainder of the gut usually ensues. Individuals, especially the mentally ill and prisoners, should be closely observed after removal because of the high incidence of reingestion while still hospitalized. Individuals with gastric bypass or partitioning procedures will frequently become obstructed. Endoscopic intervention is often necessary.[20] Coated tablets resistant to gastric digestion, such as Ecotrin, are often the cause of obstruction.

Endoscopic retrieval of gastric foreign bodies utilizes the same array of accessories helpful in the esophagus (Fig. 12–2). Considerable manipulation may be necessary to extract a foreign body from the stomach. If the patient is young or uncooperative or if the object is large, general anesthesia may be needed. As in the esophagus, it is wise to make a "dry run" with the various snares and retrieval devices at hand. The same maneuvers useful in the esophagus apply to bringing objects from the stomach through the esophagus.

THE DUODENUM AND SMALL BOWEL

There are areas below the pylorus where objects may lodge with serious consequences. The angulations of the duodenal sweep and the ligament of Treitz may arrest the progress of long, thin objects. The terminal ileum, ileocecal region, and sigmoid colon are the most frequent sites of obstruction or perforation by bones and pins (Fig. 12–1). The so-called mural withdrawal reflex partially explains how the small bowel copes with such noxious objects. Observations in animals demonstrate the ability of the bowel to locally dilate in response to mucosal contact with a sharp object.[2]

Another recent problem is the so-called "body packer syndrome." Individuals smuggling drugs may ingest packaged amounts of drugs. These usually pass uneventfully, but obstruction and drug intoxication have been reported.[21]

Periodic X-rays are useful in monitoring the progress of worrisome objects. The onset of fever, pain, distention, vomiting, or bleeding heralds a complication. Surgical intervention usually is necessary if such symptoms develop. However, sharp pointed objects such as corsage pins may penetrate the wall of the duodenum, causing only minor symptoms without signs of peritoneal irritation. Endoscopic removal may be curative but should be followed by water-soluble contrast studies to rule out a leak.[22]

Particular note should be made of a rare, but potentially hazardous event. Rupture of mercury-containing balloons may occur in the GI tract. If there is leakage of mercury outside the bowel lumen (i.e., fistula or perforation), then the potential for systemic mercury intoxication exists. If no evidence for perforation is present and little or no risk exists, cathartics should be given to hasten the elimination of the element.[23]

THE COLON AND RECTUM

Foreign bodies in the colon and rectum may cause obstruction or perforation. Ingested objects may lodge

Table 12–1. ALGORITHM FOR MANAGEMENT OF FOREIGN BODIES

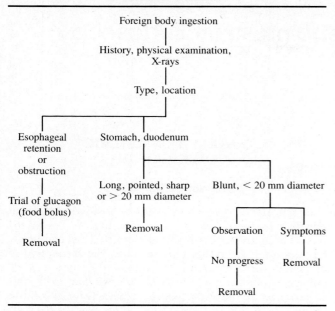

References

1. Carp, L. Foreign bodies in the gastrointestinal tracts of psychotic patients. Arch. Surg. *60*:1055, 1950.
2. Carp, L. Foreign bodies in the intestine. Ann. Surg. *85*:575, 1927.
3. McCaffery, T. D., and Lilly, J. O. The management of foreign affairs of the GI tract. Am. J. Dig. Dis. *20*:121, 1975.
4. Maleki, M., and Evans, W. E. Foreign body perforation of the intestinal tract. Arch. Surg. *101*:475, 1970.
5. Vizcarrondo, F. J., Brady P. G., and Nord H. J. Foreign bodies of the upper intestinal tract. Gastrointest. Endosc. *29*:208, 1983.
6. Brady P. G. Endoscopic removal of foreign bodies. *In* Vennes, J. (ed.). Therapeutic Endoscopy. New York, Tokyo, Igaku-Shoin, 1985.
7. Nadi, P., and Ong, G. B. Foreign body in the esophagus: Review of 2394 cases. Br. J. Surg. *65*:5, 1978.
8. Ctercteko, G., and Mok, D. K. Aorto-esophageal fistula induced by a foreign body: The first recorded survival. J. Thorac. Cardiovasc. Surg. *80*:233, 1980.
9. Litovitz, T. L.: Button battery ingestions. JAMA *249*:2495, 1983.
10. Blatnik, D. S., Toohill, R. J., and Lehman, R. H. Fatal complication from an alkaline battery foreign body in the esophagus. Ann. Oto. Rhino. Laryngol. *86*:611, 1977.
11. Ferrucci, J. R., and Long, J. A. Radiologic treatment of esophageal food impaction using intravenous glucagon. Radiology *125*:25, 1977.
12. Goldmer, F., and Danley D. Enzymatic digestion of esophageal meat impaction. Dig. Dis. Sci. *30*:456, 1985.
13. Rodgers, B. H. G. A new method for extraction of impacted meat from the esophagus utilizing a flexible fiberoptic endoscope and an overtube (abstract). Gastrointest. Endosc. *25*:47, 1979.
14. Christie, D. L., and Ament, M. E. Removal of foreign bodies from esophagus and stomach with flexible fiberoptic panendoscopes. Pediatrics *57*:931, 1976.
15. Gracia C., Frey, C. F., and Blazas, B. J. Diagnosis and management of ingested foreign bodies: A ten-year experience. Ann. Emerg. Med. *13*:30, 1984.
16. Webb, W. A., McDaniel, L., and Jones, L.: Foreign bodies of the upper gastrointestinal tract: Current management. Southern Med. J. *77*:1093, 1984.
17. Selivanov, W., Sheldon, G. F., Cello, J. P., et al. Management of foreign body ingestion. Ann. Surg. *199*:187, 1983.
18. Waye, J. D. Removal of foreign bodies from the upper intestinal tract with fiberoptic instruments. Am. J. Gastroenterol. *65*:557, 1976.
19. Edridge, W. W. Foreign bodies in the gastrointestinal tract. JAMA *178*:665, 1961.
20. Strodel, W. E., Knol, J. A., and Eckhauser, F. E. Endoscopy of the partitioned stomach. Ann. Surg. *200*:582, 1984.
21. Caruna, D. S., Weinbach, B., Georg, D., and Gardner, L. B. Cocaine-packet ingestion. Ann. Intern. Med. *100*:73, 1984.
22. Dagradi, A. E., and Severance, S. R. Fiberoptic endoscopic extraction of foreign body perforating the stomach. Am. J. Gastroenterol. *65*:335, 1976.
23. Bredfeldt, J. E., and Moeller, D. P.: Systemic mercury intoxication following rupture of a Miller-Abbott tube. Am. J. Gastro. *69*:478, 1978.
24. Oehler, J. R., Dent, T. L., Mostafa, A. H., Ibrahin, M. D., and Gracie, W. A. Endoscopic identification and removal of an unusual symptomatic colonic foreign body. Dig. Dis. Sci. *24*:237, 1979.
25. Sohn, N., and Weinstein, M. A. Office removal of foreign bodies in the rectum. Surg. Gynecol. Obstet. *146*:209, 1978.
26. Eftaiha, M., Hambrik, E., and Abcarian, H. Principles of management of colorectal foreign bodies. Arch. Surg. *112*:691, 1977.
27. Barone, J. E., Sohn, M., and Nealon, T. F. Perforations and foreign bodies of the rectum: Report of 28 cases. Ann. Surg. *184*:601, 1976.

in the cecum or in the ascending or sigmoid colon. Colonoscopy may be useful in identifying and retrieving these foreign bodies.[24] Patients who develop signs of peritoneal inflammation or irritation should undergo prompt laparotomy.

Objects in the rectum and rectosigmoid usually have been inserted transanally. These include a bizarre variety of objects inserted for sexual stimulation or during criminal assault or of iatrogenic origin.[25, 26] Removal is usually feasible with the aid of the sigmoidoscope, and adequate relaxation of the anal sphincter is usually achieved with local or general anesthesia. Retrieval may be performed with the aid of a large Kocher clamp or uterine tenaculum and anal retractor. If an object is beyond the reach of the sigmoidoscope and the patient has no evidence of perforation or obstruction, observation for 12 to 24 hours will usually permit the object to descend to the rectosigmoid level, allowing transanal removal. No enema or cathartic should be used. Sigmoidoscopy should be repeated following removal of a rectal foreign body to search for mucosal injury.[27]

SUMMARY

The approach to foreign bodies can be rationally planned if the location and type are known. The algorithm provided in Table 12–1 will cover most situations encountered.

13

Complications of Gastrointestinal Endoscopy

THEODORE R. SCHROCK

Complications of diagnostic and therapeutic endoscopy of the upper and lower gastrointestinal tract in adults are discussed here. The benefits of endoscopic procedures, and all aspects of endoscopic retrograde cholangiopancreatography, laparoscopy, and percutaneous gastroscopy are considered in other chapters.

Concern about complications focuses on the patient, but the endoscopist and assistants are also exposed to hazards, including transmissible organisms, electrical devices, and heavy equipment. Informed consent must be obtained from the patient; the proposed procedure, its risks and benefits, and alternatives, if any, should be explained in simple language.[1] Table 13–1 lists some items of history that should be sought to evaluate the risk of endoscopic complications.

Much of the data on complication rates for gastrointestinal endoscopy are derived from retrospective surveys, which may suffer from underreporting. Some of the information is old, compiled in the early years of this relatively recent technologic advance. With these reservations, the overall complication rate for diagnostic upper endoscopy is less than 0.2 per cent,[2] and for diagnostic colonoscopy it is 0.3 to 0.6 per cent.[2–4] Difficult emergency situations and therapeutic endoscopic procedures are more risky. Death from complications of elective diagnostic upper endoscopy is rare, but in acute upper gastrointestinal bleeding, the mortality rate reaches 0.1 per cent.[5] Diagnostic colonoscopy results in fatal complications in 0.02 per cent of patients.[2–4]

Table 13–1. PRESENT AND PAST MEDICAL HISTORY FEATURES RELEVANT TO ENDOSCOPIC RISK

Drugs
    Current
    Allergies, reactions
Bleeding disorder
Infection
    Susceptibility
    Hepatitis
    AIDS
Glaucoma
Hypothyroidism
Pulmonary disease
Heart
    Congenital disease
    Endocarditis
    Valvular disease
    Valve prosthesis
    Pacemaker
Orthopedic implanted prosthesis

GENERAL AND SYSTEMIC COMPLICATIONS

Erroneous Diagnosis

Diagnostic errors include false positive and false negative findings and incorrect labeling of abnormalities. These mistakes must be regarded as complications, and all are potentially serious. The frequency of diagnostic errors cannot be estimated, but undoubtedly, it varies inversely with the knowledge, skill, and experience of the endoscopist. Characteristics of the patient and the indication for endoscopy also help determine the likelihood of incorrect diagnosis.

Effects of Medications

Medications administered to facilitate endoscopy may cause complications from allergic reactions or from doses that prove excessive for certain individuals. Major problems arise in about 0.02 per cent of endoscopic procedures.[4–7]

Topical Anesthetics. Anaphylactoid reactions to topical anesthetics for upper endoscopy are rare but potentially lethal. The need for pharyngeal anesthesia during endoscopy with modern small caliber instruments is debatable, and many endoscopists no longer use these agents.[6]

Antispasmodic and Antisecretory Drugs. Inhibition of motor and secretory activity of the intestinal tract can be achieved with atropine, scopolamine, dicyclomine hydrochloride, and glucagon. An important complication of atropine or scopolamine is increased intraocular pressure in patients with narrow-angle glaucoma; bradycardia, tachycardia, and atrioventricular block occur at increasing doses.[6] Dicyclomine seems to have fewer side effects, but most endoscopists do not employ any of these drugs routinely in upper endoscopy. Glucagon is used most commonly during colonoscopy; vomiting is avoided by slow administration of small doses (0.5 to 1.0 mg).[6]

Sedatives. Diazepam and midazolam are benzodiazepines with comparable sedative-hypnotic, muscle-relaxant, anxiolytic, and anticonvulsant properties.[6, 8] Paradoxic excitement occurs occasionally, but excessive depression of the central nervous system is the most serious side effect; elderly patients and those with hypoalbuminemia are especially susceptible.[6] Physostigmine (1 to 2 mg IV) may reverse central depression through a nonspecific general arousal mechanism.[6]

Diazepam causes phlebitis in 3.5 to 17 per cent of patients.[6] Tenderness may linger for a month. The drug should be injected into a large vein; flushing the vein with saline may help.

Analgesics. Meperidine is frequently given with a benzodiazepine to achieve analgesia, sedation, and euphoria.[6] Short-acting narcotics (e.g., fentanyl and phenoperidine) are new entries in this field. Side effects of meperidine include nausea and vomiting, respiratory depression, hypotension, and spasm of intestinal smooth muscle. Allergic reactions, usually urticaria or rashes, are uncommon.

Respiratory depression lasts from two to four hours on the average, but in patients who have hypothyroidism, head trauma, or chronic pulmonary disease, serious impairment of respiration can persist even longer.[6] Benzodiazepines do not seem to act synergistically with meperidine to prolong respiratory depression. Hypotension results from peripheral vasodilation; it is usually treatable by administration of intravenous fluids and by placement of the patient in Trendelenburg position.

Naloxone is a readily available antagonist of the narcotic effects of meperidine. Intravenous doses of 0.4 to 0.8 mg reverse respiratory depression, sedation, and hypotension in one to two minutes. The action of naloxone persists for one to four hours.

Cardiopulmonary Problems

Aspiration. During upper endoscopy, sedation, pharyngeal anesthesia, and supine positioning contribute to development of aspiration and its sequelae. A full stomach, active bleeding, and retained secretions due to obstructive lesions are risk factors. The elderly and any other patients who have depressed cough and gag reflexes must be handled with special care. The incidence of aspiration is 0.08 per cent, but the mortality rate of this complication may reach 10 per cent.[9] The likelihood of aspiration is minimized by turning patients and encouraging them to cough immediately after endoscopy.[10]

Hypoxemia. Medications, particularly meperidine, contribute significantly to hypoxemia, which is observed in up to 40 per cent of patients during upper endoscopy.[11, 12] A smaller percentage of patients have arterial desaturation during colonoscopy.[13] Small caliber instruments for upper endoscopy are associated with less hypoxemia than larger endoscopes.

Dysrhythmias. Disturbances of cardiac rhythm during endoscopy are most frequently seen in patients with underlying chronic heart disease, but medications and hypoxemia are deleterious influences also.[2] Transient ischemic changes are seen sometimes. Continuous monitoring of the electrocardiogram is a wise precaution.[14]

Transmission of Infection

Transmission of infection from one patient to another or to endoscopic personnel is a source of great concern. Fortunately, documented instances of this complication are rare.[15] *Salmonella* and *Pseudomonas* transmission have been reported,[16, 17] and *Clostridium difficile* infection has also been spread endoscopically in all likelihood.[18] Among the viruses, hepatitis B and HIV are the main causes for worry, but fears have not been realized to date; hepatitis B transmission is very rare, and AIDS cross-infection by endoscopy has not been reported.[15, 19, 20]

Disinfection of endoscopes and accessories is the main preventive measure. Mechanical cleansing with water and detergent, immersion in 2 per cent glutaraldehyde solution for 10 to 30 minutes, rinsing, and air-drying are the usual steps; shorter exposure to germicide has also been suggested.[18, 21] It is important that disinfection of instruments be carried out by experienced personnel and not delegated casually to just anyone who might be available.

Bacteremia

The frequency of bacteremia during endoscopy varies with the type of procedure (Table 13–2). Therapeutic endoscopy, including procedures listed in Table 13–2 and others such as laser treatment and colonoscopic polyectomy, are associated with higher rates of bacteremia than are seen with diagnostic endoscopy.[23, 24] Additional details are important, too; in variceal sclerotherapy, the incidence of bacteremia correlates with the length of the needle, site of injection, and volume of sclerosant.[25]

In normal individuals, bacteremia is transient, and bacteria are cleared without complication. Susceptible patients, however, may develop serious infection; fortunately, few examples of this problem have been documented.[22] Bacterial endocarditis may occur in patients with valvular heart disease, prosthetic valves, or pacemakers; a previous episode of endocarditis is an especially important risk factor.[22, 26–28] Mitral valve prolapse, idiopathic hypertrophic subaortic stenosis, and other uncomplicated lesions pose little threat.[28] Implanted orthopedic prostheses and peritoneal shunts are theoretical concerns, but the necessity for antibiotic prophylaxis during endoscopy has not been established in these patients.[22, 23]

Potentially pathogenic organisms isolated from peripheral blood during endoscopy include *Streptococcus viridans, Staphylococcus aureus,* and *Staphylococcus epidermidis.*[22] Gram-negative organisms have been

Table 13–2. FREQUENCY OF BACTEREMIA DURING ENDOSCOPIC PROCEDURES

Procedure	Bacteremia (Percentage of Procedures)
Upper GI endoscopy	4.2
Esophageal dilatation	45
Variceal sclerotherapy	31
Colonoscopy	2.2
Sigmoidoscopy	6.9

Data from Botoman and Surawicz.[22]

Table 13–3. ANTIBIOTIC PROPHYLAXIS FOR GASTROINTESTINAL ENDOSCOPY

If not allergic to penicillin:
    Amipicillin, 2 gm IM or IV, and gentamicin, 1.5 mg/kg IM or IV, before procedure and 6 to 8 hours postoperatively

or

    Amoxicillin, 3 gm po, one hour before procedure, then amoxicillin, 1.5 gm, five hours after procedure

If allergic to penicillin:
    Vancomycin, 1 gm IV, and gentamicin 1.5 mg/kg IV or IM, one hour before procedure and 6 to 8 hours after procedure

Data from Botoman and Surawicz.[22]

identified in some cases.[27] Current recommendations for antibiotic prophylaxis against endocarditis are listed in Table 13–3. The addition of aminoglycoside to ampicillin or amoxicillin is most relevant to lower tract procedures.[22] The decision to give prophylactic antibiotics, weighing the risks of infection against side effects of the drugs, can be difficult with so little solid data available. Today's litigious climate compounds the dilemma.

Electrosurgical Hazards

Complications from the use of electrosurgical devices during endoscopy include explosion, perforation, and bleeding—all are discussed separately later in this chapter. Burns and cardiac dysrhythmias are other accidents that may be avoided by knowledge of the principles of electrosurgery.[29]

High-frequency current from the electrosurgical generator can leak by a phenomenon called "capacitive coupling" in which the snare wire and the endoscope body form a capacitor.[29] The eyes and hands of the endoscopist can be burned by high-frequency leakage; the metallic ocular of the endoscope should be covered with an insulating eye piece, and surgical gloves should be kept intact to avoid burns through small holes. Patients are burned by contact with exposed metal. The possibility of electrical burns is increased by the use of endoscopes with metal tips that are not recessed behind insulated hoods and by the presence of metal rings on the insertion tube.[29]

A patient with a pacemaker may develop cardiac dysrhythmia if monopolar current passes through the pacemaker or the heart. Bipolar electrosurgery is safer, but if monopolar must be used, the patient ground plate should be placed as close as possible to the electrosurgical site.

Impaction of the Instrument

An endoscope may impact in the distal esophagus or in a hiatal hernia during retroversion.[2, 10] Disimpaction should be attempted by advancing the instrument under fluoroscopic guidance.[10] Endoscopic impaction in the colon is rare also, and it usually results from

volvulus. Polypectomy snares, biopsy forceps, and brushes on occasion can be difficult to withdraw. An external splinting tube can lodge in the rectum during colonoscopy if the flange is not sufficiently large.[30]

Abdominal Distention

Abdominal distention from insufflated gas is seldom a problem during routine upper endoscopy, but laser therapy can create troublesome distention because gas is used to keep the fiber tip clear and because procedures are not completed rapidly. Colonic distention during colonoscopy is expected routinely, and sometimes it causes marked discomfort. Insufflation of air also may impair mucosal blood flow.[31] Carbon dioxide is absorbed from the colon, blood flow is less affected, and the chance of ischemia is reduced.[31] Carbon dioxide is nonexplosive, an additional advantage.[32] Rapid absorption of carbon dioxide allows air contrast barium enema X-rays to be obtained later that day.[33]

COMPLICATIONS OF UPPER ENDOSCOPY

Perforation

The esophagus or stomach is perforated during diagnostic upper endoscopy in 0.03 to 0.1 per cent of procedures.[2, 4, 7] Perforation occurs most commonly where the endoscope is passed blindly (i.e., the pharynx and cervical esophagus, cardia, and superior duodenal angle).[10] Osteoarthritic spurs on the cervical spine, anastomoses, strictures, and weakening of the wall from inflammation, ischemia, neoplasm, or caustic ingestion are predisposing factors. Lack of endoscopic skill must be listed, too. Perforation of the midesophagus usually results from biopsy of a carcinoma.[2] Excessive force of endoscopic insertion or insufflation of air under high pressure can perforate tumors and ulcers. More than one-half of perforations during diagnostic upper endoscopy occur in the stomach.[7, 34]

Therapeutic endoscopy clearly carries an increased risk of perforation. Dilatation of strictures may lead to perforation at or proximal to the narrowing. Hydrostatic balloon dilatation of benign esophageal stenosis is complicated in this way in 0.4 per cent of procedures.[35] The incidence of perforation from endoscopic balloon dilatation of strictures at some other sites is as follows: pyloric stenosis (0.5 per cent), gastrojejunostomy (2.2 per cent), and gastric staple line (0.8 per cent).[35] Other causes of luminal narrowing and other methods of dilatation yield different statistics. The safest dilating device appears to be the "through the scope" (TTS) dilator.[36]

Variceal sclerotherapy in the esophagus is complicated by perforation in 1 to 2 per cent of patients.[37] Many perforations are subtle, remain localized, and heal without problems; a few end fatally.

Palliation of esophageal carcinoma by laser or bipolar coagulation leads to perforation or tracheoesophageal fistula in at least 5 per cent of patients.[38] It is sometimes difficult to determine if the complication is attributable to the carcinoma, laser treatment, other treatment, or a combination of factors.[39, 40] Endoscopic therapy of nonvariceal bleeding sites in the upper tract by laser, bipolar or monopolar coagulation, heater probe, or injection is quite safe in the hands of an expert, and perforation is very rare.[41-43]

Endoscopic perforation of the esophagus or stomach may be obvious immediately or within a few hours. Cervical pain, subcutaneous emphysema, fever, tachycardia, and characteristic radiographic appearances make the diagnosis easy, but some distal esophageal injuries are more subtle.[10] An emergency esophagogram should be obtained if perforation is suspected. A major leak, or one that occurred through tumor or an ulcer, requires immediate operation.[10, 44] Limited or absent extravasation on the radiographs allows treatment by intravenous antibiotics and close observation. Endoscopic esophageal perforation was fatal in up to 20 per cent of patients in the older literature, but that statistic probably no longer applies.[44]

Bleeding

Bleeding from diagnostic endoscopy, even with biopsy, is rare (about 0.03 per cent of procedures[2]). Coagulopathy, of course, increases the risk. The bleeding site is more often gastric than esophageal, and Mallory-Weiss tear has been reported.[45] Therapeutic procedures such as sclerotherapy, polypectomy, laser destruction of tumors, and dilatation of strictures cause bleeding more frequently.

Other

Esophageal ulcers are so common after variceal sclerotherapy that some endoscopists do not regard them as complications in the absence of bleeding or perforation.[46] Strictures may develop after variceal sclerotherapy or endoscopic destruction of esophageal cancer.[47] Aggressive interventional techniques have various other complications not discussed here (see pp. 647-649).

COMPLICATIONS OF SIGMOIDOSCOPY AND COLONOSCOPY

Perforation

Rates of perforation from sigmoidoscopy and colonoscopy are listed in Table 13-4. Mechanical perforation by the tip of the instrument occurs at sites of weakness of the colonic wall (e.g., diverticula, inflammation, radiation injury, or ischemia) and distal to obstructing points (e.g., neoplasms, strictures, flexures, or kinks). The shaft of the endoscope may act as a lead point if the instrument is flexed sharply, and perforation can

Table 13-4. INCIDENCE OF PERFORATION DURING SIGMOIDOSCOPY AND COLONOSCOPY

Procedure	Perforation (Percentage of Procedures)
Sigmoidoscopy	
Rigid	0.005 to 0.01[48]
Flexible	0.01[49, 50]
Colonoscopy	
Diagnostic	0.2 to 0.4[2, 51]
Polypectomy	0.3 to 1.0[2, 51-53]
Dilatation	4.4[35]

develop as shown in Figure 13-1. Fixation of the sigmoid colon in the pelvis by diverticular disease or previous pelvic surgery predisposes to this mechanism.

Pneumatic perforation of the colon or the ileum results from distention by insufflated air.[50, 54, 55] If the ileocecal valve is competent to retrograde flow and the colonoscope obstructs the lumen distally, the colon forms a closed loop, and pressure in the cecum may become extreme.[50, 54] Diastatic serosal tears are also the consequence of colonic distention (Fig. 13-2). The damage here is partial thickness and usually goes unrecognized unless laparotomy is performed for some other reason.

Perforation from colonoscopic polypectomy is an electrosurgical injury, either an immediate full-thickness cut through the wall by a snare or hot biopsy forceps or delayed rupture of necrotic tissue.[51, 56-58] The "postpolypectomy coagulation syndrome" of pain, peritoneal irritation, and fever may represent a microperforation.[59]

The possibility of perforation is greater in the presence of poor bowel preparation, acute bleeding, aortic or iliac aneurysms, or an uncooperative patient.[60] A biopsy forceps, brush, dilator, or other accessory may perforate the colon. Perforation of the cecum during colonoscopic decompression of nonobstructive colonic dilatation has been noted, but of course this procedure is performed in patients with pre-existing colonic distension.[61]

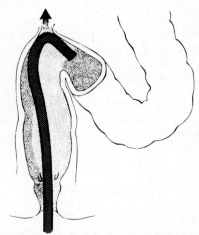

Figure 13-1. Perforation by the shaft of a sharply flexed colonoscope or sigmoidoscope. (From Katon, R. M., Keefe, E. B., Melnyk, C. S. Flexible Sigmoidoscopy. Orlando, Grune & Stratton, 1985.)

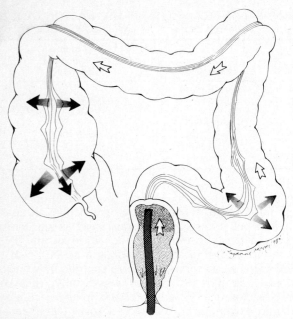

Figure 13–2. Diastatic serosal tears occur most often on the antimesocolic side of the cecum, ascending colon, or sigmoid. (From Katon, R. M., Keefe, E. B., Melnyk, C. S. Flexible Sigmoidoscopy. Orlando, Grune & Stratton, 1985.)

Free perforation into the peritoneal cavity is recognized at the time if abdominal viscera are seen through the instrument. In other situations, marked persistent abdominal distention, pain, and absence of dullness over the liver prompt the ordering of X-rays which reveal pneumoperitoneum. Symptoms of perforation may be delayed for several days if the leak is tiny and well-localized. Retroperitoneal perforation, usually a pneumatic injury, gives rise to subcutaneous emphysema and retroperitoneal and subcutaneous air on X-rays.[62] Fever and leukocytosis may develop eventually in any of these varieties of perforation.

Large lacerations seen directly through the colonoscope demand immediate operation.[63] If no defect is observed endoscopically and plain abdominal X-rays show pneumoperitoneum, a water-soluble contrast enema X-ray should be obtained.[58] Gross extravasation requires operation, but in the absence of leakage, treatment with intravenous antibiotics and close observation may be considered. Benign pneumoperitoneum is relatively asymptomatic abdominal distention, presumably from microperforation, and it responds well to antibiotics.[64] Most retroperitoneal perforations and those associated with the postpolypectomy coagulation syndrome also do not require operation initially.[50, 58, 63]

Bleeding

Bleeding from biopsy sites or mucosal tears during diagnostic colonoscopy or sigmoidoscopy is rare. The incidence of hemorrhage after colonoscopic polypectomy is 0.7 to 2.5 per cent.[2, 51, 52] Postpolypectomy bleeding may occur immediately, but in 30 to 50 per

cent of cases, it is delayed for two days to a week, when the eschar sloughs.[51]

Sessile polyps, large thick pedicles, equipment failure, and faulty technique account for some of the bleeding associated with polypectomy. Coagulopathy (including salicylate ingestion), inflammation, and hypertension are contributory. Prevention depends on recognition of potential problems and expertise in performing the procedures. A bleeding pedicle can be grasped with the snare or coagulated with a bipolar electrode in some cases. Interventional angiography or even laparotomy is necessary occasionally. Management of delayed hemorrhage begins with rapid colonic cleansing followed by colonoscopy to identify and treat the bleeding site.

Explosion

Explosive concentrations of combustible gases, mostly hydrogen but also methane in some patients, can be avoided by preparing the colon with electrolyte solution containing sodium sulfate and polyethylene glycol.[65, 66] Bacteria produce hydrogen from mannitol, and although antibiotics suppress the responsible fecal flora, there is little reason to incur even the small risk of explosion associated with this cathartic.[67–69] Carbon dioxide insufflation during colonoscopy is an additional safety precaution, but it has not been widely adopted at present.[31–33]

Fluid Shifts

Preparation of the colon with laxatives and enemas can dehydrate a patient. Peroral lavage with saline may result in fluid overload, a dangerous side effect in patients with cardiac disease. Sodium sulfate-polyethylene glycol lavage seems to escape these problems.[65, 66] Questions about potential harmful effects of absorption of polyethylene glycol have been answered in the negative thus far.[70] Ventricular ectopy has been reported following ingestion of lavage solutions, but the significance of this observation is unknown.[71, 72]

Other Complications

Extracolonic Injury. The spleen is normally tethered to the colon and may be torn by traction on the splenic flexure during colonoscopy.[73]

Volvulus. Volvulus of the colon or the ileum is a rare complication of colonoscopy.[74]

Lost Specimen. Inability to retrieve biopsy or polypectomy specimens is an important complication. Failure to recognize a malignancy is probably the greatest concern.

References

1. Plumeri, P. A. Informed consent and the gastrointestinal endoscopist. Gastrointest. Endosc. *31*:218, 1985.

2. Shahmir, M., and Schuman, B. M. Complications of fiberoptic endoscopy. Gastrointest. Endosc. 26:85, 1980.
3. Schwesinger, W. H., Levine B. A., and Ramos, R. Complications in colonoscopy. Surg. Gynecol. Obstet. 148:270, 1979.
4. Davis, R. E., and Graham, D. Y. Endoscopic complications. The Texas experience. Gastrointest. Endosc. 25:146, 1979.
5. Gilbert, D. A., Silverstein, F. F., and Tedesco, F. J. National ASGE survey on upper gastrointestinal bleeding. Complications of endoscopy. Dig. Dis. Sci. 26:1, 1981.
6. Mayer, I. E. Endoscopic premedications. Endosc. Rev. March/April, 1985, p. 38.
7. Silvis, S. E., Nebel, O., Rogers, G., et al. Endoscopic complications. Results of the 1974 American Society for Gastrointestinal Endoscopy survey. JAMA 235:928, 1976.
8. Waye, J. D. Diazepam versus midozolam (Versed) in outpatient colonoscopy: A double blind randomized study (abstract). Gastrointest. Endosc. (in press).
9. Schiller, K. F., Cotton, P. B., and Salmon, P. R. The hazards of digestive fiberendoscopy. A survey of British experience (abstract, Br. Soc. Dig. Endosc.). Gut 12:1027, 1973.
10. Cotton, P. B., and Williams, C. B. Practical Gastrointestinal Endoscopy. ed. 2, Oxford, England, Blackwell Scientific Publications, 1982.
11. Rosen, P., Fireman, Z., and Gilat, T. The causes of hypoxemia in elderly patients during endoscopy. Gastrointest. Endosc. 28:243, 1982.
12. Barkin, J. S. Abnormal breathing pattern and oxygen desaturation in patients during upper endoscopy (abstract). Gastrointest. Endosc. (in press).
13. Barkin, J. S. Abnormal breathing pattern and oxygen desaturation in patients undergoing colonoscopy (abstract). Gastrointest. Endosc. (in press).
14. Levy, N., and Abinader, E.: Continuous electrocardiographic monitoring with Holter electrocardiorecorder throughout all stages of gastroscopy. Am. J. Dig. Dis. 22:1091, 1977.
15. Vennes, J. A. Infectious complications of gastrointestinal endoscopy. Dig. Dis. Sci. 26:605, 1981.
16. O'Connor, B. H., Bennett, J. R., Alexander, J. G., et al. Salmonellosis infection transmitted by fiberoptic endoscopes. Lancet 2:864, 1982.
17. Doherty, D. E., Falko, J. M., Lefkovity, N., et al.: *Pseudomonas aeruginosa* sepsis following retrograde cholangiopancreatography. Dig. Dis. Sci. 27:169, 1982.
18. Hughes, C. E., Gebhard, R. L., Peterson, L. R., and Gerding, D. Efficacy of routine fiberoptic endoscope cleaning and disinfection for killing *Clostridium difficile*. Gastrointest. Endosc. 32:7, 1986.
19. Villa, E., Pasquinelli, C., Rigo, G., et al. Gastrointestinal endoscopy and HBV infection: No evidence for a causal relationship. A prospective controlled study. Gastrointest. Endosc. 30:15, 1984.
20. Fauci, A. S. Acquired immunodeficiency syndrome: Epidemiologic, clinical, immunologic and therapeutic considerations. Ann. Intern. Med. 100:92, 1984.
21. Gerding, D. N., Peterson, L. R., and Vennes, J. A. Cleaning and disinfection of fiberoptic endoscopes: Evaluation of glutaraldehyde exposure time and forced-air drying. Gastroenterology 83:613, 1982.
22. Botoman, V. A., Surawicz. Bacteremia with gastrointestinal endoscopic procedures. Gastrointest. Endosc. 32:342, 1986.
23. Perucca, P. J., and Meyer, G. W. Editorial: Who should have endocarditis prophylaxis for upper gastrointestinal procedures? Gastrointest. Endosc. 31:285, 1985.
24. Wolf, D., Fleischer, D., and Sivak, M. V., Jr. Incidence of bacteremia with elective upper gastrointestinal endoscopic laser therapy. Gastrointest. Endosc. 31:247, 1985.
25. Gerhartz, H. H., Sauerbruch, T., Weinzierl, R. A., and Ruckdeschel, G. Nosocomial septicemia in patients undergoing sclerotherapy for variceal hemorrhage. Endoscopy 16:129, 1984.
26. Kaye, D. Prophylaxis for endocarditis: An update. Ann. Intern. Med. 104:419, 1986.
27. Shorvon, P. J., Eykyn, S. J., and Cotton, P. B.: Gastrointestinal instrumentation, bacteraemia, and endocarditis. Gut 24:1078, 1983.
28. Shulman, S. T., Amren, D. P., Bisno, A. L., et al. Prevention of bacterial endocarditis. Circulation 70:1123A, 1984.
29. Barlow, D. E. Endoscopic applications of electrosurgery: A review of basic principles. Gastrointest. Endosc. 28:73, 1982.
30. Vazquez, D. J., Nieto, M., Galipienzo, J. M. R., and Alvarez, F. New complication of fiberoptic colonoscopy. Gastrointest. Endosc. 29:251, 1983.
31. Brandt, L. J., Boley, S. J., and Sammartano, R. Carbon dioxide and room air insufflation of the colon. Effects on colonic blood flow and intraluminal pressure in the dog. Gastrointest. Endosc. 32:324, 1986.
32. Williams, C. B. Editorial: Who's for CO_2? Gastrointest. Endosc. 32:365, 1986.
33. Phaosawasdi, K., Cooley, W., Wheeler, J., and Rice, P. Carbon dioxide-insufflated colonoscopy: An ignored superior technique. Gastrointest. Endosc. 32:330, 1986.
34. Sugawa, C., and Schuman, B. M. Primer of Gastrointestinal Fiberoptic Endoscopy. Boston, Little, Brown and Company, 1981.
35. Kozarek, R. A. Hydrostatic balloon dilation of gastrointestinal stenoses: A national survey. Gastroinest. Endosc. 32:15, 1986.
36. Lindor, K. D., Ott, B. J., and Hughes, R. W. Balloon dilatation of upper digestive tract strictures. Gastroenterology 89:545, 1985.
37. Sivak, M. V., Jr. Endoscopic injection sclerosis of esophageal varices: ASGE survey. Gastrointest. Endosc. 28:41, 1982.
38. Fleischer, D., and Sivak, M. V., Jr. Endoscopic Nd:Yag laser therapy as palliation for esophagogastric cancer. Parameters affecting initial outcome. Gastroenterology 89:827, 1985.
39. Cello, J. P., Gerstenberger, P. D., Wright, T., et al. Endoscopic neodymium-YAG laser palliation of nonresectable esophageal malignancy. Ann. Intern. Med. 102:610, 1985.
40. Ell, C. H., Riemann, J. F., Lux, G., and Demling, L.: Palliative laser treatment of malignant stenoses in the upper gastrointestinal tract. Endoscopy 18(Suppl 1):21, 1986.
41. Swain, C. P., Brown, S. G., Salmon, P. R., et al. Controlled trial of Nd:YAG laser photocoagulation in bleeding peptic ulcers. Gastrointest. Endosc. 30:137, 1984.
42. Johnston, J., Jones, J., Long, B., and Posey, E. L. Comparison of heater probe and YAG laser in endoscopic treatment of major bleeding from peptic ulcers. Gastrointest. Endosc. 31:175, 1985.
43. Jensen, D. M., Machiado, G. A., Silpa, M., et al. BICAP vs heater probe for hemostatis of severe ulcer bleeding. Gastrointest. Endosc. 32:140, 1986.
44. Chung, R. Dilation of strictures of the upper gastrointestinal tract. *In* Dent, T. L., Strodel, W. E., Turcotte, J. G., and Harper, M. L. (eds.). Surgical Endoscopy. Chicago, Year Book Medical Publishers, 1985, pp. 123–135.
45. Watts, H. D. Mallory-Weiss syndrome occurring as a complication of endoscopy. Gastrointest. Endosc. 22:171, 1976.
46. Sivak, M. V., Jr. Sclerotherapy for esophageal varices. *In* Silvis, S. (ed.): Therapeutic Gastrointestinal Endoscopy. New York, Igaku-Shoin, 1984, pp. 31–36.
47. Haynes, W. C., Sanowski, R. A., Foutch, P. G., and Bellapravalu, S. Strictures following endoscopic variceal sclerotherapy: Clinical course and response to therapy. Gastrointest. Endosc. 32:202, 1986.
48. Befeler, D. Proctoscopic perforation of the large bowel. Dis. Colon Rectum 10:376, 1967.
49. Traul, D. G., Davis, C. B., Pollock, J. C., and Scudamore, H. H. Flexible fiberoptic sigmoidoscopy. The Monroe Clinic experience. A prospective study of 5000 examinations. Dis. Colon Rectum 26:161, 1983.
50. Katon, R. M., Keefe, E. B., and Melnyk, C. S. Flexible Sigmoidoscopy. Orlando, Grune & Stratton, 1985.
51. MacRae, F. A., Tan, K. G., and Williams, C. B. Toward safer colonoscopy: A report on the complications of 5000 diagnostic or therapeutic colonoscopies. Gut 24:376, 1983.
52. Hunt, R. H., and Waye, J. D. Colonoscopy Techniques. Clinical Practice and Color Atlas. Chicago, Year Book Medical Publishers, 1981.
53. Hunt, R. H. Toward safer colonoscopy. Gut 24:371, 1983.
54. Kozarek, R. A., Earnest, D. L., Silverstein, M. E., and Smith,

R. G. Air-pressure-induced colon injury during diagnostic colonoscopy. Gastroenterology 78:7, 1980.

55. Razzak, I. A., Millan, J., and Schuster, M. M. Pneumatic ileal perforation: An unusual complication of colonoscopy. Gastroenterology 70:268, 1976.

56. Ghazi, A., and Grossman, M. Complications of colonoscopy and polypectomy. Surg. Clin. North Am. 62:889, 1982.

57. Berci, G., Panish, J. F., Schapiro, M., and Corlin, R. Complications of colonoscopy and polypectomy: Report of the Southern California Society for Gastrointestinal Endoscopy. Gastroenterology 67:584, 1974.

58. Schrock, T. R. Colonoscopic polypectomy. In Dent, T. L., Strodel, W. E., Turcotte, J. G., and Harper, M. L. (eds.): Surgical Endoscopy. Chicago, Year Book Medical Publishers, 1985, pp. 233–252.

59. Waye, J. D. The postpolypectomy coagulation syndrome. Gastrointest. Endosc. 27:182, 1981.

60. Smith, L. E., and Nivatvong, S. Complications in endoscopy. Dis. Colon Rectum 18:214, 1975.

61. Bode, W. E., Beart, R. W., Jr., Spencer, R. J., et al. Colonoscopic decompression for acute pseudoobstruction of the colon. (Ogilvie's syndrome.) Report of 22 cases and review of the literature. Am. J. Surg. 147:243, 1984.

62. Schmidt, G., Börsch, G., and Wegener, M. Subcutaneous emphysema and pneumothorax complicating diagnostic colonoscopy. Dis. Colon Rectum 29:136, 1986.

63. Vincent, M., and Smith, L. E. Management of perforation due to colonoscopy. Dis. Colon Rectum 26:61, 1983.

64. Ecker, M. D., Goldstein, M., Hoexter, B., et al. Benign pneumoperitoneum after fiberoptic colonoscopy. A prospective study of 100 patients. Gastroenterology 73:226, 1977.

65. Davis, G. R., Santa Ana, C. A., Morawski, S. G., and Fordtran, J. S. Development of a lavage solution associated with minimal water and electrolyte absorption or secretion. Gastroenterology 78:991, 1980.

66. Goldman, J., and Reichelderfer, M. Evaluation of rapid colonoscopy preparation using a new gut lavage solution. Gastrointest. Endosc. 28:9, 1982.

67. Bond, J. H., Jr., and Levitt, M. D. Factors affecting the concentration of combustible gases in the colon during colonoscopy. Gastroenterology 68:1445, 1975.

68. Taylor, E. W., Bentley, S., Young, D., and Keighley, M. R. B. Bowel preparation and the safety of colonoscopic polypectomy. Gastroenterology 81:1, 1981.

69. La Brooy, S. J., Avgerinos, A., Fendick, C. L., et al. Potentially explosive colonic concentrations of hydrogen after bowel preparation with mannitol. Lancet 1:634, 1981.

70. Brady, C. E., III, DiPalma, J. A., Marawski, S. G., et al. Urinary excretion of polyethylene glycol 3350 and sulfate after gut lavage with a polyethylene glycol electrolyte lavage solution. Gastroenterology 90:1914, 1986.

71. Marsh, W. H., Bronner, M. H., Yantis, P. L., et al. Ventricular ectopy associated with peroral colonic lavage. Gastrointest. Endosc. 32:259, 1986.

72. Reichelderfer, M. Colonoscopy preparation: Is it better from above or below? Gastrointest. Endosc. 32:301, 1986.

73. Ellis, W. R., Harrison, J. M., and Williams, R. S. Rupture of spleen at colonoscopy. Br. Med. J. 1:307, 1979.

74. Keeffe, E. B. Ileal volvulus following colonoscopy. Gastrointest. Endosc. 31:228, 1985.

14

Nausea and Vomiting

MARK FELDMAN

Although nausea and vomiting undoubtedly have some protective value, their importance stems from the large number of conditions which may cause or be associated with nausea and vomiting and from the possible serious consequences of vomiting. Vomiting may be a manifestation a wide variety of conditions including gastrointestinal obstruction, pregnancy, motion sickness, radiation sickness, drug toxicity, hepatitis, myocardial infarction, renal failure, increased intracranial pressure, asthma, Zollinger-Ellison syndrome, diabetes mellitus, thyrotoxicosis, and epilepsy.[1-6] Serious consequences of vomiting include aspiration pneumonia (a chemical pneumonitis due to aspirated gastric acid), Mallory-Weiss syndrome, esophageal rupture (Boerhaave's syndrome), volume and electrolyte depletion, acid-base imbalance, and malnutrition.

THE ACT OF VOMITING (Fig. 14–1)

Three components of vomiting are recognized: nausea, retching ("dry heaves"), and emesis (vomiting).[7] Nausea may occur without retching or vomiting and retching may occur without vomiting.[8] Characteristic, but not invariable, changes in gastrointestinal motility have been recognized for each of the three stages.

Nausea is a psychic experience of humans that defies precise definition, although attempts are being made to try to measure and quantitate nausea.[9] A variety of stimuli may produce nausea (labyrinthine stimulation, visceral pain, unpleasant memories). The neural pathways mediating nausea are not known, but evidence suggests that they are the same as pathways mediating vomiting (see below). ıt may be that mild activation of these pathways leads to nausea and that more

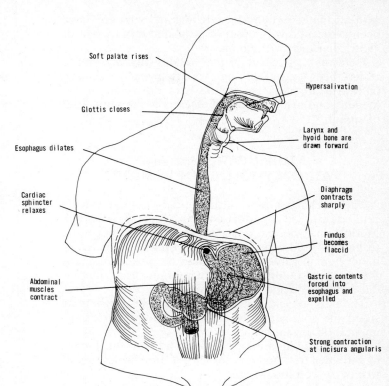

Soft palate rises

Glottis closes

Esophagus dilates

Cardiac sphincter relaxes

Abdominal muscles contract

Hypersalivation

Larynx and hyoid bone are drawn forward

Diaphragm contracts sharply

Fundus becomes flaccid

Gastric contents forced into esophagus and expelled

Strong contraction at incisura angularis

Figure 14–1. A summary of the act of vomiting in man. (From Searle: Research in the Service of Medicine *44*:2, 1956.)

intense activation leads to retching or vomiting. Recent evidence in rats suggests that the nausea pathway may also overlap with the neural pathway mediating satiety.[10]

During nausea, gastric tone is reduced and gastric peristalsis is diminished or absent. In contrast, the tone of the duodenum and proximal jejunum tends to be increased, and reflux of duodenal contents into the stomach is frequent.[11] Nausea is not caused by increased duodenal and jejunal tone, however, because these abnormalities are not always present in a nauseated person.

Retching consists of spasmodic and abortive respiratory movements with the glottis closed, during which time inspiratory movements of the chest wall and diaphragm are opposed by expiratory contractions of the abdominal musculature. During retching, the antrum of the stomach contracts, whereas the fundus and cardia relax. The mouth is closed.

Vomiting occurs as the gastric contents are forcefully brought up to and out of the mouth, which opens just prior to stomach evacuation. This occurs by virtue of a forceful sustained contraction of the abdominal muscles and diaphragm at a time when the cardia of the stomach is raised and open and the pylorus is contracted.[12] Elevation of the cardia serves the purpose of eliminating the intra-abdominal portion of the esophagus, which if present would tend to prevent the high intragastric pressure from forcing gastric contents into the esophagus. The cardia may be so high as to cause a temporary hiatal hernia. The mechanism by which the cardia opens during vomiting is not clear.

Experimental observations in cats have added to our understanding of retching and vomiting.[13] Retching was characterized by repeated herniations of the abdominal esophagus and cardia into the thorax, which coincided with negative intrathoracic pressure pulses mirrored by positive pulses in the abdomen. These pressure changes were associated with to and fro movement of gastric contents into a dilated esophagus. Vomiting (i.e., expulsion), which began with the cardia in the chest as a result of the preceding retch, was associated with a reversal of intrathoracic pressure from negative to positive. It seems, then, that retching is a preparatory maneuver in which respiratory mechanisms are used to overcome the inherent antireflux characteristics of the abdominal esophagus and cardia prior to expulsion.

Intestinal contents are frequently present in vomited material and some workers have implicated reverse peristalsis in the small intestine as the cause. Injection of apomorphine, morphine, or cisplatin leads to intense electrical spike activity which begins in the distal small intestine and migrates proximally at a rate of 2 to 3 cm/sec, reaching the duodenum and stomach just prior to emesis.[14] Whether similar retrograde electrical and motor events occur in the human small intestine prior to vomiting is unknown, but likely.

Associated Phenomena

Hypersalivation. Hypersalivation is probably due to the close proximity of the medullary vomiting and salivary centers (see below).

Cardiac Rhythm Disturbances. Nausea usually is accompanied by tachycardia, retching by bradycardia. Cardiac arrhythmias sometimes occur in animals made to vomit, and these may be prevented by pretreatment with atropine. In humans, retching and vomiting have been associated with onset of atrial and termination of ventricular tachyarrhythmias.[15, 16]

Defecation. Defecation may accompany vomiting.[17] It has been suggested that vomiting and defecation pathways are adjacent in the area postrema of the medulla and are acted on by essentially the same kind of stimuli.[18]

NEURAL PATHWAYS AND PATHOPHYSIOLOGY OF VOMITING

The mechanism of vomiting in cats was extensively studied in 1953 by Borison and Wang.[17] Although caution must be exercised in extrapolating their data to humans, the experiments can never be repeated in intact human subjects, and what little is known about the pathophysiology of vomiting in humans is compatible with the hypotheses of Borison and Wang.[19]

The pathophysiology of vomiting can best be understood and appreciated by a brief review of four experimental observations:

1. Vomiting involves a complex and reproducible set of activities that suggests some central neurologic control by a "vomiting center."

2. Vomiting can be induced by electrical stimulation of the medulla, specifically in the dorsal portion of the lateral reticular formation in the vicinity of the fasciculus solitarius. No other portion of the brain regularly produces vomiting on stimulation. Destruction of the electrically responsive region of the reticular formation (vomiting center) causes animals to become highly refractory to the emetic action of apomorphine and copper sulfate. This vomiting center is anatomically adjacent to medullary centers controlling respiration and salivation, and integrated activities mediated by all these centers are involved in vomiting. Although direct electrical stimulation of the vomiting center causes vomiting, there is no evidence that any substance which causes vomiting does so by direct stimulation of the vomiting center. Rather, the center coordinates the activities of the other medullary structures to produce a patterned response.

3. Intravenously injected apomorphine, an opiate and a dopamine agonist, induces vomiting within minutes. The emetic response to this drug can be eliminated either by ablation of the vomiting center or by ablation of the area postrema, which is located on the surface of the brain in the floor of the fourth ventricle (leaving the vomiting center intact). Direct application of apomorphine to an intact area postrema causes vomiting. Therefore, apomorphine is a centrally acting emetic agent, its site of action being the area postrema or the so-called chemoreceptor trigger zone (CTZ).[18] Unlike the vomiting center, the CTZ is not responsive to electrical stimulation. Instead, the CTZ is responsive to chemical stimuli in the circulation; the "blood-brain barrier" in the region of the CTZ is virtually nonexistent.[20] Thus, the CTZ can be regarded as an emetic chemoreceptor, as illustrated in Figure 14–2.

4. Copper sulfate is a potent emetic when ingested

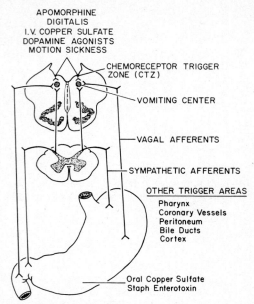

Figure 14–2. The interrelation of the vomiting center, the chemoreceptor trigger zone, and peripheral trigger areas. (Modified from Wang, S. C., and Borison, H. L. Gastroenterology 2:1, 1952.)

orally. Interruption of the abdominal vagus nerves and sympathetic nerves makes animals highly refractory to oral copper sulfate. On the other hand, ablation of the CTZ, which makes animals resistant to the emetic action of apomorphine, has no effect on the sensitivity of animals to oral copper sulfate. These experiments indicate that oral copper sulfate induces vomiting via afferent impulses that reach the medullary vomiting center via the vagus and sympathetic nerves without traversing the CTZ.* This also is illustrated in Figure 14–2.

The preceding observations indicate that the medullary emetic mechanism consists of two anatomically and functionally separate units: a vomiting center in the reticular formation, which is excited directly by visceral afferent impulses arising from the gastrointestinal tract, and a chemoreceptor trigger zone in the area postrema in floor of the fourth ventricle, which is the site of emetic action of apomorphine and intravenously injected copper sulfate. The CTZ is not able to cause vomiting without the mediation of an intact vomiting center. How many synapses exist between the CTZ and vomiting center is unknown.[18]

Cardiac glycosides and many other drugs are thought to induce emesis by acting on the CTZ. Examples include opiates, ergot derivatives, cancer chemotherapy agents, staphylococcal enterotoxin, emetine, salicylate, and nicotine.[18] Ipecac has both a central action on the CTZ and a reflex action via the gastrointestinal mucosa directly to the vomiting center. The CTZ is also important in mediating nausea and vomiting associated with uremia,[18] hypoxia,[18] and perhaps diabetic

---

*Copper sulfate is also an effective emetic when injected intravenously. Ablation of the CTZ prevents vomiting in response to intravenous copper sulfate, whereas denervation of the gut is without effect. This shows that intravenous copper sulfate is also a central emetic agent (like apomorphine) with its action on the CTZ.

ketoacidosis. Finally, the CTZ may mediate the response to nonchemical emetic stimuli such as radiation sickness[18, 21] and, in certain species, motion sickness.[18] However, in squirrel monkeys, motion sickness can induce vomiting even after ablation of the area postrema.[22]

There is strong evidence that dopamine receptors in the CTZ play a role in mediating vomiting.[23] Thus, dopamine agonists such as apomorphine, L-dihydroxyphenylanine (L-dopa), and bromocriptine can cause vomiting, whereas dopamine antagonists, such as metoclopramide and domperidone, are effective antiemetics.[24, 25] Recent studies have suggested that, in addition to dopamine, the mammalian CTZ contains other neurotransmitters including serotonin, norepinephrine, gamma-aminobutyric acid (GABA), and the neuropeptides substance P and enkephalin.[26] Studies in dogs utilized ionophoretic application of some of these transmitters and neuropeptides to the area postrema. As expected, apomorphine and dopamine induced emesis in this model, as did serotonin, norepinephrine, glutamate, and histamine (but not acetylcholine). Several peptides also induced emesis (angiotensin II, neurotensin, thyrotropin-releasing hormone, vasoactive intestinal peptide, gastrin, substance P, vasopressin, and leucine-enkephalin), but somatostatin and cholecystokinin did not. There was a correlation between a peptide's ability to produce emesis when applied directly to the CTZ and its ability to produce emesis after intravenous administration.[27] These studies show that, in addition to responding to drugs and toxins, the CTZ may also respond to certain endogenous transmitters and neuropeptides.

Besides relaying signals to the vomiting center to initiate emesis, the CTZ and area postrema may have other functions. For example, activation of the CTZ by nausea-producing drugs or by radiation leads to a reflex delay in gastric emptying, which could contribute to vomiting.[18, 28] The CTZ has been incriminated also in conditioned taste aversions,[18] picas,[18] rumination,[18] and cardiovascular regulation.[29] Finally, activation of the CTZ with chemical agents such as apomorphine leads to release of oxytocin and vasopressin (antidiuretic hormone, or ADH) from the neurohypophysis,[10, 30-32] hormonal changes which can result in hyponatremia,[33] and alterations in hemostatic function.[34]

The anatomic structure of the area postrema in mammals and its neural connections have been reviewed recently.[35, 36] In addition to the direct afferent pathways from the gastrointestinal tract to the vomiting center, there also is evidence that the pharynx, heart, peritoneum, mesenteric vasculature, and bile ducts can be a source of afferent emetic impulses. Presumably, these peripheral receptors, like the gastrointestinal receptors stimulated by copper sulfate (Fig. 14–2), transmit impulses directly to the vomiting center. With regard to the gastrointestinal tract, it is of interest that distention of the antrum of the stomach (but not the fundus), the small bowel, colon, and biliary tree regularly leads to vomiting. Like that caused by irritation of the mucosa by copper sulfate, vomiting in response to distention is blocked by denervation of the organ in

question. Obviously there are also corticobulbar afferents to the vomiting center that mediate vomiting in response to some smells, sights, and tastes. These supramedullary receptors may influence the reactivity of the vomiting center or the CTZ, and they may play a role in psychogenic vomiting (see below). Vomiting can occur even in decerebrate animals,[13] indicating that the vomiting reflex occurs in the absence of higher, cortical influences.

After direct or indirect stimulation of the vomiting center, efferent pathways are mainly somatic, involving the vagus nerves, the phrenic nerves, and the spinal nerves (which supply the abdominal musculature). It is likely that the changes in tone and motility of the stomach during vomiting are mediated by visceral (presumably vagal) efferent neurons. Therefore, vomiting is an integrated somatovisceral process.

CLINICAL CHARACTERISTICS OF VOMITING

Although vomiting does not always signify the presence of serious illness, it may be the first manifestation of many conditions including those listed at the beginning of this chapter as well as peritonitis, cholecystitis, pancreatitis, gastric cancer, peptic ulcer, hypertensive crisis, intracranial lesion, addisonian crisis, and many other conditions. The following clinical features may help the physician in approaching a patient with nausea and vomiting.

Timing of Vomiting in Relation to Meals. Vomiting during or soon after a meal is common in patients with psychogenic vomiting and occasionally occurs in patients with peptic ulcer near the pyloric channel, presumably because of pyloric irritability, edema, and spasm. Delayed vomiting (more than one hour after eating), especially if it occurs repeatedly, is characteristic of gastric outlet obstruction or a motility disorder of the stomach, such as diabetic neuropathy or postvagotomy gastroparesis. Vomiting of material eaten 12 hours earlier is rarely, if ever, seen in patients with psychogenic vomiting and is strong evidence for gastric outlet obstruction or atony. Patients with this history will often have a succussion splash over the stomach. Nausea and vomiting in the early morning, before eating, is characteristic of nausea and vomiting of pregnancy (morning sickness) and may also be seen in postgastrectomy patients with bilious vomiting as well as in individuals with uremia, alcoholism, postnasal drip, and increased intracranial pressure.

Relief of Pain by Vomiting. Vomiting often relieves pain due to peptic ulcer disease, but not pain caused by pancreatitis or biliary tract disease.

Projectile Vomiting. Some use this term to describe vomitus which is ejected forcefully from the mouth, whereas others define it as vomiting that occurs at the peak of maximum inspiration without the rhythmic hyperactivity of the respiratory muscles noted with retching. Used in the latter sense, it may be contrasted with the "dry heaves" characterized by repeated violent and explosive rhythmic respiratory activity, leading to fatigue but to little or no vomitus. The vomiting associated with raised intracranial pressure is often referred to as projectile, is said to occur without nausea or retching, and may be precipitated by exertion or stooping. However, projectile vomiting is not a specific or sensitive indicator of intracranial hypertension.

Content of the Vomitus. The significance of old food in the vomitus suggests gastric outlet obstruction, high small bowel obstruction, or a gastric motor disorder (gastroparesis). Vomiting of undigested food suggests the possibility that the "vomitus" is from the esophagus (as in achalasia) or from an esophageal or pharyngeal (Zenker's) diverticulum. Blood or "coffee grounds" in vomitus (hematemesis) is of obvious importance (see p. 397). The presence of bile indicates an open connection between the proximal duodenum and stomach and generally excludes gastric outlet or proximal duodenal obstruction. Bilious vomiting is common after gastric surgery and is discussed below under "Specific Syndromes" as well as on page 966.

Odor of Vomitus. A feculent odor suggests intestinal obstruction, peritonitis with ileus, gastrocolic fistula, ischemic injury to the gut, or longstanding gastric outlet obstruction or stasis with secondary bacterial overgrowth of the stomach. Occasionally, feculent vomiting is seen in patients with bacterial overgrowth in the proximal small bowel.

Other Considerations. The duration of vomiting (acute versus chronic), age of the patient, presence or absence of weight loss, abdominal mass, inguinal hernia, history of prior abdominal surgery, dysphagia, chest pain, jaundice, and the presence of other diseases or conditions will weigh heavily in the initial diagnostic impression. Abdominal distention and the character of bowel sounds should be carefully evaluated in regard to the possibility of intestinal obstruction. Evidence of cardiovascular disease should suggest the possibility of intestinal ischemia.

INABILITY TO VOMIT

Certain animals, such as rats, do not vomit. In humans, a family with members who cannot vomit has been reported.[37] This autosomal dominant disorder was characterized by failure to vomit from an early age, absence of an emetic response to intravenous apomorphine, absent gag reflex, and late-onset ataxia. This constellation of findings suggests that the lesion is in the medulla and may involve the vomiting center. Many individuals develop an inability to vomit after gastric fundoplication surgery for reflux esophagitis ("gas-bloat" syndrome).

SPECIFIC SYNDROMES ASSOCIATED WITH VOMITING

Drug-Induced Nausea and Vomiting

Drugs are one of the commonest causes of nausea and vomiting. As discussed already, many drugs act on the CTZ in the area postrema to induce nausea and vomiting. The major offenders in this regard are dopamine agonists (e.g., L-dopa, bromocriptine), opiate analgesics, digitalis preparations, and cancer chemotherapy agents (e.g., cisplatin). Some drugs such as aspirin and nonsteroidal anti-inflammatory agents may induce nausea and vomiting by damaging the gastric mucosa and activating the vomiting center via ascending reflexes from the stomach. Although alcohol might induce vomiting by the same mechanism (alcoholic gastritis), a recent study has suggested that alcohol also may act centrally on the CTZ.[38] Before embarking on an expensive and possibly invasive work-up of the patient with vomiting, the physician should elicit a careful and thorough drug history, including the use of nonprescription drugs and alcohol.

Nausea and vomiting are common in cancer patients, especially those who are terminally ill,[39] and this can be exacerbated by cancer chemotherapy agents. Although many such agents are thought to act directly on the CTZ to induce nausea and vomiting, nausea and vomiting are usually delayed for two to six hours after these agents are given, suggesting that these drugs may not act directly on the CTZ.[40] It has recently been suggested that susceptibility to chemotherapy-related nausea and vomiting can be predicted if the patient has a history of motion sickness.[41] A learned anticipatory nausea and vomiting syndrome may also occur in cancer patients who receive chemotherapy[42]; this psychologic reaction can be treated in many instances by behavioral modification techniques.[43, 44]

Motion Sickness

This is a common syndrome that can occur in an automobile ("car sickness"), in an airplane ("air sickness"), at sea ("sea sickness"), or even in outer space.[45] As with drug-induced vomiting, motion sickness is readily diagnosed by history. Symptoms and signs often preceding vomiting in motion sickness include nausea, epigastric discomfort, pallor, cold sweating, headache, and hypersalivation. Of interest, these prodromal symptoms may be absent in astronauts who vomit while partaking in parabolic flight maneuvers.[45]

In motion sickness, activation of the vestibular system leads to neural activation of the vomiting center. Whether the CTZ is also involved in the emetic response to motion sickness in humans is uncertain. Motion sickness can be induced in the laboratory using a slowly rotating room or drum or a linear accelerator.[46, 47] These methods also allow laboratory evaluation of antiemetic agents for prevention of this syndrome.

A recent study used electrogastrography, a noninvasive technique which records gastric electrical activity from electrodes placed on the abdominal wall, to evaluate gastric electrical activity in 15 subjects during experimentally induced motion sickness. Ten of the subjects developed symptoms of motion sickness with a change in gastric electrical slow wave activity from the normal rate of three per minute to four to nine per minute ("tachygastria"). The other five subjects did not develop motion sickness or electrogastro-graphic changes.[47] These findings suggest that vestibular stimulation with resultant activation of the vomiting center (and perhaps the CTZ) can secondarily affect gastric motor function. Vestibular disorders other than motion sickness (e.g., labyrinthitis, Meniere's disease) are also associated with nausea and vomiting.

Gastroparesis Syndromes

Diabetic Gastroparesis. In a survey of 136 unselected patients attending a diabetes clinic, 39 (29 per cent) complained of intermittent or chronic nausea and vomiting.[48] Such patients are often labeled as having diabetic gastroparesis, implying that gastric motor dysfunction with delayed gastric emptying is the cause of vomiting. However, this term should be restricted to those patients in whom delayed gastric emptying is documented and in whom other causes of vomiting, including psychogenic vomiting,[49] can be reasonably excluded. It must also be kept in mind that diabetic gastroparesis may be present in the absence of any symptoms of nausea and vomiting. Thus, nausea and vomiting in a diabetic is not always due to gastroparesis, and conversely, gastroparesis, when present, does not always result in nausea and vomiting.

Although some diabetic patients with symptomatic gastroparesis vomit regularly, others have attacks of nausea and vomiting that last days or weeks and resolve gradually. During these attacks, glycemia becomes difficult to control, and weight loss occurs. Between attacks, few if any symptoms are present. The prototype diabetic patient with symptomatic gastroparesis is one with longstanding, insulin-dependent diabetes that has been poorly controlled for many years. Peripheral neuropathy, manifestations of autonomic neuropathy (bladder dysfunction, sweat disorder, orthostatic hypotension, impotence), nephropathy, and retinopathy are frequently found. However, there are patients in whom gastroparesis is the only diabetic complication, in whom diabetes is of fairly recent onset, or in whom diabetes is relatively easy to control.

If gastroparesis is suspected by history, an upper gastrointestinal series can be done. Findings may include residual gastric secretions or retained food despite a prolonged fast, mild gastric dilatation, poor or no peristalsis, prolonged retention of barium, patulous pylorus, and atonic duodenal bulb. To exclude pyloric obstruction as a cause of poor emptying of barium from the stomach, it may be necessary to compress the abdomen manually to express barium through the patent pylorus or, alternatively, to do an endoscopic examination. Gastric scanning after ingestion of a radiolabeled meal appears to be more a sensitive diagnostic test than an upper gastrointestinal series. It is possible to quantitate emptying of the liquid component or the solid component of the meal (or both) with this technique. Recent studies using indigestible radiopaque solid markers suggest that this radiographic technique may be even more sensitive than radio-nuclide scanning for detection of diabetic gastroparesis.[50]

There is evidence that diabetics with symptomatic gastroparesis have abnormal gastric motor function in both the fasted and postprandial states. For example, during fasting there is a reduction or absence of phase III migrating motor complexes.[51, 52] On the other hand, fasting and postprandial contractile activity of the pylorus appear to be increased in diabetics with recurrent nausea and vomiting.[53] How reduced interdigestive migrating motor activity and pylorospasm are related to gastric emptying abnormalities or symptoms of nausea and vomiting is uncertain.

Current evidence supports the notion that vagal autonomic neuropathy may be responsible for gastric motor disturbance in diabetic patients with gastroparesis. In addition to the radiologic and gastric manometric similarities between patients with diabetes and patients who have had vagotomies (see pages 939–952 and 965–966), there is also histologic[54] and physiologic[55] evidence of vagal dysfunction in diabetic patients with gastroparesis.

Diabetic ketoacidosis itself also may cause nausea, vomiting, and abdominal pain.[56] In this setting, acute gastric dilatation and gastroparesis may develop and resolve rapidly as ketoacidosis clears. In addition, some patients with diabetic ketoacidosis develop acute hemorrhagic gastritis that can cause vomiting, abdominal pain, or upper gastrointestinal bleeding.[57]

Nondiabetic Gastroparesis. It has been speculated that other conditions associated with neuropathy, such as uremia, may also produce gastroparesis. Although one study has suggested that some patients with end-stage renal disease have gastroparesis,[58] other studies have found normal gastric emptying in renal failure patients either before or after they are on chronic dialysis.[59, 60]

Disorders of gastric smooth muscle may also be capable of producing gastroparesis and delayed gastric emptying. These include scleroderma, polymyositis, and dermatomyositis.[61]

Many otherwise healthy individuals with unexplained nausea and vomiting are referred for evaluation to gastroenterologists and internists.[62] Because disorders of gastric smooth muscle and of autonomic innervation of stomach can lead to nausea and vomiting (see above section), it has been speculated that, in at least some patients, unexplained nausea and vomiting is due to an underlying gastric neuromuscular disorder (idiopathic gastroparesis). It may be difficult, if not impossible, to distinguish this syndrome from psychogenic vomiting in many patients (see below). Idiopathic gastroparesis is discussed on page 694 but will be reviewed here briefly.

Gastric emptying tests and studies measuring gastric smooth muscle function (electrical activity, contraction) have been used to evaluate patients with unexplained nausea and vomiting. Both approaches have identified patients with abnormal gastric emptying or motor function, although it is much more difficult to document that the motor abnormality is the cause of the nausea and vomiting. As already mentioned, induction of nausea by activation of the CTZ leads to a reflex delay in gastric emptying.[18] Thus, it is possible that gastric motility disorders in patients with nausea and vomiting may be secondary to nausea rather than its cause.

Some patients with nondiabetic gastroparesis have onset of their symptoms after an apparent bout of viral gastroenteritis.[63] Radiation therapy may also produce transient gastroparesis,[23] and this may be mediated by reflexes involving the CTZ.[18] However, in most cases of gastroparesis in nondiabetics, the etiology of the motor dysfunction is unknown ("idiopathic" gastroparesis). In some instances, a functional, stress-related disorder has been proposed.[64] In other cases, "idiopathic" gastroparesis seems to be part of a more generalized syndrome of gut dysmotility with intestinal pseudo-obstruction (see p. 377–379).

Several approaches have been employed to evaluate gastric smooth muscle activity in humans. Electrical activity can be measured by electrodes implanted on the serosa of the stomach at the time of laparotomy, by peroral mucosal suction electrodes, or by electrodes placed on the abdominal surface (electrogastrogram).[65] Using these techniques, regular gastric slow-wave activity can be recorded (normal frequency, three to four cycles per minute). A few nondiabetic patients with nausea and vomiting have been described in whom slow-wave activity occurred at a higher frequency than normal (e.g., six to eight cycles per minute).[65–68] This accelerated slow-wave activity was either regular ("tachygastria") or irregular ("gastric tachyarrhythmia"). Propagation of these waves was sometimes in an oral direction rather than in the usual aboral direction, suggesting a distally located ectopic pacemaker. When measured, electrical spike activity (and hence motor activity) did not occur on the plateau phase of these slow waves. Tachygastria may also be present in diabetics during episodes of nausea, with three cycles per second activity returning when nausea abates.[65]

Recently, Geldof et al. carried out an extensive electrogastrographic study of 52 healthy individuals and 48 patients with unexplained, chronic nausea and vomiting.[69] The ratio of female to male patients was almost 2:1. Twenty-three of the patients (48 per cent) had an abnormal electrogastrogram in either the fasting or postprandial state, but only eight (16 per cent) had tachygastria. Thirty patients also underwent gastric emptying scintigraphy using a radiolabeled solid meal, and 13 (43 per cent) had delayed gastric emptying; all 13 of these patients also had an abnormal electrogastrogram. Their studies suggest that abnormal gastric motor function is common in patients with unexplained nausea and vomiting and that this abnormality is often associated with delayed gastric emptying. Of interest, follow-up of patients one year later revealed that one-third had become asymptomatic without treatment and that electrogastrograms, if abnormal initially, reverted to normal, as did gastric emptying scans in the majority of patients restudied. In the patients who were still symptomatic, abnormal electrogastrograms and gastric emptying scans persisted. These studies and others[70] suggest that many patients with unexplained nausea and vomiting have disorders of gastric smooth muscle function with associated delayed gastric emptying. Whether the motor dysfunction is the cause of or the result of the symptoms of nausea and vomiting is uncertain. A salutary clinical response to therapy with dopamine antagonists in such patients[69] is consistent with either possibility because these agents increase gastric emptying and also act centrally on the CTZ to reduce nausea and vomiting.

Epidemic Vomiting

This disorder has many synonyms, including acute infectious nonbacterial gastroenteritis, epidemic nausea and vomiting, winter vomiting disease, and epidemic collapse. The disease is characterized by sudden and explosive outbreaks of profuse vomiting, often beginning in the early hours of the morning.[71] The urge to vomit is so intense that vomiting often occurs before the patient can get out of bed.[72] Headache, giddiness, muscular pains, sweating, and feverishness may also occur. Diarrhea may be a feature of some outbreaks, but not of the majority.

Immune electron microscopy has permitted detection of viral particles in the stool of a large percentage of patients in a given epidemic. These viruses include the Norwalk agent,[72] the Hawaii agent,[73] and human reovirus-like agent.[74] Infection occurs in the small bowel and not in the stomach. Gastric emptying may be abnormally slow during the acute phase of the illness.[75] Rapid recovery is the rule, although the disorder may last up to 10 days and relapses may occur for up to three weeks.

Food poisoning may cause a similar acute vomiting syndrome of epidemic proportions. In these cases, a careful history is helpful in documenting the source of contamination and the short incubation period (usually 6 to 12 hours). Organisms involved include *Staphylococcus aureus*, *Clostridium perfringens*, and *Bacillus cereus*.[76–78] Jamaican vomiting sickness is caused by ingestion of the unripe akee fruit.[79]

In the late 1970s, an epidemic illness characterized by nausea, vomiting, and epigastric pain occurred in a laboratory involved in research on acid secretion.[80] The illness was associated with acute superficial gastritis (primarily in the oxyntic mucosa) without enteritis. Marked hypochlorhydria or achlorhydria developed with gradual recovery of acid secretory capacity over several months. The exact nature of this epidemic of gastritis was uncertain, but it has been suggested but not yet proven that the illness may have been related to infection with a gastric campylobacter-like organism.[81]

Cyclical Vomiting

This syndrome is characterized by recurring attacks of severe vomiting.[82] Vomiting may recur at regular intervals, for example, every 60 days.[83] Attacks may be associated with headache, abdominal pain, and fever.[82] The onset is usually sudden, and the attack may last several days. Recovery is usually spontaneous, although the disease can threaten life acutely by producing profound dehydration and alkalosis. Between attacks patients are asymptomatic. The onset of the disease is usually before the age of six years, and the episodes may end at puberty or persist into young adulthood.[84] In some cases episodes may begin after puberty in teenagers or young adults. In cyclic vomiting the frequency of attacks varies from more than one a month to three per year.[85]

Many theories have been invoked to explain this syndrome, including chronic appendicitis, epilepsy, and migraine. In one study, headache was associated with vomiting in 16 of the 44 patients when initially examined; 9 of the 38 patients who could be traced for follow-up had recurrent headache after the vomiting had ceased.[85] A family history of migraine was obtained in 11 of the 44 patients. Some studies suggest that perinatal and postnatal brain injury and lesions may cause the disorder.[86]

Some consider the syndrome to be of psychogenic origin.[84] Parental anxiety about the health of the child and failure of the child to separate and individuate from his parents (especially the mother) are commonly present. In some cases, previous parental losses (miscarriages, still birth, loss of parents) leads to an excessive concern for their child and to labeling the child as "ill" or "weak" at any early age. The child may become dependent and may regress easily under stress.

The diagnosis of cyclic vomiting usually can be made from the history if numerous episodes of vomiting have occurred in the past. X-ray studies of the gastrointestinal tract as well as careful neurologic evaluation (including head computerized tomography) will rule out the majority of organic lesions that may produce recurrent vomiting, such as malrotation of the midgut and intracranial tumors. It is important to reach a diagnosis early so as to avoid unnecessary surgery, such as laparotomy, which will only add to the confusion when future attacks of vomiting occur (adhesions, etc.). The physician must be alert to the possibility that an earlier diagnosis of cyclic vomiting was in error; frequent re-evaluation is necessary. One child originally included in a series of cyclic vomiting turned out to have an astrocytoma.[85] Because of resemblance to migraine, one patient with cyclic vomiting was treated successfully with propranolol.[83] However, a spontaneous remission could also have explained the end of vomiting cycles in this patient.

Vomiting in Infants and Children

Vomiting is one of the most common problems encountered in infants and children. It may indicate anything from a minor feeding upset or milk allergy to intestinal obstruction, and it can be a symptom of almost any disease system.[87] A normal baby may vomit small amounts of food during or just after a meal; this may be associated with regurgitation of milk or food. Posture has a marked effect on the tendency of a baby to vomit after a meal. In the supine position, the fundus and cardia are dependent, and food accumulates there, tending to result in regurgitation. In the prone position or on the right side, food tends not to regurgitate because it is in the antrum. In these positions, gas rises to the cardia and burping tends to occur without food. The best way to hold the baby who regurgitates or vomits is in the right antero-oblique position,[87] although from a practical standpoint placing the child in an infant seat for one hour after meals is usually sufficient.

Loss of weight, failure to gain weight, presence of bile in the vomitus, and abdominal distention in association with vomiting or regurgitation are abnormal and their presence demands a thorough evaluation. Various congenital lesions that are incompatible with life (e.g., hypertrophic pyloric stenosis) do not necessarily give symptoms immediately after birth. A diagnosis of pneumonia, vomiting caused by feeding difficulty, gastroenteritis, or "failure to thrive" in the first week of life may well be in error, with the symptoms caused in fact by congenital defects.[87] It should be recalled that vomiting is only a symptom and that renal lesions and disease of other organs (including intracranial birth injuries) may produce vomiting in infancy.

If the vomiting has any suspicious features, including persistence, it is important to inquire about the passage of meconium, to perform a rectal examination, and to look carefully for evidence of abdominal distention. Repeated physical examinations are necessary in order to make the correct diagnosis and to prevent a potentially fatal outcome. X-rays of the abdomen and in some instances of the gastrointestinal tract are often of great value in these patients. Some of the serious causes of vomiting at different ages are listed in Table 14–1.

Nausea and Vomiting during Pregnancy

Nausea and Vomiting of Pregnancy. Nausea occurs in 50 to 90 per cent of all pregnancies and vomiting in 25 to 55 per cent.[96–99] The onset is usually shortly after the first missed menstrual period (rarely before), and thus, symptoms may begin before the woman or her physician recognizes that pregnancy has occurred. Although nausea and vomiting may be caused by gallbladder disease,[96] gastritis,[96] food allergies,[96, 100] and other conditions, in the majority of women the etiology is unknown. Nausea and vomiting may be more common in primigravidas, younger women, nonsmokers, obese women, women with less than 12 years of education,[97] women who had experienced nausea and vomiting while receiving oral contraceptive medication,[96] and women with a corpus luteum primarily on the right side of the uterus rather than on the left side.[101] Nausea, sometimes accompanied by vomiting, is especially prevalent in the morning, although in

Table 14–1. SOME SERIOUS CAUSES OF VOMITING IN CHILDREN[88–95]

Age	Cause	Comments
Newborn	Tracheoesophageal fistula	Hypersalivation; cyanosis and choking with meals; abdominal distention often present
	Hypertrophic pyloric stenosis	Male predominance; symptoms onset before seven weeks but not immediately after birth; absence of bile in vomitus; palpable "olive" rarely present; high serum gastrin concentration[88]
	Duodenal atresia	Air-fluid levels in stomach and duodenum ("double-bubble")
	Intestinal atresia, stenosis, diaphragms	May produce vomiting in utero with bile-stained amniotic fluid[89]
	Meconium ileus	May signify cystic fibrosis
	Midgut volvulus with malrotation	Intermittent vomiting
	Miscellaneous	Brain injury; sepsis; adrenal insufficiency; narcotic addiction; inherited and metabolic disorders (e.g., galactosemia)
Infancy and childhood	Intussusception	"Currant jelly" stool; mass; colicky pain
	Appendicitis	See Chapter 74 (Acute Appendicitis)
	Gastroesophageal reflux	Respiratory symptoms may be prominent[90, 91]; weight loss; may be associated with antral dysmotility[92]
	Reye's syndrome	Encephalopathy and fatty liver[93]; association with viruses (e.g., influenza) and aspirin[94, 95]
	Miscellaneous	Peptic ulcer; pneumonia; viral hepatitis; intracranial tumors; inherited and metabolic disorders (e.g., fructose intolerance)

some instances these symptoms may persist throughout the day. The term "nausea and vomiting of pregnancy" implies that the woman has not developed fluid and electrolyte derangements or nutritional deficiency. The term hyperemesis gravidarium should be used if these complications are present (see below).

Nausea and vomiting during early pregnancy is often associated with sleep disturbances, fatigue, and irritability. Symptoms usually disappear by the fourth month of pregnancy, although in some cases, especially those with psychologic or psychiatric problems, the symptoms may persist into the third trimester.[98] Women who have nausea and vomiting during a particular pregnancy are more likely to have these symptoms during subsequent pregnancies,[97] but such recurrent symptoms are not invariable. Fetuses born to mothers

with "nausea and vomiting of pregnancy" have birth weights similar to fetuses born to mothers without these symptoms.[97] Furthermore, the incidence of fetal death is actually lower than normal in mothers with "nausea and vomiting of pregnancy."[99] There is no evidence that the offspring of women who have "nausea and vomiting of pregnancy" have an increased incidence of congenital malformations.[102] Thus, the prognosis for mother and child is generally excellent.

The pathogenesis of "nausea and vomiting of pregnancy" is obscure. There are two leading theories: hormonal and psychologic. Although abnormal serum levels of human chorionic gonadotropin,[103] progesterone,[104] and androgens[104] have been reported in emetic subjects, results have not been consistent from study to study. Psychologic studies suggest that women with "nausea and vomiting of pregnancy" are more likely to have had an undesired pregnancy and have negative relationships with their mothers.[98]

Treatment of nausea and vomiting of pregnancy consists primarily of reassurance that the condition is very common and temporary along with in-office supportive psychotherapy if indicated. It may be necessary to prescribe an antiemetic drug (see below).

Hyperemesis Gravidarum. Hyperemesis gravidarum, also called pernicious vomiting of pregnancy, refers to those patients who develop fluid and electrolyte disturbances or nutritional deficiency from intractable vomiting in early pregnancy. As in milder cases, the onset of symptoms tends to be soon after the first missed menstrual period. Classically the vomiting disappears during the third month, and rarely persists into the fourth month, although Guze and his colleagues reported that 60 per cent of their patients vomited during more than half of the pregnancy.[105]

The reported incidence of hyperemesis gravidarum varies considerably, with an average figure of 3.5 per 1000 deliveries. The incidence is not increased by parity, race, color, or the desire for an abortion but is markedly decreased during wartime.[106] Patients with hyperemesis gravidarum do not have an increased incidence of toxemia of pregnancy or spontaneous abortion, and their babies are not underweight or deformed.

Women with twins or with molar pregnancy (hydatidiform mole) have an increased incidence of hyperemesis gravidarum. These women have elevated concentrations of human chorionic gonadotropin (HCG). However, the relationship between elevated HCG and hyperemesis has not been convincingly demonstrated. Abnormalities of thyroid function tests are also common in hyperemesis gravidarum,[107–110] although their significance is uncertain. Because hyperthyroidism can cause vomiting *per se*,[5] including during pregnancy,[111] these observations are intriguing and deserve further study.

In a postpartum follow-up study, Guze et al. found that hysteria was present in 15 per cent of patients who had had hyperemesis gravidarum, compared with only 2 per cent of control subjects.[105] In other ways the vomiters were no different from the control subjects, and 41 per cent of the vomiters were without any psychologic illness at the time of follow-up. Harvey and Sherfey[112] regularly obtained a clear-cut history of previous vomiting in response to emotional disturbance in 19 of their 20 patients. They also reported a strikingly high incidence of emotional immaturity, undue maternal attachment, and sexual maladjustment. The facts that hyperemesis gravidarum is seen only in humans, that it is treatable by hypnosis and other forms of suggestion, that its incidence markedly decreases during wartime, and that it rarely occurs in primitive countries are further suggestive evidence of a psychosomatic etiology, although there is still controversy about the nature of and importance of psychologic derangements.[112-115]

The metabolic consequences of hyperemesis gravidarum can be severe, and the mortality rate in untreated patients is high. Salt and water depletion and potassium deficiency may be marked. Treatment of hyperemesis gravidarum is mainly directed at fluid and electrolyte replacement and supportive psychotherapy. Behavior modification techniques may also be effective.[116]

Acute Fatty Liver of Late Pregnancy.[117] This is a serious condition of unknown etiology, occurring in approximately 1 in 13,000 deliveries. Symptoms of nausea, vomiting, headache, and malaise begin in the third trimester, usually around week 35. Features of the pre-eclampsia syndrome (hypertension, edema, proteinuria) may also be present. The disease often progresses to hepatic failure complicated by disseminated intravascular coagulation. If nausea and vomiting begin in the latter part of pregnancy, serum aminotransferase activity should be measured. An elevated aminotransferase in the 200 to 500 range (Karmen units/ml) is an indication for liver biopsy (assuming coagulation tests permit). The characteristic finding on biopsy is microvesicular fat. Once this diagnosis is established, pregnancy termination is indicated to prevent maternal and fetal death. Differential diagnosis includes fulminant viral hepatitis and tetracycline hepatotoxicity.

Bilious Vomiting after Gastric Surgery

Bilious vomiting can be a crippling long-term complication of the surgical treatment of peptic ulcer.[118] In a severe case, the patient vomits clear bile-stained fluid, which does not contain food, soon after each meal. This feature distinguishes it from gastric outlet obstruction, in which case the vomitus contains food. The pathogenesis, diagnosis, and treatment of this syndrome are discussed on page 966.

Superior Mesenteric Artery (SMA) Syndrome

The SMA branches off the aorta at an acute angle and, traveling in the root of the mesentery, crosses over the duodenum, usually just to the right of the midline (see p. 1904). In rare instances the SMA may obstruct the duodenum as it crosses over it, possibly because of a more acute angle than normal between the aorta and SMA, leading to dilatation of the proximal duodenum and stomach.[119-121]

Symptoms attributed to this condition include epigastric fullness and bloating after meals, bilious vomiting, and midabdominal crampy pain that may be relieved by the prone or knee-chest position. Precipitating factors include prolonged bed rest, weight loss, previous abdominal surgery, increased lordosis (including use of body casts), and loss of tone in the abdominal wall musculature. The syndrome has been reported in conjunction with pancreatitis, peptic ulcer, and other intra-abdominal inflammatory conditions. On barium examination, the stomach and proximal duodenum may be dilated, with a sharp duodenal cut-off just to the right of the midline (Fig. 14–3). Dilatation of the proximal duodenum may also be due to atony and stasis (e.g., due to scleroderma or diabetes) rather than actual obstruction by the SMA.[122]

Treatment of the acute syndrome is decompression by nasogastric tube and intravenous fluid and electrolyte replacement. The patient with intermittent attacks is a difficult therapeutic problem. Many surgical techniques have been employed over the past 75 years, the most effective being duodenojejunostomy, based upon uncontrolled observations. Gastrojejunostomy may fail

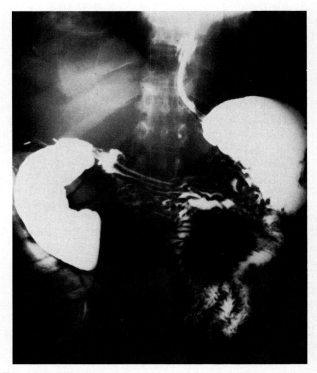

Figure 14–3. Barium examination in a 64-year-old man who developed intermittent bilious vomiting during a prolonged hospitalization for infection of a hip prosthesis. During the hospitalization he was bedridden and had lost considerable weight. Radiograph shows sharp cutoff of contrast material at the third portion of the duodenum, a finding compatible with superior mesenteric artery syndrome.

because it does not adequately decompress the duodenum.[123] Despite several reports describing the SMA syndrome, many physicians remain skeptical about its existence.[124-126]

Psychogenic Vomiting[127-130]

Chronic or recurrent vomiting, especially in young women, may be caused by underlying emotional disturbance. The latter is often related to sexual and marital conflicts, but may also be caused by health problems of relatives (e.g., alcoholism, aging, senility of parents) as well as by more deep-seated problems, such as loss of parental affection. Psychogenic vomiting may on rare occasions also be related to depression.[131]

Psychogenic vomiting may be recognized by the following features:

1. The vomiting has usually been present for years, either chronically or intermittently. Frequently, history will reveal vomiting in childhood or while in high school when under emotional strain.

2. There is often a family history of vomiting.

3. The vomiting typically occurs soon after the meal has begun (even after just a few bites) or just after it has been completed. Delayed vomiting does not occur.

4. Vomiting may be unaccompanied by preceding nausea and may be self-induced.

5. Vomiting can be suppressed if necessary. Thus, vomiting can be suppressed voluntarily until the patient reaches a toilet.

6. Vomiting may be of relatively little concern to the patient. Instead, members of the family may insist on the patient seeing a physician.

7. Despite nausea or vomiting, appetite is usually normal unless the patient also has a coexistent eating disorder such as anorexia nervosa or bulimia (see pp. 185–194). Most patients are thin and in some weight loss may be profound.

8. Vomiting may subside shortly after hospitalization, perhaps because the patient has been removed from a stressful situation.

Although organic disease must first be ruled out by appropriate tests, the history of these patients is often so typical that the diagnosis may be strongly suspected on this basis alone. It is important that the correct diagnosis be made quickly so that the patient is not subjected to unnecessary and expensive diagnostic procedures or to abdominal surgery, which may worsen and complicate the issue. It should also be recognized that patients with psychogenic vomiting may in time develop a second disease, and the physician should be alert for a change in the pattern of the illness.

Hill[127] studied 20 patients (15 females and five males) with psychogenic vomiting and compared them with a control group consisting of 22 patients suffering from abdominal pain for which no cause could be found (the abdominal pain was apparently of psychogenic origin in the control subjects). Three of the vomiting patients had suffered from paralysis, probably caused by potassium deficiency. Ten had lost 14 lb or more in weight. Only one of the patients had menstrual irregularity. Twelve of the 20 patients were living with a person to whom they were fundamentally antagonistic. The others experienced antagonism to other important people in their lives. In the control group, only two were involved in a comparable domestic situation. Nine of 20 psychogenic vomiters had lost a parent before age 15, and three others had had a significant separation experience in their lives, while this had occurred in only three of the control group. Ten of the vomiters gave a history of spells of vomiting during childhood, often at time of separation. In the control group, only one gave such a history. Nine of the vomiters gave a family history of functional or persistent organic vomiting, compared with none of the control group. Hill concluded that psychogenic vomiters are trapped in a hostile relationship, and especially significant is the fact that they often shared the same house and ate with the source of their antagonism. (In the control group, hostile relationships were less common and, more important, were outside rather than inside the family unit, so that the patient did not have to eat with the source of his or her antipathy.) The greater frequency of this disorder in women than in men may be due to the greater passivity of the female when faced with an unsatisfactory relationship. Thus, none of the vomiters had taken active steps to break off an unsatisfactory relationship, whereas two in the control series had. The experience of a major loss in childhood may have made these patients reluctant to accept another loss in later life.

Whether patients with psychogenic vomiting improve with antiemetic drugs has not been studied carefully; the impression of the author is that they do not. It is generally agreed that surgery (such as gastroenterostomy) is of no help. It has been stated that some patients may improve with verbal catharsis and psychologic support, while others have little insight and respond poorly to psychotherapy.[129] In one study most patients were still vomiting on follow-up approximately one and one-half years later, although to a lesser degree in many instances.[128]

A number of variants of the psychogenic vomiting syndrome have been described.

Self-Induced Vomiting. This is most commonly seen in young women with eating disorders such as anorexia nervosa and bulimia (see pp. 185–194). These individuals may also abuse laxatives and diuretics in order to lose weight.[132]

Concealed (Surreptitious) Vomiting.[133-135] Surreptitious vomiting is not rare, and one needs a high index of suspicion and some ingenuity to make and confirm the correct diagnosis. Patients may become highly skilled in their ability to conceal vomiting. Most have no organic cause for the vomiting, although some patients with organic disease of the stomach deny vomiting, either because of secondary gain from the medical curiosity aroused by their metabolic disturbances or in order to prevent others from knowing of their illness. Concealed vomiting may lead to metabolic derangements, suggesting the presence of serious organic disease (see below).

Erotic Vomiting. In some women with underlying psychologic aberrations, it has been suggested that vomiting is induced in order to obtain sexual gratification.[136]

CONSEQUENCES OF VOMITING

Metabolic Derangements (Fig. 14–4). Potassium deficiency results from decreased intake of potassium, from loss of potassium in the vomitus and, most important, from renal potassium wasting. Alkalosis, if severe, is associated with delivery of sodium bicarbonate to the kidneys at a rate which exceeds the renal tubular maximum (Tm) for bicarbonate reabsorption. Because of Na^+/K^+ exchange in the distal tubule, renal K^+ loss will occur (as potassium bicarbonate). Sodium and volume depletion may enhance this distal Na^+/K^+ exchange via the renin-angiotensin-aldosterone pathway. The clinical features of potassium deficiency include muscle weakness, constipation, polydipsia, nocturia, impaired urinary concentration, and cardiac arrhythmia (particularly ventricular ectopy).

Alkalosis develops because of (a) loss of hydrogen ions in the vomitus; (b) contraction of the extracellular fluid space without a commensurate loss of extracellular bicarbonate from this compartment; and (c) a shift of hydrogen ions into cells caused by potassium deficiency.

Sodium depletion develops because of loss of sodium in the vomitus and in some cases because of renal sodium loss in association with bicarbonate excretion (if the bicarbonate Tm is exceeded). The clinical features of sodium depletion may include hyponatremia (not always present), hypotension, oliguria, decreased blood volume, and hemoconcentration. Plasma renin and aldosterone levels are elevated and creatinine clearance is reduced. Recent studies indicate that nausea and vomiting stimulate release of antidiuretic hormone (ADH), presumably via a reflex mechanism.[30-34] Excessive ADH release could contribute to hyponatremia and oliguria in some patients.[33]

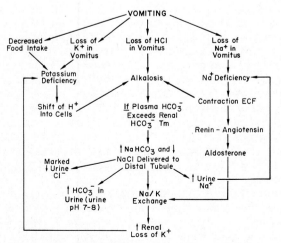

Figure 14–4. Metabolic consequences of vomiting.

Table 14–2. DIFFERENTIAL DIAGNOSIS OF UNEXPLAINED HYPOCHLOREMIC HYPOKALEMIC METABOLIC ALKALOSIS

Condition	Comments
Concealed (surreptitious) vomiting	See page 232
Surreptitious diuretic use[132]	Laxative abuse common
Bartter's syndrome[138]	Hyperplasia of juxtaglomerular apparatus*; decreased responsiveness to angiotensin*; normotension
Primary hyperaldosteronism	Hypertension; absence of weight loss and hyponatremia
Milk-alkali syndrome	Antacid ingestion; azotemia; may be complicated by vomiting
Welt's syndrome[139]	Renal wasting of potassium and magnesium; hypomagnesemia; familial disorder
Hypokalemic periodic paralysis	Familial disorder

*May be seen in patients with chronic vomiting also.

The urinary findings vary depending on whether or not the renal Tm for bicarbonate is exceeded.[137] If the Tm is not exceeded, the urine will not contain a high concentration of bicarbonate, the urinary pH will vary within the normal range, and urinary levels of Na^+, K^+, and Cl^- will be low, correctly suggesting extrarenal loss of these ions. On the other hand, if the Tm for bicarbonate is exceeded, urinary bicarbonate will be high, the urinary pH will be alkaline, and urinary Na^+ and K^+ will be high (even in the face of Na^+ and K^+ depletion); however, urinary Cl^- will still be low, accurately reflecting that the metabolic alkalosis is due to nonrenal losses.

Although the cause of these metabolic derangements will be obvious, if there is a history of vomiting, great diagnostic difficulty will arise if vomiting is concealed by the patient. The differential diagnosis is listed in Table 14–2.

Nutritional. Chronic nausea and vomiting may lead to reduced caloric intake or loss of ingested calories in vomitus. Thus, regardless of etiology, nausea and vomiting may result in malnutrition and various deficiency states (see pp. 1983–1994).

Emetic Injuries to Esophagus and Stomach. Vomiting can lead to Mallory-Weiss lacerations and upper gastrointestinal bleeding (see p. 410). Vomiting can also lead to a deeper laceration involving the wall of the esophagus with a resultant confined intramural perforation or a transmural tear of the esophagus (or rarely the stomach[140]) with free perforation (Boerhaave's syndrome). These complications may necessitate urgent surgery and can be fatal (see p. 647).

Dental Disease. Chronic vomiting may result in dental erosions and caries.[141]

Purpura. These cutaneous lesions may appear after prolonged vomiting and are acute, evanescent, pinhead-sized red macules on the face and upper neck ("mask phenomenon").[142] This eruption is probably related to a suddenly increased intrathoracic pressure. Similar skin lesions can also occur during prolonged coughing or during a Valsalva maneuver. Thus, the pathogenesis resembles that of Mallory-Weiss syndrome.

THERAPY OF VOMITING

If the cause of nausea and vomiting can be treated (e.g., gastric outlet obstruction, diabetic ketoacidosis), antiemetic drugs are not necessary. In other instances, such as morning sickness, frequent small feedings and reassurance may suffice. However, in some situations drug therapy may be indicated.

Antihistamines of the H_1 type are effective in morning sickness but some of these compounds, such as meclizine and cyclizine, are teratogenic in animals and thus should be used with caution. Antihistamines are also useful in motion sickness or vomiting due to other vestibular disorders. *Anticholinergics* such as scopolamine are also effective in motion sickness, and this compound may be given as a transdermal patch for prophylactic therapy.

Phenothiazines, such as prochlorperazine (Compazine) and chlorpromazine (Thorazine) or the structurally related butyrophenone haloperidol (Haldol), are effective in vomiting due to drugs (e.g., opioids, anesthetics, cancer chemotherapy agents), radiation, and gastroenteritis.[143] Phenothiazines have antihistaminic and anticholinergic properties; they also decrease dopamine transmission in the CTZ and reduce afferent signals to the vomiting center from the gut. The most common side effect is sedation. These drugs may have more serious side effects (blood dyscrasia, jaundice, extrapyramidal reactions) and therefore should be used cautiously.

Dopaminergic antagonists such as metoclopramide are useful in preventing vomiting induced by anesthetics or by cancer chemotherapy agents, although large doses such as 2 mg/kg IV may be required to prevent cisplatin-induced emesis.[44, 144] It is unclear whether the antiemetic action of metoclopramide, for example, in cisplatin-induced emesis, is due to a central dopamine antagonist action or, quite possibly, a peripheral action by enhancing gastric motility.[145] Metoclopramide, in an oral dose of 10 to 20 mg before meals, is also effective in some patients with diabetic gastroparesis[146] and in postvagotomy gastroparesis.[147] Another newer dopamine antagonist, domperidone, which is structurally related to phenothiazines, also enhances gastric motility and may have fewer CNS side effects than metoclopramide.[25]

Tetrahydrocannabinol (THC), the active ingredient of marijuana, is more effective than placebo in preventing nausea and vomiting after cancer chemotherapy, and in some studies THC has been more effective than a phenothiazine.[148, 149] THC has been marketed recently as dronabinol (Marinol). Commonest side effects are drowsiness, orthostatic hypotension, tachycardia, and dry mouth. Anxiety, depression, visual hallucinations, and manic psychosis may occur, especially in older individuals and patients who have never used marijuana. The antiemetic site of action of THC is uncertain.

In addition to phenothiazines, metoclopramide, and dronabinol, high-dose dexamethasone and also adrenocorticotropic hormone have been reported to be effective in preventing chemotherapy-induced emesis.[150, 151] Although these agents are less impressive as single agents, they may be useful in combination with other agents.[44] Their mechanism of action is uncertain. Thus, several drugs are useful in prevention of chemotherapy-induced emesis, and in the future, combinations of drugs may prove to be more efficacious than a single drug. A list of cancer chemotherapy agents most likely to cause nausea (e.g., cisplatin, dacarbazine, actinomycin D) and those least likely to cause vomiting (e.g., vincristine, bleomycin, chlorambucil) has been published recently,[152] as has an algorithm for choosing antiemetic agents.[153]

Although drugs represent the conventional approach to the therapy of nausea and vomiting, other nonpharmacologic approaches may be efficacious in certain settings. These include behavior modification treatment (e.g., in cancer chemotherapy-induced emesis[43, 44, 154] and in idiopathic gastric stasis[155]) and acupuncture (e.g., in perioperative vomiting[156]).

RUMINATION

Rumination is distinct from vomiting and consists of regurgitating food, one mouthful at a time, from the stomach to the mouth, chewing the food again, and reswallowing it.[157] Regurgitation is usually involuntary, effortless, and not associated with abdominal discomfort, heartburn, or nausea. Rumination usually begins 15 to 30 minutes after a meal and lasts for about one hour. During this period the patient will ruminate up to 20 times. Rumination characteristically ceases when the food becomes acid to taste. It is apparently a pleasant sensation, but often embarrassing, so that patients tend to hide the fact that they reswallow their food. Rumination can be suppressed voluntarily, at least in some instances.

The cause and mechanism of rumination in adults are unknown, although nearly all authors conclude that psychologic factors are important.[157] Recent manometric studies have demonstrated that the underlying esophageal, gastric, and upper small intestinal motility are normal. Associated with regurgitation are spike waves corresponding to increases in intra-abdominal pressure. It has been suggested that rumination is triggered by a forced inspiration against a closed glottis (Mueller maneuver).[158] Regurgitation may be associated with acid reflux, both of which may respond to biofeedback therapy.[159] Although rumination in adults is rare it is important to be aware of this entity so that needless surgery (such as hiatal hernia repair) can be avoided.

Rumination in infants is associated with failure to thrive, marasmus, and even death, if untreated.[160] Typically, previously ingested food is regurgitated, rechewed, and some is then reswallowed. The syndrome may be caused by an abnormal mother-child relationship. The mothers of these infants tend to be immature and unable to develop a close and comfortable relationship with the baby. The rumination process is interpreted as an effort to recreate the gratification of the feeding process in an emotionally deprived infant. Hospitalization will often bring improvement, provided that hospital personnel can take on the role of a loving mother.[160, 161] In one instance in which rumination and vomiting were life-threatening, an infant was treated by "conditioning therapy." Electric shock was given each time the baby ruminated, and within a few brief sessions vomiting and rumination ceased, and weight gain and other improvements were noted.[162] This observation suggests that rumination may be a learned habit (i.e., a conditioned response). Rumination is also not uncommon in mentally retarded children, and may be treated successfully by various behavior modifications.[163, 164]

The differential diagnosis of rumination in infants and children includes gastroesophageal incompetence, hiatal hernia, drug reaction (including drugs given to the mother), diencephalic seizures, hypothalamic tumors, milk allergy, and metabolic disorders such as fructose intolerance, as well as some of the conditions mentioned in Table 14–1.

References

1. Hanson, J. S., and McCallum, R. W. The diagnosis and management of nausea and vomiting: A review. Am. J. Gastroenterol. 80:210, 1985.
2. Ruscone, T. G., Guzzetti, S., Lombardi, F., and Lombardi, R. Lack of association between prodromes nausea and vomiting, and specific electrocardiographic patterns of acute myocardial infarction. Internat. J. Cardiol. 11:17, 1986.
3. Schreier, L., Cutler, R. M., and Saigal, V. The vomiting asthmatic. Ann. Allergy 53:42, 1984.
4. Mignon, M., Bonnefond, A., Gratton, J., and Bonfils, S. Repeated vomiting of gastric juice in a patient with Zollinger-Ellison syndrome. Modifying influence upon clinical features. Dig. Dis. Sci. 26:752, 1981.
5. Rosenthal, F. D., Jones, C., and Lewis, S. I. Thyrotoxic vomiting. Br. Med. J. 2:209, 1976.
6. Mitchell, W. G., Greenwood, R. S., and Messenheimer, J. A. Abdominal epilepsy: Cyclic vomiting as the major symptom of simple partial seizures. Arch. Neurol. 40:251, 1983.
7. Lumsden, K., and Holden, W. S. The act of vomiting in man. Gut 10:173, 1969.
8. Finestone, H. M., and Clifford, J. C. "Dry heaves": The sole presenting complaint in a case of ruptured abdominal aortic aneurysm. Can. Med. Assoc. J. 135:1154, 1986.
9. Melzack, R., Rosberger, Z., Hollingsworth, M. L., and Thirlwell, M. New approaches to measuring nausea. Can. Med. Assoc. J. 133:755, 1985.
10. Verbalis, J. G., McCann, M. J., McHale, C. M., and Stricker, E. M. Oxytocin secretion in response to cholecystokinin and food: Differentiation of nausea from satiety. Science 232:1417, 1986.
11. Ingelfinger, F. J., and Moss, R. E. The activity of the descending duodenum during nausea. Am. J. Physiol. 136:561, 1942.
12. Johnson, H. D., and Laws, J. W. The cardia in swallowing, eructation and vomiting. Lancet 2:1268, 1966.
13. McCarthy, L. E., Borison, H. L., Spiegel, P. K., and Friedlander, R. M. Vomiting: Radiographic and oscillographic correlates in the decerebrate cat. Gastroenterology 67:1126, 1974.
14. Akwari, O. E. The gastrointestinal tract in chemotherapy-induced emesis. A final common pathway. Drugs 25(Suppl. 1):18, 1983.
15. Wilson, C. L., and Davis, S. J. Recurrent atrial fibrillation
16. Lyon, L. J., and Nevins, M. A. Retching and termination of ventricular tachycardia. Chest 74:110, 1978.
17. Borison, H. L., and Wang, S. C. Physiology and pharmacology of vomiting. Pharmacol. Rev. 5:193, 1953.
18. Borison, H. L., Borison, R., and McCarthy, L. E. Role of the area postrema in vomiting and related functions. Fed. Proc. 43:2955, 1984.
19. Baker, P. C. H., and Bernat, J. L. The neuroanatomy of vomiting in man: Association of projectile vomiting with a solitary metastasis in the lateral tegmentum of the pons and the middle cerebellar peduncle. J. Neurol. Neurosurg. Psychiat. 48:1165, 1985.
20. Wislocki, G. B., and Putnam, T. J. Note on the anatomy of the area postrema. Anat. Rev. 19:281, 1920.
21. Rabin, B. M., Hunt, W. A., Chedester, A. L., and Lee, J. Role of the area postrema in radiation-induced taste aversion learning and emesis in cats. Physiol. Behav. 37:815, 1986.
22. Wilpizeski, C. R., Lowry, L. D., and Goldman, W. S. Motion-induced sickness following bilateral ablation of area postrema in squirrel monkeys. Laryngoscope 96:1221, 1986.
23. Souskes, T. L. Neural and neuroendocrine functions of dopamine. Psychoneuroendocrinology 1:69, 1975.
24. Pinder, R. M., Brogden, R. N., Sawyer, P. R., Speight, T. M., and Avery, G. S. Metoclopramide: A review of its pharmacologic properties and clinical use. Drugs 12:81, 1976.
25. Reyntjens, A. Domperidone as an anti-emetic; summary of research reports. Postgrad. Med. J. 55(Suppl. 1):50, 1979.
26. Pickel, V. M., and Armstrong, D. M. Ultrastructural localization of monoamines and peptides in rat area postrema. Fed. Proc. 43:2949, 1984.
27. Carpenter, D. O., Briggs, D. B., and Strominger, N. Behavioral and electrophysiological studies of peptide-induced emesis in dogs. Fed. Proc. 43:2952, 1984.
28. Layer, P., Demol, P., Hotz, J., and Goebell, H. Gastroparesis after radiation. Successful treatment with carbachol. Dig. Dis. Sci. 31:1377, 1986.
29. Barnes, K. L., Ferrario, C. M., Chernicky, C. L., and Brosnihan, K. B. Participation of the area postrema in cardiovascular control in the dog. Fed. Proc. 43:2959, 1984.
30. Rowe, J. W., Shelton, R. L., Helderman, J. H., Vestal, R. E., and Robertson, G. L. Influence of the emetic reflex on vasopressin release in man. Kidney Internat. 16:729, 1979.
31. Fisher, R. D., Rentschler, R. E., Nelson, J. C., Godfrey, T. E., and Wilbur, D. W. Elevation of plasma antidiuretic hormone (ADH) associated with chemotherapy-induced emesis in man. Cancer Treatment Reports 66:25, 1982.
32. Sorensen, P. S., and Hammer, M. Vasopressin in plasma and ventricular cerebrospinal fluid during dehydration, postural changes, and nausea. Am. J. Physiol. 248:R78, 1985.
33. Coslovsky, R., Bruck, R., Estrov, Z. Hypo-osmolal syndrome due to prolonged nausea. Arch. Intern. Med. 144:191, 1984.
34. Grant, P. J., Hughes, J. R., Dean, H. G., Davies, J. A., and Prentice, C. R. M. Vasopressin and catecholamine secretion during apomorphine-induced nausea mediate acute changes in haemostatic function in man. Clin. Sci. 71:621, 1986.
35. Brizzee, K. R., and Klara, P. M. The structure of the mammalian area postrema. Fed. Proc. 43:2944, 1984.
36. Leslie, R. A., and Gwyn, D. G. Neuronal connections of the area postrema. Fed. Proc. 43:2941, 1984.
37. McLellan, D. L., and Park, D. M. Failure to vomit in hereditary ataxia. Report of a family. Neurology 23:725, 1973.
38. Shen, W. W. Potential link between hallucination and nausea/vomiting induced by alcohol? Psychopathology 18:212, 1985.
39. Reuben, D. B., and Mor, V. Nausea and vomiting in terminal cancer patients. Arch. Intern. Med. 146:2021, 1986.
40. Borison, H. L., and McCarthy, L. E. Neuropharmacology of chemotherapy-induced emesis. Drugs 25(Suppl. 1):8, 1983.
41. Morrow, G. R. The effect of a susceptibility to motion sickness on the side effects of cancer chemotherapy. Cancer 55:2766, 1985.
42. Cella, D. F., Pratt, A., and Holland, J. C. Persistent anticipatory nausea, vomiting, and anxiety in cured Hodgkin's dis-

ease patients after completion of chemotherapy. Am. J. Psychiatry *143*:641, 1986.

43. Morrow, G. R., and Morrell, C. Behavioral treatment for the anticipatory nausea and vomiting induced by cancer chemotherapy. N. Engl. J. Med. *307*:1476, 1982.

44. Eyre, H. J., and Ward, J. H. Control of cancer chemotherapy-induced nausea and vomiting. Cancer *54*:2642, 1984.

45. Lackner, J. R., and Graybiel, A. Sudden emesis following parabolic flight maneuvers: Implications for space motion sickness. Aviat. Space Environ. Med. *57*:343, 1986.

46. Pyykko, I., Schalen, L., and Jantti, V. Transdermally administered scopolamine vs. dimenhydrinate. I. Effect on nausea and vomiting in experimentally induced motion sickness. Acta Otolaryngol. (Stockh.) *99*:588, 1985.

47. Stern, R. M., Koch, K. L., Stewart, W. R., and Lindblad, I. M. Spectral analysis of tachygastria recorded during motion sickness. Gastroenterology *92*:92, 1987.

48. Feldman, M., and Schiller, L. R. Disorders of gastrointestinal motility associated with diabetes mellitus. Ann. Intern. Med. *98*:378, 1983.

49. Berlin, R. M., and Wise, T. N. Severe vomiting in a diabetic woman. Psychological considerations. Gen. Hosp. Psychiatry *2*:313, 1980.

50. Feldman, M., Smith, H. J., and Simon, T. R. Gastric emptying of solid radiopaque markers: Studies in healthy subjects and diabetic patients. Gastroenterology *87*:895, 1984.

51. Malagelada, J.-R., Rees, W. D. W., Mazzotta, L. J., and Go, V. L. W. Gastric motor abnormalities in diabetic and postvagotomy gastroparesis: Effect of metoclopramide and bethanechol. Gastroenterology *78*:286, 1980.

52. Fox, S., and Behar, J. Pathogenesis of diabetic gastroparesis: A pharmacologic study. Gastroenterology *78*:757, 1980.

53. Mearin, F., Camilleri, M., and Malagelada, J.-R. Pyloric dysfunction in diabetics with recurrent nausea and vomiting. Gastroenterology *90*:1919, 1986.

54. Kristensson, K., Nordborg, C., Olsson, Y., and Sourander, P. Changes in the vagus nerve in diabetes mellitus. Acta Pathol. Microbiol. Scand. *79*:684, 1971.

55. Feldman, M., Corbett, D. B., Ramsey, E. J., Walsh, J. H., and Richardson, C. T. Abnormal gastric function in longstanding insulin-dependent diabetic patients. Gastroenterology *77*:12, 1979.

56. Beardwood, J. T. The abdominal symptomatology of diabetic acidosis. JAMA *105*:1168, 1935.

57. Carandang, N., Schuman, B. M., and Whitehouse, F. W. The gastric mucosa of patients in diabetic ketoacidosis. A gastrocamera study. Diabetes *17*:319, 1968.

58. McNamee, P. T., Moore, G. W., McGeown, M. G., Doherty, C. C., and Collins, B. J. Gastric emptying in chronic renal failure. Br. Med. J. *291*:310–311, 1985.

59. Freeman, J. G., Cobden, I., Heaton, A., and Keir, M. Gastric emptying in chronic renal failure. Br. Med. J. *291*:1048, 1985.

60. Wright, R. A., Clemente, R., and Wathen, R. Gastric emptying in patients with chronic renal failure receiving hemodialysis. Arch. Intern. Med. *144*:495, 1984.

61. Horowitz, M., McNeil, J. D., Maddern, G. J., Collins, P. J., and Shearman, D. J. C. Abnormalities of gastric and esophageal emptying in polymyositis and dermatomyositis. Gastroenterology *90*:434, 1986.

62. Malagelada, J.-R., and Camilleri, M. Unexplained vomiting: A diagnostic challenge. Ann. Intern. Med. *101*:211, 1984.

63. Rhodes, J. B., Robinson, R. G., and McBride, N. Sudden onset of slow gastric emptying of food. Gastroenterology *77*:569, 1979.

64. Camilleri, M., Malagelada, J.-R., Kao, P. C., and Zinsmeister, A. R. Gastric and autonomic responses to stress in functional dyspepsia. Dig. Dis. Sci. *31*:1169, 1986.

65. Hamilton, J. W., Bellahsene, B. E., Reichelderfer, M., Webster, J. G., and Bass, P. Human electrogastrograms. Comparison of surface and mucosal recordings. Dig. Dis. Sci. *31*:33, 1986.

66. Telander, R. L., Morgan, K. G., Kreulen, D. L., Schmalz, P. F., Kelly, K. A., and Szurszewski, J. H. Human gastric atony with tachygastria and gastric retention. Gastroenterology *75*:497, 1978.

67. You, C. H., Lee, K. Y., Chey, W. Y., and Menguy, R. Electrogastrographic study of patients with unexplained nausea, bloating, and vomiting. Gastroenterology *79*:311, 1980.

68. You, C. H., Chey, W. Y., Lee, K. Y., Menguy, R., and Bortoff, A. Gastric and small intestinal myoelectric dysrhythmia associated with chronic intractable nausea and vomiting. Ann. Intern. Med. *95*:449, 1981.

69. Geldof, H., Van der Schee, E. J., Van Blankenstein, M., and Grashuis, J. L. Electrogastrographic study of gastric myoelectrical activity in patients with unexplained nausea and vomiting. Gut *27*:799, 1986.

70. Camilleri, M., Brown, M. L., and Malagelada, J.-R. Relationship between impaired gastric emptying and abnormal gastrointestinal motility. Gastroenterology *91*:94, 1986.

71. Epidemic vomiting. Br. Med. J. *2*:327, 1969.

72. Dolin, R., Blacklow, N. R., Du Pont, H., Buscho, R. F., Wyatt, R. G., Kasel, J. A., Hornick, R., and Chanock, R. M. Biological properties of Norwalk agent of acute infectious nonbacterial gastroenteritis. Proc. Soc. Exp. Biol. Med. *140*:578, 1972.

73. Dolin, R., Levy, A. G., Wyatt, R. G., Thornhill, T. S., and Gardner, J. D. Viral gastroenteritis induced by the Hawaii agent. Am. J. Med. *59*:761, 1975.

74. Kapikian, A. Z., Kim, H. W., Wyatt, R. G., Cline, W. L., Arrobio, J. O., Brandt, C. D., Rodriguez, W. J., Sack, D. A., Chanock, R. M., and Parrott, R. H. Human reovirus-like agent as the major pathogen associated with "winter" gastroenteritis in hospitalized infants and young children. N. Engl. J. Med. *294*:965, 1976.

75. Meeroff, J. C., Schreiber, D. S., Trier, J. S., and Blacklow, N. R. Abnormal gastric motor function in viral gastroenteritis. Ann. Intern. Med. *92*:370, 1980.

76. Loewenstein, M. S. Epidemiology of clostridium perfringens food poisoning. N. Engl. J. Med. *286*:1026, 1972.

77. Terranova, W., and Blake, P. A. Bacillus cereus food poisoning. N. Engl. J. Med. *298*:143, 1978.

78. Carpenter, C. C. J. Acute infectious diarrhea disease and bacterial food poisoning. *In* Braunwald, E., Isselbacher, K. J., Petersdorf, R. G., Wilson, J. D., Martin, J. B., and Fauci, A. S. (eds.) Harrison's Principles of Internal Medicine. Ed. 11. New York, McGraw-Hill Book Company, 1987, p. 885.

79. Tanaka, K., and Johnson, B. Jamaican vomiting sickness. N. Engl. J. Med. *295*:461, 1976.

80. Ramsey, E. J., Carey, K. V., Peterson, W. L., Jackson, J. J., Murphy, F. K., Read, N. W., Taylor, K. B., Trier, J. S., and Fordtran, J. S. Epidemic gastritis with hypochlorhydria. Gastroenterology *76*:1449, 1979.

81. Peterson, W. L., Lee, E., and Skoglund, M. The role of campylobacter pyloridis in epidemic gastritis with hypochlorhydria. (Abstract.) Gastroenterology *92*:1575, 1987.

82. Gee, S. On fitful or recurrent vomiting. St. Bart. Hosp. Rep. *18*:1, 1882.

83. Weitz, R. Prophylaxis of cyclic vomiting with propranolol. Drug Intelligence Clin. Pharmacol. *16*:161, 1982.

84. Reinhart, J. B., Evans, S. L., and McFadden, D. L. Cyclic vomiting in children: Seen through the psychiatrist's eye. Pediatrics *59*:371, 1977.

85. Hoyt, C. S., and Stickler, G. B. A study of 44 children with the syndrome of recurrent (cyclic) vomiting. Pediatrics *25*:775, 1960.

86. Lorber, J. Causes of cyclic vomiting. Develop. Med. Child. Neurol. *5*:645, 1963.

87. MacMahon, R. A., and Grattan-Smith, P. The baby who vomits. Med. J. Aust. *2*:543, 1966.

88. Bleicher, M. A., Shandling, B., Zingg, W., Karl, H. W. A., and Track, N. S. Increased serum immunoreactive gastrin levels in idiopathic hypertrophic pyloric stenosis. Gut *19*:794, 1978.

89. Shrand, H. Vomiting in utero with intestinal atresia. Pediatrics *49*:767, 1972.

90. Euler, A. R., and Ament, M. E. Gastroesophageal reflux in children: Clinical manifestations, diagnosis, pathophysiology, and therapy. Pediatr. Ann. *5*:678, 1976.

91. Leape, L. L., Holder, T. M., Franklin, J. D., Amoury, R. A., and Ashcraft, K. W. Respiratory arrest in infants secondary to gastroesophageal reflux. Pediatrics *60*:924, 1977.

92. Byrne, W. J., Kangarloo, H., Ament, M. E., Lo, C. W., Berquist, W., Foglia, R., and Fonkalsrud, E. W. "Antral dysmotility." An unrecognized cause of chronic vomiting during infancy. Ann. Surg. 193:521, 1981.

93. Reye, R. D. K., Morgan, G., and Baral, J. Encephalopathy and fatty degeneration of the viscera: A disease entity in childhood. Lancet 2:749, 1963.

94. Davis, L. E., and Kornfeld, M. Influenza A associated Reye's syndrome in adults. J. Neurol. Neurosurg. Psych. 43:516, 1980.

95. Hurwitz, E. S., Barrett, M. J., Bregman, D., Gunn, W. J., Schonberger, L. B., Fairweather, W. R., Drage, J. S., La-Montagne, J. R., Kaslow, R. A., Burlington, D. B., et al. Public health service study on Reye's syndrome and medications. Report of the pilot phase. N. Engl. J. Med. 313:849, 1985.

96. Jarnfelt-Samsioe, A., Samsioe, G., and Velinder, G.-M. Nausea and vomiting in pregnancy—a contribution to its epidemiology. Gynecol. Obstet. Invest. 16:221, 1983.

97. Klebanoff, M. A., Koslowe, P. A., Kaslow, R., and Rhoads, G. G. Epidemiology of vomiting in early pregnancy. Obstet. Gynecol. 66:612, 1985.

98. FitzGerald, C. M. Nausea and vomiting in pregnancy. Br. J. Med. Psychol. 57:159, 1984.

99. Tierson, F. D., Olsen, C. L., and Hook, E. B. Nausea and vomiting of pregnancy and association with pregnancy outcome. Am. J. Obstet. Gynecol. 155-1017, 1986.

100. Baylis, J. M., Leeds, A. R., and Challacombe, D. N. Persistent nausea and food aversions in pregnancy. A possible association with cow's milk allergy in infants. Clin. Allergy 13:263, 1983.

101. Samsioe, G., Crona, N., Enk, L., and Jarnfelt-Samsioe, A. Does position and size of corpus luteum have any effect on nausea of pregnancy? Acta Obstet. Gynecol. Scand. 65:427, 1986.

102. Klebanoff, M. A., and Mills, J. L. Is vomiting during pregnancy teratogenic? Br. Med. J. 292:724, 1986.

103. Masson, G. M., Anthony, F., and Chau, E. Serum chorionic gonadotropin (HCG), schwangerschaftsprotein 1 (SP1), progesterone and oestradiol levels in patients with nausea and vomiting in early pregnancy. Br. J. Obstet. Gynecol. 92:211, 1985.

104. Jarnfelt-Samsioe, A., Bremme, K., and Eneroth, P. Steroid hormones in emetic and non-emetic pregnancy. Eur. J. Obstet. Gynecol. Reprod. Biol. 21:87, 1986.

105. Guze, S. B., DeLong, W. B., Majerus, P. W., and Robins, E. Association of clinical psychiatric disease with hyperemesis gravidarum. A three-and-a-half-year follow-up study of 48 patients and 45 controls. N. Engl. J. Med. 261:1363, 1959.

106. Fitzgerald, J. P. B. Epidemiology of hyperemesis gravidarum. Lancet 1:660, 1956.

107. Kauppila, A., Huhtaniemi, I., and Ylikorkala, O. Raised serum human chorionic gonadotrophin concentrations in hyperemesis gravidarum. Br. Med. J. 1:1670, 1979.

108. Bruun, Th., and Kristoffersen, K. Thyroid function during pregnancy with special reference to hydatidiform mole and hyperemesis. Acta Endocrinol. 88:383, 1978.

109. Bouillon, R., Naesens, M., Van Assche, F. A., De Keyser, L. E., De Moor, P., Render, M., De Vos, P., and De Roo, M. Thyroid function in patients with hyperemesis gravidarum. Am. J. Obstet. Gynecol. 143:922, 1982.

110. Juras, N., Banovac, K., and Sekso, M. Increased serum reverse triiodothyronine in patients with hyperemesis gravidarum. Acta Endocrinol. 102:284, 1983.

111. Dozeman, R., Kaiser, F. E., Cass, O., and Pries, J. Hyperthyroidism appearing as hyperemesis gravidarum. Arch. Intern. Med. 143:2202, 1983.

112. Harvey, W. A., and Sherfey, M. J. Vomiting in pregnancy. A psychiatric study. Psychosom. Med. 16:1, 1954.

113. Coppen, A. J. Vomiting of early pregnancy. Psychological factors and body build. Lancet 1:172, 1959.

114. Semmens, J. P. Female sexuality and life situations. An etiologic psychosocio-sexual profile of weight gain and nausea and vomiting in pregnancy. Obstet. Gynecol. 38:555, 1971.

115. Wolkind, S., and Zajicek, E. Psycho-social correlates of nausea and vomiting in pregnancy. J. Psychosom. Res. 22:1, 1978.

116. Long, M. A. D., Simone, S. S., and Tucher, J. J. Outpatient treatment of hyperemesis gravidarum with stimulus control and imagery procedures. J. Behav. Ther. Exp. Psychiat. 17:105, 1986.

117. Kaplan, M. M. Acute fatty liver of pregnancy. N. Engl. J. Med. 313:367, 1985.

118. Meshkinpour, H., Marks, J. W., Schoenfield, L. J., Bonnoris, G. G., and Carter, S. Reflux gastritis syndrome: mechanism of symptoms. Gastroenterology 79:1283, 1980.

119. Kaiser, G. C., McKain, J. M., and Shumacher, H. B. The superior mesenteric artery syndrome. Surgery 110:133, 1960.

120. Mansberger, A. R., Hearn, J. B., Byers, R. M., Fleisig, N., and Buxton, R. W. Vascular compression of the duodenum. Am. J. Surg. 115:89, 1968.

121. Rosenberg, S. A., and Sampson, A. The syndrome of mesenteric vascular compression of the duodenum. Arch. Surg. 73:296, 1956.

122. Gondos, B. Duodenal compression defect and the "superior mesenteric artery syndrome." Radiology 123:575, 1977.

123. Lee, C.-S., and Mangla, J. C. Superior mesenteric artery compression syndrome. Am. J. Gastroenterol. 70:141, 1978.

124. Burrington, J. D. Superior mesenteric artery syndrome in children. Am. J. Dis. Child. 130:1367, 1976.

125. Shandling, B. The so-called superior mesenteric artery syndrome. Am. J. Dis. Child. 130:1371, 1976.

126. Editorial Comment. Am. J. Dis. Child. 130:1373, 1976.

127. Hill, O. W. Psychogenic vomiting. Gut 9:348, 1968.

128. Rosenthal, R. H., Webb, W. L., and Wruble, L. D. Diagnosis and management of persistent psychogenic vomiting. Psychosomatics 21:722, 1980.

129. Wruble, L. D., Rosenthal, R. H., and Webb, W. L., Jr. Psychogenic vomiting: A review. Am. J. Gastroenterol. 77:318, 1982.

130. Morgan, H. G. Functional vomiting. J. Psychosom. Res. 29:341, 1985.

131. Haggerty, J. J., Jr., and Golden, R. N. Psychogenic vomiting associated with depression. Psychosomatics 23:91, 1982.

132. Killen, J. D., Taylor, C. B., Telch, M. J., Saylor, K. E., Maron, D. J., and Robinson, T. N. Self-induced vomiting and laxative and diuretic use among teenagers. Precursors of the binge-purge syndrome? JAMA 255:1447, 1986.

133. Wallace, M., Richards, P., Chesser, E., and Wrong, O. Persistent alkalosis and hypokalemia caused by surreptitious vomiting. Quart. J. Med. 37:577, 1968.

134. Wolff, H. P., Vecsei, P., Kruck, F., Roscher, S., Brown, J. J., Dvsterdieck, G. O., Lever, A. F., and Robertson, J. I. S. Psychiatric disturbances leading to potassium depletion, sodium depletion, raised plasma renin concentration, and secondary hyperaldosteronism. Lancet 1:257, 1968.

135. Wrong, O., and Richards, P. Psychiatric disturbances and electrolyte depletion. Lancet 1:421, 1968.

136. Stoller, R. J. Erotic vomiting. Arch. Sexual Behavior 11:361, 1982.

137. Seldin, D. W., and Rector, F. C., Jr. Symposium on acid-base homeostasis. The generation and maintenance of metabolic alkalosis. Kidney Int. 1:306, 1972.

138. Veldhuis, J. D., Bardin, O. W., and Demers, L. M. Metabolic mimicry of Bartter's syndrome by covert vomiting. Utility of urinary chloride determinations. Am. J. Med. 66:361, 1979.

139. Gitelman, H. J., Graham, J. B., and Welt, L. G. A new familial disorder characterized by hypokalemia and hypomagnesemia. Tr. Assoc. Am. Physicians 79:221, 1966.

140. Gapp, G. A., James, E. C., Iwen, G. W., and Siegel, M. B. Postemetic rupture of herniated cardia of the stomach. A variant of Boerhaave's syndrome. JAMA 247:811, 1982.

141. Kleier, D. J., Aragon, S. B., and Averbach, R. E. Dental management of the chronic vomiting patient. J. Am. Dent. Assoc. 108:618–621, 1984.

142. Alcalay, J., Ingber, A., and Sandbank, M. Mask phenomenon: Postemesis facial purpura. Cutis 38:28, 1986.

143. Wampler, G. The pharmacology and clinical effectiveness of phenothiazines and related drugs for managing chemotherapy-induced emesis. Drugs 25(Suppl. 1):35, 1983.

144. Gralla, R. J., Itri, L. M., Pisko, S. E., Squillante, A. E., Kelsen, D. P., Braun, D. W., Jr., Bordin, L. A., Braun, T. J., and Young, C. W. Antiemetic efficacy of high-dose meto-

clopramide: Randomized trials with placebo and prochlorperazine in patients with chemotherapy-induced nausea and vomiting. N. Engl. J. Med. *305*:905, 1981.

145. Alphin, R. S., Proakis, A. G., Leonard, C. A., Smith, W. L., Dannenburg, W. N., Kinnier, W. J., Johnson, D. N., Sancilio, L. F., and Ward, J. W. Antagonism of cisplatin-induced emesis by metoclopramide and dazopride through enhancement of gastric motility. Dig. Dis. Sci. *31*:524, 1986.

146. Snape, W. J., Battle, W. M., Schwartz, S. S., Braunstein, S. N., Goldstein, H. A., and Alavi, A. Metoclopramide to treat gastroparesis due to diabetes mellitus. Ann. Intern. Med. *96*:444, 1982.

147. McClelland, R. N., and Horton, J. W. Relief of acute, persistent postvagotomy atony by metoclopramide. Ann. Surg. *188*:439, 1978.

148. Synthetic marijuana for nausea and vomiting due to cancer chemotherapy. Med. Letter Drugs Therapeutics *27*:97, 1985.

149. Orr, L. E., McKernan, J. F., and Bloome, B. Antiemetic effect of tetrahydrocannabinol. Arch. Intern. Med. *140*:1431, 1980.

150. Markman, M., Sheidler, V., Ettinger, D. S., Quaskey, S. A., and Mellits, E. D. Antiemetic efficacy of dexamethasone. Randomized, double-blind, crossover study with prochlorperazine in patients receiving cancer chemotherapy. N. Engl. J. Med. *311*:549, 1984.

151. Colbert, N., Izrael, V., Lotz, J.-P., Stoppa-Lyonnet, D., Vannetzel, J. M., Pene, F., Schlienger, M., and Laugier, A. Adrenocorticotropic hormone in the prevention of cisplatin-induced nausea and vomiting. J. Clin. Oncol. *1*:635, 1983.

152. Laszlo, J., Gralla, R. J., Einhorn, L. H., and Wampler, G. Antiemetics: A round table discussion. Drugs *25*(Suppl. 1):74, 1983.

153. Laszlo, J. Selecting an antiemetic for the individual patient. Drugs *25*(Suppl. 1):81, 1983.

154. Stoudemire, A., Cotanch, P., and Laszlo, J. Recent advances in the pharmacologic and behavioral management of chemotherapy-induced emesis. Arch. Intern. Med. *144*:1029, 1984.

155. Latimer, P. R., Malmud, L. S., and Fisher, R. S. Gastric stasis and vomiting: Behavioral treatment. Gastroenterology *83*:684, 1982.

156. Dundee, J. W., Chestnutt, W. N., Ghaly, R. G., and Lynas, A. G. A. Traditional Chinese acupuncture: A potentially useful antiemetic? Br. Med. J. *293*:583, 1986.

157. Amarnath, R. P., Abell, T. L., and Malagelada, J.-R. The rumination syndrome in adults. Ann. Intern. Med. *105*:513, 1986.

158. Reynolds, R. P. E., and Lloyd, D. A. Manometric study of a ruminator. J. Clin. Gastroenterol. *8*:127, 1986.

159. Shay, S. S., Johnson, L. F., Wong, R. K. H., Curtis, D. J., Rosenthal, R., Lamott, J. R., and Owensby, L. C. Rumination, heartburn, and daytime gastroesophageal reflux. A case study with mechanisms defined and successfully treated with biofeedback therapy. J. Clin. Gastroenterol. *8*:115, 1986.

160. Menking, M., Wagnitz, J. G., Burton, J. J., Coddington, R. D., and Sotos, J. F. Rumination—a near-fatal psychiatric disease of infancy. N. Engl. J. Med. *280*:802, 1969.

161. Hollowell, J. G., and Gardner, L. I. Rumination and growth failure in male fraternal twin. Association with disturbed family environment. Pediatrics *36*:565, 1965.

162. Lang, P. J., and Melamed, B. G. Avoidance conditioning therapy in an infant with chronic ruminative vomiting. J. Abnorm. Psychol. *74*:1, 1969.

163. Singh, N. N., Manning, P. J., and Angell, M. J. Effects of an oral hygiene punishment procedure on chronic rumination and collateral behaviors in monozygous twins. J. Appl. Behav. Analysis *15*:309, 1982.

164. Daniel, W. H. Management of chronic rumination with a contingent exercise procedure employing topographically dissimilar behavior. J. Behav. Exp. Psychiat. *13*:149, 1982.

15

Abdominal Pain

LAWRENCE W. WAY

Pain is a subjective sensation resulting from central transmission of peripherally received noxious stimuli. It is usually a harbinger of tissue damage unless the stimulus is removed. The type of pain that is experienced is partly due to factors other than intensity of initial stimulus.

The word pain is derived from the Latin *poena,* or punishment. Punishment is usually painful, and pain, from whatever cause, may be interpreted psychologically as a form of punishment. However, pain may act as the stimulus that brings the ailing patient to a physician, and a careful analysis of the pain may help the physician to determine its cause and to outline appropriate treatment. Clinically, when pain has outlived its useful purpose, it should be allayed by drugs, specific treatment, or, occasionally, palliative neurosurgical techniques.

This chapter covers the physiology of pain, an understanding of which helps in interpreting the clinical manifestations of patients with pain. The general principles of managing patients with acute or chronic abdominal pain are also discussed, but detailed descriptions of specific conditions manifesting pain (e.g., acute appendicitis, acute cholecystitis) are presented in later chapters.

ANATOMY AND PHYSIOLOGY[1-4]

Painful stimuli activate a specific set of nocireceptors, consisting of free endings of small A-delta and C afferent fibers, which are triggered by strong mechanical stimulation or extreme heat or cold. Tissue hormones, such as bradykinin, histamine, serotonin, leukotrienes, and prostaglandins, may either activate pain receptors directly or lower their threshold to other stimuli. About 25 per cent of A-delta and 50 per cent of C fibers function as nocireceptors, having the characteristics of very high thresholds to mechanical or thermal stimuli, small receptive fields, and persistent discharges for suprathreshold stimuli. The quality of the sensation carried by A-delta and C fibers differs. The A-delta fibers, 3 to 4 μ in diameter, are distributed principally to skin and muscle. They mediate the sharp, sudden, well-localized pain that follows an acute injury (*epicritic* pain). The C fibers, 0.3 to 3 μ in diameter, are found in muscle, periosteum, parietal peritoneum, and viscera. The sensory afferents that convey intraperitoneal abdominal pain are of this type. The sensation transmitted by C fibers tends to be dull, sickening, poorly localized, and of more gradual onset and longer duration (*protopathic* pain).

The vagi do not transmit pain from the gut (despite the fact that 90 per cent of their nerve fibers are sensory), and the ability to feel pain from the abdominal viscera is unaltered after vagotomy.

Pain from the esophagus is transmitted to the spinal cord by afferents in small, unnamed sympathetic nerves. Visceral afferents from the capsule of the liver, the hepatic ligaments, the central portion of the diaphragm, the splenic capsule, and the pericardium are derived from dermatomes C3 to C5 and reach the central nervous system via the phrenic nerve. The fibers from the periphery of the diaphragm, gallbladder, stomach, pancreas, and small intestine travel through the celiac plexus and the greater splanchnic nerves, and enter the spinal cord from T6 to T9 (Fig. 15–1).

Stimuli from the colon, appendix, and pelvic viscera enter the tenth and eleventh thoracic segments by way of the mesenteric plexus and lesser splanchnic nerves. The sigmoid, rectum, renal pelvis and capsule, ureter, and testes are innervated by fibers that reach the T11 to L1 segments through the lowest splanchnic nerve. The bladder and rectosigmoid send afferents through the hypogastric plexus to enter the cord from S2 to S4.

The cell bodies of the visceral afferent neurons are located in the dorsal root ganglia (Color Fig. 15–2, p. xxxii). The fibers in the splanchnic nerves join the sympathetic chains and reach the dorsal roots via the white rami communicantes. After entering the spinal cord their fibers send branches directly into the pos-

terior horn and others through the tract of Lissauer cranially and caudally for several segments before terminating on dorsal horn cells in laminae I and V. The visceral afferent neurons synapse with marginal neurons and others at the base of the dorsal horn. Cells bodies in lamina V of the dorsal horn that mediate visceral pain also receive input from peripheral nonpain fibers, and this dual innervation sets the stage for the sensation of referred pain that accompanies visceral pain. These neurons transmit nociceptive impulses via fibers that cross through the anterior commissure, ascend in the lateral spinothalamic and spinoreticulothalamic tracts, and end in the reticular formation of the medulla and midbrain or the thalamic nuclei. In either case, the cerebral terminations receive fibers from both sides of the body. The cells in the thalamic nuclei relay the pain impulses to the postcentral gyrus of the cerebral cortex, at which point conscious sensation is perceived.

The large myelinated afferent neurons that mediate touch, vibration, and proprioception enter the dorsal column and course along the medial border of the dorsal horn. At intervals they send branches into the substantia gelatinosa that bifurcate into ascending and descending fibers, which give rise to multiple endings that terminate by synapses with gelatinosa neurons. These primary neurons of the gelatinosa have axons that join the tract of Lissauer, travel for five or six segments, and re-enter the gelatinosa to terminate on marginal neurons. These gelatinosa neurons are activated by the large afferents; their principal function is inhibitory.

Fibers originating in the ventrolateral part of the central gray substance of the mesencephalon and periventricular gray and caudate nucleus descend within the cord to end at various sites in the afferent pathway for pain. Impulses traveling in this descending system have a profound potential for inhibiting pain. The cell bodies of this system possess receptors specific for opiates; high concentrations of endorphins are present in these areas; and the morphine antagonist, naloxone, reverses the inhibition that results from activation of this system.[5, 6] Naloxone also antagonizes analgesia induced by stress, acupuncture, or administration of placebos. In addition, there is evidence for the existence of other central analgesic systems mediated, respectively, by noradrenalin, serotonin, and baclofen.[7, 8] These inhibitory mechanisms allow cerebral influences to modify afferent pain impulses.

STIMULI FOR ABDOMINAL PAIN[4, 9, 10]

Abdominal viscera are ordinarily insensitive to many stimuli that, when applied to the skin, evoke severe pain. Cutting, tearing, or crushing of viscera does not result in a perceptible sensation. The principal forces to which visceral pain fibers are sensitive are *stretching* or *tension* in the wall of the gut. This can be the result of traction on the peritoneum (neoplasm), distention of a hollow viscus (biliary colic), or forceful muscular

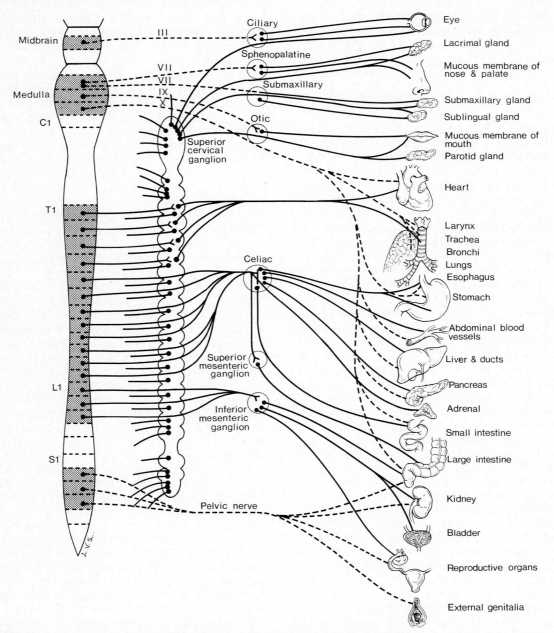

Figure 15–1. Diagram of autonomic nervous system. The visceral afferent fibers mediating pain travel with the sympathetic nerves, except for those from the pelvic organs which follow the parasympathetics of the pelvic nerve. Sympathetics are represented here by solid lines; parasympathetics, by dashed lines.

contractions (intestinal obstruction). The nerve endings of pain fibers in the hollow viscera (gut, gallbladder, and urinary bladder) are located in the muscular walls. Those in the solid viscera, such as the liver and kidney, supply the capsule and respond to stretching of the capsule from parenchymal swelling. The mesentery, parietal peritoneum, and peritoneal covering of the posterior abdomen are sensitive to pain, but the visceral peritoneum and greater omentum are insensitive. The rate at which tension develops must be fairly rapid for pain to be produced. Gradual distention, such as that in malignant biliary obstruction, may be painless.

Inflammation, whether of bacterial or chemical origin, may also produce visceral pain. Moreover, inflammation and tissue congestion sensitize the nerve endings and lower the threshold to pain from other stimuli. Effects on nerve endings of the tissue hormones, bradykinin, serotonin, histamine, leukotrienes, or prostaglandins, is the mechanism by which inflammation produces pain.

Ischemia causes abdominal pain by increasing the concentration of tissue metabolites in the region of the sensory nerves. Ischemia also lowers the threshold to other noxious stimuli. Since the adventitia of mesenteric blood vessels are also supplied with pain fibers, traction on blood vessels may cause pain.

Intra-abdominal pain can also be caused by involvement of sensory nerves by *neoplasms*. This is the mechanism for pain produced by some retroperitoneal tumors such as pancreatic carcinoma. Malignant invasion of the walls of viscera is painless unless obstruction or ulceration develops.

TYPES OF ABDOMINAL PAIN[4, 11]

Classically, abdominal pain is separated into three categories: *visceral* pain, *parietal* (somatic) pain, and *referred* pain. Although neurophysiologic differences between them are slight, the distinctions possess value for understanding patterns of clinical pain.

Visceral Pain (Fig. 15–3). Visceral pain is felt in the abdomen when noxious stimuli affect an abdominal viscus. The pain is usually dull and poorly localized in the epigastrium, periumbilical region, or lower mid-abdomen. Visceral pain is felt near the midline because, with few exceptions, the abdominal organs receive sensory afferents from both sides of the spinal cord. The site where the pain is felt corresponds roughly to the dermatomes from which the diseased organ receives its innervation. The pain is not well localized because the innervation of most viscera is multisegmental and the number of nerve endings in viscera is less than in skin. The quality is generally cramping, burning, or gnawing. Secondary autonomic effects such as sweating, restlessness, nausea, emesis, perspiration, and pallor often accompany visceral pain. The patient may move about in a vain attempt to relieve the discomfort.

Parietal (Somatic) Pain. Pain sensations that arise from noxious stimulation of the parietal peritoneum are generally more intense and more precisely localized to the site of the lesion than visceral pain. An example is the localized pain in acute appendicitis produced by inflammatory involvement of the peritoneum at Mc-Burney's point. Parietal pain is usually aggravated by movement or coughing. The nerve impulses travel in A-delta and C fibers within somatic sensory nerves. The nerve endings activated by stimulation of the parietal peritoneum are distributed in the areolar connective tissue beneath, rather than in, the mesothelium. The fibers reach the spinal cord in the peripheral nerves corresponding to the cutaneous dermatomes from T6 to L1. Lateralization of the discomfort of parietal pain is possible because at any given point the parietal peritoneum obtains innervation from only one side of the nervous system.

Pain elicited by traction on the mesentery or posterior abdominal peritoneum has the characteristics of visceral pain and is carried in splanchnic nerves.[12]

Referred Pain.[4, 11, 13] Referred pain is felt in remote areas supplied by the same neurosegment as the diseased organ and is due to the existence of shared central pathways for afferent neurons from different sites. Referred pain may be felt in skin or deeper

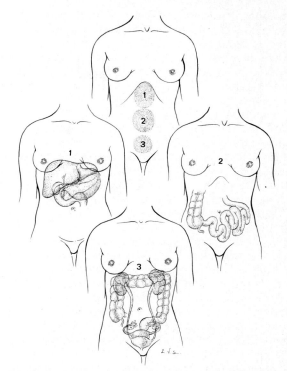

Figure 15–3. Sites where visceral pain is felt. Pain arising from organs depicted in 1, 2, and 3 is felt in the epigastrium, midabdomen, and hypogastrium, respectively.

tissues but is usually fairly well localized, much as the somatic sensory nerves themselves. As a rule, referred pain appears when the noxious visceral stimulus becomes more intense. For example, pain produced experimentally by distention of a balloon within the intestine is first entirely visceral and is then accompanied by referred pain in the back as distention is increased. In some cases referred pain may exist in the absence of visceral pain, but this is unusual.

Hyperesthesia of skin and hyperalgesia of muscle may develop in the distribution of the referred pain. When hyperesthesia and hyperalgesia are present, infiltration of the spinal nerves to that area will abolish the heightened sensitivity and may also reduce or eliminate the referred pain itself.[9]

PERCEPTION OF PAIN

Melzack and Wall[14] proposed a theory of pain that reconciled many seemingly contradictory observations in the older specificity and pattern theories. The specificity theory had postulated that pain was the result of activation of a special subsection of the nervous system in which pain was conceived as involving a specific set of receptors, peripheral fibers, and central tracts. In such a system one might suppose that any given stimulus would elicit a predictable reproducible response.

Alternatively, the pattern theory postulated that there were no specialized neural structures or centers for pain. The sensation was thought to be a result of activation of general receptors and fibers in a special pattern coded for pain, which was deciphered as such by the cerebral cortex. This theory ignored the increasing evidence for at least some specialization in transmission of pain impulses. Both theories overlooked the substantial variations in an individual's pain perception due to factors other than the intensity and nature of the noxious stimulus.

Melzack and Wall proposed what they called a "gate theory" to account for the observed phenomena. Central to their hypothesis was a complex neural system in the dorsal horn of the spinal cord that could integrate central and other peripheral impulses with the incoming ones for pain. Augmentation or inhibition of the pain impulses was possible before they reached consciousness in the cerebral cortex.

Sternbach[15] emphasized that pain should be considered a single entity, at times divisible into neural, psychologic, and secondary autonomic effects for analytic purposes, but ultimately involving all three in every case. Failure to appreciate the critical role of the psychologic component in every painful event would be shortsighted and likely to impair clinical interpretations and management of pain. Until recently the tendency to maintain a duality of thinking regarding physiologic and psychologic pain has been widespread.

It has been recognized for many years, and is now supported by the demonstration of powerful central inhibitory mechanisms, that higher cerebral function exerts a strong influence on pain perception. Psychologic traits, learning, ethnic and cultural background, personality, and events surrounding the injury are among the factors that contribute to an individual's pain experience in response to any specific stimulus. Heightened anxiety lowers the pain threshold, and relief of anxiety or depression, by any means, generally raises the threshold. Wall views pain as a phenomenon more akin to hunger and thirst than to seeing or hearing. After injury, the pain sequence may be divided into immediate, acute, and chronic stages, each possessing specific characteristics and under the strong influence of many aspects of body state, but only loosely correlated with the injury itself.[16]

It has been demonstrated repeatedly that about 30 per cent of individuals with pain (e.g., patients who have had recent major surgery) experience substantial pain relief in response to administration of a placebo.[17] In fact, the effectiveness of placebo analgesia seems to be directly related to the intensity of the pain stimulus, not the opposite, as is sometimes imagined. Virtually anyone may, in the right circumstances, respond to a placebo (i.e., individuals cannot be separated into those who do and those who do not respond), but it is not yet possible to predict which patients will respond in any specific situation. The placebo response is blocked by naloxone, which indicates that it is probably mediated by the central opioid inhibitory system. The biology of placebo analgesia is still not fully appreciated by the medical profession, for there remains a belief among some that it is possible, by giving a placebo, to distinguish between real and imagined pain (i.e., manipulative behavior).[18]

PAIN FROM SPECIFIC ORGANS[11]

Numerous observations have been made on experimental pain produced by stimulation of abdominal organs or the splanchnic nerves. These experimental observations have been compared with clinical pain patterns, and generalizations have emerged concerning the location and quality of pain from different segments of the gut (Fig. 15–3).

Esophagus. Lesions of the esophagus usually produce substernal discomfort felt at the level of the disease. Balloon distention at various levels has demonstrated the ability of the subject to indicate accurately the site of the stimulus in this organ. Upper esophageal stimulation produces pain in the neck, and stimulation in the lower third is felt near the xiphoid process. In some subjects a low esophageal stimulus is felt high in the esophagus, but the opposite pattern is uncommon. More severe stimulation produces referred pain in the middle of the back.

Stomach and Duodenum. Experimental stimulation or spontaneous visceral pain from the stomach and duodenum causes pain in the midline of the epigastrium. Disease of the duodenal bulb may cause discomfort somewhat to the right side of the upper abdomen. Stimuli farther down the duodenum produce pain that is experienced lower in the epigastrium. Radiation to the back is fairly common in experimental subjects and clinical patients.

Small Intestine. Pain originating from jejunum to distal ileum is located in the midabdomen about the umbilicus. Referred pain may appear in the middle of the back if the stimulus is of sufficient intensity or if the individual's threshold is relatively low.

Ileum. Disease or other stimuli in this area usually cause pain near the umbilicus, but sometimes in the lower abdomen or to the right of the midline.

Colon. Pain from the colon is poorly localized to the lower midabdomen. Stimulation of the rectum usually creates discomfort felt posteriorly over the sacrum.

Gallbladder and Common Bile Duct.[13, 19] Experimental dilatation of either of these structures causes pain in the midepigastrium or right upper quadrant. Both may be associated with referred pain in the back between the scapulae or to one side of the midline. The biliary system is supplied with fibers from T6 to T10, but most originate from the T9 dermatome. Although the innervation is bilateral, most of the fibers reach the cord through the right splanchnic nerves.

Pancreas. Pain from the pancreas is felt in the midline or left side of the epigastrium. The nerves arise from segments T8 to T10. Pancreatic disease is often accompanied by referred pain in the middle of the back. Somatic pain felt in the left shoulder may result from activation of pain fibers in the left diaphragm by an adjacent inflammatory process in the tail of the pancreas.

Pelvic Organs.[20] Pain sensation from the uterus passes in fibers derived from segments S2 to S4 through the hypogastric plexus. The uterus becomes painful in response to obstruction, distention, or severe contraction, much like other hollow viscera.

In contrast to other solid organs, the ovary is insensitive to most stimuli because it does not have a capsule. Ovarian inflammation or tumors are usually silent unless there is strangulation by torsion or rupture of a cyst.

PRINCIPLES OF CLINICAL MANAGEMENT: ACUTE AND CHRONIC PAIN[10, 21–23]

When abdominal pain is the presenting complaint, it must be evaluated by the usual process of obtaining historical, physical, and laboratory data, which usually suggest diagnostic hypotheses and therapeutic plans. The acuteness of the illness is a major factor in determining the clinical approach to abdominal pain. If symptoms have been present for weeks or months without recent exacerbation, the work-up may be slow and deliberate, aimed at achieving an exact diagnosis. In patients with acute pain, the goal of making a specific diagnosis remains the same, but in some cases it will be necessary to proceed with laparotomy in the face of advancing peritonitis before the cause can be determined.

History

The common innervation of many abdominal organs, the low concentration of nerve endings in the viscera, the patient's lack of previous experience with sensations arising from these organs, and the often nonspecific localization of the pain all interact to complicate the diagnostic process. The patient must be questioned carefully regarding his pain. The following dimensions of a complaint of abdominal pain must be explored.

Location. The site of the pain and the extent to which it is localized must be determined. Significant radiation of pain may be present, such as the sensation of pain in the thigh with disease in the ureter or testicle. Pain in the shoulder may signify diaphragmatic involvement. The pain in biliary, duodenal, or pancreatic disease is often referred to the back. Visceral pain tends to be poorly localized, but pain produced by irritation of the parietal peritoneum is confined to the area involved by disease.

Intensity and Character. The severity of the pain is loosely related to the magnitude of the noxious stimulus. Acute perforated duodenal ulcer or mesenteric occlusion, for example, evokes excruciating pain, and the obvious intensity of the symptom is of diagnostic value. On the other hand, estimates of severity are at times unreliable because of the interaction of the various factors that determine the response. As might be expected, the significance of the amount of pain is more obvious at the extremes of severity than in between.

Certain diseases produce pain with distinct qualities. Well-known examples are the burning or gnawing pain of duodenal ulcer or the cramping pain of intestinal obstruction. The pain in biliary colic may be constrict-ing; in ruptured aneurysm, tearing; in pancreatitis, terrifying; in acute appendicitis, aching; and so forth. Melzack and Torgerson[24] suggested that a systematic study of the taxonomy of pain may lead to a better understanding of its production. They point out the wide range of adjectives used to describe different kinds of pain and their significance in support of a pattern concept of pain production.

Chronology. The quantity and quality of pain in relationship to time are often clues as to its cause. Acute abdominal pain that has persisted for more than six hours usually indicates a surgical problem. Chronic pain of duodenal ulcer rarely occurs before breakfast but appears later in the interprandial period. Acute appendicitis evolves steadily over 12 hours without remission. Intestinal obstruction is associated with cramping pain, separated by pain-free intervals. Steady pain is produced by ischemia whether due solely to vascular disease or secondary to strangulation obstruction.

Setting. What are the circumstances in which the pain appears? Heartburn may be experienced only when abdominal pressure is increased. Emotional tension may aggravate peptic ulcer pain or that associated with the irritable colon syndrome.

Aggravating or Alleviating Factors. Numerous important diagnostic clues are discovered in this category, such as the response of peptic ulcer pain to antacids. In fact, therapeutic trials of antacids, antispasmodics, or diets are sometimes prescribed with the aim of obtaining diagnostic data as well as relieving the patient.

Associated Signs and Symptoms. Information should be obtained regarding changes in gastric function (anorexia, nausea, emesis), evacuation (diarrhea, constipation), weight, renal function, gynecologic function, and the like. Diarrhea may signify pain from gastroenteritis, whereas obstipation suggests intestinal obstruction. Bloody urine may be seen with ureteral colic caused by a ureteral stone. Jaundice can direct attention to the biliary tree in cases of upper abdominal pain.

Physical Examination

The clinical history often provides only enough information to suggest that the diagnosis is one of several possibilities. The physical examination must be carried out systematically to uncover unsuspected abnormalities as well as to test specific hypotheses formed from symptom analysis. A thorough physical examination is essential, because it may provide the answer in many a puzzling case. The examination begins with a general inspection and includes the head, neck, extremities, and chest as well as the abdomen.

The patient's appearance may provide a clue to the nature of his disease. *Tachycardia, fever,* and *perspiration* suggest sepsis from peritonitis, cholangitis, pyelonephritis, or severe bacterial enteritis. The patient with pure visceral pain may change position frequently, but if localized or general peritonitis is present he avoids movement.

The abdomen should be inspected for *distention* from intestinal obstruction or ascites. All potential hernial sites must be carefully examined in every case. Incarceration of a segment of bowel in a small femoral hernia can be easily missed if not specifically looked for. *Hyperperistalsis* may be audible with the stethoscope in intestinal obstruction or enteritis. Generalized peritonitis usually causes *decreased* or *absent peristalsis*. Vascular bruits may be clues to an aortic or splenic artery aneurysm.

Palpation of the abdomen should be performed with a mental picture of its contents. It should be especially gentle at first and started at a distance from the painful area. Otherwise the patient may lose confidence in the examiner and become so guarded that an accurate examination is impossible.

Abdominal *rigidity* or involuntary *guarding* may be the result of adjacent peritonitis. The most classic example is the board-like upper abdominal rigidity that occurs early in perforated peptic ulcer. Lesser degrees of guarding or rigidity develop over the area of an acutely inflamed gallbladder or appendix or in acute diverticulitis. If the patient's knees are drawn up, this may provide just enough relaxation to allow an examination that was otherwise impossible because of guarding. An abnormal mass may be produced by enlargement of a diseased organ, tumors, or inflammatory processes.

Pure visceral pain is usually unaccompanied by tenderness. When *tenderness* is present, the most important question is the extent of its localization. Generalized peritonitis is suggested by severe diffuse tenderness with rigidity and clinical toxicity. However, mild general tenderness without toxicity is more compatible with acute gastroenteritis, salpingitis, or some other nonsurgical condition. The early uncomplicated stage of acute cholecystitis, appendicitis, or diverticulitis is characterized by tenderness that can usually be well localized to a small area. The key to determining localization is gentle palpation with one finger until the tender area has been thoroughly mapped out. Localized tenderness over McBurney's point is by far the most important finding when making the diagnosis of acute appendicitis. Regardless of the remainder of the history, if tenderness is confined to a spot a few centimeters in diameter, acute appendicitis will nearly always be present.

Rebound pain is produced by pressing slowly and deeply over a tender area and then suddenly releasing the hand. This maneuver merely confirms the presence of peritonitis of the parietal peritoneum. Since the same information can be obtained by light percussion over the tender spot, the quest for rebound tenderness is usually unnecessary.

Hyperesthesia in response to gently touching the skin may appear in the dermatome affected by intraperitoneal parietal pain. If present, this finding is useful, but it is often absent even though significant localized peritonitis exists.

Genital, rectal, and pelvic examinations are part of the evaluation of every patient with abdominal pain. Acute pelvic inflammation or a twisted ovarian cyst or uterine fibroid may be found, or rectal examination may reveal a tumor, abscess, or occult blood in the feces.

Laboratory Findings

Routine hematologic studies should include a complete blood count and a serum creatinine. Other tests should be ordered according to clinical clues derived from symptoms and signs.

Gastrointestinal X-ray examination with barium may be required to establish the correct diagnosis. Oral cholecystography or ultrasound or HIDA scans may be indicated to verify biliary disease. Selective mesenteric angiography may reveal mesenteric arterial stenosis in patients suspected of suffering from intestinal angina. Endoscopy via the upper or lower gut orifices may be of great diagnostic value. Esophageal manometry is clinically useful in the differential diagnosis of substernal pain, and manometry may eventually earn a place in the evaluation of colonic or other intestinal disorders.

Diagnosis

The history, physical examination, and laboratory findings generally result in a correct diagnosis and treatment plan (Table 15–1). In some cases, however, the etiology of recurrent or persistent abdominal pain cannot be further defined. In this situation one must consider the long list of rare causes of pain and perform special tests if the complaint truly appears to be of clinical significance.

Prospective analyses[25–27] of symptom reliability in the diagnosis of chronic upper abdominal pain have shown that in the average case an accurate diagnosis is not possible without the help of X-rays and sometimes endoscopy. In some patients the story of peptic ulcer is so typical that the X-rays are merely confirmatory. However, the pain patterns of gallstone disease, duodenal and gastric ulcer, gastritis, esophagitis, and cancer overlap greatly.

Chronic recurrent undiagnosed abdominal pain is a significant clinical problem that often has led to repeated laparotomies.[27, 28] It is more common in women than in men. The usual patient has had recurrent attacks for years without experiencing weight loss or developing disorders other than the pain. Barium X-ray studies of the upper and lower gastrointestinal tract may be normal or may show questionable abnormal findings in the duodenal bulb, leading to gastrectomy. Other patients have had appendectomy for "chronic appendicitis," hiatus hernia repair for undocumented esophagitis, or cholecystectomy for postprandial pain despite a normal cholecystogram. Pancreatitis from pancreas division, alkaline reflux gastritis, and stenosis

Table 15–1. SOME CAUSES OF ABDOMINAL PAIN

I. Intra-abdominal
   A. Generalized peritonitis
      1. Perforated viscus: peptic ulcer, gallbladder colonic diverticulum
      2. Primary bacterial peritonitis: pneumococcal, streptococcal, enteric bacillus, tuberculous
      3. Nonbacterial peritonitis: ruptured ovarian cyst, ruptured follicle cyst
      4. Familial Mediterranean fever (familial periodic peritonitis)
   B. Localized peritonitis: many types of local peritonitis may become generalized by rupture into the free peritoneal cavity
      1. Appendicitis
      2. Cholecystitis
      3. Peptic ulcer
      4. Meckel's diverticulitis
      5. Regional enteritis
      6. Acute colonic diverticulitis
      7. Colitis: ulcerative, amebic, bacterial
      8. Abdominal abscess: postoperative, hepatic, pancreatic, splenic, diverticular, tubo-ovarian
      9. Gastroenteritis
      10. Pancreatitis
      11. Hepatitis: viral, toxic
      12. Pelvic inflammatory disease, gonococcal perihepatitis (Fitz-Hugh and Curtis syndrome)
      13. Endometritis
      14. Lymphadenitis
   C. Pain from increased tension in viscera
      1. Intestinal obstruction: adhesions, hernia, tumor, volvulus, fecal impaction, intussusception
      2. Intestinal hypermotility: irritable colon, gastroenteritis
      3. Biliary obstruction: gallstone, stricture, tumor, parasites, hemobilia
      4. Ureteral obstruction: calculi
      5. Hepatic capsule distention: acute hepatitis (toxic or viral), common duct obstruction, Budd-Chiari syndrome
      6. Renal capsule distention: pyelonephritis, ureteral obstruction
      7. Uterine obstruction: neoplasm, childbirth
      8. Ruptured ectopic pregnancy
      9. Aortic aneurysm
   D. Ischemia
      1. Intestinal angina or infarction: arterial stenosis, embolism, polyarteritis
      2. Splenic infarction
      3. Torsion: gallbladder, spleen, ovarian cyst, testicle, omentum, appendix epiploica
      4. Hepatic infarction: toxemia
      5. Tumor necrosis: hepatoma, uterine fibroid
   E. Retroperitoneal neoplasms
II. Extra-abdominal
   A. Thoracic
      1. Pneumonitis
      2. Pulmonary embolism
      3. Pneumothorax
      4. Empyema
      5. Myocardial ischemia
      6. Myocarditis, endocarditis
      7. Esophagitis, esophageal spasm
      8. Esophageal rupture
   B. Neurogenic
      1. Radiculitis: spinal cord or peripheral nerve tumors, degenerative arthritis of spine, herpes zoster
      2. Tabes dorsalis
      3. Abdominal epilepsy
   C. Metabolic
      1. Uremia
      2. Diabetes mellitus
      3. Porphyria
      4. Acute adrenal insufficiency
   D. Toxins
      1. Hypersensitivity reactions: insect bites, reptile venoms
      2. Drugs: lead poisoning, etc.
   E. Miscellaneous
      1. Muscular contusion, hematoma, or tumor

---

of the sphincter of Oddi are currently popular, but difficult to prove, diagnoses in patients with chronic abdominal pain. Many of these females have had hysterectomies.

Many of these patients are psychologically unstable, and follow-up examination usually fails to reveal an organic source of the symptom.[29] In some cases, functional disturbances characterized by spasm of the gut are responsible for pain.[30] For example, increased intraluminal pressures coincident with pain have been found in patients with the irritable colon syndrome.[31] The common syndrome of chronic episodic pain in the right lower quadrant may have a similar explanation, but no simple techniques are suitable for studying cecal peristalsis. In any event the diagnosis of chronic appendicitis to account for intermittent abdominal pain has been seriously challenged. Unless findings are fairly specific, appendectomy is unlikely to eliminate the complaint.

In perplexing cases, a question arises as to the value of diagnostic laparotomy. If there are no objective findings (fever, jaundice, mass, X-ray abnormality), laparotomy is usually negative. On the other hand, in the presence of at least one objective finding, diagnostic laparotomy may solve the puzzle.[32–36]

Treatment

The principal objective is to find a specific treatment such as antacids for peptic ulcer or cholecystectomy for gallstones. Even the use of anticholinergic agents in the irritable colon syndrome has a pathophysiologic rationale.

In patients with acute abdominal pain, one may not be able to define the condition more precisely than "acute surgical peritonitis." In such cases, laparotomy is indicated because of the protean nature of common problems such as acute appendicitis and the increased illness if perforation occurs. Treatment of the specific conditions is covered elsewhere in this book.

The care of patients with chronic pain may be extremely taxing.[37–40] Numerous treatment centers devoted primarily to this problem have been formed, where various specialists (neurosurgeons, psychiatrists, internists, and others) jointly contribute to the management plan. Therapy generally is tailored to the patient's life expectancy; patients with malignant disease and two years or less to live are treated with narcotics and mood-altering drugs without concern for the potential of addiction.[39, 40] The therapy of patients with benign disease is more complex. In these individuals the use of addicting drugs must be curtailed, and therapy must rely on attempts to adapt the patient to the problem.[41] In either case, ablative or other neurosurgical techniques may have a role in carefully selected patients.[42, 43]

THE ACUTE ABDOMEN[21–23, 44–48]

The "acute abdomen" is medical slang for sudden abdominal symptoms, consisting for the most part of pain, vomiting, constipation, and changes in genitourinary function. Because many of the conditions responsible for producing the acute abdomen are potentially lethal unless treated promptly by operation, the care of these patients is among the most challenging problems in clinical medicine.

Diagnosis is often difficult. Studies of patients seen in emergency rooms with the complaint of acute abdominal pain show that in about half the cases the final diagnosis is nonspecific pain, representing gastroenteritis, menstrual discomfort, or other disorders.[44–47] Of patients sick enough for admission to the hospital, only half had the same diagnosis on discharge as on admission.[48] The most common surgical problem is *acute appendicitis,* with *cholecystitis, small bowel obstruction, perforated ulcer,* and *diverticulitis* together constituting a group of similar size. Diagnostic error is about twice as common in women as in men and is highest (30 per cent error rate) in females between the ages of 1 and 20 years. Incorrect diagnosis is also common in patients over age 50. Elderly patients with acute abdominal pain more often have a condition requiring surgery than younger patients. The most common condition mistakenly thought to require operation is *acute salpingitis;* on initial evaluation the surgical conditions most commonly thought to be nonsurgical are *acute appendicitis* and *small bowel obstruction.*

Comparison of patients with nonspecific abdominal pain and those with surgical problems shows that many in both groups have fever and elevated leukocyte counts, and many have no fever and normal leukocyte counts.[45] One generalization that may be helpful is that in patients with surgical problems, pain nearly always precedes vomiting. The reverse sequence is common in nonsurgical diseases. Several authors, after reviewing the management of patients with acute abdominal pain cared for in their hospitals, noted that diagnostic accuracy would have been better if pelvic and rectal examinations had been performed with greater regularity.

For most conditions that produce acute abdominal pain there is no pathognomonic clinical syndrome or set of laboratory or X-ray findings. Consequently, if there is a significant possibility that the patient has a surgical condition, laparotomy is usually indicated. Inevitably this means that some diagnostic laparotomies will serve only to rule out the presence of surgical disease and will have no direct therapeutic value. For example, about 10 to 20 per cent of operations performed with the presumptive diagnosis of appendicitis

reveal a normal appendix and either some other nonsurgical cause of the symptoms or, in some cases, no abnormalities at all. Negative diagnostic laparotomies in these situations should not be considered "unnecessary operations." They reflect a deliberate choice (i.e., to reduce false negatives at the expense of increased false positives) considering the degree of diagnostic accuracy possible with the available data. On the other hand, it has been observed that when a study is made of the diagnostic accuracy of an institution's staff, the effect of the study has been to increase overall accuracy, resulting in both fewer negative laparotomies and fewer delayed operations for surgical problems.[44] Thus there usually is room for improvement even without better tests.

The differential diagnosis of the acute abdomen involves numerous conditions, most of which are discussed in later chapters in this book. Here we will cover diagnosis in a general sense.

The practice of strictly withholding analgesic drugs from patients with acute pain in the belief that to do otherwise would cloud the findings and interfere with early diagnosis is no longer accepted. After the initial examination, the patient should be given enough analgesics to provide comfort but not deep sedation. Repeated examinations may even be facilitated enough to clarify the diagnosis.

Among the most useful historical information is the speed and character of the onset of the pain (Table 15–2). The onset may be (1) sudden, (2) rapid, or (3) gradual.

Sudden severe pain will have such an abrupt and noticeable beginning that the patient can say, for example, that he was opening a letter or reaching for a book when it started. The principal causes of this kind of pain, listed in Table 15–2, are an *abdominal vascular accident, perforation of a viscus,* or *passage of a kidney stone.* The patient may collapse and become shocky. With a perforated viscus, the severity of pain and shock often diminishes during the first few hours after perforation; with intra-abdominal bleeding, pain and shock progress steadily. The degree of abdominal tenderness and guarding is determined by the extent of peritonitis, being marked with a perforated viscus and usually mild to moderate with *mesenteric occlusion* or *perforating aneurysm.* In fact, the combination of very severe pain and relatively unimpressive abdominal findings is characteristic of *acute abdominal vascular disease.*

Plain films of the chest and abdomen should be obtained in most cases.[49] Abdominal paracentesis may be indicated in some. Occasionally, abdominal arteriography may help verify a diagnosis of mesenteric vascular occlusion. Fever and leukocytosis are not often pronounced early in the course of diseases responsible for sudden severe pain. Exploratory laparotomy will usually be indicated after myocardial infarction, pulmonary embolism, and spontaneous pneumothorax have been ruled out.

Pain of *rapid* onset develops over an hour or so and is characteristic of inflammatory processes and obstruc-

Table 15–2. CLASSIFICATION OF CAUSES OF ABDOMINAL PAIN ACCORDING TO RATE OF DEVELOPMENT OF THE PAIN

1. Sudden onset (instantaneous)
   Perforated ulcer
   Rupture of abscess or hematoma
   Rupture of esophagus
   Ruptured ectopic pregnancy
   Infarct of abdominal organ, heart, or lung
   Spontaneous pneumothorax
   Ruptured or dissecting aortic aneurysm
2. Rapid onset (minutes)
   Perforated viscus
   Strangulated viscus (strangulated obstruction; torsion)
   High small intestinal obstruction
   Pancreatitis
   Acute cholecystitis; biliary colic
   Mesenteric infarction
   Ureteral or renal colic
   Ectopic pregnancy
   Pneumonitis
   Peptic ulcer
   Diverticulitis
   Appendicitis (less commonly than gradual onset)
3. Gradual onset (hours)
   Appendicitis
   Strangulated hernia
   Low mechanical small bowel obstruction
   Cholecystitis
   Pancreatitis
   Duodenal ulcer
   Gastritis
   Gastric ulcer
   Mesenteric lymphadenitis
   Terminal ileitis (regional enteritis; Crohn's disease)
   Meckel's diverticulitis
   Sigmoid diverticulitis
   Ulcerative colitis
   Perforated tumor (usually of the colon or stomach)
   Intra-abdominal abscess
   Ectopic pregnancy before rupture
   Threatening abortion
   Ureteral colic
   Cystitis or pyelitis
   Salpingitis (PID)
   Prostatitis
   Urinary retention
   Mesenteric cyst
   Small bowel tumor or infarct

tion of a hollow viscus. Most of the conditions that present with sudden pain may have this slower onset. *Appendicitis, acute cholecystitis, pancreatitis, intestinal obstruction,* and *ureteral stone* are the most common causes of pain of rapid onset, although the onset of *appendicitis* more often places it in the next category (gradual onset). The clinician's primary task is to avoid overlooking a perforated viscus, strangulation obstruction, acute appendicitis, or ruptured ectopic pregnancy. The other conditions in this group generally evolve slowly before serious complications develop.

As a rule, if the patient prefers to lie still in bed, parietal pain (peritonitis) is present; if he moves about restlessly, he has visceral pain (e.g., intestinal or ureteral obstruction, biliary colic). Upper abdominal pain usually represents *cholecystitis, pancreatitis,* or *perforated peptic ulcer;* midabdominal pain is due to *appendicitis, intestinal obstruction,* or *mesenteric vascular*

occlusion; lower abdominal pain may be from *appendicitis, diverticulitis, ureteral colic, ectopic pregnancy,* or *twisted ovarian cyst.*

Localized pain and tenderness indicate localized peritonitis, as with appendicitis, cholecystitis, diverticulitis, or pancreatitis. A tender mass may be present in some cases, representing the inflamed organ or a localized perforation (e.g., appendicitis, cholecystitis, diverticulitis). As a rule, the working diagnosis is determined more by the location of pain and tenderness than by any other finding. For example, whenever right lower quadrant pain and tenderness are confined to a small area at McBurney's point, the patient usually must be treated as if he had appendicitis, regardless of atypical details in the history or laboratory findings.

Vomiting occurs in most cases with pain of rapid onset, but the persistence and severity of vomiting are much greater with intestinal obstruction than with a primary inflammatory disorder. The vomitus may be feculent with low intestinal obstruction, bilious with mid- or high intestinal obstruction, or free of bile with pyloric obstruction. Pain nearly always precedes vomiting with surgical problems; the opposite sequence is common with nonspecific abdominal disorders (e.g., gastroenteritis).

Physical examination must include a thorough inspection of all hernial orifices, recognizing that small incarcerated hernias (especially femoral hernias) may be inconspicuous (especially in obese individuals). Nearly every experienced clinician has encountered at least one patient whose incarcerated obstructing hernia was overlooked by the first examiner.

Moderate fever (38.5° C) is characteristic of most of the diseases in this category. Higher fever (>39° C) and chills are uncommon except with *urinary infection* or *cholangitis* or late in the development of *cholecystitis, appendicitis,* or *diverticulitis* when suppurative complications have developed. A mild leukocytosis is usually present. Urinary tract infection or ureteral stone will be disclosed by the finding of white or red blood cells in the urinary sediment.

Pain of *gradual* onset, reaching a peak in 12 to 24 hours, may be a manifestation of most of the diseases discussed in the previous category with the addition of several others as listed in Table 15–2. The slower onset of symptoms may mislead the clinician into thinking that there is no urgency in establishing a diagnosis, whereas just the opposite is true. For instance, when appendicitis is seen early, the pain and abdominal findings may be deceptively unimpressive. Because of this pitfall, frequent examinations are required in the first few hours to achieve early diagnosis and optimal results.

The following is a list of caveats for the diagnostician confronted with a patient who has acute abdominal pain:

1. Acute diseases of the chest may closely mimic primary diseases of the abdomen. Always look for *pneumonia, pneumothorax, pulmonary infarction, myocardial infarction,* and *congestive heart failure.*

2. In the first 12 hours after the onset of acute

abdominal pain, *appendicitis* can almost never be completely ruled out short of laparotomy. Always reevaluate patients at frequent intervals during the initial hours of an acute abdominal illness. Whenever a patient is unexpectedly getting worse, suspend previous judgments and perform an exploratory laparotomy.

3. Regardless of the serum amylase level, *acute pancreatitis* is principally a diagnosis of exclusion. If a patient with presumed pancreatitis is becoming sicker, operation should be seriously considered. Occasionally the patient will be found at laparotomy to have some other condition that might have produced fatal complications if managed expectantly. Furthermore, pancreatitis may be a secondary manifestation of choledocholithiasis, a condition that can be definitively treated by surgery. Common duct stones should be especially suspected if the patient is icteric early in the attack of pain. Most cases of biliary pancreatitis should be managed by elective surgery following resolution of the acute symptoms, but lack of improvement calls for earlier operation. Diagnostic laparotomy by itself has no detrimental effects on the course of pancreatitis, and if necrotizing pancreatitis is encountered, pancreatic debridement may be beneficial.

4. *Acute pyelonephritis,* which occasionally produces abdominal pain out of proportion to dysuria, can masquerade as acute appendicitis, cholecystitis, or intestinal obstruction. Only the urinalysis will reveal the real cause of the symptoms.

5. Many cases (about 25 per cent) of *perforated peptic ulcer* are atypical in the sense that the onset is not abrupt or free intraperitoneal air is absent. Always obtain an abdominal plain film on patients with acute abdominal pain, unless the diagnosis is obvious (e.g., some cases of acute appendicitis, pelvic inflammatory disease, urinary tract infection, and so forth). Watch for perforations confined to the lesser sac, those into retroperitoneal tissues, or those that allow pus to travel along the right gutter and present as right lower quadrant pain. Beware of *perforated ulcer* as a cause of recent abdominal pain in a patient hospitalized for some other illness.

6. *Acute mesenteric infarction* is very difficult to diagnose early, at the stage when surgery is most likely to be effective. The paucity of abdominal findings and systemic signs and the nonspecific X-ray picture tend to contradict the patient's report of persistent progressive pain. Bloody or guaiac-positive stools are only a late finding, rarely available at the time when exploratory laparotomy can be helpful. It is difficult to select patients for angiography, and early exploratory laparotomy in elderly patients with persistent severe pain is usually the best approach.

7. Surgical conditions that present with visceral pain, no signs of intestinal obstruction, and no abdominal mass or localized tenderness are difficult to diagnose early, as this is also the clinical picture of gastroenteritis and other nonspecific causes of pain. The surgical conditions with these features are *mesenteric vascular occlusion, Richter's hernia, cecal volvulus,* and some cases of *gallstone ileus.* A significant delay in treatment

is reported in more than half the patients with each of these conditions.

8. Clinical findings will not reliably indicate if *intestinal obstruction* is complicated by strangulation.[50] Except for patients with carcinomatosis or those with repeated previous episodes of obstruction, exploratory laparotomy should be performed as soon as the diagnosis of complete small bowel obstruction has been established and the patient's fluid and electrolyte balance has been restored.

9. Be prepared to recognize pain and hypovolemic shock resulting from intra-abdominal bleeding. The conditions that present in this way are *delayed* or *spontaneous splenic rupture, ruptured hepatic tumor, ruptured arterial aneurysm, mesenteric apoplexy,* and *ruptured ectopic pregnancy.* An immediate laparotomy is required to save the patient.

10. Most patients with emetogenic rupture of the esophagus have abdominal (not chest) pain as their major complaint. The radiologic findings are subtle and will be missed unless specifically sought.

11. Special radiologic studies can be used to great advantage in selected cases. For example, a HIDA scan is of value to diagnose or exclude acute cholecystitis. An IVP may disclose a ureteral calculus. An upper gastrointestinal or small bowel series may differentiate mechanical small bowel obstruction from ileus. An upper gastrointestinal series with water-soluble contrast may be used to demonstrate an otherwise occult perforation. Barium enema may be of help in intussusception or volvulus.

The Acute Abdomen During Pregnancy[51] and the Puerperium[52]

Acute abdominal pain during pregnancy and the puerperium poses special problems. In pregnancy the enlarged uterus displaces lower abdominal organs from their usual position, compromises abdominal examination, alters the clinical manifestations, and interferes with natural mechanisms that localize infection.

Indications for exploratory laparotomy occur in 0.2 per cent of all pregnancies. Of explorations performed, one third are negative and one quarter result in spontaneous abortion. Analysis of the latter cases shows that abortion is related more to the extent of the pathologic process and the intra-abdominal procedure than to laparotomy, which by itself seldom produces abortion. For example, if *appendicitis* progresses to local perforation, the uterus forms the medial wall of the abscess, a situation that may stimulate premature delivery. After the uterus empties, it pulls away from the appendiceal abscess, resulting in free perforation and generalized peritonitis with a serious threat to survival of the mother.

Appendicitis is the most common indication for operation during pregnancy. The incidence of appendicitis is the same in pregnant as in nonpregnant women, and the cases are distributed equally among the three trimesters. The fetal mortality rate of 20 per cent in appendicitis is directly related to the stage of the disease, being 15 per cent with perforation and under 2 per cent with uncomplicated appendicitis. The overall maternal mortality rate of 5 per cent is related to the degree of peritonitis and period of gestation.

Ovarian cysts complicated by torsion, rupture, or intracystic hemorrhage are the second most frequent lesion prompting laparotomy. If oophorectomy is performed, abortion occurs in about 40 per cent of patients and is especially prone to follow oophorectomy during the first trimester.

Acute cholecystitis complicating pregnancy will usually subside without complications if managed expectantly. However, cholecystectomy is tolerated well by both fetus and mother, so if the disease progresses there should be no reluctance to proceed with operation.

In general, diagnosis of the acute abdomen is considerably less reliable during pregnancy than at other times and the mortality rate of peritonitis is greater. If a surgical condition is strongly suspected, operation should be scheduled without delay. Negative explorations are well tolerated by fetus and mother; but when a preoperative diagnosis of appendicitis is unsubstantiated at operation, removal of the normal appendix is contraindicated, as this triples the risk of fetal loss. Oophorectomy in pregnant women, particularly in the first trimester, should be performed only when absolutely necessary.

Acute abdominal pain in the first few days after childbirth may be misdiagnosed because intercurrent disease is unexpected and abdominal examination is confusing owing to laxity of the abdominal wall, which eliminates voluntary and involuntary guarding. *Acute appendicitis* and *intestinal obstruction* are the most frequent conditions of surgical significance. Obstruction may be from adhesions following previous operations or may be directly related to the changes of pregnancy. Pseudo-obstruction of the colon with dilatation proximal to the splenic flexure is occasionally seen in post-partum women. The cecum may rupture if it gets too big and cecostomy is delayed. Occasionally, as it re-enters the pelvis, the big uterus obstructs the sigmoid colon at the pelvic brim.

In general, the normal puerperium should not entail much pain; when pain does appear, diagnostic laparotomy may be required for less clear-cut indications than at other times.

References

1. Fields, H. L. *Pain*. New York, McGraw-Hill Book Company, 1987.
2. Ignelzi, R. J., and Atkinson, J. H. Pain and its modulation. Neurosurgery *6*:577, 584, 1980.
3. Mendelson, G. Pain. Med. J. Aust. *1*:106, 213, 285, 1981.
4. Almy, T. P. Basic considerations in the study of abdominal pain. *In* Melinkoff, S. M. (ed.). The Differential Diagnosis of Abdominal Pain. New York, McGraw-Hill Book Company, 1959, pp. 1–33.
5. Hill, R. G. Endogenous opioids and pain: A review. J. R. Soc. Med. *74*:448, 1981.
6. Jeffcoate, W. J. Brain peptides in pain sensation. Am. Heart J. *99*:1, 1980.
7. Yaksh, T. L., and Ramana Reddy, S. V. Studies in the primate on the analgetic effects associated with intrathecal actions of opiates, α-adrenergic agonists and baclofen. Anesthesiology *54*:451, 1981.
8. Liebeskind, J. C. Multiple mechanisms of pain inhibition intrinsic to the central nervous system. Anesthesiology *54*:445, 1981.
9. Menacker, G. J. The physiology and mechanism of acute abdominal pain. Surg. Clin. North Am. *42*:241, 1962.
10. Wolff, H. G., and Wolf, S. Pain. Ed. 2. Springfield, Illinois, Charles C Thomas, Publisher, 1958.
11. Jones, C. M. Digestive Tract Pain. New York, The Macmillan Company, 1938.
12. Doran, F. S. A. Observations on referred pain from the posterior abdominal wall and pelvis. Br. J. Surg. *49*:376, 1962.
13. Doran, F. S. A. The sites to which pain is referred from the common bile duct in man and its implication for the theory of referred pain. Br. J. Surg. *54*:599, 1967.
14. Melzack, R., and Wall, P. D. Pain mechanisms: A new theory. Science *150*:971, 1965.
15. Sternbach, R. A. Pain. A Psychophysiological Analysis. New York, Academic Press, 1968.
16. Wall, P. D. On the relation of injury to pain. Pain *6*:253, 1979.
17. Fields, H. L., and Levine, J. D. Biology of placebo analgesia. Am. J. Med. *70*:745, 1981.
18. Goodwin, J. S., Goodwin, J. M., and Vogel, A. V. Knowledge and use of placebos by house officers and nurses. Ann. Intern. Med. *91*:106, 1979.
19. Schrager, V. L., and Ivy, A. C. Symptoms produced by distention of the gallbladder and biliary ducts. Surg. Gynecol. Obstet. *47*:1, 1928.
20. Jeffcoate, T. N. A. Pelvic pain. Br. Med. J. *3*:431, 1969.
21. Beal, J. M., and Raffensperger, J. G. Diagnosis of Acute Abdominal Disease. Philadelphia, Lea & Febiger, 1979.
22. Currie, D. J. Abdominal Pain. New York, Hemisphere, 1979.
23. Silen, W. Cope's Early Diagnosis of the Acute Abdomen. Ed. 16. New York, Oxford University Press, 1983.
24. Melzack, R., and Torgerson, W. S. On the language of pain. Anesthesiology *34*:50, 1971.
25. Rinaldo, J. A., Jr., Scheinok, P., and Rupe, C. E. Symptom diagnosis. A mathematical analysis of epigastric pain. Ann. Intern. Med. *59*:145, 1963.
26. Edwards, F. C., and Coghill, N. F. Clinical manifestations in patients with chronic atrophic gastritis, gastric ulcer, and duodenal ulcer. Q. J. Med. *37*:337, 1968.
27. Ingram, P. W., and Evans, G. Right iliac fossa pain in young women. Br. Med. J. *2*:149, 1965.
28. Rang, E. H., Fairbairn, A. S., and Acheson, E. D. An enquiry into the incidence and prognosis of undiagnosed abdominal pain treated in hospital. Br. J. Prev. Soc. Med. *24*:47, 1970.
29. Hill, O. W., and Blendis, L. Physical and psychological evaluation of "nonorganic" abdominal pain. Gut *8*:221, 1967.
30. Chaudhary, N. A., and Truelove, S. C. The irritable colon syndrome. Q. J. Med. *31*:307, 1962.
31. Holdstock, D. J., Misiewicz, J. J., and Waller, S. L. Observations on the mechanism of abdominal pain. Gut *10*:19, 1969.
32. Bourke, J. B., Cannon, P., and Ritchie, H. D. Laparotomy for jaundice. Lancet *2*:521, 1967.
33. Keller, J. W., and Williams, R. D. Laparotomy for unexplained fever. Arch. Surg. *90*:494, 1965.
34. Piedrahita, P., and Butterfield, W. C. Abdominal exploration as a diagnostic procedure. Am. J. Surg. *131*:181, 1976.
35. Sarfeh, I. J. Abdominal pain of unknown etiology. Am. J. Surg. *132*:22, 1976.
36. Scott, P. J., Hill, R. S., Fook, A. L. S., and Bensley, K. E. Benefits and hazards of laparotomy for medical patients. Lancet *2*:941, 1970.
37. Reuler, J. B., Girard, D. E., and Nardone, D. A. The chronic pain syndrome: misconceptions and management. Ann. Intern. Med. *93*:588, 1980.
38. Long, J. C., and Webb, W. L., Jr. Improving diagnostic strategies for pain patients. Neurosurgery *7*:225, 1980.
39. Shimm, D. S., Logue, G. L., Maltbie, A. A., and Dugan, S.

Medical management of chronic cancer pain. JAMA *241*:2408, 1979.

40. Foley, K. M. The treatment of cancer pain. N. Engl. J. Med. *313*:84, 1985.
41. Maruta, T., Swanson, D. W., and Finlayson, R. E. Drug abuse and dependency in patients with chronic pain. Mayo Clin. Proc. *54*:241, 1979.
42. Long, D. M. Surgical therapy of chronic pain. Neurosurgery *6*:317, 1980.
43. Fields, H. Pain II: New approaches to management. Ann. Neurol. *9*:101, 1981.
44. Blacklock, A. R. E., and Gunn, A. A. The "acute abdomen" in the accident and emergency department. J. R. Coll. Surg. Edinb. *21*:165, 1976.
45. Brewer, R. J., Golden, G. R., Hitch, D. C., Rudolf, L. E., and Wangensteen, S. L. Abdominal pain. An analysis of 1,000 consecutive cases in a university hospital emergency room. Am. J. Surg. *131*:219, 1976.

46. Thomson, H. J., and Jones, P. F. Active observation in acute abdominal pain. Am. J. Surg. *152*:522, 1986.
47. Yajko, R. D., and Steele, G., Jr. Exploratory celiotomy for acute abdominal pain. Am. J. Surg. *128*:773, 1974.
48. Adams, I. D. et al. Computer aided diagnosis of acute abdominal pain: A multicentre study. Br. Med. J. *293*:800, 1986.
49. Lee, P. W. R. The plain x-ray in the acute abdomen. Br. J. Surg. *63*:763, 1976.
50. Shatila, A. H., Chamberlain, B. E., and Webb, W. R. Current status of diagnosis and management of strangulation obstruction of the small bowel. Am. J. Surg. *132*:299, 1976.
51. Saunders, P., and Milton, P. J. D. Laparotomy during pregnancy: an assessment of diagnostic accuracy and fetal wastage. Br. Med. J. *3*:165, 1973.
52. Munro, A., and Jones, P. F. Abdominal surgical emergencies in the puerperium. Br. Med. J. *4*:691, 1975.

16

The Management of Abdominal Pain

ROGER B. TRAYCOFF

The treatment of abdominal pain may be a source of frustration to both physicians and patients. Most data relating to therapy deal with well-defined pain syndromes in which management is usually disease-oriented rather than symptom-oriented. Therapy is most successful when the pathophysiologic process is well understood and treatment is directed at the underlying disease. Most therapeutic failures arise from errors in diagnosis or poor patient compliance.

In contrast, there is little information on the treatment of chronic abdominal pain of undefined etiology. Many of these patients are labeled as psychoneurotic or as having somatoform disorders based on the inability to identify an underlying disease. Therapy is empiric and symptom-directed, with many patients obtaining little or no relief. Failures in management relate to a lack of knowledge and understanding. In these cases, approaching pain as a disease rather than a symptom will do much to decrease suffering.

This chapter deals with pain as both a symptom and a disease. Emphasis is on the use of analgesics and adjuvant drugs for treating pain. Because pain is most effectively managed by treating the underlying disease, the reader is encouraged to refer to the appropriate chapters for information relating to specific diseases. Empiric therapy is seldom appropriate.

The optimal management of abdominal pain requires an understanding that pain is as much an experience as a sensation. It is an elusive concept that is difficult to define because it is multidimensional, having affective, cognitive, and sensory components.[1] In a practical sense it is a personal private sense of hurt expressed through verbal descriptors and physical posturing which are interpreted as suffering.

The two major determinants of pain behavior are the intensity of the nociceptive stimulus and the interpretation of the meaning of the pain. One's response to a painful stimulus is determined in part by age, sex, ethnic origin, mood, and potential for secondary gain. In most instances, especially in chronic pain states, there is no way to measure the intensity of nociception; the patient's pain complaints must be taken at face value.[2]

Pain should be treated on the basis of an understanding of disease mechanisms and a knowledge of pharmacokinetics and pharmacodynamics rather than by empiricism. Symptomatic therapy may be appropriate in the treatment of acute pain but in most instances is contraindicated in chronic pain. Therapy should be directed at both the physical and the psychologic factors that affect pain behavior. Having a correct diagnosis and developing a logical treatment plan are prerequisites for optimal therapy

The understanding that acute and chronic pain differ

is imperative. Acute pain is usually self-limited and easily treated, whereas chronic pain is seldom responsive to treatment, often being a disease unto itself. Furthermore, one must distinguish between chronic benign pain and chronic pain associated with malignancy; they differ in treatment implications rather than amount of suffering, disability, or alteration of lifestyle. It would be incorrect to treat chronic benign pain with potent narcotics because of the development of tolerance, habituation, and addiction. Similarly, the use of lytic nerve blocks or neuroablative procedures for treating patients with chronic pain of nonmalignant origin would be inappropriate because pain relief is often of short duration, and the risks of causing deafferentation pain may be unacceptable. Nevertheless, one would err in assuming that chronic pain of nonmalignant origin is less intense than pain of carcinoma and that these patients are less deserving of treatment. The potential long-term risks of therapy must be balanced against the demands of the patient for relief. Treatment failures may result from the inappropriate use of either drugs or surgery, or a failure to use all therapeutic options.

In the most basic construct, there are three mechanisms for relieving pain. The first is to block receptor activation; the second is to block pain transmission, and the third is to alter the perception of the stimulus as being painful (Table 16–1). Drugs that decrease receptor activation should be classified as antialgesics, not analgesics.[3] True analgesics block pain transmission and are capable of eliminating the response to painful stimuli, whereas antialgesics convert a hyperalgesic state to a normal algesic state by decreasing the sensitivity of receptors to painful stimuli. Antialgesics such as nonsteroidal anti-inflammatory drugs have no intrinsic analgesic properties; they elevate the threshold for firing of free nerve endings to normal by inhibiting the synthesis of E prostaglandins.[4] Similarly, corticosteroids, having no intrinsic analgesic properties, can only relieve pain caused by inflammation or associated with the release of algesic substances such as prostaglandins and kinins.

The second group includes local anesthetics and neurolytic agents which block neurotransmission. These drugs have a limited role in treating chronic pain because most nerves that carry nociceptive impulses

Table 16–1. MECHANISMS OF ANTINOCICEPTION

1. Decreased receptor activation (antialgesics)
    Salicylates, acetaminophen, nonsteroidal anti-inflammatory
      drugs
    Corticosteroids?
    Radiation?
2. Inhibition of pain transmission
    Local anesthetics (analgesic)
    Spinal opiates (analgesic)
    Neuroablative surgery or lytic blocks
3. Decreased response to stimulus
    Opiates (analgesic)
    Antidepressants
    Major tranquilizers
    Anxiolytic sedatives

Table 16–2. TREATMENT OPTIONS

Antialgesics	Acetaminophen, nonsteroidal anti-inflammatory drugs
Opiates	
Agonists	Codeine, propoxyphene, morphine, meperidine, hydromorphone, methadone, oxycodone, levorphanol
Agonist-antagonist	Pentazocine, butorphanol, nalbuphine
Partial agonist	Buprenorphine
Antidepressants	Amitriptyline, doxepin, trazadone
Antihistamines	Hydroxyzine
Major tranquilizers	Chlorpromazine, haloperidol
Anxiolytic sedatives	Chlordiazepoxide, chlorazepate, diazepam, lorazepam, oxazepam, prazepam

also subserve motor function. The major indication for the use of local anesthetics is treating acute pain, such as that seen with trauma or surgery. Local anesthetics cannot be used chronically because of the development of tachyphylaxis with loss of efficacy. Spinal opiates which are also included in this group selectively inhibit the transmission of aversive stimuli in the dorsal horn of the spinal cord.[5]

Drugs in the third group alter pain perception. They include the antihistamines, tricyclic antidepressants, anticonvulsants, phenothiazines, butyrophenones, and benzodiazepines. These drugs are most useful in treating pain of central origin, in potentiating opiate-induced analgesia, and in treating depression associated with chronic pain. Opiates are also included in this group because they alter the affective response to an aversive stimulus as a result of their effect on the limbic system.

In general, acute pain is treated with antialgesics, opiates, or neuroblockade using local anesthetics. In contrast, patients with chronic pain of benign origin, no matter how severe, are usually treated with antialgesics, weak opiates, or psychotropic drugs. There is a reluctance to treat chronic pain of benign origin with opiates other than codeine or propoxyphene because of potential for abuse. Unfortunately, we are unable to distinguish nociceptive pain from psychogenic pain and to reliably identify the pain amplifiers in individual patients.

A knowledge of treatment options is a prerequisite for the optimal management of both acute pain and chronic pain (Table 16–2). In most instances, treatment directed at the underlying disease is preferable to empiric or symptom-directed therapy. Disease specific treatments will not be discussed herein because they are reviewed in other chapters.

SIMPLE ANALGESICS

Drugs used for treating mild to moderate pain can be classified as simple analgesics. They can be arbitrarily divided into "peripheral" and "central acting" based on their primary site of action. Central acting drugs such as codeine and propoxyphene are thought to act by binding to opiate receptors in the central nervous system.[6] Peripheral acting drugs such as salicylates, acetaminophen, and nonsteroidal anti-inflammatory drugs are generally not thought to have central effects; however, there is evidence that zomepirac (a nonsteroidal drug) may act through central as well as peripheral mechanisms. The term "simple analgesic" is an operational definition rather than a pharmacologic classification.

Acetaminophen may be the simple analgesic of choice in the treatment of abdominal pain if one chooses to use an antialgesic. It is effective in relieving mild to moderate pain, having a dose-response curve similar to aspirin.[7] In single-dose studies, maximal efficacy is seen with doses of 800 to 1000 mg. Administering doses greater than 1000 mg increases the risk of toxicity without providing additional analgesia.[8]

Hepatic injury, the major toxicity seen with excessive doses of acetaminophen, results from the accumulation of toxic metabolites.[9] Although alcoholics and patients with cirrhosis appear to be at greatest risk, hepatic necrosis has been reported with therapeutic doses in patients having no risk factors.[10] Therefore, single doses greater than 1000 mg or daily doses greater than 4000 mg should be avoided.

Data on the efficacy of salicylates and nonsteroidal anti-inflammatory drugs in the treatment of abdominal pain are lacking. Both classes of drugs have the potential for causing gastrointestinal dysfunction, which can increase rather than decrease patients' complaints. In general, salicylates and nonsteroidal anti-inflammatory drugs are avoided because of their ulcerogenic potential.

Data on the use of antialgesics in the treatment of abdominal pain are lacking. However, if one chooses to use an antialgesic, acetaminophen alone or in combination with either codeine or propoxyphene may be used in treating patients who have not responded to therapy directed at the underlying disease. Administering a combination of acetaminophen with either a salicylate or a nonsteroidal anti-inflammatory drug is to be discouraged. Combinations of peripherally acting antialgesics are not additive or synergistic in terms of analgesia but their potential for causing side effects is increased.

The use of propoxyphene is controversial. Single-dose studies have shown that 32 mg of propoxyphene is no better than placebo.[11] Higher doses of propoxyphene in the range of 90 to 120 mg are comparable to 60 mg of codeine in analgesic efficacy.[12] Although the value of lower doses is questioned, many patients may obtain significant relief because propoxyphene tends to accumulate with chronic use.[13] Analgesic blood levels may not be reached for several days following initiation of therapy.

The major problem associated with the long-term administration of propoxyphene is its potential for causing physical dependence.[14] The withdrawal syndrome following discontinuation of the drug may produce symptoms which can be mistaken for an exacerbation of pain. Usually this is not seen at doses less than 600 mg per day with the hydrochloride salt and 1000 mg per day with the napsylate form. The potential for overdose is also a major concern especially in patients who abuse alcohol.[15] Alcohol interferes with the metabolism of propoxyphene resulting in increased blood levels. It also potentiates the central nervous system effects of propoxyphene such that lethal respiratory depression can occur with daily doses of propoxyphene as low as 750 mg.

The use of codeine for treating abdominal pain is problematic. The major detractor to its use is the tendency to produce cramping and constipation. As with most centrally acting agents, it has the potential for causing physical dependence and tolerance.

In summary, a role for simple analgesics in treating abdominal pain is not well defined. Their use must be considered empiric because data on efficacy are lacking. They may be used for treating abdominal pain which has not responded to therapy directed at the underlying disease process where one hesitates to use more potent drugs. The indications for the use of codeine and propoxyphene in the treatment of chronic abdominal pain are as yet undefined. The fact that they may be used for this purpose does not validate their efficacy.

OPIATE DRUGS

A role for opiates in treating acute abdominal pain is well established. The major contraindication to their use is the situation in which masking pain might interfere with therapeutic judgments. The risk of addiction in these patients is minimal, being in the range of 1 in 7000 patients treated.[16] In contrast, using opiates to treat chronic pain has a significant, but most likely overstated, potential for abuse. Another major limitation to their use in this setting is the development of tolerance, with the need for dosage escalation to maintain analgesia. Adverse side affects such as unacceptable sedation, nausea, vomiting, constipation, and urinary retention are also potential problems with both acute and chronic use.

One's choice of opiate should be based on an understanding of pharmacokinetics and pharmacodynamics (Table 16–3). For example, it would be inappropriate to administer meperidine to patients with

Table 16–3. COMPARISON OF OPIATES*

| Drug | Route of Administration (Relative Potency mg/mg) | | Duration of Action (Hours) | Slow Half-Life (Hours) |
	IM/SQ	Oral		
Morphine	10	30–60	3–6	2–4
Meperidine	80–100	300	2–3	3–7
Methadone	10	20	3–5	25–45
Hydromorphone	1.5	7.5	4–5	2–4
Butorphanol	2	—	4–5	2–4
Nalbuphine	12	—	4–5	4–5
Buprenorphine	0.2–0.6	0.4–0.8†	4–5	2–4

*Single dose studies.
†Sublingual.

renal insufficiency, to use morphine in acute pancreatitis with volume depletion, or to use pentazocine in the drug addict. Normeperidine, the major metabolite of meperidine, may accumulate in the presence of renal insufficiency, causing myoclonus or seizures.[17] Administering morphine to volume-contracted patients can lead to hypotension due to venodilation.[18] Pentazocine, being an agonist-antagonist drug, may precipitate a narcotic withdrawal syndrome in patients tolerant of opiates.[19] An awareness of these properties will ensure the proper use of opiates in the treatment of both acute and chronic pain.

In most instances, meperidine is the drug of choice for treating patients with acute abdominal pain; yet, it is not without problems. It has poor bioavailability when taken orally, erratic absorption when administered intramuscularly, and a tendency to produce pain when injected.[20] Using meperidine intravenously by either continuous infusion or by patient demand (patient-controlled analgesia) may circumvent these problems.

The dose of meperidine required to relieve pain may vary fourfold among patients. Doses required to provide analgesia may range from 50 to 150 mg. As with all narcotics, the recommended dose should be considered a starting point, subject to change, based on the needs of the patient. The goal of therapy is to relieve pain without causing undue side effects.

Narcotics should be used with caution in patients with liver or biliary tract disease. All narcotics have the potential for precipitating hepatic encephalopathy in patients with end stage liver disease. Doses of meperidine should be decreased in patients with cirrhosis because of decreased hepatic clearance.[21] Morphine, which may be metabolized primarily in the kidney, can be used without dosage modification in most patients.[22]

Meperidine has been considered the drug of choice in treating patients with biliary tract disease because it is thought to be less spasmogenic than morphine.[23] More recent data suggest that butorphanol and possibly nalbuphine may cause less increase in biliary tone than meperidine and therefore may have a role in treating pain associated with diseases of the bile ducts and gallbladder.[24, 25]

Nalbuphine may be the preferred drug in patients who are hemodynamically unstable due to either bleeding or loss of fluid to the third space.[26] It has little effect on heart rate, preload, afterload, or myocardial contractility. Nalbuphine may have a role in treating patients with chronic obstructive pulmonary disease who require treatment with potent analgesics because of there being a ceiling on its effect on the respiratory center.[27]

Levorphanol, hydromorphone, and methadone are useful under certain circumstances. Both levorphanol and methadone have long elimination half-lives and good oral bioavailability, making them useful in treating chronic pain. Hydromorphone, because of its potency, may be the preferred drug for intramuscular injection in cachectic patients.

The role of agonist-antagonist drugs in the treatment of both acute and chronic pain is as yet not well defined. Three agonist-antagonists are currently in use: pentazocine, nalbuphine, and butorphanol. Buprenorphine, a partial agonist, is also available. The effects of agonist-antagonist drugs are dose related. At low doses the agonist properties predominate, whereas at higher doses the antagonist properties predominate. There may be a ceiling on their analgesia; for example, with buprenorphine increasing the dose beyond a point may decrease rather than increase the effects.

The route of administration is often more important than the choice of drug. In most instances opiates used for treating acute severe abdominal pain should be administered intravenously. Problems with erratic absorption and drug accumulation are minimized. Opiates can be given by intermittent bolus injection, by patient-controlled infusion pumps,[28] or by continuous intravenous infusion.[29] Intermittent bolus injections are preferred in hemodynamically unstable patients whose prognosis or disease progression is in doubt. Patient-controlled analgesia is favored in conditions in which parenteral opiates are required, assuming there are no contraindications to their use. Administration of opiates by continuous intravenous infusion is technically demanding and potentially fraught with problems such as respiratory depression and excessive sedation.

The use of opiates for treating chronic abdominal pain of nonmalignant origin is controversial. Risks of addiction, habituation, and physical dependence are major considerations. The use of opiates on a chronic basis may aggravate rather than relieve suffering. Problems such as narcotic bowel syndrome can complicate therapy, particularly when complaints of obstipation and cramping are prominent.[30] In these cases it is difficult to determine if the patient's pain is coming from the underlying disease or from therapy. If narcotic bowel syndrome is a consideration, one can administer clonidine to permit drug withdrawal.[31] Pain due to narcotic bowel syndrome will resolve once the patient stops taking opiates.

Treating chronic abdominal pain due to malignancy with opiates is appropriate in patients who do not respond to therapy with simple analgesics or adjuvant analgesics. The oral route of administration is preferred when feasible. The drugs of choice are oxycodone, hydromorphone, and methadone because of good oral bioavailability. Oxycodone combined with acetaminophen is useful for the treatment of mild to moderate pain but is frequently ineffective for treating severe pain. Hydromorphone, a very potent opiate, with high lipid solubility, has a rapid onset of action, but short elimination half-life. In contrast, methadone has a long elimination half-life. In single-dose studies, its duration of action is similar to morphine; with repetitive use, it tends to accumulate such that less frequent dosing is required.[32] The major problem with the use of methadone is the risk of respiratory depression, which may occur days after therapy has begun.

Using time-release morphine to treat pain is controversial. Problems with erratic absorption make therapy unsatisfactory in many patients.[33] Oral bioavailability is unpredictable ranging from 10 to 40 per cent. Conceptually, the time-release system ensures constant morphine blood levels with minimal risk of accumulation. Although this may be true, in practice the results are not always satisfactory. Hydromorphone or oxycodone can be administered on an as-needed basis along with time-release morphine when additional analgesia is required, particularly in cases in which the pain intensity varies with time of day.

The oral route of drug administration is preferred for treating chronic pain of malignant origin. Using oral rather than injectable drugs fosters independence and may decrease the risk of developing addiction. The use of intermittent demand parenteral analgesia tends to increase pain behavior; the patient must complain in order to get relief. The patient and the nurse are often placed in adversary roles in which the patient is demanding relief and the nurse is resisting because of the limits prescribed by the physician. Opiates, as a rule, should be administered on a time-contingent rather than a demand basis because prevention of pain not only improves the quality of analgesia but decreases pain behavior as well. The goal of treating pain is to relieve suffering and improve the quality of life. This can only be achieved by providing the patient with enough drug to control his pain. If abuse occurs, it should be handled in a thoughtful caring manner.

ADJUVANT ANALGESICS

Medications which are not truly analgesics or antialgesics can best be classified as adjuvant analgesics. These include (1) stimulants such as dextroamphetamine, (2) antihistamines such as hydroxyzine, (3) anticonvulsants such as phenytoin, clonazepam, and carbamazepine, (4) antidepressants such as amitriptyline and doxepin, (5) antipsychotics such as the chlorpromazine and haloperidol, and (6) anxiolytics such as diazepam and chlordiazepoxide. The most commonly prescribed drugs are listed; their mention does not indicate preference over other drugs in each class.

Hydroxyzine is the best studied and most commonly used antihistamine for treating pain.[34] It is useful, not only in potentiating opiate-induced analgesia, but has analgesic activity itself. Its sedative, anxiolytic, and antinauseant properties are also of clinical benefit. A 100 mg dose of hydroxyzine administered intramuscularly provides analgesia equivalent to 50 mg of meperidine.[35] There are few data to suggest that oral administration of hydroxyzine has any value in either potentiating opiate-induced analgesia or providing pain relief itself.

Stimulants are useful in potentiating the analgesia of both opiates and simple analgesics. The major use of stimulants is to counteract the sedation caused by opiates used to treat patients with terminal malignancies. Ten milligrams of dextroamphetamine combined with 12 mg of morphine when administered intramus-cularly is twice as effective as morphine alone.[36] Caffeine, another stimulant, is commonly combined with simple analgesics such as salicylates and acetaminophen. Caffeine not only potentiates the analgesia of these drugs but has analgesic properties itself when administered in doses higher than 65 mg.[37]

Anticonvulsants have little value in treating abdominal pain of visceral origin. Their major use is in treating deafferentation pain characterized by paresthesias, dysesthesias, and allodynia.[38] Anticonvulsants, which may act by suppressing epileptiform discharges in the dorsal horn of the spinal cord, are most efficacious in treating acute lancinating pain such as that seen with intercostal neuralgia involving the abdominal dermatomes.

Antidepressant drugs can be useful in treating abdominal pain. Tricyclic antidepressants may decrease complaints of pain in patients who have pain as a manifestation of their underlying depression or in whom depression is an aggravating factor. They may also act centrally to activate intrinsic antinociceptive systems.[39] Using antidepressants to potentiate opiate-induced analgesia is of questionable value. Side effects of tricyclic antidepressants such as sedation, urinary retention, and constipation may be additive to those of opiates, thus limiting their use. Antidepressants such as doxepin have potent H_2 receptor blocking activity and can be used for treating peptic ulcer disease.[40] Data on other tricyclic antidepressants are lacking.

Major tranquilizers are not widely used for treating abdominal pain in the absence of psychosis. However, they are useful as adjuncts to opiates because of their antiemetic properties. Prochlorperazine, the most commonly used drug in this class, is an effective antinauseant with minimal sedating effects; however, its use cannot be recommended. Controlled studies have shown it to be antialgesic rather than analgesic.[41] This may also be true for chlorpromazine; recent reports suggest that it has no intrinsic analgesic properties.[42] The use of chlorpromazine with narcotics may decrease pain behavior because of sedation rather than analgesia. Other than sedation, its major detractor is the risk of causing hypotension by alpha-adrenergic receptor blockade. Data on the use of haloperidol as an analgesic are contradictory.[43, 44] Nevertheless, it may be useful for treating hallucinations and nightmares associated with chronic opiate usage especially in the elderly.

Methotrimeprazine is the only phenothiazine with intrinsic analgesic properties.[45] The analgesic effect of a 15 mg dose of methotrimeprazine given intramuscularly is equivalent to 10 mg of morphine. The frequent occurrence of excessive sedation, orthostatic hypotension, and extrapyramidal effects limits its use. Its major use is in the short-term treatment of patients who have developed tolerance to the analgesic properties of opiates.

Using anxiolytic sedatives to treat pain is controversial. They may have short-term value in the treatment of acute pain where anxiety plays a role in pain behavior.[46] However, this anxiolytic effect may not persist with chronic use. Drugs such as diazepam may aggravate rather than relieve pain when used chronically by depleting brain serotonin.[47] In addition, chronic use may be associated with personality changes manifested by hostility and anger, which may compromise the doctor-patient relationship.

The major indication for their use is in treating "trait" anxiety rather than nonspecific complaints suggestive of agitation. If one chooses to use an anxiolytic drug, the selection should be based on differences in pharmacokinetics. Diazepam and clorazepate are useful in treating acute short-lived attacks of anxiety because of their having a rapid onset of action. If drug accumulation is a potential problem, oxazepam may be preferred because of its having a short elimination half-life and inactive metabolites. Diazepam and chlorazepate should be used with caution in the elderly because accumulation of active metabolites may lead to overdosage. Accumulation may also occur when chlordiazepoxide, diazepam, or alprazolam are used concurrently with cimetidine because of impaired clearance by the liver. Oxazepam and lorazepam may be the drugs of choice in this setting because their metabolism is not affected by cimetidine.

The use of anxiolytics on a chronic basis is of questionable value. Excluding the question of efficacy, issues of drug dependence and abuse remain. The development of physical dependence can complicate therapy because missed doses or discontinuation of the drug may precipitate a withdrawal syndrome with pain behavior indistinguishable from that seen with the underlying disease. The widespread use of anxiolytics in the treatment of functional bowel syndrome is to be condemned.

NEUROBLOCKADE

Nerve blocks have a limited role in treating abdominal pain in most instances. Neuroblockade is useful in the treatment of postoperative abdominal pain[48] and pain due to terminal malignancies,[49] but has a limited role in the treatment of chronic pain of nonmalignant origin. Local anesthetics cannot be used for long term treatment because of the development of tachyphylaxis. Neurolytic drugs such as alcohol and phenol destroy neural tissue, but their effects may be short lived because of the tendency for the nervous system to regenerate or to develop alternate pathways for pain transmission.

The advantage of regional anesthesia for treating abdominal pain following surgery is that it can provide excellent analgesia without causing respiratory depression.[50] Intercostal nerve blocks are of value in treating the morbidly obese patient or the patient with obstructive pulmonary disease in whom opiates may cause CO_2 retention. The major limitation to their use is the risk of pneumothorax. This risk can be circumvented by administering the local anesthetic via an indwelling epidural catheter, by either an intermittent bolus injection or continuous infusion.[51] However, problems

with urinary retention and orthostatic hypotension restrict the use of epidural anesthesia use to patients who have indwelling urinary catheters. Epidural anesthesia is also relatively contraindicated in patients who are hemodynamically unstable or volume contracted because of the risks of causing hypotension. The potential for masking a complication of surgery by blocking the warning signal of persistent pain is also a consideration. Nevertheless, epidural anesthesia may be a useful technique for managing pain in the patient who is intolerant of narcotics.

Neuroblockade also has a role in the treatment of intractable pain due to malignancy. A lytic celiac plexus block can provide partial or complete relief of pain to many patients with carcinoma of the pancreas, stomach, or liver.[52, 53] Its major limitation is that it may cause orthostatic hypotension. In most patients, the pain relief will persist until death, which usually occurs within several months. This is in contrast to chronic pancreatitis where pain relief is often short lived.[54] The problems of the patient continuing to drink and the risk of a "silent" abdomen would seem to contraindicate its use in this setting. Nevertheless, there may be an occasional patient in whom relief may be long lasting and the benefits exceed the risks.

Transsacral neurolytic blocks at the S4 level are useful in treating intractable pain associated with tumors infiltrating the perineum.[55] In the absence of infiltration of the sacral plexus, a transsacral block can afford the patient significant, albeit short-term, relief. The block is technically easy to perform and therefore can be repeated when necessary. The risks of bladder dysfunction are acceptable in this setting.

Regional anesthesia as a modality for treating abdominal pain has major limitations. First, the problem of availability limits its use to settings in which physicians knowledgeable in regional anesthesia are committed to providing care to patients in pain. Second, patients must be selected appropriately. Many patients with seemingly intractable pain can be successfully managed with opiates when used appropriately. Third, the use of lytic blocks should be limited to patients whose life expectancy is less than six months because the duration of the blocks is seldom long lasting. However, the patient should never be denied the opportunity to have a lytic procedure performed when conservative therapy has failed and the quality of life is compromised. The results are spectacular in some patients, providing pain relief without sedation in the last weeks to months of life.

Spinal opiate analgesia has developed as an acceptable method for providing relief for postoperative pain, and intractable pain due to malignancy.[56] The major limitation to its use is the risk of unexpected respiratory arrest.[57] The frequency and relative risks of sudden apnea are as yet not well defined. Therefore, the use of either epidural or intrathecal opiates should be limited to conditions in which other therapeutic options have failed or are less attractive. Treatment of intractable pain in patients with terminal malignancies is one such condition. In these cases, problems with catheter malfunction, infection, and loss of efficacy occur frequently. Nevertheless, it is a useful technique for treating patients who are unresponsive to conventional therapy.

PLACEBO THERAPY

Placebos have a role, albeit limited, in the treatment of abdominal pain. Although they may be effective, their use cannot be recommended except under unusual circumstances.[58] Placebos are a powerful tool which is subject to abuse and misunderstanding. Every drug has a placebo effect contributing to its efficacy. Thus, an apparent short-term response to "active drug" cannot be taken as evidence of efficacy. Conversely, relief of pain following administration of a placebo does not confirm that the pain is of psychogenic origin. Placebos cannot be used to distinguish "real" from psychogenic pain; over one third of all patients are potential placebo responders. The placebo response may in part be endorphin-mediated because it can be blocked by naloxone.

PSYCHIATRIC CARE

Patients who present with poorly defined pain syndromes unresponsive to conventional therapy are particularly difficult to manage. In most instances no significant underlying abnormalities can be detected, even after extensive evaluation. The inability to identify a source of nociception cannot be taken as evidence for there being a psychogenic basis for their complaints. A diagnosis of somatoform disorder is not a diagnosis of exclusion.

Treatment should be directed at behavior modification with the development of coping strategies. Relief of pain may not be an obtainable goal. Emphasis should be on wellness and avoidance of the sick role. Equally important, the physician should avoid being placed in an adversary role with the patient. The reality of the suffering should not be questioned, and therapy should be directed at behavior modification.

CONCLUSION

Relief of pain is a major goal of medicine. Successful therapy requires a knowledge of pain mechanisms, an understanding of the nature of suffering, and an awareness of treatment options. One's choice of therapy should be based on the expected duration of the pain, its intensity, and the underlying disease process. The role of the physician as friend and advisor cannot be minimized. A thoughtful caring physician can ease the burden of pain by helping the patient draw from within the strengths that separate pain from suffering.

References

1. Sternbach, R. A. Pain—A Psychophysiologic Analysis. New York, Academic Press, 1968.
2. Roy, R., and Tunks, E. Chronic Pain: Psychologic Factors in Rehabilitation. Baltimore, Williams & Wilkins, 1982.
3. Capetola, R. J., Rosenthale, M. E., Dubinsky, B., and McGuire, J. L. Peripheral antialgesics: A review. J. Clin. Pharmacol. 23:545, 1983.
4. Smith, M. J. H. Aspirin and prostaglandins: Some recent developments. Agents Actions 8:427, 1978.
5. Yaksh, T. L. Spinal opiate analgesia: Characteristics and principles of action. Pain 11:293, 1981.
6. Synder, S. H. Opiate receptors in the brain. Life Sci. 30:1443, 1982.
7. Wallenstein, S. L. Analgesic studies of aspirin in cancer patients. In Proceedings of The Aspirin Symposium. London, The Aspirin Foundation, 1975, pp. 5–10.
8. Koch-Weser, J. Drug Therapy: Acetaminophen. N. Engl. J. Med. 295:1297, 1976.
9. Mitchell, J. R., Jollow, D. J., Potter, W. Z., et al. Acetaminophen induces hepatic necrosis: Role of drug metabolism. J. Clin. Pharmacol. 187:185, 1973.
10. Bonkowsky, H. L., Mudge, G. H., and McMurtry, R. J.: Chronic hepatic inflammation and fibrosis due to low doses of paracetamol. Lancet 1:1016, 1978.
11. Smith, R. J. Federal government faces painful decision on Darvon. Science 203:857, 1971.
12. Miller, R. R., Feingold, A., and Paximos, J. Propoxyphene HCl: A critical review. JAMA 213:996, 1970.
13. Kiplinger, G. F., and Nickander, R. Pharmacologic basis for use of propoxyphene, JAMA 216:289, 1971.
14. D'Abidie, N. B., and Lenton, J. D. Propoxyphene dependence: Problems in management. South. Med. J. 77:299, 1984.
15. Young, R. J. Dextropoxyphene overdose: Considerations and clinical management. Drugs 26:70, 1983.
16. Porter, J., and Jick, H. Addiction rare in patients treated with narcotics. N. Engl. J. Med. 302:123, 1980.
17. Szeto, H. H., Inturrisi, C. E., Houde, R., et al. Accumulation of normeperidine an active metabolite of meperidine in patients with renal failure. Ann. Intern. Med. 86:738, 1977.
18. Henney, R. P., Vasko, J. S., Brawley, R. R., et al. Effects of morphine on the resistance and capacitance vessels of the peripheral circulation. Am. Heart J. 72:842, 1966.
19. Houde, R. W. The use and abuse of narcotic in the treatment of chronic pain. Adv. Neurol. 4:527, 1979.
20. Austin, K. L., Stapelton, J. V., and Mather, L. E. Multiple intramuscular injection: A major source of variability in analgesic response to meperidine. Pain 8:47, 1980.
21. Pond, S. M., Tang, T., Benowitz, N. L., et al. Presystemic metabolism of meperidine to normeperidine in normal and cirrhotic subjects. Clin. Pharmacol. Ther. 30:183, 1981.
22. Patwardan, R. V., Johnson, R. F., Hoyumpa, A., et al. Normal metabolism of morphine in cirrhosis. Gastroenterology 81:1006, 1981.
23. Radnay, P. A., Duncalf, D., and Novakovic, M. Common bile duct pressure changes after fentanyl, morphine, meperidine, butorphanol, and naloxone. Anesth. Anal. 63:441, 1984.
24. Vatashsky, E., and Haskely, R. Effects of nalbuphine compared to morphine and fentanyl on common duct pressure. Curr. Ther. Res. Clin. Exp. 37:95, 1985.
25. McCammon, R. L., Stoehting, R. K., and Madura, J. Butorphanol and the bile duct. Anesth. Analg. 63:139, 1984.
26. Lee, G., Low, R. I., Amsterdam, E. A., et al. Hemodynamic effects of morphine and nalbuphine in acute myocardial infarction. Clin. Pharmacol. Ther. 29:576, 1981.
27. Romagnoli, A., and Keats, A. S. Ceiling effect for respiratory depression by nalbuphine. Clin. Pharmacol. Ther. 27:475, 1980.
28. Church, J. J. Continuous narcotic infusion for refief of postoperative pain. Br. Med. J. 1:977, 1979.
29. Tamsen, A., Hartvig, P., Dahlstrom, B., et al. Patient controlled analgesic therapy in the early postoperative period. Acta. Anaesthesiol. Scand. 23:462, 1979.
30. Sandgren, J., McPhee, M. S., and Greenberger, N. J. Narcotic bowel syndrome: Resolution of abdominal pain and intestinal pseudo-obstruction. Ann. Intern. Med. 101:331, 1984.
31. Devenyi, P., Mitwalli, A., and Graham, W. Clonidine therapy for narcotic withdrawal. Can. Med. Assoc. J. 127:1009, 1982.
32. Gourlay, G. K., Wilson, P. R., and Glynn, C. J. Methadone

produces prolonged postoperative analgesia. Br. Med. J. *284*:630, 1982.

33. Banning, A., Schmidt, J. F., Chraemmer-Jorgersen, B., et al. Comparison of oral controlled release morphine and epidural morphine in the management of postoperative pain. Anesth. Analg. *65*:385, 1986.
34. Hupert, C., Yacoub, M., and Turgeon, L. R. Effect of hydroxyzine on morphine analgesia for the treatment of post-operative pain. Anesth. Analg. *59*:690, 1980.
35. Beaver, W. T. Comparison of analgesic effects of morphine sulfate, hydroxyzine and their combination in patients with postoperative pain. *In* Bonica, J., and Ventafridda, R. (eds.) Advances in Pain Research and Therapy. Vol. 1. New York, Raven Press, 1976, p. 553.
36. Forrest, W. H., Brown, B. W., Brown, C. R., et al. Dextroamphetamine with morphine for treatment of postoperative pain. N. Engl. J. Med. *296*:712, 1977.
37. Lasker, E. M., Sunshine, A., and Mueller, F. Caffeine as an analgesic. JAMA *251*:1711, 1985.
38. Swerdlow, M., and Cundill, J. G. Anticonvulsant drugs used in the treatment of lancinating pain. A comparison. Anesthesia *36*:1129, 1981.
39. Walsh, T. D. Antidepressants and chronic pain. Clin. Neuropharmacol. *6*:279, 1983.
40. Hoff, G. S., Ruud, T. E., Tonder, M., et al. Doxepin in the treatment duodenal ulcer: An open clinical and endoscopic study comparing doxepin to cimetidine. Scand. J. Gastroenterol. *16*:1041, 1981.
41. Moore, J., and Dundee, J. W. Alterations in response to somatic pain associated with anaesthesia: V. The effect of promethazine. Br. J. Anaesth. *33*:3, 1961.
42. Houde, R. W. On assaying analgesics in man. *In* Knighton, and Dumke. Pain. Boston, Little, Brown and Co., 1966.
43. Hanks, G. W. Psychotropic drugs. Clin. Oncol. *3*:135, 1984.
44. Maltbie, A. A., Cavenar, J. O., Sullivan, J. L., et al. Analgesia and haloperidol: A hypothesis. J. Clin. Pharmacol. *19*:323, 1979.
45. St. John, A. E., and Born, C. K. Characterization of analgesic and activity effects of methotrimeprazine and morphine. Res. Commun. Chem. Pathol. Pharmacol. *26*:25, 1979.
46. Bellantuono, C., Reggi, V., Tognoni, G., et al. Benzodiazepines: Clinical pharmacology and therapeutics. Drugs *19*:195, 1980.
47. Young, R. R., and Delwaide, P. M. Spasticity, Parts I, II. N. Engl. J. Med. *304*:28, 96, 1981.
48. Green, R., and Dawkins, C. J. M. Postoperative analgesia: The use of continuous drip epidural block. Anesthesia *21*:372, 1966.
49. Arner, S. The role of nerve blocks in the treatment of cancer pain. Acta Anaesthesiol. Scand. (Suppl. 74) *74*:104, 1982.
50. Galaway, J. E., Caves, P. K., and Dundee, J. W. Effects of intercostal nerve blocks during operation on lung function and the relief of pain following thoracotomy. Br. J. Anaesth. *47*:730, 1975.
51. Buckley, P., and Simpson, R. Relief of pain following upper abdominal operations by thoracic epidural block with etidocaine. Acta Anaesthesiol. Scand. (Suppl.) *60*:76, 1975.
52. Ischia, S., Luzzani, A., Ischia, A., et al. A new approach to the neurolytic block of the coeliac plexus: The transaortic approach. Pain *16*:333, 1983.
53. Moore, D. C. Celiac (splanchnic) plexus block with alcohol for cancer pain of the upper intra-abdominal viscera. *In* Bonica, J. J., and Ventafridda, V. (eds.) Advances in Pain Research and Therapy. Vol. 2. New York, Raven Press, 1979, p. 357.
54. Leung, J. W. C., Bowen-Wright, M., Aveling, P. J., et al. Coeliac plexus block for pain in pancreatic cancer and chronic pancreatitis. Br. J. Surg. *70*:730, 1983.
55. Robertson, D. N. Transsacral neurolytic block. Br. J. Anaesth. *55*:873, 1983.
56. Arner, S., and Arner, B. Differential effects of epidural morphine in the treatment of cancer-related pain. Acta Anaesthesiol. Scand. *29*:32–36, 1985.
57. Cristensen, V. Respiratory depression after extradural morphine. Br. J. Anaesth. *52*:841, 1980.
58. Goodman, J. S., Goodman, J. M., and Vogel, A. V. Knowledge and use of placebos by house officers and nurses. Ann. Intern. Med. *91*:106, 1979.

17

Intestinal Gas

MICHAEL D. LEVITT
JOHN H. BOND

Although gaseous complaints are extremely common, this problem has received little serious, scientific attention. As a result, diagnosis and treatment are highly unsatisfactory. For example, measurements of the volume of gas in the gut or the rate of gas elimination are seldom obtained to confirm that the patient truly has a "gas" problem. Thus, the physician nearly always relies on the patient's assessment of the problem. Treatment of these complaints seldom has a scientific basis and, therefore, usually does not alleviate the problem. This chapter first summarizes available data on the physiology of intestinal gas and then discusses the relation of these data to the clinical syndromes thought to be caused by excessive gas.

VOLUME

The volume of gas present in the intestinal tract has been measured using a plethysmorgraph[1] or a rapid intestinal infusion of gas to wash out the bowel gases.[2] The intestines of normal subjects usually contain less than 200 ml of gas, both in the fasting state and after a meal. Similar volumes were found in subjects complaining of abdominal distention, which they attributed to excessive gas.[3]

The rate of excretion of gas per rectum is highly variable, ranging from 200 to 2000 ml per day (mean, 600 ml per day).[4] The number of passages of gas per rectum averaged 13.6 ± 6 (1 SD) in a small group of male young adult control subjects.[5] Of the many foods alleged to enhance excretion of rectal gas, the bean is the only food that has been carefully studied. A diet containing 51 per cent of its calories as pork and beans increased flatus elimination from a basal level of 15 to 176 ml per hour.[6]

COMPOSITION

Five gases (N_2, O_2, CO_2, H_2, and CH_4 [methane]) account for greater than 99 per cent of gas passed per rectum. The composition of this gas is highly variable, with the following ranges reported: N_2, 11 to 92 per cent; O_2, 0 to 11 per cent; CO_2, 3 to 54 per cent; H_2, 0 to 69 per cent; and CH_4, 0 to 56 per cent.[7, 8] Periods of rapid flatus excretion are associated with high H_2 and CO_2 concentration.

The composition of gas within the intestinal tract of ten normal subjects has been measured by the washout technique (Fig. 17–1).[2] Nitrogen was usually predominant; O_2 was present in very low concentration, and the concentrations of CO_2, H_2, and CH_4 were highly variable. Nitrogen plus O_2 composed less than 50 per cent of the gas of three of the ten subjects, indicating that swallowed air was not always the major source of bowel gas.

SOURCES OF INTESTINAL GAS

Gas in the gut may be derived from three different sources: air swallowing, intraluminal production, and diffusion from the blood.

Air Swallowing

The gastric gas bubble is frequently absent in subjects who cannot swallow air, as exemplified by severe achalasia in which a liquid level in the esophagus acts as a "trap" for gas. Thus, air swallowing is the major source of gas in the stomach, and intraluminal production plays a minor role.

Although it is clear that air is swallowed, controversy exists as to how much air reaches the stomach via this route and what fraction is subsequently eructated. Gastric aspiration studies suggest that several milliliters of air are deposited in the stomach with each swallow of a bolus of food or saliva.[9] Two or 3 ml of air per swallow would lead to the daily deposition of many liters of N_2 in the stomach. Little or no N_2 is absorbed

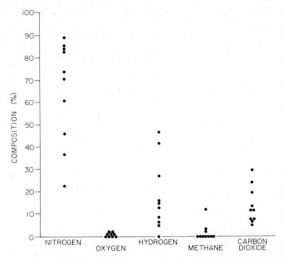

Figure 17–1. Composition of intestinal gas in ten fasting healthy subjects as determined by the gas washout technique.

during its passage through the intestine, yet only about 400 ml of N_2 is passed in flatus each day. Thus, it seems likely that most swallowed air never enters the small bowel. Subjects may subconsciously or consciously (i.e., esophageal speech) aspirate enormous quantities of air into the esophagus via a maneuver in which they relax their upper esophageal sphincter as they produce a negative intrathoracic pressure. Such aspiration can deposit air in the stomach at a rate of over 200 ml/min (personal observation).

The fraction of swallowed air passing into the duodenum is probably influenced by posture. The esophagus enters the posterosuperior aspect of the stomach. In the supine position gas becomes trapped above liquid overlaying the gastroesophageal junction and eructation is difficult, and a larger fraction of gastric air may be propelled into the small intestine. Eructation also may be markedly restricted following surgical repair of a hiatal hernia. Inability to eructate has been postulated to cause the "gas-bloat" syndrome, observed in patients following hiatal hernia repair.[10]

Intraluminal Gas Production

Three gases—CO_2, H_2, and CH_4—are produced in appreciable quantity in the bowel lumen. In the upper gut, CO_2 is liberated from the interaction of hydrogen ion and bicarbonate. In the duodenum, acid for this reaction results from gastric secretion, which averages about 30 mEq per hour after meals,[11] or from the digestion of triglycerides to fatty acids, which releases about 100 mEq per 30 g of fat. Although this reaction theoretically yields 22.4 ml of CO_2 per ml of bicarbonate neutralized, the actual volume of CO_2 liberated as gas may be far below this value owing to the slow decomposition of H_2CO_2 to CO_2 and H_2O in the absence of carbonic anhydrase and the relatively high solubility of CO_2 in water.[12] The pCO_2 of duodenal contents after a meal averaged 300 mm Hg and 500 mm Hg in control subjects and duodenal ulcer patients, respectively.[13] CO_2 therefore represents about 40 to 70 per cent of the duodenal gas of control subjects and duodenal ulcer patients. This gas is rapidly absorbed during intestinal passage, and CO_2 liberated in the upper gut contributes minimally to flatus volume. Flatus CO_2 concentration can be as high as 50 to 60 per cent, and such levels are usually associated with high concentrations of H_2. Because H_2 is produced solely by metabolism of the colonic flora, it seems likely that flatus CO_2 is derived from a similar source. It is not clear whether such CO_2 is a direct metabolic product of bacteria or whether bacterial fermentation liberates acids that interact with bicarbonate, yielding CO_2.

Hydrogen and Methane. Germ-free rats[14] and newborn infants[15] produce no H_2 nor CH_4, but such production is detected within hours of bacterial contamination of the rat. Thus, bacterial metabolism appears to be the sole source of these gases.

The site and rate of bacterial H_2 liberation in the human gut have been studied using a triple-lumen tube with an infusion site in the jejunum and collecting sites in the proximal and distal ileum.[16] During a constant infusion of N_2, negligible H_2 was found in gas aspirated from the proximal or distal ileum, both in the fasting state and after lactose instillation into the bowel (Fig. 17–2). Excretion of H_2 per rectum, which averaged 0.23 ml per minute in the fasting state, rose dramatically to 1.6 ml per minute following instillation of lactose into the colon. Thus, the H_2-producing bacteria normally are limited to the colon, and these bacteria require exogenous fermentable substrate for copious H_2 production. Human intestinal bacteria can liberate H_2 during fermentation of either carbohydrate or protein, although H_2 production from amino acids is appreciably less than from sugars.[17] Even in patients with severe overgrowth of the small bowel, H_2 produc-

tion in the small intestine was only a minor fraction of the colonic production when studied by the triple-lumen tube technique. However, high levels of fasting breath H_2 have been observed in subjects with bacterial overgrowth,[18] suggesting that H_2 can be produced in the contaminated small bowel. However, the possibility that colonic production of H_2 from malabsorbed carbohydrates has not been excluded in such patients.

Intestinal bacteria are capable of catabolizing as well as producing H_2. Less than 10 per cent of H_2 instilled into the cecum of a rat can be recovered, whereas recovery is complete in germ-free rats.[19] Thus, H_2 excretion represents the balance of production and catabolism by bacteria. The increased H_2 excretion observed in humans[20] and rats[19] after treatment with antibiotics may be due to inhibition of the H_2-catabolizing flora.

An acid pH in the colon inhibits H_2 release by fecal homogenates. One group of investigators attributed the diminution in H_2 excretion observed during chronic ingestion of the nonabsorbable carbohydrate, lactulose, to an acid colonic pH.[21] However, a second study observed no appreciable fall in cecal pH during chronic lactulose ingestion but found that the colonic bacteria adapted to malabsorption of the carbohydrate with an increased production of organic acids and a commensurate fall in H_2 production.[22] Another study of the H_2 response to prolonged exposure to a nonabsorbable carbohydrate found that long-term ingestion of a fructo-oligosaccharide enhanced H_2 production.[23] The metabolic adaptation of the colonic flora to chronic malabsorption of a carbohydrate may depend on the chemical structure of the carbohydrate.

A fraction of the H_2 liberated in the colon is absorbed and then excreted by the lungs, and a good correlation exists between simultaneous measurements of the rate of breath H_2 excretion and the rate of H_2 production in the colon.[16] Hence breath H_2 measurements provide a simple but reasonably accurate estimate of colonic H_2 production, and an increase in breath H_2 following ingestion of a test carbohydrate is widely employed as an indicator of carbohydrate malabsorption.[24, 25]

The excessive gas production noted by patients with malabsorption is probably explained by the incomplete absorption of carbohydrates and proteins which provide substrates for H_2 and CO_2 production by the colonic bacteria. In addition, a variety of fruits and vegetables (particularly beans) contain oligosaccharides and polysaccharides which cannot be digested by the enzymes of the small bowel[6] and hence are nonabsorbable. Recent studies also indicate that breath H_2 excretion increases after normal subjects ingest flours derived from whole or refined wheat, oats, corn, or potatoes.[26] Only rice flour is nearly totally absorbed.[26, 27] The production of H_2 after ingestion of these flours appears to be due to malabsorption of starch rather than fiber. In vitro studies with human fecal homogenates showed no liberation of H_2 from the fibers, cellulose, and lignin.[26] Although H_2 was released from pectin and gums, this H_2 liberation per gram of substrate was only about 15 per cent of that observed with

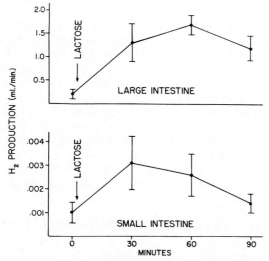

Figure 17–2. Comparison of the effect on H_2 production of instillation of 2 gm of lactose into the large and the small intestine. Production in the large intestine greatly exceeds that in the small intestine (scale for small intestine equals 1/500 that for large intestine).

soluble carbohydrates such as lactulose or glucose. Because the fiber content of the flours was insufficient to account for the H_2 production observed in in vivo studies, presumably starch must have been malabsorbed.

Like H_2, the sole source of CH_4 in humans is the metabolism of the colonic bacteria. Only about a third of the adult population excretes appreciable CH_4, and this individual tendency to produce or not to produce CH_4 usually is a fairly consistent trait when studied at intervals over a period of several years.[28] The CH_4-producing status of an individual seems to be familial and determined by early environmental rather than genetic factors. An unusual feature of subjects who produce large quantities of CH_4 is that they have stools that consistently float. Stools float because of their gas content rather than their fat content, and CH_4 becomes trapped in the stool, reducing its density below that of water.[29] Of greater clinical importance are two reports showing a higher than expected prevalence of CH_4 production in patients with colon cancer,[30, 31] although this finding was not observed in a third study.[32]

Fecal Odor. None of the quantitatively important gases has an odor, and the smell of feces is attributable to gases present in trace quantities. Surprisingly, the gases which cause the characteristic odor of feces have not been identified with certainty. Although indole and skatols were implicated in early studies,[33] a recent elegant study suggested that sulfur-containing compounds such as methanethiol and dimethyl sulfide are the gases responsible for the unpleasant odor of human feces.[34]

Diffusion of Gas between Lumen and Blood

Gases have appreciable solubility in both lipid and water and passively diffuse between the lumen and mucosal blood flow. The direction of movement is determined by the partial pressure gradient. Because the partial pressure of H_2 or CH_4 is always greater in the lumen than in blood, these gases always diffuse from the lumen into blood. In contrast, the direction of diffusion of CO_2, N_2, and O_2 is variable, and diffusion of these gases may either increase or decrease the volume of intestinal gas. For example, swallowed air contains minimal CO_2, and CO_2 diffuses from the mucosa into the stomach bubble. The pCO_2 rises dramatically in the duodenum, and CO_2 now diffuses from lumen to blood.

The pN_2 of swallowed air is slightly higher than that of venous blood, and in the stomach N_2 may be slowly absorbed. However, in the duodenum, the luminal pN_2 falls below that of the blood owing to dilution with CO_2, and N_2 diffuses into the lumen. Also, the production of CO_2, H_2, and CH_4 in the colon may reduce the pN_2 of flatus to below that of blood, with a resultant movement of N_2 from blood to lumen. When a near maximal pN_2 difference (about 400 mm Hg) is established between blood and lumen, N_2 diffuses across the mucosa of the entire human intestinal tract at a rate of about 100 ml per hour.[4] Because only about 16

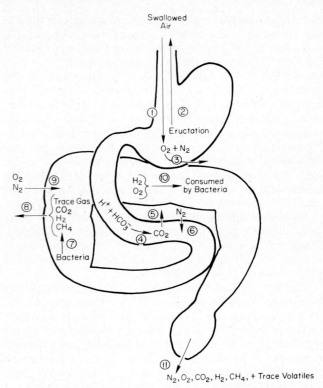

Figure 17–3. Mechanisms influencing rate of accumulation of gas in the gastrointestinal tract. Air is swallowed (1), and a sizable fraction is then eructated (2). The O_2 of gastric air diffuses into the blood draining the stomach. The reaction of H^+ and HCO_3^- yields CO_2 (4), which rapidly diffuses into the blood (5) while N_2 (6) diffuses into the lumen down a gradient established by the CO_2 production. In the colon, bacteria produce CO_2, H_2, and CH_4 (7), which diffuse into the blood perfusing the colon (8). Bacteria also consume O_2 and H_2 (9). N_2 diffuses into the colon (10) down a gradient established by bacterial production of CO_2, H_2, and CH_4. The net result of all these processes determines the composition and rate of passage of gas per rectum (11). (From Levitt, M. D., Bond, J. H., and Levitt, D. G. Physiology of the Gastrointestinal Tract. New York, Raven Press, 1981. Used by permission.)

ml of N_2 per hour is necessary to account for all the N_2 passed in flatus per day (400 ml), diffusion might account for an appreciable fraction of flatus N_2. Using presently available techniques, it is not possible to differentiate between air swallowing and diffusion as sources of luminal N_2.

The pO_2 of swallowed air is greater than that of blood, and O_2 is absorbed from the stomach. However, the pO_2 of colonic gas is very low, and O_2 constantly diffuses from blood to lumen.

Figure 17–3 shows the various mechanisms that influence the quantity and composition of bowel gas.

CLINICAL GAS SYNDROMES

Eructation

The occasional belch during or after meals expels gas from the stomach bubble. In contrast, individuals who repeatedly eructate can be shown to aspirate air into the esophagus prior to each belch. Most of this air is noisily regurgitated and never actually enters the stomach. Patients under emotional stress or who have thoracic or abdominal discomfort of any cause may complain of frequent, seemingly involuntary belching. For some reason, it appears that belching transiently relieves this distress. However, if appreciable portions of the swallowed air enter the stomach and intestines, increased discomfort may occur and a vicious circle results. Unaware that they are swallowing air, patients become convinced that they have a severe digestive abnormality and this concern further aggravates their aerophagia.

Evaluation of patients who complain of repeated belching consists of appropriate studies to rule out organic disease in those who complain of abdominal or thoracic symptoms. If no associated disease is found, counseling in which the aerophagia-belching mechanism is thoroughly explained may break the vicious circle. Although many subjects will still continue to belch, their distress is diminished when they understand the benign origin of their eructation.

Patients undergoing X-ray or minor surgical procedures in the supine position may develop diffuse distention of the entire gut over a period of minutes,[35, 36] and this distention is aggravated by ingestion of water or soda. Such distention results from air swallowing by the nervous patient, and the ingestion of liquids in the supine posture prevents subsequent eructation of the air. The ability of gas to pass rapidly through the gut with a mouth-to-anus transit time of 15 to 20 minutes accounts for rapid distention of the entire gut.

Gas and Functional Abdominal Pain

Abdominal discomfort and bloating, thought to be due to "too much gas," may be the most frequently encountered gastrointestinal complaints. Lacking objective measurements of intestinal gas volume, physicians have generally accepted their patient's conviction that excessive intestinal gas is the cause of these symptoms. However, abdominal roentgenograms seldom show excessive gas in such subjects. Studies employing the intestinal gas washout technique showed normal intestinal gas volumes in such patients in that 18 patients who thought they had excessive gas had mean fasting intestinal gas volume (176 ml) similar to that of ten control subjects (199 ml).[3] The composition of intestinal gas was also similar in the "gaseous" patients and control subjects. The bloating patients did differ from normal control subjects in that more of the infused gas refluxed back into the stomach, and they more frequently complained of severe abdominal pain during the infusion (Fig. 17–4).

Thus, complaints of pain and bloating usually result from disordered intestinal motility interfering with the orderly intestinal passage of gas rather than from excessive gas. Bloating patients also appear to have an enhanced pain response to bowel distention.[37] The

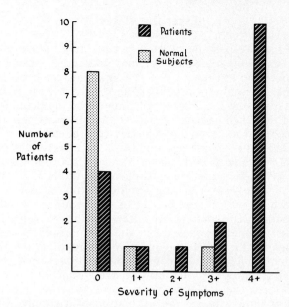

Figure 17–4. Severity of symptoms induced by infusion of gas into the intestinal tracts of normal subjects and patients with functional symptoms of abdominal pain and bloating. (From Lasser, R. B., et al.: N. Engl. J. Med. *293:*524, 1975. Used by permission.)

frequent claim that various foods "turn to gas" may represent the ability of these foods to stimulate abnormal motility rather than their tendency to gasify in the gut.

The treatment of these "gaseous" symptoms presumably should be directed toward correcting the abnormal intestinal motility. Anticholinergic agents are frequently prescribed for this purpose; however, their efficacy is yet to be proved conclusively in controlled studies. The symptoms of some bloating patients is clearly aggravated by anticholinergics.

One controlled trial suggested that the prokinetic agent, metaclopramide, improved bloating symptoms.[38] Because normal volumes of gas may serve as a painful stimulus in these patients, efforts should be made to reduce the volume of gas via counseling regarding repeated eructation (with its associated air swallowing) and elimination of foods from the diet that might serve as a substrate for colonic gas production. Lactose restriction appears to benefit some patients with functional abdominal complaints. There is contradictory evidence concerning the ability of activated charcoal to reduce the volume of gas produced during carbohydrate malabsorption, with two studies[39, 40] showing a dramatic reduction, whereas a third study[41] found that charcoal was not beneficial.

Although a variety of maneuvers to reduce air swallowing have been recommended, including chewing rather than gulping food, eating and drinking slowly, and avoidance of chewing gum, the effectiveness of such measures has never been demonstrated objectively. Massive air swallowers are almost always chronic eructators, and these patients usually improve if they can control the urge to eructate.

Excessive Flatus

Excessive passage of gas per anus may be a source of social embarrassment or may cause the patient to suspect the existence of a serious digestive derangement. The only thoroughly studied patient with excessive flatus was a 28-year-old man who meticulously recorded each passage of gas over a three-year period.[5] In contrast to seven age-matched control subjects who passed flatus an average of 13.6 ± 6 (1 SD) times per day, this man passed gas an average of 34 times daily. On his regular diet, his gas excretion (collected via a rectal tube) was 1380 ml per four hours, 82 per cent of which was H_2 and CO_2, gases produced in the intestine. The patient was lactase-deficient, and his flatus volume decreased but did not normalize when he avoided milk. By means of an elimination diet, the patient developed a low-flatus diet that was restricted in carbohydrate, particularly wheat products.[42]

Conventional blood, X-ray, or endoscopic studies are of little value in the evaluation of a patient with excessive flatus. A major problem is to determine if the patient actually passes excessive gas or is unusually sensitive to the passage of normal gas volumes. Although not very precise, the frequency of gas passage may be used as a crude indicator of normality.

Whether excessive flatus is due to air swallowing or to intraluminal production may be determined by gas chromatographic analysis of rectal gas, taking care to prevent room air contamination. In our experience, virtually every patient who complains of excessive flatus is producing this gas (H_2, CO_2, and CH_4) in his or her colon rather than swallowing excessive air (O_2 and N_2). Because flatus H_2 and CO_2 are largely derived from fermentation of malabsorbed carbohydrate, high flatus concentrations of H_2 and CO_2 may be indicative of an abnormality of carbohydrate absorption caused by either a generalized malabsorptive disorder or an isolated abnormality such as lactase deficiency. More commonly, no such absorptive problem is demonstrable and the patient apparently has a colonic flora which produces excessive gas from the fermentable substrates that normally reach the colon. A diet low in lactose, starches, and legumes will reduce flatus excretion in most subjects, although such a diet is seldom adhered to for long periods of time.

Explosions in the Colon

Two gases formed in the colon, H_2 and CH_4, are combustible and potentially explosive. Numerous explosions resulting in severe colonic trauma and perforation have been triggered by electrocauterization performed through the proctosigmoidoscope.[43–45] The usual thorough bowel cleansing prior to colonoscopy prevents the development of explosive concentrations of H_2 and CH_4.[46] The only reported explosion during electrocautery-snare polypectomy through the colonoscope occurred in a patient who received mannitol as a purgative.[47] Mannitol serves as a substrate for H_2-producing bacteria and hence is an inappropriate choice of purgative if electrocautery is contemplated. The commonly employed oral preparations now used for colonic cleaning, such as Golytely, contain electrolytes and polyethylene glycol, a nonabsorbable, osmotically active polymer, which cannot be fermented by the colonic bacteria.[48] There have been no intracolonic explosions reported when such solutions have been employed for colonic cleansing.

References

1. Bedell, G. N., Marshall, R., Dubois, A. B., and Harris, J. H. Measurement of the volume of gas in the gastrointestinal tract. J. Clin. Invest. *35*:336, 1956.
2. Levitt, M. D. Volume and composition of human intestinal gas determined by means of an intestinal washout technique. N. Engl. J. Med. *284*:1394, 1971.
3. Lasser, R. B., Bond, J. H., and Levitt, M. D. The role of intestinal gas in functional abdominal pain. N. Engl. J. Med. *293*:524, 1975.
4. Kirk, E. The quantity and composition of human colonic flatus. Gastroenterology *12*:782, 1949.
5. Levitt, M. D., Lasser, R. B., Schwartz, J. S., and Bond, J. H. Studies of a flatulent patient. N. Engl. J. Med. *295*:260, 1976.
6. Steggerda, F. R. Gastrointestinal gas following food consumption. Ann. N.Y. Acad. Sci. *150*:57, 1968.
7. Levitt, M. D., and Bond, J. H. Volume, composition and source of intestinal gas. Gastroenterology *59*:921, 1970.
8. Calloway, D. H. Gas in the alimentary canal. *In* Code, C. F. (ed.) Handbook of Physiology. Vol. V. Sect. 6, Alimentary Canal. Washington, D.C., American Physiological Society, 1967, pp. 2839–2859.
9. Maddock, W. G., Bell, J. L., and Tremaine, M. J. Gastrointestinal gas. Observations on belching during anesthesia, operations and pyleography and rapid passage of gas. Ann. Surg. *130*:512, 1949.
10. Woodward, E. R., Thomas, H. F., and McAlhany, H. P. Comparison of crural repair and Nissen fundoplication in the treatment of esophageal hiatus hernia with peptic esophagitis. Ann. Surg. *173*:782, 1971.
11. Fordtran, J. S., and Walsh, J. H. Gastric acid secretion rate and buffer content of the stomach after eating. Results in normal subjects and in patients with duodenal ulcer. J. Clin. Invest. *52*:645, 1973.
12. Fordtran, J. S., Morawski, S. G., Santa Ana, C. A., and Rector, F. C., Jr. Gas production after reaction of sodium bicarbonate and hydrochloric acid. Gastroenterology *87*:1014, 1984.
13. Rune, S. J. Acid-base parameters of duodenal contents in man. Gastroenterology *62*:533, 1972.
14. Levitt, M. D., French, P., and Donaldson, R. M. Use of hydrogen and methane excretion in the study of the intestinal flora (abstract). J. Lab. Clin. Med. *72*:988, 1968.
15. Engel, R. R., and Levitt, M. D. Intestinal tract gas formation in newborns (abstract). *In* Program for meeting of American Pediatric Society and Society for Pediatric Research, 1970, p. 266.
16. Levitt, M. D. Production and excretion of hydrogen gas in man. N. Engl. J. Med. *281*:122, 1969.
17. Calloway, D. H., Colasito, D. J., and Mathews, R. D. Gases produced by human intestinal microflora. Nature *212*:1238, 1966.
18. Perman, J. A., Modler, S., Barr, R. G., and Rosenthal, P. Fasting breath hydrogen concentration: Normal values and clinical application. Gastroenterology *87*:1358, 1984.
19. Levitt, M. D., Berggren, T., Hastings, J., and Bond, J. H. Hydrogen (H_2) catabolism in the colon of the rat. J. Lab. Clin. Med. *84*:163, 1974.
20. Murphy, E. L., and Calloway, D. H. The effect of antibiotic drugs on the volume and composition of intestinal gas from beans. Am. J. Dig. Dis. *17*:639, 1972.
21. Perman, J. A., Modler, S., and Olson, A. C. Role of pH in production of hydrogen from carbohydrates by colonic bacterial flora. J. Clin. Invest. *67*:643, 1981.

22. Florent, C., Flourie, B., Leblond, A., Rautureau, M., Bernier, J. J., and Rambaud, J. C. Influence of chronic lactulose ingestion on the colonic metabolism of lactulose in man (an in vivo study). J. Clin. Invest. 75:608, 1985.

23. Stone-Dorshow, T., and Levitt, M. D. Gaseous response to ingestion of a poorly absorbed fructo-oligosaccharide sweetener. Am. J. Clin. Nutr. (in press).

24. Levitt, M. D., and Donaldson, R. M. Use of respiratory hydrogen (H_2) excretion to detect carbohydrate malabsorption. J. Lab. Clin. Med. 75:937, 1970.

25. Bond, J. H., and Levitt, M. D. Quantitative measurement of lactose absorption. Gastroenterology 70:1058, 1972.

26. Levitt, M. D., Hirsh, P., Fetzer, C. A., Sheahan, M., and Levine, A. S. H_2 excretion after ingestion of complex carbohydrates. Gastroenterology (in press).

27. Kerlin, P., Wong, L., Harris, B., and Capra, S. Rice flour, breath hydrogen and malabsorption. Gastroenterology 87:578, 1984.

28. Bond, J. H., Engel, R. R., and Levitt, M. D. Factors influencing pulmonary methane excretion in man. J. Exp. Med. 133:572, 1971.

29. Levitt, M. D., and Duane, W. C. Floating stools—flatus versus fat. N. Engl. J. Med. 286:973, 1972.

30. Haines, A., Metz, G., Dilawari, J., Blendis, L., and Wiggins, H. Breath methane in patients with cancer of the large bowel. Lancet 2:481, 1977.

31. Pique, J. M., Pallares, M., Cuso E., Vilar-Bonet, J., and Gassull, M. A. Methane production and colon cancer. Gastroenterology 87:601, 1984.

32. Karlin, D. A., Jones, R. D., Stroeleim, J. R., Mastromarino, A. J., and Potter, G. D. Breath methane excretion in patients with unresected colorectal cancer. J. Natl. Cancer Inst. 69:573, 1982.

33. Orton, J. M., and Neuhaus, O. W. Nutrition: Digestion, absorption and energy metabolism. Chapter 13. In Orton, J. M., Neuhaus, O. W. (eds.) Human Biochemistry. 9th ed. St. Louis, C. V. Mosby Co., 1975, p. 471.

34. Moore, J. G., Jessop, L. D., and Osborne, D. N. A gas-chromatographic and mass spectrometric analysis of the odor of human feces. Gastroenterology (in press).

35. Oppenheimer, A. Gas in the bowels. Surg. Gynecol. Obstet. 70:105, 1940.

36. Begg, R. C. A rational theory of intestinal distention and its urologic application. J. Urol. 59:358, 1948.

37. Ritchie, J. Pain from distention of the pelvic colon by inflating a balloon, in the irritable colon syndrome. Gut 14:125, 1973.

38. Johnson, A. G. Controlled trial of metoclopramide in the treatment of flatulent dyspepsia. Br. Med. J. 2:25, 1971.

39. Hall, G. H., Jr., Thompson, H., and Strother, A. Effects of orally administered activated charcoal on intestinal gas. Am. J. Gastroenterol. 75:192, 1981.

40. Jain, N. K., Patel, V. P., and Pitchumoni, C. S. Activated charcoal, simethicone, and intestinal gas: A double-blind study. Ann. Intern. Med. 105:61, 1986.

41. Potter, T., Ellis, C., and Levitt, M. Activated charcoal: In vivo and in vitro studies of effect on gas formation. Gastroenterology 88:620, 1985.

42. Sutalf, L. O., and Levitt, M. D. Follow-up of a flatulent patient. Dig. Dis. Sci. 24:652, 1979.

43. Levy, E. I. Explosions during lower bowel electrosurgery. Am. J. Surg. 88:754, 1954.

44. Carter, H. G. Explosions in the colon during electrodesiccation of polyps. Am. J. Surg. 84:514, 1952.

45. Bond, J. H., Levy, M., and Levitt, M. D. Explosions of hydrogen gas in the colon during proctosigmoidoscopy. Gastrointest. Endosc. 23:41, 1976.

46. Bond, J. H., and Levitt, M. D. Factors affecting the concentration of combustible gases in the colon during colonoscopy. Gastroenterology 68:1445, 1975.

47. Bigard, M. A., Gaucher, P., and Lassalle, C. Fatal colonic explosion during colonoscopic polypectomy. Gastroenterology 77:1307, 1979.

48. Davis, G. R., Santa Ana, C. A., and Morawski, S. G. Development of a lavage solution associated with minimal water and electrolyte absorption or secretion. Gastroenterology 78:991, 1980.

18

Maldigestion and Malabsorption

TERESA L. WRIGHT
MARTIN F. HEYWORTH

Malabsorption of one or more constituents of food occurs when the normal digestion and absorption of food is interrupted. Malabsorption is a comprehensive term which includes both defective hydrolysis of large molecules and ineffective uptake of breakdown products of these molecules in the small intestine. Knowledge of the normal digestive process greatly facilitates the understanding of the pathophysiology of malabsorption (see p. 1062–1088). This chapter will discuss the mechanisms responsible for different malabsorptive states and will only briefly mention specific diseases, which are discussed in detail in other chapters.

Normal digestion and absorption can be divided into three sequential stages. The *intraluminal stage* comprises the luminal hydrolysis of fat and protein by pancreatic enzymes released into the duodenum and the solubilization of fat by bile salts. In addition, normal absorption of certain dietary components (such as iron and vitamin B_{12}) requires that they are present in the intestinal lumen in a biologically assimilable form (for example, free Fe^{2+} ions in the case of iron), or that cofactors for their absorption are present (for example, intrinsic factor in the case of vitamin B_{12} absorption). The *intestinal stage* includes (1) hydrolysis of carbohydrates by brush border disaccharidases, (2) epithelial cell transport of monosaccharides, fatty acids, monoglycerides, small peptides, and amino acids, and (3) formation of chylomicrons from triglycerides and cholesterol in epithelial cells. Finally, the *lymphatic transport stage* is important for removal of nutrients from intestinal epithelial cells to other organs for storage or metabolism. Diseases which interrupt any of these stages can lead to inefficient absorption of one or more constituents of food.

PATHOPHYSIOLOGIC MECHANISMS

A pathophysiologic classification of different causes of impaired digestion and absorption and diseases associated with these defects are summarized in Table 18–1. The mechanisms of malabsorption in different disease states are briefly discussed here in the order in which they appear in Table 18–1.

Intraluminal Stage: Impaired Hydrolysis and Solubilization of Nutrients in the Small Intestinal Lumen

Impaired Fat Absorption. Because pancreatic lipase and colipase are necessary for triglyceride hydrolysis in the duodenum, disorders that cause pancreatic enzyme deficiency lead to fat malabsorption. Furthermore, pancreatic enzymes are inactivated by a low luminal pH (as occurs in the *Zollinger-Ellison syndrome*) with consequent malabsorption of fat. The products of triglyceride hydrolysis, namely fatty acids and monoglycerides, are solubilized by bile salts to form micelles and are then absorbed in the small intestine. Disorders that interrupt the enterohepatic circulation of bile salts lead to impaired micelle formation and fat absorption and are summarized in Table 18–2. These diseases may be associated with malabsorption of fat-soluble vitamins (A, D, E, and K), which leads to clinical manifestations of vitamin deficiencies (Table 18–3).

Impaired Protein Absorption. Although protein hydrolysis begins in the stomach through the action of pepsin, it mainly occurs in the small intestine, catalyzed by pancreatic proteases. Deficiency of pancreatic proteases (trypsin, chymotrypsin, and carboxypeptidases

Table 18–1. PATHOPHYSIOLOGIC CLASSIFICATION OF MALABSORPTION

Affected Mechanism	Pathophysiology	Associated Diseases
1. *Intraluminal stage*		
a. Digestion (fat, protein)	Decreased pancreatic enzyme and bicarbonate release	Chronic pancreatitis, cystic fibrosis, pancreatic carcinoma
	Pancreatic enzyme inactivation by acid	Zollinger-Ellison syndrome
	Rapid transit of nutrients; dilution of pancreatic enzymes	Post-gastrectomy
b. Solubilization (fat)	Disruption of the enterohepatic circulation of bile (see Table 18–2)	Biliary tract obstruction, terminal ileal resection or disease, small bowel bacterial overgrowth, cholestatic liver disease (see Table 18–2)
	Decreased CCK-PZ release	Extensive small intestinal destruction
c. Availability of ingested nutrients	Deficiency of intrinsic factor promoting vitamin B_{12} absorption	Pernicious anemia
	Uptake of vitamin B_{12} by intestinal bacteria	Blind loop syndrome
	Uptake of vitamin B_{12} by tapeworms	*Diphyllobothrium latum* infection
	Binding by oxalates or fatty acids	Calcium deficiency
	Binding by phytates	Iron deficiency
2. *Intestinal stage*		
a. Epithelial cell digestion (carbohydrate)	Disaccharidase deficiency	Lactase deficiency, Crohn's disease.
b. Epithelial cell transport (fat, protein)	Loss of normal epithelial cells	Crohn's disease, celiac disease, sarcoidosis, tropical sprue, radiation enteritis, intestinal ischemia, Whipple's disease, ileal resection, eosinophilic gastroenteritis, colchicine, neomycin
	Impaired amino acid transport	Hartnup disease, cystinuria
	Impaired vitamin B_{12} transport	Inherited vitamin B_{12} deficiency
	Impaired folate transport	Congenital folate deficiency
	Nonformation of chylomicrons	Abetalipoproteinemia
	Impaired transport of bile acids	Primary bile acid malabsorption
3. *Lymphatic transport stage* (fat, protein)	Lymphatic duct obstruction	Lymphangiectasia, lymphoma, tuberculosis, carcinoid
4. *Unexplained* (multiple)		Diabetes mellitus, giardiasis, adrenal insufficiency, hyperthyroidism, hypogammaglobulinemia, amyloidosis Acquired immune deficiency syndrome

Table 18–2. CONDITIONS ASSOCIATED WITH
IMPAIRED MICELLE FORMATION

Pathophysiology	Associated Diseases
Decreased bile salt formation	Severe parenchymal liver disease
Decreased bile salt delivery to the duodenum	Cholestatic liver disease (primary biliary cirrhosis, drug-induced cholestasis), bile duct obstruction (cholangiocarcinoma, pancreatic carcinoma, gallstones, sclerosing cholangitis)
Decreased ionization of conjugated bile salts	Zollinger-Ellison syndrome
Decreased intraluminal bile salt concentration	Binding agents (cholestyramine)
Bile salt deconjugation	Bacterial overgrowth in jejunal diverticula, small intestinal fistulae and strictures in Crohn's disease, scleroderma, intestinal pseudo-obstruction, diabetes and the elderly
Increased intestinal bile salt loss	Crohn's disease, small intestinal resection, cholecystocolonic fistula

A and B) results in impaired hydrolysis of polypeptides. Therefore, *chronic pancreatitis, pancreatic carcinoma, cystic fibrosis*, and *pancreatic resection* can lead to protein malnutrition. Pancreatic proteases are also important for vitamin B_{12} absorption. These enzymes release vitamin B_{12} from R proteins, prior to binding with intrinsic factor. In profound pancreatic insufficiency, normal release of the vitamin from R proteins does not occur, so the amount of the vitamin available for binding to intrinsic factor for absorption is decreased. As pancreatic protease function tends to be preserved until there is extensive pancreatic damage, vitamin B_{12} deficiency is a rare consequence of pancreatic insufficiency.

Impaired Carbohydrate Absorption. Most diseases that cause carbohydrate malabsorption do so by affecting the intestinal stage of digestion and absorption. However, because pancreatic amylase catalyzes the hydrolysis of starch to oligosaccharides some carbohydrate malabsorption is seen in pancreatic insufficiency.

Decreased Availability of Ingested Nutrients and Cofactors for Absorption. Vitamin B_{12} malabsorption can result from intrinsic factor deficiency (following gastrectomy or antibody formation directed against gastric parietal cells or intrinsic factor in pernicious anemia). A rare inherited disorder results in the production of an abnormal intrinsic factor by gastric parietal cells which is unable to bind to vitamin B_{12} in the intestinal lumen[1, 2] and the absorption of the vitamin is therefore impaired. In addition, bacteria in the small intestinal lumen of patients with blind loop syndrome (see pp. 1106–1112) can bind vitamin B_{12}. Vitamin B_{12} deficiency also occurs in patients infected with the fish tapeworm, *Diphyllobothrium latum*, because the worm competes with the host for dietary vitamin B_{12}.

Certain dietary constituents can bind nutrients in the intestinal lumen, which then become unavailable for absorption. For example, excessive dietary oxalate binds calcium with the consequent formation of calcium oxalate. This is insoluble in the intestinal lumen, and the calcium in the calcium oxalate is unavailable for absorption. Similarly, long-chain fatty acids bind calcium (in fat malabsorption), and a high dietary phytate content binds iron.

Table 18–3. SYMPTOMS AND SIGNS OF MALABSORPTION

Clinical Features	Pathophysiology	Laboratory Findings
Diarrhea	Increased secretion and decreased absorption of water and electrolytes; unabsorbed fatty acids and bile salts	Increased fat excretion, decreased serum carotene, "osmotic gap" in stool electrolytes
Weight loss with hyperphagia	Decreased absorption of fat, protein, and carbohydrate	Increased fat excretion
Bulky, foul-smelling stools	Decreased fat absorption	Increased fat excretion
Muscle wasting, edema	Decreased protein absorption	Decreased serum albumin
Flatulence, borborygmi, abdominal distention	Fermentation of carbohydrates by intestinal bacteria	Increased fat excretion Decreased D-xylose absorption
Abdominal pain	Small intestinal stricture Infiltration of the pancreas Intestinal ischemia	Increased fat excretion
Paresthesias, tetany	Decreased vitamin D and calcium absorption	Hypocalcemia, hypomagnesemia
Bone pain	Decreased calcium absorption	Hypocalcemia, increased alkaline phosphatase
Muscle cramps, weakness	Excess potassium loss	Hypokalemia, abnormal ECG
Easy bruisability, petechiae, hematuria	Decreased vitamin K absorption	Prolonged prothrombin time, increased fat excretion
Hyperkeratosis, night blindness	Decreased vitamin A absorption	Decreased carotene, increased fat excretion
Pallor	Decreased vitamin B_{12}, folate, or iron absorption	Macrocytic anemia, microcytic anemia
Glossitis, stomatitis, cheilosis	Decreased vitamin B_{12}, folate, or iron absorption	Decreased serum vitamin B_{12}, folate, or iron
Acrodermatitis	Zinc deficiency	Decreased serum zinc

Intestinal Stage: Abnormalities of Small Intestinal Mucosa

Impaired Epithelial Cell Digestion. Oligosaccharides are hydrolyzed to monosaccharides by specific enzymes located in the brush border membrane of intestinal epithelial cells and the monosaccharides are then transported across the cells. When specific brush border enzymes are deficient, the nonabsorbed oligosaccharides are metabolized by colonic bacteria to di- and trisaccharides, carbon dioxide, and hydrogen, with consequent abdominal distention and flatulence. Although a number of disaccharidase deficiencies have been described, the most common is *lactase deficiency*, which may be either congenital or acquired. Lactase is required for the hydrolysis of lactose to glucose and galactose, which are then transported across the enterocyte by a sodium-dependent active transport mechanism. *Congenital lactase deficiency* presents in infancy and is rare. *Acquired lactase deficiency* may be either a primary decrease in the amount of the enzyme in the mucosa (see below) or may occur when there is abnormality or destruction of small intestinal epithelial cells, as seen, for example, in *celiac disease, acute infectious enteritis, Crohn's disease, tropical sprue*, or *radiation enteritis*. Other much less common genetic defects include deficiencies of other disaccharidases (trehalase and sucrase alpha-dextrinase).

Intestinal Stage: Impaired Epithelial Cell Transport

Transport of Multiple Nutrients. A number of diseases cause significant loss of intestinal surface area resulting in malabsorption of all major dietary constituents (see Table 18–1). Conditions in which intestinal epithelial surface area is reduced or remaining epithelial cells are abnormal include *celiac disease* (p. 1134), *tropical sprue* (p. 1281), *collagenous sprue* (Fig. 61–7, p. 1146), *radiation enteritis* (p. 1369), *Whipple's disease* (p. 1297), *eosinophilic gastroenteritis* (p. 1123), and *intestinal ischemia* (p. 1903). Extensive surgical resection of the small intestine also reduces the epithelial surface area available for absorption (p. 1106). Some compensatory increase in the epithelial area of the remaining small intestine occurs following surgical resection, allowing for absorption of certain nutrients, although once lost, vitamin B_{12} and bile salt transport do not return. Certain drugs may also reduce the surface area available for absorption. Colchicine inhibits cell division and reduces the number of cells available for absorption, and neomycin produces blunting of the small intestinal villi through an unknown mechanism, leading to steatorrhea. In all these disorders due to drugs, steatorrhea is typically mild (6 to 15 gm of fecal fat per day) and patients have decreased D-xylose absorption (see below).

Transport of Carbohydrates. Specific defects in the absorption of carbohydrates are usually caused by mucosal enzyme deficiencies (see above). However, there is a rare, recessively inherited disorder in which the carrier-mediated transport of glucose and galactose in the intestinal epithelial cell membrane is impaired. This presents clinically as a watery diarrhea in infants shortly after birth.

Transport of Amino Acids. There are also rare recessively inherited defects in amino acid transport. *Hartnup disease* is characterized by impaired transport of neutral amino acids (phenylalanine and tryptophan) by intestinal and renal epithelial cells. Patients have a pellagra-like dermatitis due primarily to a deficiency of tryptophan (a precursor of nicotinamide), although protein malnutrition is not seen because dipeptide absorption is normal. Similarly, patients with *cystinuria*, although unable to transport dibasic amino acids (cystine, lysine, and arginine), have few symptoms of protein malabsorption. Patients with these disorders may have diarrhea, attributed to bacterial metabolism of the excess amino acids in the intestine. They also have aminoaciduria with the formation of renal calculi in *cystinuria* (see p. 1081).

Transport of Fats. Micelles consisting of the products of triglyceride hydrolysis (monoglycerides, free fatty acids, and glycerol), phospholipids, cholesterol, and bile salts are transported from the intestinal lumen across the apical membrane of small intestinal epithelial cells. Disaggregation of micelles occurs during the transport process; diglycerides and triglycerides are resynthesized in the cells, and subsequently, chylomicrons are formed from triglycerides, phospholipids, cholesterol, and apoproteins (p. 1070). In the rare inherited disorder *abetalipoproteinemia*, chylomicron formation is impaired due to absence of apolipoprotein B. Fat malabsorption results, and fat accumulates within epithelial cells because its export across the basolateral membrane is inhibited.

Other Inherited Transport Defects. Vitamin B_{12} deficiency is occasionally due to impaired intestinal transport. The vitamin B_{12}–intrinsic factor complex can bind to ileal cells, but transport across the cells does not occur.[3] In *congenital folate deficiency*, folic acid transport is impaired as a result of a rare specific intestinal cell transport defect.[4]

Lymphatic Transport: Impaired Transport of Nutrients from the Small Intestine

Diseases that cause lymphatic obstruction can lead to fat malabsorption and a protein-losing enteropathy (p. 283). In *intestinal lymphangiectasia*, the subepithelial lymphatics are dilated and functionally obstructed. Consequently, removal of chylomicrons in the lymph is abnormally slow in this condition. In infiltrative diseases of the small intestine (for example, *tuberculous enteritis, intestinal lymphoma*, and *Whipple's disease*), mononuclear leukocytes may compress lymphatic vessels in the small intestinal wall and retard chylomicron removal. In addition, enlargement of regional lymph nodes (as in *tuberculosis, lymphoma, metastatic carcinoma*, and *metastatic carcinoid disease*) may produce lymphatic obstruction and fat malabsorption.

Unclear Mechanism

A number of diseases are associated with malabsorption, but the pathophysiologic reason for the impaired absorption is unclear. Normal enterocyte function may be impaired in *amyloidosis* and *giardiasis*, although the observed steatorrhea seems to be disproportional to the intestinal infiltration (by amyloid fibrils or organisms, respectively). Malabsorption is common in patients with acquired immune deficiency syndrome (AIDS), some of whom have intestinal *Kaposi's sarcoma* or infection with *Mycobacterium avium intracellulare*, but in some no obvious etiology for diarrhea and impaired absorption can be found (pp. 1237, 1244, and 1246). A number of endocrine disorders (*diabetes mellitus* and *thyrotoxicosis*) are associated with malabsorption which is postulated to result from intestinal dysmotility and bacterial overgrowth, although the true etiology of the malabsorption is unknown. Normal absorptive functions of the small intestine are decreased in the elderly (see below), and again, the pathophysiologic reason for this change is not well understood (p. 162).

CLINICAL MANIFESTATIONS

History. Although many of the symptoms of malabsorption are nonspecific, for example, *diarrhea, weight loss*, and *symptoms of anemia*, clinical history can provide clues to the etiology of malabsorption in some patients. Early symptoms of *intestinal* or *pancreatic disease* include fatigue, bloating, anorexia, and the passage of two to three loose stools per day. An increase in stool bulk may be the first change noticed by the patient. However, more advanced pancreatic insufficiency may be associated with classic symptoms of fat malabsorption, which include the passage of bulky, floating, malodorous stools. Although stools were considered to float because of a high fat content, they actually float because of increased gas.[5] Some common clinical features of malabsorption and their pathophysiology are summarized in Table 18–3. Both small intestinal and pancreatic disease may result in profound weight loss, although anorexia is more characteristic of small intestinal disease or *pancreatic carcinoma* than chronic pancreatitis. Patients with *chronic pancreatitis* tend to have hyperphagia, which may contribute to the marked fat excretion characteristic of this disease. Anemia (due to vitamin B$_{12}$, iron, or folate malabsorption) may present with dyspnea, dizziness, fatigue, and pallor.

Diffuse abdominal pain is not usually associated with malabsorption unless extensive small intestinal disease with partial intestinal obstruction is present (as in *Crohn's disease* or *radiation enteritis*, for example). Patients with chronic *intestinal ischemia* classically have pain 20 to 60 minutes after meals and usually have other evidence of peripheral vascular disease. The abdominal pain of chronic pancreatitis tends to be epigastric with radiation into the back. Patients with small intestinal *lymphoma* frequently have severe periumbilical or generalized abdominal pain.

Specific questions should be asked which may help to define the cause of malabsorption. Recent foreign travel may be associated with parasitic diseases, including *giardiasis*, and residence overseas may result in tropical sprue. Homosexual contact, intravenous drug abuse, or multiple blood tranfusions predispose to infection with the *human immunodeficiency virus* (HIV). Patients infected with this virus are prone to develop opportunisic infections caused by a variety of organisms, including *Mycobacterium avium intracellulare*. Alcohol is toxic to the small intestinal mucosa affecting absorption,[6] and chronic alcohol abuse may cause pancreatic insufficiency and fat malabsorption. In a child, small stature or failure to thrive are features of *celiac disease* and of *cystic fibrosis*. Malabsorption and concomitant bronchitis or bronchiectasis also suggest cystic fibrosis. Patients with disaccharidase deficiencies experience abdominal distention, nausea, and watery diarrhea 30 to 90 minutes after ingesting a particular disaccharide sugar (e.g., milk sugar in *lactase deficiency*). *Eosinophilic gastroenteritis* should be suspected in any patient with malabsorption and a history of "food allergies." A history of peptic ulcer disease and diarrhea raises the possibility of *Zollinger-Ellison syndrome*. Abdominal surgery, particularly a Billroth II partial gastrectomy, can lead to the creation of a blind loop of small intestine. As discussed on page 1289, malabsorption is a feature of the blind loop syndrome. Small intestinal resection may interrupt the enterohepatic circulation of bile salts with resulting fat malabsorption and, if extensive, may impair the absorption of other nutrients. In patients with malabsorption, nondeforming arthritis, neurologic symptoms, or valvular heart disease, *Whipple's disease* should be considered (p. 1297). *Scleroderma* can lead to small intestinal dysmotility and bacterial overgrowth. Certain small intestinal diseases have dermatologic manifestations (for example, *dermatitis herpetiformis* in *celiac disease*). Some endocrine disorders (*diabetes mellitus, Addison's disease, hypoparathyroidism*, and *thyrotoxicosis*) are also associated with malabsorption, and symptoms suggestive of these disorders should be sought in the patient's history (p. 488). Finally, a careful drug history should be taken because certain drugs (for example, colchicine, cholestyramine, neomycin, and cathartics) may cause malabsorption.

Physical Examination. If malabsorption is not severe, the physical examination may be normal, or there may be minor physical abnormalities including smooth lateral margins of the tongue and hyperactive bowel sounds. With more severe malabsorption, patients may show evidence of malnutrition, with muscle wasting particularly in the temporal areas. *Pallor* of mucous membranes suggests anemia (which may result from malabsorption of iron, vitamin B$_{12}$, or folate). Deficiencies of fat-soluble vitamins can produce *hyperkeratosis* of the skin (vitamin A), *ecchymoses* and *hematuria* (vitamin K), and *paresthesias, tetany, positive Chvostek* and *Trousseau signs*, and *bone pain* with vertebral collapse (vitamin D and calcium). Patients with intestinal disease may have malabsorption of water-soluble vitamins (notably B vitamins) with resulting *glossitis* (riboflavin and niacin deficiency), *cheilosis, dermatitis* (pellagra from niacin deficiency), and *peripheral neuropathy* (vitamin B_{12} deficiency).

The prognosis of patients with malabsorption is determined by the nature of the underlying disease (diseases which cause malabsorption are summarized in Table 18–1).

SPECIFIC DISEASE STATES

Diseases that impair digestion and absorption are summarized in Tables 18–1 and 18–2. Many of these diseases are discussed in detail in other portions of the book. The clinical features and investigation of specific diseases will now be considered according to their pathophysiologic classification.

Intraluminal Stage: Digestion

Pancreatic Disease. Pancreatic proteases, lipase, and amylase are essential for the normal digestion of nutrients, and diseases of the pancreas typically produce significant fat malabsorption (commonly > 25 gm of fecal fat excretion per day). Pancreatic bicarbonate secretion neutralizes gastric acid and maintains the duodenum at the alkaline pH required for pancreatic enzyme activity. Profound destruction of the pancreas must occur before significant steatorrhea results.[7, 8]

Although chronic *alcoholic pancreatitis* is the commonest cause of pancreatic exocrine insufficiency, in one study 75 per cent of patients with *pancreatic carcinoma* had fat malabsorption, some of whom improved with exogenous pancreatic enzyme replacement.[9] Symptoms of fat malabsorption predominate in patients with pancreatic exocrine insufficiency, but symptoms of impaired protein absorption (for example, *muscle wasting* and *edema*) also occur. Patients typically have hyperphagia and are able to maintain their body weight despite significant malabsorption. Impaired vitamin B_{12} absorption is common but true vitamin B_{12} deficiency is rare. Symptoms result from malabsorption of the fat-soluble vitamins (A, D, E, and K, see Table 18–3) and from hypocalcemia caused by chelation of calcium by excess fatty acids in the intestine. For further discussion of the clinical features and causes of pancreatic disease see pages 1814 to 1872.

Pancreatic disease should be suspected in any patients with steatorrhea (determined by fecal fat excretion), normal small intestinal function (determined by D-xylose absorption), and without evidence of *terminal ileal disease* (determined by a small intestinal barium contrast radiograph). Pancreatic dysfunction may be confirmed by a bentiromide test (see below). The specific pancreatic disease (*chronic pancreatitis, pancreatic resection*, or *carcinoma*) may be diagnosed by computerized tomography, endoscopic retrograde cho-

langiopancreatography, and if necessary, fine needle aspiration of the gland. If patients with known pancreatic disease fail to improve after pancreatic enzyme replacement, coexisting small intestinal disease should be sought.[10]

Pancreatogenous malabsorption in children is most commonly associated with *cystic fibrosis* (see p. 1789). Rare syndromes of pancreatic exocrine insufficiency and a sideroblastic anemia[11] or neutropenia (Schwachman syndrome)[8] have been described (p. 1801).

Zollinger-Ellison Syndrome (see p. 909). High gastric acid production stimulated by gastrin-secreting tumors of the pancreas or duodenum results in impaired fat absorption. Excess acid in the duodenum has a dual effect on fat digestion by (1) inactivating pancreatic enzymes and (2) decreasing bile salt ionization. Acid suppression (by cimetidine or surgery) results in reversal of the malabsorption.[12, 13]

Surgery for Peptic Ulcer Disease (see p. 962). Malabsorption of fats and carbohydrates occurs after *total* or *partial gastrectomy* and is multifactorial in etiology. Gastric emptying rate is increased and gastric antral function is lost, resulting in inadequate grinding of food particles and inadequate mixing of nutrients with gastric secretions, as well as dilution of pancreatic enzymes with decreased proteolysis and lipolysis.[14] Effective pancreatic enzyme concentration is reduced by the increased solute load in the duodenum. Because the pancreas is innervated by the vagus, absolute levels of pancreatic enzymes are reduced after vagotomy, and fat malabsorption results. Rapid gastric emptying after a *partial gastrectomy* or *vagotomy and pyloroplasty* causes a 10 to 50 per cent reduction in glucose absorption.[15] Following a *Billroth II* anastomosis, bacterial overgrowth in the jejunal loop causes both bile salt and vitamin B_{12} malabsorption (see p. 1289). Such intestinal loops are prone to become colonized with bacteria because the contents of the loops are stagnant and are not transported by peristalsis, and because the intraluminal pH in the loops may become abnormally high in patients who have had a partial gastrectomy. Nutritional consequences of peptic ulcer surgery are discussed more completely on pages 962 to 987.

Intraluminal Stage: Solubilization

Disruption of the Enterohepatic Circulation of Bile. Bile salts are necessary for the effective solubilization of fats in the small intestinal lumen (p. 144), and any disease that interrupts the normal enterohepatic circulation of bile can result in decreased micelle formation and fat malabsorption (Table 18–2). Whether low bile salt concentrations in the duodenum are due to decreased production (severe *parenchymal liver disease*), decreased delivery (*cholestatic liver disease, biliary tract obstruction*), bile salt deconjugation to free bile acids (*bacterial overgrowth*), or increased bile salt loss (*terminal ileal disease* or *resection*), symptoms relate to impaired absorption of fat and fat-soluble vitamins (Table 18–3). In these disorders, protein and carbohydrate absorption remain normal. The absorption of vitamin B_{12} is impaired in *bacterial overgrowth*, as intestinal bacteria compete with intrinsic factor for binding to vitamin B_{12},[16] and in terminal ileal disease when receptors for the vitamin B_{12}–intrinsic factor complex are lost.

Regardless of the cause, patients with reduced bile salt concentrations have significant steatorrhea (15 to 20 gm excreted fat per day). The specific disorder resulting in decreased bile salts may be identified by routine liver function tests, small intestinal contrast radiographs, and sonographic imaging of the biliary tract and pancreas. An abnormal ^{14}C-D-xylose breath test is diagnostic of small intestinal bacterial overgrowth, and an abnormal cholyl-^{14}C-glycine breath test is suggestive of *terminal ileal disease or resection* or *bacterial overgrowth* (p. 1289). The clinical features, diagnostic evaluation, and therapy of the following diseases are discussed elsewhere in the book: *scleroderma* (p. 505), *Crohn's disease* (p. 1327), *sclerosing cholangitis* and *biliary tract obstruction* (p. 1722).

Finally, cholecystokinin-pancreozymin (CCK-PZ), a gut hormone secreted by I cells in the proximal small intestinal mucosa, is essential for normal gallbladder contraction. Any disease that destroys the intestinal mucosa (for example, *celiac disease*) may reduce CCK-PZ release, reduce gallbladder contraction, reduce bile salt and pancreatic enzyme delivery to the duodenum, and hence result in impaired fat absorption.

Intestinal Stage: Epithelial Cell Digestion

Disaccharidase Deficiency. *Acquired lactase deficiency* is the most common disorder of carbohydrate absorption in humans. Lactase in intestinal brush border epithelial cells is important for lactose hydrolysis in neonates, but levels decline after weaning[17] so that by adulthood, most humans are lactase deficient.[18] The rate of fall of lactase levels differs in different ethnic groups,[19] and there is considerable variation in the prevalence of *lactase deficiency* among different races, occurring in more than 65 per cent of people of Asian and African origin.

Symptoms of abdominal *distention, flatulence,* and *diarrhea* after ingestion of milk products commonly begin in adolescence. Diagnosis is best made by measurement of breath hydrogen after ingestion of lactose (see below). Lactase levels in a small intestinal mucosal biopsy may be measured directly, although this is rarely necessary clinically.[20] As the symptoms of lactose intolerance are nonspecific, and *lactase deficiency* is very prevalent, diagnosis ultimately depends on the resolution of symptoms after elimination of milk from the diet (see p. 1997). Lactose can be more readily absorbed from yogurt as intraintestinal lactase is released by bacilli in yogurt, facilitating digestion of lactose.[21]

Lactase deficiency also results from diseases that damage the small intestinal mucosa (*celiac disease, tropical sprue, radiation enteritis*).[22] Chronic alcoholics have reduced levels of intestinal lactase, which improves with abstinence.[23] Improvement of the primary disease is often associated with a return of mucosal lactase levels to normal. Although lactose malabsorption was thought to influence the severity of symptoms in children with inflammatory bowel disease,[24, 25] a recent study of breath hydrogen elimination after lactose ingestion in 70 children with inflammatory bowel disease found no increased incidence of lactose intolerance.[26] Milk intolerance may contribute to symptoms in patients with irritable bowel syndrome.[25]

Congenital lactase deficiency is a rare disorder in which mucosal lactase levels are low at birth. Infants have watery diarrhea, irritability, and weight loss from the first feed of breast milk[27] and improve on a lactose-free diet.

Other rare inherited disorders of brush border enzymes include *sucrase alpha-dextrinase deficiency*[28] and *trehalase deficiency*. The latter enzyme is necessary for the metabolism of trehalose, a disaccharide found in mushrooms. In all these disorders, the nonabsorbed carbohydrates are fermented by colonic bacteria to produce short-chain fatty acids, carbon dioxide, and hydrogen, which result in symptoms of abdominal distention, flatulence, and diarrhea after ingestion of the relevant sugar.

Intestinal Stage: Epithelial Transport

Many small intestinal diseases result in destruction of epithelial cells and loss of normal absorptive function. Patients with *celiac sprue* (gluten-sensitive enteropathy) may have profound malnutrition secondary to mucosal destruction (p. 1134). Elimination of gluten from the diet usually reverses the small intestinal damage with improvement of enterocyte absorption. A variant of *celiac disease* has recently been described in six patients with loss of small intestinal villi, atrophy of the spleen and "cavitation" of mesenteric lymph nodes.[29] All patients had abnormal D-xylose absorption, and four had steatorrhea.

Small intestinal involvement in *sarcoidosis* is rare but can cause malabsorption with increased fecal fat excretion and abnormal D-xylose absorption.[30] Small intestinal biopsy reveals villous atrophy and multinucleate giant cells in the mucosa which resolves with steroid therapy. Other disorders causing loss of intestinal surface area for absorption are summarized in Tables 18–1 and 18–6 and are discussed elsewhere in this book (*Crohn's disease*, p. 1327; *radiation enteritis*, p. 1369; *Whipple's disease*, p. 1297; *tropical sprue*, p. 1281; *eosinophilic gastroenteritis*, p. 1123. For discussion of specific defects in amino acid transport (*Hartnup disease, cystinuria*) and vitamin B_{12} and folate transport, see above.

Alcohol. Acute and chronic alcohol ingestion directly damages the small intestinal mucosa with resulting altered absorption of nutrients. Acute alcohol administration produces hemorrhagic erosion of the intestinal villous tips in alcoholic volunteers.[31] Chronic alcohol ingestion in alcoholics produces ultrastructural changes in the mitochondria and endoplasmic reticulum of the crypt and villous epithelial cells but no light microscopic changes to the intestinal mucosa.[32]

Steatorrhea in alcoholics is primarily due to *pancreatic insufficiency* rather than mucosal disease. Alcohol administration in healthy volunteers causes impaired absorption of methionine, thiamine, and D-xylose,[6] presumably due to intestinal epithelial cell damage. Small intestinal motility is also increased[33] and may contribute to the diarrhea seen in alcoholics.

Small Intestinal Resection or Bypass (p. 1106). Resection of the small intestine is most commonly performed in patients with *Crohn's disease* with severe mucosal damage and stricture formation. *Jejunoileal bypass* was frequently used for the treatment of morbid obesity before the severe metabolic consequences were appreciated.[34] Surgical resection of the small intestine decreases the surface area available for absorption. The affected nutrient and degree of malabsorption depend on a number of factors: (1) the extent and site of intestine resected, (2) the absorptive function of the remaining small intestine and the functional integrity of the liver and pancreas, (3) adaptive responses of the remaining intestine, and (4) the presence of the ileocecal valve.[35]

1. Patients who have had more than 75 per cent of their small intestine resected have severe malabsorption with diarrhea caused by the rapid transit of nutrients into the colon. If the jejunum alone is resected, steatorrhea is typically mild (approximately 10 gm of fecal fat per day) and the specific functions of the terminal ileum (vitamin B_{12} and bile salt absorption) are maintained. However, after terminal ileal resection, the bile salt pool is reduced and micelle formation is inhibited, resulting in marked steatorrhea (20 to 40 gm of fecal fat daily). In addition, the unabsorbed fats and bile salts which reach the colon inhibit colonic water and electrolyte absorption and may stimulate colonic electrolyte secretion, causing watery diarrhea.[36, 37] Bile salt–induced diarrhea occurs after as little as 100 cm of ileum is resected, but steatorrhea is usually mild (see pp. 153 and 296).[38]

2. Patients who have disease in the remaining small intestine have major difficulties in absorbing nutrients (for example, *Crohn's disease*). Similarly, patients with concomitant liver or pancreatic disease may have reduced bile salt or pancreatic enzyme secretion with aggravation of steatorrhea. In patients who have a total colonic as well as ileal resection, water and electrolyte absorption in the colon is lost, and fluid losses in the ileostomy may become unmanageable.

3. There is good evidence from animal studies that after resection of the jejunum, adaptive changes occur in the remaining ileum. As early as one week after the resection, transit time is decreased.[39] The height of the intestinal villi and mucosal enzyme content increase and intestinal absorption improves.[40]

4. Nutrient malabsorption and diarrhea seem to be less in patients who do not have resection of the ileocecal valve. Intestinal transit time is prolonged and small intestinal contamination by colonic bacteria is reduced with preservation of the ileocecal valve.[35]

Following intestinal resection or bypass, patients may have impaired absorption of trace elements (calcium, magnesium) and vitamins (A, D, E, K, and B_{12}). In normal individuals, oxalate in the diet is precipitated by calcium and little is absorbed. In patients with severe steatorrhea, calcium binds to the excess fats and is unavailable for binding to oxalate, which remains soluble. Hence, oxalate absorption from the colon is increased, explaining the high incidence of oxalate renal stones in patients with terminal ileal disease.

For the management of patients with extensive small intestinal resection, see Table 18–7, p. 1109, and an excellent review by Weser.[35] Although long-term survival of patients with only 6 to 18 inches of remaining jejunum, in addition to duodenum, is reported,[41] lifelong intravenous hyperalimentation is usually necessary (see pp. 1994–2027).

Abetalipoproteinemia. A group of rare inherited defects in chylomicron formation have been described. Following lipolysis, fatty acids are passively transported into the enterocyte where chylomicrons are formed from phospholipids, cholesterol, triglycerides, and apoproteins in the endoplasmic reticulum prior to transport to the Golgi apparatus. Children with *abetalipoproteinemia* or with homozygous *hypobetalipoproteinemia* are unable to synthesize chylomicrons.[42, 43] The enterocytes become filled with fat and patients have fat malabsorption with steatorrhea (see Fig. 18–1). A

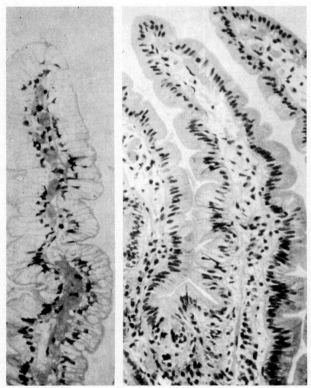

Figure 18–1. Small intestinal mucosal biopsy from a patient with abetalipoproteinemia *(left)* and from a normal subject *(right)*. Small intestinal mucosal cells are dilated and filled with lipid, although villi are usually normal. (Reproduced by kind permission of Dr. W. M. Weinstein).

progressive sensory neuropathy, ataxia, and retinitis pigmentosa are also characteristic of these diseases. *Chylomicron retention disease* is a recently described variant of *abetalipoproteinemia*, with similar features of steatorrhea and neurologic impairment.[44] Both diseases have an autosomal recessive mode of inheritance and can be distinguished by the lipoprotein profiles in the serum.[44] Treatment consists of substituting medium-chain triglycerides for dietary fat and supplementing with fat-soluble vitamins, particularly vitamin E.

Adult Familial Hyaline Membrane Disease. A familial syndrome of progressive hyalinosis of capillaries, veins, and arteries has recently been described.[44a] Clinical manifestations include diarrhea, malabsorption, and intestinal protein loss. Extraintestinal manifestations include hypertension, retinal ischemia, and subarachnoid hemorrhage.

Abnormalities of Lymphatic Transport

Intestinal lymphoma should be considered in any patient with profound steatorrhea and hypoalbuminemia (p. 1550). Lymphatic transport of chylomicrons and proteins is obstructed with consequent fat malabsorption and protein loss into the intestine. In developed countries, the disease is usually a localized ileal tumor, which may present with obstructive symptoms; whereas in third world countries, intestinal involvement is often diffuse, and symptoms of malabsorption predominate.[45]

Other causes of obstruction of mesenteric lymphatics include *tuberculosis,*[46] *metastatic carcinoma, metastatic mesothelioma,*[47] and *metastatic carcinoid.*[48, 49] *Retractile mesenteritis* and *retroperitoneal fibrosis* are diseases of unknown etiology which cause lymphatic obstruction.[50] Lymphatic duct obstruction of any etiology is frequently associated with chylous ascites. *Primary intestinal lymphangiectasia* is a genetically determined structural disorder of the lymphatics. Intestinal biopsy characteristically shows dilated lymphatics (p. 287), and the villi may also be distended or may appear normal.

Differentiation between these different causes of lymphatic obstruction may be difficult. Lymph nodes in *tuberculous enteritis* may be calcified, small intestinal biopsy may show malignant lymphocytes in *primary lymphoma*, and urinary 5-hydroxyindole acetic acid levels are usually increased in *metastatic carcinoid disease*, but often definitive diagnosis is only made at laparotomy (p. 1560).

Diseases of Unexplained Mechanism

Enteropathy of the Acquired Immune Deficiency Syndrome. Diarrhea and weight loss occur in approximately two thirds of male homosexuals with the *acquired immune deficiency syndrome* (AIDS), many of whom have malabsorption[51, 52] (p. 1242). Although enteric pathogens may be present (*Giardia, Cryptosporidium, Isospora belli*), in one recent study, no identifiable pathogen could be identified by stool culture in 20 of 72 patients with AIDS and diarrhea.[51] D-Xylose absorption was impaired in all patients and fat malabsorption was common. Intestinal biopsy revealed *Mycobacterium avium intracellulare* in 5 of the 20 patients and nonspecific inflammation without pathogens in 13 of 20. Jejunal biopsy in some patients revealed partial villous atrophy, but the causative agent was not identified. Thus, there seems to be an enteropathy associated with AIDS which presents with diarrhea and symptoms of malabsorption but without an identifiable etiology.

Even when organisms are seen on intestinal biopsy, the pathophysiologic mechanism of the malabsorption in these patients is unexplained. Infection with *Cryptosporidium* in immunocompetent hosts causes an acute self-limited diarrhea. However, in AIDS patients, *Cryptosporidium* produces a severe incapacitating diarrhea with major fluid and electrolyte loss and occasionally nutrient malabsorption.[53] *Isospora belli* may be identified by acid-fast stains of stool specimens or by electron microscopy of a small intestinal biopsy[54] (p. 1165). Light microscopy of the small intestine typically reveals partial villous atrophy. *Microsporidia* have been found in the intestinal mucosa of patients with AIDS and diarrhea, but malabsorption has not been associated with the organisms, and their importance in the pathogenesis of diarrhea is unclear.[53]

Mycobacterium avium intracellulare is an important pathogen in patients with AIDS and is known to produce PAS-positive inclusions in intestinal macrophages similar to the lesions identified in *Whipple's disease.*[55, 56] Although malabsorption is commonly associated with this pathogen, the pathophysiologic mechanism is unknown.[51]

Cytomegalovirus infection in AIDS patients typically causes diarrhea and occasionally colonic perforation. Although small intestinal involvement has been described, diffuse colonic ulceration is seen more commonly[53] and malabsorption has not been reported. AIDS patients with gastrointestinal *Kaposi's sarcoma* are usually asymptomatic.[57] The gastrointestinal manifestations of AIDS are discussed further in Chapter 65 (p. 1242).

Endocrinopathies. A number of endocrine disorders are associated with malabsorption. Abnormalities of gastrointestinal motility have been documented in patients with thyroid disease, and rapid intestinal transit may cause the impaired fat absorption which is frequently associated with thyrotoxicosis.[58, 59] Steatorrhea is increased by the high dietary fat intake in these patients, but malabsorption resolves with treatment of the underlying disease. Similarly, the steatorrhea observed in patients with *Addison's disease* improves with steroid replacement. Mild steatorrhea is also reported in patients with deficient parathyroid function, in whom diagnosis may be made by measuring parathormone levels. Treatment with vitamin D and calcium will improve the steatorrhea as well as other symptoms of the disease (p. 490).

Patients with long-standing *diabetes mellitus* frequently have diarrhea and may have mild steatorrhea.[60] Although a few patients have associated *pancreatic exocrine insufficiency* and some have intestinal *bacterial overgrowth*, in most diabetics, small intestinal histologic findings and pancreatic exocrine function are normal. Autonomic neuropathy is common in these patients, and dysmotility may predispose to *bacterial overgrowth*, but small intestinal cultures rarely reveal increased organisms and steatorrhea rarely improves with antimicrobial therapy (p. 494).

Malabsorption in the Elderly. Malabsorption in the elderly is increasingly recognized as contributing to the poor nutrition commonly seen in this population. Poor intake is probably the major cause of malnutrition, but in a recent study 45 per cent of elderly patients were found to have *bacterial overgrowth* of the small intestine.[61] Impaired absorption of fat[62] and carbohydrate[63] has been reported in patients over 65 years of age, although the mechanism is unclear. Investigation of these patients may reveal unsuspected anatomic abnormalities (for example, jejunal diverticula) (p. 162).

Other Disorders. Both primary and secondary *amyloidosis* may involve the small intestine and cause malabsorption (p. 509). Proposed mechanisms include small intestinal ischemia from amyloid infiltration of mesenteric arterioles, amyloid deposition in the lamina propria inhibiting transport of nutrients, and altered intestinal motility. Of note, as only 50 per cent of patients with intestinal *amyloidosis* have impaired D-xylose absorption, damage to the small intestine seems to be variable.[64] *Giardiasis* is known to cause steatorrhea, but the mechanism is uncertain. However, there is evidence that *Giardia lamblia* trophozoites can take up bile salts and may thus reduce intraluminal bile salt concentrations, leading to fat malabsorption.[65] *Giardia* infection is frequent in patients with *hypogammaglobulinemia* and may in part explain the malabsorption associated with this disorder.

Drug-Induced Malabsorption. *Colchicine*, a drug commonly used in the treatment of gout, inhibits epithelial crypt cell division.[66] Mild steatorrhea and impaired D-xylose absorption may result. *Neomycin* can produce partial villous atrophy and impaired D-xylose and fat absorption in doses as low as 4 gm per day. The pathophysiologic mechanism is unclear, although lipolysis of fats is reduced and bile salts in the intestinal lumen may be precipitated by the drug.[67] *Bacitracin, polymyxin*, and *kanamycin* may cause malabsorption. *Clindamycin* in therapeutic doses inhibits jejunal water and electrolyte absorption, which may, in the absence of *pseudomembranous colitis*, contribute to the diarrhea that occurs during *clindamycin* therapy.[68] *Methotrexate*[69] and *irritant laxatives* appear to impair absorption by directly damaging small intestinal epithelial cells. *Cholestyramine*, in doses of 12 gm or more per day, binds bile salts in the intestinal lumen and impairs fat absorption. The oral anticoagulant *phenindione* also causes steatorrhea by an unknown mechanism. *Aluminum-containing antacids* bind dietary phosphate and can lead to hypophosphatemia, hypercalciuria, and nephrolithiasis.

CLINICAL TESTS OF DIGESTION AND ABSORPTION

Numerous tests are available for evaluating patients with symptoms of maldigestion and malabsorption. Not all these tests are necessary, however, in any given patient. A logical approach to investigating such patients can be made if attention is given to clinical features suggestive of specific etiologies during a careful history and physical examination (for example, excess alcohol intake causing small intestinal or pancreatic disease). Routine laboratory tests may also be helpful. Thus, a macrocytic or microcytic anemia would suggest deficiency of vitamin B_{12}, folate, or iron, respectively, and hypoalbuminemia might indicate protein malabsorption or a protein-losing enteropathy. A low serum carotene level would suggest impaired fat absorption, which would then be investigated directly by a qualitative Sudan stain and then measurement of quantitative fecal fat.

Fat excretion is increased in most malabsorptive states, and although severe fat malabsorption is indicative of pancreatic rather than intestinal disease, the specific defect in absorption must be defined by other tests. In patients with *chronic pancreatitis*, a plain abdominal X-ray may demonstrate pancreatic calcification (this is present in 30 per cent of such patients[70]), whereas an abdominal CT scan may demonstrate a pancreatic mass in patients with pancreatic carcinoma. If fat malabsorption is due to small intestinal disease, carbohydrate absorption as determined by D-xylose absorption, a hydrogen breath test, or a bile acid breath test is likely to be abnormal (see p. 1294).

Small intestinal barium X-rays may show evidence of previous intestinal surgery (e.g., subtotal gastrectomy or massive small bowel resection), or may show partial intestinal obstruction in a patient with *Crohn's disease* or *lymphoma*. Distortion of the second portion of the duodenum by *pancreatic carcinoma* may also be seen on barium contrast radiographs. A small intestinal biopsy may provide diagnostic information in patients with specific mucosal diseases and occasionally may be used to measure disaccharidase activities in patients with suspected disaccharidase deficiencies. In general, these various tests tend to be complementary in defining the defective stage of digestion or absorption.

Investigation of each patient should be directed toward the most likely diseases associated with his or her clinical presentation. A schematic approach to investigating the patient with suspected malabsorption is summarized in Figure 18–2. The range of normal values for the different tests is given in Table 18–4. Some of the more frequently used tests will now be considered in further detail.

Tests of Fat Absorption

Qualitative Fecal Fat. This simple test is useful for screening individuals with suspected fat malabsorption and correlates well with the quantitative fecal fat.[71-73] The qualitative fecal fat test is most useful in patients

SELECTION OF TESTS IN THE EVALUATION OF MALABSORPTION

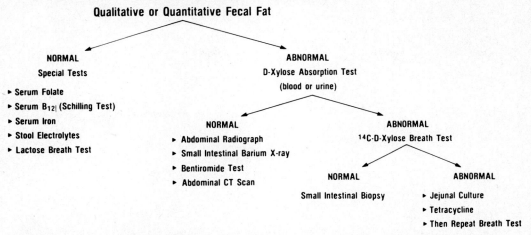

Figure 18–2. Algorithm for selecting tests in the evaluation of patients with suspected malabsorption.

with moderate to severe fat malabsorption (excreting more than 10 per cent of a daily intake of 60 gm of fat) in whom it is positive in 94 to 100 per cent of cases. In patients with mild to moderate fat malabsorption (excreting 6 to 10 per cent of dietary fat), the test is less sensitive and will be positive in only 75 per cent of cases. In addition, 14 per cent of fecal specimens from healthy individuals (excreting <7 per cent of dietary fat) will have a slight increase in microscopic estimates of fecal fat.[71]

The test is performed on a stool specimen, which is placed on a glass slide and mixed with two drops of glacial acetic acid and two drops of Sudan III in 95 per cent alcohol. After a coverslip is placed over the specimen, it is gently heated to boiling and examined by light microscopy while still warm. Acetic acid and heat are required for hydrolysis of esterified fats to free fatty acids, which are stained with Sudan III. Normally, only a few red-staining fat globules (slightly smaller than an erythrocyte) are seen (see Fig. 18–3).

Table 18–4. TESTS FOR MALABSORPTION IN COMMON CLINICAL USE

Test	Test Reflects	Normal Values	Abnormal Results Indicate	Factors Affecting Interpretation of the Test
Serum carotene		>0.06 mg/dl	Pancreatic insufficiency, small intestinal disease, see Table 18–2	Inadequate dietary fat
Qualitative fecal fat	Fat digestion and	A few fat globules/hpf		
Quantitative fecal fat	absorption	<6 gm/day		Incomplete collection, inadequate dietary fat
Schilling test	Vitamin B_{12} absorption	>7%/24 hours	See Table 18–5	Renal insufficiency
D-Xylose (25 gm orally)	Carbohydrate absorption	>4 gm/5 hours	Small intestinal mucosal dysfunction, bacterial overgrowth	Renal insufficiency, age, ascites
Lactose tolerance test (50 gm orally)	Lactase activity of enterocytes	>20 mg/dl rise in blood	Acquired lactase deficiency, congenital lactase deficiency, Crohn's disease, radiation enteritis, celiac sprue	
Bentiromide test (PABA) (500 mg orally)	Pancreatic secretion	>57% arylamine excretion/6 hours	Pancreatic insufficiency, extensive small intestinal wall damage	Renal or liver disease, diabetes
Breath tests				
a. ^{14}C-Xylose	Carbohydrate digestion and absorption	<0.0013% of administered dose at 30 min	Bacterial overgrowth	Delayed gastric emptying
b. Cholyl-^{14}C-glycine	Enterohepatic circulation of bile acids	<1% of administered dose any time within 4 hours	Bacterial overgrowth, terminal ileal disease/resection	
c. Lactose H_2 (50 gm orally)	Lactase activity of enterocytes	<20ppm rise in breath H_2 any time within 3 hours	Lactase deficiency (see above)	
Small intestinal culture	Bacteria in the small intestine	<10^5 organisms/ml	Bacterial overgrowth	Unrepresentative sampling of the small intestine, inadequate culture techniques
Small intestinal biopsy	Small intestinal morphology	See Figure 18–1	See Table 18–6	Unrepresentative sampling of the small intestine

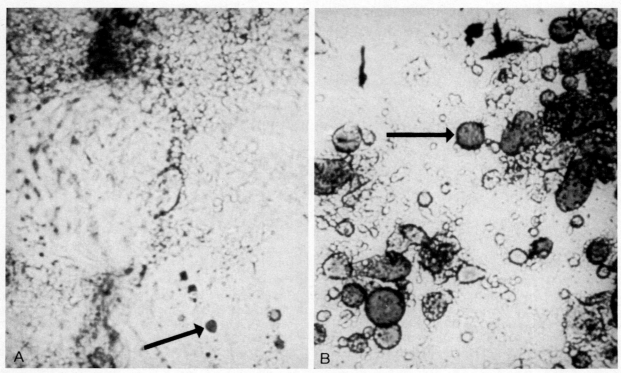

Figure 18–3. Sudan stain of stool from a control subject *(A)* and from a patient with steatorrhea *(B)*. A few fat globules, smaller than an erythrocyte (arrow, A), may be seen in normal individuals. Many fat globules greater in size than erythrocytes are indicative of impaired fat absorption (arrow, B).

In moderate steatorrhea, many fat globules the size of erythrocytes are present, and in severe steatorrhea, many fat globules greater in size than erythrocytes are seen. In patients with a positive test, the degree of fat malabsorption should be further evaluated with a quantitative fecal fat measurement. Patients ingesting mineral oils may have a false positive test. False negative qualitative fecal fat tests arise in patients with inadequate dietary fat intake, or only mild steatorrhea (6 to 10 gm excreted fat per day). If fat malabsorption is suspected, further evaluation of the patient with a quantitative fecal fat is necessary.

Quantitative Fecal Fat. Measurement of the amount of fat in the stool excreted in three days by a patient on a daily diet containing 80 to 100 gm of fat is the best method for evaluating fat malabsorption. The stool specimen is analyzed by the van de Kamer method,[74] which is based on extraction and titration of long-chain fatty acids by NaOH. Fecal fat levels greater than 6 gm per day are abnormal and suggest underlying *small intestinal, pancreatic*, or *hepatobiliary disease* (see Table 18–1). If the patient is on a 100 gm per day fat diet and a complete three-day stool specimen is collected, the test provides a useful measure of the amount of fat which is not absorbed by the small intestine, and it remains the "gold standard" to which all other tests of fat absorption are compared. Small errors arise in patients taking medium-chain triglycerides[75] or mineral oils[71] which interfere with fecal fat analysis. In addition, the test does not localize the pathophysiologic defect in absorption (diminished digestion, uptake, or trans-

port of fat), and thus, further evaluation is necessary. Moreover, it must be remembered that fecal fat levels may be normal in patients with advanced destruction of the pancreas, since pancreatogenous steatorrhea will not usually appear until the enzyme output of the gland has been reduced to <2 per cent of normal values.[8]

Recent attempts have been made to introduce less cumbersome tests of fat absorption which avoid the problem of inadequate dietary fat intake and inadequate collection of excreted fat. The most widely used of such tests is the ^{14}C-triolein breath test (see below). A new double-isotope method using radiolabeled triglycerides and free fatty acids, as well as a nonabsorbable marker to assess the adequacy of the fecal collection, promises to overcome some of the deficiencies of the quantitative fecal fat test but requires further evaluation.[76]

^{14}C-Triolein Breath Test. Triolein is a triglyceride (glyceryl trioleate) that normally is hydrolyzed by pancreatic lipase in the small intestine and, after absorption and further metabolism, contributes to the CO_2 in exhaled air. Following oral administration of glyceryl tri(1-^{14}C)oleate, exhaled $^{14}CO_2$ is trapped by hyamine, then quantitated by scintillation counting. In patients with impaired fat absorption, the amount of $^{14}CO_2$ exhaled in six hours after an oral dose of ^{14}C-labeled triolein is reduced. This test has been validated in patients with steatorrhea.[77, 78] It is easier to perform than the 72 hour fecal fat test but, as with other tests of fat absorption, provides little information about the cause of malabsorption in any particular patient. In addition, results may be misleading in patients with altered metabolism of absorbed ^{14}C-triolein or impaired excretion of $^{14}CO_2$ in breath (for example, in patients with *diabetes, obesity, thyroid disease, pulmonary disease,* and *liver disease,* conditions which are often associated with *chronic pancreatitis*). It is also insensitive in detecting early pancreatic insufficiency and is a qualitative rather than a quantitative test. A variant of this test employs triolein labeled with the nonradioactive isotope ^{13}C, which is quantitated by mass spectrometry.

In an attempt to differentiate patients with pancreatic and small intestinal disease, Goff has repeated the test after pancreatic enzyme replacement (the two-stage triolein breath test) and found an increase in $^{14}CO_2$ excretion in patients with pancreatic insufficiency.[79] At present, the triolein breath test is available only in research laboratories, and its major disadvantages for clinical use are the false negative results in patients with mild steatorrhea and false positive results in healthy individuals.

Specific Pancreatic Function Tests

Radiographic techniques (ultrasound, computerized tomography, and cholangiopancreatography) have greatly improved our ability to diagnose *chronic pancreatitis*, but tests of pancreatic function are helpful in establishing whether structural abnormalities of the pancreas are the cause of the patient's symptoms. Pancreatic function tests measure the ability of pancreatic acinar cells to secrete enzymes and bicarbonate into the duodenum following certain stimuli. However, most of these tests are insensitive in detecting pancreatic insufficiency, as they are only abnormal when enzyme secretion is reduced to <10 per cent of normal levels.[80] As few of these tests are in general clinical use, they will be discussed only briefly here but are dealt with in greater detail on pages 1849 to 1851.

Bentiromide Test. The underlying principle of this noninvasive test of pancreatic function is that an adequate duodenal concentration of chymotrypsin is nec-essary to cleave free para-aminobenzoic acid (PABA) from the synthetic peptide N-benzoyl-L-tyrosyl-para-aminobenzoic acid (bentiromide).[81, 82] After a 500 mg oral dose of bentiromide, free PABA is released in the duodenum, absorbed, conjugated in the liver, and excreted in the urine, where it is measured in a 6 hour urine sample (Table 18–4). PABA excretion is reduced in severe pancreatic insufficiency when enzyme output is less than 5 per cent of normal. In addition, patients with *defective intestinal absorption, renal disease, diabetes,* or *severe liver disease* may have diminished urinary PABA excretion in the absence of pancreatic insufficiency.[7, 83] Modifications of the test, involving measurement of plasma PABA levels, have increased its accuracy.[82]

Pancreatic Stimulation Tests. In these tests, the duodenum is intubated and the duodenal contents are aspirated after a specific stimulus (intravenous secretin or cholecystokinin or a liquid meal containing fat, protein, and carbohydrate, known as the Lundh meal). Duodenal fluid is analyzed for pancreatic enzymes (lipase, colipase, trypsin, or chymotrypsin) and bicarbonate content. Although these tests remain the "gold standard" by which other pancreatic tests are measured, they are cumbersome to perform, are uncomfortable for the patient, and are rarely used clinically.[8]

Schilling Test. Approximately 50 per cent of patients with pancreatic exocrine insufficiency have impaired absorption of vitamin B_{12}, as measured by the standard Schilling test.[84] The standard Schilling test measures vitamin B_{12} absorption and is used to detect the intrinsic factor (IF) deficiency in patients with *pernicious anemia.* The test is also abnormal in patients with *genetic defects in vitamin B_{12} absorption, bacterial overgrowth of the small intestine, extensive mucosal destruction, resection or bypass of the terminal ileum,* and *pancreatic insufficiency* (for which the dual label Schilling test was developed). Results in different disease states are summarized in Table 18–5.

In the standard Schilling test, an oral dose of vitamin B_{12} (0.5 to 2.0 µg radiolabeled with either ^{57}Co or ^{58}Co) is given with a simultaneous intramuscular injection of 1 mg of nonradioactive vitamin B_{12} (which

Table 18–5. ABSORPTION OF ^{57}CO- OR ^{58}CO-LABELED VITAMIN B_{12} IN DIFFERENT DISEASES

Test	Pernicious Anemia or Total Gastrectomy	Celiac Disease	Intestinal Bacterial Overgrowth	Primary Vitamin B_{12} Malabsorption or Ileal Resection	Pancreatic Insufficiency
Vitamin B_{12}* (stage 1 Schilling test)	Low	Low-normal	Low	Low	Low**
Vitamin B_{12} + intrinsic factor (stage 2 Schilling test)	Normal	Low-normal	Low	Low	Low
Vitamin B_{12} after antibiotic therapy	Low	Low-normal	Normal	Low	Low
Vitamin B_{12} after gluten-free diet	Low	Normal	Low	Low	Low
Vitamin B_{12} + pancreatic enzyme replacement	Low	Low-normal	Low	Low	Normal

*In severe vitamin B_{12} deficiency, tests should be performed after one week of vitamin B_{12} therapy to allow recovery of normal epithelial function.

**Vitamin B_{12} malabsorption is common in pancreatic insufficiency, although vitamin B_{12} deficiency is rare.

saturates hepatic binding sites for vitamin B_{12} and reduces the amount of radioactive vitamin B_{12} retained by the liver). The urine is collected for 24 hours following the administration of vitamin B_{12} and the amount of radioactivity determined. Patients with normal absorption and normal renal function excrete >7 per cent of the radioactive vitamin B_{12} in 24 hours, and those with impaired absorption excrete <7 per cent during the period of collection. The low level of urinary radiolabeled vitamin B_{12} in patients with pernicious anemia is corrected when the test is repeated and 60 mg of intrinsic factor is given orally with the test dose of labeled vitamin B_{12} (second-stage Schilling test). Patients with small intestinal bacterial overgrowth often show malabsorption of vitamin B_{12} with the first-stage Schilling test because of bacterial utilization of the vitamin, which, however, is not corrected in the second-stage test by administration of intrinsic factor. In such patients, the absorption of vitamin B_{12} plus intrinsic factor remains low, but usually a week of antibiotic treatment (for example, metronidazole, 250 mg three times a day) eliminates the intestinal bacteria and restores the vitamin B_{12} absorption of the first-stage test to normal.

The dual-label Schilling test was developed to provide information about pancreatic exocrine function because proteases are required for the release of vitamin B_{12} from so-called R proteins of gastric juice which preferentially bind the vitamin.[85] For vitamin B_{12} to become bound to intrinsic factor the action of proteases in the duodenum is essential. The vitamin B_{12} thus released will then be bound to intrinsic factor in the duodenum. This test compares the absorption of [58]Co-labeled vitamin B_{12} given orally bound to R protein and [57]Co-labeled vitamin B_{12} given orally bound to intrinsic factor. In pancreatic insufficiency, the [58]Co-labeled vitamin B_{12} is malabsorbed and the ratio of [58]Co: [57]Co in a urine specimen is lower than if pancreatic function is normal.[84] In patients with bacterial overgrowth of the small intestine or distal ileal disease, both forms of vitamin B_{12} are malabsorbed, but the ratio of the cobalt isotopes in the urine is normal. Although theoretically attractive, the dual-label Schilling test is no longer in clinical use because attempts to standardize this test by different laboratories have not been successful. Normalization of vitamin B_{12} absorption after pancreatic enzyme replacement as measured by the standard Schilling test, suggests pancreatogenous malabsorption.

Tests of Carbohydrate Absorption

Hydrogen Breath Test. In normal individuals, hydrogen is produced exclusively by the bacterial metabolism of carbohydrates. This test measures the hydrogen exhaled at timed intervals during the first three hours after ingestion of the carbohydrate under investigation (for example, lactose, lactulose, fructose, or sucrose).[86, 87] Patients who are unable to digest or absorb carbohydrates in the small intestine have increased delivery of carbohydrate to the colon and hence increased production of hydrogen, which is then absorbed in the colon and exhaled by the lungs. Patients with small intestinal *bacterial overgrowth* have increased hydrogen production by the intestinal bacteria. The peak excretion is early, i.e., within 3 hours. Patients with *small intestinal disease* and carbohydrate malabsorption have a later peak of hydrogen release, as do patients with *disaccharidase deficiency* who have ingested the appropriate disaccharide (Table 18–4).

The hydrogen breath test is now the most commonly used test to diagnose *lactase deficiency*[88] and is more sensitive than the lactose tolerance test (see below). After measurement of basal breath hydrogen levels, an oral dose of lactose (1 gm per kg of body weight) is given. A rise of >20 ppm in exhaled hydrogen is diagnostic of lactose malabsorption. Patients with *bacterial overgrowth* of the small intestine have increased production of hydrogen by the intestinal bacteria in response to ingested carbohydrate (50 or 80 gm of glucose or 10 gm of lactulose) (see p. 1295) and an early peak of hydrogen exhalation after carbohydrate ingestion. The hydrogen breath test appears to be complementary to other breath tests in diagnosing small intestinal bacterial overgrowth (see below).[89] A controlled diet on the day before the test affects fasting breath hydrogen levels and may improve the accuracy of this test.[87, 90] Because it is simple to perform and does not involve radioisotopes, this test is commonly used to study carbohydrate absorption in children.[87] Of note, patients with severe pancreatic insufficiency may have impaired carbohydrate absorption and a positive hydrogen breath test.[90]

D-Xylose Absorption Test. Xylose is a five-carbon sugar that is incompletely absorbed in the small intestine by the same transport mechanism as glucose and galactose. Intestinal uptake of xylose occurs by both passive diffusion and active transport, but unlike glucose and galactose, xylose is not completely metabolized after it is absorbed but is largely excreted unchanged in the urine. The xylose absorption test has been used extensively to assess the functional integrity of the small intestinal mucosa. After an overnight fast, a 25-gm (less commonly, 5 gm) dose of D-xylose is given orally, and the patient is encouraged to drink fluids to maintain a good urinary output. Approximately 25 per cent of the administered dose is excreted in the urine (normal values in a five hour urinary collection after a 25-gm oral dose, ≥ 5 gm). In patients with fat malabsorption, this test is useful to differentiate between small intestinal disease (in which xylose absorption is diminished) and pancreatic insufficiency (in which xylose absorption is normal). However, xylose absorption may be normal in patients with only mild impairment of small intestinal mucosal function and in patients with predominantly distal small intestinal disease.[91] The accuracy of the test is increased by measuring serum D-xylose levels one or two hours after the oral dose (normal levels >20 mg/dl two hours after a 25-gm dose, or 11 to 22 mg/dl one hour after a 5-gm dose).[92–94] After an oral dose, serum D-xylose levels should be normal in patients with impaired renal function (elderly individuals or patients with renal parenchymal disease in whom urinary xylose levels will be diminished) and in patients with ascites (in whom xylose is retained in the ascitic fluid). Serum D-xylose levels will also be decreased in more than 85 per cent of patients with bacterial overgrowth of the small intestine, as bacterial metabolism of xylose in the intestinal lumen decreases the amount available for absorption.[94] In patients with bacterial overgrowth and normal small intestinal mucosal function, D-xylose absorption and urinary excretion are likely to increase after oral administration of antibiotics.

In summary, the D-xylose absorption test is useful for evaluating patients with steatorrhea. If serum and urinary levels are reduced, the patient should be further investigated with a jejunal biopsy or tests for bacterial overgrowth (see below). If D-xylose absorption is normal, steatorrhea is most likely to be due to pancreatic insufficiency. However, because the test may be inaccurate (particularly if urinary xylose excretion alone is measured) further investigation of the patient should be influenced by the clinical situation.

Lactose Tolerance Test. This test is performed to identify patients with either a specific defect in lactose absorption (*congenital* or *acquired lactase deficiency*) or a more generalized defect in carbohydrate absorption (for example, mucosal abnormalities associated with Crohn's disease). After oral administration of 50 gm of lactose, plasma glucose is measured at one and two hours. In normal subjects, the plasma glucose rises by >20 mg/dl, whereas little increase in plasma glucose level is seen in most patients with lactase deficiency. The lactose tolerance test may not detect certain patients with biopsy-proved lactase deficiency (6 of 25 patients in one study),[88] and has largely been replaced by the more sensitive breath hydrogen test (Table 18–4).

Ileal Intubation Tests. Although not commonly in clinical use, intubation tests have recently been described which directly quantify the unabsorbed carbohydrate reaching the ileocecal valve.[95, 96] These tests are easier to interpret than the D-xylose absorption or hydrogen breath tests as carbohydrate fermented by colonic bacteria is not measured by the tests. Intubation tests provide promise in the investigation of carbohydrate absorption, but further validation and comparison with other tests are necessary.

Tests for Bacterial Overgrowth

Quantitative Bacterial Culture. To quantify bacteria in the small intestine, the jejunum is intubated either with a peroral small intestinal tube passed under fluoroscopy or with a tube passed through an endoscope and the intestinal aspirate cultured for both aerobic and anaerobic bacteria. There are no data comparing these two techniques, but with both methods care should be taken to use nonbacteriostatic saline for flushing the tube, and fresh specimens should be taken

directly to the laboratory for anaerobic and aerobic culture. In normal individuals, $<10^3$ bacteria per milliliter (usually streptococci and staphylococci) are cultured. The presence of $\geq 10^5$ bacteria per milliliter (commonly coliforms and anaerobes) has been used as the minimum concentration for diagnosis of small intestinal bacterial overgrowth. However, this test requires special culture techniques to detect anaerobic bacteria and is not as useful for diagnosing bacterial overgrowth as the breath tests listed below.[97] False positive cultures result when the jejunal specimen is contaminated with saliva.[98]

Breath Tests. Bacteria in the small intestine metabolize orally administered carbohydrates or bile salts with the release of CO_2 in exhaled air. This is the underlying principle of the ^{14}C-D-xylose and cholyl-^{14}C-glycine tests. Both these tests are in clinical use, and the relative merits of the two are discussed below. Hydrogen in exhaled air is also increased in patients with bacterial overgrowth after oral administration of carbohydrate (see above) and may be diagnostically elevated in patients with a normal cholyl-^{14}C-glycine test. For a more extensive discussion of the breath tests, see pages 1294 to 1295.

[14]C-D-Xylose Breath Test. This clinical breath test[99] measures [14]CO_2 in exhaled air following oral administration of 1 gm of ^{14}C-labeled D-xylose. In patients with small intestinal bacterial overgrowth, gram-negative aerobic bacteria metabolize ^{14}C-D-xylose to [14]CO_2 which, following absorption, is exhaled. Eighty-five per cent of these patients will have a diagnostic elevation of exhaled [14]CO_2 within 60 minutes of ingesting ^{14}C-D-xylose.[100] In patients with delayed gastric emptying and small intestinal bacterial overgrowth (for example, in *scleroderma*), the release of [14]CO_2 may be delayed until three hours. Confirmation of bacterial overgrowth is obtained by the normalization of this test and resolution of the malabsorption after antibiotic administration. The labeled xylose breath test has been shown to be more reliable than quantitative bacterial culture for diagnosing bacterial overgrowth because multiple tests of xylose absorption give reproducible results in 95 per cent of patients compared to only 38 per cent for bacterial culture.[97] In addition, because xylose is absorbed in the proximal small intestine, little is available for metabolism by colonic bacteria and [14]CO_2 release is not increased in patients with small intestinal resections. This contrasts with the bile acid breath test (see below), in which false positive results are obtained in patients with distal small intestinal resections (p. 1294).

Cholyl-^{14}C-Glycine Breath Test. The bile acid breath test is based on the normal enterohepatic circulation of bile salts (p. 144). In contrast to the normal situation, following the oral administration of cholyl-^{14}C-glycine, anaerobic bacteria in the small intestine of patients with bacterial overgrowth deconjugate the bile salt with the release of glycine. The glycine is then absorbed and after further metabolism, [14]CO_2 is released, resulting in an early peak of radioactivity in the expired air. Unfortunately, this test cannot easily differentiate between bacterial overgrowth and small intestinal disease or resection, in which unabsorbed cholyl-glycine is metabolized by colonic bacteria with a delayed release of $^{14}CO_2$. Comparisons of the radio-labeled cholyl-glycine and D-xylose breath tests in patients with culture-proved bacterial overgrowth have shown that the latter test more accurately identifies patients with *blind loop syndrome*.[101, 102] The ^{14}C-D-xylose test is commonly used by clinical laboratories.

Tests of Bile Salt Absorption

The cholyl-^{14}C-glycine breath test may also be used to identify patients with impaired ileal absorption of bile salts,[100] although it cannot reliably differentiate patients with bile salt deconjugation due to small intestinal bacterial overgrowth from patients with bile salt malabsorption secondary to small intestinal disease or resection. The usefulness of this test is further limited for even in normal subjects there is a significant metabolism of (^{14}C-labeled) bile salts by colonic bacteria, with generation of $^{14}CO_2$ in the breath.[100] ^{14}C excretion in the stool (after ingestion of cholyl-^{14}C-glycine) is increased in patients with impaired ileal or colonic bile salt absorption, and measurement of fecal ^{14}C may increase the accuracy of the cholyl-glycine breath test, but it also decreases the facility with which this test is performed.[103] The recently developed ^{75}SeHCAT test overcomes some of these difficulties and attempts to measure the total "bile salt balance" in patients.

^{75}**SeHCAT Test.** This radioactive taurocholic acid analogue (23-selena-25-homotaurocholic acid) undergoes a similar enterohepatic circulation to taurocholic acid and has recently been used to detect patients with increased bile acid loss. After oral administration of the compound, the patient is scanned under a gamma camera on sequential days and the amount of retained bile acid is quantitated. Patients who retain less than 34 per cent of the administered dose after three days are considered abnormal.[104] This test has been used to identify patients with bile acid malabsorption secondary to vagotomy or ileal resection, many of whom have improvement in their diarrhea when treated with cholestyramine.[104, 105] In these small studies, 20 to 50 per cent of patients with idiopathic diarrhea had decreased retention of ^{75}SeHCAT suggesting bile acid malabsorption, and 75 to 100 per cent of these patients had symptomatic improvement when taking cholestyramine. Although the ^{75}SeHCAT test is not in general clinical use, it is simple to perform and promises to be helpful for identifying patients who have *idiopathic bile acid malabsorption*[105a] who may respond to cholestyramine therapy.

Radiographs of the Small Intestine

The primary role of barium contrast radiographs of the small intestine is to define anatomic abnormalities which may be associated with bacterial overgrowth. *A true blind loop, small intestinal strictures* (as in patients with *Crohn's disease* or those who have undergone abdominal surgery), *multiple jejunal diverticula*, or marked small intestinal hypomotility (as in *scleroderma*) all cause stasis, which leads to *bacterial colonization* and *overgrowth* with serious impairment of digestion and absorption (see p. 1289). On occasion, hitherto unsuspected massive resection of the small intestine with a jejunocolic anastomosis may be found by radiographs to be the cause of malabsorption. Other anatomic abnormalities may be associated with malabsorption of nutrients. *Pancreatic carcinoma* or *pseudocyst* in patients with *chronic pancreatitis* may be detected by distortion of the sweep of the descending duodenum. Radiographs are less important in the diagnosis of infiltrative diseases of the small intestine, although subtle changes (thickening and nodularity) may be seen in patients with *amyloidosis* (see p. 509), *lymphoma* (see p. 1550), and *lymphangiectasia* (see p. 287). In patients with *celiac sprue*, barium X-rays typically show intestinal dilatation with little mucosal thickening (see p. 1144).

Mucosal Biopsy of the Small Intestine*

Mucosal biopsy is essential for the diagnosis of many diseases of the intestinal mucosa. Characteristic histologic changes in different diseases are summarized in Table 18–6. A normal small intestinal mucosal biopsy is shown in Figure 18–1. In contrast, the small intestinal mucosal biopsy in *abetalipoproteinemia* reveals dilated, lipid-filled enterocytes (Fig. 18–1). Although many diseases affect the small intestine diffusely (for example, *abetalipoproteinemia, Whipple's disease*), it is important to remember that certain diseases may be patchy in their distribution (for example, *Crohn's disease*) and that random small intestinal biopsy may sample a relatively normal area of mucosa. Small intestinal biopsy is important for identifying specific infectious causes of impaired digestion and absorption (for example, *tropical sprue* and *giardiasis*), and additional information may be obtained if the specimen is processed for electron microscopy (for example, demonstration of *microsporidia*, or bacilli in *Whipple's disease*) (see pp. 1169 and 1298).

In the past, most peroral small intestinal biopsies were performed with a Quinton-Rubin tube or Crosby capsule and the suction technique. The procedure is safe and reliable when the tube is positioned fluoroscopically at the duodenojejunal junction.[106] With a Quinton-Rubin tube, multiple biopsy samples can be taken. More recently, small intestinal biopsy specimens have been obtained endoscopically using a 1.5-m instrument (for example, a pediatric colonoscope passed orally). There are no comparative studies of these two techniques, but endoscopic sampling appears to yield adequate biopsy specimens and has the advantage of

---

*Representative illustrations of biopsy samples taken from patients with different disease states may be found in the relevant chapters.

Table 18–6. HISTOLOGIC FEATURES OF SMALL INTESTINAL DISEASES CAUSING MALABSORPTION

Disease	Pathologic Features	Pattern of Distribution
Celiac sprue	Villous flattening, crypt hyperplasia, increased lymphocytes and plasma cells in lamina propria	Diffuse in proximal jejunum
Tropical sprue	Shortened villi, increased lymphocytes and plasma cells in lamina propria	Diffuse in proximal jejunum
Crohn's disease	Noncaseating granulomas with or without giant cells	Patchy lesions particularly affecting terminal ileum
Collagenous sprue	Subepithelial collagen deposits	Diffuse
Primary lymphoma	Malignant lymphocytes or histiocytes in lamina propria, variable villous flattening	Patchy
Whipple's disease	Lamina propria laden with PAS-staining foamy macrophages, bacilli in macrophages	Diffuse
Amyloidosis	Amyloid deposition in blood vessels, muscle layers	Diffuse in muscularis mucosae, mucosal sparing
Abetalipoproteinemia	Lipid-laden, vacuolated epithelial cells, normal villi	Diffuse
Radiation enteritis	Flattened villi, mucosal inflammation, fibrosis, ulceration	Patchy
Lymphangiectasia	Dilated lymphatics in lamina propria	Patchy
Eosinophilic gastroenteritis	Eosinophilic infiltrate in the intestinal wall	Patchy
Hypogammaglobulinemia	Villous flattening, *Giardia* trophozoites often present, few plasma cells	Patchy
Giardiasis	Trophozoites may be present, variable villous flattening	Patchy
Opportunistic infections	Organisms may be seen (*Isospora belli*, cryptosporidia, microsporidia), PAS-staining macrophages (*Mycobacterium avium intracellulare*)	Patchy

directly visualizing the small intestine, avoiding the need for fluoroscopy. With both techniques, it is important that the small intestinal mucosal samples are properly oriented and rapidly fixed in formalin. The muscularis mucosae of the biopsy samples tends to contract, orienting the villi outward. The tissue can be reoriented by placing it on the index finger and rolling the muscularis outward with a needle.

Finally, if a specific *disaccharidase deficiency* is suspected, an unfixed small intestinal biopsy can be analyzed for disaccharidase activity.[107] Decreased disaccharidase levels may be secondary to small intestinal disease or may represent a primary disaccharidase deficiency.

MANAGEMENT OF PATIENTS WITH MALABSORPTION

Nutritional Supplements

Mineral and vitamin supplements commonly used in the treatment of malabsorption are summarized in Table 18–7. Therapy should be directed toward correcting known deficiencies. For example, patients with *pancreatic exocrine insufficiency* require enzyme replacement, bicarbonate supplements, and fat-soluble vitamins, but not vitamin B_{12}, folate, or iron. A histamine-2 receptor antagonist (for example, cimetidine) reduces acid output, preventing degradation of the nonenteric-coated enzyme supplements in the stomach.[108] In contrast, patients with *terminal ileal resection* require vitamin B_{12} injections monthly, but fat-soluble vitamins are not necessary unless steatorrhea is significant. Following limited ileal resections, *cholestyramine* is used to bind bile salts and reduce the irritant effects of bile salts on the colon. However, following extensive ileal resection, *cholestyramine* increases fat malabsorp-

tion by further reducing the bile salt pool.[38] Medium-chain triglycerides (comprising 50 to 75 per cent of the total dietary fat) have been shown to improve fat absorption in patients following *small intestinal resection*.[35] The importance of maintaining these patients on a low-fat diet is controversial.[109] Enteral and parenteral supplementation are discussed on pages 1983 to 2027. Medium-chain triglycerides are important in the

Table 18–7. DIETARY SUPPLEMENTS IN PATIENTS WITH MALABSORPTION*

1. Calcium, oral: requires 1200 mg elemental calcium daily as (a) calcium gluconate (93 mg Ca^{2+}/gm), 5–10 gm three times a day, or (b) calcium carbonate (200 mg Ca^{2+}/500 mg tablets), 1–2 gm per day
   Intravenous: calcium gluconate (10% solution, 9.3 mg Ca^{2+}/ml), 10–30 ml administered slowly
2. Magnesium, oral: magnesium gluconate (20 Mg^{2+}/500 mg tablet), 1–4 gm per day
   Intramuscular: magnesium sulfate (50% solution) 2 ml two to three times daily
3. Iron, oral: ferrous sulfate 325 mg three times a day
   Intramuscular (Imferon): adjust to the severity of the anemia
4. Vitamin B_{12}, intramuscular: 100 μg daily for two weeks, then 100 μg monthly
5. Folic acid, oral: 5 mg daily for 1 month; 1 mg/d maintenance
6. Fat-soluble vitamins
   a. Vitamin A: water-soluble vitamin A capsules, USP (25,000 units per capsule), 100,000–200,000 units daily in severe deficiencies; maintenance 25,000–50,000 units daily
   b. Vitamin D: 50,000 units daily (25,000 units/capsule); increase dose as necessary to raise serum calcium to normal
   c. Oral: menadione, USP 4–12 mg/d
      Intravenous: vitamin K_1 (Mephyton), 10 mg ampule *slowly* over 10 minutes for acute bleeding episodes only
7. Cholestyramine: 4 gm dose three times a day before meals
8. Antidiarrheal agents, oral: diphenoxylate hydrochloride (2.5 mg) with atropine sulfate (0.025 mg) (Lomotil), two tablets, two or three times daily; deodorized tincture of opium, 10 drops two to three times per day; loperamide (Imodium) (2 mg capsules), 4 mg followed by 2 mg for each unformed stool (max. 16 mg/d)

*See also pages 1983 to 2027 for more detailed information.

management of patients with *abetalipoproteinemia*, as they can be absorbed without apoproteins and chylomicron formation.

Antidiarrheal agents have a role in controlling the symptoms of patients with malabsorption if the diarrhea is uncontrolled after nutritional supplement and specific therapy is given. These medications are particularly useful in patients with massive *small intestinal resection, jejunileal bypass*, or *AIDS enteropathy*, in whom no specific infectious agent is identified.

Therapy of the Underlying Disease

The specific treatment of different diseases associated with malabsorption is discussed in detail in the relevant chapters. Corticosteroids are used to treat patients with *Crohn's disease* (p. 1350) and *celiac sprue* refractory to a gluten-free diet (p. 1149), antimicrobial therapy (for example, tetracycline or Flagyl) is used to treat patients with documented *bacterial overgrowth* (p. 1295) and patients with documented parasitic infections (pp. 1153–1191); immune serum globulin injections (0.165 gm per ml) are used for treating patients with *hypogammaglobulinemia* and recurrent infections (0.05 ml per kg intramuscularly, every three to four weeks).

References

1. Yang, Y. M., Ducos, R., Rosenberg, A. J., Catron, P. G., Levine, J. S., Podell, E. R., and Allen, R. H. Cobalamin malabsorption in three siblings due to an abnormal intrinsic factor that is markedly susceptible to acid and proteolysis. J. Clin. Invest. 76:2057, 1985.
2. Levine, J. S., and Allen, R. H. Intrinsic factor within parietal cells of patients with juvenile pernicious anemia. A retrospective immunohistochemical study. Gastroenterology 88:1132, 1985.
3. Burman, J. F., Jenkins, W. J., Walker-Smith, J. A., Phillips, A. D., Sourial, N. A., Williams, C. B., and Mollin, D. L. Absent ileal uptake of IF-bound vitamin B_{12} in vivo in the Imerslund-Grasbeck syndrome (familial vitamin B_{12} malabsorption with proteinuria). Gut 26:311, 1985.
4. Corbeel, L., Van den Berghe, G., Jaeken, J., Van Tornout, J., and Eeckels, R. Congenital folate malabsorption. Europ. J. Pediatr. 143:284, 1985.
5. Levitt, M. D., and Duane, W. C. Floating stools—flatus versus fat. N. Engl. J. Med. 286:973, 1972.
6. Green, P. H. R. Alcohol, nutrition and malabsorption. Clin. Gastroenterol. 12:563, 1983.
7. Di Magno, E. P. Diagnosis of chronic pancreatitis: Are noninvasive tests of exocrine pancreatic function sensitive and specific? Gastroenterology 83:143, 1982.
8. Gaskin, K. J., Durie, P. R., Lee, L., Hill, R., and Forstner, G. G. Colipase and lipase secretion in childhood onset pancreatic insufficiency: Delineation of patients with steatorrhea secondary to relative colipase deficiency. Gastroenterology 86:1, 1984.
9. Perez, M. M., Newcomer, A. D., Moertel, C. G., Go, V. L., and Dimagno, E. P. Assessment of weight loss, food intake, fat metabolism, malabsorption and treatment of pancreatic insufficiency in pancreatic cancer. Cancer 52:346, 1983.
10. Lembcke, B., Kraus, B., and Lankische, P. G. Small intestinal function in chronic relapsing pancreatitis. Hepatogastroenterology 32:145, 1985.
11. Pearson, H. A., Lobel, J. S., Kocoshis, S. A., Naiman, J. L., Windmiller, J., Lammi, A. T., Hoffman, R., and Marsh, J. C. A new syndrome of sideroblastic anemia with vacuolization of marrow precursors and exocrine pancreatic dysfunction. J. Pediatr. 95:976, 1979.
12. King, C. E., and Toskes, P. P. Nutrient malabsorption in the Zollinger-Ellison syndrome. Arch. Intern. Med. 143:349, 1983.
13. Kingham, J. G., Levison, D. A. and Fairclough, P. D. Diarrhea and reversible enteropathy in Zollinger-Ellison syndrome. Lancet 2:610, 1981.
14. MacGregor, I. L., Martin, M. S., and Meyer, J. H. Gastric emptying of solid food in normal man and after subtotal gastrectomy and truncal vagotomy with pyloroplasty. Gastroenterology 72:206, 1977.
15. Radziuk, J., and Bondy, D. C. Abnormal oral glucose tolerance and glucose malabsorption after vagotomy and pyloroplasty. Gastroenterology 83:1017, 1982.
16. Giannella, R. A., Broitman, S. A., and Zamcheck, N. Competition between bacteria and intrinsic factor for vitamin B_{12}: Implications for vitamin B_{12} malabsorption in intestinal bacterial overgrowth. Gastroenterology 62:255, 1972.
17. Kretschmer, N. The significance of lactose intolerance: An overview. In Paige, D. M., and Bayless, T. M. (eds.) Lactose Digestion: Clinical and Nutritional Implications. Baltimore, Johns Hopkins University Press, 1981, pp. 3–7.
18. Huang, S. S., and Bayless, T. M. Milk intolerance in healthy orientals. Science 160:83, 1968.
19. Ravich, W. J., and Bayless, T. M. Carbohydrate absorption and malabsorption. Clin. Gastroenterol. 12:335, 1983.
20. Hyams, J. S., Stafford, R. J., Grand, R. J., and Watkins, J. B. Correlation of lactose breath hydrogen test, intestinal morphology and lactase activity in young children. J. Pediatr. 97:609, 1980.
21. Kolars, J. C., Levitt, M. D., Aouji, M., and Savaiano, D. A. Yogurt—an autodigesting source of lactose. N. Engl. J. Med. 310:1, 1984.
22. Weiss, R. G., and Styker, J. A. ^{14}C-lactose breath tests during pelvic radiotherapy: The effect of the amount of small bowel irradiated. Radiology 142:507, 1982.
23. Perlow, W., Baraona, E., and Lieber, C. S. Symptomatic intestinal disaccharidase deficiency in alcoholics. Gastroenterology 71:680, 1977.
24. Pena, A. S., and Truelove, S. C. Hypolactasia and ulcerative colitis. Gastroenterology 64:400, 1973.
25. Sciaretta, G., Giacobazzi, G., Verri, A., Zanirato, P., Garuti, G., and Malaguti, P. Hydrogen breath test quantification and clinical correlation of lactose malabsorption in adult irritable bowel syndrome and ulcerative colitis. Dig. Dis. Sci. 12:1098, 1984.
26. Kirschner, B. S., DeFararo, M. V., and Jensen, W. Lactose malabsorption in children and adolescents with inflammatory bowel disease. Gastroenterology 81:829, 1981.
27. Freiburghaus, A. U., Schmitz, J., Schindler, M., Rotthauwe, H. W., Kuitunen, P., Launiala, K., and Hadorn, B. Protein patterns of brush border fragments in congenital lactose malabsorption and in specific hypolactasia in the adult. N. Engl. J. Med. 294:1030, 1976.
28. Gray, G. M., Townley, R. R. W., and Conklin, K. A. Sucrase-isomaltase deficiency. Absence of an inactive enzyme variant. N. Engl. J. Med. 274:750, 1976.
29. Matuchansky, C., Colin, R., Hemet, J., Touchard, G., Babin, P., Eugene, C., Bergue, A., Zeitoun, P., and Barboteau, M. A. Cavitation of mesenteric lymph nodes, splenic atrophy and a flat small intestinal mucosa. Gastroenterology 87:606, 1984.
30. Sprague, R., Harper, P., McClain, S., Trainer, T., and Beeken, W. Disseminated gastrointestinal sarcoidosis. Gastroenterology 87:421, 1984.
31. Gottfried, E. B., Korsten, M. A., and Lieber, C. S. Gastritis and duodenitis induced by alcohol: An endoscopic and histologic assessment. Gastroenterology 70:890, 1976.
32. Rubin, E., Rybak, B. J., Lindenbaum, J., Gerson, C. D., Walker, G., and Lieber, C. S. Ultrastructural changes in the small intestine induced by ethanol. Gastroenterology 63:801, 1972.
33. Robles, E. A., Mezey, E., Halsted, C. H., et al. Effect of ethanol on motility of the small intestine. Johns Hopkins Med. J. 135:17, 1974.
34. Adibi, S. A., and Stanko, R. T. Perspectives on gastrointestinal

surgery for treatment of morbid obesity: The lesson learned. Gastroenterology 89:1381, 1984.

35. Weser, E. The management of patients after small bowel resection. Gastroenterology 71:146, 1976.

36. Mekhjian, H. S., Phillips, S. F., and Hofmann, A. F. Colonic secretion of water and electrolytes induced by bile acids: Perfusion studies in man. J. Clin. Invest. 50:1569, 1971.

37. Ammon, H. V., and Phillips, S. F. Inhibition of colonic water and electrolyte absorption by fatty acids in man. Gastroenterology 65:744, 1973.

38. Hofmann, A. F., and Poley, J. R. Role of bile acid malabsorption in pathogenesis of diarrhea and steatorrhea in patients with ileal resection. Gastroenterology 62:918, 1972.

39. Curtis, K. J., Sleisenger, M. H., and Kim, Y. S. Protein digestion and absorption after massive small bowel resection. Dig. Dis. Sci. 29:834, 1984.

40. McCarthy, D. M., and Kim, Y. S. Changes in sucrase, enterokinase, and peptide hydrolase after intestinal resection. The association of cellular hyperplasia and adaptation. J. Clin. Invest. 52:942, 1973.

41. Winawer, S. J., and Zamcheck, N. Pathophysiology of small intestinal resection in man. In Glass, G. B. J. (ed.) Progress in Gastroenterology. Vol. 1. New York, Grune & Stratton, 1968, p. 334.

42. Isselbacher, K. J., Scheig, R., Plotkin, G. R., and Caulfield, J. B.: Congenital β-lipoprotein deficiency: an inherited disorder involving a defect in the absorption and transport of lipids. Medicine 43:347, 1974.

43. Cottrill, C., Glueck, C. J., Leuba, V., Millett, F., Puppione, D., and Brown, W. V. Familial homozygous hypobetalipoproteinemia. Metabolism 23:779, 1974.

44. Roy, C. C., Levy, E., Green, P. H. R., Sniderman, A., Letarte, J., Buts, J.-P., Orquin, J., Brochu, P., Weber, A. M., Morin, C. L., Marcel, Y., and Deckelbaum, R. J. Malabsorption, hypercholesterolemia and fat-filled enterocytes with increased intestinal apoprotein B. Chylomicron retention disease. Gastroenterology 92:390, 1987.

44a. Rambaud, J. C., Galian, A., Touchard, G., Morel-Maroger, L., Mikol, J., van Effenterre, G., LeClerc, J.-P., Le Charpentier, Y., Haut, J., Matuchansky, C., and Zittouin, R. Digestive tract and renal small vessel hyalinosis, idiopathic nonarteriosclerotic intracerebral calcifications, retinal ischemic syndrome, and phenotypic abnormalities. A new familial syndrome. Gastroenterology 90:930, 1986.

45. Mondhiry, H. A. Primary lymphomas of the small intestine: East-West contrast. Am. J. Hematol. 22:89, 1986.

46. Hanson, R. D., and Hunker, T. B. Tuberculous peritonitis: CT appearance. Am. J. Roentgenol. 144:931, 1985.

47. Raptopoulos, V. Peritoneal mesothelioma. CRC Crit. Rev. Diagn. Imaging 24:293, 1985.

48. Case records of the Massachusetts General Hospital (Case 20—1986). N. Engl. J. Med. 314:1369, 1986.

49. Seigel, R. S., Kuhns, L. R., Borlaza, G. S., McCormick, T. L., and Simmons, J. L. Computed tomography and angiography in ileal carcinoid tumor and retractile mesenteritis. Radiology 134:437, 1980.

50. Case records of the Massachusetts General Hospital (Case 21—1984). N. Engl. J. Med. 310:1374, 1984.

51. Gillin, J. S., Shike, M., Alcock, N., Urmacher, C., Krown, S., Kurtz, R. C., Lightdale, C. J., and Winawer, S. J. Malabsorption and mucosal abnormalities of the small intestine in the acquired immunodeficiency syndrome. Ann. Intern. Med. 102:619, 1985.

52. Kotler, D. P., Gaetz, H. P., Lange, M., Klein, E. B., and Holt, P. R. Enteropathy associated with the acquired immunodeficiency syndrome. Ann. Intern. Med. 101:421, 1984.

53. Rodgers, V. D., and Kagnoff, M. F. Gastrointestinal manifestations of the acquired immunodeficiency syndrome. Western J. Med. 146:57, 1987.

54. Schein, R., and Gelb, A. Isospora belli in a patient with acquired immunodeficiency syndrome. J. Clin. Gastroenterol. 6:525, 1984.

55. Strom, R. L., and Gruninger, R. P. AIDS with Mycobacterium avium-intracellulare lesions resembling those of Whipple's disease. N. Engl. J. Med. 309:1323, 1983.

56. Gillin, J. S., Urmacher, C., West, R, and Shike, M. Disseminated Mycobacterium avium-intracellulare infection in acquired immunodeficiency syndrome mimicking Whipple's disease. Gastroenterology 85:1187, 1983.

57. Friedman, S. L., Wright, T. L., and Altman, D. F. Gastrointestinal Kaposi's sarcoma in patients with acquired immunodeficiency syndrome—Endoscopic and autopsy findings. Gastroenterology 89:102, 1985.

58. Shafer, R. B., Prentiss, R. A., and Bond, J. H. Gastrointestinal transit in thyroid disease. Gastroenterology 86:852, 1984.

59. Thomas, F. B., Caldwell, J. H., and Greenberger, N. J. Steatorrhea in thyrotoxicosis: Relationship to hypermotility and excessive dietary fat. Ann. Intern. Med. 78:669, 1973.

60. Wruble, L. D., and Kalser, M. H. Diabetic steatorrhea: A distinct entity. Am. J. Med. 37:118, 1964.

61. McEvoy, A., Dutton, J., and James, O. F. Bacterial contamination of the small intestine is an important cause of occult malabsorption in the elderly. Br. Med. J. 287:789, 1983.

62. Webster, S. G. P., Wilkinson, E. M., and Gowland, E. A comparison of fat absorption in young and old subjects. Age Ageing 6:113, 1977.

63. Feibusch, J. M., and Holt, P. R. Impaired absorptive capacity for carbohydrate in the aging human. Dig. Dis. Sci. 27:1095, 1982.

64. Steen, L. E., and Ek, B. O. Familial amyloidosis with polyneuropathy. Aspects of the relationship between gastrointestinal symptoms, EMG findings, and malabsorption studies. Scand. J. Gastroenterol. 19:480, 1984.

65. Farthing, M. J. G., Keusch, G. T., and Carey, M. C. Effects of bile and bile salts on growth and membrane lipid uptake by Giardia lamblia. J. Clin. Invest. 76:1727, 1985.

66. Race, T. F., Paes, K., and Faloon, W. W. Intestinal malabsorption induced by oral colchicine. Comparison with neomycin and cathartic agents. Am. J. Med. Sci. 259:32, 1970.

67. Rogers, A. I., Vloedman, D. A., Bloom, E. C., and Kalser, M. H. Neomycin-induced steatorrhea. JAMA 197:185, 1966.

68. Spiller, R. C., Higgins, B. E., Frost, P. G., and Silk, D. B. Inhibition of jejunal water and electrolyte absorption by therapeutic doses of clindamycin in man. Clin. Sci. 67:117, 1984.

69. Gwavava, N. J., Pinkerton, C. R., Glasgow, J. F., Sloan, J. M., and Bridges, J. M. Small bowel enterocyte abnormalities caused by methotrexate treatment in acute lymphoblastic leukaemia of childhood. J. Clin. Pathol. 34:790, 1981.

70. Reber, H. A. Chronic pancreatitis. In Sleisenger, M. H. and Fordtran, J. S. (eds.) Gastrointestinal Disease. 2nd ed. Philadelphia, W. B. Saunders Co., 1978, p. 1439.

71. Drummey, G. D., Benson, J. A., Jr., and Jones, C. M. Microscopical examination of the stool for steatorrhoea. N. Engl. J. Med. 264:85, 1961.

72. Ghosh, S. K., Littlewood, J. M., Goddard, D., and Steel, A. E. Stool microscopy in screening for steatorrhea. J. Clin. Pathol. 30:749, 1977.

73. Bin, T. L., Stopard, M., Anderson, S., Grant, A., Quantrill, D., Wilkinson, R. H., and Jewell, D. P. Assessment of fat malabsorption. J. Clin. Pathol. 36:1362, 1983.

74. van de Kamer, J. H., ten Bokkel Huinink, H., and Weijers, H. A. A rapid method for the determination of fat in feces. J. Biol. Chem. 177:347, 1949.

75. Braddock, L. I., Fleisher, D. R., and Barbera, G. J. A physical chemical study of the van de Kamer method for fecal fat analysis. Gastroenterology 55:165, 1968.

76. Thorsgaard Pedersen, N., and Halgreen, H. Simultaneous assessment of fat maldigestion and fat malabsorption by a double isotope method using fecal radioactivity. Gastroenterology 88:47, 1985.

77. Newcomer, A. D., Hofmann, A. F., Di Magno, E. P., Thomas, P. J., and Carlson, G. L. Triolein breath test: A sensitive and specific test for fat malabsorption. Gastroenterology 76:6, 1979.

78. Butler, R. N., Gehling, N. J., Lawson, M. J., and Grant, A. K. Clinical evaluation of the ^{14}C triolein breath test: A critical analysis. Aust. N. Z. J. Med. 14:111, 1984.

79. Goff, J. S. Two-stage triolein breath test differentiates pancreatic insufficiency from other causes of malabsorption. Gastroenterology 83:44, 1982.

80. Di Magno, E. P., Go, V. L. W., and Summerskill, W. H. J.

Relations between pancreatic enzyme outputs and malabsorption in severe pancreatic insufficiency. N. Engl. J. Med. *288*:813, 1973.

81. Toskes, P. P. Bentiromide as a test of exocrine pancreatic function in adult patients with pancreatic exocrine insufficiency: Determination of appropriate dose and urinary collection interval. Gastroenterology 85:565, 1983.

82. Weizman, Z., Forstner, G. G., Gaskin, J., Kopelman, H., Wong, S., and Durie, P. R. Bentiromide test for assessing pancreatic dysfunction using analysis of para-amino benzoic acid in plasma and urine. Gastroenterology *89*:596, 1985.

83. Niederau, C., and Grendell, J. Diagnosis of chronic pancreatitis. Gastroenterology 88:1973, 1985.

84. Brugge, W. R., Goff, J. S., Allen, N. C., Podell, E. R., and Allen, R. H. Development of a dual label Schilling test for pancreatic exocrine function based on the differential absorption of cobalamin bound to intrinsic factor and R protein. Gastroenterology 78:937, 1980.

85. Allen, R. H., Seetharam, B., Podell, E., and Alpers, D. H. Effect of proteolytic enzymes on the binding of cobalamin to R protein and intrinsic factor. In vitro evidence that a failure to partially degrade R protein is responsible for cobalamin malabsorption in pancreatic insufficiency. J. Clin. Invest. *61*:47, 1978.

86. Levitt, M. D. Production and excretion of hydrogen gas in man. N. Engl. J. Med. *281*:122, 1969.

87. Perman, J. A., Madler, S., Barr, R. G., and Rosenthal, P. Fasting breath hydrogen concentration: Normal values and clinical application. Gastroenterology 87:1358, 1984.

88. Newcomer, A. D., McGill, D. B., Thomas, P. J., and Hofmann, A. F. Prospective comparison of indirect methods for detecting lactase deficiency. N. Engl. J. Med. *293*:1232, 1975.

89. Metz, G., Gassull, M. A., Drasar, B. S., Jenkins, D. J. A., and Blendis, L. M. Breath-hydrogen test for small intestinal bacterial colonisation. Lancet *1*:668, 1976.

90. Kerlin, P., Wong, L., Harris, B., and Capra, S. Rice flour, breath hydrogen and malabsorption. Gastroenterology 87:578, 1984.

91. Ryan, M. E., and Olsen, W. A. A diagnostic approach to malabsorption syndromes. A pathophysiological approach. Clin. Gastroenterol. *12*:533, 1983.

92. Finlay, J. M., Hogarth, J., and Wightman, K. J. R. A clinical evaluation of the D-xylose tolerance test. Ann. Intern. Med. *61*:411, 1964.

93. Sladen, G. E., and Kumar, P. J. Is the xylose test still a worthwhile investigation? Br. Med. J. *3*:223, 1973.

94. Haeney, M. B., Culank, L. S., Montgomery, R. D., and Sammons, H. G. Evaluation of xylose absorption as measured in blood and urine: A one-hour blood xylose screening test in malabsorption. Gastroenterology 75:393, 1978.

95. Stephen, A. M., Haddal, A. C., and Phillips, S. F. Passage of carbohydrate into the colon. Direct measurements in humans. Gastroenterology 85:589, 1983.

96. Higuchi, S., Fukushi, G., Baba, T., Sasaki, D., and Yoshida, Y. New method of testing for carbohydrate absorption in man. Dig. Dis. Sci. *31*:369, 1986.

97. Tillman, R. T., King, C. E., and Toskes, P. P. Continued experience with the xylose breath test: Evidence that the small bowel culture as the gold standard for bacterial overgrowth may be tarnished. Gastroenterology 80:1304, 1981.

98. Hamilton, I., Worsley, B. W., Cobden, I., Cooke, E. M., Shoesmith, J. G., and Axon, A. T. Simultaneous culture of saliva and jejunal aspirate in the investigation of small bowel bacterial overgrowth. Gut 23:847, 1982.

99. Toskes, P. P., King, C. E., Spivey, J. C., and Lorenz, E. Xylose catabolism in the experimental rat blind loop syndrome. Studies including use of a newly-developed D-^{14}C-xylose breath test. Gastroenterology 74:691, 1978.

100. King, C. E., and Toskes, P. P.: The use of breath tests in the study of malabsorption. Clin. Gastroenterol. *12*:591, 1983.

101. King, C. E., Toskes, P. P., Guilarte, T. R., Lorenz, E., and Welkos, S. L. Comparison of the one-gram D-^{14}C xylose breath test to the ^{14}C bile acid breath test in patients with small-intestine bacterial overgrowth. Dig. Dis. Sci. 25:53, 1980.

102. Schneider, A., Novis, B., Chen, V., and Leichtman, G. Value of the ^{14}C-D-xylose breath test in patients with intestinal bacterial overgrowth. Digestion 32:86, 1985.

103. Rutgeerts, P., Ghoos, Y., and Vantrappen, G. Bile acid studies in patients with Crohn's colitis. Gut 20:1072, 1979.

104. Sciaretta, G., Vicini, G., Fagioli, G., Verri, A., Ginevra, A., and Malaguti, P. Use of 23-selena-25-homocholyltaurine to detect bile acid malabsorption in patients with ileal dysfunction or diarrhea. Gastroenterology 91:1, 1986.

105. Merrick, M. V., Eastwood, M. A., and Ford, M. J. Is bile acid malabsorption underdiagnosed? An evaluation of accuracy of diagnosis by measurement of SeHCAT retention. Br. Med. J. *290*:665, 1985.

105a. Popovic, O. S., Kostic, K. M., Milovic, V. B., Milutinovic-Djuric, S., Miletic, V. D., Sesic, L., Djordjevic, M., Bulajic, M., Bojic, P., Rubinic, M. and Borisavljevic, N. Primary bile acid malabsorption. Gastroenterology 92:1851, 1987.

106. Brandborg, L. L., Rubin, C. E., and Quinton, W. E. A multipurpose instrument for suction biopsy of the esophagus, stomach, small bowel and colon. Gastroenterology 37:1, 1959.

107. Dahlqvist, A. Assay of intestinal disaccharidase. Anal. Biochem. *22*:99, 1968.

108. Regan, P. T., Malagelada, J. R., DiMagno, E. P., Glanzman, S. L., and Go, V. L. W. Comparative effects of antacids, cimetidine and enteric coating on the therapeutic response to oral enzymes in severe pancreatic insufficiency. N. Engl. J. Med. *297*:854, 1977.

109. Woolf, L. G. M., Kurian, R., and Jeejeebhoy, K. N. Diet for patients with a short bowel: high fat or high carbohydrate? Gastroenterology *84*:823, 1983.

19

Protein-Losing Gastroenteropathy

GRAHAM H. JEFFRIES

Protein-losing gastroenteropathy describes a wide range of gastrointestinal disorders that are associated with an excessive loss of plasma protein into the gut.

HISTORICAL PERSPECTIVE

A syndrome of hypoproteinemia unexplained by external loss of plasma protein (e.g., in urine) or by decreased plasma protein synthesis (e.g., liver disease) was described in several early clinical studies.[1-3] Measurements of albumin metabolism following intravenous injection of ^{131}I-albumin in these patients documented an increased rate of albumin catabolism but did not define the mechanism or site of this protein degradation. The term "idiopathic hypercatabolic hypoproteinemia" was used to describe the condition in these patients.

In 1957, Citrin and coworkers first documented enteric loss of plasma protein in a patient with giant hypertrophic gastritis; the patient's hypoproteinemia and increased ^{131}I-albumin catabolism were explained by the albumin content of gastric aspirates.[4] In subsequent studies, the role of the gut in the metabolism of plasma proteins both physiologically and in disease states was clarified by the development of methods to identify plasma proteins in gastrointestinal secretions and by the introduction of ^{131}I-labeled polyvinylpyrrolidone (PVP) and ^{51}Cr-labeled albumin.[5-9] It was found that the normal loss of plasma proteins in gastrointestinal secretions accounted for up to 10 per cent of plasma protein degradation and that a variety of gastrointestinal diseases were associated with excessive enteric protein loss.[9] The term "exudative enteropathy"[5] replaced "idiopathic hypercatabolic hypoproteinemia" and was soon replaced by the term "protein-losing gastroenteropathy."[10]

METHODS FOR MEASURING GASTROINTESTINAL LOSS OF PLASMA PROTEINS

Analysis of Gastrointestinal Secretions for Plasma Proteins. Attempts to measure enteric protein loss by direct analysis of aspirated gastrointestinal contents have been limited by the rapid proteolytic digestion of plasma proteins.[9] In the stomach, peptic digestion can be inhibited by neutralizing gastric juice to pH 7 either with phosphate buffer instilled by nasogastric tube or with alkali following aspiration. When the volume of gastric secretion is measured accurately in perfusion studies with a reference marker to correct for incomplete collection, the clearance of plasma proteins in the stomach (ml of plasma cleared per unit of time) can be estimated from measurements of individual plasma proteins in both plasma and secretion. Excessive protein loss due to gastric mucosal disease can thus be measured directly. Using this technique, Kelly et al. observed that the gastric clearance of albumin in normal subjects ranged from 14 to 39 ml per 24 hours; in four patients with Menetrier's disease and hypoalbuminemia (< 2.75 gm per dl) gastric albumin clearance was increased to an average value of 225 ml per 24 hours.[11]

In the intestine, protein-losing enteropathy is usually associated with diffuse lesions; thus, although an analysis of perfusates from localized segments might document increased segmental loss of plasma protein, particularly when intraluminal plasma protein is protected by protease inhibitor, the estimation of protein loss throughout the length of the intestine requires other methods.

Alpha₁-antitrypsin (α_1-AT) has the properties of an ideal molecule for studies of enteric protein loss; it is a natural plasma protein that is not selectively secreted into the gut, it resists proteolytic digestion, and its concentration in both plasma and intestinal secretions or stool can be measured simply and accurately by immunologic methods.[12, 13] Furthermore, measurements of alpha₁-antitrypsin loss do not require the use of radioisotopes. In a study of normal subjects and patients with protein-losing enteropathy, it has been shown that the clearance of alpha₁-antitrypsin correlates significantly with protein loss measured with [51]CrCL;[14] the lower clearance values obtained with α_1-AT may have been due to digestion of this protein in acid gastric juice.

Studies With Radiolabeled Serum Proteins and Macromolecules. The ideal labeled macromolecule for measuring enteric loss of plasma protein is one that has a normal metabolic behavior that permits simultaneous measurements of endogenous metabolism and enteric loss. The label should be excreted into the gastrointestinal tract only when bound to the injected protein and should not be reabsorbed from the gastrointestinal tract when released from the protein by proteolytic digestion.[15] In addition, the injected tracer molecule should be safe and its label easy to measure in plasma, stool, or urine.

Radioiodinated Serum Proteins. Serum proteins carefully labeled with ^{125}I or ^{131}I retain their normal metabolic behavior. Thus, after an intravenous injection of ^{131}I-albumin or ^{131}I-gamma globulin, the tracer protein is distributed throughout the intravascular and extravascular pools of protein and is catabolized at the same rate as the recipient's plasma protein. Under steady-state conditions (when the volumes of distribution are constant and the protein synthesis and degradation are equal), tracer protein studies provide measurements of the distribution volumes, the total pool, and the catabolism of the protein.[16–18] Kinetic studies suggest that albumin is normally catabolized from the intravascular pool at a rate that is related to the pool size.[19]

Although plasma proteins labeled with radioiodine are ideal for studying plasma protein kinetics, they are not suitable for measuring enteric protein loss. Inorganic iodine is concentrated and secreted by salivary glands and gastric mucosa and is reabsorbed in the intestine; thus, radioiodine recovered from the gut after injection of ^{131}I-protein may reflect not only the loss of labeled protein but also the excretion and absorption of free radioiodine.

Plasma protein leakage into the gut has been estimated in experimental animals by collecting secretions from isolated segments of the intestine and by measuring their content of injected radioiodinated albumin or gamma globulin.[20] These studies have suggested that between 40 and 60 per cent of plasma protein catabolism takes place in the gut. This is difficult to reconcile with observations in eviscerated animals; removal of the gut prolongs the survival of injected iodinated albumin by less than 10 per cent.[21] Several factors may have contributed to an overestimation of enteric protein loss in animal studies. Study periods were brief compared with the turnover time of the plasma protein; only short segments of the gut were used at one time; and operative injury to the gut may have caused excessive leakage of plasma of lymph.

In some patients with gastric mucosal disease, the measurement of albumin-bound ^{131}I in gastric juice collected after intragastric instillation of neutral buffer solution to prevent proteolysis has been of clinical value in demonstrating an excessive loss of plasma protein.[4, 7] With this exception, radioiodinated albumin has not been of value in measuring gastrointestinal protein loss in humans.

A technique in which an ion-exchange resin (Amberlite) was given orally in an attempt to chelate ^{131}I that entered the gut after an intravenous injection of labeled protein did not provide a measure of enteric protein loss as was initially claimed;[22] radioiodine excreted with resin in the feces was derived not only from ^{131}I-albumin leakage but also from free iodide secreted by salivary glands and stomach.

^{51}*Cr-Labeled Albumin.* Proteins labeled with ^{51}CrCL$_3$ are unsuitable for measuring plasma protein kinetics; the half-life of the labeled protein is shortened by elution of chromium from the protein. The properties of the ^{51}Cr label, however, make it ideal for enteric studies; chromium salts are neither secreted into nor absorbed from the gastrointestinal tract in significant amounts. Thus, ^{51}Cr-albumin loss into the gut following an intravenous injection is reflected by excretion of ^{51}Cr label in the stool.[23]

When stools, uncontaminated with urine, are collected for a period of several days after an intravenous injection of ^{51}Cr-albumin and the daily fecal radioactivity is related to the corresponding plasma radioactivity, the loss of albumin into the gut may be expressed as a fraction of the plasma pool or as milliliters of plasma excreted per day. In normal subjects tested by this procedure, between 5 and 25 ml of plasma, or less than 1 per cent of the plasma albumin pool, was cleared daily by the gastrointestinal tract.[23, 24] Evidence that ^{51}Cr may exchange between albumin and other plasma proteins, particularly transferrin, reduces the value of this label in physiologic studies.

^{51}Cr-albumin is no longer commercially available in the United States. Alternatively, ^{51}Cr-chloride may be given as a direct intravenous injection to label plasma proteins; the injected isotope binds rapidly to both albumin and transferrin.[25, 26] Fecal radioactivity reflecting loss of labeled protein has been expressed as a percentage of the injected dose, or as the volume of plasma cleared by the gut per day.[25–27]

^{67}*Cu-Labeled Ceruloplasmin.* ^{67}Cu-labeled ceruloplasmin has biologic advantages as a labeled macromolecule for physiologic studies of enteric protein loss; the isotopic label is an integral part of the molecule, and the ^{67}Cu label is absorbed poorly from the gut. Estimates of plasma protein loss in normal subjects, based on fecal excretion of ^{67}Cu following intravenous administration of ^{67}Cu-ceruloplasmin, correspond to the values obtained with ^{51}Cr-albumin.[28] Unfortunately, the short half-life of ^{67}Cu and the expense of preparing ^{67}Cu-ceruloplasmin make this molecule unsuitable for clinical studies.

Other Labeled Macromolecules. ^{131}I-labeled polyvinylpyrrolidone (^{131}I-PVP), with molecular weight corresponding to that of serum proteins, provided early information on enteric protein loss.[5, 8] The fecal excretion of ^{131}I was greater in patients with idiopathic hypoproteinemia than in control subjects. Instability of the iodine-PVP bond with excretion of free iodine and the heterogeneity of different preparations of ^{131}I-PVP were the major disadvantages of this molecule.

^{59}Fe-labeled iron-dextran (Imferon) was introduced in 1966 for measurements of enteric protein loss.[29] After oral administration, 80 to 100 per cent of the radioactive label was recovered in the stool. After intravenous injection of ^{59}Fe iron-dextran, there was an increased fecal excretion of ^{59}Fe in patients with gastrointestinal protein loss; the results of fecal excretion studies using this labeled macromolecule corresponded to those obtained with ^{51}Cr-albumin.

ENTERIC LOSS OF PLASMA PROTEIN IN NORMAL SUBJECTS

Serum proteins have been identified by immunologic methods in a variety of gastrointestinal secretions.[9, 30]

Studies of gastrointestinal plasma protein loss in normal subjects using ^{51}Cr-albumin, [67]Cu-ceruloplasmin, or alpha$_1$-antitrypsin clearance methods indicate that the daily enteric loss of plasma protein corresponds to less than 1 to 2 per cent of the plasma pool; in the case of albumin, this corresponds to less than 10 per cent of the protein catabolized daily.[24]

The route of plasma protein loss across the normal mucosa has not been well defined. With the exception of secretory IgA, there is no evidence that intestinal epithelial cells actively transport plasma proteins from the lamina propria to the lumen; indeed, it is more likely that the epithelium represents a normal barrier in which cell membranes and apical junctional complexes limit the passage of plasma proteins either through or between the epithelial cells. The rapid shedding of epithelial cells from the mucosal surface is likely to be accompanied by a loss of plasma proteins from the lamina propria at the site of cell extrusion; in the small intestine, this takes place at the tips of the villi. In an experimental study using albumin labeled with Evans blue dye, it was shown that the mucosa at the villus tip was more permeable to protein than were other sites; although no protein extravasation was observed physiologically, with an increase in venous pressure, labeled protein was detected within intraepithelial and interepithelial spaces at the villus tips.[31]

EXCESSIVE ENTERIC LOSS OF PLASMA PROTEINS

Pathophysiology

Excessive transmucosal efflux of plasma proteins may result from mucosal cell damage with increased permeability to protein, from an increase in epithelial cell shedding, from mucosal erosion or ulceration with loss of inflammatory exudate containing protein, or by direct leakage of lymph from obstructed lacteals. Changes in vascular permeability may influence mucosal protein loss by altering the concentration of plasma protein in the interstitial fluid within the lamina propria; topical irritation of the gastric mucosa is accompanied by the release of histamine and an increase in vascular permeability.[32] Gastrointestinal diseases that are associated with increased plasma protein loss may be classified into three groups: (1) those with increased mucosal permeability to protein because of surface cell damage or increased cell loss, (2) those with mucosal erosion or ulceration, and (3) those causing lymphatic obstruction (Table 19–1).

In patients with protein-losing gastroenteropathy, the leakage of individual plasma proteins appears to be independent of their molecular weight (in contrast to urinary protein losses in the nephrotic syndrome). Changes in the pool and plasma concentration of individual plasma proteins will be influenced not only by the magnitude of enteric losses but also by varying rates of hepatic synthesis and endogenous catabolism of the protein. Studies of hepatic plasma protein syn-

Table 19–1. DISEASES ASSOCIATED WITH PROTEIN-LOSING GASTROENTEROPATHY

Mucosal Disease Without Ulceration
(Mechanism: increased permeability with cell damage or cell loss)
 Giant hypertrophic gastritis (Menetrier's disease)[4]
 Hypertrophic hypersecretory gastropathy[36]
 Acute viral enteritis[37, 38, 43]
 Parasitic infestation[41, 42]
 Intestinal bacterial overgrowth[39]
 Whipple's disease[40] (see also under Lymphatic Obstruction)
 Allergic enteropathy[44, 45]
 Eosinophilic gastroenteritis[71]
 Celiac sprue[46]
 Tropical sprue[70]
 Systemic lupus erythematosus[47, 48, 72]
Mucosal Erosion or Ulceration
(Mechanism: inflammatory exudation)
 Erosive gastritis or multiple benign ulcers[7]
 Gastric carcinoma and lymphoma[7]
 Crohn's disease[50] (see also under Lymphatic Obstruction)
 Idiopathic ulcerative jejunoileitis[51]
 Chronic ulcerative colitis[50]
 Pseudomembranous enterocolitis
Lymphatic Obstruction
(Mechanism: direct leakage of intestinal lymph)
 Congenital intestinal lymphangiectasia[60]
 Lymphenteric fistula[57]
 Mesenteric tuberculosis and sarcoidosis[53]
 Intestinal lymphoma[59]
 Chronic pancreatitis and pseudocyst
 Constrictive pericarditis[54, 55]
 Congestive heart failure[56]
 Whipple's disease[40]
 Crohn's disease[50]

thesis in normal subjects and patients with enteric protein loss indicate that the capacity of the liver to increase protein synthesis is limited; hepatic albumin synthesis increased only 25 per cent above control levels in patients with enteric loss.[33] Adaptive changes in the endogenous catabolism of individual plasma proteins may compensate partially or completely for excessive enteric loss. Excessive protein loss will cause a greater increase in the fractional catabolic rate of proteins with a long survival (albumin, gamma globulin) than of those with a short survival (clotting factors); plasma albumin levels are thus more likely to be depressed than are the plasma levels of clotting factors. Impaired hepatic protein synthesis in patients with malabsorption (e.g., celiac sprue) or liver disease (e.g., fatty liver) and increased endogenous catabolism of plasma proteins will augment the plasma protein depletion that results from excessive enteric loss.

Clinical Manifestations

Hypoproteinemia caused by excessive enteric loss of plasma protein may be manifested by dependent edema resulting from a lowered colloidal osmotic pressure of plasma with increased fluid transudation from the capillaries; patients with edema will usually exhibit secondary hyperaldosteronism with sodium retention. Analysis of the plasma proteins usually shows a decrease not only in albumin but also in gamma globulin, fibrinogen, lipoproteins, α_1-antitrypsin, transferrin, and ceruloplasmin. A depression of the levels of thyroid and cortisol-binding proteins will lower the total plasma level of these hormones, although normal levels of free hormone will maintain normal hormone function. The excessive enteric losses of plasma proteins other than albumin rarely lead to clinical problems; secondary hypogammaglobulinemia in these patients does not predispose them to infection, and the loss of blood clotting factors is rarely sufficient to impair hemostasis.

In patients with intestinal lymphatic obstruction, the leakage of intestinal lymph into the gut is associated not only with loss of plasma proteins but also with impaired absorption and/or loss of long-chain triglyceride and fat-soluble vitamins in chylomicrons and a depletion of small lymphocytes (see pp. 287–288))

Diagnosis of Protein-Losing Gastroenteropathy

The possibility of protein-losing enteropathy is usually considered in patients who exhibit hypoproteinemia with or without edema; other causes for hypoproteinemia (proteinuria, protein malnutrition, and liver disease) should be excluded. In some patients, hypoproteinemia with edema may be the only indication of a gastrointestinal lesion; in most patients, however, there are other manifestations of gastrointestinal disease (e.g., diarrhea with bleeding in those with inflammatory bowel disease).

In many patients with suspected protein-losing gastroenteropathy, quantitative assessments of plasma protein metabolism and enteric loss are of limited clinical value and do not modify treatment. In some patients, however, serial measurements of protein loss have been valuable both in diagnosis and in monitoring of treatment. Although studies with ^{51}Cr-albumin or ^{51}Cr-chloride have been widely used since 1961, studies of alpha$_1$-antitrypsin clearance now provide a measure of enteric protein loss without the need for radioisotopes.

The diagnosis of mucosal lesions causing excessive plasma protein loss is based on radiologic, endoscopic, and histopathologic studies.

Diseases Associated with Protein-Losing Gastroenteropathy

As noted previously, the diseases that are associated with excessive enteric loss of plasma protein fall into three categories: diseases in which there is damage to the surface epithelium with increased shedding of surface epithelial cells, diseases in which there is mucosal erosion or ulceration, and diseases causing obstruction to the flow of intestinal lymph (Table 19–1).

Mucosal Disease Without Ulceration. Giant hypertrophic gastritis[4] (Menetrier's disease) is the most com-

mon gastric lesion causing severe protein loss (Fig. 19–1). Normal gastric glands are replaced by hyperplastic glands of mucus-secreting cells; a decrease in the number of parietal cells leads to hypochlorhydria or achlorhydria. The efflux of plasma protein across the mucosal epithelium has been related to a widening of the tight junctions between epithelial cells.[34] In experimental protein-losing gastropathy in dogs, protein loss was observed via an intercellular route.[35] In both the experimental model and in patients with hypertrophic gastritis, antisecretory agents may decrease mucosal permeability and protein loss;[34-36] Kelly et al. observed that propantheline bromide reduced gastric albumin loss in patients with Menetrier's disease and concurrently decreased the width of tight junctions between mucosal epithelial cells, whereas cimetidine was without effect.[11] In hypertrophic, hypersecretory protein-losing gastropathy,[36] giant rugal hypertrophy of the stomach is associated with acid hypersecretion and protein loss without hypergastrinemia (Fig. 19–2). In patients with chronic gastritis, either superficial or atrophic, enteric protein loss is usually mild and of no clinical significance.

Lesions of the small intestine that cause acute or chronic malabsorption are usually also associated with leakage of plasma protein. These lesions may be due to viral infection,[37, 38] bacterial overgrowth (stasis syndrome),[39] bacterial colonization of the mucosa (Whipple's disease[40]), or parasitic infestation (giardiasis[41] and intestinal capillariasis[42]). Enteric protein loss measured by fecal clearance of α_1-AT in children with diarrhea due to *Shigella*, enterotoxigenic *E. coli*, or rotavirus infection was significantly increased when the enteric infection had been preceded by measles infection during the prior two weeks. This enteric protein loss in poorly nourished children with enteric infections may contribute to the development of kwashiorkor.[43]

Mucosal injury with protein loss may result from

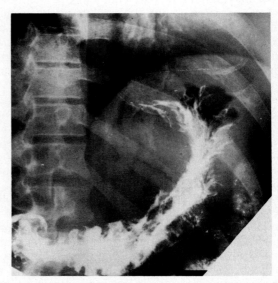

Figure 19–1. Menetrier's disease, as demonstrated by an upper gastrointestinal series in a patient with protein-losing enteropathy. These patients usually are hyposecretors of acid.

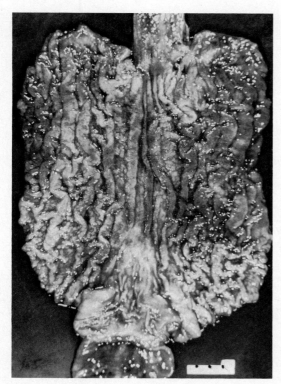

Figure 19–2. Gross surgical specimen of stomach in a patient with protein-losing enteropathy. Although the folds are enormous, mucous cell hyperplasia was not present and hypersecretion of acid was noted. Thus, it is not Menetrier's disease but hypertrophic, hypersecretory protein-losing gastropathy. (From Overholt, B. F., and Jeffries, G. H.: Gastroenterology 58:80, 1970. Used by permission.)

sensitization to dietary antigens or may be due to systemic disease. Allergic enteropathy in children is often due to cow's milk protein sensitivity; occult bleeding and protein loss lead to anemia and hypoproteinemia.[44, 45] In patients with celiac sprue, both malabsorption and enteric losses contribute to hypoproteinemia.[46] In systemic lupus erythematosus, intestinal loss of plasma protein may be associated with hypoalbuminemia in the absence of proteinuria; vascular injury with an increase in permeability to plasma protein may be the mechanism for this enteric loss.[47, 48] Graft-versus-host disease in bone marrow transplant patients is a severe diarrheal illness; fecal clearance of α_1-AT is markedly increased in these patients.[49]

The diagnosis and treatment of these diseases causing protein loss are discussed in the chapters that deal with each specific disease.

Mucosal Erosion or Ulceration. Mucosal erosion or ulceration may be localized or diffuse and may be due to either benign or malignant disease. The severity of plasma protein leakage in individual patients will depend upon the extent of epithelial cell loss and the degree of associated inflammation or lymphatic obstruction. Diffuse ulceration of the small intestine or colon or both causes severe protein loss in patients with Crohn's disease,[50] idiopathic ulcerative jejunoilei-

tis,[51] ulcerative colitis,[50] and pseudomembranous enterocolitis.

Intestinal Lymphatic Obstruction (Intestinal Lymphangiectasia). Obstruction to the flow of lymph from the small intestine causes dilatation of intestinal lymphatic vessels in the mesentery, serosa, submucosa, and villi. The intestinal lymph that may leak from ruptured lacteals contains plasma proteins, chylomicrons, and small lymphocytes.

Etiology and Pathogenesis. Congenital intestinal lymphangiectasia is due to a malformation of the lymphatic system; patients with intestinal lesions often exhibit peripheral lymphedema (Milroy's disease).[52] The diseases causing secondary obstruction to intestinal lymphatic vessels include retroperitoneal fibrosis, chronic pancreatitis, mesenteric tuberculosis or sarcoidosis,[53] Crohn's disease, and retroperitoneal neoplasms, particularly pancreatic carcinoma and lymphoma.

The flow of lymph from the thoracic duct is decreased by elevated pressure in the left subclavian vein. Constrictive pericarditis,[54, 55] chronic congestive heart failure,[56] and obstruction of the left subclavian vein cause secondary intestinal lymphangiectasia with enteric protein loss that will contribute to the patient's hypoproteinemia and edema.

The sites of intestinal lymph efflux in intestinal lymphangiectasia include major lymphenteric fistulas[57] as well as multiple distended lacteals in the intestinal villi. The mild steatorrhea of intestinal lymphangiectasia is probably due to the leakage of chylomicrons into the intestinal lumen; histologic studies show retention of chylomicrons within dilated lymphatic vessels and in the lamina propria.[58] Peripheral lymphocytopenia is explained by sequestration or loss of small lymphocytes in the gut,[59] these cells normally undergo a rapid recirculation from blood through the intestinal mucosa and intestinal lymphatic system. Lymphocytopenia in patients with congenital intestinal lymphangiectasia is associated with anergy to skin test antigens and impaired homograft rejection.[60] Thymic hypoplasia in a child with intestinal lymphangiectasia has been attributed to the loss of regulatory T cells from the intestine.[61]

Clinical Features. The most common presenting symptom of intestinal lymphangiectasia is peripheral edema, either asymmetric in the presence of peripheral lymphatic lesions, or generalized in patients with severe hypoproteinemia. Patients with lymphedema may have dystrophic, yellow nails on the affected extremities.[62] Gastrointestinal symptoms are usually mild, but some patients may have considerable disability from abdominal pain and distention, nausea, vomiting, and diarrhea. Chylous ascites due to leakage of lymph from mesenteric or serosal lymphatic vessels is a complication of both congenital and secondary intestinal lymphangiectasia.[63] Lymphedema predisposes to bacterial infection. In spite of lymphocyte depletion and impaired cell-mediated immunity, opportunistic infections occur infrequently; patients with extensive warts and severe chickenpox have been described.[64]

In children with severe intestinal lymphangiectasia, a decreased food intake and protein loss with hypoproteinemia contribute to growth retardation; hypocalcemia with tetany are explained by vitamin D malabsorption deficiency.

Diagnosis. Intestinal lymphangiectasia should be considered in the differential diagnosis of hypoproteinemia whenever this is accompanied by lymphocytopenia. The diagnosis is usually established by a peroral biopsy of the jejunal mucosa, which exhibits dilated submucosal lymphatics and lacteals (Fig. 19–3); multiple biopsies may be necessary to demonstrate the lymphatic lesion. Dilated lacteals within the villi are visible at duodenoscopy as opalescent white lesions.[65] Radiographic studies of the small intestine usually show only a nonspecific coarsening of the jejunal mucosal folds as a result of edema.

In patients with congenital lymphatic lesions, peripheral lymphangiography demonstrates hypoplastic peripheral lymphatic vessels, retention of contrast material in retroperitoneal lymph nodes, and thoracic duct lesions;[66] the intestinal lymphatic system usually remains unfilled. In patients with acquired lesions, contrast material may reflux into dilated mesenteric lymphatics with extravasation into the gut[57] or peritoneal cavity.[63]

In the presence of ascites or pleural effusions or both, a diagnostic tap should be performed and the fluid examined for protein, cells, enzymes (LDH and amylase), chylomicrons (by centrifugation), acid-fast bacteria, and malignant cells.

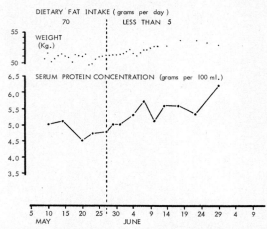

Figure 19–4. Patient with lymphangiectasia and protein-losing enteropathy. ^{131}I-Albumin turnover study also revealed diminution of enteric protein loss during low-fat diet. (From Jeffries, G. H., Chapman, A., and Sleisenger, M. H.: N. Engl. J. Med. *270:*761, 1964. Used by permission.)

Treatment. Enteric protein loss in patients with intestinal lymphangiectasia usually decreases during treatment with a low-fat diet (Fig. 19–4).[67, 68] The absorption of long-chain triglycerides stimulates intestinal lymph flow; in their absence there is probably a decrease in the pressure within intestinal lymphatic vessels. Medium-chain triglycerides (C 6:0 to C 12:0), which do not require intestinal lymphatic transport, can be substituted for long-chain triglycerides; for infants, a commercially available liquid formula (Portagen) provides total nutrition, while for older children and adults, medium-chain triglyceride oil can be used in cooking as a dietary supplement.

Peripheral lymphedema should be treated with external elastic support; diuretics are of limited benefit in patients with lymphedema. The involved extremity should be protected from skin injury to reduce the risk of cellulitis, and established infection should be treated vigorously with antibiotics; recurrent infection increases the severity of the peripheral edema.

Surgery is of limited value in patients with intestinal lymphangiectasia. Major lymphenteric fistulas can be resected, and dilated intestinal lymphatic ducts might be decompressed by lymph venous anastomosis.[69] Patients with constrictive pericarditis respond to pericardiectomy.[55]

When intestinal lymphangiectasia is secondary to inflammatory or neoplastic disease (tuberculosis, sarcoidosis, and lymphoma), specific treatment of the primary condition may relieve the lymphatic obstruction and decrease enteric protein loss.

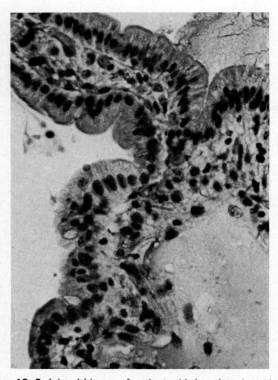

Figure 19–3. Jejunal biopsy of patient with lymphangiectasia and protein-losing enteropathy. Note very dilated lacteal at the base of the villus. Villous epithelium is normal. × 200.

References

1. Albright, F., et al. Studies on fate of intravenously administered plasma proteins in idiopathic hypoproteinemia and osteoporosis. *In* Youmans, Y. B. (ed.) Symposia on Nutrition of the Robert

Gould Research Foundation. Vol. 2. Springfield, Illinois, Charles C Thomas, Publisher, 1950, p. 352.

2. Schwartz, M., and Thomsen, B. Idiopathic or hypercatabolic hypoproteinaemia: Case examined by ^{131}I-labelled albumin. Br. Med. J. *1*:14, 1957.

3. Holman, H., Nickel, W. F., Jr., and Sleisenger, M. H. Hypoproteinemia antedating intestinal lesions and possibly due to excessive serum protein loss into the intestine. Am. J. Med. *27*:963, 1959.

4. Citrin, Y., Sterling, K., and Halsted, J. A. Mechanism of hypoproteinemia associated with giant hypertrophy of gastric mucosa. N. Engl. J. Med. *257*:906, 1957.

5. Gordon, R. S., Jr. Exudative enteropathy: Abnormal permeability of gastrointestinal tract demonstrable with labelled polyvinylpyrrolidone. Lancet *1*:325, 1959.

6. Gordon, R. S., Jr., Bartter, F. C., and Waldmann, T. Idiopathic hypoalbuminemias: Clinical staff conference at the National Institutes of Health. Ann. Intern. Med. *51*:553, 1959.

7. Schwartz, M., and Jarnum, S. Protein-losing gastroenteropathy: Hypoproteinemia due to gastrointestinal protein loss of varying aetiology, diagnosed by means of ^{131}I-albumin. Danish Med. Bull. *8*:1, 1961.

8. Waldmann, T. A., Steinfeld, J. L., Dutcher, T. F., Davidson, J. D., and Gordon, R. S., Jr. The role of the gastrointestinal system in "idiopathic hypoproteinemia." Gastroenterology *41*:197, 1961.

9. Jeffries, G. H., Holman, H. R., and Sleisenger, M. H. Plasma proteins and the gastrointestinal tract. N. Engl. J. Med. *266*:652, 1962.

10. Editorial. Protein-losing gastroenteropathy. Lancet *1*:351, 1959.

11. Kelly, D. G., Miller, L. J., Malagelada, J.-R., Huizenga, K. A., and Markowitz, H. Giant hypertrophic gastropathy (Menetrier's disease): Pharmacologic effects on protein leakage and mucosal ultrastructure. Gastroenterology *83*:581, 1982.

12. Bernier, J. J., Florent, C., Desmazures, C., Aymes, C., and L'Hirondel, C. Diagnosis of protein-losing enteropathy by gastrointestinal clearance of alpha_1-antitrypsin. Lancet *2*:763, 1978.

13. Thomas, D. W., Sinatra, F. R., and Merritt, R. J. Random fecal alpha_1-antitrypsin concentration in children with gastrointestinal disease. Gastroenterology *80*:776, 1981.

14. Florent, C., L'Hirondel, C., Desmazures, C., Aymes, C., and Bernier, J. J. Intestinal clearance of α_1-antitrypsin. A sensitive method for the detection of protein-losing enteropathy. Gastroenterology *81*:777, 1981.

15. Waldmann, T. A. Protein-losing enteropathy. Gastroenterology *50*:422, 1966.

16. Sterling, K. Turnover rate of serum albumin in man as measured by I[131] tagged albumin. J. Clin. Invest. *30*:1228, 1951.

17. Berson, S. A., Yalow, R. S., Schreiver, S. S., and Post, J. Tracer experiments with I[131] labeled serum albumin: Distribution and degradation studies. J. Clin. Invest. *32*:746, 1953.

18. MacFarlane, A. S. The behavior of I[131]-labelled plasma proteins in vivo. Ann. N. Y. Acad. Sci. *70*:19, 1957.

19. Andersen, S. B. Intravascular or extravascular degradation of γ_{ss}-globulin. *In* Physiology and Pathophysiology of Plasma Protein Metabolism. Berne, Hans Huber, 1964, pp. 105–115.

20. Glenert, J., Jarnum, S., and Reimer, S. Albumin transfer from blood to gastrointestinal tract in dogs. Acta Chir. Scand. *124*:63, 1962.

21. Gitlin, D., Klinenberg, J. R., and Hughes, W. L. Site of catabolism of serum albumin. Nature *181*:1064, 1958.

22. Jeejeebhoy, K. N., and Coghill, N. F. The measurement of gastrointestinal protein loss by a new method. Gut *2*:123, 1961.

23. Waldmann, T. A. Gastrointestinal protein loss demonstrated by ^{51}Cr-labelled albumin. Lancet *2*:121, 1961.

24. Waldmann, T. A., Wochner, R. D., and Strober, W. The role of the gastrointestinal tract in plasma protein metabolism. Studies with ^{51}Cr-albumin. Am. J. Med. *46*:275, 1969.

25. Rootwelt, K. Direct intravenous injection of [51]chromic chloride compared with ^{125}I-polyvinylpyrrolidone and ^{131}I-albumin in the detection of gastrointestinal protein loss. Scand. J. Clin. Lab. Invest. *18*:405, 1966.

26. Walker-Smith, J. A., Skyring, A. P., and Mistilis, S. P. Use of [51]CrCl_3 in the diagnosis of protein-losing enteropathy. Gut *8*:166, 1967.

27. van Tongeren, J. H. M., and Majoor, C. L. H. Demonstration of protein-losing gastroenteropathy. The disappearance rate of ^{51}Cr from plasma and the binding of ^{51}Cr to different serum proteins. Clin. Chim. Acta *14*:31, 1966.

28. Waldmann, T. A., Morell, A. G., Wochner, R. D., and Sternlieb, I. Quantitation of gastrointestinal protein loss with copper[67]-labeled ceruloplasmin. J. Clin. Invest. *44*:1107, 1965.

29. Andersen, S. B., and Jarnum, S. Gastrointestinal protein loss measured with ^{59}Fe-labelled iron-dextran. Lancet *1*:1060, 1966.

30. Soergel, K. H., and Ingelfinger, F. J. Proteins in serum and rectal mucus of patients with ulcerative colitis. Gastroenterology *40*:37, 1961.

31. Granger, D. N., Cook, B. H., and Taylor, A. E. Structural locus of transmucosal albumin efflux in canine ileum. A fluorescent study. Gastroenterology *71*:1023, 1976.

32. Wood, J. G., and Davenport, H. W. Measurement of canine gastric vascular permeability to plasma proteins in the normal and protein-losing states. Gastroenterology *82*:725, 1982.

33. Wochner, R. D., Weissman, S. M., Waldmann, T. A., Houston, D., and Berlin, N. I. Direct measurement of the rates of synthesis of plasma proteins in control subjects and patients with gastrointestinal protein loss. J. Clin. Invest. *47*:971, 1968.

34. Krag, E., Frederiksen, H.-J., Olsen, N., and Henriksen, J. H. Cimetidine treatment of protein-losing gastropathy (Menetrier's disease). A clinical and pathophysiological study. Scand. J. Gastroenterol. *13*:635, 1978.

35. Munro, D. R. Route of protein loss during a model protein-losing gastropathy in dogs. Gastroenterology *66*:960, 1974.

36. Overholt, B. F., and Jeffries, G. H. Hypertrophic, hypersecretory protein-losing gastropathy. Gastroenterology *58*:80, 1979.

37. Dossetor, J. F. B., and Whittle, H. C. Protein-losing enteropathy and malabsorption in acute measles enteritis. Br. Med. J. *2*:592, 1975.

38. Schreiber, D. S., Blacklow, N. R., and Trier, J. S. The mucosal lesion of the proximal small intestine in acute infectious nonbacterial gastroenteritis. N. Engl. J. Med. *288*:1318, 1973.

39. King, C. E., and Toskes, P. P. Protein-losing enteropathy in the human and experimental rat blind-loop syndrome. Gastroenterology *80*-504, 1981.

40. Laster, L., Waldman, T. A., Fenster, L. F., and Singelton, J. W. Reversible enteric protein loss in Whipple's disease. Gastroenterology *42*:762, 1962.

41. Sherman, P., and Liebman, W. M. Apparent protein-losing enteropathy associated with giardiasis. Am. J. Dis. Child. *134*:893, 1980.

42. Whalen, G. E., Strickland, G. T., Cross, J. H., Uylangco, C., Rosenberg, E. B., Gutman, R. A., Waten, R. H., and Dixon, J. J. Intestinal capillariasis. A new disease in man. Lancet *1*:13, 1969.

43. Sarker, S. A., Wahed, M. A., Rahaman, M. M., Alam, A. N., Islam, A., and Jahan, F. Persistent protein losing enteropathy in post measles diarrhoea. Arch. Dis. Child. *61*:739, 1986.

44. Wilson, J. F., Heiner, D. C., and Lahey, M. E. Milk-induced gastrointestinal bleeding in infants with hypochromic microcytic anemia. JAMA *189*:568, 1964.

45. Waldmann, T. A., Wochner, R. D., Laster, L., and Gordon, R. S. Allergic gastroenteropathy. A cause of excessive gastrointestinal protein loss. N. Engl. J. Med. *276*:761, 1967.

46. Gordon, R. S., Jr. Protein-losing enteropathy in the sprue syndrome. Lancet *1*:55, 1961.

47. Chase, G. J., O'Shea, P. A., Collins, E., and Brem, A. S. Protein-losing enteropathy in systemic lupus erythematosus. Hum. Pathol. *13*:1053, 1982.

48. Wood, M. L., Foulds, I. S., and French, M. A. Protein losing enteropathy due to systemic lupus erythematosus. Gut *25*:1013, 1984.

49. Weisdorf, S. A., Salati, L. M., Longsdorf, J. A., Ramsay, N. K. C., and Sharp, H. L. Graft-versus-host disease of the intestine: A protein losing enteropathy characterized by fecal-antitrypsin. Gastroenterology *85*:1076, 1983.

50. Steinfeld, J. L., Davidson, J. D., Gordon, R. S., Jr., and Greene, F. E. Mechanism of hypoproteinemia in patients with regional enteritis and ulcerative colitis. Am. J. Med. *29*:405,1961.

51. Jeffries, G. H., Steinberg, H., and Sleisenger, M. H. Chronic

ulcerative (nongranulomatous) jejunitis. Am. J. Med. *44*:47, 1968.

52. Eustace, P. W., Gaunt, J. I., and Croft, D. N. Incidence of protein-losing enteropathy in primary lymphoedema using chromium-51 chloride technique. Br. Med. J. *2*:737, 1975.

53. Popovic, O. S., Brkic, S., Bojic, P., Kenic, V., Jojic, N., Djuric, V., and Djordjevic, N. Sarcoidosis and protein losing enteropathy. Gastroenterology *78*:119, 1980.

54. Petersen, V. P., and Hastrup, J. Protein-losing enteropathy in constrictive pericarditis. Acta Med. Scand. *173*:401, 1963.

55. Wilkinson, P., Pinto, B., and Senior, J. R. Reversible protein-losing enteropathy with intestinal lymphangiectasia secondary to chronic constrictive pericarditis. N. Engl. J. Med. *273*:1178, 1965.

56. Davidson, J. D., Waldmann, T. A., Goodman, D. S., and Gordon, R. S., Jr. Protein-losing enteropathy in congestive heart-failure. Lancet *1*:899, 1961.

57. Mistilis, S. P., Skyring, A. P., and Stephen, D. D. Intestinal lymphangiectasia. Mechanism of enteric loss of plasma protein and fat. Lancet *1*:77,1965.

58. Dobbins, W. I., III. Electron microscopic study of the intestinal mucosa in intestinal lymphangiectasia. Gastroenterology *51*:1004, 1966.

59. Douglas, A. P., Weetman, A. P., and Haggith, J. W. The distribution and enteric loss of ^{51}Cr-labelled lymphocytes in normal subjects and in patients with coeliac disease and other disorders of the small intestine. Digestion *14*:29, 1976.

60. Strober, W., Wochner, R. D., Carbone, P. P., and Waldmann, T. A. Intestinal lmphangiectasia. A protein-losing enteropathy with hypogammaglobulinemia, lymphocytopenia and impaired homograft rejection. J. Clin. Invest. *46*:1643, 1967.

61. Sorensen, R. U., Halpin, T. C., Abramowsky, C. R., Hornick, D. L., Miller, K. M., Naylor, P., and Incefy, G. S. Intestinal lymphangiectasia and thymic hypoplasia. Clin. Exp. Immunol. *59*:217, 1985.

62. Dhura, P. M., Quigley, E. M. M., and Marsh, M. N. Chylous ascites, intestinal lymphangiectasia and the "yellow-nail" syndrome. Gut *26*:1266, 1985.

63. Camiel, M. R., Benninghoff, D. L., and Herman, P. G. Chylous ascites with lymphographic demonstration of lymph leakage into the peritoneal cavity. Gastroenterology *47*:188, 1964.

64. Ross, I. N., Chesner, I., Thompson, R. A., Parker, R. G., and Asquith, P. Cutaneous viral infection as a presentation of intestinal lymphangiectasia. Br. J. Derm. *107*:357, 1982.

65. Donzelli, F., Norberto, L., Marigo, A., Barbato, A., Tapparello, G., Basso, G., and Zachello, G. Primary intestinal lymphangiectasia. Comparison between endoscopic and radiological findings. Helv. Paediatr. Acta *35*:169, 1980.

66. Pomerantz, M., and Waldman, T. A. Systemic lymphatic abnormalities associated with gastrointestinal protein loss secondary to intestinal lymphangiectasia. Gastroenterology *45*:703, 1963.

67. Jeffries, G. H., Chapman, A., and Sleisenger, M. H. Low-fat diet in intestinal lymphangiectasia: Its effect on albumin metabolism. N. Engl. J. Med. *270*:761, 1964.

68. Tift, W. L., and Lloyd, J. K. Intestinal lymphangiectasia. Long term results with MCT diet. Arch. Dis. Child. *50*:269, 1975.

69. Mistilis, S. P., and Skyring, A. P. Intestinal lymphangiectasia. Therapeutic effect of lymph venous anastomosis. Am J. Med. *40*:634, 1966.

70. Rubini, M. E., Sheehy, T. W., Meroney, W. H., and Louro, J. Exudative enteropathy. II. Observations in tropical sprue. J. Lab. Clin. Med. *58*:902, 1961.

71. Klein, N. C., Hargrove, R. L., Sleisenger, M. H., and Jeffries, G. H. Eosinophilic gastroenteritis. Medicine *49*:299, 1970.

72. Trentham, D. E., and Masi, A. T. Systemic lupus erythematosus with a protein-losing enteropathy. JAMA *236*:287, 1976.

20

Diarrhea

KENNETH D. FINE
GUENTER J. KREJS
JOHN S. FORDTRAN

DEFINITIONS

Normal Stools

In a recent study from our laboratory, stools were collected quantitatively for 72 hours in 11 normal young adults (students or their spouses).[1] The results are shown in Table 20–1. Average stool weight in seven men was 142 gm per day, but was only 55 gm per day in four women. Water content varied from 59 to 82 per cent. Total solid output averaged 35 gm per day in the men and 16 gm per day in women. Qualitatively similar results, also shown in Table 20–1, were obtained previously in 11 normal men from Scotland.[2] The upper limit of normal frequency of defecation has not been definitely established. The highest average stool frequency during a three-day collection in our 11 normal subjects was 1.3 per day. For purposes of this discussion, we will assume that more than an average of two bowel movements per day during a three-day period is abnormal.

The factors which account for variation in stool weight, percentage of water content, and frequency among various people without gastrointestinal disease

Table 20–1. STOOL WEIGHT AND WATER AND
SOLID CONTENT IN NORMAL ADULTS

Study	Stool Weight (gm/day)	Wet Weight (%)	Total Water (gm/day)	Total Solids (gm/day)
Dallas, Texas[1]				
Men, n = 7				
Average	142	75	107	35
Range	102–195	73–80	74–156	27–47
± 2 SD	76–208	70–80	53–161	21–49
Women, n = 4				
Average	55	70	39	16
Range	31–81	59–82	18–56	11–25
Edinburgh, Scotland[2]				
Men, n = 11				
Average	107	.74	79	27
Range	60–182	63–81	NA	15–43
± 2 SD	27–187	63–85	NA	12–42

NA = Data not available.

have not been fully elucidated. In one study,[3] when male volunteers were on a control diet containing 8 to 12 gm of fiber per day, stool weight averaged 100 gm per day (±2 SD = 15 to 185 gm per day). When fiber intake was increased to about 26 gm per day with wheat bran, average stool weight was 149 gm per day (±2 SD = 71 to 227 gm per day). When fiber increases daily stool weight, stool frequency also tends to increase.[3] The authors of this study suggested that personality factors influenced stool output about as much as dietary fiber ("personality factors predispose some persons to low stool output"). In another study,[4] fecal weight, consistency, and form were correlated with dietary fiber intake; men produced a greater quantity of stool and softer stools than women, probably because they ingested more fiber. During the luteal phase, women have less and harder stools, whereas during the first few days of menses they have larger and looser stools.[4]

Diarrhea

The word "diarrhea" originates from the Greek terms *dia* (through) and *rhein* (to flow). Diarrhea is present when one or more of the following are present: (1) abnormal increase in daily stool weight; (2) abnormal increase in stool liquidity; (3) abnormal increase in stool frequency. Diarrhea is often accompanied by urgency, perianal discomfort, incontinence, or a combination of all three.

Stool weight and frequency are easy to measure, but a quantitative method for measuring stool liquidity apparently has not been developed. The "rheology" of normal stools, dependent on the degree of penetration into the stool of a cone of standard weight, has been used in normal people[4] but apparently has not been applied to the stools of patients with diarrhea.

To a major extent, however, liquidity is dependent on the percentage of water content of the stool. It is clear from the results shown in Table 20–1 that stool water content could increase markedly in some people, especially women, before stool weight would exceed the upper limits of normal. For example, a person's normal stool weight might be 50 gm per day, with a wet weight of 75 per cent. If 100 gm of water were added to this stool because of abnormal intestinal fluid absorption, stool weight would be 150 gm per day, which is still within the normal range; however, wet weight would now be 92 per cent—clearly an abnormally liquid stool.

Figure 20–1 shows an analysis of 72-hour stool collections carried out in 58 consecutive patients referred to Baylor Hospital in Dallas for an evaluation of chronic or recurrent diarrhea. Stool weight per day is plotted against percentage of wet weight. Normal values (from Table 20–1) are indicated by the rectangle inside the plot. Most of the patients had abnormally high stool weights or increased percentage of water content. Ten patients fell into the normal range for both these variables. However, six of these had increased stool frequency (three to nine stools per day). Thus, only four of 58 patients referred to us for chronic diarrhea had normal stools during a three-day stool collection.

As also shown in Figure 20–1, steatorrhea tends to be associated with reduced percentage of water content of stool, for a given stool weight. Some patients with steatorrhea have a marked increase in stool weight, yet have a normal percentage of water content of stool.

Goy et al.[2] claim that the consistency of feces depends not only on water content but probably also on the physical and chemical properties of the stool matrix. ("This is created by fiber and water bound to it both on the surface and interstitially with an additional component that is 'free' water.")

Figures 20–2 and 20–3 show, in our 58 patients with chronic diarrhea, that there is not a close correlation

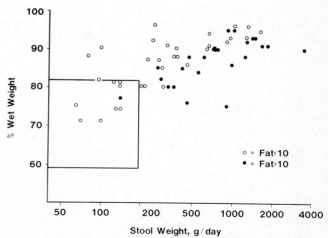

Figure 20–1. Stool weight and percentage of wet weight (percentage of water content) in 58 consecutive patients referred to Baylor Hospital for evaluation of chronic or recurrent diarrhea. Normal values are taken from the range of values given in Table 20–1 and are indicated by the rectangle. Note log scale for stool weight. Patients with steatorrhea (>10 gm of fat per day) are indicated by the solid symbols.

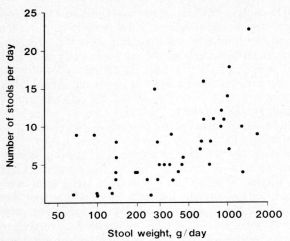

Figure 20–2. Stool weight and number of stools per day in the 58 patients described in Figure 20–1.

between stool frequency and either stool weight or percentage of wet weight of stools.

It should be remembered that the stools of a diarrhea patient may vary considerably from day to day and week to week. When evaluating the results of stool analysis, one needs to know if the sample was collected during a time that the patient was having what he or she considers to be a problem with diarrhea.

NORMAL PHYSIOLOGY

Fluid Absorptive Capacity

When perfused with a balanced electrolyte solution at high rates of flow, average rates of fluid absorption in normal people are 107 ml per hour per 30 cm in the jejunum and 76 ml per hour per 30 cm in the ileum.[5] Taking into account the fact that the length of the intubated small bowel is about 250 cm, these values correspond to an average small intestinal absorption rate of about 750 ml per hour. When figured on a 24-

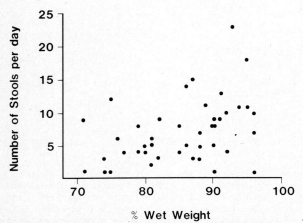

Figure 20–3. Percentage of wet weight and number of stools per day in the 58 patients described in Figure 20–1.

hour basis, the capacity of the small bowel to absorb a balanced electrolyte solution amounts to about 18 liters per day. Moreover, if one considers the fact that glucose and other actively absorbed nonelectrolytes stimulate small bowel fluid absorption, the fluid absorptive capacity of the normal small bowel is enormous. By contrast, the normal colon has an average daily absorptive capacity of 3.8 liters per day,[5] and this is not enhanced by glucose. On the other hand, the colon (and the ileum to a lesser extent) can absorb ions against steep electrochemical gradients, although the jejunum cannot.[6-8] To illustrate the importance of this last point, if one were to perfuse an isotonic solution with half of the osmolality accounted for by mannitol and half by sodium chloride, the colon would absorb fluid, whereas there would be net fluid secretion by the jejunum.

Flow Rates and Gut Volume During a Fast

Studies carried out in the 1950s indicated that the fasting intestine of normal people contains very little fluid.[9] This is consistent with the impression of surgeons at laparotomy and with barium contrast studies, which usually reveal no evidence of dilution of ingested barium in the small bowel. However, perfusion studies using slow marker infusion methods have suggested average fasting flow rates of 2.5 ml per minute (3.6 liters per day) through the upper jejunum,[10] 1.2 ml per minute (1.7 liters per day) through the midileum,[10] and 0.4 to 0.9 ml per minute (about 0.6 to 1.3 liters per day) through the ileocecal valve area.[11, 12] These results might seem to contradict the concept that the fasting small bowel contains almost no fluid in normal people. However, the volume of a tube cannot be calculated from flow rates through the tube. For example, one can infuse fluid at a rate of 20 ml per minute (28.8 liters per day) through a 300 cm long, small bore tube, which has a volume capacity of only 5 ml. To reconcile fasting intestinal flow rates of several liters per day with the concept of a near empty small intestine requires only that the flow take place through a near collapsed or air-distended intestine. Under such conditions, the fluid traveling through the intestine would be exposed to only a very small fraction of the intestinal epithelial cells. This limited exposure to epithelial cells, plus rapid movement in boluses rather than a steady flow, are two possible explanations for why fasting intestinal fluid is not completely absorbed by an intestine with a relatively enormous absorptive capacity.

The origin of the fluid which flows through the fasting intestine is unknown; presumably it originates at least in part from fasting secretions by the digestive glands. It might originate in part from active secretion by specialized epithelial cells in the intestine (crypt cells, for example), but such an hypothesis is speculative.

As noted above, data on the quantitative aspects of such fasting flow comes from slow marker perfusion studies; since these involve intestinal intubation, it is at least theoretically possible that fluid flow under these conditions is nonphysiologic, being somehow enhanced by the experimental procedure. We were not able to find data on the 24-hour fluid output of well-functioning ileostomies in fasting people for comparison, but even such data wouldn't settle the issue with certainty because ileostomies are not physiologic either.

Flow Rates While Eating

When people eat three normal meals per day, about 9 liters of fluid per day are delivered to the proximal duodenum (Fig. 20–4).[13, 14] Approximately 2 liters of this fluid are from ingested food and liquids, the rest being from digestive secretions. The volume of chyme that passes through different segments of the small bowel depends on the type of food that has been eaten.[14] For example, meals containing high concentrations of sugar are hypertonic, and, when such meals are ingested, the volume of material passing through the jejunum is even greater than the volume that enters the proximal duodenum. On the other hand, after isotonic or hypotonic meals (such as a meal of steak, potatoes, and tea), the volume of fluid traversing the jejunum is much less than was delivered to the duodenum. (These considerations are especially important in patients who have had gastric surgery or intestinal resection.) In either case, the osmolality of chyme is adjusted toward that of plasma as fluid travels through the duodenum and upper jejunum. For example, after a meal of milk and doughnuts, peak osmolality in the antrum of the stomach was about 540 mOsm per kilogram, whereas peak osmolality of fluid collected 5 cm distal to the ligament of Treitz peaked at about 360 mOsm per kilogram.[15] By the time chyme reaches the ileum, most of the dietary sugars, amino acids and fats have been absorbed (the completeness of starch digestion and absorption depends upon the kind of starch ingested). Fluid passing through the middle small bowel is mainly an isotonic salt solution, roughly similar in its ionic make-up to plasma.[14] The ileum absorbs much, but not all, of this solution, altering the electrolyte make-up as shown in Figure 20–4.

The volume of unabsorbed ileal fluid which is delivered to the colon under physiologic conditions has not been settled to everyone's satisfaction. Slow marker perfusion studies in normal subjects eating regular food suggest this volume to be about 1.5 to 2.0 liters per day.[11, 12] The significance of possible artifacts of such methodology have been debated,[16] but most investigators seem content with the method. Another way to look at the issue is to examine the volume of ileostomy drainage (colectomy done for ulcerative colitis). Such drainage averages about 600 ml per day after full recovery from surgery. However, the ileostomy data probably are not representative of normal ileal delivery to the colon, because of postulated adaptive changes (hyperabsorption) in the terminal ileum after colectomy.[11, 12] Uncertainty on the question of the normal volume of fluid delivered to the colon makes it impossible to know the amount of fluid normally absorbed by the colon. The volume of water not absorbed by the colon (passed in stools) varies from 18 to 156 ml, as shown in Table 20–1.

Summary of Flow Rates (Fig. 20–4)

To summarize in ballpark figures, for normal people eating three meals per day, the daily volume of fluid traversing the duodenum is 9 liters, traversing the ileocecal valve area is uncertain (probably 1 to 1.5 liters), and traversing the anal sphincter is 0.1 liter. Stated in another way, the small bowel absorbs about 8 liters of fluid per day and empties 1.0 to 1.5 liters into the colon, and the colon absorbs 0.9 to 1.4 liters per day.

Reserve Capacity and Margin for Error

The colonic absorptive capacity for isotonic salt solution, measured under high flow and steady-state conditions, averages 3.8 liters per day in normal people.[5] It is important to point out that these experimental conditions (high flow, steady state) maximize epithelial cell exposure to an absorbable solution and thus allow absorption rate to approach maximal values. This is not the case normally, and probably is not the case in any diarrheal disease. Moreover, to the extent

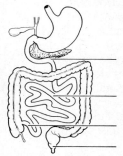

| FLOW RATE | ION CONCENTRATIONS meq/L | | | | OSMO-LALITY |
ml/day	Na	K	Cl	HCO₃	mOsm/kg
9000	60	15	60	15	Variable
3000	140	6	100	30	Isotonic
1000	140	8	60	70	Isotonic
100	40	90	15	30	Isotonic

Colon absorption capacity 3–4 L/day

Figure 20–4. Normal human physiology. Approximate flow rates per day and ionic constituents of fluid passing through different levels of the intestine. There is some uncertainty about the volume of fluid delivered from the terminal ileum to the colon, as discussed in the text.

that the fluid delivered to the colon contains poorly absorbable solutes or inhibitors of ion transport, colonic epithelial cell absorption rate would be depressed.

The normal colonic absorptive capacity (for isotonic salt solutions) of 3.8 liters per day corresponds to an absorptive capacity of 2.7 ml per minute. Delivery of unabsorbed ileal fluid to the colon is estimated by slow marker perfusion to peak at 2 to 7 ml per minute after meals in normal subjects.[11] Thus, temporarily after meals, perhaps lasting as long as one to two hours, the inflow rate may exceed the absorptive capacity. Diarrhea does not result, presumably because the periods of high flow are too brief and the colon (being more or less closed at the lower end and not prone to frequent peristaltic contractions) can hold excessive fluid for subsequent absorption. However, quantitatively small abnormalities in crucial segments of the gut can cause diarrhea. For example, resection of the ileocecal valve area (without resection of substantial absorptive surface) frequently results in mild but persistent diarrhea.[17] For another example, cecal infusion of saline at a rate of 8.3 ml per minute for 60 minutes (500 ml total) results in diarrhea in normal subjects.[18] It thus appears that the margin of safety is small; given the frequency of chronic diarrhea and chronic constipation, it seems likely that normal bowel habit is a fine line that is easily crossed in either direction.

Electrolyte Composition of Gut Fluid

This is summarized in Figure 20–4 for fluid passing through different segments of the intestine.[13, 14] The low chloride concentration in ileal and fecal fluid[19] results in part from an exchange of luminal chloride with plasma bicarbonate across ileal and colonic mucosa.[7, 20–22] Therefore, a very high (relative to plasma) bicarbonate concentration in stool water would be expected. However, the bicarbonate concentration is only about 30 meq per liter. The remaining anions in stool water are organic and consist, among others, of acetate, propionate, butyrate, and lactate that result from bacterial fermentation of unabsorbed carbohydrates.[23, 24] The chemical reaction of these organic acids with bicarbonate lowers the concentration of bicarbonate. Sodium is absorbed across colonic mucosa against steep electrochemical gradients, generating a lumen negative potential difference, which retards potassium absorption or stimulates potassium secretion. This is the major explanation for the high potassium and low sodium (relative to plasma) concentrations in fecal fluid. Pages 1022 to 1045 contain a more complete discussion of ion transport mechanisms in the intestine.

Because the gastrointestinal tract does not have a significant diluting or concentrating mechanism, the osmolality of fecal fluid should be similar to the osmolality of plasma. In fact, collected fecal fluid usually has an osmolality higher than that of plasma, often about 350 mOsm per kilogram.[19] This is related to colonic bacteria, which split one unabsorbed carbohydrate molecule into two or more smaller solutes. If

this happens in the colon, water should be retained or secreted and the osmolality should not rise, unless colonic or rectal mucosal permeability to bulk water flow is so low in relation to the generation rate of additional solute that osmotic equilibration cannot occur. Probably some, if not all, of the hyperosmolality of fecal fluid develops outside the body during storage of fecal samples prior to analysis. If antibiotics are given to normal subjects, stool osmolality is the same as that of plasma.[25]

For sake of completion, fecal NH_3 and NH_4^+ also need to be considered, although their clinical importance is uncertain. Ammonia is generated in the human colon by the action of bacteria, the main precursor being endogenous urea. Most is reabsorbed and reconverted into urea in the liver. A small amount may be incorporated into bacterial proteins. Only 1 to 2 mmol per day, representing 1 per cent of total colonic production, is passed unchanged in feces. The bicarbonate concentration in stool water influences the fraction of total ammonia in the ionized and nonionized state.

$$NH_4^+ + HCO_3^- \rightleftarrows NH_3 + H_2CO_3$$

The pK of this reaction is about 9.0. The relative concentration of NH_3 increases tenfold for every unit increase in pH. Because the colon absorbs ammonia mainly by passive nonionic (NH_3) diffusion, an increase in pH increases ammonia absorption, and a fall in pH has the opposite effect. Thus, the concentration of total ammonia in stools increases if the stools have an acidic reaction. Fecal total ammonia concentration varies widely in normal stool water, from 2 to 50 mmol per liter, with most values between 5 and 20 mmol per liter. Because stools have a pH of less than 9 (the pK), NH_4^+ predominates over NH_3.[26]

PATHOPHYSIOLOGY

There are five major mechanisms of diarrhea[13]: (1) the presence in the gut lumen of unusual amounts of poorly absorbable, osmotically active solutes; (2) intestinal ion secretion; (3) deletion or inhibition of a normal active ion absorptive process; (4) deranged intestinal motility, with disordered contact between luminal contents and mucosal surface; and (5) outpouring into the bowel lumen of mucus, blood, and protein from sites of inflammation.

Osmotic Diarrhea

Osmotic diarrhea is caused by ingestion of a poorly absorbable solute, usually a carbohydrate or a divalent ion (Mg or SO_4, for example). A hypothetical example (which, in part, is based on observations reported in references 14 and 27) is shown in Figure 20–5. The patient ingests 250 ml of fluid containing 150 mM of a nonabsorbable solute, X. The ingested material is hypertonic, 600 mOsm per kilogram. As fluid passes

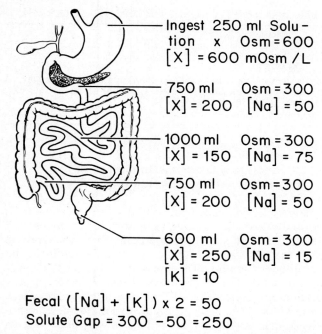

Ingest 250 ml Solution x Osm = 600
[X] = 600 mOsm / L

750 ml   Osm = 300
[X] = 200   [Na] = 50

1000 ml   Osm = 300
[X] = 150   [Na] = 75

750 ml   Osm = 300
[X] = 200   [Na] = 50

600 ml   Osm = 300
[X] = 250   [Na] = 15
[K] = 10

Fecal ([Na] + [K]) x 2 = 50
Solute Gap = 300 − 50 = 250

Figure 20–5. Hypothetic example of osmotic diarrhea caused by ingestion of a nonabsorbable and nonfermentable solute, X. (For further explanation, see text.)

the ligament of Treitz, its volume has expanded to 750 ml, the concentration of X has been reduced to 200 mOsm per kilogram, sodium has accumulated, and the osmolality is the same as that of plasma.* The volume of fluid passing through the middle small bowel is even larger (1000 ml), the concentration of X even lower, and the concentration of Na even higher. In the ileum, some of the luminal fluid and sodium are reabsorbed, which reduces the volume delivered to the colon to 750 ml, raises [X] and reduces [Na]. Further absorption of sodium and water takes place in the colon, and fluid leaving the rectum has a volume of 600 ml, a [X] of 250 mOsm per kilogram, a sodium concentration of 15 mEq per liter, and a K concentration of 10 mEq per liter.

This pattern of flow through the gut is caused by different permeability and ion transport mechanisms in different segments of the intestine. The proximal small bowel is highly permeable to water and NaCl[28] (but not to solute X). Therefore, water influx across the duodenum rapidly adjusts the osmolality of luminal fluid toward that of plasma and dilutes X. Sodium diffuses from plasma to lumen down the steep concentration gradient. However, even after the osmolality

of the luminal fluid is reduced to 300 mOsm per kilogram, the effective osmotic pressure[28] of luminal fluid (across the jejunum) is higher than that of plasma. This is because the jejunum is highly permeable to NaCl in plasma, but not to solute X in the lumen. Therefore, the proximal small bowel continues to secrete water even after the osmolality values of luminal contents and plasma are identical. In the ileum and colon, the mucosa has a very low permeability to NaCl and to X; therefore, the effective osmotic pressure of luminal fluid, across ileal and colonic mucosa, is similar to that of plasma.[28] Furthermore, the ileum and colon have efficient active ion transport mechanisms that allow them to reabsorb NaCl (and therefore water), even against steep electrochemical gradients. Therefore, fluid is absorbed as it traverses the ileum and colon. The end result of ingesting 250 ml of fluid containing solute X is diarrhea of 600 ml. The diarrheal fluid has a sodium concentration that is much lower than the sodium concentration of plasma, but the osmolality is the same as that of plasma.

It is easy to see that osmotic diarrhea is reduced in its severity by the ileum and colon. Were these missing, the diarrheal volume would have been 1000 instead of 600 ml, and the sodium loss would have been 75 mEq rather than 9 mEq.

In the example shown in Figure 20–5, the nonabsorbable solute was not metabolizable by colonic bacteria. If, instead of a nonmetabolizable solute X, the subject had ingested a solution containing a comparable amount of lactulose, the situation in the small bowel would be the same (lactulose cannot be digested by intestinal mucosal enzymes), but differences would occur in the colon. Specifically, colonic bacteria would metabolize the unabsorbable sugar to component monosaccharides, and these would be further metabolized by bacteria to short-chain fatty acids (proprionate, butyrate, and others) and to CO_2, H_2, and CH_4. The short-chain fatty acids would be absorbed across the colonic mucosa,[29] and to some extent this would help the body reclaim energy that otherwise would be lost in the stool.[30] Bacterial metabolism of unabsorbed carbohydrates and absorption of short-chain fatty acids thus reduce the severity of diarrhea. For example, in one carefully studied subject, oral ingestion of 73 mmol of magnesium sulfate resulted in 647 ml of diarrhea, whereas ingestion of 73 mmol of lactulose did not cause diarrhea. On the other hand, when 146 mmol of lactulose was ingested, the protective role of colonic bacteria and absorption of short-chain fatty acids was overwhelmed, and the subject had 849 ml of diarrhea.[31] Accumulation of carbohydrate moieties in fecal water, and not short-chain fatty acids, probably determines the severity of diarrhea when ingested carbohydrates are not absorbed by the small bowel.[30, 31]

Clinically, osmotic diarrhea is distinguished by the fact that diarrhea stops when the patient fasts (or stops ingesting the poorly absorbable solute).[13] Stool analysis reveals an osmotic gap; that is, ($[Na^+]$ + $[K^+]$) × 2 (multiplied by 2 to account for anions) is less than the osmolality of fecal fluid. The size of the osmotic gap

---

*That the osmolality at the ligament of Treitz would be the same as that of plasma is supported by references 27 and 14. On the other hand, data in reference 15 suggest that the osmolality of fluid arriving at the ligament of Treitz after a hypertonic carbohydrate meal would peak at an average of about 360 mOsm per kilogram rather than be 300, as shown in the figure. This slight discrepancy does not alter the general validity of the figure or the concepts described in the text.

is approximately equivalent to the concentration of poorly absorbable solute(s) in fecal water (see Fig. 20–5).

Two clinical aspects of osmotic diarrhea are quite uncertain at the present time. First, how does one deal with fecal osmolalities that are higher than the osmolality of plasma? At least in part, such high values probably represent bacterial action on unabsorbed carbohydrates after the stool specimen was evacuated from the rectum. It is, therefore, our current belief that a fecal fluid osmolality higher than 290 mOsm per kilogram (the actual osmolality of plasma by freezing point depression) reflects mainly bacterial metabolism outside the body, and thus indicates malabsorption of carbohydrates but not necessarily osmotic diarrhea. In calculating the clinically significant osmotic gap, insofar as diarrhea is concerned, we use the osmolality of plasma rather than the measured osmolality of stool unless the measured osmolality of the stool is less than 290 mOsm per kilogram, in which case the measured value is used. For example, if a stool specimen contained 100 mM sodium and 45 mM potassium and had an osmolality of 400 mOsm per kilogram, we would interpret this as evidence for carbohydrate malabsorption but not osmotic diarrhea. The carbohydrates that were malabsorbed could have been large or even insoluble moieties that did not exert a significant osmotic effect on colonic fluid in vivo. On the other hand, if sodium were 40 mM, potassium were 40 mM, and osmolality were 400 mOsm per kilogram, we would calculate an osmotic gap of 130 mOsm per kilogram and interpret this as evidence for osmotic diarrhea as well as carbohydrate malabsorption (the latter inferred from the high osmolality). Examination of spot stool specimens immediately after collection and the effect of a 48-hour fast may be needed to resolve uncertainties.

The second unanswered problem about osmotic diarrhea concerns the correlation of the size of the osmotic gap with the severity of diarrhea. This has not been well studied in patients or in normal subjects with experimentally induced osmotic diarrhea. Currently, we disregard gaps of less than 50 mOsm per kilogram. Gaps may be as high as 230 mOsm per kilogram[32]; in the hypothetical example shown in Figure 20–5, the gap was 250 mOsm per kilogram.

If osmotic diarrhea is due to carbohydrate malabsorption, the stool pH is low, usually around 5 (normal, around pH 7) because of short-chain fatty acids (see earlier); stool osmolality is higher than that of plasma; total reducing substances and total carbohydrate content of the stool will be high;[33] and the patient will usually complain of flatulence as well as (or instead of) diarrhea. In osmotic diarrhea caused by poorly absorbable salts and mineral ions, such as magnesium and sulfate in Glauber's and Epsom salts, stool pH will not be lowered. Milk of magnesia will cause an osmotic diarrhea with high stool pH (up to 8.0).

Some of the causes of osmotic diarrhea are shown in Table 20–2.

Table 20–2. SOME CAUSES OF OSMOTIC DIARRHEA

Disaccharidase deficiencies
Glucose-galactose malabsorption, fructose malabsorption[34]
Mannitol, sorbitol ingestion ("Chewing gum diarrhea")[35, 36]
Lactulose therapy
Magnesium sulfate (Epsom salt), sodium sulfate (Glauber's salt, Carlsbad salt), sodium phosphate, sodium citrate, some antacids (MgO, $Mg[OH]_2$)
Generalized malabsorption

Secretory Diarrhea (Inhibition of Ion Absorption and Stimulation of Ion Secretion)

Some physiologists believe that small intestinal cells normally secrete as well as absorb electrolytes and water, with the secretion rate being of less magnitude than the absorption rate (see p. 1022); therefore, the net effect of small bowel transport processes is absorption of fluid. The putative small bowel secretion may originate in crypt cells, whereas absorption takes place from villous cells. According to this concept, a pathophysiologic event might reduce absorption rate in either of two ways: (1) by stimulating secretion or (2) by inhibiting absorption. In either case, there is less difference between the greater absorption and the lower secretion rate, and the observed effect is reduced absorption. Similarly, a pathophysiologic event might cause secretion by stimulating active secretion so that it overwhelms the normal absorptive process, or it could cause secretion by inhibiting absorption so that the normal secretion is unmasked.

Current evidence suggests that mediators of intestinal ion secretion also inhibit normal ion absorption simultaneously. Either or both could result in secretory diarrhea, and it is usually difficult, if not impossible, to ascertain which of these two factors is predominant. Therefore, at the present time and for clinical purposes, it seems best to consider inhibition of ion absorption and stimulation of ion secretion together. Regardless of the cause, in secretory diarrhea either the rate of fluid absorption is reduced or the intestine secretes when perfused with a balanced electrolyte solution (the former is much more common), and the intestinal lumen and stool contain an excess of monovalent ions and water. Divalent ions are not actively secreted by intestinal mucosa, nor are they present in large enough amounts in digestive secretions to influence gut luminal and fecal volumes.

It is important to note that reduced ion absorption or intestinal ion secretion are often superimposed upon an otherwise intact epithelium (histologic features and permeability to large molecules are usually normal) and that some absorptive events continue at a normal rate. For example, glucose absorption and the basolateral membrane sodium pump are intact, and the addition of glucose to luminal contents causes a normal increment in sodium chloride and water absorption (and thus may stimulate absorption or reduce the secretion rate).

Secretory diarrhea is characterized clinically by three features.[13] First, stool osmolality can be accounted for by normal ionic constituents. For practical purposes, the extent to which these ions contribute to stool osmolality can be determined by $([Na^+] + [K^+]) \times 2$ (multiplied by 2 to account for anions). In secretory diarrhea this value is close to the osmolality of plasma and stool (measured by freezing point depression). If, on the other hand, there is a large osmotic gap, secretory diarrhea cannot be the only mechanism of diarrhea. Second, since the diarrhea is caused by abnormalities in ion transport that have nothing to do with food, the diarrhea usually persists during a 48- to 72-hour period of fasting. Ingestion of food would add about a 9-liter load per day of water and electrolytes to the proximal small bowel, so why wouldn't the diarrhea increase by about 9 liters when patients change from fasting to eating status? The fact that nutrients (carbohydrate, protein, and fat) are absorbed normally and the fact that absorption of monosaccharides and amino acids stimulates net absorption of NaCl and water across jejunal mucosa probably explain why eating does not markedly increase stool volume in patients with secretory diarrhea. Third, patients with a pure secretory diarrhea usually do not have pus, blood, or excess fat in their stool; some exceptions to this generalization are the secretory diarrhea than can occur in some patients with celiac sprue and with intestinal lymphoma.

Having made these important generalizations, the following qualifications are in order: First, some secretory diarrheas stop when the patient fasts. These types include secretory diarrhea secondary to fatty acid malabsorption. In addition, secretory diarrhea resulting from surreptitious laxative ingestion may stop during fasting if patients simultaneously stop taking the laxative, which some of them do. Second, the fecal electrolyte pattern described above applies to a pure secretory diarrhea. In some diseases, osmotic and secretory mechanisms are both at play, and the characteristic clinical features may become blurred. For example, a patient with malabsorption might have diarrhea because of the osmotic effects of unabsorbed carbohydrates and because of inhibition of colonic absorption by unabsorbed fatty acids. Fecal electrolytes would reflect both these mechanisms. Third, absence of an osmotic gap and persistence of diarrhea during a fast does not always indicate a reduced capacity of the gut to absorb fluid and electrolytes.[37] Since, by definition, secretory diarrhea implies a reduction in absorptive function of epithelial cells, it is therefore not possible to identify secretory diarrhea with certainty using the clinical information described in the previous paragraph. To be certain, intestinal perfusion must be carried out to prove that ion and fluid absorption rates are abnormally low, and this is usually impractical.

The major mediators of secretory diarrhea are listed in Table 20–3, along with some of the gastrointestinal diseases or syndromes which have been associated with the clinical features of secretory diarrhea. In some of these (but not in all), intestinal perfusion studies have

Table 20–3. SOME CAUSES OF SECRETORY DIARRHEA

Major Mediators
1. Enterotoxins (see pp. 1037 and 1192 and reference 38)
2. Tumor elaboration of secretagogues—VIP, calcitonin, peptide histidine methionine, helodermin, serotonin, etc. (see pp. 78 and 1884 and reference 39)
3. Laxatives (ricinoleic acid, phenolphthalein, oxyphenisatin, dioctyl sodium sulfosuccinate, aloe, senna, danthron)[40]
4. Bile acids (see pp. 144 and 1038 and reference 41)
5. Fatty acids (see pp. 309 and 1030 and reference 42)
6. Congenital defects (see p. 303)

Some Disorders That May Have Clinical Features of Secretory Diarrhea*
1. Inflammatory bowel disease
2. Microscopic colitis
3. Secretory villous adenoma of the rectum
4. Small bowel total villous atrophy
5. Intestinal lymphoma
6. Giardiasis, strongyloidiasis
7. Chronic infections (granulomatous)
8. Pseudopancreatic cholera syndrome (see text)
9. Ileocolic resection
10. Hyperthyroidism
11. Zollinger-Ellison syndrome
12. VIPoma
13. Malignant carcinoid syndrome
14. Medullary carcinoma of thyroid
15. Collagen vascular diseases (systemic lupus erythematosus, scleroderma, mixed connective tissue disease

*Secretory diarrhea suggested by fasting diarrhea and absence of significant fecal osmotic gap. Not all these diseases and syndromes have been studied by intestinal perfusion to prove decreased absorption or intestinal secretion (see p. 296).

revealed reduced ion and fluid absorption in some part of the intestine (thus confirming that the pathogenesis of diarrhea was mediated at least in part by inhibition of ion absorption or ion secretion). See page 1035 for a further discussion of agents which inhibit ion absorption.

It should be noted that while endocrine tumors may cause diarrhea via release of secretagogues such as vasoactive intestinal polypeptide or by release of agents which cause hypermotility, others produce diarrhea entirely or in part by other mechanisms, such as somastatinoma by steatorrhea because of inhibition of pancreatic enzyme secretion or gastrinoma by gastric HCl secretion, for example.

Deranged Motility

That alteration in motility *can* affect absorption in humans is quite evident from previous work. Three examples will be cited. First, reduced motility, induced by atropine, increases xylose absorption.[43] Second, codeine, which has no effect on mucosal cell absorptive rate but which delays fluid movement through the jejunum, increases fluid absorption and reduces diarrhea after a bolus of salt solution is infused into the stomach.[44] Third, slowing intestinal transit time by infusing fat into the ileum increases carbohydrate absorption from a test meal.[45]

However, *proving* that abnormal motility *is* the cause of diarrhea in a given patient or in a given group of patients is difficult, if not impossible. Measurements of transit time are, generally speaking, inconclusive in this regard because diarrhea itself (with increased luminal fluid content) would decrease transit time secondarily.[45, 46] Additional methodology will be required to prove or disprove the concept that deranged motility can cause diarrhea, and even with new methodology there will remain problems concerning the proper control group for comparison.

In the meantime, motility derangements are suspected to be the cause of diarrhea when other measurable causes such as osmotic and secretory diarrhea seem to have been excluded. For example, we have seen patients with no demonstrable X-ray or histologic abnormality, who absorb dietary fat normally, who absorb fluid normally (at all levels of the small bowel and in the colon) during steady-state intestinal perfusion of a balanced electrolyte solution, and yet who have mild, moderate, or severe diarrhea—even when they are fasting.[37] The fact that such patients absorb fluid normally during steady-state perfusion of a balanced electrolyte solution at high rates of flow indicates that absorptive function by their epithelial cells is normal. Deranged motility does not influence absorption rate under such high flow, steady-state conditions. However, under normal conditions, eating or fasting, there is no steady state, and motility determines the rate of movement of boluses of fluid through the gut and therefore the time of contact between epithelial cells and luminal contents. Defective motility could, therefore, result in diarrhea—even though absorptive function by epithelial cells is normal. This could occur by reduction in contact time between luminal contents and epithelial cells. For example, small intestinal "hurry" might reduce contact time between small bowel mucosa and its contents, and thus result in delivery of abnormally large and qualitatively abnormal boluses of fluid to the colon. Or premature emptying of the colon could result in reduced contact between luminal fluid and colonic mucosa and, therefore, increased volume and liquidity of the stools.

Some chronic diarrheal diseases possibly or probably caused mainly or in part by deranged motility are irritable bowel syndrome, malignant carcinoid syndrome, medullary carcinoma of the thyroid, postvagotomy and postgastrectomy diarrhea, diarrhea due to diabetic neuropathy, diarrhea due to thyrotoxicosis, diarrhea due to bile acid malabsorption, diarrhea after ileocecal valve resection, and diarrhea after ileal resection. Abnormal motility may also contribute to the acute diarrhea caused by infections.

As already mentioned, currently there is no way, either clinically or by research, to prove that abnormally increased motility is the cause of diarrhea. If one accepts the notion that motility is the cause of nonosmotic diarrhea in patients who absorb fluid normally during steady-state perfusion at high flow rates, then abnormal motility can cause voluminous diarrhea, and the diarrhea can persist during a 48-hour period of fasting. The fecal electrolyte pattern in such patients can resemble that described for secretory diarrhea, or it can show evidence of a moderate osmotic gap when patients eat food. Some such patients have mild steatorrhea.

Abnormally reduced motility may allow bacterial overgrowth in the small bowel and thereby cause diarrhea and steatorrhea (see pp. 111 and 1289). It has been suggested that disorders of the anorectum may enhance stool frequency without altering stool weight or consistency[45] (see p. 317).

Exudation

Disruption of the integrity of the intestinal mucosa owing to inflammation and ulceration may result in discharge of mucus, serum proteins, and blood into the bowel lumen. In affected patients (with shigella dysentery or ulcerative colitis, for example) bowel movements may at times consist only of mucus, exudate, and blood. This exudation probably is not voluminous enough to account for excessive loss of water and electrolytes in the stool. When that occurs in a patient with exudation, it most likely reflects one of the other mechanisms of diarrhea. For example, colonic absorption of water and electrolytes is severely impaired in ulcerative colitis[47] and when ileal flow is diverted from the colon, it is unusual to have any appreciable fluid discharge from the colon even though it may remain intensely inflamed.[48] These findings strongly suggest that malabsorption of water and electrolytes is the major cause of abnormal losses of water and electrolytes in ulcerative colitis (and probably also in other patients with exudation).

DIAGNOSIS

This section is concerned with a diagnostic approach to the patient with diarrhea in whom the cause is unknown. We will first review the help that can be obtained from a careful history and physical examination, then consider the most likely diagnostic possibilities for particular clinical situations, and conclude with a discussion of some diagnostic tests.

History

The degree to which different aspects of the history are emphasized will naturally vary, depending on the duration of diarrhea, the presence or absence of evidence of systemic disease, the age of the patient, and other factors. We will not deal with such considerations here; rather, we present those aspects of the history that will help localize the disease process and help establish its nature.

The site of the underlying disorder within the bowel is suggested by the character of the stools and by the location and quality of any accompanying pain.[49] It is helpful to distinguish between large stool and small stool diarrhea. When the stools are consistently large, the underlying disorder or disease is likely to be in the small bowel or the proximal colon. Such stools are likely to be light in color; to be watery, soupy, or greasy; to be foul; to be free of gross blood; and to contain undigested food particles. When pain accompanies this large stool diarrhea, it is likely to be periumbilical or localized to the right lower quadrant. These areas have been recognized as zones of pain reference from the small intestine and the cecum. The pain in such instances is often intermittent, cramp-like, and accompanied by audible borborygmi.

In small stool diarrhea, the patient has frequent urges to defecate but passes small quantities of feces. In its extreme form he or she, despite a great sense of urgency, may pass only flatus or a small quantity of mucus. This syndrome is likely to be associated with disease or disorder of the left colon and rectum. The increase in irritability of that section results in the premature discharge of a quantity of stool otherwise insufficient to trigger a defecation reflex. When fecal matter in any quantity is passed, it is mushy or jelly-like, and in some diseases it is often mixed with visible mucus or blood. It is usually dark in color and rarely excessively foul. Pain, when present, is likely to be in the hypogastrium, in the left or right lower quadrant, or in the sacral region, reflecting the established zones of pain reference from the colon and rectum. It is usually gripping, aching, or with a quality of tenesmus. It may be continuous, but it is usually relieved to some extent by an enema, a bowel movement, or even the passage of flatus.

These two patterns of diarrhea are, of course, not mutually exclusive. With widespread inflammation or dysfunction of the intestines, they may occur at different times in the same patient, even on the same day.

The history also may provide valuable information about the nature of the disorder or disease process. Passage of blood indicates an inflammatory, infectious, or neoplastic disease and rules out psychogenic diarrhea. (Of course, hemorrhoidal or vaginal bleeding may confuse the issue, but bleeding from these sources can usually be distinguished by history.) Passage of pus or exudate in the stools indicates inflammation or infection, although exudate is often incorrectly assumed to be mucus. Lack of odor and presence of blood-tinged mucus is characteristic of shigellosis, whereas green, slimy "pea soup" stools are usually associated with salmonellosis (and in infants with enteropathogenic *Escherichia coli* infection). Passage of nonbloody mucus is suggestive of irritable bowel syndrome. Mushy stools that are frothy or contain oil suggest malabsorption. Intermittent diarrhea and constipation suggest irritable bowel syndrome, especially if the stools are pellet-like during the constipation phase. Intermittent diarrhea and constipation are also frequent in diabetic autonomic neuropathy and may be the first sign of carcinoma of the colon. Diarrhea that stops when the patient fasts suggests osmotic diarrhea and only very rarely food allergy. Diarrhea

at night favors organic disease over irritable bowel syndrome, but this is not always specific. Complaints of nocturnal diarrhea and fecal soiling are especially frequent in patients with neurologic problems or rectal sphincter dysfunction and in those with diabetic autonomic disorders. The occurrence currently or in the past of a perianal fistula or abscess is suggestive of Crohn's disease. Diarrhea associated with a patient's desire to reduce weight suggests abuse of laxatives or diuretics. Other general symptoms that may help suggest the etiology of diarrhea are listed in Table 20–4.

The family history of any diarrheal disease may be helpful. Hereditary pancreatitis and multiple endocrine neoplasia with medullary carcinoma of the thyroid are autosomal dominantly inherited diseases associated with steatorrhea or diarrhea. The incidence of regional enteritis, ulcerative colitis, and irritable bowel syndrome may be high within a family or kinship.

The probability of exposure to infectious agents must be estimated, sexual activity determined (see Table 20–5, item 3), and the duration of the symptoms, their mode of onset, and variable occurrence or progression

Table 20–4. CLUES TO DIAGNOSIS OF DIARRHEA FROM OTHER SYMPTOMS, SIGNS, AND LABORATORY TESTS

Symptom or Sign Associated with Diarrhea	Diagnoses to Be Considered
Arthritis	Ulcerative colitis, Crohn's disease, Whipple's disease, enteritis due to *Yersinia enterocolitica*, gonococcal proctitis
Liver disease	Ulcerative colitis, Crohn's disease, bowel malignancy with metastases to liver
Fever	Ulcerative colitis, Crohn's disease, amebiasis, lymphoma, tuberculosis, Whipple's disease, other enteric infections
Marked weight loss	Malabsorption, inflammatory bowel disease, cancer, thyrotoxicosis
Eosinophilia	Eosinophilic gastroenteritis, parasitic disease (particularly *Strongyloides*)
Lymphadenopathy	Lymphoma, Whipple's disease, AIDS
Neuropathy	Diabetic diarrhea, amyloidosis
Postural hypotension	Diabetic diarrhea, Addison's disease, idiopathic orthostatic hypotension
Flushing	Malignant carcinoid syndrome, pancreatic cholera syndrome
Erythema	Systemic mastocytosis, glucagonoma syndrome
Proteinuria	Amyloidosis
Collagen vascular disease	Mesenteric vasculitis
Peptic ulcers	Zollinger-Ellison syndrome
Chronic lung disease	Cystic fibrosis
Systemic arteriosclerosis	Ischemic injury to gut
Frequent infections	Immunoglobulin deficiency
Hyperpigmentation	Whipple's disease, celiac disease, Addison's disease
Good response to corticosteroids	Ulcerative colitis, Crohn's disease, Whipple's disease, Addison's disease, eosinophilic gastroenteritis, celiac disease
Good response to antibiotics	Blind loop syndrome, tropical sprue, Whipple's disease

Table 20–5. MOST LIKELY CAUSES OF DIARRHEA IN SEVEN DIFFERENT CLINICAL CATEGORIES

1. *Acute Diarrhea (<2–3 weeks' duration)*
   Viral, bacterial, parasitic, and fungal infections
   Food poisoning
   Drugs* and food additives
   Fecal impaction
   Pelvic inflammation
   Heavy metal poisoning (acute or chronic)

2. *Traveler's Diarrhea*
   Bacterial infections
       Mediated by enterotoxins, e.g., LT and/or ST producing *E. coli*
       Mediated mainly by invasion of mucosa and inflammation, e.g., invasive *E. coli, Shigella*
       Mediated by combination of invasion and enterotoxins, e.g., *Salmonella*
   Viral and parasitic infections

3. *Diarrhea in Homosexual Men without AIDS*
   Amebiasis
   Giardiasis
   Shigellosis
   Campylobacter
   Rectal syphilis
   Rectal spirochetosis other than syphilis
   Rectal gonorrhea
   Chlamydia trachomatis (lymphogranuloma venereum and non-LG serotypes D–K)
   Herpes simplex

4. *Diarrhea in Patients with AIDS*
   Cryptosporidium
   Amebiasis
   Giardiasis
   Isospora belli
   Herpes simplex, *Cytomegalovirus*
   Mycobacterium avium intracellulare
   Salmonella typhimurium
   Cryptococcus
   Candida
   AIDS enteropathy

5. *Chronic and Recurrent Diarrhea*
   Irritable bowel syndrome
   Inflammatory bowel disease
   Parasitic and fungal infections
   Malabsorption syndromes
   Drugs,* food additives, sorbitol
   Colon cancer
   Diverticulitis
   Fecal impaction
   Heavy metal poisoning (acute or chronic)
   Raw milk–related diarrhea

6. *Chronic Diarrhea of Unknown Origin (previous work-up had failed to reveal diagnosis)*:
   Surreptitious laxative abuse
   Defective anal incontinence masquerading as severe diarrhea
   Microscopic colitis syndrome
   Previously unrecognized malabsorption
   Pseudopancreatic cholera syndrome
   Idiopathic fluid malabsorption
   Hypermotility-induced diarrhea
   Neuroendocrine tumor

7. *Incontinence*
   Cause of sphincter dysfunction (see also p. 324)
       Anal surgery for fissures, fistulas, or hemorrhoids
       Episiotomy or tear during childbirth
       Anal Crohn's disease
       Diabetic neuropathy
   Cause of diarrhea—same as under items 5 and 6.

---

*Digitalis, propranolol, quinidine, diuretics, colchicine, antibiotics, lactulose, antacids, laxatives, chemotherapeutic agents, bile acids, meclomen, and many others (see *Physicians' Desk Reference* for any specific drug the patient has been taking).

in severity, as well as the age of the patient when the symptoms began, should be taken into account. Any correlation with diet, especially milk, should be noted.

The temporal association of diarrhea and emotional conflict should be sought if the pattern of diarrhea and other features are compatible with irritable bowel syndrome. It is important to find out why the patient is seeking medical help—whether he or she is worried about what might be causing symptoms (fear of cancer) or is primarily interested in relief of symptoms.

Physical Examination

A complete physical examination may reveal important clues to the cause of diarrhea, including abdominal mass, abdominal bruit, perianal fistula or abscess, anemia, fever, edema, postural hypotension, lymphadenopathy, hyperpigmentation, skin lesions, purpura, neuropathy, bone and soft tissue tumors, goiter, clubbing of the fingers, liver enlargement, ascites, gaseous abdominal distention, and a rectal mass or impaction. The nutritional status of the patient and any evidence of fluid and electrolyte depletion should be carefully noted.

Some other signs that may suggest the correct diagnosis are given in Table 20–4.

The Most Likely Diagnostic Possibilities

If the cause of diarrhea is not apparent after the history and physical examination, it is helpful to consider a list of the most likely diagnostic possibilities as provided in Table 20–5. Diagnostic tests designed to establish or refute the most likely causes of diarrhea are a good way to begin a further evaluation.

Diagnostic Tests

Patients with diarrhea in whom the diagnosis is not evident should usually have a hemogram, chemical profile, and urinalysis. In chronic diarrhea, a case can also be made for obtaining an early sonogram of the abdomen, looking for evidence of hepatic, biliary, pancreatic, retroperitoneal, and pelvic disease.

The order in which other tests are carried out, assuming that further tests are necessary, will vary according to the most likely diagnostic possibilities (see Table 20–5) and according to the physician's intuition about a particular patient. Obviously, as few tests as possible should be used in order to avoid unnecessary expense and discomfort. One should remember to do simple things first and not be seduced by sophisticated new or old tests that have little discriminatory value. A shotgun approach is wasteful and usually reflects the lack of a careful history, lack of understanding of pathophysiology, or lack of knowledge about which diseases are likely and which are very unlikely in a particular clinical situation. In some patients with severe diarrhea, it is much more important initially to correct dehydration than to do diagnostic studies. Certain diagnostic tests deserve brief discussion here.

Routine Examination of Stool. Unless the diagnosis is apparent from the history and physical examination, some relatively simple studies on the stool should be carried out. These are a stain for pus, a search for occult blood, a Sudan stain for excess fat, and alkalinization to test for phenolphthalein. The information obtained will usually narrow the diagnostic possibilities. For example, the presence of blood and pus will suggest inflammatory disease, blood without pus will suggest neoplastic disease, and excess fat will suggest one of the diseases that cause malabsorption syndrome.

Stain For Pus. The presence or absence of intestinal inflammation often can be ascertained by examination of a stained stool specimen.[50, 51] Wright's or methylene blue stains are satisfactory. The presence of large numbers of white blood cells is diagnostic of inflammation. The presence of rare, scattered white blood cells is within normal limits.

In patients with acute or traveler's diarrhea, pus in the stool suggests invasion of the mucosa by *Shigella*, *E. coli*, *E. histolytica*, salmonella, gonococci, *Campylobacter*, or other invasive organisms. In general, shigellosis, *Campylobacter*, and invasive *E. coli* infections cause more pus than salmonella and *E. histolytica*. Pseudomembranous colitis often is associated with pus.

In patients with chronic and recurrent diarrhea or in diarrhea of unknown etiology, pus suggests colitis of some type, be it idiopathic ulcerative colitis, Crohn's colitis, antibiotic-associated colitis, amebic colitis, ischemic colitis, tuberculous colitis, or some other form. Pus is especially abundant in idiopathic ulcerative colitis and tends to be less so in amebic colitis. Absence of pus on a single examination does not, of course, absolutely rule out any of these entities. Radiation-induced disease of the large or small bowel and Crohn's disease limited to the small intestine may or may not be associated with pus in the stool. Pus is not present in the stools of patients with irritable bowel syndrome, with diarrhea caused by noninvasive organisms that produce enterotoxins (toxigenic *E. coli*, for example), with most types of malabsorption syndrome, laxative abuse, viral gastroenteritis, or giardiasis, and sometimes pus is not present in patients with amebic colitis.

Occult Blood. Occult (or gross) blood in association with diarrhea usually indicates inflammation and, therefore, usually has the same significance as pus in the stools (see above). When blood is present in diarrheal stools that do not contain pus, one should think of amebiasis, neoplasms of the colon, heavy metal poisoning, and acute ischemic damage to the gut.

Sudan Stain for Fat. If excess fat is present on Sudan stain,[52] steatorrhea is probably present, and the various causes of malabsorption syndromes should be considered (see p. 272). Acute infections from giardiasis to viral gastroenteritis can cause steatorrhea transiently, so it is not always necessary to proceed immediately with a "malabsorption workup."

Alkalinization. A pink or red color indicates phenolphthalein ingestion as the cause of diarrhea. The test is so easily and quickly done, and the significance of a positive result so great, that it should be carried out routinely in patients with unexplained chronic diarrhea. (See p. 307 for a further discussion of phenolphthalein testing.)

Proctosigmoidoscopy. This is a very important part of the examination in most patients with chronic and recurrent diarrhea. It will not be helpful in most patients with malabsorption syndrome. If stool specimens are accurately examined (see earlier), proctosigmoidoscopy is usually of little help in patients with acute and traveler's diarrhea. Exceptions are in antibiotic-associated diarrhea in which pseudomembranes might be revealed, and in amebiasis in which typical discrete ulcers may be found. Proctoscopy also affords an easy opportunity to obtain fresh stool specimens necessary to demonstrate motile trophozoites.

During proctosigmoidoscopy, the mucosa should be carefully examined for ulceration, friability, polyps, and tumors (secretory villous adenomas of the rectum are often missed for suprisingly long periods of time). The anal region also can be well visualized with the sigmoidoscope as it is withdrawn. The specific findings in amebic colitis, Crohn's disease of the colon, and ulcerative colitis by proctoscopy are covered in detail on pages 1159, 1341, and 1439 to 1442, respectively. Shigellosis, *Campylobacter* infection, and occasionally salmonellosis may mimic exactly the sigmoidoscopic findings of ulcerative colitis. Proctitis due to infection with chlamydia also mimics ulcerative colitis at proctosigmoidoscopy, as may gonococcal proctitis. Melanosis coli should always be interpreted as a consequence of heavy use of anthracene cathartics.

As emphasized by Anthonisen and Riis,[50] rectal and sigmoid mucosal smears (prepared by Wright stain) for pus are helpful. The presence or absence of pus on mucosal smear has the same significance as in the stool (see previous section). Mucosal smears are especially useful in distinguishing mild ulcerative colitis (mucosa appears normal but mucosal smears contain many pus cells) from irritable bowel syndrome (no pus).

In most patients with diarrhea, smears are preferable to biopsy, especially initially, because they can be taken from multiple areas, never produce serious bleeding, will not delay barium enema examination, and are much less expensive. In our opinion, mucosal smears should be a routine procedure in the evaluation of any patient who receives a proctosigmoidoscopy for evaluation of diarrhea, unless mucosal biopsies are done.

Rectal Biopsy. The main disorders that might be detected by biopsy but not by smears and stool examination are amyloidosis, Whipple's disease, granulomatous inflammation, melanosis coli, schistosomiasis in its chronic form, rectal spirochetosis other than syphilis, and microscopic colitis or collagenous colitis. It has been suggested that serial sections of rectal biopsy specimens, to reveal granulomas, might aid in the diagnosis of Crohn's colitis[53] and that biopsy may aid in the diagnosis of *Campylobacter* colitis.[54] Criteria for distinguishing acute self-limited colitis from chronic ulcerative colitis have been proposed.[55] Biopsy is indicated in patients with diarrhea of unknown origin in search of disorders that might otherwise be overlooked, including melanosis coli.

Rectal biopsy in the presence of a diffuse lesion is best done with small forceps (colonoscopy type rather than with the large forceps that come with most rigid proctoscopy sets). When using the large forceps, mucosal biopsy specimens should be taken from the posterior wall of the distal rectum on a valve. Although the risk is uncertain, some clinicians believe that a rectal biopsy with large forceps predisposes to a colonic perforation if a barium enema is done within ten days of the biopsy.

Search for Infections and Parasitic Organisms. It is important to complete the examination for parasites and to have adequate bacterial cultures in progress prior to examination of the patient with radiologic contrast medium because barium interferes with successful demonstration of some pathogens. It should be recognized that failure to find *Giardia* or *Strongyloides* in stool samples is not strong evidence against disease caused by these parasites; sometimes it is necessary to examine duodenal fluid in order to demonstrate these organisms. The importance of *Candida* as a cause of acute and chronic diarrhea has been emphasized by some authors.[56] Special culture methods are required if the presence of gonococcal, *Yersinia*, and *Campylobacter* infections is to be established. Serologic tests for amebas and lymphogranuloma venereum may assist in the diagnosis in some patients. Finally, tests for clostridial toxin are helpful in the evaluation of antibiotic-associated diarrhea.

Quantitative Stool Collection. For reasons indicated in the preceding sections on Definition and History, knowledge of stool volume may help clarify the nature of the patient's problem and help localize the region of the intestine most likely responsible for the diarrhea.

In some instances, knowledge of stool volume is of direct help in diagnosis and management. For example, stool volumes greater than 500 ml per day are rarely, if ever, seen in patients with irritable bowel syndrome,[2, 57] and stool volumes of less than 1000 ml per day are evidence against pancreatic cholera syndrome. Also, very large stool volumes will alert the physician to the possible need for vigorous fluid replacement. Stool volumes cannot be accurately estimated by stool frequency (Fig. 20–2).

Some simple equipment is necessary to make stool collection easy. This consists of a preweighed metal can (or plastic bucket) with an airtight lid that holds at least 3 liters, and a disposable collection unit (Fig. 20–6) that allows separation of stool and urine. Stools should be kept refrigerated during the collection period. Several days prior to and during the collection, the patient should have been eating three regular meals per day of known (approximate) fat content. During the several days that stools are collected, the patient should miss no meals, and there should be no diagnostic test (lactose tolerance test, D-xylose test, or barium studies) that would disturb the normal eating pattern, add foreign material to the gut, or risk an episode of incontinence. All but essential medications are avoided. There is no a priori reason why this cannot be done at home. We provide the patient with the equipment shown in Figure 20–6, a Styrofoam box, and liquid refrigerant that can be frozen and reused. We have the patient keep a diary so that stool weight per movement can be estimated and so that fat intake can be estimated from dietary tables.

In addition to weight, stool examinations may include fat content, electrolyte concentrations and osmolality, pH, glucose, reducing substances, and tests for laxatives (to be discussed later). Electrolytes, os-

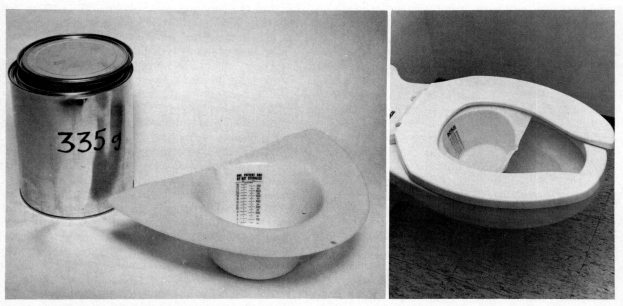

Figure 20–6. Utensils for quantitative stool collection. Preweighed metal can (3 to 4 L) with airtight lid. The disposable collection unit (Specipan TM Collection Unit, Patent No. 3,654,638, The Kendall Co., Boston, Massachusetts) is put into the posterior half of the seat of the commode (right). It allows easy separation of urine and stool. A second unit can be placed anteriorly for urine collection.

molality, and so on are determined in supernatant stool water obtained after centrifugation (30 minutes at 2000 g). In special instances, it is useful to determine whether or not diarrhea persists during a 48-hour fast (while the patient is given glucose and salt solutions intravenously). Interpretation of fecal electrolytes, osmolality, and persistence of diarrhea during a fast are discussed under secretory, osmotic, and motility diarrheas.

Evaluating the Patient for Bile Acid Malabsorption. It is believed that bile acid malabsorption can be a cause of diarrhea even in the absence of ileal disease or ileal resection and even when other tests of ileal absorption (e.g., the Schilling test) give normal results (see p. 310). Therefore, methods for accurate measurement of bile acid absorption are required for a complete assessment of patients with chronic diarrhea.

The bile acid breath test does not appear to be a reliable clinical test for bile acid malabsorption because results are frequently normal in patients who have bile acid malabsorption as assessed by more specific methods[58, 59] and because an abnormal breath test does not constitute strong evidence for bile acid malabsorption (abnormal results are also caused by bacterial overgrowth of the small bowel). Probably the best clinical method for measuring bile acid absorption is quantitative measurement of ^{14}C excretion in stool after an oral dose of ^{14}C-cholylglycine. The main disadvantages of this method, aside from the fact that it requires special equipment not available in most institutions, is the radiation hazard. This has been estimated to be comparable to that of a barium enema examination.[58] The isotope should not be used in children or pregnant women. The results of any test of bile acid absorption must be interpreted in light of the patient's stool volume.[1] Other tests of bile acid absorption are discussed on pages 144 to 161 and in reference 41.

Given the general unavailability of an accurate method for measuring bile acid absorption, many clinicians use a therapeutic trial of cholestyramine. To what extent a good therapeutic response to cholestyramine signifies bile acid malabsorption as the main cause of diarrhea, and to what extent failure to improve on cholestyramine denotes the absence of bile acid malabsorption as the main cause of diarrhea, are unsettled issues that have been recently discussed.[1] Cholestyramine does not reduce diarrhea in patients with ulcerative colitis[60] or idiopathic tropical diarrhea[61] and actually increases stool water output in control subjects.[60] Thus, it is not a nonspecific antidiarrheal agent. However, cholestyramine could bind diarrhea-producing substances other than bile acids, so reduction of diarrhea by cholestyramine suggests but does not prove that the diarrhea is due to bile acid malabsorption. Looked at from another vantage point, many patients with diarrhea and bile acid malabsorption do not respond to cholestyramine;[1] presumably, this means that many patients with diarrhea have bile acid malabsorption but that the diarrhea is not caused by the bile acid malabsorption. It is clear, therefore, that the result of a cholestyramine trial does not establish whether or not bile acid malabsorption is present or not; a good response to cholestyramine suggests but does not prove that bile acid malabsorption is the cause of the diarrhea. From a practical standpoint clinicians are just as interested in controlling diarrhea as in understanding its mechanism, so cholestyramine trials are proper in patients with unexplained and troublesome diarrhea even though the meaning of the response is uncertain.

Vasoactive Intestinal Polypeptide (VIP) and Other Secretagogues. If diarrhea of unknown origin has lasted longer than four weeks, has the clinical features of secretory diarrhea, and is severe (> 1 liter per day or associated with hypokalemia and salt and water depletion); if surreptitious laxative and diuretic abuse and organic disease of the gastrointestinal tract have been excluded; and if severe steatorrhea is not present, then such patients may have pancreatic cholera syndrome or one of its variants (see pp. 1890 to 1892). It is only in this rare subgroup of patients that serum assay for VIP, calcitonin, and so on is likely to be helpful. Because these assays are imperfect, and because pancreatic cholera syndrome is a very rare disorder (one new case per 10 million population per year), high values should be interpreted with caution. The role of circulating agents and prostaglandins in diarrhea have been recently reviewed.[39, 62]

Urine Examination. A 24-hour urine collection is useful in detecting polydipsia, which occurs in some patients with chronic diarrhea. Whether or not the polydipsia contributes to the diarrhea in such patients is unclear,[63, 64] but in our experience with three patients, it did not. Urine collections also may be used for drug identification (to be discussed), for measurement of 5-hydroxyindoleacetic acid or metanephrins, and to see whether renal conservation of electrolytes is appropriate for the apparent clinical situation (see p. 306 for discussion of factitious and self-induced diarrhea).

Other Tests. Some other tests that are often or sometimes indicated in the evaluation of patients with diarrhea are included in Table 20–6. This list is useful in attempting to make sure that all indicated tests have been carried out when the cause of diarrhea is difficult to establish.

SPECIAL CONSIDERATIONS

Congenital Secretory Diarrheas

Figure 20–7 shows the major ion transport mechanisms in the ileum. A congenital deletion of the glucose-sodium entry carrier is presumably the cause of glucose-galactose malabsorption, which is manifested by osmotic diarrhea that is treatable by substitution of fructose and elimination of dietary carbohydrates that contain glucose and galactose.

Congenital defects in the neutral NaCl entry mechanism result in secretory diarrhea. The mechanism of the neutral NaCl entry mechanism is shown in Figure 20–7. This model was worked out in normal human subjects in vivo by measuring absorption and secretion

Table 20–6. CHECKLIST FOR DIARRHEA WORK-UP

Stool	*Gastric Analysis*
Consistency	
Frequency/24 hr	*Imaging Studies*
Volume/24 hr	Upper GI, small bowel, barium
WBCs by Wright stain	enema
Blood	Abdominal and pelvic
Sudan	sonogram, CT scan
Quantitative fat/24 hr	Abdominal angiogram
NaOH, other laxatives	
Cultures for enteric pathogens	*Small Bowel Studies*
Ova and parasites	Aspirate (O&P, colony count,
Clostridium difficile toxin	cultures)
Osmolality	Biopsy
Na, K, Cl	Mucosal disaccharidase assays
pH	D-Xylose
Reducing substances	Schilling test with IF
Mg, SO_4, PO_4	Bile acid absorption
α_1-Antitrypsin (protein-losing	Carbohydrate tolerance tests
enteropathy)	Carbohydrate breath tests
Proctoscopy	*Exocrine Pancreatic Function*
Mucosal appearance	
Biopsy	*Upper Endoscopy*
Melanosis	
	Colonoscopy with Biopsies
Blood	
Electrolytes	*Urine*
Immunoglobulins, albumin	Volume, Na, K
T_3, T_4	5-HIAA
Ameba serology	Metanephrines. VMA
Folate, vitamin B_{12}	NaOH (for phenolphthalein)
Cortisol	Heavy metals, drug screen
Ca, Mg, PO_4	
Erythrocyte sedimentation rate	*Room Search for Drugs*
Eosinophil count	
	Rectal Manometry
Special Assays	
VIP	*Intestinal Perfusion Studies*
Calcitonin	
Gastrin	*Therapeutic Trials*
Other	(see text)

of Na^+, K^+, Cl^- and HCO_3^- during perfusion of a variety of carefully selected test solutions.[6, 7] The model has more recently been verified by in vitro studies using vesicles of the brush border membrane.[65, 66] This neutral mechanism for NaCl absorption is based on coupled exchange carriers, one that exchanges Na^+ for H^+ and another that exchanges Cl^- for HCO_3^-. If the

exchangers work at the same rate, sodium and chloride enter the cell and are absorbed across the basolateral membrane at the same rate. Likewise, hydrogen and bicarbonate are secreted in equal amounts; they react with each other in the gut lumen with the formation of CO_2 and water (which are free to diffuse across the mucosa), and there is no net absorption or secretion of hydrogen or bicarbonate. Net absorption or secretion of bicarbonate will result if the exchangers work at different rates.[6, 7] Further details of ion transport are reviewed on pages 1022 to 1045.

Two congenital defects in ion transport have been recognized and are believed to be due to defects in the two exchangers. The first is an autosomal recessive disease called congenital chloridorrhea; it is due to defective Cl^-/HCO_3^- exchange in the ileum and colon.[67] As a result, chloride cannot be absorbed actively in the ileum and colon. The Na^+/H^+ exchanger is normal, but sodium absorption is accomplished at the expense of net hydrogen secretion owing to the fact that secreted hydrogen in exchange for sodium is not balanced by secreted bicarbonate in exchange for chloride. The overall result of this defect is reduced rate of fluid absorption, acidification of the luminal contents, and a high chloride concentration in the fluid remaining in the lumen of the ileum and colon. This is expressed clinically by a diarrheal fluid with a chloride concentration equal to or greater than the sum of the sodium and potassium concentrations (this does not occur in any other disease). The cation gap, if any, is usually made up by NH_4^+, which may accumulate in fecal water because of the low fecal pH (see p. 294). Because of loss of acid in the stools, these patients characteristically develop metabolic alkalosis. The diarrhea may persist (at a reduced rate) during fasting. If the intestinal losses are not replaced, death usually supervenes. However, because passive chloride permeability in the jejunum is normal, it is usually possible to treat these patients successfully with NaCl and KCl by the oral route. If so, development is normal in spite of continuing chronic diarrhea.

The second disease, only recently described, is due to defective Na^+/H^+ exchange.[67, 68] This defect has

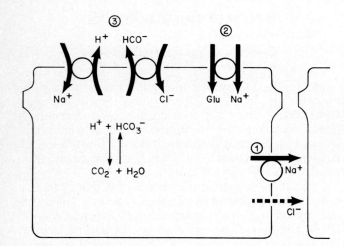

Figure 20–7. Active ion transport mechanisms in the human ileum. The illustration represents an epithelial cell from the human ileum, with the brush border membrane at the top and the intercellular space (bordered by two adjacent lateral cell membranes) on the right. The basolateral sodium pump (1), the glucose-Na^+ entry mechanism (2), and the neutral NaCl entry mechanism (3) are shown. (See text for other details.)

been specifically proved only in the jejunum,[68] but it seems likely on clinical grounds that the ileal Na^+/H^+ exchanger is also defective. As would be anticipated from the model, sodium absorption is defective and stool sodium concentration is high. Because of continued Cl^-/HCO_3^- exchange (without concomitant hydrogen secretion via the Na^+/H^+ exchanger), stool bicarbonate is high, stool chloride is low, and the patient develops metabolic acidosis. (These findings are just the opposite of congenital chloridorrhea.) Treatment consists of oral sodium citrate (absorbed citrate is metabolized to bicarbonate) and glucose-electrolyte replacement solution. With this, growth and development are normal, although diarrhea persists.

These diseases attest to the physiologic importance of these two exchangers in the human intestine. In both diseases, as expected, the sodium-glucose carrier is intact. Both diseases begin in utero with diarrhea manifested by hydramnios. In one instance abdominal sonogram performed one month prior to delivery showed the fetal abdomen to be distended by fluid-filled loops of intestine. Profuse watery diarrhea begins immediately after birth.

Several other causes of congenital diarrhea have also been described and are discussed in reference 69.

Chronic Diarrhea of Unknown Origin

This refers to patients in whom a more or less complete diagnostic evaluation in the recent past by another physician has failed to reveal the cause of troublesome chronic diarrhea. Referral of such patients to a gastroenterologist is common, because undiagnosed and untreated chronic diarrhea constitutes a major clinical problem. In addition to their physical and social disability, these patients and their families and physicians often begin to wonder if the diarrhea is caused by a psychologic disturbance. When such patients are re-evaluated at institutions with special interests and special facilities, a specific diagnosis is forthcoming in only about half the cases.[1, 37, 70-72] Although it is obvious that almost any cause of diarrhea could have been missed during a previous evaluation, the most common diagnoses we have made in such patients are surreptitious abuse of laxatives (almost always in women) or ingestion of other drugs that cause diarrhea, defective anal continence with incontinence masquerading as severe diarrhea, irritable bowel syndrome, microscopic/collagenous colitis syndrome, and various causes of previously unrecognized malabsorption syndrome. Although many of the patients were referred with a suspected diagnosis of neuroendocrine tumor, this turned out to be a very rare final diagnosis.

Many remain in whom a satisfactory diagnosis cannot be made. This is not to say that abnormalities are not discovered in such patients, but rather that the demonstrated abnormalities do not seem to be the cause of the diarrhea in many instances. For example, lac-tose-free diets often fail to improve chronic diarrhea in patients with lactase deficiency; patients with abnormal numbers of bacteria in their jejunal contents often continue to have diarrhea when bacterial counts are made normal by antibiotics; diarrhea often persists after questionable pathogens are no longer present in stool cultures; and even though bile acid malabsorption is common, it appears that this is usually not the primary cause of idiopathic chronic diarrhea.[1]

The pathogenesis of idiopathic diarrhea (i.e., diarrhea that is unexplained even after an exhaustive evaluation) is a continuing problem. Recently we studied seven patients in whom we could discover no etiology for chronic diarrhea, and in whom perfusion studies were carried out in all segments of the intestine as well as total gut perfusion.[37] Two of these seven patients had normal fluid and electrolyte absorption in all areas of the gut, and we therefore believe their diarrhea was not caused by defective absorption; we speculate that their diarrhea was mediated by an idiopathic motility disturbance. The other five patients had abnormal absorption at one or more levels of the intestine. Thus, idiopathic chronic diarrhea in these seven patients seems to have been caused by malabsorption of water and electrolytes, or abnormal motility. Unfortunately, such complete perfusion studies are not practical in most patients. In a large group of patients with chronic idiopathic diarrhea most patients were found to have bile acid malabsorption.[1] Because these patients did not respond favorably to cholestyramine, bile acid malabsorption was probably not the cause of their diarrhea. More likely, abnormal bile acid absorption reflects an underlying defect in ileal fluid absorption or motility; this postulated defect may be the cause of diarrhea in some of these patients.

The extent to which it helps patients to undergo such a thorough evaluation is debatable. To do all this and come up with a diagnosis of idiopathic bile acid malabsorption, a motility defect, or idiopathic colonic malabsorption is of dubious value to the patient, and in other instances the disease or syndrome identified may have no specific therapy. On the other hand, the discovery of surreptitious laxative abuse may help spare such patients destructive surgical therapy (many of our patients had already had it) or useless and potentially dangerous therapy with prednisone. In addition, in some patients a fairly specific medical or surgical therapy is suggested by the diagnosis that is reached. Another benefit is the substantial satisfaction some patients obtain from understanding the pathogenesis of their diarrhea. Everything considered, we believe that about 55 per cent of our patients have been benefited to a significant degree, and that the benefit to the other 45 per cent is marginal or minimal. It is our tentative opinion that such a complete evaluation is worthwhile provided that the patient is severely disabled by the diarrhea, and provided that he or she understands that even such an involved and expensive work-up may not reveal a diagnosis or suggest a satisfactory therapy in every particular case.

Pseudopancreatic Cholera Syndrome

Pseudopancreatic cholera syndrome refers to patients with chronic severe diarrhea (stool weights >750 gm per day) that persists (sometimes in a reduced amount) during a fast, with no evidence of endocrine tumor by plasma radioimmunoassay or by CT scan. Although it was initially believed that all such patients had diarrhea due to defective ion and water absorption or actual intestinal secretion, this did not always turn out to be the case when a series of such patients was studied by intestinal perfusion.[37] This syndrome can result from idiopathic secretory diarrhea[37, 73] and apparently from a motility disturbance.[37] In either case, the cause of the intestinal malfunction is unknown. The severity varies widely. Some patients have seemingly endless severe chronic diarrhea, some have persistent diarrhea of moderate severity, and still others have a complete resolution of diarrhea after several months to a few years. Some patients are remarkably benefited by opiates. We have tried several patients (the more severely ill ones) on prednisone in doses of 60 to 80 mg per day, with benefit seen in only an occasional instance. In one such patient we observed complete and reproducible resolution of severe secretory diarrhea during treatment with a new somatostatin analogue (SMS 201-995, Sandostatin) given subcutaneously.[74] One of our patients died, and the autopsy was negative.

Decisions in such patients about angiography in search of endocrine tumor are difficult. We would tend to do angiography in patients with more severe diarrhea who have an ion absorptive defect as measured by intestinal perfusion. Usually the results are negative. We do not advocate blind pancreatic resection, and we have little or no experience with reversed segments of small intestine, but we do seriously consider (in patients who require fluids intravenously) insertion of a jejunostomy feeding tube that can subsequently be used for infusion of glucose-containing electrolyte solutions. One of our patients with isolated colon malabsorption and incontinence was benefited by ileostomy.

In our opinion, the major lesson to be learned from these case studies is that patients may have severe "secretory" diarrhea that mimics most, if not all, of the clinical features of the pancreatic cholera syndrome, and yet have no evidence of an endocrine tumor, surreptitious laxative ingestion, or any other known cause of secretory diarrhea. This syndrome is much more common than pancreatic cholera syndrome itself.

Self-Induced and Factitious Diarrhea

Factitious disorders have been classified into four subgroups: self-induced infections, simulated illnesses, chronic wounds, and self-medication.[75] Patients may induce or simulate diarrhea in several different ways, including ingestion of laxatives that produce either secretory or osmotic diarrhea depending on the agent, or by adding water, urine, or other liquid to their feces. Almost all patients reported to have self-induced and factitious diarrhea have been women and are not infrequently associated in some way with the medical profession. In a variant of this syndrome, mothers induce diarrhea in their children with either laxatives or frequent hypertonic feedings.[76-79] Surreptitious laxative ingestion is the most common identifiable cause of chronic diarrhea of unknown origin.[71]

After the diagnosis of surreptitious laxative abuse has been established, it becomes obvious that such patients are severely neurotic. However, in many instances this is not evident to the physicians who were taking care of the patients before the diagnosis was established. The lack of obvious emotional disturbance is one of the reasons there is usually such a delay in correct diagnosis. The diagnosis is usually as shocking to the referring physician as it is to the patient and family.

The underlying psychologic factors that lead patients to this behavior are not well understood. From our own experience, we believe there are two major groups of patients who surreptitiously ingest laxatives. The first consists of women from about 18 to 40 years of age who have a variant of anorexia nervosa with a severe preoccupation with body weight and an altered self-image. Prior to using laxatives, many use self-induced vomiting as a method of weight control. They then begin to take laxatives (frequently along with diuretics), often in large quantities under the assumption that laxatives will cause food to be flushed through the gut unabsorbed. Actually, in a controlled study, 10 to 50 Correctol tablets decreased calorie absorption by only about 5 per cent.[80] Weight loss after such purging is due almost entirely to fluid depletion; of course, this is transient, leading to the need for repeated use of laxatives. Although this behavior seems logical to the patients, they apparently do not perceive the relationship between laxatives and their diarrhea, hypokalemia, lassitude, abdominal discomfort, and other symptoms. At last, they present to a physician with these problems and fail to mention that they are taking laxatives. Furthermore, they submit to any requested diagnostic test or surgical procedure in hopes of regaining their health. However, when confronted with evidence that they are ingesting laxatives, they usually admit it. When the laxatives are discontinued, they may become quite edematous, possibly due in part to persisting hyperreninemia and secondary hyperaldosteronism.[81] This edema may cause them to return to laxatives or to start using diuretics. If they do nothing, the edema will subside spontaneously in three to six weeks.

The second group consists of older women, usually 40 to 60 years of age, who have no features suggestive of anorexia nervosa and who totally deny laxative ingestion as the cause of their diarrhea, even when confronted with undeniable evidence. The underlying psychologic factors that motivate such women are complex. Secondary gain of attention is probably a factor. Some investigators believe that surreptitious laxative ingestion in these patients represents one of the presentations of hysteria.[82] Many features of hysterical behavior are present, including the capacity for self-deception, lack of insight, and manipulation of relatives, friends, and physicians, often in the absence of an obvious motive for gain. The denial that they make when presented with evidence that they are taking laxatives is not simply deliberate lying. They do not admit this even to themselves. This allows them to continue to take purgatives even after being told of their physician's conclusion, and it helps explain why they suffer such severe symptoms and undergo prolonged and uncomfortable diagnostic tests or surgical procedures.

In addition to chronic diarrhea, the clinical picture of surreptitious laxative ingestion includes abdominal pain, usually cramping in nature, rectal pain associated with bowel movements, nausea, vomiting, weight loss, muscle weakness, lassitude, hypokalemia (sometimes with its attendant nephropathy), skin pigmentation, bone pain, finger clubbing (reported with senna preparations), abnormalities on barium enema,[83] rectal biopsy that may simulate inflammatory bowel disease,[84, 85] cyclic edema,[81] and kidney stones consisting of ammonium urate.[86] These symptoms and findings may have persisted for years without specific diagnosis despite multiple admissions for diagnostic studies, fluid therapy, and surgical procedures. The surgical procedures have included exploratory laparotomy, gastric resection, vagotomy, cholecystectomy, hysterectomy, reversal of intestinal loops, partial pancreatectomy, adrenalectomy, and colectomy with ileostomy.

Melanosis coli,[87, 88] a dark pigmentation of the colorectal mucosa, develops as a consequence of anthracene laxative use (senna, cascara, aloe) but not with use of diphenolic laxatives (phenolphthalein, bisacodyl) or osmotic agents. At sigmoidoscopy, this discoloration is seen to spare lymphoid follicles and polyps. The pigment is not melanin, but is derived from lipofuscin and anthraquinone. The lipofuscin is formed from damaged cell organelles incorporated into lysosomes of macrophages located primarily in the lamina propria. In less severe cases, the mucosa is grossly normal while the above histologic changes may be the only findings. Although mainly affecting the rectosigmoid region, the entire colon may be involved. Melanosis coli starts to develop as early as four months after starting anthracene laxatives and goes away within one year of discontinuance.

Characteristic roentgenologic findings, known as cathartic colon,[82] are most marked in the right colon, but can affect the entire colon and ileum. The large bowel is dilated with loss of haustrations and with focal areas of transient narrowing ("pseudostrictures"). The ileocecal valve is frequently incompetent and the ileal plicae may be lost. These radiologic changes are due to structural alterations in the bowel wall, seen histologically as degeneration and loss of myenteric neurons,[89, 90] atrophy of smooth muscle, increased submucosal fat, and fibrosis and hypertrophy of the muscularis mucosae.[88]

Diagnosis depends upon a high index of suspicion, chemical tests of stool and urine, and if necessary, a search of the patient's hospital room, home, and belongings. Chemical tests include analysis of stool in search of nonphysiologic (and therefore suspicious) constituents, and analysis of stool and urine for specific laxatives.[82, 91] Finally, as mentioned previously, sigmoidoscopy with a rectal biopsy may reveal the characteristic changes of melanosis coli.

The simplest test, one that should be part of the routine examination in any patient with chronic idiopathic diarrhea, is alkalinization of stool and urine. This will result in a pink or red color if phenolphthalein is present. Phenolphthalein is colorless up to pH 8.5, whereas a pink to red color develops above pH 9. A large excess of alkali will result in the formation of the trisodium salt which, again, is colorless. Thus, if too much alkali is added, one might fail to detect the presence of phenolphthalein. The absorption maximum of phenolphthalein is 550 to 555 μm. So far, we have never seen a pink color develop upon alkalinization of the stool that did not prove to be phenolphthalein, although it is possible that a Bromsulphalein (BSP) test, ingestion of beet root or rhubarb might result in a false positive result. Aloes and aloin also are said to turn alkaline urine red.[82] To specifically test for phenolphthalein, we add one drop of 1 N NaOH to about 3 ml of fecal supernatant or urine. If a pink or red color develops, we measure absorption in a spectrophotometer to see if maximum absorption occurs at 550 to 555 μm, and we add 10 N NaOH to see if the color disappears at very high pH levels. Although free phenolphthalein is excreted in the urine and is detected by the above described method, the predominant urinary metabolites, the sulfated and glucuronated forms, may yield a positive test only after boiling with HCl, liberating free phenolphthalein via hydrolysis.[88]

Fecal fluid also should be analyzed for osmolality and electrolytes. If findings suggest secretory diarrhea, one of the laxatives capable of causing secretory diarrhea and sodium sulfate ingestion should be suspected. If findings suggest osmotic diarrhea, magnesium laxatives should be ruled out.[32] If the osmolality is significantly lower than the osmolality of plasma, water in some form has been added to the stool. For example, if stool osmolality is 100 mOsm per kilogram, the stool has been diluted about threefold with water. If the osmolality is far above that of plasma, urine may have been added to stool. This can be confirmed by finding a high monovalent cation concentration (e.g., sodium concentration higher than in plasma) and high concentration of urea or creatinine in stool.

Additional tests that can be done include a qualitative test for senna in urine, chromatography for bisacodyl, and measurement of sulfate and phosphate in diarrheal stool.[82, 91] Diarrhea caused by sodium sulfate or sodium phosphate ingestion is osmotic diarrhea (due to sulfate and phosphate), but it would appear clinically as secretory because there would be no solute gap by analysis of Na+, K+, and osmolality. Therefore, sulfate and phosphate must be considered when diarrhea is apparently secretory in type. Unfortunately, the normal upper limits for sulfate and phosphate concentration in stool water have not been reliably established.

Measurement of urine volume and electrolytes is also helpful because a sodium and potassium diuresis associated with diarrhea suggests the possibility of surreptitious ingestion of diuretics. Diuretics can, of course, also cause hypokalemia; if they are ingested surreptitiously, the physician may think the hypokalemia is caused by the diarrhea and consider pancreatic cholera syndrome.

Some physicians think it is unethical to search a patient's room for laxatives and diuretics.[92] Others feel it should be viewed as a diagnostic study, requiring informed consent and including a discussion with the patient of the procedure, its risks and benefits, and alternatives.[93] Although these are respectable opinions, they seem impractical. Furthermore, we feel a room search is not unethical, for if the diagnosis of surreptitious laxative ingestion is missed, the patient most likely will be subjected to needless hazardous tests and therapies. Three patients in our series had previously undergone partial pancreatectomy and one had undergone total colectomy; recently this cause of diarrhea in a four-year-old patient (via the mother) hospitalized in Dallas was discovered shortly after the patient's death. In some series, a room search had a higher diagnostic yield for surreptitious laxative ingestion than any other test.[94] No hospital has analytic methods available for all the drugs that can cause diarrhea.

If a diagnosis of surreptitious laxative ingestion is made, should the patient and family be confronted with the discovery? In most instances, we think the answer is yes. The main thing to hope for is prevention of useless and harmful tests and therapies in the future. With the anorexia nervosa type of patient, the confrontation usually goes relatively well; she is thankful that this habit is now out in the open, but she nevertheless frequently continues to take laxatives. With older women who do not take laxatives for weight control, one should expect vehement denial and early self-discharge from the hospital. We have not had a patient become violent or attempt suicide after confrontation, but such events have been recorded,[94] and one must consider this and be ready to prevent such occurrences. Every effort must be made to be gentle and considerate with the patient and her family.

Follow-up of 11 patients from Cleveland over a six- to 57-month interval, conducted by telephone interview, revealed that six patients felt improved; five felt they received no benefit, commenting that the opinions were conflicting and the explanations were not understood or were dissatisfying. It is interesting that two of the patients with subjective improvement "never heard a definite cause" and "didn't recall the explanation." Finally, as is typical of this disorder, four of these patients were known to have sought further medical attention at other facilities.[95]

Collagenous Colitis

Collagenous colitis was first described by Lindström in 1976.[96] Its name stemmed from the histologic finding of excessive subepithelial collagen deposition in colonic mucosa. Most patients with this histologic abnormality have chronic diarrhea that begins in middle age (mean age, 56 years; range of 23 to 86 years); women are affected at least four times as often as men.[97, 98] The syndrome is characterized clinically by a history of chronic watery diarrhea (months to years) without frank or occult blood and variably associated colicky abdominal pain, nausea, vomiting, and weight loss. The diarrhea may be persistent or intermittent, may be nocturnal and urgent with incontinence, and may have the clinical features of secretory diarrhea on stool analysis.[99] By colonoscopy and barium enema the colon is normal or exhibits only minor nonspecific changes. Collagenous colitis has not been consistently linked with other systemic diseases, although an association with inflammatory polyarthritis (including rheumatoid arthritis) and thyroid disease has been suggested.[97, 100]

The excessive collagen band has been immunotyped and found to be mainly type III;[101] it has a variable thickness in different parts of the colon, ranging from 7 to 100 µm, compared to normal values of 1 to 7 µm.[102] The abnormal collagen deposition may be focal or diffuse; in one report it was patchy proximally and more continuous distally,[103] and in another it was more severe in the proximal colon and occasionally absent from the rectum.[104] Abnormal collagen is present only under the surface epithelium; the pericryptal areas are normal. The surface epithelium is also abnormal with somewhat flattened cells, microscopic erosions, occasional separation from underlying structures, and even focal loss of the epithelium.[103] Capillary blood vessels with some abnormal features have been seen to lie within the collagenous fibrous tissue in several instances.[102, 103, 105] Excessive mast cells in the lamina propria were noted in one report.[101]

Although not emphasized in early reports, most patients with diarrhea associated with excessive subepithelial collagen have increased numbers of inflammatory cells in the lamina propria of the colonic mucosa. These are primarily chronic inflammatory cells (lymphocytes, plasma cells, and eosinophils), although acute inflammation has been described in as high as 83 per cent of some series.[104] Crypt abscesses have been described only rarely, and granulomas have not been found. This inflammation may precede the development of an abnormally thickened collagen plate. The regularity of inflammatory reaction in collagenous colitis, along with its presence antedating an abnormally thick subepithelial collagen plate, suggests that collagenous colitis and microscopic colitis may be variations of the same syndrome.[97, 104]

The pathogenesis of these histologic abnormalities is unknown. It is known that normal collagen is laid down in the subepithelial lamina propria by fibroblasts that originate in the pericryptal fibroblastic sheath and migrate toward the surface. It has been suggested that a primary abnormality of this process may be involved in the production of this disorder. Another possibility is that collagen deposition may occur as part of a reparative process, caused by inflammation. Some evidence for this view lies in the fact that type III collagen is produced in tissue repair.[98] The cause of diarrhea is presumably reduced colonic absorption, which is probably mainly due to surface epithelial abnormalities and inflammation rather than the thickened subepithelial collagen band.[104]

No consistent therapeutic benefit has been produced by any single agent or combination of agents, but spontaneous resolution has been reported.[98] Some patients have improved during treatment with sulfasalazine[98] or local or systemic corticosteroids,[102, 106] but others have not.[100, 102] Isolated reports of improvement with mepacrine hydrochloride[107] and psyllium hydrophilic mucilloid and loperamide[108] have been published.

Microscopic Colitis Syndrome

The term microscopic colitis denotes a nonspecific inflammation of colonic mucosa in patients who have a normal appearance of the colon by colonoscopy and barium enema. This was noted and named by Read and associates in 1980[71] and subsequently was studied in more detail by Kingham and colleagues in 1982[109] and by Bo-Linn and associates in 1985.[5] Abnormalities on light microscopy include excessive acute and chronic inflammatory cells in the lamina propria and occasionally within the surface epithelium, and reactive changes in the surface epithelium, including loss of cellular polarity, nuclear irregularity, and decreased mucus. Cryptitis and crypt abscesses are sometimes present. The lesion tends to be diffuse throughout the colon, although severity is variable, and occasionally a given region of the colon may be spared. Some patients have mild thickening of the subepithelial collagen band, although serial biopsies (when available) have indicated that inflammatiion precedes increased collagen band thickening.[104]

Colonic perfusion studies have revealed a marked decrease in colonic absorption of fluid and electrolytes. Small bowel absorption of fluid during perfusion with a balanced electrolyte solution was also reduced in a few of the patients, suggesting that the disease may in some instances involve the small as well as the large intestine.[4]

The etiology of microscopic colitis is unknown. Women are affected more commonly than men. Mean daily stool output in Bo-Linn's patients was 672 gm (range of 401 to 1105 gm). The stools are nonbloody and do not have occult blood. Fecal fat excretion is normal, and fecal leukocytes are absent. Other than the diarrhea, most patients remain in good health, although many lose weight. No treatment is of proven benefit, although some patients have improved while taking sulfasalazine or indocin. Progression of the disease to ulcerative colitis or Crohn's colitis has not been noted.

After a joint review of case material from Baltimore and Dallas, it was concluded that microscopic and collagenous colitis are variations of the same entity and that mucosal inflammation and surface epithelial changes are more likely than subepithelial collagen to be responsible for reduced colonic absorption.[104]

Diarrhea and Steatorrhea

Hydroxy fatty acids inhibit colonic fluid absorption under experimental conditions (see pp. 1022–1045), and this is probably one reason for excessive fecal fluid losses in patients with malabsorption syndrome. However, most causes of malabsorption syndrome result in malabsorption of carbohydrates and proteins as well as fat; because unabsorbed carbohydrate and probably unabsorbed proteins can inhibit intestinal fluid absorption, it is unclear how much fecal fluid loss is attributable to steatorrhea per se. Recently, stool fat excretion was measured in a group of patients with primary biliary cirrhosis.[110] Steatorrhea in such patients is the result of luminal bile acid deficiency, and this would not be expected to cause malabsorption of protein or carbohydrate. In fact, fecal nitrogen excretion is known to be normal in patients with steatorrhea (up to 50 gm of fat per day) due to bile acid deficiency caused by obstructive jaundice.[111] Data on stool weight were not reported on the patients with primary biliary cirrhosis, but were kindly supplied to us by Dr. Eugene DiMagno. In Figure 20–8 we have plotted fecal fat excretion versus stool weight, and it is evident from these results that fat malabsorption is associated with only a modest increase in stool weight. For example, in patients whose fecal fat excretion was about 50 gm per day, stool weight ranged from about 225 to about 500 gm per day, with an average of about 350 gm per day. Of this 350 gm stool, 50 gm was fat, so nonfat weight averaged about 300 gm per day. Assuming a stool weight of 100 gm per day if there was no steatorrhea, 50 gm of steatorrhea increased fecal fluid losses by about 200 gm per day.

Because fecal fluid losses rise only modestly with increasing fecal fat excretion in people with primary biliary cirrhosis, the concentration of fat in feces is high. Fecal fat concentration also tends to be high in

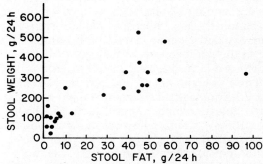

Figure 20–8. Stool weight as a function of stool fat excretion in patients with primary biliary cirrhosis. (Data supplied by Dr. E. P. DiMagno, on patients reported in reference 110.)

patients with pancreatic insufficiency (often over 9 per cent) and tends to be lower in patients with steatorrhea due to gastric resection or small bowel disease.[112] Exceptions to these generalizations clearly occur, but when they occur they provide useful pathophysiologic insight. For example, if a patient with pancreatic exocrine insufficiency had steatorrhea and relatively large fecal fluid losses (evident from a low fecal fat concentration), we would suspect that something other than exocrine pancreatic insufficiency was also contributing to the diarrhea (such as the effect of alcohol if the patient had alcoholic pancreatitis). If a patient with celiac disease had a high fecal fat concentration (and some of them do), we would suspect that they may have secondary deficiency in exocrine pancreatic secretion as a second cause of their steatorrhea. In any case, looking at fecal fat concentration provides an interesting and easy way to compare fecal fat and fluid losses. Clearly, fecal fat concentration is not an accurate method for *making* a diagnosis. Other observations on fecal fat concentration in patients with other causes of steatorrhea are available in references 113 and 114.

As already mentioned, some patients with severe steatorrhea have severe diarrhea, and their fecal fat concentrations are not high. Stools in such patients may not look fatty. Unless fecal fat output is quantitated, the presence of fat malabsorption is easily overlooked in such patients. (Sudan stains are mainly abnormal when fecal fat concentration is high.)

Diarrhea Due to Bile Acid Malabsorption

Bile acid malabsorption has been divided into three types.[41] Type I, the most common, is caused by ileal disease, resection, or bypass (see p. 153). Type II, the rarest, is known as idiopathic bile acid diarrhea or primary choleric enteropathy. Type III is the bile acid malabsorption that may follow truncal vagotomy or cholecystectomy.

Unabsorbed bile acids, if present in the aqueous phase, exert a cathartic effect on colonic mucosa. The dihydroxy bile acids are more potent than trihydroxy bile acids. Solubility of bile acids is pH dependent; the dihydroxy bile acids are fully water soluble at pH 6.8 to 7.0[41, 115] but precipitate at lower pH levels. Concentration in aqueous colonic contents is also influenced by the amount of colonic fluid (dilution effect) as well as by the binding of bile acids by intraluminal particulate matter.[41] Thus, bile acid malabsorption can be present and may even be severe, yet may not be playing a role in the pathogenesis of diarrhea.

Diarrhea due to bile acid malabsorption is typically mild (stool weight about 300 gm per day), follows meals, does not wake the patient at night, and responds well to cholestyramine. Clinical features which would argue strongly against bile acid malabsorption as the cause of diarrhea are large stool volume, fecal fat excretion greater than 20 gm per day, and an acid pH of fecal fluid.[41]

In Denmark, idiopathic bile acid catharsis has been reported to be a common cause of chronic idiopathic diarrhea.[116, 117] It was suggested that such patients either have a selective abnormality in ileal active transport of bile acids or that they have increased production of bile acids and thereby overwhelm the normal ileal bile acid transport system. In contrast to the experience in Denmark, primary bile acid malabsorption is an extremely rare cause of idiopathic diarrhea in the United States.[1, 41] Bile acid malabsorption also has been reported as a cause of protracted diarrhea of infancy.[118]

Care must be exercised in interpreting the results of bile acid absorption tests; rapid intestinal transit and high stool volume per se (independent of intestinal disease or dysfunction) accelerate bile acid losses into stool.[1]

Postcholecystectomy Diarrhea

Increased fecal loss of bile acids is found in a significant number of patients following cholecystectomy, one form of type III bile acid malabsorption. How cholecystectomy predisposes to bile acid malabsorption has not been clearly elucidated, but the mechanism may involve increased enterohepatic cycling of bile acids due to the loss of the normal reservoir function of the gallbladder. This in turn may overcome what had been a marginal and clinically silent defect in ileal uptake of bile acids.

Some patients develop diarrhea after cholecystectomy, and catharsis due to bile acid malabsorption has been suspected as the cause. However, fecal bile acids are only moderately increased, and in only a minority of instances is the aqueous concentration high enough to inhibit colonic absorption.[41, 119] This probably explains the inconsistent therapeutic response to cholestyramine.[119] Although some patients do respond to cholestyramine,[120] it appears that mechanisms other than bile acid malabsorption are usually involved in the etiology of postcholecystectomy diarrhea;[119] their nature remains a mystery at this time.

Postvagotomy Diarrhea

Diarrhea is an accepted complication of truncal vagotomy and gastric drainage, occurring to some degree in up to 25 per cent of patients.[121] It is severe and incapacitating in 2 to 8 per cent of vagotomized patients.[121, 122] The diarrhea is commonly episodic, although 11 per cent of patients in one large series had continuous diarrhea.[122] When the diarrhea is episodic, it can be explosive, with urgency and fecal incontinence.

The mechanisms by which truncal vagotomy and drainage procedures produce diarrhea are unclear. The incidence of diarrhea following proximal or selective vagotomy is much less than with truncal vagotomy,[123] suggesting denervation of organs other than the proximal stomach or involvement of the accompanying pyloroplasty.[124] Careful preservation of the hepatic branches of the vagus nerve apparently reduces the incidence of diarrhea after truncal vagotomy, implying that denervation of the small intestine does not play a role.[125] Rapid intestinal transit,[121, 126] possibly secondary to an early increase in postprandial jejunal osmolality, plus increased ileal fluid secretion rate,[121] have been implicated as contributors to postvagotomy diarrhea. Whether gastric emptying is faster in patients with vagotomy and diarrhea than in those with vagotomy but without diarrhea is controversial.

Bile acid malabsorption may develop following truncal vagotomy.[127, 128] Although the fecal loss of bile acids is increased, it is not known whether the concentrations of bile acids in the aqueous phase reach levels high enough to interfere with colonic fluid absorption. Lada et al. found no significant difference in the bile acid malabsorption in postvagotomy patients with diarrhea compared with those without.[121] Cholestyramine may or may not be beneficial.[121, 129, 130] As a last resort, surgical therapy may be attempted.[130, 131]

Diarrhea in Patients with Diabetes

Diarrhea complicating diabetes mellitus, first recognized as a clinical entity in 1936,[132] has since become well known as one of the many gastrointestinal manifestations of diabetes (see p. 496). The affected patients are usually insulin-dependent type I diabetics, with a mean age of 36 to 42 years, and have been affected by their illness for an average of eight years.[133] This syndrome has been reported to affect anywhere from 0.1 to 7 per cent of diabetics, although up to 22 per cent of diabetics in one series complained of diarrhea.[133, 134] Typical "diabetic diarrhea" consists of frequent (usually 10 to 30 per day) passages of watery brown stool, often occurring at night or while supine, and usually associated with fecal incontinence.[135, 136] (If fecal incontinence is not present, some cause of diarrhea other than diabetes should be highly suspected.) Stool weights in one series varied from 211 to 1605 gm per day.[137] The diarrhea may be intermittent and recurrent, with attacks that last hours, weeks, or months, or it may be continuous. If intermittent, it may alternate with bouts of constipation. The diarrhea is often refractory to antidiarrheal drugs or regimens. Occasionally the diarrhea may spontaneously and permanently cease. Mild steatorrhea is often present. However, some patients develop an unusual form of steatorrhea in which they malabsorb up to 70 gm of fat per day yet do not manifest weight loss, cachexia, or biochemical abnormalities typically seen with other malabsorption syndromes. This steatorrhea is also intractable to usual therapies, although it must be remembered that diabetics are at greater risk than normal subjects for some forms of treatable steatorrhea (see below).

Research in this area has been influenced by the consistent coexistence of diabetic diarrhea and steatorrhea with autonomic neuropathy, e.g., orthostatic hypotension, impotence, neurogenic bladder, pupillary dysfunction, anhidrosis, retrograde ejaculation, and gustatory sweating. Originally and classically, it was believed that autonomic neuropathy caused deranged motility, which in turn led to diarrhea. Recently, it has been pointed out that the link between autonomic nervous dysfunction and diabetic diarrhea might be by virtue of enterocyte secretion rather than by an effect on intestinal motility. The background for this hypothesis is the fact that enterocytes contain alpha$_2$-adrenergic receptors, and that their stimulation promotes electrolyte absorption or inhibits anion secretion in vitro.[138, 139] Chang, Field, and their associates postulated that diabetic diarrhea might be due to reduced electrolyte absorption by enterocytes, secondary to loss of normally present noradrenergic innervation. This hypothesis was tested in rats made diabetic by treatment with streptozocin.[140] Such rats develop diarrhea, and in vivo, loop experiments have shown that the ileum and colon secrete rather than absorb when the lumen is in contact with an isotonic saline solution. By contrast, jejunal loops absorbed saline normally. Furthermore, clonidine, an alpha$_2$-agonist, reversed abnormal ileal and colonic secretion in diabetic rats.[141] These results support the hypothesis that diabetic diarrhea in streptozocin-treated rats is mediated by loss of normal adrenergic stimulation, which results in ileal and colonic fluid secretion and therefore diarrhea.

The relevance to human diabetic diarrhea of this important work in diabetic animals is unclear at the present time. One essential component of the pathogenesis of diarrhea in the animal model is reduced enterocyte absorption rate or enterocyte secretion. In human diabetic diarrhea, jejunal and ileal absorption of isotonic saline is known to be normal.[137] To the best of our knowledge, colonic absorption has not been studied in patients with diabetic diarrhea, so it is possible that colonic secretion might be present, as in diabetic animals. Another essential feature of the animal model is stimulation of enterocyte absorption by clonidine. This has apparently not been studied in human diabetic diarrhea. Clonidine did reduce stool weight in three patients,[142] but this could have been because of its prominent antimotility effect.[143] Hopefully, future work will prove that the animal model is correct for humans, because it offers such promising therapeutic possibilities.

Although the concept of abnormal motility as the cause of human diabetic diarrhea has been de-emphasized recently, in our view it remains the most likely explanation. Abnormal motility could explain diarrhea, steatorrhea, bile acid malabsorption (see next paragraph), the intermittent nature of the diarrhea in some patients and the alteration with constipation in some others, and the normal enterocyte absorption rate during saline perfusion of the jejunum and ileum. The fact that other gastrointestinal manifestations of diabetes (including constipation, abnormal anal continence mechanisms, and gastroparesis) are apparently due to abnormal motility seems to strengthen this concept. Although rapid bolus movement could explain most, if not all, aspects of diabetic diarrhea, Soergel's group found delayed fluid movement through the ileum rather than accelerated bolus flow.[137] On the other hand, some (but not all) patients have been shown to have extremely rapid mouth-to-anus transit times with dye markers, and rapid small bowel and colon transit on barium X-ray is often noted.[145] Such a defect, if present only intermittently during the day (perhaps mainly in the interdigestive periods), would be very difficult to detect consistently with any current methodology. It is possible that delayed flow (as noted in Soergel's study with a test meal) causes luminal pooling and that this alternates with rapid bolus propulsion that causes diarrhea. Proof of this hypothesis is clearly not at hand. In other instances, intestinal stasis due to hypomotility seems likely to play a role because some patients have bacterial overgrowth or respond dramatically to tetracycline.

Molloy and Tomkin have described increased bile acid pool size with concomitant abnormally high fecal bile acid excretion in diabetics with autonomic neuropathy but no diarrhea;[144] they proposed decreased intestinal motility and gallbladder atony, with reduced bile acid recycling frequency, as the explanation. In contrast, they found a reduced bile acid pool with increased fecal bile acid excretion in those diabetics with diarrhea.[144] Although this represented a theoretic mechanism for diabetic diarrhea, no consistent therapeutic benefit has been reported with cholestyramine, arguing against bile acid malabsorption as a major etiologic factor in this diarrhea syndrome.

Treatment of diabetic diarrhea is usually disappointing and therapy that is initiated is hard to interpret because of the sometimes episodic nature of the diarrhea. Clonidine reduced stool weight in half in three diabetic patients;[142] although stool frequency was not reduced, the patients perceived benefit. Lidamidine (an experimental alpha$_2$-agonist) was shown in another three patients to decrease stool frequency by 30 to 60 per cent and improve "stool consistency."[146] The side effects of clonidine (especially hypotension and sedation) limit its usefulness. Tsai et al. in one isolated report found that the long-acting somatostatin analogue, SMS 201-995 (Sandostatin), benefited one patient whose diarrhea was refractory to other conventional treatments.[147] Cholestyramine, antibiotics (for possible bacterial overgrowth), and opiates deserve a therapeutic trial. Finally, because of the association of a history of poor diabetic control with diabetic diarrhea, as well as observed relapses during periods of poor control, tight control of blood glucose is recommended.

There are several nondiabetic and treatable causes of diarrhea or steatorrhea that may affect diabetics with increased frequency. One of these is an osmotic diarrhea resulting from the frequent consumption of gum and snack foods sweetened with nonabsorbable hexitols such as sorbitol. Although this type of diarrhea can affect anybody, it must be looked for in diabetics as they often use artificially sweetened dietetic foods. Other possible causes of diarrhea or steatorrhea in diabetic patients are exocrine pancreatic insufficiency (chronic pancreatitis or cancer),[148] blind loop syndrome,[149] and celiac disease,[150] as discussed in Chapter 29 (p. 497).

Diarrhea and Alcohol

Diarrhea is a common complaint of those who consume large amounts of alcohol, whether acutely or chronically. As has been shown in numerous in vivo and in vitro studies, alcohol has a multitude of effects on the small intestine that are probably important in the precipitation of diarrhea in this population. Rapid intestinal transit has been seen in patients after exposure to ethanol, shown to be due to enhanced propulsive movements.[151, 152] Another study used a breath H_2 test following consumption of lactulose to show shortened mouth-to-cecum transit times in alcoholics while drinking.[153] Other factors that contribute to the diarrhea of drinkers are decreased activity of intestinal disaccharidases,[155, 156] decreased bile secretion in those alcoholics with liver disease,[155, 156] and decreased pancreatic exocrine function (that can be reversible) leading to steatorrhea.[157] As many as one-third of binge drinkers have steatorrhea. In addition to malabsorption of fat, both normal subjects exposed to alcohol acutely as well as chronic alcoholics have been shown to variably malabsorb vitamin B_1,[158] vitamin B_{12},[159] folate,[160-162] glucose,[163] amino acids,[164] and sodium and water.[162, 165, 166] In one study,[166] jejunal perfusion revealed absorption of water and electrolytes to be reduced from a normal value of 205 to 51 ml per hour per 30 cm (p < 0.001). It seems likely that this jejunal absorption defect, possibly coupled with ileal and colonic malabsorption, may contribute to the diarrhea associated with alcohol ingestion. Several reviews on the effects of alcohol on the gastrointestinal tract have been published.[162, 167, 168]

Raw Milk–Associated Diarrhea

Systemic illness caused by streptococci, *Brucella*, corynebacteria, and *Listeria* have been linked to raw milk drinking. Genera known to cause enteritis with associated diarrhea (usually self-limited) include *Campylobacter*, *Salmonella*, and *Yersinia*.[169]

In the summer of 1984, physicians in Brainerd, Minnesota, a community of about 14,000 residents, noticed an increased number of patients presenting with chronic diarrhea.[170] This information reached the U.S. Centers for Disease Control, and a formal report was made public.[171] Based on epidemiologic association, drinking raw milk from an implicated dairy during the three weeks prior to the onset of the diarrhea was added to the case definition. The median age of the case patients was 41 years, with the range being one to 91 years. Fifty-one per cent were male. The median incubation period was 15 days, with a range of four to 23 days. The attack rate was 8 per cent, calculated from a survey of 94 families who drank raw milk. The illness was characterized by the acute onset of watery diarrhea, frequently with 10 to 20 stools per day. Weight loss occurred in 51 per cent of patients, but other systemic symptoms were rare. The diarrhea had lasted at least 18 months for most patients, although a gradual decrease in stool frequency was noticed by most over time; the average numbers of stools decreased from 11 during the first 50 days to three by day 500 of the illness.

No etiology for this raw milk–associated diarrheal illness has been uncovered, although an infectious agent is suspected. A similar illness associated with raw milk has been reported in at least seven states,[170] and a chronic diarrhea syndrome with many striking parallels was identified in San Antonio, Texas, to be epidemiologically associated with eating at a local Mexican restaurant.[172] It is interesting that no unpasteurized dairy products were ever used by this restaurant, and the victims denied raw milk consumption.

Although the above-mentioned facts constitute evidence for an infectious etiology for this illness, the empiric use of conventional antimicrobial agents including metronidazole, erythromycin, tetracycline, trimethoprim sulfamethoxazole, and cephalexin brought no relief to affected patients.

Chronic Diarrhea in Infants and Young Children

Chronic diarrhea in young children poses special management problems because large fluid and electrolyte losses are tolerated poorly. A complete discussion of diarrhea in the pediatric age group would go beyond the scope of this chapter, but a checklist of diarrheal and malabsorptive diseases in young children is given in Table 20–7. In the absence of histologic, endoscopic, radiographic, or other abnormalities that would explain the diarrhea, poisoning by drugs or heavy metals should be suspected, particularly in a child that previously had normal bowel movements. Toxicology tests should then be done and the child should be separated

from the parent or guardian to see whether the diarrhea persists.

Table 20–7. CAUSES OF CHRONIC DIARRHEA IN YOUNG CHILDREN

Celiac disease
Disaccharidase deficiencies
Milk allergy and other food allergies
Glucose-galactose malabsorption
Congenital chloridorrhea
Congenital sodium diarrhea
Primary bile acid malabsorption
Lethal protracted secretory diarrhea (idiopathic secretory diarrhea)
Surreptitious administration of laxatives by parents
Poisoning by drugs, heavy metals or other substances
Familial dysautonomia
Blind loop syndrome
Short bowel syndrome (e.g., after massive resection for necrotizing enterocolitis)
Amino acid disorders (e.g., cystinuria, Hartnup disease, "blue diaper" syndrome)
Intestinal lymphangiectasia
Abetalipoproteinemia
Ganglioneuroma, ganglioneuroblastoma
Nesidioblastosis (islet cell microadenomatosis containing vasoactive intestinal polypeptide)
Enterokinase deficiency
Immunodeficiency states
Giardiasis

References

1. Schiller, L. R., Hogan, R. B., Morawski, S. G., Santa, C. A., Bern, M. J., Norgaard, R. P., and Fordtran, J. S. The incidence and significance of bile acid malabsorption in patients with chronic idiopathic diarrhea. Gastroenterology 92:151, 1987.
2. Goy, J. A. E., Eastwood, M. A., Mitchell, W. D., Pritchard, J. L., and Smith, A. N. Fecal characteristics contrasted in the irritable bowel syndrome and diverticular disease. Am. J. Clin. Nutr. 29:1480, 1976.
3. Tucker, D. M., Sandstead, H. H., Logan, G. M., Klevay, L. M., Mahalko, J., Johnson, L. K., Inman, L., and Inglett, G. E. Dietary fiber and personality factors as determinants of stool output. Gastroenterology 81:879, 1981.
4. Davies, G. S., Crowder, M., Reid, B., and Dickerson, T. W. T. Bowel function measurements of individuals with different eating patterns. Gut 27:164, 1986.
5. Bo-Linn, G. W., Vendrell, D. D., Lee, E., and Fordtran, J. S. An evaluation of the significance of microscopic colitis in patients with chronic diarrhea. J. Clin. Invest. 75:1559, 1985.
6. Turnberg, L. A., Fordtran, J. S., Carter, N. W., and Rector, F. C., Jr. Mechanism of bicarbonate absorption and its relationship to sodium transport in the human jejunum. J. Clin. Invest. 49:548, 1970.
7. Turnberg, L. A., Bieberdorf, F. A., Morawski, S. G., and Fordtran, J. S. Interrelationship of chloride, bicarbonate, sodium, and hydrogen transport in the human ileum. J. Clin. Invest. 49:557, 1970.
8. Billich, C. O., and Levitan, R. Effects of sodium concentration and osmolality on water and electrolyte absorption from the intact human colon. J. Clin. Invest. 48:1336, 1969.
9. Gotch, F., Nadell, J., and Edelman, I. S. Gastrointestinal water and electrolytes. IV. The equilibration of deuterium oxide (D_2O) in gastrointestinal contents and the proportion of total body water (T.B.W.) in the gastrointestinal tract. J. Clin. Invest. 36:289, 1957.
10. Soergel, K. H. Flow measurements of test meals and fasting contents in the human small intestine. In Gastrointestinal Motility. International symposium on motility of the GI tract. Erlangen, West Germany, July 15 and 16, 1969. Stuttgart, Georg Thieme Verlag, and New York, Academic Press, 1969.
11. Phillips, S. F., and Giller, J. The contribution of the colon to electrolyte and water conservation in man. J. Lab. Clin. Med. 81:733, 1973.
12. Ladas, S. D., Isaacs, P. E. T., Murphy, G. M., and Sladen, G. E. Fasting and postprandial ileal function in adapted ileostomates and normal subjects. Gut 27:906, 1986.
13. Fordtran, J. S. Speculations on the pathogenesis of diarrhea. Fed. Proc. 26:1405, 1967.
14. Fordtran, J. S., and Locklear, T. W. Ionic constituents and osmolality of gastric and small intestinal fluids after eating. Am. J. Dig. Dis. 11:503, 1966.
15. Ladas, S. D., Isaacs, P. E. T., and Sladen, G. E. Post-prandial changes of osmolality and electrolyte concentration in the upper jejunum of normal man. Digestion 26:218, 1983.
16. Fordtran, J. S., and Phillips, S. F. Letters to the Editor, Effect of PEG on absorption. Gastroenterology 80:212, 1981.
17. Gazet, J. C. The surgical significance of the ileocecal junction. Ann. R. Coll. Surg. Eng. 43:19, 1968.
18. Debongnie, J. C., and Phillips, S. F. Capacity of the human colon to absorb fluid. Gastroenterology 74:698, 1978.
19. Wrong, O., Metcalfe-Gibson, A., Morrison, R. B. I., Ng, S. T., and Howard, A. V. In vivo dialysis of faeces as a method of stool analysis. I. Technique and results in normal subjects. Clin. Sci. 28:357, 1965.
20. Davis, G. R., Morawski, S. G., Santa Ana, C. A., and Fordtran, J. S. Evaluation of chloride/bicarbonate exchange in the human colon in vivo. J. Clin. Invest. 71:201, 1983.
21. Turnberg, L. A. Electrolyte absorption from the colon. Gut 11:1049, 1970.

22. Levitan, R., Fordtran, J. S. Burrows, B. A., and Ingelfinger, F. J. Water and salt absorption in the human colon. J. Clin. Invest. 41:1754, 1962.

23. Rubinstein, R., Howard, A. V., and Wrong, O. M. In vivo dialysis of faeces as a method of stool analysis. IV. The organic anion component. Clin. Sci. 37:549, 1969.

24. Bjork, J. T., Soergel, K. H., and Wood, C. M. The composition of "free" stool water. Gastroenterology 70:864, 1975.

25. Wrong, O., and Metcalfe-Gibson, A. The electrolyte content of feces. Proc. R. Soc. Med. 58:1007, 1965.

26. Down, P. F., Agostini, L., Murison, J., and Wrong, O. M. The interrelations of faecal ammonia, pH and bicarbonate: Evidence of colonic absorption of ammonia by non-ionic diffusion. Clin. Sci. 43:101, 1972.

27. Christopher, N. L., and Bayless, T. M. Role of the small bowel and colon in lactose-induced diarrhea. Gastroenterology 60:845, 1971.

28. Fordtran, J. S., Rector, F. C., Ewton, M. F., Soter, N., and Kinney, J. Permeability characteristics of the human small intestine. J. Clin. Invest. 44:1935, 1965.

29. Ruppin, H., Bar-Meir, S., Soergel, K. H., Wood, C. M., and Schmitt, M. G. Absorption of short-chain fatty acids by the colon. Gastroenterology 78:1500, 1980.

30. Bond, J. H., Currier, B. E., Buchwald, H., and Levitt, M. D. Colonic conservation of malabsorbed carbohydrate. Gastroenterology 78:444, 1980.

31. Saunders, D. R., and Wiggins, H. S. Conservation of mannitol, lactulose and raffinose by the human colon. Am. J. Physiol. 241:G397, 1981.

32. Krejs, G. J., Hendler, R. S., and Fordtran, J. S. Diagnostic and pathophysiologic studies in patients with chronic diarrhea. In Field, M., Fordtran, J. S., and Schultz, S. G. (eds.). Secretory Diarrhea. Bethesda, Maryland, American Physiological Society, 1980, pp. 141–151.

33. Ameen, V. Z., Powell, G. K., and Jones, L. A. Quantitation of fecal carbohydrate excretion in patients with short bowel syndrome. Gastroenterology 92:493, 1987.

34. Andersson, D. E. H., and Nygren, A. Four cases of long-standing diarrhoea and colic pains cured by fructose-free diet. A pathogenetic discussion. Acta Med. Scand. 203:87, 1978.

35. Goldbert, L. D., and Ditchek, N. D. Chewing gum diarrhea. Am. J. Dig. Dis. 23:568, 1978.

36. Ravry, M. J. R. Dietetic food diarrhea. JAMA 244:270, 1980.

37. Fordtran, J. S., Santa Ana, C. A., Morawski, S. G., Bo-Linn, G. W., and Schiller, L. R. Pathophysiology of chronic diarrhoea: Insights derived from intestinal perfusion studies in 31 patients. Clin. Gastroenterol. 15:477, 1986.

38. Moriarty, K. J., and Turnberg, L. A. Bacterial toxins and diarrhea. Clin. Gastroenterol. 15:529, 1986.

39. Rambaud, J. C., Hautefeville, M., Ruskone, A., and Jacquenod, P. Diarrhoea due to circulating agents. Clin. Gastroenterol. 15:603, 1986.

40. Binder, H. J. Pharmacology of laxatives. Annu. Rev. Pharmacol. Toxicol. 17:355, 1977.

41. Fromm, H., and Malavolti, M. Bile acid–induced diarrhoea. Clin. Gastroenterol. 15:567, 1986.

42. Binder, H. J. Pathophysiology of bile acid and fatty acid induced diarrhea. In Field, M., Fordtran, J. S., and Schultz, S. G. (eds.). Secretory Diarrhea. Bethesda, Maryland, American Physiological Society, 1980, pp. 159–178.

43. Fordtran, J. S., Soergel, K. H., and Ingelfinger, F. J. Intestinal absorption of D-xylose in man. N. Engl. J. Med. 267:274, 1962.

44. Schiller, L. R., Davis, G. R., Santa Ana, C. A., Morawski, S. G., and Fordtran, J. S. Studies of the mechanism of the antidiarrhea effect of codeine. J. Clin. Invest. 70:999, 1982.

45. Read, N. W. Diarrhée Motrice. Clin. Gastroenterol. 15:657, 1986.

46. Dillard, R. L., Eastman, H., and Fordtran, J. S. Volume-flow relationship during the transport of fluid through the human small intestine. Gastroenterology 49:58, 1965.

47. Harris, J., and Shields, R. Absorption and secretion of water and electrolytes by the intact human colon in diffuse untreated proctocolitis. Gut 11:27, 1970.

48. Gooptu, D., Truelove, S. C., and Warner, G. T. Absorption of electrolytes from the colon in cases of ulcerative colitis and in control subjects. Gut 10:555, 1969.

49. Almy, T. P. Chronic and recurrent diarrhea. Disease-a-Month, October, 1955.

50. Anthonisen, P., and Riis, P. A new diagnostic approach to mucosal inflammation in protocolitis. Lancet 2:81, 1961.

51. Harris, J. C., DuPont, H. L., and Hornick, R. B. Fecal leukocytes in diarrheal illness. Ann. Intern. Med. 76:697, 1972.

52. Masomune, O., Takahashi, T., Nagasaki, A., Iwabuchi, S., and Ishikawa, M. Diagnostic significance of the Sudan III staining for fecal fat. Tohoku J. Exp. Med. 122:397, 1977.

53. Surawicz, C. M., Meisel, J. L., Ylvisaker, T., Saunders, D. R., and Rubin, C. E. Rectal biopsy in the diagnosis of Crohn's disease: Value of multiple biopsies and serial sectioning. Gastroenterology 80:66, 1981.

54. Price, A. B., Jewkes, J., and Sanderson, P. J. Acute diarrhoea: Campylobacter colitis and the role of rectal biopsy. J. Clin. Pathol. 32:990, 1979.

55. Nostrant, T. T., Kumar, N. B., and Appleman, H. D. Histopathology differentiates acute self-limited colitis from ulcerative colitis. Gastroenterology 92:318, 1987.

56. Kane, J. G., Chretien, J. H., and Garagusi, V. F. Diarrhoea caused by Candida. Lancet 1:335, 1976.

57. Pimparkar, B. D., Tulsky, E. G., Kalser, M. H., and Bockus, H. L. Correlation of radioactive and chemical fecal fat determinations in the malabsorption syndrome. I. Studies in normal man and in functional disorders of the gastrointestinal tract. Am. J. Med. 30:910, 1961.

58. Thaysen, E. H. Diagnostic value of the ¹⁴C-cholylglycine breath test. Clin. Gastroenterol. 6:227, 1977.

59. Heaton, K. W. Bile salt tests in clinical practice. Br. Med. J. 1:644, 1979.

60. Miettinen, T. A. The role of bile salts in diarrhoea of patients with ulcerative colitis. Gut 12:632, 1971.

61. McCloy, R. M., and Hofmann, A. F. Tropical diarrhea in Vietnam. A controlled study of cholestyramine therapy. N. Engl. J. Med. 284:139, 1971.

62. Rask-Madsen, J. Eicosanoids and their role in the pathogenesis of diarrheal diseases. Clin. Gastroenterol. 15:545, 1986.

63. Low-Beer, T. S., and Read, A. E. Progress report. Diarrhoea: Mechanisms and treatment. Gut 12:1021, 1971.

64. Crohnheim, J. Lectures on General Pathology. Vol. 3. New Sydenham Society Publications, Vol. 133. London, New Sydenham Society, 1882, p. 967.

65. Liedtke, C. M., and Hopfer, U. Mechanism of Cl⁻ translocations across small intestinal brush border membrane. I. Absence of Na⁺-Cl⁻ cotransport. Am. J. Physiol. 5:G263, 1982.

66. Liedtke, C. M., and Hopfer, V. Mechanism of Cl⁻ translocation across small intestinal brush border membrane. II. Demonstration of Cl⁻OH exchange and Cl⁻ conductance. Am. J. Physiol. 5:G272, 1982.

67. Holmberg, C. Congenital chloride diarrhea. Clin. Gastroenterol. 15:583, 1986.

68. Booth, I. W., Murer, H., Strange, G., Fenton, T. R., and Milla, P. J. Defective jejunal brush border Na⁺/H⁺ exchange: A cause of congenital secretory diarrhoea. Lancet 1:1066, 1985.

69. Kanof, M. E., Rance, N. E., Hamilton, S. R., Luk, G. D., and Lake, A. M. Congenital diarrhea with intestinal inflammation and epithelial immaturity. J. Pediatr. Gastroenterol. Nutr. 6:141, 1987.

70. Krejs, G. J., Walsh, J. H., Morawski, S. G., and Fordtran, J. S. Intractable diarrhea. Intestinal perfusion studies and plasma VIP concentrations in patients with pancreatic cholera syndrome and surreptitious ingestion of laxatives and diuretics. Am. J. Dig. Dis. 22:280, 1977.

71. Read, N. W., Krejs, G. J., Read, M. G., Santa Ana, C. A., Morawski, S. G., and Fordtran, J. S. Chronic diarrhea of unknown origin. Gastroenterology 78:264, 1980.

72. Read, N. W., Harford, W. V., Schmulen, A. C., Read, M. G., Santa Ana, C., and Fordtran, J. S. A clinical study of patients with fecal incontinence and diarrhea. Gastroenterology 76:747, 1979.

73. Read, N. W., Read, M. G., Krejs, G. J., Hendler, R. S., Davis, G., and Fordtran, J. S. A report of five patients with

large-volume secretory diarrhea but no evidence of endocrine tumor or laxative abuse. Dig. Dis. Sci. *27*:193, 1982.

74. Santangelo, W. C., Dueno, M. I., and Krejs, G. J. Pseudopancreatic cholera syndrome: Effect of a synthetic somatostatin analogue (SMS 201-995). Am. J. Med. *82*(suppl. 5B):84, 1987.

75. Reich, P., and Gottfried, L. A. Factitious disorders in a teaching hospital. Ann. Intern. Med. *99*:240, 1983.

76. Ackerman, N. B., Jr., and Strobel, C. T. Polle syndrome: Chronic diarrhea in Munchausen's child. Gastroenterology *81*:1140, 1981.

77. Pickering, L. K., and Kohl, S. Munchausen syndrome by proxy. Am. J. Dis. Child. *135*:288, 1981.

78. Forbes, D. A., O'Loughlin, E. V., Scott, R. B., and Gall, D. G. Laxative abuse and secretory diarrhoea. Arch. Dis. Child. *60*:58, 1985.

79. Volk, D. Factitious diarrhea in two children. Am. J. Dis. Child. *136*:1027, 1982.

80. Bo-Linn, G. W., Santa Ana, C. A., Morawski, S. G., and Fordtran, J. S. Purging and calorie absorption in bulimic patients and normal women. Ann. Intern. Med. *99*:14, 1983.

81. Ullrich, I., and Lizarralde, G. Amenorrhea and edema. Am. J. Med. *64*:1080, 1978.

82. Morris, A. I., and Turnberg, L. A. Surreptitious laxative abuse. Gastroenterology *77*:780, 1979.

83. Plum, G. E., Weber, H. M., and Sauer, W. G. Prolonged cathartic abuse resulting in roentgen evidence suggestive of enterocolitis. Am. J. Roentgenol. *83*:919, 1960.

84. Morson, B. C. Histopathology of cathartic colon. Gut *12*:867, 1971.

85. Meisel, J. L., Bergman, D., Saunders, D. R., and Graney, D. Human rectal mucosa: Proctoscopic and morphologic changes caused by laxatives. Gastroenterology *70*:918, 1976.

86. Lingeman, J. E., Dick, W. H., and Sherrill, W. L. Ammonium urate urolithiasis—a marker for laxative abuse? J. Urol. *137*:158A, 1987.

87. Wittoesch, J. H., Jackman, R. J., and McDonald, J. R. Melanosis coli: General review and a study of 887 cases. Dis. Colon Rectum *1*:172, 1958.

88. Ewe, K., and Karbach, U. Factitious diarrhoea. Clin. Gastroenterol. *15*:723, 1986.

89. Smith, B. Pathologic changes in the colon produced by anthraquinone purgatives. Dis. Colon Rectum *16*:455, 1973.

90. Dufour, P., and Gendre, P. Ultrastructure of mouse intestinal mucosa and changes observed after long term anthraquinone administration. Gut *25*:1358, 1984.

91. de Wolff, F. A., de Haas, E. J. M., and Verweij, M. A screening method for establishing laxative abuse. Clin. Chem. *27*:914, 1981.

92. McGill, D. B., Miller, L. J., Carney, J. A., Phillips, S. F., Go, V. L. W., and Schutt, A. J. Hormonal diarrhea due to pancreatic tumor. Gastroenterology *79*:571, 1980.

93. Plumeri, P. A. Gastroenterology and the law. J. Clin. Gastroenterol. *6*:181–185, 1984.

94. Cummings, J. H., Sladen, G. E., James, O. F. W., Sarner, M., and Misiewicz, J. J. Laxative-induced diarrhoea: A continuing clinical problem. Br. Med. J. *1*:537, 1974.

95. Slugg, P. H., and Carey, W. D. Clinical features and follow-up of surreptitious laxative users. Cleveland Clin. Q. *51*:167, 1984.

96. Lindström, C. G. "Collagenous colitis" with watery diarrhea: A new entity? Pathol. Eur. *11*:87, 1976.

97. Giardiello, F. M., Bayless, T. M., Jessurun, J., Hamilton, S. R., and Yardley, J. H. Collagenous colitis: Physiologic and histopathologic studies in seven patients. Ann. Intern. Med. *106*:46, 1987.

98. Rams, H., Rogers, A. I., and Ghandur-Mnaymneh, L. Collagenous colitis. Ann. Intern. Med. *106*:108, 1987.

99. Rask-Madsen, J., Grove, O., Hansen, M. G. J., Bukhave, K., Scient, C., and Henrik-Nielsen, R. Colonic transport of water and electrolytes in a patient with secretory diarrhea due to collagenous colitis. Dig. Dis. Sci. *28*:1141, 1983.

100. Palmer, K. R., Berry, H., Wheeler, P. J., Williams, C. B., Fairclough, P., Morson, B. C., and Silk, D. B. Collagenous colitis—a relapsing and remitting disease. Gut *27*:578, 1986.

101. Flejou, J. F., Grimaud, J. A., Molas, G., Baviera, E., and Potet, F. Collagenous colitis. Arch. Pathol. Lab. Med. *108*:977, 1984.

102. Kingham, J. G. C., Levison, D. A., Morson, B. C., and Dawson, A. M. Collagenous colitis. Gut *27*:570, 1986.

103. Guarda, L. A., Nelson, R. S., Stroehlein, J. R., Korinek, J. K., and Raymond, A. K. Collagenous colitis. Am. J. Clin. Pathol. *80*:503, 1983.

104. Jesserun, J., Yardley, J. H., Lee, E. L., Vendrell, D. D., Schiller, L. R., and Fordtran, J. S. Microscopic and collagenous colitis: Different names for the same condition? Gastroenterology *91*:153, 1986.

105. Teglbjaerg, P. S., Thaysen, E. H., and Jensen, H. H. Development of collagenous colitis in sequential biopsy specimens. Gastroenterology *87*:703, 1984.

106. Pariente, E. A., and Maitre, F. Collagenous colitis. Dig. Dis. Sci. *31*:222, 1986.

107. Pieterse, A. S., Hecker, R., and Rowland, R. Collagenous colitis: A distinctive and potentially reversible disorder. J. Clin. Pathol. *35*:338, 1982.

108. Yeshaya, C., Novis, B., Bernheim, J., Leichtmann, G., Samara, M., and Griffel, B. Collagenous colitis. Dis. Colon Rectum *27*:111, 1984.

109. Kingham, J. G. C., Levison, D. A., Ball, J. A., and Dawson, A. M. Microscopic colitis—a cause of chronic watery diarrhoea. Br. Med. J. *28*:1601, 1982.

110. Lanspa, S. S., Chan, A. T. H., Bell, J. S., Go, V. L. W., Dickson, E. R., and Dimagno, E. P. Pathogenesis of steatorrhea in primary biliary cirrhosis. Hepatology *5*:837, 1985.

111. Atkinson, M., Nordin, B. E. C., and Sherlock, S. Malabsorption and bone disease in prolonged obstructive jaundice. Q. J. Med. *25*:299, 1956.

112. Bo-Linn, G. W., and Fordtran, J. S. Fecal fat concentration in patients with steatorrhea. Gastroenterology *87*:319, 1984.

113. Letters to the Editor. Gastroenterology *88*:857, *89*:230, *89*:231, 1985.

114. Pedersen, N. T., Halgreen, H., and Worning, H. Estimation of the three days fecal fat concentration as a test of exocrine pancreatic insufficiency. Scand. J. Gastro. *20*(suppl. 113):28, 1985.

115. McJunkin, B., Fromm, H., Sarva, R. P., and Amin, P. Factors in the mechanisms of diarrhea in bile acid malabsorption: Fecal pH—a key determinant. Gastroenterology *80*:1454, 1981.

116. Thaysen, E. H., and Pederson, L. Idiopathic bile acid catharsis. Gut *17*:965, 1976.

117. Thaysen, E. H. Idiopathic bile acid diarrhoea reconsidered. Scand. J. Gastroenterol. *20*:452, 1985.

118. Balistreri, W. F., Partin, J. C., and Schubert, W. K. Bile acid malabsorption—a consequence of terminal ileal dysfunction in protracted diarrhea of infancy. J. Pediatr. *89*:21, 1977.

119. Fromm, F., Tunuguntla, A. K., Malavolti, M., Sherman, C., and Ceryak, S. Absence of significant role of bile acids in diarrhea of a heterogeneous group of postcholecystectomy patients. Dig. Dis. Sci. *32*:33, 1987.

120. Hutcheon, D. F., Bayless, T. M., and Gadacz, T. R. Postcholecystectomy diarrhea. JAMA *241*:823, 1979.

121. Ladas, S. D., Isaacs, P. E. T., Quereshi, Y., and Sladen, G. Role of the small intestine in postvagotomy diarrhea. Gastroenterology *85*:1088, 1983.

122. Raimes, S. A., Wheldon, E. J., Smirniotis, V., Venables, C. W., and Johnston, I. D. A. Postvagotomy diarrhoea put into perspective. Lancet *2*:851, 1986.

123. Clark, C. G., Karamanolis, D., and Ward, M. W. N. Preference for proximal gastric vagotomy combined with cholecystectomy. Br. J. Surg. *71*:185, 1984.

124. Duncombe, V. M., Bolin, T. D., and David, A. E. Double-blind trial of cholestyramine in postvagotomy diarrhoea. Gut *18*:531, 1977.

125. Burge, H., Hutchison, J. S. F., Longland, C. J., McLennan, I., Miln, D. C., Rudick, J., and Tompkin, A. M. B. Selective nerve section in the prevention of post-vagotomy diarrhoea. Lancet *1*:577, 1964.

126. Wingate, D. L. Postvagotomy diarrhea. Gastroenterology *87*:250, 1984.

127. Allan, J. G., Gerskowitch, V. P., and Russell, R. I. The role of bile acids in the pathogenesis of post-vagotomy diarrhoea. Br. J. Surg. *61*:516, 1974.

128. Blake, G., Kennedy, T. L., and McKelvey, S. T. D. Bile acids and post-vagotomy diarrhoea. Br. J. Surg. *70*:177–179, 1983.

129. Taylor, T. V., Lambert, M. E., and Torrance, H. B. Value of bile-acid binding agents in post-vagotomy diarrhoea. Lancet *1*:635, 1978.

130. Cuschieri, A. Surgical management of severe intractable post-vagotomy diarrhoea. Br. J. Surg. *73*:981, 1986.

131. Herrington, J. L., and Sawyers, J. L. A new operation for the dumping syndrome and post-vagotomy diarrhea. Ann. Surg. *175*:790, 1972.

132. Bargen, J. A., et al. Diarrhea of diabetes and steatorrhea of pancreatic insufficiency. Mayo Clin. Proc. *2*:737, 1936.

133. Miller, L. J. Small intestinal manifestations of diabetes mellitus. Yale J. Biol. Med. *56*:189, 1983.

134. Rundles, R. W. Diabetic neuropathy: General review with report of 125 cases. Medicine *24*:111, 1945.

135. Schiller, L. R., Santa Ana, C. A., Schmulen, A. C., Hendler, R. S., Harford, W. V., and Fordtran, J. S. Pathogenesis of fecal incontinence in diabetes mellitus. N. Engl. J. Med. *307*:1666, 1982.

136. Malins, J. M., and French, J. M. Diabetic diarrhoea. Q. J. Med. *104*:467, 1957.

137. Whalen, G. E., Soergel, K. H., and Geenen, J. E. Diabetic diarrhea. Gastroenterology *56*:1021, 1969.

138. Field, M., Fromm, D., and McColl, I. Ion transport in rabbit ileal mucosa. I. Na and Cl fluxes and short-circuit current. Am. J. Physiol. *220*:1388, 1971.

139. Chang, E. B., Field, M., and Miller, R. J. Alpha$_2$-adrenergic receptor regulation of ion transport in rabbit ileum. Am. J. Physiol. *242*:G237, 1982.

140. Chang, E. B., Bergenstal, R. M., and Field, M. Diarrhea in streptozocin-treated rats. J. Clin. Invest. *75*:1666, 1985.

141. Chang, E. B., Fedorak, R. N., and Field, M. Experimental diabetic diarrhea in rats. Gastroenterology *91*:564, 1986.

142. Fedorak, R. N., Field, M., and Chang, E. B. Treatment of diabetic diarrhea with clonidine. Ann. Intern. Med. *102*:197, 1985.

143. Schiller, L. R., Santa, C. A., Morawski, S. G., and Fordtran, J. S. Studies of the antidiarrheal action of clonidine. Gastroenterology *89*:982, 1985.

144. Molloy, A. M., and Tomkin, G. H. Altered bile in diabetic diarrhoea. Br. Med. J. *2*:1462, 1978.

145. Vinnik, I. E., Kern, F., Jr., and Struthers, J. E. Malabsorption and the diarrhea of diabetes mellitus. Gastroenterology *43*:507, 1962.

146. Goff, J. S. Diabetic diarrhea and lidamidine. Ann. Intern. Med. *101*:874, 1984.

147. Tsai, S. T., Vinik, A. I., and Brunner, J. F. Diabetic diarrhea and somatostatin. Ann. Intern. Med. *104*:894, 1986.

148. Blumenthal, H. T., et al. Interrelationships of diabetes mellitus and pancreatitis. Arch. Surg. *87*:844, 1963.

149. Goldstein, F., et al. Diabetic diarrhea and steatorrhea. Microbiologic and clinical observations. Ann. Intern. Med. *72*:215, 1970.

150. Maki, M., Hallstrom, O., Hunpponen, T., Vesikari, T., and Visakorpi, J. K. Increased prevalence of coeliac disease in diabetes. Arch. Dis. Child. *59*:739, 1984.

151. Robles, E. A., Mezey, E., Halsted, C. H., et al. Effect of ethanol on motility of the small intestine. Johns Hopkins Med. J. *135*:17, 1974.

152. Martin, J. L., Justus, P. G., and Mathias, J. A. Altered motility of the small intestine in response to ethanol (ETOH): An explanation for the diarrhea associated with the consumption of alcohol. Gastroenterology *78*:1218, 1980.

153. Keshavarzian, A., Iber, F. L., Dangleis, M. D., and Cornish, R. Intestinal transit and lactose intolerance in chronic alcoholics. Am. J. Clin. Nutr. *44*:70, 1986.

154. Perlow, W., Baraona, E., and Leiber, C. S. Symptomatic intestinal disaccharidase deficiency in alcoholics. Gastroenterology *72*:680, 1977.

155. Roggin, G. M., Iber, I. L., and Linscheer, W. G. Intraluminal fat digestion in the chronic alcoholic. Gut *13*:107, 1972.

156. Linscheer, W. G. Malabsorption in cirrhosis. Am. J. Clin. Nutr. *23*:488, 1970.

157. Mezey, E., Jow, E., Slavin, R. E., et al. Pancreatic function and intestinal absorption in chronic alcoholism. Gastroenterology *59*:657, 1970.

158. Thompson, A. L., Baker, M., and Leevy, C. M. Patterns of 35 S-thiamine hydrochloride absorption in the malnourished alcoholic patient. J. Lab. Clin. Med. *76*:34, 1970.

159. Lindenbaum, J., and Leiber, C. S. Effect of chronic ethanol administration on intestinal absorption in man in the absence of nutritional deficiency. Ann. N.Y. Acad. Sci. *252*:228, 1975.

160. Halsted, C. H., Robles, E. A., and Mezey, E. Decreased jejunal intake of folic acid in alcoholic patients: Roles of alcohol and nutrition. N. Engl. J. Med. *285*:701, 1971.

161. Halsted, C. H., Robles, E. A., and Mezey, E. Intestinal malabsorption in folate deficient alcoholics. Gastroenterology *64*:526, 1973.

162. Geokas, M. C., Lieber, C. S., French, S., and Halsted, C. H. Ethanol, the liver, and the gastrointestinal tract. Ann. Intern. Med. *95*:198, 1981.

163. Dinda, P. K., and Beck, I. T. On the mechanism of the inhibitory effect of ethanol on intestinal glucose and water absorption. Dig. Dis. Sci. *22*:529, 1977.

164. Chang, T., Lewis, J., and Glazko, A. J. Effect of ethanol and other alcohols on the transport of amino acids and glucose by everted gut sacs of rat small intestine. Biochim. Biophys. Acta *135*:1000, 1967.

165. Mekhjian, H. S., and May, E. S. Acute and chronic effects of ethanol on fluid transport in the human small intestine. Gastroenterology *72*:1280, 1977.

166. Krasner, N., Cochran, K. M., Russell, R. I., et al. Alcohol and absorption from the small intestine. I. Impairment of absorption from the small intestine in alcoholics. Gut *17*:245, 1976.

167. Burbige, E. J., Lewis, D. R., Jr., and Halsted, C. K. Alcohol and the gastrointestinal tract. Med. Clin. North Am. *88*:77, 1984.

168. Van Thiel, D. H., Lipsitz, H. D., Porter, L. E., Schade, R. R., Gottlieb, G. P., and Graham, T. O. Gastrointestinal and hepatic manifestations of chronic alcoholism. Gastroenterology *81*:594, 1981.

169. Blaser, M. J. Brainerd diarrhea: A newly recognized raw milk–associated enteropathy. JAMA *256*:510, 1986.

170. Osterholm, M. T., MacDonald, K. L., White, K. E., Wells, J. G., Spika, J. S., Potter, M. E., Forfang, J. C., Sorenson, R. M., Milloy, P. T., and Blake, P. A. An outbreak of a newly recognized chronic diarrhea syndrome associated with raw milk consumption. JAMA *256*:484, 1986.

171. Centers for Disease Control. Chronic diarrhea associated with raw milk consumption—Minnesota. JAMA *252*:1996, 1984.

172. Martin, D. L., and Hoberman, L. J. A point source outbreak of chronic diarrhea in Texas: No known exposure to raw milk. JAMA *256*:469, 1986.

21

Fecal Incontinence

LAWRENCE R. SCHILLER

Fecal continence is the ability to defer defecation until an appropriate time at an appropriate place. Most people can take fecal continence for granted. Those who cannot experience lives of quiet desperation characterized by anxiety and fear and punctuated by episodes of embarrassment and shame. For fear of an episode of incontinence in a public place, patients often become reclusive, venturing out of their homes only when absolutely necessary. In many ways it is among the most disabling of gastrointestinal symptoms.

Incontinence is a problem that affects society, too. Fecal incontinence is often the major factor in the decision to institutionalize an elderly family member. These patients require two to three times the amount of nursing care as similar, but continent, patients. The care of institutionalized, incontinent patients costs an estimated $8 billion in the United States each year.[1]

PREVALENCE

Reliable data on the prevalence of fecal incontinence in the United States is not available. One study suggests that approximately 5 per cent of the general population may have some problem with fecal soiling, but it is likely that most of these individuals had only a very slight problem.[2] In England, the prevalence of fecal incontinence in the general population has been estimated to be as high as 0.4 per cent and in the elderly population (>65 years old) at between 1.0 and 1.3 per cent.[3] In one study of residents of homes for the elderly in England, approximately 10 per cent of the residents had fecal incontinence at least once weekly.[4] In other studies as many as 50 per cent of institutionalized patients had fecal incontinence.[5, 6]

In analyzing these reports of the prevalence of fecal incontinence, one must realize that incontinence is an intermittent symptom and may be the result of physical barriers placed in the way of defecation in an appropriate place, not just a loss of the ability to control defecation. An "accident" may result from an unanswered call to the nurse for assistance as well as from a true problem with the patient's continence mechanisms. Alternatively, a mobile patient with a continence problem may not have any episodes of incontinence if he stays at home or in a hospital room only a few steps away from a toilet. Thus, the presence or absence of incontinence must be judged against the opportunity for it to occur in a certain situation. This is particularly important to bear in mind when evaluating the results of therapy for incontinence.

Another factor which can alter the occurrence of incontinence is the stress placed on the continence mechanisms. Liquid stools put a great stress on the continence mechanisms and this may bring out latent problems with the neuromuscular machinery regulating continence. Paradoxically, this leads to underreporting of incontinence because many of these patients (and their doctors) view incontinence as just a manifestation of particularly severe diarrhea. Patients with incontinence presenting as chronic diarrhea rarely volunteer a history of incontinence and must be asked specifically about it.[7, 8]

MECHANISMS OF CONTINENCE AND INCONTINENCE

Continence is the result of a series of barriers to the aboral movement of feces. These barriers are reversible and can be removed to allow for defecation. The barriers are redundant; under ordinary conditions incontinence usually results only when more than one of the barriers are compromised. To understand the physiology of continence one must understand the anatomic arrangements that produce these barriers and the dynamic responses that reinforce these barriers when stressed and remove them when defecation is appropriate. Disruption of the anatomic arrangements or dysfunction of the dynamic responses can lead to incontinence.[9-18]

Functional Anatomy

The structures basic to continence include (1) the rectum, (2) the internal anal sphincter, (3) the external anal sphincter, (4) the pelvic diaphragm including the puborectalis muscle, and (5) the innervation of this area which coordinates the activity of these structures.

As the colon enters the pelvis, the longitudinal muscle layer becomes continuous around the circumference of the rectum. The rectal mucosa is thrown up into a series of bands, the valves of Houston (Fig. 21–1). At the distal end of the rectum, the circular muscle layer becomes two to three times thicker than usual, forming the internal anal sphincter (Fig. 21–2). The sphincter is a typical smooth muscle sphincter and is able to maintain tonic contraction for extended periods of time. The columnar epithelium of the colon joins the squamous epithelium of the anal canal at the dentate line (Fig. 21–1). The anal canal is not circular

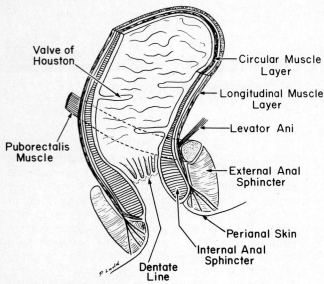

Figure 21–1. Anatomy of the rectum and anus.

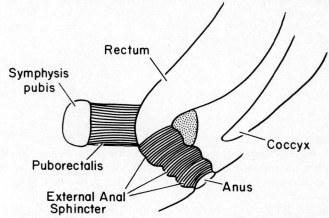

Figure 21–3. Relationship of external anal sphincter, puborectalis muscle, and rectum.

in cross section, but rather is slit-like, with the slit oriented in the anterior-posterior direction. In the anal canal, spongy vascular tissue underlies the mucosa forming the so-called anal cushions.[19]

The external anal sphincter, a voluntary striated muscle, surrounds the internal sphincter and extends distally to the subcutaneous tissue surrounding the anus (Fig. 21–3). It is composed of both "red" and "white" fibers and shares some of the electromechanical properties of antigravity muscles elsewhere in the body.[20]

As the distal rectum passes inferiorly through the pelvis on its way to join the anal canal, it passes through a muscular layer, the pelvic diaphragm. This striated muscle and its central ligament form a continuous sheet dividing the abdominal cavity from the perineum, closing off the base of the pelvis. The pelvic diaphragm is pierced by orifices for the rectum, vagina, and urethra and surrounds each of these structures. It is composed of the same type of skeletal muscle fibers

as the external anal sphincter and shares similar physiologic properties (e.g., the ability to generate continuous contraction).[21] Named components of the pelvic diaphragm include the levator ani, pubococcygeus, iliococcygeus, and the puborectalis muscle.[22]

The puborectalis muscle consists of a group of fibers in the pelvic diaphragm which extend from the pubic arch around the posterior part of the rectum and back to the pubic arch (Fig. 21–4). When this muscle is contracted, it draws the rectum forward, producing an angulation between the axis of the rectum and the axis of the anal canal of approximately 90 degrees (Fig. 21–4A). This angle seems to be crucial for maintaining continence for solid stool. This probably has to do with several factors. First, the rheologic characteristics of a bolus of solid stool would make it difficult to negotiate a sharp curve. Second, the angulation occludes the lumen, increasing drag on the fecal bolus. Third, the orientation of this angle makes it likely that increases in intra-abdominal pressure, which might threaten continence, result in compression of the anterior wall of the rectum against the posterior wall, further occluding the lumen.[9] When defecation is imminent, the puborectalis muscle relaxes, straightening out the rectoanal angle and allowing increases in intra-abdominal and intraluminal pressure to expel feces (Fig. 21–4B). Of all the voluntary muscles responsible for maintaining continence, the puborectalis muscle is thought to be the most important. Transection of this muscle (as occasionally happens accidentally during anorectal surgical procedures) usually results in incontinence for solid stool. Weakness of this muscle and straightening of the anorectal angle are frequent findings in idiopathic fecal incontinence (see below).

The innervation of the muscles in this region and the nerves supplying sensory structures in the area are also important in maintaining continence (Fig. 21–5).[11, 23] The skeletal muscle of the pelvic diaphragm and of the external anal sphincter is absolutely dependent on the somatic nerve supply from sacral levels of the spinal cord. The puborectalis is supplied by direct branches from the third and fourth sacral nerves, which

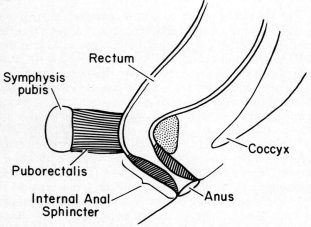

Figure 21–2. Lateral schematic view of relationships of the rectum, internal anal sphincter, and puborectalis muscle.

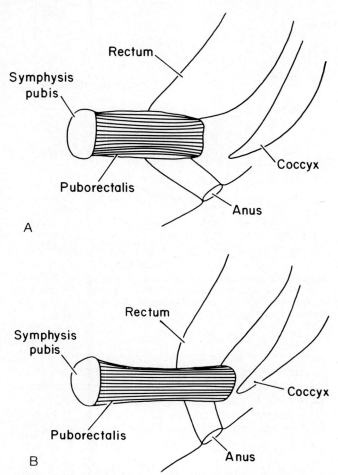

Figure 21–4. *A*, Puborectalis muscle contracting to maintain the rectoanal angle at approximately 90 degrees. *B*, Puborectalis muscle relaxing to allow straightening of the rectoanal angle for defecation.

receptors, including those for pain, touch, and temperature. The voluntary muscles of the pelvic diaphragm have the usual array of stretch receptors, but these receptors may be of unusual importance in generating conscious feelings from this area.

Dynamics of Continence

Although the structures just discussed mediate continence, the mechanisms of continence are related to the dynamic responses of these structures to the movement of feces. The dynamic components of continence include (1) the delivery of colon contents to the rectum, (2) rectal compliance and accommodation, (3) internal anal sphincter responses, (4) rectal and pelvic sensation, and (5) skeletal muscle responses. Abnormalities in any of these dynamic components can impair continence.

The delivery of colon contents to the rectum depends on the function of the more proximal bowel. The more proximal bowel determines not only the amount of feces presented to the rectum but also the consistency of the feces and the rate at which material enters the rectum (see p. 292). Because the rectum is usually empty in most people,[28] it appears that feces are retained in the sigmoid colon and are presented to the rectum only intermittently. The motility patterns underlying this process are not well understood (see p. 1090). Some have postulated a special motility pattern or sphincter at the rectosigmoid junction, but this idea is controversial.[29] It seems likely that the sigmoid colon controls the presentation of material to the rectum and

ramify on the superior surface of the pelvic diaphragm.[24] The external anal sphincter is supplied by branches from the pudendal nerve.

The rectum and internal anal sphincter are supplied by extrinsic autonomic nerves arising from the lumbosacral spinal cord and distributed through the pelvic plexus.[25] These nerves include both elements of the sympathetic and parasympathetic nervous systems and both efferent and afferent fibers. These extrinsic nerves probably mediate their effects at least in part through the intrinsic nerves of the myenteric plexus, but the details of this innervation are not yet known in humans. Ganglia of the intrinsic nervous system of the gut are present in the rectum but are not found in the internal anal sphincter. It is likely though that nerve fibers originating in the myenteric plexus in the rectum also innervate the internal anal sphincter.

The sensory innervation of this area also appears to be important to the preservation of continence.[26, 27] The rectal mucosa and muscle are innervated like the rest of the intestine (see pp. 38–46) and are sensitive only to distention. In contrast, the epithelium of the anal canal is richly supplied with a variety of sensory

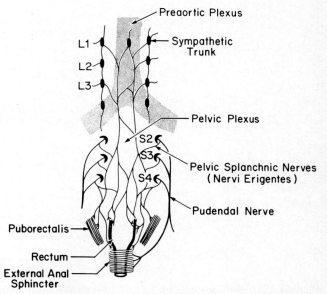

Figure 21–5. Innervation of structures involved with continence. Sympathetic fibers from the lumbar cord and preaortic plexus descend to join parasympathetic nerves from the sacral cord in the pelvic plexus. These nerves supply the sigmoid colon, rectum, and internal anal sphincter. Somatic nerves from sacral roots supply the puborectalis directly and the external anal sphincter via the pudendal nerves.

that the continence mechanisms are designed to best handle delivery of the normal amount of solid stool each day (about 100 gm). Otherwise normal individuals can usually maintain continence for liquid stools as well, but in some situations voluminous phasic flows of liquid stool may produce urgency and incontinence by overwhelming the continence mechanisms.[7]

When feces enter the rectum, they must be accommodated there if defecation is to be delayed. This is accomplished by the process of rectal compliance.[30-34] The muscle of the rectum is capable of relaxing, reducing intraluminal pressure to a level that will not threaten continence and maintaining a relatively low intraluminal pressure while filling (Fig. 21–6A and B). The rectum can serve as a reservoir much like the proximal stomach. Rectal accommodation to distention appears to depend on an intact intrinsic nervous system and on viable smooth muscle; it is impaired in both Hirschsprung's disease, in which the intrinsic neural plexus is abnormal,[31] and chronic rectal ischemia (Fig. 21–7), in which fibrosis produces a rigid rectal wall.[34] A similar mechanism may underlie urgency and incontinence in patients with inflammatory bowel disease.[32, 33]

The internal anal sphincter is responsible for the bulk of the resting pressure in the anal canal.[35-37] This tonic contraction is probably due in part to intrinsic myogenic properties of the smooth muscle[38] and also to the action of intrinsic and extrinsic autonomic

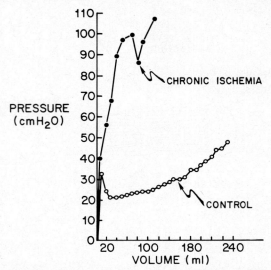

Figure 21–7. Rectal compliance in a normal subject and in a patient with chronic rectal ischemia. Patients tolerated a much lower volume than normal individuals. (After Devroede, G. Dis. Colon Rectum 25:90, 1982.)

nerves.[25, 39–41] When the rectum is distended, pressure in the upper anal canal (reflecting mainly internal anal sphincter contraction) decreases transiently, indicating relaxation of the internal anal sphincter (Fig. 21–8).[11, 23] In general, this decrease in pressure is proportional to the distending volume and is only a partial relaxation

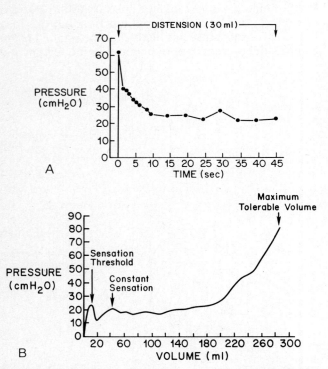

Figure 21–6. Rectal compliance in a normal subject. *A,* Viscous properties of the rectum. An intrarectal balloon was inflated with 30 ml of air, and pressures were monitored. The pressure in the balloon decreased, indicating relaxation of the rectal wall. *B,* Elastic properties of the rectum. An intrarectal balloon was gradually inflated and pressures were monitored. The intraballoon pressure was maintained at a low level until a substantial volume had been introduced. (After Devroede, G. Dis. Colon Rectum 25:90, 1982.)

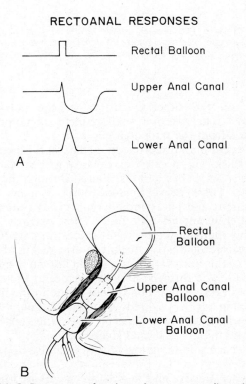

Figure 21–8. Responses of anal canal pressure to distention of a balloon in the rectum. The upper anal canal (reflecting largely the internal anal sphincter) relaxes and the lower anal canal (reflecting largely the external anal sphincter) contracts transiently.

unless very large distending volumes are used. This reflex is mediated by the intrinsic neural plexus of the rectum and is missing in Hirschsprung's disease (see p. 337).[11, 42, 43]

The importance of the internal anal sphincter in maintaining continence is controversial. Some cite the reflex relaxation of the internal sphincter or the fact that transection of the internal sphincter (i.e., sphincterotomy) results in only a modest compromise of continence as evidence that the internal anal sphincter is of little or no importance to the preservation of continence.[9] Others note that the internal anal sphincter regains its tone as the rectum accommodates to distention and suggest that the internal anal sphincter provides the bulk of the pressure barrier at the anus, even with rectal distention.[44] Weakness of the internal sphincter has been implicated in fecal incontinence occurring in diabetics[45] and in patients who have had anal dilatation for the treatment of hemorrhoids.[46, 47]

Rectal or pelvic sensation is central to continence because it initiates the dynamic responses to threats to continence and brings awareness of the need for defecation to consciousness. Autonomic and somatic responses to rectal distention have different thresholds, are affected differently by disease states, and may involve different receptors and pathways.[48] Autonomic responses (e.g., internal sphincter relaxation in response to rectal distention) are organized within the myenteric plexus and may also involve reflex arcs to the spinal cord. Whether information from autonomic stretch receptors in the rectal wall reaches consciousness is not known but seems likely.[23] The perception of rectal distention may also be mediated by stretch receptors in the muscle of the pelvic diaphragm and requires intact somatic nerves as well as intact pathways from the spinal cord to brain.[16] Some mechanism like this probably accounts for reflex activation of the pelvic diaphragm during acute increases in intra-abdominal pressure as with coughing.[15]

Most people can differentiate solid, liquid, and gas in the rectum. The mechanism of this awareness is not certain. Some investigators have postulated that internal anal sphincter relaxation at the time of rectal distention allows a small amount of rectal contents to come in contact with the sensitive lining of the anal canal.[13] Whether this so-called sampling response is important or not cannot be decided at present.[16]

Defective rectal or pelvic sensation or perception may contribute to the incontinence seen in patients with altered mental status (i.e., stroke, encephalopathy, dementia) who may not recognize or respond to threats to continence. This may also be a factor in patients with neurologic diseases or sensory neuropathy. For instance, patients with diabetes mellitus and fecal incontinence have higher than normal thresholds for conscious perception of rectal distention, which may contribute to incontinence.[48] Abnormal anorectal sensation may also contribute to incontinence in patients with fecal impaction.[49] Some patients with incontinence have been reported to have a delay in the recognition of rectal distention, which may promote fecal soiling.[50] These studies need to be interpreted

with caution, however. Anorectal sensation is a subjective phenomenon and often studies have not been adequately controlled or blinded.

Skeletal muscle responses cued by rectal and pelvic sensation are central to the defense of continence. Tension in the puborectalis muscle is under reflex control, increasing when increases in intra-abdominal or intrarectal pressure threaten continence, but also maintaining tonic activity.[15] The origin of this tonic activity must be at a spinal level, but details of its control or its inhibition during defecation are unknown.

The external anal sphincter is under similar control with both tonic and phasic activity. Rectal distention induces an increase in lower anal canal pressure attributed to contraction of the external anal sphincter (Fig. 21–8).[11] This has been thought to be a spinal reflex but may be a learned response.[51] The phasic increase in external anal sphincter contraction lasts only a few seconds, and voluntary external anal sphincter contraction fatigues after approximately one minute. Consequently, external anal sphincter contraction can only delay defecation for a short time, while the rectum accommodates to an increase in volume.

Abnormal skeletal muscle function is a frequently encountered problem in patients with fecal incontinence. Histopathologic[52, 53] and electromyographic[54–63] studies show that many patients with idiopathic fecal incontinence have evidence of denervation of the puborectalis and external anal sphincter muscles. This situation is often seen as part of the "perineal descent syndrome" in which weakness of the entire pelvic diaphragm can be demonstrated, with straightening of the rectoanal angle and ballooning of the perineum with straining. It has been postulated that repeated stretching of the pelvic diaphragm injures the motor nerves that run on the surface of these muscles, causing progressive denervation and weakness.[62] Some have questioned whether progressive weakness alone accounts for incontinence in patients with perineal descent, however.[63] In general, both the puborectalis and external anal sphincter must be weakened for incontinence to complicate the course of perineal descent syndrome.[64] More severe impairment of the external anal sphincter seems to predispose these patients to incontinence of solid as well as liquid stools.[65] A similar mechanism of neuropathic injury has been postulated to contribute to incontinence following childbirth.[66] Prolonged labor may damage the motor nerves to the skeletal muscle of the pelvic diaphragm and sphincter and this, rather than perineal tears alone, may result in defective continence in multiparous women.[66, 67]

Defecation

For stool to be ejected from the rectum, the barriers that constitute the continence mechanisms must be removed. The process of defecation begins when sufficient material enters the rectum and evokes a "call to stool."[16] This can be duplicated by distention of a balloon in the rectum with approximately 50 to 60 ml of air or water. The physiologic equivalent of this is

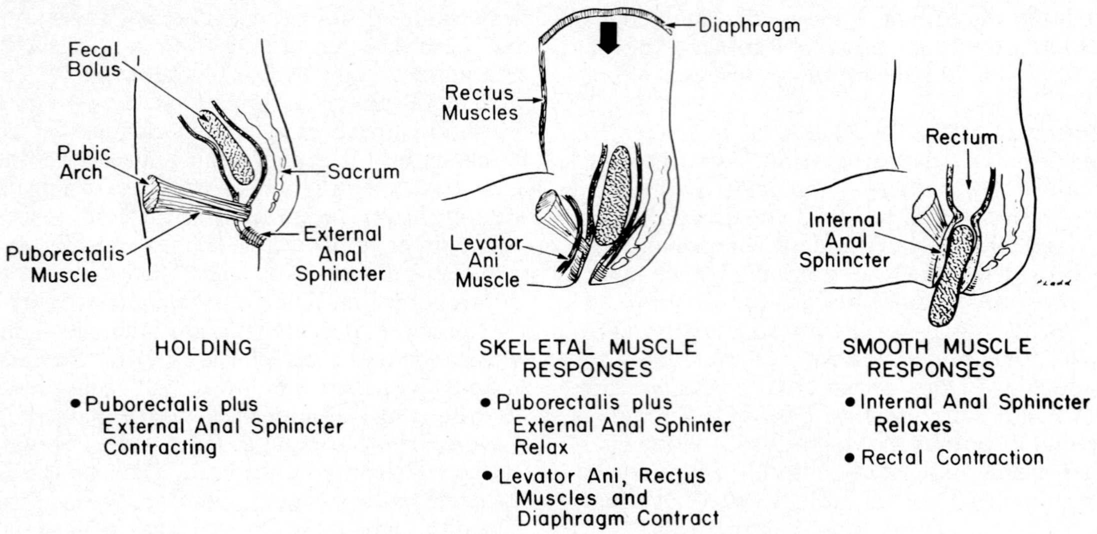

HOLDING

• Puborectalis plus
  External Anal Sphincter
  Contracting

SKELETAL MUSCLE
RESPONSES

• Puborectalis plus
  External Anal Sphinter
  Relax
• Levator Ani, Rectus
  Muscles and
  Diaphragm Contract

SMOOTH MUSCLE
RESPONSES

• Internal Anal Sphincter
  Relaxes
• Rectal Contraction

Figure 21–9. Mechanism of defecation.

not well defined. If continence mechanisms are intact, defecation can be delayed until the person reaches a place appropriate for defecation (Fig. 21–9). At that time the person sits or squats and the puborectalis muscle and external anal sphincter are inhibited, allowing the rectoanal angle to straighten out. The levator ani muscle contracts, limiting inferior movement of the pelvic floor and anus with straining. Internal sphincter tone is inhibited, the person performs a Valsalva maneuver and contracts the muscles of the anterior abdominal wall, thus increasing intra-abdominal pressure. This tends to force stool distally and may help to initiate a contraction in the sigmoid colon and proximal rectum, ejecting stool through the anus.[12] It has been postulated that a defecation reflex organized in the spinal cord results in persistence of the colonic and rectal contraction as long as stool is in contact with the sensitive epithelium of the anal canal.[12] Defecation can occur as a coordinated response even in paraplegics and thus can be organized by the lumbosacral cord without intact connections to the brain.[23] Disturbances of the continence mechanisms can lead to incomplete removal of the barriers to defecation and the syndrome of obstructed defecation, manifested as the complaint of constipation (see pp. 331–368).

DIFFERENTIAL DIAGNOSIS

With the complexity of the mechanisms preserving continence, it is no wonder that a variety of diseases have been associated with incontinence (Table 21–1). In general these diseases compromise the anatomic integrity of the structures of the continence mechanisms or impair one or more of the dynamic factors maintaining continence. For most of these entities our understanding of the pathophysiology leading to incontinence is incomplete. In most of these diseases, multiple defects in the continence mechanisms have been identified.

Neurologic diseases are prominent causes of incontinence because continence depends on the perception of threats to continence and is defended by neurally mediated reflexes and responses. In addition, neuropathic weakness of the skeletal muscle of the pelvic floor and external anal sphincter appears to be an important cause of "idiopathic" fecal incontinence. The variety of neurologic diseases associated with incontinence includes all those that cause a depressed sensorium, affect the brainstem or spinal cord, or affect the peripheral nerves (Table 21–1).

Skeletal muscle diseases such as myasthenia gravis have been associated with fecal incontinence. Other skeletal muscle diseases which result in muscle weakness may also predispose to fecal incontinence, but the extent to which they do so is not certain from the literature because only scattered cases have been described.

Smooth muscle of the rectum or internal anal sphincter can be dysfunctional and lead to incontinence. This can be related to abnormal rectal compliance, such as is seen with proctitis[32, 33] or ischemia,[34] or to weakness of the internal anal sphincter, causing low basal sphincter pressures. For most of these entities it is unclear whether the defect is within the smooth muscle itself or its autonomic innervation.

A variety of anatomic derangements can be responsible for fecal incontinence. Although the pathogenesis of incontinence is obvious in most of these problems, multiple mechanisms may be present. For instance, rectal prolapse is complicated by incontinence only when sphincteric function is compromised.[56, 60, 68] Another example of multiple mechanisms is childbirth injury in which direct tears of the sphincter are only part of the problem; a traumatic neuropathy may also be present in many patients with postpartum incontinence.[66, 67]

The miscellaneous category includes conditions in which the delivery of stool to the rectum may be abnormal (e.g., overwhelmingly voluminous diarrhea

Table 21–1. DIFFERENTIAL DIAGNOSIS OF FECAL INCONTINENCE BY TYPE OF DISEASE AND AREA OF DYSFUNCTION

Neurologic Diseases
Central nervous system processes
    Dementia, sedation, mental retardation
    Stroke, brain tumors, spinal cord lesions
    Multiple sclerosis
    Tabes dorsalis
Peripheral nervous system processes
    Cauda equina lesions
    Polyneuropathies
        Diabetes mellitus[45, 48]
        Shy-Drager syndrome
        Toxic neuropathy
    Traumatic neuropathy
        ? "Idiopathic" incontinence[52–63]
        Perineal descent[53, 62, 64]
        Postpartum[66, 67]
Altered rectal sensation (site of lesion not known)
    Fecal impaction[49]
    "Delayed sensation" syndrome[50]

Skeletal Muscle Diseases
  Myasthenia gravis
  ? Myopathies

Smooth Muscle Dysfunction
Abnormal rectal compliance
    Proctitis due to inflammatory bowel disease[32, 33]
    Radiation proctitis[69]
    Rectal ischemia[34]
    ? Fecal impaction
Internal anal sphincter weakness
    Radiation proctitis[69]
    Diabetes mellitus[45]
    Childhood encopresis[70]

Anatomic Derangements
  Congenital anomalies of the anorectum
  Fistula
  Rectal prolapse/procidentia
  Anorectal trauma
    Injury
    Surgery (including hemorrhoidectomy)
    Childbirth injury
  Sequelae of anorectal infections, Crohn's disease

Miscellaneous
  ? Severe diarrhea
  ? Irritable bowel syndrome
  ? Idiopathic hypoparathyroidism
  ? Acute myocardial infarction

or irritable bowel syndrome). Incontinence should be attributed to these causes only when careful investigation reveals no impairment of the continence mechanisms.

EVALUATION OF PATIENTS WITH FECAL INCONTINENCE

The objectives of the evaluation of patients with fecal incontinence are (1) to understand the severity of the problem, (2) to discover treatable diseases that may be causing incontinence, and (3) to understand the pathophysiology of the incontinence problem so that appropriate therapy can be instituted, if possible. These objectives can be reached by a careful history and physical examination and appropriate selection of objective tests.

History. The key to understanding the patient's symptoms is to establish the fact that the patient is incontinent. Few patients will volunteer this symptom and the interviewer must ask about it directly, particularly in patients in whom the chief complaint is chronic diarrhea.[7, 8] A history of fecal incontinence should also be sought in patients with complaints of urgency, constipation, other defecation problems, urinary incontinence, neurologic diseases, muscle diseases, and diabetes mellitus. It may be necessary to use such terms as "leakage," "soiling," or "accidents" to facilitate communication.

Once a history of incontinence is elicited, questioning should be directed at the circumstances under which incontinence occurs. The presence or absence of physical problems or barriers to defecating in an appropriate place (such as the need for assistance to get to the toilet or the need to climb a flight of stairs) should be defined. The frequency with which incontinence is occurring can only be judged against any adaptations that the patient may have made to limit the possibility of an accident. It is also essential to know whether or not loose stools are present, how long incontinence has been present, whether incontinence is occurring only during sleep or some other alteration of consciousness (such as after taking sedatives), or whether it is occurring while the patient is fully awake. Other important information includes what degree of warning the patient has before defecation, whether the patient can defer defecation for any period of time, and when the patient senses that an accident is happening: while it is occurring or only after the fact.

Questioning should then be directed at possible causes of incontinence. The patient should be asked about anorectal trauma, infections, and operations; about straining at stool and difficult childbirth; about problems with skeletal muscle function or symptoms of neuropathy elsewhere in the body; about spinal cord or back injury and stroke; and about the presence of diabetes mellitus. The temporal relationship between any of these conditions and incontinence should be developed, realizing that years may separate an inciting event from the occurrence of fecal incontinence, especially if the patient has recently developed diarrhea and incontinence.

Physical Examination. A careful physical examination can yield important clues as to the integrity of the neuromuscular machinery of continence and can help with the selection of objective tests. For this examination the patient should be made as comfortable as possible and should be placed in the left lateral decubitus position.

The perineum should be inspected for evidence of dermatitis or infection, the presence of scars, and the ability of the patient to maintain local hygiene. A careful search for hemorrhoids, skin tags, or deformity of the anus should be made while the patient is at rest. The anus and perineum should also be inspected while the patient is bearing down to look for rectal prolapse or leakage and ballooning of the perineum, which would suggest perineal descent (devices can be used to measure the degree of perineal descent with straining, but their accuracy has been questioned[71]). The perianal skin should be stroked with a pin to induce the cutaneo-anal contractile reflex in each quadrant.[17] In response to the pin, the subcutaneous external anal sphincter should contract and produce a visible puckering at the anal margin. Failure to elicit this reflex suggests a problem with either the sensory or motor nerves or central connections mediating this reflex.

The gloved examining finger should then be lubricated and inserted into the anal canal. The examiner can gain an impression of the length of the anal canal, the bulk of the perianal tissues, and the tone of the anal sphincter. Although it is impossible to estimate anal sphincter pressure accurately by digital assessment,[7] a frankly patulous anal canal can be recognized by most examiners. The patient should then be asked to squeeze down as if to prevent defecation, and an increase in anal pressure should be appreciated. The cutaneo-anal reflex can again be elicited and the contraction of the external sphincter should be felt by the examining finger. Attention should then be focused on the puborectalis muscle. This muscle can be palpated in the posterior midline as an extrinsic transverse bar. The muscle should be stretched by pulling the examining finger posteriorly; gaping of the anus during this maneuver indicates weakness of the skeletal muscles in the area.[72] The patient should then be asked to try to prevent the passage of stool again, and the puborectalis should move briskly anteriorly. Each quadrant of the anus should then be carefully palpated for the presence of fluctuation or scar. The presence of a fecal impaction or rectal mass should then be sought, and stool should be retrieved for occult blood testing.

Objective Tests. Several tests have been developed which can supply objective information about rectoanal function and capabilities (Table 21–2). Not all these studies need to be done in every patient. The selection of studies should be based on how the results of the study will alter the management of a given patient. In some cases none of the studies will be needed before trying a course of therapy. In most cases, one or more of these will prove useful in defining defects that may be responsible for incontinence or in designing a therapeutic plan. It is essential that these studies be done correctly in centers where enough control studies have been done to define normal results.

Anal manometry can be used to provide a direct measure of the pressures generated in the anal canal under basal conditions and with squeezing. Several different recording devices have been described, and there can be important artifacts with some of them. Perfusion manometry using a small diameter catheter with radially arranged ports and a station pull-through technique is one standard method for recording anal pressures.[7] Other devices include intraluminal transducer arrays and balloon devices.[11, 72] Intraluminal transducer arrays may be as accurate as perfused catheters but care must be taken that the probe on which they are placed is not very stiff or large, because this may alter the measured pressure. Balloon devices are generally inappropriate for measuring absolute pressures in the anal canal because the recorded pressure depends on the geometry of the balloon.[11] Important artifacts in pressure recordings may result from radial and longitudinal variations in pressure in the anal canal.[73] Most investigators also recognize important differences in pressure measured in men and women and in young and old patients,[7] although there is some dispute as to the effect of age on anal pressures.[74] Normal values ($\pm$ SE) for basal and squeeze pressure in our laboratory are 66 ± 6 and 218 ± 18 mm Hg in men and 58 ± 3 and 135 ± 15 mm Hg in women.[7]

Basal anal pressure is thought to be largely due to tonic contraction of the internal anal sphincter because it is well maintained even with nerve blocks that paralyze the external anal sphincter.[35-37] Tonic contraction of the internal anal sphincter has been attributed to rhythmic electrical activity in the smooth muscle (slow wave).[38] The component of squeeze pressure that exceeds basal pressure is due to active contraction of the external anal sphincter; it is abolished by nerve blocks.[35-37] Because the sphincters are coaxial over most of their length, one does not find segments representing only the internal or only the external anal sphincters except at the anal verge where the subcutaneous external anal sphincter may sometimes be recorded by itself.

As a group, patients with fecal incontinence have significantly lower basal and squeeze pressures than age- and sex-matched control subjects.[7] However, there is a considerable range of pressures among incontinent patients, and many have normal sphincter pressures recorded. Anal manometry is most valuable when it demonstrates abnormally low pressures and confirms the presence of a sphincter defect. An isolated decrease in basal pressure or squeeze pressure suggests a problem with internal or external anal sphincter dysfunction, respectively.

Balloon manometry, in which a three-balloon assembly (Fig. 21–8) or a balloon-tipped manometry device is inserted into the rectum and anal canal, can provide

Table 21–2. OBJECTIVE TESTS OF RECTOANAL FUNCTION

Test	Purpose
Anal manometry	Measurement of basal and squeeze pressures in anal canal
Balloon manometry	Measurement of rectal sensation, rectal compliance, rectoanal inhibitory reflex, and rectoanal contractile response
Electromyography of puborectalis and external anal sphincter	Assessment of motor nerve supply and skeletal muscle responses
Defecography	Assessment of perineal descent and puborectalis function
Test of continence for solid sphere	Assessment of active and passive resistance to passage of a solid bolus
Test of continence for rectally infused saline	Quantitative assessment of ability to maintain continence against a reproducible stress

information about several physiologic functions.[11] By inflating the rectal balloon with increasing volumes of air, one can determine the threshold for conscious sensation of rectal distention. Most normal individuals can sense as little as 10 ml of air in the rectal balloon. Some incontinent patients (especially diabetics) have higher sensory thresholds.[48] Other incontinent patients have delayed perception of rectal distention.[50]

By monitoring pressure in the upper anal canal, the rectoanal inhibitory reflex can be evaluated.[11] The threshold amount of rectal distention to elicit reflex relaxation of the internal anal sphincter averages about 20 ml in normal subjects and is usually higher than the threshold for conscious sensation. In general, the amplitude and duration of relaxation are related to the volume of rectal distention. Because these measurements are usually made with an air- or fluid-filled balloon, the pressures recorded may have only a distant relationship to the pressures measured by perfused catheters.[11] This response is absent in patients with Hirschsprung's disease.[42, 43]

The increase in pressure in the lower anal canal after rectal distention reflects contractile activity in the external anal sphincter, the rectoanal contractile response.[11] The manometric record shows a sharp inflection simultaneous with internal anal sphincter relaxation but usually of shorter duration. This appears to be a learned response[51] and is missing in many patients with fecal incontinence of a variety of causes.[75] Relearning this response is an important aspect of biofeedback training for the treatment of fecal incontinence (see below).

Balloon manometry provides important information about the integrity of the neural pathways mediating sensation (both to consciousness and as a trigger for the rectoanal relaxation reflex) and mediating the motor responses of the internal and external anal sphincters. Interpretation must be cautious, however, because problems with perception or with the effector muscles can also produce an abnormal test result.

Balloon manometry can also be used to estimate rectal compliance. By gradually inflating a balloon placed in the rectum and simultaneously recording pressure within the balloon, a compliance curve can be generated.[72, 76] This should be corrected for the elastic properties of the balloon itself by subtracting the pressure-volume curve obtained outside the body. This test is of most value in investigating incontinence associated with diseases that alter rectal compliance (Table 21–1).

Electromyography with standard concentric needles or with more sophisticated, single fiber EMG techniques can provide information about the innervation and responses of the skeletal muscles of continence.[77–82] It has been most useful as a research tool in discovering unexpected neuropathic injury in "idiopathic" incontinence. Clinically, its utility is limited at present because the information to be gained in an individual case is not often worth the discomfort involved; the effects of neuropathy can be assessed by tests of muscle function. EMG can be useful in designing operations to improve continence by identifying viable, innervated muscle that can be used in reconstruction.

Radiographic imaging of the angle between the rectum and anus is a relatively new method of visualizing the action of the puborectalis muscle. Several techniques have been developed. In one technique a small amount of barium is injected into the rectum, a metal chain is placed through the anal canal, and well-penetrated lateral views of the pelvis are made while the patient relaxes and then strains.[64, 83] On these static images, the angle made between the axis of the rectum and the axis of the anal canal can be measured. Normally, this angle is maintained at 90 degrees at rest and when straining by the action of the puborectalis muscle (Fig. 21–10). It becomes more obtuse with weakness of the puborectalis muscle. The degree of perineal descent can be judged by relating the vertex of the rectoanal angle to a line drawn between the pubic arch and the tip of the coccyx. Normally the vertex of the rectoanal angle is within 1 cm of the pubococcygeal line both at rest and when straining. Pelvic descent is diagnosed when the vertex of the angle is distinctly below the pubococcygeal line at rest or with straining.

Defecography is another technique for evaluating the rectoanal angle which also allows for assessment of the movements of the pelvic floor.[84, 85] The patient is seated in a chair and a small amount of barium is introduced into the rectum and is left to coat the anal canal. Rapid sequence radiograms (one per second) or videofluoroscopy are used to image the rectum and anal canal at rest, with straining (and attempted holding) and with defecation. The rectoanal angle can be seen and measured, and in addition the movements of the barium-containing rectum can be used to infer the movements of the pelvic floor. Weakness of the puborectalis and pelvic floor can be readily appreciated with this technique.

Other radiographic techniques for assessing the anorectum and the act of defecation have been described as well.[85, 86] The importance of any of these radiographic tests in the evaluation of patients with incontinence is that they allow the physician to visualize the activity and assess the integrity of the puborectalis muscle and pelvic floor. This information is not readily available by other techniques at present.

Two other tests—the *test of continence for a solid sphere*[7, 87] and the *test of continence for rectally infused saline*[7]—have been used as objective measures of continence for solids and liquids, respectively. In the first of these tests, a small sphere attached to a string is inserted into the rectum. The patient is seated on a chair with a central aperture and a bucket is attached to the string. Steel shot are then poured into the bucket until the sphere is pulled from the rectum. The weight of the filled bucket is recorded. The study is done once while the patient is making no special effort to retain the sphere (to measure passive resistance) and once while the patient is making a maximal effort to retain the sphere (to measure active continence). Incontinent patients require less weight to pull the sphere from the

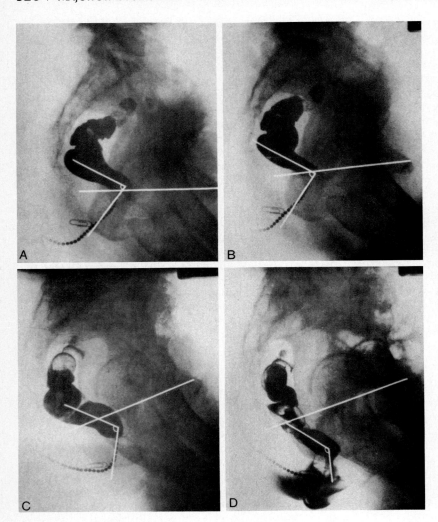

Figure 21–10. Lateral radiographs of the pelvis in a normal individual at rest (A) and while straining (B). The normal relationships between the rectoanal angle and pubococcygeal line are indicated. The same views are shown in a patient with perineal descent at rest (C) and while straining (D). Note the obtuse rectoanal angle and its relation to the pubococcygeal line. (From Bartolo et al.[64] and used with permission.)

rectum than control subjects, both basally and while making maximal effort.[7] The weight required to pull the sphere through the contracted sphincter correlates well with maximum squeeze pressure and probably relates to the strength of the skeletal muscles of continence (puborectalis and external anal sphincter).

The other objective test of continence is the test of continence for rectally infused saline.[7] In this test the patient is again seated in a chair with a central aperture, a fine catheter is inserted into the rectum and 1500 ml of saline is pumped into the rectum over 25 minutes. The patient is instructed to try to retain all the infused fluid. A funnel and graduated cylinder are placed under the chair to catch any leakage. Most normal individuals do not leak at all during this test. During the infusion the fluid progressively fills the colon from rectum to cecum.[44] There is a pattern of regular rectal pressure peaks and internal sphincter relaxations, but at no time does the highest rectal pressure exceed the lowest pressure in the anal canal in normal individuals. Most incontinent patients leak a fair amount of fluid during the test.[7, 88] Leaks coincide with peaks in rectal pres-

sure, and incontinent patients can be divided into two groups.[88] The first group includes those patients with low basal sphincter pressure that is overcome by even modest increases in rectal pressure. The second group includes patients in whom normal basal sphincter pressure is overcome by abnormally high peak rectal pressures. It seems likely that patients in the second group have a problem with colon or rectal compliance. Results on this test are not dependent upon mucosal sensation because continence is maintained during rectal infusion even after topical anesthetics have been applied to the anal canal.[89]

The value of these objective tests of continence is that they place a fixed and reproducible stress on the continence mechanisms. Variation in the occurrence of incontinence due to variation in stool consistency, the proximity of toilet facilities, or adaptations that the patient may have made is eliminated. These tests can be used to reproducibly challenge the continence mechanisms and to judge the effect of therapy for incontinence. They can also be used to assess latent defects in continence. As a clinical "test for incontinence" they are only of limited value because the presence or absence of incontinence can usually be judged by history alone.

TREATMENT

General Principles

Fecal incontinence is either curable or preventable in most patients. Even in elderly, institutionalized patients incontinent episodes can be substantially reduced or eliminated by proper management in over half of the affected patients.[4] Success in treatment is primarily due to recognizing the problem and doing something about it.

If a specific, underlying cause for incontinence can be discovered, therapy directed against that cause may help to alleviate incontinence. For instance, it has been claimed that diabetics with incontinence on the basis of underlying neuropathy might benefit from more vigorous therapy for control of glycemia.[90] Progression of problems may be limited if the patient can prevent further damage. For instance, it has been postulated that the neuropathy related to perineal descent syndrome may not progress if the patient can reduce straining at stool by modifying his or her defecation habits.[91]

One nonspecific but effective strategy for treating incontinence is to stimulate defecation at regular intervals by use of enemas to keep the colon and rectum empty of feces.[92] This strategy is particularly useful in patients who are incontinent of solid stool and has been used extensively in children with chronic constipation and encopresis. For patients with diarrhea, intensive efforts to make a diagnosis and to treat the patient may result in a solid stool that can be more readily controlled by the continence mechanisms. Bulking agents or nonspecific antidiarrheal drugs may help to achieve this aim.

Much of the disability from fecal incontinence is due to psychologic problems that develop in response to the fear of an accident in a public place and lead to reclusiveness. These patients often need a great deal of support in attempting to return to society. Advice on the use of continence aids such as adult-sized training pants can help these patients return to a more normal existence.[92-94] The best help that these patients can receive is to do something that will prevent or reduce the chance of incontinence. Three such approaches are available: drug therapy, biofeedback training, and surgery.

Drug Therapy

The only two drugs that have been scientifically assessed for an effect on fecal incontinence are Lomotil (diphenoxylate and atropine) and loperamide, both opioid antidiarrheals. One double-blind, crossover study of incontinent patients with diarrhea evaluated the effects of Lomotil and placebo on stool frequency, stool weight, anal sphincter pressure, and tests of continence for a solid sphere and for rectally infused saline.[95] Lomotil reduced stool frequency and weight but had no effect on any of the other tests. Incontinent episodes occurred too infrequently under observation in the hospital with both treatments to draw any conclusion as to the effectiveness of Lomotil in preventing incontinence.

A similar study of the effect of loperamide suggested that loperamide, 4 mg three times daily, significantly reduced the frequency of incontinent episodes and urgency, increased basal anal sphincter pressure slightly, and improved the results of the test of continence to rectally infused saline.[96] However, only 11 of 26 patients had any episodes of incontinence during the trial, and the median number of episodes of incontinence was 0 with both placebo and loperamide. Nonetheless, these findings suggest that loperamide may have some direct effect on the continence mechanisms over and above its antidiarrheal effect. When faced with a patient with chronic diarrhea and fecal incontinence, loperamide may be the nonspecific antidiarrheal agent of choice. It is unclear, however, whether use of loperamide is justified in patients with incontinence for solid stool. If tried in this setting, patients should be carefully observed for development of constipation.

Biofeedback Training

Biofeedback training is a form of operant conditioning or instrumental learning in which information about a physiologic process which would otherwise be unconscious is presented to a subject with the aim of having the subject modify that physiologic process.[97] In the case of patients with fecal incontinence, the balloon manometry device (Fig. 21–8) is used to help the patient improve the conscious threshold for sensation of rectal distention and to coordinate external anal sphincter contraction with rectal distention (two mechanisms that are frequently defective in these patients).[98] To do this, the device and the proper responses on the physiograph are described to the patient and the patient is shown how he or she can squeeze the external anal sphincter and alter the physiograph record. The patient is then instructed to do this every time the rectal balloon is distended, an event that the patient can feel (if the balloon is inflated above the sensory threshold) and see by observing the pressure tracing from the rectal balloon. The appropriate response (external anal sphincter contraction) is rewarded verbally, and the procedure is repeated again and again. The volume in the rectal balloon is gradually reduced as the patient is able to sense rectal distention consistently. After a while the physiograph display is removed from the sight of the trainee and the extent to which he or she has learned to perceive rectal distention and to coordinate external anal sphincter contraction can be evaluated.

In general, reports from centers experienced with this technique suggest that about 70 per cent of patients in whom training can be done (i.e., cooperative patients with some degree of perception of rectal distention and the ability to generate a squeeze pressure; in all, perhaps two-thirds of incontinent patients[99]) have either a disappearance or substantial reduction of spontaneous incontinence.[98-101] Most patients responded after a single session, and in most the results were long-lasting. Responders differed from nonresponders in that responders had improvement in their threshold for conscious sensation (from approximately 40 ml to 15 ml), whereas nonresponders had no improvement in sensation.[99, 102]

Although these reports are impressive, they must be interpreted with caution. Biofeedback has not been tested in a blinded fashion. One study suggests that the components of biofeedback (i.e., sensory training alone and muscle training alone) can be done independently with equivalent results.[103] Another study suggests that behavioral modification is as successful as biofeedback training in incontinent children with spina bifida.[104] Finally, there has been no evidence of improvement in objective tests of continence with biofeedback. Thus, we cannot say how biofeedback works to improve continence or even that it does work better than placebo treatment would.

Nevertheless, biofeedback is an inexpensive, quick, and safe procedure for treating fecal incontinence. Until better studies are available, it should be offered to patients with incontinence who are appropriate candidates. To be a reasonable candidate, a patient must have some ability to sense rectal distention (albeit at a higher than normal threshold), good motivation, the ability to understand instructions, and the ability to contract the external anal sphincter voluntarily. Patients with dementia, absence of rectal sensation, or inability to contract the external anal sphincter cannot be expected to respond to biofeedback therapy. Biofeedback training has been applied mostly to patients with incontinence for solid stools; it may be less effective in incontinent patients with diarrhea.

Techniques other than balloon manometry have been used for biofeedback training in small groups of patients.[105-107] In one uncontrolled study, supplementing biofeedback training with muscle exercises improved continence and increased measured squeeze pressure.[108]

Surgery

Operative management of fecal incontinence should be considered in patients who fail to respond to medical therapy or who have altered anatomy in the anorectal region.[109-112] The large number of surgical procedures advocated for fecal incontinence (Table 21–3) indicates the lack of any one procedure that is suitable for most patients. None of these procedures is easy or free of complications, and they should always be done by skilled colon and rectal surgeons. Patients should be meticulously evaluated before planning surgery so that

Table 21–3. SURGICAL TREATMENT OF FECAL INCONTINENCE

1. Use of pelvic floor muscles
   Anal sphincter repairs
   Reefing (plication) of sphincter muscle
   Mobilization of scar tissue to narrow anus
   Use of nonsphincteric perineal muscle
   Puborectalis repair (postanal perineorrhaphy)
   Pubococcygeus repair
2. Use of flaps of other muscles
   Gluteus
   Adductor longus
   Gracilis
3. Circumanal fascial strips connected to gluteal muscles
4. Thiersch procedures (circumanal wire, Teflon, Marlex, or elastic band)

the best approach can be planned for each individual. Few long-term studies and no randomized comparative studies are available to choose between these procedures. Much interest has been focused lately on the use of a postanal repair or levatorplasty to reconstruct the rectoanal angle in patients with pelvic floor weakness.[113-116] Collected series of what must be highly selected patients show good to excellent results, with success related to the ability of the surgeon to restore normal anatomic relationships or to improve anal sphincter pressure.[113] As a last resort, fecal diversion (ileostomy or colostomy) can be considered if no direct approach is feasible.

Surgery has a special role to play in the restoration of continence after colectomy and ileoanal anastomosis for the management of ulcerative colitis. In this procedure, care is taken to preserve the voluntary muscles of continence and a cuff of muscle from the distal rectum. The ileum is directed through the muscular tunnel, and thus, many of the barriers to the aboral movement of feces are preserved. An ileal pouch is created to serve as a reservoir for stool. Physiologically, anal pressures and pouch compliance are close to that of the normal anal canal and rectum, and clinically, results with this operation often have been satisfactory.[117-121]

References

1. Ehrman, J. S. Use of biofeedback to treat incontinence. J. Am. Geriatr. Soc. *31*:182, 1983.
2. Drossman, D. A., Sandler, R. S., Broom, C. M., and McKee, D. C. Urgency and fecal soiling in people with bowel dysfunction. Dig. Dis. Sci. *31*:1221, 1986.
3. Thomas, T. M., Egan, M., Walgrove, A., and Meade, T. W. The prevalence of faecal and double incontinence. Community Med. *6*:216, 1984.
4. Tobin, G. W., and Brocklehurst, J. C. Faecal incontinence in residential homes for the elderly: Prevalence, aetiology and management. Age Aging *15*:41, 1986.
5. McLaren, S. M., McPherson, F. M., Sinclair, F., and Ballinger, B. R. Prevalence and severity of incontinence among hospitalized, female psychogeriatric patients. Health Bull. *39*:157, 1981.
6. Smith, R. G. Fecal incontinence. J. Am. Geriatr. Soc. *31*:694, 1983.
7. Read, N. W., Harford, W. V., Schmulen, A. C., Read, M. G., Santa Ana, C., and Fordtran, J. S. A clinical study of patients with fecal incontinence and diarrhea. Gastroenterology *76*:747, 1979.

8. Leigh, R. J., and Turnberg, L. A. Faecal incontinence: The unvoiced symptom. Lancet *1*:1349, 1982.

9. Phillips, S. F., and Edwards, D. A. W. Some aspects of anal continence and defaecation. Gut *6*:396, 1965.

10. Tagart, R. E. B. The anal canal and rectum: Their varying relationship and its effect on anal continence. Dis. Colon Rectum *9*:449, 1966.

11. Schuster, M. M. Motor action of rectum and anal sphincters in continence and defecation. *In* Code, C. F. (Ed.). Handbook of Physiology. Section 6. Volume IV. Motility. Washington, American Physiology Society, 1968, Chap. 103, p. 2121.

12. Scharli, A. F., and Kiesewetter, W. B. Defecation and continence: Some new concepts. Dis. Colon Rectum *13*:81, 1970.

13. Duthie, H. L. Dynamics of the rectum and anus. Clin. Gastroenterol. *4*:467, 1975.

14. Schuster, M. M. The riddle of the sphincters. Gastroenterology *69*:249, 1975.

15. Dickinson, V. A. Maintenance of anal continence: A review of pelvic floor physiology. Gut *19*:1163, 1978.

16. Duthie, H. L. Defaecation and the anal sphincter. Clin. Gastroenterol. *11*:621, 1982.

17. Wunderlich, M., and Parks, A. G. Physiology and pathophysiology of the anal sphincters. Internat. Surg. *67*:291, 1982.

18. Schiller, L. R. Faecal incontinence. Clin. Gastroenterol. *15*:687, 1986.

19. Gibbons, C. P., Trowbridge, E. A., Bannister, J. J., and Read, N. W. Role of anal cushions in maintaining continence. Lancet *1*:886, 1986.

20. Fay, D. F., Jones, N. B., and Porter, N. H. Spectral analysis of the myoelectric activity of the pelvic floor during voluntary contractions. Electromyogr. Clin. Neurophysiol. *16*:525, 1976.

21. Vereecken, R. L., Puers, B., and Van Mulders, J. Spectral analysis of perineal muscles EMG. Electromyogr. Clin. Neurophysiol. *22*:321, 1982.

22. Shafik, A. New concept of the anatomy of the anal sphincter mechanism and the physiology of defecation. II. Anatomy of the levator ani muscle with special reference to puborectalis. Investigative Urol. *13*:175, 1975.

23. Denny-Brown, D., and Robertson, E. G. An investigation of the nervous control of defaecation. Brain *58*:256, 1935.

24. Percy, J. P., Neill, M. E., Swash, M., and Parks, A. G. Electrophysiological study of motor nerve supply of pelvic floor. Lancet *1*:16, 1980.

25. Frenckner, B., and Ihre, T. Influence of autonomic nerves on the internal anal sphincter in man. Gut *17*:306, 1976.

26. Garry, R. C. The responses to stimulation of the caudal end of the large bowel in the cat. J. Physiol. *78*:208, 1933.

27. Goligher, J. C., and Hughes, E. S. R. Sensibility of the rectum and colon: Its role in the mechanism of anal continence. Lancet *1*:543, 1951.

28. McNeil, N. I., and Rampton, D. S. Is the rectum usually empty? A quantitative study in subjects with and without diarrhea. Dis. Colon Rectum *24*:596, 1981.

29. Ballantyne, G. H. Rectosigmoid sphincter of O'Beirne. Dis. Colon Rectum *29*:525, 1986.

30. Ihre, T. Studies on anal function in continent and incontinent patients. Scand. J. Gastroenterol. *9*(suppl 25):1, 1974.

31. Arhan, P., Devroede, G., Danis, G., Dornic, C., Faverdin, C., Persoz, B., and Pellerin, D. Viscoelastic properties of the rectal wall in Hirschsprung's disease. J. Clin. Invest. *62*:82, 1978.

32. Denis, P., Colin, R., Galmiche, J. P., Geffroy, Y., Hecketsweiler, P., LeFrancois, R., and Pasquis, P. Elastic properties of the rectal wall in normal adults and in patients with ulcerative colitis. Gastroenterology *77*:45, 1979.

33. Suzuki, H., and Fujioka, M. Rectal pressure and rectal compliance in ulcerative colitis. Jap. J. Surg. *12*:79, 1982.

34. Devroede, G., Vobecky, S., Masse, S., Arhan, P., Leger, C., Duguay, C., and Hemond, M. Ischemic fecal incontinence and rectal angina. Gastroenterology *83*:970, 1982.

35. Duthie, H. L., and Watts, J. M. Contribution of the external anal sphincter to the pressure zone in the anal canal. Gut *6*:64, 1965.

36. Frenckner, B., and Euler, C. V. Influence of pudendal block on the function of the anal sphincters. Gut *16*:482, 1975.

37. Schweiger, M. Method for determining individual contributions of voluntary and involuntary anal sphincters to resting tone. Dis. Colon Rectum *22*:415, 1979.

38. Ustach, T. J., Tobon, F., Hambrecht, T., Bass, D. D., and Schuster, M. M. Electrophysiological aspects of human sphincter function. J. Clin. Invest. *49*:41, 1970.

39. Meunier, P., and Mollard, P. Control of the internal anal sphincter (manometric study with human subjects). Pflugers Arch. *370*:233, 1977.

40. Burleigh, D. E., D'Mello, A., and Parks, A. G. Responses of isolated human internal anal sphincter to drugs and electrical field stimulation. Gastroenterology *77*:484, 1979.

41. Parks, A. G., Fishlock, D. J., Cameron, J. D. H., and May, H. Preliminary investigation of the pharmacology of the human internal anal sphincter. Gut *10*:674, 1969.

42. Schnaufer, L., Talbert, J. L., Haller, J. A., Reid, N. C., Tobon, F., and Schuster, M. M. Differential sphincteric studies in the diagnosis of anorectal disorders of childhood. J. Pediatr. Surg. *2*:538, 1967.

43. Lawson, J. O. N., and Nixon, H. H. Anal canal pressures in the diagnosis of Hirschsprung's disease. J. Pediatr. Surg. *2*:544, 1967.

44. Haynes, W. G., and Read, N. W. Ano-rectal activity in man during rectal infusion of saline: A dynamic assessment of the anal continence mechanism. J. Physiol. *330*:45, 1982.

45. Schiller, L. R., Santa Ana, C. A., Schmulen, A. C., Hendler, R. S., Harford, W. V., and Fordtran, J. S. Pathogenesis of fecal incontinence in diabetes mellitus: Evidence for internal-anal-sphincter dysfunction. N. Engl. J. Med. *307*:1666, 1982.

46. Hancock, B. D. Lord's procedure for hemorrhoids: A prospective anal pressure study. Br. J. Surg. *68*:729, 1981.

47. Snooks, S., Henry, M. M., and Swash, M. Faecal incontinence after anal dilatation. Br. J. Surg. *71*:617, 1984.

48. Wald, A., and Tunuguntla, A. K. Anorectal sensorimotor dysfunction in fecal incontinence and diabetes mellitus: Modification with biofeedback therapy. N. Engl. J. Med. *310*:1282, 1984.

49. Read, N. W., and Abouzekry, L. Why do patients with faecal impaction have faecal incontinence. Gut *27*:283, 1986.

50. Buser, W. D., and Miner, P. B., Jr. Delayed rectal sensation with fecal incontinence: Successful treatment using anorectal manometry. Gastroenterology *91*:1186, 1986.

51. Whitehead, W. E., Orr, W. C., Engel, B. T., and Schuster, M. M. External anal sphincter response to rectal distention: Learned response or reflex. Psychophysiology *19*:57, 1981.

52. Beersiek, F., Parks, A. G., and Swash, M. Pathogenesis of ano-rectal incontinence: A histometric study of the anal sphincter musculature. J. Neurol. Sci. *42*:111, 1979.

53. Henry, M. M., Parks, A. G., and Swash, M. The pelvic floor musculature in the descending perineum syndrome. Br. J. Surg. *69*:470, 1982.

54. Neill, M. E., and Swash, M. Increased motor unit fibre density in the external anal sphincter muscle in ano-rectal incontinence: A single fibre EMG study. J. Neurol. Neurosurg. Psychiatr. *43*:343, 1980.

55. Henry, M. M., Parks, A. G., and Swash, M. The anal reflex in idiopathic faecal incontinence: An electrophysiological study. Br. J. Surg. *67*:781, 1980.

56. Neill, M. E., Parks, A. G., and Swash, M. Physiological studies of the anal sphincter musculature in faecal incontinence and rectal prolapse. Br. J. Surg. *68*:531, 1981.

57. Bartolo, D. C. C., Jarratt, J. A., Read, M. A., Donnelly, T. C., and Read, N. W. The role of partial denervation of the puborectalis in idiopathic faecal incontinence. Br. J. Surg. *70*:664, 1983.

58. Kiff, E. S., and Swash, M. Normal proximal and delayed distal conduction in the pudendal nerves of patients with idiopathic (neurogenic) faecal incontinence. J. Neurol. Neurosurg. Psychiatr. *47*:820, 1984.

59. Kiff, E. S., and Swash, M. Slowed conduction in the pudendal nerves in idiopathic (neurogenic) faecal incontinence. Br. J. Surg. *71*:614, 1984.

60. Snooks, S. J., Henry, M. M., and Swash, M. Anorectal incontinence and rectal prolapse: Differential assessment of the innervation to puborectalis and external anal sphincter muscles. Gut *26*:470, 1985.

61. Snooks, S. J., Swash, M., and Henry, M. M. Abnormalities in

central and peripheral nerve conduction in patients with ano-rectal incontinence. J. Roy. Soc. Med. 78:294, 1985.

62. Swash, M., Snooks, S. J., and Henry, M. M. Unifying concept of pelvic floor disorders and incontinence. J. Roy. Soc. Med. 78:906, 1985.

63. Womack, N. R., Morrison, J. F. B., and Williams, N. S. The role of pelvic floor denervation in the aetiology of idiopathic faecal incontinence. Br. J. Surg. 73:404, 1986.

64. Bartolo, D. C. C., Read, N. W., Jarratt, J. A., Read, M. G., Donnelly, T. C., and Johnson, A. G. Differences in anal sphincter function and clinical presentation in patients with pelvic floor descent. Gastroenterology 85:68, 1983.

65. Read, N. W., Bartolo, D. C. C., and Read, M. G. Differences in anal function in patients with incontinence to solids and in patients with incontinence to liquids. Br. J. Surg. 71:39, 1984.

66. Snooks, S. J., Henry, M. M., and Swash, M. Faecal incontinence due to external anal sphincter division in childbirth is associated with damage to the innervation of the pelvic floor musculature: A double pathology. Br. J. Obstet. Gynecol. 92:824, 1985.

67. Snooks, S. J., Setchell, M., Swash, M., and Henry, M. M. Injury to innervation of pelvic floor sphincter musculature in childbirth. Lancet 2:546, 1984.

68. Keighley, M. R. B., and Shouler, P. J. Abnormalities of colonic function in patients with rectal prolapse and faecal inconti-nence. Br. J. Surg. 71:892, 1984.

69. Varma, J. S., Smith, A. N., and Busuttil, A. Function of the anal sphincters after chronic radiation injury. Gut 27:528, 1986.

70. Loening-Baucke, V. A. Abnormal rectoanal function in chil-dren recovered from chronic constipation and encopresis. Gas-troenterology 87:1299, 1984.

71. Oettle, G. J., Roe, A. M., Bartolo, D. C. C., and Mortensen, N. J. M. What is the best way of measuring perineal descent? A comparison of radiographic and clinical methods. Br. J. Surg. 72:999, 1985.

72. Devroede, G. Anal incontinence. Dis. Colon Rectum 25:90, 1982.

73. Taylor, B. M., Beart, R. W., Jr., and Phillips, S. F. Longitu-dinal and radial variations of pressure in the human anal sphincter. Gastroenterology 86:693, 1984.

74. Loening-Baucke, V., and Anuras, S. Effects of age and sex on anorectal manometry. Am. J. Gastroenterol. 80:50, 1985.

75. Alva, J., Mendeloff, A. I., and Schuster, M. M. Reflex and electromyographic abnormalities associated with fecal inconti-nence. Gastroenterology 53:101, 1967.

76. Varma, J. S., and Smith, A. N. Reproducibility of the proc-tometrogram. Gut 27:288, 1986.

77. Henry, M. M., and Swash, M. Assessment of pelvic-floor disorders and incontinence by electrophysiological recording of the anal reflex. Lancet 1:1290, 1978.

78. Swash, M. Early and late components in the human anal reflex. J. Neurol. Neurosurg. Psychiatr. 45:767, 1982.

79. Pedersen, E., Klemar, B., Schroder, H. D. A. A., and Torring, J. Anal sphincter responses after perianal electrical stimulation. J. Neurol. Neurosurg. Psychiatr. 45:770, 1982.

80. Bartolo, D. C. C., Jarratt, J. A., and Read, N. W. The use of conventional electromyography to assess external sphincter neuropathy in man. J. Neurol. Neurosurg. Psychiatr. 46:1115, 1983.

81. Bartolo, D. C. C., Jarratt, J. A., and Read, N. W. The cutaneo-anal reflex: A useful index of neuropathy? Br. J. Surg. 70:660, 1983.

82. Swash, M. Anorectal incontinence: Electrophysiological test. Br. J. Surg. 72:S14, 1985.

83. Kuypers, J. H. C. Fecal incontinence and the anorectal angle. Netherlands J. Surg. 36:20, 1984.

84. Kuijpers, H. C., and Strijk, S. P. Diagnosis of disturbances of continence and defecation. Dis. Colon Rectum 27:658, 1984.

85. Mahieu, P. H. G., and Bartram, C. Contribution of radiology to the study of defecation disorders. Acta Gastro-Enterol. Belg. 48:11, 1985.

86. Preston, D. M., Lennard-Jones, J. E., and Thomas, B. M. The balloon proctogram. Br. J. Surg. 71:29, 1984.

87. Ling, L., Malmfred, S., and Thesleff, P. Solid-sphere test for examination of anal sphincter strength. Scand. J. Gastroen-terol. 19:960, 1984.

88. Read, N. W., Haynes, W. G., Bartolo, D. C. C., Hall, J., Read, M. G., Donnelly, T. C., and Johnson, A. G. Use of anorectal manometry during rectal infusion of saline to inves-tigate sphincter function in incontinent patients. Gastroenter-ology 85:105, 1983.

89. Read, M. G., and Read, N. W. Role of anorectal sensation in preserving continence. Gut 23:345, 1982.

90. Feldman, M., and Schiller, L. R. Disorders of gastrointestinal motility associated with diabetes mellitus. Ann. Intern. Med. 98:378, 1983.

91. Swash, M. New concepts in the prevention of incontinence. Practitioner 229:895, 1985.

92. Brocklehurst, J. C. Management of anal incontinence. Clin. Gastroenterol. 4:479, 1975.

93. Beber, C. R. Freedom for the incontinent. Am. J. Nurs. 80:482, 1980.

94. Morton, G. Management of the incontinent patient: Practical guidelines for home care. Aust. Fam. Physician 10:40, 1981.

95. Harford, W. V., Krejs, G. J., Santa Ana, C. A., and Fordtran, J. S. Acute effect of diphenoxylate with atropine (Lomotil) in patients with chronic diarrhea and fecal incontinence. Gastro-enterology 78:440, 1980.

96. Read, M., Read, N. W., Barber, D. C., and Duthie, H. L. Effects of loperamide on anal sphincter function in patients complaining of chronic diarrhea with fecal incontinence and urgency. Dig. Dis. Sci. 27:807, 1982.

97. Marzuk, P. M., Biofeedback for gastrointestinal disorders: A review of the literature. Ann. Intern. Med. 103:240, 1985.

98. Engel, B. T., Nikoomanesh, P., and Schuster, M. M. Operant conditioning of rectosphincteric responses in the treatment of fecal incontinence. N. Engl. J. Med. 290:646, 1974.

99. Wald, A. Biofeedback therapy for fecal incontinence. Ann. Intern. Med. 95:146, 1981.

100. Cerulli, M. A., Nikoomanesh, P., and Schuster, M. M. Prog-ress in biofeedback conditioning for fecal incontinence. Gastro-enterology 76:742, 1979.

101. Goldenberg, D. A., Hodges, K., Hersh, T., and Jinich, H. Biofeedback therapy for fecal incontinence. Am. J. Gastroen-terol. 74:342, 1980.

102. Wald, A. Biofeedback for neurogenic fecal incontinence: Rec-tal sensation is a determinant of outcome. J. Pediatr. Gastro-enterol. Nutr. 2:302, 1983.

103. Latimer, P. R., Campbell, D., and Kasperski, J. A components analysis of biofeedback in the treatment of fecal incontinence. Biofeedback Self-Regulation 9:311, 1984.

104. Whitehead, W. E., Parker, L., Bosmajian, L., Morrill-Corbin, E. D., Middaugh, S., Garwood, M., Cataldo, M. F., and Freeman, J. Treatment of fecal incontinence in children with spina bifida: Comparison of biofeedback and behavior modifi-cation. Arch. Phys. Med. Rehab. 67:218, 1986.

105. Schiller, L. R., Santa Ana, C., Davis, G. R., and Fordtran, J. S. Fecal incontinence in chronic diarrhea: Report of a case with improvement after training with rectally-infused saline. Gastroenterology 77:751, 1979.

106. Constantinides, C. B., and Cywes, S. Fecal incontinence: A simple pneumatic device for home biofeedback training. J. Pediatr. Surg. 18:276, 1983.

107. MacLeod, J. H. Biofeedback in the management of partial anal incontinence. Dis. Colon Rectum 26:244, 1983.

108. Melange, M., Heuchamps, Y., and Vanheuverzwyn, R. The medical treatment of anorectal incontinence. Acta Gastro-enterol. Belg. 48:53, 1985.

109. Corman, M. L. The management of anal incontinence. Surg. Clin. North Am. 63:177, 1983.

110. Keighley, M. R. B., and Fielding, J. W. L. Management of faecal incontinence and results of surgical treatment. Br. J. Surg. 70:463, 1983.

111. Schoetz, D. J. Operative therapy for anal incontinence. Surg. Clin. North Am. 65:35, 1985.

112. Cohen, M., Rosen, L., Khubchandani, I., Sheets, J., Stasik, J., and Riether, R. Rationale for medical or surgical therapy in anal incontinence. Dis. Colon Rectum 29:120, 1986.

113. Browning, G. G. P., and Parks, A. G. Postanal repair for neuropathic faecal incontinence: Correlation of clinical result and anal canal pressures. Br. J. Surg. 70:101, 1983.
114. Keighley, M. R. B. Postanal repair for faecal incontinence. J. Roy. Soc. Med. 77:285, 1984.
115. Henry, M. M., and Simson, J. N. L. Results of postanal repair: A retrospective study. Br. J. Surg. 72:S17, 1985.
116. Kottmeier, P. K., Velcek, F. T., Klotz, D. H., Coren, C. V., Hansbrough, F., and Price, A. P. Results of levatorplasty for anal incontinence. J. Pediatr. Surg. 21:647, 1986.
117. Heppell, J., Kelly, K. A., Phillips, S. F., Beart, R. W., Jr., Telander, R. L., and Perrault, J. Physiologic aspects of continence after colectomy, mucosal proctectomy, and endorectal ileo-anal anastomosis. Ann. Surg. 195:435, 1982.
118. Pescatori, M., and Parks, A. G. The sphincteric and sensory components of preserved continence after ileoanal reservoir. Surg. Gynecol. Obstet. 158:517, 1984.
119. Taylor, B. M., Beart, R. W., Jr., Dozois, R. R., Kelly, K. A., Wolff, B. G., and Ilstrup, D. M. The endorectal ileal pouch-anal anastomosis: Current clinical results. Dis. Colon Rectum 27:347, 1984.
120. Martin, L. W., Sayers, H. J., Alexander, F., Fischer, J. E., and Torres, M. A. Anal continence following Soave procedure. Ann. Surg. 203:525, 1986.
121. Pemberton, J. H., and Kelly, K. A. Achieving enteric continence: Principles and applications. Mayo Clin. Proc. 61:586, 1986.

22

Constipation

GHISLAIN DEVROEDE

The economic aspects of constipation are staggering: in the United States alone, $368 million was spent on laxatives in 1982.[1, 2]

Constipation is a symptom. It is not a disease, nor a sign. As a symptom, constipation may be indicative of many diseases, and a differential diagnosis should be made as would be done for abdominal pain. A symptom is also the experience of a sign by a patient: not only is the subjective appreciation highly variable from patient to patient, but previous unpleasant experiences of the same nature, both physical and emotional, interfere with the perception of the present experience. The difference between sign and symptom is that the scientific method, which relies upon observation and measurement, is applicable only to the sign. Dismissing the symptom as unimportant as compared with the sign, dismissing the emotions as marginally relevant, is bound to lead to an oversimplified approach to constipation. Thus, our understanding of the mechanisms of constipation and our approach to treatment is plagued by the highly variable definition of constipation used in different studies.

CLINICAL DEFINITION AND ETHNOLOGIC CONSIDERATIONS

Constipation has different meanings for different patients. The term may imply that stools are too small, too hard, too difficult to expel, or too infrequent, or that patients have a feeling of incomplete evacuation after defecation. These symptoms are difficult to quantify.

Size cannot be recorded accurately because of the deformity imposed upon stools by the anorectal structures and by gravity during the act of defecation. Normal stool weight has a wide range (35 to 225 gm per stool).[3] If a patient passes lighter stools, this suggests constipation, although stool weight does not necessarily correlate well with stool size and deformability, factors that are probably also important. There are geographic variations in stool weight.[4, 5] In England and in the United States, stool weight is usually 100 to 200 gm, but may be much less. In contrast, healthy adult Indians defecate stools of an average 311 gm,[6] and the stools of rural Ugandans average 470 gm.[7] Age also exerts influence on stool output.[8, 9] Thus, this parameter of constipation is probably not very practical in a clinical situation.

The complaint of hard stools is unreliable, because two studies have demonstrated a wide range of subjective ratings in normal individuals.[3, 10] Stool consistency may be measured objectively,[11, 12] but again this is not very practical clinically. Stool consistency is determined by the liquid content of stools, which is 40 to 60 per cent in hard stools, 70 per cent in normal stools and over 95 per cent in liquid stools.[13]

Stool frequency is the easiest parameter of constipation to quantify. To avoid potential exaggeration of the problem,[14] it should be measured through a meticulous counting of stools over a period of weeks. Four studies of stool frequency[3, 10, 15, 16] show that normal subjects in Western countries pass at least three stools per week. However, normal men defecate more than five times per week when eating a high-residue diet,[10] and a recent study confirms that less than five stools per week may be considered as a sign of constipation.[17] In addition, whites defecate more often than blacks, and males more often than females[17] (Fig. 22–1). In Senegal, people usually defecate in the morning and evening, and consider themselves constipated if they only have one stool per day; while over three stools per day is considered abnormal in the West, it is considered quite physiologic for many of these people.[18] Thus, in spite of quantitative studies, the question of what is a normal stool frequency is unresolved. One third of "normal" Western subjects complain of symptoms that could be attributed to irritable bowel:[19] 6 per cent (20 per cent in elderly subjects) suffer from painless constipation and another 14 per cent have the attributes of a spastic type of irritable bowel syndrome, including incomplete relief at defecation; at times 50 per cent complain of the latter symptom, and 38.5 per cent must strain to expel the stool. Moreover, frequency *per se* is not of much concern to people, who worry more about efforts to defecate, excessive stool consistency, and incapacity to defecate at will[17] (Fig. 22–2). Normality is not necessarily what most people do. Normal bowel function should be evaluated not in terms of epidemiology but of state of well being: thus, any complaint of constipation, even within the "normal" range, should be listened to.

The feeling of incomplete evacuation cannot be used for diagnosis, because most normal subjects who refrain from defecating have no rectal sensation, although they can defecate at will stools that remain in the rectum.[20] The rectal wall can accommodate itself to stool contents. These compliance properties are

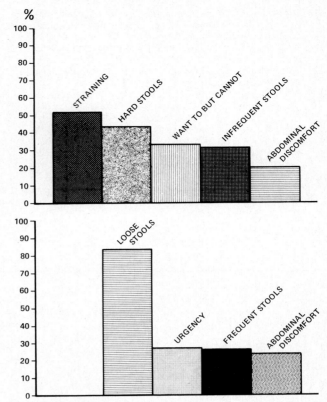

Figure 22–2. Perception of abnormal bowel habits by healthy subjects: constipation (above) and diarrhea (below). (Data from Sandler and Drossman.[17])

partly viscoelastic in nature—that is, purely mechanical. Rapid distention leads to a quick increase in tension with an exponential decrease in time (the viscous properties), and the residual tension after accommodation is due to the elastic properties.[21] There is a wide range of pressure levels between that at which rectal sensation is perceived and that at which it becomes intolerable.[22] Differences between normal subjects and patients in this regard have scarcely been explored. Moreover, the relationship between defecation dynamics, residual stool content in the rectum, and viscoelastic properties of the rectal wall has not been explored in patients who complain of feeling residual stools in their bowel after defecation.

Difficulties in expelling stools are not measurable.

ASSOCIATED SYMPTOMS

Fecal Incontinence and Encopresis as Presenting Symptoms of Constipation

Leakage or involuntary passage of feces in children can force parents to consult a physician; this leakage may result from constipation. For the sake of clarity the term fecal incontinence should probably be reserved to indicate the leakage of small amounts of liquid or soft stool, and the term encopresis to designate the involuntary passage of an entire stool. Al-

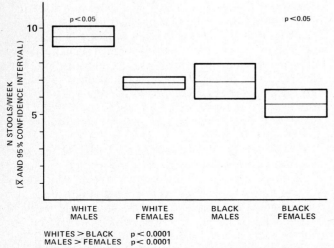

Figure 22–1. Bowel habits of young adults. (Data from Sandler and Drossman.[17])

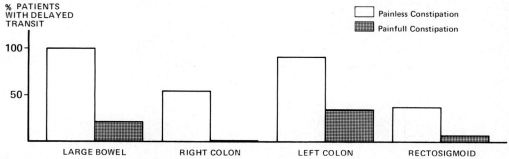

Figure 22–3. The transit time through the large bowel is shorter in patients who complain of both constipation and pain. (Data from Lanfranchi et al.[25])

though no good data are available to distinguish the two conditions in terms of clinical function and pathophysiologic mechanisms, encopresis as defined above is probably not related to constipation. In a large series of children who could not maintain continence, 57 per cent had enormous-caliber stools when defecating that needed to be mechanically broken up prior to flushing the toilet; this probably suggests underlying constipation.[23] Similarly, among 119 patients with intervals of 4 days or longer between bowel movements, soiling occurred in 64 per cent.[24]

The Relationship between Constipation and the Irritable Bowel Syndrome

Patients with constipation may or may not have abdominal pain, and the presence of pain is associated with shorter transit times[25] (Fig. 22–3).

Bloating may simulate pregnancy, because of bowel distention and lumbar lordosis with forward tipping of the pelvis.[26] This can occur with the irritable bowel syndrome, but patients with colonic inertia or slow-transit constipation retain gas and do not pass flatus apart from bowel movements.[26] Less severe forms of constipation can be part of the spectrum of the irritable bowel syndrome. In this syndrome, there are more associated symptoms with constipation than with diarrhea[27] (Fig. 22–4).

EPIDEMIOLOGY

Depending on the definition, the prevalence of constipation varies from 20 per cent, if straining is considered as evidence, to less than 5 per cent if constipation is defined as a stool frequency of less than two per week.

The ratio of females to males varies along the lifespan (Fig. 22–5). Young boys are more often constipated than young girls,[24, 29–35] but a reversal of the ratio occurs later in life and women are much more often constipated than men.[36, 37]

When constipation is defined as delayed transit in the ascending colon, women are found to be in an overwhelming majority of patients with constipation.[37,]

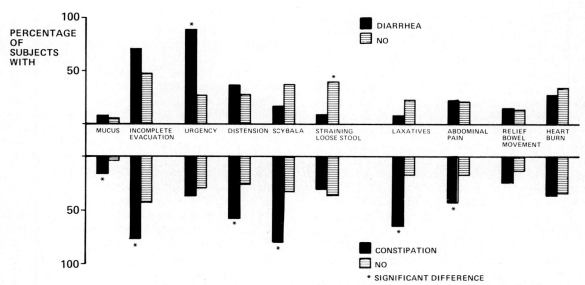

Figure 22–4. In the irritable bowel syndrome, symptoms are associated with constipation more often than with diarrhea. (Data from Thompson and Heaton.[19])

SEX RATIO IN CONSTIPATED CHILDREN

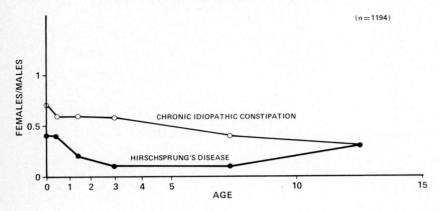

PREVALENCE OF CONSTIPATION AMONG ADULTS

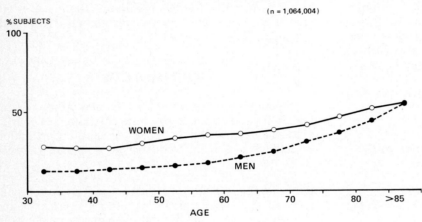

Figure 22–5. In childhood, constipation is a problem more frequently among boys; in adulthood, it is more common among women. (Date on children provided by P. Arhan, Paris. Data on adults from Hammond.[28])

[38] In addition, all patients with a colon of normal size at barium enema are women.[26] The female to male ratio also varies according to anorectal function. It is 6:1 among patients with normal motility, 3.4:1 among those with anal hypertonicity, and 2.3:1 among those with a rectoanal inhibitory reflex that is of less than normal amplitude.[39]

Elderly individuals are said to be more frequently constipated, and indeed the incidence of complaints increases with age[19] (Fig. 22–5). Yet 94 per cent of elderly persons have a stool frequency between three per day and three per week.[16] Half of elderly people living at home defecate at least once a day, and over 90 per cent have at least three stools per week. In contrast, 23 per cent of these people complain of constipation, and this percentage increases to 55 per cent in those attending a geriatric day hospital.[40]

The natural history of constipation is not known. Longitudinal studies have never been performed to see what happens to a single constipated individual over a lifespan. Constipation may be part of the irritable bowel syndrome, which is a chronic relapsing condition.[27, 41–43] It is also more prevalent among subjects who do not report: pain, not constipation, pushes patients to seek help.[44]

RISKS

Constipation is associated with numerous symptoms, which are a source of discomfort.[36] It is not innocuous and carries some risks.

Urinary tract infections may be associated with constipation and disappear after treatment.[45] In children, constipation is also associated with enuresis and vesicoureteral reflux.[46–48] Constipation and abnormal accommodation properties of the rectum are associated with uninhibited bladder contractions;[47, 48] treatment of constipation abolishes fecal incontinence, enuresis, and urinary tract infections and improves bladder function. It should be remembered, however, that association is not causation and that the pelvic floor is one neuromuscular unit, traversed by the urinary, genital, and intestinal tract.[49] Prostatorrhea has also been related to the presence of constipation and hemorrhoids.[50]

Constipation is associated with obesity: its incidence is tripled for overweight men and doubled for women.[51] Whether this is related to accelerated gastric emptying, which is known to occur in obese subjects, or another motor disorder of the gastrointestinal tract has not been studied.

Potentially hazardous dilated loops of sigmoid are

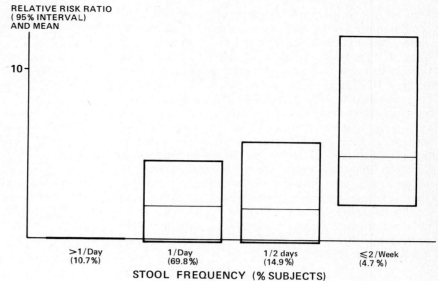

Figure 22–6. Constipation is associated with an increased incidence of epithelial dysplasia in breasts. (Data from Petrakis and King.[63])

often associated with constipation.[52] Stercoraceous perforation is a potentially lethal consequence of prolonged storage of hard feces.[53-56]

Four controlled studies[57-60] establish a link between cancer of the colon and rectum and constipation, particularly in women. In two studies[59, 60] having only three stools per week for a long period of time was considered a risk factor. However, the magnitude of risk for a given patient to develop cancer of the bowel is not known. In studies investigating geographic differences of cancer risk, a low prevalence of cancer of the large bowel was associated with greater stool weight but not with differences in rates of transit.[4, 5]

A socially inconvenient complication may result from chronic straining. Stretching of the pudendal nerve results in a weak and lax pelvic floor where striated muscles are denervated,[61] and this is conducive to fecal incontinence.

Benign and even malignant breast disease has been said to be a consequence of constipation,[62] and the incidence of epithelial dysplasia in mammary secretions is in reverse correlation with stool frequency[63] (Fig. 22–6).

Constipated patients are at high risk for unnecessary surgery. Young women undergo appendectomy more often than young men,[64-67] in a ratio comparable to the greater frequency of constipation in women. Few constipated subjects present with acute abdominal pain, but a history of long-standing constipation in such a patient should encourage the physician not to rush to surgery. Unnecessary laparotomy is also performed much more often in constipated patients than in controls.[68, 69] This is particularly evident in those with slow-transit constipation, who are all women, and who have, as compared with controls, an increased incidence of ovarian cystectomy and hysterectomy[26] (Fig. 22–7).

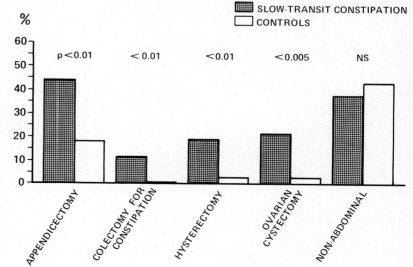

Figure 22–7. Constipation exposes the patient to the risk of unnecessary surgery. (Data from Preston and Lennard-Jones.[26])

Similarly, women with megarectum who were not constipated at birth also often undergo hysterectomy after which the specimen is found to be normal.[70] This has also been pointed out in patients with the irritable bowel syndrome, who are at high risk for unnecessary surgery.[71, 72] The error is easy to explain because of the frequent association of chronic lower abdominal pain with constipation. Thus, a real danger exists of converting a functional problem into a real iatrogenic disease, or even into Munchausen syndrome with multiple unnecessary laparotomies. Many physicians are unaware that psychiatric illness is often present in subjects with the irritable bowel syndrome.[73] This precludes optimal treatment. For example, hysteria seems not to be recognized by internists,[73] and since it is a polysymptomatic illness, unnecessary surgery is often performed[73–75] and more medications and more hospitalizations prescribed.[73]

ETIOLOGY

Constipation may be secondary to diseases that are inborn or acquired during life. The most widely recognized congenital disease producing constipation is, of course, Hirschsprung's disease. But it is not the only one. For instance, when one of two twins is constipated, the chance is four times as high in monozygotic as compared with dizygotic twins that the other member of the pair will also be constipated; this genetic predisposition increases when a parent or a sibling is affected.[76] Diseases producing constipation may run in kindreds,[77, 78] and the onset of constipation sometimes occurs after the first decade of life.[78]

Diseases producing constipation may be systemic in nature, or they may afflict the gastrointestinal tract solely.

Table 22–1. DRUGS INDUCING CONSTIPATION

Analgesics
Anesthetic agents
Antacids (calcium and aluminum compounds)
Anticholinergics
Anticonvulsants
Antidepressive agents
Barium sulfate
Bismuth
Diuretics
Drugs for parkinsonism
Ganglionic blockers
Hematinics (iron especially)
Hypotensives
Laxative addiction (?)
MAO inhibitors
Metallic intoxication
    (arsenic, lead, mercury, phosphorus)
Muscle paralyzers
Opiates
Psychotherapeutic drugs

Table 22–2. METABOLIC AND ENDOCRINE DISORDERS INDUCING CONSTIPATION

Metabolic Disorders
Diabetes: acidosis, neuropathy
Porphyria
Type I (Portuguese) and type II (Indiana) amyloid neuropathy; sporadic primary amyloidosis
Uremia
Hypokalemia
Endocrine Disorders
Panhypopituitarism
Hypothyroidism
Hypercalcemia: hyperparathyroidism, milk-alkali syndrome, carcinomatosis
Pseudohypoparathyroidism
Pheochromocytoma
Enteric glucagon excess

Systemic Causes

Many drugs induce constipation (Table 22–1). The chronic use of laxatives itself has been incriminated in the production of organic constipation, by inducing damage to the nervous structures of the colon.[79–82] The retrospective character of these studies, at least in human beings, casts some doubt on the causal relationship.

Metabolic and endocrine abnormalities may induce constipation (Table 22–2). Some patients suffering from hypothyroidism present with constipation as the primary complaint,[83] and megacolon may develop because of myxedematous infiltration.[84] Severe constipation may be the presenting symptom of pseudohypoparathyroidism and disappears after return of calcium to normal levels.[85] Pheochromocytoma may produce constipation.[86, 87] Glucagon-producing tumors cause severe constipation,[88, 89] and glucagon alone has been found to decrease bowel motility.[90]

Menstruation may be associated with interference with bowel function and constipation.[91]

The effect of pregnancy on bowel habit is uncertain. Conflicting data from different countries reveal that pregnancy is associated with a low incidence of constipation in Israeli women.[92] but that as many as 38 per cent of British women suffer from constipation at some time during pregnancy and 20 per cent in the third trimester.[93] Although there is no difference in dietary fiber intake between matched groups of nonconstipated and constipated British women in their third trimester of pregnancy,[94] the addition of 10 gm of dietary fiber supplements per day increases the number and decreases the consistency of stools.[95] These data indicate a difference between constipated and nonconstipated pregnant women, unrelated to dietary intake, that may be overcome by an increased intake of fiber.

In some families, a visceral myopathy causes thinning and extensive collagen replacement of the longitudinal muscle layer of the bowel. It may be conducive to constipation after the first decade of life. There is generalized smooth muscle disease, and esophagus, bladder, and eyes are afflicted.[78]

Smooth muscle cells of both small and large bowel can be replaced by collagen, and this may cause severe constipation in systemic sclerosis.[96] Muscle atrophy may also be noted in varying degrees with myotonic dystrophy and dermatomyositis.[97]

Lack of exercise and long-distance travel are vague factors said to be related to bowel habits: it is known that a change in posture alters the motility of the pelvic colon.[98] Elderly subjects with arthritis complain of infrequent bowel movements and need to strain at defecation; poor mobility is also associated with a frequent complaint of constipation and increased use of laxatives.[40] How much of this is due to lack of exercise, diet, medications, and underlying disease? For instance, some elderly people suffer from chronic ischemic proctitis as an underlying cause of constipation.[99]

Position modifies the anorectal angle.[100] In addition, the distance between the anterior and posterior margins of the anus increases as hips are flexed and walls are drawn apart.[13] The influence of this on bowel habits is not known.

Neurogenic Causes

Constipation is often associated with diseases of the nervous system, both peripheral and central (Table 22–3).

Hirschsprung's Disease

In Hirschsprung's disease,[101] neurons are absent in the diseased segment,[102–106] the affected bowel is spastic,[107] and there is no rectoanal inhibitory reflex (the reflex relaxation of internal anal sphincter induced by rectal distention and recorded in the upper anal canal).[108–112] This disease is discussed in detail on pages 1390 to 1395.

Hirschsprung's disease may involve only a very short aganglionic segment.[113–116] Two pitfalls in diagnosis must then be avoided. The first is to fail to recognize Hirschsprung's disease, which should be treated surgically, and make an erroneous diagnosis of chronic idiopathic constipation, because the typical features of the disease are not all present. The second, conversely, is to make an erroneous diagnosis of Hirschsprung's disease because the rectoanal inhibitory reflex is absent. Since the absence of the reflex is the only way by which a diagnosis can be made in patients with ultra-short-segment Hirschsprung's disease, it becomes critical to make sure that this absence is not due to another disease, or to a technical error. Thus, the presence of feces in the rectum may falsely suggest Hirschsprung's disease, and a rectoanal inhibitory reflex may appear only after rectal washout.[117] There may likewise be no reflex in patients with chronic rectal ischemia[99] and systemic sclerosis.[96] Surgery, such as full-thickness sphincterotomy[117] or a very low rectal resection,[118] may abolish the reflex. Finally, there is no reflex in neonates weighing less than 2.7 kg and following gestation of less than 39 weeks.[119] In such infants, it may take up to two weeks to appear.[120–122] To avoid making the wrong diagnosis of Hirschsprung's disease in premature normal neonates who have no rectoanal inhibitory reflex or, conversely, missing the diagnosis in the occasional patient who has one, the measurement of acetylcholinesterase activity has been recommended: patients with high levels in the mucosa have Hirschsprung's disease; those with low levels are normal if hypoganglionosis has been ruled out.[123–125]

Hypoganglionosis and Hyperganglionosis

Hypoganglionosis causes constipation,[126, 127] but the diagnosis is difficult because we do not know the normal range of neuronal concentration.[116, 126]

The diagnosis of hyperganglionosis is also difficult to quantify on biopsy[128–130] and may be overlooked because of the mere presence of ganglia. Hyperganglionosis is associated with severe symptoms of bowel dysfunction, present from early infancy and varying from severe constipation to intestinal obstruction. Fluid, electrolyte, and protein loss from the colon may cause rapid deterioration in the patient's condition. Segmental contractions of the colon with poor peristalsis are typical findings on barium enema, and the rectoanal inhibitory reflex may be absent as in Hirschsprung's disease.[131] Hyperganglionosis may exist alone, be associated to pheochromocytoma,[132] or be part of the Sipple syndrome, which involves multiple endocrine neoplasia.[129, 130, 133, 134]

Not only does the number of neurons matter but also their appearance and function, as well as that of the surrounding structures. Neurons mature after birth,[135] but the process is difficult to assess.

Constipation from birth may also be associated with a decreased content of enterochromaffin cells in the rectal mucosa.[136]

Table 22–3. NEUROGENIC CONSTIPATION

Peripheral
Aganglionosis (Hirschsprung's disease)
Hypoganglionosis
Hyperganglionosis
Ganglioneuromatosis
  Primary
  von Recklinghausen's disease
  Multiple endocrine neoplasia, type 2B
Autonomic neuropathy: paraneoplastic, pseudo-obstruction
Chagas' disease

Central
Medulla
  Trauma to nervi erigentes
  Cauda equina tumor
  Meningocele (anterior or posterior)
  Shy-Drager syndrome
  Tabes dorsalis
  Multiple sclerosis
  Trauma to the medulla
Brain
  Parkinson's disease
  Tumors
  Cerebrovascular accidents

Autonomic Neuropathy

Infection by *Trypanosoma cruzi* is responsible for Chagas' disease. This is an acquired form of denervation. Periganglionitis and degeneration of neurons produce dilated segments of colon and constipation.[137] Of note, there is no such neuronal loss with an extrinsic autonomic neuropathy, such as in chronic autonomic failure.[138]

Neurofibromatosis is also a cause of megacolon.[139]

Autonomic neuropathy may also be found in the bowel wall of some patients, who suffer from severe constipation as a paraneoplastic manifestation.[140]

Some patients with pseudo-obstruction complain of severe constipation. Scanty, swollen, or shrunken neurons and a reduction in axons with swollen processes are found to be associated with inflammatory cells and a considerable increase in Schwann cells. This is found in the small and large bowel.[141-145] The progression of symptoms in these patients may result from increasing dependence on laxatives, which induces secondary colonic damage. Occasionally a small granuloma is found between the muscular layers, associated with the nervous plexuses, and unrelated to Crohn's disease.[38, 146]

There are many technical difficulties in the evaluation of bowel wall with regard to constipation. Cut sections should be taken tangentially to the gut wall and not, as customarily done, transversely. Silver stains reveal the presence of argyrophilic nerves, and their respective proportion to argyrophobic cells is probably important in terms of neuropathology. Surprisingly little information, using this technique, is available from the literature.[143, 145, 147] Thus, little correlation is available between histopathologic evaluation of specimens and preoperative functional evaluation. Some patients with megarectum and megasigmoid have severe abnormalities of the myenteric plexus on silver staining: there are only occasional normal argyrophil ganglion cells and most neurons are abnormal, with small dark nuclei without nucleoli or visible chromatin structure, with ballooned cytoplasm and no stainable processes.[148, 149]

Central Nervous System Lesions

Bowel habits and mechanisms of constipation in patients with brain lesions have not been well studied. However, elderly subjects with cerebrovascular disease or parkinsonism do not complain of constipation.[40]

Patients with high cord transection and those with low cord lesions are constipated.[150] Trauma to the cauda equina also causes constipation.[151-153]

The diagnosis of anterior sacral meningocele, another cause of chronic constipation, may be delayed up to 20 years.[154, 155]

In primary autonomic insufficiency, postural hypotension is associated with bladder dysfunction and severe constipation.[156, 157] Some patients with Shy-Drager syndrome also suffer from severe constipation (unpublished observation).

Gastrointestinal Lesions

Upper Gastrointestinal Tract

Patients with celiac sprue may present with fecaloma[158] or megacolon.[159] Stenosing duodenal ulcers, gastric cancer, and cystic fibrosis may also be accompanied by constipation.

Large Bowel

The most common disorders of the colon associated with constipation are the irritable bowel syndrome and diverticular disease, but there are many lesions to rule out (Table 22–4).

There is some evidence that diverticular disease is the long-term result of the irritable bowel syndrome.[160] Symptoms regress in the first condition during dietary therapy simply by placebo effect.[161-163] This raises the possibility of a psychosomatic element in both conditions.

Megacolon may or may not be an entity. Its selection criteria are rather vague and its pathophysiologic mechanisms have not been thoroughly investigated. In particular, patients with megacolon should be compared with those having slow-transit constipation[26] or colonic

Table 22–4. DISEASES OF THE LARGE BOWEL ASSOCIATED WITH CONSTIPATION

Lesions of the Colon
Stenotic Obstructions
Extraluminal
  Tumors
  Chronic volvulus
  Hernias
Luminal
  Tumors
  Strictures
  Diverticulitis
  Chronic amebiasis
  Lymphogranuloma venereum
  Syphilis
  Tuberculosis
  Ischemic colitis
  Endometriosis
  Corrosive enemas
  Surgery
Muscular Abnormalities
Diverticular disease
Segmental dilatation of the colon
Myotonic dystrophy
Systemic sclerosis
Dermatomyositis

Lesions of the Rectum
Tumors
Ulcerative proctitis
Rectocele
Internal rectal prolapse
Surgical stricture (EEA anastomosis)

Lesions of the Pelvic Floor
Descending perineum syndrome

Lesions of the Anal Canal
Stenosis
Anterior ectopic anus
Anal fissure
Mucosal prolapse

inertia.[38] A comparison has been done between patients with idiopathic megacolon and those with megacolon because of Hirschsprung's disease.[164, 165] Surprisingly, 30 per cent of the former group have a history of constipation from birth and 57 per cent have one with onset during the first year of life.

Diaphragmatic hernia should be ruled out in patients who present with chronic constipation and have chronic respiratory symptom, particularly if a history of blunt abdominal trauma is elicited.[166]

Another poorly characterized disorder is segmental dilatation of the colon. This occurs in children, and the only recognized abnormality is hypertonicity of the muscle layers.[167, 168]

Anal Canal

Anterior ectopic anus is a cause of constipation in children.[169, 170]

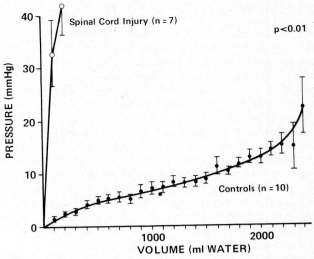

Figure 22–9. Less fluid can be accommodated by the large bowel of male patients with complete spinal cord injury. (Data from Glick et al.[177])

MECHANISMS OF CONSTIPATION SECONDARY TO AN ORGANIC DISEASE

Gastrointestinal transit time, from mouth to cecum, is prolonged in the second and third trimesters of pregnancy,[171, 172] and in the luteal phase of the menstrual cycle, where progesterone levels are increased.[173]

In patients with hypothyroidism, transit time to the cecum decreases after adequate treatment.[83]

The normal postprandial increase in motor activity of the sigmoid colon[174, 175] does not occur in diabetic patients who complain of severe constipation, presumably because of autonomic neuropathy.[176] Those with mild constipation do have a postprandial response, but it is delayed.

The integrity of the nervous system is essential to maintain normal defecation. In patients with traumatic transection of the spinal cord, above the level of the first lumbar vertebra, there is no colonic response to a meal (Fig. 22–8), while response to prostigmin indicates the muscle itself is normal. Colonic compliance and tolerance to fluid filling is also markedly reduced[177] (Fig. 22–9). The reverse occurs in patients with lower lesions of the spinal cord and destruction of the cauda equina: pressure-volume curves within the colon are flat during filling and the compliance is markedly enhanced.[178, 179]

Fifty per cent of multiple sclerosis patients are constipated,[180] and their colonic compliance is decreased.[181] Those who have urinary bladder dysfunction are almost all constipated, and many have fecal incontinence. Transit time through the colon is delayed in different segments of large bowel. Some patients have spontaneous rectal contractions and many manometric abnormalities in the anorectal area suggestive of outlet obstruction: hypertonicity of the anal canal, unstable anal canal pressure, or decreased amplitude of the rectoanal inhibitory reflex. The activity of the striated

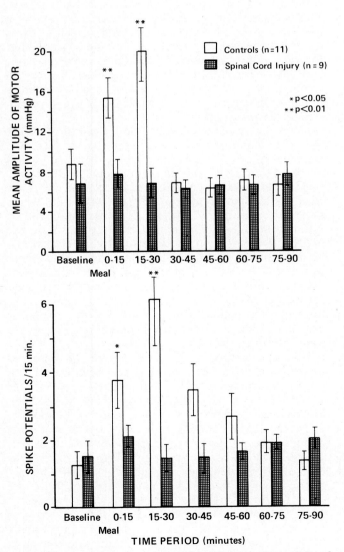

Figure 22–8. There is no postprandial increase in motor activity of the left colon in male patients with complete thoracic spinal cord injury. (Data from Glick et al.[177])

pelvic floor is also impaired.[182] Thus, in patients with multiple sclerosis, colonic propulsion and defecation are impaired. One third of these patients have symptoms of gastric retention, and in some, delayed gastric emptying can be demonstrated.[180] The fact that many have postural lightheadedness and that constipated patients, in contrast to the others, have urinary symptoms points to a similarity to chronic idiopathic constipation by colonic inertia.[38]

Although it is classically said that sympathectomy exerts no influence on colon, rectal, and anal motility, this really has not been studied adequately. In contrast, parasympathetic innervation has been repeatedly found to be essential for normal bowel function.[151-153] Resection of the nervi erigentes leads to obstipation, loss of rectal sensation, and delayed transit through the large bowel. Rectal sensation is lost and rectal capacity to distention increased after bilateral sacrifice of sacral nerves, but not after unilateral sacrifice.[183] The loss of rectal sensation may be neurogenic, through damage of the afferent nerves, but conceivably could also be due simply to a loss of rectal muscle tone. Bypass of the hindgut restores transit,[152] suggesting that sacral parasympathetic outflow exerts no influence on the ascending colon. Pathologic evaluation of the resected specimen of distal colon demonstrates neuronal loss, decrease in size of remaining neurons, and focal Schwann cell hyperplasia.

Trauma to the cauda equina also results in constipation even in the absence of paraplegia. Transit time is prolonged in the large bowel.[153] The anal canal becomes hypertonic. The rectoanal inhibitory reflex persists,[153, 183] but its amplitude is maximal for minimal levels of rectal distention,[153] and the normal correlation[10] between relaxation of the internal sphincter and rectal distention. The rectoanal contractile reflex of the external anal sphincter is much weaker than normal.[153] An internal anal sphincter relaxing in the presence of minimal rectal distention, and associated with a poorly functioning external anal sphincter, of course offers little protection against fecal incontinence if laxatives or enemas are used to overcome constipation.

MECHANISMS OF CHRONIC IDIOPATHIC CONSTIPATION

Constipation as a Body Clue: Disease of the Person

The relationship between emotions, the psyche, and bowel habits is poorly understood. That there could be one involved in constipation was proposed over 50 years ago by Groddeck.[184] There is some support for the idea that a conflict between parent and child over bowel function may modify bowel habits.[185] Voluntary repression of defecation is said to lead to chronic rectal distention and megarectum, but this is simplistic, because some children with chronic idiopathic constipation may pass infrequent stools even before they reach the age of toilet training.

There is a relationship between stool output and personality. Healthy individuals, who display a greater degree of self-esteem and are more outgoing, tend to produce more frequent and heavier stools.[186] As frequency decreases, wet weight also decreases because of reabsorption of water.

Megacolon is found in psychotic patients,[187-189] and this also suggests the possibility of a link between mind and body. Schizophrenics appear to be particularly at risk; this should be placed in perspective with the fact that, in patients with constipation by colonic inertia, transit time in the ascending colon correlates with the score of paranoia in the Minnesota Multiphasic Personality Inventory.[190] In early observations, tonicity and motility of the colon were decreased in the acutely ill, hallucinating paranoid schizophrenics, and normal in the chronic, deteriorated paranoid patients,[191] but this was not confirmed.[187]

There is a very close relationship between the levels of anxiety and transit time in the ascending colon in patients with constipation by delayed colonic transit. This suggests the possibility that constipation, as a mirror, simply reflects in some patients anxiety, that is not expressed via the mind but through physical dysfunction. Cure from constipation by a psychologic approach demonstrates that the basic mechanism in some people is not organic.[27, 192] Conversely, any emotional problem must be channeled through a pathophysiologic mechanism.

Constipated patients with delayed transit through the ascending colon have a different personality than arthritic controls.[190] They score higher on several scales of the Minnesota Multiphasic Personality Inventory (MMPI): Hypochondria, Hysteria, Control, and Low Back Pain. They score lower on the MF scale, which means they are more feminine. The two groups can be differentiated by discriminant analysis: use of the MMPI data alone yields 83 per cent correct answers; addition of age raises this to 97 per cent! This means the computer can recognize a constipated patient versus an arthritic one just with personality and age, regardless of medical investigation! Of course, this does not prove that constipation leads to personality disorder or the contrary, but it demonstrates there is a link between the two.

Several studies have also demonstrated an increased incidence of neurotic traits in patients with the irritable bowel syndrome.[73, 193-196] Constipation is part of this syndrome. However, neurotic patients score even higher than these patients,[197] and some colonic motility measurements are similar in irritable bowel syndrome patients and psychoneurotic controls without the syndrome.[196] Patients with gastrointestinal disorders other than the irritable bowel syndrome may also be depressed and phobic, and somatize abnormally to the same extent as irritable bowel syndrome patients.[198] This suggests that the psychologic profile of irritable bowel syndrome patients is not specific. Many patients with an irritable bowel syndrome do not consult a physician.[19, 44, 199] The possibility has been raised that anxious or depressed patients are more likely to seek treatment for gastrointestinal illness,[19] but reporters and nonreporters are similar in terms of psychometric evaluation. Despite this lack of difference, women tend to consult more than men.[200] Is it because they seek help more easily, when needed, than men? Is it because they are more aware of their needs? Does this explain the marked preponderance of women among adult constipated subjects? American outpatients with an irritable bowel syndrome have a significantly higher level of performance difficulty (which corresponds to obsessive compulsion) than their New Zealand counterparts, while healthy controls score in the same way in both countries.[200] This suggests geographic differences in the irritable bowel syndrome and points to a need for an ethno-physiopathologic evaluation.

Is the presence of a functional abnormality in patients with chronic idiopathic constipation proof that they suffer from an organic lesion? Most children with chronic idiopathic constipation have functional abnormalities in the anal canal and, in 40 per cent, constipation can be traced back to the first month of life.[201] Such data need to be evaluated before the syndrome is labeled psychogenic. Conversely, the finding of these functional abnormalities does not necessarily imply that the patient has an organic lesion. If the root of the problem is emotional in nature, it must be expressed via a circulating substance and/or neurologic circuits. Many patients who complain of constipation used to be dismissed summarily and sent to the psychiatrists. Today, it is said that since functional abnormalities are found in most patients, there must be an organic disease. This pendulum movement between psychiatric and organic approaches simply reflects a dualistic attitude of physicians toward difficulties about mind-body interactions.

Can Chronic Idiopathic Constipation Be Ascribed to a Single Pathophysiologic Mechanism?

It is highly unlikely that a single mechanism is responsible for chronic idiopathic constipation. When more than one functional test is performed, an abnormality is found in almost all patients[31, 202] (Fig. 22–10). In addition, common abnormal mechanisms are found in apparently very different groups of constipated patients. They have difficulties in expelling rectal balloons whether they suffer from slow or normal transit constipation or megarectum, but with different sex ratios in the three groups.[203] At this stage of our understanding, it is difficult to do more than simply describe the different abnormalities at different levels of the colon, rectum, and anus.

Studies in the Stomach and Small Bowel

Transit time to the cecum is slightly prolonged in constipated patients,[204] but this is not of major clinical importance. Within 24 hours, swallowed radiopaque markers are in the large bowel.[10, 13, 36, 205, 206] Any delay in the small bowel points to an organic lesion at that level or to chronic idiopathic pseudo-obstruction. Gastrin and motilin levels rise to a lesser extent than normal, when constipated subjects drink water.[13]

Large Bowel Absorption

The contribution of the colonic mucosa to constipation is minimal, and purely induced by delayed transit and prolonged storage.[207]

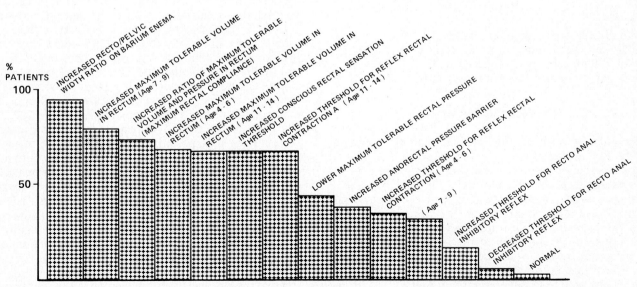

Figure 22–10. A functional abnormality may be found in practically all children with chronic idiopathic constipation. (Data from Meunier et al.[31])

Colorectal Transit Studies

Mechanisms of constipation can be approached in two different ways: following the progress of feces along the large bowel, or evaluating the bowel wall muscular activity and tone. The first method of course provides an estimate of the end results induced by abnormalities demonstrated by the second method.

On the basis of radiopaque marker studies, patients with constipation may be divided into three different groups. In the first, there is delay in the colon.[36, 38, 205, 208–210] In the second, feces pass normally along the colon but are stored too long in the rectum.[70, 211–213] In the third, transit time of the radiopaque markers is normal.

Relatively few patients have a delayed transit in the ascending colon. Thus, a study had to cover a ten-year period to yield 54 subjects.[38] In a recent study of 21 patients with less than two stools per week, 38 per cent were found to have a prolonged transit in all three segments of large bowel.[37]

Patients with hindgut dysfunction have normal right colon transit but a distal delay. Some patients with delayed transit in the ascending colon, however, have clear evidence of reflux from left to right colon,[38] and in some the delay is not reproducible.[190] One of the explanations for these two observations is that distal spasm slows down transit through the ascending colon. These patients probably belong to the group of subjects constipated by hindgut dysfunction. Thirty-three per cent of patients with less than two stools per week have normal transit through the right colon but distal delay, and they are subdivided roughly in half with delay in the left colon and rectosigmoid area, and another half with outlet obstruction.[37]

It is not clear whether these two groups of patients should be pooled together and classified under the broader term of distal constipation.

Some patients clearly have normal colonic function with rectal stasis and suffer from outlet obstruction.[36, 70]

Finally, 29 per cent of patients with less than two stools per week have normal transit in the large bowel.[37] Similarly, half of those with less than three stools per week also have normal transit.[214]

Colonic Constipation

In patients with colonic inertia, markers stagnate along the entire large intestine because the bowel muscle is ineffective.[38] However, delayed transit in the ascending colon may be merely secondary to a distal obstacle, which counteracts an effective colonic musculature in the ascending colon.[215] The term constipation by delayed colonic transit has been proposed for this situation. Dysfunction of the hindgut (the embryologic distal bowel, which goes from the left third of the transverse colon to the anorectal junction) may exist as an isolated congenital abnormality.[215] It probably also exists on a functional basis and provokes delayed transit proximally. Retrograde movement of

feces may be shown objectively with radiopaque marker studies: the markers can be seen to travel back and forth from right to left colon, and in the ascending colon, they disappear not in an exponential but in a bumpy fashion. In a recent study, two groups of patients with delayed transit in the ascending colon were identified. In the first, the abnormality was reproducible one year apart and there was no observable reflux of markers from descending to ascending colon. In the second, there was reflux or the abnormality was not reproducible, suggesting the possibility of distal spasm.[190] One should thus probably reserve the term colonic inertia for the situation in which transit time in the ascending colon is prolonged and no reflux of markers from the left colon is demonstrated.

Some patients suffer from slow-transit constipation:[26] transit time is prolonged in the large bowel, which is of normal size and configuration. This resembles the situation of colonic inertia or constipation by delayed colonic transit.[38, 215] It is probably this kind of subject who, at the beginning of the century, underwent colectomy for protracted obstipation.[63, 216]

Slow-transit constipation and colonic inertia are found almost exclusively in women, regardless of bowel size at barium enema. In contrast, megacolon is found in both sexes, suggesting that proportionally more constipated men have an easily distensible colon.[164, 165] This is in contrast to the incidence of megarectum, which is found more often in women.[70]

Very little is known about the mechanisms conducive to delayed passage of feces through the colon. In women with slow-transit constipation and those with colonic inertia, decreased bowel frequency is severe (one stool per week) and, together with other symptoms, begins around the age of puberty.[26, 38] In a few patients, symptoms begin suddenly after an abdominal operation or accident, and are the consequence of a physical or emotional trauma. The latter possibility is rendered more plausible because these subjects have cold hands—a clear sign of anxiety—and blackouts.[26]

Colonic motility, as measured with miniature balloons, does not differ between patients with slow-transit constipation and controls.[217] However, the introduction of bisacodyl into the colonic lumen, which stimulates the appearance of powerful peristaltic waves in normal subjects, does not in slightly less than half of those with slow transit constipation[217] (Fig. 22–11). The response or absence of response of colonic motility to bisacodyl may perhaps help in the future in recognition of patients who have a very inert colonic musculature. In some constipated subjects, motor activity of the sigmoid colon increases to an abnormal degree after a meal, suggesting spasticity; in others, it is the reverse, and hypomotility is observed postprandially.[174] This again suggests two groups of constipated subjects who have delayed transit in the colon: the hypomotor and the hypermotor subjects.

Myoelectric spiking activity of the descending and sigmoid colon has been measured in patients with constipation who have prolonged transit time in the right colon. The number of propagating electrical po-

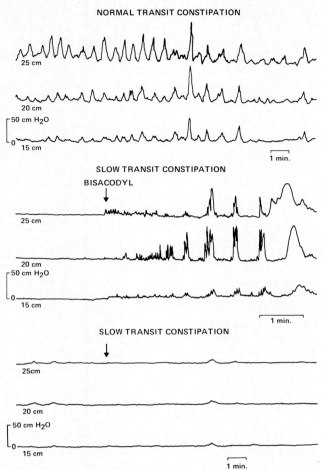

Figure 22–11. In some women with slow transit constipation, bisacodyl exerts no influence on colonic intraluminal pressure. (From Preston, J. E., and Lennard-Jones, J. E. Dig. Dis. Sci. *30*:289, 1985. Used by permission.)

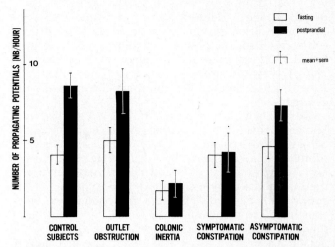

Figure 22–12. Patients with colonic inertia have little propagating electrical activity in the distal colon, and it does not increase after a meal. For definition of the other groups of subjects, see Schang.[214]

pass urine in patients with slow-transit constipation.[26] Finally, there is a high incidence of galactorrhea with normal prolactin levels in these two groups of constipated women.[26, 38] Reproductive hormones may be involved since these women often complain of irregular painful menstruation, have difficulties in becoming

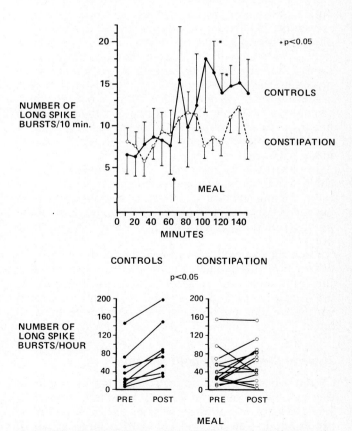

Figure 22–13. In patients with irritable bowel syndrome who complain of painful constipation (<3 stools/week), there is little increase of the propagating electrical activity in the distal colon after ingestion of a meal. (Data from Dapoigny et al.[218])

tentials is significantly decreased in the fasting conditions, and no postprandial increase in their number is observed[214] (Fig. 22–12). Unfortunately, this study did not distinguish patients with colonic inertia from those with constipation by delayed colonic transit. No abnormality was found in the number of rhythmic spike potentials, which are repetitive and stationary, nor in terms of the sporadic spike potentials, which are long spike bursts but do not propagate. Similarly, there is no postprandial increase in long spike bursts in patients with the irritable bowel syndrome who have less than three stools per week[218, 219] (Fig. 22–13).

Dysphagia and gastroesophageal reflux are associated with hypertonicity of the pharyngoesophageal sphincter and a weak gastroesophageal sphincter in patients with colonic inertia.[38] There is also a high incidence of simultaneous contractions of the esophagus (tertiary contractions) together with hypersensitivity of the bladder to urecholine. Thus, there is evidence for abnormal function of esophagus, colon, rectum, anus, and bladder in these patients.[38] There is also a high incidence of nocturia and difficulty in starting to pregnant, and undergo a lot of gynecologic surgery.[26] In some, raised serum prolactin levels, low urinary estrogens, and low plasma estradiol levels have been found.[220] Stress[221] and the circadian rhythms[222] may be involved. Motor disorders in the gastrointestinal tract may also have altered the enterohepatic circulation of estrogens.

This all points to a systemic disease[38] or disorder. Some patients who undergo surgery have abnormalities of neurologic structures in the bowel, whether on a primary or a secondary basis,[141-149] but evidence has also been produced of a correlation between transit time in the ascending colon and anxiety levels.[190] Together with markedly different personalities between constipated women with colonic inertia and controls,[190] this may indicate the presence of a disorder of the person rather than a diseased body. The mechanism, whether pharmacologic or neurogenic, remains to be clarified. These patients often resent any implication that their symptoms are psychologically determined, yet they have a high incidence of unhappy childhood and psychosocial problems.[223] More studies are clearly in order to grasp the roots of this major problem.

Constipation by Outlet Obstruction

The existence of a mechanism of constipation by outlet obstruction was originally postulated because retrograde movement of radiopaque markers could be observed during transit studies in constipated patients.[224] Increase in stool frequency and decrease in transit time in the distal large bowel after anorectal myectomy gave further support to the existence of such a mechanism.[36] The existence of a hypertonic anal canal, of an unstable resting pressure in the anal canal, or of a poor relaxation of the upper anal canal during rectal distention[36] has now been confirmed to exist in many patients.[39]

In patients in whom markers are retained in the left colon and/or the rectosigmoid area, the level of sporadic spiking electrical activity is normal or slightly elevated; the most striking feature is an increase in the number of retrograde, orally moving propagating bursts.[225]

On a theoretical basis, several mechanisms of outlet obstruction are possible: a hyperactive rectosigmoid junction, increased storage capacity of the rectum, rectal spasticity, and hypertonicity of the anal canal with incoordination of the reflexes between rectum and anus.

Hyperactive Rectosigmoid Junction

Under basal conditions, pressure changes greatly in the sigmoid colon from minute to minute and from week to week,[226] and this increases difficulties of interpretation. In the sigmoid colon of a large group of patients with severe (one stool per week or less), persistent constipation, motor activity was present for a greater proportion of time in normal subjects, but the mean amplitude of pressure waves was decreased. Younger patients had a more active bowel than older ones. In the upper rectum, duration and mean amplitude of pressure were decreased in constipated subjects.[227] Other investigators found little change in motor activity during or after a meal.[228, 229] Of note, stool frequency is often used as a selection criterion, but it does not correlate with transit time in the bowel.[70, 230] Under basal conditions, no difference is usually found between normal and constipated subjects after prolonged fasting; food, however, exerts various effects in constipated patients, and this makes it possible to separate them into hypomotor responders, normal responders, and hypermotor responders.[174]

With a pull-through technique, a zone of complex wave activity 1.5 to 2 cm in length, at 9 to 15 cm from the anal margin, is found in most severely (less than two stools per week) constipated patients but not in healthy subjects.[231] Neither secretin nor cholecystokinin influences the wave activity of the hyperactive segment, but atropine and glucagon inhibit markedly all wave activity and decrease the motility index of this segment significantly, suggesting overactivity of the muscarinic effector cells.[231] Patients with mild constipation show slightly greater pressure changes at 15 cm than normal subjects, but no difference at 20 and 25; moreover, there is no difference between patients with constipation and those with diarrhea.[226] The rectosigmoid area is a key area in the mechanism of constipation of at least some patients. Normally, there is a circadian rhythm of motor activity in the large bowel. Large meals increase myoelectrical activity,[222] and sleep[222] or rest[221] decrease it, but the rectosigmoid junction remains in a state of constant activity.[222] Surgeons know empirically that the rectosigmoid area must be removed in patients operated upon for diverticulitis for fear of recurrent disease, and O'Beirne long ago had postulated the existence of a sphincter in this area, which was later found not to be existent.[232] Is the presence of constant activity in the rectosigmoid area a subtle indication of the presence of a mild irritable bowel syndrome?

Anorectal Motility

The function of the anorectal junction is often abnormal in patients with chronic idiopathic constipation. In a pilot study, manometric findings in subjects with chronic idiopathic constipation included a decreased amplitude of the rectoanal inhibitory reflex, a hypertonic anal canal relaxing more than normally when the rectum is distended, and unstable resting pressure in the upper anal canal[36] (Fig. 22–14). Those various patterns of response have been recognized in other laboratories.

Resting pressure in the anal canal of patients with chronic idiopathic constipation has been found to be increased,[36, 38, 39, 201, 233] normal,[234] or decreased.[32] These differences probably result from the criteria used in patient selection and the modalities of recording, which, in a sphincter, only reflects its resistance to

ANORECTAL MANOMETRY IN IDIOPATHIC CONSTIPATION

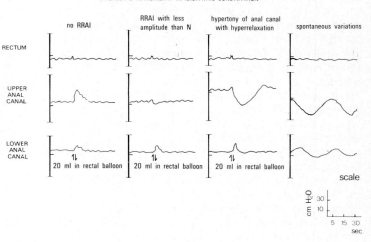

Figure 22–14. Four patterns of anorectal motility in patients with chronic idiopathic constipation. In those with spontaneous variations, the mean level of pressure may be normal or increased; it is difficult to recognize the presence of a rectoanal inhibitory reflex (RRAI) unless the rectum is distended while the resting pressure is on a decreasing slope. (Reprinted with permission from: Mechanisms of idiopathic constipation: outlet obstruction, by Martelli, H., Devroede, G., Arhan, P., and Duguay, C. Gastroenterology 75:623. Copyright 1978 by The American Gastroenterological Association.)

distention. Water perfusion systems, for instance, produce errors because the rate of perfusion influences recording: it is the pressure within the artificially produced water-filled compartment that is measured. In addition, leakage of fluid modifies external anal sphincter activity and can even abolish the presence of a normal rectoanal inhibitory reflex (P. Denis: unpublished observations). Finally, the anal canal of constipated patients who also complain of pain is hypertonic, but it is not when constipation is painless[25] (Fig. 22–15). The finding of normal basal pressure thus does not, as has been suggested, rule out outlet obstruction as a mechanism of constipation.[234]

Constipated children with encopresis have a hypotonic anal canal.[32] Since they also have a very low stool frequency, they may suffer from an enlarged rectal capacity. Indeed, patients with megarectum have a lower resting pressure than controls.[70] Of note, patients with congenital megarectum have a similar pressure in the upper and lower parts of the anal canal, in contrast to healthy subjects and patients with acquired megarectum.

Instability of the anal pressure may take the appearance of ultraslow waves of low frequency and high amplitude, or of slow waves of higher frequency and low amplitude. Pudendal block may abolish these abnormalities, and this suggests that they are probably due in part to external rather than internal sphincter activity. These fluctuations have been described in other laboratories[39, 235] and may or may not be associated with a higher than normal level of pressure.

In patients with chronic idiopathic constipation, the rectoanal inhibitory reflex may be normal or absent, or an abnormality such as a lesser than normal or an excessive amplitude may be found.[36] Other abnormalities, such as prolonged duration of the reflex, have been described in chronic ischemia of the rectum with or without constipation.[99] Several other laboratories have described the existence of a rectoanal inhibitory reflex decreased[235, 236] or increased[235] in amplitude. An increase in threshold of the rectoanal inhibitory reflex has also been recognized.[35, 233, 237]

Anismus

A mechanism of outlet obstruction, well identified recently, has been labeled anismus, spastic pelvic floor syndrome, or sphincteric disobedience syndrome. A broader term without implication of etiology (psychologic or organic) might be that of rectosphincteric dyssynergia, similar to the term vesicourethral dyssynergia used by urologists who deal with similar problems in the bladder and urethra.

Normally during defecation, the pelvic floor, which at rest is in a state of constant activity and contraction, relaxes completely.[238–240] This does not always occur. Some subjects indeed contract the external anal sphincter during straining. Records of electromyographic activity show a transient increase in activity at onset and end of straining, or a highly increased level of activity during the entire duration of the act of defecation. A few subjects exhibit bursts of repetitive tetanic-like grouped action potentials succeeding each other in a fast (8 per second) rhythm, and completely different from those recorded during voluntary contraction of the perianal musculature.[241] The clinical

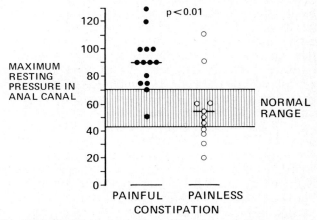

Figure 22–15. The anal canal is hypertonic in constipated patients who complain of pain but not in those who do not. (Data from Lanfranchi et al.[25])

counterpart of this abnormality was initially labeled the puborectalis syndrome: constipation, incomplete evacuation of the rectum, and anorectal pain were the presenting symptoms;[242] the length of the anal canal was increased, and spasm was present at the level of the puborectalis muscle; the posterior rectal pouch was unusually deep because of the angulation at the anorectal ring, and any attempt to pull the puborectalis sling posteriorly triggered more spasm and pain.

An association between constipation and abnormal external anal sphincter activity was also reported in patients with megarectum.[243] A larger volume of rectal distention, enough to cause abdominal pain but no rectal sensation, was needed to produce total inhibition of the striated muscle activity of the pelvic floor, and occasionally, an attempt to defecate caused an intense contraction of the floor.

Defecation straining was also found to induce a grossly abnormal overactivity in the puborectalis muscle, usually with little change in the superficial external anal sphincter, in two other groups of patients: those with the solitary rectal ulcer syndrome and those with the descending perineum syndrome.[240] Patients with the solitary rectal ulcer syndrome have an internal rectal prolapse and complain of obstructed defecation: they feel a complete blockage of the anal canal. Patients with the descending perineum syndrome have a weak pelvic floor, and when they strain, it can easily be seen to bulge; they may at least in the early stages of dysfunction contract the pelvic floor at the same time they push it out. Patients with either condition thus must defecate through an unrelaxed puborectalis sling. It must be noted that the puborectalis muscle is innervated in part by a branch of the sacral nerve that lies above the pelvic floor; the pudendal nerve supplies only the ipsilateral external anal sphincter muscle. There may be distinct pathologies of the puborectalis muscle (and its associated iliococcygeus and pubococcygeus muscles) and of the external anal sphincter.[244] Pudendal block, indeed, does not abolish the increase in resting pressure of the upper and lower anal canal that results from maximal voluntary contraction.[245]

Recent studies have explored these relationships in depth. In patients with anismus, no inhibition of electrical activity occurs in either the puborectalis or external anal sphincter muscles during straining, but rather there is increased activity in one or both of these muscles, associated with a rise in anal canal pressure[246] (Fig. 22–16). In a few subjects this excess activity may persist up to two minutes after the straining effort has ceased. Thus, despite a rise in intrarectal pressure conducive to defecation, the anorectal pressure barrier persists, and patients are unable to defecate a 50-ml water-filled balloon placed in the rectum. The term anismus is quite appropriate because of its analogy with vaginismus, where a spasm of the pelvic floor muscles occurs, the difference of course being that vaginismus is resistance to penetration and anismus to expulsion. The findings have been confirmed in patients complaining of severe difficulty to pass formed stools who have no megarectum.[247] A similar

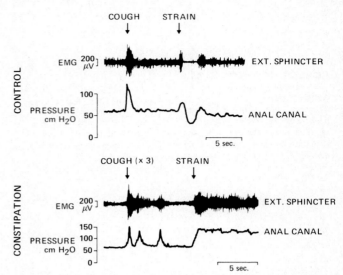

Figure 22–16. In anismus, patients who complain of constipation contract their anal canal while they strain. (From Preston, D. M., and Lennard-Jones, J. E. Dig. Dis. Sci. *30*:413, 1985. Used by permission.)

pathology exists in the anterior part of the pelvic floor. Vesicourethral dyssynergia is conducive to bladder retention and infection: patients contract the external urethral sphincter when they try to void.[248] Chronic pelvic tensions have been said to result from psychologic conflicts during childhood and lead to urinary control problems and diminished orgasmic response.[249, 250] In an interesting study of a large group of predominantly heterosexual college graduate women, the contractile strength of the pelvic floor muscles has been demonstrated to be in relationship with both urinary control and orgasmic response.[49] The participation of the posterior section of the pelvic floor to these relationships has not been investigated yet, but preliminary data suggest sexual difficulties in severely constipated women (unpublished observation). Therefore, the old suggestion of gynecologists that the pelvic floor should be treated as a neuromuscular unit that takes into account the interrelationships between muscular motility and supportive, sphincteric, sensorimotor and sexual functioning, may be pertinent for physicians dealing with patients complaining of constipation and found to have outlet obstruction.

The cause of anismus is not known. Malfunction of the anorectal structure, on an organic basis, is a possibility. However, the only successful treatment found to date for this disorder has been biofeedback,[251] and this suggests the nature of it to be an abnormal learning process rather than a disease. Moreover, in a large series of constipated children who did not have Hirschsprung's disease, one quarter were found to strain when asked to squeeze, one quarter to squeeze when asked to strain, like in anismus, and five per cent to do both and thus reverse the command—therefore the labeling of a sphincteric disobedience syndrome.[252] It is not known if the child does not want to do what is asked or does not understand what is asked.

Defecography is a radiologic technique used to observe the dynamics of defecation, the morphology of the anorectal structures during this process, and the anorectal angle at rest, during squeezing, and during straining. In some constipated patients, the anorectal angle does not increase during straining but remains at 90 degrees and the barium paste in the rectum cannot be excreted. The term spastic pelvic floor syndrome has been proposed to describe this abnormality.[253] This is not, as originally described in anismus,[246] found exclusively in women.[247, 253, 254] The clinical counterpart of the spastic pelvic floor syndrome is a sensation of perineal fullness and urge, straining for prolonged periods of time, and difficult and painful evacuation. Several patients insert a finger into the anal canal to initiate defecation. Pressure in the anal canal is normal at rest and during squeezing, but electromyographic studies of both external anal sphincter and puborectalis sling demonstrate a marked increase in activity during straining.

The relationship between anismus and large bowel transit time is not clear. In one study,[246] all patients had delayed transit of radiopaque markers. In others, however, some patients had normal segmental transit time in all areas of the large bowel.[253, 254] In patients with congenital megarectum, colonic transit is normal, and stasis occurs only in the rectum and is alleviated by rectal bypass.[70] This suggests that isolated mechanisms of outlet obstruction exist. If this is so for anismus, it is not known.

The demonstration of anismus may be done in several ways. At defecography, the anorectal angle may be narrow and does not open during straining to defecate; on rare occasions it becomes more narrow during straining. The patient may also be unable to defecate a rectal balloon. Also, electromyographic evidence of pelvic floor contraction may be found during attempted defecation. Very few constipated patients have all three of these abnormalities.[202] However, external anal sphincter activity decreases during the act of bearing down for defecation in 100 per cent of controls, in 58 per cent of constipated children with encopresis able to defecate balloons, and in only 7 per cent of patients unable to defecate balloons.[35] This suggests a very strong association between increased external anal sphincter activity during defecation attempts, as recorded by electromyography, and failure to defecate a rectal balloon filled with 30 to 100 ml of water.

A fourth way to search for anismus is to record the anal resting pressure during a Valsalva maneuver; control subjects have an anal relaxation, but 75 per cent of constipated children without fecal incontinence, on the contrary, have an increase in pressure.[255] This abnormality is often associated with other rectoanal disorders: anal hypertonia, increased rectal compliance, and impaired rectal conscious sensitivity. A fifth method is to evaluate the configuration of the rectoanal inhibitory reflex during rectal distention: occasionally, it is possible to record an external anal sphincteric contraction in the midst of the reflex.[192] This is also found in 45 per cent of encopretic children who exhibit external anal sphincter contraction during expulsion, and this, of course, is thought to contribute to fecal retention.[256] A final way to detect anismus is to ask the patient to strain while doing a rectal examination. No study has been done to compare this clinical sign with the other diagnostic modalities of anismus.

Descending Perineum Syndrome. In some constipated patients, the perineum descends during straining. The level of this descent can be measured by defecography.[256] Anismus may be associated with it.[240, 254] In about half of patients, it is the reverse that occurs, with prolonged inhibition of the pelvic floor muscles.[240, 256, 257] Mean motor unit potential duration is prolonged, indicating neuropathic changes.[257] When it occurs, there is no anismus as judged by defecography, but on the contrary the anorectal angle opens more than in controls during straining efforts.[257] It is possible that the descending perineum syndrome is the consequence of anismus, and that the long-term result of denervation[257, 259, 260] abolishes the pelvic floor muscle activity, but this has not been studied longitudinally to learn the natural history of anismus and the descending perineum syndrome.

Megarectum. The association of megarectum with constipation has long been recognized.[261–264] When the rectum is distended, electrical activity increases in the external anal sphincter and the puborectalis muscle, but as distention progresses, complete inhibition eventually occurs. The pressure at which this inhibition occurs is much higher and induced by a larger distending volume.[262] The rectal wall of these patients has little elasticity and can easily be distended to accommodate large amounts of fluid.[70] Although impaired rectal sensation has been reported in these patients,[29] the level of pressure at which sensation occurs is the same regardless of rectal volume, and this suggests that the nature of the problem is not impaired rectal sensation but inelasticity of the musculature: a greater stretch is needed before sufficient tension occurs and sensation begins.[70] The rectoanal inhibitory reflex is also impaired, since it is triggered by rectal accommodation;[265] the amplitude is less than normal, and the reflex can even be abolished at lesser levels of distention. It is easy to understand that rectal deformation by a rectal balloon distended with air is much less if the rectal wall is flaccid. When the reflex is absent, this should not be mistaken for the absence of reflex found in Hirschsprung's disease. Patients with constipation from birth who are found to have a megarectum seem to differ from those who became constipated later in life; colonic transit is normal and storage exists exclusively in the rectum, which accommodates huge volumes and is more flaccid than in any other situation. Rectal bypass offers some hope of surgical cure in patients with congenital megarectum, but it should be discouraged in patients with acquired megarectum. In patients with acquired megarectum, a greater recorded as compared with recalled stool frequency, clinical improvement by vastly different treatment modalities such as surgery or psychotherapy, delayed transit at the colonic as well as rectal level, and absence of correlation between colonic transit and rectal capacity all point to a functional problem akin to the irritable bowel syndrome, but without spasticity.

The relationship between anismus and megarectum is not known. It is possible that children with megarectum and fecal soiling have a disorder of anorectal sphincteric function. This indeed often occurs in encopretic children, with or without megarectum.[256] No specific study of anismus has been done in patients with megarectum, but there is anecdotal observation of an association, as demonstrated by electromyography.[243] In most patients with megarectum, in addition, the volume necessary to produce reflex inhibition of the pelvic floor is high: 700 ml or more is necessary to distend the rectum before this occurs, and no sensation is yet present.[243] This is also found in chronically constipated children with encopresis who pass episodically very large amounts of stools, sufficient to clog the toilet; they are likely to have a megarectum.[35] Thus, a rectoanal dyssynergia occurs at least in terms of nonrelaxation. Whether this is akin to anismus, in which active sphincteric contraction occurs, is not known.

Anorectal Structures during Defecation

Sigmoido-rectal intussusception can occur in patients with constipation, and may be accompanied by such abnormalities as enterocele, internal rectal prolapse, rectocele, and anterior mucosal rectal prolapse. It is uncertain which are primary and which are secondary abnormalities, and the same is true of the descending perineum syndrome, megarectum, and anismus. There is an urgent need to understand normal dynamics of defecation. In subjects without clinical evidence of a defecatory problem, the pelvic floor may be seen at defecography to descend as much as 5 cm during straining, and this is more than can be detected clinically (up to 2 cm).[266] At rest, the anorectal angle is 94 ± 19 degrees, and lies less than 2 cm above the plane of the ischial tuberosities. The anal canal is closed and the puborectalis impression is clearly defined. The angle opens at defecation to 113 ± 16 degrees. In women, posterior folds of the distal rectum and small anterior rectoceles are common; there is also frequent inversion of the anterior wall over the anal canal, with a guttering effect of the rectal folds at the end of evacuation but this does not correlate absolutely with the proctoscopic finding of anterior mucosal prolapse.[266] In perfectly asymptomatic healthy volunteers not responsive in any way to stress, we twice found an internal rectal prolapse (unpublished observation). Thus, although observable abnormalities should be searched for, they should always be correlated with clinical findings. This approach to management is comparable to that for hiatal hernia of the stomach, which is not always symptomatic and should not *per se* be an indication for surgery.

Rectal Sensation

Rectal sensation is decreased in patients with megarectum.[29, 70] It is also decreased in some children[35, 233] and adults[234, 237] with chronic idiopathic constipation. Fifty per cent of severely constipated women who have a normal barium enema do not have rectal sensation, in contrast to only 13 per cent of controls; 10 per cent do not even have an abdominal sensation as indicative of an urge to defecate.[13] Impaired rectal sensation is not related to the capacity to defecate balloons placed in the rectum.[35] It is common thinking among clinicians that some children and adults may block out rectal sensation. The recent finding that sensation occurs at a given level of rectal pressure, regardless of rectal volume, suggests that this may be entirely secondary to inelasticity of the rectum,[70] rather than to a relative rectal anesthesia. Sensation possibly may also be present but ignored; this has not been evaluated.

Constipation with Normal Transit Times

A large proportion of constipated patients have normal transit time of radiopaque markers.[37, 214, 254] The exact percentage of patients in whom this finding is made depends on the modalities of patient selection. It has been shown to exist in those who defecate less than two stools per week[37] as well as those with megarectum.[70] Of interest is the observation that these patients are for the most taking psychotropic agents, particularly antidepressants, are receiving psychiatric counseling, or are involved in medical or nonmedical litigation, in contrast to what is observed in patients with delayed transit in part or all of the large bowel.[37]

The mechanisms of constipation with normal transit time are beginning to be elucidated. For instance, patients with this type of constipation are found to have a colonic motor activity much in excess of controls,[217] and they have a postprandial increase in the number of rhythmic and stationary potentials.[214]

Some of these patients clearly deny that they defecate as often as they do; markers disappear from plain films of the abdomen, while the patient fails to report any stool.[208] There is no way to recognize this unless marker studies are performed.

In some other patients, the transit is really normal. However, in a recent study of patients with megarectum, it has been shown that some have transit times that fall within the normal range of healthy controls, but that are prolonged as compared with controls whose bowel habits are not modified by stress.[70] The irritable bowel syndrome is highly prevalent in the healthy population, and thus great care should be taken in the selection of control subjects in studies of constipation.

The severity of the problem is less in patients with normal transit than in those patients with delayed transit throughout the large bowel. Follow-up studies also show that improvement varies according to mechanisms; clinical improvement during follow-up is seen in almost all patients with distal slowing, in two thirds of those with normal transit times, and only 25 per cent of those with delayed transit in the ascending colon.[37] An appealing hypothesis, in view of the psychosocial disturbances in patients with normal transit, would be that the more distal is the mechanism of constipation, the greater is the influence of the mental component in the disorder.[27, 267] This hypothesis, if true, would help explain the greater frequency of improvement with more distal slowing, since emotional conflicts are more amenable to resolution than physical complaints. An exception to this hypothesis would be the patient who denies any bowel movement even though a marker study gives evidence of defecation. One such patient, found repeatedly to have transit times throughout the gastrointestinal tract of only 48 hours, managed to find a surgeon who performed an ileosigmoid anastomosis. There was a subsequent increase in symptoms. Four years later, after dismantling of the anastomosis, this patient again denied defecation with a normal transit time (unpublished observation). Similarly, out of six patients with colonic transit within normal limits, those who claimed no improvement on a high-fiber diet, reassurance and encouragement without any hint of accusation of misrepresenting the complaints, declined to undergo repeated transit studies.[37]

An Overview of the Mechanism of Chronic Idiopathic Constipation

A distinction should be made between constipated patients who have an atonic bowel and those with a spastic bowel, and this can be evaluated by compliance studies. The extent of the lesion should be appreciated; megacolon may coexist or exist apart from megarectum. A second distinction should be made as far as the level of functional abnormality; marker studies may be used for that purpose.

Finally, an important distinction should be made between striated muscle dysfunction and smooth muscle disorder. Pelvic floor dysfunction is definitely an abnormality that should be distinguished.

EVALUATION

The evaluation of constipated patients should be a three-stage process.

Morphologic Evaluation

History

The key question to ask at first visit is about the onset of constipation. Most patients who have constipation due to congenital diseases, such as Hirschsprung's disease or meningocele, have had difficulties with their bowel habits from birth. When constipation occurs later in life, the symptom, at presentation, may

be of chronic or recent onset. Constipation of recent onset is frequently due to significant pathology. The most important disease to rule out is, of course, colonic malignancy. A history of two years or more is a safe cut-off point.[27, 43]

It is also important to have the patients define what they mean by constipation.

Physical Examination

Cutaneous sensations around the anus may be absent in patients with neurogenic disorders; this may indicate the level and side of the abnormality. At rest, the anal canal tone can be evaluated grossly and correlates fairly well with the incidence of incontinence.[268] The anus may be too tight. The distinction between internal and external sphincter hypertonicity can be appreciated if the rectal examination is prolonged; talking to the patient and inducing relaxation or even hypnosis may abolish the hypertonicity, suggesting that tightness was due to striated muscle hyperactivity. A reliable sign of disordered innervation of the anus is the gaping of the canal when the puborectalis muscle is grasped by the examining finger and pulled posteriorly. In some patients, anal tone is normal but does not resist traction. In some others, a return to the resting position is very slow. The incidence of these abnormalities and their significance in terms of pathways and etiology remain to be ascertained. Spinal lesions are probably present if these abnormalities are demonstrated. In cervical transection, the anus remains closed and a balloon can be retained in the rectum, whereas in low, flaccid lesions of the medulla, the anus is patulous and unable to contract to prevent extrusion of the balloon.[150] A mechanism of rectoanal dyssynergia has been recognized; this can also be appreciated grossly during rectal examination, after organic lesions have been ruled out. The patient is asked to strain, while the clinician keeps his or her finger in the rectum. Patients with anismus will squeeze, and this is easy to recognize. Some will have intermittent contractions.[241] Descent of the perineum is also easy to recognize during this examination step. It is often associated with the presence of a rectocele; curbing the finger through the anterior rectal wall makes it appear in the vagina, on the other side of the perineal body. Posteriorly, pain can be triggered by pulling the levator ani.

Finally, in Hirschsprung's disease, after rectal examination a profuse fecal discharge occurs.

Endoscopy

Endoscopy is usually performed with flexible instruments. This serves the purpose of ruling out organic lesions, but the instrument has a superior value in demonstrating the presence of internal rectal prolapse and anterior mucosal prolapse, as there is no air pressure to counteract the dynamics of the rectal wall during straining efforts to defecate.

Melanosis coli is a term used to describe the appearance of the colonic mucosa after abuse of laxatives, mainly those of the anthraquinone family. The mucosa has a brown-black spotty coloration owing to deposits of lipofuscin, both free and in macrophages in the lamina propria. The distal rectum may be spared by the melanosis; this suggests that the colon functions normally to the junction between melanotic and amelanotic bowel and that the abnormality lies in the distal bowel, free from melanosis (unpublished observations). The lumen may be of enormous size and contain stools of much smaller caliber. Atony of the bowel wall may be demonstrated by the fact that the rectum remains wide open when it is exposed to atmospheric pressure. Whether this atony is primary or secondary to outlet obstruction cannot be inferred from the proctosigmoidoscopy.

Radiographic Studies

In constipation of recent origin, a barium enema is mandatory in order to determine whether obstruction due to organic narrowing, particularly carcinoma, underlies the change in bowel habit. In chronic constipation the size of the distal bowel is greater than normal, but on a single examination the radiologist is unable to distinguish constipated from nonconstipated patients, and the change in bowel size after treatment does not correlate well with its outcome.[114] There is also no correlation between rectal size, as determined radiologically, and rectal elastic properties, as determined by manometric studies.[31] Nevertheless, a useful measure to remember is 6.5 cm, the upper limit of normal rectosigmoid width on lateral view at the pelvic brim.[269] At present, the barium enema is essential to diagnose megacolon.

In patients with long-segment Hirschsprung's disease, a narrow rectum can be demonstrated at barium enema, and in children with this problem it is thus not necessary to complete the investigation to the cecum. However, barium enema is useless in short-segment Hirschsprung's disease, because there is no narrow segment.

There is no quantitative clinical way to recognize large bowel length or volume, and dye dilution curves have not been used outside of a research setting.[224, 270] A diagnosis of redundant colon, as defined when an enema-filled pelvic loop rises above the iliac crest, is found much more often in patients with long-standing constipation than in controls.[271] Colonmetrograms are probably superior in this regard.[177, 181] The volume of fluid that can be infused into the large bowel of healthy subjects may reach up to 2400 ml.

Plain films of the abdomen are useful, especially in large bowel pseudo-obstruction. When patients complain of acute abdominal pain and distention, they may exhibit gaseous distention of the colon to monstrous proportions, up to 20 cm.

Biopsies

Some of the limitations of histologic diagnosis have been pointed out. Abnormal histopathologic findings are significant, but normal histology does not necessarily rule out disease and should be interpreted in the context of history, examination, and radiologic and manometric findings.

In the infant, the absence of neurons in a rectal suction biopsy specimen, taken at least 25 mm above the distal edge of the internal sphincter, is suggestive of Hirschsprung's disease.

In young children at the age of bowel training with a normal rectoanal inhibitory reflex, the treatment of choice is not clearly established. In this group of patients, it is probably best to wait until it becomes evident that the problem persists beyond the age of toilet training. In this group of patients, a suction biopsy specimen may be obtained about 3 cm above the distal edge of the internal sphincter to rule out aganglionosis.

Rectal biopsies should not be used to evaluate adult patients who complain of long-standing idiopathic constipation.

Functional Evaluation

Studies of Colonic Transit Times

The next major step in the evaluation of patients with chronic idiopathic constipation is the measurement of colonic transit times. The subject ingests radiopaque markers, remains on a high-residue diet, and refrains from laxatives, enemas, and all nonessential drugs. The markers are not commercially available and are simply cut from a radiopaque nasogastric tube. Stools may be visualized radiographically,[272–274] or, to distinguish between the different types of constipation, the progression of markers along the colon may be followed by daily radiographs of the abdomen.[10, 36, 207, 208, 275] Films are taken until total expulsion of markers, for a maximum of seven days after ingestion. Markers are counted in the right colon, left colon, and rectosigmoid area by using the bony landmarks of the spine and pelvic contours. Occasionally a large cecum overlaps the pelvis, or a transverse colon is sagging into the abdomen; this can be recognized either by gaseous shadows or by barium enema in the same patient on another day.

Segmental transit time is probably the safest and most practical measure to obtain. A simplified formula can be obtained if the patient swallows 20 markers and a film is obtained every 24 hours; markers are counted in the segment of colon, each day, until distal total progression; these numbers are added and the sum is multiplied by 1.2.[206]

Normal values in adults have been obtained under strict dietary conditions (Table 22–5).[36, 206] These values have been used by other authors as a standard of normality.[37] Although acceptable for gross motor abnormalities and severe constipation, this practice is misleading when used to compare healthy controls and subjects complaining of minor constipation. Transit

Table 22–5. MAXIMUM NUMBER (N) OF MARKERS FOUND IN DIFFERENT SEGMENTS OF LARGE BOWEL, IN HEALTHY SUBJECTS WHO INGESTED 20 MARKERS WHILE EATING A HIGH-RESIDUE DIET, AND UPPER LIMIT OF SEGMENTAL COLONIC TRANSIT TIME

Site	Days After Ingestion (N Markers)							Mean Transit Time (Hours)
	1	2	3	4	5	6	7	
Adults								
Right colon	20	10	4	1	0	0	0	38
Left colon	15	11	8	4	3	1	0	37
Rectosigmoid	9	12	10	7	3	1	0	34
Large bowel	20	20	18	10	5	3	0	93
Children								
Right colon	14	1	0	0	0	0	0	18
Left colon	12	4	0	0	0	0	0	20
Rectosigmoid	20	12	7	5	0	0	0	34
Large bowel	20	13	7	4	0	0	0	62

times of controls, whose bowels are not influenced by stress, are shorter; the longest transit time through the large bowel is only 34 hours (instead of 93), and segmental transit times in the ascending and descending colon and rectosigmoid are a maximum of 18, 13, and 20 hours, respectively, instead of 38, 37, and 34.[70] More studies on normality are needed.

This test permits detection of patients who lie or misrepresent their complaint. In such an event, it is best to use the discovery of misrepresentation as encouragement and relate the information back to the patient as evidence of improvement. Transit studies may also be used to evaluate segmental colonic transit time in order to detect specific areas of the bowel that are not functioning properly; results of these studies may be abnormal even though patients have more than three stools per week. For all these reasons, it is probably safer to do marker studies in all constipated patients. During follow-up, marker studies also serve the purpose of providing objective data reflecting the clinical course.

Markers can also be counted in stools. This approach is useful to evaluate mouth-to-anus transit time, but cannot be used to detect segmental abnormalities along the gastrointestinal tract. Thus, patients with constipation by delayed colonic transit or colonic inertia cannot be separated from those with outlet obstruction with this method. In severe chronic constipation, stools are not frequent, and markers may not be excreted in the preset time of study. The first marker should be excreted by the end of the third day after ingestion, and 80 per cent within five days.[10, 224, 274] This is also true in elderly subjects,[275] which indicates that age *per se* exerts little influence on fecal propulsion.

Other methods of estimating transit time have been used but have not gained wide clinical popularity. A radioactive point source can be used alone[209, 210] or with a telemetering capsule so that the site can be determined from characteristic pressure waves.[205, 228, 229, 276] Liquid unabsorbed markers can also be used. First appearance is usually the only practical measurement that can be obtained, unless chemical analyses are performed.

Colorectal Pressure Studies

There is a pressure gradient from proximal to distal colon in normal subjects,[270, 277] but it has not been studied in patients with constipation. There are also technical difficulties that prevent pressure studies from being of practical value in clinical practice. Open-ended perfused tubes or tubes mounted with pressure-sensitive membranes measure accurately absolute levels of pressure, but these do not necessarily reflect local colonic muscular activity; local contraction against distal resistance and movement elsewhere in the colon are also transmitted via the lumen. Balloons do not suffer such handicap but they record not only pressure but artifacts induced by contact with the bowel wall and solid feces.

Electromyography of the Colon

Recording the electrical activity of the bowel smooth muscle is of interest, because spike bursts are the electrical counterpart of smooth muscle contraction.[277, 278] Little is known about the myoelectrical activity of the colon because of difficulties in access, presence of feces, as well as weakness and complexity of signals recorded at this level. Studies have been done with suction electrodes,[280] electrodes clipped onto the colonic mucosa,[279] and surgically implanted electrodes.[281] A major advance has been the use of the intraluminal tube introduced by flexible colonoscopy and equipped with ring electrodes that can pick up the signals by simple contact with the bowel wall.[175, 282, 283]

In health, slow waves are not always present and there is a gradient along the large bowel of both frequency and percentage of electrical activity.[284] Data are scarce in constipation and have focused on slow wave frequency, with conflicting results[279, 285] and frequencies at 2 to 3 cpm, 6 cpm, and 10 to 12 cpm.[279, 284, 285]

The recording of myoelectrical activity appears more promising when signals are filtered with short time constants and spiking activity only is recorded.[285] This consists basically of two types. The first type, the "rhythmic and stationary bursts," are of short duration and occur in sequences lasting for several minutes. They are also called "short spike bursts"[285] and "discrete electrical response activity."[286] In healthy subjects they occur at a rhythm of 11 to 80 per hour, but they may go beyond 100 in constipated patients who complain of pain. The second type, the "sporadic bursts," is made of bursts with much more variable duration, ranging from 5 to 120 seconds. They are also called "long spike bursts"[285] and "continuous electrical response activity."[286] These sporadic spike bursts can be divided into two subgroups. Some show evidence of propagation from one recording site to another over long distances[175] or even the entire length of the colon.[285] The others do not seem to propagate and are seen at only one or two electrode sites. The sporadic bursts, particularly when propagating, are associated with both intraluminal pressure waves and significant propulsion on bowel content; the rhythmic bursts, on the other hand, do not seem to be involved in colonic propulsive activity[287] (Fig. 22–17).

Bisacodyl and vasopressin increase considerably the number of propagating spike bursts,[288, 289] and morphine is associated with their disappearance.[290] Physiologic conditions also significantly affect colonic motility. Food seems to be the most powerful stimulant of propulsive activity.[175] In contrast, rest considerably inhibits all types of myoelectrical spiking activity.[221] These parameters are modified in chronic idiopathic constipation.

Anorectal Pressure Studies

Several probes are available for studying pressure profile and anorectal reflexes.[10, 109–111, 262, 291] It is essential to remember that, although qualitative results can be compared from series to series, regardless of instrumentation and technique, these must be standardized to compare results on a quantitative basis. Under the same conditions, and using the same probe, similar data have been obtained in two independent laboratories.[10]

There are two kinds of anorectal pressure studies. A pressure profile from rectum to anal margin can be recorded by withdrawing an open-tipped recording catheter.[232] When the normal rectum is transiently distended, a sampling reflex occurs in the anal canal. It consists in the conjunction of a rectoanal inhibitory reflex (internal sphincter relaxation) and a rectoanal contractile reflex (external sphincter contraction).[10, 291] As a result of these reflexes the anorectum assumes the shape of a funnel. Rectal contents that triggered the reflexes descend into the cloacogenic zone, at the dentate line and just above, which can sample their nature, while continence is preserved because of the tight closure of the external sphincter. This does not occur in Hirschsprung's disease. Thus, the most commonly performed type of anorectal manometry investigates resting tones in the anal and rectoanal reflexes.

Viscoelastic properties of the rectum differ in health and disease[99, 107, 292, 293] and should be studied to distin-

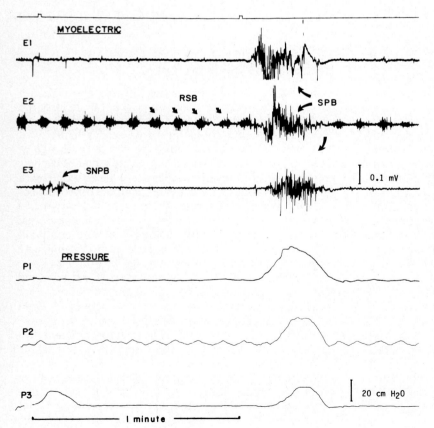

Figure 22–17. Electrical activity in the distal human colon. RSB, rhythmic and stationary bursts; SNPB, sporadic nonpropagating bursts; SPB, sporadic propagating bursts. SNPB and SPB correspond to intraluminal pressure waves. (From Schang, J. C., Hemond, M., Herbert, M., and Pilote, M. Dig. Dis. Sci. *31*:1331, 1986. Used by permission.)

guish outlet obstruction induced by a hypo- or hypertonic rectum from simple anal achalasia. This type of studies investigates the accommodation properties of the rectum to rapid (with air) or slow (with water) distention. Viscous properties reflect accommodation of the rectum to distention, and elastic properties the residual tension after accommodation. These properties correlate poorly to rectal size at barium enema.[31]

Anal Sphincter Electromyography

The search for anismus has provided some impetus to more routine performance of electromyography of the external anal sphincter and the puborectalis muscle. This can be performed with needle electrodes or with a less invasive method of plug electrodes. Reflexes between the perineal skin and the pelvic muscle floor can also be investigated to determine the integrity of the innervation to and from the cauda equina.

Dynamic Evaluation of Defecation

Balloon defecation is a new method to investigate the rectoanal dynamics during defecation. Impaired expulsion correlates to the mechanisms of constipation.[35, 203, 246]

The balloon proctogram permits evaluation of the anorectal angle and its relationship with the pubococcygeal level.[294] Balloon topography, in addition to this, yields opening pressures of the anal canal during distention, and anal canal length.[295]

Defecography is another practical way to investigate anorectal morphology and dynamics during defecation. The most popular technique uses a barium paste that reproduces stool consistency.[296, 297]

The Colon Is within a Person

With some humor, one could say that constipated patients may constipate some physicians. The scientific approach to medicine does not take into account the often imaginary elements in the patient's unconscious representation of his or her own body.[298] Physicians must constantly keep in mind that constipation is not

only the passage of hard and infrequent stools via different investigable mechanisms, but what this does subjectively to the patient. Not to be forgotten are the areas where physicians still find selfish pleasure in the practice of medicine: curiosity for interesting "cases," control of disease and patient, and thoroughness of investigation.[299] Often the constipated patient is not a "good" obedient patient, and this may trigger unpleasant feelings, frustration, or even anger in the physician. This may lead to a break in the doctor-patient relationship or even to unnecessary surgery.[26, 70]

Recording a life history as well as a case history is essential. An interview reviewing in depth major life experiences serves this purpose.[192, 300] It may trigger marked emotional responses, which contribute to the release of long-repressed conflicts.[192] A cruder approach consists in using the Minnesota Multiphasic Personality Inventory and relating to the patient the findings and profile interpretation.[190] Some patients resent even the idea of having a psychologic problem, and caution must be exercised in this regard or the patient may go shopping for another doctor.[37]

TREATMENT

Warning

The nonspecificity of all therapeutic approaches to constipation is exemplified in a report describing the effects of staying in a spa station for 94 patients with the irritable bowel syndrome. Evaluation of the total gastrointestinal transit time was done before, one month after, and six months after this stay. In the group of constipated subjects, there was a significant reduction in transit time from 76 to 56 hours, but six months later this effect had disappeared[301] (Fig. 22–18). Drinking water with alleged therapeutic properties in a relaxing environment thus serves a temporary useful purpose. Even if patients remain clinically improved, functional disorders may persist over long periods[302, 303] (Fig. 22–19). These two observations must be kept in mind to evaluate critically all available data on the treatment of constipation. No random study of any kind of treatment has been done taking into

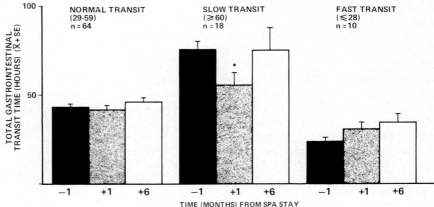

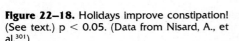

Figure 22–18. Holidays improve constipation! (See text.) $p < 0.05$. (Data from Nisard, A., et al.[301])

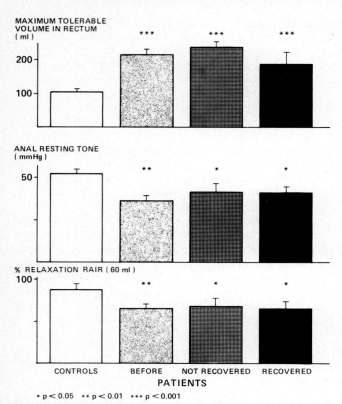

Figure 22–19. Anorectal motility may remain persistently abnormal despite clinical improvement. (Data from Loening-Baucke.[302])

account the natural history of constipation, which is unknown, and the possibility of symptom displacement into another system. Long-term results with evaluation of the total person are needed.

The irritable bowel syndrome is a chronic recurrent disorder, with at least a 50 per cent failure rate at five years,[42, 43] and its precursor is recurrent abdominal pain in childhood.[71] Most patients with chronic idiopathic constipation complain of a lifelong history, with frequent onset at an early age[201] or at adolescence.[26, 38, 165] The prognosis is just as poor for constipation or even worse; out of 200 patients with functional abdominal complaints, 34 were found to suffer from constipation and only one had become asymptomatic at follow-up two years later.[251]

Management begins when the patients walk into the consultation room for the first time.[71] Over 80 per cent of patients with an irritable bowel syndrome have cool, clammy hands, a higher percentage than is found in a control population, and most have an abnormally tender and palpable colon.[69, 71] The percentage with a scar of previous appendectomy is also in excess of that found in controls.[69, 71] A lot of attention must be directed to nonverbal communication; patients are often described as exhibiting inappropriate behavior and voicing many concerns without showing corresponding facial and bodily expressions.[71] It is during this history-taking and physical examination that the quality of the doctor-patient relationship is determined. Patients have often been dismissed as being "not sick"

or "sick in their head," or been told that "nothing can be done." The problem-solving approach to constipation is a highly effective way to achieve a correct diagnosis, but is limited in laying the groundwork for successful management. Functional disorders are not synonymous with no disorders.[299] Too often, the patient leaves the clinician with a high level of frustration, after having been told there was nothing wrong with him or her. Making a positive diagnosis that there *is* something wrong and relating the findings of the functional evaluation of constipation serves an important purpose to establish a therapeutic alliance with the patient. When trust is present, it becomes easier to relate the message that the basis for functional abnormality is not necessarily organic.

Some patients are noncompliant in terms of both diagnostic tests and treatment. The key element here is to have a reasonable clinical opinion that there is no organic lesion. If this is so, patients should be accepted in their noncompliance. A patient with a 20-year history of one stool per week was cured simply by accepting her refusal to undergo testing and treatment and her request to come back a month later; it turned out it was the first time in her life that someone had granted her a demand (unpublished data). Thus, paradoxically, not being a doctor was a better treatment than being one.

An extensive effort should be made to find a specific cause of constipation and treatment, of course, should be aimed at that cause.

The approach to a patient who consults for chronic idiopathic constipation varies according to the level of medical resources. The same attitude should not be taken when the patient has already seen numerous general practitioners, general internists, gastroenterologists and colorectal surgeons, who are the professionals most likely to be consulted. Clinical judgment is needed here to determine the depth of investigation prior to treatment. If an organic lesion has been ruled out, a minimum evaluation should include marker studies and a minimum treatment an increase in dietary fiber, if the intake is inadequate.

Diet

Short gastrointestinal transit times become longer, when subjects eat more fiber;[161, 304, 305] long ones become shorter.[306–309] Dietary fibers increase stool weight,[161, 310] frequency,[161] and water content;[161] different fibers have a different effect. Thus, vegetarians have been found to have a more rapid transit than non-vegetarians. Men, for unknown reasons, have faster transit than women, and the difference is more profound in non-vegetarians.[311] This sex difference is even more striking in constipated patients. Transit time does not correlate to age, even if dietary fiber intake is controlled;[311] thus, in elderly subjects, there is no correlation between dietary fiber intake and constipation.[40]

The effectiveness of indigestible residues is not due primarily to the mechanical stimulus of distention, but rather to chemical stimuli that arise from the destruction of hemicelluloses and cellulose by the intestinal bacterial flora. One of these stimulating products is the lower volative fatty acids.[310] The increase in stool weight correlates with the increased intake of pentose-containing polymers present in the fiber.[309, 310] This is not related, as originally thought, to the water-holding capacity of the fiber; in fact, those fibers that take up most water in vitro—that is, the gel-forming polysaccharides such as guar and pectin—have the least effect on bowel habit, while the most effective fecal bulkers, such as bran, hold very little water on a weight to weight basis.[310] Virtually all fiber is broken down in the gut, but the cellulosic fraction tends to survive digestion better than the noncellulosic polysaccharides and fiber from cereals survives better than that from fruit and vegetables. This is a further argument against the water-holding hypothesis as a mechanism of action of fiber. Fecal microbial mass increases when dietary fiber is fed and composes up to half of the fecal solids in subjects eating typical Western diets; this is surely one of the mechanisms of action of fiber.[310, 312]

On a basal diet, pronounced individual differences in fecal weight occur, and from these, the response of subjects to the fiber preparations can be predicted: the increase in fecal weight is proportional to fecal weight on the basal diet. This is particularly important in constipation. A poor response to dietary fiber can be expected because subjects who start out with the smallest stool weight also produce the smallest increase in fecal weight. Similarly, people with the longest transit times show the smallest response in fecal weight.[310] Thus, in patients with constipation much more dietary fiber is required, and in some fiber alone will not overcome the disability.

The individual differences in stool output and response to dietary fiber are as much related to personality as they are to diet: Outgoing individuals with a good self-esteem produce more frequent and heavier stools.[186] This recent finding, of paramount importance, has been ignored in all studies of diet and bowel habit relationship. Dietary fiber induces a faster passage of stools through the rectosigmoid part of the bowel,[314] where motility can be influenced by a stressful interview.[300, 314]

The diet ingested by Africans is often cited as a model for avoidance of Western civilization diseases,[315] because it contains a lot of fiber. Rural Africans have a daily stool output of 400 to 500 gm, in contrast to people in the Western world who only excrete 100 to 200 gm per day.[7, 310, 316] Yet Africans also live in a different environment and have a different culture. In the Ivory Coast, only 2 per cent of cancers occur in the colon and rectum; and the administration of hot pepper enemas is very common, probably because 95 per cent of people consider themselves "constipated."[317]

Despite these considerations, a trial with a high-fiber diet is in order in all constipated patients. Adequate amounts (30 gm of dietary fiber or 14.4 gm of crude fiber) should be taken daily. This may increase stool weight and frequency and decrease stool consistency. It should be remembered, however, that there is a strong placebo effect to dietary fiber[161–163, 318, 319] and that it has no prophylactic value to prevent constipation in hospitalized patients.[320] A difference in stool frequency may be found between recalled and recorded data; many subjects defecate more often than they say.[14, 70] This may be because of diet, because of unconscious or conscious exaggeration of the problem, or simply because taking care of the patient has already modified bowel function.

The use of a diary is important because quite often constipation may vary with time and patients may then be taught to look for coincidences or associations with events in their life. The physician should refrain from telling the patient what he or she has noted in the relationships with stress of any kind, because this would deprive the patient of the emotional impact of finding out; just understanding a link will not change behavior and bowel function.[192] The patient should carefully note the number of stools each day and their consistency. Patients with large bowel pseudo-obstruction may pass watery, at times colorless, stools, and patients with short-segment Hirschsprung's disease sometimes suffer from overflow incontinence. It is essential to instruct the patient to stop taking laxatives and non-essential drugs (particularly those for pain) and not to use enemas. Some effort is required to make this regimen acceptable to patients. A useful approach is to laud its therapeutic advantage. The ideal duration of this treatment should probably be a month, because some patients have an irregular type of constipation, in which a week with daily stools is followed by a week without any. Prolonging the dietary trial reduces the chances of counting stools only during a good week, but clinical judgment must be used to determine the length of trial.

Dietary fiber is no panacea in the treatment of adult constipation. Increase in symptomatology may occur and point to the presence of slow-transit constipation.[26] It may also indicate the presence of anismus.[321] Patients with constipation from birth found to have a megarectum also fail to respond to a high-fiber diet.[70]

Behavioral Approach

The re-education of patients in regard to bowel habits, in terms of spending time on the toilet at regular intervals, is seldom prescribed as a sole treatment. Its value is therefore debatable.

The initial and probably very important step is to completely evacuate the bowel. Fecal impactions should be treated prior to the evaluation of the patient. This can be done with multiple oil or saline enemas.[24, 322] A good combination is to give one of each, morning and evening. One may also give colonic washouts with a balanced solution or tap water (20 ml/kg/day),[322] or perform a complete gastrointestinal washout with Golytely.[323] This preparation contains sodium and potassium salts as well as polyethylene glycol 3350 and is administered in a volume of 3 to 6 liters. It takes generally one week to clean the colon and rectum completely and eliminate fecal soiling.[322] Lactulose (10 ml twice a day) may on rare occasion be useful. Digital fragmentation is unpleasant to both patient and physician, and may be dangerous because traumatic ulcerations are easy to induce.

Thereafter, the patient is asked to take milk of magnesia (0.5 to 1 ml/kg/day), mineral oil (0.5 ml/kg/day), or docusate sodium (Colace) (3 to 5 mg/kg/day), enough to produce one to three stools per day. Some authors do not use laxatives, but rely solely upon a daily or every other day enema (Fleet sodium phosphate enema; aqueous enema 20 ml/kg) for a month, then decrease its frequency as progress is noted.[48, 322] The objective is to create an artificial regularity. Simultaneously, the patient eats a high-fiber diet, with or without bran cereal or a bulk laxative. The patient is requested to go to the toilet for 5 to 15 minutes after breakfast each day.[24, 322, 324] Negative reinforcement may be useful in the behavioral approach to children with constipation;[325] if the patient does not defecate in the morning, he or she is requested to go for longer periods of time at noon without engaging in any other activity (e.g., reading) while seated on the toilet, and if still unsuccessful, for even longer periods of time in the evening. This in effect deprives a child of constantly increasing periods of play time.

This approach results in about a 50 to 75 per cent rate of success over long-term periods.[24, 322] The effect of aging and natural history versus treatment is not known. The medical approach should not be a fight to force a child to behave, and the office should never become a battleground between parents and child. On two occasions, respecting the desire of a child not to be forced to have an endoscopy and take enemas, when the child's preference was in opposition to the will of the parent, resulted in permanent cure of constipation and encopresis on the basis of megarectum (unpublished observations). Moreover, there are data showing the beneficial effect of paradoxical instruction in the treatment of encopresis and chronic constipation: if an individual is anxious regarding successful performance of "normal" bowel habits, instructing him or her *not* to try to have these "normal" bowel habits may reduce his or her anxiety and thereby facilitate the disappearance of the undesired symptoms.[326] Thus, caution is needed to interpret data on behavioral approaches to constipation. The fact that so many adult patients consult for constipation with childhood onset leads one to suspect that laxative therapy is wishful thinking. If a battle is considered to be won, it will be lost. Finally, the psychologic effects over a lifetime of giving multiple enemas and *forcing* a child to defecate and become continent is not known. This has been argued against,[322] but the question to ask is what constitutes a successful outcome: it certainly should not be restricted to the defecation pattern but to what happens overall to the child.

There is no good study on the effect of exercise, swimming, and massages on constipation.

A final point to make is that the behavioral approach may be useful in children but its value in independent adults remains to be substantiated. In one series of 71 adult subjects, only 38 adhered strictly to the regimen for at least two months: although 80 per cent of these subjects by then had a bowel movement at least every two days without laxatives or complaints, the dropout rate is impressive and indicative of more difficulties than with children.[327]

Biofeedback Approach

Biofeedback techniques may be used in a nonspecific way to bring relaxation. This is useful in patients with the irritable bowel syndrome.[328]

Biofeedback techniques may also be aimed at specific measurable functional abnormalities found in patients with chronic idiopathic constipation, such as the spastic pelvic floor syndrome. It cured eight of ten such patients with a prolonged history of constipation, impossibility to defecate without enemas or laxatives, no defecation urge, and difficult and painful defecation once every 4 to 14 days.[251] An anal-plug electrode is inserted to record the electromyographic activity of the external anal sphincter. Numeric and graphic feedback is produced to the patient asked to strain: this, in anismus or the spastic pelvic floor syndrome, increases muscular activity. To help the patient understand that straining must be carried out in a different manner, without pelvic floor contraction, a balloon is inserted into the rectum, distended with 60 ml of air, and slowly pulled out to have the patient recognize the feeling that the pelvic floor is relaxing and stool is coming. The next step, when he or she correctly relaxes the pelvic floor during straining, consists in learning to defecate artificial feces introduced into the rectum. Another approach uses anorectal pressures at rest and during rectal distention as a modality of feedback source.[27, 192, 303]

There are predictors of outcome. For instance, a depression score above 67 and a psychasthenia score above 57 on the Minnesota Multiphasic Personality Inventory are highly predictive of a failure of biofeedback-relaxation training outcome.[329] Individuals who tend to like responsibility and are more executive and independent generally benefit more than doubtful, obedient, and depressed individuals.

Psychologic Approach

Over the past five years, several studies have demonstrated the merits of using a psychologic approach to patients with constipation and the irritable bowel syndrome. What can safely be said today is that these patients may improve apart from any organic treatment, and that the functional results can be measured so that success can be evaluated objectively.[27, 192]

A comparison of a classic organic approach to patients with the irritable bowel syndrome, and the same approach with additional individual psychotherapy aimed at modifying maladaptive behavior has revealed the superiority of the latter[330] (Fig. 22–20). Both ap-

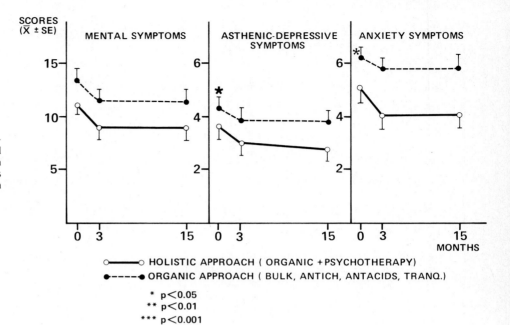

Figure 22–20. A classic organic approach to patients with irritable bowel syndrome has a therapeutic value in reducing mental symptoms, and thus *is* a type of psychotherapy. (Data from Svedlund.[330])

proaches reduce to a similar extent anxiety and mental symptoms; the paradoxical conclusion to be drawn from these data is that a purely medical approach, without consideration of the importance of psyche in diseases, has a psychotherapeutic value! It is in the area of abdominal symptoms (pain, bowel dysfunction) that the combined physical-mental approach is superior. The major flaw in this study is that subjective ratings rather than functional measurements were taken as measures of outcome. In another comparative study, the same medical regimen was compared with psychologic treatment alone.[331] The latter was based on the hypothetic model that symptoms of the irritable bowel syndrome and anxiety both result from a common underlying autonomic reactivity, with the resulting manifestations (anxiety or physical symptoms) determined by vicarious learning, and maintained by environmental contingencies.[332] The treatment included an educational phase to change any misconceptions about bowel function and provide a rationale for psychologic intervention, and stress management training based on progressive muscle relaxation and self-instructional training.[333] Psychologic intervention reduced both anxiety and symptoms of irritable bowel syndrome; anxiety levels were not reduced by the medical treatment.

Hypnotherapy and psychotherapy have been compared in a random fashion.[334] Hypnotherapy was aimed at general relaxation and control of intestinal motility, while psychotherapy centered on discussion of symptoms and exploration of emotional problems and stressful life events. Hypnotherapy was found to be superior in reducing abdominal pain and distention and improving bowel habits (Fig. 22–21). However, a three-month follow-up is far too short in a condition known for its remissions and relapses and its sensitivity to placebo treatment.[335] Another difficulty is the possible im-

portance of transference between patient and therapist.[336, 337]

Group therapy has been tested.[71, 338] This approach, aimed at changing the tendency of patients to dichotomize their illness into organic factors and emotional components, reduced constipation in only 15 per cent of subjects but resulted in marked psychometric improvement on several dimensions.[338]

In children, constipation may be part of a constellation of familial difficulties. They may be symptom free in the hospital on repeated visits but constipated at home. This suggests a conflict between one or both parents and the child. Physicians have a tendency to ally with the parents, but this may not be the best approach for the child.

Pharmacologic Approach

Attempts to modify measurable functional abnormalities have been scarce. Bethanechol has been tried without success in patients with delayed transit in the ascending colon.[37] Cisapride is an investigational gastrointestinal prokinetic drug which has no antidopaminergic or cholinergic effects. In severely constipated patients (one bowel movement every 4 to 14 days) it reduces the level of constant rectal sensation by 33 per cent.[237] Other preclinical studies suggest that cisapride may improve symptoms of constipation, particularly in the setting of more widespread gastrointestinal motility disorders.

A combined treatment with adrenergic blockage and cholinergic drugs may help patients with malignant pheochromocytoma who suffer from intractable constipation.[339]

Two patients with severe constipation were success-

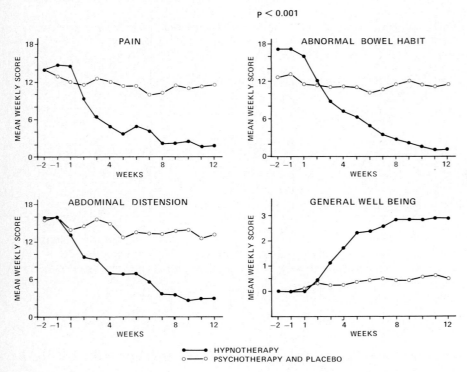

$p < 0.001$

Figure 22–21. Hypnosis modifies bowel habits in patients with irritable bowel syndrome. (Data from Whorwell et al.[334])

HYPNOTHERAPY
PSYCHOTHERAPY AND PLACEBO

fully treated with naloxone, a specific opioid antagonist.[340] This effect may be modulated via an acceleration of gastric emptying and small bowel transit times.[341]

Surgical Approach

Hirschsprung's Disease

Hirschsprung's disease should be treated surgically, and this is discussed on page 1394.

Anismus

This is an area in which surgery should be abandoned. Puborectalis resection was advocated a long time ago to treat patients who had a *clinical* diagnosis of anorectal spasm.[242] Initial gratifying results were confirmed in subsequent uncontrolled observations.[342] However, in a group of women who had surgery with the preoperative *functional* diagnosis of anismus, posterior division of the puborectalis muscle provided no benefit; incontinence for solid stool was not reported, but there was some leakage of flatus, liquid stool, and mucus.[343] A more drastic approach, subtotal colectomy, also failed to cure patients with anismus.[243, 254]

Biofeedback therapy, in contrast, cures constipation by spastic pelvic floor in most subjects.[251] There is no reason, therefore, at this stage of our understanding, to prefer a surgical approach for patients with any kind of rectoanal dyssynergia (anismus, spastic pelvic floor syndrome, disobedient sphincter syndrome).

Chronic Idiopathic Constipation

Anorectal Myectomy. Anorectal myectomy is a procedure that has both diagnostic and therapeutic value. It involves the section of the internal anal sphincter and the full thickness of distal rectal musculature, with excision of a strip of muscle. This may help patients who undergo this procedure not only for Hirschsprung's disease, but also for chronic idiopathic constipation.[36, 127, 236, 344–349] In a recent study, 73 constipated children were classified into three groups, according to anorectal manometry: those who had a hypertonic anal canal at rest and a rectoanal inhibitory reflex, those who had no rectoanal inhibitory reflex but no radiologic evidence of Hirschsprung's disease, and those with normal pressure in the anal canal at rest and a rectoanal inhibitory reflex. Surgery was limited to 25 patients of the first and second groups, and only eight had daily bowel movements on their own postoperatively. The authors observed a reduction in resting pressure in patients with a hypertonic anal canal and the appearance of a rectoanal inhibitory reflex in the second group.[350] Thus, the role of anorectal myectomy in treating patients with chronic idiopathic constipation is far from clear, and anorectal manometry is mandatory before surgery. Surprisingly, the occurrence of one of the feared consequences of this procedure, fecal incontinence, is rare[36] or absent[345, 346, 349, 350] in most series. Correction of constipation by this procedure is a strong argument that preoperatively the mechanism of constipation was outlet obstruction.

Anorectal myectomy has also a diagnostic value because it produces a strip of rectal muscle, which can be examined to provide a basis upon which a diagnosis of Hirschsprung's disease can be made[36, 127] or ruled out.[127, 350] In a large series of 105 myectomies, Hirschsprung's disease was diagnosed in 29 patients and normal structure recognized in 46. Fibrosis or hyperplasia of the internal sphincter were the other diagnosis. Fifty-nine per cent of patients with Hirschsprung's disease and 78 per cent of those with idiopathic constipation were improved.[349]

In a group of 60 patients consulting for severe constipation, 20 were diagnosed as suffering from hypoganglionosis. Seventeen were relieved from constipation by anorectal myectomy.[127] This indicates that myectomy may relieve patients with a-, hypo-, or normoganglionosis and is thus not specific therapy. Success of anorectal myectomy does not imply in any way that there was an organic lesion that was cured. This procedure has never been the subject of a randomized controlled trial, and success should thus be placed in perspective of successes by other therapeutic modalities, which have not been evaluated properly either. An exception, to date, is that if aganglionosis is present, improvement is almost guaranteed if the diseased segment lies within the length of the excised specimen.

Colectomy. Anorectal myectomy fails to cure patients with colonic inertia and those who became constipated after the age of 10 years.[36] In this group of patients, better results may be obtained with total colectomy and ileorectal anastomosis. Removal of the large bowel was advocated at the beginning of the century by surgical enthusiasts, who were good clinical observers[62, 216] but were living at a time when the colon was considered as a sewage organ.[351, 352] The preservation of the caecum does not seem to provide better functional results[353] and may even be worse.[354] Total colectomy seems to be superior to more limited resections.[347, 353–359] However, anterior resection[347] or rectal bypass[70] may produce good results when the dilatation as seen on barium enema studies is confined to the rectosigmoid.[347]

No less than 50 per cent of patients undergoing colectomy and ileorectal anastomosis for functional constipation subsequently require further intervention because of acute small bowel obstruction; in contrast, in the same institution, the incidence of small bowel obstruction after resection for large bowel tumors was only 2 per cent and for inflammatory bowel disease it was 9 per cent.[360] Other authors confirm these findings.[353] It is not clear why there are such enormous differences after identical surgical procedures.

Laxatives

When definitive therapy of a specific disease cannot be offered, then and only then should laxatives be prescribed (Table 22–6). The patient's preference and tolerance should be followed. Bulk laxatives may increase symptoms if the cause of constipation is organic or if there is a delayed transit through the colon,[26] but

are recommended for long-term therapy of chronic idiopathic constipation. The other laxatives are used for short-term therapy of acute conditions or when the bowel needs to be emptied prior to an examination.

Very little work has been done on the mechanisms of action of laxatives in the large bowel using modern techniques of investigation, such as measurements of pressure or electrical activity, bowel tone, or fecal propulsion as reflected by radiopaque marker studies. Propulsive waves are rarely identified in the colon or rectum under normal condition. They are not induced by distention[361] but are induced by topically active laxatives, such as bisacodyl, oxyphenisatin[362] and rhein-anthrone,[361] once the bowel has been sensitized, physical stimuli cause fresh contractions. These drugs stimulate increased pressure waves in the rectum, usually fast low-amplitude waves, but not true peristalsis. Many patients complain that chemical laxatives lose their effectiveness over the years. In some patients with delayed transit in the colon, bisacodyl is unable to exert an influence on motor activity of the descending colon, but there is *no* correlation between this and the anatomy of the myenteric plexus.[217] There is, however, a correlation with duration of the disease; the disorder may thus either be spontaneously progressive or become nonresponsive to laxatives with long continued use.[13] It should, however, be kept in mind that placebo responders consume more laxatives than nonresponders.[363] Thus, some of the effects of laxatives may be purely of a placebo nature, such as has been demonstrated for methylcellulose.[364]

Basically all laxatives work by promoting some of the mechanisms involved in the pathogenesis of diarrhea. These involve active electrolyte secretion, decreased water and electrolyte absorption, increased intraluminal osmolarity, increased hydrostatic pressure in the gut, and motor effects. Laxatives can be divided into several groups.[2]

Bulk-forming agents consist of foods that are high in fiber as well as commercially available products that contain polysaccharides or cellulose derivatives. Intended results may be achieved in 12 to 24 hours but can take several days. Preparations are multiple and dosage varies with product. If taken without water, these products may cause obstruction.

Emollient laxatives are surfactants that facilitate the mixture of aqueous and fatty substances in the fecal mass to soften it. They may also increase water secretion in the gastrointestinal tract. They are primarily not absorbed, but they may increase the absorption of other agents if they are administered concurrently; this is suspected to be the mechanism of hepatotoxicity of laxatives such as danthron. Dioctyl potassium sulfosuccinate may be used rectally.

The major lubricant laxative is mineral oil, and this may be given orally or rectally. It allows easier passage of coated feces and may also decrease colonic absorption of water. When given orally, it induces an effect within 8 hours. It may have some adverse effects, such as causing foreign body reaction in lymphoid tissue after absorption of small amounts, or lipoid pneumonia

Table 22–6. LAXATIVES

Class	Agent	Brand Names	Adult Daily Dosage	Class	Agent	Brand Names	Adult Daily Dosage
Bulk	Methylcellulose	Cologel Hydrolose	4–6 gm orally	Saline	Magnesium citrate	Citrate of magnesium Citroma Citronesia Evac-Q-Mag	11–18 gm in 10 oz orally
	Malt soup extract	Maltsupex	12 gm orally		Magnesium hydroxide	Milk of magnesia Haley's M-O Phillips' Milk of Magnesia	2.4–4.8 gm orally
	Polycarbophil	Mitrolan	4–6 gm orally				
	Plantgo seed (psyllium)	Konsyl Casyllium* Effersyllium Hydrocil instant Saraka Prompt* Syllact Metamucil Mucilose Nuggets Petro-Syllium no. 1* Perdiem* Siblin	Varies with product		Magnesium sulfate	Various brands	10–30 gm orally
					Sodium phosphates	Fleet Enema Phospho-Soda Saf-tip phosphate enema	Varies
				Stimulant	Bisacodyl	Carter's Little Pills Dulcolax Theralax	5–15 mg orally 10 mg rectally
	Plant gums	Gentlax-B* Kondremul*			Cascara sagrada	Caroid tablets Cas-Evac Stimulax*	Varies
Emollient	Docusate sodium	Afko-lube Coloctyl Constiban* Dio-Medicone Diosate Dorbantyl* Gentlax-S* Modane Soft Regul-Aid Senokap DSS* Stimulax* Colace Comfolax Correctol* Dio-Sul Doctate Doxinate Kasof Peri-Colace* Regutol Softenex Unilax*	50–360 mg orally		Castor oil	Purge Evacuant Neoloid	15–60 mg orally
					Casanthranol	Black Draught Constiban* Dialose-Plus* Diothron* Lanes Pills Disanthrol* Peri-Colace*	
					Danthron	Doctate-P* Dorbane Dorbantyl Modane Doxidan Tonelax Unilax	75–150 mg orally
					Phenolphthalein	Alophen Correctol* Disolan* Phenolax Feen-a-Mint Espotabs Evac-U-Gen Ex-lax	30–270 mg orally
	Docusate calcium	Doxidan* Surfak	50–360 mg orally				
	Docusate potassium	Dialose	100–300 mg orally		Senna	Fletcher's Castoria Gentlax-S* Glycerin ID Nytilax Senokot	Various dosages
Lubricants	Mineral oil	Agoral Plain* Fleet enema oil retention Haley's M-O Kondremul* Milkinol Neo-cultol Petrogalar Saf-tip oil retention enema	15–45 ml orally or enemas	Hyperosmotic	Lactulose Glycerin	3 gm suppository

*Mixed active ingredients.
Data from Tedesco and Di Piro.[2]

if the agent is aspirated. Its chronic use reduces absorption of fat-soluble vitamins A, D, and K.

Magnesium, sulfate, phosphate, and citrate ions are the principal active ingredients in saline laxatives. They exert an osmotic effect that causes increased intraluminal volume but may also have other actions. They are used orally and act within three hours of administration, or intrarectally and act within 15 minutes. Use of laxatives may lead to mineral imbalances: patients with renal dysfunction may accumulate toxic amounts of magnesium; those who restrict sodium intake must be careful; and young children may develop hypocalcemia.

Stimulant laxatives consist of the anthraquinone derivatives such as cascara sagrada, sennosides, danthron, casanthranol, and the diphenylmethane derivatives such as bisacodyl and phenolphthalein. The action of the anthraquinone derivatives is limited to the colon and distal ileum, and is not fully understood. Bisacodyl has been shown to stimulate the mucosal nerve plexus of the colon, producing contractions of the entire colon and decreasing water absorption in the small and large bowel. Phenolphthalein inhibits glucose absorption, which causes accumulation of intraluminal fluid, and inhibits active sodium absorption. Castor oil is also classed in this group; it is metabolized into ricinoleic acid, which stimulates active secretory processes, decreases glucose absorption, and promotes intestinal motility. These products may act by mouth or as suppositories; action occurs within 12 hours and 60 minutes, respectively. Phenolphthalein acts longer, because it undergoes enterohepatic recirculation. Stimulant laxatives may cause severe cramping or fluid and electrolyte imbalance with chronic use, inducing metabolic acidosis or alkalosis. The anthraquinone derivatives may cause melanosis coli all along the gastrointestinal tract, but mainly in the cecum and rectum. This is harmless; the pigment accumulates within 4 to 13 months and disappears within 3 to 6 months after discontinuation. Phenolphthalein may cause dermatologic reactions such as erythema multiforme, or may mimic Bartter's syndrome with hyperaldosteronism and hypokalemia. Danthron may cause hepatotoxicity similar to chronic active hepatitis when combined with docusate.

Glycerin and lactulose are hyperosmotic laxatives. Glycerin is absorbed when given by mouth and therefore is used rectally only; it acts within 30 minutes. Lactulose exerts an osmotic effect and is metabolized by bacteria in the colon to low molecular weight acids, which lower the pH of the colon and increase colonic peristalsis. It acts within 48 hours and may cause flatulence, cramps, diarrhea, and electrolyte imbalances.

References

1. Glaser, M., and Chi, J. Thirty-fifth annual report on consumer spending. Drug Topics, July 4, 18–20, 1983.
2. Tedesco, F. J., and Di Piro, J. T. American College of Gastroenterology's Committee on FDA-related matters. Laxative use in constipation. Am. J. Gastroenterology *80*:303, 1985.
3. Rendtorff, R. C., and Kashgarian, M. Stool patterns of healthy adult males. Dis. Colon Rectum *10*:222, 1967.
4. Report from the International Agency for Research on Cancer Intestinal Microecology Group. Dietary fibre, transit time, faecal bacteria, steroids, and colon cancer in two Scandinavian populations. Lancet *2*:207, 1977.
5. Glober, G. A., Nomura, A., Kamiyama, S., Shimada, A., and Abba, B. C. Bowel transit-time and stool weight in populations with different colon-cancer risks. Lancet *2*:110, 1977.
6. Tandon, R. K., and Tandon, B. N. Stool weights in North Indians. Lancet *2*:560, 1975.
7. Burkitt, D. P., Walker, A. R. P., and Painter, N. S. Effect of dietary fiber on stools and transit times, and its role in the causation of disease. Lancet *2*:1408, 1972.
8. Colon, A. R., and Jacob, L. J. Defecation patterns in American infants and children. Clin. Pediatr. *16*:999, 1977.
9. Lemoh, J. N., and Brooke, O. G. Frequency and weight of normal stools in infancy. Arch. Dis. Child. *54*:719, 1979.
10. Martelli, H., Duguay, C., Devroede, G., Arhan, P., Dornic, C., and Faverdin, C. Some parameters of large bowel function in normal man. Gastroenterology *75*:612, 1978.
11. Patel, P. D., Picologlou, B. F., and Lykoudis, P. S. Biorheological aspects of colonic activity. II. Experimental investigation of the rheological behavior of human feces. Biorheology *10*:441, 1973.
12. Exton-Smith, A. N., Bendall, M. J., and Kent, F. A new technique for measuring the consistency of feces: a report on its application to the assessment of Senokot therapy in the elderly. Age Ageing *4*:58, 1975.
13. Lennard-Jones, J. E. Constipation: pathophysiology, clinical features and treatment. *In* Henry, M. M., and Swash, M. (eds.). Coloproctology and the Pelvic Floor. Pathophysiology and Management. London, Butterworth, 1985, pp. 350–375.
14. Manning, A. P., Wyman, J. B., and Heaton, K. W. How trustworthy are bowel histories? Comparison of recalled and recorded information. Br. Med. J. *2*:213, 1976.
15. Connell, A. M., Hilton, C., Irvine, G., Lennard-Jones, J. E., and Misiewicz, J. J. Variation of bowel habit in two population samples. Br. Med. J. *2*:1095, 1965.
16. Milne, J. S., and Williamson, J. Bowel habit in older people. Gerontol. Clin. *14*:56, 1972.
17. Sandler, R. S., and Drossman, D. A. Bowel habits in apparently healthy young adults. Dig. Dis. Sci., in press.
18. Epelboin, A. Selles et urines chez les Fulbe Bande du Sénégal Oriental. Un aspect particulier de l'ethnomédecine. Cah. O.R.S.T.O.M., Ser. Sci. Hum. 18: no. 4, 515–530, 1981–1982.
19. Thompson, W. S., and Heaton, K. W. Functional bowel disorders in apparently healthy people. Gastroenterology *79*:283, 1980.
20. Edwards, D. A. W., and Beck, E. R. Movement of radiopacified feces during defecation. Am. J. Dig. Dis. *16*:709, 1971.
21. Arhan, P., Faverdin, C., Persoz, B., Devroede, G., Dubois, F., Dornic, C., and Pellerin, D. Relationship between viscoelastic properties of the rectum and anal pressure in man. J. Appl. Physiol. *41*:677, 1976.
22. Ihre, T. Studies on anal function in continent and incontinent patients. Scand. J. Gastroenterol. *9*(Suppl. 25):1, 1974.
23. Levine, M. D. Children with encopresis: a descriptive analysis. Pediatrics *56*:412, 1975.
24. Davidson, M., Kugler, M. M., and Bauer, C. H. Diagnosis and management in children with severe and protracted constipation and obstipation. J. Pediatr. *62*:261, 1963.
25. Lanfranchi, G. A., Bazzoichi, G., Brignola, C., Campieri, M., and Labo, G. Different patterns of intestinal transit time and anorectal motility in painful and painless chronic constipation. Gut *25*:1352, 1984.
26. Preston, D. M., and Lennard-Jones, J. E. Severe chronic constipation in young women: idiopathic slow transit constipation. Gut *27*:41, 1986.
27. Devroede, G. The irritable bowel syndrome: clinical and therapeutical aspects. *In* Poitras, P. (ed.). Proceedings of the First International Symposium on Small Intestinal and Colonic Motility. Centre de Recherche Cliniques, Hôpital Saint-Luc, and Jouveinal Laboratoires/Laboratories Inc. Montreal, 1985, pp. 129–139.

28. Hammond, E. C. Some preliminary findings on physical complaints from a prospective study of 1,064,004 men and women. Am. J. Public Health 54:11, 1964.

29. Meunier, P., Mollard, P., and Marechal, J-M. Physiopathology of megarectum: the association of megarectum with encopresis. Gut 17:224, 1976.

30. Meunier, P., Marechal, J-M, and Jaubert de Beaujeu, M. Rectoanal pressures and rectal sensitivity studies in chronic childhood constipation. Gastroenterology 77:330, 1979.

31. Meunier, P., Louis, D., and Jaubert de Beaujeu, M. Physiologic investigation of primary chronic constipation in children: comparison with the barium enema study. Gastroenterology 87:1351, 1984.

32. Loening-Baucke, J. A., and Younorzai, M. K. Abnormal anal sphincter response in chronically constipated children. J. Pediatr. 100:213, 1982.

33. Loening-Baucke, V. A., and Younorzai, M. K. Effect of treatment on rectal and sigmoid motility in chronically constipated children. Pediatrics 73:199, 1984.

34. Loening-Baucke, V. A. Sensitivity of the sigmoid colon and rectum in children treated for chronic constipation. J. Pediatr. Gastroenterol. Nutr. 3:454, 1984.

35. Loening-Baucke, V. A., and Cruikshank, B. M. Abnormal defecation dynamics in chronically constipated children with encopresis. J. Pediatr. 108:562, 1986.

36. Martelli, H., Devroede, G., Arhan, P., and Duguay, C. Mechanisms of idiopathic constipation: Outlet obstruction. Gastroenterology 75:623, 1978.

37. Wald, A. Colonic transit and anorectal manometry in chronic idiopathic constipation. Arch. Intern. Med. 146:1713, 1986.

38. Watier, A., Devroede, G., Duranceau, A., Abdel-Rahman, M., Duguay, C., Forand, M., Tetreault, L., Arhan, P., Lamarche, J., and Elhilali, M. Constipation with colonic inertia. A manifestation of systemic disease? Dig. Dis. Sci. 28:1025, 1983.

39. Ducrotte, P., Denis, P., Galmiche, J. P., Hellot, M. F., Deschalliers, J. P., Colin, R., Pasquis, P., and Hecketsweiler, P. Motricité anorectale dans la constipation idiopathique. Etude de 200 patients consécutifs. Gastroenterol. Clin. Biol. 9:10, 1985.

40. Donald, I. P., Smith, R. G., Cruikshank, J. G., Elton, R. A., and Stoddart, M. E. A study of constipation in the elderly living at home. Gerontology 31:112, 1985.

41. Waller, S. L., and Misiewiecz, J. J. Prognosis in the irritable-bowel syndrome. Lancet 2:753, 1969.

42. Holmes, K. M., and Slater, R. H. Irritable bowel syndrome—a safe diagnosis? Br. Med. J. 2:1533, 1982.

43. Kruis, W., Thieme, C., Weinzierl, M., Schussles, P., Holl, J., and Paulus, W. A diagnosis score for the irritable bowel syndrome. Its value in the exclusion of organic disease. Gastroenterology 87:1, 1984.

44. Sandler, R. S., Drossman, D. A., Nathan, H. P., and McKee, D. C. Symptom complaints and health care seeking behaviour in subjects with bowel dysfunction. Gastroenterology 87:314, 1984.

45. Neumann, P. A., De Domenico, I. J., and Nogrady, M. B. Constipation and urinary tract infection. Pediatrics 52:241, 1973.

46. Shopfner, C. E. Urinary tract pathology associated with constipation. Radiology 90:865, 1968.

47. O'Regan, S., and Yazbeck, S. Constipation: a cause of enuresis, urinary tract infection and vesico-ureteral reflux in children. Med. Hypotheses 17:409, 1985.

48. O'Regan, S., Yazbeck, S., and Schick, E. Constipation, bladder instability, urinary tract infection syndrome. Clin. Nephrol. 23:152, 1985.

49. Meier, E. Pubococcygeal strength: relationship to urinary control problems and to female orgasmic response. PhD thesis 1977, California School of Professional Psychology. Ann Arbor, MI, University Microfilms International.

50. Shafik, A. Urethral discharge, constipation and hemorrhoids. New syndrome with report of 7 cases. Urology 18:155, 1981.

51. Percora, P., Suraci, C., Antonelli, M., De Maria, S., and Marrocco, W. Constipation and obesity: a statistical analysis. Bull. Soc. It. Biol. Sper. 57:2384, 1981.

52. Riedl, P. Radiological morphology of the sigmoid colon in the Ethiopian population with reference to the occurrence of volvulus. E. Afr. Med. J. 55:470, 1978.

53. Huttunen, R., Heikkinen, E., and Larmi, T. K. I. Stercoraceous and idiopathic perforations of the colon. Surg. Gynecol. Obstet. 140:756, 1975.

54. Shatila, A. H., and Ackerman, N. B. Stercoraceous ulcerations and perforations of the colon: report of cases and survey of the literature. Dis. Colon Rectum 20:524, 1977.

55. Verhaeghe, P., Stoppa, R., Largueche, S., and Lesueur, P. Les perforations stercorales du côlon. Med. Chir. Dig. 8:125, 1979.

56. Gekas, P., and Schuster, M. M. Stercoral perforation of the colon: case report and review of the literature. Gastroenterology 80:1054, 1981.

57. Bjelke, E. Epidemiologic studies of cancer of the stomach, colon and rectum. Scand. J. Gastroenterol. 9(Suppl.):31, 1974.

58. Higginson, J. Etiological factors in gastrointestinal cancer in man. J. Natl. Cancer Inst. 37:527, 1966.

59. Wynder, E. L., and Shigematsu, T. Environmental factors of cancer of the colon and rectum. Cancer 20:1520, 1967.

60. Vobecky, J., Caro, J., and Devroede, G. A case control study of risk factors for large bowel carcinoma. Cancer 51:1958, 1983.

61. Kiff, E. S., Barnes, P. R. H., and Swash, M. Evidence of pudendal neuropathy in patients with perineal descent and chronic straining at stool. Gut 25:1279, 1984.

62. Lane, W. A. Chronic intestinal stasis. Br. Med. J., Nov. 1, 1913, p. 1125.

63. Petrakis, N. L., and King, E. B. Cytological abnormalities in nipple aspirates of breast fluid from women with severe constipation. Lancet, 2:1203, 1981.

64. Lee, J. A. H. "Appendicitis" in young women. Lancet 2:815, 1961.

65. Register General: Hospital in-patient inquiry 1976. Department of Health and Social Security. London, H.M. Stationery Office 1979.

66. West, R. R., and Carey, M. J. Variation in rates of hospital admission for appendicitis in Wales. Br. Med. J. 1:1662, 1978.

67. Creed, F. Life events and appendicectomy. Lancet 1:1381, 1981.

68. Chaudhary, N. A., and Truelove, S. C. The irritable colon syndrome. A study of clinical features, predisposing causes, and prognosis in 130 cases. Q.J. Med. 31:307, 1962.

69. Keeling, P. W. N., and Fielding, J. F. The irritable bowel syndrome. A review of 50 consecutive cases. J. Irish Coll. Phys. Surg. 4:91, 1975.

70. Verduron, A., Devroede, G., Bouchoucha, M., Arhan, P., Schang, J. C., Poisson, J., Hemond, M., and Hebert, M. Megarectum. Dig. Dis. Sci., in press.

71. Fielding, J. F. The irritable bowel syndrome. Clin. Gastroenterol. 3:607, 1977.

72. Fielding, J. F. Surgery and the irritable bowel syndrome: the singer as well as the song. Irish Med. J. 1:33, 1983.

73. Young, S. J., Alpers, D. H., Norland, C. C., and Woodruff, R. A., Jr. Psychiatric illness and the irritable bowel syndrome. Practical implications for the primary physician. Gastroenterology 70:162, 1976.

74. Purtell, J. J., Robins, E., and Cohen, M. E. Observations on clinical aspects of hysteria; a quantitative study of 50 hysteria patients and 156 control subjects. JAMA 146:902, 1951.

75. Woodruff, R. A., Goodwin, D. W., and Guze, S. B. Hysteria (Briquet's syndrome). In Psychiatric Diagnosis. New York, Oxford University Press, 1974, pp. 58–74.

76. Bakwin, H., and Davidson, M. Constipation in twins. Am. J. Dis. Child. 121:197, 1971.

77. Teixdor, H. S., and Heneghan, M. A. Idiopathic intestinal pseudo-obstruction in a family. Gastrointest. Radiol. 3:91, 1978.

78. Faulk, D. L., Anuras, S., Gardner, G. D., Mitros, F. A., Summers, R. W., and Christensen, J. A familial visceral myopathy. Ann. Intern. Med. 89:600, 1978.

79. Bodin, F., Le Guillant, F., Cheinisse, C., Conte, M., Frumusan, P., Goiffon, B., and Fouet, P. Iléocolite grave, avec atteinte rénale, par prise prolongée de laxatifs. Arch. Fr. Mal. App. Dig. 56:703, 1967.

80. Lemaitre, G., L'Hermine, C., Decoulx, M., Houcke, M., and Linquette, M. Les lésions coliques par abus de laxatifs. Etude anatomo-radiologique de deux observations. Presse Med. 77:393, 1969.
81. Plum, G. E., Weber, H. M., and Sauer, W. G. Prolonged cathartic abuse resulting in roentgen evidence suggestive of enterocolitis. AJR 83:919, 1960.
82. Smith, B. Effect of irritant purgatives on the myenteric plexus in man and the mouse. Gut 9:139, 1968.
83. Shafer, R. B., Prentiss, R. A., and Bond, J. H. Gastrointestinal transit in thyroid disease. Gastroenterology 86:852, 1984.
84. Burrell, M., Cronan, J., Megna, D., Toffler, R. Myxedema megacolon. Gastrointest. Radiol. 5:181, 1980.
85. Margulies, A., Metman, E. H., Girard, J. J., Dorval, E. D., and Bertrand, J. Constipation sévère révélatrice d'une pseudo-hypoparathyroïdie et résolutive après normalisation de la calcémie. Ann. Gastroenterol. Hepatol. 22:271, 1986.
86. Duffy, T. J., Erickson, E. E., Jordan, G. L., and Bennet, H. D. Megacolon and bilateral pheochromocytoma. Am. J. Gastroenterol. 38:555, 1962.
87. Short, I. A., and Padfield, P. L. Malignant phaeochromocytoma with severe constipation and myocardial necrosis. Br. J. Med. 2:793, 1976.
88. Gleeson, M. H., Bloom, S. R., Polak, J. M., Henry, K., and Dowling, R. H. Endocrine tumour in kidney affecting small bowel structure, motility, and absorptive function. Gut 12:773, 1971.
89. Bloom, S. R. An enteroglucagon tumor. Gut 13:520, 1972.
90. Kock, N. G., Darle, N., and Dotevall, G. Inhibition of intestinal motility in man by glucagon given intraportally. Gastroenterology 53:88, 1967.
91. Rees, W. D. W., and Rhodes, J. Altered bowel habit and menstruation. Lancet 289:475, 1976.
92. Levy, N., Lemberg, E., and Sharf, M. Bowel habit in pregnancy. Digestion 4:216, 1971.
93. Anderson, A. S. Constipation during pregnancy. Incidence and methods used in its treatment in a group of Cambridgeshire women. J. Health Visitor, 57:363, 1984.
94. Anderson, A. S. Dietary factors in the aetiology and treatment of constipation during pregnancy. Br. J. Obstet. Gynecol. 3:245, 1985.
95. Anderson, A. S., and Whichelow, M. J. Constipation during pregnancy: dietary fibre intake and the effect of fibre supplementation. Hum. Nutr. Appl. Nutr. 39A:202, 1985.
96. Hamel-Roy, J., Devroede, G., Arhan, P., Tetreault, J. P., Duranceau, A., and Menard, H. A. Comparative esophageal and anorectal motility in scleroderma. Gastroenterology 88:1, 1985.
97. Swenson, W. M., Witkowski, L. J., and Roskelley, R. C. Total colectomy for dermatomyositis. Am. J. Surg. 115:405, 1968.
98. Connell, A. M., Gaafer, M., Hassanein, M. A., and Khayal, M. A. Motility of the pelvic colon. III. Motility responses in patients with symptoms following amoebic dysentery. Gut 5:443, 1964.
99. Devroede, G., Vobecky, S., Masse, S., Arhan, P., Leger, C., Duguay, C., and Hemond, M. Ischemic fecal incontinence and rectal angina. Gastroenterology 83:970, 1982.
100. Tagart, R. E. B. The anal canal and rectum. Their varying relationship and its effect on anal incontinence. Dis. Colon Rectum 9:449, 1966.
101. Hirschsprung, H. Stuhlträgheit Neugeborener in Folge von Dilatation und Hypertrophie des Colons. Jahrb. Kinder. 27:1, 1888.
102. Tittel, K. Ueber einer angeborne Missbildung des Dickdarmes. Wien. Klin. Wschr. 14:903, 1901.
103. Dalla Valle, A. Ricerche istologiche su di un caso di megacolon congenito. Pediatria 28:740, 1920.
104. Cameron, J. A. M. On aetiology of Hirschsprung's disease. Arch. Dis. Child. 3:210, 1928.
105. Tiffin, M. E., Chandler, L. R., and Faber, H. K. Localized absence of myenteric plexus in congenital megacolon. Am. J. Dis. Child. 59:1071, 1940.
106. Whitehouse, F. R., and Kernohan, J. W. Myenteric plexus in congenital megacolon. Study of eleven cases. Arch. Intern. Med. 82:75, 1948.
107. Arhan, P., Devroede, G., Danis, K., Dornic, C., Faverdin, C., Persoz, B., and Pellerin, D. Viscoelastic properties of the rectal wall in Hirschsprung's disease. J. Clin. Invest. 62:82, 1978.
108. Lawson, J. O. N., and Nixon, H. H. Anal canal pressures in the diagnosis of Hirschsprung's disease. J. Pediatr. Surg. 2:544, 1967.
109. Schuster, M. M., Tobon, F., Reid, N. C. R. W., and Talbert, J. L. Nonsurgical test for the diagnosis of Hirschsprung's disease. N. Engl. J. Med. 278:188, 1968.
110. Suzuki, H., Watanabe, K., and Kasai, M. Manometric and cineradiographic studies on anorectal motility in Hirschsprung's disease before and after surgical operations. Tohoku J. Exp. Med. 102:69, 1970.
111. Frenckner, B. Anorectal manometry in the diagnosis of Hirschsprung's disease in infants. Acta Paediatr. Scand. 67:187, 1978.
112. Faverdin, C., Dornic, C., Arhan, P., Devroede, G., Jehannin, B., Revillon, Y., and Pellerin, D. Quantitative analysis of anorectal pressures in Hirschsprung's disease. Dis. Colon Rectum 24:422, 1981.
113. Nissan, S., and Bar-Maor, J. A. Further experience in the diagnosis and surgical treatment of short-segment Hirschsprung's disease and idiopathic megacolon. J. Pediatr. Surg. 6:738, 1971.
114. Patriquin, H., Martelli, H., and Devroede, G. Barium enema in chronic constipation: is it meaningful? Gastroenterology 75:619, 1978.
115. Mahboubi, S., and Schnaufer, L. The barium-enema examination and rectal manometry in Hirschsprung's disease. Pediatr. Radiol. 130:643, 1979.
116. Aldridge, R. T., and Campbell, P. E. Ganglion cell distribution in the normal rectum and anal canal. A basis for the diagnosis of Hirschsprung's disease by anorectal biopsy. J. Pediatr. Surg. 3:475, 1968.
117. Devroede, G., Arhan, P., Schang, J. C., and Heppell, J. Orderly and disorderly fecal continence. In Kodner, I. J., Fry, R. D., and Roe, J. P. (eds.). Colon, Rectal and Anal Surgery: Current Techniques and Controversies. St. Louis, C. V. Mosby Co., 1985, pp. 40–62.
118. Schuster, M. M. Motor action of rectum and anal sphincters in continence and defecation. In Code, C. F. (ed.). Handbook of Physiology, Section 6, Alimentary Canal, Vol. 4, Motility. Washington, D.C., American Physiological Society, 1968, p. 2121.
119. Verder, H., Krasilnikoff, P. A. and Scheibel, E. Anal tonometry in the neonatal period in mature and premature children. Acta Paediatr. Scand. 64:592, 1974.
120. Boston, V. F., and Scott, J. E. S. Anorectal manometry as a diagnostic method in the neonatal period. J. Pediatr. Surg. 11:9, 1976.
121. Holschneider, A. M., Kellner, E., Streibl, P., and Sippell, W. G. The development of anorectal continence and its significance in the diagnosis of Hirschsprung's disease. J. Pediatr. Surg. 11:151, 1976.
122. Morikawa, P., Donahoe, P. D., and Hendren, W. H. Manometry and histochemistry in the diagnosis of Hirschsprung's disease. Pediatrics 63:865, 1979.
123. Meier-Ruge, W., Lutterbeck, P. M., Herzog, B., Morger, R., Moser, R., and Scharli, A. Acetylcholinesterase activity in suction biopsies of the rectum in the diagnosis of Hirschsprung's disease. J. Pediatr. Surg. 7:11, 1972.
124. Dale, G., Bonham, J. R., Lowdon, P., Wagget, J., Rangecroft, L., and Scott, D. J. Diagnostic value of rectal mucosal acetylcholinesterase levels in Hirschsprung's disease. Lancet 1:347, 1979.
125. Garrett, J. R., Howard, E. R., and Nixon, H. H. Autonomic nerves in rectum and colon in Hirschsprung's disease. A cholinesterase and catecholamine histochemical study. Arch. Dis. Child. 44:406, 1969.
126. Weinberg, A. G. The anorectal myenteric plexus: its relation to hypoganglionosis of the colon. Am. J. Clin. Pathol. 54:637, 1970.
127. Howard, E. R., Garrett, J. R., and Kidd, A. Constipation and congenital disorders of the myenteric plexus. J. R. Soc. Med. 77(Suppl. 3):13, 1984.
128. Nezelof, C., Guy-Grand, D., and Thomine, E. Les mégacolons

avec hyperplasie du plexus myentérique. Une entité anatomo-clinique, à propos de 3 cas. Presse Med. 78:1501, 1970.

129. Aidan Carney, J., Go, V. L. M., Sizemore, G. W., and Hayles, A. B. Alimentary tract ganglioneuromatosis. A major component of the syndrome of multiple endocrine neoplasia type 2B. N. Engl. J. Med. 295:1287, 1976.

130. Cuthbert, J. A., Gallagher, N. D., and Turtle, J. R. Colonic and esophageal disturbance in a patient with multiple endocrine neoplasia, type 2B. Aust. N.Z. J. Med. 8:518, 1978.

131. Scharli, A. F., Meier-Ruge, W. Localized and disseminated forms of neuronal intestinal dysplasia mimicking Hirschsprung's disease. J. Pediatr. Surg. 16:164, 1981.

132. Duffy, T. J., Erikson, E. E., Jordan, G. L., Jr., and Bennett, H. D. Megacolon and bilateral pheochromocytoma. Am. J. Gastroenterol. 38:555, 1962.

133. Le Marec, B., Roussey, M., Cornec, A., Calmettes, C., Kerisit, J., and Allanic, H. Cancer de la thyroïde à stroma amylouïde, syndrome de Sipple, mégacolon congénital avec hyperplasie des plexus: une seule et même affection autosomique dominante à pénétrance complète. J. Genet. Hum. 28:169, 1980.

134. Verdy, M., Weber, A. M., Roy, C. C., Morin, C. L., Cadotte, M., and Brochu, P. Hirschsprung's disease in a family with multiple neoplasia type 2. J. Pediatr. Gastroenterol. Nutr. 1:603, 1982.

135. Yunis, E. J., Dibbins, A. W., and Sherman, F. E. Rectal suction biopsy in the diagnosis of Hirschsprung's disease in infants. Arch. Pathol. Lab. Med. 100:329, 1976.

136. Lassman, G. Diminished content of enterochromaffin cells in the rectal mucosa of an infant. Virchows Arch. A. Pathol. Anat. Histol. 372:253, 1976.

137. Ferreira-Santos, R. Megacolon and megarectum in Chagas' disease. Proc. R. Soc. Med. 54:1047, 1961.

138. Long, R. G., Bishop, A. E., Barnes, A. J., Albuquerque, R. H., O'Shaughnessy, D. J., McGregor, G. P., Bannister, R., Polak, J. M., and Bloom, S. R. Neural and hormonal peptides in rectal biopsy specimens from patients with Chagas' disease and chronic autonomic failure. Lancet 1:559, 1980.

139. Feinstat, T., Tesluk, H., Schuffler, M. D., Krishnamurthy, S., Verlenden, L., Gilles, W., Frey, C., and Trudeau, W. Megacolon and neurofibromatosis: a neuronal intestinal dysplasia. Gastroenterology 86:1573, 1984.

140. Ahmed, M. N., and Carpenter, S. Autonomic neuropathy and carcinoma of the lung. Can. Med. Assoc. J. 113:410, 1975.

141. Coste, T., Bernades, P., Molas, G., Glaser, J., Vallin, J., and Dupuy, R. Syndrome pseudo-obstructif chronique de l'intestin grêle avec anomalies des plexus mésentériques. Nouv. Presse Med. 1:447, 1972.

142. Phat, V. N., Chousterman, M., Bloch, F., Petite, J. P., and Camilleri, J. P. Lésions des plexus myentériques dans la pseudo-obstruction intestinale chronique idiopathique et certaines maladies générales. Ann. Anat. Pathol. (Paris) 23:131, 1978.

143. Schuffler, M. D., and Jonak, Z. Chronic idiopathic intestinal pseudo-obstruction caused by a degenerative disorder of the myenteric plexus: the use of Smith's method to define the neuropathology. Gastroenterology 82:476, 1982.

144. Preston, D. M., Butler, M. G., Smith, B., and Lennard-Jones, J. E. Neuropathology of slow transit constipation. (Abstract.) Gut 24:A997, 1983.

145. Krishnamurthy, S., Schuffler, M. D., Rohrmann, C. A., and Pope, C. E., II. Severe idiopathic constipation is associated with a distinctive abnormality of the colonic myenteric plexus. Gastroenterology 88:26, 1985.

146. Henley, F. A. Pelvic colectomy for obstinate constipation. Proc. R. Soc. Med. 60:806, 1967.

147. Smith, B. The neuropathology of the alimentary tract. London, Edward Arnold, 1972.

148. Dyer, N. H., Dawson, A. M., Smith, B. F., and Todd, I. P. Obstruction of bowel due to lesion in the myenteric plexus. Br. Med. J. 1:686, 1969.

149. Smith, B., Grace, R. H., and Todd, I. P. Organic constipation in adults. Br. J. Surg. 64:313, 1977.

150. Connell, A. M., Frankel, H., and Guttman, L. The motility of

151. Kettlewell, M. G. W. Surgical management of the bowel in cauda equina lesions. Proc. R. Soc. Med. 65:69, 1972.

152. Devroede, G., and Lamarche, J. Functional importance of extrinsic parasympathetic innervation to the distal colon and rectum in man. Gastroenterology 66:273, 1974.

153. Devroede, G., Arhan, P., Duguay, C., Tetreault, L., Akoury, H., and Perey, B. Traumatic constipation. Gastroenterology 77:1258, 1979.

154. Anderson, F. M., and Burke, B. L. Anterior sacral meningocele. A presentation of three cases. JAMA 237:39, 1977.

155. Oren, M., Lorber, B., Lee, S. H., Truex, R. C., and Gennaro, A. R. Anterior sacral meningocele. Report of five cases and review of the literature. Dis. Colon Rectum 20:492, 1977.

156. Hickler, R. B., Thompson, G. R., Fox, L. M., and Hamlin, J. R. Successful treatment of orthostatic hypotension with 9-alpha-fluorohydrocortisone. N. Engl. J. Med. 261:788, 1959.

157. Caronna, J. J., and Plum, F. Cerebrovascular regulation in preganglionic and postganglionic autonomic insufficiency. Stroke 4:12, 1973.

158. Egan-Mitchell, B., and McNicholl, B. Constipation in childhood coeliac disease. Arch. Dis. Child. 47:238, 1972.

159. Kappelman, N. B., Burrell, M., and Toffler, R. Megacolon associated with celiac sprue: report of four cases and review of the literature. AJR 128:65, 1977.

160. Havia, T. Diverticulosis of the colon. A clinical and histological study. Acta Chir. Scand. (Suppl.) 415:1, 1971.

161. Ornstein, M. H., Littlewood, E. R., Baird, I. M., Fowler, J., North, W. R. S., and Cox, A. G. Are fiber supplements really necessary in diverticular disease of the colon? A controlled clinical trial. Br. Med. J. 282:1353, 1981.

162. Devroede, G. Roving critic. In Reilly, R. W., and Kirsner, J. B. (eds.). Fiber Deficiency and Colonic Disorders. New York, Plenum Press, 1974, p. 120.

163. Devroede, G., Vobecky, J. S., Vobecky, J. M., Beaudry, R., Haddad, H., Navert, H., Perey, B., and Poisson, J. Medical management of diverticular disease: a random trial. (Abstract.) Gastroenterology 72:1157, 1977.

164. Tobon, F., and Schuster, M. M. Megacolon: special diagnostic and therapeutic features. Johns Hopkins Med. J. 135:91, 1974.

165. Barnes, P. R. H., Lennard-Jones, J. E., Hawley, P. R., and Todd, I. P. Hirschsprung's disease and idiopathic megacolon in adults and adolescents. Gut 27:534, 1986.

166. Nehme, A. E. Constipation: an uncommon etiology. Dis. Colon Rect. 27:819, 1984.

167. Swenson, O., Rathauser, F. Segmental dilatation of colon: new entity. Am. J. Surg. 97:734, 1959.

168. Etzioni, A., Benderly, A., and Bar-Maor, J. A. Segmental dilatation of the colon, another cause of chronic constipation. Dis. Colon Rectum 23:580, 1980.

169. Leape, L. L., and Ramenofsky, M. L. Anterior ectopic anus: a common cause of constipation in children. J. Pediatr. Surg. 13:627, 1978.

170. Hendren, W. H. Constipation caused by anterior location of the anus and its surgical correction. J. Pediatr. Surg. 13:505, 1978.

171. Wald, A., Van Thiel, D. H., Hoechstetter, L., Gavaler, J. S., Egler, K. S., Verm, R., Scott, L., and Lester, R. Effect of pregnancy on gastrointestinal transit. Dig. Dis. Sci. 27:1015, 1982.

172. Lawson, M., Kern, F., Jr., and Everson, G. T. Gastrointestinal transit time in human pregnancy: prolongation in the second and third trimesters followed by post-partum normalization. Gastroenterology 89:996, 1985.

173. Wald, A., Van Thiel, D. H., Hoechstetter, L., Gavaler, J. S., Egler, K. M., Verm, R., Scott, L., and Lester, R. Gastrointestinal transit: the effect of the menstrual cycle. Gastroenterology 80:1497, 1981.

174. Meunier, P., Rochas, A., and Lambert, R. Motor activity of the sigmoid colon in chronic constipation: comparative study with normal subjects. Gut 20:1095, 1979.

175. Schang, J. C., and Devroede, G. Fasting and postprandial

myoelectric spiking activity in the human sigmoid colon. Gastroenterology 85:1048, 1984.

176. Battle, W. M., Snape, W. J., Jr., Alair, A., Cohen, S., and Braunstein, S. Colonic dysfunction in diabetes mellitus. Gastroenterology 79:1217, 1980.

177. Glick, M. E., Meshkinpour, H., Haldeman, S., Hoehler, F., Downey, N., and Bradley, W. E. Colonic dysfunction in patients with thoracic spinal cord injury. Gastroenterology 86:287, 1984.

178. White, J. C., Verlot, M. G., and Ehrentheil, O. Neurogenic disturbances of the colon and their investigation by the colon-metrogram. Ann. Surg. 112:1042, 1940.

179. Scott, H. W., Jr., and Cantrell, J. R. Colonmetrographic studies of the effects of section of the parasympathetic nerves of the colon. Bull. Johns Hopkins Hosp. 85:310, 1949.

180. Sullivan, S. N., and Ebers, G. C. Gastrointestinal dysfunction in multiple sclerosis. Gastroenterology 84:1640, 1983.

181. Glick, M. E., Meshkinpour, H., Haldeman, S., Bhatia, N. N., and Bradley, W. E. Colonic dysfunction in multiple sclerosis. Gastroenterology 83:1002, 1982.

182. Weber, J., Grise, P., Roquebert, M., Hellot, M. F., Mihout, B., Samson, M., Beuret-Blanquart, F., Pasquis, P., and Denis, P. Radio-opaque markers transit and anorectal manometry in 16 patients with multiple sclerosis and urinary bladder dysfunction. Dis. Colon Rectum, 30:95, 1987.

183. Gunterberg, B., Kewenter, J., Petersen, I., and Stener, B. Anorectal function after major resections of the sacrum with bilateral or unilateral sacrifice of sacral nerves. Br. J. Surgery 63:546, 1976.

184. Groddeck, G. Verstopfung als Typus des Widerstands. Die Arche No. 8/9, 1926.

185. Pinkerton, P. Psychogenic megacolon in children: the implications of bowel negativism. Arch. Dis. Child. 33:371, 1958.

186. Tucker, D. M., Sandstead, H. H., Logan, G. M., Jr., Klevay, L. M., Mahalko, J., Johnson, L. K., Inman, L., and Inglett, G. E. Dietary fiber and personality factors as determinants of stool output. Gastroenterology 81:879, 1981.

187. Ehrentheil, O. F., and Wells, E. P. Megacolon in psychotic patients. A clinical entity. Gastroenterology 29:285, 1955.

188. Johnston, I. D. A., and Gibson, J. B. Megacolon and volvulus in psychotics. Br. J. Surg. 47:394, 1960.

189. Watkins, G. L., and Oliver, G. A. Giant megacolon in the insane: further observations in patients treated by subtotal colectomy. Gastroenterology 48:718, 1965.

190. Devroede, G., Roy, T., Bouchoucha, M., Pinard, G., Camerlain, M., Girard, G., Black, R., Schang, J. C., and Arhan, P. Constipation as a mirror of anxiety? Constipated women with colonic dysfunction have a distinct personality. Dig. Dis. Sci., in revision.

191. Henry, G. W., Gastrointestinal motor functions in schizophrenia. Roentgenological observations. Schizophrenia (Dementia Praecox) Research Publ. A Nerv. Ment. Dis. 5:280, 1928.

192. Devroede, G. La constipation: du symptôme à la personne. Psychol. Med. 17:1515, 1985.

193. Hislop, I. G. Psychological significance of the irritable bowel syndrome. Gut 12:452, 1971.

194. Liss, J. L., Alpers, D., and Woodruff, R. A. The irritable colon syndrome and psychiatric illness. Dis. Nerv. Syst. 34:151, 1973.

195. Latimer, P. Psychophysiologic disorders: a critical appraisal of concept and theory illustrated with reference to the irritable bowel syndrome (IBS). Psychol. Med. 9:71, 1979.

196. Latimer, P., Sarna, S., Campbell, D., Latimer, M., Waterfall, W., and Daniel, E. E. Colonic motor and myoelectrical activity: a comparative study of normal subjects, psychoneurotic patients and patients with irritable bowel syndrome. Gastroenterology 80:893, 1981.

197. Palmer, R. L., Stonehill, E., Crisp, A. H., Waller, S. L., and Misiewicz, J. J. Psychological characteristics of patients with irritable bowel syndrome. Postgrad. Med. 50:416, 1974.

198. Welch, G. W., Stace, N. H., and Pomare, E. W. Specificity of psychological profiles of irritable bowel patients. Aust. N.Z. J. Med. 14:101, 1984.

199. Bommelaer, G., Rouch, M., Dapoigny, M., Pair, D., Loisy, P., Gualino, M., and Tournut, R. Epidemiologie des troubles fonctionnels intestinaux dans une population apparemment saine. Gastroenterol. Clin. Biol. 10:7, 1986.

200. Welch, G. W., Hillman, L. C., and Pomare, E. W. Psychoneurotic symptomatology in the irritable bowel syndrome: a study of reporters and non-reporters. Br. Med. J. 291:1382, 1985.

201. Arhan, P., Devroede, G., Jehannin, B., Faverdin, C., Revillon, Y., Lefebvre, D., Gignier, P., and Pellerin, D. Idiopathic disorders of fecal continence in children. Pediatrics 71:774, 1983.

202. Shouler, P., and Keighley, M. R. B. Changes in colorectal function in severe idiopathic chronic constipation. Gastroenterology 90:414, 1986.

203. Barnes, P. R. H., and Lennard-Jones, J. E. Balloon expulsion from the rectum in constipation of different types. Gut 26:1049, 1985.

204. Cann, P. A., Read, N. W., Brown, C., Hobson, N., and Holdsworth, C. C. Irritable bowel syndrome: relationship of disorders in the transit of a single solid meal to symptom pattern. Gut 24:405, 1983.

205. Waller, S. L. Differential measurement of small and large bowel transit times in constipation and diarrhoea: a new approach. Gut 16:372, 1975.

206. Arhan, P., Devroede, G., Jehannin, B., Lanza, M., Faverdin, C., Dornic, C., Persoz, B., Tetreault, L., Perey, B., and Pellerin, D. Segmental colonic transit time. Dis. Colon Rectum 24:625, 1981.

207. Devroede, G., and Soffie, M. Colonic absorption in idiopathic constipation. Gastroenterology 64:552, 1973.

208. Hinton, J. M., and Lennard-Jones, J. E. Constipation: definition and classification. Postgrad. Med. J. 44:720, 1968.

209. Kirwan, W. O., and Smith, A. N. Gastrointestinal transit estimated by an isotope capsule. Scand. J. Gastroenterol. 9:763, 1974.

210. Kirwan, W. O., and Smith, A. N. Postprandial changes in colonic motility related to serum gastrin levels. Scand. J. Gastroenterol. 11:145, 1976.

211. Hinton, J. M., Lennard-Jones, J. E. Constipation: definition and classification. Postgrad. Med. J. 44:720, 1968.

212. Eastwood, M. A., Kirkpatrick, J. R., Mitchell, W. D., Bone, A., and Hamilton, T. Effects of dietary supplements of wheat bran and cellulose on faeces and bowel function. Br. Med. J. 4:392, 1973.

213. Melkersson, M., Andersson, H., Bosaeus, I., and Falkheden, T. Intestinal transit time in constipated and non constipated geriatric patients. Scand. J. Gastroenterol. 18:593, 1983.

214. Schang, J. C. Colonic motility in subgroups of patients with the irritable bowel syndrome. In Poitras, P. (ed.). Proceedings of the first international symposium on small intestinal and colonic motility. Centre de Recherches Cliniques, Hôpital Saint-Luc, and Jouveinal Laboratoires/Laboratories Inc. Montreal, 1985, pp. 101–112.

215. Likongo, Y., Devroede, G., Schang, J. C., Arhan, P., Vobecky, S., Navert, H., Carmel, M., Lamoureux, G., Strom, B., and Duguay, C. Hindgut dysgenesis as a cause of constipation with delayed colonic transit. Dig. Dis. Sci. 31:993, 1986.

216. Lane, W. A. The results of the operative treatment of chronic constipation. Br. Med. J., Jan. 18, p. 126, 1908.

217. Preston, J. E., and Lennard-Jones, J. E. Pelvic motility and response to intraluminal bisacodyl in slow-transit constipation. Dig. Dis. Sci. 30:289, 1985.

218. Dapoigny, M., Tournut, D., Trolese, J. F., Bommelaer, G., and Tournut, R. Activité myoélectrique colique à jeûn et en période post-prandiale chez le sujet sain et chez le colopathe. Gastroenterol. Clin. Biol. 9:223, 1985.

219. Dapoigny, M., Trolese, J. F., Tournut, D., Moncharmont, L., Bommelaer, G., and Tournut, R. Analyse automatique de l'activité myoélectrique rapide du côlon à l'aide d'un micro-ordinateur. Gastroenterol. Clin. Biol. 9:371, 1985.

220. Preston, D. M., Rees, L. H., and Lennard-Jones, J. E. Gynaecological disorders and hyperprolactinaemia in chronic constipation. Gut 24:A480, 1983.

221. Schang, J. C., Devroede, G., Hebert, M., Hemond, M., Pilote,

M., and Devroede, L. Effects of rest, stress and food on myoelectric spiking activity of the left and sigmoid colon in man. Dig. Dis. Sci., in press.

222. Frexinos, J., Bueno, L., and Fioramonti, J. Diurnal changes in myoelectric spiking activity of the human colon. Gastroenterology *88*:1104, 1985.

223. Preston, D. M., Pfeffer, J. M., and Lennard-Jones, J. E. Psychiatric assessment of patients with severe constipation. Gut *25*:A582, 1984.

224. Devroede, G., and Soffie, M. Colonic absorption in idiopathic constipation. Gastroenterology *64*:552, 1973.

225. Schang, J. C., Devroede, G., Duguay, C., Hemond, M., Hebert, M. Constipation par inertie colique et obstruction distale: étude électromyographique. Gastroenterol. Clin. Biol. *9*:480, 1985.

226. Dinoso, V. P., Jr., Murphy, S. N. S., Goldstein, J., and Rosner, B. Basal motor activity of the distal colon: a reappraisal. Gastroenterology *85*:637, 1983.

227. Connell, A. M. The motility of the pelvic colon. Part II. Paradoxical motility in diarrhoea and constipation. Gut *3*:342, 1962.

228. Waller, S. L., and Misiewicz, J. J. Colonic motility in constipation or diarrhoea. Scand. J. Gastroenterol. *7*:93, 1972.

229. Waller, S. L., Misiewicz, J. J., and Kiley, N. Effect of eating on motility of the pelvic colon in constipation or diarrhoea. Gut *13*:805, 1972.

230. Devroede, G. Dietary fiber, bowel habits and colonic function. Am. J. Clin. Nutr. *31*(10 Suppl): 157, 1978.

231. Chowdhury, A. R., Dinoso, V. P., and Lorber, S. H. Characterization of a hyperactive segment of the rectosigmoid junction. Gastroenterology *71*:584, 1976.

232. Hill, J. R., Kelley, M. L., Jr., Schlegel, J. F., and Code, C. F. Pressure profile of the rectum and anus of healthy persons. Dis. Colon Rectum *33*:203, 1960.

233. Meunier, P., Marechal, J. M., and Joubert De Beaujeu, M. Rectoanal pressures and rectal sensitivity studies in chronic childhood constipation. Gastroenterology *77*:330, 1979.

234. Baldi, F., Ferrarini, F., Corinaldesi, R., Balestra, R., Cassan, M., Ferati, G. P., and Barbara, L. Function of the internal anal sphincter and rectal sensitivity in idiopathic constipation. Digestion *24*:14, 1982.

235. Orr, W. C., and Robinson, M. G. Motor activity of the rectosigmoid in patients with chronic constipation. Gastroenterology *80*:1244, 1981.

236. Holschneider, A. M. Differential Diagnose und chirurgische Therapie des chronischen Obstipation im Kindesalter. Klin. Pädiat. *186*:208, 1974.

237. Reboa, G., Arnulfo, G., Frascio, M., Di Somma, C., Pitto, G., Berti-Riboli, E. Colon motility and coloanal reflexes in chronic idiopathic constipation. Effects of a novel enterokinetic agent cisapride. Eur. J. Clin. Pharmacol. *26*:745, 1984.

238. Parks, A. G., Porter, N. H., and Melzack, J. Experimental study of the reflex mechanism controlling the muscles of the pelvic floor. Dis. Colon Rectum *5*:407, 1962.

239. Fry, I. K., Griffiths, J. D., and Smart, P. J. G. Some observations on the movement of the pelvic floor and rectum with special reference to rectal prolapse. Br. J. Surg. *53*:784, 1966.

240. Rutter, K. R. P. Electromyographic changes in certain pelvic floor abnormalities. Proc. R. Soc. Med. *67*:53, 1974.

241. Kerremans, R. Morphological and Physiological Aspects of Anal Continence and Defecation. Brussels, Editions Arscia SA, Presses Académiques Européennes, 1969.

242. Wasserman, I. F. Puborectalis syndrome (rectal stenosis due to anorectal spasm). Dis. Colon Rectum *7*:87, 1964.

243. Jennings, P. J. Megarectum and megacolon in adolescents and young adults: result of treatment at St. Marks's Hospital. Proc. R. Soc. Med. *60*:805, 1967.

244. Percy, J. P., Swash, M., Neill, M. E., and Parks, A. G. Electrophysiological study of motor nerve supply of pelvic floor. Lancet *1*:16, 1981.

245. Hamel-Roy, J., Devroede, G., Arhan, P., Tetreault, J. P., Lemieux, B., and Scott, H. Functional abnormalities of the anal sphincters in patients with myotonic dystrophy. Gastroenterology *86*:1469, 1984.

246. Preston, D. M., and Lennard-Jones, J. E. Anismus in chronic constipation. Dig. Dis. Sci. *30*:413, 1985.

247. Womack, N. R., Williams, N. S., Holmfield, J. M. M., Morrison, J. F. B., and Simpkins, K. C. New method for the dynamic assessment of anorectal function in constipation. Br. J. Surg. *72*:994, 1985.

248. Pavlakis, A., Wheeler, J. S., Jr., Krane, R. J., and Siroky, M. B. Functional voiding disorders in females. Neurourology and Urodynamics *5*:145, 1986.

249. Reich, W. The Function of the Orgasm: Sex-economic Problems of Biological Energy. New York, Farrar, Straus and Giroux, 1943.

250. Lowen, A. Love and Orgasm. New York, New American Library, 1967.

251. Bleijenberg, G., and Kuijpers, H. C. Treatment of the spastic pelvic floor syndrome with biofeedback. Dis. Colon. Rectum, *30*:108, 1987.

252. Hero, M., Arhan, P., Devroede, G., Jehannin, B., Faverdin, C., Babin, C., and Pellerin, D. Measuring the anorectal angle. J. Biomed. Eng. *7*:321, 1985.

253. Kuijpers, H. C., and Bleijenberg, G. The spastic pelvic floor syndrome. A cause of constipation. Dis. Colon Rectum *28*:669, 1985.

254. Kuijpers, H. C., Bleijenberg, G., and De Morree, H. The spastic pelvic floor syndrome. Large bowel outlet obstruction caused by pelvic floor dysfunction: a radiological study. Int. J. Colorectal Dis. *1*:44, 1986.

255. Meunier, P. Rectoanal dyssynergia in constipated children. (Abstract.) Dig. Dis. Sci. *30*:784, 1985.

256. Wald, A., Chandra, R., Gabel, S., and Chiponis, D. Anorectal manometry and continence studies in childhood encopresis. (Abstract.) Dig. Dis. Sci. *29*:554, 1984.

257. Bartolo, D. C. C., Roe, A. M., Virjee, J., and Mortensen, N. J. Evacuation proctography in obstructed defaecation and rectal intussuception. Br. J. Surg. *72*:S111, 1985.

258. Parks, A. G., Porter, N. H., and Hardcastle, N. D. The syndrome of the descending perineum. Proc. R. Soc. Med. *59*:477, 1966.

259. Bartolo, D. C. C., Read, N. W., Jarratt, J. A., Read, M. G., Donnelly, T. C., and Johnson, A. G. Differences in anal sphincter function and clinical presentation in patients with pelvic floor descent. Gastroenterology *85*:68, 1983.

260. Kiff, E. J., Barnes, P. R. H., and Swash, M. Evidence of pudendal neuropathy in patients with perineal descent and chronic straining at stool. Gut *25*:1279, 1984.

261. Porter, N. H. Megacolon: a physiological study. Proc. R. Soc. Med. *54*:1043, 1961.

262. Callaghan, R. P., and Nixon, H. H. Megarectum: physiological observations. Arch. Dis. Child. *39*:153, 1964.

263. Bard, L. Le mégarectum, dilatation idiopathique d'origine congénitale. La Semaine Médicale 30, no. 48, p. 565, Nov. 30, 1910.

264. Hillemand, B. Mégarectum: étiologie, pathogénie, clinique, traitement médical. Arch. Mal. Appar. Dig. *54*:3, 1965.

265. Arhan, P., Devroede, G., Persoz, B., Faverdin, C., Dornic, C., and Pellerin, D. Response of the anal canal to repeated distension of the rectum. Clin. Invest. Med. *2*:83, 1979.

266. Bartram, C. I., Turnbull, G. K., and Lennard-Jones, J. E. Evacuation proctography—a study of 20 subjects without defaecation disturbance. Gastrointest. Radiol., in press.

267. Bonfils, S., Hachette, J. C., and Danne, O. L'abord psychosomatique en gastroentérologie. Paris, Masson, 1982.

268. Stewart, E. T., and Dodds, W. J. Predictability of rectal incontinence on barium enema examination. AJR *132*:197, 1979.

269. Preston, D. M., Lennard-Jones, J. E., and Thomas, B. M. Toward a radiologic definition of idiopathic megacolon. Gastrointest. Radiol. *10*:167, 1985.

270. Chauve, A., Devroede, G., and Bastin, E. Intraluminal pressures during perfusion of the human colon in situ. Gastroenterology *70*:336, 1976.

271. Brummer, P., Seppala, P., and Wegelius, U. Redundant colon as a cause of constipation. Gut *3*:140, 1962.

272. Cummings, J. H., Jenkins, D. J. A., and Wiggins, H. S.

Measurement of the mean transit time of dietary residue through the human gut. Gut *17*:210, 1976.

273. Cummings, J. H., and Wiggins, H. Transit through the gut measured by analysis of a single stool. Gut *17*:219, 1976.

274. Hinton, J. M., Lennard-Jones, J. E., and Young, A. C. A new method for studying gut transit times using radiopaque markers. Gut *10*:842, 1969.

275. Eastwood, H. D. H. Bowel transit studies in the elderly: radiopaque markers in the investigation of constipation. Gerontol. Clin. *14*:154, 1972.

276. Holdstock, D. J., Misiewicz, J. J., Smith, T., and Rowlands, E. N. Propulsion (mass movements) in the human colon and its relationship to meals and somatic activity. Gut *11*:91, 1970.

277. Wangel, A. G., and Deller, J. D. Intestinal motility in man. III. Mechanisms of constipation and diarrhea with particular reference to the irritable colon syndrome. Gastroenterology *48*:69, 1965.

278. Daniel, E. E., Wachter, B. T., Honour, A. J., and Bogoch, A. The relationship between electrical and mechanical activity of the small intestine of dog and man. Can. J. Biochem. Physiol. *38*:777, 1961.

279. Snape, W. J., Jr., Carlson, G. M., and Cohen, S. Colonic myoelectric activity in the irritable bowel syndrome. Gastroenterology *70*:326, 1976.

280. Couturier, D., Roze, C., Couturier-Turpin, M. H., and Debray, C. Electromyography of the colon in situ: an experimental study in man and in the rabbit. Gastroenterology *56*:317, 1969.

281. Sarna, S. K., Waterfall, W. E., Bardakjian, B. L., and Lind, J. F. Types of human colonic electrical activities recorded postoperatively. Gastroenterology *81*:61, 1981.

282. Fleckenstein, P. A probe for intraluminal recording of myoelectric activity from multiple sites in the human small intestine. Scand. J. Gastroenterol. *73*:767, 1978.

283. Fioramonti, J., Bueno, L., and Frexinos, J. Sonde endoluminale pour l'exploration électromyographique de la motricité colique chez l'homme. Gastroenterol. Clin. Biol. *4*:546, 1980.

284. Taylor, I., Darby, C., Hammond, P., and Basu, P. Is there a myoelectrical abnormality in the irritable colon syndrome? Gut *19*:391, 1978.

285. Bueno, L., Fioramonti, J., Ruckebusch, Y., Frexinos, J., and Coulom, P. Evaluation of colonic myoelectrical activity in health and functional disorders. Gut *21*:480, 1980.

286. Sarna, S. K., Latimer, P., Campbell, D., and Waterfall, W. E. Electrical and contractile activities of the human rectosigmoid. Gut *23*:698, 1982.

287. Schang, J. C., Hemond, M., Hebert, M., and Pilote, M. Myoelectrical activity and intraluminal flow in human sigmoid colon. Dig. Dis. Sci. *31*:1331, 1986.

288. Schang, J. C., Hemond, M., Hebert, M., and Pilote, M. Changes in colonic myoelectric spiking activity during stimulation by bisacodyl. Can. J. Physiol. Pharmacol. *64*:39, 1985.

289. Schang, J. C. Effects of naloxone and pitressin on colonic myoelectric spiking activity in acute constipation. Gastroenterology *88*:A1573, 1985.

290. Schang, J. C., Hemond, M., Hebert, M., and Pilote, M. How does morphine work on colonic motility? An electromyographic study in the human left and sigmoid colon. Life Sci. *38*:671, 1986.

291. Schuster, M. M., Hookman, P., Hendrix, T. P., and Mendeloff, A. I. Simultaneous manometric recording of internal and external sphincteric reflexes. Bull. Johns Hopkins Hosp. *116*:79, 1965.

292. Farthing, M. J. G., and Lennard-Jones, J. E. Sensibility of the rectum to distension and the anorectal reflex in ulcerative colitis. Gut *19*:64, 1978.

293. Colin, R., Galmiche, J. P., Geoffroy, Y., Hecketsweiler, P., Denis, P., Lefrancois, R., and Pasquis, P. Elastic properties of the rectal wall in normal adults and patients with ulcerative colitis. Gastroenterology *77*:45, 1979.

294. Preston, D. M., Lennard-Jones, J. E., and Thomas, B. M. The balloon proctogram. Br. J. Surg. *71*:29, 1984.

295. Lahr, C. J., Rothenberger, D. A., Jensen, L. L., and Goldberg, S. M. Balloon topography. A simple method of evaluating anal function. Dis. Colon Rectum *29*:1, 1986.

296. Mahieu, P., Pringot, J., and Bodart, P. Defecography. I. Description of a new procedure and results in normal patients. Gastrointest. Radiol. *9*:247, 1984.

297. Mahieu, P., Pringot, J., and Bodart, P. Defecography. II. Contribution to the diagnosis of defecation disorders. Gastrointest. Radiol. *9*:253, 1984.

298. Sami-Ali Corps réel, corps imaginaire. Paris, Dunod ed., 1984.

299. Sapir, M. De soignant à soigné: le corps à corps. Mythe ou champ de recherche? Evol. Psychiatr. *48*:989, 1983.

300. Almy, T. P., Hinkle, L. E., Jr., Berle, B., and Kern, F., Jr. Alterations in colonic function in man under stress. III. Experimental production of sigmoid spasm in patients with spastic constipation. Gastroenterology *12*:437, 1949.

301. Nisard, A., Jian, R., Chevalier, J., and Lefrant, L. Effet d'une cure thermale à Châtel-Guyon sur le temps de transit intestinal total de patients atteints de colopathie fonctionnelle. Rev. Fr. de Gastroenterologie *175*:5, 1982.

302. Loening-Baucke, V. A. Abnormal rectoanal function in children recovered from chronic constipation and encopresis. Gastroenterology *87*:1299, 1984.

303. Denis, P., Cayran, G., and Galmiche, J. P. Biofeedback: the light at the end of the tunnel? Maybe for constipation. Gastroenterology *80*:1089, 1981.

304. Harvey, R. F., Pomare, E. W., and Heaton, K. Effects of increased dietary fibre on intestinal transit. Lancet *1*:1278, 1973.

305. Payler, D. K., Pomare, E. W., Heaton, K. W., and Harvey, R. F. The effect of wheat bran on intestinal transit. Gut *16*:209, 1975.

306. Holmgren, G. O., and Mynors, J. M. The effect of diet on bowel transit times. S. Afr. Med. J. *46*:918, 1972.

307. Kirwan, W. O., Smith, A. N., McConnell, A. A., Mitchell, W. D., and Eastwood, M. A. Action of different bran preparations on colonic function. Br. Med. J. *4*:187, 1974.

308. Walker, A. R. P. Effect of high crude fiber intake on transit time and the absorption of nutrients in South African Negro school children. Am. J. Clin. Nutr. *28*:1161, 1975.

309. Cummings, J. H., Southgate, D. A. T., Branch, W., Houston, H., Jenkins, D. J. A., and James, W. P. T. Colonic response to dietary fibre from carrot, cabbage, apple, bran, and guar gum. Lancet *1*:5, 1978.

310. Cummings, J. H. Constipation, dietary fibre and the control of large bowel function. Postgrad. Med. J. *60*:811, 1984.

311. Gear, J. S. S., Brodribb, A. J. M., Ware, A., and Mann, J. I. Fibre and bowel transit times. Br. J. Nutr. *45*:77, 1981.

312. Cummings, J. H. Fermentation in the human large intestine: evidence and implications for health. Lancet *1*:1206, 1983.

313. Anderson, H., Bosaeus, I., Falkheden, T., and Melkersson, M. Transit time in constipated geriatric patients during treatment with a bulk laxative and bran: a comparison. Scand. J. Gastroenterol. *14*:821, 1979.

314. Almy, T. P. Experimental studies on the irritable colon. Am. J. Med. *10*:60, 1951.

315. Burkitt, D. P. Large bowel cancer—an epidemiologic jigsaw puzzle. J. Natl. Cancer Inst. *54*:3, 1975.

316. Burkitt, D. P. Epidemiology of cancer of the colon and rectum. Cancer *28*:3, 1971.

317. Soubeyrand, J., Condat, J. M., and Niamkey, E. Constipation africaine. Nouv. Presse Méd. *9*:2083, 1980.

318. Brodribb, A. J. M. Treatment of symptomatic diverticular disease with a high-fibre diet. Lancet *1*:664, 1977.

319. Sóltoft, J., Gudmand-Hoyes, E., Krag, B., Kristensen, E., Wulfe, M. R. A double-blind trial of the effect of wheat bran on symptoms of irritable bowel syndrome. Lancet *1*:270, 1976.

320. Kochen, M. M., Wegscheider, K., and Abholz, H. H. Prophylaxis of constipation by wheat bran: a randomized study in hospitalized patients. Digestion *31*:220, 1985.

321. Turnbull, G. K., Lennard-Jones, J. E., and Bartram, C. I. Failure of rectal expulsion as a cause of constipation: why fibre and laxatives sometimes fail. Lancet *1*:767, 1986.

322. Sarahan, T., Weintraub, W. H., Coran, A. G., and Wesley, J. R. The successful management of chronic constipation in infants and children. J. Pediatr. Surg. *17*:171, 1982.

323. Brandt, D. J. Gastrointestinal disorders of the elderly. New York, Raven Press, 1984.

324. Yonace, A. H., and Faulkner, J. E. Behavioral management of intractable constipation. Lancet 2:1371, 1980.
325. Rolider, A., Van Houten, R. Treatment of constipation-caused encopresis by a negative reinforcement procedure. J. Behav. Ther. Exp. Psychiatry 16:67, 1985.
326. Bornstein, P. H., Sturm, C. A., Retzlaff, P. D., Kirby, K. L., and Chong, H. Paradoxical instruction in the treatment of encopresis and chronic constipation: an experimental analysis. J. Behav. Ther. Exp. Psychiatry 12:167, 1981.
327. Eshchar, J., and Cohen, L. Re-education of constipated patients. A non-medicinal treatment. Am. J. Proctol. Gastroenterol. Colon Rectal Surg. 32:16, 1981.
328. Ford, M. R. Biofeedback treatment for headaches, Raynaud's disease, essential hypertension, and irritable bowel syndrome: a review of the long-term follow-up literature. Biofeedback Self-Regul. 7:521, 1982.
329. Ford, M. R. Interpersonal stress and style as predictors of biofeedback/relaxation training outcome: preliminary findings. Biofeedback Self-Regul. 10:223, 1985.
330. Svedlund, J. Psychotherapy in irritable bowel syndrome: a controlled outcome study. Acta Psychiatr. Scand. 306:67, 1981.
331. Bennett, P., and Wilkinson, S. A comparison by psychological and medical treatment of the irritable bowel syndrome. Br. J. Clin. Psychol. 24:215, 1985.
332. Latimer, P. R. Colonic psychophysiology. Implications for functional bowel disorders. In Hölzl, R., and Whitehead, W. E. (eds.). Psychophysiology of the Gastrointestinal Tract. Experimental and Clinical Applications. New York, Plenum Press, 1983.
333. Meichenbaum, D. Cognitive Behavior Modification: An Integrative Approach. New York, Plenum Press, 1977.
334. Whorwell, P. J., Prior, A., and Faragher, E. B. Controlled trial of hypnotherapy in the treatment of severe refractory irritable-bowel syndrome. Lancet 2:1232, 1984.
335. Clare, A. Stress management and irritable bowel syndrome. Lancet 2:719, 1985.
336. Freud, S. An outline of psychoanalysis. Int. J. Psychoanal. 21:27, 1940.
337. Searles, H. F. Countertransferance and Related Subjects. Selected Papers. New York, International University Press, 1979.
338. Wise, T. N., Cooper, J. N., and Ahmed, S. The efficacy of group therapy for patients with irritable bowel syndrome. Psychosomatics 23:465, 1982.
339. Thurtle, O. A., Allen, A. P., Walters, M. T., Kitchen, J. V., Smith, C. L., and Cawley, M. I. D. Intractable constipation in malignant phaeochromocytoma: combined treatment with adrenergic blockade and cholinergic drugs. J. R. Soc. Med. 77:327, 1984.
340. Kreek, M. J., Schaeffer, R. A., Hahn, E. F., and Fishman, J. Naloxone, a specific opioid antagonist, reverses chronic idiopathic constipation. Lancet 1:261, 1983.
341. Schang, J. C., and Devroede, G. Beneficial effects of naloxone in a patient with intestinal pseudoobstruction. Am. J. Gastroenterol. 80:407, 1985.
342. Wallace, W. C., and Madden, W. M. Experience with partial resection of the puborectal muscle. Dis. Colon Rectum 12:196, 1969.
343. Barnes, P. R. H., Hawley, P. R., Preston, D. M., and Lennard-Jones, J. E. Experience of posterior division of the puborectalis muscle in the management of chronic constipation. Br. J. Surg. 72:475, 1985.
344. Shandling, B., and Desjardins, J. G. Anal myomectomy for constipation. J. Pediatr. Surg. 4:115, 1969.
345. Holschneider, A. M., Shauer, A., and Meister, P. Ergebnisse der Sphincteromyotomie bei Analsphincterachalasien. Chirurgie 47:294, 1976.
346. Clayden, G. S., and Lawson, J. O. N. Investigation and management of long-standing chronic constipation in childhood. Arch. Dis. Child. 51:918, 1976.
347. McCready, R. A., and Beart, R. W. The surgical treatment of incapacitating constipation associated with idiopathic megacolon. Mayo Clin. Proc. 54:779, 1979.
348. Mitrofanoff, P., Grise, P., Lefort, J., and Borde, J. Intérêt de la sphinctérotomyectomie dans le traitement de la constipation idiopathique et des formes courtes de la maladie de Hirschsprung. Chir. Pediatr. 22:267, 1981.
349. Rush, F., Leenders, E., Canter, C., Capesius, C., and Lamesh, A. Intérêt de la sphincteromyectomie anorectale pour le diagnostic et le traitement des constipations chroniques de l'enfant. Acta Chir. Belg. 83:261, 1983.
350. Mishalany, H. G., and Woolley, M. G. Chronic constipation. Manometric patterns and surgical considerations. Arch. Surg. 119:1257, 1984.
351. Metchnikoff, E. Etudes sur la nature humaine. Essai de philosophie optimiste., 5th ed. Paris, A. Maloine, 1917, p. 239.
352. Metchnikoff, E. Mémoires publiées à l'occasion du jubilé de Elie Metchnikoff. Paris, Masson et Cie. 1921, pp. 8–12.
353. Preston, D. M., Hawley, P. R., Lennard-Jones, J. E., and Todd, I. P. Results of colectomy for severe idiopathic constipation in women (Arbuthnot Lane's disease). Br. J. Surg. 71:547, 1984.
354. Fasth, S., Hedlund, H., Svaninger, G., Oresland, T., and Hulten, L. Functional results after subtotal colectomy and caecorectal anastomosis. Acta Chir. Scand. 149:623, 1983.
355. Lane, R. H. S., and Todd, I. P. Idiopathic megacolon: a review of 42 cases. Br. J. Surg. 64:305, 1977.
356. Schuffler, M. D., and Deitch, E. A. Chronic idiopathic intestinal pseudo-obstruction—a surgical approach. Ann. Surg. 192:752, 1980.
357. Belliveau, P., Goldberg, S. M., Rohtenberger, D. A., and Nivatvongs, S. Idiopathic acquired megacolon: the value of subtotal colectomy. Dis. Colon Rectum 25:118, 1982.
358. Loening-Baucke, V., Anuras, S., and Shirazi, S. Severe idiopathic constipation. (Abstract.) Gastroenterology 90:1525, 1986.
359. Roe, A. M., Bartolo, D. C. C., Mortensen, N. J. Diagnosis and surgical management of intractable constipation. Br. J. Surg. 73:854, 1986.
360. Hughes, E. S. R., McDermott, F. T., Johnson, W. R., Polglase, A. L. Surgery for constipation. Aust. N. Z. J. Surg. 51:144, 1981.
361. Hardcastle, J. D., and Wilkins, J. C. The action of sennosides and related compounds on human colon and rectum. Gut 11:1038, 1970.
362. Hardcastle, J. D., and Mann, C. V. Study of large bowel peristalsis. Gut 9:512, 1968.
363. Lasagna, L., Mosteller, F., Von Felsinger, J. M., and Beecher, H. K. A study of the placebo response. Am. J. Med. 16:770, 1954.
364. Hodgson, W. J. B. The placebo effect. Is it important in diverticular disease? Am. J. Gastroenterol. 67:157, 1977.

Intestinal Obstruction, Pseudo-Obstruction, and Ileus

23

R. SCOTT JONES
BRUCE D. SCHIRMER

INTESTINAL OBSTRUCTION

Intestinal obstruction exists when there is any pathologic impediment to the aboral progression of intestinal luminal content. It may be produced by occlusion of the bowel lumen in mechanical obstruction or by lack of peristalsis of the intestinal muscle (paralytic ileus).

Clinical Picture

Abdominal pain, vomiting, obstipation, abdominal distention, and failure to pass flatus characterize the syndrome of intestinal obstruction.[1] Typically, *mechanical intestinal obstruction* produces crampy pain, with paroxysms occurring at four- to five-minute intervals in proximal obstruction and less frequently in distal obstruction. After a longer period of mechanical obstruction, the crampy pain may subside because bowel distention may inhibit motility. *Intestinal strangulation* should be suspected when continuous severe abdominal pain succeeds crampy abdominal pain. Proximal jejunal obstruction can cause profuse vomiting unassociated with abdominal distention. In distal obstruction, the vomiting will be less frequent and may become feculent owing to a greatly increased bacterial population of intestinal contents during obstruction. Obstipation and failure to pass gas from the rectum characterize complete obstruction, but occur only after evacuation of the bowel distal to the obstruction. Patients with distal small bowel obstruction, colonic obstruction, or paralytic ileus often develop increased abdominal girth resulting from accumulation of fluid and gas in the intestine (Table 23–1). A complete physical examination is indicated, but certain points should receive particular attention.

Tachycardia and hypotension may indicate severe

Table 23–1. CHARACTERISTICS OF PROXIMAL AND DISTAL OBSTRUCTION

High Small Bowel Obstruction	Low Small Bowel Obstruction
Onset acute	Onset less acute
Vomiting prominent	Vomiting present, less prominent
Vomiting not feculent	Vomiting often feculent
Pain at frequent intervals	Pain at less frequent intervals
Distention minimal or absent	Distention noticeable

dehydration, peritonitis, or both. The status of hydration should also be estimated by examination of skin turgor and moisture of the mucous membranes. Fever suggests the possibility of bowel necrosis or gangrene resulting from strangulation. The abdomen is usually distended, and the examiner must determine whether abdominal distention is due to bowel obstruction or ascites. A fluid wave, shifting dullness, and fullness in the flanks characterize ascites. Peristaltic waves, characteristic of small bowel obstruction, are sometimes visible through the abdominal wall of thin patients with longstanding obstruction. Abdominal surgical scars should be noted because of the etiologic implication of previous surgery. Incarcerated hernias may be obscure, particularly in obese patients. Abdominal masses and organomegaly should be sought. Patients with intestinal obstruction characteristically exhibit abdominal tenderness; however, localized tenderness, rebound tenderness, and guarding suggest the possibility of strangulation with bowel necrosis and its sequelae. Abdominal auscultation in the patient with mechanical intestinal obstruction will occasionally reveal periods of increasing or "crescendoing" bowel sounds separated by relatively quiet periods. The quality of bowel sounds in intestinal obstruction is usually high-pitched or musical in character. In prolonged obstruction, the sounds will often disappear as bowel motility decreases. Rectal examination should be done to detect masses. The presence or absence of feces should be noted; if feces are present, examination for occult blood should be done. Blood in the feces suggests an alimentary mucosal lesion, as may occur in cancer, intussusception, or infarction. Sigmoidoscopic examination should be done if colonic obstruction is suspected.

Acute intestinal obstruction can usually be diagnosed on the basis of history and physical examination. Any patient having acute onset of crampy abdominal pain, vomiting, obstipation, abdominal distention, and abdominal tenderness should be considered to have intestinal obstruction until that diagnosis can be confidently excluded.

Radiologic Examination

X-rays usually confirm the clinical diagnosis. Plain abdominal X-ray examination in patients with intestinal obstruction usually reveals abnormally large quantities of gas in the bowel. One can usually determine whether

369

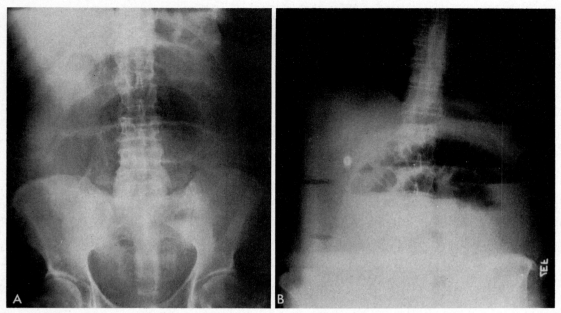

Figure 23–1. *A*, This plain X-ray was taken with the patient in the supine position. Note the excessive amount of gas in the small intestine. The small intestine is identified in this film by its central location in the abdomen and the presence of valvulae conniventes. There is little or no colonic gas seen on this film. *B*, An upright film, showing air-fluid levels in the small intestine. The films in *A* and *B* were obtained on a 61-year-old man with a history of cramping abdominal pain, vomiting, obstipation, failure to pass gas, and abdominal distention. After a period of fluid replacement, surgical exploration revealed complete mechanical obstruction of the ileum caused by Crohn's disease with infarction of a segment of bowel proximal to the point of obstruction. This patient had an uncomplicated recovery following resection of the involved bowel.

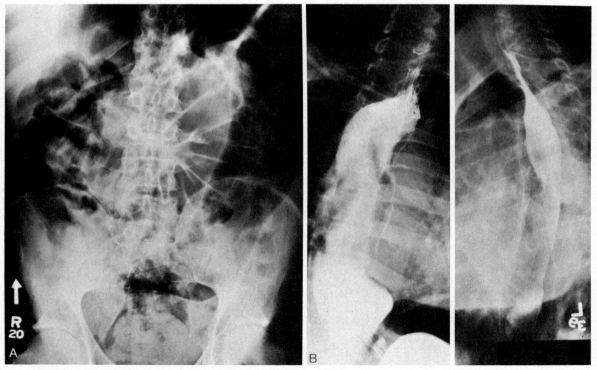

Figure 23–2. *A*, This plain abdominal X-ray depicts distention of the colon and small intestine in a young woman with familial idiopathic intestinal pseudo-obstruction. *B*, This barium swallow discloses esophageal dilatation from an esophageal motility disorder accompanying familial idiopathic intestinal pseudo-obstruction in the same patient shown in *A*. (Courtesy of Dr. Hubert Shaffer.)

small intestine, colon, or both are distended. Gas in the small bowel outlines the valvulae conniventes, which usually occupy the entire transverse diameter of the bowel image. Colonic haustral markings, on the other hand, occupy only a portion of the diameter of the bowel. Typically, the small bowel pattern occupies the more central portion of the abdomen, whereas the colonic shadow resides on the periphery of the abdominal film or in the pelvis. Patients with mechanical small intestinal obstruction usually have minimal or no colonic gas (Fig. 23–1). Radiographs from patients who have colonic obstruction with a competent ileocecal valve will show colonic distention but little small bowel gas (Fig. 23–2). Patients with colonic obstruction and an incompetent ileocecal valve usually have radiographic evidence of small bowel and colonic distention (Fig. 23–3A). Films taken in the upright or lateral decubitus position in patients with mechanical small bowel obstruction usually show multiple gas-fluid levels with distended bowel resembling an inverted U. Plain films may be misleading in patients with proximal jejunal obstruction or proximal closed loop obstruction by failing to show dilated loops and air-fluid levels. This is noteworthy because the risk of strangulation with closed loop obstruction is high. Occasionally, ordinary X-ray films fail to distinguish colonic from small intestinal obstruction, and the administration of a radiographic contrast agent may help. In that instance a carefully performed barium enema constitutes the safest and quickest means to distinguish colonic from small bowel obstruction preoperatively (Fig. 23–3B).

It is often difficult to distinguish paralytic ileus from mechanical obstruction by radiography. Uniform gaseous distention of the stomach, small bowel, colon, and rectum radiographically characterizes paralytic ileus. Gas-fluid levels develop in both mechanical intestinal obstruction and paralytic ileus (Fig. 23–4). Examination after a barium meal may assist in distinguishing between paralytic ileus and mechanical obstruction, but use of barium by mouth should be avoided if colonic obstruction cannot be excluded.

Laboratory Tests

Any patients suspected of having intestinal obstruction with vomiting or evidence of intra-abdominal fluid loss should have laboratory measurements of serum sodium, chloride, potassium, bicarbonate, and creatinine concentrations. The hematocrit, white blood cell count, and serum electrolytes should be measured serially to assess adequacy of therapy and to detect the earliest evidence of tissue necrosis.

Categories of Mechanical Obstruction

Three categories of abnormalities produce mechanical bowel obstruction (Table 23–2): obturation obstruction, intrinsic bowel lesions, and extrinsic lesions.
Obturation Obstruction. Obturation of the intestinal lumen may have many causes. *Intussusception* is an

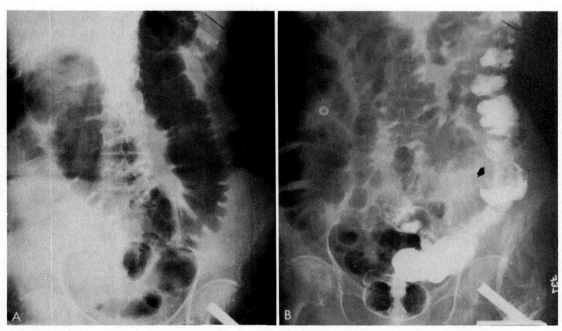

Figure 23–3. *A,* A plain abdominal film on a 71-year-old woman with a several-day history of increasing abdominal distention and failure to pass gas or feces from the rectum. The presence of a large quantity of gas in the transverse and descending colon and a small amount of small intestinal gas suggests the diagnosis of obstruction of the descending colon. *B,* Barium enema on the same patient, revealing an obstructing carcinoma of the descending colon. Note the presence of small bowel gas on this film, compatible with incompetent ileocecal valve. Note the haustral markings on the colon in both *A* and *B.* This patient was treated by right transverse colostomy. After she recovered from the effects of the episode of obstruction, she was reoperated upon and underwent a left colectomy and colocolostomy. After recovery from that procedure, her colostomy was closed.

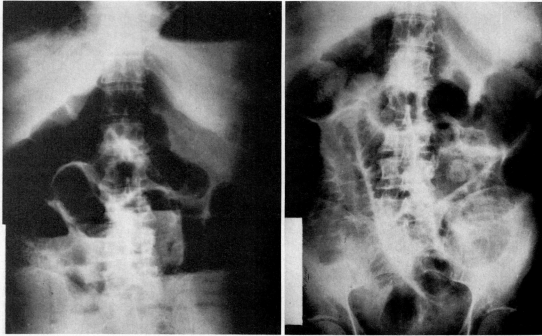

Figure 23–4. Paralytic ileus is frequently difficult to distinguish from mechanical obstruction. The presence of gas in stomach, small bowel, and colon suggests ileus, as shown in these films.

invagination of the bowel lumen with the invaginated portion (the intussusceptum) passing distally into the ensheathing outer portion (the intussuscipiens) by peristalsis (Fig. 23–5). In adults, an abnormality in the bowel wall, such as a tumor or Meckel's diverticulum,

Table 23–2. MECHANICAL INTESTINAL OBSTRUCTION

I. Obturation obstruction
    A. Polypoid tumors
    B. Intussusception
    C. Gallstones
    D. Foreign bodies
    E. Bezoars
    F. Feces
II. Intrinsic bowel lesions
    A. Atresia
    B. Stenosis
    C. Strictures
        1. Neoplastic
        2. Inflammatory
        3. Chemical
        4. Anastomotic
    D. Vascular abnormality
        1. Arterial occlusion
        2. Venous occlusion
III. Extrinsic bowel lesions
    A. Adhesions
        1. Previous surgery
        2. Previous peritonitis
    B. Hernias
        1. Internal
        2. External
    C. Neoplasm
    D. Abscesses
    E. Volvulus
    F. Congenital bands

usually causes intussusception; however, in infants and children, intussusception may occur without apparent anatomic cause. Large gallstones, which can enter the intestinal lumen via a cholecystoenteric fistula, may cause obturation obstruction. This produces a rare condition called *gallstone ileus.* Feces, meconium, or bezoars may also obstruct the intestine. Bezoars occur most frequently in children, the mentally retarded, the toothless, and postgastrectomy patients.

Intrinsic Bowel Lesions. Intrinsic bowel lesions producing intestinal obstruction are often congenital, as in *atresia* or *stenosis,* and occur most commonly in infants and small children. *Strictures* of the intestine may result from neoplasm or from inflammation, as in Crohn's disease. Rarely, one may encounter iatrogenic strictures following intestinal anastomosis or *radiation therapy.* Mesenteric vascular occlusion occasionally produces the syndrome of intestinal obstruction.

Extrinsic Lesions. Extrinsic lesions comprise the most important cause of small bowel obstruction. Occlusion of the intestine by *adhesions* from previous surgery leads all causes of small intestinal obstruction. Adhesions may produce obstruction by kinking or angulation or by creating bands of tissue that compress the bowel. Other important causes of mechanical small intestinal obstruction include external hernias such as inguinal, femoral, umbilical, and incisional hernias. The risk of intestinal obstruction constitutes the principal reason for the elective repair of hernias. *Internal hernias* resulting from congenital abnormalities or surgical defects in the mesentery occasionally cause bowel obstruction. Extrinsic masses such as neoplasms and abscesses may sometimes cause mechanical bowel obstruction. A *volvulus* is an extrinsic abnormality in

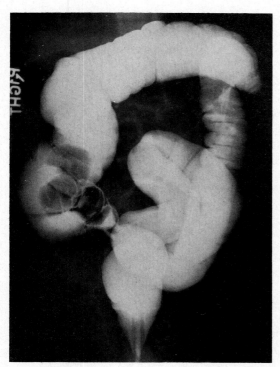

Figure 23–5. Barium enema on a young child with severe abdominal pain and the passage of dark bloody material from the rectum. The radiolucent filling defect in the cecum and ascending colon with a pattern suggestive of mucosa and failure to reflux barium into the small bowel are the typical findings of an ileocecal intussusception. Because this intussusception could not be reduced hydrostatically with the barium enema, the patient was operated upon and underwent resection of the terminal ileum.

plasms and hernias. *Neoplasms* are the most common cause of colonic obstruction (Table 23–3).

Pathophysiology

Simple Mechanical Small Intestinal Obstruction. Mechanical obstruction of the small intestine results in accumulation of fluid and gas proximal to the obstruction, producing distention of the intestine. Intestinal gas, ingested fluid, and digestive secretions initiate distention. Peristalsis normally propels intestinal gas aborally for expulsion from the rectum as flatus. Swallowed air provides the most important source of gas in intestinal obstruction because its nitrogen content is very high and nitrogen is not well absorbed by the intestinal mucosa. Consequently, intestinal gas is primarily made up of nitrogen. Five gases—N_2, O_2, H_2, CO_2, and CH_4 (methane)—constitute 99 per cent of intestinal gas in normal subjects. N_2 predominates, followed by H_2 and CO_2. The neutralization of HCl or fatty acids by bicarbonate releases large quantities of CO_2 into the upper intestine; thus, CO_2 represents the predominant duodenal gas. The bowel rapidly absorbs most of this CO_2; therefore, little if any of this CO_2 appears in the distal intestine.[3] Intestinal bacteria that produce hydrogen and methane are normally limited to the colon. However, probably the abnormally increased flora in the small bowel during obstruction produce some hydrogen or methane that contributes to the distention.

Loss of water and electrolytes from the body's intra-

which a portion of the alimentary canal rotates or twists about itself, occasionally involving the blood supply of the twisted portion of the bowel. This abnormality kinks the gut producing mechanical obstruction, frequently with occlusion of the blood supply to the bowel. A volvulus usually accompanies some underlying abnormality; for example, the mesenteric abnormality of malrotation allows midgut volvulus to develop. *Cecal volvulus* occurs when the cecum or right colon possesses a mesentery rather than being retroperitoneal (Fig. 23–6). Cecal volvulus may occur at any age between adolescence and the eighth decade, but the average age for cecal volvulus is in the fifth decade. The average duration of symptoms is about two days, and a history of chronic constipation is infrequent.[2]

An abnormally long or redundant sigmoid colon allows sigmoid volvulus to develop (Fig. 23–7). The majority of patients with sigmoid volvulus are elderly, and many have associated medical or psychiatric problems. A history of chronic constipation characterizes patients with sigmoid volvulus. A third type of volvulus occurs when adhesions produce a pivot about which the intestine can twist. The most common cause of small intestinal obstruction in adults is adhesions, usually resulting from previous surgery, followed by neo-

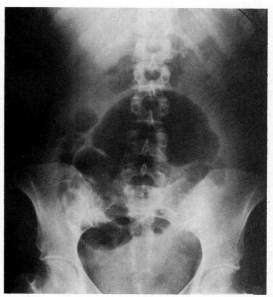

Figure 23–6. Plain X-ray obtained on a patient who developed severe abdominal pain and distention. This film shows a large amount of gas which appears to be in the cecum situated in the midabdomen; there is a paucity of gas in the transverse, descending, and sigmoid colon and in the rectum. This patient had a cecal volvulus.

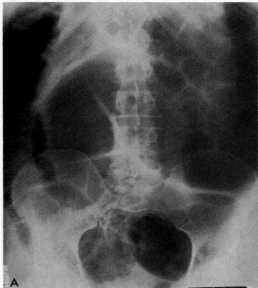

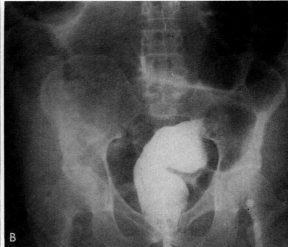

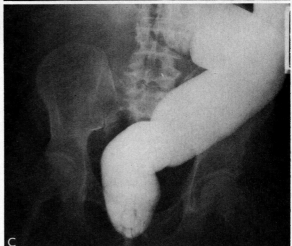

Figure 23–7. *A,* A plain abdominal X-ray obtained on a patient who developed marked abdominal distention, abdominal pain, and tenderness while convalescing from a neurosurgical operation. *B,* Barium enema performed on this patient, illustrating the typical "bird's beak" picture of sigmoid volvulus. This patient was treated by passing a fiberoptic colonoscope through the narrowed area and decompressing the colon. *C,* A barium enema performed on the day following reduction of the sigmoid volvulus.

vascular space, caused mainly by intestinal distention and its sequelae, constitutes one of the most important events during mechanical obstruction. First, reflex vomiting may result from intestinal distention. In addition, intestinal distention is self-perpetuating in the obstructed small bowel, because distention increases intestinal secretion of water and electrolytes in the

Table 23–3. RELATIVE CAUSES OF MECHANICAL INTESTINAL OBSTRUCTION IN ADULTS*

Small Bowel	Percentage
Adhesions	74
Hernia	8.1
Malignancy	8.6
Inflammatory bowel disease	5.2
Other	4.1
Colon	**Percentage**
Cancer	67
Volvulus	9
Diverticulitis	7
Fecal impaction	4.6
Miscellaneous	12.5

*Data from Bizer, L. S., et al. Surgery *89:*407, 1981; and Carden, A. B. G. Med. J. Aust. *1:*662, 1966.

obstructed segment.[4] Also, obstructed segments of intestine may harbor water owing to edema, which develops following a period of obstruction. Finally, transudation of water through the wall of the obstructed bowel leads to the development of peritoneal fluid.

The metabolic sequelae of fluid loss in simple mechanical obstruction of the small bowel depend upon the site and duration of the obstruction. Proximal small bowel obstruction causes relatively greater vomiting and less intestinal distention than distal obstruction. Distal small bowel obstruction may entail loss of large quantities of fluid into the bowel and metabolic acidosis. Oliguria, azotemia, and hemoconcentration may accompany the resultant dehydration. If dehydration persists, circulatory changes such as tachycardia, low central venous pressure, and reduced cardiac output may lead to hypotension and hypovolemic shock. Other sequelae of intestinal distention accompany increased intra-abdominal pressure, resulting in decreased venous return from the legs and elevation of the diaphragm with impaired pulmonary ventilation. In addition, when intestinal obstruction occurs, intestinal bacteria proliferate rapidly. Normally, the small intestine contains very small quantities of bacteria. Several factors cause the sparse bacterial population of the small intestine, but normal peristalsis with continued aboral progression of luminal content minimizes small intestinal flora. During small intestinal stasis, however, bacteria proliferate rapidly, and this phenomenon is particularly notable in intestinal obstruction. The small intestinal contents will thus become feculent during obstruction owing to large quantities of bacteria. The bacteria in the small intestine probably play no role in the ill effects of simple mechanical small bowel obstruction, as the bacteria or bacterial toxins do not cross the normal intestinal mucosa.

Strangulation Obstruction. *Strangulation* exists during any impairment of the circulation to the obstructed intestine. Occlusion of the bowel lumen at two points along its length produces closed-loop obstruction, which is noteworthy because this type of obstruction may proceed more rapidly to strangulation than simple obstruction. Sustained increase in intraluminal pressure may also impair circulation to the bowel. Pressure necrosis can develop if unyielding adhesive bands or hernial rings hold the obstructed distending bowel. Deformity or twisting of the mesentery can also occlude the mesenteric vessels, as in volvulus or intussusception. As a result, the patient may suffer all the ill effects of simple obstruction in addition to the effects of strangulation. Strangulation causes loss of blood or plasma from the strangulated segment, and such losses may be severe if venous vascular obstruction predominates. The loss of blood or plasma can cause shock, particularly in previously dehydrated patients. If strangulation produces gangrene, peritonitis will follow. Rupture or perforation of a strangulated segment produces devastating complications. The strangulated intestine may release toxic material into the peritoneum and then into the blood stream. The luminal fluid from the strangulated intestinal segment and the bloody malodorous peritoneal fluid are both lethal when experimentally administered to normal animals. Both bacteria and necrotic tissue appear necessary for the development of the toxic fluid. Apparently the lethal factor forms in the lumen of the strangulated intestine and passes through the intestinal wall when distention, vascular compromise, and bacteria injure the gut. The peritoneal cavity may then absorb the toxic material to produce systemic effects.[5]

It is extremely important to recognize the clinical features suggesting strangulation in a patient with intestinal obstruction. The findings of tenderness, tachycardia, leukocytosis, constant pain, fever, and abdominal guarding should alert the clinician to the possibility of strangulation. One study of 235 patients with small bowel obstruction examined four findings: leukocytosis (WBC count greater than 10,000 cells per cu mm), fever (temperature greater than 37°C orally), tachycardia (pulse rate greater than 96 beats per minute), and localized tenderness. Nearly 90 per cent of the patients with gangrenous bowel exhibited two or more of these findings. When all the classic findings were absent, no patient had gangrenous bowel.[6]

Although the clinical signs of strangulation must be sought, there is no infallible method of detecting strangulation preoperatively. For that reason, most patients with intestinal obstruction should be managed operatively to prevent the development of this serious complication and to avoid overlooking an undetected instance of strangulation.

Colonic Obstruction. In general, colonic obstruction produces less fluid and electrolyte disturbance than mechanical small bowel obstruction. If the patient has a competent ileocecal valve, there may be little or no small bowel distention, and gas will accumulate within the colon. As the colon becomes massively distended by gas, it may perforate; in this situation, because of its spherical shape and large diameter, the cecum is the likely site for perforation. However, the most common cause of colonic obstruction is cancer, and the most common site of perforation with an obstructing cancer is adjacent to the tumor rather than in the cecum. In patients with an incompetent ileocecal valve, signs of small bowel distention may accompany colonic obstruction. The colon, of course, is also subject to strangulation when obstruction compromises the blood supply.

Treatment

With few exceptions the appropriate treatment for mechanical intestinal obstruction is surgical relief of the obstruction. Because severe metabolic derangements may accompany prolonged bowel obstruction, the decision of when to operate requires careful judgment. The overlapping sequence of events in managing patients with intestinal obstruction should be *investigation, resuscitation* and *operation.*[7]

The timing of operation depends upon three factors: (1) duration of obstruction, e.g., the severity of fluid, electrolyte, and acid-base abnormalities; (2) improvement of vital organ function, i.e., management of concomitant cardiac and pulmonary disorders; and (3) consideration of the risk of strangulation. The mortality rate of intestinal obstruction with intestinal strangulation ranges from 4.5 per cent to 38 per cent,[6, 8] whereas in simple mechanical obstruction, when the operation is done within 24 hours of onset, the mortality rate is less than 8 per cent.[9, 10] Because no method reliably detects strangulation preoperatively, operation should be performed as soon as is reasonable if the diagnosis of *acute complete mechanical obstruction* is secure. Patients with bowel obstruction are likely to be depleted of water, sodium, chloride, and potassium so that intravenous therapy usually should begin with intravenous isotonic sodium chloride solution. After adequate urine formation occurs, potassium chloride should be added to the infusion. In severely dehydrated patients, sufficient fluids should be given to elevate and maintain the central venous pressure between 5 and 10 cm of saline. In all patients a minimum parameter of urine output equal to 0.5 ml per kilogram per hour must be achieved to demonstrate adequate organ perfusion. Administration of blood, plasma, or both should be considered if the patient is in shock and if strangulation is suspected. Severe metabolic acidosis, reflecting ischemia, may also require vigorous corrective measures. Concomitant cardiac and pulmonary disorders should be assessed but should not be allowed to delay operation unduly. After pulse, blood pressure, central venous pressure, and urinary output return to normal, surgery should be considered. If marked hemoconcentration and severe electrolyte imbalance were present initially, laboratory studies should be repeated. If the values are returning to normal, the patient should be operated upon. Antibiotics should be given during the period of resuscitation, if strangulation is suspected.

In addition to fluid therapy, another important adjunct to the supportive care of patients with intestinal obstruction is nasogastric or intestinal suction. Nasogastric suction with a Levin tube will empty the stomach, reducing the hazard of pulmonary aspiration of vomitus and minimizing further intestinal distention from swallowed air during the preoperative period. A nasogastric tube is not effective in decompressing distended intestine.

Operative treatment may be delayed for a short trial period of conservative nonoperative therapy under the following circumstances:

1. The patient who develops intestinal obstruction in the period immediately following an abdominal operation initially may be treated nonoperatively with a Cantor or other intestinal type tube. However, overlooked strangulation is a risk in this instance.

2. The patient with obstruction caused by documented disseminated intra-abdominal cancer may be treated with passage of a Cantor tube.

3. Infants with ileocecal intussusception may be managed by hydrostatic reduction of the intussusception, which avoids operation entirely. Adults with intussusception should be operated upon because of the high frequency of underlying causes for the intussusception.

4. Some patients with Crohn's disease or radiation enteritis may develop symptoms of intestinal obstruction that will abate with a period of conservative treatment.

5. Patients with partial small bowel obstruction resulting from adhesions may respond to conservative treatment without increased risk of strangulation.[11]

6. In patients with sigmoid volvulus, decompression can be performed with the sigmoidoscope or colonoscope, but elective operation should be performed later to prevent recurrent volvulus.

It should be emphasized that the patient must show continuous significant clinical improvement during a 12- to 24-hour period, or operation must be performed. A prolonged trial of unsuccessful conservative therapy results in significantly increased morbidity and mortality.[12, 13] Nonoperative treatment must also be carried out with the realization that strangulating obstruction cannot be diagnosed accurately prior to operation. The development of any clinical evidence of strangulation mandates operation.

The nature of the problem often determines the surgical management of mechanical intestinal obstruction. Five general approaches are commonly employed:

1. Procedures not requiring opening of the bowel with removal of external causes of obstruction: an example is obstruction caused by peritoneal adhesions, which is relieved by division of the adhesion.

2. Procedures requiring an enterotomy to remove an obturating obstruction: an example would be an enterotomy to remove a large obstructing gallstone.

3. The creation of an intestinal bypass: an example of this therapy is the treatment of a terminal ileal or ileocecal valve obstruction by ileotransverse colon anastomosis.

4. The placement of an enterocutaneous fistula, such as a colostomy, proximal to an obstruction.

5. Excision of a lesion or nonviable intestine with restoration of intestinal continuity: an example of this approach is the excision of the right colon with ileotransverse colostomy for obstructing carcinoma of the cecum.

With few exceptions, operation for intestinal obstruction should be performed under general anesthesia, administered with an endotracheal tube. The risks in operating on patients with intestinal obstruction include vomiting and tracheobronchial aspiration of the feculent vomitus. In the absence of an external hernia in patients with small bowel obstruction, abdominal exploration should be performed through a midline incision. The obstructed point can be located by following the distended bowel distally to find collapsed unobstructed intestine. Preoperative decompression facilitates the operative manipulation of obstructed intestine. To empty distended bowel during the operation, one can frequently manipulate the tip of a long intestinal tube from the stomach into the intestine. In operating on patients with multiple intra-abdominal adhesions, the surgeon should verify that no additional site of obstruction persists distal to the clinically obvious one. It may be desirable to express luminal content distally to prove patency of the entire intestinal lumen.

It is sometimes difficult to establish viability of a segment of bowel. Color, motility, and arterial pulsation generally can determine intestinal viability. If questionable, the bowel segment can be completely released, placed in a saline-moistened sponge for 15 to 20 minutes, and then re-examined. The use of fluorescein dye can accurately predict the viability of small intestine following ischemic injury should there be any question of bowel viability based on clinical criteria.[14] Return of normal color and peristalsis predict recovery and safety in retaining the bowel. Reasonable doubt of the bowel's viability indicates its removal.

Recurrent Intestinal Obstruction

An occasional unfortunate patient will exhibit recurrent small bowel obstruction by dense intraperitoneal adhesions. This is generally managed by reoperation if the obstruction is complete. Most surgeons simply free the obstructed intestine as described previously. There have been efforts to prevent reobstruction by plicating either the small bowel or its mesentery to permit its reintroduction into the peritoneal cavity in an orderly manner without kinks. Another method that has been employed to minimize postoperative obstruction is passage of a long intestinal tube through the length of the intestine and to permit it to remain there for two weeks while healing occurs, to ensure an adequate intestinal lumen. One report described the results of the treatment of intestinal obstruction due to extrinsic intra-abdominal adhesions by plication or tube stenting. The transmesenteric plication technique had a 10.7 per cent mortality rate, and 14.2 per cent of surviving patients required reoperation before discharge. In this group there were no late recurrent obstructions. When the intraluminal tube stent was used, there was a 2.7 per cent mortality rate, and 2.7 per cent of patients required reoperation for subsequent recurrent obstruction.[15]

Colonic Obstruction

The approach to colonic obstruction differs somewhat from that for small bowel obstruction. The classic method of treating obstruction of the left colon entails three separate operative steps: (1) relief of gaseous distention by colostomy proximal to the obstruction; (2) removal of the diseased segment of colon and anastomosis, leaving the colostomy intact; and (3) closure of the colostomy when healing of the anastomosis is complete.

The staged procedures are performed for the following reasons:

1. Intestinal obstruction and its sequelae are significant and immediate threats to life and should be treated as simply as possible. Colonic resection may be a formidable operation and is more safely performed electively.

2. Surgical anastomosis of distended colon is hazardous. A technically excellent colonic anastomosis is difficult with distended, thin-walled bowel filled with fluid and feces. Colostomy can be performed where the colon is mobile with a mesentery, such as in the sigmoid or transverse colon. In most instances, transverse colostomy is the best choice in treating left-sided colonic obstruction. In elderly, poor-risk patients with colon distention, a tube cecostomy inserted with local anesthesia may be appropriate. Obstructive lesions of the cecum and right colon are managed differently. In treating cecal or right colon obstruction caused by cancer, one must usually choose between right colectomy with ileotransverse colostomy and a bypassing operation (ileotransverse colostomy) to relieve the obstruction, with later elective resection of the right colon. The bypass operation should be reserved for poor-risk patients. Right colectomy can be done safely in patients with obstruction because the obstructed colon can be removed and the dilated small bowel can

usually be sutured safely to normal colon. Patients with cecal volvulus should be operated upon, but the treatment depends on the viability of the cecum. If the cecum is not judged viable, it should be resected and intestinal continuity restored with an ileocolonic anastomosis if conditions are ideal. Otherwise an ileostomy should be done. When the cecum is viable, the volvulus should be reduced, and the cecum should be fixed to the abdominal wall by cecopexy. The overall operative mortality rate for cecal volvulus is about 12 per cent. In the presence of cecal gangrene the mortality rate is about 33 per cent and in the absence of gangrene it is about 7 per cent.[16] In one series of patients treated by cecopexy, no recurrent volvulus occurred during a five-year follow-up period.

The initial approach to the patient with sigmoid volvulus should be nonoperative if the colon is thought to be viable. Eighty-five per cent of patients with sigmoid volvulus can have the volvulus reduced satisfactorily using the proctoscope and a rectal tube, or in some cases using a colonoscope. Most patients who have undergone successful decompression in this manner should undergo elective sigmoid resection after suitable preparation, because the sigmoid volvulus will recur in 50 to 90 per cent of cases. When the patient with sigmoid volvulus is suspected of having gangrenous bowel, operation should be performed to remove the sigmoid colon.[17]

INTESTINAL PSEUDO-OBSTRUCTION

Patients who develop a chronic clinical picture of intermittent to persistent bowel obstruction, and whose barium contrast studies exclude mechanical obstruction, probably have *chronic intestinal pseudo-obstruction*. In fact, this term generally describes a variety of states with different pathologic etiologies whose only common feature is the clinical picture described. Ileus can result from intrinsic defects in intestinal smooth muscle, intestinal innervation, or disturbances of neurohumoral controls of otherwise normal intestine. Reversible perturbations of these cause the acute self-limited condition called *paralytic ileus*. Chronic intestinal pseudo-obstruction syndromes have irreversible intrinsic muscle or nerve damage, either as a result of a systemic disease, or as a *primary* disease.

Primary Chronic Intestinal Pseudo-Obstruction

In 1948, Ogilvie described intestinal colic on the basis of a pseudo-obstruction syndrome.[18] Since then, an increasing number of reports have shown a familial relationship to some cases of this syndrome, while sporadic cases with no familial history have also been reported with regularity.

Faulk used the term "familial visceral myopathy"[19] to describe a syndrome of a variably inherited autosomal dominant trait resulting in smooth muscle degeneration of gastrointestinal tract as well as bladder and iris. Histologic examination of resected specimens revealed smooth muscle fibrosis with predominant longitudinal layer involvement and also revealed sparing of the intrinsic intestinal nerves. The same organs tend to be involved within each kindred, while patterns of organ involvement vary between families. Patients with familial visceral myopathy tend to have a very slow, almost imperceptible progression of their disease process over the course of years. Similar gastrointestinal smooth muscle pathologic changes occur in patients without other affected family members; "sporadic visceral myopathy" describes the syndrome in such patients.[20] Patients with this form of pseudo-obstruction tend to have generalized involvement of the gastrointestinal tract smooth muscle and a more rapidly progressive course of their disease than their familial myopathy counterparts.[21]

Familial visceral neuropathy and sporadic visceral neuropathy describe cases of primary chronic intestinal pseudo-obstruction with and without familial patterns. Histologic studies in such patients reveal abnormalities of the myenteric plexus of the intestine.[20] Pathognomonic intranuclear inclusions characterize the neurons of the myenteric plexus. Silver-staining of the longitudinal sections of the intestinal wall remains the best technique currently available for demonstrating the degenerative changes in the myenteric plexus.[22] Degeneration of other portions of the nervous system may also produce this syndrome because simultaneous calcification of the basal ganglia is accompanied by pseudo-obstruction in a kindred of mentally retarded siblings.[23] The symptoms of chronic intestinal pseudo-obstruction vary as a result of the extent of involvement of different areas of the gastrointestinal tract as well as the intermittent nature of the disease. Most patients develop their first symptoms early in life and usually relate a history of years of intermittent vomiting, distention, and crampy abdominal pain. Most patients will complain of diarrhea, but some will instead have constipation or a mixture of the two. Diarrhea commonly accompanies the steatorrhea produced by the intraluminal bacterial overgrowth from intestinal stasis and responds to treatment with antibiotics.

A subset of patients with chronic intestinal pseudo-obstruction manifests primarily isolated duodenal enlargement and motility disorders,[23] and consequently less severe systemic symptoms. Although dysphagia is rarely a significant complaint in these patients, esophageal manometry has shown most of them to have poor peristalsis of the esophagus and incomplete relaxation of the lower esophageal sphincter. Specifically, patients with familial visceral myopathy have low amplitude, simultaneous contractile waves, while patients with familial visceral neuropathy exhibit spontaneous diffuse esophageal activity.

Radiographic examination with plain films of the abdomen reveals distended large and small bowel in pseudo-obstruction patients (Fig. 23–8). Barium swallow and cineradiographic studies of the remainder of the alimentary tract help to characterize the areas of

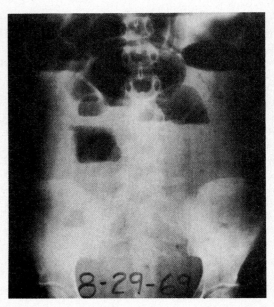

Figure 23–8. Flat film of the abdomen in a patient with pseudo-obstruction of the large bowel, with air-fluid levels. Small bowel distention is evident. (Courtesy of Dr. H. I. Goldberg.)

motility dysfunction in individual patients. Barium swallow confirms the abnormal peristalsis in the esophagus demonstrated by manometry, particularly in patients with familial visceral neuropathy where numerous spastic contractions greatly delay emptying. Gastric enlargement and delay in emptying is present in about one-third of all patients.[23]

Barium studies uniformly reveal small intestine motility dysfunction in chronic intestinal pseudo-obstruction. Duodenal enlargement is common, especially in visceral myopathy. Some portion of the small intestine is always dilated. Visceral neuropathy patients tend to have somewhat less distention and more uncoordinated intestinal contractions, resulting in faster intestinal transit times than patients with visceral myopathy (whose intestinal contractions are infrequent). Recent studies revealed normal duodenal electromyographic slow wave activity in these disorders but showed impaired physiologic motor response to intestinal distention.[24]

Barium enema may be normal in some cases of intestinal pseudo-obstruction but more frequently demonstrates distention and poor colonic contractility in patients with myopathy and diverticulosis and spasm in patients with neuropathy.

Laboratory assessment of these patients reveals the biochemical manifestations of malabsorption and steatorrhea in varying degrees. Folate or vitamin B_{12} deficiency, hypoalbuminemia, and iron deficiency anemia may be present.

Other than antibiotics to alleviate the symptoms of steatorrhea and malabsorption, there are currently no good available medical treatments for patients with chronic primary intestinal pseudo-obstruction. Elemental diets, steroids, indomethacin, a variety of hormones, cholinergic agents, metoclopramide, and prostaglandins have all been tried without significant success.[24, 25]

Surgical treatment should be avoided in patients with a confirmed diagnosis of chronic intestinal pseudo-obstruction, based on the generally mixed results reported thus far.[26, 27] Nonoperative treatment with nasogastric suction and intravenous fluids avoids the problem of whether recurrence of obstructive symptoms in the postoperative period in this patient population represents mechanical obstruction from adhesions or simply further symptoms of their underlying motility disorder. The occasional patient with localized stable disease, such as the subset of patients with isolated duodenal dilatation and motility disorder, may benefit from a surgical bypass procedure. Venting enterostomy and home TPN is an alternative in managing patients with malnutrition resulting from chronic intestinal pseudo-obstruction.[28]

Secondary Intestinal Pseudo-Obstruction

Secondary intestinal pseudo-obstruction denotes the group of illnesses with clinical manifestations similar to those of primary intestinal pseudo-obstruction. However, secondary pseudo-obstruction can follow several identifiable factors (Table 23–4).

Table 23–4. CHRONIC INTESTINAL PSEUDO-OBSTRUCTION: SECONDARY CAUSES*

I. Diseases involving the intestinal smooth muscle
  A. Collagen vascular disease
    1. Scleroderma
    2. Dermatomyositis/polymyositis
    3. Systemic lupus erythematosus
  B. Amyloidosis
  C. Primary muscle disease
    1. Myotonic dystrophy
    2. Progressive muscular dystrophy
  D. Ceroidosis
  E. Nontropical sprue
II. Endocrine disorders
  A. Myxedema
  B. Diabetes mellitus
  C. Hypoparathyroidism
  D. Pheochromocytoma
III. Neurologic diseases
  A. Parkinson's disease
  B. Hirschsprung's disease
  C. Chagas' disease
  D. Familial autonomic dysfunction
IV. Pharmacologic causes
  A. Phenothiazines
  B. Tricyclic antidepressants
  C. Antiparkinsonian medications
  D. Ganglionic blockers
  E. Clonidine
  F. Amanita (mushroom) poisoning
V. Miscellaneous
  A. Jejunoileal bypass
  B. Diverticulosis (jejunal)
  C. Psychosis
  D. Cathartic colon

*From Faulk, D. L., Anuras, S., and Christensen, J. Gastroenterology 74:922, 1978.

Collagen vascular diseases, particularly scleroderma, can cause gastrointestinal motor dysfunction as an important symptom. Approximately half of patients with scleroderma or progressive systemic sclerosis (PSS) will develop gastrointestinal motor dysfunction. The esophagus is most frequently involved, in contrast to patients with primary intestinal pseudo-obstruction where intestine, particularly small intestine, is usually the area of most marked disease. In PSS the gastrointestinal circular smooth muscle, rather than the longitudinal layer, undergoes fibrosis, and muscle vacuolization fails to occur.[21] These histologic differences in gastrointestinal disease and dysfunction, as well as the extraintestinal manifestations of PSS, usually serve to differentiate secondary intestinal pseudo-obstruction due to PSS from primary pseudo-obstruction syndromes. Other collagen vascular diseases, such as dermatomyositis and lupus erythematosus, have an even lower incidence of gastrointestinal motor dysfunction and their own collection of extraintestinal symptoms and signs that usually serve to avoid confusion as to the diagnosis.

Muscle disorders, including myotonic dystrophy and progressive muscular dystrophy, can affect gastrointestinal muscle function as well as other muscles throughout the body. In myotonic dystrophy, abnormal small intestinal motility is common and better detected by jejunal manometry than barium radiographic studies.[29]

Certain endocrine disorders produce symptoms of gastrointestinal motility dysfunction. Diabetes mellitus has a high accompanying rate of constipation in long-standing disease. Diabetic gastroparesis responds to peripheral dopamine antagonists—both metoclopramide and domperidone.[30] Myxedema ileus is a potentially reversible form of intestinal pseudo-obstruction that usually presents with colonic hypomotility and severe constipation.[31]

Primary disorders of nerves, including Hirschsprung's disease, achalasia, and Chagas' disease, produce characteristic gastrointestinal motility symptom complexes. Similarly, numerous drugs can induce profound ileus and, over a protracted course of administration, a syndrome resembling pseudo-obstruction. Psychotropic drugs, such as phenothiazines in particular, can produce marked colonic atony with resulting dilatation. However, the etiology of this atony is as yet undefined. Similarly, the exact pathogenesis of clinically observed ileus or pseudo-obstruction following antineoplastic agents, chronic laxative use, anti-Parkinson drugs, and other medications is as yet undefined.[21]

The treatment for all forms of secondary intestinal pseudo-obstruction is based upon treating, wherever possible, the primary disease leading to the syndrome.

PARALYTIC ILEUS

Paralytic ileus is a common disorder, occurring to some extent in most patients undergoing abdominal surgery. Several neural, humoral, and metabolic factors probably interact to cause this abnormality. There are reflexes that inhibit intestinal motility, such as the intestinointestinal reflex, resulting from prolonged intestinal distention. In the immediate postoperative period, circulating catecholamines and the resultant relative neuroendocrine-mediated dysfunction of the upper intestinal tract, particularly the stomach, may result in passage of abnormally large quantities of swallowed air, triggering such reflexes.

After an uncomplicated laparotomy, the small intestine will usually resume contractile activity within one day in the absence of complicating factors such as peritonitis. Paralytic ileus may accompany spinal fractures, retroperitoneal hemorrhage, trauma, myocardial infarction, or severe infection, including pneumonia. The administration of large quantities of enteral nutrition to the intestine immediately after abdominal operation has been reported to restore postoperative gastrointestinal function and motility rapidly.[32]

Postoperative ileus is most persistent in the left colon compared to other bowel segments, and recovery of normal peristaltic patterns occurs by about the third or fourth postoperative day.[33] Recent studies on monkeys suggested that adrenergic tone present in the colon may delay return of left colon function.[34]

Other humoral factors influence postoperative or posttraumatic paralytic ileus. Experiments in dogs in which the motility of transplanted (denervated) intestinal loops was inhibited during experimental peritonitis suggests humoral factors influence paralytic ileus. The substances responsible for this phenomenon remain unknown. Certain gastrointestinal peptide hormones can influence human gastrointestinal motor function. Neurotensin stimulates colonic motility,[35] but its physiologic role in regulating colonic activity is as yet unproved. Impaired release of the peptide hormone motilin accompanies the clinical syndrome of idiopathic delay in gastric emptying and clinical dyspepsia.[36]

Electrolyte imbalances, particularly hypokalemia, contribute to paralytic ileus by interfering with normal ionic movements during smooth muscle contractions. The intestinal ileus resulting from severe electrolyte depletion can be extremely profound, resulting in loss of not only contractile activity, but the normal small intestinal slow wave activity as well. Certain drugs, such as phenothiazines and narcotics, can also inhibit bowel motility. Finally, ischemia of the intestine rapidly inhibits motility (Table 23–5).

Paralytic ileus is treated by nasogastric suction and intravenous fluid administration. Correction of electrolyte imbalance, especially hypokalemia, is particularly important in managing this disorder. In some cases of paralytic ileus, particularly with extreme distention, passage of a Cantor tube into the intestine should be tried, because this method of suction provides intestinal decompression superior to that achieved with a nasogastric tube. In cases of transient acute colonic distention in the setting of paralytic ileus, rectal tube decompression, or if unsuccessful, colonoscopic decompression of the acute colonic dilatation can usually avoid laparotomy to avoid cecal perforation from distention.

Most often, ileus develops after abdominal surgery and is transient, lasting two to three days. When ileus persists or appears without obvious cause, one should endeavor to rule out mechanical obstruction, intraabdominal sepsis, or peritonitis. A laparotomy may be necessary to exclude these factors with confidence. Occasionally bowel distention secondary to ileus will be sufficient to threaten viability of the bowel, and operation may be necessary to decompress the intestine.

Table 23–5. CAUSES OF ILEUS

Surgical operations
Peritonitis
Unrelieved mechanical obstruction
Gram-negative sepsis
Electrolyte imbalance
Retroperitoneal hemorrhage
Spinal or pelvic fractures

References

1. Wangensteen, O. H. Intestinal Obstruction, 3rd ed. Springfield, Ill., Charles C Thomas, Publisher, 1955.
2. O'Mara, C. S., Wilson, T. H., Stonesifer, G. L., and Cameron, J. Cecal volvulus: Analysis of 50 patients with long-term follow-up. Curr. Surg. 37:132, 1980.
3. Levitt, M. D. Volume and composition of intestinal gas determined by means of an intestinal wash out technique. N. Engl. J. Med. 284:1394, 1971.
4. Wright, H. K., O'Brien, J. J., and Tilson, M. D. Water absorption in experimental closed segment obstruction of the ileum in man. Am. J. Surg. 121:96, 1971.
5. Miller, L. D., Mackie, J. A., and Rhoads, J. E. The pathophysiology and management of intestinal obstruction. Surg. Clin. North Am. 42:1285, 1962.
6. Stewardson, R. H., Bombeck, T., and Nyhus, L. M. Critical operative management of small bowel obstruction. Ann. Surg. 187:189, 1978.
7. Moore, F. D. Metabolic Care of the Surgical Patient. Philadelphia, W. B. Saunders Company, 1959.
8. Lo, A. M., Evans, W. E., and Carey, L. L. Review of small bowel obstruction at Milwaukee County General Hospital. Am. J. Surg. 111:884, 1966.
9. Turner, D. M., and Croom, R. D., III. Acute adhesive obstruction of the small intestine. Am. Surg. 49:126, 1983.
10. Hofstetter, S. R. Acute adhesive obstruction of the small intestine. Surg. Gynecol. Obstet. 152:141, 1981.
11. Pertz, D. J., Jr., Gomelli, R. L., and Pilcher, D. B. Intestinal intubation in acute mechanical small bowel obstruction. Arch. Surg. 117:334, 1982.
12. Becky, W. F. Intestinal obstruction: an analysis of 1007 cases. South. Med. J.48:41, 1955.
13. Silen, W., Hein, M. F., and Goldman, L. Strangulation obstruction of the small intestine. Arch. Surg. 85:137, 1962.
14. Bulkley, G. B., Zuidema, G. D., Hamilton, S. R., et al. Intraoperative determination of small intestinal viability following ischemic injury: A prospective, controlled trial of two adjuvant methods compared with standard clinical judgment. Ann. Surg. 193:628, 1981.
15. Close, M. B., and Christensen, N. M. Transmesenteric small bowel plication or intraluminal tube stenting. Indications and contradictions. Am. J. Surg. 138:89, 1979.
16. O'Mara, C. S., Wilson, T. H., Stonesifer, G. L., Cameron, J. L. Cecal volvulus—analysis of 50 patients with long-term follow-up. Ann. Surg. 189:724, 1979.
17. Anderson, J. R., and Lee, D. The management of acute sigmoid volvulus. Br. J. Surg. 68:117, 1981.

18. Ogilvie, H. Large-intestine colic due to sympathetic deprivation. A new clinical syndrome. Br. Med. J. 2:671, 1948.
19. Faulk, D. L., Anuras, S., et al. A familial visceral myopathy. Ann. Intern. Med. 29:600, 1978.
20. Schuffler, M. D., and Deitch, E. A. Chronic idiopathic intestinal pseudo-obstruction. A surgical approach. Ann. Surg. 192:752, 1980.
21. Christensen, J. Intestinal pseudo-obstruction and paralytic ileus. In Moody, F. G., Carey, L. C., et al. Surgical Treatment of Digestive Disease. Chicago, Year Book Publications, 1986, pp. 565–579.
22. Schuffler, M. D., and Jonak, Z. Chronic idiopathic intestinal pseudo-obstruction caused by a degenerative disorder of the myenteric plexus: The use of Smith's method to define the neuropathology. Gastroenterology 82:476, 1982.
23. Schuffler, M. D. Chronic intestinal pseudo-obstruction syndromes. Med. Clin. North Am. 65:1331, 1981.
24. Sullivan, M. A., Snape, W. J., Jr., et al. Gastrointestinal myoelectrical activity in idiopathic intestinal pseudo-obstruction. N. Engl. J. Med. 297:233, 1977.
25. Faulk, D. L., Anuras, S., Christensen, J. Chronic intestinal pseudo-obstruction. Gastroenterology 74:922, 1978.
26. Golladay, E. S., and Byrne, W. T. Intestinal pseudo-obstruction. Surg. Gynecol. Obstet. 153:257, 1981.
27. Anuras, S., Shirazi, S., Faulk, D. L., et al. Surgical treatment in familial visceral myopathy. Ann. Surg. 189:306, 1979.
28. Pitt, H. A., Mann, L. L., Berquist, W. E., Ament, M. E., Fonkalsrud, E. W., and DenBesten, L. Chronic intestinal pseudo-obstruction. Management with total parenteral nutrition and a venting enterostomy. Arch. Surg. 120:614, 1985.
29. Nowak, T. V., Anuras, S., et al. Small intestinal motility in myotonic dystrophy patients. Gastroenterology 86:808, 1984.
30. Horowitz, M., Harding, P. E., et al. Acute and chronic effects of domperidone on gastric emptying in diabetic autonomic neuropathy. Dig. Dis. Sci. 30:1, 1985.
31. Abbas, A. A., Douglass, R. C., Bissell, G. W., and Chen, Y. Myxedema ileus. JAMA 234:181, 1975.
32. Moss, G. Maintenance of gastrointestinal function after bowel surgery and immediate full enteral nutrition. II. Clinical experience with objective demonstration of intestinal absorption and motility. JPEN 5:215, 1981.
33. Condon, R. E., Frantzides, C. T., Cowles, V. E., et al. Resolution of postoperative ileus in humans. Ann. Surg. 203:574, 1986.
34. Mahoney, J. L., Condon, R. E., and Cowles, V. E. Effects of adrenergic agents on colonic motility. Gastroenterology 91:1061, 1986.
35. Thor, K., and Rossell, S. Neurotensin increases colonic motility. Gastroenterology 90:27, 1986.
36. Labo, G., Bortolotti, M., et al. Interdigestive gastroduodenal motility and serum motilin levels in patients with idiopathic delay in gastric emptying. Gastroenterology 90:20, 1986.

Abdominal Abscesses and Gastrointestinal Fistulas

24

HOWARD A. REBER
JAMES L. AUSTIN

ABDOMINAL ABSCESSES

Abdominal abscesses may be classified as intraperitoneal, retroperitoneal, and visceral. They occur with approximately equal frequency.

Intraperitoneal abscesses are localized collections of pus that may follow either *generalized* peritonitis or a more *localized* intra-abdominal disease process or injury. In the former case the normal barriers that limit the inflammatory process are inadequate, and the abscess may occur at some distance from the original source of contamination. In the latter case the spread of peritonitis is limited by contiguous viscera, omentum, and peritoneum, and the abscess develops closer to the source of contamination.

Posterior retroperitoneal abscesses (perinephric abscesses) are found between the layers of the renal fascia and arise from primary renal disease (70 per cent) or from unknown sources (25 per cent). Peri-nephric abscesses will not be discussed in this chapter. Abscesses in the anterior retroperitoneum (between the posterior parietal peritoneum and the anterior layer of the renal fascia) are usually caused by gastrointestinal lesions such as appendicitis, diverticulitis, pancreatitis, and perforated duodenal ulcer.

Visceral abscesses may be hepatic, pancreatic, splenic, renal, cholecystic, and pericholecystic. Only hepatic and splenic abscesses will be discussed in this chapter (see pp. 1691–1714 and 1814–1842).

Etiology

Most intraperitoneal abscesses arise from another identifiable intra-abdominal cause, such as *trauma, perforation, infection,* or *inflammation* of an intra-abdominal viscus. Peritonitis is frequently present, along with fluid containing bacteria and blood or bile.

Less frequently, intraperitoneal abscesses are cryptogenic—i.e., no intra-abdominal cause can be found. The organisms are spread by the blood or lymph, or by the female reproductive tract.

Postoperative abscesses follow intra-abdominal operations involving direct bacterial contamination and/or postoperative leakage of an anastomosis. Although the presence of intraperitoneal bacteria is important to the development of abscess, the peritoneal defenses usually destroy the organisms and an abscess does not result. The presence of foreign material, necrotic tissue, and inadequately drained collections of fluid impair the peritoneal defenses and make abscess formation more likely.

Bacteriology[1]

Regardless of where the intraperitoneal abscess is located, the kinds of organisms it contains are similar. Five bacterial species (two aerobes and three anaerobes) are present in the average abscess. Of the aerobic bacteria, the gram-negative enteric bacilli (*Escherichia coli, Klebsiella, Proteus,* and *Pseudomonas*) are most common. The anaerobes most frequently encountered are *Bacteroides fragilis, Clostridium* species, and anaerobic cocci (peptostreptococci and peptococci). Anaerobic organisms are recoverable in over 90 per cent of intraperitoneal abscesses when sufficient attention is given to their fastidious culture requirements.

A variety of studies has led to the recognition of synergism among aerobic and anaerobic bacteria within abdominal abscesses. For example, coliforms can change the oxidation-reduction potential of the environment to permit the proliferation of anaerobes. At the same time, anaerobic strains frequently produce exotoxins that favor the localization of an abscess. Some anaerobic organisms can inhibit bacterial phagocytosis by cells involved with host defenses. Thus, accurate identification of organisms in an abscess is important in selecting antibiotic coverage to accompany drainage.[2] The importance of enterococci in patients with abdominal abscess has been recognized with increasing frequency. Debilitated patients who have been on prolonged antibiotic therapy are at greatest risk for infection with this organism.[3]

Anterior retroperitoneal abscesses have similar bacteriologic characteristics, but posterior retroperitoneal abscesses related to renal disease (usually pyelonephritis) reveal a single organism in 75 per cent of cases.

Abscess Localization

Physical factors determine the site of abscesses. Radiographic contrast medium injected anywhere into the peritoneal cavity spreads into the pelvis and the subphrenic and subhepatic spaces, primarily along the paracolic gutters.[4] The transverse colon acts as an effective barrier, because sepsis rarely spreads over it to involve the central peritoneal cavity. In addition to the anatomic factors that govern the patterns of spread, negative upper abdominal pressure from diaphragmatic excursion and increased lower abdominal pressure in the erect position are also thought to foster spread to the subphrenic and subhepatic areas.

Abscesses also frequently localize close to the disease process from which they arise (Table 24–1). This is because most of the primary disease processes evolve slowly, and the peritoneal defenses have time to confine the developing abscess. Following appendicitis, abscesses tend to localize in the right paracolic gutter and pelvis. *Diverticulitis* of the rectosigmoid may be associated with abscesses in the left paracolic gutter and pelvis. Lesser sac abscesses usually are secondary to pancreatic disease or perforated posterior duodenal or gastric ulcer. When abscesses occur in association with *Crohn's disease* of the small bowel, they frequently are found between adherent loops of intestine in the central peritoneal cavity.

Clinical Features

The clinical manifestations of an abdominal abscess depend on its site and the primary disease responsible for it. For this reason, certain abscesses (e.g., subphrenic, pelvic) will be discussed separately. The first sign of an abscess, regardless of site, is fever that persists or begins a stepwise rise. The fever may be remittent, intermittent, or continuous and is usually associated with other signs of intra-abdominal inflammation. Shaking chills are common. Sinus tachycardia is frequent and may persist in the absence of fever. Accurate abdominal examination may be hampered by the presence of a healing abdominal incision, but a localized area of persistent tenderness may offer a clue to diagnosis. A palpable mass, especially if it is tender and gradually increases in size, is a reliable finding. These signs are unusual with intraperitoneal abscesses, in which physical findings may be minimal or absent. Leukocytosis ranging from 15,000 to 30,000 per μl and a left shift are usually present, and a normocytic anemia is common. If perforation or spread of the abscess is imminent, the fever may increase, the physical findings may become more impressive, and hypotension may supervene. Especially in protracted cases, weight loss may be severe, and evidence of malnutrition may be present.

Occasionally, patients present with isolated remote organ failure as the initial manifestation of an intra-

Table 24–1. LOCATION OF ABSCESS ACCORDING TO PRIMARY DISEASE

Primary Disease	Usual Location of Abscess
Appendicitis	Right paracolic gutter, pelvis
Sigmoid diverticulitis	Left paracolic gutter, pelvis
Pancreatitis; perforated posterior gastric or duodenal ulcer	Lesser sac
Crohn's disease of small bowel	Central peritoneal cavity

abdominal abscess. Acute renal failure may develop in association with abscess. Therapy with antibiotics, especially the aminoglycosides, may make the problem worse. Renal failure requiring dialysis may continue after abscess drainage, and return of normal renal function is unpredictable. The mortality rate of renal failure in patients with abdominal abscess is as high as 80 per cent.[5] Respiratory failure occurs in about a third of patients with intra-abdominal abscess.[6] This may be manifest only as a requirement for an increasing proportion of oxygen in the inspired air, or it may progress to the respiratory distress syndrome. Characteristically, the functional residual capacity and lung compliance are decreased, and arteriovenous shunting is increased. Pulmonary function may be slow to improve after abscess drainage, and the patient may be left with significant pulmonary fibrosis.[7] Glucose intolerance is common in septic hospitalized patients in whom there may be inadequate insulin secretion in response to glucose.[8] Such glucose intolerance may be an early sign of an abdominal abscess, especially in a postoperative patient.

Radiologic Features[9]

Primary signs of abdominal abscess which may be seen in plain X-rays of the abdomen include a soft tissue mass representing the abscess, viscus displacement by the abscess, fixation of a normally mobile organ, and a collection of gas outside the bowel lumen. Extraluminal bowel gas may be seen as a discrete rounded lucency with or without an air-fluid level, multiple small lucencies ("soap bubbles") (Fig. 24–1), or linear radiolucent shadows which follow fascial planes. These are all reliable signs of abscess, but after abdominal surgery there may be confusion with normal postoperative intraperitoneal air that has not yet been reabsorbed. Normally postoperative intra-abdominal air is reabsorbed in five to seven days, but may be present for as long as ten days in some patients. Beyond this time intra-abdominal air is usually associated with abscess.

Other signs of abscess are scoliosis, concave toward the side of involvement, particularly with retroperitoneal abscesses; elevation or limitation in movement of a hemidiaphragm, particularly with subdiaphragmatic abscesses; and localized ileus. A localized segment of bowel distended with gas ("sentinel loop") may be an early sign. Chest fluoroscopy should be done to observe the motion of the diaphragms, since motion is often impaired by an upper abdominal abscess. Chest X-ray may reveal pleural effusion on the affected side.

In the search for abdominal abscess, plain X-rays of the abdomen must include supine, upright, and both decubitus projections. The multiple views help to outline the size and contour of an abscess cavity with an air-fluid level (Fig. 24–2). Because the air in an abscess is usually fixed in position and bowel gas is mobile, views with the patient in different positions also help to distinguish the two. Sequential examinations on

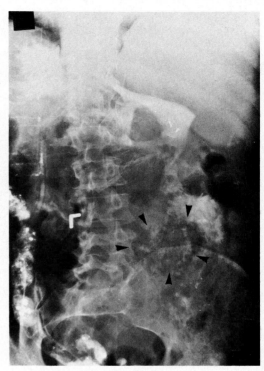

Figure 24–1. Gas bubbles *(arrowheads)* in an abscess cavity in a patient with abdominal abscess secondary to an inadequately drained gastrointestinal fistula.

different days are important, because abnormalities that persist or progress usually indicate abscesses.

Contrast studies of the gastrointestinal tract may also be helpful. The bowel may be distorted or displaced by an abscess. Injection of a fistulous tract with a water-soluble contrast agent may outline an abscess cavity.

Special Diagnostic Procedures

Radioisotope Scans. Radioisotope scanning methods depend upon the localization and concentration of a suitable radioactive nuclide within the parenchyma of an organ (liver, spleen, lung) or within an abscess itself. A photograph is made which demonstrates the region of nuclide uptake. When the nuclide concentrates within the parenchyma of an organ, abscesses are revealed as space-occupying lesions (in or near the organ) without radioactivity ("cold spots"). When the nuclide is taken up by the abscess itself, the scan reveals "hot spots" indicative of a suppurative process.

Hepatic Scanning.[10] These methods involve concentration of nuclides in hepatocytes or reticuloendothelial (Kupffer) cells, which are evenly distributed throughout the liver. A variety of agents have been used, including sodium rose bengal ^{131}I, Gold ([198]Au), and technetium sulfur colloid (^{99m}Tc) (Fig. 24–3). The use of both [198]Au and ^{99m}Tc colloids has been associated with an overall diagnostic accuracy of about 80 per

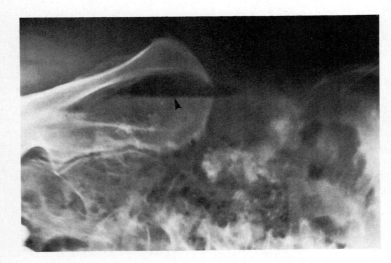

Figure 24–2. Air-fluid level in a right lower quadrant abscess cavity. Multiple views showed that this was not within the lumen of the colon, and operation confirmed the diagnosis of abscess.

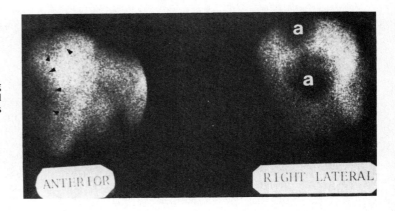

Figure 24–3. Technetium sulfur colloid liver scan, showing lateral and superior defects *(arrowheads)* on anterior view and large filling defects (a) on lateral view. Amebic liver abscess was subsequently confirmed.

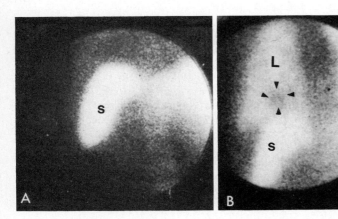

Figure 24–4. *A,* Liver-spleen scan (posterior view), showing uniform uptake in the spleen (s). *B,* [131]I albumin macroaggregates have been given to image the lungs (L), and a defect *(arrowheads)* is evident between the lung and spleen. This left-sided diaphragmatic abscess was subsequently drained.

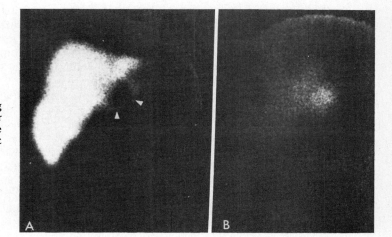

Figure 24–5. *A*, Technetium sulfur colloid liver scan showing uniform uptake except for defect *(arrowheads)* along inferior liver edge. *B*, ⁶⁷Ga liver scan shows concentration of nuclide within this same area, suggesting the diagnosis of pyogenic hepatic abscess. The abscess was drained.

cent, and both false positive and false negative results occur. Because other space-occupying lesions within the parenchyma (e.g., metastatic tumor, hepatoma) also show up as cold spots, the entire clinical picture must be correlated with the information derived from the scan. Today these techniques have been largely supplanted by the use of ultrasound and CT scanning.

Combined Lung-Liver Scanning.[11, 12] Combined scanning of the lung, liver, and spleen has been used to detect subdiaphragmatic abscess. The liver and spleen are scanned using ^{99m}Tc. The lung is simultaneously imaged with ¹³¹I albumin macroaggregates (particle size 10 to 100 μm in diameter), which wedge in the lung capillaries. An abscess appears as a defect that separates the normally indistinguishable borders between the lungs and the liver or spleen (Fig. 24–4). The accuracy of liver-lung scanning to detect subdiaphragmatic abscess approaches 90 per cent. The total incidence of false positives and false negatives is about 10 per cent. Today the use of ultrasound and CT scanning is generally preferred to this technique.

Gallium-67 Citrate (⁶⁷Ga), Indium-111 (¹¹¹In) Scintiscans.[13–17] Both ⁶⁷Ga and ¹¹¹In bind *in vivo* to granulocytes, concentrating within intracellular organelles. Granulocytes enter pus, which explains the concentration of these nuclides in abscesses. Following intravenous injection of ⁶⁷Ga, satisfactory scans may be obtained in six hours, although scans made after 24 to 72 hours may be superior. The delay may be a disadvantage in a critically ill patient in whom diagnostic information is needed immediately. Because the nuclide is also phagocytized by the reticuloendothelial system, the liver and spleen are also imaged (Fig. 24–5). Difficulties in interpretation may arise, as the nuclide is also taken up by soft tissue tumors, and tumor may be indistinguishable from abscess. Because about 15 per cent of an injected dose is excreted into the intestinal lumen, fecal radioactivity in the colon may obscure areas of diagnostic concern. ¹¹¹In may be better than ⁶⁷Ga for the detection of abscesses because it is neither taken up by tumors nor excreted into the colon, and satisfactory scans can usually be obtained 24 hours after injection. About 10 per cent of Ga or In scans are false negative or false positive; the overall diagnostic accuracy is 80 to 90 per cent. Because these nuclides specifically concentrate in inflammatory tissue, they are the only radioactive substances that can be used to detect intra-abdominal abscess remote from the liver and spleen (Fig. 24–6).

Ultrasound.[18–20] Ultrasonic images can distinguish

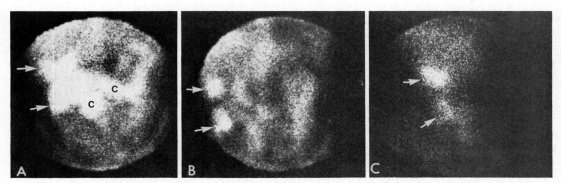

Figure 24–6. *A*, The patient had an appendectomy for perforated appendix and had right lower quadrant tenderness, fever, and chills two weeks later. Scan done 24 hours after injection of ⁶⁷Ga revealed diffuse uptake in the colon (c) as well as in areas *(arrows)* that corresponded to the areas of tenderness. *B* and *C*, Posteroanterior and right lateral views of scan performed after 96 hours. The persistent areas of uptake *(arrows)* are now distinct from the colon. The patient had a right paracolic abscess drained.

clearly between solid tissue and fluid-filled structures (abscesses), because fluid is echo-free and conducts sound well (Fig. 24–7). A solid mass contains echoing elements. Because air, bowel gas, and barium sulfate reflect the sonic energy and prevent it from reaching deeper structures, this may prevent a satisfactory examination. Minimal patient preparation or cooperation is required, and most studies can be completed in less than an hour.

Because complete ultrasound examination may require an intact abdominal wall, its use in some patients with recent operations or open abdominal wounds is limited. As with most other diagnostic modalities, ultrasound scanning cannot distinguish sterile fluid collections from pus. However, the fluid may be aspirated percutaneously under ultrasonic guidance to clarify its nature. When an abscess is present, drainage through a catheter placed percutaneously may be definitive therapy (see later discussion). Transabdominal passage of the needle appears to be safe, although complications do occur.

Ultrasonic scanning for the diagnosis of intra-abdominal abscess is associated with both false positives and false negatives, but an overall accuracy rate of about 90 per cent is claimed. Because it is noninvasive and safe and requires a minimum of patient inconvenience, it is a useful diagnostic procedure in many cases in which abscess is suspected.

CT Scan[21] (Fig. 24–8). Computed tomography is extremely sensitive in detecting both fluid collections and extraluminal gas. It is the most accurate single examination for the detection of abdominal abscesses (over 90 per cent). Its use is not limited by the presence of luminal gas overlying abscess cavities or the condition of the abdominal wall. Diagnostic accuracy may be enhanced by the use of oral, intravenous, or rectal contrast agents.

Diagnostic percutaneous needle aspiration with CT guidance is also valuable in differentiating uninfected phlegmon from abscess. Because of sampling error, a negative aspiration may not be helpful. On the other hand, a positive aspiration with recovery of organisms seen on Gram strain of the aspirate may be used as a guide for further therapy. In some cases a drainage catheter can be placed in the cavity using CT guidance.

CT scanning has now supplanted other conventional diagnostic methods as the first and often the only diagnostic test necessary. When multiple tests have been performed on the same patient, CT scan is more accurate than ultrasound and Ga scanning. Results agree in about 70 per cent of cases, and multiple tests are redundant. When results disagree, the CT scan is consistently the most accurate test.[22]

Miscellaneous. Abscesses are avascular structures that may displace, stretch, or otherwise distort the normal vascular pattern. Selective angiography may therefore occasionally demonstrate abscesses. However, because it is an invasive procedure associated with significant complications and expense, angiography is indicated to diagnose abdominal abscesses only in rare cases.

Many patients with intra-abdominal abscess are septic and critically ill, so that a diagnosis is urgently needed. The tests mentioned above may be employed singly or in combination as the clinical situation dictates. Repetitive use of single examinations may also be helpful, as persistence of an abnormality or increase in its size may help to confirm the diagnosis. Ultimately the decision for operation (percutaneous drainage) must rest on clinical judgment, weighing many factors, in addition to the results of special diagnostic procedures. Occasionally, surgery is advisable even in the presence of equivocal information.

Subdiaphragmatic Abscess[23]

Because the clinical presentation and problems of diagnosis and treatment are similar, subphrenic and subhepatic abscesses are considered together. The ma-

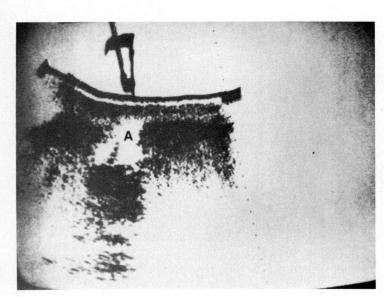

Figure 24–7. Abdominal ultrasound—longitudinal scan. A 4 × 4 cm trans-sonic area (A) in the right flank, 8 cm to the right of the umbilicus, was consistent with the diagnosis of abdominal abscess. (Same patient as in Figure 24–6.)

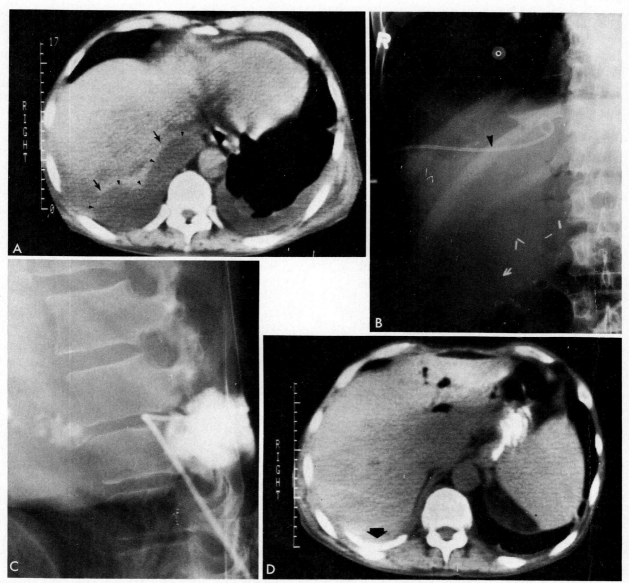

Figure 24–8. *A*, CT scan reveals a subdiaphragmatic abscess on the right side. The arrows and arrowheads outline the abscess, which is displacing the liver anteriorly and inferiorly. *B*, Guided by this information, a catheter *(arrowhead)* has been introduced percutaneously into the region of the abscess. *C*, Proper placement is confirmed by injection of contrast material through the catheter. Dye pools in the abscess cavity. *D*, A repeat CT scan shows that the abscess is drained. Note the catheter *(arrow)* containing contrast material.

jority of these are associated with gastroduodenal or biliary disease or follow upper abdominal surgery.

Anatomy.[24] Subhepatic abscesses are found on either side of the falciform ligament between the liver and the transverse colon. On the right side they may be anterior or posterior. On the left side, posterior subhepatic abscesses are synonymous with lesser sac abscesses. Left anterior subhepatic abscesses occur between the left lobe of the liver and the stomach or spleen. Some clue to localization is afforded by a knowledge of the primary disease process. After appendicitis, right-sided abscesses are more frequent. Perforated duodenal ulcer may be complicated by right anterior subhepatic collections. Pancreatic disease is more likely to result in a lesser sac abscess.

Subphrenic abscesses occur between the dome of the liver and the diaphragmatic surface, and are called right or left according to their relation to the falciform ligament. On the right side, abscesses tend to localize either anteriorly or posteriorly, and are designated right anterior or right posterior subphrenic. On the left side no such distinction is made.

Diagnosis.[23] In most patients there are few localizing signs. Far advanced cases may be associated with intercostal edema, erythema, and tenderness. Dyspnea, cough, and chest pain are frequent. X-ray demonstration of a pleural effusion with a subphrenic air-fluid level (or a focal collection of gas bubbles) is diagnostic of subphrenic abscess. More frequently, only diaphragmatic elevation, limitation of diaphragmatic motion, and pleural effusion are seen. Subhepatic abscesses are less likely to be associated with pleural or diaphragmatic abnormalities, and usually present with symptoms referable to the abdomen. They are most difficult to diagnose. Abdominal pain and tenderness are usually present and a mass is occasionally found. The liver may or may not be palpable. Liver function is usually normal. In addition to chest X-ray and fluoroscopy, special diagnostic studies are useful. Ultrasound examination on the right side may show the liver displaced medially and inferiorly by an echo-free abscess. When the abscess is small, diagnosis may be difficult because of interference from overlying ribs. On the left side, subdiaphragmatic abscesses are particularly difficult to diagnose by ultrasound because of interference from aerated lung above, gas-filled stomach and colon anteriorly, and ribs laterally. The spleen itself is of variable size and shape, and normally contains few echoes. Information about splenic size and configuration derived from radionuclide scan may help with the interpretation of the ultrasonic picture. CT scans generally provide the most accurate information about the presence and extent of abscesses in these areas. They should be done early if an abscess is suspected. If a pleural effusion is present, it may be tapped and will usually be sterile.

Complications.[25] Serious thoracic complications, which occur in 25 per cent of patients with subdiaphragmatic abscess, include *empyema, diaphragmatic perforation, bronchial fistula,* and *lung abscess.* Abdominal complications, such as *perforation* of the abscess and generalized *peritonitis,* occur in 10 per cent of patients, principally those with subhepatic abscess.

Prognosis. The mortality rate for surgically drained subphrenic abscess is 20 per cent. The mortality rate increases with incomplete drainage or complications. Multiple operations and prolonged hospitalization may be necessary.

Midabdominal Abscesses[26, 27]

Midabdominal abscesses form in the peritoneal cavity anywhere between the transverse colon and the pelvis. They are frequent in the paracolic gutters, but may localize between the leaves of the small bowel mesentery. Because they may be separated from the anterior abdominal wall by intervening viscera, physical findings may be minimal. In addition they may distort adjacent structures only minimally, as the abdominal viscera are quite mobile. For both reasons, diagnosis of midabdominal abscesses is particularly difficult.

In addition to the usual clinical evidence of a septic abdominal process (e.g., fever, tachycardia, abdominal tenderness), repeated abdominal examination may reveal a gradually enlarging abdominal mass. X-ray examinations may show an air-fluid level whose position does not change. Although unusual, this finding is diagnostic. A barium contrast study may indicate displacement of the bowel by the abscess mass. Ultra-sound, radionuclide, and especially CT scanning may be valuable in the diagnosis and localization of these lesions.

When the abscess is found, it should be drained. Even without a firm diagnosis, a progressively enlarging, painful, tender abdominal mass in a febrile patient is an indication for drainage, because perforation of the abscess may be imminent. Occasionally in a gravely ill patient with no localizing findings, abdominal exploration may be necessary to find and drain an abscess. At laparotomy the abdomen must be explored thoroughly, as these abscesses are frequently multiple. If the clinical picture does not promptly improve, re-exploration may be necessary for missed or new abscesses. As with other intra-abdominal abscesses, antibiotic therapy effective against both aerobic and anaerobic enteric organisms should also be instituted (see below).

Pelvic Abscess[25, 26]

Pelvic abscess occurs most frequently following acute perforated *appendicitis, pelvic inflammatory disease,* and *diverticulitis* of the colon. In addition to the usual signs of sepsis, pelvic abscess may be associated with lower abdominal discomfort and diarrhea. Rectal examination may reveal a tender mass on the anterior rectal or posterior vaginal wall. Repeated daily examination may be necessary as the abscess develops.

When the mass is fluctuant, the diagnosis may be confirmed under general anesthesia by needle aspiration of pus through the rectum or vagina, and the abscess incised and drained. Laparotomy is usually unnecessary, and recovery is generally prompt. Antibiotics effective against aerobic and anaerobic enteric organisms are appropriate.

Treatment of Abdominal Abscesses[21, 23, 28–33]

Antibiotics. The polymicrobial nature of abdominal abscesses is important in choosing antibiotic regimens. Single agent therapy is acceptable in certain cases of generalized primary and even secondary peritonitis. Examples are perforated appendix or perforated duodenal ulcer when the systemic manifestations of sepsis are minimal, contamination is limited, and host defenses have not been overwhelmed. In this setting, a second or third generation cephalosporin may be appropriate. However, when sepsis is life-threatening or its origin is obscure, more comprehensive treatment should be chosen.

Most antibiotics penetrate the normal peritoneal cavity and reach therapeutic concentrations in abdominal fluid. Clindamycin is a notable exception and may achieve levels in peritoneal fluid only half of that in serum.[34] However, the normal function of the peritoneum is altered during abdominal sepsis, and antibiotic delivery is unpredictable. Individual antibiotics also may be rendered ineffective as a result of local conditions within the abscess cavity.[35]

Therapy is usually instituted on a presumptive basis prior to drainage, for it is unrealistic to wait for culture and sensitivity information. If percutaneous aspiration is done, this material can be gram stained, and important information gained to guide therapy. Aminoglycosides are highly effective against enteric bacteria that infect most abscesses. Gentamicin or tobramycin is given in a loading dose of 1.5 to 2.0 mg per kg and repeated every eight hours. Nephrotoxicity and ototoxicity are probably equivalent with both of these agents, and peak and trough serum concentrations must be monitored during therapy to prevent complications. Anaerobic coverage must be instituted as well because of the frequent recovery of these organisms from abscess material. The widest experience in this country has been with clindamycin. However, metronidazole has been shown to be as effective as clindamycin when either is given in combination with an aminoglycoside. Finally, ampicillin (1.5 to 2.0 gm per kg) is given routinely for coverage of enterococci.

Antibiotic treatment should be started before drainage if possible but should not delay it. Because intestinal function is unreliable and musculocutaneous circulation may be impaired, the preferred route of administration is by intravenous infusion. Antibiotics should be continued until the patient is afebrile and the white blood cell count is in the normal range. Nevertheless, 6 per cent of the patients with a normal white blood cell count, and 19 per cent of patients with a normal rectal temperature experience recurrence of sepsis at the conclusion of antibiotic therapy. The rates of recurrent sepsis are much higher if the patient is febrile, has an elevated white blood cell count, and has immature white blood cell forms on smear of peripheral blood when the antibiotics are stopped.[36]

Nutrition. Nutritional management (usually total parenteral nutrition) is an important part of the management of these patients, especially if complications such as respiratory or renal failure occur, and multiple operations are required. Nevertheless, if drainage of an abscess is indicated, it should not be delayed while parenteral nutrition is provided in an attempt to improve the patient's nutritional status.

Drainage. Drainage of the infected material is the most important aspect of abdominal abscess treatment. In the past, this was done exclusively by operative methods. Today CT or ultrasound guided percutaneous drainage is a safe and effective method that avoids surgery in many patients. Each approach has limitations.[37, 38]

Percutaneous drainage should not be used when there is a continued source of peritoneal contamination such as a perforated viscus. The technique is less successful when the material in the abscess cavity is too viscous to aspirate or the wall of the cavity is emphysematous. The percutaneous drainage route should not traverse the wall of another organ or uncontaminated space. When repeat scanning of the abscess cavity reveals residual material, additional catheters may be placed. If this is again unsuccessful in eradicating the material, the patient should have

operative drainage. It is claimed that as many as 90 per cent of abdominal abscesses will be managed by the percutaneous route as experience increases and capabilities expand.[39, 40]

There are two methods of operative drainage of abdominal abscesses. Extraserous drainage is used when the abscess is adjacent to the abdominal wall or when the abscess cavity can be drained without entering the peritoneal space. Thus, contamination of the peritoneal cavity can be avoided, and in some cases, a general anesthetic is not necessary. The disadvantage of the approach is that the underlying problem causing the abscess cannot be treated and may be overlooked.

The advantage of the transperitoneal approach is that the entire abdomen can be explored, multiple abscesses detected and drained, and other associated conditions treated. However, even with scrupulous technique, uninfected areas are contaminated. The rate of abscess recurrence and fistula formation is equal with both methods.[41, 42]

Pyogenic Hepatic Abscess

Hepatic abscess is an infrequent disease, accounting for less than 0.02 per cent of all hospital admissions.[43] In the United States, over 90 per cent are pyogenic, the remainder being due to *Entamoeba histolytica* (see pp. 1162 to 1165 for discussion of amebic abscess).

Etiology. Twenty-five years ago, pyogenic hepatic abscess was predominantly a disease of young adults and usually followed appendicitis complicated with portal vein pylephlebitis. Today it is usually seen in elderly patients in association with *biliary tract infection, malignant disease,* or *bacteremia,* and as a complication of major *abdominal surgery* or *trauma.* Because the majority of cases appear in such a clinical setting, the symptoms of the abscess are frequently overshadowed by those of the associated disease, and diagnosis may be difficult.

Classification.[25, 44] Hepatic abscesses have been classified according to the portal of entry of the responsible organisms. Biliary tract infections are associated with the most cases (40 to 50 per cent). The organisms probably enter the hepatic parenchyma from the infected bile through the biliary radicles. Another 20 per cent are associated with identifiable sources of sepsis in other abdominal viscera, whose venous drainage is via the portal vein. About 10 per cent are the result of infection in areas contiguous to the liver where the organisms can enter the hepatic parenchyma directly. Examples include subhepatic or pericholecystic abscess. Probably fewer than 5 per cent are the result of dissemination through the hepatic artery during bacteremia. The cause of the remaining 10 to 20 per cent, termed cryptogenic abscesses, remains obscure.

Hepatic abscesses may be solitary (50 per cent) or multiple, and when multiple they may involve one or both lobes. The solitary lesions usually are in the right lobe. The reason for right lobe localization is probably the more extensive arborization of the bile ducts in that lobe. Abscesses that result from bacteremia with organisms entering the liver via the hepatic artery tend to be multiple and bilateral.

Hepatic abscesses can be separated into two groups, one amenable to surgical drainage (60 per cent) and the other not. In the former group the abscesses are 1.5 cm in diameter or larger, the lesions are more often solitary, and bacteremia with multiple abscesses in other organs is usually absent. In the latter group the abscesses are smaller and multiple, and bacteremia with abscesses in other organs is frequent. Until recently, both groups required surgery to make the distinction. However, CT scans now allow more reliable preoperative diagnosis. For this reason as well as the availability of new nonoperative drainage methods, surgery may be avoided in some patients.

Clinical Features.[43, 45] The clinical setting of the disease varies according to the age of the patient and the primary problem. In infants and children under four years, hepatic abscess is usually associated with generalized infection and septicemia and with diseases in which immunologic defense mechanisms are impaired. In older children and young adults, trauma is more frequently responsible. In middle age and beyond, hepatic abscess is usually associated with biliary tract infection, another focus of abdominal sepsis, or systemic bacteremia. Malignant disease is not uncommon, especially in the elderly. In those cases associated with biliary infection, a distinction must be made between acute obstructive suppurative cholangitis (see pp. 1714–1729), which may produce multiple *microscopic* hepatic abscesses, and chronic partial common duct obstruction with infected bile, which causes macroscopic abscesses. Each requires surgical decompression of the common duct, but only in the latter are the hepatic lesions amenable to drainage. Suppurative cholangitis is associated with abdominal pain, chills, jaundice, fever, bacteremia, and shock, and tends to run a rapid and severe course (one to two days). With macroscopic hepatic abscess secondary to infection and partial biliary obstruction, the patients are generally less ill and the course is more protracted (weeks). The clinical picture, however, may occasionally be identical regardless of the size of the abscess.

Regardless of the cause of the abscess, the symptoms reflect a systemic febrile illness of a week or more. Over 90 per cent have fever between 38.9 and 41.1°C; shaking chills and temperatures over 40°C appear more frequently in those with bacteremia and multiple small abscesses. In patients with large abscesses, shaking chills and high fevers are less frequent and the disease is associated with more chronic constitutional symptoms, such as anorexia, weakness, malaise, and weight loss. Some patients have symptoms of a primary intrathoracic process, such as cough, dyspnea, pleuritic pain, or hemoptysis.

About 50 per cent have hepatomegaly, and an equal number complain of abdominal pain. Clinically evident jaundice is present only in a third of patients, mainly those with associated biliary infection and multiple small abscesses. Jaundice is often a manifestation of extrahepatic biliary obstruction rather than of the abscess itself. As a rule the clinical picture associated with multiple small hepatic abscesses consists of nonspecific signs of sepsis or of a remote primary disease process. Large lesions are more likely to produce localizing clues.

Laboratory Findings. A marked leukocytosis (average, 20,000 per μl) is found in most instances. A mild normocytic anemia is common. The liver function studies that are most frequently abnormal are elevated alkaline phosphatase (75 per cent), serum albumin less than 3 gm per dl (75 per cent), and elevated total bilirubin (50 per cent). Alkaline phosphatase and bilirubin levels are generally highest in those with biliary tract obstruction. Serum protein abnormalities are greatest in those with serious underlying disease or longstanding (more than two months) infection. SGOT and SGPT measurements are usually normal.

Diagnosis. About half the patients with macroscopic hepatic abscesses have some abnormality of the chest film, such as *pleural effusion, basilar atelectasis* and/or *pneumonitis,* and *elevated diaphragm.* An upper gastrointestinal series may reveal displacement of the stomach, especially when the abscess is situated in the left lobe. Oral or intravenous cholangiography is rarely helpful, because the biliary tree rarely opacifies in this clinical setting.

The liver can be examined by ultrasound or CT, and abscesses larger than 2 or 3 cm identified. CT scan is preferred. Because multiple hepatic abscesses may be present, it is important to examine the entire organ even when a large abscess is identified early in the study.

In all patients with liver abscess, hemagglutination and/or complement fixation tests for amebiasis are indicated. Although amebic abscesses are usually associated with less fever and toxicity, lower WBC, and a more chronic course than pyogenic abscesses, amebic and pyogenic abscesses are often clinically indistinguishable.

Treatment. Drainage is indicated in the management of all pyogenic hepatic abscesses; both percutaneous and standard surgical techniques have been used. Most amebic abscesses are treated medically (see pp. 1162–1165). Amebic abscesses that have become secondarily infected, are unresponsive to drugs, or are in danger of imminent rupture also require drainage. In addition, all patients with pyogenic abscess should be treated with antibiotics effective against aerobic and anaerobic bacteria (see later discussion). In chronically ill, debilitated patients parenteral hyperalimentation may be useful.

Bacteriology.[46–48] In the past, bacteria usually implicated as a cause of pyogenic hepatic abscesses included *Escherichia coli,* aerobic streptococci, and *Staphylococcus aureus.* Moreover, up to 60 per cent of cultures of pus from these lesions were reported as sterile, almost certainly reflecting faulty transport and culture techniques. More recently, the important role of anaerobic organisms in the pathogenesis of this disease has been stressed. With anaerobic culture techniques, fastidious anaerobes *(Bacteroides fragilis,* anaerobic streptococci, fusobacteria, and clostridia) have been recovered in 50 to 75 per cent of cases. Blood cultures are positive for anaerobes in over half the cases. The majority of patients have mixed infections that include coliforms.

Chemotherapy. The choice of antibiotic therapy initially should be based on statistical probability of a mixed gram-negative and anaerobic infection, and ultimately on the isolation of organisms from blood in patients with bacteremia and on the Gram staining and culture of pus when the abscess is drained. Coliforms can be treated with an aminoglycoside, and the anaerobic coverage should include an agent active against *B. fragilis;* clindamycin or chloramphenicol is satisfactory. The dose of metronidazole that is effective against amebic liver abscess is also effective against anaerobes (see below). The efficacy of metronidazole against anaerobes may account for the temporary clinical improvement occasionally seen in patients with pyogenic hepatic abscess who are treated mistakenly for amebic abscess with this drug.

After drainage has been instituted, appropriate antibiotic therapy should continue for one to two months in patients with a single hepatic abscess and for at least four months if multiple abscesses were present.

The place of percutaneous drainage of amebic liver abscess for primary therapy is uncertain. However, percutaneous aspiration of liver abscess may be done for diagnosis when amebic abscess is strongly suspected and hemagglutination or complement fixation titers are not available. Amebic abscesses contain a reddish brown material, which on Gram stain reveals few cellular elements. Trophozoites of *E. histolytica* are difficult to identify in pus, but are more easily seen in material from the abscess wall. Pyogenic abscesses typically contain yellow or green pus, and Gram staining usually reveals organisms. Neither aspiration nor drainage of amebic abscess(es) for therapy is usually necessary, as it (they) can usually be cured with one of the following drug regimens:[32] metronidazole, 750 mg by mouth three times a day for five days; emetine or dehydroemetine, 1 to 1.5 mg per kg per day intramuscularly for ten days; or chloroquine, 1 gm per day for two days and 500 mg daily for three weeks (see pp. 1162–1165).

Surgery. In most cases a pyogenic abscess should be drained as soon as the diagnosis is reasonably certain. Percutaneous catheter drainage appears to be a safe and effective way to accomplish this in most cases. When it is not, surgical drainage should be done. Comparison of percutaneous and surgical methods of hepatic abscess drainage have shown both to be acceptable and associated with similar morbidity and mortality rates in appropriately selected patients.[49, 50]

Goals of surgery include the identification and dependent drainage of all abscesses. The pus should be examined by Gram stain and promptly transported in anaerobic containers to the bacteriology laboratory for aerobic and anaerobic cultures and drug sensitivities to help guide antibiotic therapy. Rarely the abscess

may be situated so that hepatic lobectomy may eradicate the entire process. Because hepatic abscess is usually a complication of another infectious process, a thorough exploration of the abdomen should be performed and other appropriate surgical therapy instituted. When the common duct is obstructed, it should be drained. Even when multiple small hepatic abscesses not amenable to surgical drainage are found, an obstructed common bile duct must be drained.

Complications. About 15 per cent of abscesses rupture into the subphrenic space, into the free peritoneal cavity, or through the diaphragm into the pleural space. Subdiaphragmatic diseases, spreading peritonitis, or empyema can result. Hemobilia has been reported. With these complications, the mortality rate increases.

Prognosis. Because diagnosis of hepatic abscess is difficult and frequently delayed, and because the patients often have serious coexisting disease, the mortality rate is high. Unrecognized hepatic abscess is invariably fatal. Reported mortality rates in diagnosed and treated cases range from 28 to over 90 per cent, with the higher figures found in the elderly and in those with multiple abscesses and complications. Improved diagnostic and therapeutic methods and use of appropriate antibiotics may improve these results.

Splenic Abscess[51–53]

Although the spleen is not part of the gastrointestinal tract, splenic abscesses produce signs and symptoms of intra-abdominal disease. Splenic abscesses are rare. In 75 per cent of cases they are multiple and are associated with abscesses in one or more other organs as part of a generalized septic process. There may be few clinical findings to indicate that the spleen is involved, and the diagnosis is usually made at autopsy. In the remaining 25 per cent of cases, the splenic abscess is solitary. Diagnosis is especially important in these patients since splenectomy is usually curative.

In the past, splenic abscess was seen more commonly in patients with typhoid fever, malaria, bacterial endocarditis, and various hemoglobinopathies. Most cases seen today arise from direct spread of infection to the spleen from adjacent structures, from splenic trauma resulting in a secondarily infected splenic hematoma, and from hematogenous seeding of the spleen in intravenous drug abusers. Both gram-negative and gram-positive organisms have been isolated; *Bacteroides, Pseudomonas, Serratia,* and *Staphylococcus aureus* are the most common.

The diagnosis of splenic abscess may be difficult. The patient may present with unexplained sepsis and abdominal pain, and the spleen may be enlarged. Frequently it is not palpable because of left upper quadrant tenderness and guarding. The pain may be pleuritic and a friction rub may be heard. Fever and leukocytosis are usually present. Because the clinical picture can be similar, the distinction between a splenic and left subphrenic abscess may be difficult. When the diagnosis is suspected, CT scan, spleen scan, or ultrasound should be done. When present, the finding of gas in the spleen on a plain abdominal X-ray is diagnostic.

Most splenic abscesses periodically seed the blood stream with bacteria, causing intermittent systemic symptoms. Occasionally spontaneous rupture may occur. When the diagnosis is strongly suspected, operation is indicated. Splenectomy can be done in most patients, and usually results in cure if the abscess is confined to the spleen. Occasionally the abscess is quite large and splenectomy is hazardous. Then splenic drainage (splenotomy) should be done.

GASTROINTESTINAL FISTULAS[54–58]

Gastrointestinal fistulas are abnormal communications between the gastrointestinal tract and another segment of bowel, another intra-abdominal organ (internal fistula), or the skin (external fistula). External fistulas may be intentionally created by the surgeon (e.g., gastrostomy, colostomy); but unless drainage from these is persistent and of high volume, there are no problems in management. This discussion will include external fistulas that appear as complications of trauma, underlying disease, or gastrointestinal operations. Such patients represent difficult problems in management, as fluid and electrolyte derangements, infection, and impaired nutrition are frequent.

Classification. External fistulas are often classified according to the volume of fluid lost through the fistulous opening, because problems in management are related to the magnitude of this loss. *High-output* fistulas are defined as those producing more than 200 ml per day, and many produce several liters of electrolyte-rich fluid. *Low-output* fistulas, which produce less than 200 ml per day, are more easily managed. In general the level of the gastrointestinal tract from which the fistula arises influences the volume of fistula drainage. Gastric, duodenal, or proximal small bowel fistulas are usually high output, as salivary, gastric, biliary, pancreatic, and small bowel secretions may contribute to the drainage. Pancreatic fistulas are usually high output, and some produce as much as 1500 ml a day. Distal small bowel and colonic fistulas are usually low output, because considerable fluid absorption may occur proximal to the fistulous opening.

Etiology. The majority of external gastrointestinal fistulas follow abdominal operations when an anastomosis fails to heal. In most cases contributory factors can be identified. A foreign body (e.g., a rubber drain) close to the suture line, tension on the anastomosis, nearby infection, ischemia, and radiation enteritis all impair healing and, singly or in combination, may be responsible for fistula formation. Other factors include inadequate resections for malignant disease with anastomosis through tumor tissue, Crohn's disease, bowel injury during dissection, and technical error in performance of the anastomosis. Rarely an intra-abdominal abscess may erode into an adjacent segment of bowel to create a fistula. Fistulas may follow unrec-

ognized traumatic perforation of a viscus; they also may originate from devitalized tissue surrounding a sutured perforation.

In the past most proximal high-output fistulas were located in the duodenum and followed operations for duodenal ulcer disease. They usually resulted from inadequate healing of a badly inflamed duodenum after a Billroth II gastrectomy. When the duodenum is in this condition, a fistula can be avoided by choosing operations (e.g., vagotomy and pyloroplasty or gastrojejunostomy, parietal cell vagotomy) that do not involve duodenal dissection and closure.

Clinical Features. Postoperative fistula formation is characterized by a complicated course with fever and abdominal pain until fistula fluid escapes through the abdominal incision or drain tract. Fistulas that develop spontaneously have a more indolent course, and an area of progressive abdominal tenderness is the eventual site of skin breakdown with discharge of fistula fluid. Because most fistulas are associated either primarily or secondarily with intraperitoneal infection, abscesses frequently coexist. These may be intra-abdominal and are usually close to the fistula tract, but others may be some distance from the fistula. Abscesses may also develop extraperitoneally along the fistula tract as it courses through the abdominal wall. In either location they may recur unless the fistula is adequately drained. The clinical features of abscesses have already been discussed, and sepsis from abdominal abscesses is usually present in the patient with a fistula. The skin around the opening of the fistula may be severely excoriated by activated pancreatic enzymes in the discharge. With high-output fistulas, fluid and

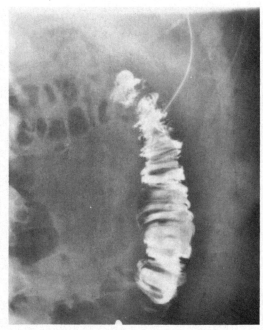

Figure 24–9. Sinus tract injection using water-soluble contrast medium in a patient with a colocutaneous fistula. The colon is opacified.

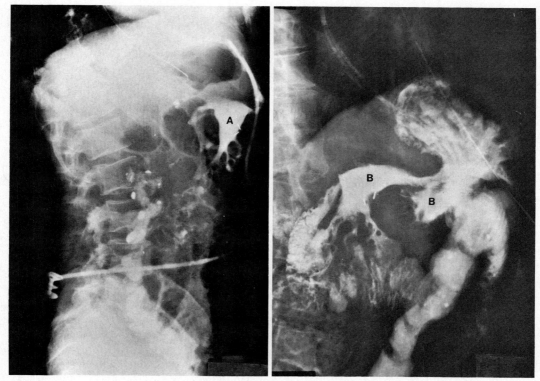

Figure 24–10. *Left,* Sinus tract injection in a patient who developed fever and a gastrojejunocutaneous fistula following surgery. The poorly drained abscess cavity *(A)* is outlined. *Right,* The same patient was given water-soluble contrast material through a nasogastric tube. The dye leaked from the gastrojejunostomy and pooled in the peritoneal cavity *(B).*

electrolyte losses may be severe. Dehydration and electrolyte imbalance demand first priority in management of patients with established fistulas which have been inadequately treated.

Extreme weight loss and protein-calorie malnutrition may result if caloric needs have not been satisfied. Caloric requirements are frequently greater than normal, as recent operative trauma and sepsis increase basal needs. Since the fistula may bypass most of the functioning intestine, the maintenance of adequate nutrition represents a major problem.

Laboratory Findings. The hematocrit will reflect the degree of hemoconcentration, and the white blood cell count may be elevated with sepsis. Anemia and hypoproteinemia reflect malnutrition and chronic disease. With high-output proximal small bowel or pancreatic fistulas, the patients may be acidotic, because the lost pancreatic and biliary secretions are alkaline. In the rarer gastric fistula, hypokalemic, hypochloremic alkalosis may result.

X-ray pictures of the fistulous tract opacified with contrast material show the source of the fistula and its anatomy (Figs. 24–9 and 24–10). Communicating abscess cavities may be seen. Contrast material administered orally or rectally may reveal associated bowel disease or distal bowel obstruction.

Treatment. The treatment of patients with external gastrointestinal fistula requires attention to multiple coexisting problems. These include fluid and electrolyte abnormalities, sepsis, malnutrition, control of fistula drainage, and protection of the skin. In addition, the underlying disease process responsible for the fistula may require specific therapy. These patients must be approached systematically with an awareness of certain treatment priorities in order to achieve a satisfactory result (Table 24–2).

General Considerations.[54, 55] The initial priority in management is the restoration of blood volume and the correction of fluid and electrolyte imbalances. Frequently whole blood transfusions are indicated. This part of the management may take up to 48 hours,

Table 24–2. TREATMENT PRIORITIES IN FISTULA MANAGEMENT

1. Up to two days
    Restore fluid and electrolyte losses
    Drain abscesses
    Antibiotics
    Control fistula drainage
2. By second or third day
    Begin nutritional support (total parenteral nutrition)
3. By end of first week
    Determine fistula anatomy
    Drain additional abscesses if evident
    Consider alternative forms of nutrition
4. Beyond two weeks
    Maintain nutrition
    Drain additional abscesses if evident
    After one to two months, operative intervention is necessary

and subsequent intravenous replacement must satisfy basal needs as well as replace continuing fluid losses. In addition, abscesses should be promptly drained as soon as they have been located. Frequently abscesses are superficial, in the abdominal wall adjacent to the fistulous tract, and they may be drained under local anesthesia. In other cases laparotomy under general anesthesia may be necesary to drain intra-abdominal abscesses. The eradication of all infection is necessary before specific therapy to close the fistula can be effective. Many of these patients are already receiving antibiotics when definitive therapy of the fistula is begun. Changes in antibiotics or choice of initial therapy should reflect culture and sensitivity reports from drained abscesses. Usually broad-spectrum coverage of enteric organisms will be appropriate.

The fistulous drainage must be controlled—i.e., it must be recovered quantitatively so that its volume and composition can be accurately determined. The surrounding skin must be protected from excoriation and digestion. An ileostomy bag fastened to the skin around the opening usually accomplishes these objectives. A suction catheter in the bag carries away the fluid. In general, suction catheters should not be inserted into the depths of the fistula tract, because pressure necrosis may enlarge the fistula or create new ones.

Next, attention must be given to nutritional management.[59-61] Total parenteral nutrition (TPN) through a central vein is almost always the best initial method, and should begin by the second or third day of treatment. Even with low-output distal fistulas TPN is preferred, because the gastrointestinal tract may not be functional when treatment is begun. Caloric intake should be at least 3000 kcal per day in adults, and more may be necessary in patients with hypermetabolic states (see pp. 2007–2027).

The third priority is to determine the anatomy of the fistula. Fistulous tracts may be multiple and communicate with each other and the bowel at more than one point. They may be inadequately drained, and side pockets off the main tract may be a focus of persistent sepsis. Roentgenograms of the upper gastrointestinal tract and small intestine, barium studies of the colon, and injection of the fistula (fistulagram) with water-soluble contrast material may all be useful. If any inadequately drained abscesses are discovered, they should be drained. Knowledge of fistula anatomy may also allow more effective control of drainage.

By the end of the first week, when sepsis is no longer present and bowel ileus has resolved, oral or tube feeding may be possible. This may supplement or replace parenteral nutrition, but at least 3000 kcal per day must be supplied to most patients until the fistula has resolved. With some proximal fistulas it may be possible to advance a feeding tube past the fistula. Occasionally the fistula fluid can be reinfused distal to the fistula opening, simplifying fluid and electrolyte management. If a feeding tube cannot be inserted, a feeding jejunostomy may be constructed. Nevertheless, although the gastrointestinal tract is generally the preferred route for alimentation, clinical experience in patients with fistula suggests that TPN may be preferable. Even when oral or tube feeding is possible, the requirement for large fluid volumes, which may produce diarrhea, frequently makes it impossible to give sufficient calories. The exception is the patient with a colonic fistula, in whom oral feeding is usually adequate.

During the second week and beyond, the objectives are to maintain nutritional support and search for and drain abdominal abscesses. In most cases by four to six weeks the fistula will begin to close and its output will progressively decrease. If it does not, then surgical correction must be considered.

Surgical Considerations. Several factors can be identified which make the spontaneous closure of fistulas unlikely. Fistulas that arise from irradiated bowel or bowel involved with Crohn's disease will usually require an operation on the involved bowel segments. When the bowel is obstructed distal to a fistula, relief of the obstruction is a prerequisite for fistula closure. In this circumstance a definitive operation should be performed once infection has been controlled and the fistula has begun to mature, usually during the second or third week. An operation is always necessary to close end fistulas in which the continuity of the gastrointestinal tract has been totally disrupted.

Even though none of these factors is present, when the fistula has persisted for one to two months after infection has been eradicated, operative closure of the fistula is usually necessary. Optimal nutritional management and attention to the other problems already mentioned ensures the greatest chance for operative success. At operation the opening in the bowel cannot be simply oversewn; the fistula will always recur. The fistulous segment should be resected if possible, and continuity restored with end-to-end anastomosis (Fig. 24–11). In some cases the segment cannot be resected,

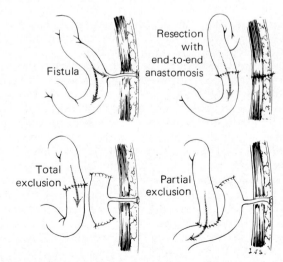

Figure 24–11. Surgical procedures that may be used to treat small bowel fistulas. Resection with end-to-end anastomosis is the preferred method. (Reproduced, with permission, from Way, L. W. [editor]: Current Surgical Diagnosis and Treatment, 7th ed. Copyright 1985 by Lange Medical Publications, Los Altos, California.)

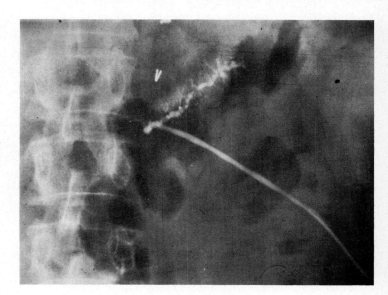

Figure 24–12. Sinus tract injection in a patient with a pancreatic fistula. The distal main pancreatic duct was opacified.

either because dissection would be hazardous or because it must be preserved (e.g., the duodenum). In such a case, partial exclusion of the involved bowel with its distal end anastomosed to the side of normal intestine is satisfactory. Rarely total exclusion of the fistulous segment, exteriorizing one end as a mucous fistula, is done. Distal obstruction must be relieved.

Pancreatic Fistula.[62, 63] Virtually all pancreatic fistulas that are clinically significant are external, and follow pancreatic trauma, external drainage of a *pseudocyst,* or *operations* on the pancreas. Traumatic fistulas usually result from pancreatic duct injury that was overlooked or inadequately treated. After external drainage of a pseudocyst, the cyst fails to obliterate about 30 per cent of the time, and a pancreatic fistula may develop (Fig. 24–12) (see pp. 1842–1872). With fistulas that arise after trauma or pseudocyst drainage, the morbidity rate may be significant, because fistula drainage may be prolonged, but the mortality rate is usually not increased. Pancreatic fistulas that complicate pancreatic surgery (usually for pancreatic cancer) do increase the mortality rate. Fistulas occur in these patients when the anastomosis between the remaining pancreas and the small bowel fails to heal (see pp. 1872–1884). Sepsis from abdominal infection and major hemorrhage from erosion of adjacent blood vessels by the enzymes in the pancreatic juice are frequent terminal events. These fistulas complicate 10 per cent of pancreaticoduodenectomies for pancreatic cancer, but are rare after pancreatic operations for chronic pancreatitis.

Pancreatic fistulas usually close spontaneously, and operative intervention is rarely needed. Most close within five months, but some persist for over a year. If the output is low, patients may be easily managed at home, provided nutrition is adequate and there is no infection.

Prognosis. The morbidity rate of external gastrointestinal fistula is high, with the average duration of hospitalization one to three months. Nevertheless, about 75 per cent of fistulas close spontaneously if properly managed. Of those requiring operation, about 90 per cent can be permanently closed. Surgical closure is less likely to be successful (75 per cent) in proximal high-output fistulas than in distal or low-output fistulas (more than 95 per cent). The mortality rate (15 to 30 per cent) is also higher in those with high-output fistulas. Recent advances in parenteral nutrition have been important in decreasing mortality and improving the outlook for these patients.

References

Abdominal Abscesses

1. Gorbach, S. L., and Bartlett, J. G. Anaerobic infections. N. Engl. J. Med. *290*:1177, 1974.
2. Mackowiack, P. A. Microbial synergism in human infections. N. Engl. J. Med. *298*:21, 1978.
3. Dougherty, S. H., Flohr, A. B., and Simmons, R. L. "Breakthrough" enterococcal septicemia in surgical patients: 19 cases and a review of the literature. Arch. Surg. *118*:232, 1983.
4. Autio, V. The spread of intraperitoneal infection. Studies with roentgen contrast medium. Acta Chir. Scand. (Suppl.)*321*:1, 1964.
5. Fischer, R. P., and Polk, H. C. Changing etiologic patterns of renal insufficiency in surgical patients. Surg. Gynecol. Obstet. *180*:85, 1975.
6. Richardson, J. D., DeCamp, M. M., Garrison, R. N., et al. Pulmonary infection complicating intra-abdominal sepsis: Clinical and experimental observations. Ann. Surg. *195*:732, 1982.
7. Rinaldo, J. E., and Rogers, R. M. Adult respiratory distress syndrome: Changing concepts of lung injury and repair. N. Engl. J. Med. *306*:900, 1982.
8. Dahn, M. D., Jacobs, L. A., Smith, S., et al. The relationship of insulin production to glucose metabolism in severe sepsis. Arch. Surg. *120*(2):166–172, 1985.
9. Meyers, M. A., and Whalen, J. P. Radiologic aspects of intra-abdominal abscess. *In* Ariel, I. M., and Kazarian, K. K. (eds.): Diagnosis and Treatment of Abdominal Abscesses. Baltimore, Williams & Wilkins Co., 1971, p. 87.
10. Gottschalk, A., and Ariel, M. Hepatic scanning in the diagnosis of liver abscess. *In* Ariel, I. M., and Kazarian, K. K. (eds.): Diagnosis and Treatment of Abdominal Abscesses. Baltimore, Williams & Wilkins Co., 1971, p. 226.

11. Brown, D. W. Combined lung-liver radioisotope scan in the diagnosis of subdiaphragmatic abscess. Am. J. Surg. *109*:521, 1965.
12. Gold, R. P., and Johnson, P. M. Efficacy of combined liver-lung scintillation imaging. Radiology *117*:105, 1975.
13. Littenberg, R. L., Taketa, R. M., Alazraki, N. P., et al. Gallium-67 for localization of septic lesions. Ann. Intern. Med. *79*:403, 1973.
14. Burleson, R. L., Holman, B. L., and Tow, D. E. Scintigraphic demonstration of abscesses with radioactive gallium labeled leukocytes. Surg. Gynecol. Obstet. *141*:379, 1975.
15. Ascher, N. L., Forstrom, L., and Simmons, R. L. Radiolabeled autologous leukocyte scanning in abscess detection. World J. Surg. *4*:395, 1980.
16. Rovekamp, M. H., Hardeman, M. R., van der Schoot, J. B., and Belfer, A. J. [111]Indium-labelled leucocyte scintigraphy in the diagnosis of inflammatory disease—first results. Br. J. Surg. *68*:150, 1981.
17. Thakur, M. L., Segal, A. W., Louis, L., Welch, M. J., Hopkins, J., and Peters, T. J. Indium-111-labeled cellular blood components: Mechanism of labeling and intracellular location in human neutrophils. J. Nucl. Med. *18*:1022, 1977.
18. Maklad, N. F., Doust, B. D., and Baum, J. K. Ultrasonic diagnosis of postoperative intra-abdominal abscess. Radiology *133*:417, 1974.
19. Doust, B. D., and Doust, V. L. Ultrasonic diagnosis of abdominal abscess. Dig. Dis. *21*:569, 1976.
20. Filly, R. A. Detection of abdominal abscesses: A combined approach employing ultrasonography, computed tomography and gallium-67 scanning. J. Assoc. Can. Radiol. *30*:202, 1979.
21. Gerzof, S. G., Robbins, A. H., and Birkett, D. H. Computed tomography in the diagnosis and management of abdominal abscesses. Gastrointest. Radiol. *3*:287, 1978.
22. Dobrin, P. B., Gully, P. H., Greenlee, H. B., et al. Radiologic diagnosis of an intra-abdominal abscess: Do multiple tests help? Arch. Surg. *121*(1):41–46, 1986.
23. Ariel, I. M., and Kazarian, K. K.: Classification, diagnosis, and treatment of subphrenic abscesses. *In* Ariel, I. M., and Kazarian, K. K. (eds.): Diagnosis and Treatment of Abdominal Abscesses. Baltimore, Williams & Wilkins Co., 1971, p. 174.
24. Boyd, D. P. Annual discourse: The subphrenic spaces and the emperor's new robes. N. Engl. J. Med. *275*:911, 1966.
25. Altemeier, W. A., Culbertson, W. R., and Fullen, W. D. Intra-abdominal sepsis. Adv. Surg. *5*:281, 1971.
26. Altemeier, W. A., Culbertson, W. R., Fullen, W. D., and Shook, C. D. Intra-abdominal abscesses. Am. J. Surg. 125:70, 1973.
27. Altemeier, W. A., Hummel, R. P., Hill, E. O., and Lewis, S. Changing patterns in surgical infections. Ann. Surg. *178*:436, 1973.
28. Haaga, J. R., and Weinstein, A. J. CT-guided percutaneous aspiration and drainage of abscesses. Am. J. Roentgenol. *135*:1187, 1980.
29. Johnson, W. C., Gerzof, S. G., Robbins, A. H., and Nasbeth, D. C. Treatment of abdominal abscesses: Comparative evaluation of operative drainage versus percutaneous catheter drainage guided by computed tomography or ultrasound. Ann. Surg. *194*:511, 1981.
30. Welch, C. E. Catheter drainage of abdominal abscesses. N. Engl. J. Med., *305*:694, 1981.
31. Gerzof, S. G., Robbins, A. H., Johnson, W. C., Birkett, D. H., and Nasbeth, D. C. Percutaneous catheter drainage of abdominal abscesses: A five-year experience. N. Engl. J. Med. *305*:653, 1981.
32. Halasz, N. A. Subphrenic abscess: Myths and facts. JAMA *214*:724, 1970.
33. Halliday, P. The surgical management of subphrenic abscess: A historical study. Aust. N. Z. J. Surg. *45*:235, 1975.
34. Gerding, D. N., Hall, W. H., and Schierl, E. A. Antibiotic concentrations in ascitic fluid of patients with ascites and bacterial peritonitis. Ann. Intern. Med. *86*:708, 1977.
35. Hau, T., Haaga, J. R., and Aeder, M. I. Pathophysiology, diagnosis, and treatment of abdominal abscesses. Curr. Probl. Surg. *21*:1–82, 1984.

36. Stone, H. H., Bourneuf, A. A., and Stinson, L. D. Reliability of criteria for predicting persistent or recurrent sepsis. Arch. Surg. *120*:17–20, 1985.
37. Walters, R., Herman, C. M., Neff, R., et al. Percutaneous drainage of abscesses in the postoperative abdomen that is difficult to explore. Am. J. Surg. *149*:623–626, 1985.
38. Porter, J. A., Loughry, C. W., and Cook, A. J. Use of the computerized tomographic scan in the diagnosis and treatment of abscesses. Am. J. Surg. *150*:257–262, 1985.
39. Haaga, J. R., and Weinstein, A. J. CT-guided percutaneous aspiration and drainage of abscesses. AJR *135*:1187, 1980.
40. Gerzof, S. G., Johnson, W. C., Robbins, A. H., and Nabseth, D. C. Expanded criteria for percutaneous abscess drainage. Arch. Surg. *120*:227–232, 1985.
41. Stone, H. H., Mullins, R. J., Dunlog, W. E., and Strom, P. R. Extraperitoneal versus transperitoneal drainage of the intra-abdominal abscess. Surg. Gynecol. Obstet. *159*:544–549, 1984.
42. Olak, J., Christou, N. V., Stein, L. A., Casola, G., and Meakins, J. L. Operative vs percutaneous drainage of intraabdominal abscesses. Arch. Surg. *121*:141–146, 1986.
43. Rubin, R. H., Schwartz, M. N., and Malt, R. Hepatic abscess: Changes in clinical, bacteriologic, and therapeutic aspects. Am. J. Med. *57*:601, 1974.
44. Altemeier, W. A., Schowengerdt, C. G., and Whiteley, D. H. Abscesses of the liver: Surgical considerations. Arch. Surg. *101*:258, 1970.
45. Ariel, I. M., and Kazarian, K. K. Intrahepatic abscesses—clinical features and treatment. *In* Ariel, I. M., and Kazarian, K. K. (eds.): Diagnosis and Treatment of Abdominal Abscesses. Baltimore, Williams & Wilkins Co., 1971, p. 207.
46. Sabbaj, J., Sutter, V. L., and Finegold, S. M. Anaerobic pyogenic liver abscess. Ann. Intern. Med. *77*:629, 1972.
47. Anderson, C. B., Marr, J. J., and Ballinger, W. F. Anaerobic infections in surgery; Clinical review. Surgery *79*:313, 1976.
48. Gorbach, S. L. Intra-abdominal infections. *In* Syllabus for AGA Postgraduate Course, Section 12. Miami, Florida, May 1976, pp. 1–14.
49. Bertel, C. K., van Heerden, J. A., and Sheedy, P. F. Treatment of pyogenic hepatic abscesses: Surgical vs percutaneous drainage. Arch. Surg. *121*:554–558, 1986.
50. Gerzof, S. G., Johnson, W. C., Robbins, A. H., and Nabseth, D. C. Intrahepatic pyogenic abscesses: Treatment of percutaneous drainage. Am. J. Surg. *149*:487–494, 1985.

Splenic Abscess

51. Gadacz, T., Way, L. W., and Dunphy, J. E. Changing clinical spectrum of splenic abscess. Am. J. Surg. *128*:182, 1974.
52. Fry, D. E., Richardson, J. D., and Flint, L. M. Occult splenic abscess: An unrecognized complication of heroin abuse. Surgery *84*:650, 1978.
53. Gadacz, T. R. Splenic abscess. World J. Surg. *9*:410, 1985.

Gastrointestinal Fistulas

54. Reber, H. A., Roberts, C., Way, L. W., and Dunphy, J. E. Management of external gastrointestinal fistulas. Ann. Surg. *188*:460, 1978.
55. Reber, H. A. Enterocutaneous fistulas. *In* Cameron, J. (ed.): Current Surgical Therapy 1984–1985. Philadelphia and St. Louis, B. C. Decker, Inc., and C. V. Mosby, 1984, p. 80.
56. Geersden, J. P., Pedersen, V. S., and Kjaergard, H. K. Small bowel fistulas treated with somatostatin: Preliminary results. Surgery *100*:811–814, 1986.
57. Mulvihill, S., Pappas, T. N., Passaro, E., and Debas, H. T. The use of somatostatin and its analogs in the treatment of surgical disorders. Surgery *100*:467–475, 1986.
58. Pederzoli, P., Bassi, C., Falconi, M., Albrigo, R., Vantini, I., and Micciolo, R. Conservative treatment of external pancreatic fistulas with parenteral nutrition alone or in combination with continuous intravenous infusion of somatostatin, glucagon or calcitonin. Surg. Gynecol. Obstet. *163*:428–432, 1986.

59. Aguirre, A., Fischer, J. E., and Welch, C. E. The role of surgery and hyperalimentation in therapy of gastrointestinal-cutaneous fistulae. Ann. Surg. *180*:393, 1974.
60. MacFadyen, B. V., Dudrick, S. J., and Ruberg, R. L. Management of gastrointestinal fistulas with parenteral hyperalimentation. Surgery *74*:100, 1973.
61. Kaminsky, V. M., and Deitel, M. Nutritional support in the management of external fistulas of the alimentary tract. Br. J. Surg. *26*:100, 1975.
62. Papachristou, D. N., and Fortner, J. G. Pancreatic fistula complicating pancreatectomy for malignant disease. Br. J. Surg. *68*:238, 1981.
63. Jordan, G. L., Jr. Pancreatic fistula. *In* Howard, J. M., Jordan, G. L., and Reber, H. A. (eds.): Surgical Diseases of the Pancreas. Philadelphia, Lea & Febiger, 1987, p. 898.

25

Gastrointestinal Bleeding

WALTER L. PETERSON

Management of gastrointestinal (GI) bleeding is straightforward and logical. The patient must be hemodynamically stabilized, the bleeding stopped, and therapy begun with the hope that further episodes of bleeding can be prevented. Most patients cease bleeding spontaneously. For those who do not, interventional measures are often invasive and not always effective; mortality is disproportionately high in these patients. Furthermore, recurrent bleeding during the first few days after hospitalization is frequent and carries with it increased mortality. In the past 5 years, several new endoscopically delivered treatments have been developed that offer promise for the cessation of active bleeding and the prevention of recurrent bleeding. However, accurate assessment of the patient as to the severity of bleeding, followed by vigorous and prompt resuscitation remains the cornerstone of managing GI bleeding and must not be overshadowed by attempts at early diagnosis and treatment of a specific bleeding lesion.

MANNER OF PRESENTATION

Patients manifest blood loss from the GI tract in five ways. *Hematemesis* is bloody vomitus, either fresh and bright red or older and "coffee-ground" in character. *Melena* is shiny, black, sticky, foul-smelling stool. It results from degradation of blood and must not be confused with the effects of exogenous stool darkeners such as iron or bismuth. *Hematochezia* is the passage of bright red or maroon blood from the rectum in the form of pure blood, blood intermixed with formed stool, or bloody diarrhea. Frequently, GI blood loss is

occult, that is, detected only by testing the stool with a chemical reagent. Finally, patients may present without any objective sign of bleeding but rather with *symptoms of blood loss,* such as dizziness, dyspnea, angina cordis, or even shock.

ASSESSMENT OF THE PATIENT

When GI bleeding is suspected, rapid assessment of the patient is carried out to gauge the urgency of the situation. Is bleeding acute or chronic? Is the patient hemodynamically stable or unstable? It is helpful to confirm objectively the presence of GI bleeding with inspection of the stool or nasogastric aspirate, but the first goal is to stabilize the patient. Vital signs are taken, the patient's skin and mucous membranes are inspected for pallor or signs of shock, and blood is sent to the laboratory for complete blood count, clotting studies, and routine chemistry studies. Blood for typing and crossmatching is sent to the blood bank so that if transfusions are necessary, they can be given without delay.

Presenting Manifestations

Hematemesis, melena, or hematochezia indicates an acute episode of bleeding, whereas occult bleeding is generally chronic. Hematemesis results from a combination of large amounts of blood filling the stomach plus nausea, which often accompanies vascular collapse.[1] Hematemesis of fresh blood, then, generally indicates a more severe bleeding episode than melena, which occurs when bleeding is slow enough to allow time for degradation of blood.[2–4] However, there is individual variation, and it would be unwise to assess severity solely on this basis. Hematochezia is usually a manifestation of a lower GI source of bleeding, and in that situation can occur with major or minor bleeding episodes. If hematochezia is from an *upper* GI source, it usually reflects a massive bleed (i.e., greater than 1000 ml).

Hematocrit

If a patient bleeds slowly and chronically, many liters of blood may be lost before bone marrow iron stores are depleted and the hematocrit begins to fall. At this time, a peripheral blood smear will usually reveal hypochromic, microcytic red blood cells and the mean corpuscular volume (MCV) of the cells may be low. If blood loss is acute, the hematocrit will reflect the magnitude of the loss, but not right away. As shown in Figure 25–1, the hematocrit does not change during the first few hours after hemorrhage, since proportionate reductions occur in both plasma and red cell volumes. During this time, caution must be used not to underestimate the severity of bleeding just because the hematocrit is normal. Only as extravascular fluid enters the vascular space to restore volume does the hematocrit fall. This process begins shortly after bleeding occurs, but is not complete until total blood volume is restored, often some 24 to 72 hours later.[1] At this point, plasma volume is larger than normal and the hematocrit is at its lowest point. The MCV will be normal unless there has been prior, chronic blood loss. This sequence is modified by administration of exogenous fluids or blood and is not as pronounced in patients with pre-existing blood volume deficiency who have less extravascular fluid to mobilize.

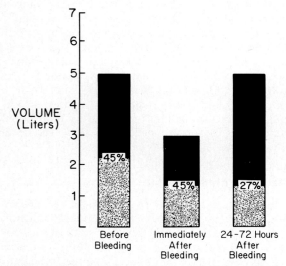

Figure 25–1. Plasma volumes (solid bars), red blood cell volumes (stippled bars), and hematocrits before bleeding and after 2 liters of blood loss. Assume a baseline hematocrit of 45 per cent.

Blood Pressure and Heart Rate

Careful attention to vital signs is the best way to judge a patient's stability, regardless of the hematocrit. The blood pressure and heart rate depend upon the amount of blood loss, the suddenness of blood loss, and the extent of cardiac and vascular compensation. Early on, or after partial compensation, the only physical finding may be postural hypotension. In this instance, blood pressure is maintained when the patient is recumbent but falls when the patient sits up. With greater losses, tachycardia and vasoconstriction ensue to compensate, and finally recumbent hypotension results. At this point, vascular collapse has occurred and the patient is "shocky" (i.e., pale to ashen gray, sweating, distressed).[1] Many patients experience a vasovagal reaction with bradycardia, vasodilation, and profound constitutional symptoms.[1, 5, 6] The individual patient's ability to manifest any or all of these findings depends on cardiac function, vascular integrity, state of hydration, and whether or not the autonomic nervous system is intact. As a rule, a systolic blood pressure under 100 mm Hg, or a postural drop in blood pressure of 10 to 15 mm Hg reflects a blood loss of 1000 ml or more.

Management after Assessment

The urgency of management depends upon the results of initial assessment. Hemodynamically stable patients with chronic bleeding are managed electively, whereas those with acute bleeding or an unstable condition must be resuscitated immediately.

RESUSCITATION

Patients who have had important acute bleeding or who are hemodynamically unstable should be admitted to an intensive care unit. Venous access is achieved using large-bore cannulas, and fluids are started. To restore vascular volume, normal saline or lactated Ringer's solution should be infused as rapidly as the patient's cardiopulmonary system will allow; measurement of central venous or pulmonary capillary wedge pressures may be used in selected fragile patients to prevent overly rapid fluid administration. The goal of fluid therapy is to improve quickly the circulation of remaining red blood cells; administration of supplemental oxygen by nasal cannula or face mask permits optimal red cell oxygen saturation. Vital signs, urine output, and electrocardiogram are monitored frequently. A flow sheet is helpful to document resuscitative measures and the patient's responses to them.

When to Transfuse

There are no hard and fast rules to tell a physician when to administer a transfusion to a patient with GI bleeding. Common sense dictates that patients who continue to bleed despite therapy, who are in shock, who have very low hematocrits (e.g., less than 25 per cent), or who have symptoms related to poor tissue oxygenation (e.g., angina cordis) should receive transfusions. For asymptomatic, stable patients with hematocrits above 25 to 30 per cent, other factors must be considered. Is the hematocrit likely to drop further as vascular repletion occurs? From what hematocrit level could the patient withstand a recurrent episode of bleeding? Is bleeding acute (more likely to need transfusion) or chronic (less likely to warrant transfusion)? If transfusions are deemed unnecessary, iron supplements should be prescribed after diagnostic tests have been completed.

What to Transfuse

Blood is transfused to (1) improve oxygenation (with red blood cells), and (2) improve coagulation (with plasma and platelets). The relative necessity of fulfilling these goals varies among patients and determines the type of blood product(s) transfused. For example, patients who are bleeding massively have both needs and should be given whole blood if available. Patients whose bleeding has ceased and whose vascular volume has been replenished with saline or lactated Ringer's solution require predominantly red blood cells. Administration of packed red blood cells to these patients not only spares the resources of blood banks but reduces the volume of fluid transfused. This is especially important in patients with marginal cardiac or renal function. Fresh frozen plasma is not required in most patients unless there is a clinically important disturbance in coagulation and should not be given prophylactically.[7] However, since deficiency of coagulation factors is a pre-existing phenomenon in many patients with cirrhosis, consideration should be given to provide these patients with fresh frozen plasma after every second or third unit of packed red blood cells.[8] Platelets are usually needed only with very large hemorrhages (10 or more units). Banked blood is anticoagulated with calcium-binding agents. However, supplemental calcium is usually necessary only if there is an important fall in serum calcium levels.

How Much to Transfuse

Patients should receive blood until their vital signs are stable, bleeding ceases, and enough red blood cells are circulating to provide adequate oxygenation. A hematocrit of 30 per cent is a reasonable goal in most patients and provides a buffer if recurrent bleeding ensues. It must be remembered that plasma volume is often overexpanded after GI bleeding (see p. 398) and the hematocrit shortly after transfusion may underestimate the actual quantity of red blood cells present.

UPPER VERSUS LOWER GI TRACT BLEEDING

As resuscitation is being carried out, the source of bleeding must be localized to the upper or lower GI

tract to direct further management. As shown in Figure 25–2, the manner of presentation is largely determined by the level of the GI tract from which bleeding occurs. Hematemesis, either alone or in combination with other manifestations, indicates an upper GI source of bleeding (above the ligament of Treitz). Melena occurs if enough hemoglobin in the GI tract is converted to hematin or other hemochromes to blacken the stool.[9] This is most likely related to degradation of hemoglobin by bacteria as blood from an upper GI source slowly enters the bacteria-laden colon. Therefore, the farther away the bleeding site is from the rectum, the more likely melena will ensue. Although melena can be produced experimentally with as little as 100 to 200 ml of blood,[10] in clinical practice larger amounts have usually been lost. Bleeding colonic lesions may occasionally produce melena,[3, 9, 11] but only if three conditions are met. First, there must be enough blood degraded to blacken the stool. Second, bleeding must not be too brisk or hematochezia will ensue. Third, colonic motility must be sluggish to allow enough time for degradation of blood to occur. Most colonic lesions either bleed in such small amounts that only occult blood is present in stool, or bleed so briskly that hematochezia occurs. Hematochezia usually represents a lower GI source of bleeding, although an upper GI lesion may occasionally bleed so briskly that blood does not remain in the bowel long enough to become melena. Lesions of the small bowel may present as either hematochezia or melena, although small bowel lesions are unusual sources of GI bleeding.

Whenever a question arises as to the location of bleeding, a nasogastric tube should be placed. A bloody aspirate confirms an upper GI source, while a negative aspirate virtually excludes active upper GI bleeding.[12] Interpretation (by guaiac reaction) of aspirates that are not grossly bloody is of little clinical

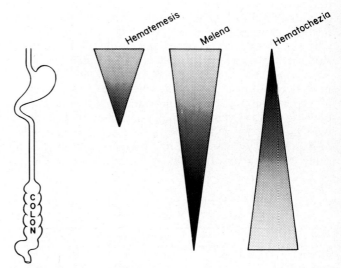

Figure 25–2. Diagrammatic representation of the likelihood of a bleeding lesion from any part of the gastrointestinal tract to produce hematemesis, melena, or hematochezia. More proximal lesions produce hematemesis and/or melena, whereas more distal lesions are more likely to produce hematochezia.

practicality and should be done with caution, since both false positive and false negative results may occur.[13] Occasionally, a postpyloric upper GI lesion will bleed (even massively) without reflux into the stomach and the aspirate will be negative. Endoscopy is the only sure way of detecting such occurrences, but other findings suggestive of upper GI bleeding include hyperactive bowel sounds and elevation of the blood urea nitrogen (BUN) out of proportion to creatinine.[14] Such rises in the BUN occur after major upper GI bleeding episodes (1000 ml or more)[14, 15] and are the result of volume depletion plus absorbed blood proteins.[16] Either factor alone will usually not result in elevation of the BUN to an important degree. A summary of differentiating features of upper and lower GI bleeding is shown in Table 25–1.

INITIAL MANAGEMENT AND DIAGNOSIS OF ACUTE UPPER GI BLEEDING

It may be estimated that over 350,000 people are admitted with acute upper GI bleeding each year in the United States.[17, 18] Despite widespread availability of accurate diagnostic techniques, sophisticated intensive care units, and new therapeutic modalities, mortality from upper GI bleeding remains at about 10 per cent,[19] a figure little different from figures reported previously.[20–23] There are several ways to interpret these data. First, mortality in patients over 60 years of age has been well recognized to be higher by several fold than mortality in younger patients.[21, 23, 24] Since the proportion of bleeding patients who are over age 60 has increased during the last 40 years from about 30 per cent to over 50 per cent,[20, 22] it might have been expected that overall mortality would also have risen. The fact that it has instead remained constant implies one of two things. Either more deaths in older patients have been offset by fewer deaths in younger patients, or mortality in older patients has in fact decreased.[23] Second, many patients who bleed have other important illnesses. Death often occurs primarily as a result of these other problems, rather than bleeding *per se.*[19] Thus, improvement in management of bleeding might not result in important reduction in mortality. Finally, it is possible that overall mortality has not declined because therapy remains inadequate for those patients who account for a disproportionate share of the mortality. These patients are, in general, those who continue bleeding or experience recurrent bleeding after

admission to hospital[21, 24–28] and, in particular, patients bleeding from esophageal and/or gastric varices.[20–28]

Gastric Lavage

If gastric aspiration discloses an actively bleeding upper GI source, gastric lavage should be carried out prior to diagnostic studies. Rinsing the bleeding stomach with iced saline is a time-honored technique. There occurs during gastric lavage at least temporary cessation of bleeding in about 90 per cent of patients, regardless of diagnosis. Whether this is a direct result of gastric lavage is unknown. However, even if it were of no help in controlling bleeding, lavage gives a good indication of the rapidity of bleeding, serves to cleanse the stomach for possible later endoscopy, and, in patients with cirrhosis, removes blood to lessen the likelihood of hepatic encephalopathy. A large-bore (No. 34 to 36 French) orogastric tube is placed after removal of the smaller-diameter nasogastric tube used for localization of bleeding. Aliquots of fluid (500 to 1000 ml) are instilled and then removed by gentle suction and gravity drainage. Iced saline is traditionally used because cold fluids reduce blood flow more effectively than room-temperature fluids.[29] On the other hand, cold fluids may impair coagulation.[30] Experimental evidence suggests that room-temperature tap water lavage is as effective as iced saline lavage.[30–32] Lavage is continued until bleeding stops (at which time the tube should be removed) or until it becomes evident that other measures will be necessary. If bleeding persists, it has been suggested that the vasoconstrictor levarterenol (Levophed, 8 mg in 100 to 250 ml saline) be instilled into the stomach. However, this agent does not reduce gastric blood flow any more than cold lavage alone,[29] and reports extolling the virtue of this technique are based on studies done without adequate controls.[33–35]

Diagnostic Approach to Acute Upper GI Bleeding

Patients who continue to bleed despite gastric lavage virtually always require a specific diagnosis. Patients who cease bleeding may or may not require a diagnosis, depending upon the clinical situation. For example, search for a diagnosis may not be necessary in a patient with a terminal illness who experiences a minor bleeding episode. The following section proceeds under the assumption that a specific diagnosis (Table 25–2) is desired in a given patient.

History and Physical Examination. As the initial steps of management are being carried out, it is important to take a history and perform a physical examination. Although a specific diagnosis can be made this way only occasionally, helpful clues may be obtained. Have there been prior episodes of bleeding? Is there a family history of diseases that cause bleeding? Does the patient have other illnesses that may lead to bleeding, such as cirrhosis, cancer, coagulopathies, connective tissue disorders, or amyloidosis? Has there

Table 25–1. DIFFERENTIATING FEATURES OF UPPER GI AND LOWER GI BLEEDING

	Upper GI	Lower GI
Presenting manifestation	Hematemesis and/or melena	Hematochezia
Nasogastric aspirate	Bloody	Clear
Blood urea nitrogen	Elevated	Normal
Bowel sounds	Hyperactive	Normal

Table 25–2. CAUSES OF GASTROINTESTINAL BLEEDING

Upper GI	Upper or Lower GI	Lower GI
Duodenal ulcer	Neoplasms	Hemorrhoids
Gastric ulcer	Carcinoma	Anal fissure
Marginal ulcer	Leiomyoma	Small intestinal or colonic diverticula
Cushing's ulcer	Sarcoma	Meckel's diverticulum
Esophageal or gastric varices	Hemangioma	Ischemic bowel disease
Mallory-Weiss tear	Lymphoma	Inflammatory bowel disease
Gastritis	Melanoma	Solitary colonic ulcer
Esophagitis	Polyps	Intussusception
Barrett's ulcer	Arterial-enteric fistulas	
Hematobilia	Vascular anomalies	
Menetrier's disease	Rendu-Osler-Weber syndrome	
	Blue rubber bleb nevus syndrome	
	CRST syndrome	
	Arteriovenous malformations	
	Angiodysplasia (vascular ectasia)	
	Hematologic diseases	
	Elastic tissue disorders	
	Pseudoxanthoma elasticum	
	Ehlers-Danlos syndrome	
	Vasculitis syndromes	
	Amyloidosis	

been prior surgery, such as for peptic ulcer or for the placement of arterial bypass grafts? Does the patient drink alcohol to excess or take drugs such as aspirin? Has there been caustic ingestion? Was the bleeding episode preceded by abdominal pain, dyspepsia, or retching? Has the patient had nosebleeds?

Examination of the skin is potentially the most helpful aspect of the physical examination (see pp. 535–537). Stigmata of cirrhosis, evidence of underlying malignancy (acanthosis nigricans, Kaposi's sarcoma), or hereditary vascular anomalies may be found. Findings of pseudoxanthoma elasticum or Ehlers-Danlos syndrome may be diagnostic. Further physical findings include lymphadenopathy or abdominal masses (malignancy), abdominal tenderness (peptic ulcer), and splenomegaly (cirrhosis or splenic vein thrombosis). Cutaneous lesions of some systemic diseases are shown in Figures 30–2 and 30–3.

Barium X-Rays and Endoscopy. Since the history and physical examination are rarely diagnostic, other techniques are necessary to define the bleeding lesion. The two most frequently employed techniques, barium X-ray and endoscopy, each have their place. In the patient with active bleeding, endoscopy is the procedure of choice. In this situation, urgent clinical decisions must be made and endoscopy is, overall, more accurate than barium X-rays, even if double contrast is used.[36–43] In addition, certain bleeding lesions may lend themselves to endoscopic therapy. Because barium introduced into the stomach makes investigation soon after by either endoscopy or arteriography difficult, it should never be given to the active bleeder.

In the patient whose bleeding has ceased, and in whom a diagnostic procedure can be performed electively, the issue of which diagnostic procedure to employ is not so clear-cut. In the best of hands, high-quality double-contrast barium studies will, in most instances, detect potential bleeding lesions as well as endoscopy.[44] Mallory-Weiss tears are not seen well with X-ray, but such lesions are rarely a clinical problem, usually being self-limited and associated with low mortality. Thus, if X-ray discloses a single lesion such as a duodenal or gastric ulcer, endoscopy often need not be performed (except for biopsy of a suspicious lesion or a gastric ulcer—see p. 893). The advantage of X-ray over endoscopy is lower cost, with X-ray usually being several-fold less expensive.

There are, however, certain settings where endoscopy is preferred to barium X-ray as the diagnostic test in patients whose bleeding has ceased. First, high-quality double-contrast X-rays are not readily available in some centers. Second, patients with portal hypertension and varices may be bleeding from a lesion other than varices in at least a third of cases.[45] Even if barium X-ray detects the second lesion, it cannot reliably determine which lesion has actually bled. Since further therapy will differ depending on which lesion is responsible, endoscopy is a better test in patients with evidence of liver disease. Third, X-ray is notoriously unreliable in patients with prior gastric resection. Fourth, patients with prior aortic bypass grafts require the more accurate diagnostic test, endoscopy, since failure to demonstrate another bleeding lesion will usually prompt exploratory laparotomy (see p. 411). Finally, some physicians believe that prophylactic endoscopic coagulative therapy of certain peptic ulcers will reduce the incidence of rebleeding (see p. 405). Endoscopy is the only way to identify these lesions. Because one or more of these conditions pertain in so many patients, it is not surprising that endoscopy is the generally employed diagnostic test.

Other Diagnostic Tests. The need for arteriography as a diagnostic tool in upper GI bleeding is rare, since endoscopy provides direct mucosal inspection. Occasionally, bleeding may be so massive that endoscopy cannot be safely or satisfactorily performed. If time permits, selective mesenteric arteriography will localize the site of bleeding (usually from the left gastric artery) in about 75 per cent of such patients.[46–48] It is widely accepted that blood loss must be at a rate of about 0.5 ml per minute for extravasated dye to be seen by X-ray.[49] Arteriography will be negative if flow rates are less than this or if the patient is bleeding from a venous lesion.

There is also little need for radionuclide imaging studies in upper GI bleeding. If bleeding has ceased, radionuclide studies cannot be helpful. If bleeding is too copious for endoscopy, then arteriography is a better test. Radionuclide imaging should be reserved for lower GI bleeding (see p. 412) or for patients with an obscure source of blood loss (see p. 416).

Overall Diagnostic Approach. Patients who continue to bleed despite gastric lavage should promptly undergo endoscopy to find the specific lesion for which specific therapy is needed. For example, a patient with bleeding esophageal varices may require sclerotherapy, while a patient with a bleeding duodenal ulcer may require thermal coagulation or urgent surgery. If bleeding is too brisk and endoscopy cannot be performed, and if urgent surgery can be delayed, arteriography is warranted.

The approach to the patient who ceases bleeding is less straightforward but, as with the patient who continues to bleed, usually includes routine early endoscopy for the reasons noted on page 401. The rationale is that making a prompt diagnosis will aid in the patient's management. Several controlled trials involving diverse patient populations suggest that, at least in terms of objective measurements of outcome, this is not the case.[26, 37, 39, 43, 50–53] Routine performance of endoscopy in patients whose bleeding has ceased has not been shown to improve survival, reduce transfusion requirements, or shorten hospital stay. Furthermore, prior knowledge of the source of bleeding does not improve the outcome of patients who rebleed, and, in one study, 12-month follow-up did not disclose a benefit to patients in whom endoscopy was performed routinely.[26] There is at least one good explanation for these observations. A diagnosis is only as good as the therapy to which it leads, and, for patients who cease bleeding, therapeutic options have, until recently, been limited. It is possible that use of newer endoscopic modalities of therapy (e.g., thermal coagulation of bleeding ulcers, sclerotherapy of varices) would change the results if these studies were repeated today.

APPROACH TO SPECIFIC UPPER GI BLEEDING LESIONS

Peptic Ulcers

Duodenal, gastric, or anastomotic (postgastrectomy) ulcers as a group are the most common cause of upper GI bleeding. Overall mortality from bleeding peptic ulcer is generally regarded to be 5 to 10 per cent,[20, 21, 28, 54] although in some series, mortality even in older patients is only about 2 per cent.[23] In general, mortality

with bleeding gastric ulcer is somewhat greater than that which occurs with bleeding duodenal ulcer. Furthermore, mortality differs depending upon the course of bleeding. First, if bleeding ceases and no rebleeding occurs, the situation with about 70 per cent of patients, mortality is very low, probably less than 2 per cent. Second, rebleeding after initial cessation occurs in about 25 per cent of patients,[26, 27, 54, 55] and mortality in this group of patients rises substantially, to well above 10 per cent.[21, 25–27, 56] Finally, about 5 per cent of patients will experience continued active bleeding despite initial medical management, and in them mortality is highest of all, perhaps as high as 30 per cent.[21, 25] Thus, therapy for bleeding peptic ulcer is directed toward (a) cessation of continuing bleeding and (b) prevention of recurrent bleeding.

Determinants of Severe Ulcer Bleeding. Continuing or recurrent bleeding is more likely to occur when an ulcer erodes one wall of a large artery coursing under the base of the ulcer.[55, 57] This produces an eccentric breach in the vessel (Fig. 25–3A) as opposed to a complete transection of the vessel. Whereas vessels, particularly smaller vessels, that are transected can constrict to aid cessation of bleeding, arteries with disruption only of one lateral wall cannot constrict. Anatomically, ulcers on the high lesser curve of the stomach or in the posteroinferior half of the duodenal bulb are more prone to bleed severely,[58] most likely because of proximity to large vessels (i.e., left gastric and gastroduodenal arteries, respectively). Recent reports suggest that use of nonsteroidal anti-inflammatory drugs increases the risk of and mortality from bleeding peptic ulcer.[58a, 58b, 58c]

Predictors of Severe Ulcer Bleeding. Clinically, the likelihood after initial cessation of a recurrent bleeding

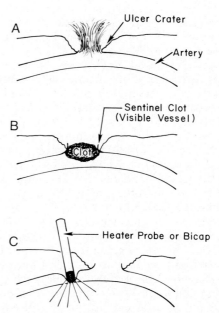

· **Figure 25–3.** *A,* Diagrammatic representation of a bleeding ulcer. *B,* An ulcer with a sentinel clot (visible vessel). *C,* The means by which a heater probe or Bicap electrode seals a bleeding artery.

episode is directly proportional to the severity of the initial episode, as manifested by degree of anemia[59] or by hemodynamic instability.[60] Endoscopically, ulcers with active bleeding or ulcers with "stigmata of recent hemorrhage"[61, 62] are more likely to result in a severe rebleeding episode (Color Fig. 25–4, p. xxxiii). Such stigmata, found in about two-thirds of ulcers that have bled, include a dark stain or spot, an adherent clot, or a "visible vessel." The latter, also called a "sentinel clot," is produced when the lateral defect in the arterial wall protrudes (often with a small plug of fibrin or clot) above the ulcer crater (Fig. 25–3B). There is general agreement that ulcers with a clean base rebleed less than 5 per cent of the time, ulcers with a spot 5 to 10 per cent of the time, and ulcers with a clot, visible vessel, or active oozing more than 20 per cent of the time. The precise incidence of recurrent bleeding from ulcers with one of these latter three stigmata, as well as their prevalence, varies enormously from study to study.[25, 56, 61, 63–70] For example, while one investigator finds visible vessels in 50 per cent of all ulcers, with a 50 per cent incidence of rebleeding,[56] another investigator may find these stigmata in only 20 per cent of ulcers with an incidence of rebleeding of less than 30 per cent.[69] Such variability may be explained by differences in definitions of stigmata, differences in the time at which endoscopy is performed, differences in the clinical severity of the initial bleeding episode, and differences in the definition of rebleeding. Of interest, one recent paper suggests that endoscopic Doppler testing can determine the patency of the involved vessel and predict which ulcers with stigmata of recent hemorrhage will rebleed.[70]

Non-Endoscopic Therapy for Continuing Ulcer Bleeding. A number of *pharmacologic agents,* including intravenous vasopressin, secretin, H_2-receptor antagonists, and somatostatin, have been tried as means of stopping active ulcer bleeding.[71–75] None has been clearly shown to be effective. It is not surprising that these agents, which act to reduce gastric acidity and/or constrict the bleeding vessel, are ineffective when one remembers that the cause of bleeding is an eccentric breach in the wall of a large vessel (Figure 25–3A). Results with prostaglandins[76, 77] and tranexamic acid,[78, 79] an antifibrinolytic agent, have also not been impressive in terms of cessation of bleeding, although there is some evidence that surgical intervention may be required less often in patients treated with tranexamic acid than those treated with placebo.

Because use of these pharmacologic agents has been unrewarding, the traditional nonendoscopic approach to continued ulcer bleeding remains *urgent surgery* (see pp. 925–952). However, since such surgery carries with it relatively high mortality,[21, 80–84] other means of controlling hemorrhage have been sought. One such approach is via *arteriography.* Because of success in using selective arterial infusion of vasopressin in acute mucosal lesions (see p. 410), this approach has also been tried in acute peptic ulcers. Perhaps as a consequence of large, complex vasculature around peptic ulcers,[85, 86] intra-arterial vasopressin is not often effec-

tive.[86–91] Another angiographic technique is embolization of the bleeding artery with autologous clot or some foreign material such as Gelfoam or small coils (Fig 25–5).[88, 89, 91–97] Although this procedure can provide dramatically successful results, the technique requires much expertise and is associated with important complications.[93, 96–99] While embolization therapy for peptic ulcers may be lifesaving in patients who could not survive surgery, it should be performed only by skilled angiographers and only when the clinical situation is desperate.

Pharmacologic Therapy to Prevent Recurrent Ulcer Bleeding. Most drug regimens that have been designed to prevent recurrent ulcer bleeding have used as a mechanism the reduction of gastric acidity. This makes sense in that *in vitro* data suggest that coagulation and platelet function are inhibited at low pH levels.[100] However, dissolution of a clot is not strictly an acid phenomenon. If a clot is placed in a solution of 0.1 N hydrochloric acid alone, no dissolution will occur.[101] On the other hand, if the clot is placed in gastric juice at the same pH, rapid and progressive dissolution occurs.[101] This is most likely due to the fact that gastric juice possesses pepsin, a fibrinolytic agent. It is well known that the activity of pepsin is pH-dependent, with reduced activity at higher pH levels.[102, 103] As pH is raised, the ability of gastric juice to dissolve a clot is markedly retarded.[104]

Analysis of clinical trials assessing the effect of H_2-receptor antagonists on recurrent ulcer bleeding suggests that the incidence of recurrent bleeding from gastric ulcers may be reduced (albeit only slightly) with such drugs, whereas there is no benefit in duodenal ulcers,[54] even if antacid is added.[72] There are two possible reasons why reduction of gastric acidity has not been shown to have an important impact on the incidence of recurrent bleeding. First, it may well be that *in vitro* data regarding clot function[100, 101, 104] are not relevant to the human model. Secondly, it is possible that previously tested regimens have failed to reduce gastric acidity to low enough levels.[105, 106] Indeed, it is possible that prevention of recurrent bleeding via reduction of gastric acidity requires reduction to levels near achlorhydria.[100] This may be achieved with a constant intravenous infusion of an H_2-receptor antagonist, especially with supplemental administration of antacids.[106, 107] It is also possible that administration of omeprazole, a hydrogen-potassium ATPase inhibitor, may raise gastric pH to levels near achlorhydria (see p. 846). Whether such regimens will actually result in reduction of recurrent ulcer bleeding must be proved by controlled clinical trials.

Recent studies have also evaluated the effect of somatostatin,[108] prostaglandins,[77] and tranexamic acid[109] as means of preventing recurrent ulcer bleeding. None of these agents has been proved effective.

Endoscopic Therapy of Bleeding Ulcer. Because nonendoscopic forms of therapy have, in general, proved of little use, and because surgical therapy carries with it substantial mortality and morbidity, it is not surprising that endoscopic techniques have been

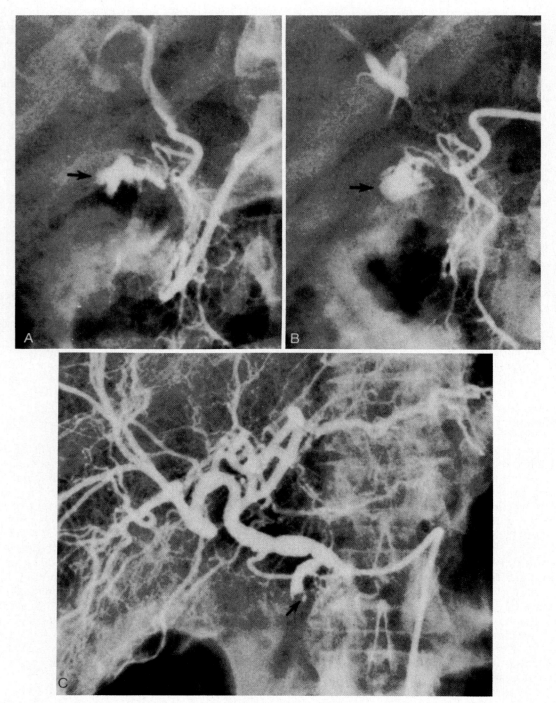

Figure 25–5. Selective injection of contrast material into the inferior *(A)* and superior *(B)* branches of the pancreaticoduodenal artery, showing extravasation from both of the branches *(arrows)* into a duodenal ulcer. *C,* Follow-up selective angiogram demonstrates occlusion of the gastroduodenal artery and both pancreaticoduodenal branches with Gelfoam *(arrow).* (Reprinted with permission from: Arterial embolization for massive upper gastrointestinal tract bleeding in poor surgical candidates, by Lieberman, D. A., Keller, F. S., Katon, R. M., and Rosch, J. Gastroenterology *86:*876. Copyright 1984 by The American Gastroenterological Association.)

developed to control peptic ulcer bleeding.[110] The advantage of these techniques is that they can be applied at the time of diagnostic endoscopy. Endoscopic modalities can be divided into two groups—those that do and those that do not produce heat. Nonthermal methods include spraying crystalline collagen, clotting factors, or cyanoacrylate tissue glues onto a bleeding lesion.[111–114] Only the latter has been studied adequately in man and was shown to be of no benefit in experimental patients as compared with control subjects.[114] Another technique consists of injection of the bleeding ulcer with a necrotizing solution, much like the procedure for esophageal varices (see p. 407).[115] These solutions include hypertonic saline, epinephrine, and pure ethanol. While this technique is, in theory, very attractive because of its simplicity and lack of expense, controlled trials have not yet been performed to document efficacy and safety. A controlled trial showed a significant reduction in blood transfusions and need for urgent surgery with injection therapy of actively bleeding ulcers.[114a]

Thermal methods of endoscopic therapy include laser photocoagulation, electrocoagulation, and the heater probe. Laser photocoagulation occurs when heat is generated by interaction of laser light with tissue. Two sources of laser light, argon and neodymium–yttrium aluminum garnet (Nd-YAG) have been well studied both in animals and man.[63–66, 116–125] While results in controlled clinical trials are at variance, the majority suggest that for all but the most severe bleeding ulcers, laser therapy will at least temporarily stop active bleeding.[63–65, 123–125] However, the impact on other parameters of outcome, such as need for blood transfusions or surgery, is less clear. It has also been suggested that prophylactic laser treatment of ulcers in which the bleeding has ceased, will prevent recurrent bleeding. Once again, results are contradictory,[63–66] but if any lesion is to be benefitted, it is the ulcer with a visible vessel.[64, 65] Ulcers with other stigmata of hemorrhage do not benefit from prophylactic treatment with laser therapy.

Whether laser therapy is or is not effective for bleeding ulcers has become a moot point. The machines are very expensive and, in general, the patient must be moved to the machine. Of more practical potential benefit are two other techniques of delivering heat to the tissue. These are electrocoagulation and the heater probe,[67, 68, 126–132] techniques that can be applied endoscopically at the patient's bedside. These techniques act by first directly tamponading the bleeding vessel to produce temporary cessation of bleeding, following which heat is generated to seal shut the two walls of the vessel (Fig. 25–3C). Techniques of electrocoagulation raise tissue temperature by passing an electric current through the tissue. This can be achieved either with a monopolar electrode, which uses a patient plate for exit of the current, or a bipolar electrode. The latter has been shown in animals to be safer and more effective.[126, 130] The bipolar electrode that has been studied most carefully in humans is the Bicap electrode. Results of randomized controlled trials of

the Bicap[67, 68, 131, 132] are at variance, but suggest that active bleeding is stopped at least temporarily[68, 132] and that prophylactic therapy of ulcers with visible vessels may reduce the incidence of recurrent bleeding.[68, 132] Treatment of ulcers with other stigmata is of no benefit.[67, 68, 131] The heater probe is the newest endoscopic technique. As with electrocoagulation, it acts by first occluding the bleeding vessel. As opposed to electrocoagulation, in which heat is generated by an electric current, the heater probe is a device that itself becomes very hot. Controlled studies are under way to determine the effectiveness of the heater probe. A large randomized trial suggests that the heater probe is no better than control and not as good as the Nd-YAG laser in preventing recurrent bleeding and improving survival in patients who have bled from peptic ulcers.[132a]

It is likely that the Bicap electrode and the heater probe will gain increased acceptance in the treatment of bleeding ulcer. It is important that further studies quantitate the effect of these modalities on survival, need for blood transfusions, hospital stay, and hospital costs.

Esophageal and Gastric Varices

Management of patients with bleeding esophageal and gastric varices (Color Fig. 25–6, p. xxxiv) remains the largest stumbling block to the reduction of overall mortality from upper GI bleeding. Mortality during the initial hospitalization is at least 30 per cent,[26, 133, 134] which is due in no small part to the fact that approximately 50 to 70 per cent of patients will experience a rebleeding episode during hospitalization.[26, 134] Mortality in patients who have bled from esophageal varices is significantly higher than in those who have bled from gastric varices.[134] Additionally, at least a third will rebleed within 6 weeks of discharge from hospitalization,[133] and no more than a third will survive beyond one year.[133, 135] It is no wonder that a number of therapeutic techniques have been proposed whose goals are to improve this outlook; the fact that a new one has surfaced each decade implies that none has been overwhelmingly successful.

There are two key factors in determining whether esophageal varices will develop and whether they will bleed. First, portal pressure must reach an hepatic vein pressure gradient of about 12 mm Hg (normal = 3 to 6 mm Hg) for varices to develop.[136] Above this level there is poor correlation between the portal pressure and the propensity of varices to bleed,[137, 138] although portal pressure tends to be higher in bleeders than in patients with varices who have not bled.[136] Second, a more important determinant of variceal bleeding is the size of the varices.[136, 138] When they reach a large size (over 5 mm in diameter), they are more likely to burst. Wall tension of varices is directly proportional to the radius of the vessel and inversely proportional to the wall thickness. Thus, at any given pressure, the wall of a large varix will be under greater tension than that of a small varix, and must be thicker to withstand the pressure.[136] While transient large increases in portal pressure (as a result of coughing, straining, or blood volume overload[139-144]) may play a contributing role in variceal bleeding, mucosal inflammation from gastroesophageal reflux appears to be unimportant.[144, 145]

Most patients with varices have cirrhosis, usually alcoholic in origin, although splenic vein thrombosis or hypersplenic states may also result in portal-venous hypertension.[146-148] Such patients often have gastric varices out of proportion to esophageal varices. It is important to differentiate such patients from patients with cirrhosis, since splenectomy alone may be curative.

When patients with suspected esophageal varices present with bleeding, it is important to perform endoscopy as soon as is practical (usually within 12 hours) to document the source of hemorrhage. Perhaps one third of patients with esophageal varices will be bleeding from some other lesion.[45, 149-151] Other causes of bleeding in patients with varices include Mallory-Weiss tears, gastritis,[152-154] peptic ulcers, and a noninflammatory vascular lesion peculiar to patients with portal hypertension that is termed "congestive gastropathy."[155, 155a]

Therapy of Actively Bleeding Varices. In patients with actively bleeding varices, the first line of therapy has traditionally been the parenteral use of *vasopressin*.[156, 157] This agent, which reduces portal venous pressure by reducing splanchnic blood flow, was used originally as an intravenous bolus.[158, 159] In this form, it appeared to stop variceal bleeding (albeit often only temporarily) but at a cost of systemic side effects such as hyponatremia, hypertension, cardiac arrhythmias, and decreased cardiac output. It was hoped that constant infusion of a lower dose directly into the superior mesenteric artery[160] would have the desired result on splanchnic blood flow (and portal pressure) without producing side effects. Although controlled trials suggested that intra-arterial infusion of vasopressin was as effective as an intravenous bolus,[161, 162] systemic complications remained. In addition, there occurred local vascular complications related to arterial puncture. It was ultimately recognized that a similar low-dose infusion of vasopressin given intravenously also reduced portal pressure.[163] Controlled trials have since demonstrated that an intravenous infusion of vasopressin controls variceal bleeding as well as selective arterial infusion,[164, 165] but without the vascular complications. Unfortunately, it is still not clear whether vasopressin, however administered, results in cessation of bleeding more often than with placebo.[166]

Several alternatives to vasopressin therapy have recently been reported. First, it has been suggested that simultaneous administration of nitroglycerin, either sublingually or intravenously, will enhance the reduction of portal pressure,[167] lower the incidence of complications with vasopressin[168, 169] and perhaps improve efficacy in controlling variceal bleeding.[169, 170] Second, a synthetic analog of vasopressin (terlipressin, glypressin), was reported in an unblinded study to be more effective than vasopressin itself in stopping variceal

bleeding.[171] Finally, intravenous somatostatin has been suggested by early studies to be more effective[172] and/or safer,[172, 173] than vasopressin in the treatment of variceal bleeding. Further data are needed before terlipressin or somatostatin can be considered effective therapy for bleeding varices.

If intravenous infusion of vasopressin fails, what should be tried next? Although there is a suggestion that intra-arterial vasopressin may succeed when an intravenous infusion does not, the evidence does not justify the delay required to obtain the services of an expert angiographer. Traditionally, the next approach has been to use balloon tamponade.

Balloon tamponade of esophageal varices is performed using one of two basic systems (Fig. 25–7). The Sengstaken-Blakemore (S-B) tube is a double-balloon system with an extra tube for gastric suction. One balloon is for inflation in the stomach and the other is for the esophagus. The Linton-Nachlas (L-N) tube uses a single large gastric balloon that has aspiration tubes both above and below the balloon. Bleeding ceases in 75 to 90 per cent of patients if balloon tamponade is used as primary therapy, although it is of interest that more recent series report a much lower incidence of success.[174] Major complications of balloon tamponade (esophageal perforation, pulmonary aspiration) occur in almost 15 per cent of patients, resulting in death in 3 per cent. The problem of pulmonary aspiration with S-B tubes has been addressed by employing a separate nasogastric tube situated above the esophageal balloon[175] or by using a four-lumen balloon system in which the extra aspiration tube is built in.[176, 177] Even these measures do not always prevent aspiration, and some investigators suggest routine endotracheal intubation before placement of the tube.[178] The L-N tube offers no advantage over the S-B tube, except possibly in patients with gastric varices.[179]

Endoscopic injection sclerotherapy was originally described in 1939,[180] but fell out of favor with the advent

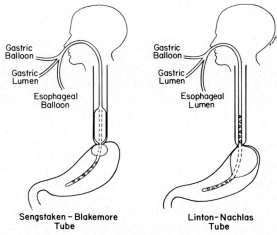

TWO TUBES FOR TAMPONADE OF VARICES

Gastric Balloon
Gastric Lumen
Esophageal Balloon
Sengstaken – Blakemore Tube

Gastric Balloon
Gastric Lumen
Esophageal Lumen
Linton-Nachlas Tube

Figure 25–7. Sengstaken-Blakemore and Linton-Nachlas tubes.

of balloon tamponade and vasopressin. Since it has become clear that vasopressin and balloon tamponade do not control all episodes of variceal bleeding, and that complications and recurrent bleeding after these procedures are frequent, sclerotherapy is being used once again. With this technique, a skilled endoscopist injects one of several formulations of a sclerosing solution into and/or around the bleeding varix.[181, 182] There is rapid occlusion of the varix by thrombosis or by perivariceal edema,[183] such that active bleeding ceases in 80 to 90 per cent of patients.[184–189] In one trial, immediate cessation of bleeding with sclerotherapy was superior to that achieved with a combination of vasopressin and nitroglycerin.[189]

Percutaneous obliteration is another technique to stop actively bleeding varices (Fig. 25–8). This is accomplished by cannulating the portal vein either transhepatically or by a transjugular approach.[190–192] Once the catheter is in the coronary vein (which feeds esophageal varices) a sclerosing agent or some substance such as Gelfoam is injected. The procedure will successfully obliterate the varices and stop active bleeding in 80 to 85 per cent of patients. Unfortunately, recanalization or collateral formation is frequent, and rebleeding occurs in 70 per cent. Complications occur in 20 per cent and include intraperitoneal bleeding, pleural effusions, and portal vein thrombosis. Because endoscopic sclerosis of varices accomplishes the same goals in actively bleeding patients without the requirement of a special radiologist, the percutaneous approach should be employed infrequently.

Urgent surgery, during which either a portal-systemic shunt or esophageal transection is performed, carries with it high operative mortality and morbidity in patients who are unstable with actively bleeding varices. Such mortality and morbidity is too high in most (but not all[193, 194]) surgeons' experience to justify a surgical

approach.[195–198] Urgent surgery should be considered only if the less invasive forms of therapy previously described fail to control bleeding. The role of surgical therapy is more appropriate as a long-term measure to prevent recurrent bleeding.

The overall approach to a patient with actively bleeding varices should begin with injection sclerotherapy at the time of diagnostic endoscopy. If bleeding is not controlled, a trial of vasopressin and, if necessary, balloon tamponade is warranted. Percutaneous transhepatic obliteration, a more invasive procedure, is reserved for those who continue to bleed despite other measures, and urgent surgery should be the intervention of last resort.

Prevention of Recurrent Bleeding from Esophageal Varices. Once initial control of bleeding has been accomplished attention is turned to prevention of recurrent bleeding, both during hospitalization and over the long term. Until recently, the only available option was surgical decompression of the portal system.

Variceal-systemic shunts are designed to divert blood in esophageal and/or gastric veins from the high-pressure portal circulation to the low-pressure systemic circulation (Fig. 25–9). Experience with elective portacaval, splenorenal and mesocaval shunts (shunts that totally divert portal flow from the liver) has shown that the incidence of recurrent bleeding after shunt is substantially lower than if the shunt is not done. However, long-term survival does not improve,[199–202] even if the procedure is done prophylactically (with no prior history of bleeding).[203–205] Instead of dying with bleeding, patients who have shunts die with liver failure and encephalopathy, especially if they are poor-risk patients initially.[206] It has been suggested that those patients whose hepatic arterial circulation does not compensate for the loss of hepatic portal flow after shunting do less well than those in whom hepatic blood

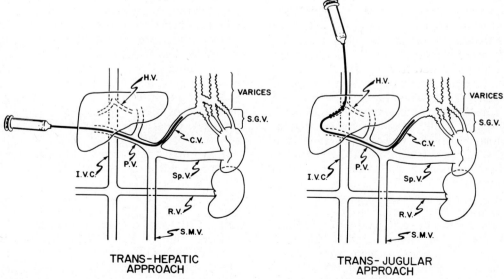

TRANS-HEPATIC
APPROACH

TRANS-JUGULAR
APPROACH

Figure 25–8. Diagrammatic representation of percutaneous transhepatic obliteration of esophageal varices. For key to abbreviations, see Color Figure 25–6 on page xxxiv.

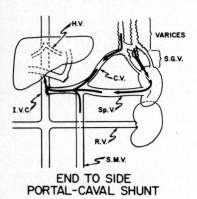

END TO SIDE
PORTAL-CAVAL SHUNT

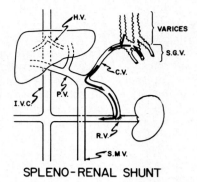

SPLENO-RENAL SHUNT

Figure 25–9. Variceal-systemic shunts. For key to abbreviations, see Figure 25–6.

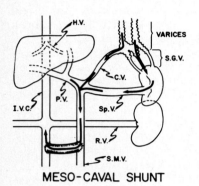

MESO-CAVAL SHUNT

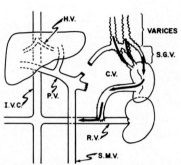

DISTAL SPLENO-RENAL SHUNT

flow is maintained after shunting.[207] Because total hepatic flow may be important, another type of shunt (the distal splenorenal shunt) was developed that decompresses only the veins of the esophagus and stomach.[208] Results with the selective distal splenorenal shunt (DSRS) have been mixed. As compared with mesocaval shunts, the DSRS is associated with fewer episodes of recurrent bleeding and postoperative encephalopathy.[209, 210] However, as compared with proximal splenorenal[211] or end-to-side portacaval[212, 213] shunts or with a variety of nonselective shunts,[214] there appears to be little advantage of the DSRS either in the incidence of recurrent variceal bleeding or in the development of encephalopathy. Indeed, in one study, the incidence of recurrent bleeding was *higher* in patients who had undergone DSRS.[213] In all six of these studies, survival was comparable between the two types (i.e., selective vs. nonselective) of shunts.[209–214] The primary factor in the development of encephalopathy and in survival is not the type of shunt, but rather the status of liver function, and, of course, consumption of or abstinence from alcohol in patients with alcoholic cirrhosis.

Repeated injection sclerotherapy has gained wide acceptance as an alternative to shunt surgery, offering the potential of prevention of recurrent variceal bleeding without the need for surgery and without the development of encephalopathy, which occurs when portal blood is diverted from the liver. Obliteration of varices occurs as repeated injections of sclerosant, using a variety of techniques[215, 216] and treatment sched-

ules,[217, 218] induce necrosis and fibrosis of variceal walls.[219] Analysis of randomized, controlled trials comparing repeated sclerotherapy to other nonsurgical regimens provides the following conclusions:

1. Recurrent variceal bleeding during the first two weeks of hospitalization appears to be reduced following sclerotherapy.[186, 220]

2. Complete obliteration of varices occurs only after a number of sessions of sclerotherapy, perhaps up to six weeks; before this occurs, recurrent variceal bleeding remains frequent.[221] Alterations in the frequency of sclerotherapy sessions (every week vs. every three weeks),[217, 218] use of supplemental variceal compression after sclerotherapy[216] or use of supplemental propranolol[222] does not reduce the frequency of bleeding prior to variceal obliteration.

3. Long-term follow-up of patients suggests that the incidence of recurrent variceal bleeding is moderately reduced, especially if variceal obliteration is accomplished.[221, 223–225]

The impact on survival of repeated sclerotherapy remains a point of contention.[186, 221, 223–226] When compared with results of "standard," nonsurgical therapy, early mortality with sclerotherapy was reduced in one study,[186] but not in two others.[220, 221] Late mortality (after variceal obliteration) was significantly improved in three studies[186, 221, 225] but not in two others.[223, 226] In the first group of studies,[186, 221, 225] recurrent variceal bleeding in the control group was managed without urgent sclerotherapy, whereas in the latter pair[223, 226] urgent sclerotherapy was included as therapy for all patients with rebleeding varices. In a sixth study,[224] control subjects who rebled were offered shunt surgery, and long-term survival in the sclerotherapy and control groups was not significantly different.

Three studies have compared results of sclerotherapy with those obtained with shunt surgery.[227–230] In one study,[227, 228] poor-risk (Child's Classification C) patients with severe bleeding were treated with sclerotherapy or early portacaval shunt. Although patients with shunts required more blood products during initial hospitalization and stayed in the hospital longer, patients who had sclerotherapy experienced late rebleeding more frequently, requiring frequent rehospitalization and transfusion. Survival, early and late, was similar in the two groups. In another study,[229] patients were stratified to "good risk" or "poor risk" groups based on modified Child's criteria and randomly assigned to medical/shunt therapy or sclerotherapy. Early and late prognoses were significantly dependent on severity of liver disease, but not on treatment. Results with sclerotherapy were comparable to those with medical/shunt therapy in good-risk patients, while outcome in patients with poor prognosis was somewhat worse in the sclerotherapy group. Finally, the originator of the DSRS is conducting a trial comparing DSRS against sclerotherapy followed by DSRS if sclerotherapy fails.[230] Preliminary results suggest that sclerotherapy backed up by DSRS provides significantly greater survival than DSRS alone.

Sclerotherapy is not without side effects.[230a] These include bacteremia,[231] acute respiratory failure,[232] pleural effusions,[233] esophageal ulcers,[234] at times leading to hemorrhage or fistulas,[235] and esophageal strictures.[236, 237] Strictures develop after repeated injections, and may be related in part to poor esophageal clearance of acid following sclerotherapy.[238, 239] Therapy to reduce gastric acidity may lower the incidence of stricture formation.[240]

Propranolol, a beta-adrenergic blocking agent, has been shown to lower portal pressure,[241, 242] most likely because of combined effects on both β_1 and β_2 adrenergic receptors. Selective blockade of β_1[243–245] or β_2[245] receptors alone has less influence on portal pressure than when both receptors are blocked. A randomized, controlled trial of propranolol (a nonselective blocking agent) in good-risk patients who had bled from varices suggested that both recurrent bleeding and mortality were reduced substantially.[246] Unfortunately, these results have not been confirmed in two other studies using propranolol[247, 248] and in one study using metoprolol, a β_1 selective antagonist.[249] One possible explanation for these results is that there may be marked variation from patient to patient in the portal-pressure response to propranolol.[250] Unless further data are more convincing, propranolol should not be used in patients who have bled from varices. An uncontrolled study suggests that propranolol reduces bleeding from congestive gastropathy.[250a]

Prophylactic Treatment to Prevent Variceal Bleeding. Because mortality after even one episode of variceal bleeding is so high, several prophylactic measures have been tried in an attempt to prevent bleeding and improve long-term survival. Prophylactic portacaval shunts prevented bleeding, but did not improve survival.[203–205] Operative mortality and postoperative hepatic dysfunction offset any benefit from the reduced incidence of bleeding. Prophylactic sclerotherapy was reported in two controlled studies to be remarkably effective in preventing initial variceal bleeding and reducing mortality.[251, 252] However, others have not found such good results,[253, 254] or imply that such results may depend on other factors such as hepatic reserve[255] or abstinence from alcohol.[256] Preliminary results in selected patients treated with prophylactic beta-adrenergic receptor blockade are promising,[257, 258] but require confirmation.[259]

In summary, therapeutic interventions to prevent bleeding or rebleeding have been shown in only a few instances to improve long-term survival of patients with esophageal or gastric varices, and such benefit is usually modest. In most patients, it is continuing liver failure that ultimately claims the patient, especially those with alcoholic cirrhosis who continue to drink. Recurrent bleeding and hepatic encephalopathy are issues more relative to quality of life, days spent in the hospital, and the drain on blood banks than to long-term survival. Until a more direct approach to the liver disease itself is devised, efforts at reducing recurrent variceal bleeding will provide only minimal long-term benefit to the patient.

Acute Hemorrhagic Gastritis

There are two common settings in which acute bleeding gastritis occurs. First, some patients present with bleeding gastritis caused by aspirin or other nonsteroidal anti-inflammatory agents (see p. 775), although recent series suggest that drug-induced gastritis is uncommon as a cause of major upper GI bleeding.[26, 260, 261] Recent case-controlled studies suggest that the overall increased risk of upper GI bleeding from nonsteroidal anti-inflammatory drugs is small.[261a, 261b, 261c] If bleeding does occur, it usually ceases spontaneously and mortality is relatively low.[152] A more important problem is that form of hemorrhagic gastritis which occurs in patients already hospitalized with some other underlying illness.[262] This entity ("stress gastritis"—see p. 785) has been reported to occur in about 20 per cent of patients in the face of sepsis, shock, burns, postoperative states, respiratory failure, and other major systemic disorders.[263–266] In patients admitted to medical intensive care units, there is a direct correlation between the need for, and duration of, ventilatory assistance and the incidence of bleeding gastritis.[267] Most patients who bleed from diffuse gastritis cease bleeding spontaneously, thus avoiding the need for invasive therapy.[263] If a patient continues to bleed from gastritis, surgery should be avoided if at all possible, since total gastrectomy is required and mortality with this operation is very high.[268] Medical therapy reported in uncontrolled observations to stop active bleeding from diffuse gastritis included antacids in enough volume to maintain gastric pH of 7.0[269] and prostaglandins,[270] although the latter are available only from pharmaceutical companies as investigational drugs. The preferred form of therapy for this entity is selective infusion of vasopressin or embolization of particulate matter via the left gastric artery.[87, 88, 91, 271–272] These procedures will produce cessation of bleeding in over 75 per cent of patients. It is re-emphasized that embolization and vasopressin, even selectively infused, are not without side effects, including gastric infarction.[273]

More important than the treatment of actively bleeding diffuse gastritis is the prevention of this lesion with prophylactic therapy. A number of well-performed studies have suggested that if antacids are given in sufficient doses to maintain gastric pH at a level of 4.0 to 5.0, the incidence of bleeding gastritis is virtually abolished.[263, 264, 274, 275] With the exception of studies treating patients with head trauma[266] or thermal injury,[276] trials using an H_2 receptor antagonist to reduce gastric acidity have yielded results that are less impressive than those reported with antacids.[264, 275, 277] This may relate to the definitions used for bleeding or may be because traditional regimens of H_2 blockers do not reliably raise and keep gastric pH above 4.0 to 5.0, especially in patients with sepsis.[105, 278–280] Constant infusions of H_2 blockers have been shown to achieve this goal[106, 107, 278] and, if so studied, might be as effective as antacids in preventing stress gastritis. A recent review suggests that cimetidine and antacids are equal in preventing clinically overt bleeding from stress ulcers.[280a]

A relatively inexpensive approach to prophylaxis is hourly administration of a potent magnesium and aluminum hydroxide antacid by nasogastric tube for patients at risk for stress bleeding. To ease the strain on nursing personnel this can be given as a constant drip at a rate of 20 to 60 ml per hour. If the pH cannot be maintained at 4.0 to 5.0, or if unacceptable levels of diarrhea ensue, an infusion of H_2 blocker can be begun in order to reduce the dose of antacids necessary to keep the pH at the desired level. It must be emphasized that even if bleeding from diffuse gastritis is prevented with such a prophylactic regimen, overall mortality in these patients in quite high because of their underlying illness.

Recent reports suggest that yet another approach to prevention of stress gastritis involves the use of sucralfate, 1 gm every 4 to 6 hours. Not only does such therapy appear to be as effective as antacid titration[281] but the incidence of nosocomial pneumonia in such patients may be lower than when antacids are used.[282, 283] Agents that raise gastric acidity may predispose to overgrowth, in the stomach, of bacteria, which can then be aspirated and lead to pneumonia.

Mallory-Weiss Tears

Arterial bleeding from an acute laceration of gastro-esophageal mucosa (Color Fig. 25–10, p. xxxiv)[284] accounts for at least 10 to 15 per cent of upper GI bleeding episodes.[260, 261, 285–287] Retching is often, but not always, implicated in Mallory-Weiss tears. An excessive intake of alcohol (with or without concomitant nonsteroidal anti-inflammatory drug ingestion) is noted in the majority of patients with this lesion. In most patients, bleeding ceases spontaneously and rebleeding is unusual. Unless rebleeding occurs, no specific therapy is necessary. For continuing bleeding, endoscopic thermal or angiographic therapy will succeed in many instances.[86–88, 288, 289] Rarely, direct oversewing of the bleeding lesion at surgery is necessary.

A similar syndrome, without a laceration but with mucosal erosions, has been described in a group of non-alcoholic patients who have an enhanced propensity to retch.[290]

Hematobilia

Causes of vascular-biliary fistulas include trauma, liver biopsy, cancer, hepatic artery aneurysm, hepatic abscess, and gallstones. The classic presentation is with upper GI bleeding accompanied by biliary colic and jaundice. The diagnosis is made endoscopically by the appearance of blood from the ampulla of Vater and/or by diagnostic hepatic arteriography. Therapy is with selective arterial catheterization[291, 292] or, if that fails, by hepatic artery ligation.

Neoplasms

Upper GI neoplasms are responsible for a very small proportion of acute upper GI bleeding episodes.[26, 260, 261] Occasionally, such lesions will continue to bleed and in some instances will prompt surgical intervention. Alternative therapy for patients with bleeding tumors include selective arterial embolization[293] (vasopressin will not work) or perhaps endoscopic thermal therapy.

Arterial-Enteric Fistulas

Aneurysms of the aorta or branches of the celiac artery may occasionally form a fistulous connection to the upper GI tract.[244, 295] Aortic aneurysms usually involve the duodenum, whereas aneurysms of the celiac branches (such as the splenic artery)[296] involve the stomach, duodenum, and liver. Aorto-enteric fistulas often produce a premonitory episode, or "herald bleed," hours to (occasionally) weeks before catastrophic hemorrhage,[294] and fistulas between smaller vessels and the intestine may cause recurrent bleeding for years.[295] Diagnosis of an aneurysm can be made only with a high index of suspicion and careful arteriography. Surgical resection is the therapy.

A more frequent circumstance is a fistula between a prosthetic aortic graft and the intestine (primarily duodenum, Fig. 25–11). These most commonly involve the proximal anastomosis of the graft and often have associated false aneurysms; localized infection may also play a role in some patients. As with primary aorto-duodenal fistulas, a "herald bleed" is common and may be accompanied by back pain.[296–299] Any patient with a prosthetic graft in place who presents with upper

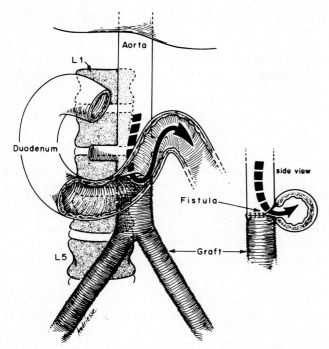

Figure 25–11. Schematic drawing of an aortoduodenal fistula communicating at the proximal anastomosis of an aortic graft. (From Case Records of the Massachusetts General Hospital #41–1977. Reprinted by permission of The New England Journal of Medicine 297:833, 1977.)

(or lower) GI bleeding must be assumed to have a fistula until proved otherwise. Endoscopy should be performed as soon as possible, although the fistula will be seen only occasionally.[300] More importantly, another bleeding lesion is sought; if none is found, it must be assumed that a fistula is present and surgery should be performed. Arteriography will only occasionally diagnose aorto-enteric fistulas (i.e., visualization of a false aneurysm or active bleeding) and therefore has no role in such patients if endoscopy reveals no other lesions. A positive arteriogram will only confirm the clinical decision to operate, while a negative examination is too unreliable to change the decision. It may be worth the effort to perform arteriography (even with a low yield) or radionuclide scanning[301] in patients in whom endoscopy detects another lesion, and a tentative decision has been made not to operate. In this case, a positive arteriogram would change the decision.

Vascular Anomalies

These are unusual causes of acute upper GI bleeding except in patients with chronic renal disease. They are discussed specifically on pages 413 to 415.

INITIAL MANAGEMENT AND DIAGNOSIS OF ACUTE LOWER GI BLEEDING

Three diagnostic techniques—colonoscopy, arteriography, and radionuclide scanning—have, during the

past 30 years, markedly changed the approach to the patient with lower GI bleeding. From the mid 1950s to the late 1960s, patients with acute massive or recurrent lower GI bleeding often underwent segmental left colectomy. This was based on the belief that diverticulosis accounted for most bleeding episodes and for the fact that most diverticula are in the left colon. This approach resulted in a 50 per cent incidence of recurrent bleeding and, in patients with massive bleeding, a mortality of about 20 per cent.[302, 303] Obviously, many patients were bleeding from the right colon or above. Therefore, surgeons turned to more radical subtotal colectomy with ileoproctostomy. While the incidence of recurrent bleeding fell, mortality was still about 10 per cent.[302, 303] Today, precise localization obtained from newer diagnostic procedures allows the surgeon once again to perform segmental resections, but now many of them involve the right colon and often the lesion is not a diverticulum. Postoperative rebleeding is negligible and mortality with massive bleeding is 5 per cent or lower.[304]

Improved management of patients with lower GI bleeding has come about for several reasons:

1. *Selective mesenteric arteriography* in patients with massive, continuing hemorrhage localizes the precise area of the bowel that is bleeding. In the case of diverticula, this is from the right colon in a majority of cases,[303-312] one reason that segmental left hemicolectomy in the past was often unsuccessful. In other instances, bleeding is from a colonic lesion other than a diverticulum, or from a noncolonic lesion such as a duodenal ulcer or small bowel tumor.[311] Blind subtotal colectomy should seldom be performed to control lower GI bleeding; blind left hemicolectomy should never be done.

2. *Infusion of vasopressin* or embolization of a substance such as Gelfoam through an angiographic catheter will, in many instances, stem the tide of active bleeding.[306, 312-314] In some patients this cessation is permanent, obviating the need for surgery, while in others it at least stabilizes the patient until an elective operation can be performed.

3. A previously unappreciated entity, *angiodysplasia,* has been increasingly detected by arteriography and colonoscopy. These often subtle vascular anomalies, which occur most frequently in the cecum, undoubtedly accounted for many cases of acute or chronic bleeding that were attributed in the past to diverticulosis. They are another reason that blind left hemicolectomy was associated with such a high incidence of failure.

4. In patients with lower GI bleeding in whom a barium enema is negative or shows only diverticulosis, *colonoscopy* detects a lesion, including carcinoma, about 40 per cent of the time.[315-319] Before the widespread use of colonoscopy, such patients may have been sent home with no diagnosis or a diagnosis of bleeding diverticula; some would have undergone blind left hemicolectomy. Colonoscopy also permits the option of applying thermal coagulative therapy to certain vascular anomalies.[319]

Diagnostic Approach to Acute Lower GI Bleeding

History and Physical Examination. Important information includes a history of hemorrhoids or inflammatory bowel disease. Has there been pain or diarrhea (colitis)? Has there been weight loss or change in bowel habits (colon cancer)? Physical examination should include a search for skin lesions associated with inflammatory bowel disease, or an abdominal mass. Is there a mass on rectal examination? It has recently been suggested that the presence of perianal skin tags is predictive of colorectal adenomas, although this remains controversial (see pp. 1483–1518).

Anoscopy and Sigmoidoscopy. Every patient with presumed lower GI bleeding should undergo early anoscopy (an often underutilized diagnostic tool)[320, 321] and sigmoidoscopy for the detection of obvious, low-lying lesions such as bleeding hemorrhoids, anal fissure, rectal ulcer, colitis, or rectal cancer. The procedure is difficult when bleeding is brisk, and it is often impossible to tell whether blood is coming from above the sigmoidoscope or is refluxing from a lesion below. Because most patients with lower GI bleeding will undergo colonoscopy (see below), use of the longer 60-cm flexible sigmoidoscope is seldom indicated.

Exclusion of Upper GI Source. If a definite diagnosis is not made on anoscopy/sigmoidoscopy, an upper GI lesion should be sought by nasogastric aspiration before more invasive lower GI procedures are undertaken. It should be remembered that an actively bleeding duodenal ulcer or aortoduodenal fistula may produce hematochezia without a positive nasogastric aspirate. Even when bowel sounds are not hyperactive and the BUN is not elevated, any suspicion of an upper GI source should prompt endoscopy, especially if arteriography is imminent.

Barium Enema. Contrast studies of the colon have no place in the management of ongoing lower GI bleeding. Not only may the bleeding lesion be missed, but the results may be misleading if only diverticula are seen. Furthermore, a colon full of barium makes subsequent arteriography difficult. If bleeding ceases, which is the usual case, a double-contrast barium enema several days later may be a helpful procedure, although most physicians now believe that colonoscopy is the preferred diagnostic procedure. There are three reasons for such a preference: First, barium enema does not detect vascular anomalies, a frequent cause of lower GI bleeding. Second, the barium enema may occasionally fail to diagnose the presence of a malignant lesion.[315–317, 322] Third, even if a suspicious lesion is seen, colonoscopy is often required to provide biopsy material and seek synchronous lesions. Thus, in most patients, colonoscopy will be performed regardless of the results of a barium enema.

Colonoscopy. Colonoscopy is the procedure of choice in patients with lower GI bleeding, unless bleeding is too massive or unless anoscopy or sigmoidoscopy has disclosed an obvious actively bleeding lesion. Presence of non-bleeding hemorrhoids must not deter the physician from seeking another, more proximal lesion, especially in patients over the age of 40.[322, 323] Colonoscopy offers the most direct way to visualize the colonic mucosa and can even be performed in patients who are actively, although not massively, bleeding.[324] It has been clearly shown that colonoscopy in patients with acute lower GI bleeding that has ceased, and in whom a barium enema is negative or shows only diverticulosis, will detect a substantial number of important lesions.[315–319, 322, 323] These lesions include cancer, colitis, and angiodysplasia.

Arteriography. There are two situations in which diagnostic arteriography is helpful. First, in the patient who is hemorrhaging massively, arteriography can reveal the site of bleeding (i.e., right or left colon, small bowel, upper GI tract) and in some instances can indicate whether the lesion is a diverticulum, a vascular anomaly, a cancer, or peptic ulcer. Beyond directing the surgeon to the correct location for the correct operation, selective arteriography permits infusion of vasopressin or embolization of particulate material directly into the bleeding artery. The most common causes of lower GI bleeding diagnosed by arteriography are diverticulosis and angiodysplasia.[303, 304, 308–314, 325, 326] Other lesions include peptic ulcer disease in 5 to 10 per cent of massive lower GI bleeding, Meckel's diverticula, neoplasms, and vascular-enteric fistulas.

Second, arteriography may define lesions with abnormal vasculature even if extravasation of contrast material is not noted. This is useful in patients with acute massive bleeding that has slowed by the time of arteriography or in patients with recurrent bouts of acute bleeding in whom a diagnosis has been difficult to define. Lesions likely to be found in this situation include ileocolic angiodysplasia, small bowel vascular anomalies, and small bowel tumors.[310, 311]

Radionuclide Scanning. An increasingly utilized diagnostic test in patients with acute lower GI bleeding consists of the use of an external gammacounter to detect intestinal extravasation of intravenously administered technetium-99 (Tc-99). Tc-99 sulfur colloid is an effective means of detecting ongoing bleeding, even if the rate of bleeding is slower than would be detected by arteriography.[327–329] It is thus a good screening technique before a patient is sent for visceral angiography. Tc-99 sulfur colloid, however, is cleared rapidly, by the liver and spleen, which makes it a poor means of detecting intermittent bleeding or bleeding in the upper abdomen.[330] Therefore, Tc-99 has been employed to label albumin[331] or red blood cells,[332–339] which then act as a blood pool scan. The benefit of this approach is that the abdomen can be scanned over a prolonged period of time to permit accumulation at a bleeding site of enough isotope to be detected by the counter. As with Tc-99 sulfur colloid, bleeding can be detected at rates that are too slow for detection by traditional angiography. Furthermore, many physicians use the Tc-99–labeled red cell scan prior to arteriography. If there is no evidence of bleeding by this study, the yield of arteriography is very low.[334] If an active site of bleeding is seen, it directs the arteriographer to the most likely source of bleeding. If subsequent arteriography is negative, implying that bleeding has slowed substantially, the radionuclide scan will provide clues for subsequent colonoscopy and even, at times, for surgical therapy.

Another use of radionuclide scanning is to detect Meckel's diverticula. In this situation, Tc-99 pertechnetate is taken up by ectopic gastric mucosa present in most Meckel's diverticula that bleed[340–343] (see p. 416).

Overall Diagnostic Approach. Anoscopy, sigmoidoscopy, and nasogastric aspiration should be performed. If no obvious bleeding site is found, and if the patient continues to bleed, the following sequence is recommended:

1. Perform upper GI endoscopy to exclude an upper GI lesion.

2. Perform a Tc-99–tagged red cell scan.

3. If bleeding slows sufficiently, perform colonoscopy after a fluid purge.

4. If bleeding remains brisk, perform mesenteric arteriography beginning with the artery most likely to be bleeding based on the tagged red cell scan. If the tagged red cell scan is unrevealing and bleeding continues, begin with the superior mesenteric artery since most lesions will be found in the right colon. If necessary, the inferior mesenteric and celiac arteries must also be injected.

5. If extravasation of contrast is seen, infuse vasopressin or consider embolization therapy. If bleeding continues despite vasopressin or embolization, surgery should be performed before blood losses become too great. If bleeding ceases, the decision regarding elective surgery can be made after further evaluation.

6. If no extravasation is noted but severe bleeding continues, exploratory laparotomy may be needed. In this instance, the results of a tagged red cell may be of help in leading the surgeon to the correct location.

If bleeding ceases spontaneously (which occurs the majority of the time) a different approach is warranted:

1. Colonoscopy should be performed at the earliest possible time.

2. If colonoscopy discloses no lesion, consideration should be given to performing a barium enema.

3. If results of colonoscopy and barium enema are negative, an upper GI or small bowel source must be excluded. This can be done with upper endoscopy and a small bowel series. If no source is found, and this is the patient's first episode of lower GI bleeding, no further diagnostic tests should be performed at this time (see p. 416).

APPROACH TO SPECIFIC LOWER GI BLEEDING LESIONS

Diverticulosis

Bleeding occurs in only a small proportion of patients with diverticulosis,[302] but because the entity itself is so common, diverticulosis accounts for about 50 per cent of the cases of lower GI bleeding severe enough to warrant arteriographic examination.[314] Bleeding is ab-

rupt in onset, painless, usually massive, and often from the right colon.[307, 308] In 20 per cent of patients bleeding will continue; in 20 per cent bleeding will cease, but subsequently recur in the hospital; and in the remaining 60 per cent, bleeding will cease and not recur.[311] For those with active bleeding, selective mesenteric arteriography locates the site and, if vasopressin is infused, the bleeding will cease at least temporarily in the majority of patients (Fig. 25–12).[306, 312, 314] About 50 per cent of these patients will rebleed and require further therapy.[314] Surgery (segmental resection) is reserved for patients who do not respond to angiographic therapy, who rebleed in the hospital, or who have had prior episodes of documented diverticular bleeding. Caution must be used in operating on such patients without angiographic or colonoscopic documentation of the precise bleeding site.

Bleeding from diverticula is believed to occur after years of pressure on a penetrating colonic artery by the dome of the diverticular pouch (see pp. 1424–1426). With time, there is eccentric breakthrough of the vessel, which ruptures into the diverticular sac. Since the artery is large, bleeding tends to be copious. Since the artery is single, bleeding usually does not recur if a thrombus forms and becomes firmly affixed to the vessel wall. Chronic, minor bleeding is not a feature of diverticulosis.[344]

Angiodysplasia

Angiodysplasias (or vascular ectasias) have become an increasingly well-recognized cause of acute lower GI bleeding.[345–350] They occur almost exclusively in older patients (thus they are probably acquired rather than congenital lesions) and they are most often noted in the cecum and ascending colon. There is a well-recognized association between such lesions and aortic stenosis.[348, 351, 352]

The arteriographic criteria of angiodysplasia include clusters of small arteries, visualization of a vascular tuft, and early and prolonged opacification of a draining vein, usually the ileocolic vein (Fig. 25–13).[345] Only occasionally will bleeding be brisk enough or persistent enough for extravasation of contrast material to be noted.[313] Colonoscopically, angiodysplasias are flat, bright red, and fern-like (Color Fig. 25–14, p. xxxiv).[349, 350]

Angiodysplasias are seen grossly and histologically at the pathology table only with meticulous examination and careful sectioning, and even then lesions may be overlooked. Determination of histologic characteristics has necessitated injection of the blood vessels of resected specimens with silicone rubber.[353] Most prominent, and earliest, findings are submucosal where there are ectatic and tortuous veins.[354] Submucosal arteries are usually normal. In most instances there are also abnormal mucosal vessels, from just a few ectatic capillary rings surrounding the crypts to large "coral reef–like" lesions. In the most advanced lesions these ectatic vessels constitute the bulk of the mucosa and are not protected by colonic epithelium from potential rupture.

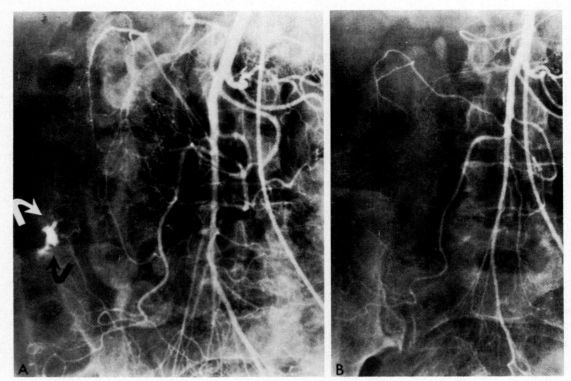

Figure 25–12. Massive bleeding from diverticulum of the right colon controlled with vasopressin infusion into the mesenteric artery. *A,* Superior mesenteric arteriogram shows extravasation in the ascending colon *(arrow)* from a branch of the ileocolic artery. *B,* Repeat mesenteric arteriogram after 20 minutes of vasopressin infusion at 0.2 units per minute into the mesenteric artery shows constriction of the mesenteric arterial branches and no extravasation. (From Athanasoulis, C. A., Waltman, A. C., Novelline, R. A., et al. Radiol. Clin. North Am. *14*:275, 1976. Used by permission.)

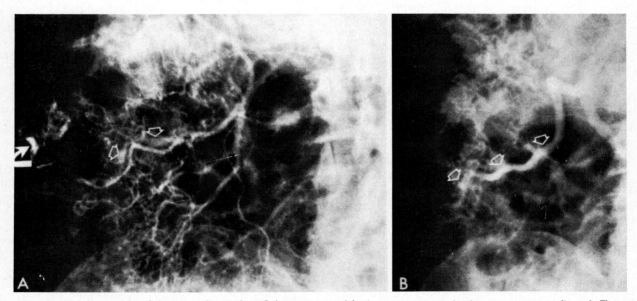

Figure 25–13. Vascular ectasia of the ascending colon. Colonoscopy and barium enema examinations were unrevealing. *A,* The arterial phase of a superior mesenteric arteriogram shows accumulation of contrast medium in a vascular space along the antimesenteric border of the ascending colon *(curved arrow)* and early opacification of a draining vein *(straight open arrows)*. *B,* During the late phase of the mesenteric arteriogram there is persistent intense opacification of the same draining vein *(arrows)*. (From Athanasoulis, C. A., Waltman, A. C., Novelline, R. A., et al. Radiol. Clin. North Am. *14*:277, 1976. Used by permission.)

There is no proven etiology for angiodysplasia. According to one theory, there is chronic low-grade obstruction of submucosal colonic veins where they traverse the muscularis propria.[346] This results in, first, ectasia of submucosal vessels, followed by dilatation of mucosal venules and capillaries, and finally loss of precapillary sphincters, producing small arterial-venous shunts. However, the suggestion that replacement of stenotic aortic valves results in resolution of angiodysplasia casts doubt on the theory.[355]

Clinically, bleeding from angiodysplasias is usually self-limited, but chronic or recurrent. Those few patients who bleed massively may demonstrate extravasation of arteriographic contrast material and may respond to vasopressin or transcatheter embolization.[356] In most situations, however, there is no evidence of active bleeding and no proof that arteriographically documented angiodysplasia is the actual source of bleeding. Boley and coworkers found submucosal ectasias in 8 of 15 elderly patients without GI bleeding, and in 4 of these 8 there were also mucosal ectasias.[346] Thus, these lesions are probably very common, producing bleeding only in those individuals with more striking mucosal involvement.

How, then, should these patients be managed? Other lesions (such as carcinoma of the colon, small bowel tumors, or upper GI lesions) must be excluded, and bleeding must be important enough to warrant therapy (i.e., chronic anemia, transfusion requirements). If treatment is indicated, there are three approaches. First, if aortic stenosis is present, and if valve replacement is to be performed, other measures to treat angiodysplasia should be postponed until it can be seen if the lesions regress. Second, isolated lesions can be ablated with endoscopic thermal coagulation.[349, 357–359] Third, patients in whom endoscopic therapy cannot be performed or fails, and in whom right-sided colonic bleeding has been documented by tagged red cell scan or by arteriography, should undergo right hemicolectomy. Even if the bleeding site has not been clearly documented, and even if left-sided diverticula are present, right hemicolectomy in patients with right colon angiodysplasia will usually prevent further bleeding.[345, 347]

Neoplasms

Neoplasms do not often produce exsanguinating hemorrhage, but rather tend to present with chronic, occult bleeding or with intermittent bouts of acute, self-limited bleeding. Small bowel tumors are rare and relatively inaccessible; arteriography is needed in many cases. Colon cancer is common and is usually diagnosed by colonoscopy or barium enema (see pp. 1519–1560).

Other Lesions

Hemorrhoids are probably the most common cause of lower GI bleeding. However, bleeding usually occurs only in the form of intermittent episodes, producing small amounts of bright red blood on the outside of formed stool or on toilet tissue. Only occasionally will massive bleeding occur. Treatment for hemorrhoids is with sitz baths, lubricating suppositories, and stool softeners. If problems continue, definitive therapy may be required. *Meckel's diverticulum* is a frequent cause of acute lower GI bleeding in children, although the lesion may also be a cause of bleeding in young adults.[360] Bleeding is usually a result of ulceration of intestinal mucosa adjacent to an area of ectopic gastric mucosa that produces hydrochloric acid. Diagnosis is made at surgery, prompted primarily by the results of radionuclide scanning,[340–343] although occasionally arteriography will disclose active bleeding[360] or a small bowel series will disclose the diverticulum.[361] Management of bleeding from *ischemic bowel disease* or *inflammatory bowel disease* is individualized and, depending on the clinical course and the severity of the basic disease, may require surgery. *Solitary ulcers of the rectum and cecum,* the latter especially in patients with renal failure,[362, 363] occasionally cause lower GI bleeding. Nonprosthetic *arterial enteric fistulas* occur in the small bowel and colon;[364] as with upper GI lesions, diagnosis is by arteriography. *Intussusception* is almost always accompanied by crampy abdominal pain, during which a plain film of the abdomen or small bowel barium x-ray may be helpful. Stools in such patients have color and consistency reminiscent of currant jelly.

OCCULT GI BLEEDING

For purposes of this discussion, occult bleeding refers to bleeding manifested only by a positive chemical test for stool blood, iron deficiency anemia, or an iron deficiency state. A discussion of fecal occult blood testing can be found on page 1538.

One important cause of chronic occult bleeding is gastroduodenal damage by various drugs (see p. 775). While it is true that a number of nonsteroidal anti-inflammatory drugs can produce occult gastrointestinal bleeding, one must be cautious, for two reasons, in ascribing bleeding to these drugs. First, the degree of bleeding produced by nonsteroidal anti-inflammatory drugs is usually mild, producing amounts of blood loss that are usually undetectable by standard fecal occult blood tests such as Hemoccult.[365, 366] Second, it has been shown that thorough evaluation of patients who are taking nonsteroidal anti-inflammatory drugs and have Hemoccult-positive stools will often disclose important lesions such as colonic carcinoma.[366, 367] Because such cancers are potentially curable, it is important that they not be overlooked. It should also be remembered that patients who bleed while taking anticoagulant drugs are often bleeding from important intestinal lesions.[367a]

Unless a patient has upper gastrointestinal symptoms, evaluation of occult bleeding should begin with evaluation of the colon. This usually consists of early colonoscopy, a more sensitive diagnostic test than barium enema.[368, 369] At the least, work-up should consist of sigmoidoscopy, preferably using a 60-cm flexible sigmoidoscope to exclude rectosigmoid lesions, in addition to a high-quality double-contrast barium enema.[370] If evaluation of the colon is unrewarding, evaluation of the upper GI tract should be performed, employing endoscopy and/or barium contrast studies of the stomach and small bowel.

GI BLEEDING OF "OBSCURE" ORIGIN

Obscure bleeding may be defined as recurrent bouts of acute bleeding or chronic bleeding for which no definite source has been discovered by routine endoscopic and x-ray contrast studies.[371, 371a] There are at least four reasons why such a source of bleeding may be difficult to discover. First, a lesion may be found by standard diagnostic techniques but cannot be said with assurance to be the definite source of bleeding. This occurs when a lesion is found in conjunction with other potential lesions. For example, angiodysplasia of the cecum may be found in a subject with widespread colonic diverticula. In these situations, it is essential that before therapeutic decisions are made, the lesion be documented to bleed by direct inspection (endoscopy/colonoscopy), arteriography, or a radionuclide scan. Second, a bleeding lesion may be in an area that is difficult to evaluate by standard diagnostic tests. This situation includes lesions that may be present in long afferent loops following gastrojejunostomy or lesions that are present in the small bowel. Third, some lesions are difficult to diagnose because their appearance is subtle, because the lesion is an unusual one with which a physician may not be familiar, or because the lesion is in an atypical location. Finally, lesions with minimal mucosal extension may be virtually impossible to detect unless active bleeding is seen endoscopically or there is a characteristic angiographic pattern.

In patients with a suspected upper GI source of bleeding in whom standard endoscopy fails to disclose a lesion, it may at times be helpful to utilize a longer endoscope, such as a pediatric-size colonoscope. This will permit inspection of the entire duodenum and part of the jejunum. In addition, this procedure enables a complete view of the afferent loop in patients with gastrojejunostomy.

If no upper GI or colonic source of bleeding has been found, a small bowel tumor or Meckel's diverticulum should next be sought. In younger patients a Tc-99 pertechnetate scan will often disclose the presence of ectopic gastric mucosa in a Meckel's diverticulum.[340–343] A small bowel infusion X-ray[372–373] is performed to exclude a malignancy, although it will occasionally also detect Meckel's diverticula. At this point asymptomatic patients with bleeding that requires no blood transfusion or who respond to oral iron supplements need not undergo further investigations.

If a patient has recurrent acute or chronic bleeding such that transfusions are necessary or there is need for repeated hospitalization, further investigative procedures are warranted. Radionuclide scanning is noninvasive and readily available. It can be used either in the chronic bleeder or in the patient who is repeatedly admitted to the hospital with acute bleeding episodes.[374–376] Mesenteric arteriography should be carried out in every patient for whom exploratory laparotomy is being considered.[377–379] Not only can arteriography confirm a positive radionuclide scan, but it may disclose vascular anomalies or tumor vessels even if bleeding is not active.

Surgery is usually reserved for removal of a previously diagnosed bleeding lesion that has not responded to, or cannot be treated by, nonoperative measures. Occasionally, however, exploratory laparotomy must be utilized as a diagnostic tool. If so, intraoperative endoscopy or radionuclide scanning may assist the surgeon.[376, 380–382]

Causes of Obscure Bleeding

Causes of obscure GI bleeding include neoplasms of the small bowel, vascular anomalies, elastic tissue disorders such as pseudoxanthoma elasticum[383] and Ehlers-Danlos syndrome,[384] vasculitis syndromes, and amyloidosis (Table 25–2). It is now recognized that vascular anomalies (excluding hemangiomas, which are neoplasms) are the most frequent cause of obscure GI bleeding.[377, 379] There is confusion over nomenclature of these lesions, but for clinical purposes they may be divided into two broad groups, those with and those without associated skin lesions.

Vascular Anomalies with Associated Skin Lesions. These include rare entities such as the hereditary syndromes of Rendu-Osler-Weber (hereditary hemorrhagic telangiectasia),[385–387] the blue rubber bleb nevus syndrome, and the acquired CRST syndrome. Lesions are found throughout the GI tract and are usually visible endoscopically. Surgical resection is at times performed, but since the lesions are often multiple and diffuse, endoscopic thermal coagulation may be a safer way to proceed.[385, 387, 388] However, even with such therapy, it is often impossible to ablate all such lesions. Furthermore, these procedures are not without complications and at times the endoscopic therapy may actually induce bleeding.

Vascular Anomalies without Associated Skin Lesions. The frequency of these lesions was unappreciated until the advent of selective mesenteric angiography.[389] It appears that there are two subgroups of vascular anomalies without associated skin lesions.[390] They are similar arteriographically, and each is difficult to see with the naked eye. They differ in terms of histology, typical location in the GI tract, age of patients in whom they are found, and probable etiology.[354, 391, 392]

The more common of the two vascular anomalies are the *vascular ectasias* (angiodysplasias), which have been discussed on pages 413 to 415. When they are present in the cecum and ascending colon, they are somewhat easier to diagnose, although proof that they have actually bled is sometimes not at hand. Such lesions are found less often in the stomach and small bowel[385, 393, 394] and at times, therefore, present a diag-

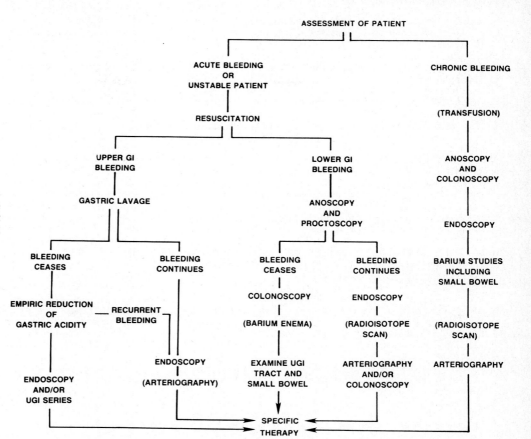

ASSESSMENT OF PATIENT

Figure 25–15. Algorithm of management after assessment of the patient. Parentheses indicate that procedure is optional depending on the clinical situation.

nostic dilemma. Therapy is similar to that for lesions found in the colon.[385, 387, 393] Vascular ectasias are frequently found in bleeding patients with underlying chronic renal failure,[395] and preliminary data suggest that estrogen and progesterone may be used to treat such patients.[396, 397]

A variant of antral vascular ectasias is the "watermelon stomach."[398–400] This lesion gives a distinctive endoscopic picture (Fig. 25–14) and appears to be successfully treated only with antrectomy. A recent abstract reports 12 patients with "watermelon stomach" who were successfully treated with the heater probe.[400a] A lesion similar in endoscopic appearance, but not a vascular anomaly, has been described in proximal gastric folds of patients with large hiatal hernias.[401]

The less common of the vascular anomalies without associated skin lesions, accounting for less than 20 per cent of vascular anomalies, are the true *arteriovenous malformations*. These consist of dilated, thick-walled arteries and nondilated, thick-walled ("arterialized") veins that communicate with each other.[354] They may be found throughout the GI tract but are most frequent in the upper intestine.[402–404] Because they are often found in younger patients, their etiology is believed to be congenital. Diagnosis is by arteriography and, at times, endoscopy. Although poor-risk patients may respond to arterial embolization, most are treated with segmental resection. Endoscopic transillumination of the bowel may assist the surgeon in localizing the lesion.

A lesion that is similar endoscopically to an arteriovenous malformation is *Dieulafoy's ulcer*.[405–408] This lesion is a single, small, superficial, easily overlooked defect of the mucosa that involves an otherwise normal, but ectatic, submucosal artery. Although there is some polymorphonuclear leukocyte infiltration, the lesion is not felt to represent a primary ulcerative process. Rather, the vessel over time produces pressure erosion of the epithelium and ultimately ruptures into the stomach. Although this lesion is rare, bleeding can be massive and surgical intervention is usually needed. Similar lesions have been found in the small intestine and the colon.[409]

OVERALL APPROACH TO THE PATIENT WITH GASTROINTESTINAL BLEEDING

Figure 25–15 is an algorithm of management based upon the results following initial patient assessment and summarizes the approach discussed in previous sections.

References

1. Ebert, R. V., Stead, E. A., and Gibson, J. G. Response of normal subjects to acute blood loss. Arch. Intern. Med. *68*:578, 1941.
2. Northfield, T. C., and Smith, T. Haematemesis as an index of blood loss. Lancet *1*:990, 1971.
3. Hilsman, J. H. The color of blood-containing feces following the instillation of citrated blood at various levels of the small intestine. Gastroenterology *15*:131, 1950.

4. Wara, P., and Stodkilde, H. Bleeding pattern before admission as guideline for emergency endoscopy. Scand. J. Gastroenterol. 20:72, 1985.

5. Howarth, S., and Sharpey-Schafer, E. P. Low blood-pressure phases following haemorrhage. Lancet 1:18, 1947.

6. Sander-Jensen, K., Secher, N. H., Bie, P., Warberg, J., and Schwartz, T. W. Vagal slowing of the heart during haemorrhage: observations from 20 consecutive hypotensive patients. Br. Med. J. 292:364, 1986.

7. Martin, D. J., Lucas, C. E., Ledgerwood, A. M., Hoschner, J., McGonigal, M. D., and Grabow, D. Fresh frozen plasma supplement to massive red blood cell transfusion. Ann. Surg. 202:505, 1985.

8. Sampliner, R. E., Mobarhan, S., King, D. M., Greenberg, M. S., Iber, F. L., and Grace, N. D. Use of blood component therapy for gastrointestinal bleeding in patients with cirrhosis of the liver. Johns Hopkins Med. J. 136:163, 1975.

9. Luke, R. G., Lees, W., and Rudick, J. Appearances of the stools after the introduction of blood into the caecum. Gut 5:77, 1964.

10. Schiff, L., Stevens, R. J., Shapiro, N., and Goodman, S. Observations on the oral administration of citrated blood in man. Am. J. Med. Sci. 203:409, 1942.

11. Tedesco, F. J., Pickens, C. A., Griffin, J. W., Sivak, M. V., and Sullivan, B. H. Role of colonoscopy in patients with unexplained melena: Analysis of 53 patients. Gastrointest. Endosc. 26:78, 1980.

12. Luk, G. D., Bynum, T. E., and Hendrix, T. R. Gastric aspiration in localization of gastrointestinal hemorrhage. JAMA 241:576, 1979.

13. Layne, E. A., Mellow, M. H., and Lipman, T. O. Insensitivity of guaiac slide tests for detection of blood in gastric juice. Ann. Intern. Med. 94:774, 1981.

14. Snook, J. A., Holdstock, G. E., and Bamforth, J. Value of a simple biochemical ratio in distinguishing upper and lower sites of gastrointestinal haemorrhage. Lancet 2:1064, 1986.

15. Pumphrey, C. W., and Beck, E. R. Raised blood urea concentration indicates considerable blood loss in acute upper gastrointestinal haemorrhage. Br. Med. J. 1:527, 1980.

16. Stellato, T., Rhodes, R. S., and McDougal, W. S. Azotemia in upper gastrointestinal hemorrhage. Am. J. Gastroenterol. 73:486, 1980.

17. Elashoff, J. D., and Grossman, M. I. Trends in hospital admissions and death rates for peptic ulcer in the United States from 1970 to 1978. Gastroenterology 78:280, 1980.

18. Cutter, J. A., and Mendeloff, A. I. Upper gastrointestinal bleeding: nature and magnitude of the problem in the U. S. Dig. Dis. Sci. 26(Suppl):90, 1981.

19. Silverstein, F. E., Gilbert, D. A., Tedesco, F. J., Buenger, N. K., and Persing, J. The national ASGE survey on upper gastrointestinal bleeding. I. Study design and baseline data. Gastrointest. Endosc. 27:73, 1981.

20. Allan, R., and Dykes, P. A study of the factors influencing mortality rates from gastrointestinal haemorrhage. Q. J. Med. 180:533, 1976.

21. Schiller, K. F. R., Truelove, S. C., and Williams, D. G. Haematemesis and melaena, with special reference to factors influencing the outcome. Br. Med. J. 2:7, 1970.

22. Schiller, K. F. R., and Cotton, P. B. Acute upper gastrointestinal haemorrhage. Clin. Gastroenterol. 7:595, 1978.

23. Kang, J. Y., and Piper, D. W. Improvement in mortality rates in bleeding peptic ulcer disease. Med. J. Aust. 1:213, 1980.

24. Jones, F. A. Hematemesis and melena. With special reference to causation and to factors influencing the mortality from bleeding peptic ulcers. Gastroenterology 30:166, 1956.

25. Fleischer, D. Etiology and prevalence of severe persistent upper gastrointestinal bleeding. Gastroenterology 84:538, 1983.

26. Peterson, W. L., Barnett, C. C., Smith, H. J., Allen, M. H., and Corbett, D. B. Routine early endoscopy in upper-gastrointestinal-tract bleeding. N. Engl. J. Med. 304:925, 1981.

27. Jones, P. F., Johnson, S. J., McEwan, A. B., Kyle, J., and Needham, C. D. Further haemorrhage after admission to hospital for gastrointestinal haemorrhage. Br. Med. J. 3:660, 1973.

28. Silverstein, F. E., Gilbert, D. A., Tedesco, F. J., Buenger, N.

K., and Persing, J. The national ASGE survey on upper gastrointestinal bleeding. II. Clinical prognostic factors. Gastrointest. Endosc. 27:80, 1981.

29. Waterman, N. G., and Walker, J. L. Effect of a topical adrenergic agent on gastric blood flow. Am. J. Surg. 127:241, 1974.

30. Ponsky, J. L., Hoffman, M., and Swayngim, D. S. Saline irrigation in gastric hemorrhage: The effect of temperature. J. Surg. Res. 28:204, 1980.

31. Gilbert, D. A., Saunders, D. R., Peoples, J., Sillery, J., and Gulascik, C. Failure of iced saline lavage to suppress hemorrhage from experimental bleeding ulcers. Gastroenterology 76:1138, 1979.

32. Bryant, L. R., Mobin-Uddin, K., Dillon, M. L., and Griffen, W. O. Comparison of ice water with iced saline solution for gastric lavage in gastroduodenal hemorrhage. Am. J. Surg. 124:570, 1972.

33. Kiselow, M. C., and Wagner, M. Intragastric instillation of levarterenol. Arch. Surg. 107:387, 1973.

34. Douglass, H. O. Levarterenol irrigation. Control of massive gastrointestinal bleeding in poor-risk patients. JAMA 230:23, 1974.

35. Wapnick, S., Leveen, E., Grosberg, S., and Leveen, H. H. Levarterenol for gastrointestinal and intraoperative bleeding. N.Y. State J. Med. 76:1963, 1976.

36. Katon, R. M., and Smith, F. W. Panendoscopy in the early diagnosis of acute upper gastrointestinal bleeding. Gastroenterology 65:728, 1973.

37. Keller, R. T., and Logan, G. M. Comparison of emergent endoscopy and upper gastrointestinal series radiography in acute upper gastrointestinal haemorrhage. Gut 17:180, 1976.

38. McGinn, F. P., Guyer, P. B., Wilken, B. J., and Steer, H. W. A prospective comparative trial between early endoscopy and radiology in acute upper gastrointestinal haemorrhage. Gut 16:707, 1975.

39. Morris, D. W., Levine, G. M., Soloway, R. D., Miller, W. T., and Marin, G. A. Prospective, randomized study of diagnosis and outcome in acute upper-gastrointestinal bleeding: endoscopy versus conventional radiography. Am. J. Dig. Dis. 20:1103, 1975.

40. Allan, R. N., Dykes, P. W., and Toye, D. K. M. Diagnostic accuracy of early radiology in acute gastrointestinal haemorrhage. Br. Med. J. 4:281, 1972.

41. Fraser, G. M. The double contrast barium meal in patients with acute upper gastrointestinal bleeding. Clin. Radiol. 29:625, 1978.

42. Stevenson, G. W., Cox, R. R., and Roberts, C. J. C. Prospective comparison of double-contrast barium meal examination and fiberoptic endoscopy in acute upper gastrointestinal hemorrhage. Br. Med. J. 2:723, 1976.

43. Dronfield, M. W., Langman, M. J. S., Atkinson, M., Balfour, T. W., Bell, G. D., Vellacott, K. D., Amar, S. S., and Knapp, D. R. Outcome of endoscopy and barium radiography for acute upper gastrointestinal bleeding: controlled trial in 1037 patients. Br. Med. J. 284:545, 1982.

44. Thoeni, R. F., and Cello, J. P. A critical look at the accuracy of endoscopy and double-contrast radiography of the upper gastrointestinal (UGI) tract in patients with substantial UGI hemorrhage. Radiology 135:305, 1980.

45. Gilbert, D. A., Silverstein, F. E., Tedesco, F. J., Buenger, N. K., and Persing, J. The national ASGE survey on upper gastrointestinal bleeding. III. Endoscopy in upper gastrointestinal bleeding. Gastrointest. Endosc. 27:94, 1981.

46. Irving, J. D., and Northfield, T. C. Emergency arteriography in acute gastrointestinal bleeding. Br. Med. J. 1:929, 1976.

47. Kelemouridis, V., Athanasoulis, C. A., and Waltman, A. C. Gastric bleeding sites: an angiographic study. Radiology 149:643, 1983.

48. Hietala, S. O., Ghahremani, G. C., Crampton, A. R., and Wirell, M. Arteriographic evaluation of postsurgical stomach. Gastrointest. Radiol. 10:31, 1985.

49. Nusbaum, S., and Baum, S. Radiographic demonstration of unknown sites of gastrointestinal bleeding. Surg. Forum 14:374, 1963.

50. Allan, R., and Dykes, P. A comparison of routine and selective

endoscopy in the management of acute gastrointestinal hemorrhage. Gastrointest. Endosc. *20*:154, 1974.

51. Sandlow, L. J., Becker, G. H., Spellberg, M. A., Allen, H. A., Berg, M., Berry, L. H., and Newman, E. A. A prospective randomized study of the management of upper gastrointestinal hemorrhage. Am. J. Gastroenterol. *61*:282, 1974.

52. Graham, D. Y. Limited value of early endoscopy in the management of acute upper gastrointestinal bleeding. Am. J. Surg. *140*:284, 1980.

53. Weissberg, J. I., Stein, D. E. T., Andres, L. L., Kemeny, M. J., Rinki, M., Walker, J., Roller, P., Miller, R., Fogel, M. R., Knauer, C. M., and Gregory, P. B. Immediate endoscopic diagnosis in acute upper gastrointestinal bleeding: does it alter diagnosis, outcome, management, or patient satisfaction? Gastroenterology *84*:1349, 1983.

54. Collins, R, and Langman, M. Treatment with histamine H₂ antagonist in acute upper gastrointestinal hemorrhage. N. Engl. J. Med. *313*:660, 1985.

55. Swain, C. P., Storey, D. W., Bown, S. G., Heath, J., Mills, T. N., Salmon, P. R., Northfield, T. C., Kirkham, J. S., and O'Sullivan, J. P. Nature of the bleeding vessel in recurrently bleeding gastric ulcers. Gastroenterology *90*:595, 1986.

56. Storey, D. W., Bown, S. G., Swain, P., Salmon, P. R., Kirkham, J. S., and Northfield, T. C. Endoscopic prediction of recurrent bleeding in peptic ulcers. N. Engl. J. Med. *305*:915, 1981.

57. Shuttleworth, R. D., and Falck, V. G. The bleeding gastric ulcer—will it bleed again, and if so, why? A case for repeat endoscopy in evaluating stigmata. S. Afr. Med. J. *66*:95, 1984.

58. Swain, C. P., Salmon, P. R., and Northfield, T. C. Does ulcer position influence presentation or prognosis of acute gastrointestinal bleeding? Gut *27*:A632, 1986.

58a. Somerville, K., Faulkner, G., and Langman, M. Non-steroidal anti-inflammatory drugs and bleeding peptic ulcer. Lancet *1*:462, 1986.

58b. Somerville, K., Pritchard, P. J., Faulkner, G., and Langman, M. Aspirin and bleeding peptic ulcer. (Abstract.) Gastroenterology *92*:1649, 1987.

58c. Armstrong, C. P., and Blower, A. L. Non-steroidal anti-inflammatory drugs and life threatening complications of peptic ulceration. Gut *28*:527, 1987.

59. Northfield, T. C. Factors predisposing to recurrent haemorrhage after acute gastrointestinal bleeding. Br. Med. J. *1*:26, 1971.

60. Bornman, P. C., Theodorou, N. A., Shuttleworth, R. D., Essel, H. P., and Marks, I. N. Importance of hypovolaemic shock and endoscopic signs in predicting recurrent haemorrhage from peptic ulceration: a prospective evaluation. Br. Med. J. *291*:245, 1985.

61. Foster, D. N., Miloszewski, K. J. A., and Losowsky, M. S. Stigmata of recent haemorrhage in diagnosis and prognosis of upper gastrointestinal bleeding. Br. Med. J. *1*:1173, 1978.

62. Griffiths, W. J., Neumann, D. A., and Welsh, J. D. The visible vessel as an indicator of uncontrolled or recurrent gastrointestinal hemorrhage. N. Engl. J. Med. *300*:1411, 1979.

63. Vallon, A. G., Cotton, P. B., Laurence, B. H., Armengol Miro, J. R., and Salord Oses, J. C. Randomised trial of endoscopic argon laser photocoagulation in bleeding peptic ulcers. Gut *22*:228, 1981.

64. Swain, C. P., Storey, D. W., Northfield, T. C., Bown, S. G., Kirkham, J. S., and Salmon, P. R. Controlled trial of argon laser photocoagulation in bleeding peptic ulcers. Lancet *2*:1313, 1981.

65. Swain, C. P., Salmon, P. R., Kirkham, J. S., Bown, S. G., and Northfield, T. C. Controlled trial of Nd-YAG laser photocoagulation in bleeding peptic ulcers. Lancet *1*:1113, 1986.

66. Krejs, G. J., Little, K. H., Westergaard, H., Hamilton, J. K., and Polter, D. E. Laser photocoagulation for the treatment of acute peptic ulcer bleeding: a randomized controlled clinical trial. N. Engl. J. Med. *316*:1618, 1987.

67. Kernohan, R. M., Anderson, J. R., McKelvey, S. T. D., and Kennedy, T. L. A controlled trial of bipolar electrocoagulation in patients with upper gastrointestinal bleeding. Br. J. Surg. *71*:889, 1984.

68. O'Brien, J. D., Day, S. J., and Burnham, W. R. Controlled trial of small bipolar probe in bleeding peptic ulcers. Lancet *1*:464, 1986.

69. Wara, P. Endoscopic prediction of major rebleeding—a prospective study of stigmata of hemorrhage in bleeding ulcer. Gastroenterology *88*:1209, 1985.

70. Beckly, D. E., and Casebow, M. P. Prediction of rebleeding from peptic ulcer experience with an endoscopic Doppler device. Gut *27*:96, 1986.

71. Carstensen, H. E., Bulow, S., Hart Hansen, O., Hamilton Jakobsen, B., Krarup, T., Pedersen, T., Raahave, D., Svendsen, L. B., and Backer, O. Cimetidine for severe gastroduodenal haemorrhage: a randomized controlled trial. Scand. J. Gastroenterol. *15*:103, 1980.

72. Zuckerman, G., Welch, R., Douglas, A., Troxell, R., Cohen, S., Lorber, S., Melnyk, C., Bliss, C., Christiansen, P., and Kern, F. Controlled trial of medical therapy for active upper gastrointestinal bleeding and prevention of rebleeding. Am. J. Med. *76*:361, 1984.

73. Kayasseh, L., Keller, U., Gyr, K., Stalder, G. A., and Wall, M. Somatostatin and cimetidine in peptic-ulcer haemorrhage. A randomised controlled trial. Lancet *1*:844, 1980.

74. Limberg, B., and Kommerell, B. Somatostatin for cimetidine-resistant gastroduodenal haemorrhage. Lancet *2*:916, 1980.

75. Magnusson, I., Ihre, T., Johansson, C., Seligson, U., Torngren, S., and Uvnas-Moberg, K. Randomised double blind trial of somatostatin in the treatment of massive upper gastrointestinal haemorrhage. Gut *26*:221, 1985.

76. Lauritsen, K., Laursen, L. S., Havelund, T., Bytzer, P., and Rask-Madsen, T. Controlled trial of arbaprostil in bleeding peptic ulcer. Br. Med. J. *291*:1093, 1985.

77. Raskin, J. B., Camara, D. S., Levine, B. A., Akdamar, K., Redlhammer, D. E., Gaskill, H. V., and Euler, A. R. Effect of 15(R)-15-methyl prostaglandin E₂ on acute upper gastrointestinal hemorrhage. Gastroenterology *88*:1550, 1985.

78. Biggs, J. C., Hugh, T. B., and Dodds, A. J. Tranexamic acid and upper gastrointestinal haemorrhage: a double blind trial. Gut *17*:719, 1976.

79. Engqvist, A., Brostrom, O., von Feilitzen, F., Halldin, M., Nystrom, B., Ost, A., Reichard, H., Sandqvist, S., Torngren, S., and Wedlund, J. E. Tranexamic acid in massive haemorrhage from the upper gastrointestinal tract: a double-blind study. Scand. J. Gastroenterol. *14*:839, 1979.

80. Immediate results of emergency operation for massive upper gastrointestinal hemorrhage. A cooperative study by the Connecticut Society of American Board of Surgeons. Am. J. Surg. *122*:387, 1971.

81. Kim, U., Dreiling, D. A., Kark, A., and Rudick, J. Factors influencing mortality in surgical treatment for massive gastroduodenal hemorrhage. Am. J. Gastroenterol. *62*:24, 1974.

82. Hunt, P. S., Elliott, B., Freidin, J., McCann, W., Marshall, R., and Peck, G. Mortality trends in the surgical management of chronic peptic ulceration: 25 years experience. Aust. N.Z. J. Surg. *48*:147, 1978.

83. Peck, G. S., and McCann, W. J. Bleeding duodenal ulcer: reduction in mortality with a planned approach. Br. J. Surg. *66*:633, 1979.

84. Hunt, P. S., Hansky, J., Korman, M. G., Francis, J. K., Marshall, R. D., and McCann, W. The management of bleeding gastric ulcer: a prospective study. Aust. N.Z. J. Surg. *50*:41, 1980.

85. Ring, E. J., Oleaga, J. A., Freiman, D. B., Husted, J. W., Waltman, A. C., and Baum, S. Pitfalls in the angiographic management of hemorrhage—hemodynamic considerations. AJR *129*:1007, 1977.

86. Twiford, T. W., Goldstein, H. M., and Zornaza, J. Transcatheter therapy for gastrointestinal arterial bleeding. Am. J. Dig. Dis. *23*:1046, 1978.

87. Johnson, W. C., and Widrich, W. C. Efficacy of selective splanchnic arteriography and vasopressin perfusion in diagnosis and treatment of gastrointestinal hemorrhage. Am. J. Surg. *131*:481, 1976.

88. Eckstein, M. R., Kelemouridis, V., Athanasoulis, C. A., Waltman, A. C., Feldman, L., and van Breda, A. Gastric

bleeding: therapy with intraarterial vasopressin and transcatheter embolization. Radiology *152*:643, 1984.

89. Clark, R. A., Cooley, D. P., and Eggers, F. M. Acute arterial gastrointestinal hemorrhage: efficacy of transcatheter control. AJR *136*:1185, 1981.

90. Sherman, L. M., Shenoy, S. S., and Cerra, F. B. Selective intraarterial vasopressin: clinical efficacy and complications. Ann. Surg. *189*:298, 1979.

91. Gomes, A. S., Lois, J. F., and McCoy, R. D. Angiographic treatment of gastrointestinal hemorrhage: comparison of vasopressin infusion and embolization. AJR *146*:1031, 1986.

92. Reuter, S. R., Chuang, V. P., and Bree, R. L. Selective arterial embolization for control of massive upper gastrointestinal bleeding. AJR *125*:119, 1975.

93. Eisenberg, H., and Steer, M. L. The nonoperative treatment of massive pyloroduodenal hemorrhage by retracted autologous clot embolization. Surgery *79*:414, 1976.

94. Matolo, N. M., and Link, D. P. Selective embolization for control of gastrointestinal hemorrhage. Am. J. Surg. *138*:840, 1979.

95. Keller, F. S., Rosch, J., Baur, G. M., Taylor, L. M., Dotter, C. T., and Porter, J. M. Percutaneous angiographic embolization: a procedure of increasing usefulness. Am. J. Surg. *142*:5, 1981.

96. Bookstein, J. J., Chlosta, E. M., Foley, D., and Walter, J. F. Transcatheter hemostasis of gastrointestinal bleeding using modified autogenous clot. Radiology *113*:277, 1974.

97. Lieberman, D. A., Keller, F. S., Katon, R. M., and Rosch, J. Arterial embolization for massive upper gastrointestinal tract bleeding in poor surgical candidates. Gastroenterology *86*:876, 1984.

98. Jacob, E. T., Shapira, Z., Morag, B., and Rubinstein, Z. Hepatic infarction and gallbladder necrosis complicating arterial embolization for bleeding duodenal ulcer. Dig. Dis. Sci. *24*:482, 1979.

99. Shapiro, N., Brandt, L., Sprayregen, S., Mitsudo, S., and Glotzer, P. Duodenal infarction after therapeutic Gelfoam embolization of a bleeding duodenal ulcer. Gastroenterology *80*:176, 1981.

100. Green, F. W., Kaplan, M. M., Curtis, L. E., and Levine, P. H. Effect of acid and pepsin on blood coagulation and platelet aggregation. Gastroenterology *74*:38, 1978.

101. Berstad, A., Holm, H. A., and Kittang, E. Experience with antipeptic agents. Scand. J. Gastroenterol. *14* (Suppl. 55):121, 1979.

102. Piper, D. W., and Fenton, B. H. pH stability and activity curves of pepsin with special reference to their clinical importance. Gut *6*:506, 1965.

103. Goldberg, H. I., Dodds, W. J., Gee, S., Montgomery, C., and Zboralske, F. F. Role of acid and pepsin in acute experimental esophagitis. Gastroenterology *56*:223, 1969.

104. Berstad, A. Management of acute upper gastrointestinal bleeding. Scand. J. Gastroenterol. *17*(Suppl. 75):103, 1982.

105. Peterson, W. L., and Richardson, C. T. Intravenous cimetidine or two regimens of ranitidine to reduce fasting gastric acidity. Ann. Intern. Med. *104*:505, 1986.

106. Ostro, M. J., Russell, J. A., Soldin, S. J., Mahon, W. A., and Jeejeebhoy, K. N. Control of gastric pH with cimetidine: boluses versus primed infusions. Gastroenterology *89*:532, 1985.

107. Peterson, W. L., and Richardson, C. T. Sustained fasting achlorhydria: a comparison of medical regimens. Gastroenterology *88*:666, 1985.

108. Somerville, K. W., Davies, J. G., Hawkey, C. J., Henry, D. A., Hine, K. R., and Langman, M. J. S. Somatostatin in treatment of haematemesis and melaena. Lancet *1*:130, 1985.

109. Barer, D., Ogilvie, A., Henry, D., Dronfield, M., Coggon, D., French, S., Ellis, E., Atkinson, M., and Langman, M. Cimetidine and tranexamic acid in the treatment of acute upper-gastrointestinal-tract bleeding. N. Engl. J. Med. *308*:1571, 1983.

110. Fleisher, D. Endoscopic therapy of upper gastrointestinal bleeding in humans. Gastroenterology *90*:217, 1986.

111. Linscheer, W. G., and Fazio, T. L. Control of upper gastrointestinal hemorrhage by endoscopic spraying of clotting factors. Gastroenterology *77*:642, 1979.

112. Protell, R. L., Silverstein, F. E., Gulacsik, C., Martin, T. R., Dennis, M. B., Auth, D. C., and Rubin, C. E. Failure of cyanoacrylate tissue glue (flucrylate, MBR 4197) to stop bleeding from experimental canine gastric ulcers. Am. J. Dig. Dis. *23*:903, 1978.

113. Martin, T. R., Onstad, G. R., and Silvis, S. E. Endoscopic control of massive upper gastrointestinal bleeding with a tissue adhesive (MBR 4197). Gastrointest. Endosc. *24*:74, 1977.

114. Peura, D. A., Johnson, L. R., Brukhalter, E. L., Hogan, W. J., LoGuidice, J. A., Schapiro, M., Klasky, I., Belsito, A. A., Butler, M. L., and Silvis, S. E. Use of trifluoroisopropyl cyanoacrylate polymer (MBR 4197) in patients with bleeding peptic ulcers of the stomach and duodenum: a randomized controlled study. J. Clin. Gastroenterol. *4*:325, 1982.

114a. Chung, S. S. C., Leung, J. W. C., Steele, R. J. C., and Crofts, T. J. Epinephrine injection for actively bleeding ulcers: a randomised controlled study. (Abstract.) Gastrointest. Endosc. *33*:146, 1987.

115. Chen, P., Wu, C., and Liaw, Y. Hemostatic effect of endoscopic local injection with hypertonic saline-epinephrine solution and pure ethanol for digestive tract bleeding. Gastrointest. Endosc. *32*:319, 1986.

116. Silverstein, F. E., Protell, R. L., Piercey, J., Rubin, C. E., Auth, D. C., and Dennis, M. Endoscopic laser treatment. II. Comparison of the efficacy of high and low power photocoagulation in control of severely bleeding experimental ulcers in dogs. Gastroenterology *73*:481, 1977.

117. Silverstein, F. E., Protell, R. L., Gulacsik, C., Auth, D. C., Deltenre, M., Dennis, M., Piercey, J., and Rubin, C. Endoscopic laser treatment. III. The development and testing of a gas-jet-assisted argon laser waveguide in control of bleeding experimental ulcer. Gastroenterology *74*:232, 1978.

118. Dixon, J. A., Berenson, M. M., and McCloskey, D. W. Neodymium-YAG laser treatment of experimental canine gastric bleeding. Gastroenterology *77*:647, 1979.

119. Johnston, J. H., Jensen, D. M., Mautner, J. W., and Elashoff, J. YAG laser treatment of experimental bleeding canine gastric ulcers. Gastroenterology *79*:1252, 1980.

120. Johnston, J. H., Jensen, D. M., Mautner, J. W., and Elashoff, J. Argon laser treatment of bleeding canine gastric ulcers: limitations and guidelines of endoscopic use. Gastroenterology *80*:708, 1981.

121. Rutgeerts, P., Vantrappen, G., Geboes, K., and Broeckaert, L. Safety and efficacy of neodymium-YAG laser photocoagulation: an experimental study in dogs. Gut *22*:38, 1981.

122. Silverstein, F. E., Protell, R. L., Gilbert, D. A., Gulacsik, C., Auth, D. C., Dennis, M. B., and Rubin, C. E. Argon vs. neodymium YAG laser photocoagulation of experimental canine gastric ulcers. Gastroenterology *77*:491, 1979.

123. Rutgeerts, P., Vantrappen, G., Broeckaert, L., Janssens, J., Coremano, G., Geboes, K., and Schurmans, P. Controlled trial of YAG laser treatment of upper digestive hemorrhage. Gastroenterology *83*:410, 1982.

124. Ihre, T., Johansson, C., Seligson, U., and Torngren, S. Endoscopic YAG-laser treatment in massive upper gastrointestinal bleeding. Scand. J. Gastroenterol. *16*:633, 1981.

125. MacLeod, I. A., Mills, P. R., Mackenzie, J. F., Joffe, S. N., Russell, R., and Carter, D. C. Neodymium yttrium aluminium garnet laser photocoagulation for major haemorrhage from peptic ulcers and single vessels: a single blind controlled study. Br. Med. J. *286*:345, 1983.

126. Protell, R. L., Gilbert, D. A., Silverstein, F. E., Jensen, D. M., Hulett, F. M., and Auth, D. C. Computer-assisted electrocoagulation: bipolar vs. monopolar in the treatment of experimental canine gastric ulcer bleeding. Gastroenterology *80*:451, 1981.

127. Johnston, J. H., Jensen, D. M., and Mautner, W. Comparison of endoscopic electrocoagulation and laser photocoagulation of bleeding canine gastric ulcers. Gastroenterology *82*:904, 1982.

128. Johnston, J. H., Jensen, D. M., and Mautner, W. Comparison

of laser photocoagulation and electrocoagulation in endoscopic treatment of UGI bleeding. Gastroenterology 76:1162, 1979.

129. Protell, R. L., Rubin, C. E., Auth, D. C., Silverstein, F. E., Terou, F., Dennis, M., and Piercey, J. R. A. The heater probe: a new endoscopic method of stopping massive gastrointestinal bleeding. Gastroenterology 74:257, 1978.

130. Swain, C. P., Mill, T. N., Shemesh, E., Dark, J. M., Lewin, M. R., Clifton, J. S., Northfield, T. C., Cotton, P. B., and Salmon, P. R. Which electrode? A comparison of four endoscopic methods of electrocoagulation in experimental bleeding ulcers. Gut 25:1424, 1984.

131. Goudie, B. M., Mitchell, K. G., Birnie, G. G., and Mackay, C. Controlled trial of endoscopic bipolar electrocoagulation in the treatment of bleeding peptic ulcers. Gut 25:A1185, 1984.

132. Laine, L. Multipolar electrocoagulation in the treatment of active upper gastrointestinal tract hemorrhage. N. Engl. J. Med. 316:1613, 1987.

132a. Matthewson, K., Swain, C. P., Bland, M., Kirkham, J. S., Bown, S. G., and Northfield, T. C. Randomized comparison of Nd YAG laser, heater probe (HP) and no endoscopic therapy for bleeding peptic ulcer. (Abstract.) Gastroenterology 92:1522, 1987.

133. Graham, D. Y., and Smith, J. L. The course of patients after variceal hemorrhage. Gastroenterology 80:800, 1981.

134. Weissberg, J., Stein, D. T., Fogel, M., Knauer, C. M., and Gregory, P. B. Variceal bleeding: does it matter to the patient whether his gastric or esophageal varices bleed? Gastroenterology 86:1296, 1984.

135. Ratnoff, O. D., and Patek, A. J. The natural history of Laennec's cirrhosis of the liver: an analysis of 386 cases. Medicine 21:207, 1941.

136. Garcia-Tsao, G., Groszmann, R. J., Fisher, R. L., Conn, H. O., Atterbury, C. E., and Glickman, M. Portal pressure, presence of gastroesophageal varices and variceal bleeding. Hepatology 5:419, 1985.

137. Smith-Laing, G., Camilo, M. E., Dick, R., and Sherlock, S. Percutaneous transhepatic portography in the assessment of portal hypertension. Gastroenterology 78:197, 1980.

138. Lebrec, D., Defleury, P., Rueff, B., Nahum, H., and Benhamou, J. Portal hypertension, size of esophageal varices, and risk of gastrointestinal bleeding in alcoholic cirrhosis. Gastroenterology 79:1139, 1980.

139. Boyer, J. L., Chatterjee, C., Iber, F. L., and Basu, A. K. Effect of plasma-volume expansion on portal hypertension. N. Engl. J. Med. 275:750, 1966.

140. Zimmon, D. S., and Kessler, R. E. The portal pressure-blood volume relationship in cirrhosis. Gut 15:99, 1974.

141. Markey, W., Payne, J. A., and Straus, A. Hemorrhage from esophageal varices after placement of the LeVeen shunt. Gastroenterology 77:341, 1979.

142. Reding, P., Urbain, D., Grivegnee, A., and Frere, D. Portal venous–esophageal luminal pressure gradient in cirrhosis. Hepatology 6:98, 1986.

143. Staritz, M., Porallo, T., and Buschenfelde, K-H. Intravascular oesophageal variceal pressure (IOVP) assessed by endoscopic fine needle puncture under basal conditions, Valsalva's manoeuvre and after glyceryltrinitrate application. Gut 26:525, 1985.

144. Liebowitz, H. R. Pathogenesis of esophageal varix rupture. JAMA 175:138, 1961.

145. Eckardt, V. F., and Grace, N. D. Gastroesophageal reflux and bleeding esophageal varices. Gastroenterology 76:39, 1979.

146. Keith, R. G., Mustard, R. A., and Saibil, E. A. Gastric variceal bleeding due to occlusion of splenic vein in pancreatic disease. Can. J. Surg. 25:301, 1982.

147. Moossa, A. R., and Gadd, M. A. Isolated splenic vein thrombosis. World J. Surg. 9:384, 1985.

148. Glynn, M. J. Isolated splenic vein thrombosis. Arch. Surg. 121:723, 1986.

149. Waldram, R., Davis, M., Nunnerley, H., and Williams, R. Emergency endoscopy after gastrointestinal haemorrhage in 50 patients with portal hypertension. Br. Med. J. 4:94, 1974.

150. Teres, J., Bordas, J. M., Bru, C., Diaz, F., Bruguera, M., and Rodes, J. Upper gastrointestinal bleeding in cirrhosis: clinical and endoscopic correlations. Gut 17:37, 1976.

151. Franco, D., Durandy, Y., Deporte, A., and Bismuth, H. Upper gastrointestinal hemorrhage in hepatic cirrhosis: causes and relation to hepatic failure and stress. Lancet 1:218, 1977.

152. Sarfeh, I. J., Tabak, C., Eugene, J., and Juler, G. L. Clinical significance of erosive gastritis in patients with alcoholic liver disease and upper gastrointestinal hemorrhage. Ann. Surg. 194:149, 1981.

153. Sarfeh, I. J., Tarnawski, A., Malki, A., Mason, G. R., Mach, T., and Ivey, K. J. Portal hypertension and gastric mucosal injury in rats. Gastroenterology 84:987, 1983.

154. Sankary, H., Sarfeh, I. J., Tarnawski, A., Maeda, R., Ivey, K. J., and Mason, G. R. Propranolol reduces ethanol-induced gastric mucosal damage in portal hypertensive rats. Dig. Dis. Sci. 31:162, 1986.

155. McCormack, T. T., Sims, J., Eyre-Brook, I., Kennedy, H., Goepel, J., Johnson, A. G., and Triger, D. R. Gastric lesions in portal hypertension: inflammatory gastritis or congestive gastropathy? Gut 26:1226, 1985.

155a. Sarfeh, I. J., and Tarnawski, A. Gastric mucosal vasculopathy in portal hypertension. Gastroenterology 93:1129, 1987.

156. Rector, W. G. Drug therapy for portal hypertension. Ann Intern. Med. 105:96, 1986.

157. Hussey, K. P. Vasopressin therapy for upper gastrointestinal tract hemorrhage. Arch. Intern. Med. 145:1263, 1985.

158. Shaldon, S., and Sherlock, S. The use of vasopressin ('pitressin') in the control of bleeding from esophageal varices. Lancet 2:222, 1960.

159. Merigan T. C. Jr., Plotkin, G. R., and Davidson, C. S. Effect of intravenously administered posterior pituitary extract on hemorrhage from bleeding esophageal varices. A controlled evaluation. N. Engl. J. Med. 266:134, 1962.

160. Nusbaum, M., Baum, S., Sakiyalak, P., and Blakemore, W. S. Pharmacologic control of portal hypertension. Surgery 62:299, 1967.

161. Conn, H. O., Ramsby, G. R., Storer, E. H., Mutchnick, M. G., Joshi, P. H., Phillips, M. M., Cohen, G. A., Fields, G. N., and Petroski, D. Intraarterial vasopressin in the treatment of upper gastrointestinal hemorrhage: a prospective, controlled clinical trial. Gastroenterology 68:211, 1975.

162. Mallory, A., Schaefer, J. W., Cohen, J. R., Holt, S. A., and Norton, L. W. Selective intra-arterial vasopressin infusion for upper gastrointestinal tract hemorrhage. Arch. Surg. 115:30, 1980.

163. Barr, J. W., Lakin, R. C., and Rosch, J. Similarity of arterial and intravenous vasopressin on portal and systemic hemodynamics. Gastroenterology 69:13, 1975.

164. Johnson, W. C., Widrich, W. C., Ansell, J. E., Robbins, A. H., and Nabseth, D. C. Control of bleeding varices by vasopressin: a prospective randomized study. Ann. Surg. 186:369, 1977.

165. Chojkier, M., Groszmann, R. J., Aterbury, C. E., Barmeir, S., Blei, A. T., Frankel, J., Glickman, M. G., Kniaz, J. L., Schade, R., Taggart, G. J., and Conn, H. O. A controlled comparison of continuous intraarterial and intravenous infusions of vasopressin in hemorrhage from esophageal varices. Gastroenterology 77:540, 1979.

166. Fogel, M. R., Knauer, C. M., Ljudevit, L. A., Mahal, A. S., Stein, D. E. T., Kemeny, M. J., Rinki, M. M., Walker, J. E., Siegmund, D., and Gregory, P. B. Continuous intravenous vasopressin in active upper gastrointestinal bleeding. Ann. Intern. Med. 96:565, 1982.

167. Groszmann, R. J., Kravetz, D., Bosch, J., Glickman, M., Bruix, J., Bredfeldt, J., Conn, H. O., Rodes, J., and Storer, E. H. Nitroglycerin improves the hemodynamic response to vasopressin in portal hypertension. Hepatology 2:757, 1982.

168. Tsai, Y-T., Lay, C-S., Lai, K-H., Ng, W-W., Yeh, Y-S., Wang, J-Y., Chiang, T-T., Lee, S-D., Chiang, B. N., and Lo, K-J. Controlled trial of vasopressin plus nitroglycerin vs. vasopressin alone in the treatment of bleeding esophageal varices. Hepatology 6:406, 1986.

169. Gimson, A. E. S., Westaby, D., Hegarty, J., Watson, A., and Williams, R. A randomized trial of vasopressin and vasopressin plus nitroglycerin in the control of acute variceal hemorrhage. Hepatology 6:410, 1986.

170. Conn, H. O. Vasopressin and nitroglycerin in the treatment of bleeding varices: the bottom line. Hepatology 6:523, 1986.

171. Freeman, J. G., Lishman, A. H., Cobden, I., and Record, C. O. Controlled trial of terlipressin ('glypressin') versus vasopressin in the early treatment of oesophageal varices. Lancet 2:66, 1982.

172. Jenkins, S. A., Baxter, J. N., Corbett, W., Devitt, P., Ware, J., and Shields, R. A prospective randomised controlled clinical trial comparing somatostatin and vasopressin in controlling acute variceal haemorrhage. Br. Med. J. 290:275, 1985.

173. Kravetz, D., Bosch, J., Teres, J., Bruix, J., Rimola, A., and Rodes, J. Comparison of intravenous somatostatin and vasopressin infusions in treatment of acute variceal hemorrhage. Hepatology 3:442, 1984.

174. Chojkier, M., and Conn, H. O. Esophageal tamponade in the treatment of bleeding varices, a decadal progress report. Dig. Dis. Sci. 25:267, 1980.

175. Boyce, H. W., Jr. Modification of the Sengstaken-Blakemore balloon tube. N. Engl. J. Med. 267:195, 1962.

176. Edlich, R. F., Lande, A. J., Goodale, R. L., and Wangensteen, O. H. Prevention of aspiration pneumonia by continuous esophagogastric aspiration during esophagogastric tamponade and gastric cooling. Surgery 2:405, 1968.

177. Mitchell, K., Silk, D. B. A., and Williams, R. Prospective comparison of two Sengstaken tubes in the management of patients with variceal haemorrhage. Gut 21:570, 1980.

178. Mandelstam, P., and Zeppa, R. Endotracheal intubation should precede esophagogastric balloon tamponade for control of variceal bleeding. J. Clin. Gastroenterol. 5:493, 1983.

179. Teres, J., Cecelia, A., Bordas, J. M., Rimola, A., Bru, C., and Rodes, J. Esophageal tamponade for bleeding varices. Controlled trial between the Sengstaken-Blakemore tube and the Linton-Nachlas tube. Gastroenterology 75:566, 1978.

180. Crafoord, C., and Frenckner, P. New surgical treatment of varicose veins of the esophagus. Acta Otolaryngol. 27:422, 1939.

181. Conn, H. O. Endoscopic sclerotherapy: an analysis of variants. Hepatology 3:769, 1983.

182. Grobe, J. L., Kozarek, R. A., Sanowski, R. A., LeGrand, J., and Kovac, A. Venography during endoscopic injection sclerotherapy of esophageal varices. Gastrointest. Endosc. 30:6, 1984.

183. Soderlund, C., Backman, L., Erwald, R., Forsgren, L., Marions, O., and Wiechel, K-L. Sclerotherapy of esophageal varices: an endoscopic and portographic study. Hepatology 4:877, 1984.

184. Terblanche, J., Northover, J. M. A., Bornman, P., Kahn, D., Barbezat, G. O., Sellars, S. L., and Saunders, S. A. A prospective evaluation of injection sclerotherapy in the treatment of acute bleeding from esophageal varices. Surgery 85:239, 1979.

185. Spence, R. A., Anderson, J. R., and Johnston, G. W. Twenty-five years of injection sclerotherapy for bleeding varices. Br. J. Surg. 72:195, 1985.

186. Paquet, K-J., and Feussner, H. Endoscopic sclerosis and esophageal balloon tamponade in acute hemorrhage from esophagogastric varices: a prospective controlled randomized trial. Hepatology 5:580, 1985.

187. Wright, P. D., Loose, H. W., Carter, R. F., and James, O. F. Two-year experience of management of bleeding esophageal varices with a coordinated treatment program based on injection sclerotherapy. Surgery 99:604, 1986.

188. Crotty, B., Wood, L. J., Willett, I. R., Colman, J., and McCarthy, P. The management of acutely bleeding varices by injection sclerotherapy. Med. J. Aust. 145:130, 1986.

189. Westaby, D., Hayes, P. C., Gimson, A. E. S., Polson, R., and Williams, R. Injection sclerotherapy for active variceal bleeding: a controlled trial. Gut 27:A1246, 1986.

190. Lunderquist, A., and Vang, J. Transhepatic catheterization and obliteration of the coronary vein in patients with portal hypertension and esophageal varices. N. Engl. J. Med. 291:646, 1974.

191. Bengmark, S., Borjesson, B., Hoevels, J., Joelsson, B., Lunderquist, A., and Owman, T. Obliteration of esophageal varices by PTP. Ann. Surg. 190:549, 1979.

192. Smith-Laing, G., Scott, J., Long, R. G., Dick, R., and Sherlock, S. Role of percutaneous transhepatic obliteration of varices in the management of hemorrhage from gastroesophageal varices. Gastroenterology 80:1031, 1981.

193. Orloff, M. J., and Bell, R. H. Long-term survival after emergency portacaval shunting for bleeding varices in patients with alcoholic cirrhosis. Am. J. Surg. 151:176, 1986.

194. Bell, R. H., Miyai, K., and Orloff, M. J. Failure of operative liver biopsy to predict survival in 195 patients undergoing emergency portacaval shunt. Gastroenterology 80:1109, 1981.

195. Malt, R. A., Szczerban, J., and Malt, R. B. Risks in therapeutic portacaval and splenorenal shunts. Ann. Surg. 184:279, 1976.

196. Malt, R. A., Abbott, W. M., Warshaw, A. L., Vander Salm, T. J., and Smead, W. L. Randomized trial of emergency mesocaval and portacaval shunts for bleeding esophageal varices. Am. J. Surg. 135:584, 1978.

197. Warren, W. D. Control of variceal bleeding. Am. J. Surg. 145:8, 1983.

198. Gouge, T. H., and Ranson, J. H. Esophageal transection and paraesophagogastric devascularization for bleeding esophageal varices. Am. J. Surg 151:47, 1986.

199. Jackson, F. C., Perrin, E. B., Felix, W. R., and Smith, A. G. A clinical investigation of the portacaval shunt: V. Survival analysis of the therapeutic operation. Ann. Surg. 174:672, 1971.

200. Resnick, R. H., Iber, F. L., Ishihara, A. M., Chalmers, T. C., and Zimmerman, H. A controlled study of the therapeutic portacaval shunt. Gastroenterology 67:843, 1974.

201. Rueff, B., Degos, F., and Degos, J. D. A controlled study of therapeutic portacaval shunt in alcoholic cirrhosis. Lancet 1:655, 1976.

202. Reynolds, T. B., Donovan, A. J., Mikkelsen, W. P., Redeker, A. G., Turrill, F. L., and Weiner, J. M. Results of a 12-year randomized trial of portacaval shunt in patients with alcoholic liver disease and bleeding varices. Gastroenterology 80:1005, 1981.

203. Conn, H. O., Lindenmuth, W. W., May, C. T., and Ramsby, G. R. Prophylactic portacaval anastomosis. A tale of two studies. Medicine 51:27, 1972.

204. Resnick, R. H., Chalmers, T. C., Ishihara, A. M., Garceau, A. J., Callow, A. D., Schimmel, E. M., and O'Hara, E. T. A controlled study of the prophylactic portacaval shunt. Ann. Intern. Med. 70:675, 1969.

205. Jackson, F. J. A clinical investigation of the portacaval shunt. Survival analysis of the prophylactic operation. Am. J. Surg. 115:22, 1968.

206. Cello, J. P., Deveny, K. E., Trunkey, D. D., Heilbron, D. C., Stoney, R. J., Ehrenfeld, W. K., and Way, L. W. Factors influencing survival after therapeutic shunts. Am. J. Surg. 141:257, 1981.

207. Zimmon, D. S., and Kessler, R. E. Effect of portal venous blood flow diversion on portal pressure. J. Clin. Invest. 65:1388, 1980.

208. Warren, W. D., Zeppa, R., Foman, J. J. Selective trans-splenic decompression of gastroesophageal varices by distal splenorenal shunt. Ann. Surg. 166:437, 1967.

209. McInnes, I. E., Gibson, P. R., Rosengarten, D. S., and Dudley, F. J. Long term follow-up of patients following successful selective and non-selective portasystemic shunt surgery. Aust. N.Z. J. Surg. 55:355, 1985.

210. Millikan, W. J., Warren, W. D., Henderson, J. M., Smith, R. B., Salam, A. A., Galambos, J. T., Kutner, M. H. and Keen, J. H. The Emory prospective randomized trial: selective versus nonselective shunt to control variceal bleeding. Ann. Surg. 201:712, 1985.

211. Fischer, J. E., Bower, R. H., Atamian, S., Welling, R. Comparison of distal and proximal splenorenal shunts. Ann. Surg. 194:531, 1981.

212. Langer, B., Taylor, B. R., Mackenzie, D. R., Gilas, T., Stone, R. M., and Blendis, L. Further report of a prospective randomized trial comparing distal splenorenal shunt with end-to-side portacaval shunt. Gastroenterology 88:424, 1985.

213. Harley, H. A. J., Morgan, T., Redeker, A. G., Reynolds, T. B., Villamil, F., Weiner, J. M., and Yellin, A. Results of a randomized trial of end-to-side portacaval shunt and distal

splenorenal shunt in alcoholic liver disease and variceal bleeding. Gastroenterology 91:802, 1986.

214. Conn, H. O., Resnick, R. H., Grace, N. D., and Boston–New Haven Collaborative Liver Group. Distal splenorenal shunt (DSRS) vs portal-systemic shunt (PSS) in patients who bled from varices: results of a randomized controlled trial. Hepatology 5:965, 1985.

215. Sarin, S. K., Nanda, R., Sachdev, G., Chari, S., Anand, B. S., and Broor, S. L. Intravariceal versus paravariceal sclerotherapy: a prospective, controlled, randomised trial. Gut 28:657, 1987.

216. Rhodes, J. M., Dawson, J., Cockel, R., Hawker, P., Dykes, P., Bradby, G. V. H., Hillenbrand, P., and Elias, E. A randomized controlled trial of variceal compression as an adjunct to endoscopic variceal sclerosis. Scand. J. Gastroenterol. 21:1217, 1986.

217. Westaby, D., Melia, W. M., MacDougall, B. R. D., Hegarty, J. E., and Williams, R. Injection sclerotherapy for oesophageal varices: a prospective randomised trial of different treatment schedules. Gut 25:129, 1984.

218. Sarin, S. K., Sachdev, G., Nanda, R., Batra, S. K., and Anand, B. S. Comparison of the two time schedules for endoscopic sclerotherapy: a prospective randomised controlled study. Gut 27:710, 1986.

219. Ayres, S. J., Goff, J. S., and Warren, G. H. Endoscopic sclerotherapy for bleeding esophageal varices: effects and complications. Ann. Intern. Med. 98:900, 1983.

220. Larson, A. W., Cohen, H., Zweiban, B., Chapman, D., Gourdji, M., Korula, J., and Weiner, J. Acute esophageal variceal sclerotherapy. JAMA 255:497, 1986.

221. Sorensen, T. I. A. Sclerotherapy after first variceal hemorrhage in cirrhosis. N. Engl. J. Med. 311:1594, 1984.

222. Westaby, D., Melia, W., Hegarty, J., Gimson, A. E. S., Stellon, A. J., and Williams, R. Use of propranolol to reduce the rebleeding rate during injection sclerotherapy prior to variceal obliteration. Hepatology 6:673, 1986.

223. Terblanche, J., Kahn, D., Campbell, J. A. H., Bornman, P. C., Jonker, M. A. T., Wright, J., and Kirsch, R. Failure of repeated injection sclerotherapy to improve long-term survival after oesophageal variceal bleeding. Lancet 2:1328, 1983.

224. Korula, J., Balart, L. A., Radvan, G., Zweiban, B. E., Larson, A. W., Kao, H. W., and Yamada, S. A prospective, randomized controlled trial of chronic esophageal variceal sclerotherapy. Hepatology 5:584, 1985.

225. Westaby, D., MacDougall, B. R. D., and Williams, R. Improved survival following injection sclerotherapy for esophageal varices: final analysis of a controlled trial. Hepatology 5:827, 1985.

226. Burroughs, A. K., D'Heygere, F., Phillips, A., Dooley, J., Epstein, O., and McIntyre, N. Prospective randomised trial of chronic sclerotherapy to prevent variceal rebleeding using the same protocol to treat bleeding. Interim analysis. Gut 27:A1246, 1986.

227. Cello, J. P., Grendell, J. H., Crass, R. A., Trunkey, D. D., Cobb, E. E., and Heilbron, D. C. Endoscopic sclerotherapy versus portacaval shunt in patients with severe cirrhosis and variceal hemorrhage. N. Engl. J. Med. 311:1589, 1984.

228. Cello, J. P., Grendell, J. H., Crass, R. A., Weber, T. E., and Trunkey, D. D. Endoscopic sclerotherapy versus portacaval shunt in patients with severe cirrhosis and acute variceal hemorrhage. N. Engl. J. Med. 316:11, 1987.

229. Silpa, J. M., Reedy, T., and Elashoff, J. Controlled trial of sclerotherapy for bleeding esophageal varices in alcoholic cirrhosis. Gastroenterology 90:1476, 1986.

230. Warren, W. D., Henderson, J. M., Millikan, W. J., Galambos, J. T., Brooks, W. S., Riepe, S. P., Salam, A. A., and Kutner, M. H. Distal splenorenal shunt versus endoscopic sclerotherapy for long-term management of variceal bleeding. Ann. Surg. 203:454, 1986.

230a. Schuman, B. M., Beckman, J. W., Tedesco, F. J., Griffin, J. W., and Assad, R. T. Complications of endoscopic injection sclerotherapy: a review. Am. J. Gastroenterol. 82:823, 1987.

231. Cohen, L. B., Korsten, M. A., Scherl, E. J., Velez, M. E., Fisse, R. D., and Arons, E. J. Bacteremia after endoscopic injection sclerosis. Gastrointest. Endosc. 29:198, 1983.

232. Monroe, P., Morrow, C. F., Jr., Millen, J. E., Fairman, R. P., and Glauser, F. L. Acute respiratory failure after sodium morrhuate esophageal sclerotherapy. Gastroenterology 85:693, 1983.

233. Bacon, B. R., Bailey-Newton, R. S., and Connors, A. F., Jr. Pleural effusions after endoscopic variceal sclerotherapy. Gastroenterology 88:1910, 1985.

234. Ayres, S. J., Goff, J. S., Warren, G. H., and Schaefer, J. W. Esophageal ulceration and bleeding after flexible fiberoptic esophageal vein sclerosis. Gastroenterology 83:131, 1982.

235. Carr-Locke, D. L. and Sidky, K. Broncho-oesophageal fistula: a late complication of endoscopic variceal sclerotherapy. Gut 23:1005, 1982.

236. Sorensen, T. I. A., Burcharth, F., Pedersen, M. L., and Findahl, F. Oesophageal stricture and dysphagia after endoscopic sclerotherapy for bleeding varices. Gut 25:473, 1984.

237. Tabibian, N., and Alpert, E. Refractory sclerotherapy-induced esophageal strictures. Ann. Intern. Med. 106:59, 1987.

238. Sauerbruch, T., Wirsching, R., Leisner, B., Weinzierl, M., Pfahler, M., and Paumgartner, G. Esophageal function after sclerotherapy of bleeding varices. Scand. J. Gastroenterol. 17:745, 1982.

239. Cohen, L. B., Simon, C., Korsten, M. A., Scherl, E. J., Skorniky, J., Guelrud, M. B., and Way, J. D. Esophageal motility and symptoms after endoscopic injection sclerotherapy. Dig. Dis. Sci. 30:29, 1985.

240. Snady, H. and Korsten, M. A. Prevention of dysphagia and stricture formation after endoscopic sclerotherapy. Gastroenterology 86:1258, 1984.

241. Lebrec, D., Corbic, M., Nouel, O., and Benhamou, J-P. Propranolol—a medical treatment for portal hypertension? Lancet 2:180, 1980.

242. Lebrec, D., Hillon, P., Munoz, C., Goldfarb, G., Nouel, O., and Benhamou, J-P. The effect of propranolol on portal hypertension in patients with cirrhosis: a hemodynamic study. Hepatology 2:523, 1982.

243. Hillon, P., Lebrec, D., Munoz, C., Jungers, M., Goldfarb, G., and Benhamou, J-P. Comparison of the effects of a cardioselective and a nonselective β-blocker on portal hypertension in patients with cirrhosis. Hepatology 2:528, 1982.

244. Westaby, D., Bihari, D. J., Gimson, A. E. S., Grossley, I. R., and Williams, R. Selective and non-selective beta receptor blockade in the reduction of portal pressure in patients with cirrhosis and portal hypertension. Gut 25:121, 1984.

245. Kroeger, R. J., and Groszmann, R. J. Effect of selective blockade of B₂-adrenergic receptors on portal and systemic hemodynamics in a portal hypertensive rat model. Gastroenterology 88:896, 1985.

246. Lebrec, D., Poynard, T., Bernuau, J., Bercoff, E., Nouel, O., Capron, J-P., Poupon, R., Bouvry, M., Rueff, B., and Benhamou, J-P. A randomized controlled study of propranolol for prevention of recurrent gastrointestinal bleeding in patients with cirrhosis: a final report. Hepatology 4:355, 1984.

247. Burroughs, A. K., Jenkins, W. J., Sherlock, S., Dunk, A., Walt, R. P., Osuafor, T. O. K., Mackie, S., and Dick, R. Controlled trial of propranolol for the prevention of recurrent variceal hemorrhage in patients with cirrhosis. N. Engl. J. Med. 309:1539, 1983.

248. Villeneuve, J-P., Pomier-Layrargues, G., Infante-Rivard, C., Willems, B., Huet, P-M., Marleau, D., and Viallet, A. Propranolol for the prevention of recurrent variceal hemorrhage: a controlled trial. Hepatology 6:1239, 1986.

249. Westaby, D., Melia, W. M., MacDougall, B. R. D., Hegarty, J. E., Gimson, A. E., and Williams, R. β₁ selective adrenoreceptor blockade for the long term management of variceal bleeding. A prospective randomised trial to compare oral metoprolol with injection sclerotherapy in cirrhosis. Gut 26:421, 1985.

250. Garcia-Tsao, G., Grace, N. D., Groszmann, R. J., Conn, H. O., Bermann, M. M., Patrick, M. J. C., Morse, S. S., and Alberts, J. L. Short-term effects of propranolol on portal venous pressure. Hepatology 6:101, 1986.

250a. Hosking, S. W., Kennedy, H. J., Seddon, I., and Triger, D. R. The role of propranolol in congestive gastropathy of portal hypertension. Hepatology 7:437, 1987.

251. Paquet, K. J. Prophylactic endoscopic sclerosing treatment of the esophageal wall in varices—a prospective controlled randomized trial. Endoscopy 14:4, 1982.

252. Witzel, L., Wolbergs, E., and Merki, H. Prophylactic endoscopic sclerotherapy of oesophageal varices. Lancet 1:773, 1985.

253. Sauerbruch, T., Wotzka, R., Kopcke, W., Harlin, M., Kuhner, W., Sander, R., Heldwein, M., Ultsch, B., Ansari, H., and Paumgartner, G. Endoscopic sclerotherapy (ST) for prophylaxis of first variceal bleeding in liver cirrhosis. Early results of a prospective randomized trial. Gastroenterology 90:1765, 1986.

254. Gregory, P., Hartigan, P., Amodeo, D., Baum, R., Camara, D., Colcher, H., Fye, C., Gebhard, R., Goff, J., Kruss, D., McPhee, M., Meier, P., Rankin, R., Reichelderfer, M., Sanowski, R., Shields, D., Silvis, S., Weesner, R., Winship, D., and Young, H. Prophylactic sclerotherapy for esophageal varices in alcoholic liver disease: results of a VA cooperative randomized trial. Gastroenterology 92:1414, 1987.

255. Koch, H., Henning, H., Grimm, H., and Soehendra, N. Prophylactic sclerosing of esophageal varices—results of a prospective controlled study. Endoscopy 18:40, 1986.

256. Triger, D. R., and Johnson, A. G. Prophylactic sclerotherapy of oesophageal varices: a preliminary report. Gut 26:A1102, 1985.

257. Pascal, J.-P., and Cales, P. Propranolol in the prevention of first upper gastrointestinal tract hemorrhage in patients with cirrhosis of the liver and esophageal varices. N. Engl. J. Med. 317:856, 1987.

258. Lebrec, D., Poynard, T., Capron, J. P., Hillon, P., Geoffroy, P., Arsene, D., Roulot, D., Chaput, J. C., and Benhamou, J-P. A randomized trial of nadolol for prevention of gastrointestinal bleeding in patients with cirrhosis. Results at one year. Gastroenterology 90:1740, 1986.

259. Burroughs, A. K., D'Heygere, F., and McIntyre, N. Pitfalls in studies of prophylactic therapy for variceal bleeding in cirrhotics. Hepatology 6:1407, 1986.

260. Graham, D. Y., and Davis, R. E. Acute upper-gastrointestinal hemorrhage: new observation on an old problem. Am. J. Dig. Dis. 23:76, 1978.

261. Webb, W. A., McDaniel, L., Johnson, R. C., and Haynes, C. D. Endoscopic evaluation of 125 cases of upper gastrointestinal bleeding. Ann. Surg. 193:624, 1981.

261a. Carson, J. L., Strom, B. L., Soper, K. A., West, S. L., and Morse, M. L. The association of nonsteroidal anti-inflammatory drugs with upper gastrointestinal tract bleeding. Arch. Int. Med. 147:85, 1987.

261b. Beard, K., et al. Arch. Int. Med. 147:1621, 1987.

262. Sanford, C. H., Hughes, J. D., and Weems, J. Pneumonia complicated by acute pneumococcic hemorrhagic ulcerative gastroenteritis (Dieulafoy's erosion). Arch. Intern. Med. 62:597, 1938.

263. Hastings, P. R., Skillman, J. J., Bushnell, L. S., and Silen, W. Antacid titration in the prevention of acute gastrointestinal bleeding. N. Engl. J. Med. 298:1041, 1978.

264. Zinner, M. J., Zuidema, G. D., Smith, P. L., and Mignosa, M. The prevention of upper gastrointestinal tract bleeding in patients in an intensive care unit. Surg. Gynecol. Obstet. 153:214, 1981.

265. Czaja, A. J., McAlhany, J. C., and Pruitt, B. A. Acute gastroduodenal disease after thermal injury. N. Engl. J. Med. 291:925, 1974.

266. Halloran, L. G., Zfass, Z. M., Gayle, W. E., Wheeler, C. B., and Miller, J. D. Prevention of acute gastrointestinal complications after severe head injury: a controlled trial of cimetidine prophylaxis. Am. J. Surg. 139:44, 1980.

267. Schuster, D. P., Rowley, H., Feinstein, S., McGue, M. K., and Zuckerman, G. R. Prospective evaluation of the risk of upper gastrointestinal bleeding after admission to a medical intensive care unit. Am. J. Med. 76:623, 1984.

268. Hubert, J. P., Kiernan, P. D., Welch, J. S., ReMine, W. H., and Beahrs, O. H. The surgical management of bleeding stress ulcer. Ann. Surg. 191:672, 1980.

269. Simonian, S. J., and Curtis, L. E. Treatment of hemorrhagic gastritis by antacid. Ann. Surg. 184:429, 1976.

270. Weiss, J. B., Peskin, G. W., and Isenberg, J. I. Treatment of hemorrhagic gastritis with 15(R)-15 methyl prostaglandin E_2: report of a case. Gastroenterology 82:558, 1982.

271. Rosch, J., Keller, F. S., Kozak, B., Niles, N., and Dotter, C. T. Gelfoam powder embolization of the left gastric artery in treatment of massive small-vessel gastric bleeding. Radiology 151:365, 1984.

272. Athanasoulis, C. A., Baum, S., Waltman, A. C., Ring, E. J., Imbembo, A., and Vander Salm, T. J. Control of acute gastric mucosal hemorrhage. N. Engl. J. Med. 290:597, 1974.

273. Alves, M., Patel, V., Douglas, E., and Deutsch, E. Gastric infarction: a complication of selective vasopressin infusion. Dig. Dis. Sci. 24:409, 1979.

274. McAlhany, J. C., Czaja, A. J., and Pruitt, B. A. Antacid control of complications from acute gastroduodenal disease after burns. J. Trauma 16:645, 1976.

275. Priebe, H. J., Skillman, J. J., Bushnell, L. S., Long, P. C., and Silen, W. Antacid versus cimetidine in preventing acute gastrointestinal bleeding. N. Engl. J. Med. 302:426, 1980.

276. McElwee, H. P., Sirinek, K. R., and Levine, B. A. Cimetidine affords protection equal to antacids in prevention of stress ulceration following thermal injury. Surgery 86:620, 1979.

277. Groll, A., Simon, J. B., Wigle, R. D., Taguchi, K., Todd, R. J., and Depew, W. T. Cimetidine prophylaxis for gastrointestinal bleeding in an intensive care unit. Gut 27:135, 1986.

278. Stothert, J. C., Simoniwitz, D. A., Dellinger, E. P., Farley, M., Edwards, W. A., Blair, A. D., Cutler, R., and Carrico, C. J. Randomized prospective evaluation of cimetidine and antacid control of gastric pH in the critically ill. Ann. Surg. 192:169, 1980.

279. Martin, L. F., Max, M. H., and Polk, H. C. Failure of gastric pH control by antacids or cimetidine in the critically ill: a valid sign of sepsis. Surgery 88:59, 1980.

280. More, D. G., Raper, R. F., Munro, I. A., Watson, C. J., Boutagy, J. S., and Shenfield, G. M. Randomized, prospective trial of cimetidine and ranitidine for control of intragastric pH in the critically ill. Surgery 97:215, 1985.

280a. Shuman, R. B. Schuster, D. P., and Zuckerman, G. R. Prophylactic therapy for stress ulcer bleeding: a reappraisal. Ann. Int. Med. 106:562, 1987.

281. Bresalier, R. S., Grendell, J. H., Cello, J. P., and Meyer, A. A. Sucralfate suspension versus titrated antacid for the prevention of acute stress-related gastrointestinal hemorrhage in critically ill patients. Am. J. Med., 83(Suppl. 3B):110, 1987.

282. Tryba, M. The risk of acute stress bleeding and nosocomial pneumonia in ventilated ICU-patients: sucralfate vs antacids. Am. J. Med., 83(Suppl. 3B):117, 1987.

283. Driks, M. R., Craven, D. E., Celli, B. R., Manning, M., Burke, R. A., Garvin, G. M., Kunches, L. M., Farber, H. W., Wedel, S. A., and McCabe, W. R. Nosocomial pneumonia in intubated patients given sucralfate as compared with antacids or histamine type 2 blockers. The role of gastric colonization. N. Engl. J. Med. 317:1376, 1987.

284. Mallory, G. K., and Weiss, S. Hemorrhages from lacerations of the cardiac orifice of the stomach due to vomiting. Am. J. Med. Sci. 178:506, 1929.

285. Foster, D. N., Miloszewski, K., and Losowsky, M. S. Diagnosis of Mallory-Weiss lesions: a common cause of upper gastrointestinal bleeding. Lancet 2:483, 1976.

286. Graham, D. Y., and Schwartz, J. T. The spectrum of the Mallory-Weiss tear. Medicine 57:307, 1977.

287. Knauer, C. M. Characterization of 75 Mallory-Weiss lacerations in 528 patients with upper gastrointestinal hemorrhage. Gastroenterology 71:5, 1976.

288. Davis, G. B., Bookstein, J. J., and Coel, M. N. Advantage of intraarterial over intravenous vasopressin infusion in gastrointestinal hemorrhage. AJR 128:733, 1971.

289. Carsen, G. M., Casarella, W. J., and Speigel, R. M. Transcatheter embolization for treatment of Mallory-Weiss tears of the esophagogastric junction. Radiology 128:309, 1978.

290. Shepherd, H. A., Harvey, J., Jackson, A., and Colin-Jones, D. G. Recurrent retching with gastric mucosal prolapse. Dig. Dis. Sci. 29:212, 1984.

291. Fagan, E. A., Allison, D. F., Chadwick, V. S., and Hodgson,

H. J. F. Treatment of haemobilia by selective arterial embolisation. Gut *21*:541, 1980.

292. Wagner, W. H., Lundell, C. J., and Donovan, A. J. Percutaneous angiographic embolization for hepatic arterial hemorrhage. Arch. Surg. *120*:1241, 1985.

293. Goldstein, H. M., Medellin, H., Ben-Menachem, Y., and Wallace, S. Transcatheter arterial embolization in the management of bleeding in the cancer patient. Radiology *115*:603, 1975.

294. Steffes, B. C., and O'Leary, P. Primary aortoduodenal fistula: a case report and review of the literature. Am. Surg. *46*:121, 1980.

295. Case records of the Massachusetts General Hospital. N. Engl. J. Med. *304*:1533, 1981.

296. Busutil, R. W., Rees, W., Baker, D., and Wilson, S. E. Pathogenesis of aortoduodenal fistula: experimental and clinical correlates. Surgery *85*:1, 1979.

297. Buchbinder, D., Leather, R., Shah, D., and Karmody, A. Pathologic interactions between prosthetic aortic grafts and the gastrointestinal tract. Am. J. Surg. *140*:192, 1980.

298. Case records of the Massachusetts General Hospital. N. Engl. J. Med. *297*:828, 1977.

299. Purdue, G. D., Smith, R. B., Ansley, J. D., and Costantino, M. J. Impending aortoenteric hemorrhage. Ann. Surg. *192*:237, 1980.

300. Brand, E. J., Sivak, M. V., and Sullivan, B. H. Aortoduodenal fistula. Dig. Dis. Sci. *24*:940, 1979.

301. Makhija, M., Schultz, S. Imaging of an actively bleeding aortoduodenal fistula. Clin. Nucl. Med. *10*:372, 1985.

302. McGuire, H. H., and Haynes, B. W. Massive hemorrhage from diverticulosis of colon. Ann. Surg. *175*:847, 1972.

303. Drapanas, T., Pennington, D. G., Kappelman, M., and Lindsey, E. S. Emergency subtotal colectomy: preferred approach to management of massively bleeding diverticular disease. Ann. Surg. *177*:519, 1973.

304. Wright, H. K., Pelicci, O., Higgins, E. F., Sreenivas, V., and Gupta, A. Controlled, semielective, segmental resection for massive colonic hemorrhage. Am. J. Surg. *139*:535, 1980.

305. Bar, A. H., DeLaurentis, D. A., Parry, C. E., and Keohane, R. B. Angiography in the management of massive lower gastrointestinal tract hemorrhage. Surg. Gynecol. Obstet. *150*:226, 1980.

306. Athanasoulis, C. A., Baum, S., Rosch, J., Waltman, A. C., Ring, E. J., Smith, J. C., Sugarbaker, E., and Wood, W. Mesenteric arterial infusions of vasopressin for hemorrhage from colonic diverticulosis. Am. J. Surg. *129*:212, 1975.

307. Casarella, W. J., Kanter, I. E., and Seaman, W. B. Right-sided colonic diverticula as a cause of acute rectal hemorrhage. N. Engl. J. Med. *286*:450, 1972.

308. Casarella, W. J., Galloway, S. J., Taxin, R. N., Follett, D. A., Pollock, E. J., and Seaman, W. B. Lower gastrointestinal tract hemorrhage; new concepts based on arteriography. AJR *121*:357, 1974.

309. Nath, R. L., Sequeira, J. C., Weitzman, A. F., Birkett, D. H., and Williams, L. F. Lower gastrointestinal bleeding. Am. J. Surg. *141*:478, 1981.

310. Talman, E. A., Dixon, D. S., and Gutierrez, F. E. Role of arteriography in rectal hemorrhage due to arteriovenous malformations and diverticulosis. Ann. Surg. *190*:203, 1979.

311. Boley, S. J., DiBiase, A., Brandt, L. J., and Sammartano, R. J. Lower intestinal bleeding in the elderly. Am. J. Surg. *137*:57, 1979.

312. Welch, C. E., Athanasoulis, C. A., and Galdabini, J. J. Hemorrhage from the large bowel with special reference to angiodysplasia and diverticular disease. World J. Surg. *2*:73, 1978.

313. Britt, L. G., Warren, L., and Moore, O. F. Selective management of lower gastrointestinal bleeding. Am. Surg. *49*:121, 1983.

314. Browder, W., Cerise, E. J., and Litwin, M. S. Impact of emergency angiography in massive lower gastrointestinal bleeding. Ann. Surg. *204*:530, 1986.

315. Swarbrick, E. T., Fevre, D. I., Hunt, R. H., Thomas, B. M., and Williams, C. B. Colonoscopy for unexplained rectal bleeding. Br. Med. J. *2*:1685, 1978.

316. Teague, R. H., Thornton, J. R., Manning, A. P., Salmon, P. R., and Read, A. W. Colonoscopy for investigation of unexplained rectal bleeding. Lancet *1*:1350, 1978.

317. Tedesco, F. J., Waye, J. D., Raskin, J. B., Morris, S. J., and Greenwald, R. A. Colonoscopic evaluation of rectal bleeding. Ann. Intern. Med. *89*:907, 1978.

318. Brand, E. J., Sullivan, B. H., Sivak, M. V., and Rankin, G. B. Colonoscopy in the diagnosis of unexplained rectal bleeding. Ann. Surg. *192*:111, 1980.

319. Brandt, L. J., and Boley, S. J. The role of colonoscopy in the diagnosis and management of lower intestinal bleeding. Scand. J. Gastroenterol. *102*:61, 1984.

320. Jaques, P. F., and Fitch, D. D. Anal verge and low rectal bleeding. A diagnostic problem. J. Clin. Gastroenterol. *8*:38, 1986.

321. Kelly, S. M., Sanowski, R. A., Foutch, P. G., Bellapravalu, S., and Haynes, W. C. A prospective comparison of anoscopy and fiberendoscopy in detecting anal lesions. J. Clin. Gastroenterol. *8*:658, 1986.

322. Bat, L., Pines, A., Rabau, M., Niv, Y., and Shemesh, E. Colonoscopic findings in patients with hemorrhoids, rectal bleeding and normal rectoscopy. Isr. J. Med. Sci. *21*:139, 1985.

323. Goulston, K. J., Cook, I., and Dent, O. F. How important is rectal bleeding in the diagnosis of bowel cancer and polyps? Lancet *2*:261, 1986.

324. Jensen, D. M., and Machicado, G. A. Emergent colonoscopy in patients with severe lower gastrointestinal bleeding. Gastroenterology *80*:1184, 1981.

325. Koval, G., Benner, K. G., Rosch, J., and Kozak, B. E. Aggressive angiographic diagnosis in acute lower gastrointestinal hemorrhage. Dig. Dis. Sci. *32*:248, 1987.

326. Uden, P., Jiborn, H., and Jonsson, K. Influence of selective mesenteric arteriography on the outcome of emergency surgery for massive, lower gastrointestinal hemorrhage. Dis. Colon Rectum *29*:561, 1986.

327. Alavi, A., Dann, R. W., Baum, S., and Biery, D. N. Scintigraphic detection of acute gastrointestinal bleeding. Radiology *124*:753, 1977.

328. Alavi, A., and Ring, E. J. Localization of gastrointestinal bleeding: superiority of ^{99m}Tc sulfur colloid compared with angiography. AJR *137*:741, 1981.

329. Winn, M., Weissmann, H. S., Sprayregen, S., and Freeman, L. M. The radionuclide detection of lower gastrointestinal bleeding sites. Clin. Nucl. Med. *8*:389, 1983.

330. Lecklitner, M. L. Pitfalls of gastrointestinal bleeding studies with 99mTc sulfur-colloid. Semin. Nucl. Med. *16*:155, 1986.

331. Miskowiak, J., Nielsen, S. L., Munck, O., Burcharth, F., Bichert-Toft, M., and Nadel, M. S. Acute gastrointestinal bleeding detected with abdominal scintigraphy using technetium-99m-labeled albumin. Scand. J. Gastroenterol. *14*:389, 1979.

332. Winzelberg, G. G., McKusick, K. A., Strauss, H. W., Waltman, A. C., and Greenfield, A. J. Evaluation of gastrointestinal bleeding by red blood cells labeled in vivo with technetium-99m. J. Nucl. Med. *20*:1080, 1979.

333. Winzelberg, G. G., Froelich, J. W., McKusick, K. A., Waltman, A. C., Greenfield, A. J., Athanasoulis, C. A., and Strauss, H. W. Radionuclide localization of lower gastrointestinal hemorrhage. Radiology *139*:465, 1981.

334. Markisz, J. A., Front, D., Royal, H. D., Sacks, B., Parker, A. J., and Kolodny, G. M. An evaluation of ^{99m}Tc-labeled red blood cell scintigraphy for the detection and localization of gastrointestinal bleeding sites. Gastroenterology *83*:394, 1982.

335. Kester, R. R., Welch, J. P., and Sziklas, J. P. The 99mTc-labeled RBC scan. A diagnostic method for lower gastrointestinal bleeding. Dis. Colon Rectum *27*:47, 1984.

336. Landry, A., Hartshorne, M. F., Bunker, S. R., Bauman, J. M., Cawthon, M. A., Karl, R. D., and Howard, W. H. Optimal technetium-99m RBC labeling for gastrointestinal hemorrhage study. Clin. Nucl. Med. *10*:491, 1985.

337. Orecchia, P. M., Hensley, E. K., McDonald, P. T., and Lull, R. J. Localization of lower gastrointestinal hemorrhage. Experience with red blood cells labeled in vitro with technetium Tc99m. Arch. Surg. *120*:621, 1985.

338. Bunker, S. R., Lull, R. J., Tanasescu, D. E., Redwine, M.

D., Rigby, J., Brown, J. M., et al. Scintigraphy of gastrointestinal hemorrhage: superiority of 99mTc red blood cells over 99mTc sulfur colloid. AJR *143*:543, 1984.

339. Siddiqui, A. R., Schauwecker, D. S., Wellman, H. N., and Mock, B. H. Comparison of technetium-99m sulfur colloid and in vitro labeled technetium-99m RBCs in the detection of gastrointestinal bleeding. Clin. Nucl. Med. *10*:546, 1985.

340. Kilpatrick, Z. M., and Aseron, C. A. Jr. Radioisotope detection of Meckel's diverticulum causing acute rectal hemorrhage. N. Engl. J. Med. *287*:653, 1972.

341. Ho, J. E., and Konieczny, K. M. The sodium pertechnetate Tc 99m scan: an aid in the evaluation of gastrointestinal bleeding. Pediatrics *56*:34, 1975.

342. Sfakianakis, G. N., and Conway, J. J. Detection of ectopic gastric mucosa in Meckel's diverticulum and in other aberrations by scintigraphy: I. Pathophysiology and 10-year clinical experience. J. Nucl. Med. *22*:647, 1981.

343. Fries, M., Mortensson, W., and Robertson, B. Technetium pertechnetate scintigraphy to detect ectopic gastric mucosa in Meckel's diverticulum. Acta Radiol. *25*:417, 1984.

344. Kewenter, J., Hellzen-Ingemarsson, A., Kewenter, G., and Olsson, U. Diverticular disease and minor rectal bleeding. Scand. J. Gastroenterol. *20*:922, 1985.

345. Athanasoulis, C. A., Galdabini, J. J., Waltman, A. C., Novelline, R. A., Greenfield, A. J., and Ezpeleta, M. L. Angiodysplasia of the colon: a cause of rectal bleeding. Cardiovasc. Radiol. *1*:3, 1978.

346. Boley, S. J., Sammartano, R., Adams, A., DiBiase, A., Kleinhaus, S., and Sprayregen, S. On the nature and etiology of vascular ectasias of colon. Gastroenterology *72*:650, 1977.

347. Boley, S. J., Sammartano, R., Brandt, L. J., and Sprayregen, S. Vascular ectasias of the colon. Surg. Gynecol. Obstet. *149*:353, 1979.

348. Weaver, G. A., Alpern, H. D., Davis, J. S., Ramsey, W. H., and Reichelderfer, M. Gastrointestinal angiodysplasia associated with aortic valve disease: part of a spectrum of angiodysplasia of the gut. Gastroenterology *77*:1, 1979.

349. Howard, O. M., Buchanan, J. D., and Hunt, R. H. Angiodysplasia of the colon. Lancet *2*:16, 1982.

350. Richter, J. M., Hedberg, S. E., Athanasoulis, C. A., and Schapiro, R. H. Angiodysplasia—clinical presentation and colonoscopic diagnosis. Dig. Dis. Sci. *29*:481, 1984.

351. Williams, R. C. Aortic stenosis and unexplained gastrointestinal bleeding. Arch. Intern. Med. *108*:103, 1961.

352. Greenstein, R. J., McElhinney, A. J., Reuben, D., and Greenstein, A. J. Colonic vascular ectasias and aortic stenosis: coincidence or causal relationship? Am. J. Surg. *151*:347, 1986.

353. Aldabagh, S. M., Trujillo, Y. P., and Taxy, J. B. Utility of specimen angiography in angiodysplasia of the colon. Gastroenterology *91*:725, 1986.

354. Mitsudo, S. M., Boley, S. J., Brandt, L. J., Montefusco, C. M., and Sammartano, R. J. Vascular ectasias of the right colon in the elderly: a distinct pathologic entity. Hum. Pathol. *10*:585, 1979.

355. Cappell, M. S., and Lebwohl, O. Cessation of recurrent bleeding from gastrointestinal angiodysplasias after aortic valve replacement. Ann. Intern. Med. *105*:54, 1986.

356. Tisnado, J., Cho, S. R., Beachley, M. C., and Margolius, D. A. Transcatheter embolization of angiodysplasia of the rectum. Report of a case. Acta Radiol. *26*:677, 1985.

357. Rogers, B. H. Endoscopic diagnosis and therapy of mucosal vascular abnormalities of the gastrointestinal tract occurring in elderly patients and associated with cardiac, vascular, and pulmonary disease. Gastrointest. Endosc. *26*:134, 1980.

358. Rutgeerts, P., Van Gompel, F., Geboes, K., Vantrappen, G., Broeckaert, L., and Coremans, G. Long term results of treatment of vascular malformations of the gastrointestinal tract by neodymium Yag laser photocoagulation. Gut *26*:586, 1985.

359. Jensen, D. M., and Machicado, G. A. Bleeding colonic angioma: endoscopic coagulation and follow-up. Gastroenterology *88*:1433, 1985.

360. Geelhoed, G. W., Druy, E. M., and Steinberg, W. M. Recurrent bleeding from Meckel's diverticulum in an adult: angiographic demonstration after normal scans. South. Med. J. *79*:65, 1986.

361. Gebarski, K. S., Byrne, W. J., Gebarski, S. S., Wesley, J. R., and Coran, A. G. Hematochezia and the false negative Meckel's scan: a continued need for barium studies. Am. J. Gastroenterol. *80*:781, 1985.

362. Sutherland, D. E. R., Chan, F. Y., Foucar, E., Simmons, R. L., Howard, R. J., and Najarian, J. S. The bleeding cecal ulcer in transplant patients. Surgery *86*:386, 1979.

363. Mills, B., Zuckerman, G., and Sicard, G. Discrete colon ulcers as a cause of lower gastrointestinal bleeding and perforation in end-stage renal disease. Surgery *89*:548, 1981.

364. Case records of the Massachusetts General Hospital. N. Engl. J. Med. *298*:208, 1978.

365. Norfleet, R. G. 1,300 mg. of aspirin daily does not cause positive fecal Hemoccult tests. J. Clin. Gastroenterol. *5*:123, 1983.

366. Bahrt, K. M., Korman, L. Y., and Nashel, D. J. Significance of a positive test for occult blood in stools of patients taking anti-inflammatory drugs. Arch. Intern. Med. *144*:2165, 1984.

367. Pye, G., Ballantyne, K. C., Armitage, N. C., and Hardcastle, J. D. Influence of non-steroidal anti-inflammatory drugs on the outcome of faecal occult blood tests in screening for colorectal cancer. Br. Med. J. *294*:1510, 1987.

367a. Jaffin, B. W., Bliss, G. M., and Lamont, J. T. Significance of occult gastrointestinal bleeding during anticoagulation therapy. Am. J. Med. *83*:269, 1987.

368. Aldridge, M. C., and Sim, A. J. W. Colonoscopy findings in symptomatic patients without x-ray evidence of colonic neoplasms. Lancet *2*:833, 1986.

369. Maxfield, R. G., and Maxfield, C. M. Colonoscopy as a primary diagnostic procedure in chronic gastrointestinal tract bleeding. Arch. Surg. *212*:401, 1986.

370. Thoeni, R. F., and Venbrux, A. C. The value of colonoscopy and double-contrast barium-enema examinations in the evaluation of patients with subacute and chronic lower intestinal bleeding. Radiology *146*:603, 1983.

371. Thompson, J. N., Salem, R. R., Hemingway, A. P., Rees, H. C., Hodgson, H. J. F., Wood, C. B., Allison, D. J., and Spencer, J. Specialist investigation of obscure gastrointestinal bleeding. Gut *18*:47, 1987.

371a. Lau, W. Y., Fan, S. T., Wong, S. H., Wong, K. P., Poon, G. P., Chu, K. W., Yip, W. C., and Wong, K. K. Preoperative and intraoperative localisation of gastrointestinal bleeding of obscure origin. Gut *28*:869, 1987.

372. Selink, J. L. Radiologic examination of the small intestine by duodenal intubation. Acta Radiol. *15*:318, 1974.

373. Maglinte, D. D., Elmore, M. F., Chernish, S. M., Miller, R. E., Lehman, G., Bishop, R., Blitz, G., Kohne, J., and Isenberg, M. T. Enteroclysis in the diagnosis of chronic unexplained gastrointestinal bleeding. Dis. Colon Rectum *28*:403, 1985.

374. Szasz, I. J., Morrison, R. T., and Lyster, D. M. Technetium-99m-labelled red blood cell scanning to diagnose occult gastrointestinal bleeding. Can. J. Surg. *28*:512, 1985.

375. Tumeh, S. S., Parker, J. A., Royal, H. D., Uren, R. F., and Kolodny, G. M. Detection of bleeding from angiodysplasia of the jejunum by blood pool scintigraphy. Clin. Nucl. Med. *8*:127, 1983.

376. Yamamoto, Y., Sano, K., and Shigemoto, H. Detection of the bleeding source from small intestine: intraoperative endoscopy and preoperative abdominal scintigraphy by technetium 99m pertechnetate. Am. Surg. *51*:658, 1985.

377. Sheedy, P. F., Fulton, R. E., and Atwell, D. T. Angiographic evaluation of patients with chronic gastrointestinal bleeding. AJR *123*:338, 1975.

378. Best, E. B., Teaford, A. K., and Rader, R. H. Angiography in chronic-recurrent gastrointestinal bleeding: a nine year study. Surg. Clin. North Am. *59*:811, 1979.

379. Athow, A. C., Sheppard, L., and Sibson, D. E. Selective visceral angiography for unexplained acute gastrointestinal bleeding in a district general hospital. Br. J. Surg. *72*:120, 1985.

380. Llau, W. Y., Fan, S. T., Chu, K. W., Yip, W. C., Poon, G. P., and Wong, K. K. Intraoperative fiberoptic enteroscopy for bleeding lesions in the small intestine. Br. J. Surg. *73*:217, 1986.

381. Navab, F., Westbrook, K. C., Slaton, G., and Boyd, C. M.

Use of intraoperative radionuclide study and colonoscopy in gastrointestinal hemorrhage. Clin. Nucl. Med. *10*:188, 1985.

382. Williamson, M. R., Boyd, C. M., McGuire, E. L., Angtuaco, T., Westbrook, K. C., Lang, N. P., Alston, J., Broadwater, J. R., Navab, F., and Bersey, M. L. Precise intraoperative location of gastrointestinal bleeding with a hand-held counter. Work in progress. Radiology *159*:272, 1986.

383. Case records of the Massachusetts General Hospital. N. Engl. J. Med. *308*:579, 1983.

384. Case Records of the Massachusetts General Hospital. N. Engl. J. Med. *300*:129, 1979.

385. Quintero, E., Pique, J. M., Bombi, J. A., Ros, E., Bordas, J. M., Rives, A., Tores, J., and Rodes, J. Upper gastrointestinal bleeding caused by gastroduodenal vascular malformations. Dig. Dis. Sci. *31*:897, 1986.

386. Vase, P., and Grove, O. Gastrointestinal lesions in hereditary hemorrhagic telangiectasia. Gastroenterology *91*:1079, 1986.

387. Bown, S. G., Swain, C. P., Storey, D. W., Collins, C., Matthewson, K., Salmon, P. R., and Clark, C. G. Endoscopic laser treatment of vascular anomalies of the upper gastrointestinal tract. Gut *26*:1338, 1985.

388. Waitman, A. M., Grant, D. Z., and Chateau, F. Endoscopic laser photocoagulation of bleeding upper gastrointestinal telangiectasia. Am. J. Gastroenterol. *74*:97, 1980.

389. Baum, S., Nusbaum, M. H., and Blakemore, W. S. The preoperative radiographic demonstration of intra-abdominal bleeding from undetermined sites by percutaneous selective celiac and superior mesenteric arteriography. Surgery *58*:797, 1965.

390. Moore, J. D., Thompson, N. W., Appelman, H. D., and Foley, D. Arteriovenous malformation of the gastrointestinal tract. Arch. Surg. *111*:381, 1976.

391. Richardson, J. D., Max, M. H., Flint, L. M., Schweisinger, W., Howard, M., and Aust, J. B. Bleeding vascular malformations of the intestine. Surgery *84*:430, 1978.

392. Meyer, C. T., Troncale, F. J., Galloway, S., and Sheahan, D. G. Arteriovenous malformations of the bowel: an analysis of 22 cases and a review of the literature. Medicine *60*:36, 1981.

393. Clouse, R. E., Costigan, D. J., Mills, B. A., and Zuckerman, G. R. Angiodysplasia as a cause of gastrointestinal bleeding. Arch. Intern. Med. *145*:458, 1985.

394. Duray, P. H., Marcal, J. M., LiVolsi, V. A., Fisher, R., Scholhamer, C., and Brand, M. H. Small intestinal angiodysplasia in the elderly. J. Clin. Gastroenterol. *6*:311, 1984.

395. Zuckerman, G. R., Cornette, G. L., Clouse, R. E., and Harter, H. R. Upper gastrointestinal bleeding in patients with chronic renal failure. Ann. Intern. Med. *102*:588, 1985.

396. Bronner, M. H., Pate, M. B., Cunningham, J. T., and Marsh, W. H. Estrogen-progesterone therapy for bleeding gastrointestinal telangiectasias in chronic renal failure. Ann. Intern. Med. *105*:371, 1986.

397. Livio, M., Mannucci, P. M., Vigano, G., Mingardi, G., Lombardi, R., Mecca, G., and Remuzzi, G. Conjugated estrogens for the management of bleeding associated with renal failure. N. Engl. J. Med. *315*:731, 1986.

398. Jabbari, M., Cherry, R., Lough, J. O., Daly, D. S., Kinnear, D. G., and Goresky, C. A. Gastric antral vascular ectasia: the watermelon stomach. Gastroenterology *87*:1165, 1984.

399. Gilliam, J. H., Geisinger, K. R., Wu, W. C., Richter, J. E., and Scharyj, M. The "watermelon stomach." Gastroenterology *88*:1394, 1985.

400. Rawlinson, W. D., Barr, G. D., and Lin, B. P. Antral vascular ectasia—the "watermelon" stomach. Med. J. Aust. *144*:709, 1986.

400a. Petrini, J. L., and Johnston, J. H. Definitive heater probe therapy for the watermelon stomach. (Abstract.) Gastrointest. Endosc. *33*:176, 1987.

401. Cameron, A. J., and Higgins, J. A. Linear gastric erosion. A lesion associated with large diaphragmatic hernia and chronic blood loss anemia. Gastroenterology *91*:338, 1986.

402. Sherman, L., Shenoy, S. S., Satschidanand, S. K., Neumann, P. R., Barrios, G. G., and Peer, R. M. Arteriovenous malformation of the stomach. Am. J. Gastroenterol. *72*:160, 1979.

403. Case records of the Massachusetts General Hospital. N. Engl. J. Med. *305*:211, 1981.

404. Vaccaro, P., Zollinger, R. W., Sharma, H., and Cooperman, M. Massive upper gastrointestinal hemorrhage from an arteriovenous malformation of the stomach. J. Clin. Gastroenterol. *7*:285, 1985.

405. Strong, R. W. Dieulafoy's disease—a distinct clinical entity. Aust. N.Z. J. Surg. *54*:337, 1984.

406. Hoffmann, J., Beck, H., and Jensen, H. E. Dieulafoy's lesion. Surg. Gynecol. Obstet. *159*:537, 1984.

407. Veldhuyzen van Zanten, S. J. O., Bartelsman, J. F. W. M., Schipper, M. E. I., and Tytgat, G. N. J. Recurrent massive haematemesis from Dieulafoy vascular malformations—a review of 101 cases. Gut *27*:213, 1986.

408. Bakka, A., and Roselland, A. R. Massive gastric bleeding from exulceratio simplex (Dieulafoy). Acta Chir. Scand. *152*:285, 1986.

409. Barbier, P., Luder, P., Triller, J., Ruchti, C., Hassler, H., and Stafford, A. Colonic hemorrhage from a solitary minute ulcer. Gastroenterology *88*:1065, 1985.

26

Ascites

MICHAEL D. BENDER
ROBERT K. OCKNER

GENERAL ASPECTS

Clinical Features of Ascites

Ascites, the accumulation of fluid within the peritoneal cavity, is a common clinical finding with a wide range of causes. Its pathophysiology varies with the cause and will be considered in detail for specific disease entities in this chapter and on pages 1932 to 1967.

Small amounts of ascites may be asymptomatic, but as the amount of fluid increases, the patient becomes aware of abdominal distention and a sense of fullness and discomfort. Larger amounts of ascites, especially when the abdomen is tensely distended, may cause respiratory distress, anorexia, nausea, early satiety, pyrosis, or frank pain. Body weight may increase as fluid accumulates, but if ascites is associated with alcoholism, poor nutrition, or neoplasm, weight may remain stable or actually drop.

On physical examination relatively large amounts of ascites cause abdominal distention, with bulging flanks which are dull to percussion. As the amount increases, flank dullness can be shown to shift as the patient is turned from side to side. When ascites is massive, a fluid wave can be elicited by striking one flank and feeling the transmitted wave on the opposite flank. Although it is difficult to detect less than 1.5 to 2 liters of fluid, placing the patient on hands and knees and percussing flatness over the dependent abdomen ("puddle sign") may permit demonstration of as little as 300 to 400 ml of fluid. Indirect evidence, such as penile or scrotal edema, umbilical herniation, and pleural effusion, may suggest the presence of ascites.

Although the physical diagnosis of large amounts of ascites may be fairly easy, physical examination has definite limitations in the diagnosis of small amounts of ascites. Two recent studies reveal that overall physical assessment is accurate in only 50 per cent of patients with equivocal ascites, resulting primarily in a high incidence of false positive results. Flank dullness is the most sensitive sign, and a fluid wave is the most specific sign.[1, 2] Measurements of *abdominal girth* to monitor changes in ascites may also be fraught with error, as wide individual variations have been noted with changes in intra-abdominal fluid volume.[3]

Because of the nonspecificity of the physical signs of ascites, it may be difficult to differentiate ascites from other causes of abdominal distention such as obesity, intestinal distention, or large tumors. Large intra-abdominal cysts may easily simulate ascites,[4] as may excessive intra-abdominal fat deposition in the mesentery (see p. 1952). When the physical diagnosis of ascites is uncertain, other techniques are available for definitive diagnosis.

Diagnosis

The presence of ascites can be further evaluated or confirmed by imaging techniques (radiology, ultrasonography, CT scan) or paracentesis. These methods may also provide information about the etiology of ascites, as will ascitic fluid analysis, peritoneal biopsy, and peritoneoscopy.

Conventional Radiology. Large amounts of fluid, readily detectable on plain abdominal films, are manifested by abdominal haziness, increased density shifting to the pelvis on upright films, separation of bowel loops, and obliteration of the psoas shadows. Smaller amounts of fluid (800 to 1000 ml) may be detected by widening of the flank stripe (the line formed by the lateral colonic wall and peritoneum, visible between the air-filled bowel lumen and the extraperitoneal fat layer) to more than 2 mm and by obliteration of the hepatic angle (the right lateral inferior margin of the liver).[5, 6] A displaced lateral edge of the liver may be visualized on plain films owing to a difference in density between the liver and fluid, which is detectable by conventional radiography. By using low kilovolt technique and placing the patient in the right posterior oblique position, the volume of liver bordering the fluid is increased and the visibility of the interface is enhanced. Generally more than 2 liters is present if the liver edge is visualized on plain films.[7]

The interposition of fluid in the right paracolic gutter (flank stripe sign) and obliteration of the liver tip (hepatic angle sign) are the most sensitive radiographic signs of a small amount of peritoneal fluid (less than 100ml). However, radiographic demonstration of these small amounts requires special attention to details of positioning and interpretation.[5]

Ultrasonography. Ultrasonography is noninvasive, can readily detect as little as 100 to 300 ml of intraperitoneal fluid, and can differentiate between free and loculated fluid.[8] Furthermore, loculated fluid usually can be distinguished from both normal fluid-containing structures and cystic masses that may mimic ascites, such as large ovarian cysts, abscesses, or hematomas.[8]

Therefore, although plain X-ray films have diagnostic limitations, ultrasonography offers better sensitivity and specificity in the diagnosis of equivcoal ascites.[6]

With the patient supine, minimal ascites is usually manifested by fluid in the flanks, more often on the right and at the superior end of the paracolic gutter around the right inferior lateral tip of the liver (i.e., usually the most dependent portion). Subtle collections around the liver, in the pelvis, and in Morison's pouch may also be present.[9] With larger amounts of ascites, fluid may be found lateral and anterior to the liver.[10, 11] Bowel loops normally float freely within the ascitic fluid. Loculated ascites is surrounded by bowel loops or organs without a smooth rounded configuration; real time ultrasonography may show peristaltic movement of bowel loops within the ascites.

Ancillary ultrasonographic features may give important information suggesting the etiology of ascites; these same features may be found on computed to-

mography, as noted below. Matted loops of bowel, loculation of fluid, debris within the fluid, or septations suggest an inflammatory or malignant process (Fig. 26–1),[9, 12] as do other features such as hepatic metastases, abdominal masses, or lymphadenopathy. Ultrasonography is occasionally helpful in guiding paracentesis when fluid is difficult to obtain.

Computed Tomography. Computed tomography also can readily demonstrate ascites and permit its differentiation from solid or cystic masses, since ascitic fluid is less radiodense than adjacent solid structures. CT can help distinguish hemoperitoneum from other types of ascites because the attenuation coefficient of blood is greater than that of most other forms of ascites[13] (see Fig. 26–1). CT scans may permit detection of small amounts of ascites, and have the added advantage of clearly delineating the retroperitoneal area.

As in ultrasonography, small amounts of fluid may

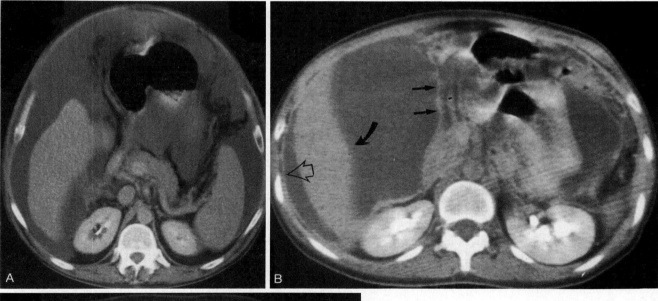

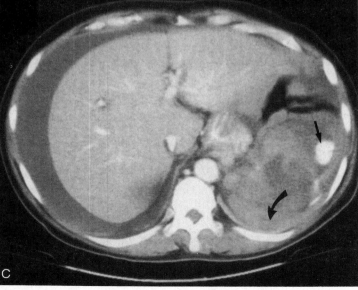

Figure 26–1. CT diagnosis of ascites. *A,* Cirrhosis with massive ascites. The fluid is homogeneous, dispersed in all compartments, and the viscera are floating in the ascites. The ascites is low density, with an attenuation coefficient near water (0–10), consistent with transudative ascites. *B,* Tuberculous peritonitis with exudative ascites. Ascites is loculated and shows displacement of the liver *(curved arrow).* There is septation within the ascites *(small arrow),* and the peritoneum is enhanced with contrast material *(open arrow).* Ascites is higher density, with an attenuation coefficient of 18. *C,* Splenic trauma with hemorrhagic ascites. The smooth liver is surrounded by unclotted blood with an attenuation coefficient of 30, i.e., above that of transudative and most exudative ascites. The spleen is heterogeneous, showing extravasated blood *(small arrow).* High-density clotted blood surrounds the spleen, with an attenuation coefficient over 40 *(curved arrow).* (Courtesy of Fay Laing, M.D., and Michael Federle, M.D., Department of Radiology, San Francisco General Hospital.)

be detected in the region of the liver tip and the right paracolic gutter. Larger amounts of fluid are seen in the left paracolic gutter and the pelvic cul-de-sacs. Fluid in the lesser sac is not typical of ascites, and its presence should suggest disease in organs surrounding the lesser sac or peritoneal carcinomatosis.[14] The mesentery (outlined by fat) appears to radiate into the fluid collection, and the bowel loops float centrally. Careful evaluation of the retroperitoneum, mesentery, intra-abdominal organs, and masses provides further indications of the presence of neoplastic or inflammatory processes.[15]

Magnetic Resonance Imaging. Magnetic resonance imaging (MRI) appears to provide similar information about the presence and extent of fluid, but currently is more expensive than other imaging techniques. Attempts have been made to distinguish various types of fluid by analyzing "relaxation times," but the value of this technique is still unproved. At present, MRI is rarely indicated to diagnose ascites.[16]

Abdominal Paracentesis and Ascites Fluid Analysis. After the diagnosis of ascites is made by examination, imaging techniques, or paracentesis, laboratory analysis of the peritoneal fluid is essential to determine its cause. Diagnostic paracentesis for obvious or suspected ascites is easily performed at the bedside and may provide valuable information with little risk. The procedure may be performed with the patient supine or sitting, after making certain that the bladder is empty. With sterile technique and under local anesthesia, the needle or catheter is introduced in the midline between the umbilicus and pubis. By entering through the avascular linea alba, the risk of hemorrhage is reduced, but the catheter may be introduced laterally, if necessary. If only a small amount of fluid is needed for diagnosis, a 22-gauge needle may be sufficient and will minimize subsequent leaking of fluid from the puncture site. If larger volumes are to be withdrawn, a larger-gauge needle or catheter-needle assembly should be used. In that situation, leakage will be minimized by using a "Z-track" entry, keeping the patient supine for several hours, and applying a pressure dressing.

The risk of complications of diagnostic paracentesis is low, but complications may occur in patients with bowel obstruction, surgical scars (suggesting possible fixation of underlying bowel to the abdominal wall), or severe coagulopathy. For instance, a recent retrospective study of 242 patients with liver disease disclosed a major complication rate of 2.9 per cent, due to hemorrhage and bowel perforation.[17] Thus, it is essential that proper precautions be employed. The avascular midline or the left lower quadrant should be used, whereas the rectus muscles, upper abdomen, collateral venous channels, and areas of surgical scars should be avoided. In patients with coagulopathy, paracentesis is possible if small-gauge needles in the vascular midline are used. In certain circumstances, however, it may be advisable to postpone paracentesis if coagulopathy is severe and there are no indications of a condition requiring prompt diagnosis or treatment. When performed by experienced personnel, paracen-

tesis should rarely result in complications; a recent prospective study of 1578 paracenteses resulted in only a 0.6 per cent incidence of bowel perforation and a 0.06 per cent incidence of clinical peritonitis; in a related study significant hemorrhage occurred in 0.9 per cent.[18, 19]

Determination of the cause of ascites consists of routine studies to characterize the fluid, and other studies which may be chosen depending on the clinical situation (Table 26–1). The protein concentration has been used to classify fluid as exudative or transudative. Fluids with protein concentrations above 3 gm per dl have been designated exudates, and those with values below these are transudates.[20] Diseases usually but not invariably associated with transudative ascites include congestive heart failure, constrictive pericarditis, inferior vena cava obstruction, Budd-Chiari syndrome, hypoalbuminemia, cirrhosis, Meigs' syndrome, and nephrotic syndrome. Exudates are common in peritoneal neoplasm, tuberculous peritonitis, pancreatic ascites, myxdema, and vasculitis. However, it is important to emphasize that strict reliance on this arbitrary division may be misleading. For example, fluid from patients with congestive heart failure may contain more than 3 gm per dl of protein.[21] In cirrhotic ascites, protein may exceed 3 gm per dl in up to 30 per cent of patients,[22] depending on the location of the resistance to portal blood flow,[23] and tuberculous peritonitis and malignancy are occasionally associated with "transudates." Despite these caveats, the protein concentration is useful as a guide to diagnostic approach, and exceptions to the aforementioned generalizations are unusual when values are found to be at the high or low extremes. Other characteristics which may help separate transudates from exudates include ascites LDH, ascites:serum protein and LDH ratios, and the *serum ascites:albumin gradient*. The latter reflects the oncotic pressure gradient between the vascular bed and the ascitic fluid. It is high in association with increased portal pressure, whereas a low gradient is found in conditions in which portal hypertension is not a factor in the genesis of ascites.[24]

Table 26–1. TESTS USED IN LABORATORY ANALYSIS OF ASCITIC FLUID

Red blood cell count
White blood cell count and differential
Total protein[1]
LDH[1]
Albumin (gradient)[2]
Bacterial culture
Mycobacterial, fungal culture
Cytology
Amylase[3]
Glucose[3]
Triglyceride[3]
Starch granules (polarizing microscopy)
pH
Lactate
Carcinoembryonic antigen
Hyaluronic acid

[1]Simultaneous blood value for ratio.
[2]Gradient = (serum albumin) − (ascites albumin) (see text).
[3]Simultaneous blood value for comparison.

Although a high ascites LDH, LDH ratio >0.6, and protein concentration ratio >0.5 suggest malignancy, these factors alone do not reliably identify malignant ascites because they may also be found in 10 to 15 per cent of patients with cirrhotic ascites. However, if all three criteria are met, the diagnosis of malignant ascites is more likely.[25] The albumin gradient has been reported to offer the best diagnostic discrimination between cirrhotic and neoplastic ascites, with a 95 per cent efficiency, but only small numbers of patients have been reported.[26] Other new studies reported to differentiate malignancy include fibronectin and cholesterol. *Fibronectin*, a glycoprotein associated with extracellular matrix, may be shed by neoplastic cells. In a study of 104 patients, an ascitic fluid fibronectin concentration >75 mg per ml distinguished the benign from the malignant ascites.[27] A later study has questioned the specificity of fibronectin.[27a] Ascitic fluid *cholesterol* in 99 patients also was highly discriminatory, with a 92 per cent diagnostic efficiency for malignancy for cholesterol concentrations >48 per 100 ml.[28] The high cholesterol may be due to a macromolecular protein-lipid complex derived from cell membranes.[29] Whether these new tests will improve the diagnosis of malignant ascites will not be clear until more data are available.

More specific *tumor markers* also have been measured in ascitic fluid. The most widely studied is carcinoembryonic antigen (CEA). Ascitic fluid CEA concentration >10 ng per ml or an ascites-serum CEA ratio >2 is 50 to 60 per cent accurate in the diagnosis of malignant ascites, with very low false positive rates.[30–32] This test is more often positive with tumors of the GI tract and breast than with others, such as ovary or lung tumors.[30] Thus far, other biochemical markers such as histaminase, beta-2-microglobulin, and beta-human chorionic gonadotropin (HCG) have not been reported to add much to the clinical diagnosis of malignant ascites.[20, 33] The newer area of immunohistochemical techniques is discussed on pages 1942 to 1943. If mesothelioma is suspected, *hyaluronic acid levels* >0.25 mg per ml may be diagnostic.[34]

Other chemical determinations may also help in diagnosis. Glucose values of <60 mg per dl may suggest neoplastic effusion with a large number of free cells.[35] Blood:ascites glucose ratios have been reported to be useful in assessing the etiology of ascites; in peritoneal lesions the ratio is said to be >1, whereas in nonperitoneal lesions it is <1.[36] This test may warrant further evaluation, but its value at present is unclear. Ascitic glucose has also been reported to be low in secondary bacterial peritonitis occurring in patients with ascites[37] (see p. 439). Peritoneal fluid *amylase* is greatly increased in pancreatic ascites; in chylous ascites, *triglyceride* concentrations will exceed those in plasma. *Ascitic fluid pH* and *lactate* may be measured to help diagnose spontaneous bacterial peritonitis; they may also be abnormal in neoplastic, tuberculous, or pancreatic ascites (see p. 439). Bilirubin is elevated in bile ascites.

A large number of red blood cells, >50,000 per cu mm, and especially grossly bloody ascites suggest the diagnosis of neoplasm, particularly hepatocellular or ovarian carcinoma. Tuberculous peritonitis, pancreatitis, endometriosis, mesenteric cysts, hepatic or mesenteric vein thrombosis, abdominal trauma, cirrhosis, and perforated viscus may also be associated with bloody ascites.[38, 39] An ascitic fluid *leukocyte count* of more than 500 per cu mm is strongly suggestive of a peritoneal inflammatory process, such as infection, or tumor infiltration. A predominance of polymorphonuclear leukocytes usually suggests acute bacterial infection, whereas lymphocytes and monocytes characterize chronic inflammatory disease, especially tuberculosis, but there are exceptions. In ascites associated with eosinophilic enteritis and peritonitis, the eosinophil count is increased.

Cytologic examination is 50 to 80 per cent accurate in the diagnosis of malignant ascites, especially when adequate volumes of fluid (at least several hundred milliliters) are obtained. False positive results of cytologic studies are rare in skilled hands.[20] The greatest source of confusion in the cytologic interpretation of ascitic fluid is the differentiation of malignant cells from atypical mesothelial cells. Newer techniques of diagnosing malignant cells in ascites are discussed further on pages 1942 to 1944. Occasionally, cytologic examination may suggest an unusual diagnosis such as the finding of plasma cells in multiple myeloma, "hairy cells" in leukemic reticuloendotheliosis, or megakaryocytes in myeloid metaplasia or hematologic malignancies.[40] Cholesterol crystals may be found in cirrhosis[41] and starch granules are found (using polarizing microscopy) in postoperative granulomatous peritonitis. All the above processes involve the peritoneum, and are discussed further on pages 1935 to 1952.

Samples of fluids should be cultured for bacteria, mycobacteria, and fungi in all cases in the appropriate clinical setting, such as the presence of fever, undiagnosed abdominal pain, or clinical deterioration in a patient with cirrhosis and portal hypertension (see later discussion).

Peritoneal Biopsy. Peritoneal biopsy may be considered when peritoneal disease is a possible cause of ascites. The peritoneum can be examined histologically by means of blind percutaneous biopsy with a Cope or Vim-Silverman needle. Blind peritoneal biopsy is a safe bedside technique with little associated morbidity, but it should not be done in the absence of ascites. Hemorrhage is the major complication, especially in the patient with portal hypertension and enlarged intraabdominal veins. Perforation of abdominal viscera and infection are uncommon complications. Most data have been accumulated using the Vim-Silverman needle. Adequate tissue is obtained in 80 to 85 per cent of attempts, and diagnosis may be made in 25 to 50 per cent in most series, with a higher diagnostic accuracy in tuberculosis than in neoplastic ascites.[42–44]

Peritoneoscopy (Laparoscopy). Peritoneoscopy is an accurate, safe, and simple technique for direct inspection of the peritoneal cavity and biopsy of suspected disease. It often permits a specific diagnosis to be made without the need for general anesthesia or laparotomy. The major *indications* for peritoneoscopy are unexplained ascites and evaluation of liver disease. In various series with different clinical emphases, unexplained ascites has been the indication in 6 to 32 per cent of patients.[45–50] The major indication is usually assessment of hepatic disease, e.g., to help exclude malignancy, assess benign disease, or define abnormal hepatic imaging studies. Other less common indications include the evaluation of chronic abdominal pain, abdominal masses, and the operability of patients with neoplasms.

During peritoneoscopy, the liver usually is well seen if there are no adhesions present in the right upper quadrant and if the liver is not covered by omentum or ascites. With the use of a tilt table, about 70 to 80 per cent of the liver surface is visible. The medial and left portions of the anterior surface of the right lobe are well seen, as is the leading edge and a small portion of the posterior surface of the right lobe. The dome and the most lateral segment of the right lobe in addition to the majority of its posterior surface are seen poorly or not at all through the peritoneoscope. The anterior portion of the left lobe, its leading edge, and a small portion of its posterior surface are well seen. The gallbladder, the falciform ligament, and the peritoneum covering the diaphragm, anterior abdominal wall, pelvis, and visceral organs usually can be seen with ease, as can the pelvic organs, omentum, and portions of the stomach and small and large bowel. Retroperitoneal structures and the porta hepatis are not seen. Some investigators have developed the expertise to see and biopsy the pancreas,[50] but this procedure is rarely attempted by most endoscopists. Peritoneoscopy is completed successfully in over 90 per cent of cases. When done by skilled endoscopists, a definitive diagnosis is possible in over 90 per cent of patients with ascites, focal liver disease, and abdominal masses, but this success rate is much lower in patients with chronic abdominal disease.[44, 46–48] It should be noted that in many cases peritoneoscopy is not necessary because of the use of CT scans with directed percutaneous biopsy, but the two techniques have not been compared in a definitive study.

Relative *contraindications* to peritoneoscopy include suspected acute bacterial peritonitis, a history of prior peritonitis, known adhesions, intestinal obstruction, abdominal wall infection, severe coagulation defects, and poor patient cooperation.

The patient is fasted overnight prior to the procedure and is medicated with Demerol, atropine, and valium. The abdomen is prepared as for exploratory laparotomy. The peritoneoscope may be inserted at any point between the umbilicus and 3 to 4 cm above or below the umbilicus and to its left. A 3-cm diameter area is infiltrated with 1 per cent procaine down to the peritoneum, and a 1-cm incision is made from skin through subcutaneous tissue. The pneumoperitoneum needle is then inserted, and pneumoperitoneum is produced with an insufflation unit using carbon dioxide or nitrous oxide. Usually 2 to 3 liters produces adequate distention, and the insufflation unit can then be set to "automatic" to maintain the desired pressure throughout the examination. Pneumoperitoneum tenses the abdominal wall and provides free space for safe insertion of the examining cannula with its trocar in place. The peritoneoscope is then passed through the cannula, and systematic examination is undertaken.

Biopsies of the liver or peritoneum may be performed through the peritoneoscope. Alternatively, one can insert a long biopsy needle through the abdominal wall at a point near where the biopsy is to be performed. The needle is then guided under direct vision into the area of interest.

Peritoneoscopy is a safe procedure with a very low mortality rate. Retrospective studies in the literature document a minor complication rate of 1 per cent, a major complication rate (bleeding or perforation) of 0.3 per cent, and a mortality rate of 0.03 per cent. However, a recent prospective study suggests that these rates may be higher, with a minor complication rate of 5.1 per cent, a major complication rate of 2.3 per cent, and a mortality rate of 0.49 per cent.[51] Minor complications include ascites leakage, pain, dehiscence, hematoma, subcutaneous emphysema, cellulitis, ileus, and hypotension. The risks of peritoneoscopy still compare quite favorably with alternative methods of direct visualization, particularly exploratory laparotomy.[50] Although recent advances in radiology may reduce the number of patients who require diagnostic peritoneoscopy, this technique will still prove useful in the diagnosis and management of many patients.[50a]

Treatment: General Considerations

Although small or moderate amounts of ascites are often only aesthetically displeasing, ascites frequently has a detrimental effect on the overall sense of well-being of the patient. Although the underlying condition should be treated by standard approaches, treatment for the purpose of removal or reduction of the ascites itself should be considered only when necessary and only when it can be done safely.

Massive ascites may require urgent removal because of severe abdominal discomfort, respiratory distress, cardiac dysfunction, or ulceration and impending rupture of an umbilical hernia. Paracentesis is the method of choice for rapid removal of fluid. In patients with tense ascites, removal of fluid will significantly reduce intra-abdominal pressure.[52, 53] Removal of a relatively small fraction of the total ascitic volume, by reducing total intra-abdominal pressure, induces symptomatic relief.[54] In the patient with tense ascites and respiratory distress or cardiac disease, removal of as little as 250 ml increases cardiac output, stroke volume, and ventricular ejection rate and decreases inferior vena caval and right atrial pressures; these changes result from increased venous return and increased cardiac filling pressures.[52, 53] Paracentesis has been reported to restore systemic perfusion when ascites is associated with circulatory shock.[55]

Although the concern has been expressed that removal of large volumes of fluid incurs the risk of hypovolemia and hypotension, studies in both cirrhotic patients and those with malignant ascites have shown that blood pressure, heart rate, electrolyte levels, blood volume, and hematocrit may remain stable.[53, 56-58] Two recent studies confirm that patients with tense ascites and edema undergoing a single paracentesis of 4 to 5 liters have no adverse effects such as orthostatic hypotension, renal dysfunction, encephalopathy, or electrolyte imbalance.[59, 60] Patients with edema appear able to safely undergo paracenteses of up to 5 liters, but in patients without edema the volume removed should probably be limited to 1000 to 1500 ml.[52, 61]

Because the successful treatment of ascites depends on management of the underlying cause, the appropriate dietary, pharmacologic, and surgical approaches will be considered in the following sections for each of the associated conditions.

CAUSES OF ASCITES

Causes of ascites may be grouped into those conditions in which the pathologic process does not directly involve the peritoneum (Table 26–2) and those in which the peritoneum itself is diseased. The former group of conditions will be discussed in this chapter, whereas the latter will be covered subsequently on pages 1935 to 1952. Despite the sizable differential diagnosis of ascites, it has been the general experience that over 90 per cent of cases are caused by one of four conditions: cirrhosis, neoplasm, congestive heart failure, or tuberculosis. The relative frequency of these causes vary, depending on the patient population selected for study,[62-66] as is evident in Table 26–3.

Portal Hypertension

Cirrhosis

The reported incidence of ascites in cirrhosis varies, but in a well-documented hospital-based series one third of cirrhotic patients presented with ascites and two thirds developed it during the course of their disease. Ascites is a poor prognostic sign; it is associated with an increase in the five-year mortality rate in otherwise uncomplicated alcoholic cirrhosis from 11 to 48 per cent in those who stop drinking, whereas in continuing drinkers it increases to 32 to 68 per cent.[67]

Pathophysiology of Ascites in Cirrhosis. In general, extravascular accumulation of fluid reflects the balance between opposing intravascular and extravascular hydrostatic and colloid osmotic pressures. In the special case of cirrhotic ascites, however, two additional factors must be considered: (1) the unique anatomic relationship of the hepatic sinusoids to the Disse space and hepatic lymphatics, and (2) the fact that portal hypertension in cirrhosis is associated with increased pressure in the hepatic sinusoids. As will be discussed below, this leads directly to a greatly increased rate of hepatic lymph formation, and at least a portion of the ascites fluid originates as lymph directly from the surface of the liver. Moreover, cirrhotic ascites is associated with profound changes in the renal metab-

Table 26–2. CAUSES OF ASCITES NOT ASSOCIATED WITH PERITONEAL DISEASE[1]

I. Portal hypertension
  A. Cirrhosis
  B. Hepatic congestion
    1. Congestive heart failure
    2. Constrictive pericarditis
    3. Inferior vena cava obstruction
    4. Hepatic vein obstruction (Budd-Chiari syndrome)
  C. Portal vein occlusion
II. Hypoalbuminemia
  A. Nephrotic syndrome
  B. Protein-losing enteropathy
  C. Malnutrition
III. Miscellaneous disorders
  A. Myxedema
  B. Ovarian disease
    1. Meigs' syndrome
    2. Struma ovarii
    3. Ovarian overstimulation syndrome
    4. Ovarian edema
  C. Pancreatic ascites
  D. Bile ascites
  E. Chylous ascites
  F. Urine ascites and dialysis-associated ascites

[1]Ascites associated with disease of the peritoneum is discussed on pages 1935 to 1952.

olism of sodium and water, the mechanism of which remains poorly understood.

The brief summary of the pathophysiology of cirrhotic ascites which follows will emphasize the changes in portal hemodynamics and hepatic lymph formation, the renal retention of sodium and water, and the relationship between these two essential components of the syndrome. The intent is to provide the reader

Table 26–3. ETIOLOGY OF ASCITES IN SELECTED SERIES

	Municipal Hospitals, U.S.[a]	Consultative Practice, U.S.[b, c]	Third World[d, e]
Number of cases	342	48	151
Method of diagnosis	Microscopy, peritoneoscopy	Peritoneoscopy	Peritoneoscopy
Diagnosis (% of cases)			
Cirrhosis	47	30	35
Neoplasm	32	41	13
Tuberculosis	12	17	45[f]
Cardiac failure	6	—	<1
Pancreatitis	1.2	—	—
Nephrotic syndrome	<1	—	<1
Chronic peritonitis	<1	2	6[f]
Chylous ascites	<1	—	—
Constrictive pericarditis	<1	2	—
Myxedema	<1	—	—
Vasculitis	—	8	—

[a]See references 21, 62, and 63.
[b]See reference 45.
[c]"Exudative" ascites only.
[d]See references 64 and 65.
[e]Overt cardiac and renal disease excluded.
[f]Possible tuberculosis in some.

with an overview upon which an understanding of the pathogenesis of ascites and its rational clinical management may be based.

Portal Hemodynamics and Hepatic Lymph Formation. In cirrhotic portal hypertension, functional resistance to flow appears to reside in the region of the central veins and smaller tributaries of the hepatic vein. Thus, it can be viewed as being at the level of the sinusoid or distal (downstream) to it (i.e., "sinusoidal" or "postsinusoidal") and reflects a general impedance to hepatic outflow secondary to extensive disruption of the hepatic architecture with fibrosis, nodular regeneration, and altered vascular flow patterns.[68] In addition, in established cirrhosis, splanchnic blood flow is increased.[69] As a consequence, hydrostatic pressure is increased in the sinusoids and throughout the entire portal system. Secondarily, there is vascular congestion in the spleen and other viscera and the development of collateral venous channels between portals and systemic circulation.

The sinusoidal endothelium normally is fenestrated and highly permeable to water and solutes (Fig. 26–2).[70–72] Thus, a rise in sinusoidal pressure drives protein-rich fluid from the sinusoid into the Disse space and thence into the hepatic lymphatics, in which flow is substantially increased. As would be expected, sinusoidal permeability (and thus lymph/plasma concentration ratio) is greater for smaller than for larger solutes under normal circumstances. However, studies in cats have shown that when sinusoidal pressure and lymph flow are increased, there is a loss of this selectivity so that the lymph/plasma concentration ratio even of larger macromolecules approaches 1.0 (Fig. 26–3).[70] The reason for this change in permselectivity is not known, but it may be related to changes in hydration, and thus of restrictive properties, of the interstitium. The increase in hepatic lymph flow has been documented clinically[71] as well as in experimental animals, in which there is a direct and linear relationship between experimentally induced increases in hepatic venous (and sinusoidal) pressure and the rate of hepatic lymph formation.[70]

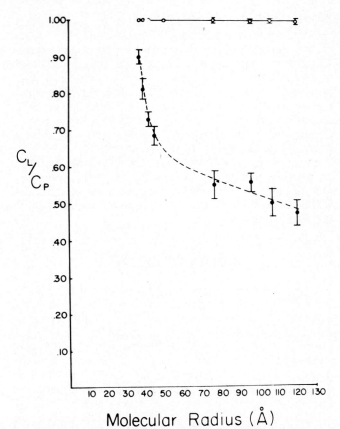

Figure 26–3. Lymph/plasma concentration ratio as a function of molecular radius and hepatic lymph flow in cats. ● = control lymph flow; ○ = lymph flow ≥ tenfold greater than control. At high flow rates, permselectivity is lost (i.e., the lymph/plasma concentration ratios for both large and small molecules remain at 1.0). (Reprinted by permission of the publisher from: Permselectivity of cat liver blood-lymph barrier to endogenous macromolecules, by Granger, D. M., Miller, T., Allen, R., et al. Gastroenterology 77:103–109. Copyright 1979 by The American Gastroenterological Association.)

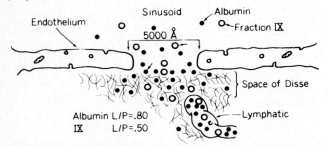

Figure 26–2. Diagram of the highly fenestrated endothelium of the hepatic sinusoid, demonstrating ready access of fluid as well as albumin and other macromolecular solutes to the space of Disse and lymphatics. The molecular radius of albumin is 3.7 nm (37 Å), and that of fraction IX is 12.0 nm (120 Å). The normal permselectivity of the blood-lymph barrier may reside in the interstitium rather than in the endothelial fenestra (see text and reference 70). (Reprinted by permission of the publisher from: Permselectivity of cat liver blood-lymph barrier to endogenous macromolecules, by Granger, D. M., Miller, T., Allen, R., et al. Gastroenterology 77:103–109. Copyright 1979 by The American Gastroenterological Association.)

At higher levels of sinusoidal pressure, excess fluid escapes the hepatic lymphatics to enter the peritoneal cavity, in part via surface lymphatics.[70] In ascitic cirrhotics, then, newly synthesized albumin can enter the abdominal cavity directly from the liver rather than via the systemic vascular compartment.[73] In cats, experimentally induced increases in hepatic venous (and, therefore, sinusoidal) pressures in excess of 10 mm Hg (relatively modest, compared with those commonly observed in cirrhotic portal hypertension) are associated with visible loss of fluid (hepatic lymph) from the surface of the liver.[70]

Thus, in cirrhosis, a progressive increase in sinusoidal pressure leads to increased formation of hepatic lymph (protein-rich, relative to lymph from other sources), which in part enters the abdominal cavity directly. In addition, increased portal venous pressure results in an expanded splanchnic blood volume and increased lymph formation in other viscera, although the latter may not contribute directly to ascites formation. Accordingly, splanchnic extracellular (intra- and extravascular) fluid volume is expanded. This expansion is obvious when it is manifest by grossly detectable ascites. However, it must also be present to a lesser extent even before ascites becomes appreciable, as the cirrhotic process and its hemodynamic consequences evolve.

The simplistic mechanical hydrodynamic model thus far described does not take into account a number of important modifying factors. For example, although "liver function," as customarily assessed by routine laboratory tests, correlates poorly with the presence of ascites,[74] hypoalbuminemia is an important predisposing factor,[75] as would be predicted by the usual Starling considerations. Also, as chronic liver disease progresses, collagen may be deposited in the Disse space[76-78] and the permeability of the sinusoidal endothelium may decrease. This so-called "capillarization" of the sinusoids would be expected to diminish the rate of formation and protein concentration of hepatic lymph at any given sinusoidal pressure.[70] Moreover, although the protein concentration in cirrhotic ascites is quite variable and occasionally in the "exudative" range,[22, 79] it usually is low, suggesting that mere extravasation of hepatic lymph probably is not its only source. Finally, the formation of ascites in cirrhotics is regularly associated with profound abnormalities in the renal metabolism of sodium and water.

Renal Function in Cirrhotic Ascites. The accumulation of ascites in patients with cirrhosis is accompanied by avid renal retention of Na^+ and water, usually with relative sparing of other indices of renal function such as glomerular filtration rate, creatinine clearance, and effective renal plasma flow, which may be normal or moderately diminished.[68, 74] Thus, although renal function in this setting may resemble that in volume-depleted subjects, its occurrence despite normal or expanded total body sodium and water stores is inappropriate. The mechanism is not completely understood, and there is evidence that it either may be secondary to the changes in hepatic hemodynamics discussed above, or may reflect a primary abnormality in renal sodium metabolism. In either case, plasma renin activities and secretion rates and plasma aldosterone concentrations are increased in most patients with cirrhotic ascites, and in some, this system may be maximally activated.[80]

In studies of the renin-angiotensin-aldosterone system in cirrhotics with ascites,[81-83] it was found that those with elevated renin levels not only had higher aldosterone concentrations and lower sodium clearance, but also had higher wedged hepatic venous pressures and a poorer prognosis compared with cirrhotic patients with normal plasma renin activity. These two groups otherwise were similar clinically and in glomerular filtration rate, effective renal plasma flow, and liver "function." Thus, plasma renin activity in this study seemed to correlate with the severity of the abnormality in hepatic hemodynamics.

Increased secretion of renin in cirrhotic portal hypertension has been attributed to sequestration of volume in the splanchnic blood and lymph vascular compartments, together with a decrease in systemic vascular resistance. The result is that some fraction of the total plasma volume is unavailable for systemic and renal perfusion (i.e., a diminished "effective" plasma volume).[84] In this circumstance, the expected renal response would be increased renin secretion and activation of the renin-angiotensin-aldosterone mechanism, leading to sodium retention. Activation of an α-adrenergic response, as reflected by increased plasma norepinephrine levels[85] and a nonosmotic stimulus to the secretion of vasopressin also suggest relative hypovolemia. Moreover, norepinephrine levels correlate directly with vasopressin levels and inversely with sodium excretion.[86] That this sequence of events may indeed be operative in the ascitic cirrhotic patient is supported by several lines of evidence. First, acute expansion of central vascular volume in ascitic cirrhotic patients by intravenous infusion of saline or albumin is associated with prompt decreases in plasma renin activity and aldosterone concentration,[87] and often diuresis.[88, 89] Second, immersion up to the neck of ascitic cirrhotic patients, resulting in central redistribution of fluid, is accompanied by similar changes.[90] Finally, peritoneovenous shunting, which effects a central venous infusion of ascites fluid, is frequently accompanied by decreased plasma renin activity and aldosterone, and increased creatinine clearance.[91-93] Thus, in three diverse clinical settings in which central vascular volume is expanded in the cirrhotic patient with ascites there is prompt suppression of renin secretion. It appears reasonable to infer, therefore, that renin and aldosterone secretion, as well as adrenergic responses, are activated in response to a real or perceived deficit in systemic plasma volume.

However, it is also clear that aldosterone can be dissociated from renal sodium metabolism in cirrhosis, suggesting that the renin-angiotensin-aldosterone mechanism alone cannot account for the abnormalities observed. For example, aminoglutethimide inhibits aldosterone secretion but does not regularly induce diuresis in cirrhotic patients,[80] and despite their general efficacy, aldosterone antagonists (e.g., spironolactone) may not induce a diuresis in some patients. Moreover, although head-out immersion and peritoneovenous shunting regularly induce fluid shifts and central volume expansion in cirrhotic patients, and thereby diminish plasma renin activity and aldosterone concentrations, these measures may fail to induce natriuresis or diuresis without the addition of diuretic agents.[90, 92]

To explain this dissociation, it has been suggested that in the ascitic cirrhotic patient the critical determinant of renal sodium and water excretion is the delivery of tubular urine to the distal nephron.[74, 88, 94, 95] If, because of hemodynamic factors or volume depletion, proximal tubular absorption is maximal, distal delivery is inadequate, and sodium and water will be retained whether or not aldosterone levels are increased. Thus, expression of the aldosterone effect seems to depend on delivery of tubular urine to the distal nephron, where it modulates but does not absolutely control sodium excretion.

Renal Hemodynamics and the Prostaglandin System. It seems clear, therefore, that in cirrhotic patients with ascites some other factor(s) must account for inappropriate aldosterone-independent sodium retention, despite what may otherwise be well-preserved overall renal function. In this context, certain recent findings are of particular interest. First, it has been shown by a variety of invasive and noninvasive techniques, including renal angiography,[96] xenon washout,[97, 98] and I-131-hippuran scanning,[99, 100] that marked renal cortical vasoconstriction is often present in patients with cirrhosis, with preferential perfusion of medullary and juxtamedullary areas. Although total renal perfusion does not appear to correlate precisely with plasma renin or aldosterone concentration,[82] there is evidence that the changes in intrarenal hemodynamics are related to plasma renin activity.[100] These changes in renal hemodynamics are labile and therefore difficult to quantify,[98] but their demonstration by several groups of investigators employing different methods suggests that the observation is valid. It has been suggested that this preferential shunting of blood to the medulla might result in a relative overperfusion of the juxtamedullary nephrons, which have been thought to be "sodium-retaining" and that this redistribution of renal blood flow might in itself explain the retention of sodium. However, juxtamedullary nephrons may actually be no more sodium-retaining than are cortical nephrons. In fact, it has been suggested that perfusion of the medullary and juxtamedullary nephrons may serve a "compensatory" or "protective" role for the kidney in which there is cortical vasospasm.[101] Thus, preservation or enhancement of medullary perfusion under these conditions would both spare this relatively hypoxic region of the kidney from further diminution in oxygen supply, and at the same time permit the juxtamedullary nephrons to perform some of the excretory functions otherwise handled in the cortex.

Available evidence suggests that this medullary compensation is mediated or modulated by locally produced prostaglandins. Renal synthesis of the vasodilator prostaglandins PGE_2 and PGI_2 is increased in states associated with decreased blood volume, renal vasoconstriction, and ischemia and by the direct effects of vasopressin, angiotensin II, and catechols. These prostaglandins effect a compensatory increase in renal blood flow, glomerular filtration, and free water clearance, the latter via promotion of "washout" of the renal medulla and in direct opposition to the hydroosmotic effect of vasopressin.[102–105] Thus, it is not surprising that in cirrhotics with ascites[106, 107] and under other circumstances in which there is renal sodium retention,[108, 109] inhibitors of prostaglandin synthesis such as indomethacin have several adverse effects on renal function, including decreased renal plasma flow and creatinine clearance. Loop diuretic agents such as furosemide appear to increase renal PGE_2 production, and it has been shown that furosemide is protective against the adverse renal effects of salicylates in cirrhotic ascites.[110] Conversely, nonsteroidal anti-inflammatory agents impair or block the diuretic effect of furosemide.[110, 111] Although certain agents such as sulindac appear to be renal-sparing,[112] the use of nonste-

roidal anti-inflammatory agents should, in general, be avoided in cirrhotic subjects with ascites (also see Treatment of Cirrhotic Ascites).

The Overflow Hypothesis. An alternative model of the interaction between cirrhosis and renal sodium retention has been proposed.[113–115] In this model, renal sodium retention is viewed as the primary abnormality, albeit set in motion by the liver disease. For unclear reasons, the kidney retains sodium and water, which leads to formation of ascites as the result of an "overflow." This concept is supported by both clinical evidence and experimental animal models of cirrhotic portal hypertension and ascites. Clinically, the "overflow" theory is consistent with the finding that ascites may accumulate in cirrhotic patients treated with mineralocorticoid[116] and that, unlike normal subjects, these subjects often fail to demonstrate "mineralocorticoid escape."[117] Also, renal cortical vasoconstriction can be demonstrated in cirrhotic subjects who do not have ascites and presumably, therefore, antedates the ascites.[97] In dogs and rats with experimental cirrhosis, renal retention of sodium and water precedes accumulation of detectable ascites[113, 118] and occurs even when expansion of splanchnic blood volume is prevented by prior formation of an end-to-side portal-systemic shunt[114] or elimination of the "third space" by peritoneovenous shunt.[115] Significantly, a side-to-side shunt, which decompresses the hepatic sinusoids in this model, prevents these changes. This has been interpreted as suggesting that increased sinusoidal pressure activates an intrahepatic baroreceptor mechanism, which leads to renal functional changes via unidentified pathways.[119]

The "overflow" model and the concept of decreased "effective" plasma volume may not be mutually exclusive. Because sequestration of volume in the splanchnic region need not be manifest by grossly evident ascites, nor dependent solely on an expanded splanchnic blood volume, it may not easily be determined which event is truly primary. In fact, in dogs with portal-systemic venous shunts, lymph flow is increased to the same extent as in nonshunted dogs, suggesting that sequestration of volume in extravascular compartments may not be diminished by the shunt.[114] Nonetheless, the possibility that excessive sodium and water retention in cirrhosis is not related to diminished "effective" plasma volume cannot be excluded. It has been suggested that the early phases of ascites formation might reflect a hepatic baroreceptor-mediated overflow phenomenon and that more advanced stages of ascites are maintained by the changes proposed to result from diminished effective plasma volume.[119–121] The disturbance could also reflect, or be modulated by, deficiency of a natriuretic factor,[122, 123] a neural reflex,[124] or abnormalities in the kinin system.[125]

Atrial Natriuretic Factor. Recent studies have called attention to the renal effects of atrial natriuretic factor, a recently discovered hormone which is synthesized and stored in the right atrial myocytes.[126–130] The prohormone, consisting of 126 amino acids, is cleaved to a 28 amino acid active hormone at the time of release, under influence of atrial volume expansion and increased right atrial transmural pressure, vasopressin, and various autonomic mediators. The active hormone has several effects which potentially would be advantageous in the cirrhotic patient with ascites, including increased glomerular filtration rate, diuresis, natriuresis, decreased secretion of renin and vasopressin, and opposition to the renal tubular effects of aldosterone and vasopressin. Several, but not all, of the actions of atrial natriuretic peptide result from its induced relaxation of vascular smooth muscle. The possible role of this very important hormone in the pathophysiology and management of cirrhotic ascites is under active investigation.

Reabsorption of Ascites Fluid. Although this discussion has almost exclusively emphasized factors involved in the formation of ascites, the amount of ascites present at any given time reflects the balance between rates of formation and reabsorption. Information regarding the latter process is more limited. However, it appears that the lymphatics on the undersurface of the diaphragm are especially important in this process because scarification of this area, which is uniquely suited to fluid transfer,[131, 132] substantially impedes the removal of fluid from the peritoneal cavity in experimental animals.[133, 134] Intraperitoneal hydrostatic pressure promotes reabsorption and exerts an important influence on the rate of accumulation of ascites under experimental conditions,[135, 136] but clinically, this countering force does not appear to be of major significance during the active phase of ascites accumulation. Also, fluids higher in protein concentration are absorbed more slowly.[137] Finally, recent studies in patients with chronic renal failure suggest that maximal rates of removal of fluid from the abdominal cavity are quite variable, ranging from approximately 25 to 130 ml per hour.[138] Although the rate may thus significantly exceed earlier estimates of 30 to 37 ml per hour,[139, 140] these more recent studies involved subjects being maintained on either peritoneal dialysis or hemodialysis, and for this reason it is difficult to compare the studies directly.

Tentative Summary of the Pathophysiology of Ascites in Cirrhosis. Although many questions remain unanswered, the currently available information can be reasonably summarized. First, the clinical syndrome occurs in the setting of advanced liver disease with sinusoidal portal hypertension, expanded splanchnic vascular and interstitial volume, and increased hepatic lymph formation. The renin-aldosterone and alpha-adrenergic systems are usually activated, there is non-osmotic release of vasopressin, major alterations occur in intrarenal hemodynamics, and sodium retention is avid, as reflected by urine [Na+], which often is less than 10 mEq per liter. Expansion of central volume regularly reduces renin and aldosterone concentrations but may not induce natriuresis or diuresis, indicating the importance of some mediator other than aldosterone in the retention of sodium. Induction of diuresis and natriuresis seems to depend more on the adequate delivery of sodium to the distal tubule than on interruption of the aldosterone or vasopressin effects. In-

hibition of prostaglandin synthesis leads to a more general deterioration of renal function, suggesting that prostaglandins play an important role in the regulation of intrarenal hemodynamics.

Several fundamental questions stand unresolved. First, although it seems clear that some effect of the underlying liver disease is responsible, it remains unclear whether it is mechanical and hemodynamic (decreased "effective" systemic plasma volume), humoral, neural, or a combination of factors. Second, although the degree of renal cortical vasoconstriction has been correlated in some studies with the severity of the portal hypertension and plasma renin activity, its cause remains unknown. Third, sodium excretion can be dissociated from the activity of the renin-aldosterone system, and its relationship to the changes in intrarenal hemodynamics is unclear. Fourth, the full significance of changes in renal prostaglandin metabolism is not understood. Finally, the possible role of atrial natriuretic peptide in the pathophysiology and treatment of ascites is being examined. The answers to these and other important questions must await new advances in the understanding of both renal and hepatic physiology, and of their aberrations in chronic liver disease.

Characteristics of Ascites Fluid in Cirrhosis. Some characteristics of ascites fluid have already been discussed (p. 430). Although ascites in cirrhosis is typically a "transudate" with relatively few cells, recent studies have shown that in a substantial proportion of patients the findings do not fit this pattern. Protein may be >3 gm per deciliter in up to 30 per cent of cirrhotic patients.[22, 25, 141] Ascites in the noninfected states usually has fewer than 300 to 500 white blood cells per cu mm, but 10 to 15 per cent may have more than 500 cells and 5 per cent may have more than 1000 cells.[25, 79, 141] In "noninfected" ascites most of these cells are mononuclear leukocytes.[79, 142] The reason that protein concentrations and leukocyte counts are higher in some patients is often unclear, and special tests to exclude spontaneous bacterial peritonitis or other superimposed disorders may be required (see later discussion). It has recently been recognized that protein concentration, mononuclear cell count, and red blood cell count may rise significantly after diuresis and may reach levels that suggest a diagnosis of infection or malignancy.[143]

Cirrhotic ascites has been found to have lower bactericidal activity, opsonizing activity, and complement levels than noncirrhotic peritoneal fluid such as cardiac, neoplastic, and tuberculous ascites in which levels are adequate.[144–147] The reduced complement levels could be due to dilution by the large volume of ascitic fluid or to activation and consumption by immune complexes, which have been identified in cirrhotic ascites.[148] However, ascites does possess humoral antimicrobial activity for gram-negative organisms, *Bacteroides fragilis*, and *Candida* but not for gram-positive organisms. This activity has not been completely characterized but may be due to complement, antibodies, lysozyme, and other non-complement-dependent mechanisms.[149] Alterations in the coagulation-related proteins in ascites have recently been noted. Compared with plasma, the ascites in cirrhotic and malignant diseases contain less fibrinogen and plasminogen and increased fibrin split products and fibrin monomer.[150–151] Ascites may have an important influence on the blood coagulation profile and fibrinogen consumption in liver disease, as well as in other disease states.[151, 152] The intravenous infusion of ascitic fluid can produce subclinical and clinical coagulation disorders (see discussion of peritoneovenous shunts, below).

Cirrhotic ascites contains macrophages capable of producing prostaglandins and leukotrienes, but the significance and effect of these locally produced eicosanoids is not yet clear.[153]

Typical cholesterol crystals have been described in the microscopic analysis of the ascites of a small number of patients with cirrhosis.[41, 154] These patients appear to have typical signs and symptoms of cirrhosis with ascites, and they have normal serum cholesterol and triglyceride levels. The serosal surfaces of the peritoneal cavity are thickened and opacified, and cholesterol plaques are found on them. This probably reflects a subclinical serositis or spontaneous bacterial peritonitis that has compromised lymphatic drainage of the peritoneum, but the mechanism is unknown. Cholesterol pulmonary embolization leading to fatal respiratory failure has been reported; thus, the presence of cholesterol crystals may be a contraindication to peritoneovenous shunting.[155]

Complications of Cirrhotic Ascites

Spontaneous Bacterial Peritonitis in Cirrhotic Patients. Spontaneous peritonitis may occur in almost 10 per cent of cirrhotic patients with portal hypertension and overt ascites.[156–159a] It also may occur in association with acute liver disease.[160] In 80 per cent of patients a single aerobic organism is identified, and in contrast to spontaneous peritonitis in noncirrhotics, about 60 per cent of causative organisms in cirrhotics are enteric, primarily *Escherichia coli*.[156–162] Among nonenteric organisms, pneumococci are most frequently seen but infections caused by *Listeria monocytogenes*,[163] *Neisseria meningitidis*,[164] *Pasteurela multocida*,[165] and *Haemophilus influenzae*[166] have also been reported. *Pseudomonas, Proteus, Aerobacter, Klebsiella, Bacteroides, Aeromonas,* and *Salmonella* are other, less frequently cultured gram-negative organisms. Anaerobic or microaerophilic organisms were present, in one report, in 8 of 125 cases.[167] Among these, *Bacteroides* species were the most common. Of interest, four of the eight cases had polymicrobial infections (versus 10 of 118 aerobic infections), and only one of the eight had bacteremia.

The pathogenesis of the syndrome is not established, but the predominance of enteric organisms has implicated local factors. Congested lymphatics and splanchnic vessels, an edematous bowel wall, and perhaps a change in the intestinal flora may all play a part in allowing passage of bacteria through the intestinal wall. Gross intestinal lesions such as erosion or infarction are uncommon. Recent demonstration of *Neisseria gonorrhoeae* infection suggests that a transfallopian route may be involved in some cases.[168] Hematogenous spread with seeding of ascites, perhaps aided by failure of the cirrhotic liver to effectively remove bacteria from the blood stream, or direct introduction during paracentesis,[169] may also play a role. The observation that cases in which anaerobes are present are more often polymicrobial and less often associated with bacteremia[167] suggests that in these cases bacteria may have gained access to the peritoneum from the bowel transmurally rather than hematogenously. Foci of infection in the biliary tract, urine, lungs, skin, or indwelling catheters are present in about 25 per cent of patients. As noted above, relative deficiency of antimicrobial activity in cirrhotic ascites[144, 145, 149] and serum[170] has also been demonstrated and may play a role. Consistent with this concept, Runyon has presented evidence that a low ascites protein concentration predisposes to spontaneous bacterial peritonitis,[171] and Runyon and Van Epps have proposed that diuresis may increase the ascites fluid protein concentration and opsonic activity and thereby help to prevent spontaneous bacterial peritonitis.[172] Finally, a possible local effect of systemic metabolic changes seen in cirrhosis, such as alkalosis, hypokalemia, and hypoxia, has not been documented, but conceivably these factors may contribute. In two cases, infection of cirrhotic ascites with multiple organisms, including anaerobes, was attributed to intra-arterial vasopressin therapy.[173]

Clinical and Laboratory Features. Spontaneous peritonitis usually occurs in the setting of decompensated hepatic function; ascites is present in virtually all cases, and jaundice and portal-systemic collaterals are seen in most. Azotemia is commonly observed. As with tuberculous peritonitis, spontaneous peritonitis may be masked by the signs of cirrhosis or hepatic failure. About one half of patients may have no abdominal pain, although only about 7 per cent develop completely silent peritonitis. Although spontaneous peritonitis is associated with abdominal pain, fever, hypotension, and encephalopathy in many patients, its manifestations may be quite protean in individual patients. For practical purposes, any deterioration of a cirrhotic patient with ascites should alert the clinician to the possibility of bacterial peritonitis. Pleural fluid also may become infected in cirrhotics;[174] in the patient described, the ascites was sterile.

Liver function studies are nearly always abnormal. Leukocytosis is the rule, but up to 25 per cent of patients have a normal white blood cell count. Blood cultures are positive in 31 to 76 per cent. Paracentesis, with cell count and culture of the ascites fluid, remains the most important diagnostic procedure. Although virtually all patients with spontaneous peritonitis have more than 250 polymorphonuclear cells per cu mm, both total leukocyte and polymorphonuclear cell counts may be surprisingly low.[79] Moreover, patients with noninfected ascites may have total counts over 250 polymorphonuclear cells per cu mm.[162, 175] Although Gram stain of the fluid is positive in only about 40 per cent, culture is positive in 80 per cent and depends critically on immediate bedside inoculation of the culture medium. The ascites protein usually remains under 3 gm per 100 ml. The pH of infected ascites is lower than that of blood or sterile ascites, and an arterial blood-ascites gradient of > 0.1 pH may be of diagnostic value.[176]

The relative usefulness of peritoneal fluid leukocyte count, pH, and lactate concentration has been assessed in several reports,[177–180] but the role of pH and lactate determinations in the routine clinical diagnosis of spontaneous bacterial peritonitis remains unclear.[181] Analysis of ascitic fluid appears helpful in distinguishing spontaneous bacterial peritonitis from visceral perforation in that the latter group tends to have higher leukocyte count, protein concentration, and lactate dehydrogenase activity and a lower glucose concentration than the former.[182, 183]

A number of cirrhotic patients have been described in whom organisms were present in the ascites fluid but who lacked other characteristic clinical features of bacterial peritonitis.[162, 173] This so-called "asymptomatic bacterascites" may represent a stage in the evolution of the fully developed syndrome. Also unclear is the significance of so-called "culture-negative neutrocytic ascites" on which organisms are not identified in patients who otherwise exhibit clinical and laboratory features of spontaneous bacterial peritonitis.[184] Perhaps these included some subjects with false negative cultures of ascites fluid.

Treatment and Prognosis. A bacteriologic response may be achieved with appropriate antibiotics in about 60 per cent of patients. Gram-positive cocci are most successfully treated, but there are no other clinical or laboratory features that predict successful treatment. However, delayed recognition and institution of antibiotic therapy may influence the outcome. Antibiotic concentrations in ascitic fluid in the presence of peritonitis rapidly achieve bactericidal levels after parenteral administration, and intraperitoneal instillation is unnecessary.[185] Although drainage of the peritoneal fluid has not been well evaluated, it probably adds little to the management of spontaneous peritonitis.

In view of the fact that many noninfected patients may have ascites fluid cell counts in the bacterial peritonitis range (i.e., > 250 polymorphonuclear cells per cu mm), a decision regarding anitibotic therapy before culture results are available may be difficult. Under these conditions, it is probably advisable to administer broad-spectrum antibiotics after cultures are obtained, with the expectation that they will be discontinued if the cultures are negative. One reasonable regimen in this setting would include a cephalosporin to cover gram-positive organisms and an aminoglycoside to cover gram-negative organisms. Depending on the agents selected and the clinical circumstances, an additional drug effective against anaerobes may be used. Dosages should be adjusted, if necessary, if renal function is impaired. Rimola et al.[186] have suggested that prophylactic administration of oral nonabsorbable antibiotics in cirrhotics with gastrointestinal hemorrhage may prevent spontaneous bacterial peritonitis; confirmation of this interesting observation will be important.

Despite the successful bacteriologic response in over half the patients with spontaneous peritonitis, prognosis is grave. Overall survival was initially reported to be less than 5 per cent,[156] although more recent studies suggest that survival rates may be higher.[157, 158, 161, 162]

Hepatic Hydrothorax. Approximately 6 per cent of cirrhotic patients develop pleural effusions, which occasionally may be massive, and appear to result from transdiaphragmatic passage of fluid through defects in the diaphragm and via diaphragmatic lymphatics.[187] Of interest, hydrothorax also occurs in approximately the same percentage of noncirrhotic patients who undergo chronic ambulatory peritoneal dialysis, probably indicating the congenital predisposition of the population to develop diaphragmatic defects with peritoneal fluid loads.[188] This complication is usually associated with ascites, but it may occur in the absence of ascites when negative intrathoracic pressure provides an alternative route for the clearance of fluid through the defect, and the abdominal lymphatics continue to adequately drain the peritoneal cavity.[189] In two thirds of the cases the effusions are right-sided, but they may occur on the left or bilaterally.

The diagnosis is most easily confirmed by intraperitoneal injection of 5 mCi of ^{99m}Tc-sulfur colloid in 1 ml of saline and observation of its passage into the pleural cavity at one-fourth, one, two, four, or 24 hours later. Occasionally fluid may need to be removed from the pleural cavity first.[189–191]

Management of these patients may be difficult. Dietary and diuretic therapy should be tried but often fails, and thoracentesis is usually temporary. Tetracycline-induced pleurodesis, using 500 to 1000 mg of tetracycline after tapping the chest dry, may be curative.[188, 190, 192] Chest tube insertion has been reported to lead to life-threatening fluid depletion and should be closely monitored.[193] Peritoneovenous shunting alone often fails because of continued preferential drainage of ascites into the chest[194]; combining shunting with tetracycline is often successful.[195] Lastly, surgical closure of the diaphragmatic defect and surgical pleurodesis (with or without shunting) are often successful, but entail higher risk in these sick patients.[189, 196]

Umbilical Hernias. Umbilical hernias occur in more than 20 per cent of cirrhotic patients and are the result of increased intra-abdominal pressure causing herniation of abdominal contents through a congenital patent ring. Complications include pain, incarceration, strangulation, leakage, and rupture.[197] These complications are associated with a mortality rate of up to 15 per cent, especially in patients with uncontrolled ascites and poor hepatic function. The best approach to prevent complications and decrease postoperative morbidity and mortality rates is to decrease ascites, optimize nutrition, and improve hepatic function.[197–199] If medical management is not sufficient, peritoneovenous shunting may prevent complications and postoperative recurrence.[200, 201] Consideration should be given to elective repair when the operative risk is low, rather than waiting for an urgent indication with its attendant increased morbidity.

Other Complications. The other complications of ascites have been alluded to earlier in this chapter. Large volumes of ascites may produce immobilization and have profound adverse psychosocial as well as physical effects. Elevation of the diaphragm produces respiratory distress and atelectasis, and increased abdominal pressure may cause abdominal pain, anorexia, inguinal herniation, gastroesophageal reflux, and scrotal edema. Hemodynamic changes may impair cardiac function.

Medical Treatment. Paracentesis for massive ascites and its complications has been discussed earlier (p. 430). It is used mainly to relieve pain, respiratory distress, or complicated umbilical herniation caused by tense ascites. Paracentesis does not significantly improve portal hypertension or renal function, nor does it decrease the likelihood of variceal bleeding.[56] After paracentesis of more than 2 liters, about half the volume usually reaccumulates within 24 hours, and the remainder reaccumulates over three to four days.[140] Two recent studies have demonstrated that repeated paracenteses, alone or combined with albumin or ascites reinfusion, is as effective as and more rapid and less subject to complications than salt restriction plus diuretics.[202, 203] However, if intravenous albumin is not given, there is a higher incidence of renal impairment.[203a, 203b] Although this may be applicable to certain hospitalized patients, more data are needed before this can become accepted therapy.[157, 204]

Bed rest may be useful in the treatment of ascites, particularly if there is an unsatisfactory response to the measures discussed below. Upright posture in patients with ascites and cirrhosis is associated with activation of the renin-angiotensin system and sympathetic nervous system, a reduction in glomerular filtration rate, and an increase in tubular sodium reabsorption.[205, 206]

The mainstays of treatment of cirrhotic ascites are *sodium restriction* and *diuretics.* Sodium restriction is the initial step to prevent further expansion of the extracellular fluid volume. Restriction to 20 mEq or even 10 mEq per day may be employed in hospitalized patients, although it is rarely feasible to achieve these levels in ambulatory patients. An initial period of bed rest and sodium restriction may lead to diuresis in only 5 to 15 per cent of cirrhotic patients, and generally it will be a much smaller diuresis than can be achieved with diuretic agents.[207–209] Therefore, there is little role for a trial of bed rest and sodium restriction alone except in those outpatients with minimal ascites.[157] However, sodium restriction initially provides an important adjunct to diuretics,[210] and once mobilization of ascites occurs, many patients may be maintained on less restrictive sodium diets with no or minimal diuretics. Some workers have advocated a more liberal sodium intake, placing major reliance on the use of diuretic agents,[211] but subsequent studies have not found any advantage to the liberal sodium diet in terms of improved nutritional status, electrolyte abnormalities, or other complications.[203, 210] It is of note, however, that patients on liberal salt diets often do as well as salt-restricted patients, and this allows some leeway in managing patients who cannot or will not maintain salt restriction.[212]

Impaired excretion of water is a frequent finding in cirrhotic patients[213] and appears to be due to a diminished distal delivery of filtrate, alterations of prostaglandin metabolism in the kidney, and nonosmotic hypersecretion of antidiuretic hormone (see above, pp. 435 to 436). Water intake should be restricted to 1000 to 1500 ml daily if the serum sodium concentration falls below 130 mEq per liter, or if there is progressive weight gain despite severe sodium restriction.

Whether or not salt and water are restricted, most cirrhotic patients with moderate to marked ascites will require some diuretic therapy to diminish ascites volume appreciably. The goal is to reduce renal sodium retention and increase the delivery of sodium and water to the distal tubule.[207, 214] Prior to and during diuretic therapy, it is important to monitor patients carefully with regard to electrolyte and acid-base status, renal function, and the presence of encephalopathy.

Spironolactone has been recommended as the first diuretic agent to employ because potassium stores frequently are depleted in cirrhotic patients, and this agent, in addition to sparing potassium, is mild and relatively free of side effects.[203, 205, 209, 214–217] Spironolactone alone has been reported to produce substantial diuresis in 40 to 90 per cent of patients.[207, 209, 214, 215] However, the onset of diuresis may not occur for days, the dose required may be large (up to 600 mg per day), and several weeks may be required to accomplish a substantial diuresis. Avid proximal salt and water retention may explain the lack of response in some patients, for the site of action of spironolactone is in the distal nephron. The usual starting dose is 100 to 200 mg per day, with an increase of 100 mg every two to four days as necessary. The urinary sodium:potassium ratio may help define the need for dosage increase; dosage can be increased until the urinary sodium:potassium ratio is greater than 1.[218] Whereas increased urinary concentrations of sodium and decreased concentrations of potassium reflect aldosterone antagonism, their concentrations are also influenced by acid-base status and distal tubular flow rates, and therefore may not necessarily reflect adequacy of spironolactone dosage. Volume depletion, encephalopathy, and hypokalemia are rarely seen following diuresis with spironolactone, but hyperkalemia and metabolic acidosis may occur.[215, 219] All potassium supplements should be avoided or given carefully in conjunction with spironolactone.

In patients with an inadequate response to spironolactone, an agent that acts on more proximal portions of the nephron may be added to the regimen. This may be required in 25 to 50 per cent of patients.[217, 220] The most potent diuretics in general use are the "loop" agents furosemide and bumetanide, which may cause excretion of up to 20 to 25 per cent of the filtered sodium load. They are thus quite potent by increasing the delivery of sodium to the distal convoluted tubule at a rate that exceeds its capacity to reabsorb it. By using spironolactone to further block distal sodium reabsorption, natriuresis can be promoted even further.[214] Some patients may show an impaired natriuretic response to furosemide; it has recently been suggested that this is due to impaired furosemide transport into the renal tubule.[220a] A loop diuretic given alone, however, has proved the most difficult to use because it often fails to increase sodium excretion and can cause severe hypokalemia regardless of diuretic response.[212, 216, 217] In addition, it has recently been reported that furosemide may cause a transient, rapid reduction in renal perfusion, which may contribute to azotemia in some patients with ascites.[220b] The initial dosage of furosemide is 40 mg per day, and this may be increased every one to two days up to 240 mg per day.

The thiazides and metolazone act at the cortical diluting site and proximal tubule and are also more potent than spironolactone. Initial dosages are 50 to 100 mg of hydrochlorthiazide or 5 to 10 mg of metolazone. In extremely diuretic-resistant ascites, addition of a thiazide or metolazone to a loop diuretic produces a superadditive synergistic effect.[221] Profound responses leading to massive fluid and electrolyte losses may occur, so one should add low doses cautiously to the initial agent. Patients on these regimens should be observed closely, with hospitalization if necessary, to assure this.

The most common complications of the diuretic management of ascites are azotemia, hypokalemia, hyponatremia, and encephalopathy. In one recent study, electrolyte disturbances were reported in 23 per cent of patients, azotemia in 14 per cent, and encephalopathy in 12 per cent; even higher figures have been reported.[222] However, ascites can be managed successfully and without complication if a careful stepwise plan is employed and if large and abrupt volume shifts, which may compromise intravascular volume, are avoided. Reasonable estimates of optimal diuresis have been provided from studies of the kinetics of endogenous ascites mobilization in cirrhotic patients. In a study of cirrhotic individuals with or without edema, only about 300 ml of total daily urine volume was derived from spontaneous mobilization of ascites; diuretics increased this component to only about 350 ml. With coexisting edema, a maximum of about 900 ml of ascites appear to be removed by diuretics.[140] These guidelines were recently re-examined, and it was found that the maximum rate of ascites mobilization was 1440 ml per day, although the maximum amount that could be safely removed was 750 ml per day. Mobilization of more than 750 ml per day of ascites led to volume contraction in patients without edema; edema protected against volume contraction and azotemia.[223] Patients without edema are able to mobilize more than 1 liter per day, but at the expense of volume contraction and azotemia; patients with peripheral edema appear to be protected from these effects because of preferential mobilization of edema, and may safely undergo diuresis at a more rapid rate until edema disappears.

These findings provide a rational basis for management. Thus, diuresis should be limited to a weight loss of 1 to 2 kg per day in patients with edema, and 0.5 to 0.75 kg per day in patients without edema. The reduced likelihood of a decrease in plasma volume under these conditions will help avoid the aforementioned complications.[207–209, 214, 215] If diuresis consistently exceeds these guidelines or complications develop, diuretics may be tapered or discontinued for a few days to allow volume expansion and electrolyte repletion. Further, there is no need to "dry out" the patient as completely as possible; the small amount of residual ascites in selected patients is consistent with patient comfort and may decrease the incidence of drug-induced complications.

Certain drugs may inhibit diuresis and should be used cautiously in cirrhotics with ascites. *Prostaglandin inhibitors* diminish renal synthesis of prostaglandins and may impair renal function and natriuresis. In addition, they have been shown to markedly reduce the natriuretic response to furosemide, but have little effect on the response to spironolactone and thiazides. Among the drugs evaluated, indomethacin has the most deleterious effect, ibuprofen and naproxen an intermediate effect, and aspirin and sulindac have the least deleterious effect.[224] Propranolol,[225] metoclopramide,[225a] and captopril[224, 226] have also been shown to reduce sodium excretion in cirrhotic patients with ascites and should therefore also be used under careful observation.

Abstinence from alcohol is also a very important part of the medical treatment of ascites in alcoholic cirrhosis. In alcoholic cirrhotic patients, ascites carries a poor prognosis. However, one half to two thirds of the patients may improve with alcohol abstention and treatment, and those who continue to abstain from alcohol may remain ascites-free and enjoy extended survival.[227] Powell and Klatskin documented a 68 per cent five-year mortality rate after the onset of ascites with continued drinking, and a 48 per cent five-year mortality rate in abstainers with ascites.[67]

Much of the initial enthusiasm for *ascites ultrafiltration and reinfusion* has been lost, since patients were subjected to large fluid loads even when given with diuretics, improvement was transient, and febrile and other reactions were not uncommon.[228] A new technique, *dialytic ultrafiltration* with peritoneal reinfusion of ascites, removes fluid without protein loss or intravenous contamination, but its efficacy remains to be determined.[229]

Surgical Treatment. Ascites fails to respond to appropriate medical therapy in only 5 per cent of cirrhotic patients with stable or improving liver function.[214, 230] These patients with so-called intractable ascites have not been studied extensively but appear to have less portal-systemic shunting and somewhat lower hepatic blood flow and higher postsinusoidal resistance than otherwise comparable patients in whom there is satisfactory response to medical treatment within several weeks to a few months.[231] In other patients, hepatic pressure abnormalities seem less important than altered renal responses; these patients manifest increased sodium retention due to enhanced proximal tubular reabsorption and a fall in glomerular filtration rate.[232] Patients with intractable ascites have been considered to be candidates for two major types of surgical treatment, the side-to-side portacaval shunt, which decreases production of ascitic fluid by lowering intrahepatic sinusoidal and mesenteric capillary pressure, and the peritoneovenous shunt, which increases drainage of ascitic fluid.[233]

A side-to-side *portacaval shunt* may relieve intractable ascites in 90 per cent of cases.[234] However, because there is a 12 per cent operative mortality rate and a 33 per cent incidence of encephalopathy, this and other portacaval shunt procedures are rarely used solely for relief of ascites. In selected cases, such as associated bleeding varices or the Budd-Chiari syndrome, a side-to-side portacaval shunt might be considered.[233]

The *peritoneovenous shunt* has become widely used since the development of a technically simple valve by LeVeen in 1974, which permits unidirectional flow of ascitic fluid to the venous system. The shunt can be placed under local anesthesia and consists of a tube inserted into the peritoneal cavity, a one-way valve placed extraperitoneally in the anterior abdominal wall, and a silicone rubber tube extending from the valve subcutaneously over the chest wall and into the internal jugular vein and superior vena cava (Fig. 26–4). Fluid flows because of the abdominal-thoracic pressure gradient generated during inspiration.[235] More recent modifications (the Denver shunt) include a manually activated pump mechanism. Although each

type of shunt has its proponents, a recent randomized prospective trial concluded that although both shunts were similar in most respects, the LeVeen shunt had superior patency.[236] New shunt designs are being developed, particularly to reduce the complication of shunt occlusion.

Initial *indications* for the use of peritoneovenous shunts include (1) intractable and disabling ascites, unresponsive to strict in-hospital medical therapy; (2) ascites persisting despite volume depletion and azotemia; and (3) complicated abdominal hernias.[230] Increasing experience has added to the number of *contraindications* to its use, however. These include encephalopathy, severe liver injury with hyperbilirubinemia, coagulopathy, bacterial peritonitis, acute tubular necrosis, cardiac failure, and previous bleeding esophageal varices.[230, 235, 237–239] Preoperative evaluation should thus include complete blood count, serum electrolytes, BUN and creatinine concentrations, liver function studies, full coagulation studies, including fibrin degradation products, chest X-ray, and diagnostic paracentesis to evaluate cellular content and bacteriologic cultures. The patient must have been treated optimally with standard approaches, including sodium restriction and diuretics, and failed to respond despite several weeks to months of such therapy.

Postoperatively, large volumes of ascitic fluid are rapidly introduced into the vascular system, leading to plasma volume expansion, increased cardiac output and creatinine clearance, rapid suppression of renin and aldosterone, hypokalemia, and dilutional anemia.[91, 92, 230, 235, 240] To avoid fluid overload during the period of massive fluid mobilization, furosemide, 40 to 80 mg four to six times daily, is given and fluids are restricted. Potassium supplements and spironolactone are used to control hypokalemia. After the initial few days, an abdominal binder and breathing exercises help to augment shunt flow.

Although there is often an immediate and dramatic diuresis with weight loss and improved renal function and nutrition.[91, 92, 230, 235, 240–243] increasing experience with the procedure has served to identify a disappointingly high incidence of complications and shunt failure. The postoperative complication rate may be as high as 60 to 70 per cent, with mortality rates as high as 20 to 25 per cent.[236, 244] The most serious postoperative problems are coagulopathy and infection, but the list of potential complications includes variceal hemorrhage, fever, hypokalemia, shunt occlusion or migration, ascites leak, bowel obstruction, heart failure, air embolism, central venous thrombosis, and sclerosing peritonitis (see p. 1949).

Consumption coagulopathy is a worrisome complication encountered after shunt insertion and is manifested by decreased platelet count and fibrinogen concentration and elevated prothrombin time and fibrin degradation products. Clinical manifestations include ecchymoses, diffuse oozing from venipuncture and tube insertion sites, and possibly overt bleeding. Clinically significant disseminated intravascular coagulation (DIC) has occurred in up to 33 per cent of patients, and almost all patients may have laboratory evidence

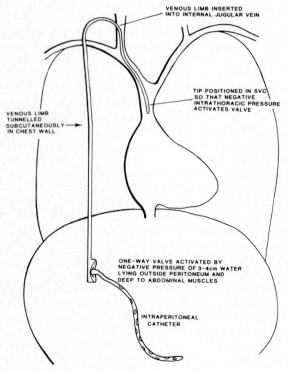

VENOUS LIMB INSERTED INTO INTERNAL JUGULAR VEIN

TIP POSITIONED IN SVC SO THAT NEGATIVE INTRATHORACIC PRESSURE ACTIVATES VALVE

VENOUS LIMB TUNNELLED SUBCUTANEOUSLY IN CHEST WALL

ONE-WAY VALVE ACTIVATED BY NEGATIVE PRESSURE OF 3–4cm WATER LYING OUTSIDE PERITONEUM AND DEEP TO ABDOMINAL MUSCLES

INTRAPERITONEAL CATHETER

Figure 26–4. Schematic representation of the LeVeen peritoneovenous shunt. (From Wood, L. J., Willett, I. R., and Dudley, F. J. Austr. N.Z. J. Med. *15*:469, 1985.)

of coagulopathy.[244-248] However, bleeding complications may be related more to the severity of liver disease and its attendant DIC than to the severity of postshunt coagulopathy.[249] If DIC proceeds uninterrupted, life-threatening hemorrhage may ensue. Treatment includes decreasing shunt flow by simple hydrostatic measures, support with platelets and fresh frozen plasma, or shunt ligation, but the best approach for the asymptomatic patient has not been established.

The mechanism of peritoneovenous shunt–associated DIC involves the transfer from ascites to the systemic circulation of an activated procoagulant, plasmin, plasminogen activator, cellular thromboplastin, or fibrin degradation products.[246-248] It recently has been proposed that ascitic fluid collagen leads to platelet aggregation and subsequent DIC.[250] Removal and replacement of ascitic fluid with saline at operation and careful selection of patients, particularly excluding patients with severe hepatic failure and pre-existing coagulation disorders, seem to have markedly reduced the incidence of coagulopathy.[236, 239, 251-253]

Infection is a common complication of peritoneovenous shunting. Bacteremia or peritonitis may occur in up to 25 per cent of patients,[237, 244, 254, 255] although some series report a lower incidence.[251, 253] *Staphylococcus aureus*, gram-negative enteric organisms, or streptococci are usually isolated. Treatment should include both antibiotic therapy and shunt removal, although despite this, the mortality rate may be very high (50 to 80 per cent).[237, 254, 255] It is unclear if prophylactic antibiotics are helpful, but in some series these antibiotics seem to have decreased the rate of infections and probably should be used.[251, 253]

In the postoperative period, *persistent or recurrent ascites* indicates a technical error, undetected cardiac or renal failure, inadequate shunt flow, or shunt occlusion caused by a plug of precipitated protein in the valve or venous tubing.[256] *Shunt occlusion* can be diagnosed by Doppler flowmeter, injection of radionuclide into the ascites with visualization of liver or lung uptake, or direct injection of radiopaque dye or radionuclide into the lumen of the outflow tubing.[257, 258] Shunt occlusion due to central venous thrombosis has been increasingly recognized with more experience, and may occur in approximately 20 per cent of patients. It may present with recurrent ascites, superior vena cava syndrome, upper limb swelling, or pulmonary emboli.[259, 260]

Long-term follow-up in a small number of patients indicates that they maintain the acites-free state, increased creatinine clearance, and normal renin and aldosterone, but they continue to be sodium retainers when challenged with a sodium load and often continue to require sodium restriction and diuretics.[95] Although the peritoneovenous shunt is effective in the initial relief of ascites, its long-term efficacy is less well defined. Ascites is controlled in about 50 per cent of patients followed for one to two years,[245, 261] but the uncertain long-term effect is emphasized by the fact that shunt occlusion is not necessarily associated with recurrent ascites.[262] Results of a larger uncontrolled study reveals a mean survival rate of 44 per cent in

four years, with improved nutrition and relief from chronic disabling ascites; however, the characteristics of this group are not well described.[263] Patient selection significantly influences survival, and a carefully designed, randomized trial to determine whether there is a prolongation of survival has not been reported.[264, 265] Most of the published data suggest that the shunt has little influence on survival. In summary, it is clear that peritoneovenous shunting has a role in the treatment of the cirrhotic patient with medically refractory tense ascites. However, the high complication rate makes it imperative that patients be chosen carefully. A recent French multicenter controlled trial emphasized these points.[265a]

Peritoneovenous shunting has also been used in the smaller number of patients with hepatorenal syndrome and noncirrhotic ascites, including Budd-Chiari syndrome, chylous ascites, malignant ascites, pancreatic ascites, nephrogenic ascites, and cardiac ascites. Its use in some of these conditions will be discussed below. A recent randomized study concluded that shunting may stabilize renal function but does not prolong life in patients with hepatorenal syndrome.[265b]

Cardiac Causes of Portal Hypertension

Diseases that cause mechanical or functional impedance to hepatic venous flow are often associated with ascites. Among these, congestive heart failure, particularly right-sided, is the most frequent. Constrictive pericarditis deserves special emphasis and should always be considered in cases of ascites of obscure origin. It usually presents with fatigue, ascites, and tender hepatomegaly, often with little peripheral edema. In the evaluation of the patient with ascites, the physical findings characteristic of this entity should be sought: jugular venous distention with early diastolic collapse and inspiratory swelling, a diastolic knock that may be confused with a third heart sound, and pulsus paradoxus. Clear lung fields and low voltage of the electrocardiogram are often present. The diagnosis may be confirmed by echocardiography, computed tomography, or cardiac catheterization.[266]

Inferior Vena Cava and Hepatic Vein Obstruction (Budd-Chiari Syndrome)

Inferior vena cava and hepatic vein obstruction characteristically causes ascites and hepatomegaly. The Budd-Chiari syndrome may present with a varied course as an acute, subacute, or chronic illness and may result from thrombi, intimal fibrosis, or tumor involving the hepatic veins or vena cava.[267] Thrombosis may be secondary to polycythemia vera (and other causes of hyperviscosity or thrombocytosis), hemoglobinopathy such as sickle cell disease, or the use of oral contraceptives. A surgically remediable condition of unknown etiology, membranous obstruction of the inferior vena cava, has been reported as a causative factor, particularly in the Far East and South Africa, but this condition recently has been reported to be responsible for 23 per cent of cases of hepatic outflow obstruction in a series from Los Angeles.[268]

Presenting signs and symptoms include abdominal pain in 55 per cent, ascites in 90 to 95 per cent, and tender hepatomegaly in 70 per cent; splenomegaly and jaundice are seen in only 30 per cent. Liver function may be only mildly abnormal, with a high alkaline phosphatase level. Femoral venous pressure may be elevated in the face of normal pressure in the tributaries of the superior vena cava. The diagnosis may be suggested by Tc-99m sulfur colloid imaging, which may show an enlarged caudate lobe, or by computed tomography or ultrasonography, which demonstrate caudate lobe hypertrophy, narrowing of the inferior vena cava, and lack of visualization of the major hepatic veins. Contrast uptake in the parenchyma shows prolonged opacification at the periphery and more rapid clearing of the caudate lobe.[269] MRI scanning may become a major diagnostic tool; it displays hepatic veins very well because of its excellent depiction of blood vessels as regions of absent signals.[270] Liver biopsy shows centrilobular necrosis, hepatic congestion, and eventually fibrosis and cirrhosis, but definitive diagnosis usually depends upon direct demonstration of venous occlusion. Hepatic venography may show vena cava obstruction or a narrow, occluded hepatic vein with a "network pattern" of neighboring veins.

Medical treatment with diuretics and anticoagulants is rarely successful, and peritoneovenous shunting does nothing to decompress the congested liver. Early portal-systemic shunting is often the best approach.[267, 271]

Hypoalbuminemia

Ascites is uncommon in patients with uncomplicated hypoalbuminemia, although it may be present in up to 12 per cent of those with nephrotic syndrome. Nephrotic patients with ascites have a serum albumin of <2.5 mg per dl and often <1.5 mg per dl. Protein-losing enteropathy and malnutrition are infrequent causes of hypoalbuminemic ascites in North America (see pp. 283–290).

MISCELLANEOUS DISORDERS

Myxedema

Myxedema is an unusual but treatable cause of clinically significant ascites (about 3 to 4 per cent of cases of myxedema) and presents with intractable exudative ascites that may respond poorly to diuretics.[272] Patients frequently have only impaired mentation and ascites. Mild systemic changes of myxedema may be overlooked, and a number of these patients are subjected to an unnecessary laparotomy. The fluid is yellow and gelatinous and generally has a protein concentration of over 4 gm per dl. Although the pathophysiology is poorly understood, it is postulated that there is increased capillary permeability with the escape of protein-rich fluid. Intravenous fluorescein causes tissue staining before, but not after, treatment with thyroxine, and protein electrophoresis of ascitic fluid is similar to the serum pattern.[273] The ascites is rapidly cleared within two to three weeks after the start of thyroid replacement therapy.

Ovarian Disease

Ovarian causes of ascites, aside from carcinoma, include Meigs' syndrome and the ovarian overstimulation syndrome. *Meigs' syndrome* consists of ascites and hydrothorax with various benign ovarian tumors. Initially, the syndrome was described specifically with fibromas, but it appears that cystadenomas are more common.[274] The formation of ascites in this condition has variously been ascribed to either an interrupted ovarian venous drainage with transudation, or large tumors with edematous myxoid stroma. *Ovarian edema*, presumably due to torsion of the ovary, is unassociated with neoplastic changes but may also cause ascites and hydrothorax by the same mechanism.[275] Torsion of other pelvic structures, such as large uterine leiomyomas, has also been reported to cause ascites.[276] A rare tumor of the ovary, *struma ovarii*, is a unilateral ovarian teratoma containing thyroid tissue. Patients may present with symptoms of hyperthyroidism, ascites, or an ovarian mass. About one third may have ascites, and about one third demonstrate hyperthyroidism; 10 per cent have both.[277, 278] Tumors associated with ascites are larger than 6 cm in diameter. The rich blood supply of thyroid tissue, together with edema and hemorrhage of the capsule caused by repeated twisting of the stalk, may acount for the ascites. The diagnosis should be suspected if ovarian calcification is noted on abdominal X-rays or if there is uptake of I-131 in the abdomen.

Massive ascites, pleural effusion, and hypovolemia have developed in association with enlarged ovaries after treatment with clomiphene or human menopausal gonadotropin. This severe form of *ovarian hyperstimulation syndrome* only occurs in 1 to 2 per cent of patients but may be serious and can lead to electrolyte imbalance, oliguria, and shock. The syndrome is caused by increased capillary permeability of ovarian vessels, possibly mediated by estrogenic metabolites or prostaglandins.[279]

Pancreatic Ascites

Pancreatic ascites is a syndrome in which massive amounts of abdominal fluid, rich in pancreatic enzymes, accumulate in association with chronic pancreatic disease.[280, 281] Reliable data on the incidence of pancreatic ascites are not available, but it may approach 3 per cent of cases of pancreatitis in Veterans Administration and municipal hospital populations.[282] Most commonly, the patients are males between the ages of 20 and 50 years who are alcoholic or have sustained abdominal trauma. Rarely, pancreatic disease of other causes may be seen, but pancreatitis secondary to biliary tract disease or carcinoma is conspicuous by its absence. Characteristically, the patient presents with increasing abdominal girth and weight loss; abdominal pain is variable, and can be either severe or entirely absent. These patients seem to have little in the way of steatorrhea, diabetes, or pancreatic calcifications. Subcutaneous fat necrosis is present in some. Associated pleural effusions may be present in 15 to 20 per cent. Most patients appear chronically ill, with massive ascites and little or no abdominal tenderness.

Laboratory studies are of particular importance diagnostically. In virtually all cases, serum and especially ascites fluid amylase values are dramatically increased. Ascitic fluid amylase has recently been reported in more detail. In ascites of nonpancreatic origin, the normal range is similar to that of the normal serum amylase; only 8 per cent had an ascitic amylase greater than serum, and none had an ascitic amylase greater than twice their serum value.[282a] In the rare patient in whom ascites fluid amylase is not significantly elevated, ascites fluid lipase determinations may be of value.[283] The elevated serum enzyme levels result from absorption of enzymes from the ascitic fluid, not from active inflammation in the gland. In addition, inasmuch as the enzymes are not activated, an acute peritonitis does not occur, and ascites is painless. The high protein concentrations (usually exceeding 3 gm per dl) in the ascitic fluid are probably due to a combination of enzyme-rich pancreatic fluid and protein-rich exudate from the inflamed pancreas, rather than to peritonitis.[284] The fluid may be serous, serosanguineous, turbid, or chylous. A pseudocyst is often demonstrable by upper GI series, ultrasonography, or computed tomography. Endoscopic retrograde pancreatography may demonstrate a duct lesion, pseudocyst, or actual point of leakage into the peritoneal cavity, and thus provides anatomic evidence for the diagnosis and pathogenesis of pancreatic ascites. If the patient should require surgery, operative time will be shortened by this information, for the need to perform transduodenal pancreatography will be obviated.[285, 286] At operation, most patients are found to have a pancreatic pseudocyst or rupture of the pancreatic duct, suggesting that leakage of pancreatic secretions into the peritoneal cavity is important in pathogenesis.

Treatment depends on the cause. In cases in which trauma is implicated, early surgical repair of the duct or pseudocyst drainage is recommended. Results in this setting appear to be quite favorable. For alcoholic pancreatic ascites, a more conservative approach seems indicated, in view of the fact that the operative mortality rate is approximately 20 per cent and there is a recurrence rate of 15 per cent. In general, it appears reasonable to rest the pancreas while attempting to improve the patient's nutritional status by means of total parenteral nutrition or the feeding of elemental diets. Success with this conservative trial may approach 40 per cent.[287] If ascites worsens, or if it fails to improve

after at most a few weeks, endoscopic retrograde pancreatography or operative pancreatography should be performed with drainage or resection of the pseudocyst or leak.[280, 281, 287] For patients who are particularly poor operative risks, radiation of the pancreas has been reported to be of value.[280, 288] Peritoneovenous shunting has been done in small numbers of patients, was well tolerated, and allowed very sick patients to improve for definitive surgical repair; this approach should be used only in a few selected patients.[289]

Bile Ascites

It is now well recognized that extravasated bile may lead to chronic peritoneal fluid accumulation.[290, 291] The cause of the extravasated bile may be trauma, spontaneous perforation of the gallbladder, procedures such as transhepatic cholangiography or liver biopsy, and biliary tract surgery.[292–295] Patients develop abdominal distention as a result of accumulation of bile in the peritoneal cavity, but may have no fever, leukocytosis, or peritoneal signs. Nausea, malaise, jaundice, and acholic stools are usually present. Bile ascites may be noted as long as two months following the onset of biliary tract leakage from any cause. Analysis of ascitic fluid bilirubin in patients without bile ascites gives a mean of 0.7 mg/dl. Patients with bile ascites all had an ascitic bilirubin >6 mg/dl with an ascitic:serum ratio >1.0.[295a]

Paracentesis is diagnostic if it yields a bilious fluid, and it may be therapeutic if the leak is slow and closes spontaneously. Most often surgical exploration is necessary to repair the leak. The difference between this group and the more dramatic course of acute bile peritonitis may reflect the sterility of the extravasated bile. Experiments using germ-free animals and antibiotics show that bacteria play a major role in determining the severity of acute experimental bile peritonitis.[291, 296] The rate of leakage may also play a role.

Chylous Ascites

Etiology. Chylous ascites is due to the accumulation of lipid-rich lymph in the peritoneal cavity and is the result of lymphatic obstruction or leakage. The etiology varies with the age of the patient and its acuteness of onset. A large retrospective review of chylous ascites going back to the early years of the century indicated the cause in adults to be neoplastic in 30 per cent, inflammatory in 35 per cent, traumatic in 11 per cent, congenital in 1 per cent, and "idiopathic" in 23 per cent.[297] However, in more recent years, neoplastic disease is the cause in 87 per cent of cases.[298, 299] Lymphomas constitute about half of these; the other half are caused by a variety of primary and metastatic neoplasms. The inflammatory causes of chylous ascites are quite varied, including pancreatitis, tuberculosis, portal vein thrombosis, mesenteric adenitis, adhesions with intestinal obstruction, radiation, and pulmonary fibrosis with thoracic duct obstruction.[297, 300, 301] Chylous ascites may also be seen rarely (0.5 per cent) in otherwise uncomplicated cirrhosis.[302] In these cases, the chyle is derived from intestinal lymph, apparently because of high lymphatic pressures, which lead to subserosal intestinal lymphangiectasis and subsequent rupture.[303] Chylous ascites may also be present in over half the patients with ascites caused by the nephrotic syndrome.[304]

Trauma is usually surgical in nature, and has been reported following extensive abdominal or retroperitoneal surgery such as portal-systemic shunt, aortic aneurysmectomy, retroperitoneal lymph node dissection, and vagotomy.[305] Congenital etiologies among adults are rare, but chylous ascites may be associated with lymphangiectasia, lymphangiomyomatosis, and other generalized dysplastic disorders of the lymphatic system.[306-308]

The etiology in pediatric patients differs, with 40 to 60 per cent being due to congenital malformations; these include lymphatic stenosis, atresia, hypoplasia, mesenteric cysts, and lymphangiomas.[297, 309, 310] Neoplasms are very rare in pediatric patients.

Acute chylous ascites (peritonitis) also has a different distribution of etiologies. In 50 per cent of patients the syndrome is idiopathic, and laparotomy is negative except for chylous fluid, dilated lymphatics, and edematous, inflamed mesentery and peritoneum. Another 20 per cent demonstrate intestinal obstruction, with distention of the lacteal glands and weeping of chyle from the bowel surface. Trauma, including operative trauma, accounts for 15 per cent, with disruption of the cisterna chyli, and a final 15 per cent are due to rupture of chyle-containing cysts.[311, 312]

Clinical Features. The symptoms and signs of chylous ascites are nonspecific, related to the accumulation of peritoneal fluid with increased intra-abdominal pressure, or to an underlying neoplasm. Laboratory analysis is also nonspecific, with hypoproteinemia and lymphocytopenia due to exudation of lymph into the abdomen. Acute chylous peritonitis presents with the sudden onset of crampy abdominal pain in up to one third of patients, often after a heavy meal, which is localized in the right lower quadrant. Occasionally, a soft swelling may be noted in the supraclavicular areas, presumably caused by lymph extravasation in the neck.

Diagnosis. Paracentesis recovers a turbid fluid from the abdomen that separates into layers on standing or stains positively for fat. Its significant lipid content differentiates it from "pseudochyle." The opalescence of the latter, which does not contain excess triglyceride, is accounted for by phospholipid-protein material from degenerating neoplastic, inflammatory, or mesothelial cells. In addition, the gross milkiness of the fluid correlates poorly with absolute triglyceride levels, because turbidity also reflects chylomicron size.

Triglycerides are often greater than 1000 mg per dl, but even when low, ascitic levels exceed those in plasma. Leukocyte counts are high and show marked lymphocytic predominance. Protein content is variable, but usually is greater than 3 gm per dl.

CT scans may help diagnose neoplasms or other causes of lymphatic obstruction. Lymphangiography may localize a site of obstruction, leakage, or dysplasia. Exploratory laparotomy is often necessary to definitively diagnose the etiology of chylous ascites.[299, 310]

Treatment. Once treatment for the underlying problem is undertaken, supportive measures are often needed to relieve the symptoms of chylous ascites. Diuretics and salt restriction are usually unsuccessful, and repeated paracentesis gives only short-term relief. A trial of low-fat diet with medium chain triglyceride supplementation should be used, but not all patients respond to this. Total parenteral nutrition is used as a means of achieving total bowel rest, particularly in traumatic or pediatric cases; this allows leaky or traumatized lymphatics to heal and may reduce lymphatic flow by 43 per cent.[313] Peritoneovenous shunts have been used successfully in some patients[314] but may occlude or predispose to complications. Finally, if supportive measures do not allow resolution of ascites, laparotomy may permit correction of leaky or obstructed lymphatics, especially in children.[309, 310, 312]

Prognosis. The prognosis depends on the underlying etiology, and thus is better in children than in adults. The one-year mortality rate is 12 per cent in children but 77 per cent in adults.[299, 310] Idiopathic or acute cases often clear spontaneously, but chronic chylous ascites contributes to the debilitation associated with the primary disease.

Urine Ascites and Dialysis-Associated Ascites

The intraperitoneal accumulation of extravasated urine is uncommon. Isolated cases have been reported following trauma to the urinary tract during abdominal surgery, with formation of ureteroperitoneal fistula.[315] Traumatic rupture of the bladder usually is extraperitoneal but occasionally occurs intraperitoneally and presents with abdominal pain, tenderness, oliguria, and urine ascites.[316] In neonates and children, urine ascites has been described secondary to rupture of congenital bladder diverticula, or "spontaneous bladder rupture."[317] Ascites may also follow renal transplantation, apparently reflecting extravasation or transudation of fluid from the transplanted kidney, although this cannot always be demonstrated and may occasionally be due to other mechanisms.[318-320] In these circumstances, the extravasated fluid may not have the characteristic appearance of urine because of solute equilibration across the peritoneal membranes, but comparison of urea nitrogen, creatinine, and electrolyte concentrations in peritoneal fluid and serum usually clarifies the nature of the fluid.[321]

An interesting form of urine ascites occurs in the neonate. This is most often seen in males within five weeks of birth and is heralded by abdominal distention associated with high-grade urinary tract obstruction, usually due to posterior urethral valves.[322, 323] Intravenous pyelography defines the site of perforation in two thirds of the cases; it is often located at the calyceal fornix, and fluid collects in the perirenal fascia. A subsequent tear in the thin peritoneal layer covering the retroperitoneum allows the formation of urine ascites. Ascites does not occur in adults with a urinary obstruction, probably owing to the relative strength of Gerota's fascia and other fascial structures that will contain extravasated urine. Urine ascites accounts for 25 per cent of the cases of neonatal ascites.[324, 325]

Ascites may become a severe problem in 3 to 12 per cent of patients maintained on chronic hemodialysis.[326–328] These patients have ascites without concomitant edema or other overt signs of cardiac failure or fluid overload. Serum albumin level is not always depressed, and ascitic fluid protein is usually greater than 3 gm per dl. Peritoneal biopsies have rarely shown more than modest inflammation or fibrosis.

The diagnosis of *dialysis associated ascites* is one of exclusion, so that it is important to rule out other etiologies of ascites in these patients. The pathophysiology of ascites in these patients appears to be multifactorial. A large proportion have had prior peritoneal dialysis or infection, hypertension, fluid overload, or poor nutrition and hypoalbuminemia. Overhydration coupled with serosal inflammation and increased vascular permeability (possibly caused by some uremic factor) may explain most cases.[329] Decreased peritoneal fluid drainage may also be a factor.[330]

The treatment of ascites in these patients may be very difficult. Special attention should be paid to enforcing sodium and fluid restriction and ensuring adequate intake of proteins and calories. Administration of albumin or blood and multiple paracenteses are often fruitless. Removal of excess fluid by aggressive dialysis with ultrafiltration may be helpful, but often must be stopped because these patients are prone to develop hypotension during dialytic ultrafiltration. Should this occur, isolated ultrafiltration without dialysis may be more successful.[331]

Nephrectomy has been advocated, but ascites has developed or recurred following nephrectomy. Renal transplantation, when possible, seems to afford the best chance of relieving chronic ascites. Peritoneovenous and chronic ambulatory peritoneal dialysis have been used successfully on a number of patients, but more experience and longer follow-up will be needed before the efficacy of these more recent therapeutic measures can be assessed.[329, 332–335]

References

1. Callan, E. L., Jr., Benjamin, S. B., Knuff, T. E., et al. The accuracy of the physical examination in the diagnosis of suspected ascites. JAMA 247:1164, 1982.
2. Cummings, S., Papadakis, M., Melnick, J., et al. The predictive value of physical examinations for ascites. West. J. Med. 142:633, 1985.
3. Aitken, R. J., and Clifford, P. C. Girth measurement is not a reliable investigation for the detection of intraabdominal fluid. Ann. R. Coll. Surg. 67:241, 1985.
4. Grobe, J. L., Kozarek, R. A., Sanowski, R. A., et al. "Pseudoascites" associated with giant ovarian cysts and elevated cyst fluid amylase. Am. J. Gastroenterol. 78:421, 1983.
5. Jurolf, H. Roentgen diagnosis of intraperitoneal fluid. Acta Radiol. (supplement) 343:1, 1975.
6. Bundrick, T. J., Cho, S., Brewer, W. H., et al. Ascites: Comparison of plain film radiographs with ultrasonograms. Radiology 152:503, 1984.
7. Love, L., Demos, T. C., Reynes, C. J., et al. Visualization of the lateral edge of the liver in ascites. Radiology 122:619, 1977.
8. Goldberg, B. Ultrasonic evaluation of intraperitoneal fluid. JAMA 235:2427, 1976.
9. Gooding, G. A., and Cummings, S. R. Sonographic detection of ascites in liver disease. J. Ultrasound Med. 3:169, 1984.
10. Proto, A. V., Lane, E. J., and Maringola, J. P. A new concept of ascitic fluid distribution. Am. J. Roentgenol. 126:974, 1976.
11. Yeh, H. C., and Wolf, B. S. Ultrasonography in ascites. Radiology 124:783, 1977.
12. Edell, S. L., and Gefter, W. B. Ultrasonic differentiation of types of ascitic fluid. Am. J. Roentgenol. 133:111, 1979.
13. Federle, M. P., and Jeffrey, R. B., Jr. Hemoperitoneum studied by computed tomography. Radiology 148:187, 1983.
14. Gore, R. M., Callen, P. W., and Filly, R. A. Lesser sac fluid in predicting the etiology of ascites: CT findings. Am. J. Roentgenol. 139:71, 1982.
15. Jolles, H., and Conlam, C. M. CT of ascites: Differential diagnosis. Am. J. Roentgenol. 135:315, 1980.
16. Cohen, J. M., Weinreb, J. C., and Maravilla, K. R. Fluid collections in the intraperitoneal and extraperitoneal spaces: Comparison of MR and CT. Radiology 155:705, 1985.
17. Mallory, A., and Schaefer, J. W. Complications of diagnostic paracentesis in patients with liver disease. JAMA 239:628, 1978.
18. Runyon, B. A., Hoefs, J. C., and Kanawati, H. N. Polymicrobial bacterascites. Arch. Intern. Med. 146:2173, 1986.
19. Runyon, B. A. Paracentesis of ascitic fluid; a safe procedure. Arch. Intern. Med. 146:2259, 1986.
20. Cheson, B. D. Clinical utility of body fluid analysis. Clin. Lab. Med. 5:195, 1985.
21. Tavel, M. Ascites: Etiological considerations, with emphasis on the value of several laboratory findings in diagnosis. Am. J. Med. Sci. 237:727, 1959.
22. Sampliner, R., and Iber, F. High protein ascites in patients with uncomplicated hepatic cirrhosis. Am. J. Med. Sci. 267:275, 1974.
23. Witte, M., Witte, C., and Dumont, A. Progress in liver disease. Physiological factors involved in the causation of cirrhotic ascites. Gastroenterology 61:742, 1971.
24. Rector, W. G., Jr., and Reynolds, T. B. Superiority of the serum-ascites albumin difference over the ascites total protein concentration in separation of transudative and exudative ascites. Am. J. Med. 77:83, 1984.
25. Boyer, T. B., Kahn, A. M., and Reynolds, T. B. Diagnostic value of ascitic fluid lactic dehydrogenase, protein and WBC levels. Arch. Intern. Med. 138:1103, 1978.
26. Pare, P., Talbot, J., and Hoefs, J. C. Serum-ascites albumin concentration gradient: The physiological approach to the differential diagnosis of ascites. Gastroenterology 185:240, 1983.
27. Scholmerich, J., Volk, B. A., Kottgen, E., et al. Fibronectin concentration in ascites differentiates between malignant and nonmalignant ascites. Gastroenterology 87:1160, 1984.
27a. Runyon, B. A. Elevated ascitic fluid fibronectin concentration: a nonspecific finding. J. Hepatol. 3:219, 1986.
28. Jungst, D., Gerbes, A. L., Martin, R., et al. Value of ascitic lipids in the differentiation between cirrhotic and malignant ascites. Hepatology 6:239, 1986.
29. Caselmann, W. H., and Jungst, D. Isolation and characterization of a cellular protein-lipid complex from ascites fluid caused by various neoplasms. Cancer Res. 46:1547, 1986.
30. Lowenstein, M. S., Rittgers, R. A., Feinerman, A. E., et al. Carcinoembryonic antigen assay of ascites and detection of malignancy. Ann. Intern. Med. 88:635, 1978.
31. Booth, S. N., Lakin, G., Dykes, P. W., et al. Cancer associated proteins in effusion fluids. J. Clin. Pathol. 30:537, 1977.
32. Nystrom, J. S., Dyce, E., Wada, J., et al. Carcinoembryonic antigen titers in effusion fluid. Arch. Intern. Med. 137:875, 1977.
33. Lynn, C. W., Inglis, N. R., and Rule, A. H. Histaminase and other tumor markers in malignant effusion fluid. Cancer Res. 39:4894, 1979.

34. Roboz, J., Greaves, J., Silides, D., et al. Hyaluronic acid content of effusions as a diagnostic aid for malignant mesothelioma. Cancer Res. *45*:1850, 1985.

35. Clarkson, B. Relationship between cell type, glucose concentration, and response to treatment in neoplastic effusions. Cancer *17*:914, 1964.

36. Polak, M., and Torres de Costa, A. Diagnostic value of the estimation of glucose in ascitic fluid. Digestion *8*:347, 1973.

37. Runyon, B. A., and Hoefs, J. C. Ascitic fluid analysis in the differentiation of spontaneous bacterial peritonitis from gastrointestinal tract perforation into ascitic fluid. Hepatology *4*:447, 1984.

38. Hacker, J. F., Richter, J. E., Pyatt, R. S., et al. Hemorrhagic ascites: An unusual presentation of primary splenic lymphoma. Gastroenterology *83*:470, 1982.

39. DeSitter, L., Rector, W. G., Jr. The significance of bloody ascites in patients with cirrhosis. Am. J. Gastroenterol. *79*:136, 1984.

40. Kumar, N. B., and Naylor, B. Megakaryocytes in pleural and peritoneal fluids. J. Clin. Pathol. *33*:1153, 1980.

41. Liss, M., Brandt, L. J., and Wolf, E. L. Cholesterol crystal pseudoascites: An unusual presentation of ovarian cyst. Am. J. Gastroenterol. *77*:245, 1982.

42. Viranuvatti, V., Hitanant, S., Boonyapaknavig, V., et al. Peritoneal biopsy: Experience with blind and direct vision biopsy. Am. J. Proctol. *17*:489, 1966.

43. Levine, H. Needle biopsy of the peritoneum and exudative ascites. Arch. Intern. Med. *120*:542, 1967.

44. Jenkins, P. F., and Ward, M. J. The role of peritoneal biopsy in the diagnosis of ascites. Postgrad. Med. J. *56*:702, 1980.

45. Trujillo, N. P. Peritoneoscopy and guided biopsy in the diagnosis of intraabdominal disease. Gastroenterology *71*:1083, 1976.

46. Hall, T. J., Donaldson, D. R., and Brennen, T. G. The value of laparoscopy under local anesthesia in 250 medical and surgical patients. Br. J. Surg. *67*:751, 1980.

47. Kistler, L. A., Reichelderfer, M., Hanson, J. T., et al. Laparoscopic evaluation of hepatic and peritoneal disease. Wisc. Med. J. *81*:19, 1982.

48. Salky, B., Bauer, J., Gelernt, I., et al. Laparoscopy for gastrointestinal diseases. Mt. Sinai J. Med. *52*:228, 1985.

49. Coupland, G. A. E., Townsend, D. M., and Martin, C. J. Peritoneoscopy—use and assessment of intraabdominal malignancy. Surgery *89*:645, 1981.

50. Ishida, H., Dohzono, T., Furukawa, Y., et al. Laparoscopy and biopsy in the diagnosis of malignant intraabdominal tumors. Endoscopy *16*:140, 1984.

50a. De Groen, P. C., Rakela, J., Moore, S. C., et al. Diagnostic laparoscopy in gastroenterology: a 14-year experience. Dig. Dis. Sci. *32*:677, 1987.

51. Cain, M. G., and Krejs, G. J. Complications of diagnostic laparoscopy in Dallas: A 7 year prospective study. Gastrointest. Endosc. *30*:237, 1984.

52. Knauer, C. M., and Lowe, H. M. Hemodynamics in the cirrhotic patient during paracentesis. N. Engl. J. Med. *276*:491, 1967.

53. Guazzi, M., Polese, A., Magrini, F., et al. Negative influence of ascites on the cardiac function of cirrhotic patients. Am. J. Med. *59*:165, 1975.

54. Buhac, I., Flesh, L., and Kishore, R. Intraabdominal pressure and ascitic fluid volume in decompensated liver cirrhosis. Am. J. Gastroenterol. *79*:569, 1984.

55. McCullough, K. I., Issener, J. M., Pandian, M. G., et al. Circulatory shock due to ascites and responsive to paracentesis. Am. J. Cardiol. *6*:500, 1985.

56. Materson, D. Hemodynamic implications of ascites in abdominal paracentesis. *In* Epstein, M. (ed.): The Kidney and Liver Disease. New York, Elsevier-North Holland, 1978, p. 337.

57. Halpin, T. F., and McCann, T. O. Dynamics of body fluids following the rapid removal of large volumes of ascites. Am. J. Obstet. Gynecol. *110*:103, 1971.

58. Kruikshank, D. P., and Buchsbaum, H. J. Effects of rapid paracentesis. JAMA *225*:1361, 1973.

59. Carey, W. D., Cohn, J. C., Leatherman, J., et al. Ascitic fluid

60. Kao, H. W., Rakov, N. E., Savage, E., et al. The effect of large volume paracentesis on plasma volume—cause of hypovolemia? Hepatology *5*:403, 1985.

61. Racco, V. K., and Ware, A. J. Cirrhotic ascites: Pathophysiology, diagnosis and management. Ann. Intern. Med. *105*:573, 1986.

62. Berner, C., Fred, H. L., Riggs, S., et al. Diagnostic probabilities in patients with conspicuous ascites. Arch. Intern. Med. *113*:687, 1964.

63. Hyman, S., Villa, F., and Steigmann, F. Mimetic aspects of ascites. JAMA *183*:651, 1963.

64. Nafeh, M. A., Shahwan, M. M., Mohammed, S. S., et al. Endoscopic diagnosis of ascites in Assiut province, upper Egypt. Endoscopy *15*:347, 1983.

65. Menzies, R. I., Fitzgerald, J. M., and Mulpeter, K. Laparoscopic diagnosis of ascites in Lesotho. Br. Med. J. *291*:473, 1985.

66. Falkner, M. J., Reeve, P. A., and Locket, S. The diagnosis of tuberculous ascites in a rural African community. Tubercle *66*:55, 1985.

67. Powell, W. J., and Klatskin, G. Duration of survival in patients with Laennec's cirrhosis. Am. J. Med. *44*:406, 1968.

68. Ring-Larsen, H., and Henriksen, J. H. Pathogenesis of ascites formation and hepatorenal syndrome: Humoral and hemodynamic factors. Semin. Liver Dis. *6*:341, 1986.

69. Benoit, J., and Granger, D. N. Splanchnic hemodynamics in chronic portal hypertension. Semin. Liver Dis. *6*:287, 1986.

70. Granger, D. N., Miller, T., Allen, R., Parker, R. E., Parker, J. C., and Taylor, A. E. Permselectivity of cat liver bloodlymph barrier to endogenous macromolecules. Gastroenterology *77*:103, 1979.

71. Witte, C. L., Witte, M. H., and Dumont, A. E. Lymph imbalance in the genesis and perpetuation of the ascites syndrome in hepatic cirrhosis. Gastroenterology *78*:1059, 1980.

72. Witte, M. H., Witte, C. L., and Dumont, A. E. Estimated net transcapillary water and protein flux in the liver and intestine of patients with portal hypertension from hepatic cirrhosis. Gastroenterology *80*:265, 1981.

73. Zimmon, D., Oratz, M., and Kessler, R. Albumin to ascites: Demonstration of a direct pathway bypassing the systemic circulation. J. Clin. Invest. *48*:2074, 1969.

74. Epstein, M. Deranged sodium homeostasis in cirrhosis. Gastroenterology *76*:622, 1979.

75. Atkinson, M., and Losowsky, M. The mechanism of ascites formation in chronic liver disease. Quart. J. Med. *30*:153, 1961.

76. Schaffner, F., and Popper, H. Capillarization of hepatic sinusoids in man. Gastroenterology *44*:239, 1963.

77. Orrego, H., Blendis, L. M., Crossley, J. R., Medline, A., MacDonald, A., Ritchie, S., and Israel, Y. Correlation of intrahepatic pressure with collagen in the Disse space and hepatomegaly in humans and in the rat. Gastroenterology *80*:546, 1981.

78. Huet, P.-M., Pomier-Layrargues, G., Villenneve, J.-P., Varin, F., and Fiallet, A. Intrahepatic circulation in liver disease. Semin. Liver Dis. *6*:277, 1986.

79. Bar-Meir, S., Lerner, E., and Conn, H. O. Analysis of ascitic fluid in cirrhosis. Dig. Dis. Sci. *24*:136, 1979.

80. Rosoff, L., Zia, P., Reynolds, T., and Horton, R. Studies of renin and aldosterone in cirrhotic patients with ascites. Gastroenterology *69*:698, 1975.

81. Arroyo, V., Bosch, J., Mauri, M., Viver, J., Mas, A., Rivera, F., and Rodes, J. Renin, aldosterone and renal hemodynamics in cirrhosis with ascites. Eur. J. Clin. Invest. *9*:69, 1979.

82. Bosch, J., Arroyo, V., Betrin, A., Mas, A., Carrilho, F., Rivera, F., Navarro-Lopes, F., and Rodes, J. Hepatic hemodynamics and the renin-angiotensin-aldosterone system in cirrhosis. Gastroenterology *78*:92, 1980.

83. Arroyo, J., Bosch, J., Gaza-Beltran, J., Kravetz, D., Estrada, L., Rivera, F., and Rodes, J. Plasma renin activity and urinary sodium excretion as prognostic indicators in nonazotemic cirrhosis with ascites. Ann. Intern. Med. *94*:198, 1981.

84. Schroeder, E. T., and Anderson, Jr., G. H. Relation of the

renin-angiotensin system to hemodynamic abnormalities in cirrhosis: Studies using blockade of angiotensin II. *In* Epstein, M. (ed.): The Kidney in Liver Disease. New York, Elsevier-North Holland, 1978, p. 239.

85. Bichet, D. G., Szatalowicz, V., Chaimovitz, C., and Schrier, R. W. Role of vasopressin in abnormal water excretion in cirrhotic patients. Ann. Intern. Med. *96*:413, 1982.

86. Bichet, D. G., Van Putten, V. J., and Schrier, R. W. Potential role of increased sympathetic activity in impaired sodium and water excretion in cirrhosis. N. Engl. J. Med. *307*:1552, 1982.

87. Wong, P. Y., Carroll, R. E., Lipinski, T. L., and Capone, R. R. Studies on the renin-angiotensin-aldosterone system in patients with cirrhosis and ascites: Effect of saline and albumin infusion. Gastroenterology *77*:1171, 1979.

88. Vlahcevic, Z. R., Adham, N. F., Jick, H., Moore, E. W., and Chalmers, T. C. Renal effects of acute expansion of plasma volume in cirrhosis. N. Engl. J. Med. *272*:387, 1965.

89. Vlahcevic, Z. R., Adham, N. F., Chalmers, T. C., Clermont, J. R., Moore, E. W., Jick, H., Curtis, G. W., and Morrison, R. S. Intravenous therapy of massive ascites in patients with cirrhosis. I. Short-term comparison with diuretic treatment. Gastroenterology *53*:211, 1967.

90. Epstein, M., Levinson, R., Sancho, J., Haber, E., and Re, R. Characterization of the renin-aldosterone system in decompensated cirrhosis. Circ. Res. *41*:818, 1977.

91. Berkowitz, H. D., Mullen, J. L., Miller, L. D., and Rosato, E. F. Improved renal function and inhibition of renin and aldosterone secretion following peritoneovenous (LeVeen) shunt. Surgery *84*:120, 1978.

92. Blendis, L. M., Greig, P. C., Langer, B., Baigrie, R. S., Ruse, J., and Taylor, B. R. The renal and hemodynamic effects of the peritoneovenous shunt for intractable hepatic ascites. Gastroenterology *77*:250, 1979.

93. Greig, P. D., Blendis, L. M., Langer, B., Taylor, B. R., and Colapinto, R. F. Renal and hemodynamic effects of the peritoneovenous shunt. II. Long-term effects. Gastroenterology *80*:119, 1980.

94. Resnick, R. K., Langer, B., Taylor, B.R., Seif, S., and Blendis, L. M. Hyponatremia and arginine vasopressin secretion in patients with refractory ascites undergoing peritoneovenous shunting. Gastroenterology *84*:713, 1983.

95. Epstein, M. E.: Derangements of renal water handling in liver disease. Gastroenterology *89*:1415, 1985.

96. Epstein, M., Berk, D., Hollenberg, N., Adams, D., Chalmers, T., Abrams, H., and Merrill, J. Renal failure in the patient with cirrhosis: The role of active vasoconstriction. Am. J. Med. *49*:175, 1970.

97. Kew, M. C., Varma, R. R., Williams, H. S., Brunt, P. W., Hourigan, K. J., and Sherlock, S. Renal and intrarenal blood flow in cirrhosis of the liver. Lancet *2*:504, 1971.

98. Epstein, M., Schneider, N., and Befeler, B. Relationship of systemic and intrarenal hemodynamics in cirrhosis. J. Lab. Clin. Med. *89*:1175, 1977.

99. Wilkinson, S. P., Smith, I. K., Clarke, M., Arroyo, V., Richardson, J., Moodie, H., and Williams, R. Intrarenal distribution of plasma flow in cirrhosis as measured by transit renography: Relationship with plasma renin activity, and sodium and water excretion. Clin. Sci. Molec. Med. *52*:469, 1977.

100. Rosoff, L., Williams, J., Moult, P., Williams, H., and Sherlock, S. Renal hemodynamics and the renin-angiotensin system in cirrhosis: Relationship to sodium retention. Dig. Dis. Sci. *24*:25, 1979.

101. Stokes, J. B., III. Liver disease and the renal prostaglandin system. Gastroenterology *77*:391, 1979.

102. Dibona, G. F. Prostaglandins and nonsteroidal anti-inflammatory drugs. Effects on renal hemodynamics. Am. J. Med. *80*:12, 1986.

103. Raymond, K. H., and Lifschitz, M. D. Effect of prostaglandins on renal salt and water excretion. Am. J. Med. *80*:22. 1986.

104. Dunn, M. J. Role of eicosanoids in the control of renal function in severe hepatic disease. Gastroenterology *87*:1392, 1984.

105. Epstein, M. Renal prostaglandins and the control of renal function in liver disease. Am. J. Med. *80*:46, 1986.

106. Boyer, T. D., Zia, P., and Reynolds, T. B. Effect of indomethacin and prostaglandin A_1 on renal function and plasma

renin activity in alcoholic liver disease. Gastroenterology *77*:215, 1979.

107. Zipser, R. D., Hoefs, J. C., Speckart, P. F., Zia, P. K., and Horton, R. Prostaglandins: Modulators of renal function and pressor resistance in chronic liver disease. J. Clin. Endocrinol. Metab. *48*:895, 1979.

108. Walshe, J. J., and Venuto, R. C. Acute oliguric renal failure induced by indomethacin: Possible mechanism. Ann. Intern. Med. *91*:47, 1979.

109. Muther, R. S., Potter, D. M., and Bennett, W. M. Aspirin-induced depression of glomerular filtration rate in normal humans: Role of sodium balance. Ann. Intern. Med. *94*:317, 1981.

110. Planas, R., Arroyo, V., Rimola, A., Perez-Arzuro, R. M., and Rodes, J. Acetylsalicylic acid suppresses the renal hemodynamic effect and reduces the diuretic action of furosemide in cirrhosis with ascites. Gastroenterology *84*:247, 1983.

111. Mirouze, D., Zipser, R. D., and Reynolds, T. B. Effect of inhibitors of prostaglandin synthesis on induced diuresis in cirrhosis. Hepatology *3*:50, 1983.

112. Laffi, G., Daskalopoulos, G. D., Kronborg, I., Hsueh, W., Gentilini, P., and Zipser, R. D. Effects of sulindac and ibuprofen in patients with cirrhosis and ascites. An explanation for the renal-sparing effect of sulindac. Gastroenterology *90*:182, 1986.

113. Levy, M. Sodium retention and ascites formation in dogs with experimental cirrhosis. Am. J. Physiol. *233*:F572, 1977.

114. Levy, M., and Wexler, M. J. Renal sodium retention and ascites formation in dogs with experimental cirrhosis but without portal hypertension or increased splanchnic vascular capacity. J. Lab. Clin. Med. *91*:520, 1978.

115. Levy, M., Wexler, M. J., and McCaffrey, C. Sodium retention in dogs with experimental cirrhosis following removal of ascites by continuous peritoneovenous shunting. J. Lab. Clin. Med. *94*:933, 1979.

116. Denison, E. K., Lieberman, F. L., and Reynolds, T. B. 9-α-Fluorohydrocortisone induced ascites in alcoholic liver disease. Gastroenterology *61*:497, 1971.

117. Wilkinson, S. P., Moodie, H., Alam, A., and Williams, R. Renal retention of sodium in cirrhosis and fulminant hepatic failure. Postgrad. Med. J. *51*:527, 1975.

118. Lopez-Novoa, J. M., Rengel, M. A., and Hernando, L. Dynamics of ascites formation in rats with experimental cirrhosis. Am. J. Physiol. *238*:F353, 1980.

119. Unikowsky, B., Wexler, M. J., and Levy, M. Dogs with experimental cirrhosis of the liver but without intrahepatic hypertension do not retain sodium or form ascites. J. Clin. Invest. *72*:1594, 1983.

120. Epstein, F. H. Underfilling versus overflow in hepatic ascites. N. Engl. J. Med. *307*:1577, 1982.

121. Henriksen, J. H. The "overflow" theory of ascites formation: A fading concept? Scand. J. Gastroenterol. *18*:833, 1983.

122. Naccarato, R., Messa, P., D'Angelo, A., Fabris, A., Messa, M., Chiaramonte, M., Gregolin, L., and Zanon, G. Renal handling of sodium and water in early chronic liver disease. Evidence for a reduced natriuretic activity of the cirrhotic urinary extracts in rats. Gastroenterology *81*:205, 1981.

123. Epstein, M. Natriuretic hormone and the sodium retention of cirrhosis. Gastroenterology *81*:395, 1981.

124. Anderson, R. J., Cronin, R. E., McDonald, K. M., and Schreier, R. W. Mechanisms of portal hypertension-induced alterations in renal hemodynamics, renal water excretion and renin secretion. J. Clin. Invest. *58*:964, 1976.

125. Wong, P. Y., Talamo, R. C., and Williams, G. H. Kallikrein-kinin and renin-angiotensin systems in functional renal failure of cirrhosis of the liver. Gastroenterology *73*:1114, 1977.

126. de Bold, A. J. Atrial natriuretic factor: A hormone produced by the heart. Science *230*:767, 1985.

127. Muack, T., Atlas, S. A., Camargo, M. J. F., and Cogan, M. G. Renal hemodynamic and natriuretic effects of atrial natriuretic factor. Fed. Proc. *45*:2128, 1986.

128. Atlas, S. A., and Laragh, J. H.: Atrial natriuretic peptide: A new factor in hormonal control of blood pressure and electrolyte homeostasis. Ann. Rev. Med. *37*:397, 1986.

129. Anderson, J. V., Millar, N. D., O'Hare, J. P., MacKenzie, J.

C., Corrall, R. J. M., and Bloom, S. R. Atrial natriuretic peptide: Physiological release associated with natriuresis during water immersion in man. Clin. Sci. 71:319, 1986.

130. Jimenez, W., Martinez-Pardo, A., Arroyo, V., Gaya, J., Rivera, F., and Rodes, J. Atrial natriuretic factor: Reduced cardiac content in cirrhotic rats with ascites. Am. J. Physiol. 250:F749, 1986.

131. French, J. E., Florey, H. W., and Morris, B. The absorption of particles by the lymphatics of the diaphragm. Quart. J. Exp. Physiol. 45:88, 1960.

132. Tsilibary, E. C., and Wissig, S. L. Absorption from the peritoneal cavity: SEM study of the mesothelium covering the peritoneal surface of the muscular portion of the diaphragm. Am. J. Anat. 149:127, 1977.

133. Raybuck, H. E., Allen, L., and Harms, W. S. Absorption of serum from the peritoneal cavity. Am. J. Physiol. 199:1021, 1960.

134. Lill, S. R., Parsons, R. H., and Buhac, I. Permeability of the diaphragm and fluid resorption from the peritoneal cavity in the rat. Gastroenterology 76:997, 1979.

135. Zink, J., and Greenway, C. V. Intraperitoneal pressure in formation and reabsorption of ascites in cats. Am. J. Physiol. 233:H185, 1977.

136. Henriksen, J. H., Stage, J. G., Schlichting, P., and Winkler, K. Intraperitoneal pressure: Ascitic fluid and splanchnic vascular pressures, and their role in prevention and formation of ascites. Scand. J. Clin. Lab. Invest. 40:493, 1980.

137. Luttwak, E. M., Fabian, R. P., and Mordochovich, D. Role of peritoneal absorption in ascites. Surg. Gynecol. Obstet. 141:693, 1975.

138. Daugirdas, J. T., Ing, T. S., Gandhi, V. C., Hano, J. E., Chen, W.-T., and Yuan, L. Kinetics of peritoneal fluid reabsorption in patients with chronic renal failure. J. Lab. Clin. Med. 95:351, 1980.

139. Shear, L., Swartz, C., Shinaberger, J. H., and Barry, K. G. Kinetics of peritoneal fluid absorption in adult man. N. Engl. J. Med. 272:123, 1965.

140. Shear, L., Ching, S., and Gabuzda, G. J. Compartmentalization of ascites and edema in patients with hepatic cirrhosis. N. Engl. J. Med. 282:391, 1970.

141. Wilson, J. A. P., Seguitan, E. A., Cassidy, W. A., et al. Characteristics of ascitic fluid in the alcoholic cirrhotic. Dig. Dis. Sci. 24:645, 1979.

142. Jones, S. R. Absolute granulocyte count in ascites. West. J. Med. 126:344, 1977.

143. Hoefs, J. C. Increase in ascites white blood cell count and protein concentrations during diuresis in patients with chronic liver disease. Hepatology 1:249, 1981.

144. Fromkes, A. J., Thomas, F. B., Mekhjian, H. S., et al. Antimicrobial activity of human ascitic fluid. Gastroenterology 73:668, 1977.

145. Simberkoff, M. S., Molover, N. H., and Weiss, G. Bacteriocidal and opsonic activity of cirrhotic ascites and nonascitic peritoneal fluid. J. Lab. Clin. Med. 91:831, 1978.

146. Runyon, B. A., Morrissey, R. L., Hoefs, J. C., et al. Opsonic activity of human ascitic fluid; a potentially important protective mechanism against spontaneous bacterial peritonitis. Hepatology 4:634, 1984.

147. Akalin, H. E., Laleli, Y., and Telatar, H. Bacteriocidal and opsonic activity of ascitic fluid from cirrhotic and noncirrhotic patients. J. Infect. Dis. 147:1011, 1983.

148. Quismorio, F. P., Kaufman, R. L., Halle, P., et al. Immune complexes and cryoproteins in ascitic fluid of patients with alcoholic liver disease. Int. Arch. Allergy Appl. Immunol. 64:190, 1981.

149. Michel, J., Bercovici, B., and Sacks, T. Comparative studies on the antimicrobial activity of peritoneal and ascitic fluid in human beings. Surg. Gynecol. Obstet. 151:55, 1980.

150. Henderson, J. M., Stein, S. F., Kutner, M., et al. Analysis of 23 plasma proteins in ascites. Ann. Surg. 192:738, 1980.

151. Hoefs, J., Barnes, T., and Halle, P. Intraperitoneal coagulation in chronic liver disease ascites. Dig. Dis. Sci. 26:518, 1981.

152. Johnson, C. A., Sobrinko, T. C., Aziz, E. M., et al. Refractory coagulopathy in an infant with loss of clotting proteins into ascitic fluid. Acta Pediatr. Scand. 65:773, 1976.

153. Ouwendijk, R. J., Zijlstra, F. J., Wilson, J. H. P., et al. Production of leukotrienes and prostaglandins by human ascites cells. Eur. J. Clin. Invest. 15:327, 1985.

154. Lo Iudice, T., Mishkin, F. R., Piziak, V., et al. Cholesterol ascites in alcoholic cirrhosis. Am. J. Gastroenterol. 72:428, 1979.

155. Eckhauser, F. E., Strodel, W. E., Girardy, J. W., et al. Bizarre complications of peritoneovenous shunts. Ann. Surg. 193:180, 1981.

156. Conn, H., and Fessel, M. Spontaneous bacterial peritonitis in cirrhosis: Variations on a theme. Medicine 50:161, 1971.

157. Stassen, W. N., and McCullough, A. J. Management of ascites. Semin. Liver Dis. 5:291, 1985.

158. Hoefs, J. C., and Runyon, B. A. Spontaneous bacterial peritonitis. Disease-A-Month 31:1, 1985.

159. Crossley, I. R., and Williams, R. Spontaneous bacterial peritonitis. Gut 262:325, 1985.

159a. Wilcox, C. M., and Dismukes, W. E. Spontaneous bacterial peritonitis. A review of pathogenesis, diagnosis and treatment. Medicine 66:447, 1987.

160. Thomas, F. B., and Fromkes, J. J. Spontaneous bacterial peritonitis associated with acute viral hepatitis. J. Clin. Gastroenterol. 4:259, 1982.

161. Curry, N., McCallum, R. W., and Garth, P. H. Spontaneous peritonitis in cirrhotic ascites. Am. J. Dig. Dis. 19:685, 1974.

162. Kline, M. M., McCallum, R. W., and Guth, P. H. The clinical value of ascitic fluid culture and leukocyte count in studies of alcoholic cirrhosis. Gastroenterology 70:408, 1976.

163. Rheingold, O. J., Chiprut, R. O., Dickinson, G. M., and Schiff, E. R. Spontaneous peritonitis of cirrhosis due to Listeria monocytogenes. Ann. Intern. Med. 87:455, 1977.

164. Bar-Meir, S., Chojkier, M., Groszman, R. J., Atterbury, C. E., and Conn, H. O. Spontaneous meningococcal peritonitis. A report of two cases. Am. J. Dig. Dis. 23:119, 1978.

165. Jacobson, J. A., Miner, P., and Duffy, O. Pasteurella multocida bacteremia associated with peritonitis and cirrhosis. Am. J. Gastroenterol. 68:489, 1977.

166. Stephens, C. G., Meadows, J. G., Kerkering, T. M., Markowitz, S. W., and Wisman, R. M. Spontaneous peritonitis due to Hemophilus influenzae in an adult. Gastroenterology 77:1088, 1979.

167. Targan, S. R., Chow, A. W., and Guze, L. B. Role of anaerobic bacteria in spontaneous peritonitis of cirrhosis. Am. J. Med. 62:397, 1977.

168. Stassen, W. N., McCullough, A. J., and Hilton, P. Spontaneous bacterial peritonitis caused by Neisseria gonorrhoeae. Evidence for a transfallopian route of infection? Gastroenterology 88:804, 1985.

169. Conn, H. Bacterial peritonitis: Spontaneous or paracentetic. Gastroenterology 77:1145, 1979.

170. Fierer, J., and Finley, F. Deficient serum bactericidal activity against Escherichia coli in patients with cirrhosis of the liver. J. Clin. Invest. 63:912, 1979.

171. Runyon, B. Low protein concentration ascitic fluid is predisposed to spontaneous bacterial peritonitis. Gastroenterology 91:1343, 1986.

172. Runyon, B. A., and Van Epps, D. E. Diuresis of cirrhotic ascites increases its opsonic activity and may help prevent spontaneous bacterial peritonitis. Hepatology 6:396, 1986.

173. Bar-Meir, S., and Conn, H. O. Spontaneous bacterial peritonitis induced by intra-arterial vasopressin therapy. Gastroenterology 70:418, 1976.

174. Falum, M. A. Spontaneous bacterial empyema in cirrhosis. Gastroenterology 70:416, 1976.

175. Conn, H. O. Spontaneous bacterial peritonitis. Multiple revisitations. Gastroenterology 70:455, 1976.

176. Gitlin, N., Stauffer, J. L., and Silvestri, R. C. The pH of ascitic fluid in the diagnosis of spontaneous bacterial peritonitis in alcoholic cirrhosis. Hepatology 2:408, 1982.

177. Scemma-Clergue, J., Doutrellot-Phillipon, C., Metreau, J.-M., Teisseire, B., Capron, D., and Dhumeaux, D. Ascitic fluid pH in alcoholic cirrhosis: A reevaluation of its use in the diagnosis of spontaneous bacterial peritonitis. Gut 26:332, 1985.

178. Pinzello, G., Virdone, R., Lojacono, F., et al.: Is the acidity of ascitic fluid a reliable index in making the presumptive

diagnosis of spontaneous bacterial peritonitis? Hepatology 6:244, 1986.

179. Stassen, W. N., McCullough, A. J., Bacon, B. R., et al. Immediate diagnostic criteria for bacterial infection of ascitic fluid. Evaluation of ascitic fluid polymorphonuclear leukocyte count, pH and lactate concentration, alone and in combination. Gastroenterology 90:1247, 1986.

180. Attali, P., Turner, K., Pelletier, G., Ink, O., and Etienne, J. P. pH of ascitic fluid: Diagnostic and prognostic value in cirrhotic and noncirrhotic patients. Gastroenterology 90:1255, 1986.

181. Reynolds, T. B. Rapid presumptive diagnosis of spontaneous bacterial peritonitis. Gastroenterology 90:1294, 1986.

182. Runyon, B. A., and Hoefs, J. C. Ascitic fluid analysis in the differentiation of spontaneous bacterial peritonitis from gastrointestinal tract perforation into ascitic fluid. Hepatology 5:463, 1985.

183. Caralis, P. V., Sprung, C. L., and Schiff, E. R. Secondary bacterial peritonitis in cirrhotic patients with ascites. South. Med. J. 77:579, 1984.

184. Runyon, B. A., and Hoefs, J. C. Culture negative neutrocytic ascites: A variant of spontaneous bacterial peritonitis. Hepatology 4:1209, 1984.

185. Gerding, D. N., Kromhout, J. P., Sullivan, J. J., and Hall, W. H. Antibiotic penetrance of ascitic fluid in dogs. Antimicrobial agents and chemotherapy. 10:850, 1976.

186. Rimola, A., Bory, F., Teres, J., Perez-Arzuso, R. M., Arroyo, V., and Rodes, J. Oral, nonabsorbable antibiotics prevent infection in cirrhotics with gastrointestinal hemorrhage. Hepatology 5:463, 1985.

187. Liberman, F. L., Hidemura, R., Peters, R. L., et al. Pathogenesis and treatment of hydrothorax complicating cirrhosis with ascites. Ann. Intern. Med. 64:341, 1966.

188. Benz, R. L., and Schleifer, C. R. Hydrothorax in continuous ambulatory peritoneal dialysis: Successful treatment with intrapleural tetracycline and a review of the literature. Am. J. Kidney Dis. 5:136, 1985.

189. Rubinstein, D., McInnes, I. E., and Dudley, F. J. Hepatic hydrothorax in the absence of clinical ascites: Diagnosis and management. Gastroenterology 88:188, 1985.

190. Crawford, K. L., and McDougall, I. R. Prediction of satisfactory response to pleural sclerosis using radiopharmaceuticals. Arch. Intern. Med. 142:194, 1982.

191. Vargas-Tank, L., Escobar, C., Fernandez, G., et al. Massive pleural effusions in cirrhotic patients with ascites. Scand. J. Gastroenterol. 19:294, 1984.

192. Falchuk, K. R., Jacoby, I., Colucci, W. S., et al. Tetracycline-induced pleural synthesis for recurrent hydrothorax complicating cirrhosis. Gastroenterology 72:319, 1977.

193. Runyon, B. A., Greenblatt, M., and Ming, R. H. C. Hepatic hydrothorax is a relative contraindication to chest tube insertion. Am. J. Gastroenterol. 81:566, 1986.

194. Ikard, R. W., and Sawyers, J. L. Persistent hepatic hydrothorax after peritoneojugular shunt. Arch. Surg. 115:1125, 1980.

195. LeVeen, H. H., Piccone, V. A., and Hutto, R. B. Management of ascites with hydrothorax. Am. J. Surg. 148:210, 1984.

196. Hartz, R. S., Bomalaski, J., LoCicero, J., et al. Pleural ascites without abdominal fluid: Surgical considerations. J. Thor. Cardiovasc. Surg. 87:141, 1984.

197. O'Hara, E. T., Oliai, A., Patek, A. J., Jr., et al. Management of umbilical hernias associated with hepatic cirrhosis and ascites. Ann. Surg. 181:85, 1975.

198. Runyon, B. A., and Juler, G. L. Natural history of repaired umbilical hernias in patients with and without ascites. Am. J. Gastroenterol. 80:38, 1985.

199. Lemmer, J. H., Strodel, W. E., Knol, J. A., et al. Management of spontaneous umbilical hernia disruption in the cirrhotic patient. Ann. Surg. 198:30, 1983.

200. Leonetti, J. P., Aranha, G. V., Wilkinson, W. A., et al. Umbilical herniorrhaphy in cirrhotic patients. Arch. Surg. 119:442, 1984.

201. O'Conner, M., Allen, J. I., and Schwartz, M. L. Peritoneovenous shunt for leaking ascites in the cirrhotic patient. Ann. Surg. 200:66, 1984.

202. Quintero, E., Arroyo, V., Bory, F., et al. Paracentesis versus diuretics in the treatment of cirrhotics with tense ascites. Lancet 1:611, 1985.

203. Descos, L., Gauthier, A., Levy, V. G., et al. Comparison of 6 treatments of ascites in patients with liver cirrhosis; a clinical trial. Hepato-gastroenterology 30:15, 1983.

203a. Gines, P., Arroyo, V., Quintero, E., et al. Comparison of paracentesis and diuretics in the treatment of cirrhotics with tense ascites. Results of a randomized study. Gastroenterology 93:234, 1987.

203b. Simon, D. M., McCain, J. R., Bonkovsky, H. L., et al. Effects of therapeutic paracentesis on systemic and hepatic hemodynamics and on renal and hormonal function. Hepatology 7:423, 1987.

204. Boyer, T. D., and Goldman, I. R. Treatment of cirrhotic ascites. Adv. Int. Med. 31:359, 1986.

205. Arroyo, V., Gines, P., Planas, R., et al. Management of patients with cirrhosis and ascites. Semin. Liver Dis. 6:353, 1986.

206. Bernardi, M. Renal function impairment induced by change in posture in patients with cirrhosis and ascites. Gut 26:629, 1985.

207. Linas, S. L., Anderson, R. J., Miller, P. D., et al. Rational use of diuretics in cirrhosis. In Epstein, M. (ed.): The Kidney in Liver Disease. New York, Elsevier-North Holland, 1978, p. 313.

208. Fuller, R. K., Khambatta, P. B., and Gobezie, G. C. An optimal diuretic regimen for cirrhotic ascites. JAMA 237:972, 1977.

209. Gregory, P. B., Broekelschen, P. H., Hill, M. D., et al. Complications of diuresis in the alcoholic patient with ascites: A controlled trial. Gastroenterology 73:534, 1977.

210. Gauthier, A., Levy, V. G., Quintan, A., et al. Salt or no salt in the treatment of cirrhotic ascites: A randomized study. Gut 27:705, 1986.

211. Reynolds, T. B., Lieberman, F. L., and Goodman, A. R. Advantages of treatment of ascites without sodium restriction and without complete removal of excess fluid. Gut 19:549, 1978.

212. Kandel, G., and Diamant, N. E. Clinical view of recent advances in ascites. J. Clin. Gastroenterol. 8:85, 1986.

213. Epstein, M. Derangements of renal water handling in liver disease. Gastroenterology 89:1415, 1985.

214. Frakes, J. T. Physiological considerations in the medical management of ascites. Arch. Intern. Med. 140:620, 1980.

215. Campra, J. L., and Reynolds, T. B. Effectiveness of high dose spironolactone treatment in patients with chronic liver disease and relatively refractory ascites. Am. J. Dig. Dis. 23:1025, 1978.

216. Perez-Ayuso, R. M., Arroyo, V., Planas, R., et al. Randomized comparative study of the efficacy of furosemide versus spironolactone in nonazotemic cirrhosis with ascites. Gastroenterology 84:961, 1983.

217. Fogel, M. R., Sawhney, V. K., Neal, E. A., et al. Diruesis in the ascitic patient: Randomized control trial of three regimens. J. Clin. Gastroenterol. 3(suppl. 1):73, 1981.

218. Eggert, R. Spironolactone diuresis in patients with cirrhosis and ascites. Br. Med. J. 2:401, 1970.

219. Gabow, P. A., Moore, S., and Schrier, R. W. Spironolactone induced hyperchloremic acidosis in cirrhosis. Ann. Intern. Med. 90:338, 1979.

220. Boyer, T. D., and Warnock, D. G. Use of diuretics in the treatment of cirrhotic ascites. Gastroenterology 84:1051, 1983.

220a. Pinzani, M., Daskapoulos, G., Laffi, G., et al. Altered furosemide pharmacokinetics in chronic alcoholic liver disease with ascites contributes to diuretic resistance. Gastroenterology 92:294, 1987.

220b. Daskapoulos, G., Laffi, G., Morgan, T., et al. Immediate effects of furosemide on renal hemodynamics in chronic liver disease with ascites. Gastroenterology 92:1859, 1987.

221. Oster, J. R., Epstein, M., and Smoller, S. Combined therapy with thiazide type and loop diuretic agents for resistant sodium retention. Ann. Intern. Med. 99:405, 1983.

222. Naranjo, C. A., Pontigo, E., Valdenegro, C., et al. Furosemide-induced adverse reactions in cirrhosis of the liver. Clin. Pharmacol. Ther. 25:154, 1979.

223. Pockros, P. J., and Reynolds, T. B. Rapid diuresis in patients

with ascites from chronic liver disease: Importance of peripheral edema. Gastroenterology 90:1827, 1986.

224. Zipser, R. D. Role of renal prostaglandins and the effects of nonsteroidal antiinflammatory drugs in patients with liver disease. Am. J. Med. 81(suppl. 2b):95, 1986.

225. Richter, W. G., Jr., and Reynolds, T. B. Propranolol in the treatment of cirrhotic ascites. Arch. Intern. Med. 144:1761, 1984.

225a. D'Arienzo, A., Ambrogio, G., Di Siervi, P., et al. A randomized comparison of metoclopramide and domperidone on plasma aldosterone concentration and on spironolactone-induced diuresis in ascitic cirrhotic patients. Hepatology 5:854, 1985.

226. Pariente, E. A., Bataille, E. C., Bercoff, E., et al. Acute effects of captopril on systemic and renal hemodynamics and on renal function in cirrhotic patients with ascites. Gastroenterology 88:1255, 1985.

227. Capone, R. R., Buhac, I., Kohlberger, R., et al. Resistant ascites in alcoholic liver cirrhosis: Course and prognosis. Am. J. Dig. Dis. 23:867, 1978.

228. Levy, V. G., Pauleauo, N., Opolon, P., et al. Treatment of ascites by reinfusion of concentrated peritoneal fluid—a review of 318 procedures in 210 patients. Postgrad. Med. J. 51:564, 1975.

229. Raju, S. F., and Achord, J. L. The effects of dialytic ultrafiltration and peritoneal reinfusion in the management of diuretic-resistant ascites. Am. J. Gastroenterol. 79:308, 1984.

230. Stanley, M. M. Treatment of intractable ascites in patients with alcoholic cirrhosis by peritoneovenous shunting. Med. Clin. North Am. 63:523, 1979.

231. Lebrec, D., Kotelanski, B., and Cohn, J. N. Splanchnic hemodynamic factors in cirrhosis with refractory ascites. J. Lab. Clin. Med. 93:301, 1979.

232. Rector, W. G., Jr. "Diuretic-resistatnt" ascites: Observations on pathogenesis. Arch. Intern. Med. 146:1597, 1986.

233. Wood, L. J., Willett, I. R., and Dudley, F. J. Treatment of refractory ascites in patients with liver disease. Aust. N. Z. J. Med. 15:469, 1985.

234. Burchell, A. R., Rousselot, L. M., and Panke, W. F. A seven year experience with side-to-side portacaval shunt for cirrhotic ascites. Ann. Surg. 168:655, 1968.

235. LeVeen, H. H., Wapnick, S., Diaz, S., et al. Ascites, its correction by peritoneovenous shunting. Curr. Probl. Surg. 16:1, 1979.

236. Fulenwider, J. T., Galambos, J. D., Smith, R. B., et al. LeVeen versus Denver peritoneovenous shunt for intractable ascites of cirrhosis: A randomized prospective trial. Arch. Surg. 121:351, 1986.

237. Fulenwider, J. T., Smith, R. B., Redd, S. C., et al. Peritoneovenous shunts; lessons learned from an eight year experience with 70 patients. Arch. Surg. 119:1133, 1984.

238. Turner, W. W., and Pate, R. M. The Denver peritoneovenous shunt: Relationship between hepatic reserve and successful treatment of ascites. Am. J. Surg. 144:619, 1982.

239. Gleysteen, J. J., and Klamer, T. W. Peritoneovenous shunts: Predictive factors of early treatment failure. Am. J. Gastroenterol. 79:654, 1984.

240. Ansley, J. D., Bethel, R. A., Bowen, T. A., et al. Effect of peritoneovenous shunting with the LeVeen valve on ascites, renal function, and coagulation in 6 patients with intractable ascites. Surgery 83:181, 1978.

241. Wapnick, S., Grosberg, S. J., and Evans, M. I. Randomized prospective matched pair study comparing peritoneovenous shunt and conventional therapy in massive ascites. Br. J. Surg. 66:667, 1979.

242. Blendis, L. M., Harrison, J. E., Russell, D. N., et al. Effects of peritoneovenous shunting on body composition. Gastroenterology 90:127, 1986.

243. Franco, D., Charra, M., Jeambrun, P., et al. Nutrition and immunity after peritoneovenous drainage of intractable ascites in cirrhotic patients. Am. J. Surg. 146:652, 1983.

244. Greig, P. D., Langer, B., Blendis, L. M., et al. Complications after peritoneovenous shunting for ascites. Am. J. Surg. 139:125, 1980.

245. Fry, P. D., Hallgren, R., and Robertson, M. E. Current status

of the peritoneovenous shunt for the management of intractable ascites. Can. J. Surg. 22:557, 1979.

246. Tawes, R. L., Sydorak, S. R., Kennedy, P. A., et al. Coagulopathy associated with peritoneovenous shunting. Am. J. Surg. 142:51, 1981.

247. Harmon, D. C., Demirgian, Z., Ellman, L., et al. Disseminated intravascular coagulation with the peritoneovenous shunt. Ann. Intern. Med. 90:774, 1979.

248. Stein, S. F., Fulenwider, J. T., Ansley, J. D., et al. Accelerated fibrinogen and platelet destruction after peritoneovenous shunting. Arch. Intern. Med. 141:1149, 1981.

249. Ragni, M. V., Lewis, J. H., and Spero, J. A. Ascites induced LeVeen shunt coagulopathy. Ann. Surg. 198:91, 1983.

250. Salem, H. H., Dudley, F. J., Merrett, A., et al. Coagulopathy of peritoneovenous shunts: Studies on the pathogenic role of ascitic fluid collagen and value of antiplatelet therapy. Gut 24:412, 1983.

251. Smadja, C., and Franco, D. The LeVeen shunt in the elective treatment of intractable ascites in cirrhosis: A prospective study of 140 patients. Ann. Surg. 201:488, 1985.

252. Biagini, J. R., Belghiti, J., and Fekete, F. Prevention of coagulopathy after placement of peritoneovenous shunt with replacement of ascitic fluid by normal saline solution. Surgery 163:315, 1986.

253. LeVeen, H. H. The LeVeen shunt. Ann. Rev. Med. 36:453, 1985.

254. Prokesch, R. C., and Rimland, D. Infectious complications of the peritoneovenous shunt. Am. J. Gastroenterol. 78:235, 1983.

255. Wormser, G. P., and Hubbard, R. C. Peritonitis in cirrhotic patients with LeVeen shunts. Am. J. Surg. 71:358, 1981.

256. LeVeen, H. H., Vujic, I., D'Ovidio, N. G., et al. Peritoneovenous shunt occlusion: Etiology, diagnosis, therapy. Ann. Surg. 200:212, 1984.

257. Rosenthall, L., Arzoumanian, A., Hampson, L. G., et al. Observations on the radionuclide assessment of peritoneovenous shunt patency. Clin. Nucl. Med. 9:227, 1984.

258. Steward, C. A., Sakimura, I. T., Applebaum, D. M., et al. Evaluation of peritoneovenous shunt patency by intraperitoneal Tc-99m macroaggregated albumin: Clinical experience. Am. J. Roentgenol. 147:177, 1986.

259. Foley, W. J., Elliot, J. P., Jr., Smith, R. F., et al. Central venous thrombosis and embolism associated with peritoneovenous shunts. Arch. Surg. 119:713, 1984.

260. Smadja, C., Tridard, D., and Franco, D. Recurrent ascites due to central venous thrombosis after peritoneojugular shunt. Surgery 100:535, 1986.

261. Bernhoft, R. A., Pellegrini, C. A., and Way, L. W. Peritoneovenous shunt for refractory ascites: Operative complications and long term results. Arch. Surg. 117:631, 1982.

262. Grischkan, D. M., Cooperman, A. V., Hermann, R. E., et al. Failure of LeVeen shunting in refractory ascites—a view from the other side. Surgery 89:3, 1981.

263. Greenlee, H. B, Stanley, M. M., and Reinhardt, G. F. Intractable ascites treated with peritoneovenous shunts. Arch. Surg. 116:518, 1981.

264. Epstein, M. Peritoneovenous shunt in the management of ascites and the hepatorenal syndrome. Gastroenterology 82:790, 1982.

265. Smith, R. E., Nostrant, T. T., Eckhauser, F. E., et al. Patient selection and survival after peritoneovenous shunting for nonmalignant ascites. Am. J. Gastroenterol. 79:659, 1984.

265a. Bories, P., Compean, D. G., Machel, H., et al. The treatment of refractory ascites by the LeVeen shunt: a multi-centre controlled trial. J. Hepatol. 3:212, 1986.

265b. Kinas, S. L., Schaefer, J. W., Moore, E. E., et al. Peritoneovenous shunt in the management of the hepatorenal syndrome. Kidney Int. 30:736, 1986.

266. Nishimura, R. A., Connelly, D. C., Parkin, T. W., et al. Constrictive pericarditis: Assessment of current diagnostic procedures. Mayo Clinic Proc. 60:397, 1985.

267. Mitchell, M. C., Boitnott, J. K., Kaufman, S., et al. Budd-Chiari syndrome: Etiology, diagnosis, management. Medicine 61:199, 1982.

268. Rector, W. G., Jr., Xu, Y., Goldstein, L., et al. Membranous

obstruction of the inferior vena cava in the United States. Medicine 64:134, 1985.

269. Baert, A. L., Fevery, I. J., Marchal, G., et al. Early diagnosis of Budd-Chiari syndrome by computed tomography and ultrasonography: Report of 5 cases. Gastroenterology 84:587,1983.

270. Friedman, A. C., Ramchandani, P., Black, M., et al. Magnetic resonance imaging diagnosis of Budd-Chiari syndrome. Gastroenterology 91:1289, 1986.

271. McCarthy, P. M., Van Heerden, J. A., Adson, M. A., et al. Budd-Chiari syndrome: Medical and surgical management of 30 patients. Arch. Surg. 120:657, 1985.

272. Danilewitz, M., Barbezat, G. O., and Helman, C. A. Myxedema presenting with ascites. S. Afr. Med. J. 52:895, 1977.

273. Clancy, R., and MacKay, I. Myxedematous ascites. Med. J. Aust. 2:415, 1970.

274. Morell, M. D., Frost, D., and Ziel, H.K. Pseudo Meigs' syndrome. J. Reproduc. Med. 25:88, 1980.

275. Fukuda, O., Munemura, M., Tohya, T., et al. Massive edema of the ovary associated with hydrothorax and ascites. Gynecol. Oncol. 17:231, 1984.

276. Gal, D., Buchsbaum, H. J., Voet, R., et al. Massive ascites with uterine leiomyomas and ovarian vein thrombosis. Am. J. Obstet. Gynecol. 144:729, 1982.

277. Kempers, R., Dockerty, M., Hoffman, D., et al. Struma ovarii—ascitic, hyperthyroid, and asymptomatic syndromes. Ann. Intern. Med. 72:883, 1970.

278. Lenehan, P. M., Colgan, T., and Vernon, C. P. Struma ovarii presenting with ascites: A difficult diagnostic problem. Eur. J. Gynecol. 6:89, 1985.

279. Schenker, G. J., and Weinstein, D. Ovarian hyperstimulation syndrome: A current survey. Fertil. Steril. 30:255, 1978.

280. Donowitz, M., Kerstein, M. D., and Spiro, H. Pancreatic ascites. Medicine 53:183, 1974.

281. Cameron, J. L. Chronic pancreatic ascites and pancreatic pleural effusions. Gastroenterology 74:134, 1978.

282. Mann, S. K., and Mann, N. S. Pancreatic ascites. Am. J. Gastroenterol. 71:186, 1979.

282a. Runyon, B. A. Amylase levels in ascitic fluid. J. Clin. Gastroenterol. 9:172, 1987.

283. Sileo, A. F., Chawla, S. K., and LoPresti, P. A. Pancreatic ascites: Diagnostic importance of ascitic lipase. Am. J. Dig. Dis. 20:1110, 1975.

284. Satz, N., Uhlschmid, G., Pei, T., et al. On the pathogenesis of pancreatic ascites. Eur. J. Surg. Res. 16:170, 1984.

285. Sankaran, S., Sugawa, C., and Walt, A. J. Value of endoscopic retrograde pancreatography in pancreatic ascites. Surg. Gynecol. Obstet. 148:185, 1979.

286. Weaver, D. W., Walt, A. J., Sugawa, C., et al. A continuing appraisal of pancreatic ascites. Surg. Gynecol. Obstet. 154:845, 1982.

287. Cameron, J. L., Kieffer, R. S., Anderson, W. J., et al. Internal pancreatic fistulas: Pancreatic ascites and pleural effusions. Ann. Surg. 184:587, 1976.

288. Morton, R. E., Deluca, R., Reisman, T. N., et al. Pancreatic ascites: Successful treatment with pancreatic radiation. Am. J. Dig. Dis. 21:333, 1976.

289. Jones, A. M., Jacobs, L. A., Bouwman, D. L., et al. Outcome after peritoneojugular shunting of pancreatic ascites. Am. Surg. 50:386, 1984.

290. Rosato, E., Berkowitz, H., and Roberts, B. Bile ascites. Surg. Gynecol. Obstet. 130:494, 1970.

291. Ackerman, N. B., Sillin, L. F., and Suresh, K. Consequences of intraperitoneal bile: Bile ascites versus bile peritonitis. Am. J. Surg. 149:244, 1985.

292. Frank, D. J., Pereires, R., Souza-Lima, M. S., et al. Traumatic rupture of the gallbladder with massive biliary ascites. JAMA 240:252, 1978.

293. Stein, J. A., and Price, J. B. Asymptomatic biliary ascites after percutaneous transhepatic cholangiogram. Gastroenterology 64:1013, 1973.

294. Avner, D. L., and Berinson, M. M. Asymptomatic bilious ascites following percutaneous liver biopsy. Arch. Intern. Med. 139:245, 1979.

295. Avner, D. L., West, H. C., and Rikkers, L. F. Bilious ascites simulating tuberculous peritonitis. West. J. Med. 137:241, 1982.

295a. Runyon, B. A. Ascitic fluid bilirubin concentration as a key to choleperitoneum. J. Clin. Gastroenterol. 9:543, 1987.

296. Cain, J., Labat, J., and Cohn, I. Bile peritonitis in germ free dogs. Gastroenterology 53:600, 1967.

297. Vasko, J. S., and Tapper, R. I. Surgical significance of chylous ascites. Arch. Surg. 95:355, 1967.

298. Kelley, M. L., Jr., and Butt, H. R. Chylous ascites: An analysis of its etiology. Gastroenterology 30:161, 1960.

299. Press, O. W., Press, N. O., and Kaufmann, S. D. Evaluation and management of chylous ascites. Ann. Intern. Med. 96:358, 1982.

300. Goldfarb, J. P. Chylous effusion secondary to pancreatitis: Case report and review of the literature. Am. J. Gastroenterol. 79:133, 1984.

301. Sipes, S. L., Newton, M., and Lurain, J. R. Chylous ascites: A sequel of pelvic radiation therapy. Obstet. Gynecol. 66:832, 1985.

302. Rector, W. G., Jr. Spontaneous chylous peritonitis of cirrhosis. J. Clin. Gastroenterol. 6:369, 1984.

303. Malagelada, J., Iber, F., and Linscheer, W. Origin of fat in chylous ascites in patients with liver cirrhosis. Gastroenterology 67:878, 1974.

304. Lindenbaum, J., and Scheidt, S. Chylous ascites in the nephrotic syndrome. Am. J. Med. 44:830, 1968.

305. Sarazin, W. G., and Sauter, K. E. Chylous ascites following resection of a ruptured abdominal aneurysm. Arch. Surg. 121:246, 1986.

306. Calabrese, P. R., Frank, H. D., and Tarber, H. L. Lymphangiomyomatosis with chylous ascites. Cancer 40:895, 1977.

307. Duhra, P. M., Quigleye, M. M., and Marsh, M. N. Chylous ascites, intestinal lymphangiectasia and the "yellow nail syndrome." Gut 26:1266, 1985.

308. Carini, L., Meregaglia, L. D., Galli, C., et al. Retroperitoneal nodal aplasia, asplenia, chylous effusion and lymphatic dysplasia: An acquired immunodeficiency syndrome? Lymphology 18:31, 1985.

309. Unger, S. W., and Chandler, A. G. Chylous ascites in infants and children. Surgery 93:455, 1983.

310. Cochran, W. J., Klish, W. J., Brown, M. R., et al. Chylous ascites in infants and children: A case report and literature review. J. Pediatr. Gastroenterol. Nutr. 4:668, 1985.

311. Thompson, P. A., Halpern, N. B., and Aldrete, J. S. Acute chylous peritonitis. J. Clin. Gastroenterol. 3(suppl. 1):51, 1981.

312. Krizek, T., and Davis, J. Acute chylous peritonitis. Arch. Surg. 91:253, 1965.

313. Kroczek, R. A. Congenital chyloperitoneum: Direct comparison of medium chain triglyceride treatment with total parenteral nutrition. Eur. J. Pediatr. 144:77, 1985.

314. Kerr, S. C., Powis, S. J. A., Ross, J. R., et al. Peritoneovenous shunt in the management of pediatric chylous ascites. Br. J. Surg. 72:443, 1985.

315. Bordeau, G., Indal, S., Gillies, R., et al. Urinary ascites secondary to ureteroperitoneal fistula. Urology 4:209, 1974.

316. Carswell, J. Intraperitoneal rupture of the bladder. Br. J. Urol. 46:425, 1974.

317. Redman, J. F., Seibert, J. J., and Watson, A. Urinary ascites in children owing to extravasation of urine from the bladder. J. Urol. 122:409, 1979.

318. Clark, W., Sullivan, S. N., Lindsay, R., et al. Ascites secondary to transudation from a renal cadaveric transplant. JAMA 235:635, 1976.

319. Singh, S., Aoaki, S., Mitra, S., et al. Ascites: An unusual manifestation of urinary leak in a renal allograft recipient. JAMA 226:777, 1973.

320. Marcel, B. R., Koff, R. S., and Chou, S. I. Ascites following renal transplantation. Am. J. Dig. Dis. 22:137, 1977.

321. Arnold, W. C., Redman, J. F., and Seibert, J. J. Analysis of peritoneal fluid in urinary ascites. South. Med. J. 79:591, 1986.

322. Mann, C., Leape, L., and Holder, T. Neonatal urinary ascites. J. Urol. 111:124, 1974.

323. Greenfield, S. P., Hensle, T. W., Burdon, W. E., et al. Urinary extravasation in the new born male with posterior urethral valves. J. Pediatr. Surg. 17:751, 1982.

324. Criscomb, N. T., Colodney, A. M., Rosenberg, H. K., et al.

Diagnostic aspects of neonatal ascites: Report of 27 cases. Am. J. Roentgenol. *128*:961, 1977.

325. Hadlock, F. P., Deter, R. L., Garcia-Pratt, J., et al. Fetal ascites not associated with RH incompatibility: Recognition and management with sonography. Am. J. Roentgenol. *134*:1225, 1980.

326. Arismendi, G., Izard, M., Hampton, W. R., et al. The clinical spectrum of ascites associated with maintenance dialysis. Am. J. Med. *60*:46, 1976.

327. Singh, S., Mitra, S., and Berman, L. Ascites in patients with maintenance hemodialysis. Nephron *12*:114, 1974.

328. Craig, R., Sparberg, M., and Avanovich, P. Nephrogenic ascites. Arch. Intern. Med. *134*:276, 1974.

329. Popli, S., Daugardis, J. T., and Ing, T. S. Dialysis ascites. Int. J. Artif. Organs *3*:257, 1980.

330. Morgan, A. G., and Terri, S. I. Impaired peritoneal fluid drainage in nephrogenic ascites. Clin. Nephrol. *15*:61, 1981.

331. Shin, K. D., Ing, T. S., Popli, S., et al. Isolated ultrafiltration in the treatment of dialysis ascites. Int. J. Artif. Organs *2*:120, 1979.

332. Rubin, J., Kiley, J., Wray, R., et al. Continuous ambulatory peritoneal dialysis: Treatment of dialysis related ascites. Arch. Intern. Med. *141*:1093, 1981.

333. Giannone, G., Glabman, N. S., Burroughs, L. et al. Treatment of refractory ascites in hemodialysis patients with peritoneovenous shunt. Mt. Sinai J. Med. *50*:256, 1983.

334. Morgan, A. G., Sivapragasam, S., and Fletcher, P. Hemodynamic improvement after peritoneovenous shunting in nephrogenic ascites. South. Med. J. *75*:373, 1982.

335. Hobar, P. C., Turner, W. W., and Valentine, R. J. Successful use of the Denver peritoneovenous shunt in patients with nephrogenic ascites. Surgery *101*:161, 1987.

27

Jaundice
BRUCE F. SCHARSCHMIDT

Jaundice is a condition in which the scleras, mucous membranes, and skin become abnormally yellow as a result of an increased concentration of bilirubin in the blood, usually greater than 3 mg per dl. It can result from a variety of disorders ranging from life-threatening disease of the liver and biliary tract to innocuous impairment of hepatic bilirubin transport. Its differential diagnosis is, therefore, one of the most interesting and challenging problems encountered by the clinician. In most instances, jaundice reflects the presence of cholestasis. Cholestasis may be defined as impaired hepatic excretion or bile flow. It results from either hepatic parenchymal disease or biliary tract obstruction and is usually manifested clinically by an elevated serum alkaline phosphatase level and accumulation in the blood stream of substances, such as bilirubin, bile acids, and cholesterol, which are normally secreted in bile. Less commonly, jaundice results from increased bilirubin production, from an isolated defect in hepatic bilirubin transport or conjugation, or from a combination of bilirubin overproduction and defective bilirubin excretion. In these instances, hyperbilirubinemia is typically present as an isolated abnormality unaccompanied by other clinical or laboratory evidence of hepatic or biliary dysfunction.

The purposes of this chapter are to describe the pathophysiology of jaundice due to disordered bilirubin metabolism or cholestasis and to outline the clinical approach to the jaundiced patient.

BILIRUBIN METABOLISM

In order to better understand the differential diagnosis of jaundice, it is helpful to briefly review current concepts regarding bilirubin metabolism (Fig. 27–1).[1,2] Bilirubin IXα, the predominant naturally occurring isomer, is a metabolic waste product formed during the catabolism of heme. Daily bilirubin production in normal adults averages approximately 4 mg per kg, of which about 70 per cent results from degradation of hemoglobin heme from senescent erythrocytes. A minor fraction of bilirubin is produced from premature destruction of newly formed erythrocytes in the bone marrow or circulation, i.e., *ineffective erythropoiesis,* but most of the remaining 30 per cent is formed from breakdown of nonhemoglobin hemoproteins in the liver such as catalase and cytochrome P-450. Although hemoproteins (e.g., cytochromes) are present also in all other mammalian cells, the tissue concentration of these hemoproteins is so low or their turnover rate so slow (e.g., myoglobin) that their overall contribution to bilirubin production is minimal.

Heme is converted to *biliverdin* by *heme oxygenase,*

Figure 27–1. Overview of normal bilirubin metabolism and transport. Heme from hemoglobin and other hemoproteins is converted to biliverdin and then to bilirubin in extrahepatic tissues, predominantly the reticuloendothelial cells of the spleen and bone marrow. The unconjugated bilirubin (UCB) released into the plasma, which normally is tightly but reversibly bound to albumin, is taken up by hepatocytes and converted very efficiently to bilirubin monoglucuronide (BMG) and bilirubin diglucuronide (BDG). Both BMG and BDG can reflux into plasma and normally account for less than 5 per cent of total serum bilirubin. BMG in the liver is largely converted to BDG, which is then excreted in bile. Trace amounts of conjugated bilirubin are also deconjugated back to UCB. BMG and BDG in plasma also bind reversibly to albumin, but less tightly than UCB. When present in abnormally high concentrations for a long period of time, BMG and BDG bind irreversibly with albumin to form BR-albumin conjugates. Although UCB, BMG, BDG, and BR-

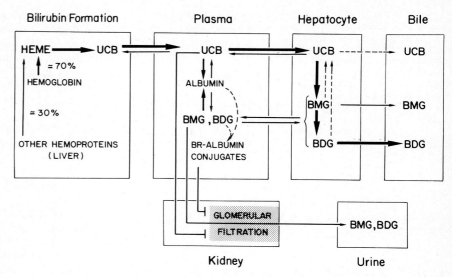

albumin conjugates all enter the kidney via the blood stream, only BMG and BDG appear in urine, presumably becuse they are most loosely bound to albumin and therefore most able to be filtered at the glomerulus. (From Scharschmidt, B. F.: Bilirubin metabolism and hereditary hyperbilirubinemia. *In* Wyngaarden, J. B., and Smith, L. H. (eds.). *Textbook of Medicine.* 18th ed. Philadelphia, W. B. Saunders Co., 1988.)

a microsomal enzyme. Hemoglobin heme from senescent erythrocytes is converted to biliverdin primarily by mononuclear phagocytic cells of the spleen, liver, and bone marrow. In contrast, free hemoglobin, haptoglobin-bound hemoglobin, and methemalbumin are catabolized predominantly in hepatic parenchymal cells. Biliverdin is converted to bilirubin by *biliverdin reductase.* The enzymes heme oxygenase and biliverdin reductase appear to exist as a single complex inside the cell, an arrangement which presumably allows for tightly coordinated and rapid conversion of heme to bilirubin. Biliverdin therefore does not normally appear in plasma. The observation that bilirubin crosses the placenta but biliverdin does not may explain why mammals convert water-soluble, nontoxic biliverdin into water-insoluble, potentially toxic bilirubin.[3]

Unconjugated bilirubin circulates in plasma bound tightly (3×10^7 M^{-1}) to *albumin.* Hepatic *uptake* of bilirubin across the sinusoidal membrane shows several features characteristic of carrier-mediated transport including saturation and competition with other organic anions such as sulfobromophthalein.[4] Fenestrations in the sinusoidal lining cells (see Chapter 87) permit albumin free access to the space of Disse and undoubtedly facilitate transfer of bilirubin to sinusoidal membrane carriers. Indeed, recent studies suggest that bilirubin uptake may be facilitated by physical interaction between the bilirubin-albumin complex and the liver cell surface.[5]

Once inside the hepatocyte, bilirubin appears to bind to cytosolic proteins, such as ligandin, which may decrease the free concentration of bilirubin in the cell available for reflux back into plasma, thereby enhancing net hepatic bilirubin uptake.[6]

Bilirubin is *conjugated* in the endoplasmic reticulum by UDP-glucuronyltransferase, which joins glucuronic acid, and occasionally other sugars, to one or both propionic acid groups on the parent compound. Conjugation thus converts unconjugated bilirubin, which is lipid-soluble and readily diffuses across biologic membranes such as the gallbladder and intestinal epithelium, into a water-soluble product that can be readily excreted. Conjugated bilirubin is then transported across the canalicular membrane into bile. In humans, approximately 80 per cent of bilirubin excreted in bile is in the form of diglucuronides, with nearly all the rest being monoglucuronides and only trace amounts being unconjugated. Reabsorption of conjugated bilirubin from the gallbladder and proximal small intestine is negligible. However, bilirubin is deconjugated by bacterial enzymes in the terminal ileum and colon and converted to a series of colorless tetrapyrroles collectively called *urobilinogens.* Up to about 20 per cent of urobilinogen is reabsorbed. Most of the reabsorbed urobilinogen is re-excreted in bile, with much of the remainder appearing in urine.

DIFFERENTIAL DIAGNOSIS OF HYPERBILIRUBINEMIA (Table 27–1)

Plasma bilirubin concentration reflects a state of dynamic equilibrium between bilirubin production and hepatic bilirubin clearance, and hyperbilirubinemia results from bilirubin overproduction, decreased bilirubin clearance, or some combination of the two.[1, 2, 7, 8]

Increased Bilirubin Production

Bilirubin overproduction is most commonly caused by hemolysis, and certain guidelines are useful in assessing the role of hemolysis in hyperbilirubinemia.[7] First, chronic steady-state hemolysis does not, by itself,

Table 27–1. CAUSES OF HYPERBILIRUBINEMIA*

I. *Increased bilirubin production*
  Examples: hemolysis, ineffective erythropoiesis, reabsorption of hematomas, transfusion
II. *Decreased bilirubin clearance*
  A. Hereditary defects in hepatic bilirubin clearance
    Examples: Gilbert's syndrome, Crigler-Najjar syndrome, Dubin-Johnson syndrome, Rotor's syndrome
  B. Cholestasis
    1. Hepatocellular disease
      Examples: drug-induced or viral hepatitis, pregnancy, sepsis
    2. Biliary tract obstruction
      Examples: choledocholithiasis, tumor, sclerosing cholangitis, pancreatitis

*From Lake, J. R., and Scharschmidt, B. F. *In* Conn, R. B. (ed.): Current Diagnosis. Vol. 7. Philadelphia, W. B. Saunders Co., 1985, p. 56.

produce a sustained bilirubin concentration greater than 4 to 5 mg per dl. Concentrations consistently above this level usually indicate the additional presence of hepatic dysfunction. In contrast, acute hemolysis can result in a bilirubin production rate that transiently exceeds the excretory capacity of even a normal liver and may cause striking bilirubin elevation. Transfusions are another important and often overlooked cause of increased bilirubin production. For example, 20 per cent of a unit (250 ml) of bank blood stored for three weeks or more hemolyzes within 24 hours of transfusion, thus acutely releasing as much bilirubin as is normally produced in a single day.[2] Resorption of large hematomas represents another cause of increased bilirubin production. Ineffective erythropoiesis may also be increased in certain disease states and can cause hyperbilirubinemia. Examples of this include megaloblastic anemia from either vitamin B_{12} or folic acid deficiency, iron deficiency anemia, sideroblastic anemia, thalassemia minor, polycythemia vera, aplasia, and lead poisoning.[1, 2]

Hereditary Hyperbilirubinemia (Table 27–2)

Hyperbilirubinemia and, less frequently, jaundice may also result from decreased hepatic bilirubin clearance due to hereditary defects in the hepatic metabolism or transport of bilirubin. Since these defects are selective for bilirubin and certain other organic anions, the hyperbilirubinemia is unaccompanied by other clinical or laboratory manifestations of cholestasis. Of the hereditary unconjugated hyperbilirubinemias (*Crigler-Najjar syndrome types I and II* and *Gilbert's syndrome*), only Gilbert's syndrome, which is present in up to 5 to 7 per cent of white adults in the United States and Western Europe, is commonly encountered. Gilbert's syndrome results from a decreased hepatic clearance of unconjugated bilirubin, probably related to diminished hepatic UDP-glucuronyltransferase activity.

Table 27–2. HEREDITARY DISORDERS OF HEPATIC BILIRUBIN METABOLISM AND TRANSPORT*

	Gilbert's Syndrome	Type I Crigler-Najjar Syndrome	Type II Crigler-Najjar Syndrome	Dubin-Johnson Syndrome	Rotor's Syndrome
Incidence	≤7% of population	Very rare	Uncommon	Uncommon	Rare
Inheritance	Autosomal dominant	Autosomal recessive	Autosomal dominant	Autosomal recessive	Autosomal recessive
Defect(s) in bilirubin metabolism	UDP-glucuronyl transferase activity, ↓ (?) hepatic uptake	Absent UDP-glucuronyl transferase activity	↓ ↓ Or undetectable UDP-glucuronyl transferase activity	Impaired excretion of conjugated bilirubin	(?) Impaired excretion or storage of conjugated bilirubin
Plasma bilirubin concentration (mg/dl)	≤3 in absence of fasting or hemolysis, essentially all unconjugated	Usually >20 (range 17–50), essentially all unconjugated	Usually <20 (range 6–45), essentially all unconjugated	Usually <7 (range 1–25), about half conjugated	Usually <7, about half conjugated
Plasma BSP disappearance	Usually normal, mild 45 min (<15%) retention in some patients	Normal	Normal	Slow initial disappearance (retention <20% at 45 min) with frequent secondary rise at 1.5 to 2 hours	Very slow disappearance (30–50% 45 min retention) without secondary rise
Oral cholecystography	Normal	Normal	Normal	Faint or nonvisualization	Usually normal visualization
Hepatic histology	Normal	Normal	Normal	Coarse pigment in centrilobar hepatocytes	Normal
Other distinguishing features	Bilirubin concentration with phenobarbital	No response to phenobarbital	Bilirubin concentration with phenobarbital	Bilirubin concentration with estrogens, characteristic urinary coproporphyrin pattern	—
Prognosis	Normal	Usually death in infancy	Usually normal	Normal	Normal

*From Scharschmidt, B. F., and Gollan, J. L. *In* Popper, H., and Scahfner, F. (eds.): Progress in Liver Disease. Vol. 6. New York, Grune & Stratton, 1979, pp. 187–212.

Serum bilirubin concentration in these patients may rise two- to threefold with fasting or dehydration, or following the administration of nicotinic acid. Serum bilirubin concentration decreases following the administration of phenobarbital due to the induction of UDP-glucuronyltransferase. Gilbert's syndrome may present as mild scleral icterus in the second or third decade of life. More commonly, though, the bilirubin elevation is insufficient to produce clinical jaundice and patients with Gilbert's syndrome present with unconjugated hyperbilirubinemia identified first on routine multiphasic biochemical screening or following fasting, as occurs pre- or postoperatively. Although a wide variety of symptoms have been associated with the disorder, they are very nonspecific and probably not attributable to Gilbert's syndrome itself. The diagnosis of Gilbert's syndrome can be established by the repeated demonstration of normal liver function tests in an asymptomatic individual with a mild elevation in the serum concentration of unconjugated bilirubin and no evidence of overt hemolysis. Liver biopsy and visualization of the biliary tract are unnecessary in routine cases. Normal fasting and postprandial concentrations of bile acids have been shown to be helpful in excluding liver disease.[9] The major reason to establish the diagnosis of Gilbert's syndrome is to reassure the patient and to avoid unnecessary surgical procedures (e.g., cholecystectomy, splenectomy).

Crigler-Najjar syndrome (congenital nonhemolytic jaundice) is an uncommon cause of unconjugated neonatal hyperbilirubinemia caused by the absence of glucuronyltransferase activity (type I) or markedly reduced glucuronyltransferase activity (type II). The majority of patients with the type I Crigler-Najjar syndrome develop kernicterus and die in the neonatal period. Patients with the type II Crigler-Najjar syndrome and occasional survivors with the type I syndrome may reach adulthood. These patients have bilirubin concentrations of 5 to 40 mg per dl, all of which is unconjugated (Table 27–2). Liver function is otherwise normal and patients with the type II syndrome are usually asymptomatic.

Familial unconjugated hyperbilirubinemia due to bilirubin overproduction not resulting from hemolysis has been described but is quite rare. Hereditary conjugated hyperbilirubinemia (*Dubin-Johnson* and *Rotor's syndromes*) also occurs and is more easily confused with hepatobiliary disease. Again, however, the diagnosis can be established by lack of other clinical or biochemical evidence of liver disease as well as the use of more specialized tests if necessary (Table 27–2).

Cholestasis

In most patients, jaundice reflects the presence of cholestasis, that is, impaired bile formation or bile flow resulting from extrahepatic biliary tract obstruction or hepatic parenchymal disease. Even in cholestasis, however, increased bilirubin production may be an impor-

tant contributing factor (e.g., hemolysis complicating viral hepatitis, ineffective erythropoiesis caused by folate deficiency in the alcoholic patient).

Cholestasis can be subdivided into intrahepatic and extrahepatic causes (Table 27–1). Intrahepatic causes include conditions in which the hepatocyte is unable to excrete bile even though the major ducts are patent. These causes include acute and chronic viral hepatitis of any etiology, alcoholic hepatitis, drug- or toxin-induced liver injury, primary biliary cirrhosis, congestive heart failure, sepsis, pregnancy, infiltrative diseases of the liver, and liver disease in infancy. The second major cause of cholestasis is extrahepatic biliary obstruction most commonly due to a neoplasm or gallstone.

APPROACH TO THE JAUNDICED PATIENT

The cause(s) of jaundice in an individual patient can usually be diagnosed or at least suspected based on the clinical history, physical examination, and routine laboratory tests.[8, 11, 12] Indeed, the value of clinical evaluation cannot be overemphasized. Careful history taking and physical examination, in conjunction with biochemical studies, will nearly always allow identification of hemolytic or hereditary disorders leading to hyperbilirubinemia and will permit about nine out of ten patients with cholestasis to be correctly categorized as having intrahepatic or extrahepatic disease.[10, 11] A practical approach to the patient with jaundice is outlined in Figure 27–2.[11, 12] Although useful as an illustration of a systematic approach, no algorithm is applicable to all patients, and selected exceptions will be illustrated by example in the discussion to follow.

History and Physical Examination

The patient's history may provide important diagnostic clues. The presence of itching should alert one to the presence of cholestasis. Although the identity of the "pruritogen(s)" is controversial, bile salts in the skin are the most likely candidates. A history of dark urine indicates the presence of increased levels of bilirubin conjugates in the serum (Fig. 27–1) and represents a clue to the presence of cholestasis, Rotor's syndrome, or Dubin-Johnson syndrome. The presence of gray-colored (acholic) stool implies severe cholestasis. Although commonly thought to result from diminished fecal bilirubin and urobilinogen excretion, this is probably not correct, because patients with the type I Crigler-Najjar syndrome excrete minimal bilirubin into bile but have normal colored feces. Given a patient with cholestasis, the initial task of the clinician, as outlined in Figure 27–2, is to determine whether the patient is or is not likely to have biliary obstruction. If biliary obstruction is unlikely, then an aggressive, invasive work-up usually is not indicated. Most types of hepatocellular injury leading to cholestasis are self-limited, not specifically treatable, and warrant only an

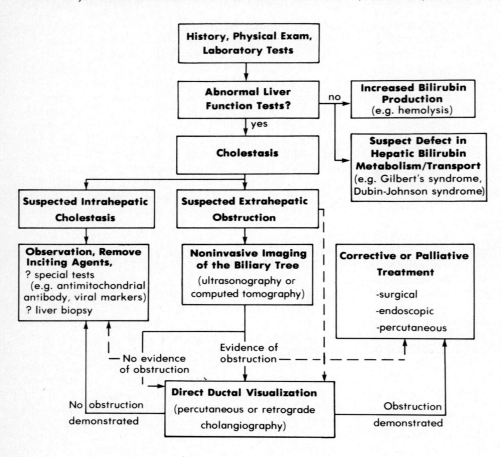

Figure 27–2. Outline of a clinical approach to the patient with jaundice. (From Scharschmidt, B. F., Goldberg, H. I., and Schmid, R. Reprinted, by permission of the New England Journal of Medicine, *308*:1515–1519, 1983.)

expectant approach with removal of inciting agents and supportive therapy as necessary. In contrast, most causes of biliary obstruction are not self-limited, and definitive or palliative treatment requires active intervention. Thus, patients with suspected biliary obstruction generally require a work-up of the sort outlined in Figure 27–2.

Clinical clues to the presence of biliary obstruction are summarized in Table 27–3. Most of the items listed in Table 27–3 are self-explanatory, but some deserve special mention. In trying to elicit a history of exposure to possible hepatotoxins, the questioner must usually be quite explicit in asking about use of nonprescription as well as prescription drugs and potential chemical toxins in the patient's home or work environment. It may occasionally be necessary to question a spouse or close friend regarding drug or alcohol use if the patient's own history is suspect. Prolonged cholestasis of more than several weeks' duration, although it can occur with certain hepatocellular disorders, also obligates the physician to seriously consider biliary disease, as does occult blood in the stool, which may represent a clue to a periampullary neoplasm or hemobilia.

Laboratory Tests

Laboratory studies are typically very helpful in the evaluation of hyperbilirubinemia. Recommended lab-

oratory studies include a complete blood count, reticulocyte count, and examination of the peripheral blood smear in cases of suspected hemolysis, and liver function tests including measurement of serum transaminase and alkaline phosphatase activities in addition to bilirubin concentration. If liver function is normal, then hemolysis, ineffective erythropoiesis, or a selective defect in hepatic bilirubin transport, such as

Table 27–3. CLINICAL CLUES TO EXTRAHEPATIC OBSTRUCTION

History
1. Abdominal pain suggestive of biliary disease or pancreatitis
2. Previous biliary surgery
3. Absence of exposure to hepatitis or potential hepatotoxins (e.g., drugs) and absence of hepatitis-like symptoms

Physical examination
1. Palpable gallbladder or abdominal mass
2. High fever suggestive of cholangitis
3. Occult blood in stool
4. Absence of stigmata of chronic liver disease
5. Abdominal tenderness

Laboratory studies
1. Disproportionate elevation of bilirubin, alkaline phosphatase
2. Elevated amylase
3. Complete normalization of a prolonged prothrombin time following parenteral administration of vitamin K
4. Negative serologic markers for viral hepatitis, chronic active hepatitis, primary biliary cirrhosis

Gilbert's syndrome, are likely diagnoses. Lactate dehydrogenase activities (particularly isoenzyme 1), decreased serum haptoglobin concentration, or the presence of urinary hemosiderin may also be useful in the evaluation of suspected hemolysis. If the patient is anemic and the reticulocyte count is inappropriately low, this should suggest ineffective erythropoiesis. If the blood count, reticulocyte count, and liver function tests are normal, Gilbert's syndrome should be considered. The increase in serum bilirubin concentration which accompanies Gilbert's syndrome and disorders associated with hemolysis or ineffective erythropoiesis is characteristically unconjugated, particularly if the new assays are employed (Fig. 27–1, see below). In contrast, the hyperbilirubinemia that accompanies the Dubin-Johnson or Rotor's syndrome or cholestasis is partially or predominantly conjugated (Table 27–2).

If liver function tests are abnormal, the jaundice is very likely a manifestation of cholestasis. Cholestasis is characteristically accompanied by increased activities of gamma glutamyltranspeptidase, 5'-nucleotidase, leucine aminopeptidase, and alkaline phosphatase in serum. Unlike bilirubin or bile acids, an elevated alkaline phosphatase activity in serum does not reflect diminished biliary excretion, but rather increased synthesis and release of this enzyme into the circulation.[15, 16] This same mechanism may be operational for the other enzymes, such as 5'-nucleotidase or leucine aminopeptidase, which are also located on the hepatocyte plasma membrane and possibly released into plasma by the detergent effects of bile acids.[16] Although increased activity of these enzymes is characteristic of cholestasis, elevations do occur in other situations.[17] Alkaline phosphatase activity may be increased in certain bone disorders and in pregnancy. Gamma glutamyltranspeptidase activity may be increased by numerous enzyme-inducing drugs, as well as alcohol, even in the absence of liver or biliary disease. It is not found in bone and an elevated value therefore suggests that an elevated alkaline phosphatase activity is of hepatic origin. Leucine aminopeptidase is also present in virtually all tissues, but elevated serum levels are seen only in hepatobiliary disease, particularly biliary obstruction, and pregnancy. Again, the primary use of this enzyme is in evaluating the significance of an elevated alkaline phosphatase activity. Other laboratory abnormalities which may accompany cholestasis include elevated concentrations of cholesterol and lipoprotein X in serum. Several additional points regarding the interpretation of biochemical tests merit emphasis. First, although disproportionate elevation of the bilirubin and alkaline phosphatase relative to serum transaminases is suggestive of biliary obstruction, exceptions to these generalizations exist. For example, infiltrative liver disease (e.g., granulomatous liver disease) may be characterized by disproportionate alkaline phosphatase elevation. Conversely, passage of a common duct stone is occasionally associated with brief but dramatic elevation (exceeding 10 to 20 times normal) of serum transaminases and amylase.[13, 14] Second, elevations of alkaline phosphatase and bilirubin do not always occur together. Tumors which selectively obstruct just a portion of the biliary tree (e.g., ductal tumors near the liver hilum, strategically located intrahepatic tumors) may cause a rise in alkaline phosphatase unaccompanied by jaundice. Finally, it is important to recognize that certain forms of clinically significant cholestasis do not invariably produce hyperbilirubinemia. For example, patients with primary biliary cirrhosis typically develop pruritus and biochemical evidence of cholestasis before hyperbilirubinemia occurs. Moreover, chronic partial or low-grade biliary obstruction sufficient to cause biliary cirrhosis may not be manifested by hyperbilirubinemia.

Specialized Laboratory Tests

Serum Bile Acids. With either parenchymal liver disease or biliary obstruction, the normally efficient hepatic clearance of *bile acids* from portal venous blood is impaired. Indeed, elevated serum bile acids are a more sensitive indicator of cholestasis than is hyperbilirubinemia.[18] Although a normal bile acid level is helpful in excluding a cholestatic disorder and may aid in making a diagnosis of Gilbert's syndrome, elevated values are nonspecific and are not useful in the differential diagnosis of cholestasis. Measurement of serum bile acid levels is presently not available in most laboratories.

Serum Bilirubin. The normal concentration of bilirubin in the serum of adults is less than 1.0 mg/dl.[1, 2, 19] Serum bilirubin is conventionally measured by a diazo reaction, in which bilirubin couples with a reagent such as diazotized sulfanilic acid to form a colored product that is quantitated spectrophotometrically. Conjugated bilirubin tends to react "directly" in this assay, that is, without the addition of an "accelerator" such as alcohol or urea. Total bilirubin is obtained by performing the assay in the presence of an "accelerator," which facilitates the reaction of unconjugated bilirubin with the diazo reagent. The indirect fraction is calculated by subtracting the direct fraction from the total bilirubin concentration.

More sensitive and specific techniques have recently become available for measuring the concentrations in serum of unconjugated bilirubin, monoconjugated bilirubin, diconjugated bilirubin, and in pathologic sera, the presence of bilirubin-albumin conjugates.[19] Clinical evaluation of these new assays, which are not yet generally available, and comparison of the results with the conventional diazo assay, has revealed certain interesting observations.

First, direct- and indirect-reacting bilirubin by the conventional diazo assay are inaccurate measures of the concentrations of conjugated and unconjugated bilirubin, respectively, in serum. Normally less than 5 per cent of total serum bilirubin is conjugated.[19, 20] *Second,* in most patients with hyperbilirubinemia due to cholestasis, fractionation of serum bilirubin by either the conventional or newer techniques is of little or no value; that is, it will not help in distinguishing paren-chymal liver disease from biliary obstruction.[20] In con-trast, when dealing with a patient who has low-level hyperbilirubinemia in whom Gilbert's syndrome, he-molysis, or subclinical hepatobiliary disease is a diag-nostic possibility, fractionation of serum bilirubin by the newer techniques is often of value. This is also a situation in which the conventional assay tends to overestimate the conjugated fraction and is particularly unreliable.[19, 20] *Third*, the sera of patients with pro-longed, conjugated hyperbilirubinemia typically has bilirubin-albumin conjugates, that is, conjugated bili-rubin bound irreversibly to albumin[21] (Fig. 27–1). These conjugates appear to form in serum by direct, nonenzymatic coupling of albumin and conjugated bilirubin (analogous to the formation of glycosylated hemoglobin in patients with diabetes mellitus), and in contrast to conjugated bilirubin, which is excreted promptly by the normal liver and appears in urine, these complexes have a serum half-life comparable to that of albumin (two to three weeks) and do not appear in urine.[21, 22] These complexes may account for up to 80 per cent of total serum bilirubin in patients with prolonged obstruction, and their presence helps to explain two important clinical observations: (1) the prolonged persistence of direct-reacting hyperbilirubi-nemia in patients with resolving liver disease or re-cently relieved obstruction, due to the long serum half-life of the complexes, and (2) the lower renal threshold for conjugated bilirubin in patients with the recent onset of hepatobiliary disease, in whom conjugates are just begining to form, as compared to patients with resolving liver disease, in whom conjugates may ac-count for most of the serum bilirubin.[22]

Thus, although total serum bilirubin measured by the conventional diazo assay remains adequate for most patients, the shortcomings of the assay are important to appreciate. The newer assays, which provide infor-mation of value in selected patients, are currently available in only a few centers.

DISTINGUISHING INTRAHEPATIC FROM EXTRAHEPATIC CHOLESTASIS

If extrahepatic obstruction is suspected based on the clinical evaluation, further investigation to determine the site and nature of the obstruction is warranted (Fig. 27–2). It also merits emphasis that certain hepatic disorders (Table 27–4) are occasionally accompanied by cholestasis which is so prominent or prolonged that extrahepatic obstruction cannot be confidently ex-cluded based on the clinical evaluation alone. More-over, the incidence of gallstones is known to be in-creased in cirrhotics, and 39 per cent of patients with primary biliary cirrhosis were found to have gallbladder stones.[23] Thus, known hepatocellular disease should not dissuade one from pursuing possible biliary disease suspected on clinical grounds.

Table 27–4. CAUSES OF LIVER DYSFUNCTION WHICH CAN MIMIC EXTRAHEPATIC OBSTRUCTION

Viral hepatitis	Parenteral nutrition
Alcoholic hepatitis	Hodgkin's disease
Benign recurrent cholestasis	Drugs (e.g., estrogens,
Pregnancy	phenothiazines, rifampin)
Sepsis	Inherited disorders (e.g.,
Infiltrative liver disease (e.g.,	arteriohepatic dysplasia)
amyloidosis, sarcoidosis)	Sickle cell disease
Hepatic neoplasia	Hereditary hyperbilirubinemia
Hepatic abscess	(e.g., Dubin-Johnson
Primary biliary cirrhosis	syndrome)
Postoperative cholestasis	

Ultrasonography and Computed Tomography

A reasonable first step is the use of a noninvasive imaging technique such as *ultrasonography* or *com-puted tomography* to determine whether the intra- or extrahepatic biliary system is dilated, implying me-chanical obstruction. Ultrasonography and computed tomography will demonstrate ductal dilatation in 85 per cent or more of patients with jaundice due to biliary obstruction.[11, 12] A common duct diameter greater than 4 to 6 mm in the area of the right branches of the portal vein and hepatic artery, as determined by ultrasonography, is generally considered abnormal. This guideline may not apply, however, to patients who have previously undergone cholecystectomy. In such individuals, ductal dilation may persist and does not, by itself, necessarily signify duct obstruction.

Both techniques may also yield additional informa-tion such as the presence of stones in the gallbladder or the presence of a pancreatic mass. Because of its lesser expense and the lack of radiation exposure, ultrasonography is generally preferred to computed tomography as a first procedure. However, for patients in whom the clinical suspicion of pancreatic cancer or other periampullary malignancy is very high, computed tomography is preferable to ultrasonography as a first test. A CT scan is at least as sensitive as ultrasonog-raphy in detecting ductal dilatation and is superior to ultrasonography in identifying the cause of the obstruc-tion and assessing resectability.[24, 25]

False negative examinations occur with both modal-ities and errors in interpretation are particularly likely to occur with ultrasonography.[12] False negative results may also occur in the presence of sclerosing cholangitis or cirrhosis, presumably because of poor distensibility of the bile ducts or hepatic parenchyma. Gallstones, which commonly produce only partial or intermittent biliary obstruction, may also fail to cause ductal dila-tation, and both techniques frequently fail to detect stones in the common duct.[26–30]

Percutaneous Transhepatic and Endoscopic Retrograde Cholangiography

If dilated bile ducts are detected, it is generally appro-priate to further define the location and perhaps nature of the obstruction with direct cholangiography, either by endoscopic retrograde cholangiography or percutaneous transhepatic cholangiography. Because false negative results from ultrasonographic or computed tomographic studies do occur, direct cholangiography is also appropriate, even if one or both of these studies is negative, if the clinical suspicion of biliary obstruction is high. Indeed, in certain selected situations such as the evaluation of recurrent symptoms suggestive of biliary disease in a patient who has previously undergone cholecystectomy, direct ductal visualization may be appropriate as a first procedure.[12, 29, 31]

In contrast to ultrasonography and computed tomography, which provide indirect evidence of ductal disease based on the presence or absence of ductal dilatation, percutaneous and retrograde cholangiography permit direct ductal visualization by injection of contrast material. *Percutaneous transhepatic cholangiography* involves passage of a needle, usually via a lateral intercostal approach, through the hepatic parenchyma and into an intrahepatic bile duct. The ductal system is then opacified by injection of contrast material through the needle. With the currently used "skinny needle" technique (23 gauge, 0.7 mm diameter), the incidence of complications following transhepatic cholangiography is less than that associated with the previously used larger, sheathed needles. In surveys of reported series totaling 1000 or more patients, skinny needle percutaneous cholangiography has been associated with serious *complications* (biliary sepsis, hemorrhage, bile peritonitis) in 3 to 10 per cent of cases and with death in 0.1 to 0.9 per cent of cases.[38, 39] Most of the serious complications have occurred in patients with biliary obstruction. The overall success rate in visualizing a dilated biliary tree by this approach has generally exceeded 90 per cent, while the success rate in visualizing nondilated intrahepatic ducts is less. The accomplished (and persistent) radiologist, who makes multiple passes, is very likely to successfully visualize the ductal system even in patients with a nondilated biliary tree.

Endoscopic retrograde cholangiography involves injection of contrast material into the biliary tree through a cannula which has been lodged in or passed through the ampulla of Vater using an endoscope. In the hands of a skilled endoscopist, this procedure visualizes the biliary tree in greater than 80 per cent of patients and is associated with about a 3 per cent incidence of serious *complications*.[40] These include *pancreatitis* (which occasionally follows overdistention of the pancreatic duct, usually in a patient with previous pancreatitis), *pancreatic abscess* (usually following injection into a pancreatic pseudocyst or obstructed panceatic duct), *cholangitis* (which typically occurs after injection into an obstructed bile duct), and *instrumental injury* (which is most common in patients with abnormal or surgically distorted anatomy).[40] In less experienced hands, the overall complication rate is higher and the success rate is much lower.[40]

The choice between *percutaneous transhepatic cholangiography* and *endoscopic retrograde cholangiography* for an individual patient depends on a number of factors, one of the most important being the local availability of skilled personnel. Clinical circumstances favoring the use of one or the other procedure, as well as their associated success rates and complications, are summarized in Table 27–5. Percutaneous transhepatic cholangiography, like liver biopsy, should not be performed in a patient with profound thrombocytopenia, marked hypoprothrombinemia, or ascites. Retrograde cholangiography, by contrast, is difficult in patients with a prior Billroth II gastrectomy and gastrojejunostomy. Other considerations are also occasionally important. For example, in a patient with a biliary tumor near the hepatic hilum, information regarding the proximal extent of the tumor may be exceedingly helpful in planning a surgical approach. This information is best provided by transhepatic cholangiography. Conversely, retrograde cholangiography may provide important visual information regarding possible peri-

Table 27–5. TECHNIQUES FOR DIRECT VISUALIZATION OF THE BILE DUCTS*

	Percutaneous Transhepatic Cholangiography	Endoscopic Retrograde Cholangiography
Success rate for satisfactory visualization of bile ducts	>90% with dilated hepatic ducts 70%; range of 25–75% with nondilated intrahepatic ducts (an average of 15 needle passes required for the higher success rates)	80–90%, regardless of presence or absence of ductal dilatation
Serious complications		
Type	Bile peritonitis, hemorrhage, cholangitis, sepsis, drug reaction, pneumothorax	Pancreatitis, pancreatic abscess, instrumental injury, sepsis, cholangitis, aspiration pneumonia
Frequency	5%; range of 3–10%	5%; range of 2–7%
Mortality rate	0.2–0.9%	0.1–0.2%
Circumstances favoring its use	Availability of skilled personnel Anticipation of a therapeutic maneuver (e.g., percutaneous drainage, stent insertion) Need to visualize proximal extent of a suspected lesion high in biliary tree Surgically distorted gastroduodenal anatomy Failed attempt at retrograde cholangiography	Availability of skilled personnel Anticipation of a therapeutic maneuver (e.g., sphincterotomy, stent insertion) Suspected periampullary neoplasm Presence of marked ascites or coagulopathy Failed attempt at percutaneous cholangiography

*From Scharschmidt, B. F., et al. Approach to the patient with cholestatic jaundice. N. Engl. J. Med. *308*:1515, 1983.

ampullary disease. It also permits biopsy of suspicious ampullary and duodenal masses, demonstration of pancreatic ductal morphologic features, and collection of fluid for cytologic evaluation. Because of possible injection into the pancreatic duct, retrograde cholangiography may be hazardous in the patient with a known pseudocyst; on the other hand, for technical reasons, transhepatic cholangiography is frequently unsuccessful in patients with sclerosing cholangitis and associated fibrosis or constriction of the intrahepatic biliary tree. Finally, anticipation of a therapeutic maneuver (percutaneous biliary drainage, sphincterotomy) may favor one or the other procedure.

Other Tests

A wide variety of other tests sometimes may be employed in the work-up of the jaundiced patient. However, because they lack sensitivity and specificity, as compared with the techniques described above, they are not indicated routinely. Some of these tests may, however, be helpful under certain circumstances.

Radionuclide Scans. *Technetium-99m sulfur-colloid scans* are useful primarily in the detection of intrahepatic mass lesions, which occasionally may produce striking cholestasis when strategically located. Overall, the diagnostic yield of a liver scan in the work-up of jaundice is low when compared to computed tomography or ultrasonography. Several reports have suggested that *hepatobiliary scintigraphy* with technetium-99m dimethyl acetanilide iminodiacetic acid (HIDA), or related biliary radionuclides (e.g., DISIDA) may be useful in the evaluation of jaundice. These compounds are taken up by hepatocytes and excreted into bile in detectable amounts even in patients with moderately severe cholestasis and hyperbilirubinemia. The detection of HIDA in the bile ducts but not in the gallbladder is a generally reliable indicator of cystic duct obstruction in the previously healthy patient, but false positive results occur frequently in alcoholic patients, patients receiving parenteral nutrition, or patients with severe systemic illness.[32, 33] Biliary scintigraphy has also been proposed as useful in the evaluation of cholestasis, with certain findings (e.g., segmental duct narrowing or duct cutoff) serving as reliable indicators of ductal obstruction. The results of prospective studies have differed, with some investigators finding biliary scintigraphy to be quite useful and others less so.[12] The more recent studies using modern scintigraphic techniques indicate that this technique may be a useful adjunct in selected patients; for example, for the further noninvasive evaluation of a patient with suspected obstruction and a negative ultrasound or computed tomographic evaluation.[34]

Intravenous Cholangiography. Although generally classified as noninvasive, intravenous cholangiography is associated with a 4 to 10 per cent incidence of adverse reactions, including a 1 per cent incidence of serious hypersensitivity reactions. Moreover, even in patients with a serum bilirubin concentration < 3 mg/ dl, duct opacification is not adequate to permit a definitive reading in up to 45 per cent of cases, and no ductal visualization is generally achieved with bilirubin concentrations exceeding 3 mg/dl. Thus, intravenous cholangiography has no role in the routine evaluation of jaundice. *Oral cholecystography* is also of no value in the work-up of the jaundiced patient. It will generally not visualize the gallbladder when the serum bilirubin concentration exceeds 3 mg/dl and provides no information about the bile ducts.

Liver Biopsy. Despite anecdotal reports suggesting that liver biopsy in patients with biliary obstruction might be associated with an inordinate risk of complications such as peritonitis, larger series suggest that the risk of liver biopsy is not greatly increased so long as the prothrombin time (< 3 seconds prolonged) and platelet count (> 80,000 per cu mm) are acceptable.[37] Nonetheless, liver biopsy is not indicated in the routine work-up of jaundice because (1) histologic findings diagnostic of obstruction are often absent in patients with proven obstruction (Table 27–6), and (2) even if histologic changes suggestive of biliary obstruction are present, the biopsy generally provides no information regarding the location or nature of the obstruction.[37] The principal role of a liver biopsy in the jaundiced patient is in the differential diagnosis of difficult or confusing cases of intrahepatic cholestasis.

Conventional X-rays. *Plain film* of the abdomen and *upper gastrointestinal x-rays*, although frequently used in the past to detect radiopaque gallstones or pancreatic disease, have largely been superseded by the more sensitive and specific tests previously described. Finally, except in unusual, urgent cases in which sepsis of suspected biliary origin precludes a work-up, *diagnostic laparotomy* should not be undertaken without evidence of biliary obstruction by ultrasonography, computed tomography, or cholangiography.

THERAPEUTIC OPTIONS FOR THE RELIEF OF BILIARY OBSTRUCTION

The treatment for patients with biliary obstruction is surgical in most instances. However, numerous ther-

Table 27–6. HEPATIC HISTOLOGIC ABNORMALITIES ASSOCIATED WITH BILIARY OBSTRUCTION

Nonspecific findings with either extra- or intrahepatic cholestasis
  Canalicular bile plugs
  Bile staining of parenchymal and Kupffer cells
Findings suggestive of biliary obstruction
  Feathery degeneration of hepatocytes
  Portal tract "edema"
  Bile duct proliferation
  Periductular fibrosis
Findings "diagnostic" of biliary obstruction
  Bile infarct
  Bile lake
  Neutrophils in the wall and lumen of interlobular bile ducts (cholangitis)
  Bile plugs in interlobular ducts

apeutic alternatives, including percutaneous or endoscopic passage of a stent and endoscopic sphincterotomy, have recently become available and have obviated the need for surgery, either emergently or altogether, in selected patients. The final sections of the chapter will briefly summarize alternatives to surgery, offer guidelines for clinical decision making, and outline the medical management of cholestasis.

Interventional Endoscopy

Endoscopic sphincterotomy involves division of the sphincter of Oddi by endoscopic passage of a sphincterotome. It is currently the procedure of choice for previously cholecystectomized patients with choledocholithiasis.[41–43] Following sphincterotomy, stones may pass spontaneously or can be extracted with special catheters. Several series report an overall success rate of about 85 per cent in clearing stones from the biliary tract when performed by an experienced endoscopist.[41] Immediate complications (bleeding, pancreatitis, cholangitis, retroperitoneal perforation) occur in 8 to 10 per cent of patients; urgent surgery is required in 1 to 2 per cent, and the overall mortality rate is about 1 per cent.[41] Follow-up of patients for up to seven years suggests that about 5 to 10 per cent of patients develop stenosis or new stones. All these figures compare favorably with the results of surgery. Endoscopic sphincterotomy is also being performed with increasing frequency in patients with symptomatic choledocholithiasis who have not previously undergone cholecystectomy and who are poor surgical candidates.[41] Although early anecdotal reports suggested that such patients had a high incidence of recurrent symptoms and acute cholecystitis, several series have now demonstrated that only about 10 per cent of patients required cholecystectomy for biliary pain or cholecystitis during a several-year follow-up.[41, 42] Less common indications for endoscopic sphincterotomy include biliary obstruction due to the "sump syndrome"[44] (obstruction in patients with previous choledochoenteric anastomosis due to reflux of food contents), sphincter of Oddi dysfunction (see p. 1662), and palliation (or diagnosis) of an obstructing distal common bile duct tumor.[45]

Endoscopic stent placement and *endoscopic dilatation* of biliary strictures are currently being evaluated at several centers.[46, 47] Although favorable results have been reported and preliminary results using a No. 10 French stent catheter in patients with inoperable periampullary malignancy appear particularly encouraging, experience is still limited and follow-up relatively short. Endoscopic stent placement appears particularly likely to find a role in the palliation of inoperable pancreatic cancer.

Interventional Radiology

Percutaneous transhepatic catheterization of the intrahepatic biliary tree has evolved from a purely diagnostic technique into a therapeutic one as well. Recent technical advances have made it possible to consistently manipulate transhepatic catheters through various types of obstruction into the duodenum, and special catheters with side holes positioned above and below the obstruction permit antegrade flow of bile.[48–51] Percutaneous insertion of a drainage catheter or stent can be used in a variety of settings and may represent adjunctive, palliative, or definitive therapy.

Preoperative biliary drainage has been proposed as a useful adjunct for jaundiced patients with malignant obstruction prior to definitive surgery; however, several randomized trials now indicate that the *routine* use of preoperative drainage does not decrease and may actually increase overall morbidity and mortality.[52, 53] In selected patients, however, with benign or malignant structures complicated by infection, drainage may represent a useful interim measure that will permit infection to be controlled and surgery delayed until the patient's condition has improved.

The most common application of interventional biliary radiologic therapy has been in the *palliative treatment* of patients with inoperable malignancy of the proximal biliary tree, most commonly cholangiocarcinoma or metastatic disease in the porta hepatis. Early approaches involved the use of an external catheter. More recently, favorable experience has been reported with an endoprosthesis, which represents less of a physical and psychologic encumbrance to the terminally ill patient.[50, 51] Satisfactory drainage can be accomplished in 85 per cent or more of patients when performed by a skilled radiologist. Percutaneous transhepatic drainage has been utilized less frequently for benign disease. There is limited experience with *dilatation of strictures,* and this technique appears to be most successful when applied to strictured choledochoenteric anastomoses.[41] Removal of common duct stones via a percutaneous approach has been successful in selected cases, but this technique (in the absence of an existing T tube) is generally inferior to endoscopic sphincterotomy and stone extraction.

These procedures are associated with both acute and long-term complications. Serious acute complications, which include sepsis and, less frequently, pneumothorax, hemothorax, intra-abdominal hemorrhage, or hemobilia, occur in 15 to 25 per cent of patients.[41, 42] Sepsis due to catheter blockage or dislodgment is the most frequent long-term complication and occurs in 25 per cent or more of patients, depending on the length of follow-up. Although an attractive option in selected patients, the use of such intraventional radiologic techniques is clearly associated with a moderately high rate of complications and should only be utilized for symptomatic patients for whom alternative approaches are inappropriate.

Examples of Clinical Decision Making

Consideration of therapeutic options should begin even before a precise diagnosis is established. If, on the basis of clinical evaluation (often coupled with a noninvasive imaging technique such as ultrasonography), biliary obstruction appears highly likely, it is reasonable to make projections regarding the most likely diagnosis and the most appropriate form of therapy. Even though such projections are occasionally incorrect and may need to be modified as further information becomes available, they help avoid the use of tests that are unnecessary, dangerous, or redundant and thus minimize risk and expense to the patient as well as the time required to establish a diagnosis and begin appropriate treatment.

This approach can be illustrated by the following examples. (1) Given an otherwise healthy patient who previously underwent cholecystectomy for gallstones and now presents with episodic right upper quadrant pain, fever, and biochemical evidence of cholestasis, a retained stone would be a very likely possibility. In this instance, endoscopic retrograde cholangiography, which could then be accompanied by sphincterotomy and stone extraction, is a reasonable first procedure. Indeed, noninvasive imaging of the biliary tract may be unnecessary in many such patients. (2) Given a similar patient without a prior history of cholescystectomy in whom a carefully performed ultrasound examination reveals gallbladder stones, a dilated common bile duct with or without stones, and no other abnormalities (e.g., no pancreatic mass), then laparotomy for an anticipated cholecystectomy with common bile duct exploration would represent a reasonable next step without further invasive evaluation. In the unusual such instance in which the preoperative diagnosis of gallstones with choledocholithiasis was incorrect, then the correct diagnosis could be made at the time of surgery and appropriate measures taken. Apart from such situations in which the diagnosis of distal common duct obstruction due to choledocholithiasis seems very likely, it is usually not appropriate to perform a laparotomy on the basis of ultrasonographic findings alone. (3) Given a debilitated elderly patient with severe, prolonged cholestasis in whom noninvasive imaging reveals dilated intrahepatic ducts without dilatation of the common duct or gallbladder, then proximal obstruction due to tumor is likely and percutaneous cholangiography would be a reasonable next step to confirm the diagnosis. If surgical resection or bypass is impossible or inappropriate, a stent could be placed as part of the same procedure. As illustrated by these selected examples, individual patients very often present special problems and considerations. Often, the most efficient approach to evaluation and treatment can best be determined using a team of individuals including the primary physician, gastroenterologist, surgeon, and radiologist.

MEDICAL TREATMENT OF CHOLESTASIS AND ITS COMPLICATIONS

Removing or bypassing the biliary obstruction is the most desirable objective, but unfortunately, this is not possible in all instances. In these patients as well as patients with prolonged cholestasis due to hepatic disease, medical measures may be necessary to deal with the consequences of cholestasis (Table 27–7).

Pruritus

Pruritus can be a particularly disturbing and disabling symptom. Although the pathogenesis is not altogether clear, use of the binding resin cholestyramine rests on the assumption that bile acids, or other substances which undergo enterohepatic circulation, are responsible.[54, 55] Therapy is typically begun with 12 to 16 gm daily, given orally in divided doses with meals. Because the resultant depletion of the bile acid pool may further impair absorption of dietary fats, particular attention must be paid to diet and vitamin supplementation. Although frequently helpful in patients with partial biliary obstruction, cholestyramine would not be expected to benefit patients with complete obstruction and therefore absence of intestinal bile acids.

Other methods of treating pruritus are generally less successful. *Phenobarbital* (120 to 250 mg per day)[56] is reportedly helpful in some patients, but controlled observation has not demonstrated relief of pruritus.[57] Neither conventional antihistamines (H_1-receptor blockade) nor H_2-receptor blockers have been found beneficial in controlled trials.[58] A variety of other modalities have been tried, including the use of 17α-alkyl substituted androgens, phototherapy, and plasma exchange or plasma perfusion through adsorbents such as charcoals.[59] Although reportedly effective in some patients, controlled observations are lacking.

In addition to these "specific" measures, simple skin care alone often provides some relief from the itching.[59] General skin care should include frequent cutting of fingernails and wearing of light clothing and few bed clothes. A lukewarm bath or shower before retiring may provide temporary relief; however, excessive bathing and the use of soaps or detergents have a drying effect on the skin which may aggravate the problem and should be avoided. Topical application of emollients should be tried even in the absence of xerosis, and lotions containing menthol or phenol may provide some additional relief by soothing the skin. Topical anesthetic agents or topical antihistamines should not be used, as they may cause sensitization. These and other approaches to the medical management of pruritus associated with cholestasis are summarized in Table 27–7.

Fat Malabsorption

Malabsorption of fat and fat-soluble vitamins is a frequent manifestation of severe cholestasis and intestinal bile acid deficiency. Such malabsorption may manifest itself as diarrhea, night blindness (vitamin A deficiency), osteomalacia (vitamin D deficiency), hypoprothrombinemia (vitamin K deficiency), and in children, possibly neurologic dysfunction (vitamin E

Table 27–7. THERAPEUTIC MEASURES USED IN TREATMENT OF CHOLESTASIS-ASSOCIATED PRURITUS*

Therapeutic Measure	Regimen	Efficacy	Adverse Effects
Drugs			
Antihistamines:			
Diphenhydramine	25–50 mg qid	Rarely provides significant relief apart from sedation	Drowsiness
hydroxyzine	25 mg tid		
Cimetidine	200 mg qid	None established	Antiandrogen effects; mental confusion; hypersensitivity reactions
Cholestyramine	12–20 gm/day: 4 gm dose 30 min before meals; double dose at breakfast; evening dose may be skipped to facilitate taking other medications	Beneficial in most patients, but may require up to 2 weeks for an effect	Fat malabsorption; decreased absorption of other medications; constipation; hyperchloremic acidosis
Phenobarbital	Starting dose: 120 mg/day in adult, 3–5 mg/day in child; dosage subsequently altered to maintain therapeutic response and plasma; concentration of drug between 10–40 µg/ml	Variable, typically incomplete relief	Drowsiness; potent inducer of hepatic enzymes involved in drug metabolism
Procedures			
Plasma perfusion or exchange	2–3 procedures on consecutive days, then prn; each procedure lasts ~4 hours and 1–6 liters of plasma are perfused	Good in the few patients tested, but limited by availability of equipment and personnel	None reported
UV-B light	2–3 treatments/week at a dose slightly below minimal erythemal dose	Good in the few patients tested, but no controlled trials to date	None reported

*From Fitz, J. G., Lake, J. R., and Scharschmidt, B. F. Cholestasis and sclerosing cholangitis. *In* Bayles, T. M. (ed.): Current Therapy in Gastroenterology and Liver Disease. Toronto, B. C. Decker, Inc., 1986, p. 400.

deficiency).[60] Symptomatic steatorrhea responds to restriction of dietary fat to less than 40 gm daily and, if necessary, supplementation with medium-chain triglycerides. The patient should also receive oral or parenteral supplementation of vitamins A, D, and K, and children should also receive vitamin E.[60]

Bone Disease

Vitamin D metabolism in patients with chronic liver disease has been intensively studied, yet remains an area of confusion. Vitamin D deficiency in patients with primary biliary cirrhosis and other chronic cholestatic disorders is probably multifactorial in origin, with poor nutrition, lack of exposure to sunlight, malabsorption of vitamin D, and increased urinary excretion of vitamin D all being possible contributing factors.[61] Osteoporosis is also present in many patients and may even be the predominant lesion in patients with primary biliary cirrhosis.[62, 63] Thus, in patients with clinically significant bone disease, a bone biopsy may be necessary to identify precisely the pathologic process and formulate a rational therapeutic approach. The dose, form, and value of vitamin D replacement in patients with *hepatic osteomalacia* remains controversial. Intramuscular vitamin D_2 did not prevent bone disease in one study, but histologic healing of bone has been reported following monthly intramuscular, 15 µg injections of 1,25-dihydroxyvitamin D_3, oral 25-hydroxyvitamin D_3 in a dose of 100 to 200 µg daily, or oral administration of 1α-hydroxyvitamin D_3.[64–67] Regardless of the approach selected, a reasonable overall goal would seem to be maintenance of normal serum levels of calcium, phosphorus, and 25-hydroxyvitamin D.

References

1. Wolkoff, A. (ed.). Bilirubin metabolism and hyperbilirubinemia. Semin. Liver Dis. *3:*1, February 1983.
2. Gollan, J. L., and Schmid, R. Bilirubin metabolism and hyperbilirubinemic disorders. *In* Wright, R. (ed.): Liver and Biliary Disease. Philadelphia, W. B. Saunders Co., 1982, pp. 255–295.
3. McDonagh, A. F., Palma, L. A., and Schmid, R. Reduction of biliverdin and placental transfer of bilirubin and biliverdin in the pregnant guinea pig. Biochem. J. *194:*273, 1981.
4. Scharschmidt, B. F., Waggoner, J. G., and Berk, P. D. Hepatic organic anion uptake in the rat. J. Clin. Invest. *56:*1280, 1975.
5. Weisiger, R., Gollan, J., and Ockner, R. Receptor for albumin on the liver cell surface may mediate uptake of fatty acids and other albumin-bound substances. Science *211:*1048, 1981.
6. Wolkoff, A. W., Goresky, C. A., Sellin, J., Gatmaitan, Z., and Arias, I. M. Role of ligandin in transfer of bilirubin from plasma into liver. Am. J. Physiol. *236:*E638, 1979.
7. Berk, P. D., Martin, J. F., Blaschke, T. F., Scharschmidt, B. F., and Plotz, P. H. Unconjugated hyperbilirubinemia. Physiologic evaluation and experimental approaches to therapy. Ann. Intern. Med. *82:*552, 1975.
8. Lake, J. R., and Scharschmidt, B. F. *In* Conn, R. B. (ed.): Current Diagnosis. Vol. 7. Philadelphia, W. B. Saunders Co., 1985, pp. 54–61.
9. Vierling, J. M., Berk, P. D., Hofmann, A. F., Martin, J. F., Wolkoff, A. W., and Sharschmidt, B. F. Normal fasting-state levels of serum cholyl-conjugated bile acids in Gilbert's syndrome. An aid to the diagnosis. Hepatology *2:*340, 1982.
10. Scharschmidt, B. F., and Gollan, J. L. Current concepts of bilirubin metabolism and hereditary hyperbilirubinemia. *In* Popper, H., and Schafner, F. (eds.): Progress in Liver Diseases. Vol. 6. New York, Grune & Stratton, Inc., 1979, pp. 187–212.
11. O'Connor, K. W., Snodgrass, P. J., Swonder, J. F., Mahoney,

S., Burt, R., Cocherill, E. M., and Lumeng, L. A blinded prospective study comparing four curent non-invasive approaches in the differential diagnosis of medical versus surgical jaundice. Gastroenterology *84:*1498, 1983.

12. Scharschmidt, B. F., Goldberg, H. I., and Schmid, R. Approach to the patient with cholestatic jaundice. N. Engl. J. Med. *308:*1515, 1983.

13. Shora, W., and Danovitch, S. H.: Marked elevation of serum transaminase activity in extrahepatic biliary tract disease. Am. J. Gastroenterol. *55:*575, 1971.

14. Ginsberg, A. L. Very high levels of SGOT and LDH in patients with extrahepatic biliary tract obstruction. Am. J. Dig. Dis. *15:*803, 1970.

15. Seetharam, S., Sussman, N. L., Komoda, T., and Alpers, D. H. The mechanism of elevated alkaline phosphatase activity after bile duct ligation in the rat. Hepatology *6:*374, 1986.

16. Debroe, M. E., Roels, F., Nouwen, E. J., Claeys, L., and Wieme, R. J. Liver plasma membrane: The source of high molecular weight alkaline phosphatase in human serum. Hepatology *5:*118, 1985.

17. Rustgi, V. K. R., and Cooper, J. N. (eds.): Gastrointestinal and Hepatic Complications in Pregnancy. New York, John Wiley and Sons, 1986.

18. Ferraris, R., Colombatti, G., Fiorentini, M. T., Caroso, R., Arossa, W., and de la Piere, M. Diagnostic value of serum bile acids and routine liver function tests in hepatobiliary disease. Dig. Dis. Sci. *28:*129, 1983.

19. Fevery, J., and Blanckaert, J. What can we learn from analysis of serum bilirubin? J. Hepatol. *2:*113, 1986.

20. Scharschmidt, B. F., Blanckaert, N., Farina, F., Kabra, P., Stafford, B., and Weisiger, R. A. Measurement of unconjugated, monoconjugated, and diconjugated bilirubin in the review of patients with hepatobiliary disease. Gut *2:*643, 1982.

21. Weiss, J. S., Gautam, A., Lauff, J. J., Lundberg, M. W., Jatlow, P., Boyer, J. L., and Seligson, D. The clinical importance of a protein-bound fraction of serum bilirubin in patients with hyperbilirubinemia. N. Engl. J. Med. *309:*147, 1983.

22. Gautam, A., Seligson, H., Gordon, D. R., Seligson, D., and Boyer, J. L. Irreversible binding of conjugated bilirubin to albumin in cholestatic rats. J. Clin. Invest. *73:*873, 1984.

23. Summerfield, J. A., Elias, E., Hungerford, G. D., Nikopata, V. L. B., Dick, R., and Sherlock, S. The biliary system in primary biliary cirrhosis. Gastroenterology *70:*240, 1976.

24. Nix, G. A. J. J., Schmitz, P. I. M., Wilson, J. H. P., Van Blankenstein, M., Groenveld, C. F. M., and Hofwizk, R. Carcinoma of the head of the pancreas. Therapeutic implications of endoscopic retrograde cholangeopancreatography findings. Gastroenterology *87:*37, 1984.

25. Jafri, S. Z. H., Aisen, A. M., Glazer, G. M., and Weiss, C. A. Comparison of CT and angiography in assessing resectability of pancreatic carcinoma. Am. J. Roentgenol. *142:*525, 1984.

26. Berk, R. N., Cooperberg, P. L., Gold, R. P., Rohrmann, C. A., Jr., and Ferrucci, J. T., Jr. Radiography of the bile ducts. Radiology *145:*1, 1982.

27. Matzen, P., Malchow-Moller, A., Brun, B., Gronvall, S., Haubek, A., Henriksen, J. H., Laussen, K., Lejerstofte, J., Stage, P., Winkler, K., and Juhl, E. Ultrasonography, computed tomography, and cholescintigraphy in suspected obstructive jaundice—a prospective comparative study. Gastroenterology *84:*1492, 1983.

28. Cronan, J. J., Mueller, P. R., Simeone, J. F., et al. Prospective diagnosis of choledocholithiasis. Radiology *146:*467, 1983.

29. Gross, B. H., Harter, L. P., Gore, R. M., et al. Ultrasonic evaluation of common bile duct stones: Prospective comparison with endoscopic retrograde cholangiopancreatography. Radiology *146:*471, 1983.

30. Laing, F. C., and Jeffrey, R. B., Jr. Choledocholithiasis and cystic duct obstruction: Difficult ultrasonographic diagnosis. Radiology *146:*475, 1983.

31. Vennes, J. A., and Bond, J. H. B. Approach to the jaundiced patient. Gastroenterology *84:*1615, 1983.

32. Shuman, W. P., Gibbs, P., Rudd, T. G., and Mack, L. A. PIPIDA scintigraphy for cholecystitis: False positive in alcoholism and total parential nutrition. Am. J. Roentgenol. *138:*1, 1982.

33. Kalff, V., Froelick, J. W., Lloyd, R., and Thrall, J. H. Predictive value of an abnormal hepatobiliary scan in patients with severe intercurrent illness. Radiology *146:*191, 1983.

34. Lieberman, D. A., and Krishnamurthy, G. T. Intrahepatic versus extrahepatic cholestasis: Discrimination with biliary scintigraphy combined with ultrasound. Gastroenterology *90:*734, 1986.

35. Osnes, M., Larsen, S., Lowe, P., Gronseth, K., Lotveit, T., and Nordshus, T. Comparison of endoscopic retrograde and intravenous cholangiography in the diagnosis of biliary calculi. Lancet *2:*230, 1978.

36. Goodman, M. W., Ansel, J. H., Vennes, J. A., Lasser, R. B., and Silvis, S. E. Is intravenous cholangiography still useful? Gastroenterology *79:*642, 1980.

37. Morris, J. S., Gallo, G. A., Scheuer, P. J., and Sherlock, S. Liver biopsy in "difficult" jaundice. Gastroenterology *68:*750, 1975.

38. Harbin, W. P., Mueller, P. R., and Ferrucci, J. T., Jr. Complications and use patterns of fine needle transhepatic cholangiography: a multi-institutional survey. Radiology *135:*15, 1980.

39. Kreek, M. J., and Balint, J. A. "Skinny needle" cholangiography—results of a pilot study of a voluntary prospective method for gathering risk data on new procedures. Gastroenterology *78:*598, 1980.

40. Bilbao, M. K., Dotter, C. T., Lee, T. G., and Katon, R. M. Complications of endoscopic retrograde cholangio-pancreatography (ERCP): A study of 10,000 cases. Gastroenterology *70:*314, 1976.

41. Cotton, P. B. Endoscopic management of bile duct stones (apples and oranges). Gut *25:*587, 1984.

42. Escourrou, J., Cordova, J. A., Lazorthes, F., Frexinos, J., and Ribet, A. Early and late complications after endoscopic sphincterotomy for biliary lithiasis with and without the gallbladder "in situ." Gut *25:*598, 1984.

43. Classen, M. Endoscopic papillotomy. *In* Sivak, M. (ed.): Gastroenterologic Endoscopy. Philadelphia, W. B. Saunders Co., 1986.

44. Katon, R. M. Sump syndrome. Gastroenterology *92:*781, 1987.

45. Nakao, N. L., Siegel, J. H., Stenger, R. J., and Gelb, A. M. Tumors of the ampulla of Vater: Early diagnosis by intraampullary biopsy during endoscopic commutation. Two case presentations and review of the literature. Gastroentrology *83:*459, 1982.

46. Marks, W. M., Freeny, P. C., Ball, T. J., and Gannon, R. M. Endoscopic retrograde biliary drainage. Radiology *152:*357, 1984.

47. Geenen, J. E., Drefus, D., and Welch, J. M. Biliary balloon dilatation: Analysis and review. Endosc. Rev. March/April 1985, pp. 10–16.

48. Ring, E. J., and Kerlan, R. K., Jr. International biliary radiology. Am. J. Roentgenol. *142:*31, 1984.

49. Neff, C. C., Mueller, P. R., Ferrucci, J. T., Jr., Dawson, S. L., Wittenberg, J., Simione, J. F., Butch, P. J., and Papanicolau, N. Serious complications following transgression of the pleural space in drainage procedures. Radiology *152:*335, 1984.

50. Kerlan, R. K., Pogany, A. C., and Ring, E. J. Biliary endoprostheses: Insertion using a combined peroral-transhepatic method. Radiology *150:*828, 1984.

51. Ring, E. J., Schwarz, W., McLean, G. K., and Freiman, D. B. A simple, indwelling biliary endoprosthesis made from commonly available catheter material. Am. J. Roentgenol. *139:*615, 1982.

52. Hatfield, A. R. W., Terblanche, J., Fataar, S., Kernoff, L., Tobias, R., Girdwood, A. H., Harris-Jones, R., and Marks, I. N. Preoperative external biliary damage in obstructive jaundice: A prospective controlled clinical trial. Lancet *2:*846, 1982.

53. McPherson, G. A. D., Benjamin, I. S., Hodgson, H. J. F., Bowley, N. B., Allison, D. J., and Blumgart, L. H. Peroperation percutaneous transhepatic biliary drainage: The results of a controlled trial. Br. J. Surg. *71:*371, 1984.

54. Carey, J. B., and Williams, G. Relief of the pruritus of jaundice with a bile-acid sequestering resin. JAMA *176:*432, 1961.

55. Schaffner, F., Klion, F. M., and Latuff, A. J. The long-term use of cholestyramine in the treatment of primary biliary cirrhosis. Gastroenterology *48:*293, 1965.

56. Bloomer, J. R., and Boyer, J. L. Phenobarbital effects in cholestatic liver disease. Ann. Intern. Med. *82:*310, 1975.
57. Metreau, J.-M., Lecompte, Y., Arondel, J., and Dhumeaux, D. Phenobarbital therapy in intrahepatic and extrahepatic cholestatis in adults. Digestion *14:*471, 1976.
58. Harrison, A. R., Littenberg, G., Goldstein, L., and Kaplowitz, N. Pruritus, cimetidine and polycythemia (letter). N. Engl. J. Med. *300:*433, 1979.
59. Fitz, J. G., Lake, J. R., and Scharschmidt, B. F. Cholestasis and sclerosing cholangitis. *In* Bayless, T. M. (ed.): Current Therapy in Gastroenterology and Liver Disease. Toronto, B. C. Decker, Inc., 1986, p. 400.
60. Rosenbaum, J. L., Keating, J. P., Prensky, A. L., and Nelson, J. S. A progressive neurologic syndrome in children with chronic liver disease. N. Engl. J. Med. *304:*503, 1981.
61. Jung, R. T., Davie, M., and Siklas, P. Vitamin D metabolism in acute and chronic cholestasis. Gut *20:*840, 1979.
62. Matloff, D. S., Kaplan, M. M., Neer, R. M., Goldberg, M. J., Bitman, W., and Wolfe, H. J. Osteoporosis in primary biliary cirrhosis: Effects of 25-hydroxyvitamin D₃ treatment. Gastroenterology *82:*97, 1982.
63. Herlong, H. F., Recker, R. R., and Maddrey, W. C. Bone disease in primary biliary cirrhosis: Histologic features and response to 25-hydroxyvitamin D₃. Gastroenterology *83:*103, 1982.
64. Long, R. G., Meinhard, E., and Skinner, R. K. Clinical, biochemical, and histologic studies of osteomalacia, osteoporosis, and parathyroid function in chronic liver disease. Gut *19:*85, 1978.
65. Long, R. G., Varghese, Z., Meinhard, E. A., Skinner, R. K., Wills, M. R., and Sherlock, S. Parenteral 1,25-dihydroxycholecalciferol in hepatic osteomalacia. Br. Med. J. *1:*73, 1978.
66. Reid, J. S., Meredith, S. C., Nemchausky, B. A., Rosenberg, I. H., and Boyer, J. L. Bone disease in primary biliary cirrhosis: Reversal of osteomalacia with oral 25-hydroxyvitamin D. Gastroenterology *78:*512, 1980.
67. Compston, J. E., Crowe, U. P., and Horton, L. W. L. Treatment of osteomalacia associated with primary biliary cirrhosis with oral 1-alpha-hydroxy vitamin D₃. Br. Med. J. *2:*309, 1979.
68. Scharschmidt, B. F. Bilirubin metabolism and hereditary hyperbilirubinemia. *In* Wyngaarden, J. B., and Smith, L. H. (eds.). Textbook of Medicine. Philadelphia, W. B. Saunders Co., 1988.

28

Evaluation of Mass Lesions in the Liver
JAMES SHOREY

Intrahepatic mass lesions most often come to attention when they are felt by the patient, palpated by the physician, or visualized on a radioisotope liver-spleen scan, abdominal sonogram, or abdominal computed tomographic (CT) scan. In another setting, the finding of abnormal "liver function tests," particularly in a patient with a known primary tumor capable of metastasis, leads to a search for hepatic mass lesions by the above-mentioned techniques.

Once a focal hepatic lesion(s) has come to attention, the physician must decide upon the most rational approach to its definitive diagnosis. This decision must be based on an optimal balance between the cost and risk of diagnostic procedures, the degree to which a given procedure will contribute to making a final diagnosis, and a consideration of how quickly that diagnosis can be made. In the hospitalized patient, it is sometimes most cost effective to go directly to a more expensive test if it leads more quickly to adequate identification of a hepatic mass, thereby shortening the hospital stay.

The first section of this chapter concerns the general approach to evaluation of focal liver lesions, the second section deals with the various imaging techniques for identifying intrahepatic masses, and the third deals with specific consideration of the principal entities which may present as focal hepatic masses.

APPROACH TO THE DIAGNOSIS OF FOCAL LIVER LESIONS

The approach to diagnosis of focal hepatic lesions will be dependent on the presenting circumstances. In recent years the number of tools available to aid the physician in this diagnostic process has increased greatly. Clearly, the objective must be to devise an optimal approach to diagnosis and treatment which best balances the minimization of the patient's risk and discomfort with greatest diagnostic accuracy and lowest cost. One must remain alert to the possibility that a currently optimal diagnostic technique may be replaced in the future by a better approach based on refinement of current methodologies as well as the introduction of entirely new diagnostic technologies.

Focal liver lesions come to attention in various ways. At times, a near certain diagnosis of intrahepatic cancer can be made from little more than the patient's complaint of weight loss and an enlarging upper abdominal mass. Further studies, usually confirming the presence of cancer, serve to define the tumor type with its implications for prognosis, to determine the need for further studies, and to provide the basis for decisions about possible therapy. In other cases, focal lesions are discovered incidentally. For example, liver lesions may be identified in a patient undergoing sonographic evaluation for suspected biliary tract disease, or on evaluation of the patient with abnormal findings on physical examination or laboratory testing noted at the time of a routine periodic health evaluation. Finally, it may be necessary to exclude, with maximal certainty, the presence of hepatic metastases in a patient with a potentially curable extrahepatic primary cancer.

The patient's history may provide initial clues for the diagnosis of a focal intrahepatic lesion. Metastatic cancer would be suspected in patients with known or probable extrahepatic primary tumor capable of metastasis or in the wasted patient with a large, hard, irregular liver palpable in the epigastrium. The likelihood of primary hepatocellular carcinoma is increased among patients with chronic liver disease, particularly alcoholic cirrhosis and hemochromatosis, and in chronic carriers of hepatitis B virus, especially Oriental immigrants. Hepatic abscess must be considered in the febrile patient with a peripheral blood leukocytosis. An amebic abscess is suggested by the history of travel, within recent months, to Mexico or other endemic areas, and by a surprisingly rapid weight loss in a previously healthy person. Echinococcal cyst must be considered in patients who have immigrated from those parts of the world where echinococcal infection is endemic, even if the patient had moved from that area several decades earlier. If the patient presents, after the abrupt onset of abdominal pain, with hypotension or shock and is found to have blood in the peritoneal cavity, rupture of an hepatic adenoma, hepatocellular carcinoma, hemangioma, or angiosarcoma must be considered. The incidental discovery of a focal intrahepatic mass(es) in a patient without symptoms or whose symptoms seem unrelated to liver disease brings to mind hepatic hemangiomas, simple cysts, or focal nodular hyperplasia. If such an unsuspected mass is found in a woman on birth control pills, the possibility of hepatic adenoma is raised, but in persons of this age, the differential diagnosis must also include focal nodular hyperplasia and the fibrolamellar variant of hepatocellular carcinoma. The latter tumor usually is found in young and middle-aged persons of either sex, without a history of liver disease or of the other features associated with the typical form of hepatocellular carcinoma (Table 28–1).

On physical examination, in a lean patient, masses located on the surface of the liver may be visible and, when viewed from the patient's side, can be seen to move with respiration. Such masses are further defined by palpation and, again, are better appreciated by noting their movement as the liver shifts with respiration. Auscultation may reveal a bruit over a highly vascular tumor such as a hepatocellular carcinoma.

Table 28–1. COMPARISON OF TYPICAL HEPATOCELLULAR CARCINOMA AND THE FIBROLAMELLAR VARIANT

	Typical Hepatocellular Carcinoma	Fibrolamellar Carcinoma
Age at time of diagnosis	Fifth decade and older	5 to 35 years
Sex ratio	More common in males (3:1)	Equally common in both sexes
Condition of uninvolved liver	Cirrhosis in 70 to 90%	Normal
Associated factors	Prior or current HBV infection; cirrhosis; anabolic male steroids; aflatoxins?	None
Tumor calcification	Uncommon	About half of cases
Laboratory tests	Elevated serum alpha-fetoprotein (90% by RIA)	Elevated serum neurotensin levels (alpha-fetoprotein usually normal)

Because such bruits may be quite localized, it is essential to listen as the diaphragm of the stethoscope is systematically moved over the entire accessible liver surface. It should be noted that cavernous hemangiomas, the most common vascular malformations found in the liver, actually have very sluggish blood flow and are not associated with a bruit.

When the presence of a focal liver lesion is suspected on the basis of abnormal liver blood tests in a patient with known extrahepatic primary cancer, or because of findings on physical examination or radionuclide liver scanning, the next decision involves determination of the solid or cystic nature of the lesion. This decision is usually made best by abdominal ultrasound, supplemented if necessary by CT scanning, and in appropriate cases by fine-needle aspiration to obtain material for cytologic examination and culture.

In the majority of cases, the final decision about the nature of a focal hepatic lesion will be based on tissue obtained by "blind" percutaneous biopsy, laparoscopic biopsy under direct vision, or fine-needle or large-bore (e.g., Klatskin, Menghini) needle biopsy performed under CT or sonographic guidance.

IDENTIFICATION OF MASSES IN THE LIVER

Imaging Techniques

Although certain information of value for identification of hepatic masses may be obtained from the chest X-ray, plain film of the abdomen, and contrast roentgenograms of the upper gastrointestinal tract and colon, most often hepatic scintigraphy, ultrasonography, computed tomography, angiography, and increasingly, magnetic resonance imaging are required for adequate evaluation of focal liver masses. These imaging modalities are considered in this section.

Ultrasonography. Ultrasonography offers the advantages of a relatively inexpensive procedure, not involving ionizing radiation, that is able at times to identify focal liver lesions as small as 1 cm in diameter and is capable also of evaluating other abdominal organs such as kidneys, adrenal glands, spleen, and retroperitoneal area. Sonography is especially useful in distinguishing solid from cystic liver masses, and often is superior to CT in defining internal cyst structure. The limitations of ultrasound include its difficulty in evaluating obese patients, patients with marked ascites, or those with a large amount of intestinal gas; inability to visualize portions of the liver or kidney because of rib or lung interference; and the demonstration of "pseudole-sions" caused by anatomic variations and poor scanning technique. Because of these problems, 5 to 25 per cent of sonographic examinations are technically unsatisfactory.[1]

The accuracy of ultrasound is optimized by use of both conventional static B-scanning and real-time scanning.[1-3] Real-time scanning, performed with current high-resolution wide field of view scanners, provides information in the manner of fluoroscopy. This procedure, usually performed by a radiologist rather than a technician, allows easier intercostal and subcostal scanning of areas that are difficult to visualize on the static B-scan.

Sonography may be better able than CT to determine whether a large right upper quadrant abdominal mass lies within or adjacent to the liver because sonography may demonstrate a cleavage plane between the mass and the liver capsule.

It is the current consensus of many radiologists and clinicians that sonography has replaced radionuclide liver-spleen scanning as the primary screening modality for suspected hepatic tumor.[1, 2] Sonography is a useful means of following the response of liver tumor to therapy. Intraoperative ultrasound scanning, using a transducer applied directly to the liver surface, may allow the surgeon to detect lesions which he cannot see or palpate and which were not found on preoperative studies.

In any patient with single or multiple lesions visible by ultrasound, further evaluation by CT, angiography, magnetic resonance imaging (MRI), or biopsy may be indicated. Ultrasound is an excellent modality for guiding percutaneous needle aspiration or biopsy, often with a long flexible fine needle (22 or 23 gauge); this is discussed further in the Biopsy Techniques section later in this chapter.

Computed Tomography. For most focal liver lesions, CT provides an imaging resolution that is as great as or greater than sonography, in a standardized and reproducible fashion and with less of a requirement for operator expertise. Lesions as small as 5 mm in diameter can be detected with current high-resolution machines, particularly with use of contrast enhancement. CT is less subject to factors such as obesity, ascites, bowel gas, or intervening ribs or lung, which often result in unsatisfactory ultrasound examinations. Unlike hepatic scintigraphy, and more effectively than sonography, CT permits identification of coexistent extrahepatic lesions, such as tumors, cysts, and ab-

scesses, or hemoperitoneum due to bleeding from hepatocellular carcinoma, hepatic adenoma, angiosarcoma, or other hepatic lesions.[5]

The most apparent disadvantage of CT is its high cost as compared to sonography or radionuclide scanning. Other disadvantages of CT include the frequent need to use intravenous iodinated contrast agents, which pose the risks of allergic reactions and renal toxicity. The air-fluid interface in the gastric fundus, or metal clips from previous surgery may cause spray-like artifacts which tend to obscure parts of the adjacent liver. Streak-like artifacts caused by cardiac pulsation are regularly seen across the dome of the liver, but similar artifacts due to respiratory movement and intestinal peristalsis have become less of a problem with current fast (two seconds or less) scanners. Because unlabeled stomach and small bowel can mimic lymphadenopathy or other abdominal mass lesions during CT examination, it is necessary to identify these organs by having the patient drink contrast medium, generally several hours before the examination so that it has time to reach the terminal ileum. Although somewhat specific CT patterns suggesting the diagnosis of metastatic carcinoma, hepatocellular carcinoma, hemangioma, focal nodular hyperplasia, abscesses, and focal fatty infiltration have been described, in most cases CT does not provide a final diagnosis for any of these lesions.

Focal fatty infiltration may simulate an intrahepatic mass.[6] If this condition cannot be diagnosed by observing normally distributed portal branches within the low-density area, further studies including hepatic scintigraphy, often demonstrating the absence of a photopenic ("cold") defect in the area of concern, or biopsy may be necessary.

It has become apparent in recent years that contrast enhancement, appropriately applied, increases the sensitivity of CT for detection of focal liver lesions. This is used to greatest advantage with the dynamic technique in which exposures are made as frequently as possible within the first two minutes after the bolus intravenous infusion of iodinated contrast medium. The exposures are made either at a fixed level of a lesion identified on prior scans or with automated incremental movement of the table between exposures. Hypervascular lesions such as some hepatocellular carcinomas, or metastases from renal cell carcinoma, islet cell tumor, or angiosarcoma, display maximal intensification within 30 seconds after contrast infusion. Hypovascular tumors as well as cystic lesions become apparent by two minutes after infusion begins as areas less dense than the surrounding hepatic parenchyma. Abscesses and some tumor foci may display a peripheral halo of intensification early in the course of infusion.

The organ-specific CT contrast agent ethiodized oil emulsion 13 (EOE-13) is an emulsion of iodinated ester of poppy seed oil in a phosphate buffer.[7] After intravenous infusion, the labeled emulsion particles are cleared from the circulation primarily by phagocytic cells in the hepatic sinusoids and spleen, diffusely increasing the CT density of these organs beyond that which can be achieved with conventional iodinated contrast media. The increased density persists for 24 to 48 hours so that scanning time is not crucial. In a manner analogous to technetium sulfur colloid scintigraphy, most discrete hepatic masses, lacking phagocytic cells, are visualized as low-density foci. Although EOE-13 has been under study for several years, it has not yet been approved for general use by the Food and Drug Administration because of uncertainty about its safety and its stability in storage.[8] Although some radiologists feel that CT scanning should be the primary screening modality for focal liver lesions, sonography is generally regarded as the most appropriate means for such screening, having replaced radionuclide scintigraphy in this role.[9]

Hepatic Scintigraphy. The current standard approach to hepatic scintigraphy is gamma camera scanning of the liver and spleen after the intravenous injection of ^{99m}Tc-labeled sulfur colloid.[10] This radiochemical is selectively taken up by the Kupffer cells and other phagocytic littoral cells of these organs. Most intrahepatic masses are relatively devoid of such phagocytes and so appear as "cold" (photopenic) areas in the hepatic scintigram.

With the general availability of ultrasonography and CT, which are more effective means of evaluating focal liver lesions, relatively few indications remain for the use of hepatic scintigraphy. When a mass identified by ultrasonography or computed tomography is not visualized on the sulfur colloid scan, the diagnosis of focal nodular hyperplasia, or occasionally hepatic adenoma, is suggested. This occurs because the vascular spaces of these lesions retain a normal complement of phagocytic lining cells. In a patient who almost certainly has advanced primary or metastatic cancer in the liver, the liver scan may provide useful verification of a focal mass prior to confirmatory biopsy.[11] In the long-term follow-up of cirrhotic patients, a baseline scintigram may subsequently, by comparison, provide useful evidence of the later development of hepatocellular carcinoma. Hepatic scintigraphy may be the simplest and least expensive way to follow the response of hepatic metastases to chemotherapy or to monitor the resolution of amebic abscesses after effective medical therapy.

A "filling defect" in the scintigram of a liver which also displays evidence of cirrhosis (i.e., "patchy uptake" of isotope within the liver, disproportionate diversion of isotope to an enlarged spleen and to the bone marrow) suggests the presence of hepatocellular carcinoma. Finally, the absence of a scintigraphic defect in a liver in which irregular defects are shown by CT or ultrasound is consistent with focal fatty infiltration.

The earliest (hepatogram) phase of iminodiacetic acid biliary visualization studies (HIDA, PIPIDA, DISIDA) also constitutes a "liver scan," produced in this case by hepatocellular uptake of the radiochemical. Whether this type of liver scan may, at times, provide information beyond that provided by the conventional ^{99m}Tc sulfur colloid scan remains to be explored.

Angiography. Only one fourth to one third of the blood supply to normal liver is derived from the hepatic artery, the remainder coming from the portal vein. On the other hand, the blood supply to primary and metastatic tumor implants is almost entirely arterial. Accordingly, these tumors may be effectively imaged by arteriography. This is especially true for hypervascular lesions such as hepatocellular carcinoma and hemangioendothelioma, and vascular metastases from renal, adrenal, thyroid, and islet cell carcinomas, cystadenocarcinoma of the pancreas and ovary, carcinoid tumor, choriocarcinoma, and leiomyosarcoma as well as liver cell adenoma, focal nodular hyperplasia, arteriovenous malformations, and aneurysms.[12, 13]

With the advent of ultrasound, CT, and MRI scanning, diagnostic angiography is no longer commonly performed.[8] Angiography still plays an important role in the preoperative evaluation of patients who are candidates for excision of hepatocellular carcinoma or localized liver metastases. In this setting the arteriogram not only provides further assurance that all lesions are confined to a resectable region of the liver but also clarifies the often anomalous hepatic vascular anatomy for guidance of the surgeon.[13, 14]

In the preoperative study of hepatocellular carcinoma, visualization of the portal vein is important to rule out tumor invasion. The portal vein is opacified during the venous phase of a superior mesenteric or splenic artery contrast medium injection. Similarly, if there is reason to suspect invasion of the inferior vena cava, this is evaluated with a cavagram following infusion of contrast medium through a femoral vein catheter whose tip lies just above the confluence of the iliac veins. The major deficiencies of arteriography are its invasive nature and high cost, its requirement for great technical expertise on the part of the angiographer, and its weakness in demonstrating lesions in the left hepatic lobe.[15]

A recent report indicates that intra-arterial digital subtraction angiography (IADSA) may offer the advantage over conventional angiography of improved contrast resolution of hepatic tumors and of the portal vein branches. This is accomplished despite a significant reduction in the dose of contrast medium required, of particular importance for patients with impaired renal function. Because only selected images are recorded on film, the cost and time of film processing are reduced and the examination time is reduced. The major limitation of IADSA is its restricted field of view so that the left and right hepatic lobes must be studied separately.[16]

Magnetic Resonance Imaging. The technical principles on which magnetic resonance imaging is based are described in several reviews concerning this imaging modality.[17-21] Optimal definition of focal liver masses by MRI is accomplished by taking advantage of differences in the so-called longitudinal (T1) and transverse (T2) relaxation times of these lesions and the surrounding liver tissue. Increases in T1 and T2 are seen in a variety of pathologic processes in which the water content of a lesion is increased (e.g., inflammation, edema, and many tumors), and a relative decrease in

T1 is seen in such conditions as subacute hemorrhage and fibrotic and fatty lesions.[19]

Tumors have prolonged T1 and T2 times which vary in different types of tumors and within regions of a single tumor. It is not possible to ascribe a specific T1 or T2 value to any particular tumor. By MRI one cannot reliably distinguish between primary and metastatic tumor in the liver.[22, 23]

MRI may prove to be useful in staging hepatocellular carcinoma (see Fig. 28–4). The extent of these tumors may not be well defined on CT examination because of uncertainty in distinguishing tumor from the frequently coexisting cirrhosis. This differentiation can often be made with greater confidence on an NMR image,[23] and invasion or occlusion of major vessels may be demonstrated.

At present, the greatest value of hepatic NMR imaging is in the identification of cavernous hemangiomas, and T2-weighted MRI may become the procedure of choice for distinguishing hemangioma from liver cancer (see Fig. 28–7).[24] The sensitivity and specificity of MRI for identifying hemangiomas have been reported to exceed those of technetium-tagged red blood cell flow study, sonography, or dynamic contrast-enhanced CT.[24] MRI may be particularly useful for diagnosing hemangiomas less than 2 cm in diameter, for such small hemangiomas are especially difficult to diagnose by other means.

NMR shares with sonography and CT the ability to produce high-quality tomographic images. At the commonly used magnetic field strengths, MRI does not appear to pose any biologic risk.[20] Additional advantages include the ability to produce multiple images in any desired plane, without the use of ionizing radiation. For example, an NMR image in the sagittal plane may permit the differentiation of intrahepatic tumor from retroperitoneal tumors protruding into the liver parenchyma, a distinction which can be extremely difficult or even impossible to make by CT.[23] In comparison with CT, internal architecture and the relationship of tumors to hepatic vascular structures are better displayed on MRI.[21] MRI offers superior contrast sensitivity, clear differentiation of vascular and nonvascular structures without the need for intravenous contrast administration, and significantly less artifact from metal and dense calcification.[25] The lack of artifact from the air-fluid interface in the stomach is an advantage over CT in detecting metastases within the left lobe of the liver.[19] If MRI becomes as widely available as CT and can be performed at comparable cost, it is likely in most cases to replace CT for evaluation of intrahepatic masses.

Biopsy Techniques

Percutaneous Biopsy Techniques. Decisions concerning whether to do a needle biopsy of a focal liver mass and, if so, which technique to employ must be based on the probable nature of the lesion. For example, there is a significant risk of serious hemorrhage if a cavernous hemangioma or liver cell adenoma is punctured with the standard biopsy needle (Klatskin, Menghini, or similar needle). Although this risk is reduced when a fine needle is used, the amount of tissue obtained with such needles from these particular lesions is not likely to be of diagnostic value, and if tissue diagnosis is considered essential, the biopsy should be obtained under direct vision—at laparoscopy or at time of surgery, in the latter case sometimes with resection of the lesion.

When the liver is massively involved with probable tumor, primary or metastatic, percutaneous blind biopsy with a Klatskin or similar type of needle may be the most expeditious means of obtaining diagnostic tissue. In patients with prominent (apparent) tumor involvement of the left hepatic lobe, who have a firm irregular mass palpable in the epigastrium, direct biopsy into this area is appropriate; to minimize the risk of puncturing the superior epigastric artery, the needle should enter the abdominal wall in the midline. With the operator at the left side of the bed, the needle can be directed rightward if greater tumor mass is believed to lie in that direction. Because the liver surface lies closer to the skin in the epigastrium, the needle need not be passed as deeply as when the intercostal approach is used.

If the apparent tumor is of a size or in a location such that it is not likely to be reached with the standard blind needle technique, which is limited in the approaches by which the needle safely can be introduced, sonography- or CT-guided biopsy may be more appropriate. The choice between these two imaging techniques is based on the characteristics of the lesion(s) to be biopsied. In general, it is reasonable to use the simplest imaging method which adequately delineates tumor; lesions more than 3 cm in diameter, peripherally located, may be biopsied with sonographic guidance. Smaller, deeper lesions or those in relatively inaccessible locations are better biopsied under CT guidance.[2]

The imaging techniques, in addition to defining the spatial position of an intrahepatic mass, can demonstrate the optimal needle path for access to the lesion, often by way of an approach one would not feel safe in taking "blindly." Use of the fine needle is necessary for lesions located more deeply or in otherwise inaccessible locations. An additional advantage of the fine needle is the probable reduced risk of hemorrhage. This is of particular importance if there is concern about the presence of a hypervascular lesion or a marginal bleeding diathesis.

With the fine needle one obtains a cellular aspirate and often, in addition, small tissue fragments. With the growing popularity of guided fine-needle biopsy technique, pathologists are becoming increasingly skilled in the interpretation of specimens obtained by this means. The cytopathologist should be present as the procedure is being done to receive the specimen and immediately prepare appropriate smears of the cellular aspirate. Any tissue fragments are placed directly in formalin. Alternatively, after instruction by the pathologist, the physician performing the aspiration may also handle the tissue preparation.[26]

Laparoscopy. Laparoscopy (peritoneoscopy) should be considered when abnormal laboratory data or hepatomegaly lead to concern about liver metastases or when results of screening with sonography and CT have been inconclusive. Laparoscopy may be particularly useful in determining the resectability of hepatocellular carcinoma by helping define the extent of tumor as well as the condition of the uninvolved portion of the liver.[28] Peritoneoscopy may obviate the need for laparotomy in a number of patients being staged for Hodgkin's disease. Laparoscopy permits detection of metastases as small as a few millimeters in diameter, both on the liver surface and on the peritoneum; these lesions may be biopsied under direct vision. Laparoscopy is especially useful in identification and biopsy of lesions in the left hepatic lobe and left portion of the right lobe when these portions of the liver are not enlarged to the extent that blind percutaneous biopsy can be done.[27]

It is estimated that 80 per cent of the liver surface can be inspected at peritoneoscopy.[28] Autopsy and surgical data indicate that in about 90 per cent of livers containing metastatic cancer metastases are visible on the liver surface.[29, 30] In addition, some subcapsular tumor masses produce a visible bulge on the liver surface. In the case of hypervascular tumors, a biopsy site can be selected away from large surface vessels.

SPECIFIC DISEASES AND CONDITIONS PRESENTING AS FOCAL HEPATIC LESIONS

In the following sections the diagnosis and management of the most common conditions which may present as masses in the liver are discussed.

Metastatic Cancer in the Liver

Recognition of neoplastic disease in the liver may significantly influence the patient's treatment and prognosis. Ideally, evaluation begins with the less invasive and less costly of the several methods available for detection of liver neoplasms. The work-up proceeds to more risky and expensive tests only when they are essential for arriving at a definitive diagnosis. Because unequivocal diagnosis usually requires a tissue biopsy, this should be done as early in the investigation as possible—for example, before undertaking studies to identify a primary extrahepatic tumor.[31]

It is nearly inevitable that this search for cancer will cause the patient anxiety. Clearly, the physician should do whatever possible, short of offering unrealistic assurances, to alleviate this fear.

A few tumor types, such as colorectal cancer, carcinoid, and of course, hepatocellular carcinoma, may present with metastases confined to the liver. Most tumors that metastasize to the liver, such as breast and lung cancer, often spread at the same time to other sites.[32] In the past, preoperative staging of colorectal cancer was not considered necessary because surgery was usually indicated to remove the primary tumor and intraoperative staging was adequate. Now, however, preoperative documentation of liver metastases can alter the planned surgery by demonstrating the feasibility of resection of isolated liver metastases or, in some centers, to facilitate plans for placement of an hepatic artery catheter and chemotherapy infusion pump.[33]

If the history, physical examination, and routine liver blood tests suggest metastatic tumor in the liver, an ultrasound or CT examination is then done. The latter modalities have largely replaced hepatic scintigraphy as means of identifying hepatic tumors because of the equal or better sensitivity and greater specificity of these techniques. Sulfur colloid scintigraphy remains a useful technique for assessing the tumor size response to chemotherapy. Angiography, an invasive and expensive procedure, is rarely employed in the search for liver metastases. Magnetic resonance imaging is not yet widely available, and it remains to be determined whether this technique will become preferable to sonography or CT for detection of liver metastases (Fig. 28–1).

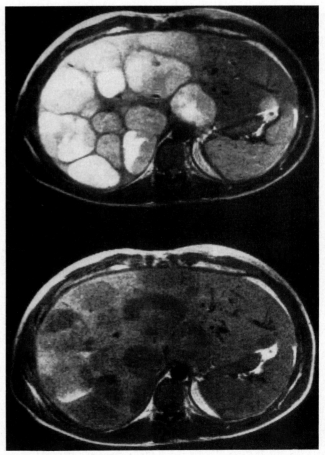

Figure 28–1. Liver metastases from small cell lung cancer; T2- *(upper)* and T1-weighted *(lower)* MRI images. The numerous round and polygonal lesions range in size from 2 to 6 cm. Areas of increased signal on both T1- and T2-weighted images represent hemorrhage within the tumors. The tumor tissue appears relatively dark on the T1 images. (Provided by Dr. Jesse Cohen.)

If focal liver lesions consistent with metastases are identified by imaging studies, a biopsy is usually required to confirm the presence of tumor and to determine its histologic type. This is discussed in detail in the Biopsy Techniques section of this chapter.

Routinely obtained blood tests may provide evidence for or against the presence of liver metastases. Most useful among these has been the alkaline phosphatase test, whose sensitivity and specificity for detection of hepatic metastases are both about 75 per cent.[34] Elevated serum levels of lactic dehydrogenase (LDH), carcinoembryonic antigen (CEA), and the aminotransaminases (aspartate aminotransferase—AST, SGOT; and alanine aminotransferase—ALT, SGPT) also increase suspicion that liver metastases are present. It has been shown that in the patient with a documented extrahepatic primary cancer and a normal alkaline phosphatase a radionuclide liver-spleen scan does not reliably identify hepatic metastases,[35, 36] but it remains to be determined whether sonography, CT, or MRI is capable of demonstrating liver metastases in such patients.

By ultrasound examination, hepatic metastases are most often hypoechoic but can display a wide spectrum of appearances, varying from relatively anechoic lesions to highly echogenic masses. The sonographic pattern has little specificity for tumor type. Necrotic areas are frequently recognized, particularly in sarcomas. Being hypoechoic, necrotic tumors sometimes simulate hepatic cysts. Truly cystic metastases sometimes arise from ovarian serous adenocarcinoma, bronchogenic carcinoma, gastric adenocarcinoma, endometrial carcinoma, choriocarcinoma, leiomyosarcoma, or soft tissue sarcoma.[37] Lymphoma tends to be very homogeneous and most often appears as hypoechoic areas with little attenuation of the sound beam. About a third of all tumors are mixed, containing areas both more and less echogenic than the surrounding liver tissue. Diffuse infiltration, as is the metastatic pattern of some lymphomas, small cell lung cancer, or breast cancer, produces subtle abnormalities in the liver sonographic image.[38]

Certain sonographic findings raise the suspicion of particular types of tumor. Calcification in a solid lesion suggests metastasis from a mucinous adenocarcinoma, such as a primary colorectal or ovarian cancer. Sonographic evidence of cirrhosis as a background for a focal hepatic mass, in the absence of detectable primary extrahepatic tumor, is typical of hepatocellular carcinoma. Dilated intrahepatic ducts, with a normal extrahepatic biliary tree, with or without a visible mass in the hilum, suggest cholangiocarcinoma of the hepatic duct confluence, i.e., a Klatskin tumor. Most regenerative nodules detected as photopenic defects on radionuclide scans have typical cirrhotic architecture on ultrasound scan, which tends to rule out tumor.

Recent studies of intraoperative sonography, performed at the time of laparotomy for abdominal cancer, suggest that this may be a very sensitive test for metastases which are not detectable on preoperative studies or revealed by the surgeon's inspection and palpation of the liver.[4]

By computed tomography most metastases appear as low attenuation lesions on plain or contrast-enhanced studies. Metastases may be hyperdense when present in a fatty liver or if they are calcified, as is the case for some metastases from papillary or mucinous adenocarcinomas or leiomyosarcomas.[37] With dynamic scanning, as many images as possible are obtained during the first two minutes or so after bolus infusion of contrast material. By this technique metastases may be of increased, mixed, or decreased attenuation, depending on lesion vascularity and the circulatory phase during which the image is obtained. Hypervascular metastases may arise from hypernephroma, endocrine neoplasms such as islet cell tumor, carcinoid tumor, choriocarcinoma, adrenal carcinoma, sarcoma, and breast carcinoma. Primary cancers of stomach, pancreas, lung, esophagus, and colon often have hypovascular metastases.[13] Dynamic CT appears to be more sensitive for detection of metastases than CT performed without contrast enhancement or after contrast equilibration with tumor foci after slow infusion of contrast material.[8, 37]

As is also true for sonography, CT may display necrotic tumors and cystic metastases and aid in distinguishing these lesions from true cysts and abscesses. More effectively than ultrasound, CT may demonstrate extrahepatic primary tumor, metastases, or lymphadenopathy.

Although it is anticipated that magnetic resonance imaging may become a powerful means for identification of liver metastases, realization of its full capability probably awaits technical advances in hardware and programming (see Fig. 28–1). It remains to be seen whether MRI can become cost competitive with sonography and CT imaging.

At laparotomy almost 90 per cent of hepatic metastases are visible on the liver surface, and larger deep tumors can be felt.[30, 39] At laparotomy, the surgeon will be able to identify metastases, by inspection and palpation, in 95 per cent of patients ultimately shown to have them.[29] As noted above, additional lesions may be identified by intraoperative real-time sonography using a transducer (enclosed in a sterile wrapping) applied directly to the surface of the liver. It is obligatory that the surgeon biopsy even the most "obvious" liver metastases because of the occasional finding of benign tumors such as adenomas, focal nodular hyperplasia, massive sarcoid or other granulomatous lesions, or unrelated, possibly treatable, malignancies—all of which may masquerade as metastases from a known primary abdominal tumor.

Hodgkin's Disease and Non-Hodgkin's Lymphoma

Demonstration of liver involvement is important in all forms of lymphoma. Extension to the liver is one criterion of stage IV Hodgkin's disease (HD), which is an indication for chemotherapy rather than radiation therapy alone. At staging laparotomy, approximately 5 per cent of untreated patients with Hodgkin's disease and 15 per cent of patients with non-Hodgkin's lymphoma (NHL) have liver involvement.[40] In HD patients a laparotomy can be avoided if hepatic tumor is demonstrated by biopsy. The mere presence of abnormal liver blood tests is not sufficient evidence for a diagnosis of HD in the liver because extrahepatic HD may, by an undefined mechanism, lead to granuloma development in the liver.[41]

Hodgkin's disease almost always invades the spleen before the liver.[42] Splenomegaly suggests the presence of tumor but approximately one third of enlarged spleens are disease-free and one third of normal-sized spleens in untreated patients are shown to contain tumor at autopsy.[40] CT is insensitive in detecting splenic involvement by HD or NHL.[40]

When the patient first presents with HD or NHL, liver involvement, if present, typically is in the form of small scattered nodules which are difficult to identify by any means other than direct inspection of the liver surface. However, CT may be useful in demonstrating hepatic hilar and retroperitoneal lymphadenopathy.[43]

If there is evidence of probable advanced tumor in the liver, percutaneous biopsy with a standard large-bore needle may be the most direct means of obtaining tissue confirmation of the diagnosis.[42] When there is no evidence of gross hepatic tumor involvement, and this remains an important issue, such as in the staging of HD, peritoneoscopy should be performed. If present, tumor implants often appear on the liver surface as multiple white macules or papules less than 3 mm in diameter. These lesions should be biopsied under direct vision. If no such lesions are seen, multiple (usually six) biopsies should be obtained from various sites in both hepatic lobes.[42] Extensive experience has shown that, overall, fewer than 10 per cent of patients with negative peritoneoscopic biopsies will be found to have hepatic HD on wedge biopsy obtained at subsequent laparotomy.[42, 43] Although peritoneoscopy also provides diagnostic information in a number of patients with non-Hodgkin's lymphoma whose preceding studies have been negative, about half of the patients with negative peritoneoscopic biopsies will have positive surgical wedge biopsies showing only rare, focal lymphomatous involvement of portal areas.[42] Peritoneoscopy is also useful for repeated abdominal examinations to evaluate the effects of treatment on liver metastases in patients with previously documented HD and NHL.[28]

Hepatocellular Carcinoma

Hepatocellular carcinoma (HCC) is an uncommon tumor in Western countries, but because of its high prevalence in the Orient, Pacific islands, and sub-Saharan Africa, it is the most common lethal tumor worldwide. In the United States, HCC is roughly three times more common in men than women, and most patients are more than 50 years old.

A major risk factor for the development of HCC is hepatitis B virus (HBV) infection. In Taiwan, Beasley et al. have demonstrated a greater than 200-fold increased risk to HBV carriers of developing this cancer.[44] Although HBV DNA, integrated into the tumor genomic DNA, is consistently demonstrable in these patients,[45] the precise means by which this virus relates to the etiology of HCC is unknown. Cirrhosis is a common, but not obligatory, intermediate in the relationship between HBV infection and HCC.

Aflatoxins, metabolites of fungi which contaminate stored grains and other foodstuffs in tropical areas, are known to be potent experimental carcinogens. Although the prevalence of HCC is also very high in some of these tropical areas, notably southern Africa, it now appears that HBV is the predominant cause of liver cancers in those areas. It remains to be determined whether aflatoxin may, in fact, be an important cocarcinogen in conjunction with HBV or other factors. There is increasing suspicion that chronic non-A, non-B virus infection may also promote the development of HCC.[46, 47] There is an increased incidence of HCC in persons who are long-term users of synthetic male hormones and anabolic steroids.

In a majority of cases—70 to 90 per cent—hepatomas develop in patients with pre-existing cirrhosis. Patients with cirrhosis, apparently regardless of its etiology, are at greatly increased risk of developing HCC. Although the relative risk of developing HCC has generally been considered lower in patients with alcoholic cirrhosis than in those with posthepatitic, cryptogenic, or hemochromatotic cirrhosis, studies comparing hepatoma prevalence at autopsy among patients with different etiologies of cirrhosis have failed to show significant differences among these groups.[48, 49] In some series as many as 27 and 30 per cent of livers from cirrhotic alcoholics were found at time of autopsy to harbor HCC.[48, 50] Owing to its great frequency, alcoholic cirrhosis is the most common predisposing factor for development of HCC in Western countries. Although this tumor has been present in up to one third of reported hemochromatosis patients at the time of death, no case of HCC has yet been reported in a precirrhotic patient with this condition.[51] It is expected, therefore, that prevention of cirrhosis by aggressive phlebotomy therapy of young hemochromatosis patients may essentially eliminate their risk of developing HCC.

The natural history of HCC is one of rapid progression, with death occurring at a median time of four to six months after onset of symptoms. This rate of progression is only modestly slowed by currently available chemotherapy regimens. A few patients, generally fewer than 10 per cent, are candidates for surgical resection, which may sometimes be curative. Five-year survival rates of 6 to 23 per cent following resection have been reported.[52, 53]

Common presenting symptoms of HCC are right upper quadrant pain, weight loss, unexplained fever, weakness, and awareness of an abdominal mass or fullness. On physical examination, often in addition to evidence of chronic liver disease, a right upper quadrant abdominal mass moving with respiration may be visible and palpable. A bruit, often highly localized, may be present over the lesion.

A number of paraneoplastic manifestations of HCC have been reported.[54] Erythrocytosis is the most common of these, occurring in up to 12 per cent of patients in some series. The increase is confined to the red blood cell mass, without changes in leukocytes or platelets. It has been speculated that, in such cases, the tumor is either secreting an erythropoietin-like substance or increased amounts of the globulin precursor of erythropoietin normally secreted by the liver and activated by renal erythropoiesis stimulating factor.[55, 56] Less frequent paraneoplastic concomitants of HCC are hypercalcemia, hypoglycemia, hypertrophic osteoarthropathy, and hypercholesterolemia.

Fibrolamellar carcinoma is a rare variant of HCC, constituting about 1 per cent of primary liver cell cancers. A number of features which distinguish this variant from typical HCC are summarized in Table 28–1. Histologically, fibrolamellar carcinoma is characterized by the presence of well-organized, layered (lamellar) collagen bands, and by prominent eosinophilic, polygonal hepatocytes, many of which contain intracytoplasmic hyaline globules and pale bodies. The importance of diagnosing this tumor lies in the likelihood that, even when large, it may be surgically resectable, thereby leading to prolonged survival or cure. The absence of complicating cirrhosis or HBV infection, and the young age and overall good health of patients with fibrolamellar carcinoma account for its frequent resectability and relatively good prognosis.

The only certain means of ruling out fibrolamellar carcinoma is by obtaining tissue. Because it may be difficult to distinguish this tumor from hepatic adenoma or focal nodular hyperplasia on a single needle biopsy specimen, it may be necessary to obtain multiple needle biopsies from different areas of the tumor at peritoneoscopy or laparotomy.[57]

The gross and histologic features of fibrolamellar carcinoma have been confused with both focal nodular hyperplasia and liver cell adenoma. Because the latter tumors, being benign, may not require resection, this diagnostic distinction is particularly important. Because of similar histologic features of fibrolamellar carcinoma and focal nodular hyperplasia, it has been suggested that the cancer may arise from this benign tumor.[58] However, current evidence indicates that malignant transformation of focal nodular hyperplasia is very rare.

The diagnosis of hepatocellular carcinoma should be suspected in patients with chronic liver disease who undergo rather abrupt and unexplained deterioration. If the history or physical examination is consistent with the presence of this tumor, tests should be done for hepatitis B surface antigen (HBsAg) and alpha-fetoprotein. Alpha-fetoprotein, an alpha-1 globulin, is present in high concentration in fetal serum, but levels become extremely low after birth; normal adult levels are less than 30 ng/ml. Prevalence of elevated serum concentrations of alpha-fetoprotein among hepatoma patients, when measured by radioimmunoassay, is in the range of 70 to 90 per cent. The serum alpha-fetoprotein concentration is less frequently elevated in patients with small hepatocellular carcinomas,[59] which detracts somewhat from its value as a screening test in areas of high HCC prevalence. Nevertheless, because of its convenience and relatively low cost, it continues to be used as a screening test in those areas. Elevated levels of alpha-fetoprotein may also be observed in patients with germ cell malignancies (teratocarcinomas) of the ovary and testis, other carcinomas or lymphomas, especially when these have metastasized to the liver, and acute and chronic hepatitis. The specificity of this test for HCC is increased when serum levels exceed 1000 ng/ml.[60] In the future assays based on monoclonal antibodies to alpha-fetoprotein may prove to be more specific for the diagnosis of hepatocellular carcinoma.[61]

By any of the commonly used imaging techniques, HCC may appear as a major solitary focus with or without a small number of additional implants, as multifocal disease with or without one or a few dominant tumors, or as diffuse infiltration. Although no completely pathognomonic features of HCC are provided by any of the imaging studies, certain characteristic features, discussed below, are recognized. By ^{99m}Tc sulfur colloid liver-spleen scan, the most typical presentation of HCC is a large hepatic mass in a patient with other scintigraphic evidence of cirrhosis—i.e., diffuse inhomogeneity of liver isotope uptake, an enlarged spleen with greater isotope concentration than the liver, and "shunting" of isotope to the marrow of bones visible on the scan—spine, ribs, and pelvis (Figs. 28–2 and 28–3). Other radionuclide scanning techniques may provide support for the diagnosis of HCC. Gallium (^{67}Ga) often concentrates in hepatoma cells,

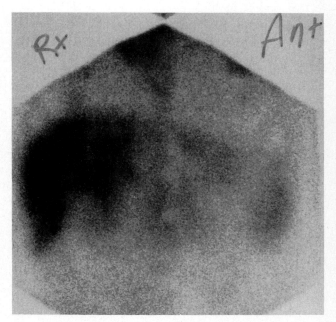

Figure 28–2. Technetium-99m sulfur colloid liver-spleen scan showing a large, irregular, photopenic ("cold") area in the left hepatic lobe due to hepatocellular carcinoma.

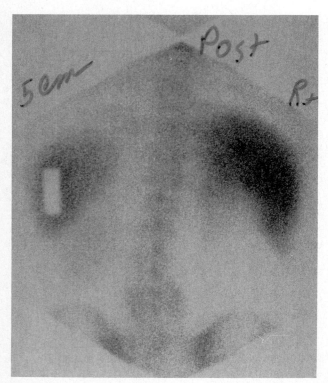

Figure 28–3. Posterior view of the sulfur colloid liver-spleen scan of the patient shown in Figure 28–2, showing diversion of radiocolloid to the spleen and to the spinal and pelvic bone marrow due to cirrhosis with portal hypertension. The hepatoma defect is obscured by the spine. (Provided by Dr. Theodore R. Simon.)

causing the tumor to appear as a "hot spot" on scintigrams made 24 to 72 hours after radionuclide injection. Abscesses, lymphomas, and some metastases may also produce a positive scan, and these must be ruled out by other means. Like normal hepatocytes, hepatoma cells may take up biliary imaging agents (^{99m}Tc-labeled iminodiacetic acid derivatives, such as DISIDA), but unlike normal liver cells, the tumor cells cannot excrete the tracer into the bile. As a result, the tumor may appear as a focus of increased density on scans made four hours or so after isotope injection.

By ultrasound examination, hepatocellular carcinoma has a widely varied appearance.[38] Small tumors tend to be hypoechoic, but as they enlarge, development of necrosis and fibrosis often leads to a mixed hyper- and hypoechoic pattern. Large tumors may show a core of low echogenicity due to central necrosis. Such a tumor is distinguished from hepatic cysts and abscesses by its thick, irregular wall. Owing to lung interference, sonography may fail to visualize tumors in the lateral dome of the right hepatic lobe.[62]

Hepatocellular carcinoma also has a variable appearance on CT scanning. A frequent appearance is an isodense mass encompassed by a narrow, low-density ring which becomes enhanced following contrast medium infusion.[63] Other hepatomas are heterogeneous in intensity prior to contrast medium infusion, and with it are enhanced in an intense inhomogeneous pattern.[64] The tumor may be shown to bulge from the

liver surface. There may be decreased attenuation of an entire hepatic lobe due to tumor occlusion of the portal vein branch to that lobe.[63]

Angiography of HCC often reveals a hypervascular mass with arteriovenous shunting, capillary staining, tumor neovascularity, encasement of large arteries, and portal venous obstruction. Although hypervascularity is the most common finding, in large tumors there are often hypo- or avascular areas resulting from vascular obstruction, necrosis, and hemorrhage in the tumor.[65] Angiography can define the hepatic vascular anatomy to aid the surgeon during tumor resection.[66]

Magnetic resonance imaging appears to be as sensitive as CT for detection of small hepatomas, without the need for contrast enhancement (Fig. 28–4). The precise role of MRI in evaluation of HCC remains to be determined.[67]

Evaluation of Patients with Suspected HCC. When the diagnosis of HCC is reasonably certain, it is of primary importance to determine whether the tumor may be surgically resectable. Patients are excluded as surgical candidates if they have clinically significant

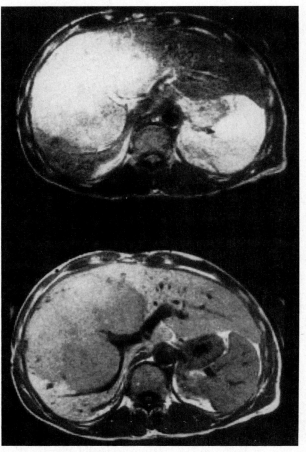

Figure 28–4. Hepatocellular carcinoma; T2- *(upper)* and T1-weighted *(lower)* MRI images. The large intrahepatic mass has prolonged T1 and T2 relaxation times. The lesion involves the right lobe and medial segment of the left lobe. This finding, which was not apparent on the CT scan, indicates that, if other conditions are appropriate, this very large tumor may be resectable by means of a trisegmentectomy procedure. (Provided by Dr. Jesse Cohen.)

cirrhosis, evidence of extrahepatic tumor spread, or other disease making them unable to tolerate major surgery. Although patients often die of HCC without clinically evident dissemination, when metastases occur they are most likely to be in local lymph nodes, the lungs, and the bones. Metastasis to these areas is reasonably excluded on the basis of a negative abdominal CT examination, chest X-ray, and radionuclide bone scan, respectively. The final criteria of resectability relate to the intrahepatic extent of tumor. For successful resection, the tumor must be confined to the right hepatic lobe or the lateral (leftmost) segment of the left lobe. In some centers, right lobe tumors extending into the medial segment of the left lobe may also be excised, with a so-called trisegmentectomy procedure.

In most cases, the patient should not be considered an operative candidate until cleared by ultrasound, CT, and angiographic studies. Each of these techniques may, in different cases, disclose foci of tumor or its extension not revealed by the other studies. Very small (less than 2 cm) tumor foci may be seen as hypoechogenic lesions at sonography. Small hypervascular tumors may be recognized when they become hyperintense after contrast infusion during dynamic CT or superselective (hepatic artery) angiography. Any of the three studies may lead to recognition of abdominal tumor metastases. CT and ultrasound have an advantage over angiography in reliably imaging the left hepatic lobe. Tumor invasion of the main portal vein or vena cava may be identified by ultrasound, dynamic CT, hepatic angiography, and MRI. Such vascular invasion precludes surgical resection.

Unless the presence of a high (greater than 1000 ng/ml) serum alpha-fetoprotein concentration makes the diagnosis of hepatoma nearly certain, biopsy should be performed for tissue confirmation. This is true regardless of whether the patient is a surgical candidate. Hepatocellular adenoma, focal nodular hyperplasia, and hemangioma, which are lesions carrying a high risk of bleeding, should be excluded with reasonable certainty before attempting biopsy. Despite the vascularity of some hepatomas, blind percutaneous large-bore (Klatskin, Menghini) needle biopsy can be performed without excessive risk, and this is the most direct means of obtaining diagnostic tissue from an accessible mass. There is little evidence that such a biopsy leads to tumor spread to the peritoneum, needle track, or other parts of the body. If blind biopsy is not feasible because of the location of the lesion(s) or concern about increased risk of bleeding, sonographic or CT-guided fine needle aspiration may provide diagnostic tissue, although in the case of well-differentiated tumors, it may be difficult for the pathologist to distinguish isolated hepatoma cells from normal or dysplastic hepatocytes.

Because of the frequency of HCC in Japan, programs have been established in that country for the regular screening of cirrhotic and HBsAg-positive patients to detect early hepatocellular carcinomas.[68] Various approaches have been taken, involving different combinations of alpha-fetoprotein testing, hepatic scintigraphy, sonography, angiography, CT (particularly with dynamic contrast technique), and MRI. The currently favored approach is the combined use of alpha-fetoprotein testing and real-time ultrasound examination.[62, 69] The patient is evaluated periodically, usually every three months. The objective is to identify hepatomas at a time when they can be curable by resection. It has been shown that, over time, the small tumors (2 to 5 cm in diameter) identified in these surveys have the same lethal potential as large hepatomas.[70]

In some cases in which HCC is suspected but the diagnosis remains uncertain after initial evaluation, it may be appropriate to perform repeat studies at short intervals, such as monthly ultrasound examination and serum alpha-fetoprotein measurement, and six-month dynamic CT, angiographic CT (CT during contrast infusion via hepatic artery catheter) or conventional hepatic angiography.[71]

Other Primary Liver Cancers

Primary sarcomas of the liver are rare. Hemangiosarcoma and hemangioendothelioma display some of the characteristics of cavernous hemangioma, but at angiography differ by having larger feeding vessels and showing arteriovenous shunts, vessel encasement, and true neovascularity.[13]

Cholangiocarcinomas may arise from the small bile ducts in the periphery of the liver, from the larger hilar ducts, or from the extrahepatic biliary tree including the papilla of Vater.[72, 73] There is little histologic difference among the tumors in these locations; they are adenocarcinomas with abundant fibrous stroma, and so may be mistaken for benign fibrous strictures. Those arising in the periphery of the liver occasionally resemble hepatocellular carcinoma in clinical features and gross morphologic appearance, while hilar (Klatskin) tumors present with obstructive jaundice with dilated intrahepatic ducts and a normal extrahepatic biliary system.

Cholangiocarcinoma is equally common in both sexes and is unassociated with cirrhosis or hepatitis B virus infection. Serum alpha-fetoprotein levels are not elevated. These tumors develop with increased frequency in patients with sclerosing cholangitis (who often have chronic ulcerative colitis) and choledochal cysts, which may be intrahepatic. The association with gallstones and, in the Far East, with liver fluke infestation is uncertain.

Peripheral cholangiocarcinoma is difficult to distinguish from HCC or other solitary liver tumors by means other than biopsy. In some cases suggestive angiographic features may be present, including arterial encasement or obstruction of vessels around the liver hilus and thin, irregular tumor vessels in the porta hepatis. Compared with HCC, cholangiocarcinoma is more invasive and less expansive and shows less neovascularity.[13] Cholangiocarcinomas often contain calcifications.[57] They do not accumulate gallium.

When the presence of a hilar (Klatskin) tumor is suggested by the sonographic findings, further definition of the tumor is provided by endoscopic retrograde cholangiography or percutaneous transhepatic cholangiography. If hilar cholangiocarcinoma is recognized early enough, it may be successfully resected. Obstructive jaundice due to unresectable tumor may be relieved ˌby transhepatic or retrograde placement of stents. Radiation therapy may be of some benefit, but chemotherapy is ineffective.

Cavernous Hemangioma

Cavernous hemangioma is considered the most common benign tumor of the liver, being found in 0.4 to 7.3 per cent of autopsy cases.[74] These vascular tumors are considered congenital hamartomas or tissue malformations, present at birth.[75] Women predominate in most series. It has been suggested that estrogens promote the growth of these lesions,[74] and rarely, they may enlarge during pregnancy.[76] Typically, cavernous hemangiomas are solitary, subcapsular, and less than 5 cm in diameter. However, multiple lesions are not uncommon, and giant hemangiomas may occupy an entire hepatic lobe.[75, 77, 78] Histologically, cavernous hemangiomas consist of a cluster of large blood spaces, some "cavernous," lined by a single row of endothelial cells and supported by fibrous septa. Central fibrosis is common, particularly in larger hemangiomas, and calcification may develop in this scar tissue.[75, 76]

The natural history of cavernous hemangioma is not clearly defined. In a series of 36 untreated patients observed for an average of 5.5 years (maximum, 15 years) three lesions became smaller and three enlarged slightly. None of the lesions bled, and none of the patients died or noted increased symptoms beyond any they may have presented with.[79, 80] It is evident that cavernous hemangiomas should be left untreated in patients with few or no symptoms unless the lesion is so large that it presents a threat of bleeding.[75, 80] However, some hemangiomas, particularly very large ones, may cause symptoms due to pressure on adjacent organs and intralesional bleeding or thrombosis. Rarely, life-threatening intraperitoneal hemorrhage occurs.[79] If technically feasible, hemangiomas producing symptoms should be surgically resected.[75, 80] If excision is not possible, irradiation, hepatic artery ligation,[81] or transcatheter arterial embolization may be attempted[82]; the value of these approaches is not well documented. In occasional cases, cavernous hemangioma has been associated with the Kasabach-Merritt syndrome, a variety of disseminated intravascular coagulation, characterized by thrombocytopenia and hypofibrinogenemia which resolves when the hemangioma is surgically removed.[81]

Diagnosis of Cavernous Hemangioma. Most often, cavernous hemangiomas are identified incidentally in the course of hepatic scintigraphy, sonography, or CT examination performed for reasons unrelated to the hemangioma. Sonography is a sensitive but nonspecific means of identifying cavernous hemangiomas. The sonographic appearance of these lesions is quite varied, but typically, they are hyperechoic, sharply marginated, and internally homogeneous subcapsular lesions. This echogenicity has been attributed to the multiple sonoreflective interfaces between the walls of the cavernous spaces and the blood within them.[75] Alternatively, they may be hypoechoic with homogeneous internal echoes or strong marginal echoes.[83, 84] Large lesions, greater than 5 cm in diameter, may have a more heterogeneous and an irregular pattern, which may be suggestive of focal nodular hyperplasia. Foci of calcification produce intense echoes and acoustic shadowing. Although small hemangiomas are often subcapsular, those deeper in the liver tend to be larger and more heterogeneous, and show areas of sonolucency apparently due to thrombosis. Most of these deeper lesions lie close to a hepatic vein tributary.[85]

The characteristic enhancement pattern of cavernous hemangioma during dynamic contrast-enhanced computed tomography is nearly pathognomonic for this lesion (Figs. 28–5 and 28–6).[8, 76, 86] Before contrast enhancement, hemangiomas typically show diminished attenuation. The dynamic technique involves the intravenous bolus infusion of iodinated contrast medium followed immediately by images taken as rapidly as the equipment permits—every 5 to 15 seconds—through the area of interest at a stationary table position. Scans made within the first two minutes first show enhancement at the periphery of the lesion. The following sequential scans demonstrate a progressive centripetal "filling in." With time, the lesion, unless it has internal scar, thrombosis, or hemorrhage, becomes isodense with the surrounding liver. This pattern of dynamic contrast enhancement is highly characteristic of cavernous hemangioma, but it is only moderately sensitive for these lesions.[86]

Radionuclide blood flow and blood pool imaging is becoming more generally recognized as a useful technique for study of suspected cavernous hemangiomas.

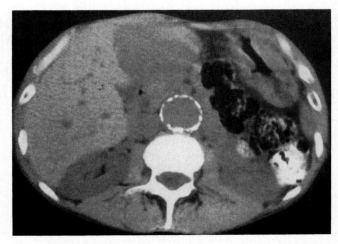

Figure 28–5. CT image of cavernous hemangioma of the left hepatic lobe prior to infusion of intravenous contrast material. The aorta is heavily calcified.

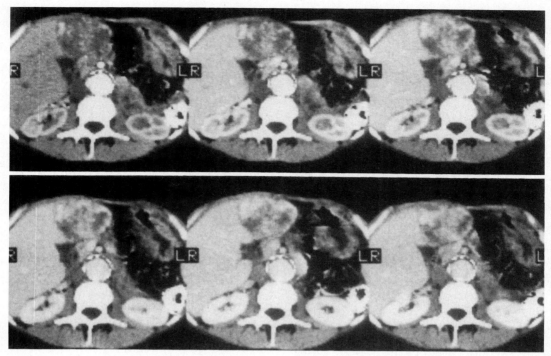

Figure 28–6. Dynamic CT scan of cavernous hemangioma of the left hepatic lobe; this is the same patient as shown in Figure 28–5. The images were made at 15-second intervals following bolus injection of intravenous contrast medium. In the first image *(upper left)* contrast intensity is beginning to increase at the periphery of the lesion at a time when the aorta is already fully opacified. On successive images contrast material progressively "fills in" the lesion. (Provided by Dr. Sheldon Blend.)

By a simple technique, the patient's red blood cells are labeled with technetium-99m. Sequential hepatic scans are made at three- to four-second intervals after infusion of the labeled cells, thus demonstrating the phase of arterial perfusion. Because of the pool of stagnant blood within the hemangioma, the lesion appears as a "cold" area in this initial phase of the study. Static images are then taken at intervals up to two hours after infusion, and on these views the hemangioma becomes a "hot spot" because the stagnant blood pool, having slowly equilibrated with the circulating pool of labeled cells, is purged of this label more slowly than is the surrounding liver tissue.[87–90] This pattern of initial hypoperfusion and delayed filling is nearly diagnostic of cavernous hemangioma. Sensitivity is diminished in complex lesions and those less than 3 cm in diameter.[89]

Angiography has long been regarded as the most sensitive and specific means of evaluating cavernous hemangiomas.[75, 78] Hemangiomas are supplied by a normal-sized hepatic artery and display lakes or puddles of contrast material, often in a ring- or C-shaped configuration, which appear during the mid to late arterial phase and persist for up to 30 seconds.[13, 82] The surrounding arteries are displaced and crowded. There is no neovascularity, arteriovenous shunting, arterial encasement, or portal venous thrombosis, which allows differentiation from metastases or hepatocellular carcinoma in the majority of cases.

Magnetic resonance imaging is becoming recognized as a highly sensitive technique for identifying cavernous hemangiomas.[24, 84, 88] Characteristically, hemangiomas

appear as very high intensity lesions on T2-weighted spin echo images (Fig. 28–7). The lesions display a rounded or lobulated shape homogeneously opacified with smooth, well-defined margins. A markedly long T2 relaxation time, exceeding 80 msec, is highly characteristic of hemangioma. They also display a prolonged T1 relaxation time leading to a greater negative contrast ratio between the lesion and normal liver on T1-weighted images. In comparison, cancers tend to have a heterogeneous appearance with poorly defined margins.[24]

When lesions characteristic of hepatic hemangioma are discovered incidentally, in a patient with normal liver blood tests and without known neoplasm, observation alone is appropriate. A typical example of such a presentation is a middle-aged woman undergoing sonographic evaluation for suspected gallstones who is noted to have a 2 cm solitary, hyperechoic, subcapsular lesion in the right lobe of the liver. It would be reasonable to repeat the ultrasound examination in such a patient a few times at intervals of two to three months.[85, 89, 91] If no change is noted during this follow-up, the diagnosis of probable hemangioma can be accepted and further studies avoided. Lesions first identified on scintigraphy or CT scan should be visualized by sonography, and if their appearance suggests hemangioma, they should be managed as discussed above. If the lesion is larger than 3 cm in diameter, a tagged red blood cell study should be done. If this displays the characteristic features of hemangioma, the investigation can be stopped at this point. If the labeled

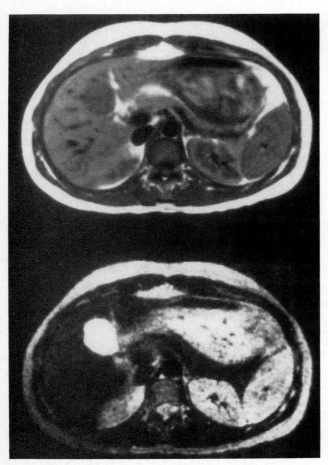

Figure 28–7. Cavernous hemangioma of the liver; the upper MRI image is T1-weighted (TR 0.5 sec/TE 30 msec), and the lower is heavily T2-weighted (TR 2.0 sec/TE 120 msec). In this 34-year-old female, who complained of right upper quadrant abdominal discomfort, MRI demonstrates a well defined, somewhat hypointense, homogeneous lesion within the medial segment of the left lobe of the liver. The lesion has a very long T2 relaxation time and a lesion-to-liver signal intensity ratio of 6:1, consistent with hemangioma. (Provided by Dr. Jesse Cohen.)

RBC study is not suggestive of hemangioma or other hypervascular lesions, percutaneous biopsy can be performed for a definitive diagnosis, as discussed below. If this scan is suggestive of hemangioma but atypical, the patient should be referred for more definitive study by dynamic contrast CT, MRI, or angiography.

If doubt about the nature of the hepatic mass persists after extensive evaluation with these imaging procedures, and there is continued concern about the presence of a malignant lesion, fine needle biopsy under CT or sonographic guidance may be attempted. Although the risk of serious hemorrhage has long been recognized as a complication of large-bore needle biopsy of cavernous hemangioma, it has been demonstrated that these lesions can be biopsied with reasonable safety using a fine needle, such as a 22 gauge Chiba needle.[8, 91, 92] In order to diminish the risk of capsular bleeding, an attempt is made to interpose normal liver tissue in the needle path between the liver surface and the lesion. The pathologist may be willing

to make a diagnosis of cavernous hemangioma if sufficiently characteristic agglomerates of capillaries or endothelial cells can be seen within the bloody aspirate. However, in general, such biopsies should be used primarily to confirm the presence of tumor rather than (with a negative biopsy) to rule out tumor or to make a confident diagnosis of hemangioma.[92] Finally, if the biopsy is nondiagnostic, and concern persists, surgical excision of the lesion may be appropriate.

Liver Cell Adenoma and Focal Nodular Hyperplasia

Liver cell adenoma (LCA) and focal nodular hyperplasia (FNH) are considered together because of the likelihood of their being confused with one another. Both commonly present as solid intrahepatic lesions in a young or middle-aged woman. It is essential to distinguish between them because their clinical significance is very different. The major features of these lesions are compared in Table 28–2.

The association between hepatic adenomas and the use of oral contraceptives is supported by several types of evidence: (1) almost all women with hepatic adenomas have been users of birth control pills, (2) hepatic adenomas were rarely reported prior to the availability of oral contraceptives, (3) hepatic adenomas often become smaller after the patient discontinues use of birth control pills, and (4) the risk of developing LCA increases progressively with the duration of contraceptive use.[93] Liver cell adenomas are more likely to grow

Table 28–2. COMPARISON OF LIVER CELL ADENOMA AND FOCAL NODULAR HYPERPLASIA

	Liver Cell Adenoma	Focal Nodular Hyperplasia
Sex	90 per cent women	80 per cent women
Age range	Predominantly women of childbearing age	All ages
Association with use of oral contraceptives	90 per cent of women	Weak association; may increase growth and vascularity of existing lesions
Number of lesions	Usually solitary (about 25 per cent are multiple)	Usually solitary (13 to 20 per cent are multiple)
Lesion diameter	Typically 8 to 15 cm	Typically 3 to 7 cm
Malignant potential	Probable, but uncommon	None?
Presenting features	Right upper quadrant abdominal pain and/or mass; acute abdominal crisis due to intraperitoneal hemorrhage	Usually asymptomatic; vague abdominal pain; usually discovered incidentally
Pathology	Large fleshy tumor; sheets of cells; no "substructure," bile ducts, or Kupffer cells; foci of hemorrhage and necrosis	Firm, nodular, cirrhosis-like; stellate fibrous core containing bile ducts; Kupffer cells line vessels

and to bleed during pregnancy.[94] LCA is also associated with type 1 glycogen storage disease (von Gierke's disease); these tumors may undergo malignant transformation but seem less prone to bleed than the adenomas associated with oral contraceptive use.[95]

Although focal nodular hyperplasia is also recognized most often among adult women, fewer patients have been users of oral contraceptives, and more of these tumors have been reported in males and children.[96] Nevertheless, there is reason to believe that contraceptive steroids may promote increased vascularity of FNH and perhaps increase the likelihood, although still very small, that they may bleed.[97]

The most important clinical feature of LCA is its propensity to bleed. Patients with LCA commonly present with right upper quadrant abdominal pain due to bleeding into the tumor. About 10 per cent of patients present with an acute abdominal crisis and hemorrhagic shock due to tumor rupture and resultant hemoperitoneum. By contrast, FNH is usually found incidentally or when the patient is being evaluated for vague and nonspecific abdominal discomfort, and only rarely is FNH complicated by hemorrhage.

An additional concern about LCA is its apparent progression to hepatocellular carcinoma in occasional cases. Alternatively, some lesions initially diagnosed as hepatic adenoma may actually be highly differentiated, slow growing malignant hepatomas from the outset.[98, 99] In a survey of 357 reported cases of FNH, none had undergone malignant transformation.[100]

On gross examination, hepatic adenomas are typically large circumscribed tumors, sometimes with large vessels coursing over the surface. The cut surface often shows areas of focal hemorrhage and central necrosis, particularly in tumors larger than 10 cm in diameter.[101] Histologically, LCA is characterized by a monotonous regular proliferation of hepatocytes, devoid of bile ducts and without lobulation. The cells are smaller and more pleomorphic than normal hepatocytes unless they have an increased content of glycogen or fat, making them larger and paler than those of the surrounding liver. No reticulin fibers are present.[93, 101]

Grossly, FNH is usually a well-circumscribed nonencapsulated, firm, nodular, cirrhosis-like mass in an otherwise normal liver. Most often it is subcapsular but is pedunculated in 20 per cent of cases. The most characteristic feature of FNH is a central fibrous core with radiating septa which subdivide the mass into nodules, but this stellate scar is not present in all cases.[101] Foci of hemorrhage and necrosis are hardly ever present. On microscopic examination, many small bile ducts are seen in the fibrous septa, and veins and arteries, particularly in the central scar, are thickened by fibromuscular hyperplasia. Kupffer cells are distributed throughout the vascular spaces.[93, 102]

The radionuclide liver-spleen scan has long been a helpful means of distinguishing hepatic adenoma from focal nodular hyperplasia. LCA is usually visualized as a "cold" area on the hepatogram while, in the classic case, FNH displays normal uptake of radiocolloid so that the lesion may not be visible. However, this approach suffers from both false positive and false negative results. Almost half of FNH cases actually show a partial or complete failure of isotope uptake, while a significant number of hepatic adenomas take up radiocolloid to some extent. Isotope uptake has also been reported in hepatoblastomas, which may be of importance in the differential diagnosis of FNH in young children.[103] A more specific finding in FNH is hyperconcentration of radionuclide (10 per cent of cases), perhaps reflecting the abundance of Kupffer cell–lined blood vessels in some of these lesions.

The sonographic patterns of both LCA and FNH are nonspecific and varied, often with a mixed pattern of hyper- or hypoechogenicity apparently related to intralesional hemorrhage in LCA or the characteristic scirrhous core of FNH.

Computed tomography is only moderately more specific than sonography for detection of LCA and FNH and it is no more sensitive, failing to detect even some large lesions.[97, 100, 104] CT may be of some value in better defining the site and extent of the tumor.[104] Hepatic adenoma ranges from homogeneously hypodense, owing to fat and glycogen content, to isodense with the surrounding liver. If a scan is done without contrast enhancement, it may show areas of increased density within a hypodense lesion, corresponding to recent intralesional hemorrhage.[101] FNH is often homogeneously isodense with surrounding liver in both unenhanced scans and in scans made after slow infusion of contrast material. Being highly vascular lesions, both LCA and FNH should become visible as hyperdense masses early in the course of a dynamic sequential contrast CT study.

Arteriography is the most sensitive means of characterizing these lesions.[13, 97] Liver cell adenomas typically are well defined, hypervascular masses with a peripheral blood supply. Vessels within the mass are tortuous and of varying caliber, but without encasement or occlusion. There is moderate capillary staining but no arteriovenous shunting or venous invasion. Avascular areas, representing intralesional hematomas, are a highly characteristic feature.[13] FNH is also a hypervascular hepatic mass with dense, tortuous vasculature. In some cases a dense septated blush appears in the capillary and early venous phase corresponding to the stellate central scar seen grossly.[102] Arteries within the mass are tortuous but without encasement, obstruction, or true neovascularity.[97] When vessels are observed to enter the lesion from the center this helps distinguish FNH from LCA, but they often enter from the periphery.[100] The angiographic features of FNH are enough like those of hepatocellular carcinoma to lead to an incorrect preoperative diagnosis of hepatoma.[101] Areas of hypovascularity due to focal hemorrhage are not seen.

Based on the thus far limited experience with magnetic resonance imaging in evaluation of LCA and FNH, it appears that LCA has an increased signal intensity on T1- and T2-weighted images, apparently due to its high glycogen and fat content (Ros, P. R., personal communication, 1986). Findings in a single patient with FNH included a mass effect with tumor nearly isointense with surrounding liver, and a central stellate region corresponding to the collagenous scar.[105]

Management of Liver Cell Adenoma and Focal Nodular Hyperplasia. The patient who presents with acute abdominal pain and hypotension due to intraperitoneal hemorrhage from a hepatic adenoma may have to be taken directly to surgery for control of bleeding. In most cases, however, a more deliberate approach to evaluation of the hepatic mass is possible. When a focal lesion(s) is identified, either incidentally as a palpable mass or by hepatic scintigraphy, sonography, CT, or MRI in evaluation of a patient complaining of abdominal pain, LCA and FNH must be considered. This possibility is further strengthened if the patient is female, is of childbearing age, has no evidence of primary extrahepatic cancer, and has no evident predisposition to develop hepatocellular carcinoma (cirrhosis, long-term HBV infection). When LCA and FNH are suspected, hepatic scintigraphy should be performed. On this study, if the lesion becomes iso- or hyperintense relative to surrounding liver parenchyma, this is useful evidence in support of the diagnosis of FNH, but cannot be taken final proof of this diagnosis. Percutaneous biopsy should be avoided, both because of the increased risk of bleeding from these very vascular lesions and because the needle biopsy specimen is likely to be too small to allow the pathologist to make a definitive diagnosis.[80, 101] Instead, hepatic angiography should be performed. In a minimally symptomatic patient with a hepatic lesion less than about 7 cm in diameter, the angiographic demonstration of intense capillary staining in stellate pattern may be sufficient evidence of FNH to permit conservative follow-up. On the other hand, if the patient complains of more than minor symptoms, or the imaging modalities show features, such as internal hemorrhage, which are suggestive of LCA, or the lesion is more than 10 cm in diameter, the patient should undergo laparotomy.[80, 101] If a frozen section wedge biopsy demonstrates FNH, in most cases the lesion should be left in place.[96, 101] Resection of FNH may be indicated if the lesion is pedunculated, and thereby subject to the complications of torsion,[100] or has behaved atypically in terms of progressive growth or internal hemorrhage.

Because of the small risk of malignant transformation of LCA, as well as the insufficient certainty of the diagnosis by any means short of biopsy, the clinician must ultimately decide if and when laparotomy should be performed. If the patient is suspected preoperatively of having a hepatic adenoma which may require excision, and her condition is stable, it would be reasonable to defer surgery, perhaps for several months. After discontinuation of oral contraceptives, in some cases the lesion will become progressively smaller and less vascular,[106] making surgical excision, if needed, safer and easier.

Cystic Lesions in the Liver

When a focal mass is identified in the liver by any means and is shown by ultrasound examination to be cystic in nature, the differential diagnosis includes simple cysts, abscesses, and cystic neoplasms. Simple cysts are either solitary, or multiple, constituting polycystic liver disease. Cysts are usually discovered incidentally. They are lined with cuboidal cells, which resemble those of bile duct epithelium. Both simple and multiple cysts are believed to arise from embryonic bile ductules which failed to establish continuity with the biliary tract.[107] Although the cyst rudiments presumably are present at birth, the patient often reaches middle age before the cyst accumulates sufficient fluid to make its presence known. The majority of patients with polycystic liver disease also have adult polycystic kidney disease and, less often, cysts in the spleen, pancreas, or lungs.

About one quarter of patients with polycystic kidney disease also have hepatic cysts. Both solitary cysts and polycystic disease are more common in women. Other benign cystic liver lesions include biliary cystadenomas, and intrahepatic choledochal cysts, which are large, rounded, well-defined anechoic lesions, with low CT attenuation.[108] Cystadenomas are rare tumors, affecting women, most often in the fifth decade.[109] Cystadenomas and choledochal cysts are of particular significance because each has the potential of malignant degeneration.

Echinococcal (hydatid) cysts are the larval stage of *Echinococcus granulosus,* for which humans serve as intermediate hosts. The definitive hosts are dogs or other carnivores in which the adult worm lives attached to the jejunal mucosa and produces eggs which are passed in the stool. Humans in the fecally contaminated environment ingest the eggs, which hatch into embryos in the intestine. The embryos pass through the gut wall into the portal blood, from which they are filtered out in the liver or other organs.[110] Here they evolve into the larval form, which is the hydatid cyst. Hydatid liver cysts, usually solitary or few in number, consist of an outer pericyst (ectocyst), which is a fibrous shell generated by the host surrounding the parasitic elements, and the parasite-derived endocyst made up of an outer laminated membrane and the innermost germinal layer.[110] The germinal layer produces brood capsules, from which scolices develop, and daughter cysts, which bud off and float in the cyst fluid.

The average diameter of echinococcal liver cysts is approximately 10 cm.[110] In about one third of cases, calcium deposits develop in the pericyst and less often in the daughter cysts. Although extensive calcification suggests that the parasite has died, moderate calcification may be seen in viable cysts. Spontaneous cessation of cyst growth is not uncommon.[111]

The diagnosis of hydatid cyst should be considered in persons who have immigrated, even many years before, from parts of the world where echinococcosis is endemic. These areas include the southern (temperate) parts of South America, Africa and Australia, Mediterranean countries, the Middle East, northern Canada, and Alaska.[110] The patient is likely to present with abdominal pain and liver tenderness, or occasionally with fever and jaundice due to passage of daughter cysts into the bile ducts.[110] Patients who have been sensitized to parasite antigens may have a peripheral blood eosinophilia.[107] If the diagnosis is suspected, before puncturing the cyst with an aspirating needle or entering it at surgery, serologic tests for echinococcal antibodies, such as complement fixation, indirect hemagglutination, latex fixation, or enzyme-linked immunosorbent (ELISA) assays, should be performed. The Casoni skin test should no longer be used because of frequent false positive and false negative results, occasional allergic reactions in hypersensitized subjects, and the possibility that the test itself may induce antibody production, leading to false positive serologic tests.[110] If cyst fluid containing free scolices and daughter cysts is spilled into the peritoneal cavity, this may not only cause a severe anaphylactic reaction if the host has been sensitized to parasitic antigens but also is likely to result in implantation of new hydatid cysts in the peritoneal cavity, which may not be resectable.

Hepatic abscesses are classified as either pyogenic or amebic. They may be solitary or few in number or, especially when complicating biliary tract sepsis, they may be multifocal. The possibility of amebic abscess should be considered in any jaundiced, febrile patient with a cystic liver mass who within the past year has traveled to an area, such as Mexico, where amebiasis is endemic. Although the parasite is believed to reach the liver via the portal blood after establishing a colonic infection, few patients give a history of severe diarrhea suggestive of amebic colitis.

The probable malignant nature of *cystic tumors* is usually evident on imaging studies. However, as discussed below, necrotic liver metastases sometimes closely mimic primary benign cysts. Cystic degeneration is most common in metastases from leiomyosarcoma, carcinoid tumors, choriocarcinoma, melanoma, small cell lung cancer, and ovarian carcinoma.[112]

Radiologic Evaluation of Cystic Liver Lesions. On plain films of the abdomen, the characteristic curvilinear or ring calcifications are present in about one third of hydatid cysts. Less often, calcified daughter cysts produce multiple small rings of calcification.[111] The chest X-ray may show pulmonary hydatid cysts.[110] Abscesses in the dome of the right lobe, particularly those due to amebic infection, may cause chest X-ray changes including elevation of the right hemidiaphragm, right-sided atelectasis, and pleural effusions.[113]

Although sulfur colloid scintigraphy is too nonspecific to be of diagnostic value for hepatic cysts, this may be the most cost-effective means of monitoring the resolution of an amebic abscess cavity over the weeks to months after definitive treatment.

By ultrasound examination, simple cysts are sharply outlined, anechoic lesions showing distal acoustic enhancement due to the high efficiency of sound trans-

mission through the clear fluid.[114] The cyst wall is thin and nonechogenic. In hydatid cysts separation of the laminated membrane from the pericyst produces a "split wall" appearance, and complete collapse results in the "water-lily sign." A fluid level due to "hydatid sand" (freed scolices and other debris) is characteristic of echinococcal cyst, but such layering in a poorly defined hydatid cyst may also indicate that it is infected.[111, 115] Multiple daughter cysts produce a multiloculated appearance simulating congenital polycystic disease.[111]

Abscesses may be difficult to distinguish from simple cysts and cannot be identified by etiology using sonography (Fig. 28–9). The abscess fluid, being thicker than simple cyst fluid and containing tissue debris, tends to show fine, homogeneous low-level echoes throughout, and distal sonic enhancement is less prominent.[115, 116] Abscesses often have irregular and echogenic walls.[38]

By sonography, biliary cystadenoma appears as anechoic masses traversed by highly echogenic septa with internal echoes representing papillary infoldings. Cystic liver metastases are suggested by the sonographic appearance of a thick, irregular echogenic cyst wall.

By computed tomography simple cysts typically are well-defined, nonenhancing spherical lesions with thin walls whose contents have attenuation values close to that of water (Fig. 28–8); unfortunately, necrotic metastases, late-stage abscesses, and chronic hematomas also may, on occasion, have attenuation coefficients in this range.[117, 120] Small or early hydatid cysts can be devoid of internal structure and, accordingly, are indistinguishable from simple cysts.[108] The abdominal scan may disclose additional intrahepatic or extrahepatic lesions.[110] Abscesses tend to be slightly less regular than simple cysts on the nonenhanced scan, with a higher average attenuation value, but the overlap of CT numbers in these two conditions is so great as to make this measurement of little diagnostic value. Abscesses may become sharply defined and show peripheral enhancement on postcontrast scans (Fig. 28–10).[112, 117] The otherwise unexplained presence of gas

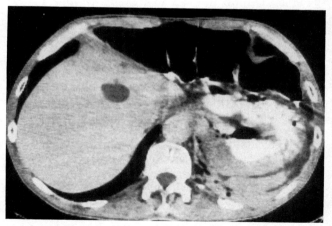

Figure 28–8. CT image of a simple hepatic cyst. Cyst fluid density was 2.0 Hausfield units (HU) near the density of water. (Provided by Dr. Sheldon Blend.)

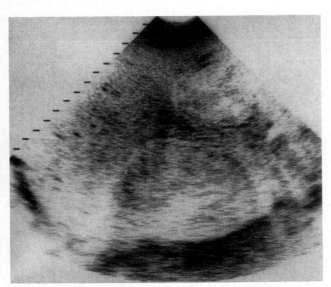

Figure 28–9. Longitudinal hepatic sonogram showing two spherical lesions later proved to be amebic abscesses. Because of their atypically high echogenicity, partially necrotic tumor, either primary or metastatic, was suspected.

in a cystic lesion is strong evidence of a pyogenic abscess due to gas-forming organisms.[104] A distinct change of lesion pattern on repeat scans done a few days apart strongly suggests hepatic abscess. Biliary cystadenoma is a smooth, thick-walled lesion with mural nodularity and internal septation. CT features of necrotic metastases include a thick rim of lower density than the surrounding hepatic parenchyma, irregular margins, mural nodules, and fluid-fluid levels.[117]

Diagnosis and Treatment of Cystic Liver Lesions. In an asymptomatic patient with ultrasound or CT defects characteristic of simple cysts, no further evaluation or treatment is needed.[115] If there are atypical features, either in the clinical presentation or on the imaging studies, without reason to suspect hydatid disease, fine-needle aspiration of the cyst should be performed and the fluid submitted for cytologic examination.[115] Unless the fluid is clear, a total and differential cell count and culture should also be performed. If solitary or polycystic lesions become so large as to cause symptoms, the treatment of choice is surgical unroofing of the larger cysts; percutaneous aspiration is of only temporary benefit.[80]

If amebic abscess is a consideration, serum should be sent for amebic serologic testing (immunodiffusion, counterelectrophoresis, indirect hemagglutination), and amebicidal therapy is initiated empirically pending the results of the amebic antibody tests (metronidazole, 750 mg, by mouth, three times a day). If the antibody test is positive, therapy should be continued for a total of 10 days. Although the majority of patients with amebic abscesses can be effectively treated with amebicidal drug therapy alone, percutaneous catheter (Fig. 28–10) or surgical drainage may be necessary for those patients with very large abscesses, those having a great

deal of pain, or those who fail to respond to drug therapy with decline in fever and improvement in symptoms within 48 to 72 hours.[113]

If a pyogenic abscess is being considered, aspiration of cyst fluid for culture, cell count, and cytologic examination should be performed shortly after initiating empirical antibiotic therapy plus metronidazole unless a negative test for amebic antibodies has been obtained. Organisms most commonly cultured from pyogenic abscesses are *E. coli, Klebsiella-Enterobacter,* and *Streptococcus, Pseudomonas,* and *Proteus* species. Anaerobes, most often microaerophilic streptococci and *Bacteroides* species, are isolated from about one fourth of pyogenic abscesses.[113] Although surgical drainage remains the primary mode of therapy for most large pyogenic liver abscesses, a number of reports of treatment by percutaneous catheter drainage plus antibiotics have appeared in the past decade.[121–124] This has been made possible by the availability of ultrasound and CT guidance for catheter placement.[5] Surgery is indicated in cases requiring biliary tract drainage or when the abscesses are inaccessible to percutaneous catheter placement.

Echinococcal cysts require surgical drainage if it is feasible. The lesion is approached in such a way as to minimize the risk of spillage of cyst contents, containing infectious scolices, into the free peritoneal cavity. When the cyst is opened, a scolicidal solution, such as hypertonic saline, 0.5 per cent silver nitrate, or 80 per cent ethanol, is infused to kill the parasite. The cyst lining is then stripped out and the pericyst cavity is collapsed by suturing. Alternatively, cysts located peripherally in a suitable area may be treated by excision of the affected hepatic segments.[110] For patients who

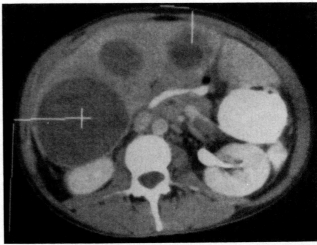

Figure 28–10. Contrast-enhanced abdominal CT scan of the patient shown in Figure 28–9. The low-density and smooth, thin walls of the hepatic lesions are more consistent with cysts or abscesses than necrotic tumor. Needle/catheter aspiration of the large right lobe cavity yielded several hundred milliliters of odorless, opaque, brownish pink fluid with the "anchovy sauce" appearance characteristic of amebic abscess contents. The fluid was sterile. The serum indirect hemagglutination titer of amebic antibody exceeded 1:4000. (Provided by Dr. Aye Aye Tin Sein.)

are not surgical candidates, or in whom there has been spillage of cyst contents during surgery, drug therapy with mebendazole or, more recently, albendazole has been used. While this treatment has caused reduction in cyst size in some cases, the full extent of its efficacy in this disease is uncertain.[111] Although needle aspiration of hydatid cysts has been considered contraindicated because of the risk of releasing cyst contents, there has been a recent report of the successful treatment of an inoperable hydatid cyst by lavage with hypertonic saline and silver nitrate via a percutaneous catheter introduced under CT guidance.[118]

In patients with cystic liver metastases fine-needle aspiration under sonographic or CT guidance may also be the most direct means of obtaining diagnostic cytologic and histologic specimens, based on cells and tissue fragments aspirated from the lesion wall and cytologic samples from the fluid center of the tumor masses.[115]

Biliary cystadenomas and choledochal cysts, because of their tendency to undergo malignant transformation, should be completely excised whenever possible.[109, 119]

References

1. Lewis, E. Screening for diffuse and focal liver disease: The case for hepatic sonography. J. Clin. Ultrasound 12:67, 1984.
2. Bernardino, M. E., Thomas, J. L., and Maklad, N. Hepatic sonography: Technical considerations and possible future applications. Radiology 142:249, 1982.
3. Mueller, P. R., and Simeone, J. F. Intraabdominal abscesses. Diagnosis by sonography and computed tomography. Radiol. Clin. North Am. 21:425, 1983.
4. Machi, J., Isomoto, H., Kurohiji, T., Yamashita, Y., and Kakegawa, T. High-resolution operative ultrasonography for screening of liver metastatic tumor from the colon and rectum. Hepatology 6:1141, 1986.
5. Wittenberg, J. Computed tomography of the body. Part I. N. Engl. J. Med. 309:1160, 1983.
6. Scott, W. W., Sanders, R. C., and Siegelman, S. S. Irregular fatty infiltration of the liver: Diagnostic dilemmas. AJR 135:67, 1980.
7. Reed, W. P., Haney, P. J., Elias, E. G., Whitley, N. O., Forsthoff, N. O., and Brown, S. Ethiodized oil emulsion enhanced computerized tomography in the preoperative assessment of metastases to the liver from the colon and rectum. Surg. Gynecol. Obstet. 162:131, 1986.
8. Zeman, R. K., Paushter, D. M., Schiebler, M. L., Choyke, P. L., Jaffe, M. H., and Clark, L. R. Hepatic imaging: Current status. Radiol. Clin. North Am. 23:473, 1985.
9. Berland, L. L. Screening for diffuse and focal liver disease: The case for hepatic computed tomography. J. Clin. Ultrasound 12:83, 1984.
10. Rothschild, M. A., Oretz, M., and Schreiber, S. S. Comments on radionuclide hepatic scanning. Semin. Liver Dis. 2:29, 1982.
11. Christensen, M., and Rodbro, P. The diagnostic value of liver scintigraphy to disclose metastases in patients with suspected or proven gastrointestinal cancer. A critical review of the literature. Dan. Med. Bull. 29:206, 1982.
12. Dittman, W. Hepatic angiography. Semin. Liver Dis. 2:41, 1982.
13. Gutierrez, O. H., and Schwartz, S. I. Relative value of imaging techniques for focal hepatic lesions. In Gutierrez, O. H., and Schwartz, S. (eds.): I. Atlas of Hepatic Tumors and Focal Lesions: Arteriographic and Tomographic Diagnosis. New York, McGraw-Hill Book Company, 1984, pp. 1–12.
14. Thompson, J. N., Gibson, R., Czerniak, A., and Blumgart, L. H. Focal liver lesions: A plan for management. Br. Med. J. 290:1643, 1985.
15. Bernardino, M. E., Thomas, J. L., Barnes, P. A., and Lewis, E. Diagnostic approaches to liver and spleen metastases. Radiol. Clin. North Am. 20:469, 1982.
16. Ariyama, J., Shimaguchi, S., Suyama, M., and Shirakabe, H. Intraarterial digital subtraction angiography in the diagnosis and treatment of gastrointestinal disorders. Gastrointest. Radiol. 11:177, 1986.
17. Smith, F. W., Mallard, J. R., Reid, A., and Hutchison, J. M. S. Nuclear magnetic resonance tomographic imaging in liver disease. Lancet 1:963, 1981.
18. Aisen, A. M., Martel, W., Glazer, G. M., and Carson, P. L. Hepatic imaging: Positron emission tomography, digital angiography, and nuclear magnetic resonance imaging. Hepatology 6:1024, 1983.
19. Steiner, R. E., and Bydder, G. M. Nuclear magnetic resonance in gastroenterology. Clin. Gastroenterol. 13:265, 1984.
20. Margulis, A. R., Moss, A. A., Crooks, L. E., and Kaufman, L. Nuclear magnetic resonance in the diagnosis of tumors of the liver. Semin. Roentgenol. 18:123, 1983.
21. Moss, A. A., Goldberg, H. I., Stark, D. B., Davis, P. L., Margulis, A. R., Kaufman, L., and Crooks, L. E. Hepatic tumors: Magnetic resonance and CT appearance. Radiology 150:141, 1984.
22. Ohtomo, K., Itai, Y., Furui, S., Yashiro, N., Yoshikawa, K., and Iio, M. Hepatic tumors: Differentiation by transverse relaxation time (T2) of magnetic resonance imaging. Radiology 155:421, 1985.
23. Vermess, M. Nuclear magnetic resonance imaging of the liver: Current status and future possibilities. In Van de Velde, J. H., and Sugarbaker, P. H. (eds.): Liver Metastasis. Boston, Martinus Nijhof Publishers, 1984, pp. 118–121.
24. Stark, D. D., Felder, R. C., Wittenberg, J., Saini, S., Butch, R. J., White, M. E., Edelman, R. R., Mueller, P. R., Simeone, J. E., Cohen, A. M., Brady, T. J., and Ferrucci, J. T. Magnetic resonance imaging of cavernous hemangioma of the liver: Tissue-specific characterization. AJR 145:213, 1985.
25. Heiken, J. P., Lee, J. K. T., Glazer, H. S., and Ling, D. Hepatic metastases studied with MR and CT. Radiology 156:423, 1985.
26. Ferrucci, J. T., Jr., Wittenberg, J., Mueller, T. R., Simeone, J. F., Harbin, W. P., Kirkpatrick, R. H., and Taft, P. D. Diagnosis of abdominal malignancy by radiologic fine-needle aspiration biopsy. Am. J. Roentgenol. 134:323, 1980.
27. Whitcomb, F. F., Jr., Gibb, S. P., and Boyce, H. W., Jr. Peritoneoscopy for the diagnosis of left lobe lesions of the liver. Arch. Intern. Med. 138:126, 1978.
28. Lightdale, C. J. Laparoscopy and biopsy in malignant liver disease. Cancer 50:2672, 1982.
29. Hogg, L., and Pack, G. T. Diagnostic accuracy of hepatic metastases at laparotomy. Arch. Surg. 72:251, 1966.
30. Ozarda, A., and Pickren, J. The topographic distribution of liver metastases: Its relation to surgical and isotope diagnosis. J. Nucl. Med. 3:149, 1962.
31. Danielson, K. S., Sheedy, P. F., Stephens, D. H., Hattery, R. R., and LaRusso, N. F. Computed tomography and peritoneoscopy for detection of liver metastases: Review of Mayo Clinic Experience. J. Comput. Assist. Tomogr. 7:230, 1983.
32. Cleton, F. J. Screening for liver metastases in daily practice. In Van de Velde, J. H., and Sugarbaker, P. H. (eds.): Liver Metastasis. Boston, Martinus Nijhof Publishers, 1984, pp. 150–153.
33. Freeny, P. C., Marks, W. M., Ryan, J. A., and Bolen, J. W. Colorectal carcinoma evaluation with CT: Preoperative staging and detection of postoperative recurrence. Radiology 158:347, 1986.
34. Read, D. R., Hambrick, E., Abcarian, H., and Levine, H. The preoperative diagnosis of hepatic metastases in cases of colorectal carcinoma. Dis. Colon Rectum 20:101, 1977.
35. Wiener, S. N., and Sachs, S. J. An assessment of routine liver scanning in patients with breast cancer. Arch. Surg. 113:126, 1978.
36. Tempero, M. A., Petersen, R. J., Zetterman, R. K., Lemon, H. M., and Gurney, J. Detection of metastatic liver disease: Use of liver scans and biochemical liver tests. JAMA 248:1329, 1982.

37. Clark, R. A., and Matsui, O. CT of liver tumors. Semin. Roentgenol. *18*:149, 1983.

38. Taylor, K. J. W. Liver imaging by ultrasonography. Semin. Liver Dis. *2*:1, 1982.

39. Schultz, W., and Hort, W. The distribution of metastases in the liver: A quantitative post-mortem study. Virchows Arch. (A) *394*:89, 1981.

40. Lee, J. K., and Balfe, D. M. Computed tomography evaluation of lymphoma patients. CRC Crit. Rev. Diagn. Imaging *18*:1, 1982.

41. Kadin, M. E., Donaldson, S. S., and Dorfman, R. F. Isolated granulomas in Hodgkin's disease. N. Engl. J. Med. *283*:859, 1970.

42. Bagley, C. M., Thomas, L. B., Johnson, R. E., Chretien, P. B., and DeVita, V. T. Diagnosis of liver involvement by lymphoma: Results of 96 consecutive peritoneoscopies. Cancer *31*:840, 1973.

43. Zornoza, J., and Ginaldi, S. Computed tomography in hepatic lymphoma. Radiology *138*:405, 1981.

44. Beasley, R. P., Hwang, L. Y., and Lin, C. C. Hepatocellular carcinoma and HBV: A prospective study of 22,707 men in Taiwan. Lancet *2*:1129, 1981.

45. Brechot, C., Nalpas, B., Courouce, A. M., Duhamel, G., Callard, P., Carnot, F., and Tiollais, B. Evidence that hepatitis B virus has a role in liver cell carcinoma in alcoholic liver disease. N. Engl. J. Med. *306*:1384, 1982.

46. Gilliam, J. H., Geisinger, K. R., and Richter, J. E. Primary hepatocellular carcinoma after chronic non-A, non-B post-transfusion hepatitis. Ann. Intern. Med. *101*:794, 1984.

47. Kiyosawa, K., Akhane, Y., Nagata, A., and Furuta, S. Hepatocellular carcinoma after non-A, non-B post-transfusion hepatitis. Am. J. Gastroenterol. *79*:777, 1984.

48. Ferenci, P., Dragosics, B., Marosi, L., and Kiss, F. Relative incidence of primary liver cancer in cirrhosis in Austria. Etiological considerations. Liver *4*:7, 1984.

49. Lehmann, F. G., and Wegner, T. Etiology of human liver cancer: Controlled prospective study in liver cirrhosis. J. Toxicol. (Environ.) *2*:281, 1979.

50. Lee, F. I. Cirrhosis and hepatoma in alcoholics. Gut *7*:77, 1966.

51. Powell, L. W. Hemochromatosis: Precirrhotic therapy restores normal life expectancy. Hepatology *6*:1423, 1986.

52. Lin, T. Y. Results of hepatic lobectomy for primary carcinoma of the liver. Surg. Gynecol. Obstet. *123*:289, 1966.

53. Foster, J. H., and Berman, M. Solid liver tumors. Major Probl. Clin. Surg. *21*:1, 1977.

54. Margolis, S., and Homcy, C. Systemic manifestations of hepatoma. Medicine *51*:381, 1972.

55. Brownstein, M. H., and Ballard, H. S. Hepatoma associated with erythrocytosis. Am. J. Med. *40*:204, 1966.

56. Jacobson, R. J., Lowenthal, M. N., and Kew, M. C. Erythrocytosis in hepatocellular cancer. S. Afr. Med. J. *53*:658, 1978.

57. Friedman, A. C., Lichtenstein, J. E., Goodman, Z., Fishman, E. K., Siegelman, S. S., and Dachman, A. H. Fibrolamellar hepatocellular carcinoma. Radiology *157*:583, 1985.

58. Vecchio, F. M., Fabiano, A., Ghirlanda, G., Manna, R., and Massi, G. Fibrolamellar carcinoma of the liver: The malignant counterpart of focal nodular hyperplasia with oncocytic change. Am. J. Clin. Pathol. *81*:521, 1984.

59. Chen, D.-S., Sung, J.-L., Sheu, J.-C., Lai, M.-Y., How, S.-W., Hsu, H.-C., Lee, C.-S., and Wai, T.-C. Serum alpha-fetoprotein in the early stage of human hepatocellular carcinoma. Gastroenterology *86*:1404, 1984.

60. Heyward, W. L., Lanier, A. P., Bender, T. R., McMahon, B. J., Kilkenny, S., Paprocki, T. R., Kline, K. T., Silimperi, D. R., and Maynard, J. E. Early detection of primary hepatocellular carcinoma by screening for alpha-fetoprotein in high-risk families. Lancet *2*:1161, 1983.

61. Bellet, D. H., Wands, J. R., Isselbacher, K. J., and Bohuon, C. Serum alpha-fetoprotein levels in human disease: Perspective from a highly specific monoclonal radioimmunoassay. Proc. Natl. Acad. Sci. USA *81*:3869, 1984.

62. Shinagawa, T., Ohto, M., Kimura, K., Tsunetomi, S., Morita, M., Saisho, H., Tsuchiya, Y., Saotome, N., Karasawa, E., Miki, M., Ueno, T., and Okuda, K. Diagnosis and clinical features of small hepatocellular carcinomas with emphasis on the utility of real-time ultrasonography: A study of 51 patients. Gastroenterology *86*:495, 1984.

63. Itai, Y., Araki, T., Furui, S., and Tasaka, A. Differential diagnosis of hepatic masses on computed tomography with particular reference to hepatocellular carcinoma. J. Comput. Assist. Tomogr. *5*:834, 1981.

64. Teefey, S. A., Stephens, D. H., James, E. M., Charboneau, J. W., and Sheedy, P. F. Computed tomography and ultrasonography of hepatoma. Clin. Radiol. *37*:339, 1986.

65. Inamoto, K., Sugiki, K., Yamasaki, H., Nakao, N., and Miura, T. Computed tomography and angiography of hepatocellular carcinoma. J. Comput. Assist. Tomogr. *4*:832, 1980.

66. LaBerge, J. M., Laing, F. C., Federle, M. P., Jeffrey, R. B., and Lim, R. C. Hepatocellular carcinoma: Assessment of resectability by computed tomography and ultrasound. Radiology *152*:485, 1984.

67. Ebara, M., Ohto, M., Watanabe, Y., Kimura, K., Saisho, H., Tsuchiya, Y., Okuda, K., Arimizu, N., Kondo, F., Ikehira, H., Fukuda, N., and Tateno, Y. Diagnosis of small hepatocellular carcinoma: Correlation of MR imaging and tumor histologic studies. Radiology *159*:371, 1986.

68. Takayasu, K., Shima, Y., Muramatsu, Y., Goto, H., Moriyama, N., Yamada, T., Makuuchi, M., Yamasaki, S., Hasegawa, H., Okazaki, N., Hirohashi, S., and Kishi, K. Angiography of small hepatocellular carcinomas: Analysis of 105 resected tumors. AJR *147*:525, 1986.

69. Sumida, M., Ohto, M., Ebara, M., Kimura, K., Okuda, K., and Hirooka, N. Accuracy of angiography in the diagnosis of small hepatocellular carcinoma. AJR *147*:531, 1986.

70. Ebara, M., Ohto, M., Shinagawa, T., Sugiura, N., Kimura, K., Matstani, S., Morita, M., Saisho, H., Tsuchiya, Y., and Okuda, K. Natural history of minute hepatocellular carcinoma smaller than 3 cm complicating cirrhosis. A study of 22 patients. Gastroenterology *90*:289, 1986.

71. Kobayashi, K., Sugimoto, T., Makino, H., Kumagi, M., Unoura, M., Tanaka, N., Kato, Y., and Hattori, N. Screening methods for early detection of hepatocellular carcinoma. Hepatology *6*:1100, 1985.

72. Mori, W., and Nagasako, K. Cholangiocarcinoma and related lesions. *In* Okuda, K., and Peters, R. (eds.): Hepatocellular Carcinoma. New York, John Wiley & Sons, 1976, pp. 227–246.

73. Okuda, K., Kubo, Y., Okazaki, N., Arishima, T., Hashimoto, M., Jinnouchi, S., Sawa, Y., Shimokawa, Y., Nakajima, Y., Noguchi, T., Nakano, M., Kojiro, M., and Nakashima, T. Clinical aspects of intrahepatic bile duct carcinoma including hilar carcinoma. Cancer *39*:232, 1977.

74. Ishak, K. G., and Rabin, L. Benign tumors of the liver. Med. Clin. North Am. *59*:995, 1975.

75. Takagi, H. Diagnosis and management of cavernous hemangioma of the liver. Semin. Surg. Oncol. *1*:12, 1985.

76. Barnett, B. H., Zerhouni, E. A., White, R. I., and Siegelman, S. S. Computed tomography in the diagnosis of cavernous hemangioma of the liver. AJR *134*:439, 1980.

77. Wiener, S. N., and Parulekar, S. G. Scintigraphy and ultrasonography of hepatic hemangioma. Radiology *132*:149, 1979.

78. Itai, Y., Furui, S., Araki, T., Yashiro, N., and Tasaka, A. Computed tomography of cavernous hemangioma of the liver. Radiology *137*:149, 1980.

79. Trastek, B. F., Van Heerden, J. A., Sheedy, P. F., and Adson, M. A. Cavernous hemangioma of the liver: Resect or observe? Am. J. Surg. *145*:49, 1983.

80. Adson, M. A. Mass lesions of the liver. Mayo Clin. Proc. *61*:362, 1986.

81. Kawarada, Y., and Mizumodo, R. Surgical treatment of giant hemangioma of the liver. Am. J. Surg. *148*:287, 1984.

82. Freeny, P. C., Vimont, T. R., and Barnett, D. C. Cavernous hemangioma of the liver; ultrasonography, arteriography, and computed tomography. Radiology *132*:143, 1979.

83. Onodera, H., Ohta, K., Oikawa, M., Abe, M., Kanno, T., Yoda, B., and Goto, Y. Correlation of the real-time ultrasonographic appearance of hepatic hemangiomas with angiography. J. Clin. Ultrasound *11*:421, 1983.

84. Itai, Y., Ohtomo, K., Furui, S., Yamauci, T., Minami, M.,

and Yashiro, N. Non-invasive diagnosis of small cavernous hemangioma of the liver: Advantage of MRI. AJR 145:1195, 1985.

85. Pen, J. H., Pelckmans, P. A., van Maercke, Y. M., Degryse, H. R., and de Schepper, A. M. Clinical significance of focal echogenic liver lesions. Gastrointest. Radiol. 11:61, 1986.

86. Freeny, P. C., and Marks, W. M. Patterns of contrast enhancement of benign and malignant hepatic neoplasms during bolus dynamic and delayed CT. Radiology 160:613, 1986.

87. Rabinowitz, S. A., McKusick, K. A., and Strauss, H. W. ^{99m}Tc red blood cell scintigraphy in evaluating focal liver lesions. AJR 143:63, 1984.

88. Sigal, R., Lanir, A., Atlan, H., Naschitz, J. E., Simon, J. S., Enat, S. R., Front, D., Israel, O., Chisin, R., Krausz, Y., Zur, Y., and Kaplan, N. Nuclear magnetic resonance imaging of liver hemangiomas. J. Nucl. Med. 26:117, 1985.

89. Ricci, O. E., Fanfani, S., Calabro, A., Milano, M., Ciatti, S., Colagrande, S., Masi, A., Casini, A., Acampora, C., Checcatelli, P., and Surrenti, C. Diagnostic approach to hepatic hemangiomas detected by ultrasound. Hepatogastroenterology 32:53, 1985.

90. Moinuddin, M., Allison, J. R., Montgomery, J. H., Rockett, J. F., and McMurray, J. M. Scintigraphic diagnosis of hepatic hemangioma: Its role in the management of hepatic mass lesions. AJR 145:223, 1985.

91. Solbiati, L., Libraghi, T., De Pra, L., Ierace, T., Misciadri, N., and Ravetto, C. Fine-needle biopsy of hepatic hemangioma with sonographic guidance. AJR 144:471, 1985.

92. Freeny, P. C., and Marks, W. M. Hepatic hemangioma: Dynamic bolus CT. AJR 147:711, 1986.

93. Ishak, K. G. Hepatic lesions caused by anabolic and contraceptive steroids. Semin. Liver Dis. 1:116, 1981.

94. Mays, E. T., and Christopherson, W. Hepatic tumors induced by sex steroids. Semin. Liver Dis. 4:147, 1984.

95. Fink, A. S., Appelman, H. D., and Thompson, N. W. Hemorrhage into a hepatic adenoma and type Ia glycogen storage disease: A case report and review of the literature. Surgery 97:117, 1985.

96. Stocker, J. T., and Ishak, K. G. Focal nodular hyperplasia of the liver: A study of 21 pediatric cases. Cancer 48:336, 1981.

97. Fishman, E. K., Farmlett, E., Kadir, S., and Siegelman, S. S. Computed tomography of benign hepatic tumors. J. Comput. Assist. Tomogr. 6:472, 1982.

98. Gordon, S. C., Reddy, K. R., Livingstone, A. S., Jeffers, L. J., and Schiff, E. R. Resolution of contraceptive-steroid-induced hepatic adenoma with subsequent evolution into hepatocellular carcinoma. Ann. Intern. Med. 105:547, 1986.

99. Goodman, Z. D., and Ishak, K. G. Hepatocellular carcinoma in women: Probable lack of etiologic association with oral contraceptive use. Hepatology 2:440, 1982.

100. Rogers, J. V., Mack, L. A., Freeny, P. C., Johnson, M. L., and Sones, P. J. Hepatic focal nodular hyperplasia: Angiography, CT, sonography and scintigraphy. AJR 137:983, 1981.

101. Kerlin, P., Davis, G. L., McGill, D. B., Weiland, L. H., Adson, M. A., and Sheedy, P. F. Hepatic adenoma and focal nodular hyperplasia: Clinical, pathologic, and radiologic features. Gastroenterology 84:994, 1983.

102. Casarella, W. J., Knowles, D. M., Wolff, M., and Johnson, P. M. Focal nodular hyperplasia and liver cell adenoma: Radiologic and pathologic differentiation. Am. J. Roentgenol. 131:393, 1978.

103. Diament, N. J., Parvey, L. S., Tonkin, I. L., Johnson, K. D., Bernstein, R., and Webber, B. Hepatoblastoma: Technetium sulfur colloid uptake simulating focal nodular hyperplasia. Am. J. Radiol. 139:168, 1982.

104. Foley, W. D., Berland, L. L., Lawson, T. L., and Varma, R. R. Computed tomography of the liver. Semin. Liver Dis. 2:14, 1982.

105. Butch, R. J., Stark, D. D., and Malt, R. A. MR imaging of hepatic focal nodular hyperplasia. J. Comput. Assist. Tomogr. 10:874, 1986.

106. Edmondson, H. A., Reynolds, T. B., Henderson, B., and Benton, B. Regression of liver cell adenomas associated with oral contraceptives. Ann. Intern. Med. 86:180, 1977.

107. Sanfelippo, P. M., Beahrs, O. H., and Weiland, L. H. Cystic disease of the liver. Ann. Surg. 179:922, 1974.

108. Kreel, L. Computed tomography in gastroenterology. Clin. Gastroenterol. 13:235, 1984.

109. Beretta, G., Spinelli, P., and Rilke, F. Sequential laparoscopy and laparotomy combined with bone marrow biopsy in staging Hodgkin's disease. Cancer Treat. Rep. 60:1231, 1976.

110. Langer, J. C., Rose, D. B., Keystone, J. S., Taylor, B. R., and Langer, B. Diagnosis and management of hydatid disease of the liver. A 15 year North American experience. Ann. Surg. 199:412, 1984.

111. Beggs, I. The radiological appearances of hydatid disease of the liver. Clin. Radiol. 34:555, 1983.

112. Araki, T. Diagnosis of liver tumors by dynamic computed tomography. CRC Crit. Rev. Diagn. Imaging 19:47, 1983.

113. Conter, R. L., Pitt, H. A., Tomkins, R. K., and Longmire, W. P. Differentiation of pyogenic from amebic hepatic abscesses. Surg. Gynecol. Obstet. 162:114, 1986.

114. Yeh, H.-C., and Rabinowitz, J. G. Ultrasonography and computed tomography of the liver. Radiol. Clin. North Am. 18:321, 1980.

115. Roemer, C. E., Ferrucci, J. T., Jr., Mueller, P. R., Simeone, J. F., vanSonnenberg, E., and Wittenberg, J. Hepatic cysts: Diagnosis and therapy by sonographic needle aspiration. AJR 136:1065, 1981.

116. Remedios, P. A., Colletti, P. M., and Ralls, P. W. Hepatic amebic abscess: Cholescintigraphic rim enhancement. Radiology 160:395, 1986.

117. Barnes, P. A., Thomas, J. L., and Bernardino, M. E. Pitfalls in the diagnosis of hepatic cysts by computed tomography. Radiology 141:129, 1981.

118. Mueller, P. R., Dawson, S. L., Ferrucci, J. T., and Nardi, G. L. Hepatic echinococcal cyst: Successful percutaneous cyst. Radiology 155:627, 1985.

119. Wheeler, D. A., and Edmondson, H. A. Cystadenoma with mesenchymal stroma (CMS) in the liver and bile ducts: A clinicopathologic study of 17 cases, four with malignant change. Cancer 56:1434, 1985.

120. Federle, N. P., Filly, R. A., and Moss, A. A. Cystic hepatic neoplasms: Complementary roles of CT and sonography. AJR 136:345, 1981.

121. Maher, J. A., Reynolds, T. B., and Yellin, A. E. Successful medical treatment of pyogenic liver abscess. Gastroenterology 77:618, 1979.

122. Gerzof, S. G., Robbins, A. H., Johnson, W. C., Birkett, D. H., and Nabseth, D. C. Percutaneous catheter drainage of abdominal abscesses: A five year experience. N. Engl. J. Med. 305:653, 1981.

123. Berger, L. A., and Osborne, D. R. Treatment of pyogenic liver abscesses by percutaneous needle aspiration. Lancet 1:132, 1982.

124. McCorkell, S. J., and Niles, N. L. Pyogenic liver abscesses: Another look at medical management. Lancet 1:803, 1985.

29

Effects of Systemic and Extraintestinal Disease on the Gut

TODD L. SACK
MARVIN H. SLEISENGER

Numerous systemic and extraintestinal diseases have gastrointestinal manifestations. Because it is impossible to discuss each entity in great detail in a single chapter, we have endeavored to emphasize frequently encountered diseases and those which may be of particular interest to the reader because of recent developments. For clarity, some diseases which result in similar manifestations are presented in tabular form. Some topics are taken up in detail in later chapters. The reader will be referred to these chapters for fuller discussion.

ENDOCRINE DISEASE

Thyroid Disease

Hyperthyroidism. For the purposes of this discussion, *thyrotoxicosis* can be considered an interchangeable term. *Hyperthyroidism* may underlie a number of important gastrointestinal symptoms owing to its effects upon almost all organs of the gastrointestinal system. In addition, these symptoms sometimes occur in the absence of the cardinal symptoms of hyperthyroidism ("apathetic" hyperthyroidism). Because hyperthyroidism may cause *myopathy,* the striated muscles of the pharynx and perhaps even the smooth muscle of the esophagus are weakened. Such patients may have dysphagia, aspirate, and develop pneumonia. Apathetic thyrotoxicosis may simulate intra-abdominal malignant disease with marked weight loss, colicky abdominal pain, and altered bowel habits.[2, 3] Another important gut complication of hyperthyroidism is intussusception.[4]

The other clinical extreme of thyrotoxicosis, *thyroid storm* (high fever, marked tachycardia, agitation, delirium), has intestinal manifestations which include acute abdominal pain, vomiting, jaundice, and diarrhea. Thyrotoxicosis associated with *ulcerative colitis* is particularly serious. It may exacerbate the diarrhea of colitis;[5, 6] conversely, active inflammatory bowel disease may aggravate hyperthyroidism; indeed, colitis may precipitate thyroid storm in patients with undiagnosed or untreated thyrotoxicosis. (Personal observations of MHS.)

Hyperthyroidism is also associated with hypergastrinemia,[7] apparently due to beta-adrenergic hyperresponsiveness or increased number of receptors, because the levels of gastrin in such patients can be reduced by propranolol.[8] Levels are also reduced to normal with successful therapy of the hyperthyroidism. Likewise, patients with Hashimoto's thyroiditis and hypothyroidism usually have normal gastrin levels.[7, 9] However, the correlation of serum T_3 and gastrin is not good—some patients with thyrotoxicosis have high and others have low levels of gastrin.[7, 9] It is curious also that acid secretion is often reduced in those with hypergastrinemia. This suggests that decreased acid secretion may be a primary effect of hyperthyroidism in some patients, and that hypergastrinemia is a secondary response to low acid output. There is no established increased incidence of peptic ulcer disease in hyperthyroidism.

Patients with hyperthyroidism are reported to have a significantly higher incidence of "superficial" and "interstitial" gastritis than an aged-matched control group, but do not show gastric atrophy.[10] Acid secretion is normal in most cases of hyperthyroidism but when acid production is low it often returns to normal after treatment, indicating no permanent damage to the mucosa.[11, 12] Contrary to older belief, hyperthyroid patients have normal gastric emptying after meals.[12] With regard to bowel habit, although diarrhea is common (15 to 20 per cent) in hyperthyroidism, constipation has been reported in 30 to 40 per cent of these patients.[13]

The effects of uncomplicated hyperthyroidism on the liver include some minor histologic changes and very little alteration of function. Occasionally, there is slight elevation of unconjugated bilirubin and of plasma glutathione-S-transferase;[14, 15] unusually prolonged disease complicated by congestive heart failure or "thyroid storm" will cause jaundice. In a small number of patients the spleen is enlarged. Conversely, cirrhosis may alter thyroid function tests of patients who are euthyroid. Thus, T_3, FT_3, T_3/thyroxine-binding globulin, T_4/thyroxine-binding globulin, and levels of TSH after TRH are all low; however, FT_4 and thyroxine binding globulin are usually elevated. Euthyroid status is usually attributed to adequate levels of FT_4.[16]

One of the striking effects of hyperthyroidism is on the small bowel, with mucosal edema and round cell infiltration of the mucosa; villi, however, are normal.[17] More than 25 per cent of such patients have mild to moderate steatorrhea.[18] With increasing fat intake, the proportion of patients with steatorrhea increases markedly, up to 60 per cent in one unselected series.[18] Although bile acid output is subnormal in these patients following a meal, the concentrations of conjugated bile acids and pancreatic enzymes in the duodenum are normal.[12] Carbohydrate absorption, as measured by D-xylose uptake, is normal in thyrotoxicosis, but calcium absorption is markedly impaired. This is because hyperthyroidism causes a decrease in parathyroid hormone levels, which leads to decreased conversion of 25-hydroxyvitamin D to 1,25-hydroxyvitamin D. Vitamin D–binding protein does not change. Serious skeletal demineralization may occur. These changes normalize with treatment of hyperthyroidism.[19, 20]

Hyperthyroidism accelerates transit through the small intestine, explaining in part the diarrhea and weight loss of this disease. The mouth-to-cecum transit time averages 29 minutes versus 72 minutes in normal subjects. This slows to normal following successful therapy and return to euthyroidism, and the slowed transit correlates with weight gain and the disappearance of diarrhea in most patients.[21, 22] Thus, hypermotility of the small bowel is still thought to be the pathophysiologic basis for the steatorrhea.[18, 21, 22] That motility may not be the sole factor, however, is shown by the amelioration of a secretory-type diarrhea in a patient with hyperthyroidism following treatment with propylthiouracil and propranolol.[23] Presumably thyroid hormone can induce intestinal secretion by increasing intracellular cyclic AMP, akin to the actions of cholera toxin and vasoactive intestinal peptide (VIP).[24]

Beta-blockade has marked cardiovascular effects in thyrotoxicosis, but it does not predictably alter transit time. Nevertheless, several patients benefited from propranolol, with marked decrement of steatorrhea.[20]

Autoimmune Thyroid Disease. *Hashimoto's thyroiditis* often causes hypothyroidism and is commonly associated with circulating parietal cell antibodies and varying degrees of gastric atrophy with hypochlorhydria, including pernicious anemia, whether the patient is hypothyroid or euthyroid.[25] Serum gastrin levels are normal in *Hashimoto's disease,* unless the mucosa is severely atrophic and the patient is achlorhydric.[8, 9] A few of these patients have both *hypothyroidism* and *pernicious anemia*; others may be achlorhydric without intrinsic factor deficiency. About 25 per cent of patients with *primary biliary cirrhosis* have circulating thyroid antibodies, half of whom have evidence of clinical thyroid disease, particularly hypothyroidism.[26] Rarely, *celiac sprue* may occur with autoimmune thyroiditis.[27]

Hypothyroidism. *Myxedema* may be associated with severe disturbances of esophageal peristalsis and gastroesophageal sphincter function causing reflux and esophagitis. Appropriate replacement therapy reverses the sphincter tone to normal and restores peristalsis.[28] Hypothyroidism also is associated with severe gastric hypomotility and the formation of *phytobezoars.*[29] Severely impaired colonic motility also may be manifested by *constipation, obstipation, sigmoid volvulus, rectal prolapse,* and *fecal impaction* (Fig. 29–1). In rare instances the patient develops *megacolon.* Even rarer, infantile myxedema may cause *microcolon* with obstipation and obstruction, apparently completely reversible with replacement therapy.[30] A clinical and radio-

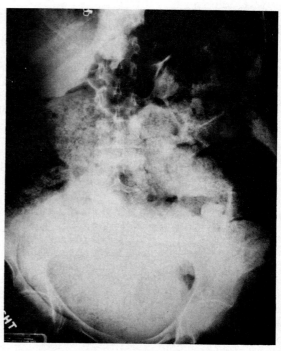

Figure 29–1. Massive fecal impaction with distended colon in a patient with myxedema. Perforation later developed.

logic picture simulating tumor of the sigmoid has been reported.[31] Hypothyroidism can be a cause of ileus and pseudo-obstruction (see pp. 377–380).[32]

Diarrhea, although rare in hypothyroidism, may occur and be associated with steatorrhea and malabsorption.[33] It has been predicted that hypomotility of the gallbladder in hypothyroidism would lead to an increased incidence of gallstones;[34] however, no such increased incidence has been documented.[35] Although excretion of indocyanine green may be delayed, and aspartate aminotransferase (AST), lactate dehydrogenase (LDH), and gamma globulins are often elevated, the liver histologic appearance is usually intact.[36] The lithogenicity of bile has not been studied in these patients so that the question of such an abnormality remains. One study of euthyroid women treated for hypothyroidism with thyroxine for many years has shown a high incidence of cholelithiasis. Perhaps a defect in bile formation persists.[37]

Inexplicably, hypothyroidism also causes other significant clinical problems, such as hyponatremia and ascites; these problems regress with proper therapy. The ascites of hypothyroidism is exudative, like the pericardial and pleural effusions of this disorder[38] (see pp. 428–454). Myxedema has been also found with the *Cronkhite-Canada* syndrome (see pp. 1511–1513).[39] Routine serum tests of liver function (LDH, AST, cholesterol, gamma globulins) are mildly elevated in approximately 50 per cent of hypothyroid patients,[36] especially in the presence of congestive heart failure or pericardial effusion.[15, 36] Changes in drug-metabolizing enzymes have been noted even in the absence of other biochemical abnormalities.[40] These abnormalities normalize with thyroid hormone replacement.[36] Patients undergoing treatment may develop elevation of the plasma activity of glutathione-S-transferase, indicating that there is subclinical hepatic thyrotoxicosis due to excessive thyroxine.[15] As noted above, hypothyroidism is encountered in about 25 per cent of patients with primary biliary cirrhosis.[25] That diminished thyroid function protects patients against liver disease is belied by rapid progression of alcoholic hepatitis in an alcoholic with untreated hypothyroidism.[41]

Tumors of the thyroid gland are discussed below with multiple endocrine neoplasms.

Adrenal Disease

An increased incidence of *cholelithiasis* in *pheochromocytoma* is recognized and appears to be related to hypertension. With fixed hypertension 10 per cent of these patients have gallstones; 30 per cent have them with intermittent hypertension. How the abnormal state of excessive catecholamines relates pathogenetically to stone formation is not clear but may be due to impairment of gallbladder contractility.[42] In patients with high serum catecholamines, basal gastrin levels and serum gastrin in response to a test meal are significantly elevated (see p. 509).[43]

Adrenal Insufficiency. *Addison's disease* involves the gut in over half of the cases, but gastrointestinal symptoms are usually overshadowed by profound fatigue, hypotension, and hyperpigmentation. Anorexia and weight loss are present in almost all patients; vomiting and abdominal pain are common.[44] Atrophic gastritis is a frequent pathologic finding, and pernicious anemia may be present in association with autoimmune Addison's disease.[45] The pancreas and small bowel are histologically normal, yet moderate to severe *fat malabsorption* and diarrhea are reported, perhaps due to a loss of the trophic effect of corticosteroids upon small intestinal brush border function.[45, 46]

Parathyroid Disease

Hyperparathyroidism. Gastrointestinal symptoms in patients with *primary hyperparathyroidism* (HPT) are estimated to be present in over 50 per cent and to constitute the presenting complaints in 10 to 15 per cent.[47, 48] The principal complaints are attributable to hypercalcemia and are roughly proportional to the degree of elevation of serum calcium. In a recent series of 100 patients with hyperparathyroidism, 33 per cent complained of constipation, 29 per cent of abdominal pain, 28 per cent of nausea, and 20 per cent of vomiting; 14 per cent had *peptic ulcer disease,* and one patient had *pancreatitis.*[48] In another series 65 per cent had abdominal complaints; 31 per cent had constipation; 23 per cent dyspepsia without ulceration, and 15 per cent had a documented peptic ulcer.[49] Most of these symptoms are alleviated upon correction of the

hypercalcemia, both acutely and following successful removal of functioning parathyroid tumors. *Cholelithiasis* is found in one fourth to one third of patients with HPT. Calcium in bile is increased; presumably, hypercalcemia underlies high concentrations of calcium in bile and accounts for the increased incidence of calcium-containing stones in HPT.[49] Anorexia is almost universal with the severe hypercalcemia of hyperparathyroidism. The abdominal pain is often epigastric (not necessarily due to peptic ulcer) but as often is described as diffuse.

The basis for these gastrointestinal symptoms due to hypercalcemia is not known, but they may be related to the damping effect of high calcium ion concentration on the neural transmission of both afferent stimuli and efferent discharges from parasympathetic ganglia, because excess calcium ion reduces neuromuscular excitability. Such effects might be responsible for decreased motor activity and may explain the constipation that may be severe in these individuals. The nausea and vomiting may be related to the gastric atony and altered motor tone of the duodenum. No likely explanation for the abdominal pain of hypercalcemia exists. It is difficult to accept hypercalcemia as the cause for all these gut troubles, however, because patients with familial hypercalcemia seem to have no abnormal incidence of these complaints.[50] Nonetheless, St. Goar's description of hyperparathyroidism as a disease characterized by "troubles with stones, bones, and abdominal groans" remains accurate.[51]

Hyperparathyroidism (HPT) and Peptic Ulcer. Peptic ulcer disease occurs in HPT when HPT is part of the *multiple endocrine neoplasia syndrome I* (MEN I) with a gastrinoma (see below). The incidence of ulcer disease has also been repeatedly reported to be increased in those with HPT alone, ranging from 5 to 30 per cent.[48, 52] Despite the reported alleviation of severe ulcer disease following removal of a functioning parathyroid tumor, and the high incidences reported in some series of patients with HPT, a statistically significant increased incidence of peptic ulcer disease in hyperparathyroidism is still not proved. The difficulty in establishing an association is compounded by the lack of solid data on the incidence of peptic ulcer disease in control populations. It is of some interest, however, that in one series of patients with duodenal ulcer disease the incidence of diagnosed hyperparathyroidism was about 10 times the predicted incidence.[53] That gastrin is responsible for ulcer disease in hyperparathyroidism is doubtful because gastrin levels are usually normal, and cure of hyperparathyroidism in many instances does not affect the course of peptic ulcer.[47]

Acutely induced hypercalcemia causes increased acid secretion via increased release of gastrin. The explanation for this effect is not clear; perhaps the autonomic nervous system plays a role.[54] However, the effect can be blocked by prior IV administration of somatostatin (SRIF).[55] Certainly, chronic hypercalcemia and hyperparathyroidism do not cause gastrin levels to rise.[56] Nevertheless, patients with hypercalcemia after renal transplantation are more likely to suffer bouts of gastrointestinal bleeding, which reportedly cease after parathyroidectomy for HPT,[57] despite little reported change in gastric acid secretion after successful transplantation (see p. 513).[58]

That hypercalcemia *per se* leads to peptic ulcer disease is certainly not established; indeed, large families with benign hypercalcemia apparently have no increased incidence of the disease.[50] Although acute elevations of serum calcium elevate gastrin and acid secretion, chronic elevations at very high calcium levels (above 15.0 mg/dl) suppress acid secretion.[59]

Hyperparathyroidism (HPT) and Pancreatitis. The possible association of elevated serum calcium due to HPT and recurrent bouts of *acute pancreatitis* has long been studied,[60-69] albeit with decreasing conviction that the incidence of pancreatitis in HPT is greater than 1.0 to 1.5 per cent.[48, 64, 68, 69] The important point is that patients with HPT will be at greatest risk for an attack of pancreatitis (usually severe and unlikely to recur after successful parathyroidectomy) when serum calcium either rises sharply or is above 14.0 mg/dl.[65, 66, 68, 70] That dramatic elevation in serum calcium may cause pancreatitis is supported by the reported incidences of the disease in patients with *vitamin D intoxication*, with *multiple myeloma*, following *IV calcium infusion*, in *renal insufficiency* with so-called rapidly progressive "secondary" HPT, *after parathyroidectomy* (if thyroidectomy is also performed), in patients receiving *total parenteral nutrition* (TPN), in *carcinoma* of the *parathyroid* with HPT, in *metastatic cancer* of *breast*, and in *familial hypercalcemia*.[70-78] The pathogenesis of pancreatitis secondary to an acutely elevated level of serum calcium is unknown. One explanation is that high Ca^{2+} levels in pancreatic ductal fluid activate trypsinogen and the "cascade" of enzymes associated with acute pancreatitis (see p. 1817).[71]

The effect of chronic hypercalcemia on the pancreas is less clear. In experimental feline chronic hypercalcemia, the fluid output and bicarbonate concentration of the pancreas are diminished in response to secretin or secretin and cholecystokinin (CCK), and the concentration of protein-independent calcium in the pancreatic juice increases markedly after stimulation. The latter effect seems due to increased ductal permeability to Ca^{2+}.[79] Of interest, after a Lundh meal, patients with HPT and chronic hypercalcemia secrete pancreatic juice which has a significantly lower volume and higher calcium content than following parathyroidectomy.[80] Perhaps the pancreatic ductal calculi occasionally seen in HPT-associated pancreatitis result from increased Ca^{2+} concentration in juice which has ample amounts of "stone" glycoprotein as a nidus (see p. 1845). Chronic disease of the pancreas may eventually lead to weight loss, steatorrhea, and diabetes mellitus. The clue to the diagnosis of underlying hyperparathyroidism in patients with pancreatitis is the normal or only slightly depressed levels of calcium in the face of rather severe clinical attacks. These levels are decidedly supernormal following recovery (see p. 1821).

Rarely, a patient with hyperparathyroidism will develop so-called *parathyroid crisis,* that is, life-threatening symptoms caused by marked elevation of serum calcium. One of the consequences of such a crisis may be *severe necrotizing pancreatitis,* an acute surgical abdomen with severe nausea, vomiting, dehydration, fever, pain, and in some instances coma due to diabetic ketoacidosis.[81] Some of the symptoms are also due to severe phosphate depletion. Acute pancreatitis of hyperparathyroidism also may be very severe during *pregnancy,* particularly in the third trimester (see p. 500).[82]

Hypoparathyroidism. Hypoparathyroidism is associated with hyposecretion of acid and is directly attributable to subnormal levels of ionized serum calcium. When these levels are raised to normal, gastric acid secretion also tends to return to normal.[59] Hypoparathyroidism also is associated with malabsorption and mild to moderate steatorrhea, leading to diarrhea, and of course, marked hypocalcemia is the hallmark (Fig. 29–2).[83] Constipation and even pseudo-obstruction may be an important gut disturbance in this disease. In the *familial polyendocrine failure syndrome (candidiasis endocrinopathy),* which features hypoparathyroidism and adrenal insufficiency, patients suffer from severe oral and esophageal *candidiasis, fat malabsorption,* and *chronic active hepatitis.*[84, 85] A defect in immunoregulation has been documented.[85]

Multiple Endocrine Neoplasms (MEN Syndromes)

A number of combinations of tumors arising from endocrine organs or from cells of neural crest, ectodermal, or ectoblastic origin which are common to the gut, pancreas, and brain (but also found in lung and other organs) are responsible for serious gastrointestinal symptoms. Their cells have in common the production of biologically active polypeptides, some of which are the classical hormones of endocrine glands. Others are known neurotransmitters, and still others are neuroendocrine or paracrine molecules. The tumors often possess ability to take up and decarboxylate amine precursors, and hence, they are called APUD tumors.* Their products may stimulate or inhibit gut functions.[86-109]

The MEN syndromes are hereditary, being transmitted in an autosomal dominant manner. Thus, 50 per cent of the children of an afflicted parent are at risk for the disease, but expression is variable. The syndromes have been divided into three major categories: MEN 1, 2A, and 2B. There is some overlap between them.

MEN 1. This syndrome is composed of *hyperparathyroidism* (in nearly 100 per cent of cases due to adenomas), *pituitary adenomas* (occasionally functional), and *islet cell tumors* of the *pancreas.* The major gastrointestinal effect of MEN 1 is *peptic ulcer disease,*

---

*Amine precursors uptake and decarboxylation tumors.

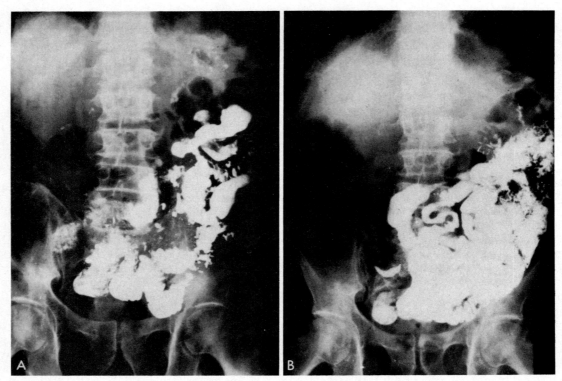

Figure 29–2. Small bowel series in a patient with hypoparathyroidism and malabsorption. *A*, Before therapy with vitamin D. *B*, After therapy. (From Clarkson, B. O., Kowlessar, O. D., Harwith, M., and Sleisenger, M. H.: Metabolism *9*:1053, 1960. Used by permission.)

due to *gastrin* released by about 25 per cent of the islet cell tumors (see pp. 909–925). Islet cell tumors of the pancreas, however, also may secrete ACTH, insulin, glucagon, serotonin, neurotensin, vasoactive intestinal peptide (VIP), and somatostatin, although somatostatinoma is not yet reported as part of MEN 1 (see pp. 1884–1900).[86] Parathyroid hormone, prolactin, and serum calcium levels are the most useful screening tests for MEN 1, although other hormones may be elevated earlier in certain families.[88, 89] The serum pancreatic polypeptide (PP) level is elevated in 50 per cent of patients with islet cell tumors and is a useful screening test in some MEN 1 families.[89, 90] Levels of PP can be elevated in other conditions (alcohol abuse, acute diarrhea, following small bowel resection, pancreatitis, and others), but intramuscular injection of atropine will identify the patients with tumors because PP release by islet cell tumors is not suppressed by atropine.[90] Serum gastrin is occasionally useful for early detection of MEN 1, although a gastrinoma is unlikely if symptoms of ulcer disease are absent and serum calcium is normal.[88, 89]

Hypoglycemia leads to a diagnosis of pancreatic insulinoma, seen in an occasional patient with MEN 1, and conversely, hyperglycemia, diabetes mellitus, skin rash, and anemia reflect the activity of yet another islet cell adenoma which may be present in MEN 1, i.e., *glucagonoma* (see below).[91] More interesting, both insulin-secreting and glucagon-secreting cells may be present in the same tumor, leading to remarkable fluctuations of blood glucose levels during the course

of the disease.[92] Also reported is the combination of excessive gastrin and glucagon secretion by an islet cell tumor, causing peptic ulcers and diabetes.[93]

An islet cell tumor in a patient with MEN 1 may cause severe diarrhea by secreting vasoactive intestinal peptide (VIP). The clinical features of this syndrome are watery diarrhea, hypokalemia, and achlorhydria (or hypochlorhydria), hence the WDHA syndrome. The WDHA syndrome more commonly is due to isolated islet cell tumors of the pancreas or to ganglioneuromas and ganglioneuroblastomas in children. Patients with MEN 1 are reported to have VIP-secreting pancreatic tumors, occasionally with hypercalcemia, and are also likely to have multiple tumors in their pancreas.[94] Other tumors that elaborate VIP and cause watery diarrhea include *bronchogenic carcinoma, ganglioneuroblastoma*, and *retroperitoneal histiocytoma* (see pp. 1890–1892).

MEN 2A. This syndrome is composed of *medullary carcinoma* of the *thyroid* (MCT), *parathyroid hyperplasia*, and *pheochromocytoma*. Pheochromocytomas are present in 25 to 50 per cent of cases and are bilateral in 80 per cent.[95] Hyperparathyroidism is present in up to 50 per cent of cases.[95, 96] The prominent gastrointestinal symptom is a watery, secretory type of diarrhea, which is due in most patients to the elaboration of calcitonin (CT).[87, 95, 96] It is contributed to by prostaglandins, VIP, and rarely, serotonin (5-HT). Additional peptide hormones produced by MCT include ACTH, somatostatin, beta-endorphin, insulin, and gastrin. The tumor also elaborates a number of bioactive amines and enzymes (including dopamine, dopa decarboxylase, and histaminase) and other substances including CEA, melanin, and nerve growth factor. All of these substances are synthesized by the C cells of the tumor.[87] Because ACTH may be produced, Cushing's syndrome occasionally is part of the clinical picture. Of interest is the finding that about 10 per cent of these patients will flush, possibly due to the release of 5-HT, prostaglandins, or CT.[87] The only gastrointestinal symptom directly attributable to tumor size is *dysphagia* due to esophageal compression. Diarrhea-induced hypokalemia is common and, if severe and persistent, may be associated with muscle weakness and *ileus* (see pp. 1890–1892).

The watery diarrhea in about 30 per cent of these patients indicates advanced disease with a high tumor burden and poor prognosis.[95, 96] The principal diagnostic test is measurement of immunoreactive serum calcitonin (iCT) after stimulation with pentagastrin, calcium, or even ethanol (whiskey).[95–97] A positive test may be obtained in asymptomatic individuals with only thyromegaly or with a family history of MCT or MEN 2A.[95, 97] Surgery, of course, is the prime mode of therapy, with the hope of complete excision of the secreting thyroid tumor. (Surgery should not be undertaken, however, until pheochromocytoma has been ruled out or, if present, properly managed.) Attempts to reduce tumor size and activity have been made by use of chemotherapeutic agents such as doxorubicin, streptozotocin, or cisplatin but with little success.[95] Symptomatic therapy consists of prostaglandin inhibitors such as indomethacin, 25.0 mg, two to three times daily by mouth to offset the effect of prostaglandins on the gut. Common antidiarrheal agents such as diphenoxylate with atropine, 5.0 mg four times daily, may be employed or, in more severe cases, codeine sulfate, 30.0 mg two to four times daily, may be given. More definitive treatment of diarrhea preoperatively or recurrent diarrhea postoperatively consists of bromocriptine or L-dopa, which inhibit CT secretion and CT synthesis, respectively. The reported effectiveness of bromocriptine and of L-dopa in the treatment of the diarrhea caused by CT in this syndrome has not been confirmed.[98]

Improvement in MEN symptoms has been reported using the somatostatin analogue, SMS 201-995, which in normal subjects inhibits the release of many substances, including insulin, glucagon, gastrin, CCK, bombesin, VIP, and growth hormone. It can also suppress the growth and secretion of unresectable endocrine tumors.[99] Side effects are unusual but can include diabetes mellitus (suppression of insulin release) and fat malabsorption (suppression of exocrine pancreatic secretion).[100]

MEN 2B (MEN 3). This syndrome is composed principally of *MCT, pheochromocytoma* (often bilateral), and multiple *mucosal neuromas* of the gastrointestinal tract, buccal mucosa, lips, tongue, and conjunctiva, plus enlarged corneal nerves seen by slit-lamp examination.[95, 96] Frequently, the abdomen is distended. The patients have distinct physical characteristics such as *marfanoid habitus*, flat bridge of the nose, and large lips. The family history is strong for the disease and the patients often develop severe gastrointestinal problems very early in life. It differs from MEN 2A in the greater virulence of the MCT, the absence of hyperparathyroidism despite parathyroid hyperplasia, and the presence of neuromas (seen on skin, lips, and tongue), as well as other somatic abnormalities as described (see Fig. 30–3 and p. 537). Symptoms include constipation, diarrhea, difficulty with feeding, projectile vomiting, crampy abdominal pain, and loud borborygmi.[101, 102] These symptoms often antedate detection of the endocrine neoplasms and thus should raise the suspicion of underlying endocrine disease, especially in those with physical characteristics suggestive of MEN 2B. The importance of early detection is the distinct possibility of curative resection of the MCT and the adrenal tumors. (For further discussion of pheochromocytomas, see pp. 490 and 509.)

It is likely, but not proved, that the neuromas scattered throughout the gastrointestinal tract in MEN 2B are responsible for some of the symptoms, such as intermittent constipation and chronic diarrhea. The constipation often is lifelong and is commonly associated with *diverticula* of the *colon* and *megacolon*. A narrowed zone in the lower sigmoid or upper rectum, suggestive of Hirschsprung's disease, has been noted, and intestinal obstruction is not rare.[95–105] Recently, MEN 2B with ganglioneuromas of the gut has been associated with *adenomatous polyposis* of the stomach, small intestine, and colon as well as with *juvenile polyposis*.[105, 106] This coincidence is very important in view of the report of *adenocarcinoma* of the *colon* in one patient with colonic ganglioneuromatosis and MEN 2B.[107] Some patients with this syndrome have severe steatorrhea and malabsorption associated with their diarrhea. Diarrhea, as in MEN 2A, also may be due to the MCT elaborating calcitonin, prostaglandins, or VIP. An inapparent MCT may be detected by stimulation of calcitonin release after administration of pentagastrin or calcium intravenously or after alcohol ingestion.[95–97] Early diagnosis is imperative for cure in view of the aggressiveness of the medullary carcinoma of the thyroid in MEN 2B. As in MEN 2A, pheochromocytoma must be ruled out or appropriately managed if discovered before thyroid surgery is undertaken. Vigorous study of asymptomatic first-degree relatives of patients afflicted with MEN 2B must be carried out early in childhood.[101–104]

MEN 1 and 2. The combination of features of MEN 1 and 2 is not rare, particularly with islet cell tumor of the pancreas and pheochromocytoma.[108] The evidence suggests that this disorder is also inherited in an autosomal dominant fashion. In some cases it is present in patients with *von Hippel–Lindau disease*; in others, it is associated with neurofibromatosis.[108] These patients become ill at an early age; the pheochromocytomas are responsible for the clinical symptoms in about 80 per cent of these cases. In contrast to the hypersecretion of the islet cell tumors in MEN 1, the islet cell tumors, although occasionally malignant, usually are nonsecreting.[109]

Diabetes Mellitus and the Gastrointestinal Tract

General Considerations. The pathogenesis of *diabetic autonomic neuropathy* (DAN) in insulin-dependent diabetics of long duration is unexplained. Several metabolic abnormalities have been demonstrated and offered as theories to explain the impaired neuron function. These include impaired neural protein synthesis, abnormal axoplasmic transport, disturbed polyol pathway activity, and abnormal myo-inositol metabolism.[110, 111] Although the molecular basis for the anatomic changes of the intrinsic innervation of the gut is not evident, it is apparent that DAN affects the gut, often severely.

The anatomic evidence of DAN of the gastrointestinal tract consists of observations from spontaneously diabetic hamsters, from rats made diabetic by streptozotocin, and from a limited number of human diabetics. While the picture of the extent of damage to the various autonomic components is not clear, some important observations emerge. Myelinated fibers of spontaneously diabetic hamsters show a significant reduction of axon diameters of vagal branches and of sympathetic ganglia with concomitant thinning of myelin sheaths. The number and densities of these fibers are also diminished.[112, 113] Rats with streptozotocin-induced diabetes have intestinal distention and diarrhea. While there is either no significant morphologic change or an increase in adrenergic, cholinergic, and serotoninergic innervation of the proximal colon, degeneration of the adrenergic nerves and of the serotoninergic innervation of the myenteric plexuses of the ileum occurs.[114, 115] Autonomic fibers containing VIP of both myenteric plexuses and of the circular muscle layer are greatly increased in number in the ileum and in the colon. The content of VIP in mucosa and smooth muscle of these segments of intestine is elevated.[116, 117] Gastric content of VIP and somastostatin is also increased.[118] On the other hand, the amount of substance P at these sites is decreased. What the increased VIP content in the autonomic nervous system of gut in diabetic rats signifies for diabetic humans is not known, but it may reflect an early stage of neuronal degeneration or an increase in VIP synthesis by these nerves. Increased activity of VIP theoretically could account for the diarrhea of some patients with diabetic neuropathy and, because of its relaxing effect on gut smooth muscle, for the colonic distention with severe constipation and even megacolon in others.[116–118]

Study of Meissner's plexuses in patients with DAN reveals unequivocal *axonal degeneration* along with thickening of the basement membrane of Schwann cells;[119] similar findings are reported in Auerbach's plexuses in streptozotocin-induced diabetes in rats in which the nerves of these plexuses in ileum and colon show axonal swelling.[120] Despite the above-noted anatomic and neuroendocrinologic findings, there is as yet no good correlation of these changes with dysfunction of the gastrointestinal tract.

A second explanation for involvement of the gut in diabetes is *microangiopathy*; however, microscopic studies have failed to show such change in the mucosa of the gastrointestinal tract.[121] A third possible mechanism is blood glucose and electrolyte imbalance, which is common in insulin-dependent diabetics. Hypokalemia, hyperkalemia, hypoglycemia, and hyperglycemia all may change gut motility. Certainly, motor abnormalities of the gut are accentuated during diabetic ketoacidosis (DKA) when there are marked abnormalities of blood sugar and electrolytes[122] (see below). Finally, there may be increased susceptibility of diabetic patients to infections such as tuberculosis and *Candida*.[122] Regardless of the exact mechanism of the gut involvement, it is clear that other evidence of diabetic neuropathy often precedes gastrointestinal symptoms. Some think that poorly controlled, insulin-dependent diabetic patients are more susceptible to both peripheral and visceral neuropathy. For good reviews of diabetes mellitus and the gut, the reader is referred to three relatively recent accounts.[123–125]

Esophageal Dysfunction. About 80 per cent of patients with diabetic neuropathy have abnormal motility of the esophagus, which in the majority of cases is asymptomatic.[126, 127] The motility disorders range from slight impairment of peristalsis to absence of coordinated peristaltic activity with many tertiary contractions upon swallowing, resembling diffuse esophageal spasm. Frequently, the resting pressure of the lower esophageal sphincter is reduced and is not increased by subcutaneous injections of bethanechol. The symptoms of the diabetic esophageal disorder are mild and consist of heartburn and rarely dysphagia. (Perhaps heartburn is less common than expected in such patients because gastric acidity is commonly reduced in long-standing diabetes.) As in any patient, such complaints demand investigation.[128–130]

Almost all insulin-dependent diabetics with or without peripheral neuropathy will have diminished esophageal motility as judged by measurement of radionuclide transit, but of these, only 50 per cent will have complaints. A number of diabetics without evidence of peripheral neuropathy have hyperperistalsis of the esophagus resembling diffuse esophageal spasm (see pp. 587–588). The severity of the manometric findings among these patients correlates best with the patients' psychiatric symptoms of depressive or anxiety disorders, though the mechanism for this relationship is not apparent.[128]

Of those with peripheral neuropathy but no symptomatic swallowing problem, 50 per cent will have delayed esophageal emptying.[126–131] In fact, esophageal dysfunction in these patients is so common that its absence in an insulin-dependent diabetic with nausea, vomiting, or diarrhea should cast doubt on the diagnosis of diabetic gastroenteropathy.[131] This dysfunction is due to defective innervation rather than disease of smooth muscle, as evidenced by damage to the vagus branches of the esophagus.[132, 133] The neurons of the esophageal myenteric plexus are largely normal in diabetics. Metoclopramide is helpful in restoring normal resting pressure to the lower esophageal sphincter and thus diminishes reflux. This drug also may improve the rate of emptying by the esophagus (see pp. 559 to 619).

Because patients with diabetes generally are more prone to *Candida* infection, *candidiasis* of the esophagus as well as of the mouth (see p. 553) is more common than in control populations. Either barium swallow or esophagoscopy may reveal characteristic findings. Yeast forms are more readily demonstrated by smears of esophageal brushings than by biopsies (see pp. 640–642).[134]

Gastric Dysfunction and Disease ("Gastroparesis Diabeticorum") (see pp. 227 and 695). Impaired motor activity of the stomach is also common in patients with diabetic neuropathy and is most common in those with orthostatic hypotension. It causes symptoms that range from vague abdominal discomfort postprandially to invariable postprandial nausea and vomiting. Like most other gastrointestinal symptoms associated with diabetic neuropathy, the nausea and vomiting are inexplicably intermittent.[125, 135] Gastric stasis may occasionally cause problems more serious than postprandial distress and vomiting, i.e., weight loss, poor diabetic control, and bezoars.[136] Diabetics stressed by constant vomiting, no matter what the cause, often develop *diabetic ketoacidosis* (DKA); conversely, hypoglycemia may be noted in those who take insulin and fail to absorb ingested food because of serious delays of gastric emptying.[125, 135]

Diabetics with DAN affecting the stomach may have profoundly delayed gastric emptying as judged by barium studies or by radionuclide scanning.[135, 137] However, sensitive studies using radiolabeled liquids and digestible solids usually show normal or nearly normal emptying of both substances in long-standing insulin-dependent diabetics with or without symptoms.[131, 137] The most consistent abnormalities seen are impaired transit of indigestible solids and absence of the antral component of the interdigestive motor complex (phase III), which normally is responsible for clearance of indigestible solids.[135, 137, 138] Other motor abnormalities seen in certain patients include postprandial antral hypomotility, continuous low-amplitude antral activity, reduced gastroduodenal-jejunal phasic pressure activity, and more commonly, nonpropagated powerful antral contractions lasting more than two minutes.[139] In addition, gastric emptying may be delayed by periods of pylorospasm before and after meals.[140]

The pathophysiology for these motor disturbances, and hence for delayed gastric emptying, is elusive. It has been attributed to defective vagal innervation, but unlike surgical vagotomy, rapid emptying of liquids in diabetic gastroparesis is uncommon (see p. 695).[135, 137] Also associated with gastroparesis and the absence of antral phase III activity is an abnormally high level of serum motilin regardless of the state of emptying.[141, 142] This observation seems paradoxic because normally motilin is believed to induce phase III activity. However, large doses of motilin in normal humans have been shown to delay gastric emptying (see pp. 88 and 91), and the success of metoclopramide in restoring more normal activity to the stomach in those with gastroparesis[138] is associated with a fall in motilin levels and the appearance of antral phase III activity.[141] Yet, motilin levels do not correlate well with the degree of motor impairment in many subjects, and there is other evidence that metoclopramide's effectiveness lies more in its augmentation of the number and height of random motor spikes (phase II) than in its effect on phase III activity (see below).[143] Another contributing factor to delayed emptying in poorly controlled insulin-dependent diabetics is hyperglycemia.[144] In summary, no single mechanism has been delineated which explains the gastric retention. Defects in vagal action, intrinsic neurons, and even smooth muscle function may all be involved.

Diagnosis. On physical examination, the diabetic patient with gastric atony may have gross gastric dilatation with a succussion splash. A saline load test may be used to quantify gastric emptying of liquids, but is considered by some to be a poor test in diabetics (see p. 685). Roentgenographic examination may reveal a significantly dilated stomach, often with retained material, and is a critical test in establishing the diagnosis and eliminating the possibility of other gastric disorders. Sluggish, ineffectual, and irregularly occurring gastric contractions are noted on barium swallow, and over 50 per cent of the barium will remain in the stomach in 30 minutes. More than 75 per cent of the patients also will have some solid gastric residue despite a prolonged fast prior to the examination.[139] Elongation of the stomach and duodenal bulb atony also may be noted. Performance of radiolabeled scintigraphy or a radiopaque marker study is the most reliable way to confirm the diagnosis of a gastric emptying disorder or to evaluate the response to therapy.[135, 137] Whether such studies should be performed depends upon their availability and the degree of uncertainty of the diagnosis in a particular patient (see above and pp. 685–689). Before one makes the diagnosis of diabetic gastric atony, the effect of prescribed anticholinergics, antidepressants like the tricyclic compounds, tranquilizers (diazepam, and so on), and ganglionic blocking agents must be excluded.

Treatment. Patients with *gastroparesis diabeticorum* may be helped by prescribing metoclopramide, 10 mg four times daily (30 minutes before meals and at bedtime). It increases the rate of gastric emptying and decreases postprandial gastric volumes.[138, 145] The effectiveness of metoclopramide in many patients with diabetic gastroparesis appears to be established. It acts favorably in a number of ways: by a direct ("prokinetic") effect on gastric motor activity, by potentiating acetylcholine release, by antagonizing dopamine and thus offsetting its inhibition of gut smooth muscle, and by stimulating the antiemetic center of the hypothalamus (possibly via its antidopamine effect).[145] Its side effects include restlessness, anxiety, dystonia, tremor, and rarely oculogyric crises. Those patients who take this medication as prescribed report subjective evidence of improvement, particularly following the ingestion of solid food. Nausea, vomiting, anorexia, fullness, and bloating are significantly ameliorated. Individual improvements in gastric emptying after parenteral or oral metoclopramide, however, cannot be correlated with symptom change during treatment.[145] The efficacy of long-term treatment is somewhat less than during the early weeks of use.[146] Bethanechol, a cholinergic agent, increases gastric emptying acutely in diabetics, but there are no reports of long-term use.[138] More recently, a metoclopramide-like compound known as domperidone, a selective peripheral dopamine antagonist, has had successful trials in Europe and Australia in the management of patients with diabetic gastroparesis and apparently has a greater margin of safety.[147, 148] Newer promotility agents, such as cisapride, are under study and may be available soon.[148a] Other therapeutic measures include strict control of blood sugar because reduction of elevated blood sugar may accelerate the rate of gastric emptying. Results of surgical procedures—e.g., gastroenterostomy or pyloroplasty—are not usually permanently successful. Because delayed gastric emptying leads to *bezoar* formation, these should be carefully sought out and, if detected, managed endoscopically (see pp. 741 to 745).

Gastritis and Gastric Atrophy (see pp. 792–813). *Acute erosive gastritis* is common in diabetic ketoacidosis and is frequently accompanied by bleeding. Management consists of the use of either antacids such as aluminum hydroxide, an H_2 blocker, or a cytoprotective agent such as sucralfate or one of the prostaglandins. If bleeding is significant, the principles of management discussed on pages 400 to 411 and 776 to 778 should be followed.

The incidence of low-grade *chronic gastritis* and *gastric atrophy* is increased in patients with long-standing diabetes. It is associated with significant titers of circulating parietal cell antibodies (approximately four times the predicted prevalence) and often with thyroid antibodies, explaining the higher incidence of *pernicious anemia* and of *hypothyroidism* in diabetics, particularly if they are female, young, and insulin-dependent.[126, 127, 136, 149] Intrinsic factor antibodies are present in about 10 per cent of diabetics, half of whom have pernicious anemia (see pp. 800–801).[126, 127, 136, 149–152]

The incidence of *duodenal ulcer* in diabetics is lower than expected, perhaps because basal and stimulated acid secretion are often significantly lower than normal.[153] In one study 17 per cent of diabetic patients were achlorhydric.[153] At least three mechanisms are at work to decrease acid output. First, gastric atrophy is present in varying degrees, though probably related more to age than to the severity or duration of the diabetes. Second, some studies show a normal response of acid secretion to pentagastrin, suggesting that there is a normal parietal cell mass, but the sensitivity to submaximal doses is diminished, akin to the diminished acid secretory response to insulin and sham feeding in

many diabetics. Such findings are compatible with defective vagal innervation.[154, 155] Finally, elevated basal and meal-stimulated levels of gastric inhibitory peptide (GIP), a potent inhibitor of acid secretion, have been reported for insulin-dependent and non–insulin-dependent diabetics.[125, 156]

Unexplained Abdominal Pain. An entity called *diabetic radiculopathy* or *diabetic plexus neuropathy* of thoracic nerve roots has been described to which is attributed otherwise unexplained upper abdominal pain in patients with diabetic neuropathy. Persisting pain causes anorexia and marked weight loss, suggesting an intra-abdominal malignancy. Inexplicably, the pain often subsides after 6 to 18 months.[157]

Small Intestinal Dysfunction. Symptomatic small bowel disorders in diabetic neuropathy are more common and bothersome than those of the esophagus or stomach. The predominant symptom is *diarrhea*, and in some instances *steatorrhea* is present. The incidence of diarrhea in diabetics ranges up to 10 per cent.[123–125, 158]

Diabetic diarrhea is particularly troublesome at night and appears to be more common in men than in women. These are usually patients with neuropathy who are insulin-dependent and often poorly controlled. Despite the diarrhea, the patient usually maintains good appetite. Fortunately, the diarrhea tends to remit at times and in some instances may disappear entirely.

Radiographically, the small intestine in diabetic diarrhea/steatorrhea shows nonspecific dilatation of loops of the small gut, segmentation, and some evidence of mucosal edema (Fig. 29–3). The transit time is variable; it may be shortened or prolonged (see below).

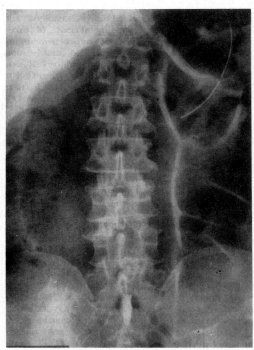

Figure 29–3. Severe intestinal dysmotility in a patient with diabetic neuropathy. A nasogastric tube is present.

Although the cause of the diarrhea and steatorrhea is not clear in most patients, several conditions must be sought. One of these, *bacterial overgrowth* of the small intestine, is probably due to impaired small bowel transit and stasis and is a cause of both the diarrhea and steatorrhea in a minority. It is ameliorated with proper use of broad-spectrum antibiotics (see pp. 1295–1296). In some patients diarrhea may be due to *chronic pancreatitis* with exocrine pancreatic insufficiency, a disease that is more common in patients with long-standing diabetes mellitus than in control populations (see p. 1848). Rarely, diarrhea is due to *adult celiac disease*, which is more common in diabetics than in the general population.[159]

What role the diabetic neuropathy plays in the diarrhea and steatorrhea is not clear. Small bowel transit times in patients with DAN do not correlate well with the presence or absence of diarrhea. Indeed, for many years studies of small bowel transit in DAN have produced conflicting results, with some reporting shortened, and others lengthened, transit times.[123, 125, 136, 158, 160–163] A recent study of small intestinal transit time determined by breath hydrogen measurements after feeding a liquid and solid meal to insulin-dependent diabetics showed normal solid meal transit in all subjects. Twenty-five per cent had rapid transit of the liquid test meal, and 25 per cent had prolonged transit. Only one of three patients with DAN and diarrhea had a shortened time; only two of four patients with nausea and bloating had delayed intestinal transit.[164]

Although a decrease in resting pressure of the upper small intestine as well as an increase in frequency of large peristaltic waves accompanies neuropathy, no known data on small bowel motility postprandially can explain the pathogenesis of the diarrhea in these patients.[158, 160–163] That a motor disturbance is very likely present, however, is supported by the recent evidence of defective cholinergic neuromuscular transmission in the myenteric plexus of the small intestine of rats in whom diabetes has been experimentally induced.[165, 166] As noted, morphologic studies in rats, hamsters, and humans show damage to (1) both adrenergic and cholinergic nervous systems of the gut, including pre- and postganglionic fibers of sympathetic ganglia; (2) the ganglia of the myenteric plexuses;[112–115, 119, 167, 168] and (3) visceral vagal fibers.[132, 167, 168] These findings probably explain the diminished responses to distention,[160–162] to cholinergic stimulation,[165] and to adrenergic stimulation in DAN.[169] However, neither deficiency of acetylcholine release nor an excess of acetylcholinesterase has been found.[114, 115] Tighter control of hyperglycemia with increased insulin dosage in diabetics with neuropathy and diarrhea may help ameliorate the diarrhea.[170] Perhaps insulin improves neuromuscular function of the gut in this situation.

Because the diarrhea of diabetic neuropathy is usually watery, intermittent, and voluminous, impaired regulation of intestinal fluid and electrolyte transport may be responsible.[171] Streptozotocin-induced diabetes in rats causes intestinal adrenergic neuropathy.[114, 115] Such neuropathy is associated with postsynaptic denervation hypersensitivity and reduced stores of mucosal norepinephrine,[169, 171] which might explain the disturbed fluid and electrolyte transport in these diabetic rats. An alpha-adrenergic agonist, clonidine, reverses this abnormality in vitro in affected loops, providing the basis for treating diabetic diarrhea in humans[172] (see below).

One additional pathophysiologic hypothesis for diabetic diarrhea is the diarrheagenic effect of bile salts on the colon. In the absence of enteric infection, it is difficult to understand how unconjugated bile acids would gain entry to the colon in sufficient amount to contribute to the diarrhea. Since the bile salt pool in diabetics with autonomic neuropathy and diarrhea may be reduced, it is possible that conjugated bile acids are not being resorbed normally by the terminal ileum, perhaps secondary to some problem with intestinal motility.[173] However, if this were an important mechanism, it is perhaps surprising that the response to cholestyramine has been so variable.[127] Further, no evidence for a primary defect in absorption of bile salts has been demonstrated.

The management of diabetic diarrhea not due to *chronic pancreatitis, bacterial overgrowth*, or *celiac sprue* is difficult, but strict control of the blood sugar levels may help.[170] Codeine sulfate, 30 mg, diphenoxylate hydrochloride with atropine (Lomotil), or loperamide, 2.0 mg, once or twice daily and at bedtime, may reduce the nocturnal movements. In some instances psyllium hydrophilic mucilloid (Metamucil) or cholestyramine, 4.0 gm every eight hours, may help. Clonidine, an alpha-adrenergic agonist, in a limited trial appeared to reduce the volume and numbers of stool in some patients with diabetic diarrhea.[172] Its principal effect may be via decreased motility because its stimulation of net fluid and electrolyte absorption in normal humans appears to be modest.[174] The dose of clonidine to treat diabetic diarrhea is 0.5 mg every 12 hours.[172] In this dosage, clonidine did not cause hypotension, and pre-existing postural hypotension was not aggravated. Diabetic control and renal function were also unaltered. If the medication needs to be withdrawn, it should be done so slowly to avoid "rebound" hypertension. Recently, severe diabetic diarrhea was shown to be controlled using the somatostatin analogue, SMS 201-995 (see p. 493).[175, 175a]

It should be emphasized that in cases in which *bacterial overgrowth* cannot be ruled out as the cause of diarrhea a two-week trial of a broad-spectrum antibiotic such as tetracycline, 0.25 gm four times a day by mouth, should be prescribed. Also, in questionable cases of *adult celiac disease* a trial of gluten-free diet should be undertaken because this disease is more common in diabetics.[159]

Colonic Involvement. *Constipation* is the most common and bothersome complaint in diabetics and appears in some cases to be related to DAN (Fig. 29–3).[123–125] Occasionally it is so severe as to cause *megacolon*. Other complications include *stercoral ulcer* or *perforation, volvulus, barium impaction* with *overflow diarrhea*, and *incontinence*. Extensive pathophysiologic studies of motility in patients with diabetes and severe constipation (defined as two or less spontaneous stools per week) revealed that although basal electrical and motor activity of the colon is normal in these patients, the myoelectrical and colonic motor responses to a test meal are blunted and delayed in diabetic patients with little or no constipation and, more important, were absent in diabetic patients with severe constipation.[176, 177] Chronic intestinal pseudo-obstruction may result late in the disease.[178, 179] These patients will respond appropriately to parenteral injections of neostigmine or metoclopramide, suggesting that the colonic muscle is capable of responding but apparently is not signaled to respond to food because of defective innervation of the colon.[176]

Therapy of constipation in these patients is usually medical. In addition to symptomatic relief, which is obtained on occasion with enemas, laxatives, and cathartics, which are taken by the majority of these individuals before they seek medical attention, metoclopramide treatment is instituted—10 mg before meals and at bedtime. High fiber diets have not proved to be of great benefit, and anorectal myectomy has not been adequately evaluated for one to have gained an impression of its possible efficacy.

A serious complication from the standpoint of patients' physical well-being is rectoanal *incontinence*, with soiling and all of its physical and psychic consequences.[125] Incontinence often coincides with the onset of diabetic diarrhea, but in most cases the total stool volume is normal.[180] Steatorrhea is present in up to 30 per cent of cases.[180] Autonomic dysfunction is thought to be responsible for the impairment of both the normal sphincteric resting tone and of the reflex which ensures internal sphincter relaxation with rectal distention. Because the internal sphincter is entirely innervated by the autonomic system, its incompetency in DAN is not surprising.[180] It is virtually axiomatic that patients with DAN and fecal incontinence will have other symptoms of DAN. Occasionally, incontinence will remit spontaneously. Management is empiric and includes biofeedback training and antidiarrheal agents (both unproven). It is important also to treat the diarrhea in these patients as an aid to the management of incontinence.

Liver and Biliary Tree. The most prominent abnormality of the liver in diabetes mellitus is *steatosis*. It has been reported to be present in 21 to 78 per cent of patients. It is common in maturity-onset diabetics but may occur in poorly controlled juvenile, insulin-dependent diabetes.[124, 126] When present, it reflects long-term poor control of the disease. The liver is enlarged and often tender. A prime factor in the appearance of fatty liver in adult patients is obesity. Loss of weight will be followed frequently by mobilization of fat from the liver as well as better control of the diabetes. The glycogen content of the liver is usually increased in diabetic patients; however, the degree of increase does not correlate with fasting blood sugar, type of diabetes, degree of ketosis, or the fat content of hepatocytes. Glycogen may be seen in the nuclei of hepatocytes in patients with or without fat; however, patients with glycogen are usually asymptomatic. Diabetics may be more susceptible to both viral and certain drug-induced hepatitis; particularly noteworthy is the cholestatic hepatitis of the oral hypoglycemic agents, especially chlorpropramide.[124]

The incidence of *cholelithiasis* is thought to be increased in patients with diabetes.[181–185] The finding of a high degree of unsaturation of cholesterol in the bile of some uncontrolled diabetics, however, casts doubt on the lithogenicity of the diabetic's bile.[184] Further, no statistically valid prospective study of the incidence of cholilithiasis in diabetics, controlled for obesity, is available for review. Bile of adult-onset diabetics (type 2) is supersaturated with cholesterol, and the concentration of bile acids is reduced.[185] Stasis of bile in the gallbladder may contribute to stone formation because many diabetics have enlarged gallbladders that contract less vigorously than normal in response to meals, particularly if DAN is present.[186, 187]

Whether or not cholelithiasis is more dangerous to future health in diabetics remains debatable.[188, 189] One need not recommend cholecystectomy for the diabetic with asymptomatic gallstones. Neither is routine screening for gallstones warranted. However, the course of the disease does not always parallel that of the nondiabetic, for acute cholecystitis and perforation are more common than in nondiabetics, and because diabetics require emergency surgery twice as often as nondiabetics.[189] It is accepted that surgery should be done for those with symptomatic gallstones or with acute cholecystitis in the absence of contraindications to surgery. Because emergency biliary tract surgery in diabetics carries a significantly higher morbidity and mortality rate, the question of elective cholecystectomy for asymptomatic cholelithiasis remains. Unfortunately it can't be answered affirmatively without consequences because elective cholecystectomy even for those diabetics with silent stones is attended by higher than normal morbidity and mortality rate (see pp. 1691–1714).[188, 189]

Gastrointestinal Manifestations of Diabetic Ketoacidosis (DKA). Nausea, vomiting, and diffuse severe abdominal pain all are part of the clinical picture of ketoacidosis with loss of metabolic control in patients with insulin-dependent diabetes. In the majority of instances these individuals are diabetics of longstanding; are often in their second, third, or fourth decades; and generally have had repeated difficulty with control of their diabetes. In such cases, the rapid control of the metabolic imbalance with administration of intravenous fluids with electrolytes and insulin will be associated with rapid disappearance (in four to six hours) of these symptoms.

The differential diagnosis of such patients on occasion may be extremely difficult when the DKA has *resulted* from an underlying inflammatory process within the abdomen and is not the primary cause of severe abdominal pain. In such instances of DKA, X-ray and scanning techniques are required to rule out *acute cholecystitis, peritonitis, acute appendicitis, is-*

chemia, acute pancreatitis, or *viscus perforation*. Correct differential diagnosis is crucial because often fatalities from DKA result from an underlying, correctable medical-surgical condition which is missed because of physician preoccupation with managing DKA, and because DKA may suppress abdominal signs and symptoms, and mental function.[190–192]

Differential diagnosis is complicated in other instances by the extreme discomfort of the gastric atony, ileus, or gastritis (occasionally hemorrhagic) or of the pancreatitis of DKA. Further, distention of the liver capsule increases discomfort.[191] Fortunately, bleeding from gastritis of DKA is usually not extensive and is limited to some coffee ground contents of the stomach which rapidly clears as the DKA is brought under metabolic control. The diagnosis of a bout of *acute pancreatitis* underlying both DKA and gastritis may be hard to pin down because serum amylase may be elevated (on occasion, as high as 1000 Somogyi units per dl) in DKA alone.[193, 194] Usually this represents nonpancreatic ("salivary-type") amylase; the presence of elevated pancreatic amylase or lipase indicates true pancreatitis.[193] Indeed, this clinical picture can be induced in the well-controlled diabetic by withdrawing insulin therapy, and it can be reversed with restoration of insulin and fluid replacement.[195] History often makes the distinction; i.e., patients with DKA will have abdominal distress after they have had hours or days of indisposition characterized perhaps by an upper respiratory infection or gastroenteritis, polydipsia, polyuria, and increasing weakness, whereas those with a severe underlying abdominal entity will refer initial symptoms to the abdomen, usually with symptoms characteristic for each entity. The physical findings in the upper abdomen are not so striking in the *pancreatitis* of DKA; that is, tenderness is usually not as well localized and dramatic as in primary pancreatitis and signs of peritoneal irritation and ileus are less likely. In doubtful instances CT or sonographic scans of the abdomen should be done to detect enlargement of the pancreas due to edema or phlegmon, or to detect evidence of distal common bile duct obstruction. In such instances the patient is likely to have jaundice and elevated alkaline phosphatase. The alcoholic diabetic with acute pancreatitis will usually be known as a heavy drinker; although metabolic imbalance in these patients supervenes quickly, pain precedes all else and always becomes severe before the symptoms of DKA appear (see p. 1820).

The diagnosis of acute inflammatory biliary tract disease—*acute cholecystitis* or *cholangitis* associated with *choledocholithiasis*—is generally more straightforward. There is right upper abdominal and back pain with fever (cholecystitis), or pain in the same area with shaking chills and higher (102 to 104°F) fever (cholangitis). Up to a day of such distress will precede the onset of DKA; dark urine may be observed. The patient often is known to have gallstones.[196] On examination the patient will invariably have tenderness in the upper right quadrant, usually with some rebound. The diagnosis of acute cholecystitis is best made by the use of nuclide scanning after the injection of HIDA type compounds (see pp. 1703–1705). Failure to visualize the gallbladder in this situation establishes the diagnosis of acute cholecystitis with a high degree of specificity. Determination of liver enzymes, particularly AST, alanine aminotransferase (ALT), and LDH, are of limited help because they frequently are abnormal in patients with DKA uncomplicated by intra-abdominal diseases. In approximately half the patients with DKA who have abnormal levels, no specific cause can be identified.[197] An enlarged liver which is somewhat tender in DKA may reflect acute enlargement due to fatty infiltration.

The most dreaded intra-abdominal disease in the diabetic is *acute mesenteric arterial ischemia*. Here pain heralds the process—it is usually severe and out of proportion to the abdominal physical findings. Small intestinal ischemia causes diffuse midabdominal pain which lessens in hours and is followed by distention due to ileus. Early diagnosis is imperative because intervention may prevent fatal gangrene. *Colonic ischemia* will often cause rectal bleeding (see pp. 1903–1916).

Fortunately, differential diagnosis is frequently facilitated by the rapid resolution of the pain, nausea, and vomiting within 12 hours of beginning intensive therapy for DKA. Symptoms persisting after this period of time must be intensively studied for a primary intra-abdominal cause. If mesenteric ischemia is suspected, action must be taken within a few hours and it must be emphasized that incompletely managed DKA should not postpone necessary surgical intervention.[192]

Diabetes and the Pancreas. Pancreatic disease and pancreatic insufficiency are common in patients with diabetes. The risks of *acute pancreatitis* and *pancreatic carcinoma* are increased. Acute pancreatitis is twice as frequent in diabetics compared with nondiabetics, particularly in young, insulin-dependent diabetics.[195–200] Acute pancreatitis causing ketoacidosis in diabetic patients has a serious prognosis, with a high mortality rate.[198] In addition, severe acute pancreatitis often leads to diabetes mellitus in the previous nondiabetic patient and exacerbates the disease in known diabetics. About 20 per cent of patients, usually those younger than 35 years old, will develop mild diabetes following bouts of acute pancreatitis.[201] These patients also may have high serum glucagon levels as a cause for hyperglycemia associated with the acute attacks.[201, 202] There is no strong correlation between the degree of hyperglycemia during the acute attack of pancreatitis and the appearance of diabetes following recovery (see p. 1819).

A higher than predicted percentage of patients with diabetes mellitus will have subnormal responses to exocrine pancreatic stimulation, especially in patients who have had juvenile diabetes for at least five years.[199, 203] However, the incidence of clinically apparent *chronic pancreatitis* is not increased. On the other hand, patients with established chronic pancreatitis (usually due to alcohol) will have an incidence of diabetes ranging from 30 per cent (those with noncalcified glands) to 70 per cent (those with pancreatic calcifications).[204] The incidence of diabetes is lower in patients with idiopathic chronic pancreatitis and much lower in those with pancreatitis due to biliary tract disease or trauma (see p. 1848).[204]

Carcinoma of the pancreas is about twice as frequent in patients with established diabetes mellitus as in the general population.[205, 206] It is often difficult to determine whether the diabetes antedates or is due to the malignancy in those recently found to have both diseases. In 80 per cent of patients with pancreatic cancer and diabetes, their diabetes is discovered within a year of the time the cancer is clinically obvious, suggesting that the malignancy is the basis for the diabetes.[207]

Glucagonoma and Non-B Islet Cell Tumors. Glucagonoma is a glucagon-secreting tumor of the A cells of the islets of Langerhans. Insulin levels are normal or reduced, depending upon how much pancreatic tissue is replaced by tumor. The diabetes that results is mild to severe, and there may be some degree of insulin resistance. Many of these patients have a skin disease called *erythema necrolytica migrans*, and they may have oral crusting, painful glossitis, loss of hair, refractory anemia, weight loss, hypoproteinemia, diminished plasma amino acids, thromboembolic disease, and elevated blood glucagon levels.[91, 208] Of great interest are giant duodenal villi sometimes noted on small bowel series or endoscopy.[209, 210] Insulinomas or gastrinomas may coexist with glucagonomas in the same tumors, giving rise to either great swings of blood sugar over many years or severe peptic ulcer disease, respectively.[92, 93] A further description of this syndrome and of the effects upon the gut of non-B islet cell tumors is on pages 1892 to 1894.

PREGNANCY

Pregnancy-related gastrointestinal disorders are due largely to decreased gut motility, the combined result of increased sex hormone levels and the bowel-displacing effects of the gravid uterus.[211] Progesterone inhibits intestinal smooth muscle activity in a number of species, including humans.[211] In pregnant women this hormone probably underlies the decreased lower esophageal sphincter pressure, increased percentage of nonperistaltic contractions of the distal esophagus, and increased gastric pressure even in the first trimester, causing *reflux esophagitis* (rarely severe) and heartburn.[212-214]

Basal and pentagastrin-stimulated acid secretion, serum gastrin,[212] and gastric emptying are all normal through most of pregnancy.[215] It is not uncommon for peptic ulcer disease to improve with pregnancy.[216]

Intestinal transit is markedly delayed, contributing to constipation and *hemorrhoids*. Nonabsorbed stool softeners, glycerine suppositories, and exercise are useful. Colonic obstruction and *pseudo-obstruction* have been reported (see pp. 369–379). Of interest is the finding that the interdigestive migratory motor complex (IMMC) of the small intestine in pregnant rats is slowed and irregular.[217]

Nausea and vomiting, quite common in the first trimester of pregnancy, and *hyperemesis gravidarum* are discussed on pages 229 to 231. *Hematemesis* may occur as a result of a *Mallory-Weiss* esophageal tear. Indeed, this is the most likely cause of bloody emesis in pregnant women, provided no other obvious disease has been diagnosed previously, such as varices associated with congenital hepatic fibrosis (see pp. 647–649).[211]

Gallbladder emptying is impaired by progesterone, and bile acid output is decreased by estrogens.[218] As a result, gallstones are more common in pregnancy, but the incidence of *cholecystitis* is not particularly increased. *Pancreatitis*, although rare, may be caused by the adverse effect of estrogens upon an underlying lipoprotein disorder[219] or as a postoperative complication;[211] it is associated with a high maternal and fetal mortality rate.[220] A rare and unexplained cause of acute upper abdominal pain and hypotension in pregnancy is *ruptured splenic artery aneurysm*.[220a]

Inflammatory bowel disease, which poses special problems in planning and managing pregnancy, is discussed on pages 1327 to 1358 and 1435 to 1477.[221]

DEFICIENCY STATES

Although nutritional deficiencies are commonly the result of gastrointestinal disease, lack of zinc or niacin is a cause of intestinal dysfunction, characterized by *diarrhea* as well as *skin lesions* and *neurologic dysfunction*. The oral and cutaneous manifestations of other deficiency states are described on pages 534 to 535. *Iron deficiency* is discussed on page 504.

Acrodermatitis Enteropathica and Zinc Deficiency

Acrodermatitis enteropathica is either an inherited disease seen in children or, more commonly, an acquired disease affecting both children and adults.[222] The clinical manifestations of both forms are due to zinc deficiency. Zinc is required by over 100 metalloenzymes, including those for the synthesis of DNA, RNA, and proteins. It is plentiful in animal protein and nuts, but its absorption is blocked by phytic acid, a chelating agent in cereals.[223] Hence, zinc deficiency is common among poor populations of the Middle East whose diets consist largely of unleavened bread (high in phytates) and vegetables.[223] Acquired deficiency also occurs with decreased intake (total parenteral nutrition), decreased enteric absorption (malabsorption syndromes, Crohn's disease with fistulas, jejunoileal bypass, geophagia), increased zincuria (hepatic cirrhosis, chronic renal failure with proteinuria, severe burns, penicillamine therapy), and increased zinc demand (sickle cell anemia, pregnancy, lactation). It affects alcoholics with *pancreatitis* as well (see also pp. 1992–1993).[222-226]

Zinc-deficient rats exhibit ultrastructural abnormalities of the small bowel enterocytes; brush border disaccharidases are depleted.[227, 228] Patients develop diarrhea in 90 per cent of cases. There may be flattening of villi, inflammatory infiltration of the lamina propria, folate malabsorption due to impairment of folate conjugase, fat malabsorption, and rarely *protein-losing enteropathy*.[222, 229, 230]

The *skin disease* symmetrically involves the face, scalp, perianal area, hands, and feet with vesiculobullous lesions that progress to chronic erythema and crusting (Fig. 29–4). Bacterial or fungal superinfection is common. Patients may have alopecia, oral erythema, and a white-coated tongue.[222]

Neurologic deterioration includes personality changes, mental lethargy, and irritability. Other manifestations of zinc deficiency include congenital defects and growth retardation in children, *male infertility*, *hypogeusea*, and *recurrent infections* (due to impaired T cell function).[222] Oral or parenteral zinc results in rapid clearing of symptoms.

Pellagra

Pellagra results from dietary deficiency or possibly impaired absorption of niacin.[231] Because niacin can be synthesized from tryptophan, concomitant protein malnutrition may be a prerequisite for development of pellagra. In Western countries, pellagra is most commonly seen in indigent alcoholics. The classic triad of the "three Ds," present in only 22 per cent of cases, includes *diarrhea*, nervous system disorders (particularly *dementia*), and *dermatitis* (see Fig. 29–4).[232]

Diarrhea occurs in 40 to 50 per cent of patients and may be associated with *steatorrhea*. Weight loss may be the first clinical sign of pellagra.[232] Small intestinal histologic findings and D-xylose absorption are usually normal unless there are coexisting multiple nutrient deficiencies.[233] Vitamin replacement causes dramatic improvement within one week.

NEOPLASTIC DISEASES

Metastatic Cancer to the Gastrointestinal Tract

Metastases to the gut may occur by direct invasion from adjacent organs, by intraperitoneal seeding, or by hematogenous or lymphangitic spread. As many as 20 per cent of malignant nongut epithelial neoplasms may involve the gastrointestinal tract.[234] Patterns of metastasis are not random but rather reflect the location and histologic type of the primary tumor, a fact of great help in characterizing a new lesion.[235] *Breast cancer, malignant melanoma*, and *bronchogenic carcinoma* are the most common tumors, usually forming

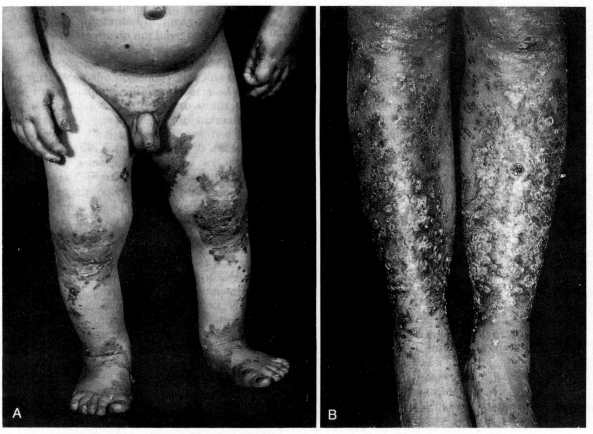

Figure 29–4. *A,* Acrodermatitis enteropathica. *B,* Pellagra. (Courtesy of Victor Newcomer, M.D.)

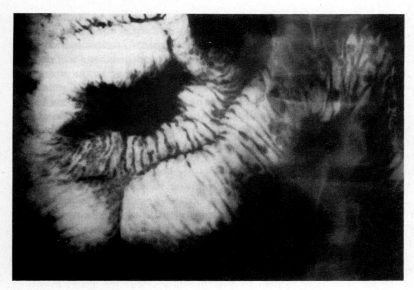

Figure 29–5. Metastatic melanoma involving the duodenum of a 21-year-old male. Multiple serosal implants are seen. (Courtesy of the Radiology Learning Center, University of California School of Medicine, San Francisco.)

implants on the serosa or mesentery. They are best detected by barium studies, which may reveal extramural masses, mucosal ulcerations, a "linitis plastica" gastric appearance (from infiltrating breast carcinoma), or ulcerating masses with a "bull's eye" appearance seen typically with metastatic melanoma (Fig. 29–5).[235] Computerized tomography is often helpful to determine the primary tumor, to stage the extent of metastases, and to detect large serosal implants.[236] Pain, fever, ascites, bleeding, obstruction, and perforation have all been described.[237]

Paraneoplastic effects can be as significant as direct metastases. Intestinal dysmotility may take the form of intestinal *pseudo-obstruction* caused by a peripheral neuropathy associated with small cell carcinoma of the lung[238] or of isolated *colonic dilatation* (Ogilvie's syndrome; see pp. 377–379). It may also result from *hypercalcemia* caused by a variety of metastatic tumors or from the MEN syndromes (see pp. 1098–1099).

Lymphoma

Lymphoma involves the gastrointestinal tract either as the primary site or secondarily from systemic lymphomas or from lymphomas originating in retroperitoneal or intra-abdominal lymphoid tissue. Lymphomas may affect any organ (see pp. 761–763 and 1545–1553)[239] and must be part of the differential diagnosis of any gastrointestinal symptom, especially in patients with the *acquired immunodeficiency syndrome (AIDS)* (see pp. 1242–1257).[240]

HEMATOLOGIC DISEASES

Leukemia

Approximately 10 per cent of leukemia patients suffer significant gastrointestinal complications, either from the leukemia itself or as the result of chemotherapy (Table 29–1).[241] Examination of autopsy specimens

reveals gastrointestinal involvement in almost half of all patients with leukemia;[242] *acute myelogenous leukemia* (AML) is the type most likely to affect the

Table 29–1. GASTROINTESTINAL COMPLICATIONS OF LEUKEMIA*

LEUKEMIC INVASION OF THE BOWEL AND RELATED STRUCTURES
  Mechanical obstruction
    Adynamic ileus
    Intussusception
  Mucosal ulceration
    Perforation, hemorrhage
  Liver and spleen enlargement
    Infarction, rupture
  Portal hypertension
    Ascites, varices, hepatorenal syndrome[256]
  Biliary and pancreatic duct obstruction
  Protein-losing enteropathy[253]
  Pneumatosis intestinalis
  Colitis[254]
IMMUNODEFICIENCY
  Necrotizing enterocolitis (leukemic typhlitis)[248–251]
  Increased susceptibility to common infections
    Appendicitis
    Wound infections
    Perianal inflammation
    Abscess, peritonitis, sepsis
  Opportunistic infections[246]
    Esophageal candidiasis
    Viruses (cytomegalovirus, herpes virus)
    Mycobacteria, protozoans
    Oral mucositis
COAGULATION DEFECTS
  Intramural hemorrhage
    Hemorrhagic necrosis
    Obstruction
  Gastrointestinal bleeding
DRUG TOXICITY
  Oral mucositis
  Nausea and vomiting
  Ileus, megacolon
  Bowel necrosis
  Hemorrhagic colitis
  Pseudomembranous colitis[252]
  Pancreatitis[255]
    Pseudocyst

*Adapted from Hunter, T. B., and Bjelland, J. C. Am. J. Roentgenol. *142*:513, 1984.

gut.[241] The lesions result from four major causes: leukemic cell infiltration, immunodeficiency, coagulation disorders, and drug toxicities (Table 29–1).

Radiologically, leukemic lesions assume many forms. Infiltration of the bowel may produce the appearance of polypoid masses, plaque-like thickenings, ulcers, and diffuse masses. Esophageal filling defects with clot and debris have been described[243] as well as typical *monilial esophagitis*. The gastric mucosal folds can assume a brainlike, deeply convoluted appearance resembling adenocarcinoma.[244] Polypoid filling defects seen in the small and large bowel may produce *obstructions* or *intussusceptions*.[245]

Immunodeficiency and immunocytopenia leads to *agranulocytic ulcers* with bacterial invasion and bleeding. Coagulation defects can produce *intramural hematomas* and hemorrhagic necrosis of bowel.[246]

Clinical syndromes are myriad (Table 29–1). Common oral symptoms are gingival bleeding, hypertrophy, and inflammation, as well as focal ulcerations. Oral *mucositis* (stomatitis) is a severe inflammatory condition which results in the setting of recent chemotherapy, radiation therapy, or bone marrow transplantation. Bacterial, fungal, or viral agents are often implicated. On examination there is diffuse ulceration of the oral mucosa, and patients complain of severe pain. Treatment consists of broad-spectrum antibiotics such as clindamycin, antifungal therapy, viscous lidocaine, and systemic analgesia. Cultures for herpes virus are obtained and acyclovir instituted. Esophageal lesions, especially due to *candidiasis* or *herpes viruses*, may cause odynophagia, dysphagia, or rarely, massive esophageal bleeding. *Gastric ulcers* have been reported in a patient with hyperhistaminemia secondary to basophilic granulocytic leukemia. *Massive gastrointestinal hemorrhage* can be caused by gastric leukemic infiltrates.[247]

An acute abdomen is especially dire for the patient with leukemia, occurring in 5 per cent of acute and 3 per cent of chronic leukemias.[248] *Acute appendicitis, abdominal abscess*, and *perforation* seemingly are noted with increased frequency. *Necrotizing enterocolitis* is a severe problem which complicates the disease in patients with neutropenia and thrombocytopenia, usually following a course of chemotherapy and antibiotics.[249] It results from bacterial invasion of neutropenic ulcers and generally is not associated with leukemic tissue infiltration. The lesion usually affects the ileocecal area (leukemic *typhlitis*), although any intestinal segment may be involved.[250] Patients present with fever, abdominal pain, and bloody diarrhea. It may progress to bowel necrosis or perforation; surgical intervention is often required.[250, 251] *Pseudomembranous colitis* may complicate antileukemia chemotherapy even in the absence of antibiotic use (see pp. 1307–1320).[252] Other rare complications are listed in Table 29–1.

Proctologic problems can include *stercoral* and *neutropenic ulcers, infection, induration* of tissues, and *perirectal abscess*.[257] Rectal pain, bleeding, and mucorrhea may result.

Bone Marrow Transplantation

Bone marrow transplantation (BMT) for the treatment of leukemia produces intestinal complications in virtually every patient.[258] The BMT begins with "conditioning" the host's marrow by high-dose radiation therapy, chemotherapy, or both. Injury to proliferating crypt cells in the gut mucosa results in cramping abdominal pain and diarrhea (usually not severe) beginning a few days after conditioning and resolving by four weeks, at which time the mucosa has recovered histologically.[258] Conditioning can also lead to *veno-occlusive disease* of the liver.[259] *Oral mucositis* is discussed above.

Graft-versus-host disease (GVHD) is an immunologic phenomenon affecting up to 50 per cent of BMT patients.[260] *Acute GVHD* occurs between the first and third months following transplantation. It consists of *skin rashes, cholestatic liver disease*, and sloughing of the intestinal mucosa, producing severe diarrhea, abdominal pain, and often, *protein-losing enteropathy*[261, 262] (see pp. 283–290). *Chronic GVHD* begins three months after engraftment and is not always preceded by acute GVHD. In its most severe form it includes *cholestatic liver disease* (with immune obliteration of the bile ducts), *upper esophageal strictures* or *webs* due to submucosal fibrosis[263] (see pp. 611–613 and 632–635), and rapidly progressing *scleroderma* which affects the gastrointestinal tract as described on pages 505 to 506. Oral mucosal atrophy, erythema, and pain are common.[264]

Finally, BMT patients are highly vulnerable to a variety of *opportunistic infections* of the gastrointestinal tract because of the immunosuppression of the conditioning regimen or the chemotherapy used to suppress GVHD. (For a recent review, see references 258 and 265 and see pp. 127–133). *Gram-negative bacterial sepsis* with enteric organisms is common because the denuded intestinal mucosa does not provide an effective barrier to their entry.[265]

Dysproteinemias

Gamma heavy chain disease, associated with abdominal pain, weight loss, and a large gastric mass composed of plasmacytoid cells, has been reported.[266] *Alpha heavy chain* disease is described on pages 131 to 132.

Multiple myeloma may affect the gastrointestinal tract in the form of *amyloidosis* (see pp. 509–510) or *plasmacytomas*. Twenty-five per cent of plasmacytomas are associated with multiple myeloma;[267] they can affect the gut from the esophagus to the rectum. Multiple masses or pyloric obstruction simulating ulcer disease can be seen radiologically. The tumors may be asymptomatic or may cause anorexia, vomiting, abdominal pain, and bleeding.[268] Involvement of the temporomandibular joint may cause difficulty in chewing. Multiple myeloma has also been reported in association with *inflammatory bowel disease*[269] and *celiac sprue*.[270]

Gastrointestinal infiltration is found in patients with *Waldenström's macroglobulinemia.* Extracellular IgM is deposited in the lamina propria and in mesenteric nodes; lacteals are dilated.[271] Thickened folds, dilatation, and filling defects are noted on small bowel X-ray studies. Symptoms may include diarrhea, abdominal pain, flatulence, and weight loss. Coagulopathy may produce retroperitoneal or gastrointestinal hemorrhage.[272] Steatorrhea, decreased D-xylose and vitamin B_{12} absorption, and intestinal protein loss have all been recorded.[271, 273]

Hemolytic-Uremic Syndrome

Hemolytic-uremic syndrome (HUS) consists of the triad of *acute renal failure, microangiopathic hemolytic anemia,* and *thrombocytopenia.*[274] Though primarily a disease of children, adults also suffer this disorder. Typically, HUS is preceded by a prodromal illness with gastrointestinal, respiratory, or systemic symptoms; severe *hemorrhagic colitis* caused by the *Escherichia coli* strain 0157:H7 has preceded several cases.[275] Once HUS appears, colonic involvement is common owing to microangiopathic thrombosis of submucosal vessels and intramural hemorrhage.[274] X-ray abnormalities include mucosal irregularity, dilatation, filling defects, bowel wall edema, and findings which may resemble idiopathic ulcerative colitis or a severe vasculitis (Fig. 29–6).[276, 277]

Clinical manifestations are primarily those of acute gastroenteritis, with crampy abdominal pain, vomiting, and diarrhea. Because HUS is usually self-limiting, therapy consists of hemodialysis and supportive gastrointestinal care. Severe complications can include *toxic megacolon, rectal prolapse,* transmural necrosis with *perforation,* or colonic stricture.[277]

Blood Coagulation Disorders

Twenty per cent of bleeding episodes in patients with *hemophilia* may originate in the gastrointestinal tract.[278] Other bleeding diatheses such as *von Willebrand's disease, heparin* or *warfarin overdose,* and other causes of *vitamin K deficiency* may also result in gastrointestinal hemorrhage.[279] Radiologically, intramural bleeding can be recognized by thickened mucosal folds, rigidity, luminal narrowing, particularly in segments of the small intestine, and intragastric masses (Fig. 29–6).[278] Intestinal obstruction and intussusception may result. Submucosal bleeding or intramesenteric hemorrhage may produce abdominal pain and signs of an acute abdomen (see pp. 1903–1916).

Thrombotic thrombocytopenic purpura (TTP) is a heterogeneous disorder consisting of thrombocytopenia, microangiopathic hemolytic anemia, fever, neurologic dysfunctions, and renal insufficiency. Twenty-four per cent of subjects have nonspecific abdominal complaints.[280] Like hemophilia, TTP can lead to gas-

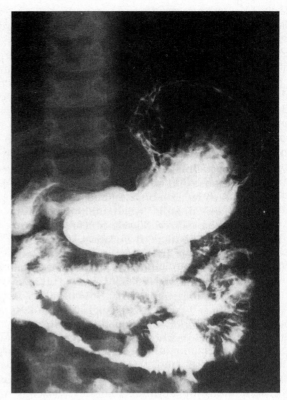

Figure 29–6. Intramural hemorrhage in Henoch-Schönlein purpura. Thickened duodenal folds and lumenal narrowing are present. Three days later, abdominal pain had resolved and repeat X-rays were normal. (Courtesy of the Radiology Learning Center, University of California School of Medicine, San Francisco.)

trointestinal bleeding, but TTP may also present with small vessel thromboses which resemble the HUS both clinically and pathologically. *Acute colitis*[281] and *cholecystitis*[282] have been reported.

Thrombocytosis of any cause (myeloproliferative diseases, reactive thrombocytosis) may be associated with vascular thrombosis or gastrointestinal hemorrhage; the latter can be especially severe in patients using aspirin or corticosteroids.[283, 284]

Miscellaneous Disorders

A number of other hematologic conditions are associated with gastrointestinal disease. Patients with *iron deficiency anemia* are reported to develop achlorhydria, atrophic gastritis, postcricoid esophageal webs (Plummer-Vinson syndrome, "sideropenic dysphagia"), and angular cheilitis (see Table 30–1 and pp. 632–635).[285] Esophageal dysmotility and painful glossitis occur with *megaloblastic anemia.*[286] Granulomatous colitis has been reported in the *Hermansky-Pudlak syndrome* (albinism, platelet aggregation defect, tissue pigment accumulation)[287] and in *chronic granulomatous disease.*[288]

Hereditary angioedema (HAE) is a disease of autosomal dominant inheritance in which deficiency of a complement cascade regulatory protein, C1 inhibitor, is associated with attacks of severe swelling of the face, airway, trunk, extremities, and abdominal viscera.[289] The deficiency appears to be due to accelerated catabolism of the inhibitor.[290] Most attacks include nausea, vomiting, and cramping abdominal pain due to bowel edema. Twenty-two per cent of patients had severe watery diarrhea in one series.[291] Similar intestinal symptoms may be seen in patients with *allergic angioedema*[289] or *chronic urticaria* (see pp. 511–512).

Gastrointestinal hemorrhage and life-threatening mesenteric vascular thrombosis may complicate *polycythemia vera*.[292] Those patients with elevated blood counts are at greatest risk, although patients with a normal red blood cell count may develop thromboses because of an underlying hypercoagulable state or coexisting *thrombocytosis* (see above).[284]

RHEUMATOLOGIC DISEASE

Rheumatic diseases commonly produce gastrointestinal abnormalities in the form of chronic inflammation with varying degrees of vasculitis and vascular obliteration. In addition, medications used to treat connective tissue disease often affect the gastrointestinal tract adversely (see below). That the gut may play an etiologic role in rheumatologic disease has been suggested by the many testimonies of patients that certain foods exacerbate their arthritis.[293, 294] Two mechanisms which have been proposed to explain these observations are an increase in small intestinal permeability, permitting the entry into the circulation of toxic food antigens, and increased patient sensitivity to normally absorbed antigens.[293]

Progressive Systemic Sclerosis (PSS, Scleroderma)

Progressive systemic sclerosis is a multisystem disorder characterized by obliterative small vessel vasculitis and proliferation of connective tissue with fibrosis of multiple organs. The gastrointestinal tract may be involved with or without evidence of the complete *CREST syndrome* (calcinosis, Raynaud's disease, esophageal involvement, sclerodactyly, telangiectasias). Most CREST patients have high serum titers of anticentromere antibodies.[295]

Oral Cavity. The perioral skin may atrophy and fibrose, restricting mandibular motion. Hypertrophy of the periodontal ligament causes characteristic X-ray changes around dental roots. The gingivae may become indurated, friable, and atrophic, and in advanced cases, the buccal mucosa thins and tongue papillae atrophy. Taste and touch perception may become severely impaired.

Esophagus. Clinical or subclinical esophageal involvement occurs in most patients with PSS.[296] The principal problems are *dysphagia* due to impaired peristalsis and strictures, *heartburn* due to reflux, and bleeding due to *ulceration* (see pp. 586–587). There is no solid evidence that the incidence of carcinoma of the esophagus in PSS is increased.

Stomach. Gastric acid secretion is increased in over 50 per cent of patients with PSS,[297] and gastric emptying of solids is delayed in 75 per cent,[298] contributing to *esophageal reflux*. Radiologic studies sometimes reveal retention of small amounts of barium or, rarely, gastric outlet obstruction and antral ulceration due to pyloric thickening.[299, 300]

Small Intestine. The pathologic changes of the small intestine in PSS consist of variable smooth muscle atrophy and deposition of collagen in submucosal, muscular, and serosal layers.[299, 301] Collagenous encapsulation of Brunner's glands has been reported in duodenal biopsies,[302] but mucosal biopsies are usually normal except for scant infiltration of the lamina propria with chronic inflammatory cells.[303]

The interdigestive migratory motor complex (IMMC) is absent or markedly diminished in amplitude in PSS patients with symptoms of intestinal dysmotility.[304] Serum levels of motilin, a peptide hormone released by the proximal small intestine and believed to be responsible for stimulating the IMMC, are elevated in these patients, perhaps as a compensatory response to the gut's end-organ insensitivity.[304]

Small bowel radiographic abnormalities have been reported in about 60 per cent of PSS subjects, sometimes unaccompanied by symptoms.[301, 305] The duodenum is often dilated, especially in the second and third portions, often with prolonged retention of barium.[306] Typically, the jejunum is dilated and foreshortened owing to mural fibrosis, but with valvulae conniventes of normal thickness, giving rise to an "accordion" appearance[306] (Fig. 29–7). *Pneumatosis intestinalis, pseudo-obstruction, pseudodiverticula, sacculations, intussusception*, and small bowel *volvulus* have also been noted.[301, 307–309]

Symptoms of intestinal PSS include abdominal discomfort, bloating, distention, postprandial borborygmi, anorexia, nausea, vomiting, and weight loss. *Thrombosis* of large mesenteric arteries has resulted in extensive bowel necrosis as well as fatal *pancreatic necrosis*.[310] *Intestinal perforation* may result from vascular thrombosis with infarction or occur in areas where extensive perivascular fibrosis leads to penetrating mucosal ulcers.[208]

Malabsorption syndrome with steatorrhea occurs in up to a third of PSS patients[297] and not uncommonly is the cause of death (see pp. 263–282).[209] Hypomotility and jejunal pseudodiverticula causing stasis contribute to bacterial overgrowth, resulting in abnormal D-xylose absorption[297] and bacterial deconjugation of bile acids. Thirty-five per cent of unselected PSS patients in one study had evidence of bacterial overgrowth by duodenal culture.[311] However, D-xylose malabsorption in scleroderma is often incompletely reversed by antibiotic therapy, suggesting that the collagen deposition in this disease may also be a cause of impaired nutrient uptake.[312] The diagnosis and management of bacterial overgrowth are described on pages 1289 to 1297.

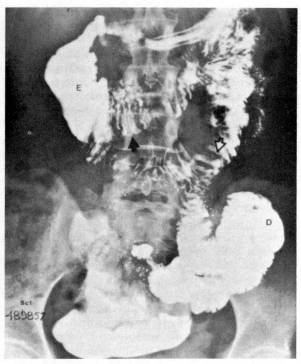

Figure 29–7. Scleroderma of the small intestine with a wide spectrum of changes: E, effacement and dilatation of the duodenum; *closed arrow*, "accordion" sign (dilatation with normal mucosal fold thickness); *open arrow*, dilatation with fold thickening; and D, jejunal dilatation. (From Meschan, I. Roentgen Signs in Diagnostic Imaging. 2nd ed. Vol. 1, Abdomen. Philadelphia, W. B. Saunders Co., 1984.)

Treatment includes courses of antibiotics and promotility agents.[303, 304] Recent trials using cisapride, which releases acetylcholine, are promising.[312a] At times, however, lifelong total parenteral nutrition may be needed.

Colon. Colonic and small bowel involvement appear to be associated. Postprandial myoelectric activity and motility are both impaired,[303, 313] suggesting a neural defect. Colonoscopy may reveal a dilated lumen with a pale, dry, and rigid mucosa. Mucosal *telangiectasias* have been described and may be a source of hemorrhage.[314] Wide-neck *pseudodiverticula* can be seen, especially on the antimesenteric border of the transverse and descending colon. Clinically, constipation is common and may lead to colonic obstruction from *fecal impaction*, to *pseudo-obstruction*, or to *volvulus*.[315]

Anorectum. Manometric studies have demonstrated decreased internal anal sphincter pressure (smooth muscle) and impaired sphincter relaxation in response to rectal distention. These defects correlate with the degree of esophageal smooth muscle dysfunction.[316] As a result, patients sometimes complain of *fecal incontinence*. The external anal sphincter (skeletal muscle) behaves normally.[316]

Pancreas. Depressed pancreatic response to standard stimulation is found in about one third of PSS patients.[317] *Calcific pancreatitis*[318] and *arteritis* leading to pancreatic necrosis[307] have been described.

Polymyositis-Dermatomyositis

Polymyositis is a syndrome characterized by weakness and inflammation primarily affecting striated muscles. When accompanied by a rash, the disease is termed *dermatomyositis*. The primary gastrointestinal symptoms are due to involvement of cricopharyngeus: *nasal regurgitation, tracheal aspiration*, and *impaired deglutition*.[319] There may be facial muscle weakness and stomatitis. However, involvement is not limited to skeletal muscle fibers. Pathologically, edema of the bowel wall, mucosal ulcers (producing *hemorrhage*), muscular atrophy, and some fibrosis can be seen at any location in the gut.[319] Significant impairment of esophageal emptying of solids and gastric emptying of liquids and solids was found in 60 per cent of patients in a recent series.[320] Most of these patients complained of *heartburn* and symptoms of *gastric retention*. Nonspecific symptoms such as bloating and constipation may be present.

The radiologic findings include disordered upper esophageal motility, barium aspiration, and barium retention in the hypopharyngeal valleculae. The esophagus may become moderately dilated, but reflux is rare and stricture unreported.[319, 321] Gastric emptying may appear normal by barium studies.[319] Dilatation, segmentation, poorly coordinated peristalsis, and delayed transit have been seen in small bowel X-ray studies.[322] *Chronic pneumoperitoneum, pneumatosis intestinalis, colonic dilatation*, and *pseudodiverticula* may be seen. *Perforations* of the *esophagus*[323] and of duodenal *diverticula* have been described as rare complications.[324]

Polymyositis and *dermatomyositis* have been associated with an increased risk of *malignancy*. In a Japanese series, over 25 per cent of males with these diseases developed gastric cancer.[325] However, another recent study failed to confirm the association and showed that this relationship, usually reported from large referral centers, is probably an artifact of patient referral bias.[326] Until better data are available, costly screening of these patients to detect cancers is unwarranted.[326]

Systemic Lupus Erythematosus (SLE)

Systemic lupus erythematosus is a multisystem disease characterized by immunologic abnormalities and the production of autoantibodies associated with tissue damage. Many of the gastrointestinal complications of SLE are due to *vasculitis* with resulting ischemia (see pp. 1916–1919).

Radiologic features of SLE are diverse and nonspecific. Abnormal motility of the esophagus and stomach, including gastric outlet obstruction, may be seen. Dilatation, thickening, and nodularity of the small bowel mucosal folds have been observed. Submucosal hemorrhage can resemble a tumor.[327] *Pneumatosis intestinalis* may be benign or the result of *necrotizing enterocolitis*.[328] Colonic findings may be indistinguishable radiologically or endoscopically from those seen in inflammatory bowel disease.[327]

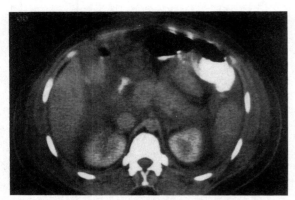

Figure 29–8. Computerized tomography demonstrating pancreatitis and diffuse serositis associated with SLE. The pancreas is enlarged and edematous. Other slices showed ascites, pleural fluid, and pericardial effusion.

Gastrointestinal symptoms are common in patients with active SLE. Anorexia, nausea, or vomiting affects about 50 per cent of patients.[317] *Oral manifestations* were reported in 40 per cent of patients in one series (see Table 30–1).[329] Heartburn or dysphagia also is reported by over half of patients.[330] Esophageal aperistalsis is detected by manometry in patients with Raynaud's phenomenon.[330]

Malabsorption of D-xylose, steatorrhea, and protein-losing enteropathy[331–332] have been described; the latter can be steroid-responsive.[332] Diarrhea is reported by 5 to 25 per cent of patients. Ascites occurs in SLE and can be due to *peritoneal or mesenteric vasculitis, pancreatitis, nephrotic syndrome*, or *cardiac failure*; bacterial peritonitis also may complicate the course (Fig. 29–8).[327] Hepatobiliary abnormalities are seen in over half of SLE patients and are reviewed elsewhere (see reference 333 and pp. 1691–1714).

Abdominal pain, common in SLE, may be perplexing diagnostically. The presence of active cutaneous disease is a clue that an abdominal symptom is due to this disease.[327] Mild, self-limited, nonlocalized pain may reflect *lupus peritonitis*, but this diagnosis can be made only after infection and other serious conditions have been carefully excluded (Fig. 29–8). Mesenteric vasculitis can cause *intestinal ischemia*, which may result in *mucosal ulceration, hemorrhage, bowel infarction*, and *perforation*.[334–336] Unfortunately, corticosteroids often mask peritoneal signs, resulting in the delay of diagnosis of serious disease. Vasculitis also can lead to *gastritis*,[327] *pancreatitis*,[337] *hemorrhagic ileitis or colitis*,[335] and *intussusception*.[337] Anti-inflammatory agents are another cause of hemorrhage.[338]

Mixed Connective Tissue Disease (MCTD)

Mixed connective tissue disease is a syndrome having features of PSS, polymyositis, and SLE, often in the presence of very high levels of antibody directed against ribonucleoprotein.[339] The term *"overlap syndrome"* is often used when not all the criteria for MCTD are present. Gastrointestinal manifestations are common and resemble those of PSS, the most frequent symptoms being esophageal regurgitation and heartburn.[330]

Rheumatoid Arthritis (RA)

In chronic RA, *temporomandibular arthritis* is common, resulting in tenderness, swelling, crepitus, and impairment of mastication.[340] *Esophageal dysmotility* is shown by low-amplitude peristaltic waves in the middle and lower esophagus, as well as reduced lower esophageal sphincter pressure in most patients. These changes are believed to be due to an intrinsic esophageal muscle abnormality.[340] However, heartburn and dysphagia are unusual complaints.

Chronic treatment of RA with nonsteroidal anti-inflammatory agents, especially high-dose aspirin therapy, produces *gastric ulcers* or erosions in 50 to 75 per cent of patients and duodenal lesions in up to 10 per cent (see pp. 885–886).[338, 341] About 33 per cent of the gastric ulcers may be present without symptoms, and it is interesting that the addition of a second anti-inflammatory drug may not increase the number or severity of lesions.[341] Basal and food-stimulated hypergastrinemia, a recently reported feature in RA, is of uncertain significance in the pathophysiology of the ulcers.[342] The incidence of gastroduodenal lesions can be reduced to about 10 per cent using enteric coated aspirin, with or without low-dose prednisone.[338, 341] It is not always necessary to discontinue aspirin when symptomatic ulcers develop because 67 per cent will heal upon addition of a standard antiulcer medication such as an H_2 blocker.[343]

Acute gastric erosions caused by high-dose aspirin in normal subjects also can be prevented with sucralfate[344] or enprostil (a prostaglandin E_2 analogue),[345] but there are as yet no persuasive studies supporting the routine use of such agents when treating rheumatoid patients with nonsteroidal anti-inflammatory agents.

Rheumatoid vasculitis is a serious complication affecting just 1 per cent of RA patients,[346] with only 10 per cent of those affected exhibiting gut manifestations.[347] Vasculitis typically occurs in the setting of severe arthritis, rheumatoid nodules, and high titers of rheumatoid factor. The patients have fever and weakness and frequently also have signs of *cutaneous vasculitis* (especially digital gangrene) and *neuropathy*. Involvement of the gut is best diagnosed by obtaining a rectal biopsy showing *necrotizing arteritis*; this finding implies a poor prognosis.[347] As in any vasculitis involving the bowel, patients may develop *ischemic bowel ulcers, pancolitis*, or *bowel infarction*, with *hemorrhage* complicating such damage (see pp. 1916–1919).[347, 348] Cholecystitis and appendicitis have been reported.[347] The response to high-dose corticosteroids is only fair;[347, 348] anecdotal reports of the benefits of cytotoxic agents or plasmapheresis are encouraging.[348]

Other complications of RA include *protein-losing enteropathy*,[349] *secondary amyloidosis* (see below),[350] and *malabsorption*.[351] *Felty's syndrome* (RA, splenomegaly, leukopenia) is associated with severe infections, including intra-abdominal *abscesses*.[352]

Sjögren's Syndrome (SS)

Sjögren's syndrome is characterized by lymphocytic tissue infiltration with the clinical findings of *keratoconjunctivitis sicca* and *xerostomia*. Patients have either a sterile or a suppurative *parotitis*.[353] Excessive dryness of the mouth and pharynx leads to fissuring and ulceration of the lips and oral mucous membranes.

Dysphagia, reported by up to three quarters of SS patients,[354] can be due to lack of saliva but also may result from connective tissue abnormalities of the esophagus. Upper esophageal webs may be seen in 10 per cent, hiatal hernia in 25 per cent, and motility abnormalities (aperistalsis, nonperistaltic contractions, or triphasic tertiary contractions) in 36 per cent of patients.[354, 355] *Atrophic gastritis* with chronic gastric mucosal inflammatory infiltrates has been found in association with SS, occasionally giving the appearance of gastric carcinoma on barium study.[356]

Pancreatic exocrine insufficiency has been found in SS patients and may or may not be associated with symptoms.

Behçet's Syndrome

Behçet's syndrome is a multisystem disease characterized pathologically by necrotizing *vasculitis* with fibrinoid degeneration. The principal manifestations include *genital* and *oral ulcerations*, skin lesions, iridocyclitis, thrombophlebitis, and arthritis (see Fig. 29–9 and Table 30–1).[357]

Other sites of gastrointestinal involvement are the *esophagus* and *colon*. *Esophageal ulcers*, *varices*, and *perforation* may occur (Fig. 29–9).[358] The colonic ulcers of Behçet's syndrome are predominantly ileocecal and often involve the colon segmentally. The endoscopic and pathologic appearance of Behçet's syndrome is strikingly similar to Crohn's disease.[359] The recent report of a family exhibiting both diseases suggests that the two may be closely related etiologically.[360] Patients will complain of *abdominal pain* and *bloody diarrhea*. Peritonitis, perforation, or death can result.[359, 360] *Anal ulcerations* have been reported.[361] Gastrointestinal involvement with Behçet's syndrome indicates a poor prognosis—the lesions may respond to corticosteroids,[360] but there is a high recurrence rate after resection of involved segments of esophagus or intestine.[358, 359]

Reiter's Syndrome (Reactive Arthritis)

Reiter's syndrome is characterized by arthritis, urethritis, conjunctivitis, and mucocutaneous lesions.[362] It is classified as a *reactive arthritis* because most cases follow a bout of infectious diarrhea (due to *Chlamydia*,

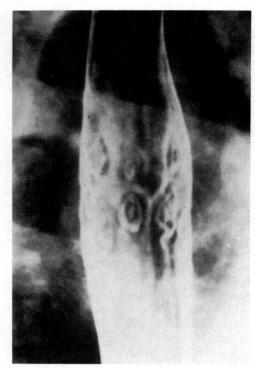

Figure 29–9. Esophageal ulcerations in Behçet's disease. (Courtesy of the Radiology Learning Center, University of California School of Medicine, San Francisco.)

Yersinia, Shigella, Salmonella, Campylobacter, or other species) or nonbacterial urethritis (usually chlamydial).[363] These patients often express the HLA-B27 antigen and have increased immune responsiveness to chlamydial antigens in vitro.[363]

Oral lesions consisting of painless, shallow, clean-based ulcers are usually seen. The *diarrhea* typically is short-lived and precedes the onset of the syndrome, but occasionally is chronic and nonbloody.[364] In a recent series, two thirds of reactive arthritis patients with no intestinal symptoms had macro- and microscopic inflammation of the colon seen during ileocolonoscopy, suggesting that subclinical *bowel inflammation* is part of the syndrome.[364] Similar findings were seen in patients with *ankylosing spondylitis*.[364] Although not considered to be a reactive arthritis, patients with *psoriatic arthritis* also express HLA-B27 more frequently than control subjects and occasionally develop inflammatory bowel disease.[362] Leukotrienes have been implicated as inflammatory mediators in both diseases,[365] but the pathophysiologic link between many forms of arthritis and the gut remains elusive.

Other Syndromes

A number of diseases which cause *necrotizing vasculitis* can have similar gastrointestinal manifestations when they involve the mesenteric vessels and are discussed on pages 1916 to 1919. These diseases include *polyarteritis nodosa (PAN), Churg-Strauss syndrome (allergic granulomatous angiitis), Takayasu's arteritis,*

Wegener's granulomatosis, and *Henoch-Schönlein purpura* (Fig. 29–6). The patients commonly complain of abdominal pain, nausea, vomiting, and diarrhea.[366] Acute abdominal symptoms can be due to *pancreatitis*,[367] *ulceration, ischemic colitis*,[368] *perforation, intussusception, cholecystitis*,[369] or *appendicitis*.[369, 370] In addition, a *chronic wasting syndrome* resembling tuberculous enteritis or neoplasm has been associated with abdominal PAN.[370] Angiography of the superior mesenteric artery often reveals characteristic small aneurysmal dilatations. In patients with upper intestinal hemorrhage, endoscopic biopsies are often useful for obtaining the correct diagnosis.[371]

NEUROHUMORAL DISEASE

Systemic Mastocytosis

Systemic mastocytosis is characterized by mast cell proliferation in skin, bones, lymph nodes, and parenchymal organs. The classic dermatologic finding of *urticaria pigmentosa* (Fig. 30–3) may be seen with or without systemic involvement. The typical symptoms in mastocytosis—pruritus, flushing, tachycardia, asthma, and headache—are believed to result from the release of histamine by mast cells.[372] In addition, several prostaglandins and thromboxanes, which also are elevated in plasma, could play a role.[373] Hyperhistaminemia can produce gastric hypersecretion as marked as in the Zollinger-Ellison syndrome, though most patients have normal or low gastric acidity.[375] Rarely, bleeding diatheses have been described and attributed to heparin released by mast cells.[376]

One fourth of patients have gastrointestinal symptoms[377] which include nausea, vomiting, diarrhea, and abdominal pain.[372] These symptoms often are provoked by ingestion of even small amounts of alcohol.[372] Gastrointestinal hemorrhage from *peptic ulcers, gastric erosions*, and *gastroesophageal varices* is also part of the syndrome.[372, 375]

Steatorrhea, hypocalcemia, and decreased absorption of D-xylose and ^{57}Co-vitamin B_{12} are found in patients with mastocytosis.[374, 378–380] Jejunal biopsy specimens may show large numbers of mast cells in the lamina propria, muscularis mucosa, and submucosa, with normal villi or mild villous atrophy.[380, 381] Endoscopy has revealed urticaria-like mucosal lesions.[382] Small bowel radiographic abnormalities may include "bull's eye" lesions resembling metastases (see p. 502), edema, thickened folds, and a nodular mucosal pattern.[383] Diffuse colonic involvement with acute inflammatory infiltrates and mucosal edema has been reported.[384]

Recently, cimetidine[385] and oral 'disodium cromoglycate[374] have been used successfully by patients with mastocytosis to relieve the diarrhea and abdominal pain, but not the malabsorption.[377] Cimetidine combined with chlorpheniramine is as effective as cromolyn;[385] ranitidine also has been approved in the United States for the treatment of ulcer disease due to mastocytosis.

The pathophysiology of the malabsorption is not clear. The lack of correlation between the degree of malabsorption and the degree of mast cell infiltration, plasma hyperhistaminemia, or gastric acidity suggests that the malabsorption is not a direct effect of histamine[377, 380, 385] and that other substances may be responsible.[373]

Pheochromocytoma

Pheochromocytomas are catecholamine-secreting tumors arising from chromaffin tissue in the adrenal medulla or other tissues. Frequently other substances are secreted and produce symptoms, including vasoactive intestinal polypeptide (VIP), somatostatin, calcitonin, gastrin, and ACTH[386, 387] (see also the discussion of the WDHA syndrome, pp. 1890–1892).

Gastrointestinal manifestations include nausea, vomiting, abdominal pain, and less frequently, watery diarrhea, steatorrhea, and gastrointestinal or retroperitoneal bleeding.[386–388] *Cholelithiasis* is increased (see p. 490).[42] Manifestations such as *paralytic ileus* and *megacolon* may result from secretion of catecholamines, for such substances inhibit gastrointestinal smooth muscle activity, and resection of the tumor may relieve these symptoms.[389] *Ischemic colitis* has been seen generally in pediatric cases in which the blood pressure has been lowered suddenly, and may be related to mesenteric vascular spasm.[390]

Carcinoid syndrome is discussed on pages 1546 to 1547 and pages 1560 to 1570.

INFILTRATIVE DISEASE

Amyloidosis

The diffuse extracellular tissue deposition of amyloid results in *systemic amyloidosis*. Amyloid is an insoluble, eosinophilic glycoprotein complex which demonstrates green birefringence under polarized light after Congo red staining. Amyloidosis has been subclassified into categories according to clinical and biochemical criteria, but all types involve the gastrointestinal tract, and all levels of the gut may be affected.[391, 392] The chief sites of intestinal amyloid deposition are blood vessel walls (producing ischemia and infarction), the muscle layers of the intestine (causing muscle atrophy and dysmotility), and the muscularis mucosa (impairing absorption).[391] The mucosa is infiltrated only in cases of massive deposition. Direct pressure damage to cells in myenteric plexuses and visceral nerve trunks also has been demonstrated.[393] Despite widespread tissue infiltration, gastrointestinal amyloidosis may be asymptomatic.

Radiography. Patients with gastrointestinal amyloidosis may have no radiographic abnormalities. *Macroglossia* from amyloid infiltration occurs in a fifth of patients[392] and has a characteric X-ray appearance.[394] Esophageal motor abnormalities are common (see below). Functional or mechanical *gastric outlet obstruc-*

tion may be due to dysmotility or to the presence of an antral amyloidoma.[395] The rugal folds may be diminished or appear rigid, simulating infiltrating submucosal adenocarcinoma.[396]

Small intestinal X-rays are often the first test to suggest the diagnosis of amyloidosis (Fig. 29–10).[396] The most common findings are sharply demarcated thickening of the valvulae conniventes, dilatation of the bowel due to replacement of the muscular layers, and the presence of multiple nodular lesions.[397] *Bowel obstruction* can occur due to amyloid infiltration of the mesentery as well.[398] Colonic studies may show multiple filling defects, ulceration due to ischemia, or narrowing and rigidity, especially in the sigmoid colon and rectum.[397]

Pathophysiology. *Dysmotility* is commonly observed but whether this is due to smooth muscle replacment or to autonomic nerve injury is uncertain. Esophageal manometry usually shows a decreased lower esophageal sphincter pressure with nonspecific dysmotility of both the skeletal and smooth muscle portions of the esophageal body.[399] A pattern resembling achalasia can also be seen. *Malabsorption* is found in about 5 per cent of patients and indicates severe disease.[392] There is evidence for several possible etiologies: bacterial overgrowth from dysmotility, mucosal ischemia, a physical barrier to absorption due to the presence of submucosal amyloid, and exocrine pancreatic insufficiency (see pp. 264–267).

Clinical Manifestations. *Macroglossia* and *temporomandibular arthritis* may cause drooling and difficulties with mastication.[401] *Gastric outlet obstruction* may

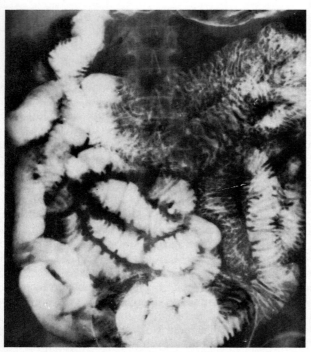

Figure 29–10. Symmetric, sharply demarcated thickening of the valvulae conniventes throughout the small intestine, producing a uniform appearance characteristic of amyloidosis. (Courtesy of Dr. R. H. Marshak.)

cause postprandial vomiting. Intestinal dysmotility can result in diarrhea, constipation, *megacolon*, fecal incontinence, *rectal prolapse*, or *pseudo-obstruction* (see pp. 377–379).[392, 402] *Gastrointestinal bleeding*[403] and *protein-losing enteropathy*[404] have been seen. A third of patients will present with *hepatosplenomegaly* or *ascites*.[392]

Diagnosis. Rectal biopsy will establish the diagnosis of gastrointestinal amyloidosis in up to 80 per cent of cases and has a low risk-benefit ratio.[392] However, recent pathologic data and clinical experience suggest that the stomach and small intestine are more sensitive sites for biopsy, especially in myeloma-associated amyloidosis (AL type).[391, 402] To be adequate, the specimen must contain a portion of submucosa.

Therapy. Colchicine can prevent amyloidosis in patients with familial Mediterranean fever,[405] but its use in other forms of amyloidosis is untested. Colorectal symptoms may be alleviated by an enterostomy.[406]

Disorders of Lipid Metabolism

Fabry's Disease. *Fabry's disease* is an X-linked disorder of glycolipid metabolism due to the deficiency or absence of the enzyme alpha-galactosidase, resulting in sphingolipid deposition in all tissues. Electron microscopic examination of the small intestine and rectum has revealed large sphingolipid-filled vacuoles in the ganglion cells of Meissner's plexus, within smooth muscle cells of the muscularis mucosae, and within endothelial cells lining blood vessels. Mucosal enterocytes are normal.[407] Clinical manifestations include characteristic skin lesions on the face (see Table 30–1), often with associated dysfunction of the renal, pulmonary, central nervous, cardiovascular, ocular, and gastrointestinal systems.

Impaired motility is the prominent gastrointestinal disorder. Patients complain of recurrent episodes of crampy abdominal pain associated with frequent liquid stools.[407, 408] Delayed gastric emptying, *secondary bacterial overgrowth*, increased fecal bile salt loss, and *cholelithiasis* have been documented.[407] One patient with these symptoms had marked improvement in diarrhea and early satiety after treatment with tetracycline and metoclopramide, confirming the role of dysmotility and bacterial overgrowth in this disorder.[407] Glycolipid deposition in small vessels can induce severe *vasculitis* and *thrombosis*, resulting in *ischemic bowel lesions*. *Ileal perforation* has been reported.[408]

Abetalipoproteinemia. *Abetalipoproteinemia* is an autosomal recessive disorder characterized by acanthocytic erythrocytes, serum lipid abnormalities, *ataxia, atypical retinitis pigmentosa*, and *steatorrhea*.[409] The typical laboratory feature is complete absence in plasma of all lipoproteins containing apolipoprotein B (chylomicrons, very low density lipoproteins or VLDL, low density lipoproteins or LDL).[410]

The histologic appearance of the small intestine is marked by mucosal epithelial cells loaded with lipid droplets (Fig. 18–1).[410] By contrast, the submucosa and lamina propria show practically no lipid, and the lymphatics are empty. The villi are normal in length and configuration.

Mild steatorrhea with onset during the first two years of life is seen. In two patients, cholesterol malabsorption with increased endogenous cholesterol synthesis was found.[411] The intestinal mucosa may appear yellowish on endoscopy, reflecting the presence of mucosal lipid.[412] Therapy consists of substituting medium-chain for long-chain dietary triglycerides (see pp. 279–280).

Hyperlipoproteinemia. In *familial hyperchylomicronemia* (type I phenotype), the plasma is lactescent, with marked elevation of chylomicrons and triglycerides due to the deficiency of lipoprotein lipase.[413] Manifestations can appear early in life and include recurrent episodes of abdominal pain, fever, signs of *peritonitis*, and *pancreatitis*. In most patients, the cause of the recurrent attacks is unknown.[413]

Patients with *familial hyperbetalipoproteinemia* (type IV phenotype) suffer from premature atherosclerosis, hyperuricemia, and attacks of *pancreatitis*, which generally occur when plasma triglycerides are above 2000 mg/dl.[414] The hyperlipidemia may mask elevated plasma amylase values. These patients also have an increased incidence of *cholelithiasis* and *cholecystitis*.[415] Patients with *familial hyperlipoproteinemia* (type V phenotype) are prone to bouts of abdominal pain with or without *pancreatitis*. Exacerbation of endogenous hypertriglyceridemia by diabetes, diet, alcohol, or medications sometimes causes pancreatitis (see pp. 1819–1821).[414]

Tangier Disease. *Tangier disease* is an autosomal recessive disorder characterized by accumulation of cholesterol esters in macrophages in tonsils, thymus, lymph nodes, marrow, liver, and the gut.[416] These patients have very low levels of plasma cholesterol and high density lipoproteins (HDL) due to a lack of apoprotein AI (apo AI) and apo AII.[416] The DNA sequence for apo AI is normal in Tangier disease, but an abnormality in post-translational processing results in rapid apo AI degradation.[416, 417]

The clinical findings include enlarged *yellow-orange "streaked" tonsils* in 80 per cent of cases,[418] *hepatosplenomegaly*, and *peripheral neuropathy*.[416] Patients may have diarrhea without steatorrhea. Colonoscopy has shown orange-brown mucosal "spots" throughout the colon and rectum in all patients reported, and laparoscopy will reveal similar yellow patches on the surface of the liver due to cholesterol esters in hepatic reticuloendothelial cells.[418]

Wolman's disease, another cholesterol ester storage disease, is caused by cholesterol ester lysosomal acid hydrolase deficiency.[419] Distinctive features are *hepatosplenomegaly*, *abdominal distention*, and calcified adrenal glands.[420]

Other Infiltrative Disorders

Eosinophilic infiltration of the gastrointestinal mucosa, in a diffuse or circumscribed pattern, pathologically characterizes *eosinophilic gastroenteritis*, the *hypereosinophilic syndrome*,[421] *allergic granulomatous vasculitis* (Churg-Strauss syndrome), and *polyarteritis nodosa*. These conditions are discussed on pages 508 to 509 and 1123 to 1131.

A familial syndrome was recently described consisting of *diarrhea, rectal bleeding, malabsorption*, and *protein-losing enteropathy*, together with poikilodermia, hair graying, and cerebrovascular calcifications.[422] This disease is called a *small vessel hyalinosis* because of the basement membrane–like deposits in the subepithelial space of intestinal capillaries, arterioles, and small veins.

MISCELLANEOUS

Cryoglobulinemia

Mixed IgG-IgM cryoglobulin complexes may circulate de novo or may complicate a variety of immune-related diseases, including ulcerative colitis.[423] These complexes can cause severe *vasculitis*, producing typical skin lesions (see Fig. 30–3) and sometimes leading to small and large bowel ischemia.[424]

Chronic Urticaria

Chronic urticaria is a heterogeneous disorder with skin biopsies characterized by a non-necrotizing perivascular lymphocytic infiltrate and an accumulation of mast cells. The most common causes are reactions to medications, foods, or food additives (see pp. 1113–1123). However, approximately 20 per cent of these patients will have a different histologic lesion consisting of *leukocytoclastic necrotizing cutaneous vasculitis*. Patients with this type of vasculitis are the most likely to experience gut symptoms: epigastric discomfort, distention, flatulence, and diarrhea.[425, 426] *Hypocomplementemia* is common in this group.[426]

The vasculitic form is often associated with a *systemic illness* such as a *malignancy, mastocytosis* (see p. 509), or one of the *rheumatologic diseases* (systemic lupus erythematosus, rheumatoid arthritis, or systemic vasculitis).[426]

Rapid gastric emptying and decreased intestinal transit time have been reported in chronic urticaria. Gastric acid secretion increases in some patients after cold immersion of the hands, presumably on the basis of histamine release.[427] Mucosal urticarial lesions can be demonstrated radiologically and on endoscopy (Fig. 29–11). Intestinal villous atrophy has been seen.[428] At times, an *acute abdomen* or *toxic megacolon* may result from intestinal urticaria.[429] There appears to be a relationship between biliary tract disease and chronic urticaria, with clearing of the latter following cholecystectomy.[430] However, the belief that chronic infection is responsible for chronic urticaria is not supported by recent reports.[425]

Chronic urticaria is managed by removing any offending agent and by the use of antihistamines. Ci-

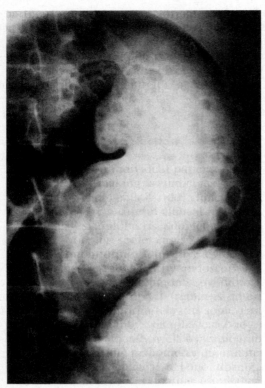

Figure 29–11. Urticaria involving the colon. The polypoid defects are unlike those seen in ulcerative colitis or Crohn's disease. (Courtesy of the Radiology Learning Center, University of California School of Medicine, San Francisco.)

metidine is helpful in a few cases.[431] Patients with *cutaneous vasculitis* often require glucocorticoid therapy.[425]

Sarcoidosis

Gastrointestinal involvement in *sarcoidosis* is unusual.[432] When present, symptoms result from granulomatous infiltration of the involved organ; hilar lymph node enlargement may cause dysphagia.

Gastric sarcoidosis, particularly of the antrum, affects about 10 per cent of patients with systemic sarcoidosis, and the stomach can be the first site to cause symptoms.[433] Histologic differentiation from *Crohn's disease, tuberculosis,* or *secondary syphilis* can be difficult (see p. 805). There may be diffuse ulceration and antral narrowing, or the disease can resemble *linitis plastica* or *Menetrier's disease.*[433] Seventy-five per cent of patients with gastric sarcoid present with pain and 25 per cent present with bleeding. Pyloric obstruction may occur. Half of the patients require surgery for bleeding or suspected malignancy; when treated with corticosteroids, 66 per cent improve symptomatically.[433] The healing of a sarcoid ulcer with antacids alone has been reported.[434]

The small intestine may be involved indirectly in sarcoid via mesenteric lymph node enlargement. Dilated lacteals seen on a small intestinal biopsy specimen are evidence of possible lymphatic obstruction. *Mal-*absorption and *protein-losing enteropathy* have been reported.[435, 436]

Colonic sarcoidosis is very rare. There may be solely the proctoscopic finding of a friable mucosa,[437] or a pattern of nodular lymphoid hyperplasia,[438] or a constricting lesion resembling carcinoma.[439] One case of *pancreatic insufficiency* associated with sarcoidosis has been reported.[440]

Down's Syndrome

Down's syndrome is associated with a high prevalence of severe *periodontal disease*[441] and congenital *duodenal atresia* with or without *annular pancreas.*[442] Clinical manifestations of duodenal obstruction include copious vomiting within hours of birth, a characteristic *"double bubble" sign* on abdominal radiographs (Fig. 96–9), and occasionally hematemesis (see pp. 1806–1807).[442]

Marfan and Ehlers-Danlos Syndromes

Owing to defective collagen synthesis, patients with Ehlers-Danlos syndrome develop skin fagility, *megaesophagus, small intestinal hypomotility, giant jejunal diverticula, bacterial overgrowth,* and *megacolon* (see Table 30–1). *Mesenteric arterial rupture* and *intestinal perforation* also may occur. A patient with the somatic features of both *Ehlers-Danlos syndrome* and *Marfan syndrome* has been described who presented with malabsorption, most likely the result of bacterial overgrowth.[443]

RENAL DISEASE

Acute Renal Failure (ARF)

Gastrointestinal *bleeding* occurs in over half of patients with ARF and is often due to multiple *gastric* or *duodenal ulcers.*[444] *Stress-related gastritis* is also common, especially when ARF is a complication of major trauma or surgery. In one series, 50 per cent of patients with ARF had elevated serum gastrin, with peak levels of 1000 to 5000 pg/ml occurring during the course of disease due to impaired renal inactivation of gastrin. Basal acid secretion is often low but maximally stimulated acid output is normal or elevated.[445]

Chronic Renal Failure (CRF)

Gastrointesinal problems frequently affect patients. Anorexia, hiccups, nausea, vomiting, epigastric pain, and heartburn are common manifestations of uremia.[446] Approximately 40 per cent of patients undergoing chronic dialysis report similar symptoms, usually in the absence of any lesions seen by endoscopy.[447]

High levels of blood urea nitrogen are associated with xerostomia, parotitis, metallic taste, and gingival bleeding.[448] *Hypogeusia* has been documented in uremic patients and may improve following dialysis[449] or zinc replacement,[450] although a relation between zinc deficiency and uremic hypogeusia has been disputed.[451] Uremic fetor probably results from microbial breakdown of salivary urea to ammonia and responds to improved oral hygiene and dialysis.[452]

Upper gastrointestinal endoscopy of stable dialysis patients reveals abnormalities in about a quarter of the patients.[447] Most of the lesions are *gastric* or *duodenal erosions*; the incidence of ulcer disease probably is not increased with chronic dialysis.[447] Gastric *angiodysplasia* is common; the lesions are smaller than the telangiectasias seen in the colon.[453, 454] Also seen are *esophagitis*, gastric fold thickening, *nodular duodenitis* (which resolves after transplantation, Fig. 29–12), and *Brunner's gland hyperplasia*.[447, 453, 455, 456] The latter may appear as multiple polyps in the duodenal bulb.[456]

The pathogenesis of uremic gastrointestinal lesions remains unclear. Attempts to correlate acid secretion with upper gastrointestinal lesions or symptoms have not been successful;[453] both basal and stimulated gastric output can be normal, high, or low.[445, 447, 457, 458] Secondary hyperparathyroidism has been implicated as a cause of bleeding ulcers (see p. 491),[57] although positive and negative correlations have been found between serum parathyoid hormone and basal acid output in patients with CRF.[459, 560]

Levels of serum gastrin correlate best with kidney function.[445] The renal cortex is responsible for clearance of gastrin and other polypeptide hormones, and the levels of these hormones often return to normal following successful renal transplantation.[456, 457, 461] However, approximately a quarter of patients will have hypoacidity and increased serum gastrin levels even after transplantation, revealing an underlying acid secretory defect. There is a close relationship between the serum creatinine, serum pepsinogen II levels, and Brunner's gland hyperplasia; pepsinogen levels fall after renal engraftment but the fate of Brunner's gland hyperplasia is not known.[456]

Clinically, gastrointestinal *hemorrhage* is a common cause of death for dialysis patients.[462] In a recent series, *angiodysplasia* was responsible for 53 per cent of the episodes of upper intestinal bleeding; peptic lesions were responsible in just 40 per cent of bleeding episodes.[453] Either an H_2-blocker at reduced doses (see pp. 845–852) or antacids can be used to treat the peptic lesions, although neither is likely to stop active hemorrhage (see p. 408).[463] Recurrent bleeding due to angiodysplasia has been treated with vasoconstrictors, endoscopic laser or heat treatment, and surgery; however, it now appears that chronic oral estrogen-progesterone therapy may prevent bleeding from both upper and lower gastrointestinal sites.[464]

A *"wasting syndrome"* is associated with CRF and is due to a number of factors including poor nutrition, endocrine abnormalities, and catabolic stresses such as infection, uremia, and the dialysis procedure.[465] *Bacterial overgrowth* has been reported in an anephric mouse model[466] and in humans.[467] The absorption of calcium, magnesium, and phosphate is decreased,[460, 468, 469] the latter probably the result of low 1,25-dihydroxyvitamin D levels and aluminum antacid therapy.[469] Brush border enzyme specific activity was found to be unchanged in uremic rats when compared with control animals.[470] Despite symptoms suggestive of delayed gastric emptying, both solids and liquids exit the stomach normally in CRF patients receiving chronic hemodialysis.[471]

Exocrine pancreatic insufficiency has been documented in a number of hemodialysis patients. The etiology of this finding is unknown, but these patients may improve clinically with pancreatic enzyme replacement.[465] The diagnosis of *pancreatitis* may be difficult to exclude in CRF patients. Both salivary-type and pancreatic amylase can be elevated to twice the upper limit of normal. The ratio of amylase clearance to creatinine clearance cannot be used in patients with CRF to identify those in whom elevated serum amylase indicates true pancreatitis because this ratio often is elevated in CRF as well as in acute pancreatitis.[472, 473]

Small intestinal ileus, ulceration, fecal obstruction leading to *perforation*, and *nonocclusive ischemic bowel disease* have been associated with uremia.[460, 474, 475]

Colonic perforation, not uncommon among dialysis

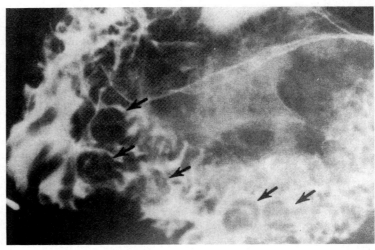

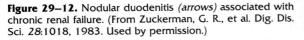

Figure 29–12. Nodular duodenitis *(arrows)* associated with chronic renal failure. (From Zuckerman, G. R., et al. Dig. Dis. Sci. *28*:1018, 1983. Used by permission.)

patients, results from *ruptured diverticula, stercoral fecalomas* (due to the use of aluminum-containing antacids or barium), or *cecal ulcers*, which may bleed profusely.[476] Life-threatening hemorrhage from rectal ulcers has occurred.[477] An association may exist between polycystic kidney disease and colonic diverticula, especially those that perforate.[478] *Colonic intussusception* and *ileus* are also encountered in CRF.[479] The *diarrhea* experienced by some patients may be related to abnormal bile acid metabolism.[480] Duodenal and fecal levels of deoxycholate are decreased, while those of ursodeoxycholate are increased.[480] It appears that uremia impairs bile acid deconjugation and dehydroxylation by normal intestinal flora, decreasing deoxycholate levels. Low ileal deoxycholate content promotes ileal bacterial overgrowth with anaerobes and colonic organisms. These species generate increased levels of unusual bile acids such as ursodeoxycholate. This pattern of bile acid abnormalities correlates with the presence of diarrhea in CRF patients.[480] The effect of cholestyramine therapy has not been reported.[480] In addition, patients undergoing hemodialysis are at increased risk for *Salmonella enteritidis* sepsis.[481]

Some hemodialysis patients develop ascites of unclear etiology that is refractory to conventional fluid restriction.[482, 483] Prior peritoneal dialysis causing chronic peritonitis has been implicated.[484, 485] Surgical removal of diseased peritoneal tissue, peritoneovenous shunts, and nephrectomy have been used successfully to reduce the excess fluid.[485]

Renal Transplantation

Gastrointestinal complications occur in 20 per cent of renal transplant recipients, mostly in the early postgraft period.[486] These problems are rare among 10-year survivors of transplantation.[487] *Esophageal candidiasis* appears frequently and has led to fatal perforation in insulin-dependent diabetics.[488]

Gastroduodenal *erosions, ulcers*, and *hemorrhage* are the most frequent problems encountered, the latter occurring in about 6 per cent of patients.[57, 447, 486] The etiology of these lesions is unclear, but stress is the most likely cause, as it is in other diseases (see pp. 772–792).[489] High-dose steroids have been implicated, but proof is lacking, and the correlation between the steroid dose and the occurrence of upper gastrointestinal bleeding is poor.[490, 491] Acid secretion is normal or somewhat depressed after successful transplantation, although occasionally it is elevated.[445, 457] Serum gastrin levels also can be normal or elevated.[457] Cytomegalovirus frequently infects the gastric and duodenal mucosa of transplant patients and is associated with seropositivity in most cases.[492] Endoscopy may reveal *multiple erosions* with cytomegalic inclusion bodies seen in the biopsy specimens. The patients can be asymptomatic or present with occult bleeding or even melena.[492, 493]

It has been suggested that the risk of hemorrhage after transplantation can be reduced using endoscopic screening to exclude candidates for transplantation who have pre-existing peptic disease[447] and by prophylactic ulcer surgery;[486] however, when studied prospectively, no correlation could be found between pretransplant gastric analysis or the presence or history of peptic ulcer and post-transplant upper gastrointesintal hemorrhage.[494] Moreover, the prophylactic use of cimetidine in the first month after transplantation has been highly effective in most,[486, 495] but not all,[496] trials. The fear that the immune-enhancing effects of cimetidine would lead to increased graft rejection, as occurs in dogs,[497] has not materialized in patients.[495]

Nonocclusive intestinal ischemia may occur following a hypotensive postoperative episode, resulting in *ischemic colitis* and frequently *perforation*.[498] Perforation may also complicate *diverticulitis* (which may bleed), *cytomegalovirus colitis*, or *isolated cecal ulcers*;[489, 498–502] *abscesses* are a common development.[500, 503] Fecalomas also can cause obstruction and perforation.[489, 501] The mortality rate from these abdominal emergencies is at least 50 per cent and may be due in part to delayed recognition of symptoms resulting from the use of high-dose steroids.[498] These facts have led some authors to advocate prophylactic segmental colectomies in transplant candidates with a history of symptomatic diverticular disease.[501] On the other hand, inflammation and *pneumatosis intestinalis* in a segment of bowel adjacent to an allograft undergoing rejection may resolve with medical management of the rejection.[504]

Necrotizing pancreatitis occurred in 1 per cent of transplant recipients in one large series.[505] All the patients were taking azathioprine and prednisone, both of which are believed to cause pancreatitis (see pp. 1820–1821), and all died.[505] Occasionally, there may be hepatobiliary complications such as *acalculous cholecystitis*[506] or *veno-occlusive disease*.[507] An increased incidence of *intestinal lymphoma* and *Kaposi's sarcoma* is suspected because of immunosuppressive therapy following renal transplantation.[508, 509]

NERVOUS SYSTEM DISEASE

Table 29–2 summarizes the gastrointestinal symptoms associated with disorders of the nervous system, including neuronal, neuromuscular, and muscular diseases. The enteric nervous system and its disorders are discussed on pages 21 to 107 and 1390 to 1395.

Impaired gut motility is responsible for the most common gastrointestinal manifestations of these diseases. As indicated in Table 29–2, many disorders may cause oropharyngeal dysphagia, characterized by lingual dyscoordination, cricopharyngeal spasm, or pharyngeal weakness. This can result in nasal regurgitation and tracheal aspiration. Esophageal dysmotility, including impaired lower esophageal sphincter function, may produce heartburn and *esophagitis*. Altered intestinal and anal motility can cause constipation, fecal impaction, and impaired defecation. Because dysmotility patterns are similar for a wide array of diseases, it is most concise to list each disease by the level of the nervous system affected and the common intestinal manifestations. Because of certain unique features,

Table 29–2. NERVOUS SYSTEM DISEASE ASSOCIATED WITH GASTROINTESTINAL DISORDERS

Disease	Gastrointestinal Manifestations	References
CENTRAL NERVOUS SYSTEM		
Cerebral and brainstem disorders		
Cerebrovascular accident	Oropharyngeal dysphagia	535–543
Huntington chorea	(lingual-cricopharyngeal dyscoordination and pharyngeal weakness)	
Multiple sclerosis		
Diphtheria	Gastroparesis	
Tetanus	Megacolon, constipation	
Pseudobulbar palsy	Anorectal dysfunction	
Other brainstem disorders	Flaccid sphincter—early	
Parkinson's disease	Spastic sphincter—late	
Pseudotumor cerebri	Nausea, emesis	
Spinal cord disorders*	Ileus, gastric atony, impaired rectal function, megacolon	511–524
Amyotrophic lateral sclerosis	Oropharyngeal dysphagia; ileus	537, 539
Poliomyelitis	Ileus, gastric atony, megacolon	539, 544
Tabes dorsalis	Abdominal pain crises, diarrhea	
Autonomic dysfunction		
Familial dysautonomia (Riley-Day syndrome)	Esophageal dysmotility, aspiration pneumonias, vomiting "crises"	547–549
	Gastric atony; rare: diarrhea, megacolon	
Shy-Drager syndrome	Postprandial orthostatic hypotension	550
	Esophageal dysmotility	
	Achlorhydria	
	Constipation	
PERIPHERAL NERVOUS SYSTEM		
Alcohol-related		
Acute intoxication†	Decreased lower esophageal sphincter pressure	
Alcoholic neuropathy	Impaired esophageal peristalsis	545
Diabetic neuropathy*	Impaired esophageal peristalsis, gastroparesis, megacolon, gallbladder dysfunction, diarrhea, steatorrhea	110–132
Myenteric plexus dysfunction		
Chagas disease†	Achalasia, megaesophagus, megacolon	
Hirschsprung disease†	Megacolon	546, 547
Achalasia‡	Achalasia	
Ganglioneuromatosis	Constipation; megacolon	
NEUROMUSCULAR JUNCTION		
Myasthenia gravis‡	Oropharyngeal dysphagia	537
MUSCLE DISEASE		
Striated muscle usually affected		
Stiff-man syndrome‡	Oropharyngeal dysphagia	551
Oculopharyngeal muscular dystrophy‡	Oropharyngeal dysphagia, aspiration	552–553
Dermatomyositis-polymyositis*‡	Oropharyngeal dysphagia, gastric atony, megacolon	319–324
Duchenne muscular dystrophy	Oropharyngeal dysphagia, gastric distention, malabsorption, megacolon, pseudo-obstruction	553, 554
Smooth muscle usually affected		
Progressive systemic sclerosis*	Lower esophageal dysmotility, gastroesophageal reflux, pseudodiverticula, malabsorption, diarrhea, bacterial overgrowth, anorectal dysfunction	295–318
Systemic amyloidosis*	Macroglossia, gastric outlet obstruction, diarrhea, constipation, megacolon, pseudo-obstruction, hemorrhage	391–406
Familial visceral myopathy	Dysphagia, pseudo-obstruction	291, 553
Smooth and striated muscle affected		
Thyroid disease		1–41
Thyrotoxicosis*	Oropharyngeal dysphagia, abdominal pain, vomiting, diarrhea	
Myxedema*	Gastric hypomotility, megacolon, pseudo-obstruction, fecal impaction, gallbladder hypotonia, ileus	
Myotonic dystrophy*‡	Oropharyngeal dysphagia, lower esophageal dysmotility, gastric atony, prolonged intestinal transit, megacolon, pseudo-obstruction, volvulus, gallbladder dysfunction	525–535

*See relevant sections of this chapter for complete discussion.
†See appropriate chapters for complete discussion.
‡See also Chapter 33, Motor Disorders of the Esophagus.

spinal cord injuries and *myotonic dystrophy* will be described in the text. Table 29–2 provides references for further reading on other specific diseases.

Upper gastrointestinal hemorrhage, often due to *gastric erosions* (Cushing ulcers), has been described in association with acute neurologic disease.[510] In one prospective study, 75 per cent of patients with severe *head trauma* had endoscopic evidence of gastroduodenal lesions, 69 per cent of which were erosive gastritis, and most were seen within one week of injury. About 45 per cent of the patients had gastrointestinal hemorrhage. There was no correlation between steroid administration in these patients and development of upper gastrointestinal lesions.[510] These are stress-related lesions and are largely preventable. Therefore, patients with acute neurologic injury due to trauma, severe strokes, neurosurgery, or other conditions should receive prophylactic therapy as described on pages 778 to 783.

Spinal Cord Injuries

Gastrointestinal complications of *spinal cord injuries* are common. In the early postinjury period, severe gastric stasis, gastric dilatation, and ileus are often present.[511] Nasogastric suction is frequently required. Promotility agents such as metoclopramide can be very effective since the enteric nervous system and smooth muscle layers are intact.[512] Another frequent problem in the first weeks after injury is *peptic ulceration*, usually in patients with no antecedent ulcer history. Upper gastrointestinal hemorrhage is more common with cervical cord injuries, with the use of anticoagulants, or when there is respiratory distress.[513–515] *Ulcer penetration, perforation,* and *peritonitis* may not be detected until late because of myelopathy involving sensory fibers or because of concomitant corticosteroid therapy.[515] When ulcer surgery is required, gastric resection or simple closure of the perforation is sufficient; truncal vagotomy is not performed because of the risk of severe gastric retention.[516] *Pancreatitis*, another early complication of spinal injuries, may also be related to steroid use.[511, 514]

Patients often face a different set of problems in the months to years following permanent spinal cord damage. With chronic loss of function, quadriplegics are more likely to have these gut complications than are paraplegics. The incidence of *hiatal hernia* and *gastroesophageal reflux* is increased.[511] There may be decreased bioavailability of orally administered drugs, perhaps due to impaired gastric emptying.[517, 518] *Secondary amyloidosis* involving the gastrointestinal tract (see pp. 509–510) and *cholelithiasis* are more common, especially when chronic renal disease complicates spinal cord disease.[511, 520] Other complications which have been reported are the *superior mesenteric artery syndrome* (see pp. 231–232), hemorrhage due to a *solitary colonic ulcer* (see pp. 1600–1603), and the precocious appearance of *diverticulosis*.[511, 519]

The Neurogenic Bowel. Chronic constipation plagues many patients with spinal cord injury. Damage to the upper motor neurons in the spinal cord eliminates both the sensation of rectal fullness and voluntary control of defecation. There may be decreased splanchnic outflow, impairing the coordination of intestinal and colonic motility. Recordings of colonic myoelectric activity in these patients show a high level of basal spike activity[521] and diminished colonic compliance.[522] These findings suggest that the spinal cord exerts an inhibitory influence upon basal colonic motility. Further, the gastrocolic reflex after feeding is often absent.[521] Fortunately, the lower motor neurons of the second, third, and fourth sacral roots, which provide the sensory and motor fibers for the defecation reflex, are usually intact.

Rehabilitation of bowel function is individualized to each patient's disability. Physical exercise, adequate fluid intake, and stool softeners are prescribed as with constipation of any origin (see pp. 353–361). Most patients learn to digitally distend the rectum on a regular schedule in order to initiate the defecation reflex. Stimulatory laxatives such as bisacodyl suppositories are occasionally necessary.

Autonomic dysreflexia, a life-threatening condition, sometimes affects patients whose lesion lies above the fifth thoracic root, the upper level of the greater splanchnic outflow (see pp. 21–52). The pathophysiology involves an abnormal autonomic reflex which is initiated by *fecal impaction* or *bladder distention* and leads to severe hypertension and tachycardia.[523, 524] If untreated, *seizures, subarachnoid hemorrhage,* and *stroke* may result.[521, 522] Routine bladder catheterization and avoidance of constipation are preventive.[523, 524]

Myotonic Dystrophy (Myotonia Dystrophica)

Myotonic dystrophy is a heredofamilial disorder characterized by myotonia (impaired muscular relaxation), muscle wasting, mental deficiencies, characteristic facies (frontal baldness, ptosis), cataracts, pulmonary and cardiac disease, and gonadal atrophy. Gastrointestinal involvement is prominent, may have its onset in adulthood, and differs from many primary muscle diseases in that both striated and smooth muscles are affected.[525]

Myotonia of the tongue and oral musculature may impair swallowing. Radiologically, there may be pooling of contrast medium in the pharynx, the valleculae, and the pyriform sinuses.[525] Esophageal involvement can be manifested by oropharyngeal dysphagia. Manometry shows a decreased amplitude of pharyngeal and upper esophageal sphincter contraction, but the peristaltic sequence is intact, consistent with striated muscle weakness.[526, 527] These abnormalities are present in most patients even in the absence of esophageal symptoms.[526] Emptying of the body of the esophagus (smooth muscle) is also slowed, but the lower esophageal sphincter behaves normally.[526]

Gastric atony, bezoar formation, impaired small intestinal motility, and *gallbladder dysfunction* with *cholelithiasis* have all been observed in this disease.[525, 528, 529] Steatorrhea has been reported[525] but is poorly documented, and malabsorption probably is not a feature of this disorder.[530] Abnormal D-glucose tolerance curves are seen, the result of poor gastric emptying.[530] Barium enemas may show *volvulus, megacolon,* and *segmental sigmoid narrowing.*[531, 532] Anorectal manometry is abnormal in most patients. The resting pressure of the internal sphincter and the relaxation with rectal distention are subnormal. Internal sphincter relaxation is followed by a characteristic high-amplitude contraction of both the internal and external sphincters.[533]

Clinical gastrointestinal symptoms in myotonic dystrophy include diarrhea, constipation, vomiting, heartburn, and *pseudo-obstruction.*[525, 534] (For discussion of these motor disorders, see pp. 377–379 and 1395–1401.)

PULMONARY DISEASE

Although nocturnal *asthma* due to tracheal aspiration is often a consequence of severe gastroesophageal reflux, asthma may also cause reflux, as suggested by a controlled trial showing that medical management of asthma improved the symptoms of esophageal reflux.[556] Pulmonary, pancreatic, and rectal lesions coexist in *cystic fibrosis* (see pp. 1789–1801).

CARDIAC DISEASE

Elevation of right atrial pressure may cause excessive enteric protein loss (see pp. 283–290).

An association has been made between *aortic stenosis* and *gastrointestinal angiodysplasia* with chronic blood loss (see pp. 413–415 and 1363–1366).

In a recent large series, 28 per cent of *cardiac transplant recipients* experienced abdominal complications.[557] *Upper gastrointestinal hemorrhage, perforated colonic diverticula, pancreatitis,* and severe *abdominal pain* of uncertain etiology were the most frequently encountered problems. One patient underwent cholecystectomy for *acalculous cholecystitis,* and one developed *gastric outlet obstruction* secondary to vagus nerve injury during heart-lung transplantation. Intestinal complications related to immunosuppressive drugs can be expected (see p. 503).[555]

References

1. Marks, P., Anderson, J., and Vincent, R. Thyrotoxic myopathy presenting as dysphagia. Postgrad. Med. J. *56*:669, 1980.
2. Dodd, M. J., and Blake, D. R. A case of apathetic thyrotoxicosis simulating malignant disease. Postgrad. Med. J. *56*:359, 1980.
3. Miller, L. J., Gorman, C. A., and Go, V. L. W. Gut-thyroid interrelationships. Gastroenterology *75*:901, 1978.
4. Lee, L. J. Hyperthyroidism and intussusception. J. Med. Assoc. Georgia *71*:83, 1982.
5. Jarnerot, G., Khan, A., and Truelove, S. The thyroid in ulcerative colitis and Crohn's disease. 2. Thyroid enlargement and hyperthyroidism in ulcerative colitis. Acta Med. Scand. *197*:83, 1975.
6. Lyer, S. K., and Karlstadt, R. G. Hyperthyroidism and ulcer-

ative colitis: Report of two cases and a review of the literature. J. Nat. Med. Assoc. *72*:127, 1980.
7. Sagara, K., Shimada, T., Fujiyama, S., and Sato, T. Serum gastrin levels in thyroid dysfunction. Gastroenterol. Jap. *18*:79, 1983.
8. Seino, Y., Miyamoto, Y., Moridera, K., Taminato, T., Matsukura, S., and Imura, H. The role of the adrenergic mechanism in the hypergastrinemia of hyperthyroidism. J. Clin. Endocrinol. Metab. *50*:368, 1980.
9. Watatani, Y., and Aoki, H. Thyroid function and gastrin levels. Nippon Naibunpi-Gakkai-Zasshi *60*:171, 1984.
10. Siurala, M., and Lamberg, B. A. Stomach in thyrotoxicosis. Acta Med. Scand. *165*:181, 1959.
11. Siurala, M., Julkunen, H., and Lamberg, B. A. Gastrointestinal tract in hyperthyroidism before and after treatment. Scand. J. Gastroenterol. *1*:79, 1966.
12. Miller, L. J., Owyang, C., Malagelada, J.-R., Gorman, C. A., and Go, V. L. W. Gastric, pancreatic, and biliary responses to meals in hyperthyroidism. Gut *21*:695, 1980.
13. Scarf, M. Gastrointestinal manifestations of hyperthyroidism. J. Lab. Clin. Med. *21*:1253, 1936.
14. Dooner, H. P., Parada, J., Aliaga, C., and Hoyl, C. The liver in thyrotoxicosis. Arch. Intern. Med. *120*:25, 1967.
15. Beckett, G. J., Kellett, H. A., Gow, S. M., Hussen, A. J., Hayes, J. D., and Toft, A. D. Raised plasma glutathione S-transferase values in hyperthyroidism and in hypothyroid patients receiving thyroxine replacement: Evidence for hepatic damage. Br. Med. J. *291*:427, 1985.
16. Borzio, M., Caldara, R., Borzio, F., Priepolio, V., Rampini, P., and Ferrari, C. Thyroid function tests in chronic liver disease: Evidence for multiple abnormalities despite clinical euthyroidism. Gut *24*:631, 1983.
17. Hellesen, C., Friis, T., Larsen, E., and Pock-Steen, O. Small intestinal histology, radiology and absorption in hyperthyroidism. Scand. J. Gastroenterol. *4*:169, 1969.
18. Thomas, F. B., Caldwell, J. H., and Greenberger, N. J. Steatorrhea in thyrotoxicosis. Relation to hypermotility and excessive dietary fat. Ann. Intern. Med. *78*:669, 1973.
19. Peerenboom, H., Keck, E., Kruskemper, H. L., and Strohmeyer, G. The defect of intestinal calcium transport in hyperthyroidism and its response to therapy. J. Clin. Endocrinol. Metab. *59*:936, 1984.
20. Boullion, R., Muls, E., and De-Moor, P. Influence of thyroid function on the serum concentration of 1,25-dihydroxyvitamin D3. J. Clin. Endocrinol. Metab. *51*:793, 1980.
21. Shafer, R. B., Prentiss, R. A., and Bond, J. H. Gastrointestinal transit in thyroid disease. Gastroenterology *86*:852, 1984.
22. Bozzani, A., Camborsi, A. G., and Tidone, L. Gastrointestinal transit in hyperthyroid patients before and after propranolol treatment. Am. J. Gastroenterol. *80*:550, 1985.
23. Culp, K. S., and Piziak, V. K. Thyrotoxicosis presenting with secretory diarrhea. Ann. Intern. Med. *105*:216, 1986.
24. Sterling, K. Thyroid hormone action at the cell level. N. Engl. J. Med. *300*:173, 1979.
25. Irvine, W. J. The association of atrophic gastritis with autoimmune thyroid disease. Clin. Endocrinol. *4*:351, 1975.
26. Crowe, J. P., Christensen, E., Butler, J., Wheeler, P., Doniach, D., Keenan, J., and Williams, R. Primary biliary cirrhosis: The prevalence of hypothyroidism and its relationship to thyroid antibodies and sicca syndrome. Gastroenterology *78*:1437, 1980.
27. Troutman, M. E., Efrusy, M. E., Bennett, G. D., Kniaz, J. L., and Dobbins, W. O., III. Simultaneous occurrence of adult celiac disease and lymphocytic thyroiditis. J. Clin. Gastroenterol. *3*:281, 1981.
28. Eastwood, G. L., Braverman, L. E., White, E. M., and Vander-Salm, T. J. Reversal of lower esophageal sphincter hypotension and esophageal aperistalsis after treatment for hypothyroidism. J. Clin. Gastroenterol. *4*:307, 1982.
29. Kaplan, L. R. Hypothyroidism presenting as a gastric phytobezoar. Am. J. Gastroenterol. *74*:168, 1980.
30. Chapoy, P., and Balzing, P. Left micro-colon syndrome and hypothyroidism. Gastroenterol. Clin. Biol. *9*:365, 1985.
31. Duks, S. Hypothyroidism simulating tumor of the sigmoid. Mayo Clin. Proc. *54*:623, 1979.

32. Wells, I., Smith, B., and Hinton, M. Acute ileus in myxoedema. Br. Med. J. *1*:211, 1977.
33. Siurala, M., Varis, K., and Lamberg, B. A. Intestinal absorption and autoimmunity in endocrine disorders. Acta Med. Scand. *184*:53, 1968.
34. Lorenzo, Y., Losada, H., Jr., Staricco, E. C., Cervino, J. M., Bellini, M. A., Maggiolo, J., de Bieno, R. B., and Fournier, J. C. M. Hypotonia of the gallbladder, of myxedematous origin. J. Clin. Endocrinol. Metab. *17*:133, 1957.
35. Morrow, L. B. How thyroid disease presents in the elderly. Geriatrics *33*:42, 1978.
36. Tajiri, J., Shimada, T., Naomi, S., Umeda, T., and Sato, T. Hepatic dysfunction in primary hypothyroidism. Endocrinol. Jpn. *31*:83, 1984.
37. Honore, L. H. A significant association between symptomatic cholesterol cholelithiasis and treated hypothyroidism in women. J. Med. *12*:199, 1981.
38. Sachdev, Y., and Hall, R. Effusions into body cavities in hypothyroidism. Lancet *I*:564, 1975.
39. Storset, O., Todnem, K., Waldum, H. L., Burhol, P. G., and Kearney, M. S. Cronkhite-Canada syndrome with myxedema and muscle atrophy. Acta Med. Scand. *205*:343, 1979.
40. Teunissen, M. W., van der Veen, E. A., Doodeman, P. J., and Breimer, D. D. Influence of mild thyroid dysfunction on antipyrine clearance and metabolite formation in man. Eur. J. Clin. Pharmacol. *27*:99, 1984.
41. Einhorn, R., Resnick, R. H., and Soff, M. Severe alcoholic hepatitis in a hypothyroid patient. Am. J. Med. *80*:991, 1986.
42. Manger, W. M., Gifford, R. W., Jr., and Hoffman, B. B. Pheochromocytoma: A clinical and experimental overview. Curr. Probl. Cancer *9*:25, 1985.
43. Tatsula, M., Baba, M., and Itoh, T. Increased gastrin secretion in patients with pheochromocytoma. Gastroenterology *84*:920, 1983.
44. Nerup, J. Addison's disease—A review of some clinical pathological and immunological features. Danish Med. Bull. *21*:201, 1974.
45. McBrien, D. J., Jones, R. V., and Creamer, B. Steatorrhoea in Addison's disease. Lancet *I*:25, 1963.
46. Miura, S., Morita, A., Erickson, R. H., and Kim, Y. S. Content and turnover of rat intestinal microvillus membrane aminopeptidase. Gastroenterology *85*:1340, 1983.
47. Gardner, E. C., Jr., and Hersh, T. Primary hyperparathyroidism and the gastrointestinal tract. South. Med. J. *74*:197, 1981.
48. Palmer, F. J. The clinical manifestations of primary hyperparathyroidism. Comp. Ther. *9*:56, 1983.
49. Layer, P., Holtz, J., Sinene, S., and Goebell, H. Bile secretion in acute and chronic hypercalcemia in the cat. Dig. Dis. Sci. *31*:188, 1986.
50. Law, W. M., Jr., and Heath, H. Familial benign hypercalcemia (hypocalciuric hypercalcemia). Clinical and pathogenetic studies in 21 families. Ann. Intern. Med. *102*:511, 1985.
51. St. Goar, W. T. Gastrointestinal symptoms as a clue to the diagnosis of primary hyperparathyroidism: A review of 45 cases. Ann. Intern. Med. *46*:102, 1957.
52. Corlew, D. S., Bryda, S. L., Bradley, E. L., III, and Di-Girolamo, M. Observations on the course of untreated primary hyperparathyroidism. Surgery *98*:1064, 1985.
53. Frame, B., and Howbrich, W. S. Peptic ulcer and hyperparathyroidism: A survey of 300 ulcer patients. Arch. Intern. Med. *105*:536, 1960.
54. Barrerea, R. Calcium and gastric secretion. Gastroenterology *64*:1168, 1973.
55. Lenz, T., Kolbel, C., Herzog, P., and Holtermuller, K. H. Effect of somatostatin on hypercalcemia stimulated gastric juice and exocrine pancreas secretion in the human. Gastroenterology *24*:74, 1986.
56. Wilson, S. D., Singh, R. B., Kalkhoff, R. K., and Go, V. L. W. Does hyperparathyroidism cause hypergastrinemia? Surgery *80*:231, 1976.
57. Sarosdy, M. F., Saylor, R., Dittman, W., Cruz, A. B., Jr., Gaskill, H. V., III, and Banowsky, L. H. Upper gastrointestinal bleeding following renal transplantation. Urology *26*:347, 1985.
58. Paimela, H. Persistence of gastric hypoacidity in uraemic patients after renal transplantation. Scand. J. Gastroenterol. *20*:873, 1985.
59. Donegan, W. L., and Spiro, H. M. Parathyroids and gastric secretion. Gastroenterology *38*:750, 1960.
60. Cope, O., Culver, P. J., Mixter, C. G., Jr., and Nard, G. L. Pancreatitis, a diagnostic clue to hyperparathyroidism. Ann. Surg. *145*:857, 1957.
61. Mixter, C. G., Jr., Keynes, W. M., and Cope, O. Further experience with pancreatitis as a diagnostic clue to hyperparathyroidism. N. Engl. J. Med. *266*:265, 1962.
62. Pyrah, L. M., Hodgkinson, A., and Anderson, C. K. Primary hyperparathyroidism. Br. J. Surg. *53*:245, 1966.
63. Schmidt, H., and Creutzfeldt, W. Calciphylactic pancreatitis and pancreatitis in hyperparathyroidism. Clin. Orthoped. *69*:135, 1970.
64. Bess, M. A., Edis, A. J., and van Heerden, J. A. Hyperparathyroidism and pancreatitis—chance or causal association? JAMA *243*:248, 1980.
65. Fink, W. I., and Finfrock, I. D. Fatal hyperparathyroid crisis associated with pancreatitis. Am. Surg. *27*:424, 1961.
66. Kelly, R. T., and Falor, W. H. Hyperparathyroid crises associated with pancreatitis. Ann. Surg. *168*:917, 1968.
67. Layer, P., Hotz, J., Eysselein, V. E., Jansen, J. B. M. J., Lamers, C. B. H. W., Schmitz-Moormann, H. P., and Goebell, H. Effects of acute hypercalcemia on exocrine pancreatic secretion in the cat. Gastroenterology *88*:1168, 1985.
68. Prinz, R. A., and Aranha, G. V. The association of primary hyperparathyroidism and pancreatitis. Am. Surg. *51*:325, 1985.
69. Carey, L. C. Pathophysiological factors in recurrent acute pancreatitis. Jpn. J. Surg. *15*:333, 1985.
70. Wang, C. A., and Gaz, R. D. Natural history of parathyroid carcinoma. Diagnosis, treatment, and results. Am. J. Surg. *149*:522, 1985.
71. Geokas, M. C., Baltaxe, H. A., Banks, P. A., and Silva, J., Jr. Acute pancreatitis. Ann. Intern. Med. *103*:86, 1985.
72. Hochgelerent, E. L., and David, S. D. Acute pancreatitis secondary to calcium infusion in a dialysis patient. Arch. Surg. *108*:218, 1974.
73. Sallman, A., Goldberg, M., and Wombolt, D. Secondary hyperparathyroidism manifesting as acute pancreatitis and status epilepticus. Arch. Intern. Med. *141*:1549, 1981.
74. Reeve, T. S., and Delbridge, L. W. Pancreatitis following parathyroid surgery. Ann. Surg. *195*:158, 1982.
75. Izsak, E. M., Shike, M., Roulet, M., and Jeejeebhoy, K. N. Pancreatitis in association with hypercalcemia in patients receiving total parenteral nutrition. Gastroenterology *79*:555, 1980.
76. Clark, O. H. Pancreatitis, hypercalcemia, and breast carcinoma. JAMA *236*:2052, 1976.
77. Gafter, U., Mandel, E. M., Har-Zahav, L., and Weiss, S. Acute pancreatitis secondary to hypercalcemia. Occurrence in a patient with breast carcinoma. JAMA *235*:2004, 1976.
78. Davies, M., Klimiuk, P. S., Adams, P. H., Lumb, G. A., Large, D. M., and Anderson, D. C. Familial hypocalciuric hypercalcaemia and acute pancreatitis. Br. Med. J. *29*:282, 1981.
79. Layer, P., Hotz, J., Schmitz-Moormann, H. P., and Goebell, H. Effects of experimental chronic hypercalcemia on feline exocrine pancreatic secretion. Gastroenterology *82*:309, 1982.
80. Cho, J. W., Seligson, U., and Sorrell, A. Pancreatic function in patients with hyperparathyroidism. A study with the Lundh test. Acta Chir. Scand. *151*:321, 1985.
81. Payne, J. E., Jr., and Tanenberg, R. J. Hyperparathyroid crisis and acute necrotizing pancreatitis presenting as diabetic ketoacidosis. Am. J. Surg. *140*:698, 1980.
82. Levine, G., Tsin, D., and Risk, A. Acute pancreatitis and hyperparathyroidism in pregnancy. Obstet. Gynecol. *54*:246, 1979.
83. Clarkson, B. O., Kowlessar, O. D., Horwith, M., and Sleisenger, M. H. Clinical and metabolic study of a patient with malabsorption and hypoparathyroidism. Metabolism *9*:1093, 1960.
84. Brun, J. M. Juvenile autoimmune polyendocrinopathy. Horm. Res. *16*:308, 1982.

85. Arulanantham, K., Dwyer, J. M., and Genel, M. Evidence for defective immunoregulation in the syndrome of familial candidiasis endocrinopathy. N. Engl. J. Med. *300*:164, 1979.

86. Krejs, G. J., Orci, L., Conlon, J. M., Ravazzoli, M., Davis, G. R., Raskin, P., Collins, S. M., McCarthy, D. M., Baetens, D., Rubenstein, A., Aldor, T. A. M., and Unger, R. H. Somatostatinoma syndrome: Biochemical, morphologic and clinical features. N. Engl. J. Med. *301*:285, 1979.

87. Lips, C. J., Vasen, H. F., and Lamers, C. B. MEN syndromes. CRC Crit. Rev. Oncol. Hematol. *2*:17, 1984.

88. Marx, S. J., Vinik, A. I., Santen, R. J., Floyd, J. C., Mills, J. L., and Green, J., III. Multiple endocrine neoplasia type I: Assessment of laboratory tests to screen for the gene in a large kindred. Medicine *65*:226, 1986.

89. Oberg, K., Walinder, O., Bostrom, H., Lundqvist, G., and Wide, L. Peptide hormone markers in screening for endocrine tumors in multiple endocrine adenomatosis type I. Am. J. Med. *73*:619, 1982.

90. Adrian, T. E., Uttenthal, L. O., Williams, S. J., and Bloom, S. R. Secretion of pancreatic polypeptide in patients with pancreatic endocrine tumors. N. Engl. J. Med. *315*:287, 1986.

91. Stacpoole, P. W. The glucagonoma syndrome: Clinical features, diagnosis, and treatment. Endocrinol. Rev. *2*:347, 1981.

92. D'Arcangues, C. M., Awoke, S., and Lawrence, G. D. Metastatic insulinoma with long survival and glucagonoma syndrome. Ann. Intern. Med. *100*:233, 1984.

93. Dawson, J., Bloom, S. R., and Cockel, R. A unique apudoma producing the glucagonoma and gastrinoma syndromes. Postgrad. Med. J. *59*:315, 1983.

94. Yamaguchi, K., Abe, K., Otsubo, K., Haniuda, C., Suzuki, M., Shimada, A., Kimura, S., Adachi, I., Kameya, T., and Yanaihara, N. The WDHA syndrome: Clinical and laboratory data on 28 Japanese cases. Peptides (Fayetteville) *5*:415, 1984.

95. Saad, M. F., Ordonez, N., Rashid, R. K., Guido, J. J., Hill, C. S., Jr., Hickey, R. C., and Samaan, N. A. Medullary carcinoma of the thyroid. A study of the clinical features and prognostic factors in 161 patients. Medicine *63*:319, 1984.

96. Pont, A. Multiple endocrine neoplasia syndromes. West. J. Med. *132*:301, 1980.

97. Fletcher, D. R., Gamvros, O., Man, W. K., Ahmed, Y., Trayner, I., and Adrian, T. Multiple endocrine neoplasia type II: The role of gastrointestinal humoral factors in calcitonin release following alcohol and pentagastrin stimulation. Aust. N.Z. J. Surg. *54*:271, 1984.

98. Spiller, I. J., Kapcala, L. P., Graze, K., Gagel, R. F., Feldman, Z. T., Biller, B., Tashjian, A. H., Jr., and Reichlin, S. Effects of L-dopa and bromocriptine on calcitonin secretion in medullary thyroid carcinoma. J. Clin. Endocrinol. Metab. *51*:806, 1980.

99. Shepherd, J. J., and Senator, G. B. Regression of liver metastases in patient with gastrin-secreting tumour treated with SMS 201-995. Lancet *2*:574, 1986.

100. Kvols, L. K., Moertel, C. G., O'Connell, M. J., Schutt, A. J., Rubin, J., and Hahn, R. G. The treatment of the malignant carcinoid syndrome. Evaluation of a long-acting somatostatin analogue. N. Engl. J. Med. *315*:663, 1986.

101. Khairi, M. R., Dexter, R. N., Burznyski, N. J., and Johnston, C. C., Jr. Mucosal neuroma, pheochromocytoma and medullary thyroid carcinoma: Multiple endocrine neoplasia type 3. Medicine *54*:89, 1975.

102. Netzloff, M. L., Garnica, A. D., Rodgers, B. M., and Frias, J. L. Medullary carcinoma of the thyroid in the multiple mucosal neuromas syndrome. Ann. Clin. Lab. Sci. *9*:368, 1979.

103. Cope, R., and Schleinitz, P. F. Multiple endocrine neoplasia, type 2b, as a cause of megacolon. Am. J. Gastroenterol. *78*:802, 1983.

104. Gardet, P., Rougier, P., Navarro, J., Schlumberger, M., Travagli, J. P., Caillou, B., Hartmann, O., Lemerle, J., and Parmentier, C. Multiple endocrine neoplasia type 2b. Clinical, diagnostic and therapeutic aspects. Bull. Cancer (Paris) *71*:172, 1984.

105. Perkins, J. T., Blackstone, M. O., and Riddell, R. H. Adenomatous polyposis coli and multiple endocrine neoplasia type 2b. A pathogenic relationship. Cancer *55*:375, 1985.

106. Weidner, N., Flanders, D. J., and Mitros, F. A. Mucosal

107. Snover, D. C., Weigent, C. E., and Sumner, H. W. Diffuse mucosal ganglioneuromatosis of the colon associated with adenocarcinoma. Am. J. Clin. Pathol. *75*:225, 1981.

108. Carney, J. A., Go, V. L. W., Gordon, H., Northcutt, R. C., Pearse, A. G. E., and Sheps, S. G. Familial pheochromocytoma and islet cell tumor of the pancreas. Am. J. Med. *68*:515, 1980.

109. Zeller, J. R., Kauffman, H. M., Komozowski, R. A., and Itskovitz, H. D. Bilateral pheochromocytoma and islet cell adenoma of the pancreas. Arch. Surg. *117*:827, 1982.

110. Clements, R. S., Jr., and Bell, D. S. Diagnostic, pathogenetic, and therapeutic aspects of diabetic neuropathy. Spec. Top. Endocrinol. Metab. *3*:1, 1982.

111. Niakan, E., Harati, Y., and Comstock, J. P. Diabetic autonomic neuropathy. Metabolism *35*:224, 1986.

112. Diani, A. R., Davis, D. E., Fix, J. D., Swartzman, J., and Gerritsen, G. C. Morphometric analysis of autonomic neuropathology in the abdominal sympathetic trunk of the ketonuric diabetic Chinese hamster. Acta Neuropathol. (Berl) *53*:293, 1981.

113. Diani, A., West, D., Vidmar, T., Peterson, T., and Gerritsen, G. Morphometric analysis of the vagus nerve in nondiabetic and ketonuric diabetic Chinese hamsters. J. Comp. Pathol. *94*:495, 1984.

114. Lincoln, J., Bokor, J. T., Crowe, R., Griffith, S. G., Haven, A. J., and Burnstock, G. Myenteric plexus in streptozotocin-treated rats. Neurochemical and histochemical evidence for diabetic neuropathy in the gut. Gastroenterology *86*:654, 1984.

115. Schmidt, R. E., Nelson, J. S., and Johnson, E. M. Experimental autonomic diabetic neuropathy. Am. J. Pathol. *103*:210–225, 1981.

116. Kishimoto, S., Kunita, S., Kambara, A., Okamoto, K., Shimizu, S., Yamamoto, M., Koh, H., Sano, K., Kajiyama, G., Miyoshi, A., et al. VIPergic innervation in the gastrointestinal tract of diabetic rats. Hiroshima J. Med. Sci. *32*:469, 1983.

117. Belai, A., Lincoln, J., Milner, P., Crowe, R., Loesch, A., and Burnstock, G. Enteric nerves in diabetic rats: Increase in vasoactive intestinal polypeptide but not substance P. Gastroenterology *89*:967, 1985.

118. Ballmann, M., and Conlon, J. M. Changes in the somatostatin, substance P and vasoactive intestinal polypeptide content of the gastrointestinal tract following streptozotocin-induced diabetes in the rat. Diabetologia *28*:355, 1985.

119. Schmidt, H., Riemann, J. F., Schmid, A., and Sailer, D. Ultrastructure of diabetic autonomic neuropathy of the gastrointestinal tract. Klin. Wochenschr. *62*:399, 1984.

120. Monckton, G., and Pekowitch, E. Autonomic neuropathy in streptozotocin-induced diabetes in rats. Can. J. Neurol. Sci. *7*:135, 1980.

121. Bojsen-Muller, F., Gronback, P., and Rostgaard, J. Light microscopic study of gastrointestinal and skin capillaries in diabetes mellitus. Diabetes *12*:429, 1963.

122. Goyal, R. K., and Spiro, H. M. Gastrointestinal manifestations of diabetes mellitus. Med. Clin. North Am. *55*:1031, 1971.

123. Feldman, M., and Schiller, L. R. Disorders of gastrointestinal motility associated with diabetes mellitus. Ann. Intern. Med. *98*:378, 1983.

124. Yang, R., Arem, R., and Chan, L. Gastrointestinal tract complications of diabetes mellitus. Pathophysiology and management. Arch. Intern. Med. *144*:1251, 1984.

125. Atkinson, M., and Hosking, D. J. Gastrointestinal complications of diabetes mellitus. Clin. Gastroenterol. *12*:633, 1983.

126. Mandelstam, P., Siegel, C. I., Lieber, A., and Siegel, M. The swallowing disorder in patients with diabetic neuropathy-gastroenteropathy. Gastroenterology *56*:1, 1969.

127. Loo, D. F., Dodds, W. J., Soergel, K. H., Arndorfer, R. C., Helm, J. F., and Hogan, W. J. Multipeaked esophageal peristaltic pressure waves in patients with diabetic neuropathy. Gastroenterology *88*:485, 1985.

128. Clouse, R. E., Lustman, P. J., and Reidel, W. L. Correlation of esophageal motility abnormalities with neuropsychiatric status in diabetics. Gastroenterology *90*:1146, 1986.

129. Stewart, I. M., Hoaking, D. J., Preston, B. J., and Atkinson,

ganglioneuromatosis associated with multiple colonic polyps. Am. J. Surg. Pathol. *8*:779, 1984.

M. Oesophageal motor changes in diabetes mellitus. Thorax *31*:278, 1976.

130. Hollis, J. B., Castell, D. O., and Braddon, R. L. Esophageal function in diabetes mellitus and its relation to peripheral neuropathy. Gastroenterology 73:1098, 1977.

131. Russell, C. O., Gannan, R., Coatsworth, J., Neilsen, R., Allen, F., Hill, L. D., and Pope, C. E., II. Relationship among esophageal dysfunction diabetic gastroenteropathy and peripheral neuropathy. Dig. Dis. Sci. 28:289, 1983.

132. Kristensson, K., Nordborg, D., Olsson, Y., and Saurander, P. Changes in the vagus nerve in diabetes mellitus. Acta Pathol. Microbiol. Scand. (section A) 79:684, 1971.

133. Smith, B. Neuropathology of the oesophagus in diabetes mellitus. J. Neurol. Neurosurg. Psychol. 37:1151, 1974.

134. Gillin, J. S., and Kurtz, R. C. Treatment of Candida esophagitis. Gastroenterology 85:971, 1983.

135. Saltzman, M. B., and McCallum, R. W. Diabetes and the stomach. Yale J. Biol. Med. 56:179, 1983.

136. Brady, P. G., and Richardson, K. Gastric bezoar formation secondary to gastroparesis diabeticorum. Arch. Intern. Med. 137:1729, 1977.

137. Feldman, M., Smith, H. J., and Simon, T. R. Gastric emptying of solid radiopaque markers: Studies in healthy subjects and diabetic patients. Gastroenterology 87:895, 1984.

138. Malagelada, J.-R., Rees, W. D. W., Mazzotta, L. J., and Go, V. L. Gastric motor abnormalities in diabetic and postvagotomy gastroparesis: Effect of metoclopramide and bethanechol. Gastroenterology 78:286, 1980.

139. Camilleri, M., and Malagelada, J.-R. Abnormal intestinal motility in diabetics with the gastroparesis syndrome. Eur. J. Clin. Invest. 14:420, 1984.

140. Mearin, F., Camilleri, M., and Malagelada, J.-R. Pyloric dysfunction in diabetics with recurrent nausea and vomiting. Gastroenterology 90:1919, 1986.

141. Achem-Karam, S. R., Funakoshi, A., Vinik, A. I., and Owyang, C. Plasma motilin concentration and interdigestive migrating motor complex in diabetic gastroparesis: Effect of metoclopramide. Gastroenterology 88:492, 1985.

142. Nakanome, C., Akai, H., Hongo, M., Imail, N., and Toyota, T. Disturbances of the alimentary tract motility and hypermotilinemia. Tohoku J. Exp. Med. 139:205, 1983.

143. Chaussade, S., Grandjouan, S., and Couturier, D. Motilin and diabetic gastroparesis: Effect of MTC. Gastroenterology 90:2039, 1986.

144. MacGregor, I. L., Gueller, R., Watts, H. D., and Meyer, J. H. The effect of acute hyperglycemia on gastric emptying in man. Gastroenterology 70:190, 1976.

145. Ricci, D. A., Saltzman, M. B., Meyer, C., Callachan, C., and McCallum, R. W. Effects of metoclopramide in diabetic gastroparesis. J. Clin. Gastroenterol. 7:25, 1985.

146. Schade, R. R., Dugas, M. C., Lhotsky, D. M., Gavaler, J. S., and Van Thiel, D. H. Effect of metoclopramide on gastric liquid emptying in patients with diabetic gastroparesis. Dig. Dis. Sci. 30:10, 1985.

147. Heer, M., Muller-Duysing, W., Benes, J., Wertzel, M., Pirovino, M., Altdorfer, J., and Schmid, N. Diabetic gastroparesis. Treatment with domperidone. Digestion 27:214, 1983.

148. Horowitz, M., Harding, P. E., Chatterton, B. E., Collins, P. J., and Shearman, D. J. C. Acute and chronic effects of domperidone on gastric emptying in diabetic autonomic neuropathy. Dig. Dis. Sci. 30:1, 1985.

148a. Horowitz, M., Maddox, A., Harding, P. E., Maddern, G. J., Chatterton, B. E., Wishart, J., and Shearman, D. J. C. Effect of cisapride on gastric and esophageal emptying in insulin-dependent diabetes mellitus. Gastroenterology 92:1899, 1987.

149. Irvine, W. J., Clarke, B. F., Scarth, L., Cullen, D. R., and Duncan, L. J. P. Thyroid and gastric autoimmunity in patients with diabetes mellitus. Lancet 2:163, 1970.

150. Leshin, H. Polyglandular autoimmune syndromes. Am. J. Med. Sci. 290:77, 1985.

151. Betterle, C., Zanette, F., Pedrini, B., Presotto, F., Rapp, L. B., Monciotti, C. M., and Rigon, F. Clinical and subclinical organ-specific autoimmune manifestations in Type I diabetic patients and their first degree relatives. Diabetologia 26:431, 1984.

152. Riley, W. J., Toskes, P. P., MacLaren, N. K., and Silverstein, J. H. Predictive value of gastric parietal cell auto antibodies as a marker for gastric and hematological abnormalities associated with insulin-dependent diabetes. Diabetes 31:1051, 1982.

153. Dotevall, G. Gastric secretion of acid in diabetes mellitus during basal conditions and after maximum histamine stimulation. Acta Med. Scand. 170:59, 1961.

154. Feldman, M., Corbett, D. B., Ramsey, E. J., Walsh, J. H., and Richardson, C. T. Abnormal gastric function in long-standing, insulin-dependent patients. Gastroenterology 77:12, 1979.

155. Hosking, D. J., Moody, F., Stewart, I. M., and Atkinson, M. Vagal impairment of gastric secretion in diabetic autonomic neuropathy. Br. Med. J. 2:588, 1975.

156. Nakanome, C., Akai, H., Umezu, M., Toyota, T., and Soto, Y. Gastric inhibitory polypeptide (GIP) response to an oral glucose load in the patients with diabetes mellitus. Tohoku J. Exp. Med. 139:287, 1983.

157. Longstreth, G. F., and Newcomer, A. D. Abdominal pain caused by diabetic radiculopathy. Ann. Intern. Med. 86:166, 1977.

158. Miller, L. J. Small intestinal manifestations of diabetes mellitus. Yale J. Biol. Med. 56:189–193, 1983.

159. Walsh, C. H., Cooper, B. T., Wright, A. D., Malins, J. M., and Cooke, W. T. Diabetes mellitus and coeliac disease: A clinical study. Q. J. Med. 185:89, 1978.

160. Whalen, G. E., Soergel, K. H., and Geenen, J. E. Diabetic diarrhea: A clinical and pathophysiological study. Gastroenterology 56:1021, 1969.

161. McNally, E. F., Reinhard, A. E., and Schwartz, P. E. Small bowel motility in diabetics. Am. J. Dig. Dis. 14:163, 1969.

162. Drewes, V. M. Mechanical and electrical activity in the duodenum of diabetics with and without diarrhea: Pressures, differential pressures and action potential. Am. J. Dig. Dis. 16:628, 1971.

163. Scarpello, J. H. B., Hague, R. V., Cullen, D. R., and Sladen, G. E. The ^{14}C-glycocholate test in diabetic diarrhea. Br. Med. J. 2:673, 1976.

164. Keshavarzian, A., and Iber, F. L. Intestinal transit in insulin-requiring diabetics. Am. J. Gastroenterol. 81:257, 1986.

165. Nowak, J. V., Harrington, B., Kalbfleisch, J. H., and Amatruda, J. M. Evidence for abnormal cholinergic neuromuscular transmission in diabetic rat small intestine. Gastroenterology 91:124, 1986.

166. Foy, J. M., and Lucas, P. D. Effect of experimental diabetes, food deprivation and genetic obesity on sensitivity of pithed rats to autonomic stimulation. Br. J. Pharmacol. 57:229, 1976.

167. Hensley, G. T., and Soergel, K. H. Neuropathologic findings in diabetic diarrhea. Arch. Pathol. 85:587, 1968.

168. Berge, K. G., Sprague, R. G., and Bennett, W. A. The intestinal tract in diabetic diarrhea: A pathologic study. Diabetes 5:289, 1956.

169. Chang, E. B., Bergenstal, R. M., and Field, M. Diarrhea in streptozotocin-treated rats. J. Clin. Invest. 75:1666, 1985.

170. White, N. H., Waltman, S. R., Krupin, T., and Santiago, J. V. Reversal of neuropathic and gastrointestinal complications related to diabetes mellitus in adolescents with improved metabolic control. J. Pediatr. 99:41, 1981.

171. Chang, E. B., Fedorak, R. W., and Field, M. Experimental diabetic diarrhea in rats. Intestinal mucosal denervation hypersensitivity and treatment with clonidine. Gastroenterology 91:564, 1986.

172. Fedorak, R. N., Field, M., and Chang, E. B. Treatment of diabetic diarrhea with clonidine. Ann. Intern. Med. 102:197, 1985.

173. Molloy, A. M., and Tomkin, G. H. Altered bile in diabetic diarrhoea. Br. Med. J. 2:1462, 1978.

174. Schiller, L. R., Santa Ana, C. A., Morawski, S. G., and Fordtran, J. S. Studies of the antidiarrheal action of clonidine. Gastroenterology 89:982, 1985.

175. Tsai, S. -T., Vinik, A. I., and Brunner, J. F. Diabetic diarrhea and somatostatin. Ann. Intern. Med. 104:894, 1986.

175a. Dudl, R. J., Anderson, D. S., Forsythe, A. B., Ziegler, M. G., and O'Dorisio, T. M. Treatment of diabetic diarrhea and orthostatic hypotension with somatostatin analogue SMS 201–995. Am. J. Med. *83*:584, 1987.

176. Battle, W. M., Snape, W. J., Jr., Alavi, A., Cohen, S., and Braunstein, S. Colonic dysfunction in diabetes mellitus. Gastroenterology *79*:1217, 1980.

177. Battle, W. M., Cohen, J. D., and Snape, W. J., Jr. Disorders of colonic motility in patients with diabetes mellitus. Yale J. Biol. Med. *56*:277, 1983.

178. Paley, R. G., Mitchell, W., and Watkinson, G. Terminal colonic dilatation following intractable diarrhea in diabetics. Gastroenterology *41*:401, 1961.

179. Anuras, S., and Shirazi, S. S. Colonic pseudo-obstruction. Am. J. Gastroenterol. *79*:525, 1984.

180. Schiller, L. R., Santa Ana, C. A., Schmulen, C., Hendler, R. S., Harford, W. V., and Fordtran, J. S. Pathogenesis of fecal incontinence in diabetes mellitus. N. Engl. J. Med. *307*:1666, 1982.

181. Lieber, M. M. The incidence of gallstones and their correlation with other diseases. Ann. Surg. *135*:394, 1982.

182. Bennion, L. J., and Grundy, S. M. Risk factors in development of cholelithiasis in man. Part II. N. Engl. J. Med. *299*:1221, 1978.

183. Foster, K. J., Griffith, A. H., Dewbury, K., Price, C. P., and Wright, R. Liver disease in patients with diabetes mellitus. Postgrad. Med. J. *56*:767, 1980.

184. Bennion, L. J., and Grundy, S. M. Effects of diabetes mellitus on cholesterol metabolism in man. N. Engl. J. Med. *296*:1365, 1979.

185. Ponz de Leon, M. P., Ferenderes, R., and Coruli, N. Bile lipid composition and bile acid pool size in diabetics. Am. J. Dig. Dis. *23*:710, 1978.

186. Gitelson, S., Oppenheim, D., and Schwartz, A. Size of the gallbladder in patients with diabetes mellitus. Diabetes *18*:493, 1969.

187. Grodzki, M., Mazurkiewicz-Rozynska, E., and Czyzyk, A. Diabetic cholecystopathy. Diabetologia *4*:345, 1968.

188. Sandler, R. S., Maule, W. F., and Baltus, M. E. Factors associated with postoperative complications in diabetics after biliary tract surgery. Gastroenterology *91*:157, 1986.

189. Pellegrini, C. A. Asymptomatic gallstones. Does diabetes mellitus make a difference? Gastroenterology *91*:248, 1986.

190. Barrett, E. J., and Sherwin, R. S. Gastrointestinal manifestations of diabetic ketoacidosis. Yale J. Biol. Med. *56*:175, 1983.

191. Beigelman, P. M. Severe diabetic ketoacidosis (diabetic coma). Diabetes *20*:490, 1971.

192. Campbell, I. W., Duncan, L. J. P., Innes, J. A., MacGuish, A. C., and Munro, J. F. Abdominal pain in diabetic metabolic decompensation: Clinical significance. JAMA *233*:166, 1975.

193. Eckfeldt, J. H., Leatherman, J. W., and Levitt, M. D. High prevalence of hyperamylasemia in patients with acidemia. Ann. Intern. Med. *104*:362, 1986.

194. Vinicor, F., Lehrner, L. M., Karn, R. C., and Merritt, A. D. Hyperamylasemia in diabetic ketoacidosis: Sources and significance. Ann. Intern. Med. *91*:200, 1979.

195. Atchley, D. W., Loeb, R. F., Richards, D. W., Jr., Benedict, E. M., and Driscoll, M. E. On diabetic acidosis. J. Clin. Invest. *12*:297, 1933.

196. Mundth, E. D. Cholecystitis and diabetes mellitus. N. Engl. J. Med. *267*:642, 1962.

197. Knight, A. H., Williams, D. W., Spooner, R. J., and Goldberg, D. M. Serum enzyme changes in diabetic ketoacidosis. Diabetes *23*:126, 1974.

198. Goyal, R. K., and Spiro, H. M. Gastrointestinal manifestations of diabetes mellitus. Med. Clin. North Am. *55*:1031, 1971.

199. Hillemeier, C., and Gryboski, J. Diabetes and the gastrointestinal tract in the pediatric patient. Yale J. Biol. Med. *56*:195, 1983.

200. Malone, J. I. Juvenile diabetes and acute pancreatitis. J. Pediatr. *85*:825, 1975.

201. Johansen, K., and Ornsholt, J. Frequency of diabetes after acute pancreatitis. Metabolism *21*:291, 1972.

202. Knight, M. Glucagon in the pathogenesis of acute pancreatitis. Br. J. Surg. *59*:912, 1972.

203. Frier, B. M., Sanders, J. H. B., Wormsley, K. G., and Bouchier, I. A. D. Exocrine pancreatic function in juvenile-onset diabetes mellitus. Gut *17*:685, 1976.

204. Bank, S., Marks, I. N., and Vinik, A. I. Clinical and hormonal aspects of pancreatic diabetes. Am. J. Gastroenterol. *64*:13, 1975.

205. Kessler, I. I. Cancer mortality among diabetics. J. Natl. Cancer Inst. *44*:673, 1970.

206. Karmody, A. J., and Kyle, J. The association between carcinoma of the pancreas and diabetes mellitus. Br. J. Surg. *56*:362, 1969.

207. Nix, G. A. J. J., Schmitz, P. I. M., Wilson, J. H. P., van Blankenstein, M., Groeneveld, C. F. M., and Hofwijk, R. Carcinoma of the head of the pancreas. Therapeutic implications of endoscopic retrograde cholangiopancreatography findings. Gastroenterology *87*:37, 1984.

208. Fujita, J., Seino, Y., Ishida, H., Taminato, T., Matsukura, S., Horio, T., Imamura, S., Naito, A., Tobe, T., Takahashi, K., Midorikawa, O., and Imura, H. A functional study of a case of glucagonoma exhibiting typical glucagonoma syndrome. Cancer *57*:860, 1986.

209. Jones, B., Fishman, E. K., Bayless, T. M., Siegelman, S. S., and Russell, H. Villous hypertrophy of the small bowel in a patient with glucagonoma. J. Comput. Assist. Tomogr. *7*:334, 1983.

210. Stevens, F. M., Flanagan, R. W., O'Gorman, D., and Buchanan, K. D. Glucagonoma syndrome demonstrating giant duodenal villi. Gut *25*:784, 1984.

211. Bynum, T. E. Hepatic and gastrointestinal disorders in pregnancy. Med. Clin. North Am. *61*:129, 1977.

212. Van Thiel, D. H., Gavaler, J. S., Joshi, S. N., Sara, R. K., and Stremple, J. Heartburn of pregnancy. Gastroenterology *72*:666, 1977.

213. Brock-Utne, J. G., Dow, T. G., Dimopoulos, G. E., Welman, S., Downing, J. N., and Moshal, M. G. Gastric and lower oesophageal sphincter pressures in early pregnancy. Br. J. Anaesth. *53*:381, 1981.

214. Bainbridge, E. T., Nicholas, S. D., Newton, J. R., and Temple, J. G. Gastro-oesophageal reflux in pregnancy. Scand. J. Gastroenterol. *19*:85, 1984.

215. Schade, R. R., Pelekuuos, M. J., Tauxe, W. N., and Van Thiel, D. H. Gastric emptying during pregnancy. Gastroenterology *86*:1234, 1984.

216. Palmer, E. D. Upper gastrointestinal hemorrhage during pregnancy. Am. J. Med. Sci. *226*:127, 1961.

217. Scott, L. D., Lester, R., Van Thiel, D. H., and Wald, A. Pregnancy-related changes in small intestinal myoelectric activity in the rat. Gastroenterology *84*:301, 1983.

218. Shaffer, E. A., Taylor, P. J., Logan, K., Gadomski, S., and Corenblum, B. The effect of a progestin on gallbladder function in young women. Am. J. Obstet. Gynecol. *148*:504, 1984.

219. Weinberg, R. B., Sitrin, M. D., Adkins, G. M., and Lin, C. C. Treatment of hyperlipidemic pancreatitis in pregnancy with total parenteral nutrition. Gastroenterology *83*:1300, 1982.

220. Jouppila, P., Mokka, R., and Larmi, T. K. I. Acute pancreatitis in pregnancy. Surg. Gynecol. Obstet. *313*:879, 1974.

220a. Salo, J. A., Salmenkivi, K., Tenhunen, A., and Kivilaakso, E. O. Rupture of splanchnic artery aneurysms. World J. Surg. *10*:123, 1986.

221. Donaldson, R. M., Jr. Management of medical problems in pregnancy—inflammatory bowel disease. N. Engl. J. Med. *312*:1616, 1985.

222. Prasad, A. S. The role of zinc in gastrointestinal and liver disease. Clin. Gastroenterol. *12*:713, 1983.

223. Navert, B., and Sandrom, B. Reduction of the phytate content of bran by leavening in bread and its effect on zinc absorption in man. Br. J. Nutr. *53*:47, 1985.

224. Fleming, C. R., Huizenga, K. A., McCall, J. T., Gildea, J., and Dennis, R. Zinc nutrition in Crohn's disease. Dig. Dis. Sci. *26*:865, 1981.

225. Atkinson, R. L., Dahms, W. T., Bray, G. A., Jacob, R., and Sandstead, H. H. Plasma zinc and copper in obesity and after intestinal bypass. Ann. Intern. Med. *89*:491, 1978.

226. Kay, R. G., Tasman-Jones, C., Pybus, J., Whiting, R., and Black, H. A syndrome of acute zinc deficiency during parenteral alimentation in man. Ann. Surg. *183*:331, 1976.

227. Elsnes, M. E., and Jones, J. G. Ultrastructural changes in the small intestine of zinc-deficient rats. J. Pathol. *130*:37, 1980.

228. Gebbhard, R. L., Karouani, R., Prigge, W. F., and McClain, C. J. The effect of severe zinc deficiency on activity of intestinal disaccharidases and 3-hydroxy-3-methylglutaryl coenzyme A reductase in the rat. J. Nutr. *113*:855, 1983.

229. Tamura, T., Shane, B., Bae, M. T., King, J. C., Margen, S., and Stokstad, E. L. R. Absorption of mono and polyglutamyl folates in zinc-depleted man. Am. J. Clin. Nutr. *31*:1984, 1978.

230. Rodin, A. E., and Goldman, A. S. Autopsy findings in acrodermatitis enteropathica. Am. J. Clin. Pathol. *51*:315, 1969.

231. Aikawa, H., and Suzuki, K. Lesions in the skin, intestine, and central nervous system induced by an antimetabolite of niacin. Am. J. Pathol. *122*:335, 1986.

232. Spivak, J. L., and Jackson, D. L. Pellagra: An analysis of 18 patients and review of the literature. Johns Hopkins Med. J. *140*:295, 1977.

233. Cook, G. C. D-Xylose absorption and jejunal morphology in African patients with pellagra (niacin tryptophan deficiency). Trans. R. Soc. Trop. Med. Hyg. *70*:349, 1976.

234. Abrams, H. S., Spiro, R., and Goldstein, N. Metastases in carcinoma: Analysis of 1000 autopsied cases. Cancer *3*:79, 1950.

235. Eisenberg, R. L. Gastrointestinal Radiology. A Pattern Approach. Philadelphia, J. B. Lippincott Co., 1983, pp. 658–666.

236. Coscina, W. F., Arger, P. H., Levine, M. S., Herlinger, H., Cohen, S., Coleman, B. G., and Mintz, M. C. Gastrointestinal tract focal mass lesions: Role of CT and barium evaluations. Radiology *158*:581, 1986.

237. Antler, A. S., Ough, Y., Pitchumoni, C. S., Davidian, M., and Thelmo, W. Gastrointestinal metastases from malignant tumors of the lung. Cancer *49*:170, 1982.

238. Schuffler, M. D., Baird, H. W., Fleming, C. R., Bell, C. E., Bouldin, T. W., Malagelada, J.-R., McGill, D. B., LeBauer, S. M., Abrams, M., and Love, J. Intestinal pseudo-obstruction as the presenting manifestation of small-cell carcinoma of the lung. Ann. Intern. Med. *98*:129, 1983.

239. Megibow, A. J., Balthazar, E. J., Naidich, D. P., and Bosniak, M. A. Computed tomography of gastrointestinal lymphoma. Am. J. Radiol. *141*:541, 1983.

240. Ioachim, H. L., Cooper, M. C., and Hellman, G. C. Lymphomas in men at high risk for acquired immune deficiency syndrome (AIDS). A study of 21 cases. Cancer *56*:2831, 1985.

241. Hunter, T. B., and Bjelland, J. C. Gastrointestinal complications of leukemia and its treatment. Am. J. Roentgenol. *142*:513, 1984.

242. Winton, R. R., Gwynn, A. M., Robert, J. C., and Thomas, L. Leukemia and the bowel. Med. J. Aust. *4*:89, 1975.

243. Stratemeier, P. H. Massive esophageal hemorrhage in leukemia. Am. J. Roentgenol. *129*:1106, 1977.

244. Cornes, J. S., and Jones, T. G. Leukemic lesions of the gastrointestinal tract. J. Clin. Pathol. *15*:300, 1962.

245. Rabin, M. S., Bledin, A. C., and Lewis, D. Polypoid leukemic infiltration of the large bowel. Am. J. Roentgenol. *131*:723, 1978.

246. Bodey, G. P., Bolivar, R., and Fainstein, V. Infectious complications in leukemic patients. Semin. Hematol. *19*:193, 1982.

247. Price, H. I., and Rabin, M. S. Gastrointestinal hemorrhage associated with leukemic infiltration of the stomach. S. Afr. Med. J. *56*:410, 1979.

248. Hawkins, J. A., Mower, W. R., and Nelson, E. W. Acute abdominal conditions in patients with leukemia. Am. J. Surg. *150*:739, 1985.

249. Kunkel, J. M., and Rosenthal, D. Management of the ileocecal syndrome. Neutropenic enterocolitis. Dis. Colon Rectum *29*:196, 1986.

250. Taylor, A. J., Dodds, W. J., Gonyo, J. E., and Komorowski, R. A. Typhlitis in adults. Gastrointest. Radiol. *10*:363, 1985.

251. Shamberger, R. C., Weinstein, H. J., Delorey, M. J., and Levey, R. H. The medical and surgical management of typhlitis in children with acute nonlymphocytic (myelogenous) leukemia. Cancer *57*:603, 1986.

252. Fainstein, V., Bodey, G. P., and Fekety, R. Pseudomembran-

ous colitis due to cancer chemotherapy. J. Infect. Dis. *143*:865, 1981.

253. Cockington, R. A. Leukemic infiltration of the gastrointestinal tract. An unusual cause of protein-losing enteropathy. Med. J. Aust. *1*:103, 1975.

254. Wilson, J. A. Richter's syndrome mimicking chronic colitis. A patient with diffuse histiocytic lymphoma complicating chronic lymphocytic leukemia. Dis. Colon Rectum *29*:191, 1986.

255. Caniano, D. A., Browne, A. F., and Boles, E. T., Jr. Pancreatic pseudocyst complicating treatment of acute lymphoblastic leukemia. J. Pediatr. Surg. *20*:452, 1985.

256. Papadakis, M. A., Busch, M. P., and Arieff, A. I. Hepatorenal syndrome complicating chronic lymphocytic leukemia. Am. J. Med. *80*:320, 1986.

257. Sehdeu, M. K., Dowling, M., Seal, S. H., and Stearns, M. W., Jr. Perianal and anorectal complications in leukemia. Cancer *31*:149, 1973.

258. McDonald, G. B. Gastrointestinal problems in bone-marrow transplant patients. *In* Bayless, T. M. (ed.): Current Therapy in Gastroenterology and Liver Disease. New York, B. C. Decker, 1984, pp. 188–194.

259. McDonald, G. B., Sharma, P., Matthews, D. E., Shulman, H. M., and Thomas, E. D. Venocclusive disease of the liver after bone marrow transplantation: Diagnosis, incidence, and predisposing factors. Hepatology *4*:116, 1984.

260. Tsoi, M. S. Immunological mechanisms of graft-versus-host disease in man. Transplantation *33*:459, 1982.

261. Fisk, J. D., Shulman, H. M., Greening, R. R., McDonald, G. B., Sale, G. E., and Thomas, E. D. Gastrointestinal radiographic features of human graft-vs.-host disease. Am. J. Roentgenol. *136*:329, 1981.

262. Weisdorf, S. A., Salati, L. M., Longsdorf, J. A., Ramsay, N. K. C., and Sharp, H. L. Graft-versus-host disease of the intestine: A protein losing enteropathy characterized by fecal α₁-antitrypsin. Gastroenterology *85*:1076, 1983.

263. McDonald, G. B., Sullivan, K. M., Schuffler, M. D., Shulman, H. M., and Thomas, E. D. Esophageal abnormalities in chronic graft-versus-host disease in humans. Gastroenterology *80*:914, 1981.

264. Schubert, M. M., Sullivan, K. M., Morton, T. H., Izkutsu, K. T., Peterson, D. E., Flournoy, N., Truelove, E. L., Sale, G. E., Buckner, D., Storb, R., and Thomas, E. D. Oral manifestations of chronic graft-v-host disease. Arch. Intern. Med. *144*:1591, 1984.

265. Winston, D. J., Gale, R. P., Meyer, D. V., and Young, L. S. Infectious complications of human bone marrow transplantation. Medicine *58*:1, 1979.

266. Kyle, R. A., Greipp, P. R., and Banks, P. M. The diverse picture of gamma heavy-chain disease. Report of seven cases and review of literature. Mayo Clin. Proc. *56*:439, 1981.

267. Rao, K. G., and Yaghmai, I. Plasmacytoma of the large bowel. Gastrointest. Radiol. *3*:225, 1978.

268. Baumgartner, B. R., and Hartmann, T. M. Extramedullary plasmacytoma of the colon. Am. J. Gastroenterol. *80*:1017, 1985.

269. Haeney, M. R., Ross, I. N., and Thompson, R. A. IgG myeloma presenting as ulcerative colitis. J. Clin. Pathol. *30*:862, 1977.

270. Ershler, W. B., Mosher, D. F., and Barreras, R. F. Multiple myeloma and adult celiac disease. Wisc. Med. J. *79*:34, 1980.

271. Mattila, J., Alavaikko, M., and Jarrentie, G. Macroglobulinemia with abdominal symptoms caused by intestinal extracellular macroglobulin. Virchow's Arch. Pathol. Histol. *389*:241, 1980.

272. Bohus, R., Waltzer, W. C., Frischer, Z., and Gonder, M. Retroperitoneal haemorrhage with abscess formation complicating Waldenstrom's macroglobulinaemia. Int. Urol. Nephrol. *17*:255, 1985.

273. Brandt, L. J., Davidoff, A., Berstein, L. H., Biempica, L., Rindfleisch, B., and Goldstein, M. L. Small intestinal involvement in Waldenstrom's macroglobulinemia. Dig. Dis. Sci. *26*:174, 1981.

274. Sun, C. C., Hill, J. L., and Combs, J. W. Hemolytic-uremic syndrome: Initial presentation mimicking intestinal intusssusception. Pediatr. Pathol. *1*:415, 1983.

275. Neill, M. A., Agosti, J., and Rosen, H. Hemorrhagic colitis with Escherichia coli 0157:H7 preceding adult hemolytic uremic syndrome. Arch. Intern. Med. *145*:2215, 1985.

276. Yates, R. S., and Osterholm, R. R. Hemolytic-uremic syndrome colitis. J. Clin. Gastroenterol. *2*:359, 1980.

277. Wallon, P., Nihoul-Fekete, C., Bouchet, J. L., Cloup, M., Gagnadoux, M. F., and Saint-Supery, G. Pseudo-surgical aspects of hemolytic-uremic syndrome in childhood. Chir. Pediatr. *22*:255, 1981.

278. Dodds, W. J., Spitzer, R. M., and Friedland, G. W. Gastrointestinal roentgenographic manifestations of hemophilia. Am. J. Roentgenol. *110*:412, 1970.

279. Prentice, C. R. M. Acquired coagulation disorders. Clin. Haematol. *14*:413, 1985.

280. Amorosi, E. L., and Ultmann, J. E. Thrombotic thrombocytopenic purpura: Report of 16 cases and review of the literature. Medicine *45*:139, 1966.

281. Lichtin, A. E., Silberstein, L. E., and Schreiber, A. D. Thrombotic thrombocytopenic purpura with colitis in an elderly woman. JAMA *255*:1435, 1986.

282. Jacobs, W. A. Acute thrombotic thrombocytopenic purpura and cholecystitis. J. Emerg. Med. *2*:265, 1985.

283. Buss, D. H., Stuart, J. J., and Lipscomb, G. E. The incidence of thrombotic and hemorrhagic disorders in association with extreme thrombocytosis: An analysis of 129 cases. Am. J. Hematol. *20*:365, 1985.

284. Davis, R. B. Acute thrombotic complications of myeloproliferative disorders in young adults. Am. J. Clin. Pathol. *84*:180, 1985.

285. Murphy, N. C., and Bissada, N. F. Iron deficiency: An overlooked predisposing factor in angular cheilitis. J. Am. Dent. Assoc. *99*:640, 1979.

286. Farrell, R. L., Nebel, O. T., McGuire, A. T., and Castell, C. O. The abnormal lower esophageal sphincter in pernicious anemia. Gut *14*:767, 1973.

287. Schinella, R. A., Greco, M. A., and Cobert, B. L. Hermansky-Pudlak syndrome with granulomatous colitis. Ann. Intern. Med. *92*:20, 1980.

288. Werlin, S. L., Chusid, M. J., Caya, J., and Oechler, H. W. Colitis in chronic granulomatous disease. Gastroenterology *82*:328, 1982.

289. Farnam, J., and Grant, J. A. Angioedema. Dermatol. Clin. *3*:85, 1985.

290. Melamed, J., Alper, C. A., Cicardi, M., and Rosen, F. S. The metabolism of C1 inhibitor and C1q in patients with acquired C1-inhibitor deficiency. J. Allergy Clin. Immunol. *77*:322, 1986.

291. Frank, M. M., Gelfand, J. A., and Atkinson, J. P. Hereditary angioedema: The clinical syndrome and its management. Ann. Intern. Med. *84*:580, 1976.

292. Myers, T. J., Steinberg, W. W., and Rickles, F. R. Polycythemia vera and mesenteric arterial thrombosis. Arch. Intern. Med. *139*:695, 1979.

293. Carini, C., and Brostoff, J. Gut and joint disease. Ann. Allergy *55*:624, 1985.

294. Wraith, D. G., Brostoff, J., and Carini, C. Adverse reactions to food. Clinical characteristics, dietary exclusion and challenge data in a group of food-sensitive patients and the role of sodium cromoglycate. Folia Allergy Immunol. Clin. *29*:456, 1983.

295. Fritzler, M. J., and Kinsella, T. D. The CREST syndrome: A distinct serologic entity with anticentromere antibodies. Am. J. Med. *69*:520, 1980.

296. Drane, W. E., Karvelis, K., Johnson, D. A., Curran, J. J., and Silverman, E. D. Progressive systemic sclerosis: Radionuclide esophageal scintigraphy and manometry. Radiology *160*:73, 1986.

297. Akesson, A., Akesson, B., Gustafson, T., and Wollhein, F. Gastrointestinal function in patients with progressive systemic sclerosis. Clin. Rheumatol. *4*:441, 1985.

298. Maddern, G. J., Horowitz, M., Jamieson, G. G., Chatterton, B. E., Collins, P. J., and Roberts-Thomson, P. Abnormalities of esophageal and gastric emptying in progressive systemic sclerosis. Gastroenterology *87*:922, 1984.

299. Peachey, R. D. G., Creamer, B., and Pierce, J. W. Sclerodermatous involvement of the stomach and the small and large bowel. Gut *10*:285, 1969.

300. Venu, R., Hogan, W. J., Geenen, J. E., Dodds, W. J., Helm, J. F., and Arndorfer, P. C. Complications of gastroesophageal reflux in scleroderma: High-risk factors associated with esophageal stricture. Gastrointest. Endosc. *26*:79, 1980.

301. Rohrmann, C. A., Jr., Ricci, M. T., Krishnamurthy, S., and Schuffler, M. D. Radiologic and histologic differentiation of neuromuscular disorders of the gastrointestinal tract: Visceral myopathies, visceral neuropathies, and progressive systemic sclerosis. Am. J. Roentgenol. *143*:933, 1984.

302. McBrien, D. J., and Lockhart-Mummery, H. E. Steatorrhea in progressive systemic sclerosis (scleroderma). Br. Med. J. *2*:1653, 1962.

303. Cohen, S. The gastrointestinal manifestations of scleroderma: Pathogenesis and management. Gastroenterology *79*:155, 1980.

304. Rees, W. D. W., Leigh, R. J., Christofides, N. D., Bloom, S. R., and Turnberg, L. A. Interdigestive motor activity in patients with systemic sclerosis. Gastroenterology *83*:575, 1982.

305. Bluestone, R., MacMahon, M., and Dawson, J. M. Systemic sclerosis and small bowel involvement. Gut *10*:185, 1969.

306. Horowitz, A. L., and Meyers, M. A. The "hide-bound" small bowel of scleroderma: Characteristic mucosal fold pattern. Am. J. Roentgenol. *119*:332, 1973.

307. Hendy, M. S., Torrance, H. B., and Warres, T. W. Small bowel volvulus in association with progressive systemic sclerosis. Br. Med. J. *1*:1651, 1979.

308. Netscher, D. T., and Richardson, J. D. Complications requiring operative intervention in scleroderma. Surg. Gynecol. Obstet. *158*:507, 1984.

309. Poirer, T. J., and Rankin, G. B. Gastrointestinal manifestations of progressive systemic scleroderma based on a review of 364 cases. Am. J. Gastroenterol. *58*:30, 1972.

310. Abraham, A. A., and Joss, A. Pancreatic necrosis in progressive systemic sclerosis. Ann. Rheum. Dis. *39*:396, 1980.

311. Cobden, I., Axon, A. T. R., and Ghoneum, A. T. Small intestinal bacterial growth in systemic sclerosis. Clin. Exp. Dermatol. *5*:37, 1980.

312. Kahn, I. J., Jeffries, G. H., and Sleisenger, M. H. Malabsorption in scleroderma: Correction by antibiotics. N. Engl. J. Med. *274*:1339, 1966.

312a. Horowitz, M., Maddern, G. J., Maddox, A., Wishart, J., Chatterton, B. E., and Shearman, D. J. C. Effects of cisapride on gastric and esophageal emptying in progressive systemic sclerosis. Gastroenterology *93*:311, 1987.

313. Battle, W. M., Snape, W. J., Jr., Wright, S., Sullivan, M. A., Cohen, S., Meyers, A., and Tuthill, R. Abnormal colonic motility in progressive systemic sclerosis. Ann. Intern. Med. *94*:749, 1981.

314. Baron, M., and Srolovitz, H. Colonic telangiectasias in a patient with progressive systemic sclerosis. Arthritis Rheum. *29*:282, 1986.

315. Frabach, R. C., Kadell, B. M., Nies, K. M., Miller, B. L., and Louie, J. S. Sigmoid volvulus in patients with progressive systemic sclerosis. J. Rheumatol. *5*:195, 1978.

316. Hamel-Roy, J., Devroede, G., Arhan, P., Tetreault, L., Duranceau, A., and Menard, H. A. Comparative esophageal and anorectal motility in scleroderma. Gastroenterology *88*:1, 1985.

317. Drieling, D. A., and Soto, J. M. The pancreatic involvement in disseminated "collagen" disorders. Am. J. Gastroenterol. *66*:546, 1976.

318. Greif, J. M., and Wolff, W. I. Idiopathic calcific pancreatitis, CREST syndrome and progressive systemic sclerosis. Am. J. Gastroenterol. *71*:177, 1979.

319. De Merieux, P., Verity, A., Clements, P. J., and Paulus, H. E. Esophageal abnormalities and dysphagia in polymyositis and dermatomyositis. Clinical, radiographic and pathologic features. Arthritis Rheum. *26*:9612, 1983.

320. Horowitz, M., McNeil, J. D., Maddern, G. J., Collins, P. J., and Shearman, D. J. C. Abnormalities of gastric and esophageal emptying in polymyositis and dermatomyositis. Gastroenterology *90*:434, 1986.

321. Jacob, H., Berkowitz, D., McDonald, E., Bernstein, L. H., and Beneventano, T. The esophageal motility disorder of polymyositis. A prospective study. Arch. Intern. Med. *143*:2262, 1983.

322. Feldman, F., and Marshak, R. H. Dermatomyositis with sig-

nificant involvement of the gastrointestinal tract. Am. J. Roentgenol. *90*:746, 1963.

323. Thompson, J. W. Spontaneous perforation of the esophagus as a manifestation of dermatomyositis. Ann. Otol. Rhinol. Laryngol. *93*:464, 1984.

324. Kaplinsky, N., Hod, C., and Gal-Sem, R. Spontaneous duodenal perforation during fulminant dermatomyositis. JAMA *33*:213, 1978.

325. Okayasu, I., Mizutani, H., Kurihara, H., and Yanagisawa, F. Cancer in collagen disease. A statistical analysis by reviewing the Annual of Pathological Autopsy Cases (Nippon Boken Shuho) in Japan. Cancer *54*:1841, 1984.

326. Lakhanpal, S., Bunch, T. W., Ilstrup, D. M., and Melton, L. J., III. Polymyositis-dermatomyositis and malignant lesions: Does an association exist? Mayo Clin. Proc. *61*:645, 1986.

327. Hoffman, B. I., and Katz, W. W. The gastrointestinal manifestations of systemic lupus erythematosus: A review of the literature. Semin. Arthritis Rheum. *9*:237, 1980.

328. Kleinman, P., Meyers, M. A., Abbott, G., and Kazam, E. Necrotizing enterocolitis with pneumatosis intestinalis in systemic lupus erythematosus and polyarteritis. Radiology *121*:595, 1976.

329. Urman, J. D., Lowenstein, M. B., Abetes, M., and Weinstein, A. Oral mucosal ulceration in systemic lupus erythematosus. Arthritis Rheum. *21*:58, 1978.

330. Gutierrez, F., Valenzuela, J. E., Ehresmann, G. R., Quismorio, F. P., and Kitridou, R. C. Esophageal dysfunction in patients with mixed connective tissue diseases and systemic lupus erythematosus. Dig. Dis. Sci. *27*:592, 1982.

331. Bazinet, P., and Marin, G. Malabsorption in systemic lupus erythematosus. Dig. Dis. Sci. *16*:460, 1971.

332. Trenthan, D. E., and Masi, A. T. Systemic lupus erythematosus with protein-losing enteropathy. JAMA *236*:287, 1976.

333. Runyon, B. A., LaBrecque, D. R., and Anuras, S. The spectrum of liver disease in systemic lupus erythematosus. Am. J. Med. *69*:187, 1980.

334. Gore, R. M., Marn, C. S., Ujiki, G. T., Craig, R. M., and Marquardt, J. Ischemic colitis associated with systemic lupus erythematosus. Dis. Colon Rectum *26*:449, 1983.

335. Helliwell, T. R., Flook, D., Whitworth, J., and Day, D. W. Arteritis and venulitis in systemic lupus erythematosus resulting in massive lower intestinal haemorrhage. Histopathology *9*:1103, 1985.

336. Zizic, T. M., Shulman, L. E., and Stevens, M. B. Colonic perforations in systemic lupus erythematosus. Medicine *54*:411, 1975.

337. Mekori, Y. A., Sheider, M., Yaretsky, A., and Klajman, A. Pancreatitis in systemic lupus erythematosus—a case report and review of the literature. Postgrad. Med. J. *56*:145, 1980.

338. Silvoso, G. R., Ivey, K. J., Butt, J. H., Lockard, O. O., Holt, S. D., Sisk, C., Baskin, W. N., Mackercher, P. A., and Hewett, J. Incidence of gastric lesions in patients with rheumatic disease on chronic aspirin therapy. Ann. Intern. Med. *91*:517, 1979.

339. Ferreiro, J. E., Busse, J. C., and Saldana, M. J. Megacolon in a collagen vascular overlap syndrome. Am. J. Med. *80*:307, 1986.

340. Sun, D. C. H., Roth, S. H., Mitchell, C. S., and England, D. W. W. Upper gastrointestinal disease in rheumatoid arthritis. Am. J. Dig. Dis. *19*:405, 1974.

341. Morris, A. D., Holt, S. D., Silvoso, G. R., Hewitt, J., Tatum, W., Grandione, J., Butt, J. H., and Ivey, K. J. Effect of anti-inflammatory drug administration in patients with rheumatoid arthritis. An endoscopic assessment. Scand. J. Gastroenterol. *67*:131, 1981.

342. Yorke, A. J., Davis, P., Salkie, M., Weinstein, W., and Thomson, A. B. Hypergastrinemia in rheumatoid arthritis. Clin. Exp. Rheumatol. *4*:49, 1986.

343. Gerber, L. H., Rooney, P. J., and McCarthy, D. M. Healing of peptic ulcers during continuing anti-inflammatory drug therapy in rheumatoid arthritis. J. Clin. Gastroenterol. *3*:7, 1981.

344. Stern, I. A., Ward, F., and Hartley, G. Sucralfate protects the normal stomach from the damaging aspects of aspirin. Gastroenterology *90*:1648, 1986.

345. Cohen, M. M., McCready, D. R., Clark, L., and Sevelius, H. Protection against aspirin-induced antral and duodenal damage with enprostil. Gastroenterology *88*:382, 1985.

346. Decker, J. L., and Plotz, P. H. Extra-articular rheumatoid disease. *In* McCarty, D. J. (ed.): Textbook of Rheumatology. Philadelphia, Lea & Febiger, 1985, p. 620.

347. Scott, D. G. I., Bacon, P. A., and Tribe, C. R. Systemic rheumatoid vasculitis: A clinical and laboratory study of 50 cases. Medicine *60*:288, 1981.

348. Burt, R. W., Berenson, M. M., Samuelson, C. O., and Cathey, W. J. Rheumatoid vasculitis of the colon presenting as pancolitis. Dig. Dis. Sci. *28*:183, 1983.

349. Plaintin, L. O., and Strandberg, O. Gastrointestinal protein loss in rheumatoid arthritis studied with ⁵¹Cr chromic chloride and ¹²⁵I albumin. Scand. J. Rheumatol. *3*:169, 1979.

350. Case records of the Massachusetts General Hospital. Case 43–1985. N. Engl. J. Med. *313*:1070, 1985.

351. Dyer, N. J., Kendall, M. J., and Hawkins, C. J. Malabsorption in rheumatoid disease. Ann. Rheum. Dis. *30*:151, 1979.

352. Dillon, A. M., Luthra, H. S., Conn, D. L., and Ferguson, R. H. Parenteral gold therapy in the Felty syndrome. Experience with 20 patients. Medicine (Baltimore) *65*:107, 1986.

353. Cohen, M., and Bankhurst, A. D. Infectious parotitis in Sjogren's syndrome: A case report and review of the literature. J. Rheumatol. *6*:185, 1979.

354. Kjellen, G., Fransson, S. G., Lindstrom, F., Sokjer, H., and Tibbling, L. Esophageal function, radiography, and dysphagia in Sjogen's syndrome. Dig. Dis. Sci. *31*:225, 1986.

355. Tsianos, E. B., Chiras, C. D., Drosos, A. A., and Moutsopoulos, H. M. Oesophageal dysfunction in patients with primary Sjogren's syndrome. Ann. Rheum. Dis. *44*:610, 1985.

356. Takasugi, M., Hayakawa, A., and Khakata, H. Gastric involvement in Sjogren's syndrome simulating early gastric cancer. Endoscopy *4*:263, 1979.

357. Wilkey, D., Yocum, D. E., Oberley, T. D., Sundstrom, W. R., and Karl, L. Budd-Chiari syndrome and renal failure in Behçet disease. Report of a case and review of the literature. Am. J. Med. *75*:541, 1983.

358. Yashiro, K., Nagasako, K., Hasegawa, K., Maruyama, M., Suzuki, S., and Obata, H. Esophageal lesions in intestinal Behçet's disease. Endoscopy *18*:57, 1986.

359. Griffin, J. W., Jr., Harrison, H. B., Tedesco, F. J., and Mills, L. R., IV. Behçet's disease with multiple sites of gastrointestinal involvement. South. Med. J. *75*:1405, 1982.

360. Yim, C. W., and White, R. H. Behçet's syndrome in a family with inflammatory bowel disease. Arch. Intern. Med. *145*:1047, 1985.

361. Iwama, T., and Utzunomiya, J. Anal complications in Behçet's syndrome. Jap. J. Surg. *7*:114, 1977.

362. Moll, J. M. H., Haslock, I., Macrae, I. F., and Wright, V. Associations between ankylosing spondylitis, psoriatic arthritis, Reiter's disease, the intestinal arthropathies and Behçet's syndrome. Medicine *53*:343, 1974.

363. Is Reiter's syndrome caused by chlamydia? Lancet *I*:317, 1985.

364. Mielants, H., Veys, E. M., Cuvelier, C., De-Vos, M., and Botelberghe, L. HLA-B27 related arthritis and bowel inflammation. Part 2. Ileocolonoscopy and bowel histology in patients with HLA-B27 related arthritis. J. Rheumatol. *12*:294, 1985.

365. Ford-Hutchinson, A. W. Leukotriene involvement in pathologic processes. J. Allergy Clin. Immunol. *74*:437, 1984.

366. Lopez, L. R., Shocket, A. L., Stanford, R. E., Claman, H. N., and Kohler, P. F. Gastrointestinal involvement in leukocytoclastic vasculitis in polyarteritis nodosa. J. Rheumatol. *7*:677, 1980.

367. Bocenagra, T., Vasey, F. B., and Espinoza, L. R. Pancreatic pseudocyst. A complication of necrotizing vasculitis (polyarteritis nodosa). Arch. Intern. Med. *140*:1356, 1980.

368. Wood, M. K., Read, D. R., Kraft, A. R., and Barreta, T. M. A rare cause of ischemic colitis—polyarteritis nodosa. Dis. Colon Rectum *22*:428, 1979.

369. Camilleri, M., Pusey, C. D., Chadwick, V. S., and Rees, A. J. Gastrointestinal manifestations of systemic vasculitis. Q. J. Med. *206*:141, 1983.

370. McCauley, R. L., Johnston, M. R., and Fauci, A. S. Surgical aspects of systemic necrotizing vasculitis. Surgery *97*:104, 1985.

371. Shepherd, H. A., Patel, C., Bamforth, J., and Isaacson, P. Upper gastrointestinal endoscopy in systemic vasculitis presenting as an acute abdomen. Endoscopy *15*:307, 1983.

372. Fishman, R. S., Fleming, C. R., and Li, R. Y. Systemic mastocytosis with review of gastrointestinal manifestations. Mayo Clin. Proc. *54*:51, 1979.

373. Ouwendijk, R. J., Zijlstra, F. J., Wilson, J. H., Bonta, I. L., Vincent, J. E., and Stolz, E. Raised plasma levels of thromboxane B2 in systemic mastocytosis. Eur. J. Clin. Invest. *13*:227, 1983.

374. Soter, N. A., Austen, K. F., and Wasserman, S. I. Oral disodium cromoglycate in the treatment of systemic mastocytosis. N. Engl. J. Med. *301*:465, 1979.

375. Keller, R. T., and Roth, H. P. Hyperchlorhydria and hyperhistaminemia in a patient with systemic mastocytosis. N. Engl. J. Med. *233*:1449, 1970.

376. Adler, S. N., Klein, R. A., and Lyon, D. T. Bleeding after liver biopsy in a patient with systemic mastocytosis and malabsorption. J. Clin. Gastroenterol. 7:350, 1985.

377. Belson, M. C., Collins, S. M., Castelli, M. F., and Qizilbash, A. H. Gastrointestinal hemorrhage in mastocytosis. Can. Med. Assoc. J. *122*:311, 1980.

378. Bredfeldt, J. E., O'Laughlin, J. C., Durham, J. B., and Blessing, L. D. Malabsorption and gastric hyperacidity in systemic mastocytosis. Am. J. Gastroenterol. *74*:133, 1980.

379. Granerus, G., Olafsson, J. H., and Roupe, G. Treatment of two mastocytosis patients with a histidine decarboxylase inhibitor. Agents-Actions *16*:244, 1985.

380. Barriere, H., Dreno, B., Pecquet, C., Le-Bodic, M. F., and Bolze, J. L. Systemic mastocytosis and intestinal malabsorption. Semin. Hop. Paris *59*:2925, 1983.

381. Jarnum, S., and Zachariae, H. P. Mastocytosis (urticaria pigmentosa) of skin, stomach and gut with malabsorption. Gut *8*:64, 1967.

382. Borda, F., Uribarrena, R., and Rivero-Puente, A. Gastroscopic findings in systemic mastocytosis. Endoscopy *15*:342, 1983.

383. Quinn, S. F., Shaffer, H. A., Jr., Willard, M. R., and Ross, S. Bull's-eye lesions: A new gastrointestinal presentation of mastocytosis. Gastrointest. Radiol. *9*:13, 1984.

384. Legman, P., Sterin, P., Vallee, C., Zag-Zag, J., Levesque, M., and Richard, J. P. Colonic involvement in systemic mastocytosis. Semin. Hop. Paris *58*:1460, 1982.

385. Frieri, M., Alling, D. W., and Metcalfe, D. D. Comparison of the therapeutic efficacy of cromolyn sodium with that of combined chlorpheniramine and cimetidine in systemic mastocytosis. Results of a double-blind clinical trial. Am. J. Med. *78*:9, 1985.

386. Viale, G., Dell Orto, P., Moro, E., Cozzaglio, L., and Coggi, G. Vasoactive intestinal polypeptide-, somatostatin-, and calcitonin-producing adrenal pheochromocytoma associated with the watery diarrhea (WDHH) syndrome. First case report with immunohistochemical findings. Cancer *55*:1099, 1985.

387. Interlandi, J. W., Hundley, R. F., Kasselberg, A. G., Orth, D. N., Salmon, W. D., Jr., and Sullivan, J. N. Hypercortisolism, diarrhea with steatorrhea, and massive proteinuria due to pheochromocytoma. South. Med. J. *78*:879, 1985.

388. Anderson, P. T., Baadsgaard, S. E., and Larsen, B. P. Repetitive bleeding from a pheochromocytoma presenting as an abdominal emergency. Case Report. Acta Chir. Scand. *152*:69, 1986.

389. Mullen, J. P., Cartwright, R. C., Tisherman, S. E., Misage, J. R., and Shapiro, A. P. Pathogenesis and pharmacologic management of pseudo-obstruction of the bowel in pheochromocytoma. Am. J. Med. Sci. *290*:155, 1985.

390. Fee, H. J., Fonkalsrud, E. W., Ament, M. E., and Bergstein, J. Enterocolitis with peritonitis in a child with pheochromocytoma. Ann. Surg. *185*:448, 1977.

391. Yamada, M., Hatakeyama, S., and Tsukagoshhi, H. Gastrointestinal amyloid deposition in AL (primary or myeloma-associated) and AA (secondary) amyloidosis: Diagnostic value of gastric biopsy. Human Pathol. *16*:1206, 1985.

392. Kyle, R. A., and Greipp, P. R. Amyloidosis (AL). Clinical and laboratory features in 229 cases. Mayo Clin. Proc. *58*:665, 1983.

393. Gilat, T., and Spiro, H. M. Amyloidosis and the gut. Am. J. Dig. Dis. *13*:619, 1968.

394. Pear, B. L. Big heart, tongue and kidneys—stiff intestines. JAMA *241*:58, 1979.

395. Dastur, K. J., and Ward, J. F. Amyloidoma of the stomach. Gastrointest. Radiol. *5*:17, 1980.

396. Pear, B. L. Radiographic studies of amyloidosis. CRC Crit. Rev. Radiol. Sci. *3*:425, 1972.

397. Seliger, G., Krassner, R. L., Beranbaum, E. R., and Miller, F. The spectrum of roentgen appearance in amyloidosis of the small and large bowel. Radiology *100*:63, 1971.

398. Raffi, F., Lerat, F., Cuilliere, P., Roudier, J. M., Le Bodic, L., and Rymer, R. Peritoneal amyloidosis in Waldenstrom's macroglobulinemia. X-ray computed tomographic aspects. J. Radiol. *66*:735, 1985.

399. Pandannath, G. S., Levine, S. M., Sorokin, J. J., and Jacoby, J. H. Selective massive amyloidosis of the small intestine mimicking multiple tumors. Radiology *129*:609, 1978.

400. Burakoff, R., Rubinow, A., and Cohen, A. S. Esophageal manometry in familial amyloid polyneuropathy. Am. J. Med. *79*:85, 1985.

401. Schwartz, Y., Tamse, A., Kissin, E., and Shani, M. An unusual case of temporomandibular joint arthopathy in systemic amyloidosis. J. Oral Med. *34*:40, 1979.

402. Case records of the Massachusetts General Hospital. Case 43–1985. N. Engl. J. Med. *313*:1070, 1985.

403. Levy, D. J., Franklin, G. O., and Rosenthal, W. S. Gastrointestinal bleeding and amyloidosis. Am. J. Gastroenterol. 77:422, 1982.

404. Hunter, A. M., Campbell, I. W., Borsey, D. D. G., and Macaulay, R. A. A. Protein-losing enteropathy due to gastrointestinal amyloidosis. Postgrad. Med. J. *55*:822, 1979.

405. Zemer, D., Pras, M., Sohar, E., Modan, M., Cabili, S., and Gafni, J. Colchicine in the prevention and treatment of the amyloidosis of familial Mediterranean fever. N. Engl. J. Med. *314*:1003, 1986.

406. Ek, B., Holmlund, D. E. W., Sjodin, J. G., and Steen, L. E. Enterostomy in patients with primary neuropathic amyloidosis. Am. J. Gastroenterol. *70*:365, 1978.

407. O'Brien, B. D., Shnitka, T. K., McDougall, R., Walker, K., Costopoulos, L., Lentle, B., Anholt, L., Freeman, H., and Thomson, A. B. Pathophysiologic and ultrastructural basis for intestinal symptoms in Fabry's disease. Gastroenterology *82*:957, 1982.

408. Bryan, A., Knauft, R. F., and Burns, W. A. Small bowel perforation in Fabry's disease. Ann. Intern. Med. *86*:315, 1977.

409. Isselbacher, K. J., Scheig, R., Plotkin, G. R., and Caulfield, J. B. Congenital β-lipoprotein deficiency: An hereditary disorder involving a defect in the absorption and transport of lipids. Medicine *43*:347, 1964.

410. Glickman, R. M., Green, P. H. R., and Lees, R. S. Immunofluorescence studies of apolipoprotein-B in intestinal mucosa. Gastroenterology *76*:288, 1979.

411. Illingworth, D. R., Connor, W. E., Lin, D. S., and Diliberti, J. Lipid metabolism in abetalipoproteinemia: A study of cholesterol absorption and sterol balance in two patients. Gastroenterology *78*:68, 1980.

412. Delpre, G., Kadish, U., and Glantz, I. Endoscopic assessment in abetalipoproteinemia (Bassen-Kornzweig syndrome). Endoscopy *10*:59, 1978.

413. Brunzell, J. D., and Bierman, E. L. Chylomicronemia syndrome. Med. Clin. North Am. *66*:455, 1982.

414. Havel, R. J. Approach to the patient with hyperlipidemia. Med. Clin. North Am. *66*:31, 1982.

415. Ahlberg, J., Angelin, B., Einarsson, K., Hellstrom, K., and Leiyd, B. Prevalence of gallbladder disease in hyperlipoproteinemia. Dig. Dis. Sci. *24*:459, 1979.

416. Malloy, M. J., and Kane, J. P. Hypolipidemia. Med. Clin. North Am. *66*:469, 1982.

417. Law, S. W., and Brewer, H. B., Jr. Tangier disease. The complete mRNA sequence encoding for preproapo-A-I. J. Biol. Chem. *260*:12810, 1985.

418. Tarao, K., Iwamura, K., Fujii, K., and Miyake, H. Japanese adult siblings with Tangier disease and statistical analysis of reported cases. Tokai J. Exp. Clin. Med. *9*:379, 1984.

419. Verola, O., de Roquancourt, A., Chanu, B., Rouffy, J., and Brocheriou, C. Hepatic cholesterolosis. Histological, histochemical and ultrastructural study of two cases. Semin. Hop. Paris 59:1753, 1983.
420. Schaub, J., Janka, G. E., Christomanou, H., Sandhoff, K., Permanetter, W., Hubner, G., and Meister, P. Wolman's disease: Clinical, biochemical and ultrastructural studies in an unusual case without striking adrenal calcification. Eur. J. Pediatr. 135:45, 1980.
421. Keshavarzian, A., Saverymuttu, S. H., Tai, P. C., Thompson, M., Barter, S., Spry, C. J. F., and Chadwick, V. S. Activated eosinophils in familial eosinophilic gastroenteritis. Gastroenterology 88:1041, 1985.
422. Rambaud, J. C., Galian, A., Touchard, G., Morel-Maroger, L., Mikol, J., Van Effenterre, G., Leclerc, J. P., Le Charpentier, Y., Haut, J., Matuchansky, C., and Zittoun, R. Digestive tract and renal small vessel hyalinosis, idiopathic nonarteriosclerotic intracerebral calcifications, retinal ischemic syndrome, and phenotypic abnormalities: A new familial syndrome. Gastroenterology 90:930, 1986.
423. Speiser, J. C., Moore, T. L., and Zuckner, J. Ulcerative colitis with arthritis and vasculitis. Clin. Rheumatol. 4:343, 1985.
424. Reya, M. J., Bennet, E. R., Pops, M., and Goldberg, L. S. Intestinal vasculitis in essential mixed cryoglobulinemia. Ann. Intern. Med. 81:632, 1974.
425. Kaplan, A. P. Chronic urticaria. Possible causes, suggested treatment alternatives. Postgrad. Med. 74:209, 1983.
426. Sanchez, N. P., Winkelmann, R. K., Schroeter, A. L., and Dicken, C. H. The clinical and histopathologic spectrums of urticarial vasculitis: Study of forty cases. J. Am. Acad. Dermatol. 7:599, 1982.
427. Lass, N., Doron, O., and Gilat, T. Gastric acid secretion in cold urticaria. Dig. Dis. Sci. 25:526, 1980.
428. Kikindjanin, V., Vukavic, T., Opric, M., and Novakov, G. Local immunodeficiency of the intestinal mucosa—a contribution to etiopathogenesis of recurrent urticaria and diarrhoea. Allerg. Immunol. (Leipzig) 31:183, 1985.
429. Jobin, G., Bourgie, J., and Girox, Y. L'urticaire du colon. Union Med. Can. 109:1030, 1980.
430. Bushkell, L. L. Chronic urticaria and gallbladder disease: Clearing after cholecystectomy. Arch. Dermatol. 115:638, 1979.
431. Singh, G. H₂ blockers in chronic urticaria. Int. J. Dermatol. 23:627, 1984.
432. Mayock, R. L., Bertrand, P., Morrison, C. E., and Scott, J. H. Manifestations of sarcoidosis. Am. J. Med. 35:67, 1963.
433. Chinitz, M. A., Brandt, L. J., Frank, M. S., Frager, D., and Sablay, L. Symptomatic sarcoidosis of the stomach. Dig. Dis. Sci. 30:682, 1985.
434. Ona, F. V. Gastric sarcoid: Unusual cause of upper gastrointestinal hemorrhage. Am. J. Gastroenterol. 75:286, 1981.
435. Popovic, O. S., Brkic, S., Bojic, P., Kenic, V., Jolie, N., Djuric, V., and Djordjevic, N. Sarcoidosis and protein-losing enteropathy. Gastroenterology 78:119, 1980.
436. Sprague, R., Harper, P., McClain, S., Trainer, T., and Beeken, W. Disseminated gastrointestinal sarcoidosis. Case report and review of the literature. Gastroenterology 87:421, 1984.
437. Mora, R. G., and Gullung, W. H. Sarcoidosis: A case with unusual manifestations. South. Med. J. 73:1064, 1980.
438. Ell, S. R., and Frank, P. H. Spectrum of lymphoid hyperplasia: Colonic manifestations of sarcoidosis, infectious mononucleosis, and Crohn's disease. Gastrointest. Radiol. 6:329, 1981.
439. Kohn, N. N. Sarcoidosis of the colon. J. Med. Soc. N.J. 77:517, 1980.
440. Chaun, H., King, D. M., Gofton, J. P., Sutherland, W. H., and Bogoch, A. Sarcoidosis of the pancreas. Am. J. Dig. Dis. 17:725, 1972.
441. Reuland-Bosma, W., vanDijk, J., and var-derWeele, L. Experimental gingivitis around deciduous teeth in children with Down's syndrome. J. Periodontol. 13:294, 1986.
442. Clark, J. F., Hales, E., Ma, P., and Rosser, S. B. Duodenal atresia in utero in association with Down's syndrome and annular pancreas. J. Natl. Med. Assoc. 76:190, 1984.
443. McLean, A. M., Paul, R. E., Jr., Kritzman, J., and Farthing, M. J. Malabsorption in Marfan (Ehlers-Danlos) syndrome. J. Clin. Gastroenterol. 7:304, 1985.
444. Ishikawa, E., Nishi, T., Matsuo, M., Yasuda, K., Shimabara, Y., Ukikusa, M., Sawanishi, K., Kawamura, J., and Yoshida, O. Clinical studies on the prognosis of 150 cases of acute renal failure. Hinyokika Kiyo 29:169, 1983.
445. Wesdorp, R. I., Falcao, H. A., Banks, P. B., Martino, J., and Fischer, J. E. Gastrin and gastric acid secretion in renal failure. Am. J. Surg. 141:334, 1981.
446. Merrill, J. P., and Hampers, C. L. Uremia, Part 1. N. Engl. J. Med. 282:953, 1970.
447. Musola, R., Franzin, G., Mora, R., and Manfrini, C. Prevalence of gastroduodenal lesions in uremic patients undergoing dialysis and after renal transplantation. Gastrointest. Endosc. 30:343, 1984.
448. Jaspers, M. T. Unusual oral lesions in a uremic patient. Oral Surg. 39:934, 1975.
449. Fornari, A. J., and Avram, M. M. Altered taste perception in uremia. Trans. Am. Soc. Artif. Intern. Organs 24:385, 1978.
450. Mahajan, S. K., Prasad, A. S., and Lambujan, J. Improvement of renal hypogeusia by zinc. Trans. Am. Soc. Artif. Intern. Organs 25:443, 1979.
451. Vreman, H. J., Venter, C., Leegwater, J., Oliver, C., and Weiner, M. W. Taste, smell, and zinc metabolism in patients with chronic renal failure. Nephron 26:163, 1980.
452. Gruskin, S. E., Tolman, D. E., and Wagoner, R. D. Oral manifestations of uremia. Minn. Med. 53:495, 1970.
453. Zuckerman, G. R., Cornette, G. L., Clouse, R. E., and Harter, H. R. Upper gastrointestinal bleeding in patients with chronic renal failure. Ann. Intern. Med. 102:588, 1985.
454. Dave, P. B., Romeu, J., Antonelli, A., and Eiser, A. R. Gastrointestinal telangiectasias. Arch. Intern. Med. 144:1781, 1984.
455. Zuckerman, G. R., Mills, B. A., Koehler, R. E., Siegel, A., Harter, H. R., and DeSchryver-Kecskemeti, K. Nodular duodenitis. Pathologic and clinical characteristics in patients with end-stage renal disease. Dig. Dis. Sci. 28:1018, 1983.
456. Paimela, H., Harkonen, M., Karonen, S.-L., Tallgren, L. G., Stenman, S., and Ahonen, J. Relation between serum group II pepsinogen concentration and the degree of Brunner's gland hyperplasia in patients with chronic renal failure. Gut 26:198, 1985.
457. Paimela, H., Harkonen, M., Karonen, S. L., Tallgren, L. G., and Ahonen, J. The effect of renal transplantation on gastric acid secretion and on the serum levels of gastrin and group I pepsinogens. Ann. Clin. Res. 17:105, 1985.
458. Gold, C. H., Morely, J. E., Vijoen, M., Tin, L. O., Fomseca, M., and Kalk, W. J. Gastric acid secretion and serum gastrin levels in patients with chronic renal failure on regular hemodialysis. Nephron 25:92, 1980.
459. Antonucci, F., Vezzadini, P., and Cecchettini, M. Gastric acid secretion, calcitonin, and secondary hyperparathyroidism in uremic patients undergoing regular dialysis therapy. Int. J. Artif. Org. 1:260, 1978.
460. Gastrointestinal symptoms and shock in a patient with chronic renal failure: Clinicopathologic conference. Am. J. Med. 69:595, 1980.
461. Hansky, J. Effect of renal failure on gastrointestinal hormones. World J. Surg. 3:463, 1979.
462. Hida, M., Saitoh, H., Shiramizu, T., Nakamura, K., Shinbo, T., Nakayama, M., and Satoh, T. Clinical report on hemodialysis in the Department of Transplantation, Tokai University School of Medicine. Tokai J. Exp. Clin. Med. 6:247, 1981.
463. Babb, R. R. Cimetidine in preventing or treating acute upper gastrointestinal tract hemorrhage. West. J. Med. 140:478, 1984.
464. Bronner, M. H., Pate, M. B., Cunningham, J. T., and Marsh, W. H. Estrogen-progesterone therapy for bleeding gastrointestinal telangiectasias in chronic renal failure. Ann. Intern. Med. 105:371, 1986.
465. Sachs, E. F., Hurwitz, F. J., Bloch, H. M., and Milne, F. J. Pancreatic exocrine hypofunction in the wasting syndrome of end-stage renal disease. Am. J. Gastro. 78:170, 1983.
466. Grunewald, K. K., Mitchell, G. E., Jr., Tucker, R. E., Langlois, B. E., and Bruckner, G. G. Influence of bilateral

nephrectomy on selected gastrointestinal bacteria in the rat. Can. J. Physiol. Pharmacol. *60*:664, 1982.

467. Mitch, W. E. Nitrogen metabolism in patients with chronic renal failure. Am. J. Clin. Nutr. *31*:1594, 1978.

468. Mountokalakis, T. D., Virvidakis, C. E., Singhellakis, P. N., Alevizaki, C. C., and Ikkos, D. C. Magnesium absorption in chronic renal failure. Gastroenterology *80*:632, 1981.

469. Davis, G. R., Zerwekh, J. E., Parker, T. F., Krejs, G. J., Pak, C. Y. C., and Fordtran, J. S. Absorption of phosphate in the jejunum of patients with chronic renal failure before and after correction of Vitamin D deficiency. Gastroenterology *85*:908, 1983.

470. Wizeman, V., Ludwig, D., Kuhl, R., and Burgmann, I. Digestive absorptive function of the intestinal brush border in uremia. Am. J. Clin. Nutr. *31*:1642, 1978.

471. Wright, R. A., Clemente, R., and Wathen, R. Gastric emptying in patients with chronic renal failure receiving hemodialysis. Arch. Intern. Med. *144*:495, 1984.

472. Pederson, E. B., Brock, A., and Koreerup, H. J. Serum amylase activity and renal amylase activity in patients treated with renal allotransplantation. Scand. J. Clin. Lab. Invest. *36*:137, 1976.

473. Keogh, B., McGeeney, K. F., Drury, M. I., Counihan, T. B., and O'Donnell, M. D. Renal clearance of pancreatic and salivary amylase relative to creatinine in patients with chronic renal insufficiency. Gut *19*:1125, 1978.

474. Rubenstein, R. B., Lantz, J., Stevens, K., and Spira, I. A. Uremic ileus. N.Y. State J. Med. *79*:248, 1979.

475. Coctney, D. R., Cutshall, W. D., and Madura, J. A. Small bowel obstruction and ileal perforation: Complications of uremia. J. Indiana State Med. Assoc. *69*:781, 1976.

476. Bischel, M. D., Reese, T., and Engel, J. Spontaneous perforation of the colon in a hemodialysis patient. Am. J. Gastroenterol. *74*:182, 1980.

477. Goldberg, M., Hoffman, G. C., and Wombolt, D. G. Massive hemorrhage from rectal ulcers in chronic renal failure. Ann. Intern. Med. *100*:397, 1984.

478. Scheff, R. T., Zuckerman, G., Harter, H., Delmey, J., and Koehler, R. Diverticular disease in patients with chronic renal failure due to polycystic kidney disease. Ann. Intern. Med. *92*:202, 1980.

479. Young, R., and Bryk, D. Colonic intussusception in uremia. Am. J. Gastroenterol. *71*:229, 1979.

480. Gordon, S. J., Miller, L. J., Haeffner, L. J., Kinsey, M. D., and Kowlessar, O. D. Abnormal intestinal bile acid distribution of azotemic man: A possible role in the pathogenesis of uremic diarrhea. Gut *17*:58, 1976.

481. Lockyer, W. A., Feifeld, D. A., Cherubin, C. E., Carvounis, G., Iancu, M., and Avram, M. M. An outbreak of Salmonella enteritis in a population of uremic patients. Arch. Intern. Med. *140*:943, 1980.

482. Arismendi, G. S., Izard, M. W., Hampton, W. R., and Maher, J. F. The clinical spectrum of ascites associated with maintenance dialysis. Am. J. Med. *60*:46, 1976.

483. Moore, E. S., Chung, E. E., and Cevallos, E. E. Intractable ascites in a child during peritoneal dialysis. J. Pediatr. *91*:949, 1977.

484. Rodriguez, H. J., Walls, J., and Slatopolsky, E. Recurrent ascites following peritoneal dialysis. Arch. Intern. Med. *124*:283, 1974.

485. Yen, M. C., and Stewart, E. E. Peritoneo-venous shunt for ascites associated with maintenance dialysis. Clin. Nephrol. *8*:446, 1977.

486. Lerut, J., Lerut, T., Grumez, J. A., Michielsen, P., and Van-Renterghem, I. Surgical gastrointestinal complications in 277 renal transplantations. Acta Chir. Belg. *79*:383, 1980.

487. Mahony, J. F., Sheil, A. G., Etheredge, S. B., Storey, B. G., and Stewart, J. H. Delayed complications of renal transplantation and their prevention. Med. J. Aust. *2*:426, 1982.

488. Jones, J. M., Glass, N. R., and Belzer, F. O. Fatal Candida esophagitis in two diabetics after renal transplantation. Arch. Surg. *117*:499, 1982.

489. Meyers, W. C., Harris, N., Steei, S., Brooks, M., Jones, R. S., Thompson, W. M., Stickel, D. L., and Seigler, H. F. Alimentary tract complications after renal transplantation. Ann. Surg. *190*:535, 1979.

490. Schweizer, R. T., and Bartus, S. A. Gastroduodenal ulceration in renal transplant patients. Conn. Med. *42*:85, 1978.

491. Conn, H. O., and Blitzer, B. L. Nonassociation of adrenocorticosteroid therapy and peptic ulcer. N. Engl. J. Med. *294*:473, 1976.

492. Pranzin, G., Muolo, A., and Griminelli, T. Cytomegalovirus inclusions in the gastroduodenal muscosa of patients after renal transplantation. Gut *22*:698, 1981.

493. Kodama, T., Fukuda, S., Takino, T., Omori, Y., and Oka, T. Gastroduodenal cytomegalovirus infection after renal transplantation. Fiberscopic observations. Endoscopy *17*:157, 1985.

494. Chisolm, C. D., Mee, A. D., and Williams, G. Peptic ulceration, gastric secretion, and renal transplantation. Br. Med. J. *1*:630, 1977.

495. Walter, S., Thorup-Andersen, J., Christensen, U., Lkkegaard, H., Kjersem, H., Dahlager-Jorgensen, J. I., and Stadil, F. Effect of cimetidine on upper gastrointestinal bleeding after renal transplantation: A prospective study. Br. Med. J. (Clin. Res.) *289*:1175, 1984.

496. Schiessel, R., Starlinger, M., Wolf, A., Pinggera, W., Zazgornik, J., Schmidt, P., Wagner, D., Schwarz, S., and Piza, F. Failure of cimetidine to prevent gastroduodenal ulceration and bleeding after renal transplantation. Surgery *90*:456, 1981.

497. Burleson, R. L., Kronhaus, R. J., Marbarger, P. D., and Jones, D. M. Cimetidine, posttransplant peptic ulcer complications, and renal allograft survival: A clinical and investigational perspective. Arch. Surg. *117*:933, 1982.

498. Mona, D., Largiader, F., Binswanger, U., and Sulser, H. Colonkomplikationen nach nierentransplantation. Langenbecks Arch. Chir. *357*:141, 1982.

499. Church, J. M., Fazio, V. W., Braun, W. E., Novick, A. C., and Steinmuller, D. R. Perforation of the colon in renal homograft recipients. A report of 11 cases and a review of the literature. Ann. Surg. *203*:69, 1986.

500. Guice, K., Rattazzi, L. D., and Marchioro, T. L. Colon perforation in renal transplant patients. Am. J. Surg., *138*:43, 1979.

501. Sawyett, O. I., Garwin, P. J., Codd, J. E., Graff, R. J., Newton, W. T., and Willman, V. L. Colorectal complications of renal allograft transplantation. Arch. Surg. *113*:84, 1978.

502. Sutherland, D. D., French, R. S., Weil, R., Najarian, J. S., and Simmons, R. L. The bleeding cecal ulcer: Pathogenesis, angiographic diagnosis, and nonoperative control. Surgery *71*:290, 1972.

503. Himal, H. S., Wise, D. J., and Cardella, C. Localized colonic perforation following renal transplantation. Dis. Colon Rectum *26*:461, 1983.

504. Polinsky, M. S., Wolfson, B. J., Gruskin, A. B., Baluarte, H. J., and Widzer, S. J. Development of pneumatosis cytoides intestinalis following transperitoneal renal transplantation in a child. Am. J. Kidney Dis. *3*:414, 1984.

505. Burnstein, M., Salter, D., Cardella, C., and Himal, H. S. Necrotizing pancreatitis in renal transplant patients. Can. J. Surg. *25*:547, 1982.

506. Hopkinson, G. B., Crowson, M. C., and Barnes, A. D. Perforation of the acalculous gallbladder following renal transplantation. Transplant. Proc. *17*:2014, 1985.

507. Read, A. E., Wiesner, R. H., LaBrecque, D. R., Tifft, J. G., Mullen, K. D., Sheer, R. L., Petrelli, M., Ricanati, E. S., and McCullough, A. J. Hepatic veno-occlusive disease associated with renal transplantation and azathioprine therapy. Ann. Intern. Med. *104*:651, 1986.

508. Coggon, D. N., Rose, D. H., and Ansell, I. D. A large bowel lymphoma complicating renal transplantation. Br. J. Radiol. *54*:418, 1981.

509. Gomez-Uribe, J. I., and Arango-Acosta, J. L. Kaposi's sarcoma in two patients after renal transplantation. Med. Cutan. Ibero. Lat. Am. *12*:215, 1984.

510. Kamada, T., Fusamoto, H., Kawano, S., Noguchi, M., Hiramatsu, K., Masuzawa, M., and Sato, N. Gastroduodenal lesions in head injury. Am. J. Gastroenterol. *68*:249, 1977.

511. Gore, R. M., Mintzer, R. A., and Calenoff, L. Gastrointestinal complications of spinal cord injury. Spine 6:538, 1981.

512. Miller, F., and Fenzl, T. C. Prolonged ileus with acute spinal cord injury responding to metaclopramide. Paraplegia 19:43, 1981.

513. Kiwerski, J. Bleeding from the alimentary canal during the management of spinal cord injury patients. Paraplegia 24:92, 1986.

514. Berlly, M. H., and Wilmot, C. B. Acute abdominal emergencies during the first four weeks after spinal cord injury. Arch. Phys. Med. Rehabil. 65:687, 1984.

515. Leramo, O. B., Tator, C. H., and Hudson, A. R. Massive gastroduodenal hemorrhage and perforation in acute spinal cord injury. Surg. Neurol. 17:186, 1982.

516. Osteen, R. T., and Barsamian, E. M. Delayed gastric emptying after vagotomy and drainage in the spinal cord injury patient. Paraplegia 19:46, 1981.

517. Segal, J. L., Brunnemann, S. R., Gordon, S. K., and Eltorai, I. M. The absolute bioavailability of oral theophylline in patients with spinal cord injury. Pharmacotherapy 6:26, 1986.

518. Halstead, L. S., Feldman, S., Claus-Walker, J., and Patel, V. C. Drug absorption in spinal cord injury. Arch. Phys. Med. Rehabil. 66:298, 1985.

519. Bernstein, L., Joseph, R., and Staas, W. E., Jr. Solitary colonic ulcer in a spinal cord injured patient. Arch. Phys. Med. Rehabil. 67:194, 1986.

520. Meshkinpour, H., Vaziri, N., and Gordon, S. Gastrointestinal pathology in patients with chronic renal failure associated with spinal cord injury. Am. J. Gastroenterol. 77:562, 1982.

521. Aaronson, M. J., Freed, M. M., and Burakoff, R. Colonic myoelectric activity in persons with spinal cord injury. Dig. Dis. Sci. 30:295, 1985.

522. Meshkinpour, H., Nowroozi, F., and Glick, M. E. Colonic compliance in patients with spinal cord injury. Arch. Phys. Med. Rehabil. 64:111, 1983.

523. McGuire, T. J., and Kumar, V. N. Autonomic dysreflexia in the spinal cord injured. What the physician should know about this medical emergency. Postgrad. Med. 80:81, 1986.

524. Bell, J., and Hannon, K. Pathophysiology involved in autonomic dysreflexia. J. Neurosci. Nurs. 18:86, 1986.

525. Kuiper, D. H. Gastric bezoar in a patients with myotonic dystrophy. Am. J. Dig. Dis. 16:529, 1971.

526. Swick, H. M., Werlin, S. L., Dodds, W. J., and Hogan, W. J. Pharyngoesophageal motor function in patients with myotonic dystrophy. Ann. Neurol. 10:454, 1981.

527. Eckardt, V. F., Nix, W., Kraus, W., and Bohl, J. Esophageal motor function in patients with muscular dystrophy. Gastroenterology 90:628, 1986.

528. Nowak, T. V., Anuras, S., Brown, B. P., Ionasescu, V., and Green, J. B. Small intestinal motility in myotonic dystrophy patients. Gastroenterology 86:808, 1984.

529. Theodor, C. H., Cornud, F., Mendez, J., Moulonguet-Doleris, D., and Pailaggi, J. A. Cholestasis and myotonic dystrophy. N. Engl. J. Med. 301:329, 1979.

530. Sjaastad, O. Intestinal absorption in myotonic dystrophy. Acta Neurol. Scand. 51:59, 1973.

531. Simpson, A. J., and Khilnani, M. T. Gastrointestinal manifestations of the muscular dystrophies. Am. J. Roentgenol. 125:948, 1975.

532. Weiner, M. J. Myotonic megacolon in myotonic dystrophy. Am. J. Roentgenol. 130:177, 1978.

533. Hamel-Roy, J., Devroede, G., Arhan, P., Tetreault, J. P., Lemieux, B., and Scott, H. Functional abnormalities of the anal sphincters in patients with myotonic dystrophy. Gastroenterology 86:1469, 1984.

534. Dabaghi, R. E., and Scott, L. D. Intestinal pseudo-obstruction in a patient with myotonic dystrophy. Tex. Med. 82:42, 1986.

535. Kilman, W. J. Disorders of pharyngeal and upper esophageal sphincter motor function. Arch. Intern. Med. 136:592, 1976.

536. Wang, L., and Karmody, C. S. Dysphagia as the presenting symptom of tetanus. Arch. Otolaryngol. 111:342, 1985.

537. Garfinkle, T. J., and Kimmelman, C. P. Neurologic disorders: Amyotrophic lateral sclerosis, myasthenia gravis, multiple sclerosis and poliomyelitis. Am. J. Otolaryngol. 3:204, 1982.

538. Robbins, J. A., Logemann, J. A., and Kirshner, H. S. Swallowing and speech production in Parkinson's disease. Ann. Neurol. 19:283, 1986.

539. Gagic, N. M. Cricopharyngeal myotomy. Can. J. Surg. 26:47, 1983.

540. Gupta, Y. K. Gastroparesis with multiple sclerosis. JAMA 252:42, 1984.

541. Glick, M. E., Meshkinpour, H., Haldeman, S., Bhatia, N. N., and Bradley, W. E. Colonic dysfunction in multiple sclerosis. Gastroenterology 83:1002, 1982.

542. Sullivan, S. N., and Ebers, G. C. Gastrointestinal dysfunction in multiple sclerosis. Gastroenterology 84:1640, 1984.

543. Rush, J. A. Pseudotumor cerebri. Clinical profile and visual outcome in 63 patients. Mayo Clin. Proc. 55:541, 1980.

544. Bosma, J. F. Residual disability of the pharyngeal area resulting from poliomyelitis: Clinical management of patients. JAMA 165:216, 1957.

545. Winship, D. H., Caflisch, C. R., Zboralski, F. F., and Hogan, W. J. Deterioration of esophageal peristalsis in patients with alcoholic neuropathy. Gastroenterology 55:173, 1968.

546. Luzzi, S., and Zilletti, L. Neurological disorders of the myenteric plexus: A review. Riv. Patol. Nerv. Ment. 104:229, 1983.

547. Vinograd, I., Udassin, R., Beilin, B., Neuman, A., Maayan, C., and Nissan, S. The surgical management of children with familial dysautonomia. J. Pediatr. Surg. 20:632, 1985.

548. Axelrod, F. B., Schneider, K. M., Ament, N. E., Kutin, N. D., and Fonkalsrud, E. W. Gastroesophageal fundoplication and gastrostomy in familial dysautonomia. Ann. Surg. 195:253, 1982.

549. Hyman, P. E., Ament, M. E., and Heyman, M. B. Congenital dysautonomia with secretory diarrhea. J. Pediatr. Gastroenterol. Nutr. 2:563, 1983.

550. Ariel, I., and Wells, T. R. Structural abnormalities of the myenteric (Auerbach's) plexus in familial dysautonomia (Riley-Day syndrome) as demonstrated by flat-mount preparation of the esophagus and stomach. Pediatr. Pathol. 4:89, 1985.

551. Sulway, M. J., Baume, P. E., and Davis, E. Stiff-man syndrome presenting with complete esophageal obstruction. Am. J. Dig. Dis. 15:79, 1970.

552. Bender, M. D. Esophageal manometry in oculopharyngeal dystrophy. Am. J. Gastroenterol. 65:215, 1976.

553. Nowak, T. V., Ionasescu, V., and Anuras, S. Gastrointestinal manifestations of the muscular dystrophies. Gastroenterology 82:800, 1982.

554. Leon, S. H., Schuffler, M. D., Kettler, M., and Rohrmann, C. A. Chronic intestinal pseudo-obstruction as a complication of Duchenne's muscular dystrophy. Gastroenterology 90:455, 1986.

555. Anuras, S., Mitros, F. A., Milano, A., Kuminsky, R., Decanio, R., and Green, J. B. A familial visceral myopathy with dilatation of the entire gastrointestinal tract. Gastroenterology 90:385, 1986.

556. Singh, V., and Jain, N. Asthma as a cause for, rather than a result of, gastroesophageal reflex. J. Asthma 20:241, 1983.

557. Steed, D. L., Brown, B., Reilly, J. J., Peitzman, A. B., Griffith, B. P., Hardesty, R. L., and Webster, M. W. General surgical complications in heart and heart-lung transplantation. Surgery 98:739, 1985.

Oral Diseases and Cutaneous Manifestations of Gastrointestinal Disease

30

TODD L. SACK
SOL SILVERMAN, JR.

The mouth, the gateway to the gastrointestinal tract, is susceptible to many diseases. The pathophysiology and management of the most common of these are discussed in this chapter. The chapter also describes and illustrates the important oral and cutaneous manifestations of intestinal diseases. Several rare conditions and diseases covered in other chapters are summarized in Table 30–1 or shown in Color Figures 30–2 and 30–3 on p. xxxv to xxxviii. (For descriptions of periodontal and salivary disease, oral cancer, and the less common disorders of the mouth, three recent oral pathology textbooks are recommended.[1–3])

ORAL DISEASES

Examination of the Mouth: Anatomy and Common Findings

The clinician should learn to examine the mouth systematically. An intraoral mirror, lighting, and knowledge of the normal anatomy are necessary for accurate examinations.

The squamous epithelium covering the tongue includes four types of papillae: the *filiform, vallate, fungiform,* and the *foliate* (Fig. 30–1). Filiform papillae are the greatest in number and have no known function. They consist of hair-like extensions of keratin which increase in length in response to a variety of stimuli such as dehydration, fever, and antibiotics and other drugs (the "coated" tongue). The vallate papillae, which contain the major taste buds, are situated posteriorly in an inverted "V" configuration on the dorsal surface of the tongue and are usually eight in number. Fungiform papillae, appearing as red mushroom-like structures interspersed among the filiform papillae, contain some taste buds as well. The foliate papillae appear in grape-like clusters located on the lateral surfaces near the base of the tongue and are composed of lymphoid tissue.

The ventral surface of the tongue includes the midline frenulum, flanked by a pair of lingual veins (Fig. 30–1). Lingual varicosities, which may undergo *thrombosis,* are common in older individuals and have no pathologic significance. The openings of Wharton's ducts, which drain the submandibular salivary glands, are located on either side of the base of the frenulum. The gingiva and dentition are inspected for inflamma-

tion, recession, and tooth mobility, which may reflect *gingivitis* or *periodontal disease.*

Most *discolorations* of the mucosa indicate the presence of melanin, the deposition of which is, for the most part, genetically regulated. Melanin deposition can also be stimulated by certain drugs or by systemic diseases such as Peutz-Jeghers syndrome (Color Fig. 30–2*I,* p. xxxvi) and Addison's disease. Heavy metal toxicity may produce a bluish-black mucosal coloration resembling melanin. Another common cause of mucosal discoloration is amalgam (silver) spillage into the mucosa during dental procedures. The oral mucosa is frequently a site of *Kaposi's sarcoma* in patients with the *acquired immunodeficiency syndrome* (see below). Oral nevi are rare, and oral melanomas extremely rare. Discolorations of teeth may be the result of genetic factors, exposure to drugs such as tetracycline during tooth development, tobacco use, or systemic disease (e.g., rickets, malabsorption). Erosion of the enamel should raise the possibility of acid injury due to excessive citrus fruit in the diet, gastric regurgitation, or chronic vomiting.[4]

The labial and buccal mucosae are normally moist with a pale, pink color. White patches on the mucosa, *leukoplakia,* may represent *dysplasia* or *oral cancer* and must be examined with biopsy (Color Fig. 30–2*A,* p. xxxv). An inflammatory or red component indicates a higher risk of dysplasia or malignancy. Furthermore, biopsy should be performed on any oral lesion that cannot be identified but persists, especially if it is enlarging or eroding. A large segment of the population has ectopic submucosal sebaceous glands, known as *Fordyce granules,* which appear as yellowish nodules, 1 to 3 mm in size, primarily on the buccal surface. The opening of the main excretory duct of the parotid gland, Stensen's duct, emerges in a papilla located on the buccal mucosa at the level of the upper first molars. The labial mucosa is often "pebbly" in appearance owing to the presence of submucosal minor salivary glands. These glands commonly become blocked, creating small painless *retention cysts* containing a mucoid secretory product. The cysts can appear as fluid-filled sacs of varying sizes; when exceeding 3 mm in size they usually require excision.[5]

Inspection of the hard and soft palate is performed after dentures are removed. Minor salivary glands are numerous, and are frequently associated with tumors as well as retention cysts. A *torus palatinus* is a smooth, often lobulated bony growth commonly seen in the

Table 30–1. ORAL AND CUTANEOUS DISEASES ASSOCIATED WITH
GASTROINTESTINAL DISORDERS*

Disease	Oral and Cutaneous Signs	Gastrointestinal Manifestations	Relevant Chapters
Primary Gastrointestinal Disease Associated with Skin Lesions			
Gastrointestinal polyposis syndromes			
Peutz-Jeghers[†]	Pigmented macules on lips, mouth, hands, and feet; clubbing	Hamartomas	80
Gardner's	Odontomas, osteomas	Adenomatous polyps	80
	Multiple sebaceous cysts	Adenocarcinomas	
	Fibromas, desmoid tumors		
Cronkhite-Canada	Alopecia, hyperpigmentation (especially of creases, hands, face), dystrophic nails, glossitis, buccal pigmentation (rare)	Hamartomatous polyps	80
		Intussusception, exocrine pancreatic insufficiency	
		Diarrhea, melena, protein-losing enteropathy	
Torre's (Muir's)	Sebaceous adenomas	Colonic adenomas	80
	Basal and squamous carcinomas	Adenocarcinomas	
	Keratoacanthomas		
Hormone-secreting tumors			
Carcinoid syndrome	Flushing, telangiectasias on face and neck	Carcinoid tumors, usually metastatic to liver	81, 82
Systemic mastocytosis[†]	Urticaria pigmentosa	Abdominal pain, diarrhea, steatorrhea, ulcer disease, hepatosplenomegaly	29
	Telangiectasias, flushing		
	Pigmented macules and papules, pruritus		
Glucagonoma syndrome	Necrolytic migratory erythema, dermographism	Pancreatic islet cell tumors, gallstones	100
Intestinal lymphoma	Ulcers, nodules, rashes	Lymphoma	29, 81
	Dermatitis herpetiformis		
Metastases	Cutaneous metastases	Carcinoma	29
Inflammatory bowel disease[‡]	See Table 30–2	See Table 30–2	71, 78
Celiac sprue[59]	Dermatitis herpetiformis	Villous flattening, malabsorption, lymphoma	18, 61
	Hyperpigmentation		
Whipple's disease[60]	Parakeratosis, hyperpigmentation, glossitis	PAS-staining macrophages, lymphatic dilation in small intestine	68
Jejunoileal bypass[61]	Papulopustular or nodular skin lesions, pyoderma gangrenosum (rare)	Enteritis, pseudo-obstruction	9
Pancreatic disease	Grey Turner sign (blue-brown flanks)	Acute pancreatitis	97
	Cullen signs (periumbilical discoloration)	Acute pancreatitis	
	Nodular fat necrosis	Acute pancreatitis	
	Erythema ab igne (pigmented truncal rash)	Chronic pancreatitis	
	Thrombophlebitis migrans	Pancreatic cancer	
Plummer-Vinson syndrome (Paterson-Brown-Kelly)	Koilonychia, glossitis	Postcricoid webs, dysphagia, esophageal squamous carcinoma	36
Familial paroxysmal polyserositis (Familial Mediterranean fever)	Erysipelas (tender, red, edema), subcutaneous nodules (panniculitis), urticaria	Peritonitis	102
Idiopathic constipation[62]	Fingerprint arches	Childhood constipation, pseudo-obstruction	
Skin Disease Affecting the Gut			
Malignant melanoma	Melanoma	Metastatic melanoma, perforation, hemorrhage, obstruction	29
Lichen planus[†‡]	"Lacy" white lesions on lips or oral mucosa; also atrophic and erosive forms	Oral and esophageal blisters, dysphagia	
	Bluish, shiny skin papules		
Erythema multiforme[‡] (Stevens-Johnson syndrome)	Oral mucosal inflammation, ulcers, blisters on lips, cheilitis, cutaneous "target" lesions, erythematous macules	Intestinal ulcers, necrosis, perforation	70
Dermatogenic enteropathy[‡]	Extensive eczema	Steatorrhea	
Gut, Oral Mucosa, and Skin Affected by the Same Disease			
Vascular disorders			
Inherited disorders associated with gastrointestinal bleeding			
Hereditary hemorrhagic telangiectasias (Osler-Weber-Rendu syndrome)[†63]	Telangiectasias on lips, mouth, palms, and soles	Mucosal telangiectasias, bleeding	72
	Oral hemorrhagic nodules, ulcers		
Blue rubber bleb nevus syndrome[†64]	Dark blue, soft, compressible, pedunculated nodules	Mucosal cavernous hemangiomas	25
		Colonic varices (rare)	
Pseudoxanthoma elasticum[†65]	Yellowish "chicken fat" papules and plaques in flexural areas	Yellowish mucosal nodules	25
		Mucosal microaneurysms, nodules, visceral ischemia	
Ehlers-Danlos syndrome	Skin fragility, paper-thin scars over bony protuberances, keloids	Diverticula, megaesophagus, megacolon, mesenteric arterial rupture, perforation, hernias, intramural hematomas	29

Table continued on opposite page

Table 30–1. ORAL AND CUTANEOUS DISEASES ASSOCIATED WITH
GASTROINTESTINAL DISORDERS* *Continued*

Disease	Oral and Cutaneous Signs	Gastrointestinal Manifestations	Relevant Chapters
Gut, Oral Mucosa, and Skin Affected by the Same Disease Continued			
Turner's syndrome	Webbing of neck skin	Mucosal cavernous hemangiomas, bleeding	
Other vascular disorders			
Polyarteritis nodosa	Palpable purpura, skin nodules	Hemorrhage, ruptured mesenteric aneurysm	29, 101
Henoch-Schönlein purpura (anaphylactoid purpura)	Palpable purpura Cutaneous edema (rare) Maculopapular rash (rare)	Abdominal pain, melena	101
Cutaneous visceral hemangiomatosis†[66]	Smooth blue dermal and subcutaneous nodules	Mucosal cavernous hemangiomas, hemorrhage	
Degos' disease† (malignant papulosis)	Dome-shaped red papules (early) White atrophic scars (late)	Endovasculitis, bowel ischemia, perforation, malabsorption	25, 101
Bullous eruptions			
Epidermolysis bullosa‡ dystrophica	Oral and cutaneous bullae Dystrophic nails	Esophageal stricture Oral and anal bullae, constipation, congenital pyloric atresia	38
acquisita	Oral and cutaneous bullae	Crohn's disease (rare)	
Bullous pemphigoid‡	Oral and skin bullae	Esophageal bullae, melena	38
Rheumatologic diseases			
Systemic lupus erythematosus	Photosensitivity, malar rash, oral ulcers, and erythema Nail splinter hemorrhages	Peritonitis Mesenteric ischemia	29
Progressive systemic sclerosis (scleroderma)	Calcinosis, Raynaud's phenomenon, sclerodactyly, telangiectasias	Gut dysmotility, bacterial overgrowth, pseudodiverticula	29, 38
Rheumatoid arthritis	Rheumatoid nodules, cutaneous vasculitis, nail splinter hemorrhages	Mesenteric vasculitis	29
Dermatomyositis	Violaceous facial rash Photosensitivity, nail fold erythema, hand edema	Oropharyngeal dysphagia Pseudodiverticula	29, 38
Behçet's syndrome†	Oral and genital ulcers	Granulomatous colitis	29
Other disorders			
Systemic amyloidosis	Small waxy amber papules on face and lips	Motility disorders, malabsorption	18, 19, 29, 78
Fabry disease	Angiokeratomas on scrotum, extremities, lips, mouth, umbilicus	Angiokeratomas, bowel ischemia	29
Kaposi's sarcoma‡	Bluish-red macules and tumors on oral mucosa and skin	Multicentric mucosal vascular tumors	64, 65
Porphyrias	Photosensitivity (blisters) Hypertrichosis, hyperpigmentation	Vomiting, abdominal pain, constipation	
Pernicious anemia[67]	Vitiligo, glossitis	Fundal atrophic gastritis, antral polyps, gastric cancer	46
Skin Disorders Associated with Increased Incidence of Gastrointestinal Tumors			
Tylosis	Hyperkeratosis of palms, soles	Esophageal adenocarcinoma Gastric adenocarcinoma (rare)	35
Erythema multiforme‡	See above	Adenocarcinoma (colon)	
Ataxia-telangiectasia	Telangiectasias on face, ears, bulbar conjunctiva, and antecubital fossa	Adenocarcinoma (stomach, pancreas)	
Sign of Leser-Trélat[68]	Sudden appearance of multiple seborrheic keratoses	Adenocarcinoma	
Acanthosis nigricans†	Pigmented verrucous and velvety plaques in axilla and groin	Adenocarcinoma	
Tuberous sclerosis[69]	Facial angiofibromas (adenoma sebaceum) Port-wine hemangiomas "Ash leaf–shaped" hypopigmentation	Hepatic angiomyolipomas (rare) Pancreatic hamartomas	
Neurofibromatosis‡	Multiple café-au-lait spots, neurofibromas, axillary freckles, skin sarcomas	Submucosal neurofibromas, hemorrhage, obstruction, megacolon, dysmotility, carcinoid tumors, malignancies	29
Hypertrichosis lanuginosa[70]	Increased lanugo hair	Adenocarcinoma	
Sister Joseph nodule	Umbilical metastases	Adenocarcinoma (gastric)	
Skin tags (acrochordons)[71]	Skin tags	Colonic adenomatous polyps	80

*Some of these manifestations are rare and not seen in every patient with the conditions described. See the relevant chapters and the references cited for further discussion.

†See Color Figure 30–2 or 30–3, pages xxxv to xxxviii.

‡Discussed in this chapter.

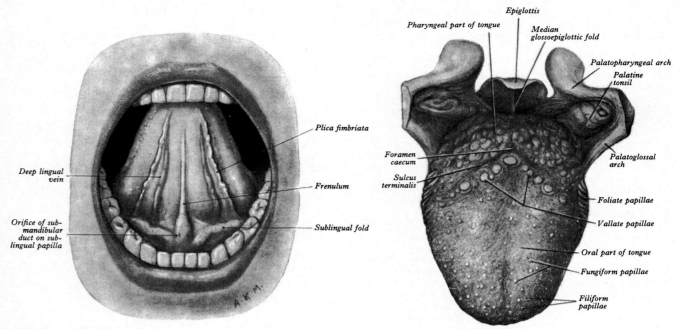

Figure 30–1. Anatomy of the floor of the mouth and tongue. *Left:* Ventral tongue and mouth floor. The tip of the tongue is turned upward; in the person from whom the drawing was made the two sublingual salivary papillae formed a single median elevation. *Right:* dorsal tongue, base of tongue, and mesopharynx. (From Warwick, R., and Williams, P. L. Gray's Anatomy. 35th British edition. Philadelphia, W. B. Saunders Co., 1973. Used by permission.)

midline of the hard palate. Tori are inconsequential unless they interfere with dentures, mastication, or phonation. Denture irritation can produce mucosal inflammation and papillomatous hyperplasia. Another entity is *"smoker's palate,"* which consists of palatal inflammation, minor salivary gland edema, and hyperkeratinization in response to tobacco.

The oropharynx is a common site for *inflammatory diseases, infections,* and *neoplasms.* The oropharynx and tonsillar fossa often exhibit accumulations of lymphoid tissue, which appear as red, papillomatous plaques that can be mistaken for signs of a pathologic process.

Halitosis. *Halitosis* (bad breath), often noted during the oral examination, is usually due to local factors, but not always. Offensive hydrogen sulfides and mercaptans are produced by the normal oral bacterial flora and accumulate between tooth brushings (e.g., "morning breath"). Halitosis, therefore, can result from the accumulation of food debris or any other condition that favors the proliferation of oral bacteria. Common causes are *poor oral hygiene, dental or tonsillar abscesses, gingivitis,* and *stomatitis. Xerostomia* of any cause (e.g. drugs, fever, dehydration, Sjögren's syndrome, radiation therapy) can produce bad breath by decreasing the clearance of oral bacteria. Another cause of halitosis is elongation of the filiform papillae (*"hairy tongue"*), which fosters local bacterial overgrowth and poor hygiene. Although hairy tongue can be idiopathic, associated conditions include antibiotic use, alcohol consumption, dehydration, and systemic illness. Certain foods and drugs, such as ethanol, garlic, isosorbide dinitrate, chloral hydrate, and dimethyl sulfoxide (DMSO), are excreted in part by the lungs and

can affect the breath adversely. Non-oropharyngeal causes of halitosis include *chronic pulmonary disease* (bronchiectasis, lung abscesses), *liver failure* ("fetor hepaticus"), *uremia,* and *diabetic ketoacidosis.*[6, 7]

The evaluation and management of halitosis begins with a careful review of the patient's medications, diet, and non-oral diseases. In most cases, reinstitution of meticulous oral hygiene and professional attention to dental pathology will be sufficient therapy. The addition of routine tongue brushing has been shown to be helpful because organisms and cellular debris collect on the tongue.[8] Dentures need to be brushed and soaked daily in a disinfecting solution. Sucking mints and chewing gum may help by increasing salivary flow, improving the removal of debris, and emitting their own flavors. Antiseptic mouthwashes are also helpful.[6, 7] For patients with xerostomia, preparations containing 1 per cent sodium carboxymethylcellulose (Xero-Lube and others) may be used to moisten the oral cavity.[8]

Oral Erosions and Ulcers

In addition to the diseases discussed below, the differential diagnosis of erosions and ulcers includes mechanical trauma and malignancy.

Aphthous Ulcers. *Aphthous ulcers* (canker sores) are painful, shallow ulcers often covered with a grayish-white exudate and surrounded by an erythematous margin (Color Fig. 30–2*B*, p. xxxv). They appear almost exclusively on unkeratinized oral mucosal surfaces (the soft palate, ventral or lateral tongue, buccal-labial mucosa, and floor of the mouth). Aphthae occur in about 25 per cent of the general population and are not infectious. Aphthous ulcers usually recur at irregular intervals with single or multiple lesions. While usually less than 5 mm in size and healed in 1 to 3 weeks, they can occur as *major aphthae* which exceed 6 mm and require months to resolve, often with scarring (Color Fig. 30–2C, p. xxxv).[10, 11]

A variety of conditions have been associated with aphthous ulcers, but most evidence points to an immunologic etiology.[11, 12] Frequently the lesions are brought on or aggravated by nuts, chocolate, or citrus products. Prolonged fever or local trauma may precipitate eruptions. Patients with severe nutritional deficiencies or *pernicious anemia* have noted improvement after treatment with iron, folate, or vitamin B_{12}, but most patients with aphthous ulcers will not benefit from vitamin or mineral supplements.[13] Morphologically identical lesions may be seen in *inflammatory bowel disease* (see below), *Behçet's syndrome*[12] (see p. 508), *Reiter's syndrome,* and *infectious mononucleosis.*

Routine aphthous ulcers are treated with a potent glucocorticoid ointment such as fluocinonide (Lidex) ointment 0.05 per cent, mixed with an equal volume of Orabase, an adhesive base. (This formulation has not been approved by the U. S. Food and Drug Administration at the time of publication.) Kenalog (triamcinolone acetonide) in Orabase is FDA approved and preformulated but is one eighth as potent as fluocinonide. Analgesics and topical anesthetics such as lidocaine ointment can be helpful. Short courses of systemic prednisone (20 to 40 mg/day) are reproducibly useful when conservative empiric approaches are not satisfactory.[14]

Herpetic Stomatitis. Infection with the herpes simplex virus (HSV) commonly produces painful vesiculoulcerative lesions affecting the genitalia, eyes, lips, mouth, and skin. Esophageal and rectal involvement are described on pages 644 and 1269 to 1270, respectively. *Herpetic meningoencephalitis* and *disseminated herpes simplex* affect neonates and immunocompromised adults, especially following bone marrow transplantation or in patients with AIDS.[15]

Primary herpetic gingivostomatitis is due to type 1 (or occasionally type 2) HSV. Primary infection occurs in 90 per cent of the population before puberty. The illness often is mild and unnoticeable but may include varying degrees of fever, malaise, and adenopathy together with oral ulcers. The lesions can also appear on the lips. They generally heal after 1 to 2 weeks upon acquisition of humoral immunity, which becomes permanent for this form of herpetic infection. Management is palliative.[15]

Recurrent herpes simplex is due to reactivation of HSV that has been dormant in regional ganglia and is not associated with an increase in anti-HSV titers. Attacks may be precipitated by almost any physical or emotional stress. About 28 per cent of patients with recurrences have attacks at least twice a year, but recurrences are variable in frequency and severity.[15] Typically, the lesions involve the lips ("cold sores") and are preceded by several hours of prodromal symptoms such as burning, tingling, or pruritus. Vesicles then appear on the lips and soon rupture, leaving small, irregular, painful ulcers. Coalescence of ulcers, crusting, and weeping are common. Serologic testing for *syphilis* should be considered in high risk patients or if there is no prior history of cold sores since chancres can have the same appearance. Intraoral recurrent herpetic ulcers are rare and are confined to keratinized mucosa, that is, mucosa which is adherent to bone—the hard palate or gingiva. They appear as shallow, irregular, small ulcerations and may coalesce. Labial and oral ulcers normally heal in less than 2 weeks.

Herpes is usually diagnosed by the history and clinical findings. A history of a prodrome or of vesicles, the site of lesions, and the appearance of lesions all help to distinguish herpes from aphthous ulcers. The diagnosis may be confirmed by a cytologic smear showing mutinucleate pseudogiant cells. Viral cultures and monoclonal antibody staining of smears are more sensitive tests but are not widely available because they are expensive and can require several days to be performed.[11]

Treatment is palliative in most cases. We have noted good symptomatic results treating adults with glucocorticoid ointment (see above) after the third day, at which time lesions are usually noninfectious. Care must be taken to avoid ocular viral inoculation. Topical acyclovir is of no reproducible benefit in recurrent labial herpes.[16] Systemic acyclovir is reserved for treatment of primary or recurrent attacks in immunosuppressed patients (1 to 2 grams daily until signs and symptoms are controlled). Oral acyclovir is used for the prevention of recurrent oral herpes associated with *bone marrow transplantation.*[17] The dose is 400 mg five times daily for five weeks beginning one week before transplantation.[17] Oral acyclovir may prevent recurrent herpes in other immunocompromised patients such as those with leukemia.[18]

Candidiasis. *Candida* species (chiefly *C. albicans*) are part of the normal oral flora in almost half the population. Illness results from impairment of the usual protective mechanisms. *Candidiasis* (moniliasis) is seen following *antibiotic* or *glucocorticoid therapy,* in *denture wearers,* and in patients with *anemia, diabetes mellitus,* or *familial hypoparathyroidism* (see p. 491). It is also associated with *xerostomia,* whatever the cause (e.g., radiation, Sjögren's syndrome, dehydration, anticholinergic drugs). Finally, *immunosuppression* due to the *acquired immunodeficiency syndrome* (see below), other debilitating illnesses, or cancer chemotherapy may lead to candidiasis.

Oral candidiasis typically appears as white, curdlike patches (thrush). However, it can present also as an erythematous, friable mucosa; as granular or eroded erythematous patches; or as angular cheilitis. Patients may complain of pain or be asymptomatic. When upper gastrointestinal bleeding or dysphagia accompanies thrush, concurrent *candida esophagitis* should be considered (see pp. 640–643).

The history and physical findings usually establish

the diagnosis. At times, a smear revealing spores and hyphae (see Figure 38–3), a culture, or a biopsy is helpful. Oral candidiasis can be treated topically (nystatin, clotrimazole) or systemically (ketoconazole, amphotericin B) using regimens similar to those for esophageal candidiasis (see pp. 642–643). Disinfectant mouthwashes available without prescription may be helpful. Causative factors should be identified and managed.

Mucositis, a severe inflammatory-ulcerative oral condition associated with cytotoxic-immunosuppressive cancer chemotherapy, is discussed on page 503.

Glossitis

Inflammation of the tongue is associated with a heterogeneous group of disorders that includes *nutritional deficiencies, chemical irritants, drug reactions, hypochromic* or *pernicious anemia, amyloidosis, sarcoidosis, microbial infections* (especially *candidiasis*), *vesiculoerosive diseases* (see below), and *systemic infection.* Sometimes no underlying cause can be detected.[19]

Patients complain of lingual pain (glossodynia) or burning (glossopyrosis). The physical examination can show any degree of filiform depapillation, ranging from mild and patchy erythema with or without erosive changes to a completely smooth, erythematous surface (Color Fig. 30–2*D*, p. xxxv). In approximately 2 per cent of the population, the disappearance of filiform papillae takes place in irregular configurations ("geographic tongue"). Geographic tongue is more common in atopic individuals and in asthmatics, but the cause is unknown.[20] It is sometimes painful and almost always self-limiting. Recurrent episodes are not uncommon.

Hypogeusia (diminished sense of taste) and *dysgeusia* (distortion of normal taste) are other complaints that can be associated with glossitis due to injury to the taste buds. Hypogeusia following radiation therapy to the mouth is often at least partially reversible.[21]

Most frequently, however, the cause of hypogeusia or dysgeusia is uncertain. There is no firm evidence that they are part of normal aging. They are common complaints among tobacco smokers, denture wearers, and patients with psychiatric disorders, especially anxiety. Hypogeusia and dysgeusia have been attributed to a variety of neurologic, nutritional, and metabolic disorders, as well as to a large number of medications, but the evidence supporting these associations is tenuous.[22, 23] The therapy is empiric. At times, patients will respond to oral zinc supplementation (440 mg zinc sulfate daily),[21] or to antianxiety or antidepressant medication.

Glossodynia in the absence of clinical or histologic evidence of glossitis is often associated with anxiety or depression. It is seen most commonly in postmenopausal women, but hormonal therapy is of no value.[24, 25]

Treatment of glossitis is based upon determining and correcting the cause. Palliative measures include viscous xylocaine, analgesics, tranquilizers, and antidepressants.

AIDS and the Mouth

Oral complications are common in patients with the acquired immunodeficiency syndrome (AIDS) or the AIDS-related complex (ARC) (see also pp. 1236–1240). These manifestations often cause significant morbidity but can provide valuable diagnostic and prognostic information.

Culture-positive oral *candidiasis* occurs in more than 75 per cent of patients with AIDS or with ARC. Most subjects are symptomatic and require specific antifungal therapy (see above).[26]

Kaposi's sarcoma (KS) is present in 20 per cent of AIDS patients, and is most common in homosexual or bisexual males. In one large series of homosexual men with AIDS, 80 per cent had KS, and over 50 per cent of those had oral mucous membrane involvement. The oral mucosa was the initial site of diagnosis in 7 per cent of cases.[26] The early lesions appear as flat, vascular-like or purpuric discolorations and are located most frequently on the palate or gingiva. They may become nodular and symptomatic, and require treatment (usually radiation). Oral *squamous carcinoma* and oral *non-Hodgkin's lymphoma* are also tumors seen with increased frequency in AIDS patients.[26]

Hairy leukoplakia (HL) is a unique lesion found on the lateral surfaces of the tongue or occasionally on the buccal mucosa.[27] It is raised and white and often has a corrugated or hairy-appearing surface (Color Fig. 30–2*J*, p. xxxvi). Histologically HL consists of epithelial hyperplasia and pseudokeratinization with little or no inflammation. The lesions are associated with the Epstein-Barr virus.[27] The clinical significance of HL is that virtually all HL patients test positively for antibody to the human immunodeficiency virus (HIV), and in one study HIV was cultured from blood in 79 per cent of cases, indicating infectivity.[28] Over half of patients presenting with HL develop AIDS within 31 months.[28]

Several other abnormalities that probably result from the immunocompromised state have been associated with AIDS or ARC. *Condyloma acuminata* (venereal warts) and *herpes simplex* (see above) are more frequent and more severe in AIDS patients; premature, progressive *periodontal disease, acute ulcerative gingivitis, erythema multiforme* (see below), and *xerostomia* are relatively frequent.[26]

Nutritional Deficiencies

Oral lesions are common with severe vitamin deficiencies (see pp. 1983–1994). Lack of vitamin B_2 (riboflavin), vitamin B_6 (pyridoxine), folate, or iron should be considered in patients with *angular cheilitis* and *atrophic glossitis* (Color Fig. 30–2*D*, p. xxxv). Iron deficiency may lead also to dysphagia and postcricoid esophageal webs in the *Plummer-Vinson syndrome* (see Table 30–1 and pp. 632–635). Tongue involvement is a prominent feature of *pernicious anemia* (vitamin B_{12} deficiency) due to sensory neuropathy and impaired mucosal cell proliferation. Glossodynia, glossopyrosis, loss of taste, and a "beefy red" inflamed tongue may be present. *Vitamin C deficiency* is associated with gingivitis and gingival bleeding (*scurvy*). Bleeding is also a feature of *vitamin K deficiency*. The oral findings in niacin deficiency (*pellagra*) may include glossodynia, atrophic glossitis, and sometimes ulcerative gingivo-stomatitis (see p. 501). Pustular, weeping perioral lesions are seen in all cases of *acrodermatitis entero-pathica* (zinc deficiency); buccal ulcers, glossitis, and candidiis can also be present (see also pp. 500–501).

DISEASES AFFECTING THE MOUTH, SKIN, AND GUT

Vesiculobullous Disorders

Epidermolysis Bullosa. *Epidermolysis bullosa* is a group of rare dermatologic diseases of the squamous epithelia in which minimal trauma results in bulla formation (Color Fig. 30–3*H*, p. xxxviii). Autosomal recessive *epidermolysis bullosa dystrophica* (EBD) is

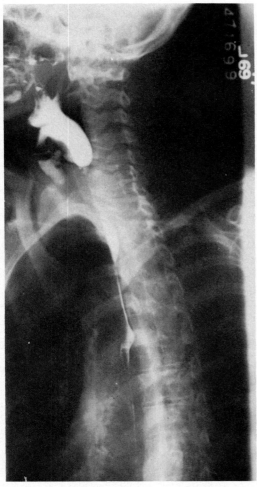

Figure 30–4. Stenotic lesions of proximal esophagus in epidermolysis bullosa. (From Schuman, B. M., and Arciniegas, E. Am. J. Dig. Dis. *17*:875, 1972. Copyright 1972, Harper & Row Publishers, Inc., Hagerstown, Md.)

the form commonly associated also with oral and gut complications.

Oral bullae are common in patients with EBD. These inevitably rupture, leaving a painful, denuded mucosa which when it heals leads to severe scarring of the tongue, microstomia, and reduced mandibular motion. Esophageal involvement (Fig. 30–4) is described on pages 645 to 646. Severe constipation, common in patients with EBD, has been attributed to low-fiber diets and defecatory pain from anal bullae.[29] The nonhereditary form of epidermolysis bullosa, *epidermolysis bullosa acquisita*, has been associated with *Crohn's disease*.[30] *Pyloric atresia* has been reported in infants with EBD.[31]

Pemphigoid. Pemphigoid is an autoimmune disorder characterized by bullae and ulcers affecting the oral mucosa, pharynx, esophagus, and anal mucosa (mucous membrane pemphigoid). When there are bullous skin lesions, with or without mucosal involvement, the term *bullous pemphigoid* is used. The patients are middle-aged or elderly and have serologic evidence of antibodies against the squamous epithelial basement membrane.[32] Immunofluorescent staining of involved mucosa shows linear deposition of antibody and complement in the basement membrane.[33] *Pemphigus* differs from pemphigoid in having more severe skin lesions (which can be life-threatening) and autoantibodies directed against antigens on the surface of squamous epithelial cells. While both conditions are associated with painful oral ulcers, only pemphigoid affects the esophagus. *Pemphigus* involving the skin can often be distinguished from other bullous diseases by eliciting the *Nikolsky sign* (easy peeling of the epidermis following gentle abrasion).

Treatment consists of various regimens of topical or systemic prednisone, sometimes supplemented with cytotoxic/immunosuppressive drugs (see also p. 646).

Erythema Multiforme. Erythema multiforme (EM) is an acute, benign mucocutaneous eruption that is associated with a diverse list of drugs, infectious agents, malignancies, and physical agents. EM is common among patients with AIDS (see above). It is often preceded or accompanied by low-grade fever, malaise, and symptoms suggesting an upper respiratory tract infection. The skin rash typically consists of red "target lesions" on the extremities, but EM can be an erythematous or vesicular eruption.[34]

Many patients with EM have only oral involvement. Any degree of nonspecific erythema may be seen, with or without ulcers. Crusting and weeping lip ulcers may be present. Severe oral and pharyngeal pain, secondary bacterial and fungal infections, and bleeding are common complications (Color Fig. 30–2*E*, p. xxxv). EM can be self-limiting or chronic, and often the inciting process goes unidentified. Management includes palliative measures and elimination of any offending allergen. Often, glucocorticoids and/or other immunosuppressive drugs are needed.[14, 34]

The term *Stevens-Johnson syndrome* (SJS) is used when there is severe, acute EM affecting the eyes, skin, and mucous membranes. Diffuse oral and pharyngeal ulceration usually prevents all oral intake (Color Fig. 30–2E, p. xxxv). At endoscopy, the esophagus may show diffuse erythema, friability, and whitish plaques that can be mistaken for candidiasis. Diffuse gastric and duodenal erythema and friability may be present without esophageal involvement.[35] The colonoscopic appearance may resemble severe ulcerative or pseudomembranous colitis; however, biopsies show extensive necrosis and lymphocytic infiltration without crypt abscesses or neutrophils. This pattern is reminiscent of *graft-versus-host disease* (see p. 503). The mucosa of large portions of bowel may slough, accounting for the reports of hematemesis, melena, and intestinal perforation in SJS.[35]

Treatment of SJS begins by removing any possible causative factors (drugs, physical agents) and treating underlying infections and malignancies. Immediately, antibiotics are provided because of the high risk for bacterial infection, and prednisone is often used empirically to suppress inflammation. Parenteral nutrition is frequently required.[35]

Other Bullous Diseases. *Dermatitis herpetiformis* is associated with *celiac sprue* and is described on page 1140.

Lichen Planus

Lichen planus (LP) is a common chronic inflammatory disorder involving the oral mucosa, the skin, and, rarely, the esophagus. The disease usually begins in adulthood, and two thirds of the patients are women.[36] The typical oral lesions consist of increased keratin formation appearing as white lace-like and/or punctate patterns on any mucosal surface (Color Fig. 30–2F, p. xxxvi). There may be associated mucosal erythema or ulceration. A slightly increased risk of developing *squamous carcinoma* is reported.[36] Approximately 20 per cent of patients with oral LP also have skin lesions consisting of flat papules, which can coalesce into large plaques covered with a charateristic fine, glistening scale. The early lesions are erythematous; chronically, they become violaceous or brownish.

The etiology of lichen planus is unknown. The patients can be asymptomatic or may develop severe oral pain. The use of topical and/or systemic glucocorticoids is helpful in decreasing the signs and symptoms in almost all cases.[36]

Two cases of *esophageal involvement* with lichen planus have been reported.[37, 38] Both patients developed progressive dysphagia and odynophagia after years of severe oral disease. The endoscopic findings included erythema, ulcers, or erosions throughout the esophagus. One case included an esophageal web 26 cm from the incisors.[37] The other case dramatically improved with a course of ACTH.[38]

Inflammatory Bowel Disease

The oral and skin complications of *Crohn's disease* and *ulcerative colitis* occur in less than 5 per cent of patients with these diseases.[39, 43] They are summarized in Table 30–2. See also Color Figures 30–2G and 30–3 on pages xxxvi to xxxviii, and pages 1338 to 1339 and 1469 to 1470.

DISEASES AFFECTING THE SKIN AND GUT

The conditions that affect both the skin and the gastrointestinal tract are summarized in Tables 30–1 and 30–2; this section describes those of interest that are not presented in another chapter.

Dermatogenic Enteropathy

The term *dermatogenic enteropathy* has been used to describe cases in which severe skin disease is believed to cause small intestinal dysfunction.[44, 45] Most of the patients have had severe *eczema* or *psoriasis* associated with diarrhea, fat malabsorption, and partial jejunal villous atrophy. In some instances, all abnormalities resolved after successful treatment of the dermatitis.[45] Similar small intestinal histologic findings

Table 30–2. ORAL AND CUTANEOUS SIGNS IN CROHN'S DISEASE (CD) AND ULCERATIVE COLITIS (UC)*

Manifestation	Disease	Features
Oral		
Oral Crohn's disease	CD	Cobblestone lesions; biopsies may show granulomas
Angular cheilitis	CD	Due to candidiasis, malnutrition
Pyostomatitis vegetans	UC	Friable, often painful; Color Fig. 30–2 (pp. xxxv and xxxvi)
Cutaneous		
Pyoderma gangrenosum	CD, UC	See pages 1469–1470; Color Fig. 30–3 (pp. xxxvii and xxxviii)
Erythema nodosum	CD, UC	On legs, painful
Erythema multiforme	CD, UC	Drug-related, especially sulfasalazine
Thrombophlebitis	CD, UC	Rare
Digital clubbing	CD, UC	
Palmar erythema	CD, UC	
Ostomy erythema	CD, UC	Cellulitis or chemical irritants
Cutaneous fistulas	CD	
Cutaneous granulomas	CD	
Rashes of malnutrition	CD	Especially zinc, niacin deficiencies; see pages 500–501
Digital ischemia	UC	With hypercoagulable state, rare

*See References 39 to 43.

have been seen with *lichen planus*[46] and with *rosacea,* a facial condition consisting of pustules superimposed upon an area of telangiectatic, congested skin.[47]

Unfortunately, most of the published examples of dermatogenic enteropathy have been incompletely studied. The villous atrophy seen in severe dermatitis may be due to folate deficiency,[48, 49] and the positive urinary D-xylose tests could be the result of decreased renal xylose clearance, which has been reported in severe dermatitis.[50] It is noteworthy that one thorough study of eight patients with extensive psoriasis failed to detect any radiographic, histologic, or physiologic small bowel abnormality.[51]

Neurofibromatosis

Gastrointestinal involvement occurs in 10 to 25 per cent of patients with *neurofibromatosis* (Von Recklinghausen's disease). The skin findings are presented in Table 30–1 and Color Figure 30–3*I*, p. xxxviii. Intestinal neurofibromas may arise at any level of the gastrointestinal tract, although small intestinal involvement is most common.[52, 53] The tumors generally are submucosal but may extend to the serosa. Dense growths known as *plexiform neurofibromatosis* of the mesentery or retroperitoneal space may lead to arterial compression or nerve injury, respectively.[54, 55]

Malignant tumors often complicate neurofibromatosis. There is an increased incidence of *pheochromocytoma,* either with or without the *multiple endocrine neoplasia type 2B syndrome* (see p. 493).[56] Duodenal and ampullary *carcinoid tumors* (producing obstructive jaundice), *malignant schwannomas, sarcomas,* and *pancreatic adenocarcinomas* are seen.[56–58]

The common clinical manifestations are abdominal pain, constipation, anemia, melena, and an abdominal mass. Serious complications that have been reported include *intestinal* or *biliary obstruction, ischemic bowel, perforation,* and *intussusception.*[52, 56, 57] Involvement of the myenteric plexus has resulted in *megacolon.*[55]

References

1. Shafer, W. G., Hine, M. K., Levy, B. M., and Tomich, C. E. A Textbook of Oral Pathology. Philadelphia, W. B. Saunders Co., 1983.
2. Kerr, D. A., Ash, M. M., Jr., and Millard, H. D. Oral Diagnosis. St. Louis, C. V. Mosby Co., 1983.
3. Jones, J. H., and Mason, D. K. Oral manifestations of systemic disease. Philadelphia, W. B. Saunders Co., 1980.
4. Stege, P., Visco-Dangler, L., and Rye, L. Anorexia nervosa: review including oral and dental manifestations. J. Am. Dent. Assoc. *104*:648, 1982.
5. Eversole, L. R. Oral sialocysts. Arch. Otolaryngol. Head Neck Surg. *113*:51, 1987.
6. Lu, D. P. Halitosis: An etiologic classification, a treatment approach, and prevention. Oral Surg. *54*:521, 1982.
7. Bogdasarian, R. S. Halitosis. Otolaryngol. Clin. North Am. *19*:111, 1986.
8. Tonzetich, J., and Ng, S. K. Reduction of malodor by oral cleansing procedures. Oral Surg. *42*:172, 1976.
9. Levine, M. J., Aguirre, A., Hatton, M. N., and Tabak, L. A. Artificial salivas: present and future. J. Dent. Res. *66*:693, 1987.
10. Axell, T., and Henricsson, V. The occurrence of recurrent aphthous ulcers in an adult Swedish population. Acta Odontol. Scand. *43*:121, 1985.
11. Olson, J. A., Greenspan, J. S., and Silverman, S., Jr. Recurrent aphthous ulcerations. J. Calif. Dent. Assoc. *10*:53, 1982.
12. Reimer, G., Luckner, L., and Hornstein, O. P. Direct immunofluorescence in recurrent aphthous ulcers and Behçet's disease. Dermatologica *167*:293, 1983.
13. Olson, J. A., Feinberg, I., Silverman, S., Jr., Abrams, D., and Greenspan, J. S. Serum vitamin B$_{12}$, folate, and iron levels in recurrent aphthous ulceration. Oral Surg. *54*:517, 1982.
14. Silverman, S., Jr., Lozada-Nur, F., and Migliorati, C.: Clinical efficacy of prednisone in the treatment of patients with oral inflammatory ulcerative diseases: A study of fifty-five patients. Oral Surg. *59*:360, 1985.
15. Straus, S. E., Rooney, J. F., Sever, J. L., Seidlin, M., Nusinoff-Lehrman, S., and Cremer, K. Herpes simplex virus infection: biology, treatment, and prevention. Ann. Intern. Med. *103*:404, 1985.
16. Shaw, M., King, M., Best, J. M., Banatvala, J. E., Gibson, J. R., and Klaber, M. R. Failure of acyclovir cream in treatment of recurrent herpes labialis. Br. Med. J. *291*:7, 1985.
17. Wade, J. C., Newton, B., Flournoy, N., and Meyers, J. D. Oral acyclovir for prevention of herpes simplex virus reactivation after marrow transplantation. Ann. Intern. Med. *100*:823, 1984.
18. Dan, M., Siegman-Igra, Y., Weinberg, M., and Michaeli, D. Long-term suppression of recurrent herpes labialis by low-dose oral acyclovir in an immunocompromised patient. Arch. Intern. Med. *146*:1438, 1986.
19. Dreizen S: Systemic significance of glossitis. Postgrad. Med. *75*(4):207, 1984.
20. Marks, R., and Czarny, D. Geographic tongue: sensitivity to the environment. Oral Surg. *58*:156, 1984.
21. Silverman, S., Jr., and Thompson, J. S. Serum zinc and copper in oral/oropharyngeal carcinoma. Oral Surg. *57*:34, 1984.
22. Schiffman, S. S. Taste and smell in disease. (First of two parts). N. Engl. J. Med. *308*:1275, 1983.
23. Schiffman, S. S. Taste and smell in disease. (Second of two parts). N. Engl. J. Med. *308*:1337, 1983.
24. Zegarelli, D. J. Burning mouth: an analysis of 57 patients. Oral Surg. *58*:34, 1984.
25. Gorsky, M., Silverman, S., Jr., and Chinn, H. Burning mouth syndrome: a review of 98 cases. J. Oral Med. *42*:7, 1987.
26. Silverman, S., Jr., Migliorati, C. A., Lozada-Nur, F., Greenspan, D., and Conant, M. A. Oral findings in people with or at high risk for AIDS: a study of 375 homosexual males. J. Am. Dent. Assoc. *112*:187, 1986.
27. Greenspan, D., Greenspan, J. S., Conant, M., Petersen, V., Silverman, S., Jr., and de-Souza, Y. Oral "hairy" leucoplakia in male homosexuals: evidence of association with both papillomavirus and a herpes-group virus. Lancet *2*:831, 1984.
28. Greenspan, D., Greenspan, J. S., Hearst, N. G., Pan, L. Z., Conant, M. A., Abrams, D. I., Hollander, H., and Levy, J. A. Relation of oral hairy leukoplakia to infection with the human immunodeficiency virus and the risk of developing AIDS. J. Infect. Dis. *155*:475, 1987.
29. Orlando, R. C., Bozymsk, E. M., Briggaman, R. A. Epidermolysis bullosa: gastrointestinal manifestations. Ann. Intern. Med. *81*:203, 1974.
30. Cheesbrough, M. J. Epidermolysis bullosa acquisita and Crohn's disease. Br. J. Dermatol. *99*:53, 1978.
31. Rabinowitz, B. W., Coldwell, J. G., and Jegathan, S. Epidermolysis bullosa and gastrointestinal anomalies. J. Pediatr. *95*:488, 1979.
32. Jordan, R. E., Kawana, S., and Fritz, K. A. Immunopathologic mechanisms in pemphigus and bullous pemphigoid. J. Invest. Dermatol. *85*:72s, 1985.
33. Daniels, T. E., and Quadra-White, C. Direct immunofluorescence in oral mucosal disease: a diagnostic analysis of 130 cases. Oral Surg. *51*:38, 1981.
34. Lozada, F., and Silverman, S., Jr. Erythema multiforme. Oral Surg. *46*:628, 1978.
35. Zweiban, B., Cohen, H., and Chandrasoma, P. Gastrointestinal involvement complicating Stevens-Johnson syndrome. Gastroenterology *91*:469, 1986.
36. Silverman, S., Jr., Gorsky, M., and Lozada-Nur, F. A prospec-

tive follow-up study of 570 patients with oral lichen planus: persistence, remission, and malignant association. Oral Surg. *60*:30, 1985.

37. Lefer, L. G. Lichen planus of the esophagus. Am. J. Dermatopathol. *4*:267, 1982.

38. Al-Shihabi, B. M. S., and Jackson, J. Dysphagia due to pharyngeal and oesophageal lichen planus. J. Laryngol. Otol. *96*:567, 1982.

39. Hansen, L. S., Silverman, S., Jr., and Daniels, T. E. The differential diagnosis of pyostomatitis vegetans and its relation to bowel disease. Oral Surg. *55*:363, 1983.

40. Estrin, H. M., and Hughes, R. W., Jr. Oral manifestations in Crohn's disease: report of a case. Am. J. Gastroenterol. *80*:352, 1985.

41. Basu, M. K., and Asquith, P. Oral manifestations of inflammatory bowel disease. Clin. Gastroenterol. *9*:307, 1980.

42. Rankin, G. B., Watts, H. D., Melnyk, C. S., and Kelley, M. L., Jr. National Cooperative Crohn's Disease Study: Extraintestinal manifestations and perianal complications. Gastroenterology *77*:914, 1979.

43. Mir-Madjlessi, S. H., Taylor, J. S., and Farmer, R. G. Clinical course and evolution of erythema nodosum and pyoderma gangrenosun in chronic ulcerative colitis: a study of 42 patients. Am. J. Gastroenterol. *80*:615, 1985.

44. Shuster, S., and Marks, J. Dermatogenic enteropathy, a new cause of steatorrhoea. Lancet *1*:1367, 1965.

45. Shuster, S. Systemic effects of skin disease. Lancet *1*:907, 1967.

46. Montagnani, A., Varotti, C., Patrone, P., Patrizi, A., Passarini, B., Corazza, G. R., Frazzoni, M., Milletti, S., Vaira, D., and Gasbarrini, G. Enteropatia dermatogenica. G. Ital. Dermatol. Venereol. *119*:287, 1984.

47. Watson, W. C., Paton, E., and Murray, D. Small-bowel disease in rosacea. Lancet *2*:47, 1965.

48. Knowles, J. P., Shuster, S., and Wells, G. C. Folic-acid deficiency in patients with skin disease. Lancet *1*:1138, 1963.

49. Bianchi, A, Chipman, D. W., Dreskin, A., and Rosensweig, N. S. Nutritional folic acid deficiency with megaloblastic changes in the small-bowel epithelium. N. Engl. J. Med. *282*:859, 1970.

50. Doran, C. K., Everett, M. A., and Welsh, J. D. The D-xylose tolerance test in patients with gluten-sensitive enteropathy and generalized dermatitis. Arch. Dermatol. *94*:574, 1966.

51. Preger, L., Maibach, H. I., Osborne, R. B., Shapiro, H. A., and Lee, J. C. On the question of psoriatic enteropathy. Arch. Dermatol. *102*:151, 1970.

52. Petersen, J. M., and Ferguson, D. R. Gastrointestinal neurofibromatosis. J. Clin. Gastroenterol. *6*:529, 1984.

53. Radhakrishnan, S., Varadarajan, V., and Narendran, S. Neurofibromatosis of the transverse colon and omentum. J. Indian Med. Assoc. *71*:287, 1978.

54. Cameron, A. J., Pairolero, P. C., Stanson, A. W., and Carpenter, H. A. Abdominal angina and neurofibromatosis. Mayo Clin. Proc. *57*:125, 1982.

55. Phat, V. N., Sezeur, A., Danne, M., Dupuis, D., and de la Vaissiera, G. Primary myenteric plexus alterations as a cause of

megacolon in von Recklinghausen's disease. Pathol. Biol. *28*:585, 1980.

56. Stamm, B., Hedinger, C. E., and Saremaslani, P. Duodenal and ampullary carcinoid tumors. A report of 12 cases with pathological characteristics, polypeptide content and relation to the MEN I syndrome and von Recklinghausen's disease. Virchows Arch. A *408*:475, 1986.

57. Nagao, T. Shigenobu, M., Teramoto, S., Fukuda, K., Mizushima, M., Nishioka, S., Mizuta, T., and Kojo, T. A case of malignant schwannoma of the mesentery in a patient with von Recklinghausen's disease. Gan No Rinsho *30*:968, 1984.

58. Keller, R. T., and Logan, G. M. Adenocarcinoma of the pancreas associated with neurofibromatosis. Cancer *39*:1264, 1977.

59. Gawkrodger, D. J., Blackwell, J. N., Gilmour, H. M., Rifkind, E. A., Heading, R. C., and Barnetson, R. S. Dermatitis herpetiformis: diagnosis, diet and demography. Gut *25*:151, 1984.

60. Weiner, S. R., and Utsinger, P. Whipple disease. Semin. Arthritis Rheum. *15*:157, 1986.

61. Callen, J. P. Acute febrile neutrophilic dermatosis (Sweet's syndrome) and the related conditions of bowel bypass syndrome and bullous pyoderma gangrenosum. Dermatol. Clin. *3*:153, 1985.

62. Gottlieb, S. H., and Schuster, M. M. Dermatoglyphic (fingerprint) evidence for a congenital syndrome of early onset constipation and abdominal pain. Gastroenterology *91*:428, 1986.

63. Bartolucci, E. G., Swan, R. H., and Hurt, W. C. Oral manifestations of hereditary hemorrhagic telangiectasia (Osler-Weber-Rendu disease). Review and case reports. J. Periodontol. *53*:163, 1982.

64. Wong, S. H., and Lau, W. Y. Blue rubber bleb nevus syndrome. Dis. Colon Rectum *25*:371, 1982.

65. Morgan, A. A. Recurrent gastrointestinal hemorrhage: an unusual cause. Am. J. Gastroenterol. *77*:925, 1982.

66. Lieberman, D. A., Krippaehne, W. W., and Melnyk, C. S. Colonic varices due to intestinal cavernous hemangiomas. Dig. Dis. Sci. *28*:852, 1983.

67. Betterle, C., Caretto, A., De-Zio, A., Pedini, B., Veller-Fornasa, C., Cecchetto, A., Accordi, F., and Peserico, A. Incidence and significance of organ-specific autoimmune disorders (clinical, latent or only autoantibodies) in patients with vitiligo. Dermatologica *171*:419, 1985.

68. Halevy, S., and Feuerman, E. J. The sign of Leser-Trelat. A cutaneous marker for internal malignancy. Int. J. Dermatol. *24*:359, 1985.

69. Roberts, J. L., Fishman, E. K., Hartman, D. S., Sanders, R., Goodman, Z., and Siegelman, S. S. Lipomatous tumors of the liver: evaluation with CT and US. Radiology. *158*:613, 1986.

70. Hegedus, S. I., and Schorr, W. F. Acquired hypertrichosis lanuginosa and malignancy. Arch. Dermatol. *106*:84, 1972.

71. Leavitt, J., Klein, I, Kendricks, F., Gavaler, J., and VanThiel, D. H. Skin tags: a cutaneous marker for colonic polyps. Ann. Intern. Med. *98*:928, 1983.

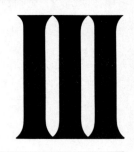

THE ESOPHAGUS: ANATOMY, PHYSIOLOGY, AND DISEASE

Anatomy and Developmental Anomalies

CHARLES E. POPE, II

ANATOMY

The esophagus is a hollow tube composed of both striated and smooth muscle, extending from the pharynx to the stomach. Its length, as measured in the cadaver, ranges from 25 to 35 cm in the adult. When measured by endoscope or with a manometric catheter, the transition from esophagus to stomach is found approximately 40 cm from the teeth. An accurate appraisal of the length of the adult esophagus can be made by measuring the distance from the lower incisor teeth to the xiphisternum with the patient lying supine with the head fully extended.[1] In infants and children, the esophageal length can be estimated by the use of regression equations employing height.[2] In its resting state the esophagus is collapsed; however, it is capable of distending to accommodate fluid and solid material. It is approximately 30 mm in lateral diameter and 19 mm in anteroposterior diameter. Both ends of the esophagus are specially modified to maintain closure under resting conditions. Only the upper portion has a clearly defined anatomic structure that marks this point of closure.

The esophagus begins as the apex of a funnel formed by the pharyngeal constrictors. When viewed from above, the mouth of the esophagus appears to be a slit running in a transverse direction. On either side of this slit are the pyriform sinuses (Fig. 31–1). This anatomic fact explains why it is important to keep a tube centered in the midline so that the tip of the tube does not stray into, and perhaps perforate, one of the laterally located pyriform sinuses.

The fibers of the cricopharyngeus muscle, traditionally considered to represent the upper esophageal sphincter, are transversely oriented and insert on the cricoid cartilage at the level of the sixth or seventh cervical vertebra. Two areas exist between the cricopharyngeus and the fibers of the inferior constrictor superiorly and the esophageal fibers inferiorly in which the muscle is attenuated and in which it is possible for diverticula to form.

Once the esophagus leaves this point of fixation, it is relatively mobile as it passes through the posterior mediastinum. It lies immediately posterior to the trachea and then close by the left main stem bronchus. However, it can be displaced relatively easily by enlargement or deviation of any of the structures. The esophagus swings slightly to the left of the mediastinum as it passes behind the heart and leaves the thorax through the diaphragmatic hiatus. During this course

through the mediastinum, impingement on the esophagus by osteophytes, an enlarged thyroid gland, an aortic aneurysm, a dilated left atrium, or hyperplastic carinal lymph nodes can be recognized during fluoroscopy by characteristic impressions on the barium-filled esophagus.

The area of the diaphragmatic hiatus has intrigued anatomists, as well as members of the other disciplines, and the names and subdivisions of this controversial 3- to 4-cm segment are indeed numerous. Many of the supposed anatomic features are an attempt to blend radiologic features with the prosector's imagination. A recent review of historical interest in this area presents evidence of international attention over the centuries.[3] Most anatomic dissections of this area show that the hiatal opening is located in the right crus of the diaphragm.[4] The hiatus has a vertical orientation, so that the esophagus enters through a 5- to 6-cm tunnel. The muscle bundles of the diaphragm are close enough to impinge on the esophagus during diaphragmatic contraction, and they may well play a role in the prevention of gastroesophageal reflux.

In its passage from the thoracic cavity to the abdominal cavity, the esophagus passes from a low-pressure area to a high-pressure area. How is this pressure differential maintained? A tight muscular seal of the diaphragm around the esophagus might lead to inability of large boluses to pass down the esophagus into the

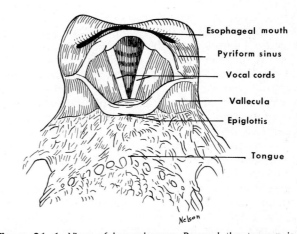

Figure 31–1. View of hypopharynx. Beyond the tongue is the epiglottis, in this view pulled forward to show the larynx. The valleculae are depressions at the base of the epiglottis. Behind the larynx is the opening of the esophagus, which appears as a crescentic slit. The pyriform sinuses are lateral to the esophageal opening.

stomach. The problem is met by allowing the diaphragm opening to be relatively large and to be filled with loose areolar tissue. The pressure seal is maintained by the phrenoesophageal membrane, a condensation of the transversalis fascia, which rises on the underportion of the diaphragm and extends up in a fibrous cone to insert on the esophagus 2 to 3 cm above the diaphragmatic opening. This phrenoesophageal ligament is in itself a source of surgical disagreement. Some surgeons believe that this ligament offers a firm anchor for sutures placed to reduce a hiatus hernia; other equally competent investigators find this wispy film of fibrous tissue difficult to locate, much less to utilize. When dissections of this area are made en bloc, there seems to be little question that in fact such a fibrous membrane does exist.[5, 6]

Until recently, most investigators thought that there was no anatomic evidence for a specialized structure that would correspond to the physiologically demonstrated lower esophageal sphincter. Yet, in a careful wax reconstruction of the lower esophageal zone, a specialized arrangement of the circular fibers was noted.[7] The circular muscle was arranged in a spiral configuration and blended with the inner oblique muscle zone of the stomach. Contraction of such spirally arranged fibers would tend to close the lower end of the esophagus.

A meticulous study of the lower end of the esophagus was performed in patients who were about to serve as organ donors and were being kept alive by artificial means.[8] In these patients, anatomic landmarks were marked *in vivo,* and distortions attendant on fixation could be corrected. This study suggests that there is, in fact, an asymmetric thickening of the circular muscle in the terminal esophagus that is above the angle of His (the junction of the tubular esophagus and the saccular stomach). The muscle fibers in the inner circular layer did not form rings but, rather, formed semicircular ovals that interdigitated both anteriorly and posteriorly with other fibers. Some of the semicircular fibers on the greater curvature side seemed to originate from the oblique gastric fibers.

Similar thickening of the circular muscle, but not the longitudinal muscle, was observed in opossums.[9] There was an increase in connective tissue in the manometrically determined sphincter zone as compared with the circular muscle in the body of the esophagus. The cell walls of the muscle within the sphincter zone were convoluted, and nerve endings contained agranular vesicles (usually thought to contain acetylcholine) and dense-core granules (thought to contain noncholinergic, nonadrenergic substances). Similar types of vesicles are reported in human material.[10]

The esophagus is lined with squamous mucosa, and the demarcation between esophageal and gastric mucosa can easily be seen as an irregular line, the ora serrata. As the esophagus is distended, this wavy line tends to straighten and become a simple circle. When viewed through an esophagoscope, the mucosa is fairly featureless, a glistening pink surface, without prominent blood vessels. At autopsy or at thoracotomy the mucosa is not firmly bound down to the underlying muscle. This leads to difficulties in precise localization of mucosal features and their relationship to other, more fixed structures.

The esophagus receives its blood supply mainly from small branches of the thoracic descending aorta. The uppermost portion of the esophagus is supplied by branches from the inferior thyroid artery. The lower portion of the esophagus is supplied from the left gastric artery. There is little overlap in the esophageal territory supplied by the left gastric artery and branches of the descending aorta, so that ischemia can be a problem in reconstructive surgery.

The venous drainage of the esophagus is also split into three portions. The upper third drains into the superior vena cava, the middle third into the azygos system, and the lower third into the portal vein via the gastric veins. All three systems have anastomotic connections that allow blood to be diverted if any one is blocked by disease processes. The most common manifestation of such blockage is esophageal varices resulting from portal hypertension. However, "upside down" varices can also be formed by blockage of the superior vena cava and dilatation of the anastomotic veins by the diverted venous flow.

The motor nerve supply to the esophagus arises in the dorsal motor nucleus of the vagus nerve and in the nucleus of the spinal accessory nerve. The latter innervates the high cervical portion of the esophagus; the vagus supplies most of the rest of the esophageal musculature. Fibers from the vagus anastomose in Auerbach's plexus with short postganglionic fibers that are distributed to the individual groups of muscle cells. The vagus nerve also carries afferent fibers; however, precise details of the afferent nerve supply of the esophagus are not well known. The esophagus receives sympathetic fibers from cervical sympathetic ganglia and from the ganglia in the thoracic sympathetic chain.

The lymphatics of the esophagus form a highly interconnected system, the upper third of the esophagus draining to the cervical nodes, the middle third to the mediastinal nodes, and the lower third to the celiac and gastric lymph nodes. The wide distribution and interconnection of the system help explain why tumors of the esophagus rarely remain localized.

Microscopic Anatomy

The esophagus is lined with stratified squamous epithelium and consists of a basal layer of two to three cells containing dark nuclei and a series of layers of squamous cells heaped upon one another (Fig. 31–2). The nuclei of these cells become pyknotic and eventually disappear before the luminal border is reached. There is no specialized structure on the free border of the squamous epithelium. Histochemical staining reveals that the squamous cells are filled with glycogen,[11] which allows staining *in vivo* with Lugol's solution, a method of demarcating squamous epithelium from transitional or gastric epithelium.[12] In addition, there

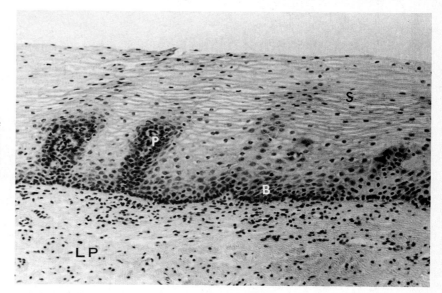

Figure 31–2. Normal esophageal mucosal biopsy. The basal layer (B) is approximately 10 per cent of the total epithelial thickness. The dermal pegs (P) extend approximately one half the distance to the epithelial surface. The lamina propria (LP) contains scattered round cells. The stratified squamous cells (S) blend with the basal layer. × 170.

are small lipid droplets and some phospholipids as well in the superficial squamous cells.[11] Scattered throughout the basal layer are a few argyrophilic cells and some melanocytes. There is a mucopolysaccharide coat on the most superficial esophageal cells that contains both neutral and acidic mucopolysaccharides and presumably serves a protective function.[13]

Into the epithelium protrude extensions of the lamina propria, the dermal pegs. These extend less than one half the way to the free luminal border. The dermal pegs often contain capillaries that are filled with erythrocytes. The lamina propria itself consists of loose connective tissue containing mononuclear cells, lymphocytes, and an occasional plasma cell. These cells may be scattered or occasionally organized into lymphoid nodules. Polymorphonuclear leukocytes are not normally seen. There are well organized mucus-producing glands, especially at the upper and lower ends of the esophagus. Ducts lead from the glands and empty onto the surface of the epithelium. A thin band of smooth muscle, the muscularis mucosae, separates the lamina propria from the underlying submucosa. The submucosa consists of loose connective tissue with fibrous and elastic elements as well as blood vessels and nerve fibers.

When the esophageal mucosa is examined with the scanning electron microscope (SEM), the squamous cells are seen as polygons with prominent intercellular ridges.[14, 15] Higher power studies by SEM show a latticework pattern of microridges on the surface of each cell.[16] When the mucosa is examined by transmission electron microscopy (TEM), the basal cells are seen to be quite close to one another, with prominent hemidesmosomes and a clearly demarcated basal lamina (Fig. 31–3). In the midzone, the cells are tightly apposed, with well-developed desmosomes (Fig. 31–4).

Underlying the submucosa are the outer muscular layers. Although the assumption has been that the top one third of the esophagus is striated muscle and the bottom two thirds are smooth muscle, recent studies

in human autopsy material reveal that only the top 5 per cent of the esophagus is exclusively striated muscle.[17] The lower half is smooth muscle, and the intervening zone varies in its composition of striated and smooth muscle among different individuals. There is manometric evidence that supports this observation: the rapid upstroke of the peristaltic wave characteristic of striated muscle is usually seen only in the first 2 to 4 cm below the upper esophageal sphincter. The muscle bands are arranged like coiled springs; the inner bands are horizontally wound and the outer bands have a steeper pitch, giving more of a longitudinal orientation. Between the two external muscle coats is the intramuscular nerve plexus named after Auerbach. Interconnections between the different plexuses form a local nerve network in the body of the esophagus. Presumably, this allows a certain degree of autonomy and allows integration of muscular activity in the esophagus without the necessity of connections with higher centers.

Unlike most of the rest of the gastrointestinal tract, the esophagus is not surrounded by serosa. This makes the surgeon's job more difficult when an anastomosis in the esophagus is being constructed, and the lack of a serosa may contribute to the more rapid spread of tumor cells outside the anatomic boundaries of the esophagus. The only serosal covering is the insertion of the phrenicoesophageal ligament, which arises from the abdomen and inserts into the lower one quarter of the esophagus.

DEVELOPMENTAL ANOMALIES

Fistulas

In embryologic development, the gut and respiratory tract start out as a single tube. However, they soon divide, so that by the second month the esophagus is in a dorsal position and the trachea and lung buds lie

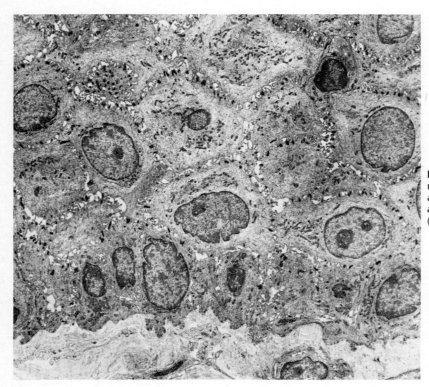

Figure 31–3. Transmission electron micrograph of normal human esophagus. The lamina propria is seen at the bottom of the picture. Cells in the basal layer are in close apposition with one another. × 8800. (Courtesy of H. T. Norris, M.D.)

Figure 31–4. Transmission electron micrograph of midzone layer of the normal human esophagus. The squamous cells are tightly bound to one another. × 8800. (Courtesy of H. T. Norris, M.D.)

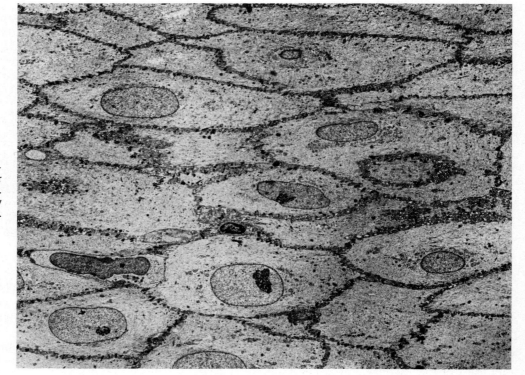

ventrally. It is therefore easy to see that the failure of these two important structures to separate completely might lead to difficulties at birth or soon thereafter. The most common abnormality is the *tracheoesophageal fistula*. In the most common type of tracheoesophageal fistula, the upper end of the esophagus ends in a blind sac and the lower end of the esophagus inserts posteriorly into the trachea (Fig. 31–5*A*). A child born with this abnormality will soon demonstrate overflow of mucus from the blind proximal pouch and will be troubled with aspiration. An X-ray of the abdomen will show the presence of air in the bowel, because it will enter freely from the connection to the trachea. This is the most common lesion and is found in from 85 to 90 per cent of tracheoesophageal fistulas presenting in the neonatal period. In the next most common lesion (Fig. 31–5*B*), the proximal portion of the esophagus is connected directly to the trachea and the distal portion of the esophagus ends as a pouch from the stomach. Those afflicted with this condition will suffer immediately from aspiration, and films of the abdomen will show no air in the bowel, as there is no pathway for air to enter the bowel. A much more uncommon type, when both trachea and esophagus are intact but connected by a fistulous tract, is the so-called H-type fistula (Fig. 31–5*C*). In childhood this is manifested as repeated bouts of pulmonary infection and abdominal distention, because crying causes air to be forced from the trachea to the esophagus.[18] Such a lesion can become manifest in adulthood and usually presents with repeated pulmonary infections.[19, 20]

Diagnosis. Diagnosis is usually easy when newborn infants have difficulty in handling secretions or when feeding provokes cyanotic coughing spells or other evidence of aspiration. A lipidol swallow with cine filming is the most helpful diagnostic maneuver. Occasionally, endoscopy will demonstrate the fistulous opening, but such openings are small and easily overlooked. Even in experienced hands, the correct classification of the type of anomaly is often made only at surgery.[21]

Diagnosis of the H-type fistula can be even more difficult in the adult than in the newborn. Probably this is because a small fistula, which only occasionally empties material into the lungs, is most compatible with survival into adult life. Occasionally, such a fistula is found during operation for an unrelated condition when positive pressure anesthesia causes massive inflation of the gastrointestinal tract. If a patient has repeated bouts of pulmonary infection and especially

if "aspiration" is seen during contrast radiography, it is sometimes necessary to employ a combination of cine studies and endoscopy of both the esophagus and the trachea with use of methylene blue to discover the site of the abnormal communication. A clever method of demonstrating an H-type fistula has been proposed, measuring the intragastric and intraesophageal oxygen concentration while ventilating the patient with 100 per cent oxygen.[22, 23] A step-up in oxygen concentration will be found as the sampling site is withdrawn from the stomach into the esophagus.

Treatment. Surgical correction is, of course, the only adequate form of therapy, but correct diagnosis of the extent of the abnormality, timing, and methods of repair are all important. In the most common type of abnormality, atresia with distal tracheoesophageal fistula (Fig. 31–5*A*), it has long been recommended to perform a gastrostomy for nutrition and then delay the procedure, especially if the child is premature or has other severe congenital abnormalities. However, improved neonatal care has now allowed definitive repair to be performed within several days of birth.[24]

There is still controversy as to whether division of the fistula and end-to-end anastomosis or ligation of the fistula and end-to-side anastomosis is the better procedure; the latter method is less apt to be followed by anastomotic stricture.[25] Regardless of the type of anastomosis, a problem always exists if the proximal and distal portions of the esophagus are widely separated. Although first handled by interposition of bowel, prolonged bougienage of the proximal esophagus can occasionally cause elongation with successful anastomosis. Even the space age has had influence on this field; the use of steel dilators, placed in proximal and distal pouches and pulled together by the field of a very strong electromagnet, has allowed successful anastomosis of widely separated proximal and distal pouches.[26]

Modern results of operative repair of tracheoesophageal fistula are quite good. An operative mortality from 3 to 5 per cent was reported in infants in relatively stable clinical condition; the presence of coexisting congenital abnormalities or severe infection raised the mortality to 41 per cent.[27] Another recent series confirms good results in uncomplicated cases; a higher mortality rate is present with coexisting malformations and other problems.[28] An arterial oxygen pressure of less than 60 mm Hg was often associated with death. Good results are probably due to the placement of a gastrostomy for alimentation, a nasogastric tube in the

Figure 31–5. Types of tracheoesophageal fistulas. *A*, The upper end of the esophagus ends in a blind sac; the lower end joins the trachea. *B*, The proximal esophagus joins the trachea; there is no connection of esophagus or trachea to the distal end of the esophagus. *C*, The trachea and esophagus are attached by a short connection, thus creating an H-fistula.

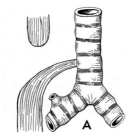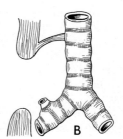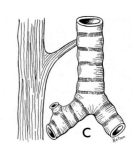

esophageal pouch to prevent aspiration, and improvement in neonatal care in general. It has been emphasized that careful preoperative evaluation for other congenital abnormalities is necessary so that coexisting abnormalities can be repaired at the same operation.[29]

Once the operative period is passed, the patient with a repaired tracheoesophageal fistula is still not free from problems. Postoperative reflux, which results in bronchitis and stricture formation, is very common.[30, 31] Abnormalities in esophageal motor function consisting of simultaneous contractions in the body of the esophagus leading to impaired clearance of intraesophageal acid are almost universal.[32] An intriguing observation that might explain these manometric findings is the relative paucity of ganglion cells in Auerbach's plexus in patients with atresia compared with control observations.[33]

An uncommon, but potentially treatable, condition found in patients who have had previous repair of a tracheoesophageal fistula is *reflex bradycardia*.[34] After apparently successful repair, these children developed attacks of apnea and cyanosis immediately after swallowing. Electrocardiographic monitoring confirmed the arrhythmia, and atropine gave a good therapeutic response.

Other Abnormalities

A much less commonly seen form of tracheoesophageal developmental anomaly is a congenital *bronchopulmonary foregut malformation*.[35] These lesions are collections of pulmonary tissue that lie either within the lung substance or are separated from the lung by another pleural covering and that, in addition, have a highly organized connection to the gut, usually to the lower end of the esophagus. Such patients commonly present either with a mediastinal mass or with repeated pulmonary infection. These lesions might arise either as a result of imperfect separation of the pulmonary and esophageal anlagen or by formation of an accessory pulmonary bud springing from the esophagus. If the communication between the pulmonary tissue and the esophagus is lost, a sequestration of pulmonary tissue will be found.

There are several types of congenital cysts that arise from or are closely applied to the esophagus[36] (Table 31–1). Congenital cysts are present in 1 in 8200 autopsies and can present with dysphagia or cough.[37] Alternatively, they can be asymptomatic and present as a mediastinal mass on a chest film taken for other reasons. Although most cysts are removed at surgery, one intrepid group first characterized the cyst with CT, then drained it transesophageally with an endoscopically placed needle.[38] The differential diagnosis of such cysts includes neuroenteric cysts. Neuroenteric cysts do not arise from the gastrointestinal tract but are derived from the primitive notochord and are associated with nonfusion of vertebral bodies. These cysts are usually lined by gastric epithelium.

Another result of a developmental quirk usually

Table 31–1. CONGENITAL CYSTS OF THE ESOPHAGUS

Type	Wall	Lining	Location
Duplication	Two muscle layers	Squamous, columnar, cuboidal, or ciliated	60% in lower one third
Bronchogenic	Cartilage	Ciliated	70% in lower one third
Gastric	Two muscle layers	Gastric	
Inclusion		Any cyst not meeting above criteria	

presenting in the neonatal period, but occasionally at an older age, is *vascular compression* of the esophagus by an *aberrant artery*. This lesion presents with dysphagia and has been dignified with the special title of *dysphagia lusoria*. This term is usually applied to an aberrant right subclavian artery springing from the descending aorta, but many other vascular abnormalities are possible, including a double aortic arch.[39] In embryologic life the aortic arch has both a right and a left arch. Failure of the right arch to resorb normally may lead to other vascular abnormalities. Diagnosis is usually made by the demonstration of an indentation on the column of barium high in the thorax. Esophagoscopy may show indentation of the esophagus but is not necessary for the diagnosis. Often such vascular abnormalities are associated with other cardiovascular abnormalities, and the prognosis of the patient is often dependent on the extent of the associated anomalies. Although aortic arch contrast injections can be performed, overlap of vessels sometimes makes interpretation difficult. Occasionally, the full extent of the abnormality is found only at the time of thoracotomy.

An additional rare congenital abnormality is a *congenital esophageal stenosis*.[40] This presents with dysphagia and is often quite resistant to dilation. On X-ray, localized linear outpouchings can sometimes be seen. When these strictures are resected, ciliated pulmonary epithelium and bronchial remnants are found.[41, 42] Another form of congenital stenosis can occur with maldevelopment of the muscularis mucosa and circular muscle.[43]

References

1. Kallor, G. J., Deshpande, A. H., and Collis, J. L. Observations on oesophageal length. Thorax *31*:284, 1976.
2. Strobel, C. T., Byrne, W. J., Ament, M. E., and Euler, A. R. Correlation of esophageal lengths in children with height: application to the Tuttle test without prior esophageal manometry. J. Pediatr. *94*:81, 1979.
3. Friedland, G. W. Historical review of the changing concepts of lower esophageal anatomy: 430 B.C.–1977. AJR *131*:373, 1978.
4. Delattre, J. F., Palot, J. P., Ducasse, A., Flament, J. B., and Hureau, J. The crura of the diaphragm and diaphragmatic passage. Anat. Clin. 7:271, 1985.
5. Strasberg, S. M., and Silver, M. D. The phrenoesophageal membrane. Surg. Forum *19*:294, 1968.
6. Friedland, G. W., Melcher, D. H., Berridge, F. R., and Gresham, G. A. Debatable points in the anatomy of the lower esophagus. Thorax *21*:487, 1966.

7. Jackson, A. J. The spiral constrictor of the gastroesophageal junction. Am. J. Anat. *151*:265, 1978.
8. Liebermann-Meffert, D., Allgöwer, M., Schmid, P., and Blum, A. L. Muscular equivalent of the lower esophageal sphincter. Gastroenterology *76*:31, 1979.
9. Seelig, L. L., and Goyal, R. K. Morphological evaluation of opossum lower esophageal sphincter. Gastroenterology *75*:51, 1978.
10. Cortesini, C., Pellegrini, M. S. F., and Romagnoli, P. The innervation of human lower esophageal sphincter. Gastroenterology *77*:819, 1979.
11. Hopwood, D., Logan, K. R., Coghill, G., and Bouchier, I. A. D. Histochemical studies of mucosubstances and lipids in normal human oesophageal epithelium. Histochem. J. *9*:153, 1977.
12. Nothmann, B. J., Wright, J. R., and Schuster, M. M. In vivo vital staining as an aid to identification of esophagogastric mucosal junction in man. Am. J. Dig. Dis. *17*:919, 1972.
13. Logan, K. R., Hopwood, D., and Milne, G. Ultrastructural demonstration of cell coat on the cell surfaces of normal human oesophageal epithelium. Histochem. J. *9*:495, 1977.
14. Carr, K. E., Shaw Dunn, J., and Toner, P. G. Scanning electron microscopy of the alimentary tract. Scott. Med. J. *19*:211, 1974.
15. Ackerman, L., Piros, J., de Carle, D., and Christensen, J. A scanning electron microscopic study of esophageal mucosa. *In* Proceedings of the Workshop on Advances in Biomedical Applications of the SEM (Part V), 1976, p. 247.
16. Goran, D. A., Shields, H. M., Bates, M. L., Zuckerman, G. R., and DeSchryver-Kecskemeti, K. Esophageal dysplasia. Gastroenterology *86*:39, 1984.
17. Meyer, G. W., Austin, R. M., Brady, C. E., III, and Castell, D. O. Muscle anatomy of the human esophagus. J. Clin. Gastroenterol. *8*:131, 1986.
18. Sundar, B., Guiney, E. J., and O'Donnell, B. Congenital H-type tracheoesophageal fistula. Arch. Dis. Child. *50*:862, 1975.
19. Lam, C. R. Diagnosis and surgical treatment of "H-type" tracheoesophageal fistulas. World J. Surg. *3*:651, 1979.
20. Enoksen, A., Lovaas, J., and Haavik, P. E. Congenital tracheo-oesophageal fistula in the adult. Scand. J. Thorac. Cardiovasc. Surg. *13*:173, 1979.
21. Hays, D. M., Wooley, M. M., and Snyder, W. H., Jr. Esophageal atresia and tracheoesophageal fistula: management of the uncommon types. Pediatr. Surg. *1*:240, 1966.
22. Korones, S. B., and Evans, L. J. Measurement of intragastric oxygen concentration for the diagnosis of H-type tracheoesophageal fistula. Pediatrics *60*:450, 1977.
23. Powers, W. F. Further experience with intragastric oxygen measurement to diagnose H-type tracheoesophageal fistula. Pediatrics *63*:668, 1979.
24. Tyson, K. R. T. Primary repair of esophageal atresia without staging or preliminary gastrostomy. Ann. Thorac. Surg. *21*:378, 1976.
25. Touloukian, R. J., Pickett, L. K., Spackman, T., and Biancani, P. Repair of esophageal atresia by end-to-side anastomosis and ligation of the tracheoesophageal fistula: a critical review of 18 cases. J. Pediatr. Surg. *9*:305, 1974.
26. Hendren, W. H., and Hale, J. R. Electromagnetic bougienage to lengthen esophageal segments in congenital esophageal atresia. N. Engl. J. Med. *293*:428, 1975.
27. Strodel, W. E., Coran, A. G., Kirsh, M. M., Weintraub, W. H., Wesley, J. R., and Sloan, H. Esophageal atresia. Arch. Surg. *114*:523, 1979.
28. Filston, H. C., Rankin, J. S., and Grimm, J. K. Esophageal atresia. Ann. Surg. *199*:532, 1984.
29. Mollitt, D. L., and Golladay, E. S. Management of the newborn with gastrointestinal anomalies and tracheoesophageal fistula. Am. J. Surg. *146*:792, 1983.
30. Dudley, N. E., and Phelan, P. D. Respiratory complications in long-term survivors of oesophageal atresia. Arch Dis. Child. *51*:279, 1976.
31. Pieretti, R., Shandling, B., and Stephens, C. A. Resistant esophageal stenosis associated with reflux after repair of esophageal atresia: a therapeutic approach. J. Pediatr. Surg. *9*:355, 1974.
32. Werlin, S. L., Dodds, W. J., Hogan, W. J., Glicklich, M., and Arndorfer, R. Esophageal function in esophageal atresia. Dig. Dis. Sci. *26*:796, 1981.
33. Nakazato, Y., Landing, B. H., and Wells, T. R. Abnormal Auerbach's plexus in the esophagus and stomach of patients with esophageal atresia and tracheoesophageal fistula. J. Pediatr. Surg. *21*:831, 1986.
34. Lukacs, V. F., Bognar, M., Jambori, M., and Denes, J. Reflex bradycardia: a grave complication of oesophageal atresia repair. Acta Paediatr. Acad. Sci. Hung. *19*:167, 1978.
35. Heithoff, K. B., Sane, S. M., Williams, H. J., Jarvis, C. J., Carter, J., Kane, P., and Brennom, W. Bronchopulmonary foregut malformations: a unifying etiological concept. AJR *126*:46, 1976.
36. Arbona, J. L., Figueroa Fazzi, J. G., and Mayoral, J. Congenital esophageal cysts: case report and review of the literature. Am. J. Gastroenterol. *79*:177, 1984.
37. Bowton, D. L., and Katz, P. O. Esophageal cyst as a cause of chronic cough. Chest *86*:150, 1984.
38. Kuhlman, J. E., Fishman, E. K., Wang, K., and Siegelman, S. S. Esophageal duplication cyst: CT and transesophageal needle aspiration. AJR *145*:531, 1985.
39. Arciniegas, E., Hakimi, M., Hertzler, J. H., Farooki, Z. Q., and Green, E. W. Surgical management of congenital vascular rings. J. Thorac. Cardiovasc. Surg. *77*:721, 1979.
40. Bluestone, C. D., Kerry, R., and Seiber, W. K. Congenital esophageal stenosis. J. Laryngol. *79*:1095, 1969.
41. Fonkalsrud, E. W. Esophageal stenosis due to tracheobronchial remnants. Am. J. Surg. *124*:101, 1972.
42. Anderson, L. S., Shackelford, G. D., Mancilla-Jimenez, R., and McAlister, W. H. Cartilaginous esophageal ring: a cause of esophageal stenosis in infants and children. Radiology *108*:665, 1973.
43. Groote, A. D., Laurini, R. N., and Polman, H. A. A case of congenital esophageal stenosis. Hum. Pathol. *16*:1170, 1985.

32

Physiology of the Esophagus

N. E. DIAMANT

Esophageal function is the result of numerous interacting control mechanisms that not only regulate those activities arising from esophageal continuity with the rest of the gut but also tie the esophagus intimately to other systems and organs, such as the central nervous system, the heart, and the lungs. Not surprisingly, therefore, esophageal function as well as dysfunction must be viewed from a much broader perspective. Several recent reviews cover the topic in detail.[1-4]

Knowledge of the more basic physiology of the esophagus has derived primarily from animal species, such as the cat, dog, sheep, and opossum, and to a lesser extent from studies in humans and nonhuman primates. There are marked between-species differences that invite some caution when applying the animal observations to normal human esophageal physiology. For example, in some species (e.g., rat, guinea pig, rabbit, dog, sheep, cow) the esophageal body is composed entirely of striated muscle, in other species (e.g., amphibians, birds) it is composed entirely of smooth muscle, and in still others, including human, opossum, cat, monkey, pig, and horse, the esophagus is a mixture of both types. This said, it is helpful to consider normal control of the human esophagus with the following more general functional characteristics in mind.

1. Functionally the esophagus can be divided into three zones: the upper esophageal sphincter (UES), the esophageal body, and the lower esophageal sphincter (LES). The function of the esophageal sphincters is coordinated not only with the activity of the esophageal body but also with the activity in the oropharynx and stomach, which abut on the UES and LES, respectively.

2. A number of control mechanisms for esophageal motor activity exist, located within the central nervous system as well as peripherally within the intramural nerves and muscles. Of particular interest, the esophagus is one region where voluntary and involuntary control mechanisms act together, and the activity of two different types of muscle is intimately coordinated.

3. Deglutition, or the act of swallowing, is the primary initiator of integrated esophageal activity. However, between swallows the esophageal body and its sphincters are not entirely passive but serve other functions.

4. In the human, normal activity of the esophagus is programmed to proceed in the aboral direction, although there is provision for necessary retrograde activity, such as in belching or vomiting.

ANATOMY OF THE ESOPHAGUS

The esophageal length is about 20 cm. Five per cent of the upper esophageal body, including the UES and the muscles involved in the buccopharyngeal phase of swallowing, is entirely striated muscle. Approximately 50 to 60 per cent of the distal esophagus, including the LES, is entirely smooth muscle, with the circular muscle layer extending more proximally than the longitudinal layer. The transition zone of striated and smooth muscle includes as much as 35 to 40 per cent of the intervening esophageal length. The area where muscle is equally striated and smooth is found about 5 cm below the proximal portion of the cricopharyngeus muscle.[5]

Striated Muscle

Pharynx

In the oropharynx and hypopharynx, the superior, middle, and inferior constrictor muscles form the lateral and posterior walls of a contractile funnel that leads to the upper end of the esophagus at the UES. Anteriorly the funnel is much less regular and is composed of numerous muscle, bony, and cartilaginous portions of such structures as the uvula, tongue, salpingopharyngeal folds, epiglottis, and larynx. As a result of this particular structural complexity and its associated functional complexity, there is ample scope for difficulty in swallowing during the buccopharyngeal stage if neural or muscular control mechanisms are disturbed.[6]

Upper Esophageal Sphincter

The UES has a length of 2 to 4.5 cm on manometry and is formed primarily by the horizontal fibers of the cricopharyngeus muscle, often with a small portion of the inferior pharyngeal constrictor muscle above. The cricopharyngeus muscle arises anteriorly from each side of the lower third of the cricoid cartilage and forms a loop posteriorly with its upper border at approximately the C6 to C7 vertebral level. The anterior wall of the UES is rigid because of the cricoid cartilage and other structures that form the posterior wall of the larynx.[2-4, 6] Owing to the anatomic features, the UES forms a transverse slit-like structure when closed, termed the lip of the esophageal mouth. The cricopharyngeus muscle can frequently be seen as a posterior indentation, the cricopharyngeal bar, on barium X-ray (Fig. 32–1). Posterolaterally, a potential separation between the cricopharyngeus muscle and the inferior constrictor is the location for a Zenker's diverticulum, which sometimes occurs.

Esophageal Body

The striated muscle portion of the esophageal body begins at the inferior border of the cricopharyngeus muscle. Generally there is a longitudinal outer layer and a circular inner layer. The longitudinal layer extends more distally than the circular layer.

Smooth Muscle

Esophageal Body

The smooth muscle in the human esophageal body also has an outer longitudinal and a thicker inner circular layer, the latter extending more proximally. Cell-to-cell contact is common,[7] particularly in the circular layer, allowing the esophageal smooth muscle to behave as a functional syncytium.

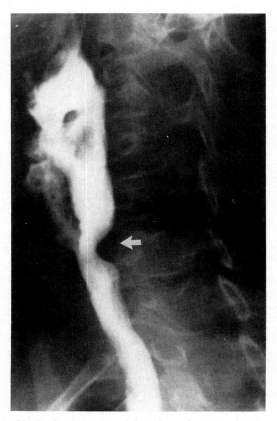

Figure 32–1. Cricopharyngeal bar *(arrow)* seen as a posterior indentation on barium X-ray of pharynx and upper esophagus.

Lower Esophageal Sphincter

At the gastroesophageal junction, which is characterized by a high-pressure zone 2 to 4 cm long and has the functional and radiologic features of a sphincter, there is a thicker ring of circular smooth muscle. The circular muscle of this sphincter zone is also intimately connected with some smooth muscle fibers of the stomach[8] and not surprisingly shares some functional characteristics with the upper stomach. For example, sphincter relaxation and receptive relaxation of the fundus occur on swallowing. In the human, many smooth muscle cells in the region of the LES show numerous branches and increased cell-to-cell contacts, which probably relate to the ability of this zone to maintain tone.[7]

INNERVATION OF THE ESOPHAGUS

The esophageal innervation provides the mechanism for excitation of the muscle at all levels and serves as the coordinating mechanism for the swallowing sequence in the buccopharyngeal region and the striated muscle portion of the esophagus. In addition, it affords at least three potential control mechanisms for coordination of peristalsis within the smooth muscle portion of the esophagus. Finally, it serves as the major control mechanism for normal function of both the UES and LES, and it includes the network for sensory and reflex modulation of the esophageal body and sphincter motor activities.

Extrinsic Innervation

Swallowing Center

Extrinsic control for esophageal motor function resides in a brainstem "swallowing center" (Fig. 32–2).[1, 4, 9, 10] This center, composed of two intimately connected half centers, is located in the medulla and pons and has three functional components: an afferent reception system, an efferent system of motor neurons, and a complex organizing or internuncial system of neurons. These components can also be conveniently subdivided topographically into buccopharyngeal (to include the UES), esophageal, and LES control functions. This latter division has some practical significance because although voluntary initiation of swallowing through activation of frontal cortical centers readily induces the buccopharyngeal stages of swallowing, the progression of the process into the esophageal phase is highly dependent on peripheral sensory input from oropharyngeal structures.

Afferent Reception. Afferent information from the periphery ultimately enters into the solitary tract, the afferent reception portion of the swallowing center. This sensory information can initiate deglutition and the swallowing sequence, alter previously initiated activity in the swallowing center and therefore modify ongoing motor activity, or function within reflexes

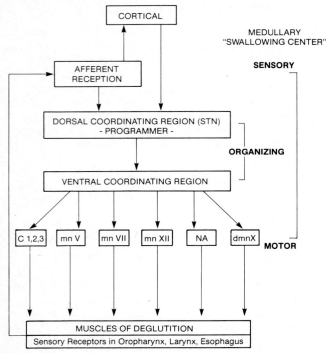

Figure 32–2. Diagram representing the central organization of swallowing. STN, Solitary tract nucleus; mn, motor nucleus; NA, nucleus ambiguus; dmnX, dorsal motor nucleus of Vagus; C1,2,3, cervical levels.

affecting the esophageal body and its sphincters independent of swallowing. Sensory information from the buccopharyngeal area and other information that is involved with this stage of the swallowing mechanism enters through extravagal cranial nerve (trigeminal, facial, hyoglossal, and glossopharyngeal) and vagal nerve pathways.[6, 9] Sensory information from the entire esophagus, including the sphincters, is carried in the vagus nerve, with the cell bodies in the nodose ganglion. However, there is also evidence for passage of sensory information via the sympathetic nerves to the spinal cord segments T3 to T12.[11] This sensory pathway may be of particular relevance when considering the differentiation of atypical chest pain of either cardiac or esophageal origin, and the effect of esophageal stimulation on the heart.

Coordinating Region. The portion of the swallowing center that programs the entire swallowing sequence is probably located in the solitary tract nucleus (STN) and the neighboring reticular substance.[10] One level of integration (dorsal) within this center is involved in the initiation of swallowing and organizing of the entire swallowing sequence, whereas a second level of organization (ventral) appears to serve as a connecting pathway to the various motor neuron pools involved in the swallowing sequence. The latter would also include integration of the swallowing sequence with the activity in other medullary centers such as the respiratory center.

Efferent Output. Motor neurons involved in the swallowing sequence lie mainly in the trigeminal, facial,

and hypoglossal nuclei; the nucleus ambiguus (for esophageal striated muscle); and the dorsal motor nucleus of the vagus (for esophageal smooth muscle).[1, 6, 9] The vagus nerve receives fibers from both the nucleus ambiguus and the dorsal motor nucleus, innervating the striated and smooth muscle portions of the esophagus, respectively, including the sphincters. Classically, in the human, the cervical esophagus is innervated by the recurrent laryngeal nerves and the more distal esophagus is innervated by the branches from the thoracic vagal trunks. In the region of the cricopharynx, fibers from the pharyngeal branches of the vagus and the superior laryngeal nerves intersect with fibers from the recurrent laryngeal nerves. Doubling of both motor and sensory innervation in this area probably serves a protective role required by the proximity of the cervical esophagus to the airway.

Sympathetic Nerves

The efferent sympathetic connections to the esophagus arise in the cervical ganglia and ganglia of the paravertebral chains and reach the esophagus by accompanying the vascular supply and, to a lesser extent, through connections to the vagus nerves. The preganglionic cell bodies are said to lie in spinal segments T5 and T6.[12] In humans, sympathetic innervation to the LES likely also occurs via the splanchnic nerves, as in the cat.

Intramural Innervation

A myenteric nerve plexus is found in both the striated and smooth muscle segments of the esophagus; this is less well developed in the striated muscle portion. The submucosal plexus is present but also sparse.[3]

Striated Muscle

In the striated muscle, the plexuses presumably serve mainly a sensory role, although an inhibitory pathway to the LES may also exist therein.[13] It is generally held that the vagal postganglionic fibers pass directly to innervate the striated muscle fibers through cholinergic, nicotinic receptors (Fig. 32–3).[1, 3, 4]

Smooth Muscle

In the smooth muscle segment, the relationships between morphology and function of the nerve plexuses are yet to be determined.[3, 14, 15] There are two important types of effector neurons within the system, one capable of mediating cholinergic excitation of both longitudinal and circular layers of smooth muscle predominantly through M2 receptors, and the other mediating nonadrenergic, noncholinergic (NANC) inhibition mainly of the circular muscle layer (Fig. 32–3).[1–4, 16–21] The neurotransmitter released by the latter type of neuron is unknown, although purine nucleotides and peptide hormones such as vasoactive intestinal

A. STRIATED MUSCLE
(UES and Esophageal Body)

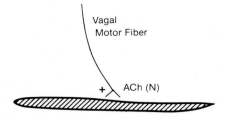

B. SMOOTH MUSCLE
(Esophageal Body and LES)

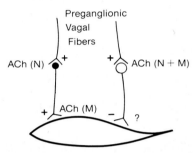

Figure 32–3. Major known motor innervation of the esophagus. Interneurons, adrenergic innervation, and other possible neurotransmitters are not shown as the circuitry is not known, a role other than modulatory is not established for adrenergic supply, and the functional role of other putative neurotransmitters is unclear. ●, Excitatory neuron; ○, inhibitory neuron; ACh, acetylcholine; N, nicotinic; M, muscarinic.

polypeptide (VIP) have been among the substances proposed.[1–4, 22, 23] Both types of neurons are excited by cholinergic input from preganglionic vagal fibers and intramural interneurons. Cholingeric excitation of the excitatory neuron is nicotinic whereas that of the NANC neuron can be muscarinic (M1 receptors) as well. Both types of neurons innervate the smooth muscle body and the LES.

Identification of various peptides, including opiates within the esophageal neural tissues, has raised questions as to the functional importance of these peptides.[24] Furthermore, it is apparent both *in vivo* and *in vitro* that the smooth muscle segment of the esophagus, especially in the region of the LES (Table 32–2), is sensitive to the action of most peptide hormones and drugs, as well as to other substances, such as histamine, prostaglandins, dopamine, and serotonin.[1–4, 22] The majority of these agents can act on muscle, nerve, or both, and there are significant species variations. Their importance awaits characterization of the various types of myenteric plexus neurons and the pharmacologic, electrophysiologic, and morphologic properties of these neurons. Also, the nature of the plexus circuitry and the interaction of all the potential modulating factors require elucidation. Until then, it is reasonable to consider that the cholinergic excitatory neuron and the NANC inhibitory neuron represent the basic effec-

tor machinery of the smooth muscle segment of the esophagus. Nevertheless, knowledge derived to date has provided some insight into potential therapeutic uses of pharmacologic agents that can act on esophageal nerve, muscle, or both.

Sympathetic Nerves

Sympathetic nerves are also present within the myenteric plexus of the striated and smooth muscle portions of the esophagus. At present there is no reason to suspect a motor function for this innervation in the striated muscle portion, although the UES may be an exception.[6] In the smooth muscle portion, these nerves make both axosomatic and axoaxonic contact with neurons of the plexuses, but only sparse contact with the smooth muscle cells themselves. Therefore, sympathetic nerves serve mainly to modulate the activity of other neurons and the release of their respective neurotransmitters. Furthermore, on swallowing, peristalsis and LES relaxation continue despite adrenergic blockade. As a result, it is unlikely that sympathetic nerves participate in central control of the peristaltic sequence or LES function with swallowing, but they act to modify features such as contraction amplitude and velocity and LES tone.[25, 26] Beta-adrenergic effect is inhibitory through both beta-1 and beta-2 receptors, the latter on the muscle, the former perhaps prejunctional in the myenteric plexus and acting to decrease acetylcholine release.[25] Alpha-adrenergic effect is excitatory, acting through receptors on the muscle (alpha-1) or on neurons (alpha-2), the latter both increasing acetylcholine release and decreasing release of the unknown inhibitory transmitter.[26]

COORDINATED ESOPHAGEAL MOTOR ACTIVITY

Accurate and reliable measurement techniques are of particular importance in assessing coordinated esophageal motility.[27–29] Furthermore, structural and functional factors affect measurements such as pressures, especially in sphincter areas. For example, marked radial asymmetry of the UES, and to a lesser extent the LES (Fig. 32–4, Table 32–1), makes pressure measurement in only one axis an unreliable index of that sphincter's true state of contraction.[30–32] These factors, along with variability introduced by the measurement techniques themselves, require that each laboratory establish normal values. Measurement techniques are not discussed further here.

At rest, the esophageal body is quiet and without motor activity, whereas the sphincters at either end maintain a contraction that can be measured manometrically as a high-pressure zone and characterized as resting tone. Tone in the UES and LES can be viewed as a protective barrier to esophagopharyngeal and gastroesophageal reflux, respectively. In addition, the sphincters also seal off the esophagus, which lies largely in a chest cavity of negative pressure. Between swal-

UES   **LES**

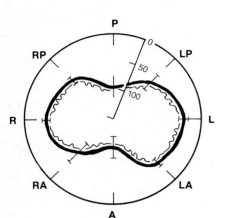   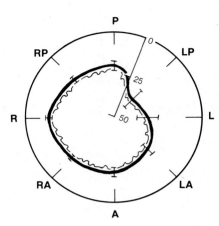

Figure 32–4. Radial asymmetry of the upper (UES) and lower (LES) esophageal sphincters. R, right; RP, right posterior; P, posterior; LP, left posterior; L, left; LA, left anterior; A, anterior; RA, right anterior. (UES profile adapted from Winans, C. Gastroenterology. *63*:738, 1972; LES profile adapted from Winans, C. Dig. Dis. Sci. *4*:348, 1977.)

lows, neither the resting tone of the sphincters nor the quiescence of the esophageal body is static and unchanging. Within the esophageal body, peristaltic or nonperistaltic esophageal contractions can arise independent of swallowing with such events as gastroesophageal reflux and stress.[33, 34] In the sphincter regions, continuous change is the rule and therefore measurement of sphincter pressure at one point in time is often misleading.

The classic coordinated motor pattern of the esophagus is initiated by the act of swallowing and is called *primary peristalsis* (Fig. 32–5). In the absence of a bolus, that is, with a dry swallow, passage of the swallow-induced activity beyond the buccopharyngeal phase occurs less frequently than when a bolus is present (wet swallow). During the buccopharyngeal phase of swallowing, the bolus is moved voluntarily into the pharynx, and the pharyngeal contractions are initiated. Thereafter, the process becomes involuntary. A rapidly progressing pharyngeal contraction transfers the bolus through a relaxed UES into the esophagus and, as the UES closes, a progressive circular contraction begins in the upper esophagus and proceeds distally along the esophageal body to propel the bolus through a relaxed LES. The LES subsequently closes

with a prolonged contraction. The esophagus shortens by about 10 per cent on swallowing, presumably through longitudinal muscle contraction, and this can be reflected in considerable transient upward movement of the LES.[35]

Secondary peristalsis is a progressive contraction in the esophageal body that is induced not by a swallow but rather by stimulation of sensory receptors in the esophageal body. Secondary peristalsis is usually attributed to distention by a bolus, such as esophageal content not completely cleared by a primary swallow, or refluxed gastric content. Secondary peristalsis occurs only in the esophagus, usually begins at or above a level corresponding to the location of the stimulus, closely resembles the peristalsis induced by a swallow, and is also mediated by a swallowing center.

In the absence of connections to the swallowing center, a local intramural mechanism can at times take over as a reserve mechanism to produce peristalsis in the smooth muscle segment of the esophagus. This has been called *tertiary peristalsis*,[36, 37] and the term should not be confused with tertiary contractions, which are incoordinate or simultaneous contractions in the esophageal body.[38]

Upper Esophageal Sphincter

At rest the UES is tonically closed owing to continuous neural excitation, and in addition there is a small passive component to the tone. The slit-like structure of the UES gives marked radial asymmetry to the profile of the intraluminal pressure[30] (Fig. 32–4). Pressures are higher anteriorly and posteriorly, corresponding to the position of the cricopharyngeus muscle sling and its action (Table 32–1). Excitatory discharge to the UES and UES pressure increase with each inspiration, providing extra protection for the airway and preventing entry of air into the esophagus. In addition, slow distention and acid in the upper esophagus cause a reflex increase in UES pressure,[32] as do a Valsalva

Table 32–1. TYPICAL MANOMETRIC PRESSURES (mm Hg)

	Mean	Range
Resting UES Pressure		
Posterior axis	101	60–142
Anterior axis	84	55–123
Lateral axis	48	30–65
Resting LES Pressure		10–26
Esophageal Contraction Amplitude		
Distal esophagus		50–110

(Data from Gerhardt, D. G., and Castell, D. O.;[32] and Benjamin, S. B., and Castell, D. O.[72])

UES, Upper esophageal sphincter; LES, lower esophageal sphincter.

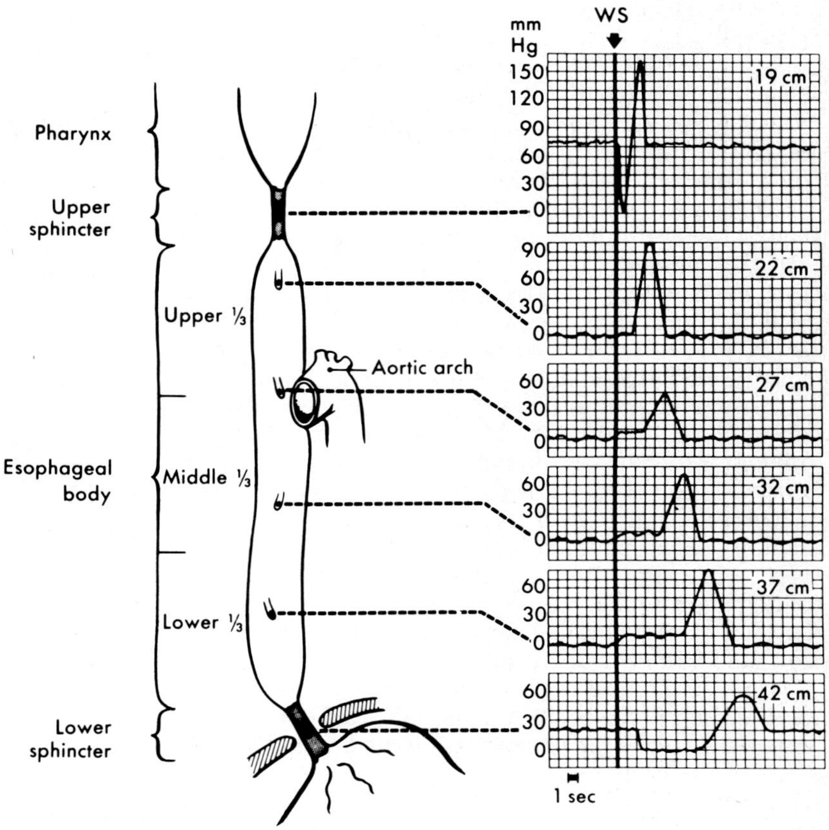

Figure 32–5. Manometric pressure changes with a swallow of an 8 cc bolus (WS). Distance (cm) from nares is shown on tracings. Proximal and distal tracings are from the upper (UES) and lower (LES) esohageal sphincters, respectively. Immediately after a swallow, UES pressure falls transiently. Shortly thereafter, LES pressure falls and remains low until the peristaltic contraction passing aborally through the UES and then the esophageal body closes the LES. (Reproduced by permission from Dodds, W. J. *In* Margulis, A. R., and Burhenne, H. J. (eds.). Alimentary Tract Radiology. 3rd ed. Vol. 1., pp. 529–603. St. Louis, 1983, The C. V. Mosby Co.)

maneuver, gagging, and secondary peristalsis.[4, 32] Some of these excitatory reflex mechanisms may explain the globus sensation in certain patients. On the other hand, belching, vomiting, and abrupt esophageal distention are associated with a fall in UES pressure to permit release of esophageal contents or decompression of the esophagus.[39]

Within 0.2 to 0.3 sec after a swallow, excitatory discharge to the UES ceases transiently in exquisite coordination with the rapid sequence of muscle activity in the buccopharyngeal phase of swallowing. This is entirely controlled by the central control mechanism. Cessation of neural excitation to the UES and elevation and forward movement of the cricoid cartilage act together to decrease the UES resting pressure for less than 1 sec and to open the sphincter on swallowing. A short burst of excitation and contraction follow.

Esophageal Body

As the peristaltic contraction passes through the esophagus, the amplitude of the waves is highest in the distal 5 cm. Waves of low pressure are seen 4 to 6 cm below the upper esophageal sphincter and over a length of 2 to 3 cm, a region where striated and smooth muscle components are approximately equal in amount. Duration of the contractions is usually less than 7 sec, and normal contraction amplitudes rarely exceed 150 mm Hg. It takes 6 to 8 sec for peristalsis

to proceed through the esophagus with an average velocity of 3 to 4 cm/sec. Proximally, the velocity is 3 to 3.5 cm/sec, increasing in the lower third to 5 cm/sec and slowing to 2 cm/sec in the very last 2 to 3 cm of the esophageal body.[1–4, 38]

Striated Muscle

The striated muscle contraction is directed and coordinated by sequential excitation through vagal fibers programmed by the central control mechanism.[1–4, 9, 40] Afferent information from the esophagus and elsewhere has a significant effect on the central program to alter the force and velocity of the peristaltic contraction in both the striated and the smooth muscle segments of the esophagus (see later discussion).

Smooth Muscle

The control mechanisms directing and modulating peristalsis in the smooth muscle segment of the esophagus have generated considerable controversy. At least four different potential mechanisms for the production of peristalsis in the smooth muscle segment are known, and these reside at different levels of control: (1) stimuli from the central program cause different efferent motor fibers to fire sequentially during both primary and secondary peristalsis in the smooth as well as the striated muscle esophagus;[40, 41] (2) there is an intramural neural mechanism that can be excited to produce peristalsis near the onset of vagal stimulation or intraluminal balloon distention—the "on-contraction";[17, 18, 20, 21, 42] (3) another intramural neural mechanism can be excited to produce peristalsis onset after the vagal or balloon stimulus is terminated—the "off-contraction" or "off-response";[17, 18, 20, 21, 42] and (4) some type of mechanism exists for myogenic propagation of a contraction, which therefore indicates that muscle properties contribute to the nature of peristalsis.[43, 44]

In the human, cat, and monkey, swallow-induced peristalsis is highly atropine-sensitive[45] and augmented by cholinergic agonists and inhibition of cholinesterase.[46, 47] Therefore, in these species direct smooth muscle excitation by the intramural cholinergic neurons is the predominant mechanism for muscle contraction during normal peristalsis. This would dictate that coordination of the excitation, and therefore of the peristaltic contraction, is primarily the result of sequencing and activation of the intramural excitatory neurons, not primarily a function of muscle characteristics. A question then arises: How does the centrally programmed sequential vagal discharge interact with the local control mechanisms to produce normal primary and secondary peristalsis?

Two main hypotheses for control of peristalsis in the smooth muscle have arisen. The first hypothesis proposes that the primary excitation and coordinating mechanism for peristalsis is the central program directing the cholinergic excitatory neurons as the final common pathway to the esophageal smooth muscle. With this hypothesis, the intramural mechanism would be viewed as normally modulating activity through local and central reflexes and providing a local mechanism for distal inhibition.

The second hypothesis proposes that the swallowing center triggers the peripheral intramural mechanism, which then is primarily responsible for coordinating the peristaltic contraction, although it is modulated by the central mechanism through temporal and frequency differences in vagal discharge. This derives from the fact that in some species, such as the opossum and cat, the intramural mechanism is perfectly capable of producing neurally mediated peristalsis on its own either in the absence of extrinsic vagal innervation or with experimental vagal stimulation that does not incorporate sequential excitation.[17, 18, 21, 22, 40–42] How muscle properties contribute to peristalsis directed by either central or intramural neural mechanisms is not clear.

Intramural Control Mechanisms. Dodds and his coworkers, using vagal stimulation with selected parameters, characterized the two intramural neural mechanisms for control of peristalsis in the opossum and cat (Fig. 32–6).[17, 18, 21] The "on-contraction" (A wave) has an apparent propagation velocity that resembles that of swallow-induced peristalsis, is atropine-sensitive, and is induced by low-frequency stimulation. On the other hand, the "off-contraction" (B wave) has a much more rapid propagation, similar to the "off-response" delays of serial muscle strips *in vitro*, is atropine-resistant, and occurs at higher stimulation frequencies. The on-contraction mechanism is attributed to the

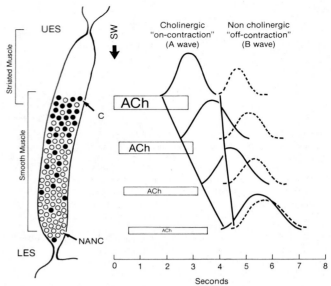

Figure 32–6. Schematic drawing of cholinergic (C, ●) and noncholinergic (NANC, ○) influences in the opossum smooth muscle esophagus, and the potential interplay of two intramural neural mechanisms for the production of peristalsis. Cholinergic influence is most prominent proximally and decreases distally; the reverse is true for the noncholinergic influence. Where the cholinergic influence is dominant, the "on-contraction" (A wave) will occur; where the noncholinergic influence is dominant, or with cholinergic blockade, contraction will occur predominantly as an "off-contraction" (B wave). Release of acetylcholine (ACh) and the noncholinergic inhibitory neurotransmitter could potentially occur through either activity of the intramural nerve plexus itself or activation of the intramural neurons by preganglionic vagal fibers. (Adapted from Crist, J, et al.: Proc. Natl. Acad. Sci. *81*:3595, 1984, and Gilbert, R. J., and Dodds, W. J.: Am. J. Physiol., *250*:G50, 1986.)

activation of the excitatory cholinergic neurons, although the nature of the circuitry dictating the progressive distal delays is not known.[16] The off-contraction mechanism of contraction has been attributed to a muscle response that follows muscle hyperpolarization through activation of the NANC inhibitory neurons, membrane depolarization, and contraction owing both to passive rebound as well as to some type of active excitation.[4, 48, 49] This supposes that the NANC inhibition is initiated almost simultaneously at all levels and that regional differences in the muscle or neural properties produce a delay to the onset of contraction that is progressively larger along the smooth muscle.

More recent studies in the opossum have shown that the cholinergic on-contraction mechanism is more prominent proximally and decreases distally,[20, 21] whereas the noncholinergic off-contraction is more prominent distally. Therefore, in the opossum, both intramural mechanisms appear to contribute to peristalsis. Furthermore, in this species, different frequencies of vagal stimulation can alter and shift the mechanisms from one to the other and therefore can change either the propagation velocity or even the direction of peristalsis.[20] In humans, there is no evidence that the off-contraction mechanism is operative normally or is of primary importance except perhaps in the

LES.[50] Therefore, in humans, if an intramural mechanism is responsible for producing peristalsis, the predominant mechanism would normally be the cholinergic on-contraction mechanism. However, it is possible that under circumstances not yet defined, the off-contraction mechanism is also called into play in humans, especially distally.

Central Control Mechanisms. The evidence for primary involvement of the central level in control of the smooth muscle peristalsis is derived mainly from experiments in animals such as the opossum, cat, and baboon, rather than in the human. There is a well-defined set of programmed neurons in the swallowing center responsible for striated muscle peristalsis.[9, 10] Presumably, similar neurons are also present for the smooth muscle portion, but this has not yet been demonstrated. However, in both the baboon and the opossum, different vagal fibers discharge with a timing corresponding to the peristaltic contractions in both striated and smooth muscle sections.[40, 41] Furthermore, in a number of animal species with intrinsic nerves intact, continuity of the intramural mechanism is not necessary for primary or secondary peristalsis to cross a level of transection regardless of whether the ends are reanastomosed or are separated with deviation of the bolus.[51] In the cat, neither primary nor secondary peristalsis occurs in the smooth muscle esophagus when the vagi are temporarily blocked in the neck.[52] Finally, afferent stimulation acting centrally has a major effect on peristalsis. Afferent stimulation from an esophageal bolus increases the duration and frequency of the efferent vagal discharges to the esophagus in animals,[40] whereas in humans the amplitude and duration of the contraction increases and the peristaltic velocity decreases.[53] A similar effect of sensory feedback also occurs from stimuli not originating in the esophagus, such as with raised intra-abdominal pressure.[54] This latter sensory effect presumably acts through the central level of control.

Integration of Central and Peripheral Mechanisms. Studies to date have not established which hypothesis explains control of peristalsis in the smooth muscle segment of the human esophagus, although this author prefers the first hypothesis giving primacy to the central control. However, regardless of which mechanism is primary, it is clear that both central and peripheral levels of control are highly integrated, and the focus of this integration is likely the excitatory cholinergic neuron. Whether this neuron reaches threshold and induces a contraction would be determined by both excitatory and inhibitory influences, and it may depend on more than one excitatory input. For example, in addition to the excitatory vagal fibers impinging on this neuron, other excitatory influences include central or local sensory reinforcement from an intraesophageal bolus, activity within the intramural peristaltic mechanism itself, and sensory information from a contraction.[55] Inhibitory influences that might act on this neuron have not yet been elucidated. In those species and circumstances under which the NANC inhibitory neuron is also present and active, the mechanism for induction of the contraction will depend on the balance between release of acetylcholine and release of the inhibitory neurotransmitter.[21]

The existence of close integration of central and peripheral mechanisms for the control of peristalsis has major clinical implications. Disease at any level can potentially cause esophageal motor abnormality. Furthermore, it is likely that similar motor abnormalities can be produced by lesions at different locations in the various control mechanisms. In other cases, a lesion in one particular location may produce a specific motor abnormality.

Deglutitive Inhibition

Deglutitive inhibition in the esophagus is primarily a function of the swallowing center. A second swallow, initiated when a previous swallow is in the striated muscle segment of the esophagus, causes rapid and complete inhibition of contractile activity induced by the first swallow. This results from cessation of excitatory discharges from the central program, and the first wave progresses no farther.[56, 57] Once the first swallow wave has reached the smooth muscle segment of the esophagus, it can proceed distally for at least 3 sec after a second swallow,[56, 58] its amplitude diminishing progressively until it disappears. With a series of swallows at short time intervals, the esophagus remains inhibited and quiescent, and the LES is relaxed. After the last swallow in the series, a normal peristaltic wave occurs. Absence of excitatory vagal activity and specific vagal activation of the NANC inhibitory neurons may both be operative to produce the quiescence in the smooth muscle portion of the esophagus.

In addition to the effect of a second swallow on a previous swallow, that is, deglutitive inhibition, the recent occurrence of a swallow or the presence of a swallow wave within the esophagus can alter the nature of a subsequent swallow wave dramatically, decreasing its amplitude, either increasing or decreasing its velocity, and at times rendering it nonperistaltic.[58–60] These effects can last for 20 to 30 sec and are highly sensitive to bolus size and therefore to afferent sensory input. The nature, location, and interplay of the different mechanisms of control that explain these phenomena await clarification. Until then, routine clinical studies of esophageal motility should include an adequate time interval between closely timed swallows. If not, interpretation of the studies must take these into account.

Lower Esophageal Sphincter

The LES is tonically closed at rest, maintaining an average pressure of about 20 mm Hg (Table 32–1). This resting tone is due to a combination of myogenic properties and active tonic neural excitation, modulated by a complex interaction of numerous other neural and hormonal factors. Radial asymmetry in the recorded pressures is less marked than in the UES (Fig. 32–3). The higher pressures are recorded in the left lateral portion of the sphincter and likely relate to the presence of gastric sling fibers in this portion of the sphincter. The myogenic component of tone is calcium-dependent, and calcium blocking agents reduce LES pressure, a potentially useful therapeutic effect in patients with achalasia.[61]

In the human, as well as in the cat, dog, and monkey, but not in the opossum, the resting tone *in vivo* is atropine-sensitive or significantly reduced by vagal interruption.[45, 62] Therefore, the majority of this tone is due to the release of acetylcholine from excitatory neurons. Some of this release is likely a result of tonically firing vagal fibers, as in the dog,[50] and perhaps some adrenergic release of acetylcholine, as in the cat.[26, 63] Beta-adrenergic antagonists also increase LES tone in the human.[64] Therefore, resting tone is regulated by a balance between excitatory and inhibitory neural influences. Both are highly centrally mediated.

A number of reflex mechanisms, physiologic alterations, and ingested substances can markedly alter resting LES tone. Every 1½ to 2 hours, LES pressure fluctuates with the migrating motor complex (MMC), with pressures highest in association with the intense phase III motor activity in the stomach.[65] LES pressure also increases after a meal, as the result of both neural and hormonal influences, and with raised intra-abdominal pressure owing to an excitatory cholinergic reflex whose afferent pathway is probably in the vagus nerves.[66] On the other hand, the transient LES relaxation (TLESR) occurs independently of swallowing, and this relaxation frequently is associated with gastroesophageal reflux in normal subjects and in patients with esophagitis.[33, 67] The mechanism for this TLESR is unknown, but presumably it is mediated neurally and can occur at least in response to intraesophageal stimuli.[68]

The large number of factors that may influence LES pressure are summarized in Table 32–2. Many of these have obvious clinical and therapeutic implications. For example, those factors that decrease sphincter pressure would tend to produce or aggravate gastroesophageal reflux on the one hand, or could be used to treat conditions such as achalasia on the other. Those factors that increase sphincter pressure would have the opposite clinical and therapeutic implications.

On swallowing, LES pressure falls within 1.5 to 2.5 sec and remains low for 6 to 8 sec as the peristaltic contraction traverses the esophageal body. The LES relaxes with virtually 100 per cent of swallows, even though the swallow may not induce esophageal body motor activity. In humans, as in other species, the swallow-induced inhibition likely includes both active inhibition of the muscle by activation of the NANC inhibitory neurons and cessation of tonic neural excitation to the sphincter.[50] In the dog, and probably in most other species, there is provision for central participation in control of this LES relaxation. However, intramural pathways within at least the smooth muscle segment of the esophageal body can also serve to inhibit the LES.[42, 69] There is reason to believe that efferent vagal fibers serving both LES excitation and

Table 32–2. FACTORS INFLUENCING LES PRESSURE*

	Increase	Decrease
Hormones	Gastrin	Secretin
	Motilin	Cholecystokinin
	Substance P	Glucagon
		Somatostatin
		Gastric inhibitory polypeptide (GIP)
		Vasoactive intestinal polypeptide (VIP)
		Progesterone
Neural Agents	Alpha-adrenergic agonists	Beta-adrenergic agonists
	Beta-adrenergic antagonists	Alpha-adrenergic antagonists
	Cholinergic agonists	Anticholinergic agents
Foods	Protein meals	Fat
		Chocolate
		Ethanol
		Peppermint
Other	Histamine	Theophylline
	Antacids	Caffeine
	Metoclopramide	Gastric acidification
	Domperidone	Smoking
		Pregnancy
	Prostaglandin (F2$_\alpha$)	Prostaglandins (E2, I2)
		Serotonin
	Coffee	Meperidine, Morphine
		Dopamine
	Migrating motor complex	Calcium blocking agents
	Raised intra-abdominal pressure	Diazepam
		Barbiturates

*When species variations occur, the dominant effect in humans is listed.

relaxation enter the esophagus at some point above the LES. Truncal vagotomy,[70] and more recently selective vagotomy,[71] which may vagally denervate up to 8 or 9 cm of the lower esophagus, have virtually no effect on LES tone, relaxation, or responsiveness to cholinergic stimulation.

PATHOGENESIS OF ESOPHAGEAL MOTOR DISORDER

Motor disorders of the smooth muscle segment of the esophagus can be considered in the perspective of the control mechanisms for peristalsis. The different types and levels of control for normal peristalsis raise the possibility of many interesting and varied effects when a control mechanism is altered or damaged.

Generally, motor disorders fall into two broad groups of abnormality, although some overlap frequently occurs. The first is characterized by hypomotility, in which decreased amplitude of contractions or the absence of a contraction in part or all of the esophagus occurs with a swallow. The sustained or transient decrease in LES pressure associated with gastroesophageal reflux could fit into this category.[33, 67] In the second group, hypermotility is predominant. In this case, swallow waves may be of high amplitude or may be prolonged or repetitive; spontaneous contractions may be frequent; intraesophageal pressure may be elevated; and the esophagus may be hypersensitive to stimulation with cholinergic and other excitatory agonists. The LES may be "hypertensive" or similarly hypersensitive to excitatory stimulation, or it may show poor or absent relaxation ability.

Another contraction characteristic that frequently is altered in either group is the pattern of coordination. This may be manifested as a significant increase or decrease in propagation velocity or as incoordination if contractions, when they occur, are aperistaltic, simultaneous, or even reversed in direction.

It is possible to imagine that when hypomotility exists, at least three mechanisms can be responsible. Either the muscle is abnormal and unable to respond to excitation (e.g., as in advanced scleroderma),[73] excitation to the muscle is diminished (e.g., as in early scleroderma),[73] or the muscle is suppressed by excessive or unopposed inhibition, such as through activity of the NANC inhibitory neuron. If the final common pathway for excitation of the smooth muscle is primarily the excitatory cholinergic neuron, diminished activity of this neuron could occur if the neuron was abnormal, if it failed to receive adequate excitatory input from central or intramural pathways, or if it was actively inhibited. However, even normal physiologic mechanisms may decrease contraction amplitude, as is seen with the second swallow in a pair of closely timed swallows.[57–60] The mechanism for this decrease in amplitude is not clear, but likely it involves refractoriness in the central or peripheral neural mechanisms for normal cholinergic excitation of the muscle (see later discussion). In the LES, low pressure or sphincter hypotension has been attributed to a number of potential disturbances, including abnormality of the muscle, lack of normal cholinergic excitation, decreased reflex excitation, decreased stimulation through low levels of or poor responsiveness to circulating substances such as gastrin, and active inhibition.[74, 75]

The hypermotility disorders can be viewed from the same perspective. The muscle may be abnormal (e.g., thickened in some patients with idiopathic diffuse esophageal spasm)[76] or hyperresponsive to excitatory neurotransmitters or circulating hormones. Alternatively, neural excitation to the muscle may be increased, or a normally active tonic neural inhibition of the muscle could be absent. It is not known if increased stimulation of the muscle can occur through excessive drive to the cholinergic neuron from a hyperactive central program or overactive afferent reflex pathways working centrally or peripherally, or if absence of inhibition of this neuron can be responsible. Perhaps the high-amplitude, prolonged, but peristaltic contractions of the "nutcracker" or "supersqueezer" esophagus have their origin in some such mechanism.[77] Alternatively, the hypermotility seen in achalasia and in some patients with diffuse esophageal spasm probably has other explanations. Classically, in achalasia, both muscle "denervation hypersensitivity" and the lack of

peristaltic progression were attributed to absence of the cholinergic neuron and its excitatory neurotransmitter acetylcholine. However, cholinergic innervation may be intact in patients with achalasia, at least to the LES, and recent attention has focused on absence or abnormality of the NANC inhibitory neurons.[16, 78] Lack of a normally present inhibitory mechanism could readily explain hypermotility and hypersensitivity of the esophagus and the LES, as well as failure of LES relaxation on swallowing.

The absence of coordination of esophageal contractions can also be viewed as resulting from more than one pathogenetic mechanism. For example, if the NANC neurons are important in determining progressive delays in the peripheral control mechanisms for peristalsis,[16] their absence might render the esophagus not only hypersensitive but also aperistaltic, such as is usually seen in achalasia. However, lack of coordinated contractions, especially associated with hypomotility, could also be explained by a number of other alterations. These include failure of the central program to discharge in a sequential pattern, refractoriness within one or other control level for peristalsis, or decreased sensory responsiveness. For example, if normally the peripheral cholinergic neurons are refractory immediately after a swallow and unable to respond to a second swallow, the second swallow might be able to call the peripheral noncholinergic off-contraction mechanism into play and produce a delayed, more or less simultaneous contraction of low amplitude. In the case of the second swallow, these changes are highly sensitive to sensory stimulation within the esophagus and can be reversed to some extent by a larger second bolus.[60]

The motor abnormalities seen in patients with esophagitis are highly reminiscent of those that can be produced with pairs of closely timed swallows.[79] Therefore, it is tempting to speculate that the motor abnormalities produced by esophagitis and perhaps other nonspecific motor abnormalities can be explained on the basis of an exaggeration of normal physiologic mechanisms or interference with these mechanisms.

References

1. Roman, C., and Gonella, J. Extrinsic control of digestive tract motility. *In* Johnson, L. R., et al. (eds.). Physiology of the Gastrointestinal Tract. Ed. 2. New York, Raven Press, 1987, pp. 507–554.
2. Christensen, J. Motor functions of the pharynx and esophagus. *In* Johnson, L. R., et al. (eds.). Physiology of the Gastrointestinal Tract. Ed. 2. New York, Raven Press, 1987, pp. 595–612.
3. Christensen, J. The esophagus. *In* Christensen, J., and Wingate, D. (eds.). A Guide to Gastrointestinal Motility. Bristol, Wright PSG, 1983, pp. 75–100.
4. Diamant, N. E. Normal esophageal physiology. *In* Cohen, S., and Soloway, R. D. (eds.). Diseases of the Esophagus. New York, Churchill Livingstone, 1982, pp. 1–33.
5. Meyer, G. W., Austin, R. M., Brady, C. E., III, and Castell, D. O. Muscle anatomy of the human esophagus. J. Clin. Gastroenterol. 8:131, 1986.
6. Bosma, J. F., Donner, M. W., Tanaka, E., and Robertson, D. Anatomy of the pharynx, pertinent to swallowing. Dysphagia 1:23, 1986.
7. Daniel, E. E., Bowes, K. L., and Duchon, G. The structural basis for control of gastrointestinal motility in man. *In* Vantrap-

pen, G. (ed.). Proceedings of the Fifth International Symposium on Gastrointestinal Motility. Herentals, Belgium, Typoff-Press, 1975, pp. 142–151.

8. Liebermann-Meffert, D., Allgower, M., Schmid, P., and Blum, A. L. Muscular equivalent of the lower esophageal sphincter. Gastroenterology 76:31, 1979.

9. Doty, R. W. Neural organization of deglutition. In Code, C. F. (ed.). Handbook of Physiology, Sec. 6, Alimentary Canal; Vol. 4. Washington, D.C., American Physiological Society, 1968, pp. 1861–1902.

10. Jean, A. Brainstem organization of the swallowing network. Brain Behav. Evol. 25:109, 1984.

11. Christensen, J. Origin of sensation in the esophagus. Am. J. Physiol. 246:G221, 1984.

12. Weisbrodt, N. W. Neuromuscular organization of esophageal and pharyngeal motility. Arch. Intern. Med. 136:524, 1976.

13. Mann, C. V., Code, C. F., Schlegel, J. F., and Ellis, F. H., Jr. Intrinsic mechanisms controlling the mammalian gastro-oesophageal sphincter deprived of extrinsic nerve supply. Thorax 23:634, 1968.

14. Yamamoto, T. Histologic studies on the innervation of the esophagus in Formosan macaque. Arch. Hist. Jpn. 18:545, 1960.

15. Seelig, L. L., Jr., and Goyal, R. K. Morphological evaluation of opossum lower esophageal sphincter. Gastroenterology 75:51, 1978.

16. Diamant, N. E., and El-Sharkawy, T. Y. Neural control of esophageal peristalsis. A conceptual analysis. Gastroenterology 72:546, 1977.

17. Dodds, W. J., Steff, J. J., Stewart, E. T., Hogan, W. J., Arndorfer, R. C., and Cohen, E. B. Responses of feline esophagus to cervical vagal stimulation. Am. J. Physiol. 235:E63, 1978.

18. Dodds, W. J., Christensen, J., Dent, J., Wood, J. D., and Arndorfer, R. C. Esophageal contractions induced by vagal stimulation in the opossum. Am. J. Physiol. 235:E392, 1978.

19. Gilbert, R., Rattan, S., and Goyal, R. K. Pharmacologic identification, activation, and antagonism of two muscarinic receptor subtypes on the lower esophageal sphincter. J. Pharmacol. Exp. Ther. 230:284, 1984.

20. Crist, J., Gidda, J. S., and Goyal, R. K. Intramural mechanism of esophageal peristalsis: roles of cholinergic and noncholinergic nerves. Proc. Natl. Acad. Sci. 81:3595, 1984.

21. Gilbert, R. J., and Dodds, W. J. Effect of selective muscarinic antagonists on peristaltic contractions in opossum smooth muscle. Am. J. Physiol. 250:G50, 1986.

22. Goyal, R. K., and Rattan, S. Neurohumoral, hormonal, and drug receptors for the lower esophageal sphincter. Gastroenterology 74:598, 1978.

23. Goyal, R. K., Rattan, S., and Said, S. I. VIP as a possible neurotransmitter of noncholinergic non-adrenergic inhibitory neurons. Nature 288:378, 1980.

24. Aggestrup, S., Uddman, R., Jensen, S. L., Sundler, F., Schaffalitzky deMuckadell, O., Holst, J. J., Høkanson, R., Ekman, R., and Sørensen, H. R. Regulatory peptides in the lower esophageal sphincter of man. Regul. Pept. 10:167, 1985.

25. Lyrenas, E., and Abrahamsson, H. Beta adrenergic influence on oesophageal peristalsis in man. Gut 27:260, 1986.

26. Gonella, J., Niel, J. P., and Roman, C. Sympathetic control of lower esophageal sphincter motility in the cat. J. Physiol. (Lond.) 287:177, 1979.

27. Dodds, W. J., Stef, J. J., and Hogan, W. J. Factors determining pressure measurement accuracy by intraluminal manometry. Gastroenterology 70:117, 1976.

28. Hollis, J. B., and Castell, D. O. Amplitude of peristalsis as determined by rapid infusion. Gastroenterology 63:417, 1972.

29. Dent, J. A new technique for continuous sphincter pressure measurement. Gastroenterology 65:557, 1972.

30. Winans, C. S. The pharyngoesophageal closure mechanism: a manometric study. Gastroenterology 63:768, 1972.

31. Winans, C. S. Manometric asymmetry of the lower-esophageal high-pressure zone. Dig. Dis. Sci. 4:348, 1977.

32. Gerhardt, D. C., and Castell, D. O. Anatomy and physiology of the esophageal sphincters. In Castell, D. O., and Johnson, L. F. (eds.). Esophageal Function in Health and Disease. New York, Elsevier Biomedical, 1983, pp. 17–29.

33. Dent, J., Dodds, W. J., Friedman, R. H., Sekiguchi, T., Hogan, W. J., Arndorfer, R. C., and Petrie, D. S. Mechanism of gastroesophageal reflux in recumbent asymptomatic human subjects. J. Clin. Invest. 65:256, 1980.

34. Stacher, G., Schmierer, G., and Landgraf, M. Tertiary esophageal contractions evoked by acoustic stimuli. Gastroenterology 77:49, 1979.

35. Dodds, W. J., Stewart, E. T., and Hodges, D. Movement of the feline esophagus associated with respiration and peristalsis. An evaluation using tantalum markers. J. Clin. Invest. 52:1, 1973.

36. Jurica, E. J. Studies on the motility of the denervated mammalian oesophagus. Am. J. Physiol. 77:371, 1926.

37. Roman, C., and Tieffenbach, L. Electrical activity of esophageal smooth muscle in vagotomized and anesthetized cats. J. Physiol. (Paris) 63:733, 1971.

38. Meyer, G. W., and Castell, D. O. Anatomy and physiology of the esophageal body. In Castell, D. O., and Johnson, L. F. (eds.). Esophageal Function in Health and Disease. New York, Elsevier Biomedical, 1983, pp. 1–15.

39. Kahrilas, P. J., Dodds, W. J., Dent, J., Wyman, J. B., Hogan, W. J., and Arndorfer, R. C. Upper esophageal sphincter function during belching. Gastroenterology 91:133, 1986.

40. Roman, C., and Tieffenbach, L. Activity of vagal efferent fibers innervating the baboon's esophagus. J. Physiol. (Paris) 64:479, 1972.

41. Gidda, J. S., and Goyal, R. K. Swallow-evoked action potentials in vagal preganglionic efferents. J. Neurophysiol. 52:1169, 1984.

42. Tieffenbach, L., and Roman, C. The role of extrinsic vagal innervation in the motility of the smooth-muscled portion of the esophagus: electromyographic study in the cat and the baboon. J. Physiol. (Paris) 64:193, 1972.

43. Bartlet, A. L. Myogenic peristalsis in isolated preparations of chicken esophagus. Br. J. Pharmacol. 48:36, 1973.

44. Sarna, S. K., Daniel, E. E., and Waterfall, W. E. Myogenic and neural control systems for esophageal motility. Gastroenterology 73:1345, 1977.

45. Dodds, W. J., Dent, J., Hogan, W. J., and Arndorfer, R. C. Effect of atropine on esophageal motor function in humans. Am. J. Physiol. 240:G290, 1981.

46. Hollis, J. B., and Castell, D. O. Effects of cholinergic stimulation on human esophageal peristalsis. J. Appl. Physiol. 40:40, 1976.

47. Humphries, T. J., and Castell, D. O. Effect of oral bethanecol on parameters of esophageal peristalsis. Dig. Dis. Sci. 26:129, 1981.

48. Chan, W. W.-L., and Diamant, N. E. Electrical off-response of cat esophageal smooth muscle: an analogue simulation. Am. J. Physiol. 230:233, 1976.

49. McKirdy, H. C., and Marshall, R. W. Effect of drugs and electrical field stimulation on circular muscle strips from human lower oesophagus. Q. J. Exp. Physiol. 70:591, 1985.

50. Miolan, J. P., and Roman, C. Activité des fibres vagales efférentes destinées à la musculature lisse du cardia du chien. J. Physiol. (Paris) 74:709, 1978.

51. Janssens, J. The Peristaltic Mechanism of the Esophagus. Leuven, Belgium, Acco, 1978.

52. Reynolds, R. P. E., El-Sharkawy, T. Y., and Diamant, N. E. Esophageal peristalsis in the cat: the role of central innervation assessed by transient vagal blockade. Can. J. Physiol. Pharmacol. 63:122, 1985.

53. Dodds, W. J., Hogan, W. J., Reid, D. P., Stewart, E. T., and Arndorfer, R. C. A comparison between primary esophageal peristalsis following wet and dry swallows. J. Appl. Physiol. 35:851, 1973.

54. Dodds, W. J., Hogan, W. J., Stewart, E. T., Stef, J. J., and Arndorfer, R. C. Effects of intra-abdominal pressure on esophageal peristalsis. J. Appl. Physiol. 37:378, 1974.

55. Mei, N. Anatomical arrangement and electrophysiological properties of sensitive vagal neurons in the cat. Exp. Brain Res. 11:465, 1970.

56. Vantrappen, G., Hellemans, J., Pelemans, W., and Janssens, J. Electromyographic and manometric studies of the deglutitive inhibition of the esophagus. Rendic R. Gastroenterol. (Abstr) 3:139a, 1971.

57. Hellemans, J., Vantrappen, G., and Janssens, J. Electromyography of the esophagus. *In* Vantrappen, G., and Hellemans, J. (eds.). Diseases of the Esophagus. New York, Springer-Verlag, 1974, pp. 270–285.
58. Meyer, G. W., Gerhardt, D. C., and Castell, D. O. Human esophageal response to rapid swallowing: muscle refractory period or neural inhibition? Am. J. Physiol. *241:*G129, 1980.
59. Ask, P., and Tibling, L. Effect of time interval between swallows on esophageal peristalsis. Am. J. Physiol. *238:*G485, 1980.
60. Vanek, A. W., and Diamant, N. E. Responses of the human esophagus to paired swallows. Gastroenterology *92:*643, 1987.
61. Bortolotti, M., and Labo, G. Clinical and manometric effects of nifedipine in patients with esophageal achalasia. Gastroenterology *80:*39, 1981.
62. Price, L. M., El-Sharkawy, T. Y., Mui, H. Y., and Diamant, N. E. Effect of bilateral cervical vagotomy on balloon-induced lower esophageal sphincter relaxation in the dog. Gastroenterology *77:*324, 1979.
63. Reynolds, R. P. E., El-Sharkawy, T. Y., and Diamant, N. E. Lower esophageal sphincter function in the cat. The role of central innervation assessed by transient vagal blockade. Am. J. Physiol. *246:*G666, 1984.
64. Thorpe, J. A. C. Effect of propanalol on the lower esophageal sphincter in man. Curr. Med. Res. Opin. *7:*91, 1980.
65. Dent, J., Dodds, W. J., Sekiguchi, T., Hogan, W. J., and Arndorfer, R. C. Interdigestive phasic control of the human lower esophageal sphincter. Gastroenterology *3:*453, 1983.
66. Crispin, J. S., McIver, D. K., and Lind, J. F. Manometric study of the effect of vagotomy on the gastro-oesophageal sphincter. Can. J. Surg. *10:*299, 1967.
67. Dodds, W. J., Dent, J., Hogan, W. J., Helm, J. F., Hauser, R., Patel, G. K., and Egide, M. S. Mechanisms of gastroesophageal reflux in patients with reflux esophagitis. N. Engl. J. Med. *307:*1547, 1982.
68. Patterson, W. G., Rattan, S., and Goyal, R. K. Experimental induction of isolated lower esophageal sphincter relaxation in anesthetized opossum. J. Clin. Invest. *77:*1187, 1986.
69. Mann, C. V., Code, C. F., Schlegel, J. F., and Ellis, F. H., Jr. Intrinsic mechanisms controlling the mammalian gastro-oeso-phageal sphincter deprived of extrinsic nerve supply. Thorax *23:*634, 1968.
70. Higgs, R. H., and Castell, D. O. The effect of truncal vagotomy on lower esophageal sphincter pressure and response to cholinergic stimulation. Proc. Soc. Exp. Biol. Med. *153:*379, 1976.
71. Temple, J. G., Goodall, R. J. R., Hay, D. J., and Miller, D. Effect of highly selective vagotomy upon the lower oesophageal sphincter. Gut *22:*368, 1981.
72. Benjamin, S. B., and Castell, D. O. Esophageal causes of chest pain. *In* Castell, D. O., and Johnson, L. F. (eds.). Esophageal Function in Health and Disease. New York, Elsevier Biomedical, 1983, pp. 86–98.
73. Cohen, S., Fisher, R., Lipshutz, W., Turner, R., Myers, A., and Schumacher, R. The pathogenesis of esophageal dysfunction in scleroderma and Raynaud's disease. J. Clin. Invest. *51:*2663, 1972.
74. Dodds, W. J., Hogan, W. J., Helm, J. F., and Dent, J. Pathogenesis of reflux esophagitis. Gastroenterology *81:*376, 1981.
75. Halter, F., and Scheurer, U. Motility abnormalities of the lower esophageal sphincter (LES) in reflux esophagitis. *In* Vantrappen, G. (ed.). Proceedings of the Fifth International Symposium on Gastrointestinal Motility. Herentals, Belgium, Typoff-Press, 1975, pp. 349–352.
76. Henderson, R. D. Primary disordered motor activity of the esophagus ("diffuse spasm"). *In* Henderson, R. D. Motor Disorders of the Esophagus. Baltimore, Williams & Wilkins, 1976, pp. 146–156.
77. Benjamin, S. B., Gerhardt, D., and Castell, D. O. High amplitude, peristaltic contractions associated with chest pain and/or dysphagia. Gastroenterology *77:*478, 1979.
78. Holloway, R. H., Dodds, W. J., Helm, J. F., Hogan, W. J., Dent, J., and Arndorfer, R. C. Integrity of cholinergic innervation to the lower esophageal sphincter in achalasia. Gastroenterology *90:*924, 1986.
79. Kahrilas, P. J., Dodds, W. J., Hogan, W. J., Kern, M., Arndorfer, R. C., and Reece, A. Esophageal peristaltic dysfunction in peptid esophagitis. Gastroenterology *91:*897, 1986.

Motor Disorders

33

RAY E. CLOUSE

Disrupted control mechanisms of the upper sphincter region, esophageal body, and lower sphincter can alter esophageal motility. Diseases of the muscles themselves will also interfere with normal contractile function. When defects are of sufficient significance to produce symptoms or measurable abnormalities on tests of motor function, a motor disorder is present. By interfering with food transit into the stomach, these disorders can be life-threatening. Some commonly observed derangements produce minimal symptoms and no apparent alteration of bolus transit. The pathologic basis for esophageal motor disorders is often not known; pathogenesis of symptoms and of manometric or radiologic findings is not fully understood in many situations. Because of this, motor disorders generally are characterized by their clinical features and manometric phenomena. The imprecision inherent in this type of descriptive nosology can certainly confuse the neophyte. Even the gastroenterologist well versed in motor disorders frequently is confronted with patients who cannot be categorized satisfactorily. For the time being, they must grapple with the fact that knowledge of disease processes in this area is quite incomplete.

DIAGNOSTIC TECHNIQUES

Clinical History

The medical history can focus the physician's attention on the esophagus as the likely organ of dysfunction and on a motor disorder as the likely cause of symptoms. Symptoms of disordered transit (dysphagia, regurgitation) and pain typify esophageal disease. Pain and other described chest discomforts (such as a burning sensation) are not specific for esophageal disease. These symptoms occur with a host of disorders ranging from cardiac angina to diseases involving the chest wall, pulmonary processes, and even intra-abdominal pathology. Transit symptoms are more typical of esophageal disease but are not specific for the motor disorders; they can readily be seen with mucosal lesions (e.g., inflammatory or neoplastic diseases).

Several aspects of the history can be useful in improving its diagnostic value. Transit symptoms should be carefully sought in the patient who complains primarily of chest discomfort. For example, episodic chest pain may be the primary symptom, but the carefully obtained history may reveal that dysphagia (noticeably less bothersome to the patient and therefore not initially mentioned) was also present over the same time period. A waxing and waning course of symptoms over a relatively long period of time is characteristic and may accompany even the more severe motor diseases. This intermittent quality of the symptoms and the presence of dysphagia for liquids as well as for solids are the two features that most strongly suggest a motor disturbance.[1] A more detailed inquiry into individual symptoms can also have some discriminatory value.

Dysphagia. Dysphagia is the cardinal symptom of motor dysfunction and is reported by nearly all patients whose disorders interfere with bolus transit. A carefully obtained history can determine the cause of dysphagia. Patients with diseases involving the pharyngoesophageal region respond positively to the question, "Do you have difficulty swallowing?" Other symptoms that typify diseases of the pharyngoesophageal region are discussed in a following section. Patients with more distal disorders may not consider their dysphagia a swallowing problem. They state that "food tends to stick" in a retrosternal location or that it tends to "hang up" before getting into the stomach. Thus, the inquiring physician should tailor questions appropriately. The dysphagia of motor disorders is often intermittent and not progressive. Although it may have an abrupt onset, it more commonly follows an insidious course. A dramatic vacillation in the severity of dysphagia is also suggestive of a motor disorder; the patient may complain of difficulty swallowing all foods

and liquids for periods of time and then report no difficulty at all. Although not all patients report such variability in their symptoms, inconsistencies help differentiate patients with motor disorders from those with structural lesions that constrict the esophageal lumen, in whom dysphagia tends to be more regular and progressively severe.

Provocation of dysphagia by liquids at the extremes of tolerated temperatures (particularly cold) is an observation that has some specificity for patients with motor disturbances.[2] This historical feature is not common in the author's experience. Patients with the more distal motor disorders (e.g., achalasia) may report alleviation of dysphagia with various physical maneuvers. Straightening of the back or raising of the arms above the head increases intraesophageal pressure and is used by some patients to effect esophageal emptying. Similar maneuvers are rarely beneficial for patients with intraluminal lesions that obstruct the esophagus and cause food impaction; regurgitation or mechanical dislodgment is often necessary in such cases.

Regurgitation. Regurgitation of solid or liquid foods into the mouth or nasopharynx occurs with great velocity. As would be expected, this is quite disturbing to the patient. Regurgitated esophageal material can be readily differentiated from vomitus if it does not have the acidic taste of gastric contents. A food bolus may taste just as it did when it left the mouth. The unprompted patient may not volunteer this seemingly unpleasant observation. Regurgitation follows the swallow immediately or may be delayed by minutes to hours if markedly abnormal transit and esophageal retention are present. Delayed regurgitation is seen only in the most severe motor disorders. In such cases, passive regurgitation when reclining or bending over may also occur. Stagnant alteration of this retained esophageal material prevents its obvious differentiation from gastric contents.

Chest Pain. Pain may be a predominant feature of the distal esophageal motor disorders. The severe pain accompanying esophageal motor disorders is gripping and frightening. It is the symptom that often precipitates medical evaluation. Stimulation of the plentiful sensory fibers in the esophagus results from a variety of processes.[3] Unusually prolonged and powerful muscle contraction, luminal distention, and mucosal acidification could potentially provoke pain, each mechanism being operational in some patients. The pain is generally midline in the retrosternal region and may be referred cephalad, toward the suprasternal notch.[4] This has been experimentally reproduced by inflating small balloons in the distal esophagus until esophageal wall distention produces discomfort.[5, 6] Mucosal lesions, including neoplasms and inflammation (e.g., from acid injury, infection, or caustic damage), and gastroesophageal reflux without mucosal damage may be associated with a central chest pain syndrome.[6] However, motor disorders should be suspected when the pain is severe and described with some angina-like characteristics. Lack of radiation into the arms helps differentiate esophageal pain from pain of cardiac origin.[7] Undependable precipitation of pain by exercise, the occurrence of frequent spontaneous episodes, and the presence of a dull, persisting discomfort once the acute pain subsides are additional features that are more indicative of an esophageal source than cardiac pain.[7] However, cardiac angina and pain of esophageal disease are sufficiently similar that differentiation on an historical basis alone often is not possible.

The onset of pain often is spontaneous but may be provoked by food ingestion. Pain as well as dysphagia may be precipitated by cold food or beverage ingestion in some cases. Episodes last from minutes to hours, and patients often report a wide variety of maneuvers used to alleviate the discomfort. Cessation of further ingestion will dependably reduce or stop the pain for some; antacids seem beneficial for others. Some patients find that quiet resting is helpful. A slow improvement in discomfort with sublingual nitroglycerin has been thought to be indicative of pain from esophageal motor disorders, but this is also an unproved clinical impression.

Heartburn. A burning retrosternal discomfort that mimics the pain of gastroesophageal reflux may also be indicative of distal motor disorders. This symptom is not necessarily related to reflux, can be reproduced with balloon distention, and may not be precipitated by acid instillation into the esophagus.[4, 5] Some motor disorders are associated with incompetency of the antireflux mechanisms (e.g., scleroderma). In such cases, heartburn may truly be related to reflux and can be intermixed with other symptoms of motor dysfunction.[4]

Other Symptoms. Tracheobronchial aspiration occurs with many types of esophageal motor disorders. Patients with diseases involving the hypopharynx and proximal esophagus may be unable to effectively transfer the ingested bolus from the pharyngeal cavity into the esophagus. Aspiration occurs immediately with swallowing attempts, and the cause of pulmonary symptoms is quite clear. Retention of food in the esophagus may occur in patients with motor disorders involving the lower sphincter. In such cases, tracheobronchial aspiration may occur at times unrelated to meals, particularly at night. Chronic cough or recurring aspiration pneumonia can be presenting symptoms. These pulmonary symptoms mandate therapy for the motor disorder itself. Systemic symptoms are rarely present with uncomplicated motor disorders unless the neuromuscular derangement is a component of a multisystem disease. Weight loss will occur if the motility derangement is severe enough to prevent transit of adequate food into the stomach to meet caloric needs or if the symptoms induced by eating are of sufficient severity to reduce oral intake.

Radiologic Evaluation

Radiologic studies are the tests used most commonly for evaluation of esophageal disorders. Fluoroscopy or, ideally, cinefluoroscopy is utilized to evaluate bolus transit. Several swallows are taken at spaced intervals, and the entire esophagus is examined. Detection of a motor derangement is optimal when the patient is studied in the horizontal position.[8] The sequence of events in the cervical region is so rapid that a more detailed evaluation of this area may be useful. Cinefluoroscopy of the cervical region while the patient is swallowing barium of various consistencies has been employed more recently.

Radiologic evaluation of the esophagus will detect the majority of severe motor disturbances[9, 10] and is readily available as a screening test. The techniques are also sensitive for other diseases producing esophageal symptoms, including superficial lesions such as esophagitis.[11, 12] Several limitations interfere with diagnostic accuracy. First, the test is evaluated subjectively as transit cannot be quantitated readily. Second, only a small number of swallows can be evaluated because of radiation exposure. This imposes a significant limitation considering the interswallow variability in normal subjects and that major derangements may be intermittent.[13] Third, techniques for taking swallows during radiologic examinations have been less standardized than for other, more quantitative diagnostic tests, an important limitation considering the impact that such variables as bolus size, bolus temperature, and time delay between swallows have on normal peristalsis.[14-16] Finally, radiologic studies cannot provide information on contraction alterations that have little or no impact on bolus transit. These limitations interfere in a lesser way with the diagnosis of more severe motor derangements. The quantitative techniques whose descriptions follow are less likely to be used as screening tests but can detect more subtle derangements in motor function before radiologic abnormalities are apparent.

Intraluminal Recording

Manometry. Except for those disorders affecting the pharyngoesophageal region, esophageal motor disorders are categorized and defined by muscle contraction characteristics. These characteristics can be identified by placing a recording probe in the lumen that is sensitive to squeeze pressures generated by the circular muscle layer. Normal or abnormal sphincter function can also be identified. Several types of intraluminal recording devices have satisfactory fidelity in measuring esophageal contraction. The most commonly utilized technique involves a probe composed of three to eight catheters of small caliber that have been fused together. The probe diameter is 5 mm or less and is well tolerated. Small side holes are spaced 3 to 5 cm apart to allow sampling of several sites in the esophagus at one time. Each catheter is perfused with water from a low-compliance perfusion device (Fig. 33–1).[17] Older perfusion systems (e.g., the Harvard pump) were too compliant to record rapid pressure events of the upper sphincter and distal esophagus accurately. Manometry probes that contain small transducers imbedded at 3-

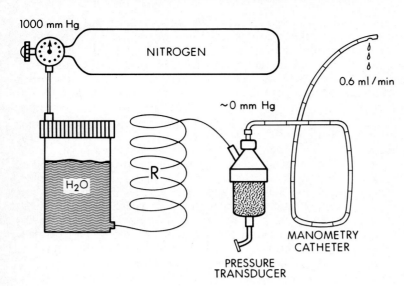

Figure 33-1. Schematic diagram demonstrating the principles of the pneumohydraulic perfusion system.[17] Nitrogen gas is used to pressurize a water reservoir. The resistance (R) imposed by a fine capillary wire reduces water pressure to nearly zero at the diaphragm of the pressure transducer. Obstruction of the catheter port by an esophageal contraction wave produces a rapid pressure increment in the dome of the transducer. Pressure in the water reservoir exceeds pressures created by typical esophageal waves sufficiently that flow of water into the transducer dome continues. Low compliance in this system produces a rapid increase in recorded pressure until perfusion pressure exceeds the contraction squeeze pressure at the catheter tip.

to 5-cm intervals are also available. This nonperfused system has excellent recording fidelity and patient tolerance, yet the perfused systems are used most commonly because of their lesser expense and disposability. Squeeze pressure and relaxation characteristics of the upper and lower sphincters are also monitored. Standard perfused catheters or imbedded microtransducers are suboptimal because of radial and axial asymmetry of contraction pressures within the sphincters. A specialized sleeve described by Dent can be attached to the distal tip of the recording probe to monitor a more circumferential lower sphincter pressure as the probe straddles this high-pressure zone.[18]

A manometric study is performed in a fasting patient in the supine position. The catheter (probe) is positioned appropriately so that recording ports sample the region of the lower sphincter as well as the esophageal body. The catheter may be left in one position throughout the study, or it may be withdrawn in a stepwise fashion so that additional areas of the esophagus are sampled by the recording ports. Often, measurement of resting lower sphincter tone is obtained first, before proceeding with evaluation of peristalsis.[19, 20] A series of swallows is then taken with at least one of the recording ports or the sleeve apparatus remaining in the lower sphincter to determine if sphincter relaxation is complete. Swallows are monitored and controlled carefully to ensure reproducibility of the study. Many factors will alter measured waves in the esophageal body, including the presence or absence of a swallowed bolus,[21] the size and temperature of the bolus,[14, 15] the interval between swallows,[16] the position of the patient,[22] and even the diameter of the recording probe.[17] The upper sphincter can be evaluated if the probe is withdrawn so that recording ports rest in this region. Measurements are more qualitative, but the presence of upper sphincter relaxation can usually be determined. A more detailed description of manometric techniques is beyond the scope of this textbook and can be found in monographs on this topic.[23]

Manometry has advantages in its quantitative approach and is the standard of diagnosis for most disorders of the esophageal body and lower sphincter. Disorders of the upper sphincter are diagnosed more satisfactorily with radiography. The limitations of manometry are primarily technical. Premedication is not used routinely because it may interfere with swallowing and also may have direct effects on motor events. Thus, the study may be poorly tolerated by some patients. In addition, the manometry probe cannot take into account alterations in longitudinal muscle contraction following the swallow.[24] Resultant axial displacement is not detected by the rigid probes and may produce artifactual results.[25] Also, the recording device measures only occlusive contraction waves that squeeze the small-diameter probes; motor events that are incompletely occlusive are unrecognized. Finally, manometry measures but the final error in the sequence of events leading to muscle contraction. Completely distinct disorders, such as one affecting intramural nerves and one affecting muscle cells, could both result in loss of esophageal peristalsis and have identical manometric diagnoses. Despite these limitations, manometry provides sufficient information to be used as a principal diagnostic tool.

Electrical Events. Electrical events underlying muscle contraction can be recorded from the esophagus as from other parts of the tubular gastrointestinal tract.[26] Myoelectric recording has been particularly useful in the understanding of gastric motor disturbances and can reveal abnormalities that are not well understood by intraluminal manometry alone. The techniques are still investigational but may overcome some of the limitations of manometry.

Radionuclide Transit Studies

Radionuclide studies examine bolus transit throughout the esophageal body, adding a quantitative capability not possible with conventional radiographic studies. A supine subject is given an oral liquid bolus labeled with technetium-99m. Radioactivity within the esophageal body and stomach is measured with a gamma camera positioned over the subject. Delayed disappearance of the label from the esophagus is typical of aperistalsis or other disorders associated with poor clearance.[27] Segments of the esophagus are so designated that sequential plots of radionuclide label movement with time can be produced (Fig. 33–2).[28] The activity-time curves generated from the different segments help distinguish aperistalsis from poorly coordinated, nonpropulsive contractions as the cause of delayed transit. Because of the intermittent nature of some motor derangements, curves are drawn from several separate swallows to enhance the detection of abnormalities.[28–30]

Transit studies of this type have certain distinct advantages. They are easy to perform, are well tolerated by patients, and produce minimal radiation exposure. Recognition of severe motor derangements exceeds that by conventional radiographic studies.[31, 32] Information regarding muscle contraction strength and sphincter tone, of course, cannot be provided. On the other hand, manometry cannot provide direct information regarding bolus transit. Thus, these two quantitative tests are complementary. The difference in the nature of measurements would explain some discrepancies between the two procedures in their ability to detect motor disturbances.[31, 32] Technical factors can produce falsely positive radionuclide transit studies in some situations.[33] It is conceivable, though, that transit errors could be present despite apparently normal manometry. At present, manometry is considered the "gold standard" in the definition of motor disorders involving all but the pharyngoesophageal region. The complementary role of transit studies is still being explored.

DISORDERS OF THE UPPER SPHINCTER AND CERVICAL ESOPHAGEAL REGION

Musculature of this region is striated and is under direct control of the swallowing center in the midbrain (see pp. 549–551). As neural control and muscle type differ from those in the remainder of the esophagus, these disorders deserve separate attention. Additionally, disorders of this proximal region are distinct in their clinical presentation.

Clinical Manifestations

Diseases affecting this area produce a distinguishing type of dysphagia. Patients truly have difficulty swallowing. The food bolus cannot be propelled successfully from the hypopharyngeal region, through the upper sphincter, and into the esophageal body. The resultant symptom is *oropharyngeal* or *transfer dysphagia*. The bolus fails to enter the esophagus with

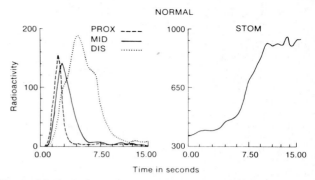

Figure 33–2. Radionuclide transit graph from normal volunteer. Vertical axes represent the radioactivity in each area and the horizontal axes indicate the time in seconds. Note sequential peaks indicating passage of the bolus in an aboral direction with early complete entry into the stomach. (Reprinted by permission of the publisher from: Radionuclide transit: a sensitive screening test for esophageal dysfunction, by Russell, C. O. H., Hill, L. D., Holmes, E. R., III, et al. Gastroenterology 80[5]:887–892. Copyright 1981 by The American Gastroenterological Association.)

repeated efforts; tracheal aspiration or nasopharyngeal regurgitation are potential outcomes. Some patients describe recurrent bolus impactions that require manual dislodgment. These disorders may be so severe that saliva cannot be swallowed and drooling occurs. Coughing episodes during a meal are indicative of concomitant tracheobroncheal aspiration. Pain is infrequent as dysphagia predominates.

Although a sense that food is lodging in the more proximal esophagus is reported not infrequently by patients with the distal motor disorders,[4] rarely is the symptom complex so focal as to be confused with the causes of oropharyngeal dysphagia (Table 33–1). The motor disorders are often representative of central nervous system disease or of striated muscle diseases with more diffuse muscle involvement. Thus, clinical manifestations that accompany such diseases should be sought. It is important to elicit the history consistent with oropharyngeal dysphagia carefully so that the diagnostic approach can be directed appropriately and so that the remainder of the esophagus is not a persistent focus of attention.

The described features of oropharyngeal dysphagia differ from the *globus sensation*. This sensation of cervical fullness or a "lump in the throat" is not necessarily accompanied by dysphagia. Bolus transfer into the esophagus is normal, and aspiration or nasopharyngeal regurgitation does not occur. The feeling of fullness may actually improve during swallowing. This symptom is no longer thought to be solely psychogenic, but rather it is believed (at least in some cases) to represent dysfunction in the region of the upper sphincter. Because of this, the term globus sensation is preferred over the original term, globus hystericus. Some evidence that alterations in cricopharyngeus muscle function can produce this sensation has been obtained from observations in gastroesophageal reflux, a disorder in which globus sensation is not uncommonly reported.[34, 35] The presumed correlate is

Table 33–1. CAUSES OF OROPHARYNGEAL
DYSPHAGIA

Structural lesions
Intrinsic pharyngoesophageal lesions
  Oropharyngeal carcinoma
  Esophageal carcinoma
  Benign esophageal tumor
  Esophageal web
  Zenker's diverticulum
  High esophageal stricture
  Inflammatory disease (e.g., pharyngitis, tonsillar abscess)
  Postsurgical change
Extrinsic lesions
  Thyroid enlargement or tumor
  Vertebral spur
  Cervical lymphadenopathy
Neuromuscular diseases
Neurologic disorders
  Central nervous system diseases
  Cerebrovascular accident
  Parkinson's disease
  Brainstem tumor
  Amyotrophic lateral sclerosis
  Huntington's chorea
  Multiple sclerosis
  Tabes dorsalis
  Diphtheria
  Cranial nerve diseases
  Poliomyelitis
  Diabetes mellitus
  Recurrent laryngeal nerve palsy (e.g., mediastinal tumor,
    postsurgical)
  Transection
Skeletal muscle diseases
  Inflammatory myopathies
    Polymyositis
    Dermatomyositis
    Scleroderma
    Mixed connective tissue disease
  Muscular dystrophies
    Oculopharyngeal muscular dystrophy
    Myotonia dystrophica
  Other muscle disorders
    Hyperthyroidism
    Myxedema
    Stiff man syndrome
Cricopharyngeus dysfunction
Other neuromuscular disorders
  Myasthenia gravis
  Amyloidosis

an increase in upper sphincter pressure that is produced by perfusing the distal esophagus with acid.[36] Balloon distention of the distal esophagus also produces a cervical symptom resembling globus sensation; reflex rise in upper sphincter pressure is recorded under these circumstances.[5, 36] Irrespective of these experimental observations and the finding of hypertension in the upper sphincter in some patients with the symptom,[37] psychologic morbidity is prevalent in patients with globus sensation alone.[38] This symptom may indicate dysfunction of the cricopharyngeus muscle but is not a typical symptom of patients with oropharyngeal dysphagia.

Neurologic Diseases

Rapid and sequential contraction of striated muscle in the pharynx and hypopharynx propel food boluses through the relaxed upper sphincter. Sequencing of neural activation in the midbrain swallowing center coordinates these events. Signals to the pharynx and proximal esophageal region travel via cranial nerves (IX, X, and XII). Diseases involving the swallowing center or the communicating nerves themselves can affect normal function.

Cerebrovascular Accidents. Oropharyngeal dysphagia can result from cerebrovascular accidents that damage the swallowing center or motor nuclei controlling striated muscles of the hypopharynx and upper esophageal region. Lesions involving the vertebrobasilar arteries or the posterior inferior cerebellar artery potentially result in motor dysfunction.[39] Severe bulbar involvement with evidence of bilateral disease is most likely to be associated with measurable motor abnormalities.[40] Unilateral involvement has also been documented to produce upper esophageal sphincter dysfunction and symptoms.[41] Oropharyngeal dysphagia occurring with cerebrovascular accidents often is abrupt in onset. Other evidence of neurologic damage is generally present, particularly in the distribution of cranial nerves. Occasionally oropharyngeal dysphagia will be the predominant complaint, and corroborating evidence of brainstem deficits will be lacking. The author has found that high-resolution studies such as CT or magnetic resonance imaging of the brainstem region can reveal evidence of multiple infarctions in such cases.

Parkinson's Disease. This degenerative lesion can affect the swallowing center. Stasis in the hypopharynx with associated upper sphincter dysfunction are prevalent findings in untreated patients.[42] Failure of upper sphincter relaxation is thought to result from an imbalance of dopaminergic and cholinergic ganglia in the brainstem region.[43] Despite the prevalence of these demonstrable abnormalities, many patients remain relatively asymptomatic.[44] The disease not only affects the upper esophageal sphincter but also influences the way the patient is able to manipulate and form the bolus in the mouth.[45] Oropharyngeal dysphagia from Parkinson's disease has a better prognosis than many other neurologic causes because improvement with conventional therapy for Parkinson's disease can occur,[46] although treatment is not uniformly successful.

Other Neurologic Causes. Although cerebrovascular accidents and Parkinson's disease are the most common neurologic causes of oropharyngeal dysphagia, this symptom and proximal esophageal dysfunction can be seen with a variety of other central and peripheral neurologic diseases as well (see Table 33–1). Oropharyngeal dysphagia is encountered infrequently in patients with multiple sclerosis, and upper sphincter dysfunction has been observed.[47] Plaque-like lesions could now possibly be detected in the brainstem by magnetic resonance imaging in such patients. As would be expected, other neurologic diseases involving the brainstem, such as amyotrophic lateral sclerosis, Huntington's chorea, and brainstem tumors, potentially result in proximal esophageal dysfunction.[40–42, 48] Cranial nerve disease may also produce similar findings. Although upper sphincter dysfunction and oropharyngeal dysphagia do not consistently result from unilateral disease, upper sphincter dysfunction has been reported from unilateral sectioning of the cranial nerves to this region.[41] The recurrent laryngeal branches of the vagus nerve innervate the upper esophagus and cricopharyngeus muscle (not the hypopharynx). Unilateral damage to these nerve branches from malignancy or accidental injury during neck surgery has been noted to produce vocal cord paralysis and oropharyngeal dysphagia simultaneously in some patients.[49] Other lesions of the cranial nerves that produce this syndrome are seen uncommonly and include bulbar poliomyelitis[50, 51] and acute neuritis.[48]

Striated Muscle Disorders

Striated muscle is found in the hypopharynx, the upper sphincter, and the proximal one third of the esophageal body and is subject to diseases that will not involve the distal esophagus. When symptomatic, these diseases produce oropharyngeal dysphagia, as occurs with neurologic disease. The onset of dysphagia may be more insidious. In contrast to neurologic disorders, in which upper sphincter relaxation is impaired, muscle diseases produce a decrease in resting sphincter tone but poor propulsion of the bolus from the pharynx into the esophagus. The end result is poorly distinguishable from neurologic causes on a clinical basis.

Inflammatory Myopathies (Dermatomyositis, Polymyositis). The inflammation of skeletal musculature observed in dermatomyositis and polymyositis also involves striated muscle of the esophagus. As would be expected, poor contraction of the pharyngeal constrictors, pooling and retention of barium in the valleculae, and nasal regurgitation of the bolus are radiographic observations.[52, 53] Manometric studies can identify decreased contractions in the pharynx with a reduction in upper sphincter resting tone;[39] contraction waves in the proximal esophageal body are also of low amplitude. It has recently been noted that motor abnormalities in the distal esophagus are also prevalent in these disorders.[54] Similar findings can be observed in some patients with scleroderma or mixed connective tissue disease. Corticosteroid therapy often improves peripheral muscle function in patients with polymyositis and dermatomyositis and has been found to improve esophageal motor function in some symptomatic patients.[55] Cricopharyngeus muscle dysfunction is also infrequently observed in association with these myopathic disorders.[56]

Muscular Dystrophies. Two uncommon forms of muscular dystrophy involve the striated muscles of the pharyngoesophageal region, and dysphagia is a common complaint in both syndromes. Myotonia dystrophica is a familial disease characterized by "myopathic facies," myotonia, swan neck, muscle wasting, frontal baldness, testicular atrophy, and cataracts. Decreased contraction pressures in the pharynx and upper esophagus, as well as decreased resting pressure of the upper esophageal sphincter, have been reported in these patients.[57, 58] Similar manometric features in the proximal esophagus are noted in patients with oculopharyngeal dystrophy.[59] This syndrome occurs later in life with ptosis and dysphagia as presenting features (the dysphagia usually preceding the ptosis) and has a dominant pattern of inheritance. Tracheobronchial aspiration is a common finding in both forms of muscular dystrophy, not infrequently being fatal.[60, 61]

Other Muscle Diseases. Oropharyngeal dysphagia occurs with other diseases that can affect the striated musculature. The symptoms are said to occur in the presence of both hyper- and hypothyroidism. Improvement in symptoms and restoration of normal upper sphincter function have been observed following treatment of myxedema.[62] Esophageal involvement has also been reported in the stiff man syndrome, a diffuse striated muscle disease resulting from uninhibited muscle stimulation by anterior horn cells in the spinal cord.[63]

Myasthenia Gravis. Myasthenia gravis, a disorder of the motor end-plate, affects striated esophageal musculature and has clinical manifestations that resemble those of myopathies and dystrophic diseases involving this same region. As is typical for other skeletal muscles in this disorder, a fatiguing effect occurs such that successive pharyngoesophageal transfer worsens with repeated swallows or as a meal progresses.[39–42] Resting to allow reaccumulation of acetylcholine in nerve endings or administration of an anticholinesterase (edrophonium chloride) will improve symptoms and pharyngoesophageal functions simultaneously.[39] Esophageal involvement with this disease is common enough that patients may present with esophageal symptoms. As is true of other muscle diseases involving this region, tracheobronchial aspiration is an important complication.

Cricopharyngeal Dysfunction

Dysfunction of the cricopharyngeus muscle can occur without other evidence of neurologic or muscle disease. This presumably primary disorder produces obstructive symptoms in the region of the upper sphincter. Oropharyngeal dysphagia, aspiration, and nasal regurgitation typify the more severe cases. In milder situations, dysphagia (generally for solid foods) may be the only complaint. Patients who have dysfunction that deserves consideration for specific therapy (i.e., myotomy) do not simply have globus sensation or an increase in upper sphincter resting pressure. Likewise, radiographic studies reveal more than simply a prominence of the normal cricopharyngeal indentation. Barium passes the cricopharyngeus muscle slowly, and the muscle appears to relax poorly during swallowing (Figs. 33–3 and 33–4). Ballooning of the pharynx may be noted and evidence of aspiration can be apparent (Figs. 33–3 to 33–5). When these radiographic findings are present, it is clear that the degree of dysfunction is medically significant. Such findings are not as pronounced in milder or earlier cases. Spasm of the

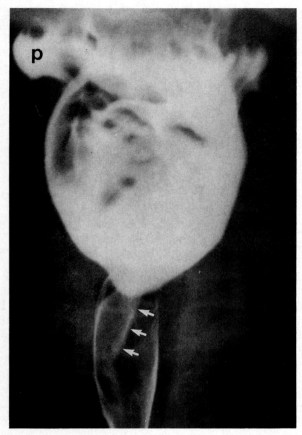

Figure 33–3. Frontal view from a barium swallow in a 40-year-old woman with cricopharyngeal dysfunction. Note the marked distention of the oropharynx with obvious presence of pharyngeal pouches (p). The cricopharyngeal indentation is only partially visualized because of overlapping barium in the distal pharynx. A jet of barium is seen passing through the region of high pressure into the proximal esophagus (arrows).

cricopharyngeus and cricopharyngeal achalasia are terms that have been applied to these phenomena.[64, 65]

No uniform manometric finding correlates with the radiographic abnormalities. In part this relates to the difficulty in studying the upper sphincter region. It has been possible to demonstrate incomplete upper sphincter relaxation in some patients with idiopathic oropharyngeal dysphagia.[48] However, this manometric feature is not found with sufficient consistency in patients with radiographs such as those shown in Figures 33–3 to 33–5 to establish satisfactory manometric criteria for diagnosis. Diagnosis rests on radiography, and the best evaluation is by cinefluoroscopy. Peculiarities in the radiographs should be clarified with direct visualization, as proximal esophageal neoplasms can produce similar clinical and radiographic features (Fig. 33–6). If flexible fiberoptic endoscopy is considered, advancement through the cricopharyngeus muscle should be performed cautiously using direct visualization rather than by blind passage through this region.

Cricopharyngeal dysfunction may represent several disorders, the cause of any being unknown. By definition no other evidence of neurologic disease in the brainstem that may be responsible for the findings is present. An increased amount of fibrous tissue has been detected in sections of the cricopharyngeus muscle obtained during myotomy for cricopharyngeal dysfunction.[66] Other myopathic features have been detected in some patients.[67] A fibrotic process that gradually restricts the maximum luminal opening of the relaxed upper sphincter would be compatible with the clinical picture in many patients. A progressive dysphagia for solid foods of decreasing caliber is a commonly obtained history.

This group of patients frequently is considered for cricopharyngeal myotomy. Simpler measures, such as bougienage, generally have little lasting effect. Muscle fibers of the cricopharyngeus are divided completely through to the level of the submucosa.[68] Relief of dysphagia occurs in the majority of patients so treated,[65, 69, 70] with reduction in resting sphincter tone.[71] This effect disarms the sphincter in its protective capacity against aspiration of refluxed material. In fact, deaths from aspiration following myotomy do occur,[65] and the procedure is reserved for patients with severe or debilitating symptoms. A preoperative evaluation for the presence of gastroesophageal reflux should be considered, if feasible, so that appropriate precautions can be taken. Myotomy remains an important treatment for a select group of patients with cricopharyngeal dysfunction as no pharmacologic therapy is available. Myotomy is also used occasionally for patients with

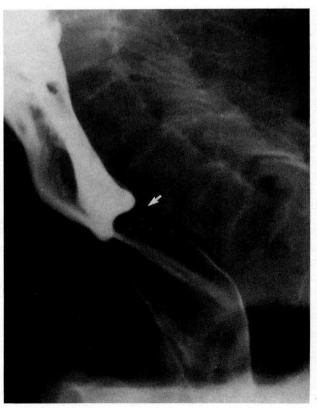

Figure 33–4. The jet effect noted in Figure 33–3 is also well demonstrated on the lateral view.

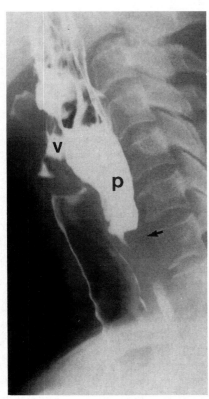

Figure 33–5. Lateral film from a barium swallow in an elderly patient with oropharyngeal dysphagia and cricopharyngeal dysfunction. The film demonstrates a prominent indentation by the cricopharyngeus muscle *(arrow)*. Dilatation of the piriform sinuses (p) is present, and aspiration of barium into the laryngeal vestibule (v) and trachea is well demonstrated on this film.

other disorders involving the pharyngoesophageal region, particularly if the cricopharyngeus muscle appears significantly obstructing as demonstrated by fluoroscopy and if no pharmacologic therapy is available for the underlying disease.[72]

ACHALASIA

Achalasia is the most recognized motor disorder of the esophagus. The term achalasia means "failure to relax" and describes a cardinal feature of this disorder, a poorly relaxing lower esophageal sphincter. Thus, the sphincter produces a functional obstruction of the esophagus and the expected symptoms of dysphagia, regurgitation, chest discomfort, and, eventually, weight loss. Transit from esophagus to stomach is further impaired by a defect involving the esophageal body that results in aperistalsis. The symptom history resembling a progressively serious, ultimately fatal disease and radiographs demonstrating a grossly contorted and dilated esophagus together produce a dramatic clinical presentation.

The first case of a patient with probable achalasia was reported more than 300 years ago by Sir Thomas Willis.[73] The disorder, then labeled cardiospasm, was

readily recognized with the advent of barium radiography in the early twentieth century. Not unreasonably, spasm in the region of the lower esophagus was thought to be responsible for the manifestations as no obstructing lesion could be detected in autopsy specimens.[74] The term achalasia was suggested by Hurst, who offered an alternative explanation—namely, that the major error was in lower sphincter relaxation.[75] This term has survived historically, and investigative techniques have confirmed failure of lower sphincter relaxation in this disease.

Etiology

The cause of achalasia, a disease with only esophageal manifestations, remains unknown. Although a viral cause has been postulated, electron microscopic examination of the vagus nerve and intramural plexus has not revealed viral particles, and epidemiologic features do not suggest an infectious cause.[76] Genetic influences also appear to contribute minimally in this disorder. Co-occurrence of the disease in first-degree family members has been reported occasionally,[77-80] but the occurrence of achalasia in only one of a pair

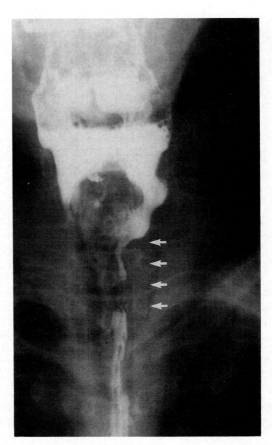

Figure 33–6. Oropharyngeal dysphagia resulted from this constricting tumor immediately distal to the upper esophageal sphincter. The tumor *(arrows)* produces some retention of barium in the hypopharynx.

of monozygotic twins speaks against strong genetic relevance of previous observations.[81] Symptoms of esophageal motor dysfunction are also uncommon among first-degree relatives of afflicted subjects.[82]

Pathology

Abnormalities in both muscle and nerve components can be detected in this disease, although the neural lesion is thought to be of primary importance.[83] Careful examination of the intramural esophageal nerve plexus has demonstrated reduction in number of ganglion cells.[84] Early autopsy series revealed a marked reduction, but this finding was thought to represent only an apparent decrease produced by mechanical separation of the plexus from esophageal dilation. An actual decrease in ganglion cells, however, has been further substantiated by the observation that neuronal bodies are less prevalent in the distal esophagus of patients with early, nondilated disease.[84] In addition, the degree of loss appears related to duration of disease; ganglion cells are nearly absent in patients with symptoms of ten years' duration or longer.[85] Lewy bodies, the characteristic histopathologic lesion in the brainstem of patients with Parkinson's disease, have been observed in the intramural plexuses of some patients with achalasia.[86]

The loss of ganglion cells within the esophageal wall itself is not the only neuropathologic abnormality detected in this disorder. By light microscopy, vagal branches to the esophagus appear normal.[87] More detailed examination by electron microscopy, however, has demonstrated degeneration of myelin sheaths and disruption of axonal membranes, the wallerian degenerative changes typical of experimental nerve transection.[88] Attention has also been directed to the brainstem in patients with achalasia. Degenerative changes, including fragmentation and dissolution of nuclear material, have been reported by Kimura in ganglia of the vagal dorsal motor nucleus.[89] Other investigators have reported a reduction in the number of ganglion cells in these nuclei.[84] These extraesophageal neuropathic changes have been demonstrated in only small numbers of achalasia patients. Nevertheless, lesions of the vagus nerve or its motor nuclei are plausible in this disease, as bilateral lesions in the feline dorsal motor nuclei can produce dysfunction resembling achalasia.[90] The interrelationship of ganglion cell loss from the esophageal wall and the vagal and brainstem lesions is not fully understood. A disorder affecting both intrinsic and extrinsic sites could be operational; on the contrary, some degree of vagal degeneration could result secondarily from ganglion cell disease. Pathophysiologic evidence supports both intrinsic and extrinsic neuropathology but also indicates that an intact intramural network is present in some patients (see later discussion). The circular muscle of the lower esophagus is thickened, but muscular changes are thought to be secondary to underlying neuropathology.

Pathophysiology

Physiologic studies have confirmed the presence of denervation of the smooth muscle segment of the esophagus in patients with achalasia. First, muscle strips from the esophageal body will contract in response to direct stimulation (acetylcholine) but not in response to ganglionic stimulation (nicotine).[91] Similarly, strips from the region of the lower esophageal sphincter do not relax in response to ganglionic stimulation in patients with achalasia, whereas they do in normal controls.[91] Second, exaggerated contractions in the esophageal body and sphincter can be measured when patients with achalasia are given parenteral injection of the acetylcholine analogue acetyl-beta-methacholine (Mecholyl).[92, 93] This response is thought to be indicative of denervation hypersensitivity. Third, cholecystokinin octapeptide (CCK-OP) produces a unexpected increase in lower esophageal sphincter pressure in the achalasia patient. This effect may represent loss of inhibitory neurons in the lower sphincter region, as these neurons normally produce the predominant response to CCK-OP stimulation.[94] These observations all support the presence of functional impairment of intramural ganglion cells in the esophageal body and lower sphincter region. In conjunction with histologic evidence that ganglion cell loss is partial, the persisting ability of lower sphincter muscle to increase sphincter pressure in response to cholinergic inhibitors provides some functional evidence that ganglion cell failure is likely not complete in this disease.[95]

There is little physiologic evidence of vagal dysfunction despite neurohistologic observations. Other aspects of vagal function might be impaired if the observed degenerative lesion were not restricted to those nuclei and fibers that innervate the esophagus. An abnormal gastric secretory response to insulin-induced hypoglycemia has been demonstrated in nearly one third of achalasia patients.[96] All with inappropriate gastric responses were found to have normal gastric acid secretion in response to a histamine analogue. This is an interesting observation, but at present there are no other data to support more generalized pathology of the vagus nerve and nuclei.

Anatomic and physiologic observations are adequate to explain the manifestations of this disease. A loss of ganglion cells in the region of the lower sphincter, particularly if the loss is predominantly of inhibitory neurons, would result in an increased basal pressure and poor relaxation under normal circumstances. Vagal changes, whether primary or secondary, could also predominantly affect inhibitory stimulation to sphincter muscle, further compounding this problem. Degeneration of ganglion cells in the esophageal body itself would eventually lead to permanent aperistalsis and allow for esophageal dilatation. The lesion in the lower sphincter region may occur first, and the aperistalsis of some early nondilated cases may be related to esophageal obstruction at the level of the sphincter.[97–99] In these patients, some peristalsis may be observed at least temporarily following reduction in lower sphincter pressure with pneumatic dilation or myotomy.

Clinical Features

Achalasia is said to occur at a rate of approximately one to two per 200,000 population per year.[100] The disease affects both sexes equally and can occur at any age.[101] Onset is usually in the third to fifth decades, and less than 5 per cent of patients have symptoms before adolescence. Symptoms rather than physical findings are the hallmarks of this disease. Dysphagia is the predominant symptom, occurring in nearly all patients.[102, 103] Dysphagia was reported by all but one of 55 consecutive subjects diagnosed with achalasia at the motility laboratory of Washington University; difficulty with solid foods was the uniform complaint (Table 33–2). The duration of symptoms at presentation averages two years, although a wide variation in duration is seen.[103, 104] As might be expected, those with mildest symptoms may have the longest histories because these patients are not bothered sufficiently to seek medical attention. The severity of dysphagia fluctuates, but for many it reaches a plateau and does not worsen with time. For others, the sense of obstruction is so severe that weight loss is pronounced.

Achalasia is the classic motor disorder for which features in the medical history may help establish the cause of dysphagia. Patients may report the use of specific maneuvers to improve esophageal emptying. Postural changes, such as raising the arms above the head, straightening the back, or standing at very erect posture, are used to increase intraesophageal pressure and improve emptying. Slow, deliberate swallowing during a meal seems to alleviate retrosternal fullness in some patients. It has been suggested that this maneuver takes advantage of the 10- to 20-mm Hg increment in intraesophageal pressure produced by swallowing a food or liquid bolus, an increment that could encourage esophageal emptying.[103] Many patients think that emotional distress worsens dysphagia and try to avoid meals in stressful situations. This observation, however, is not specific for achalasia. Chest pain is reported by one third to one half of patients with achalasia and tends to improve with the course of the disease.[102, 103] The pain is retrosternal and typical of other forms of esophageal pain.[105] Chest pain is often precipitated by eating and is the cause of decreased intake and weight loss in some patients. Persistence of pain for several years indicates the likely presence of an atypical form of achalasia, such as

Table 33–2. SYMPTOMS IN 55 CONSECUTIVE PATIENTS WITH ACHALASIA*

Symptom	Prevalence N (%)
Any dysphagia	54(98)
Dysphagia for solid food	54(98)
Dysphagia for liquids	38(69)
Regurgitation	38(69)
Chest pain	21(38)
Heartburn	15(27)

*34 male; 31 female; mean age, 46 years.

vigorous achalasia. Regurgitation of undigested foods in the esophagus is a common complaint; as many as 60 to 90 per cent of patients complain of this symptom.[102, 105] Active, unprovoked regurgitation often occurs during or shortly after a meal. Some patients induce regurgitation to relieve the uncomfortable feeling of fullness in the retrosternal region after a meal. These symptoms may be confused with those of eating disorders (e.g., anorexia nervosa or bulimia), and such incorrect diagnoses have been reported.[106] Passive regurgitation is more likely to occur from the dilated esophagus of long-standing disease and may be accompanied by aspiration.

Other symptoms relate to the complications of this disease. Weight loss is not uncommon, but when it is significant it is usually representative of advanced disease with marked food and liquid retention.[107] Pulmonary symptoms indicate aspiration of esophageal contents. In one large series, 30 per cent of patients reported nocturnal coughing spells and nearly 10 per cent had significant bronchopulmonary complications.[102] Patients with esophageal symptoms of long duration may actually come to medical attention because of pulmonary complications. In such cases, signs of esophageal motor disease, including the dilated esophageal "bag" and a thoracic air fluid level, may be detected on the screening chest films (Figs. 33–7 and 33–8).

Manometric Features

Several features are typical of the achalasia pattern on manometry. First, no sequentially propagated waves traversing the esophageal body are detected. Contraction waves that are measured are generally of low amplitude and are simultaneous in onset (Fig. 33–9). The pressure tracings from different parts of the esophageal body show remarkable similarity, indicating that the recording ports on the manometry probe are detecting pressure changes in a closed chamber, the dilated esophageal body with closed sphincters at each end. Contraction wave amplitudes in achalasia diminish with esophageal dilatation (Fig. 33–10). Some of the remaining pressure increment is simply related to the swallowed bolus entering the esophagus. Peristaltic sequences may return following successful reduction in lower sphincter pressure with pneumatic dilation or myotomy.[97, 98, 108] Repetitive contraction waves with amplitudes generally greater than 60 mm Hg are seen in the variant called *vigorous achalasia*.[109] The onsets of these waves are also simultaneous, as in typical achalasia. A rise in esophageal baseline pressure as well as the occurrence of high-amplitude, repetitive contractions in the esophageal body is observed with administration of acetyl-beta-methacholine (Mecholyl).[92] It does not provoke any meaningful peristalsis. This pharmacologic agent has been administered to patients with achalasia to add support to the diagnosis. However, the pain and unpleasant cholinergic side

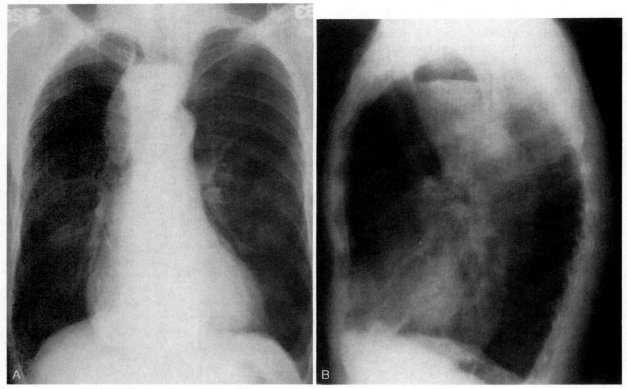

Figure 33–7. Posteroanterior *(A)* and lateral *(B)* chest films from a patient with achalasia. An air-fluid level is present in the superior mediastinal region, suggesting a fluid- and food-filled esophagus. A double density is seen in the region of the right heart border. One of the margins represents the dilated distal esophagus (see Fig. 33–8).

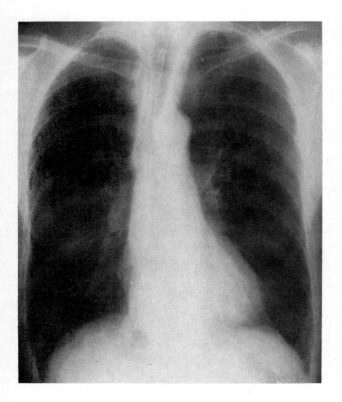

Figure 33–8. A tube was cautiously passed into the esophagus of the patient shown in Figure 33–7, and the dilated esophagus was evacuated. It is now clear that the right cardiac silhouette observed in Figure 33–7 was actually the esophagus.

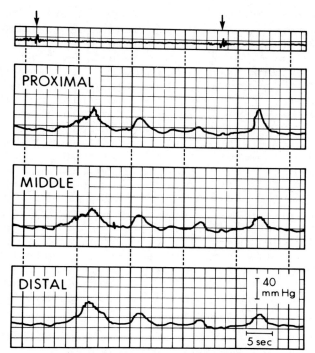

Figure 33–9. A manometric tracing from the esophageal body in a patient with idiopathic achalasia. The three esophageal recording ports (separated by 5 cm) are recording from the smooth muscle region of the esophagus. No progressive contraction waves are noted following the two swallows *(arrows)*. Monotonous similarity is noted on the pressure tracings from all three leads, indicating a "closed chamber" effect.

effects produced do not justify its routine use considering the little additional information gained.

Advancing the manometry catheter through the lower sphincter in achalasia patients may be difficult. It is important to persevere, employing fluoroscopy and contrast material when necessary,[110] as lower sphincter characteristics are important for manometric diagnosis (Fig. 33–11). An elevated resting pressure is detected in as many as 90 per cent of untreated patients.[111] (Pressure values vary considerably depending on measurement and analysis technique, making interstudy comparison of absolute pressure values difficult.) Length of the high-pressure zone is also longer than that seen in normal subjects. In addition, intraesophageal resting pressure is higher than intragastric, an opposite relationship to that seen in normal subjects. This intraesophageal pressure increment appears to be attributable to retained food and secretions within the esophagus, as it can be eliminated with esophageal evacuation. More important to the diagnosis of achalasia than resting sphincter characteristics is the demonstration of incomplete sphincter relaxation following a swallow (Fig. 33–10). This manometric finding distinguishes the achalasia pattern from other disorders with aperistalsis. Some degree of relaxation may be observed intermittently.[112] In most cases, sphincter pressure drops by only approximately 30 per cent of its elevation over gastric baseline compared with near

complete relaxation in normal subjects.[111] The combination of aperistalsis with incomplete lower sphincter relaxation (with or without an increase in resting sphincter pressure) typifies achalasia. It does not differentiate idiopathic achalasia from disorders that can closely mimic this disease (see later discussion).

Diagnosis

The disease is suspected from a compatible clinical history, and diagnosis usually is easily accomplished. Early cases may be misdiagnosed if screening radiographs fail to reveal the esophageal dilatation and distortion seen in advanced cases. Remember that some symptoms of this disease, notably chest pain and active regurgitation, may be most pronounced early in the course, before overt esophageal dilatation occurs. The diagnosis of achalasia will be made correctly in virtually all cases if a systematic approach is taken for patients with symptoms suggestive of this motor disorder.

Radiographic Studies. Radiographic studies are the primary screening tests in patients with dysphagia. Although plain films of the chest may provide important clues (Fig. 33–7), a barium swallow with fluoroscopy is the appropriate radiographic study. The barium

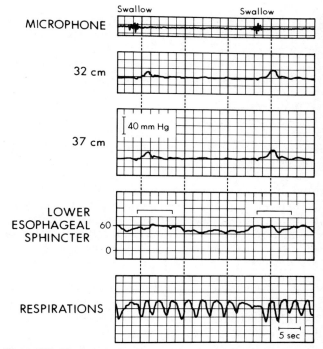

Figure 33–10. A typical manometric tracing from a patient with achalasia demonstrating failure of lower sphincter relaxation. Aperistalsis is shown by the two recording leads from the esophageal body (32 and 37 cm). Measurements from the region of the lower sphincter (at 42 cm from the nares) demonstrate an elevated basal pressure in the sphincter with no meaningful relaxation following the two swallows. The brackets indicate the time periods following the two swallows during which a drop in sphincter pressure to zero (intragastric pressure) should have been observed.

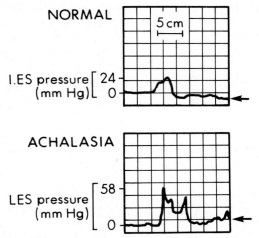

NORMAL

LES pressure [24
(mm Hg) [0

ACHALASIA

LES pressure [58
(mm Hg) [0

Figure 33–11. Measurement of the lower esophageal sphincter (LES) pressure in a patient with achalasia compared with a normal subject. Resting pressure is measured by slowly withdrawing the manometry catheter through the sphincter zone while the subject suspends respiration. In these tracings, intragastric pressure is recorded on the left, the high-pressure zone of the lower esophageal sphincter is recorded in the middle, and intraesophageal pressure is recorded on the right. Three differences in the LES characteristics are often observed: resting pressure is elevated, the length of the high-pressure zone is greater, and intraesophageal pressure exceeds intragastric pressure in patients with achalasia (arrows).

bolus enters the esophagus in a normal way, and a peristaltic contraction may travel a short distance from the upper sphincter region. In the recumbent subject, peristalsis fails to clear the bolus from the esophagus. Contrast material may be moved up and down the esophageal body by nonpropulsive, tertiary contraction or may simply lie in the atonic organ. The lower sphincter opens intermittently, allowing contrast material to escape in small quantities from the esophagus. Relaxation does not appear to be associated temporally with swallowing.

Once enough barium is swallowed to fill the esophagus, other typical features are seen (Fig. 33–12). The esophageal body is dilated, and dilatation is greatest in the distal esophagus. The barium column terminates in a tapered point, the location of the tight, nonrelaxing sphincter. This smoothly tapered projection is commonly called a "bird's beak," as the silhouette of this projection in conjunction with the dilated distal esophagus resembles the beak of common North American songbirds. The esophagus dilates with an unusual configuration in some cases (Figs. 33–13 and 33–14). As the skeletal muscle portion of the esophagus is least involved, the proximal esophagus may have a normal contour. In cases with relatively short history of symptoms, the esophageal body may be only slightly or not at all dilated (Fig. 33–15). In fact, it may take several years for esophageal dilatation to appear. In such cases, radiographic diagnosis may be incorrect, particularly if fluoroscopy is not employed. Epiphrenic diverticula rising immediately proximal to the region of the lower

sphincter can be seen in this disease. Diverticula can be massive, interfering significantly with other diagnostic tests and therapeutic maneuvers.

Endoscopy. Endoscopy is an important diagnostic tool in the patient with symptoms of achalasia and should be performed even if radiographic evaluation is typical. The purpose of endoscopy is twofold: (1) to exclude several of the diseases that mimic achalasia, and (2) to evaluate the esophageal mucosa prior to therapeutic manipulations. Typical endoscopic findings include dilatation and atony of the esophageal body and a puckered, closed lower sphincter that does not open during the procedure. The instrument passes through the sphincter and into the stomach with gentle pressure. Absence of a stricture or constricting mass is best established if an endoscope of relatively large caliber is employed. The esophagogastric junction must be examined carefully for any evidence of neoplasm.[104] As adenocarcinoma of the stomach is the most common neoplasm associated with an achalasia-like presentation, examination of the gastric cardia and fundus by

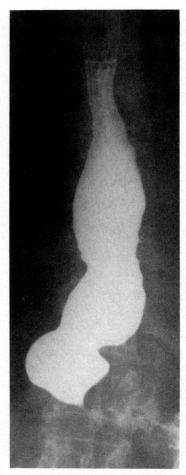

Figure 33–12. A typical barium esophagram from a patient with achalasia. The dilated esophagus ends in a pointed "beak" that represents the nonrelaxing lower esophageal sphincter. Fluoroscopy during the swallow revealed no meaningful peristalsis in the esophageal body.

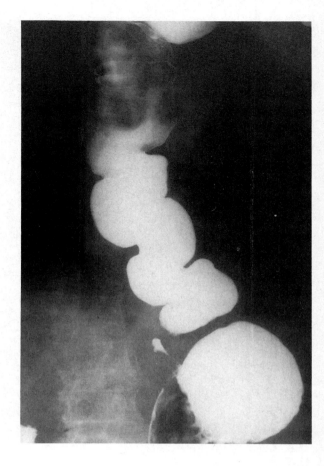

Figure 33–13. Achalasia of the esophagus with marked distortion of the esophageal body. The esophagus itself resembles colon ("sigmoid esophagus").

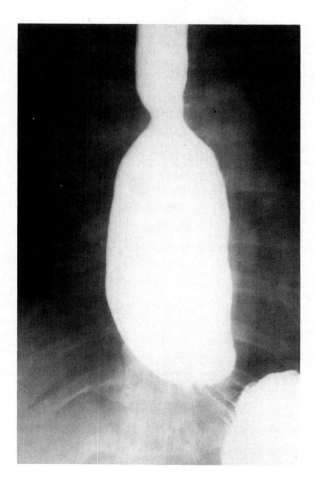

Figure 33–14. One radiogaphic appearance of achalasia in which the proximal esophagus is of completely normal caliber and the distal esophagus is grossly dilated.

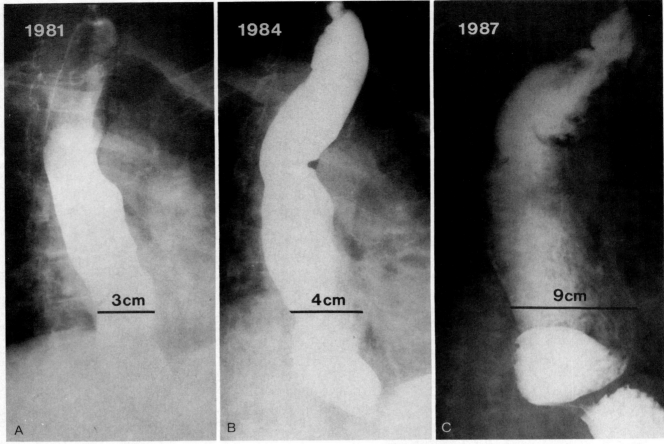

Figure 33–15. Three sequential barium esophagrams from an elderly patient with untreated achalasia. In 1977, the patient underwent a barium swallow for reasons other than esophageal symptoms and the radiographs were normal. *A*, The patient presented in 1981 with a one year history of dysphagia. Fluoroscopy demonstrated aperistalsis; mild dilatation of the distal esophagus is noted. Manometric studies confirmed the diagnosis of achalasia, and treatment was refused. *B*, The esophagram three years later showed only a slight increase in distal dilatation. *C*, The patient returned following another three years with symptoms of tracheobronchial aspiration. The X-rays reveal a marked increase in distal esophageal dilatation.

retroflexion is an essential step. The presence of a hiatus hernia should be determined simultaneously, as this finding, although uncommon in achalasia patients, may influence method of treatment.[113] If the endoscope cannot be passed into the stomach, the possibility of stricture or neoplasm in the lower sphincter region should be entertained and pneumatic dilation not contemplated. Inflammatory changes of the esophageal mucosa can be related to stasis of esophageal contents, caustic damage from medications, or *Candida* infection. If a mucosal biopsy reveals evidence of *Candida* infection, topical antifungal therapy prior to pneumatic dilation is recommended as prophylaxis against mediastinal contamination should perforation occur.

Manometry. Manometry confirms or establishes the diagnosis of achalasia and is particularly important when radiographs are normal or inconclusive. The test contributes less in advanced cases with classic radiographic findings and typical endoscopic appearance. Typical manometric findings were described earlier.

Differential Diagnosis. A group of disorders that mimic achalasia must be considered when making a diagnosis (Table 33–3). These diseases may resemble

achalasia so closely that conventional diagnostic tests are misleading. The most alarming pretenders are the malignant neoplasms, and a wide variety of tumors have been reported (Table 33–4).[104] The esophageal manifestations occur by one of two mechanisms: (1) the tumor mass encircles or compresses the distal esophagus, producing a constricting segment, or (2) malignant cells infiltrate the esophageal neural plexus,

Table 33–3. DISORDERS WITH MANOMETRIC AND RADIOLOGIC FEATURES THAT MIMIC IDIOPATHIC ACHALASIA

Disorder	Reference
Malignancy	104
Chronic idiopathic intestinal pseudo-obstruction	114
Amyloidosis	115
Chagas' disease	116
Postvagotomy disturbance	117
Familial glucocorticoid deficiency syndrome	118
Multiple endocrine neoplasia, type IIb	119
Juvenile Sjögren's syndrome with achalasia and gastric hypersecretion	120

Table 33–4. MALIGNANCIES ASSOCIATED WITH FEATURES RESEMBLING ACHALASIA

Gastric adenocarcinoma*
Esophageal squamous cell carcinoma
Lymphoma
Lung carcinoma (squamous cell, oat cell, adenocarcinoma)
Pancreatic carcinoma
Prostatic carcinoma
Hepatocellular carcinoma
Anaplastic carcinoma

*Represents over 70 per cent of reported cases.

impairing postganglionic lower sphincter innervation. Certain historical features can help the clinician suspect a malignancy.[121] A short duration of symptoms (less than six months), presentation later in life (over 50 to 60 years), and unusually great weight loss are all more typical of malignancy than of idiopathic achalasia, although these have a relatively poor specificity.[122]

Manometry cannot discriminate patients with these neoplasms from patients with achalasia.[104, 121] Apparent ulceration in the narrowed segment may suggest a tumor on barium studies, but irregularities in this region have also been noted in patients with idiopathic achalasia.[102] Amyl nitrate administration during the barium study improves the accuracy of this radiologic technique for differentiating achalasia from malignancy. The reduction in lower sphincter pressure following amyl nitrate administration in patients with idiopathic achalasia is not observed in patients with malignancies that are behaving as distal strictures.[104, 121] Computed tomography is also of value in detecting distal tumors (Figs. 33–16 and 33–17). In idiopathic achalasia, the esophageal wall may appear somewhat thickened on CT, but any thickening in the lower sphincter region should be concentric and symmetric.[123]

Chagas' disease includes esophageal involvement that resembles achalasia strikingly. This disease results from infection by the parasite *Trypanosoma cruzi*.[116] Damage to the neural plexuses of the esophagus and of other tubular organs occurs late in the course of the disease; the severity of esophageal motor dysfunction is directly related to the loss of intramural ganglion cells.[124, 125] Chagas' disease is endemic in South America, particularly in areas of Brazil, and is rarely seen in North America. Evidence of other tubular organ involvement (megaureter, megaduodenum, megacolon, megarectum) is most useful in establishing the diagnosis in a likely candidate. Differentiation from idiopathic achalasia is less critical than for malignancy as treatment in this late stage of Chagas' disease is similar. Aperistalsis and poor sphincter relaxation typical of the idiopathic disease also occur with esophageal amyloid deposition and with chronic idiopathic intestinal pseudo-obstruction.[114, 115] Successful palliation of esophageal symptoms from amyloidosis has been reported using conventional pneumatic dilation.[115]

Treatment

The degenerative neural lesion of this disease cannot be corrected. Treatment is directed at palliation of

symptoms and prevention of complications. Aggressive therapy is not necessary for a patient who has few symptoms and minimal esophageal dilatation. Once dilatation and food retention occur, treatment is enforced to prevent serious pulmonary complications. Development of carcinoma in the achalasia esophagus, although uncommon, may also be related to dilatation and chronic mucosal irritation from stasis. Further observations regarding these complications are discussed later in this chapter. Effective peristalsis is rarely restored with successful treatment, but improvement in esophageal emptying and reduction in the esophageal diameter are generally expected (Fig. 33–18).

Three palliative treatments are available, all intended to reduce lower sphincter pressure and improve emptying by gravity. Each has its place in the management of this disease.

Pharmacotherapy. Agents that have a direct relaxant effect on smooth muscle fibers of the lower esophageal sphincter alleviate symptoms and improve esophageal emptying in some patients. Nitrates have this effect, and the acute administration of amyl nitrate rapidly enhances esophageal emptying.[126, 127] Sublingual isosorbide dinitrate (Isordil), 5 to 10 mg before meals, improves symptoms as well as radionuclide transit in the majority of treated patients.[128, 129] Typical side effects, particularly headache, prevent continued use of the drug in up to one third of patients. Substitution of the oral formulation reduces the likelihood of side effects but may have a less dependable onset of action because of esophageal retention.

Calcium channel blockers (diltiazem, nifedipine, verapamil) also have recognized relaxant effects on lower esophageal sphincter muscle. These drugs interfere with calcium uptake by smooth muscle cells, cells that are dependent on intracellular calcium for contraction.

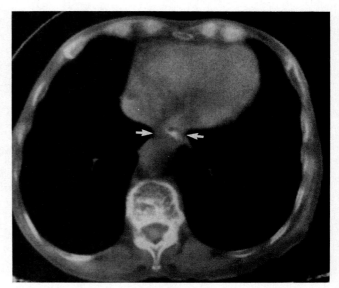

Figure 33–16. A CT section through the lower esophagus at the level of the gastroesophageal junction from a patient with idiopathic achalasia. Compare this figure with Figure 33–17C; no mass effect is seen. (The junction was unusually high in this case.)

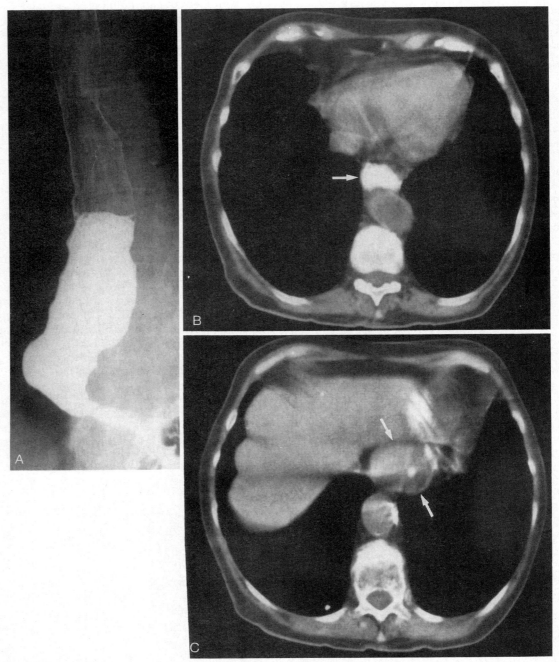

Figure 33–17. Radiographic studies from an octogenarian with a gastric adenocarcinoma mimicking achalasia. *A,* An upright film from barium radiographs of the esophagus reveals a dilated, atonic esophagus that sustains a barium column. Radiographic features were indistinguishable from those of idiopathic achalasia. *B, C,* Two CT sections of the lower chest and upper abdomen in the same patient. The more cephalad cut reveals contrast in the atonic esophagus *(B, arrow).* Contrast within the esophageal lumen narrows at the esophagogastric junction and is surrounded by a soft tissue (tumor) mass *(C, arrows).*

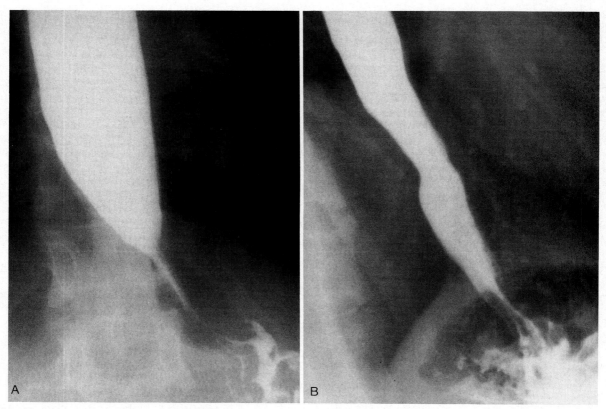

Figure 33–18. Some reduction in esophageal diameter occurs following successful pneumatic dilation. *A*, Before dilation. *B*, Twenty-four hours after dilation, showing reduced esophageal diameter and improved flow of barium into the stomach.

The lower sphincter in achalasia relaxes promptly in response to nifedipine (10 to 20 mg) (Fig. 33–19),[130, 131] and esophageal emptying improves.[129, 132] The response rate may be less than that for nitrates, but side effects limiting therapy are uncommon. Since nifedipine is not available in sublingual form, the capsule must be broken open in the patient's mouth. Reduction in pressure in the lower sphincter following nifedipine or isosorbide dinitrate is most pronounced shortly after the medication is taken (Fig. 33–19). Thus, these agents should be given in close proximity to the meal for maximum benefit.

The role of pharmacologic agents in the long-term management of achalasia remains unclear. It is not known whether continued use will prevent dilatation or complications. Some patients may not adhere to a medication schedule rigorously, but as symptom palliation is one goal, this would be the patient's prerogative. At least 70 per cent of patients can be expected to respond.[129, 132] Patients with medical conditions that interfere with pneumatic dilation or myotomy certainly are candidates.[133] The author has also found that patients are appreciative of pharmacotherapy while trying to arrange their schedules for other forms of treatment. In addition, normal nutritional status can be re-established for the patient with severe weight loss, making him or her a better candidate for other forms of treatment. Some data indicate that relief of dysphagia lasts for some time, at least a year.[129]

Dilation. Bougienage with large-caliber dilators (No. 50 French or greater) produces transient improvement, for several days at most. Forceful dilation to a diameter of approximately 3 cm is necessary to tear the circular muscle and effect lasting reduction in lower sphincter pressure. Various types of dilators have been developed for this purpose.[103] The pneumatic dilators are

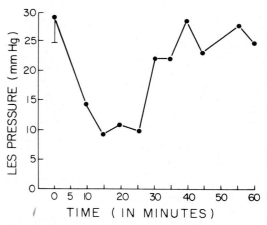

Figure 33–19. Reduction in lower esophageal sphincter pressure by nifedipine. A drop in basal sphincter pressure occurred within 10 min of sublingual administration (10 mg) in this patient with achalasia. Some effect on sphincter tone was noted for up to 40 min following the dose. (From Berger, K., McCallum, R. W. Ann. Intern. Med. *96*:61, 1982. Used by permission.)

conventionally utilized today, and several types are readily available (Fig. 33–20).

The procedure is performed on hospitalized patients, and surgical personnel and facilities capable of handling an esophageal perforation should be accessible. A liquid diet is instituted a day before dilation. Evacuation of the esophagus with a large-caliber tube (e.g., Ewald tube) may be necessary immediately before dilation for patients with persisting food and liquid retention. Limited premedication with meperidine (up to 50 mg intravenously) is utilized to reduce discomfort of the procedure. Sedation with diazepam generally is not offered as the patient should remain alert and cooperative. It is also unclear if relaxant effects of diazepam on the lower sphincter would interfere with the efficacy of dilation. Some recent evidence would suggest that successful dilation can still be obtained.[134] Atropine (0.4 mg intravenously for the average adult) will reduce oral secretions, an effect that can be quite beneficial. However, similar concerns regarding its potential influence on sphincter pressure and outcome of dilation can be raised. The dilator is passed with fluoroscopic guidance until the center of the bag is positioned at the level of the lower sphincter (Fig. 33–21). Slight inflation confirms that there is symmetric distention. The bag will have a tendency to migrate aborally with inflation; gentle tension is often necessary to maintain its proper position. Once positioning adjustments are made, the bag is inflated rapidly to a pressure of at least 6 pounds per square inch (psi) for 15 to 60 sec. The inflation pressure and duration of dilation vary considerably from author to author, and there are insufficient data at this time to say that one technique is superior to another. Beneficial results

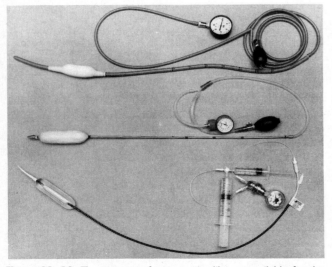

Figure 33–20. Three types of pneumatic dilators available for the treatment of achalasia. The Brown-McHardy dilator is affixed to a rubber bougie resembling a Hurst dilator *(top)*. The Rider-Moeller dilator has a semi-rigid metal post *(middle)*. A flanged tip on this dilator can be passed over a guidewire or thread. The Rigiflex dilator *(bottom)* has a double-lumen catheter that allows placement of the entire dilator over a guidewire. The catheter on this dilator is less than 5 mm in diameter.

using dilations for as brief as 4 sec have been similar to those obtained with longer (more conventional) inflation times.[135] In that report, a much larger diameter dilator (5 cm) was used than is conventionally employed (3 to 3.5 cm). The author generally uses a 3.5 cm diameter dilator inflated to 9 to 12 psi for 30 to 60 sec, a procedure similar to that reported by Bennett and Hendrix.[136]

Following dilation, a small amount of water-soluble contrast material (such as Hypaque) is given cautiously by mouth, through a small-caliber nasal tube that has been carefully placed into the midesophagus, or through the central lumen of the Rigiflex dilator that has been withdrawn into the esophagus. The purpose of the test is to examine for distal esophageal leaks near the region of the esophagogastric junction and not to determine the adequacy of dilation.[137] If no leak is seen, the patient is observed carefully over the subsequent six hours, and then the diet is gradually resumed. The patient with a small perforation and contrast material extending beyond the normal esophageal lumen can also be managed conservatively.[92] Antibiotics should be initiated, as should close observation for signs of worsening pain and fever. Clinical deterioration or presence of free-flowing barium into the mediastium mandates immediate thoracotomy and repair. If the tear is small, the repair and the myotomy can be performed in the same operation.

The success of pneumatic dilation would seemingly depend on multiple variables: the diameter of the dilator, the duration of bag inflation, the number of dilations per session.[138] Influence of these variables on outcome has not been conclusive enough for standards to have been established. Good response occurs in at least 60 per cent of patients,[102, 134, 139] and success rates exceeding 95 per cent have been reported.[138, 140] The response rate varies with patient age (younger patients do less well than older patients[139]) and duration of symptoms (those with a shorter history respond less well), but it does not seem to be related to the degree of esophageal dilatation or tortuosity.[141] Efficacy of this procedure is reduced by half for each subsequent dilation. Thus, patients who have a poor initial result or rapid recurrence of symptoms have a lesser likelihood of responding to additional dilations.[141] Response to myotomy is not influenced by previous dilation.[142] Morbidity is mostly related to esophageal perforation, a complication occurring in approximately 2 to 4 per cent of patients,[143] but surgical repair has been required in less than half of the recognized cases. Mortality from pneumatic dilation has rarely been reported.

Both pneumatic dilation and surgical myotomy offer long-lasting benefits, and the choice of one over the other depends on several factors. Assuming the dilator can be positioned, as is usually so considering the variety of dilators available, most patients would be candidates for pneumatic dilation (Table 33–5). The advantages of this procedure are its brief period of discomfort, short hospital stay, and relatively low expense. The disadvantages are its lesser efficacy compared with myotomy and the risk of serious complica-

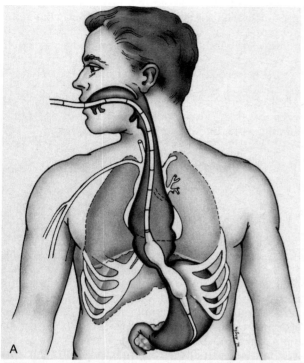

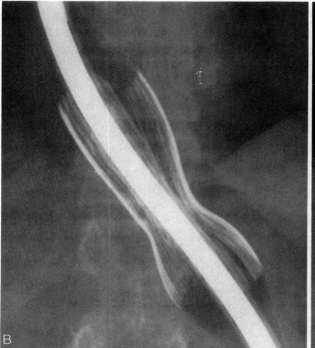

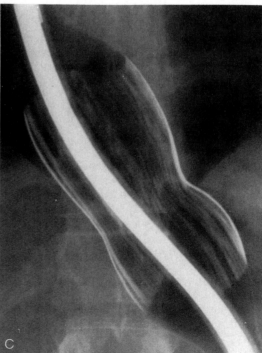

Figure 33–21. Placement of the Brown-McHardy pneumatic dilator in the treatment of achalasia. *A,* The bag is positioned so that it straddles the high-pressure region of the lower esophageal sphincter. *B,* radiopaque stays reveal the contour of the bag in its partially inflated position. The "waist" produced in the center of the bag by the lower esophageal sphincter indicates its appropriate position. *C,* A slight indentation persists while the bag is inflated to maximal pressure. This indentation nearly resolves as dilation is successfully completed.

Table 33–5. CONTRAINDICATIONS TO PNEUMATIC DILATION*

Absolute	Relative
Moribund condition	Tortuous sigmoid shape
Uncooperative patient	Previous myotomy
Recent myocardial infarction	Infancy
Inability to exclude carcinoma	Variant form of achalasia
	Epiphrenic diverticulum
	Large hiatus hernia

*Adapted from Pope, C. E., II. Motor disorders. *In* Sleisenger, M. H., and Fordtran, J. S. (eds.). Gastrointestinal Disease: Pathophysiology, Diagnosis, Management, 3rd ed. Philadelphia, W. B. Saunders Co., 1983, p. 439.

tion, albeit small. It seems unlikely that further refinements in dilation technique will reduce the perforation rate much below its current level. The author would recommend that, at institutions where skilled personnel are available for both procedures, both options be explained to the patient and pneumatic dilation encouraged based on the low likelihood of an adverse outcome.

Esophagomyotomy. The goal of surgical therapy in achalasia is to reduce lower sphincter resting pressure without completely surrendering its competency against gastroesophageal reflux. Complete disruption of the sphincter, as with cardioplasty, rapidly relieves dysphagia but promotes severe esophagitis and stricturing, negating the utility of the operation. The Heller procedure was described in 1913,[144] and a modification of this procedure is employed most commonly in the surgical management of achalasia.[145, 146] An anterior myotomy is performed by dividing the circular muscle fibers down to the level of the mucosa. The myotomy extends less than 1 cm onto the stomach and to several centimeters above the palpated region of the lower sphincter. A transthoracic approach is preferred as it allows for careful palpation and inspection of the esophagus, helps confirm the diagnosis, and allows the surgeon to extend the myotomy proximally as far as seems necessary by palpation. Patients with vigorous achalasia may have a longer region of muscular thickening and require a more extensive myotomy.[141]

Good results from myotomy occur in 80 to 90 per cent or more of patients.[102, 143, 147] Myotomy reduces lower sphincter pressure more dependably than does pneumatic dilation, and this appears responsible for its greater efficacy.[135] The most significant complication is gastroesophageal reflux. The modified Heller procedure does not destroy sphincter competency completely as long as extension of the myotomy onto the stomach is not excessive. Thus, the incidence of symptomatic reflux is less than 10 per cent, although higher rates have been noted.[148–152] Systematic measurements of reflux using 24-hour pH monitoring have not been performed routinely in follow-up. Some of the reflux-related morbidity in earlier reports was compounded by the lesser availability of effective medical management. The addition of H2 blockers to the medical

armamentarium surely will further reduce the serious nature of this complication. Persistent severe dysphagia also occurs in less than 10 per cent of patients treated surgically.[135, 143, 146, 148] Evaluation should include barium radiography and endoscopy. These two studies will demonstrate the luminal caliber at the lower sphincter, the presence of esophagitis or stricture, and change in the retention of a barium column. Improved surgical techniques and medical therapy for reflux has obviated the need for fundoplication at the time of myotomy, as has been advocated by some authors.[146, 147] Fundoplication that is too tight also results in severe dysphagia,[153] a complication requiring additional surgical intervention.[154] Although death as a result of operation is possible, the likelihood is small (less than 2 per cent).[134, 151, 155]

Complications of Achalasia

The complications of achalasia are related to retention and stasis in the esophagus. Irritation of the mucosal lining results in an endoscopically evident esophagitis. Symptoms or complications of esophagitis (e.g., stricture formation or hemorrhage) are not recognized. A more serious complication is the aspiration of esophageal contents. As many as 30 per cent of patients report nocturnal coughing spells;[102] fewer develop pulmonary infiltrates from aspiration, but this complication may be severe.[156] Severity is increased by the fact that retained esophageal contents harbor many bacteria.

Carcinoma of the Esophagus. Esophageal carcinoma has been reported in association with achalasia with rates as high as 20 per cent, but such series were contaminated by patients with primary tumors mimicking achalasia.[104] Even with more careful exclusion of patients with this presentation, it appears that the prevalence of carcinoma is higher in achalasia patients than should be observed. Rates ranging from 2 to 7 per cent have been found in the larger series.[157, 158] This possible complication may be more likely in patients who have had unsatisfactory or no treatment, suggesting that stasis and mucosal irritation may be a precipitating factor. As the tumors often arise in a greatly dilated esophagus, symptoms can be quite delayed; neoplasms can be large and advanced when detected, even in patients who have regular medical attention. Because of this, rigorous investigation with endoscopy, cytology, and random biopsy every one or several years has been advocated.[159] The likelihood of carcinoma development is small enough that a cost-benefit analysis would not support such an approach,[160] but a risk-benefit analysis would favor a regular surveillance program until more information is available. Other factors (e.g., tobacco or alcohol use) may be identified as contributing to risk of carcinoma, directing surveillance to higher risk subgroups.

SPASTIC DISORDERS OF THE SMOOTH MUSCLE SEGMENT OF THE ESOPHAGUS

Definition

Describing this group of disorders is a difficult task. Only a moderate degree of consensus exists regarding the types of dysfunction that should be included, and investigators have been diverse in their definitions of diffuse spasm.[161] In previous editions of this book, the discussion of these disorders was restricted to symptomatic patients with radiographically apparent tertiary contractions and evidence of repetitive contraction waves on manometry. All patients (symptomatic or not) who demonstrate excessive or intensified contractions by radiography or manometry in the smooth muscle portion of the esophagus—providing that at least some normally propagated peristalsis is seen—are included in the present discussion. Manifestations may range from mild to severe and result from several different underlying pathogenetic mechanisms. Grouping patients in this way seems justified on the basis of current knowledge as the clinical presentation of patients is quite similar within the group, a pathologic basis has been determined for none, management approaches are similar for all, and an outcome that appears specific to any one subset is not recognized. The cause of the spastic disorders remains unknown. Typical manometric patterns have been associated with a variety of chronic illnesses,[162, 163] including psychiatric disorders.[164] No causal relationship has been determined for these associations.

Manometric Features. Manometric findings are restricted to the smooth muscle portion of the esophagus and are most pronounced in the 5- to 10-cm segment proximal to the lower sphincter.[165] Several types of abnormalities have been included in prior descriptions of esophageal spasm, and each may have a different underlying mechanism. These findings are (1) repetitive sequences of contraction following a swallow, many or most of which are nonsequential in propaga-

tion; (2) abnormalities of the contraction wave characteristics (e.g., amplitude, duration); and (3) sporadic, long periods of intense or repetitive contraction associated with baseline pressure elevations. This third type has a distinctive onset and termination that may be associated with swallowing.

A series of repetitive contraction waves, many of which have simultaneous onset at different recording sites, typifies one description of esophageal spasm (Fig. 33–22).[166] The esophageal pressure approximates baseline pressure between contractions. Some waves with normal propagation are seen during the study, differentiating this pattern from that of vigorous achalasia.[109] Repetitive contraction sequences are seen frequently during a study and may or may not be directly associated with symptoms. The sequences are often composed of waves with intense contraction pressure (wave amplitude) and long contraction duration. It has been recognized that many patients with the clinical features of esophageal spasm have only the contraction wave abnormalities without repetitive sequences (Fig. 33–23).[167-170] These contraction abnormalities are most severe near the lower sphincter and are not observed in the skeletal muscle portion of the esophagus. The measured waves may be only mildly distorted, with a slight increase in amplitude or duration or with frequent multipeaked configurations, or they may have all of these features to an exaggerated degree (Fig. 33–23 *e*). The term "nutcracker esophagus" has been applied to that subgroup with a marked increase in contraction amplitude.[168] Sporadic events, such as the isolated occurrence of simultaneous contractions at different sites (Fig. 33–24), are also observed in conjunction with contraction abnormalities. These events are associated with disruption of radionuclide transit and may have some relation to intermittent symptoms.[161] Distinct periods of prolonged esophageal contraction with bizarre manometric appearance are seen infrequently (Fig. 33–25). These contraction episodes may last more than one minute and can be, not surprisingly, directly associated with symptoms.[171]

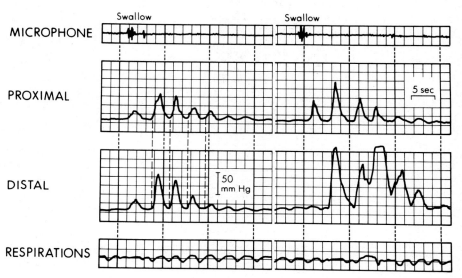

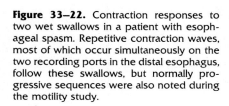

Figure 33–22. Contraction responses to two wet swallows in a patient with esophageal spasm. Repetitive contraction waves, most of which occur simultaneously on the two recording ports in the distal esophagus, follow these swallows, but normally progressive sequences were also noted during the motility study.

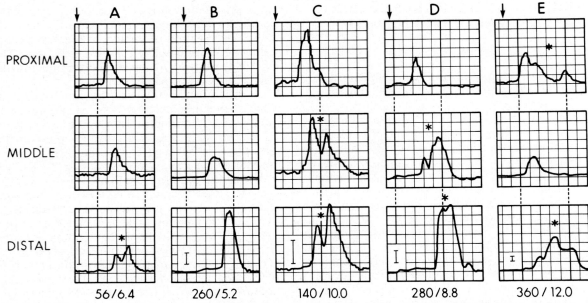

Figure 33–23. Representative contraction sequences from swallows of five different patients who presented with symptoms of esophageal spasm. The recording ports are separated by 5 cm and are located in the middle to distal portions of the esophagus. The onset of contraction is sequential in all cases. *A*, Multipeaked waves can occur in the presence of normal contraction amplitude. *B*, Increased contraction amplitude can occur without evidence of other wave abnormalities. *C–E*, Waves may be of greatly increased contraction duration.

A wide variety and combination of contraction abnormalities is observed, ranging from nearly normal *(A)* to grossly distorted *(E)* contraction responses to swallows. Calibration marks represent 50 mm Hg in amplitude. Asterisks indicate multipeaked contraction waves. The numbers under each frame represent the amplitude of the distal contraction in mm Hg and duration of contraction in secs, respectively.

These findings are rare but perpetuate the impression that muscular spasm is responsible for symptoms in these disorders, particularly pain. Prolonged pressure recording has not detected such events in most patients with typical symptoms and the other types of manometric abnormalities described above.[172, 173]

Several types of abnormalities may be seen in the same tracing,[166] and conversion of contraction abnormalities to the repetitive pattern has been observed in some patients.[174, 175] An elevation in resting lower

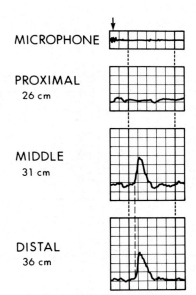

Figure 33–24. A simultaneous contraction sequence occurring without other abnormalities in wave configuration.

sphincter pressure is most certainly associated with these disorders and is seen in at least one third of patients with more severe derangements.[170, 176] Poor relaxation of the lower sphincter has been detected in some patients,[177, 178] but this is not a common feature.

Pathology and Pathophysiology

The esophageal muscles and neural plexuses are not readily accessible for routine biopsy. This, in conjunction with the fact that these motor disorders are not fatal, has resulted in little material for pathologic examination. Diffuse muscular thickening in the distal esophagus has been found in some but not all patients with more severe manometric abnormalities.[179, 180] This inconsistent finding is not thought to be a primary abnormality.[83] Little specific evidence of neuropathology has been reported. Loss of ganglion cells in the intramural plexuses has not been demonstrated. Changes in vagal fibers have been found inconsistently by electron microscopy;[83, 179, 181] some of these changes resemble wallerian degeneration. In contrast to achalasia, however, the spastic disorders do not show a progression in disease severity as might be expected from a degenerative neural process. Deterioration from more severe abnormalities to achalasia has been reported,[182, 183] but these are exceptional cases. Contraction abnormalities are prevalent in alcoholics and diabetic patients with peripheral neuropathy, but the manometric findings are independent of neuropathy.[163, 184]

Despite little evidence of neuropathology, physio-

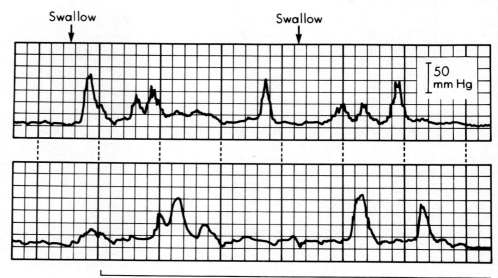

Swallow   Swallow

50 mm Hg

"Burning" Discomfort

Figure 33–25. A long period of baseline pressure elevation and spontaneous contractions in a patient with symptoms of esophageal spasm. A chest discomfort similar to the presenting complaint accompanied the episode. (Each small box represents 2.5 secs.)

logic studies indicate neural dysfunction. The esophagus in these disorders is particularly sensitive to cholinergic stimulation. Methacholine, bethanechol, or carbechol will produce an exaggeration of abnormal manometric findings in many patients.[185–189] Edrophonium chloride, a cholinesterase inhibitor, will produce similar results.[187, 190] Response to cholinergic stimulation is not completely sensitive or specific for the spastic disorders; at least 15 per cent of patients show no manometric change, and patients with achalasia are similarly hypersensitive. An exaggerated response also follows parenteral injection of ergonovine maleate.[191–193] As with cholinergic stimulation, response to this alpha-adrenergic agent is seen in some control subjects, response is more exaggerated in those with spastic disorders, and not all patients show a worsening of manometric findings. These physiologic studies do not add sufficient information to localize the pathologic process(es). Some evidence is available indicating that central nervous system disease could participate in producing the manometric abnormalities. Central stimulation with psychologic stress produces repetitive waves in normal subjects that resemble the described contraction abnormalities. Likewise, loud noise or stressful mental tasks performed during manometry increase contraction wave amplitude in the distal esophagus, although the magnitude of change is small.[194] These findings may have a relationship to observations that anxiety and affective disorders are unusually prevalent in symptomatic patients with contraction abnormalities compared with those having other manometric abnormalities or normal esophageal motility.[195]

Results from provocative testing provide the best evidence suggesting two components to these disorders, a motor component and a sensory component (Fig. 33–26). The disease process or processes involve both limbs. In the studies mentioned earlier, some degree of differential stimulation to either the motor (effector) or sensory component has been observed.

Cholinergic stimulation frequently precipitates motility change (with or without pain) but can provoke pain without significantly altering esophageal contraction. Balloon distention reproduces pain at low distending volumes without noticeable motor change.[196] This provocatory test precipitates pain in some subjects who have no abnormality or mild findings on baseline manometry and who have no dysphagia.[197] In such patients, a sensory disorder may be the predominant finding. Acid instillation may stimulate sensitive neural receptors that produce discomfort independent of mo-

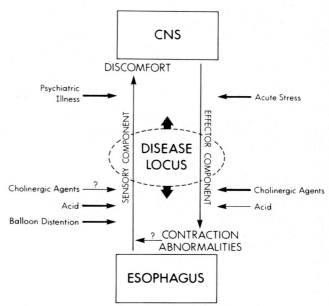

Figure 33–26. A proposed model for the spastic motor disorders. The location of pathology in these disorders (disease locus) is not known but appears to include both an effector (motor) component and a sensory component. These two limbs may not be involved equally in all cases and can be stimulated independently by various maneuvers. Contraction abnormalities measured in the esophagus are markers for the disease in this model and only occasionally provoke the sensory limb.

tor events.[198, 199] As suggested by the model in Figure 33–26, psychiatric illness may have its effect only by altering sensory perception, a concept promoted for some other chronic pain disorders.

Clinical Features

Spastic disorders appear at any age; the mean age of presentation is approximately 40 years. A female predominance may be present, particularly in persons with contraction wave abnormalities.[4] Prevalence is unknown. Various contraction abnormalities represent the most common manometric diagnoses;[170, 199] up to 50 per cent of patients referred with esophageal symptoms will have these findings. Those with severe contraction abnormalities or repetitive waves, as in Figure 33–22, represent less than 5 per cent of referred patients.[170, 171] Dysphagia is more prevalent in this latter group, but other clinical features do not appear to differentiate them from the remainder.[4]

Dysphagia is present in 30 to 60 per cent of patients.[4, 200] This symptom is intermittent, varying on a daily basis from mild to very severe. It does not usually have a direct relationship to chest pain, but it often is more severe during periods when pain is more frequent or severe. Regurgitation of a food or liquid bolus into the mouth or nasopharynx may accompany dysphagia but is infrequent compared with its occurrence in achalasia. Also in contrast to achalasia, dysphagia generally is neither progressive nor severe enough to produce weight loss. Chest pain is reported by 80 to 90 per cent of patients with these disorders. The pain generally is retrosternal, may radiate directly into the back, and often is more severe than the recurrent pain that would be expected from coronary artery disease. A dull residual discomfort persisting after the severe episode abates also differentiates the pain from angina.[7] Pain episodes may last from minutes to hours, and swallowing generally is not impaired during the episodes.

Other esophageal symptoms are less helpful in diagnosis. Heartburn is a component of the syndrome in as many as 20 per cent of patients.[4] This symptom may reflect abnormal esophageal sensation rather than pathologic reflux, as it often is not reproduced by acid instillation[4] and is poorly responsive to antireflux therapy in some patients with these motor disorders. Other gastrointestinal symptoms typical of functional bowel disorders are reported with relatively high prevalence.[201] Symptoms of psychologic dysfunction, particularly those of anxiety and depression, are also common.[164, 202]

Diagnosis

Esophageal spasm is suspected when dysphagia or chest pain (with an esophageal distribution) or both are reported with the vague and inconsistent history outlined earlier. Because of the poor specificity of

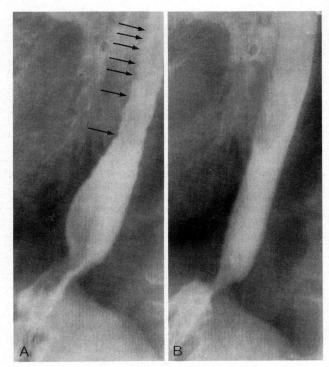

Figure 33–27. Two consecutive swallows from a patient with dysphagia and chest pain. *A,* Nonpropulsive circular muscle contractions (tertiary contractions, *arrows*) were observed with the first swallowed bolus of barium during this radiographic study. *B,* These contractions were not observed on the subsequent swallow, in which stripping of the barium bolus by primary peristalsis was normal.

manometric findings for chest pain, esophageal testing has not alleviated the need for careful consideration and exclusion of potentially coexisting disorders. The pain of esophageal spasm can mimic coronary artery disease sufficiently that extensive cardiac evaluation is not uncommonly required. Diagnosis of the spastic disorders depends on manometry, and typical features have been outlined. Other investigative tests can contribute to diagnosis.

Radiologic Findings. A barium study of the esophagus with fluoroscopy is the initial test in a patient with dysphagia and should also be considered in subjects with chest pain potentially of esophageal origin. Frequent, nonpropulsive contractions may indent the barium column in the smooth muscle portion of the esophagus (Fig. 33–27). These indentations are produced by dysfunctional circular muscle contraction. The severe extreme produces entrapment of barium between powerfully contracted segments. Transit of barium from the esophagus may be markedly delayed as the contractions produce a kneading effect. This distorted radiographic appearance has been described as a "corkscrew esophagus," a "rosary bead esophagus," or as esophageal "curling" (Fig. 33–28). In all cases, from mild to severe, the uncoordinated postswallow contractions are intermixed with swallows that have normal appearance (Fig. 33–27).[171] Sliding hiatus hernias appear to be more frequent in patients with

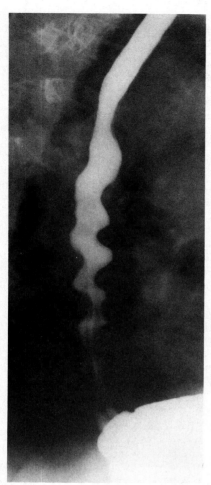

Figure 33–28. A single film from an esophagram that demonstrates broad muscular indentations, producing the configuration of "corkscrew esophagus." This patient was asymptomatic despite the fact that this configuration was observed on multiple swallows.

the spastic disorders.[203, 204] These could result from esophageal shortening during intense muscle contraction, as their prevalence is related to the severity of the motor abnormality.[203] In the spastic disorders, radiographic findings have not correlated well with manometry[205] or with symptoms.[206]

Endoscopy. Endoscopy may be employed in the evaluation of dysphagia and chest pain. No features are typical of the spastic disorders, and the endoscopic appearance should be normal. The test may detect alternative explanations for symptoms, such as esophagitis or stricture.

Other Tests. The effects of provocative agents, such as edrophonium chloride, have been described. These agents may enhance diagnostic yield, particularly in the evaluation of chest pain.[189, 190, 207] Pharmacologic provocation possibly has greatest utility in patients who have normal baseline manometric studies. The technique of 24-hour ambulatory manometry was developed to improve diagnostic accuracy of esophageal testing in patients with atypical chest pain.[173] The test is still investigational, but initial results have revealed the limitations of this technique. Radionuclide transit studies demonstrate disorganization of bolus transit,[28] but the test has not contributed sufficiently to the diagnosis of spastic disorders to be routinely utilized.

Treatment

Spastic disorders of the smooth muscle segment of the esophagus are generally not progressive or fatal, and treatment is directed at symptom reduction. In uncontrolled trials, short- and long-acting nitrate preparations have reduced symptoms and improved manometric or radiographic patterns in some patients.[208-211] Isosorbide dinitrate, 5 to 10 mg sublingually, can be tried. These medications are thought to be beneficial because of their relaxant effects on smooth muscle, although the effects on manometric parameters may actually be minimal.[211-212] Calcium channel blockers (e.g., nifedipine, diltiazem) also affect smooth muscle contraction. Anecdotal reports have indicated the potential benefits of these medications in management of spastic disorders.[213-216] A controlled trial in patients with high-amplitude contractions (the "nutcracker esophagus") did not support a benefit of nifedipine over placebo in reduction of chest pain, the major presenting symptom, despite significant effects on motility.[217] Firm evidence supporting the uniform efficacy of diltiazem is also lacking. A double-blind, controlled trial using trazodone hydrochloride (Desyrel) for symptomatic patients with esophageal contraction abnormalities has been reported.[218] A low dosage of this antidepressant (100 to 150 mg/day) was employed. Trazodone produced global improvement and reduced distress from esophageal symptoms. The overall improvement was not dependent on any change in manometric pattern during the course of the study. Successful management of symptoms from esophageal spasm has been anecdotally reported using other psychologic techniques.[219, 220]

If several different medications fail, dilation or surgical myotomy can be considered, but these treatments should be reserved for patients with severe symptoms. Bougienage is generally thought to be ineffective.[221] Pneumatic dilation helps 40 per cent of patients with severe manometric abnormalities, its greatest effect being on dysphagia.[143] Pneumatic dilation is appropriate for the subgroup with documented incomplete relaxation of the lower sphincter.[178] This subgroup may be more closely related to achalasia,[182] and there is no evidence that the complications of pneumatic dilation are more common in these patients than in those with achalasia. Long esophagomyotomy extending above the level of muscular thickening (usually to the level of the aortic arch) has been used successfully in severe cases and when manometry has revealed only contraction abnormalities.[179, 200, 222-225] Success rates exceeding 50 per cent have been reported. The author has not seen a case that has required myotomy. It has been suggested that myotomy for esophageal spasm should be reserved for patients in whom manometry has documented abnormal motor activity during an attack of pain.[171] This may be a difficult requirement to fulfill, but it carries an appropriate tone of reservation.

DISORDERS OF THE LOWER SPHINCTER

Abnormalities in resting sphincter tone and of relaxation occur without evidence of motor disturbance in the esophageal body. A *hypertensive lower sphincter* is seen most commonly in association with spastic disorders. This finding may also be observed as an isolated abnormality[170, 197, 226] and is thought to be associated with esophageal symptoms.[197] Treatment has been similar to the pharmacologic therapy for esophageal spasm. *Hypotension of the lower sphincter* is commonly associated with reflux esophagitis. The primary cause of pathologic reduction in sphincter tone is not known, but esophagitis itself is thought to have a detrimental effect on sphincter muscle function.[227] Decreased sphincter pressure has also been observed with scleroderma and other connective tissue diseases,[228, 229] diabetes mellitus,[230] and pregnancy.[231] An incompetent sphincter can be seen in association with hiatus hernia, but the hernia is not thought to be directly responsible for reduction in sphincter pressure.[232] Experimental production of hiatus hernia does not alter sphincter pressure in laboratory animals.[233] *Incomplete lower sphincter relaxation* without aperistalsis has been found early in the course of achalasia.[234] This finding is also present in some patients with Chagas' disease[235] and following vagotomy.[236] Pneumatic dilation can be offered to patients with this isolated finding if symptoms are of sufficient magnitude and obstructive lesions in the region of the lower sphincter are carefully excluded.

SYSTEMIC DISEASES ASSOCIATED WITH ESOPHAGEAL MOTOR DYSFUNCTION

Connective Tissue Diseases

Scleroderma. This disorder of connective tissue frequently involves the esophagus. As many as 74 per cent of patients with typical skin manifestations will have evidence of esophageal involvement at autopsy,[237] and clinical involvement may exceed this rate.[238] Light microscopy demonstrates muscle atrophy and fibrosis that affect predominantly the smooth muscle region of the esophagus. The end result is failure of muscle contraction in the distal esophagus and incompetency of the lower sphincter.[239] In some patients with this connective tissue disease, the esophageal muscle may still be responsive to cholinergic stimulation, suggesting that neural dysfunction has preceded muscle atrophy and fibrosis.[239] Similarly, normal reactivity of smooth muscle but impaired neural responses has been demonstrated in both the small and large intestine in early cases of scleroderma.[240, 241] Despite additional evidence in the esophagus that physiologic motor disturbances precede histologic change,[242] a distinct neuropathologic

lesion has not been described in the esophagus or other parts of the gut. Inflammatory infiltrates composed of mast cells and eosinophils are found in skin lesions early in the course of this disease and have been detected in close association with intestinal neural plexuses,[243] a finding that may have relevance to physiologic observations.

Clinical Features. Clinical features of esophageal involvement include symptoms of heartburn and dysphagia. Although the degree of motor dysfunction often is profound, these symptoms are reported by less than half of patients.[244] Gastroesophageal reflux is pronounced because of loss of lower sphincter competency in conjunction with poor esophageal clearance. Evidence of esophageal involvement may actually be present on plain films of the chest (Fig. 33–29).[245] Dysphagia may result from the motor disturbance itself or from a stricture complicating reflux.[246] Barium studies further clarify the loss of normal motility (Fig. 33–30) and also may provide evidence of esophagitis or stricture.

Manometry. Manometry will show abnormalities both in the smooth muscle portion of the esophageal body and in the lower sphincter (Fig. 33–31).[23] Dysfunction in the esophageal body becomes evident before the loss of lower sphincter tone,[242] and reduction in contraction strength precedes aperistalsis that is seen with advanced involvement.[247, 248] The combination of aperistalsis in the smooth muscle region of the esophageal body with hypotension of the lower sphincter is

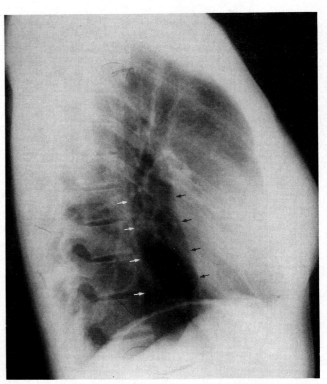

Figure 33–29. A lateral chest film from a patient with scleroderma and typical esophageal involvement. The air-filled esophagus on the upright film is outlined by arrows and results from incompetency of the lower sphincter in association with esophageal atony.

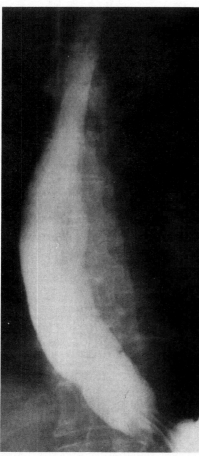

Figure 33–30. An atonic esophagus with wide patency of the lower esophageal sphincter region in a patient with scleroderma and esophageal involvement. Free reflux to the thoracic inlet was readily demonstrated, as was complete absence of a primary peristaltic stripping wave.

so typical that it has been labeled "scleroderma esophagus." From a diagnostic standpoint, the pattern is not specific, and less than 40 per cent of patients identified at a motility laboratory with these findings will have any evidence of connective tissue disease.[249] Radionuclide transit studies correlate well with manometry in scleroderma,[250] and these well-tolerated tests are useful in staging the disease.

Treatment. Treatment cannot reverse the motor findings in this disease and is directed toward gastroesophageal reflux and its complications. Dysphagia without stricture may also improve with treatment of reflux esophagitis. Conventional antireflux therapy should be employed, and typical medical maneuvers are beneficial[251, 252] (see pp. 608–616). Management should be aggressive considering the predisposition of this group to serious complications. Stricture formation also seems to be more insidious in scleroderma patients than in others with gastroesophageal reflux, occurring without a history of significant heartburn. Antireflux surgery is discouraged because of its potentially serious worsening of dysphagia. Despite this concern, good results have been reported and such management could be considered in exceptionally refractory cases.[253]

Other Connective Tissue Diseases. Esophageal features similar to those described for scleroderma have been seen in other connective tissue diseases, especially those that overlap with typical scleroderma (CREST syndrome, polymyositis, dermatomyositis, mixed connective tissue disease).[238, 254–257] Esophageal motor abnormalities are most likely when Raynaud's phenomenon is a component of the manifestations.[238, 239]

Diabetes Mellitus

Abnormalities in esophageal motility are frequently detected in patients with diabetes mellitus when they are studied by either radiography or manometry.[163, 258–260] Their direct relation to the metabolic disease remains uncertain. More than 60 per cent of diabetic persons with evidence of peripheral or autonomic neuropathy may have disordered motility, but symptoms are reported by a minority of these.[163, 258, 259] Radiographic studies reveal failure of the stripping wave in some cases and findings suggestive of a spastic disorder in others. Manometry also has demonstrated failed contraction sequences[259] and contraction abnormalities, as seen in the spastic disorders.[163] A cholinergic mechanism may be responsible for double-peaked waves noted in these patients;[261] this mechanism is not necessarily specific to diabetes. Vagal neuropathy has been proposed as the cause of these findings, but

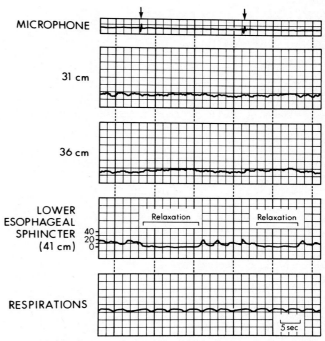

Figure 33–31. A manometric tracing from a patient with typical physical manifestations of scleroderma. Two recording ports in the distal esophagus (31 and 36 cm from the nares) show no meaningful contractions following two swallows *(arrows).* The third recording port in the region of the lower sphincter reveals appropriate relaxation of this sphincter following the swallows. The sphincter pressure drops to gastric baseline from a low resting pressure of 10 mm Hg. These features are typical of advanced esophageal involvement by this disease.

histologic evidence has been meager. In one study, contraction abnormalities correlated with the presence of psychiatric disturbances but not with neuropathy,[163] a finding similar to observations in nondiabetic subjects with esophageal spasm symptoms.[164] Reduction in contraction amplitudes and durations in the distal esophagus, on the other hand, appeared to have an independent association with neuropathy in diabetic patients.

Other Diseases

Disordered esophageal motility has been described in association with a variety of diseases that are not restricted to the esophagus. A direct relationship between the motor abnormalities and the systemic disease is often incompletely proved. A reduction in distal contraction amplitudes can be observed with hypothyroidism,[262] chronic alcoholism,[263] amyloidosis,[115] chronic idiopathic intestinal pseudo-obstruction,[264] and aging.[265] The defect can be severe enough that no measurable waves can be detected in some of these disorders. In addition to the disorders known to produce oropharyngeal dysphagia, steroid myopathy[266] and alcoholic myopathy[267] may interfere with function of the skeletal muscle portion of the esophagus.

References

1. Cattau, E. L., Jr., and Castell, D. O. Symptoms of esophageal dysfunction. *In* Castell, D. O., and Johnson, L. F. (eds.). Esophageal Function in Health and Disease. New York, Elsevier Biomedical, 1983, pp. 31–46.
2. Edwards, D. A. W. Discriminative information in the diagnosis of dysphagia. J. R. Coll. Phys. (Lond.) 9:257, 1975.
3. Christensen, J. Origin of sensation in the esophagus. Am. J. Physiol. 246:G221, 1984.
4. Reidel, W. L., and Clouse, R. E. Variations in clinical presentation of patients with esophageal contraction abnormalities. Dig. Dis. Sci. 30:1065, 1985.
5. Kramer, P., and Hollander, W. Comparison of experimental esophageal pain with clinical pain of angina pectoris and esophageal disease. Gastroenterology 29:719, 1955.
6. Jones, C. M. Digestive Tract Pain: Diagnosis and Treatment, Experimental Observations. New York, Macmillan, 1938.
7. Davies, H. A., Jones, D. B., Rhodes, J., and Newcombe, R. G. Angina-like esophageal pain: differentiation from cardiac pain by history. J. Clin. Gastroenterol. 7:477, 1985.
8. Dodds, W. J. Current concepts of esophageal motor function: clinical implications for radiology. AJR 128:549, 1977.
9. Margulis, A. R., and Koehler, R. E. Radiologic diagnosis of disordered esophageal motility. Radiol. Clin. North Am. 14:429, 1976.
10. Stewart, E. T. Radiographic evaluation of the esophagus and its motor disorders. Med. Clin. North Am. 65:1173, 1981.
11. Ott, D. J., Wu, W. C., and Gelfand, D. W. Efficacy of radiology of the esophagus for evaluation of dysphagia. Gastrointest. Radiol. 6:109, 1981.
12. Koehler, R. E., Weyman, P. J., and Oakley, H. F. Single- and double-contrast techniques in esophagitis. AJR 135:15, 1980.
13. Mandelstam, P., and Lieber, A. Cineradiographic evaluation of the esophagus in normal adults. Gastroenterology 58:32, 1970.
14. Hollis, J. B., and Castell, D. O. Effect of dry swallows and wet swallows of different volumes on esophageal peristalsis. J. Appl. Physiol. 38:1161, 1975.
15. Meyer, G. W., Gerhardt, D. C., and Castell, D. O. Human esophageal response to rapid swallowing: muscle refractory period or neural inhibition? Am. J. Physiol. 241:G129, 1981.
16. Vanek, A. W., and Diamant, N. E. Responses of the human esophagus to paired swallows. Gastroenterology 92:643, 1987.
17. Arndorfer, R. C., Stef, J. J., Dodds, W. J., Linehan, J. H., and Hogan, W. J. Improved infusion system for intraluminal esophageal sphincter pressure. Gastroenterology 68:437, 1975.
18. Dent, J. A new technique for continuous sphincter pressure measurements. Gastroenterology 71:263, 1976.
19. Stef, J. J., Dodds, W. J., Hogan, W. J., Linehan, J. H., and Stewart, E. T. Intraluminal esophageal manometry: an analysis of variables affecting recording fidelity of peristaltic pressures. Gastroenterology 67:221, 1974.
20. Welch, R. W., and Drake, S. T. Normal lower esophageal sphincter pressure: a comparison of rapid vs. slow pull-through techniques. Gastroenterology 78:1446, 1980.
21. Dodds, W. J., Hogan, W. J., Reid, D. P., Stewart, E. T., and Arndorfer, R. C. A comparison between primary esophageal peristalsis following wet and dry swallows. J. Appl. Physiol. 35:851, 1973.
22. Kaye, M. D., and Wexler, R. M. Alteration of esophageal peristalsis by body position. Dig. Dis. Sci. 26:897, 1981.
23. Hurwitz, A. L., Duranceau, A., and Haddad, J. K. Disorders of Esophageal Motility. Philadelphia, W. B. Saunders Co., 1979.
24. Dodds, W. J., Stewart, E. T., Hodges, D., and Zboralske, F. F. Movement of the feline esophagus associated with respiration and peristalsis. J. Clin. Invest. 52:1, 1973.
25. Dodds, W. J., Stewart, E. T., Hogan, W. J., Stef, J. J., and Arndorfer, R. C. Effect of esophageal movement on intraluminal esophageal pressure recoding. Gastroenterology 67:592, 1974.
26. Ouyang, A., Reynolds, J. C., and Cohen, S. Spike-associated and spike-independent esophageal contractions in patients with symptomatic diffuse esophageal spasm. Gastroenterology 84:907, 1983.
27. Tolin, R. D., Malmud, L. S., Reilley, J., and Fisher, R. S. Esophageal scintigraphy to quantitate esophageal transit. Gastroenterology 76:1402, 1979.
28. Russell, C. O. H., Hill, L. D., Holmes, E. R., III, Hull, D. A., Gannon, R., and Pope, C. E., II. Radionuclide transit: a sensitive screening test for esophageal dysfunction. Gastroenterology 80:887, 1981.
29. Netscher, D., Larson, G. M., and Polk, H. C., Jr. Radionuclide esophageal transit. A screening test for esophageal disorders. Arch. Surg. 121:843, 1986.
30. Bartlett, R. J. V. Scintigraphy of the oesophagus. *In* Robinson, P. J. A. (ed.). Nuclear Gastroenterology. Edinburgh, Churchill Livingstone, 1986.
31. DeCaestecker, J. S., Blackwell, J. N., Adam, R. D., Hannan, W. J., Brown, J., and Heading, R. C. Clinical value of radionuclide oesophageal transit measurement. Gut 27:659, 1986.
32. Mughal, M. M., Marples, M., and Bancewicz, J. Scintigraphic assessment of oesophageal motility: what does it show and how reliable is it? Gut 27:946, 1986.
33. Blackwell, J. N., Richter, J. E., Wu, W. C., Cowan, R. J., and Castell, D. O. Esophageal radionuclide transit tests: potential false positive results. Clin. Nucl. Med. 9:679, 1984.
34. Cherry, J., Siegel, C. I., Margulies, S. I., and Donner, M. Pharyngeal localization of symptoms of gastroesophageal reflux. Ann. Otol. Rhinol. Laryngol. 79:912, 1970.
35. Hallewell, J. D., and Cole, T. B. Isolated head and neck symptoms due to hiatus hernia. Arch. Otolaryngol. 92:499, 1970.
36. Gerhardt, D. C., Shuck, T. J., Bordeaux, R. A., and Winship, D. H. Human upper esophageal sphincter. Response to volume, osmotic, and acid stimuli. Gastroenterology 75:268, 1978.
37. Watson, W. C., and Sullivan, S. N. Hypertonicity of the cricopharyngeal sphincter: a cause of globus sensation. Lancet 2:1417, 1974.
38. Lehtinen, V., and Puhakka, H. A psychosomatic approach to the globus hystericus syndrome. Acta Psychiatr. Scand. 53:21, 1976.
39. Kilman, W. J., and Goyal, R. K. Disorders of pharyngeal and

upper esophageal sphincter motor function. Arch. Intern. Med. *136*:592, 1976.

40. Fischer, R. A., Ellison, G. W., Thayer, W. R., Spiro, H. M., and Glaser, G. H. Esophageal motility in neuromuscular disorders. Ann. Intern. Med. *63*:229, 1965.
41. Serebro, H. A., Mieny, C. J., Webster, A., and Jackson, H. Oesophageal manometric studies of dysphagia in Vernet's syndrome. Br. J. Surg. *58*:461, 1971.
42. Silbiger, M. I., Pikielney, R., and Donner, M. W. Neuromuscular disorders affecting the pharynx: cineradiographic analysis. Invest. Radiol. *2*:442, 1967.
43. Bramble, M. G., Cunliffe, J., and Dellipiani, A. W. Evidence for a change in neurotransmitter affecting oesophageal motility in Parkinson's disease. J. Neurol. Neurosurg. Psychiatry *41*:709, 1978.
44. Calne, D. B., Shaw, D. G., Spiers, A. S. D., and Sterne, G. M. Swallowing in Parkinsonism. Br. J. Radiol. *43*:456, 1970.
45. Cotzias, G. C., Papavasiliou, P. S., and Gellene, R. Modification of Parkinsonism: chronic treatment with L-dopa. N. Engl. J. Med. *280*:337, 1969.
46. Nowack, W. J., Hatelid, J. M., and Sohn, R. S. Dysphagia in Parkinsonism. Arch. Neurol. *34*:320, 1977.
47. Daly, D. D., Code, C. F., and Andersen, H. A. Disturbances of swallowing and esophageal motility in patients with multiple sclerosis. Neurology *12*:250, 1962.
48. Hurwitz, A. L., Nelson, J. A., and Haddad, J. K. Oropharyngeal dysphagia: manometric and cine-esophagraphic findings. Am. J. Dig. Dis. *20*:313, 1975.
49. Henderson, R. D., Boszko, A., and VanNostrand, A. W. P. Pharyngoesophageal dysphagia and recurrent laryngeal nerve palsy. J. Thorac. Cardiovasc. Surg. *68*:507, 1974.
50. Brahdy, M. B., and Lenarsky, M. Difficulty in swallowing in acute epidemic poliomyelitis. JAMA *103*:229, 1934.
51. Bosma, J. F. Residual disability of pharyngeal area resulting from poliomyelitis. JAMA *165*:216, 1957.
52. O'Hara, J. M., Szemes, G., and Lowman, R. M. The esophageal lesions in dermatomyositis: a correlation of radiologic and pathologic findings. Radiology *89*:27, 1967.
53. Feldman, F., and Marshak, R. H. Dermatomyositis with significant involvement of the gastrointestinal tract. AJR *90*:746, 1963.
54. Horowitz, M., McNeil, J. D., Maddern, G. J., Collins, P. J., and Shearman, D. J. Abnormalities of gastric and esophageal emptying in polymyositis and dermatomyositis. Gastroenterology *90*:434, 1986.
55. Pearson, C. M., and Currie, S. Polymyositis and related disorders. *In* Walton, J. N. (ed.). Disorders of Voluntary Muscle, 3rd ed. Edinburgh, Churchill Livingstone, 1974, p. 614.
56. Kagen, L. J., Hochman, R. B., and Strong, E. W. Cricopharyngeal obstruction in inflammatory myopathy (polymyositis/dermatomyositis). Report of three cases and review of the literature. Arthritis Rheum. *28*:630, 1985.
57. Siegel, C. L., Hendrix, T. R., and Harvey, J. C. The swallowing disorder in myotonia dystrophica. Gastroenterology *50*:541, 1966.
58. Eckardt, V. F., Nix, W., Kraus, W., and Bohl, J. Esophageal motor function in patients with muscular dystrophy. Gastroenterology *90*:628, 1986.
59. Duranceau, A. C., Beauchamp, G., Jamieson, G. G., and Barbeau, A. Oropharyngeal dysphagia and oculopharyngeal muscular dystrophy. Surg. Clin. North Am. *63*:825, 1983.
60. Bender, M. D. Esophageal manometry in oculopharyngeal dystrophy. Am. J. Gastroenterol. *65*:215, 1976.
61. Garrett, J. M., Dubose, T. D., Jr., Jackson, J. E., and Norman, J. R. Esophageal and pulmonary disturbances in myotonia dystrophica. Arch. Intern. Med. *123*:26, 1969.
62. Wright, R. A., and Penner, D. B. Myxedema and upper esophageal dysmotility. Dig. Dis. Sci. *26*:376, 1981.
63. Sulway, M. J., Baume, P. E., and Davis, E. Stiff-man syndrome presenting with complete esophageal obstruction. Am. J. Dig. Dis. *15*:79, 1970.
64. Asherson, N. Achalasia of the cricopharyngeal sphincter. J. Laryngol. Otol. *64*:747, 1950.
65. Hurwitz, A. L., and Duranceau, A. Upper esophageal sphinc-

ter dysfunction: pathogenesis and treatment. Am. J. Dig. Dis. *23*:275, 1978.
66. Cruse, J. P., Edwards, D. A. W., Smith, J. F., and Wyllie, J. H. The pathology of cricopharyngeal dysphagia. Histopathology *3*:223, 1979.
67. Hanna, W., and Henderson, R. D. Nemaline rods in cricopharyngeal dysphagia. Am. J. Clin. Pathol. *74*:186, 1980.
68. Ellis, F. H., Jr. Surgical management of esophageal motility disturbances. Am. J. Surgery *139*:752, 1980.
69. Ellis, F. H., Jr. Upper esophageal sphincter in health and disease. Surg. Clin. North Am. *51*:553, 1971.
70. West, E. M., Jr. and Baker, H. W. Esophageal dysphagia treated by cricopharyngeal myotomy. Ann. Surg. *43*:703, 1977.
71. Henderson, R. D., and Marryatt, G. Cricopharyngeal myotomy as a method of treating cricopharyngeal dysphagia secondary to gastroesophageal reflux. J. Thorac. Cardiovasc. Surg. *74*:721, 1977.
72. Bonavina, L., Khan, N. A., and DeMeester, T. R. Pharyngoesophageal dysfunctions. The role of cricopharyngeal myotomy. Arch. Surg. *120*:541, 1985.
73. Willis, T. Pharmaceutice rationalis sive diatribe de medicamentorum operationibus in humano corpore. London, Hagae-Comitis: A. Leers, 1674.
74. Von Mikulicz, J. Zur Pathologie und Therapie des Cardiospasmus. Dtsch. Med. Wochenschr. *30*:17, 1904.
75. Lendrum, F. C. Anatomic features of the cardiac orifice of the stomach with special reference to cardiospasm. Arch. Intern. Med. *59*:474, 1937.
76. Smith, B. The neurological lesion in achalasia of the cardia. Gut *11*:388, 1970.
77. Nagler, R. W., Schwartz, R. D., Stahl, W. M., Jr., and Spiro, H. M. Achalasia in fraternal twins. Ann. Intern. Med. *59*:906, 1963.
78. Kilpatrick, Z. M., and Milles, S. S. Achalasia in mother and daughter. Gastroenterology *62*:1042, 1972.
79. London, F. A., Raab, D. E., Fuller, J., and Olsen, A. M. Achalasia in three siblings. Mayo Clin. Proc. *52*:97, 1977.
80. Mackler, D., and Schneider, R. Achalasia in father and son. Am. J. Dig. Dis. *23*:1042, 1978.
81. Eckrich, J. D., and Winans, C. S. Discordance for achalasia in identical twins. Dig. Dis. Sci. *24*:221, 1979.
82. Mayberry, J. F., and Atkinson, M. A study of swallowing difficulties in first degree relatives of patients with achalasia. Thorax *40*:391, 1985.
83. Friesen, D. L., Henderson, R. D., and Hanna, W. Ultrastructure of the esophageal muscle in achalasia and diffuse esophageal spasm. Am. J. Clin. Pathol. *79*:319, 1983.
84. Cassella, R. R., Brown, A. L., Jr., Sayre, G. P., and Ellis, F. H., Jr. Achalasia of the esophagus: pathologic and etiologic considerations. Ann. Surg. *160*:474, 1964.
85. Csendes, A., Smok, G., Braghetto, I., Ramirez, C., Velasco, N., and Henriquez, A. Gastroesophageal sphincter pressure and histological changes in distal esophagus in patients with achalasia of the esophagus. Dig. Dis. Sci. *30*:941, 1985.
86. Qualman, S. J., Haupt, H. M., Yang, P., and Hamilton, S. R. Esophageal Lewy bodies associated with ganglion cell loss in achalasia. Similarity to Parkinson's disease. Gastroenterology *87*:848, 1984.
87. Etzel, E. Megaoesophagus and its neuropathology: a clinical and anatomo-pathological research. Guy's Hosp. Rep. *87*:158, 1937.
88. Cassella, R. R., Ellis, F. H., Jr., and Brown, A. L., Jr. Fine-structure changes in achalasia of the esophagus. I. Vagus nerves. Am. J. Pathol. *46*:279, 1965.
89. Kimura, K. The nature of idiopathic esophagus dilatation. Jpn. J. Gastroenterol. *1*:199, 1929.
90. Higgs, B., Kerr, F. W. L., and Ellis, F. H., Jr. The experimental production of esophageal achalasia by electrolytic lesions in the medulla. J. Thorac. Cardiovasc. Surg. *50*:613, 1965.
91. Misiewicz, J. J., Waller, S. L., Anthony, P. P., and Gummer, J. W. Achalasia of the cardia: pharmacology and histopathology of isolated cardiac sphincteric muscle from patients with and without achalasia. Q. J. Med. *38*:17, 1969.
92. Kramer, P., and Ingelfinger, F. J. Esophageal sensitivity to Mecholyl in cardiospasm. Gastroenterology *19*:242, 1951.

93. Heitmann, P., Espinoza, J., and Csendes, A. Physiology of the distal esophagus in achalasia. Scand. J. Gastroenterol. *4*:1, 1969.

94. Dodds, W. J., Dent, J., Hogan, W. J., Patel, G. K., Toouli, J., and Arndorfer, R. C. Paradoxical lower esophageal sphincter contraction induced by cholecystokinin-octapeptide in patients with achalasia. Gastroenterology *80*:327, 1981.

95. Holloway, R. H., Dodds, W. J., Helm, J. F., Hogan, W. J., Dent, J., and Arndorfer, R. C. Integrity of cholinergic innervation to the lower esophageal sphincter in achalasia. Gastroenterology *90*:924, 1986.

96. Woolam, G. L., Maher, F. T., and Ellis, F. H., Jr. Vagal nerve function in achalasia of the esophagus. Surg. Forum *18*:362, 1967.

97. Bianco, A., Cagossi, M., Scrimieri, D., and Greco, A. V. Appearance of esophageal peristalsis in treated idiopathic achalasia. Dig. Dis. Sci. *31*:40, 1986.

98. Lamet, M., Fleshler, B., and Achkar, E. Return of peristalsis in achalasia after pneumatic dilatation. Am. J. Gastroenterol. *80*:602, 1985.

99. Little, A. G., Correnti, F. S., Calleja, I. J., Montag, A. G., Chow, Y. C., Ferguson, M. K., and Skinner, D. B. Effect of incomplete obstruction on feline esophageal function with a clinical correlation. Surgery *100*:430, 1986.

100. Mayberry, J. F., and Atkinson, M. Studies of incidence and prevalence of achalasia in the Nottingham area. Q. J. Med. *56*:451, 1985.

101. Barrett, N. R. Achalasia of the cardia: reflections upon a clinical study of over 100 cases. Br. Med. J. *1*:1135, 1964.

102. Vantrappen, G., Hellemans, J., Deloof, W., Valembois, P., and Vandenbroucke, J. Treatment of achalasia with pneumatic dilatations. Gut *12*:268, 1971.

103. Wong, R. K. H., and Johnson, L. F. Achalasia. *In* Castell, D. O., and Johnson, L. F. (eds.). Esophageal Function in Health and Disease. New York, Elsevier Biomedical, 1983, pp. 99–123.

104. Kahrilas, P. J., Kishk, S. M., Helm, J. F., Dodds, W. J., Harig, J. M., and Hogan, W. J. Comparison of pseudoachalasia and achalasia. Am. J. Med. *82*:439, 1987.

105. Olsen, A. M., Holman, C. B., and Andersen, H. A. Diagnosis of cardiospasm. Dis. Chest *23*:477, 1953.

106. Stacher, G., Kiss, A., Wiesnagrotzki, S., Bergmann, H., Hobart, J., and Schneider, C. Oesophageal and gastric motility disorders in patients categorized as having primary anorexia nervosa. Gut *27*:1120, 1986.

107. Ellis, F. G. The natural history of achalasia of the cardia. Proc. R. Soc. Med. *53*:663, 1960.

108. Ponce, J., Miralbes, M., Garrigues, V., and Berenguer, J. Return of esophageal peristalsis after Heller's myotomy for idiopathic achalasia. Dig. Dis. Sci. *31*:545, 1986.

109. Sanderson, D. R., Ellis, F. H., Jr., Schlegel, J. F., and Olsen, A. M. Syndrome of vigorous achalasia: clinical and physiologic observations. Dis. Chest *52*:508, 1967.

110. Krevsky, B., and Fisher, R. S. Manometry in corkscrew esophagus [letter]. Gastrointest. Endosc. *32*:241, 1986.

111. Cohen, S., and Lipshutz, W. Lower esophageal sphincter dysfunction in achalasia. Gastroenterology *61*:814, 1971.

112. Katz, P. O., Richter, J. E., Cowan, R., and Castell, D. O. Apparent complete lower esophageal sphincter relaxation in achalasia. Gastroenterology *90*:978, 1986.

113. Vantrappen, G., van Goidsenhoven, G. E., Verbeke, S., van den Berghe, G., and Vandenbroucke, J. Manometric studies in achalasia of the cardia, before and after pneumatic dilations. Gastroenterology *45*:317, 1963.

114. Schuffler, M. D. Chronic intestinal pseudo-obstruction syndromes. Med. Clin. North Am. *65*:1331, 1981.

115. Costigan, D. J., and Clouse, R. E. Achalasia-like esophagus from amyloidosis: successful treatment with pneumatic bag dilatation. Dig. Dis. Sci. *28*:763, 1983.

116. Koberle, F. Chagas' disease and Chagas' syndrome: the pathology of American trypanosomiasis. Adv. Parasitol. *6*:63, 1968.

117. Greatorex, R. A., and Thorpe, J. A. Achalasia-like disturbance of oesophageal motility following truncal vagotomy and antrectomy. Postgrad. Med. J. *59*:100, 1983.

118. Stuckey, B. G., Mastaglia, F. L., Reed, W. D., and Pullan, P. T. Glucocorticoid insufficiency, achalasia, alacrima with autonomic and motor neuropathy. Ann. Intern. Med. *106*:62, 1987.

119. Cuthbert, J. A., Gallagher, N. D., and Turtle, J. R. Colonic and oesophageal disturbance in a patient with multiple endocrine neoplasia, Type 2b. Aust. N.Z. J. Med. *8*:518, 1978.

120. Similä, S., Kokkonen, J., and Kaski, M. Achalasia sicca—juvenile Sjögren's syndrome with achalasia and gastric hyposecretion. Eur. J. Pediatr. *129*:175, 1978.

121. Tucker, H. J., Snape, W. J., Jr. and Cohen, S. Achalasia secondary to carcinoma: manometric and clinical features. Ann. Intern. Med. *89*:315, 1978.

122. Sandler, R. S., Bozymski, E. M., and Orlando, R. C. Failure of clinical criteria to distinguish between primary achalasia and achalasia secondary to tumor. Dig. Dis. Sci. *27*:209, 1982.

123. Tishler, J. M., Shin, M. S., Stanley, R. J., and Koehler, R. E. CT of the thorax in patients with achalasia. Dig. Dis. Sci. *28*:692, 1983.

124. Köberle, F. Aspectos neurologicos da molestia de Chagas. Arq. NeuroPsiqiat. (São Paulo) *25*:159, 1967.

125. Bettarello, A., and Pinott, H. W. Oesophageal involvement in Chagas' disease. Clin. Gastroenterol. *5*:103, 1976.

126. Dodds, W. J., Stewart, E. T., Kishk, S. M., Kahrilas, P. J., and Hogan, W. J. Radiological amyl nitrite test for distinguishing pseudoachalasia from idiopathic achalasia. AJR *146*:21, 1986.

127. Ritvo, M., and McDonald, E. J. The value of nitrites in cardiospasm (achalasia of esophagus): preliminary report. AJR *43*:500, 1940.

128. Rozen, P., Gelfond, M., Salzman, S., Baron, J., and Gilat, T. Radionuclide confirmation of the therapeutic value of isosorbide dinitrate in relieving the dysphagia in achalasia. J. Clin. Gastroenterol. *4*:17, 1982.

129. Gelford, M., Rozen, P., and Gilat, T. Isosorbide dinitrate and nifedipine treatment of achalasia: a clinical manometric and radionuclide evaluation. Gastroenterology *83*:963, 1982.

130. Berger, K., and McCallum, R. W. Nifedipine in the treatment of achalasia. Ann. Intern. Med. *96*:61, 1982.

131. Traube, M., Hongo, M., Magyar, L., and McCallum, R. W. Effects of nifedipine in achalasia and in patients with high-amplitude peristaltic esophageal contractions. JAMA *252*:1733, 1984.

132. Bortolotti, M., and Labo, G. Clinical and manometric effects of nifedipine in patients with esophageal achalasia. Gastroenterology *80*:39, 1981.

133. Thomas, E., Lebow, R. A., Gubler, R. J., and Bryant, L. R. Nifedipine for the poor-risk elderly patient with achalasia: objective response demonstrated by solid meal study. South. Med. J. *77*:394, 1984.

134. Dellipiani, A. W., and Hewetson, K. A. Pneumatic dilatation in the management of achalasia: experience of 45 cases. Q. J. Med. *58*:253, 1986.

135. Csendes, A., Velasco, N., Braghetto, I., and Henriquez, A. A prospective randomized study comparing forceful dilatation and esophagomyotomy in patients with achalasia of the esophagus. Gastroenterology *80*:789, 1981.

136. Bennett, J. R., and Hendrix, T. R. Treatment of achalasia with pneumatic dilatation. Mod. Treat. *7*:1217, 1970.

137. Sariyannis, C., and Mullard, K. S. Oesophagomyotomy for achalasia of the cardia. Thorax *30*:539, 1975.

138. Van Goidsenhoven, G. E., Vantrappen, G., Verbeke, S., and Vandenbroucke, J. Treatment of achalasia of the cardia with pneumatic dilations. Gastroenterology *45*:326, 1963.

139. Fellows, I. W., Ogilvie, A. L., and Atkinson, M. Pneumatic dilatation in achalasia. Gut *24*:1020, 1983.

140. Lawrance, K., and Shoesmith, J. H. A review of the treatment of cardiospasm. Thorax *14*:211, 1959.

141. Olsen, A. M., Harrington, S. W., Moersch, H. J., and Andersen, H. A. The treatment of cardiospasm: analysis of a twelve-year experience. J. Thorac. Surg. *22*:164, 1951.

142. Vantrappen, G., and Janssens, J. To dilate or to operate? That is the question. Gut *24*:1013, 1983.

143. Vantrappen, G., and Hellemans, J. Treatment of achalasia and related motor disorders. Gastroenterology *79*:144, 1980.

144. Heller, E. Extramukose Cardiaplastik beim chronischen Car-

diospasmus mit Dilatation des Oesophagus. Mitt. a.d. Grenzgeb. d. Med. u. Chir. (Jena) 27:141, 1913.

145. Scott, H. W., Jr., DeLozier, J. B., III, Sawyers, J. L., and Adkins, R. B., Jr. Surgical management of esophageal achalasia. South. Med. J. 78:1309, 1985.

146. Pai, G. P., Ellison, R. G., Rubin, J. W., and Moore, H. V. Two decades of experience with modified Heller's myotomy for achalasia. Ann. Thorac. Surg. 38:201, 1984.

147. Ellis, F. H., Jr., Crozier, R. E., and Watkins, E., Jr. Operation for esophageal achalasia. Results of esophagomyotomy without an antireflux operation. J. Thorac. Cardiovasc. Surg. 88:344, 1984.

148. Sawyers, J. L., and Foster, J. H. Surgical considerations in the management of achalasia of the esophagus. Ann. Surg. 165:780, 1967.

149. Wingfield, H. V., and Karwowski, A. The treatment of achalasia by cardiomyotomy. Br. J. Surg. 59:281, 1972.

150. Black, J., Vorbach, A. N., and Collis, J. Results of Heller operation for achalasia of the esophagus: the importance of hiatal hernia. Br. J. Surg. 63:949, 1976.

151. Okike, N., Payne, W. S., Neufeld, D. M., Bernatz, P. E., Pairolero, P. C., and Sanderson, D. R. Esophagomyotomy versus forceful dilation for achalasia of the esophagus: results in 899 patients. Ann. Thorac. Surg. 28:119, 1979.

152. Douglas, K., and Nicholson, F. The late results of Heller's operation for cardiospasm. Br. J. Surg. 47:250, 1959.

153. Ellis, F. H., Jr., and Gibb, S. P. Reoperation after esophagomyotomy for achalasia of the esophagus. Am. J. Surg. 129:407, 1975.

154. Mercer, C. D., and Hill, L. D. Reoperation after failed esophagomyotomy for achalasia. Can. J. Surg. 29:177, 1986.

155. Jara, F. M., Toledo-Pereyra, L. H., Lewis, J. W., and Magilligan, D. J., Jr., Long-term results of esophagomyotomy for achalasia of esophagus. Arch. Surg. 114:935, 1979.

156. Sanderson, D. R., Ellis, F. H., Jr., and Olsen, A. M. Achalasia of the esophagus: results of therapy by dilation, 1950–1967. Chest 58:116, 1970.

157. Lortat-Jacob, J. L., Richard, C. A., Fekete, F., and Testart, J. Cardiospasm and esophageal carcinoma: report of 24 cases. Surgery 66:969, 1969.

158. Wychulis, A. R., Woolam, G. L., Andersen, H. A., and Ellis, F. H., Jr. Achalasia and carcinoma of the esophagus. JAMA 125:1638, 1981.

159. Heiss, F. W., Tarshis, A., and Ellis, F. H., Jr. Carcinoma associated with achalasia. Occurrence 23 years after esophagomyotomy. Dig. Dis. Sci. 29:1066, 1984.

160. Chuong, J. J., DuBovik, S., and McCallum, R. W. Achalasia as a risk factor for esophageal carcinoma. A reappraisal. Dig. Dis. Sci. 29:1105, 1984.

161. Richter, J. E., and Castell, D. O. Diffuse esophageal spasm: a reappraisal. Ann. Intern. Med. 100:242, 1984.

162. Bennett, J. R., and Hendrix, T. R. Diffuse esophageal spasm: a disorder with more than one cause. Gastroenterology 59:273, 1970.

163. Clouse, R. E., Lustman, P. J., and Reidel, W. L. Correlation of esophageal motility abnormalities with neuropsychiatric status in diabetics. Gastroenterology 90:1146, 1986.

164. Clouse, R. E., and Lustman, P. J. Psychiatric illness and contraction abnormalities of the esophagus. N. Engl. J. Med. 309:1337, 1983.

165. Creamer, B., Donoghue, E., and Code, C. F. Pattern of esophageal motility in diffuse spasm. Gastroenterology 34:782, 1958.

166. Vantrappen, G. R., and Hellemans, J. Motility. In Sircus, W., and Smith, A. N. (eds.). Scientific Foundations of Gastroenterology. Philadelphia, W. B. Saunders Co., 1980, pp. 227–253.

167. Herrington, J. P., Burns, T. W., and Balart, L. A. Chest pain and dysphagia in patients with prolonged peristaltic contractile duration of the esophagus. Dig. Dis. Sci. 29:134, 1984.

168. Benjamin, S. B., Gerhardt, D. C., and Castell, D. O. High amplitude, peristaltic esophageal contractions associated with chest pain and/or dysphagia. Gastroenterology 77:478, 1979.

169. Traube, M., Albibi, R., and McCallum, R. W. High-amplitude peristaltic esophageal contractions associated with chest pain. JAMA 250:2655, 1983.

170. Clouse, R. E., and Staiano, A. Contraction abnormalities of the esophageal body in patients referred for manometry: a new approach to manometric classification. Dig. Dis. Sci. 28:784, 1983.

171. Pope, C. E., II. Motor disorders. In Sleisenger, M. H., and Fordtran, J. S. (eds.). Gastrointestinal Disease, 3rd ed. Philadelphia, W. B. Saunders Co., 1983, pp. 424–448.

172. Clouse, R. E., Staiano, A., Landau, D. W., and Schlachter, J. L. Manometric findings during spontaneous chest pain in patients with presumed esophageal "spasms." Gastroenterology 85:395, 1983.

173. Janssens, J., Vantrappen, G., and Ghillebert, G. 24-hour recording of esophageal pressure and pH in patients with noncardiac chest pain. Gastroenterology 90:1978, 1986.

174. Traube, M., Aaronson, R. M., and McCallum, R. W. Transition from peristaltic esophageal contractions to diffuse esophageal spasm. Arch. Intern. Med. 146:1844, 1986.

175. Narducci, F., Bassotti, G., Gaburri, M., and Morelli, A. Transition from nutcracker esophagus to diffuse esophageal spasm. Am. J. Gastroenterol. 80:242, 1985.

176. DiMarino, A. J., Jr., and Cohen, S. Characteristics of lower esophageal sphincter function in symptomatic diffuse esophageal spasm. Gastroenterology 66:1, 1974.

177. Kaye, M. D. Anomalies of peristalsis in idiopathic diffuse oesophageal spasm. Gut 22:217, 1981.

178. Ebert, E. C., Ouyang, A., Wright, S. H., Cohen, S., and Lipshutz, W. H. Pneumatic dilatation in patients with symptomatic diffuse esophageal spasm and lower esophageal sphincter dysfunction. Dig. Dis. Sci. 28:481, 1983.

179. Gillies, M., Nicks, R., and Skyring, A. Clinical, manometric and pathological studies in diffuse oesophageal spasm. Br. Med. J. 2:527, 1967.

180. Ferguson, T. B., Woodbury, J. D., Roper, C. L., and Burford, T. H. Giant muscular hypertrophy of the esophagus. Ann. Thorac. Surg. 8:209, 1969.

181. Cassella, R. R., Ellis, F. H., Jr., and Brown, A. L. Diffuse spasm of the lower part of the esophagus. Fine structure of esophageal smooth muscle and nerve. JAMA 191:379, 1965.

182. Vantrappen, G., Janssens, J., Hellemans, J., and Coremans, G. Achalasia, diffuse esophageal spasm, and related motility disorders. Gastroenterology 76:450, 1979.

183. Kramer, P., Harris, L. D., and Donaldson, R. M., Jr. Transition from symptomatic diffuse spasm to cardiospasm. Gut 8:115, 1967.

184. Keshavarzian, A., Iber, F. L., and Ferguson, Y. Esophageal manometry and radionuclide emptying in chronic alcoholics. Gastroenterology 92:651, 1987.

185. Kramer, P., Fleshler, B., McNally, E., and Harris, L. D. Oesophageal sensitivity to Mecholyl in symptomatic diffuse spasm. Gut 8:120, 1967.

186. Kaye, M. D. Dysfunction of the lower esophageal sphincter in disorders other than achalasia. Am. J. Dig. Dis. 18:734, 1973.

187. Mellow, M. Symptomatic diffuse esophageal spasm. Manometric follow-up and response to cholinergic stimulation and cholinesterase inhibition. Gastroenterology 73:237, 1977.

188. Eckardt, V. F., Krüger, J., Holtermüller, K-H., and Ewe, K. Alteration of esophageal peristalsis by pentagastrin in patients with diffuse esophageal spasm. Scand. J. Gastroenterol. 10:475, 1975.

189. Nostrant, T. T., Sams, J., and Huber, T. Bethanechol increases the diagnostic yield in patients with esophageal chest pain. Gastroenterology 91:1141, 1986.

190. Benjamin, S. B., Richter, J. E., Cordova, C. M., Knuff, T. E., and Castell, D. O. Prospective manometric evaluation with pharmacologic provocation of patients with suspected esophageal motility dysfunction. Gastroenterology 84:893, 1983.

191. London, R. L., Ouyang, A., Snape, W. J., Jr., Goldberg, S., Hirshfeld, J. W., Jr., and Cohen, S. Provocation of esophageal pain by ergonovine or edrophonium. Gastroenterology 81:10, 1981.

192. Koch, K. L., Curry, R. C., Feldman, R. L., Pepine, C. J., Long, A., and Mathias, J. R. Ergonovine-induced esophageal

spasm in patients with chest pain resembling angina pectoris. Dig. Dis. Sci. *27*:1073, 1982.

193. Dart, A. M., Davies, H. A., Lowndes, R. H., Dalal, J., Ruttley, M., and Henderson, A. H. Oesophageal spasm and "angina": diagnostic value of ergometrine provocation. Eur. Heart J. *1*:91, 1980.

194. Richter, J. E., Dalton, C. B., Katz, P. O., Anderson, K. O., Rehberg, H. R., Young, L. D., and Bradley, L. A. Stress: a modulator of esophageal contractions. Gastroenterology *90*:1603, 1986.

195. Clouse, R. E., and Alpers, D. H. The relationship of psychiatric disorder to gastrointestinal illness. Ann. Rev. Med. *37*:283, 1986.

196. Richter, J. E., Barish, C. F., and Castell, D. O. Abnormal sensory perception in patients with esophageal chest pain. Gastroenterology *91*:845, 1986.

197. Katz, P. O., Dalton, C. B., Richter, J. E., Wu, W. C., and Castell, D. O. Esophageal testing of patients with noncardiac chest pain or dysphagia. Ann. Intern. Med. *106*:593, 1987.

198. Richter, J. E., Johns, D. N., Wu, W. C., and Castell, D. O. Are esophageal motility abnormalities produced during the intraesophageal acid perfusion test? JAMA *253*:1914, 1985.

199. Cole, M. J., Paterson, W. G., Beck, I. T., and DaCosta, L. R. The effect of acid and bethanechol stimulation in patients with symptomatic hypertensive peristaltic (nutcracker) esophagus. Evidence that this disorder may be a precursor of diffuse esophageal spasm. J. Clin. Gastroenterol. *8*:223, 1986.

200. Ellis, F. H., Jr., Olsen, A. M., Schlegel, J. F., Code, C. F. Surgical treatment of esophageal hypermotility disturbances. JAMA *188*:862, 1964.

201. Clouse, R. E., and Eckert, T. C. Gastrointestinal symptoms of patients with esophageal contraction abnormalities. Dig. Dis. Sci. *31*:236, 1986.

202. Richter, J. E., Obrecht, W. F., Bradley, L. A., Young, L. D., and Anderson, K. O. Psychological comparison of patients with nutcracker esophagus and irritable bowel syndrome. Dig. Dis. Sci. *31*:131, 1986.

203. Clouse, R. E., Eckert, T. C., and Staiano, A. Hiatus hernia and esophageal contraction abnormalities. Am. J. Med. *81*:447, 1986.

204. Texter, E. C., Jr., Lazar, H. P., Puletti, E. J., Van Derstappen, G., Danovitch, S. H., and Douglas, W. W. Hiatal hernia. *In* Thompson, C. M., Berkowitz, D., Polish, E., and Moyer, J. Y. (eds.). The Stomach Including Related Areas in the Esophagus and Duodenum. New York, Grune and Stratton, 1967, pp. 54–71.

205. Ott, D. J., Richter, J. E., Wu, W. C., Chen, Y. M., Gelfand, D. W., and Castell, D. O. Radiologic and manometric correlation in "nutcracker esophagus." AJR *147*:692, 1986.

206. Vantrappen, G., and Hellemans, J. Esophageal motor disorders. *In* Cohen, S., and Soloway, R. D. (eds.). Diseases of the Esophagus. New York, Churchill Livingstone, 1982, pp. 161–179.

207. Richter, J. E., Hackshaw, B. T., Wu, W. C., and Castell, D. O. Edrophonium: a useful provocative test for esophageal chest pain. Ann. Intern. Med. *103*:14, 1985.

208. Orlando, R. C., and Bozymski, E. M. Clinical and manometric effects of nitroglycerin in diffuse esophageal spasm. N. Engl. J. Med. *289*:23, 1973.

209. Swamy, N. Esophageal spasm: clinical and manometric response to nitroglycerine and long acting nitrites. Gastroenterology *72*:23, 1977.

210. Parker, W. A., and MacKinnon, G. L. Nitrites in the treatment of diffuse esophageal spasm. Drug. Intell. Clin. Pharm. *15*:806, 1981.

211. Mellow, M. H. Effect of isosorbide and hydralazine in painful primary esophageal motility disorders. Gastroenterology *83*:364, 1982.

212. Kikendall, J. W., and Mellow, M. H. Effect of sublingual nitroglycerin and long-acting nitrate preparations on esophageal motility. Gastroenterology *79*:703, 1980.

213. Nasrallah, S. M., Tommaso, C. L., Singleton, R. T., and Backhaus, E. A. Primary esophageal motor disorders: clinical response to nifedipine. South. Med. J. *78*:312, 1985.

214. Cargill, G., Theodore, C., and Paolaggi, J. A. Nifedipine for relief of esophageal chest pain? N. Engl. J. Med. *307*:187, 1982.

215. Nasrallah, S. M. Nifedipine in the treatment of diffuse oesophageal spasm. Lancet *2*:1285, 1982.

216. Richter, J. E., Spurling, T. J., Cordova, C. M., and Castell, D. O. Effects of oral calcium blocker, diltiazem, on esophageal contractions. Dig. Dis. Sci. *29*:649, 1984.

217. Richter, J. E., Dalton, C. B., Bradley, L. A., and Castell, D. O. Oral nifedipine in the treatment of noncardiac chest pain in patients with the nutcracker esophagus. Gastroenterology *93*:21, 1987.

218. Clouse, R. E., Lustman, P. J., Eckert, T. C., Ferney, D. M., and Griffith, L. S. Low-dose trazodone for symptomatic patients with esophageal contraction abnormalities: a double-blind, placebo-controlled trial. Gastroenterology *92*:1027, 1987.

219. Jacobson, E. D. Spastic esophagus and mucus colitis: etiology and treatment by progressive relaxation. Arch. Intern. Med. *39*:433, 1927.

220. Latimer, P. R. Biofeedback and self-regulation in the treatment of diffuse esophageal spasm: a single case study. Biofeedback Self. Reg. *6*:181, 1981.

221. Winters, C., Artnak, E. J., Benjamin, S. B., and Castell, D. O. Esophageal bougienage in symptomatic patients with the nutcracker esophagus. A primary esophageal motility disorder. JAMA *252*:363, 1984.

222. Leonardi, H. K., Shea, J. A., Crozier, R. E., and Ellis, F. H., Jr. Diffuse spasm of the esophagus. Clinical, manometric and surgical considerations. J. Thorac. Cardiovasc. Surg. *74*:736, 1977.

223. Henderson, R. D., Ho, C. S., and Davidson, J. W. Primary disordered motor activity of the esophagus (diffuse spasm): diagnosis and treatment. Ann. Thorac. Surg. *18*:327, 1974.

224. Jamieson, W. R., Miyagishima, R. T., Carr, D. M., Stordy, S. N., and Sharp, F. R. Surgical management of primary motor disorders of the esophagus. Am. J. Surg. *148*:36, 1984.

225. Horton, M. L., and Goff, J. S. Surgical treatment of nutcracker esophagus. Dig. Dis. Sci. *31*:878, 1986.

226. Code, C. F., Schlegel, J. F., Kelley, M. L., Jr., Olsen, A. M., and Ellis, F. H., Jr. Hypertensive gastroesophageal sphincter. Proc. Staff Meet. Mayo Clin. *35*:391, 1960.

227. Burns, T. W., and Venturatos, S. G. Esophageal motor function and response to acid perfusion in patients with symptomatic reflux esophagitis. Dig. Dis. Sci. *30*:529, 1985.

228. Neschis, M., Siegelman, S. S., and Rotstein, J. The esophagus in progressive systemic sclerosis. Am. J. Dig. Dis. *15*:443, 1970.

229. Ramirez-Mata, M., Reyes, P. A., Alarcon-Segovia, D., and Garza, R. Esophageal motility in systemic lupus erythematosus. Am J. Dig. Dis. *19*:132, 1974.

230. Stewart, I. M., Hosking, D. J., Preston, B. J., and Atkinson, M. Oesophageal motor changes in diabetes mellitus. Thorax *31*:278, 1976.

231. Van Thiel, D. H., Gavaler, J. S., Joshi, S. N., Sara, R. K., and Stremple, J. Heartburn of pregnancy. Gastroenterology *72*:666, 1977.

232. Cohen, S., and Harris, L. D. Does hiatus hernia affect competence of the gastroesophageal sphincter? N. Engl. J. Med. *284*:1053, 1971.

233. Meiss, J. H., Grindlay, J. H., and Ellis, F. H., Jr. The gastroesophageal sphincter mechanism: II. Further experimental studies in the dog. J. Thorac. Surg. *36*:156, 1958.

234. Meshkinpour, H., and Glick, M. E. Achalasia: is it an intermittent manometric phenomenon? Gastroenterology *90*:1550, 1986.

235. Csendes, A., Strauszer, T., and Uribe, P. Alterations in normal esophageal motility in patients with Chagas' disease. Am. J. Dig. Dis. *20*:437, 1975.

236. Guelrud, M., Zambrano-Rincones, V., Simon, C., Gomez, G., Salinas, A., Toledano, A., and Rudick, J. Dysphagia and lower esophageal sphincter abnormalities after proximal gastric vagotomy. Am. J. Surg. *149*:232, 1985.

237. Rodnan, G. P., Medsger, T. A., Jr., and Buckingham, R. B. Progressive systemic sclerosis-CREST syndrome: observations on natural history and late complications in 90 patients. Arthritis Rheum. *18*:423, 1975.

238. Stevens, M. B., Hookman, P., Siegel, C. I., Esterly, J. R.,

Shulman, L. E., and Hendrix, T. R. Aperistalsis of the esophagus in patients with connective-tissue disorders and Raynaud's phenomenon. N. Engl. J. Med. *270*:1218, 1964.

239. Cohen, S., Fisher, R., Lipshutz, W., Turner, R., Myers, A., and Schumacher, R. The pathogenesis of esophageal dysfunction in scleroderma and Raynaud's disease. J. Clin. Invest. *51*:2663, 1972.

240. DiMarino, A. J., Carlson, G., Myers, A., Schumacher, H. R., and Cohen, S. Duodenal myoelectric activity in scleroderma. Abnormal response to mechanical and hormonal stimuli. N. Engl. J. Med. *289*:1220, 1973.

241. Battle, W. M., Snape, W. J., Jr., Wright, S., Sullivan, M. A., Cohen, S., Meyers, A., and Tuthill, R. Abnormal colonic motility in progressive systemic sclerosis. Ann. Intern. Med. *94*:749, 1981.

242. Treacy, W. L., Baggenstoss, A. H., Slocumb, C. H., and Code, C. F. Scleroderma of the esophagus. A correlation of histologic and physiologic findings. Ann. Intern. Med. *59*:351, 1963.

243. DeSchryver-Kecskemeti, K., and Clouse, R. E. Gastrointestinal neuropathic changes in a group of patients with systemic connective tissue disease. Dig. Dis. Sci. *29*:549, 1984.

244. Garrett, J. M., Winkelmann, R. K., Schlegel, J. F., and Code, C. F. Esophageal deterioration in scleroderma. Mayo Clin. Proc. *46*:92, 1971.

245. Dinsmore, R. E., Goodman, D., and Dreyfuss, J. R. The air esophagram: a sign of scleroderma involving the esophagus. Radiology 87:348, 1966.

246. Zamost, B. J., Hirschberg, J., Ippoliti, A. F., Furst, D. E., Clements, P. J., and Weinstein, W. M. Esophagitis in scleroderma: prevalence and risk factors. Gastroenterology *92*:421, 1987.

247. Weihrauch, T. R., Korting, G. W., Ewe, K., and Vogt, G. Esophageal dysfunction and its pathogenesis in progressive systemic sclerosis. Klin. Wochenschr. *56*:963, 1978.

248. Stevens, M. B., Hookman, P., Siegel, C. I., Esterly, J. R., Schulman, L. E., and Hendrix, T. R. Aperistalsis of the oesophagus in patients with connective tissue disorders and Raynaud's phenomenon. N. Engl. J. Med. *270*:1218, 1964.

249. Schneider, H. A., Yonker, R. A., Longley, S., Katz, P., Mathias, J., and Panush, R. S. Scleroderma esophagus: a nonspecific entity. Ann. Intern. Med. *100*:848, 1984.

250. Drane, W. E., Karvelis, K., Johnson, D. A., Curran, J. J., and Silverman, E. D. Progressive systemic sclerosis: radionuclide esophageal scintigraphy and manometry. Radiology *160*:73, 1986.

251. Petrokubi, R. J., and Jeffries, G. H. Cimetidine versus antacid in scleroderma with reflux esophagitis. Gastroenterology *77*:691, 1979.

252. Ramirez-Mata, M., Ibanez, G., and Alarcon-Segovia, D. Stimulatory effect of metoclopramide on the esophagus and lower esophageal sphincter of patients with PSS. Arthritis Rheum. *20*:30, 1977.

253. Orringer, M. B. Surgical management of scleroderma reflux esophagitis. Surg. Clin. North Am. *63*:859, 1983.

254. Clark, M., and Fountain, R. B. Oesophageal motility in connective tissue disease. Br. J. Dermatol. *79*:449, 1967.

255. Tatelman, M., and Keech, M. K. Esophageal motility in systemic lupus erythematosus, rheumatoid arthritis and scleroderma. Radiology *86*:1041, 1966.

256. Sharp, G. C., Irvin, W. S., Tan, E. M., Gould, R. G., and Holman, H. R. Mixed connective tissue disease—an apparently distinct rheumatic disease syndrome associated with a specific antibody to an extractable nuclear antigen (ENA). Am. J. Med. *52*:148, 1972.

257. Sharp, G. C. Mixed connective tissue disease. Bull. Rheum. Dis. *25*:828, 1975.

258. Mandelstam, P., and Lieber, A. Esophageal dysfunction in diabetic neuropathy-gastroenterology. JAMA *201*:582, 1967.

259. Hollis, J. B., Castell, D. O., and Braddom, R. L. Esophageal function in diabetes mellitus and its relation to peripheral neuropathy. Gastroenterology *73*:1098, 1977.

260. Russell, C. O. H., Gannan, R., Coatsworth, J., Neilsen, R., Allen, F., Hill, L. D., and Pope, C. E., III. Relationship among esophageal dysfunction, diabetic gastroenteropathy, and peripheral neuropathy. Dig. Dis. Sci. *28*:289, 1983.

261. Loo, F. D., Dodds, W. J., Soergel, K. H., Arndorfer, R. C., Helm, J. F., and Hogan, W. J. Multipeaked esophageal peristaltic pressure waves in patients with diabetic neuropathy. Gastroenterology *88*:485, 1985.

262. Christensen, J. Esophageal manometry in myxedema. Gastroenterology *52*:1130, 1967.

263. Winship, D. H., Caflisch, C. R., Zboralske, F. F., and Hogan, W. J. Deterioration of esophageal peristalsis in patients with alcoholic neuropathy. Gastroenterology *55*:173, 1968.

264. Schuffler, M. D., and Pope, C. E., II. Esophageal motor dysfunction in idiopathic intestinal pseudoobstruction. Gastroenterology *70*:677, 1976.

265. Anuras, S., and Loening-Baucke, V. Gastrointestinal motility in the elderly. J. Am. Geriatr. Soc. *32*:386, 1984.

266. Cohen, S. Motor disorders of the esophagus. N. Engl. J. Med. *301*:184, 1979.

267. Weber, L. D., Nashel, D. J., and Mellow, M. H. Pharyngeal dysphagia in alcoholic myopathy. Ann. Intern. Med. *95*:189, 1981.

34 Gastroesophageal Reflux Disease (Reflux Esophagitis)

WALTER J. HOGAN
WYLIE J. DODDS

Symptomatic gastroesophageal reflux disease is the most common malady of the esophagus and probably the most prevalent clinical condition stemming from the alimentary tract.[1] Clinical symptoms of heartburn are reported to occur in 10 to 20 per cent of the general population.[2, 3]

In this chapter, the term "gastroesophageal reflux disease" is used to include any symptomatic clinical condition or histologic alteration that results from episodes of gastroesophageal (GE) reflux. The term "reflux esophagitis" refers to reflux changes, such as epithelial erosion or hyperplasia, accompanied by inflammation. Noninflammatory epithelial alterations associated with reflux, such as epithelial basal hyperplasia,[4–6] are referred to as "reflux changes." Generally, reflux esophagitis or reflux changes are accompanied by clinical symptoms, but these histologic alterations may be asymptomatic. In some individuals, basal cell hyperplasia of the esophageal epithelium may be unrelated to gastroesophageal reflux.[7]

PATHOGENESIS

The modern concept of reflux disease did not emerge until 1935, when Winkelstein suggested that garden-variety esophagitis was related to the digestive action of peptic gastric juice on the esophageal mucosa.[8] Before this time, the common malady of reflux peptic esophagitis was attributed to causes such as infection, chemical irritants, or a secondary effect of cardiospasm, diverticulum, or neoplasm. In the 1940s and 1950s, many workers believed that reflux esophagitis was caused mainly by abnormal mechanical factors associated with a sliding hiatal hernia. In the 1960s, the focus of attention shifted to the intrinsic lower esophageal sphincter (LES), and it was soon believed that the major villain in esophagitis production was a feeble or atonic LES.[9–11]

During the past two decades, a consensus has emerged that gastroesophageal (GE) reflux disease is not caused by a single abnormality, but rather is a multifactorial process wherein different abnormalities may predominate in a given patient.[12] The multiple factors that determine whether or not reflux esophagitis occurs include (1) efficacy of the antireflux mechanism, (2) volume of gastric contents, (3) potency of refluxed material, (4) efficiency of esophageal clearance, and (5) resistance of the esophageal tissue to injury and ability to repair. Thus, the extent and severity of reflux esophagitis does not depend on GE reflux episodes alone. Different factors or combinations of factors may predominate in causing reflux disease in a given patient.

Gastroesophageal Reflux

By definition, some episodes of GE reflux must occur for reflux disease to develop. Although some episodes of GE reflux occur in virtually everyone, the rate of reflux in patients with reflux disease generally is greater than in healthy asymptomatic subjects.[13, 14] Some symptomatic patients, however, exhibit a reflux rate within the range of normal.[15]

Evidence reported during the past decade[13, 16, 17] suggests that acid GE reflux may occur by one of three general mechanisms: (1) spontaneous reflux associated with transient LES relaxation, generally not associated with swallowing, (2) stress reflux owing to transient increases in intra-abdominal pressure caused by abdominal muscle contraction, and (3) free reflux (Fig. 34–1). Reflux associated with transient LES relaxation may occur against a background of either normal or low LES pressure, whereas stress or free reflux is invariably associated with low or absent LES tone.[13]

In normal subjects, acid GE reflux nearly always occurs secondary to transient LES relaxation, which is the mechanism involved in about two thirds of reflux episodes in patients with esophagitis as well.[13] Therefore, the major distinction between GE reflux in most esophagitis patients and controls is quantitative rather than qualitative. The patients, however, show heterogeneity with respect to the predominant reflux mechanism. Some patients (i.e., those with normal basal LES pressure) reflux virtually exclusively by LES relaxations, whereas others (i.e., those with hypotonic LES pressure) reflux mainly by the mechanisms of stress and free reflux. Still other patients show a relatively even distribution of the three generic mechanisms that underlie GE reflux.

The schema in Figure 34–1 also indicates that basal LES tone is an important constituent of the antireflux mechanism because GE reflux does not occur when basal LES pressure is above a minimal value. Moreover, it explains the apparent paradox of why sample values of LES pressure commonly are normal in many patients with reflux disease. Also explained is the

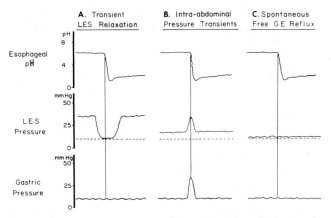

Figure 34–1. Schematic representation of three different mechanisms of gastroesophageal (GE) reflux. GE reflux events (shown as vertical lines) may accompany a transient lower esophageal sphincter (LES) relaxation *(A)*, develop as stress reflux during a transient increase in intra-abdominal pressure that overcomes LES resistance *(B)*, or occur as spontaneous free reflux across an atonic sphincter *(C)*. (From Dodds W. J., Dent J., Hogan W. J., et al. Reprinted by permission of the New England Journal of Medicine *308*:1547, 1982.)

nettlesome observation that GE reflux cannot be induced at fluoroscopic examination in half or more of patients with reflux esophagitis.[18] Even heroic stress maneuvers do not induce reflux when LES pressure is in the normal range (i.e., ≥ 10 mm Hg).

An important unanswered question is why some patients with reflux disease have hypotonic basal LES pressure. The LES hypotonia in some of these patients is undoubtedly secondary to reflux esophagitis, as has been shown in experimental animal models.[19] However, in some patients hypotonic LES pressure clearly predates the development of reflux symptoms, and LES hypotonia generally persists after therapeutic resolution of histologic esophagitis.[20, 21] A satisfactory explanation for primary LES hypotonia is not established.

A second critical question concerns the nature of the mechanism(s) that triggers an unduly high rate of reflux-associated transient LES relaxations in a high percentage of patients with reflux disease. Such LES relaxations are almost certainly mediated by the same inhibitory vagal efferent nerves that relax the LES in response to swallowing, esophageal distention, or vagal stimulation.[22]

An increased rate of nondeglutitive LES relaxations is elicited by gastric distention produced by eating, acid, gas, or gastric balloon inflation.[13, 23] Sensory stimuli from the pharynx or esophagus might also contribute. The authors hypothesize that the nondeglutitive LES relaxations associated with acid GE reflux may represent a variant of the belch reflux. Whether an abnormally high rate of LES relaxation is caused by an increase in provocative sensory stimuli, such as gastric distention, or by a decreased central threshold, or both, remains to be determined. In some cases, acid reflux may be associated with swallow-induced LES relaxation, particularly during failed peristaltic sequences.

Gastric Volume

For GE reflux to occur, clearly some gastric contents must be available to reflux. Increased gastric fluid volume not only makes more volume available for reflux but also increases the rate of nondeglutitive LES relaxations. Current findings suggest that a subset of patients with reflux disease may exhibit delayed gastric emptying of unknown cause.[24] If this is true, the increases in gastric volume could act as a contributory factor in the development of reflux disease.

Potency of Refluxate

For esophageal epithelial changes or complications of GE reflux to develop, the character of the refluxate must have some potency to cause injury. Experimentally, copious perfusion of the esophagus with saline solution or weak acid is quite harmless. Although hydrochloric acid alone at pH below 3.0 may cause esophageal injury by protein denaturization, pepsin is a major constituent of gastric juice that induces esophageal injury.[25] Pepsin, which becomes an active proteolytic enzyme in an acid milieu at a pH of less than 3.0, causes esophageal injury by digesting epithelial protein. A small amount of pepsin contributes substantially to the development of reflux "peptic" esophagitis. Other components that may be present in esophageal refluxate that can contribute to esophageal injury include both bile acids and pancreatic enzymes.[26, 27, 28] These latter components are likely to be present in patients who have undergone previous gastric surgery and have excessive reflux of bile and pancreatic juice into the stomach.

Esophageal Clearance

The obverse of acid GE reflux is esophageal acid clearance. Although reflux events determine the frequency and extent of esophageal exposure to refluxate, esophageal clearance determines the duration of esophageal exposure to the injurious effects of refluxate. Whereas a reflux event occurs in a few seconds, esophageal clearance of acid material commonly takes several minutes or longer. An understanding of esophageal clearance requires a clear distinction between volume clearance, which is a true clearance, and acid clearance, which is not a true clearance at all, but rather describes the restoration of esophageal pH to normal following an acid exposure. Although these two phenomena are related, they are not equivalent.

Current evidence indicates that esophageal acid clearance occurs normally as a two-step process.[13, 29] First, peristaltic esophageal motor activity rapidly clears fluid volume from the esophagus, and then a small amount of residual acid is neutralized by swallowed saliva (Fig. 34–2). Thus, normal peristalsis is extremely effective for volume clearance. For example, one or two peristaltic sequences generally clear all of a 15-ml fluid bolus from the esophagus.[30] Nonperistaltic contractions may promote some volume clearance but are much less effective than peristalsis. In the event that peristalsis is abnormal, gravity promotes esophageal drainage when the individual is upright, but not when he or she is supine. When peristalsis is normal, the effects of gravity are not needed to achieve normal esophageal clearance of volume.

Of interest is the fact that following acid GE reflux, primary peristalsis elicited by swallowing rather than secondary peristalsis elicited by esophageal stretch is the major type of esophageal motor activity that clears the esophagus of refluxate. Although secondary peristalsis has an ancillary protective role, about 80 per cent of the peristaltic sequences that occur during the restoration of esophageal acid to normal after acid GE reflux are primary peristaltic sequences.[16] This finding is explained by the fact that swallowing occurs about once a minute in awake subjects, regardless of whether or not reflux occurs. Such a high rate of spontaneous swallowing is elicited by saliva production of about 0.5 ml/min.[31] Thus, the protective mechanism of frequent swallow-induced peristalsis is already operative whenever GE reflux occurs. During sleep, salivation and swallowing virtually cease, thereby placing individuals at risk for prolonged esophageal exposure to acid refluxate whenever individuals sleep before esophageal clearance is complete or, less likely, when reflux occurs during sleep.

In addition to esophageal peristalsis, the second essential factor required for normal esophageal acid clearance is swallowed saliva. This fact is supported by the findings that increased salivation induced by an oral lozenge is associated with a significant decrease in acid clearance time, whereas aspiration by suction of saliva is accompanied by a marked prolongation in esophageal clearance, despite the occurrence of normal peristaltic sequences.[30, 32] Although saliva is ineffective in neutralizing a large volume of acid (e.g., 5 to 10 ml), the amount of saliva produced in several minutes is sufficient to neutralize the small amount of residual acid that normally remains in the esophagus after esophageal volume is cleared by one or more normal peristaltic sequences. The small amount of residual acid does not persist as a residual volume, but rather hydrogen ions move into the thin obligatory layer of fluid, or unstirred layer, that coats the esophageal mucosa.[33] When acidified, the mucosal fluid layer is neutralized effectively by bicarbonate ions carried within small boluses of swallowed saliva. A mini-titration occurs with each swallow, thereby accounting for the observation that an acid esophageal pH is typically restored to normal in a series of small steps, each associated with a swallow, rather than as a ramp function.

Abnormal esophageal clearance exists in a substantial subgroup of patients with reflux esophagitis.[34, 35] Delayed esophageal clearance may be caused by abnormal esophageal function, abnormal salivation, or sleep. Generally, impaired esophageal acid clearance in patients with reflux disease is caused by abnormal esophageal peristalsis. In a recent study, about 50 per cent of patients with mild to severe esophagitis exhibited some impairment of primary esophageal peristalsis.[36] In the authors' experience, only a small minority of esophagitis patients with abnormal esophageal acid clearance have impaired salivation.

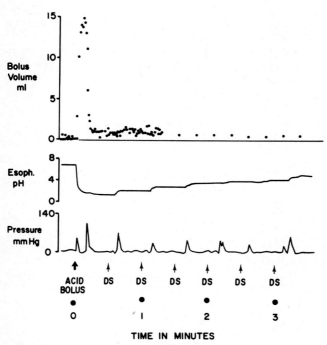

Figure 34—2. Relationship among esophageal acid clearance, motor activity, and emptying of fluid volume. Only peristaltic pressure complexes from the distal esophagus are shown. DS denotes dry swallows every 30 sec. After one swallow-induced peristaltic sequence, esophageal volume is reduced to less than 1 ml. Despite subsequent peristaltic sequences, a small number of counts persist over the esophagus owing to some adherence of the isotope to the mucosa. Although one or two peristaltic sequences clear virtually all the acid volume from the esophagus, a small amount of residual acid coats the esophageal mucosa. This acid must be neutralized, in step-wise fashion, by subsequent swallows that deliver small volumes of saliva to the esophagus. (From Helm J. F., Dodds W. J., Pelc L. R., et al. Reprinted by permission of the New England Journal of Medicine *310*:284, 1984.)

Tissue Resistance

The ability of the esophageal epithelium to withstand injury is an important determinant of whether or not a given individual develops reflux disease. The capacity of the esophageal mucosa to withstand injury and to repair following injury appears to be influenced by age and nutrition as well as other factors that are poorly understood at present.

The primary role of the stratified squamous esophageal epithelium is to provide an impermeable esophageal lining that has no requirements for secretion or absorption. Resistance of the esophageal epithelium to acid-peptic injury is governed by pre-epithelial, epithelial, and postepithelial factors.[37] For epithelial injury to occur, H^+ ions and agents such as pepsin must reach the esophageal mucosa. However, pre-epithelial defenses such as mucus, the unstirred water layer coating the mucosa, and surface bicarbonate ions may minimize or prevent such contact. The gel properties of the unstirred mucus-fluid layer serve as a barrier to large molecules such as pepsin. Although H^+ ions readily enter the mucus-fluid layer, HCO_3^- ions within the unstirred fluid layer neutralize some H^+ ions.

When H^+ penetrates the pre-epithelial defenses, several epithelial defenses must be overridden before epithelial injury occurs.[37] The stratified squamous epithelial cells and their tight intercellular junctions are initially impermeable to H^+ ions. When H^+ penetrates the intercellular junctions and reaches the deeper epithelial cells, these cells have active ionic transport mechanisms that tend to maintain a normal intracellular pH. These cellular mechanisms must be overwhelmed for cell death to occur. A compensatory mechanism for a modest rate of cell death is an increased cell turnover that leads to basal cell hyperplasia. In many cases, the latter mechanism is sufficient to present epithelial erosion or ulceration. Postepithelial factors that affect tissue resistance include mucosal blood flow and acid-base status.

Hiatus Hernia

The relationship between a sliding hiatus hernia and the genesis of esophagitis remains controversial. A consensus exists, however, that most patients with moderate to severe esophagitis have a sliding hiatus hernia, whereas the substantial majority of individuals with a sliding hiatus hernia do not have reflux disease.[12] Thus, in general, a direct causal relationship does not seem to exist between hiatus hernia and GE reflux disease. Nevertheless, the possibility remains that mechanical or functional aberrations associated with a sliding hiatus hernia may contribute to reflux disease in some patients. For example, some hernias could possibly compromise LES closure or give rise to sensory stimuli responsible for transient LES relaxations. In other instances, a hiatus hernia may act as a fluid trap that promotes GE reflux during swallow-induced LES relaxations in supine subjects.[38]

Special Conditions

A number of special-case circumstances may act as major determinants to the development of GE reflux disease. For example, reversible reflux disease occurs commonly during pregnancy. This occurrence is attributed to the depressant effects of high circulating levels of estrogen and progesterone on LES tone.[39] Other special circumstances that may provide or contribute to reflux disease include hyperemesis, anesthesia, unconsciousness, head injury, mental retardation, and nasogastric intubation. These conditions may reduce LES tone, provoke LES relaxations, or impair esophageal acid clearance. Lastly, specific diseases may affect esophageal motor function so as to favor the develop-

ment of reflux disease. Typical of such a condition is scleroderma, a disease that causes atrophy of esophageal smooth muscle and leads to excessive GE reflux, owing to feeble LES tone, and prolonged esophageal acid clearance, owing to impaired esophageal peristalsis. Additionally, some of these patients may also exhibit delayed gastric emptying and decreased salivation, impairments that may also contribute to the development of reflux disease.

CLINICAL SYMPTOMS AND NATURAL HISTORY

The most common clinical symptom of reflux disease is heartburn, or pyrosis, which generally is experienced as a retrosternal sensation of burning and discomfort. This symptom is believed to be caused by acid stimulation of sensory nerve endings located in the deeper layers of the esophageal epithelium. These nerve endings normally are protected by an impermeable epithelium, but with epithelial changes caused by reflux they may be stimulated by hydrogen ions or spicy foods.[40] Other symptoms associated with reflux disease include intermittent retrosternal chest pain, regurgitation, sour brash, water brash, dysphagia, and, rarely, odynophagia. Frank chest pain may be caused by acid stimulation of pain receptors or, less commonly, by acid-induced spastic esophageal contractions. Odynophagia, or pain with swallowing, occurs occasionally in patients with severe, erosive reflux disease but is more common in infectious esophagitis, such as candidiasis. In some patients, reflux episodes are associated with severe chest pain that may simulate angina.

Occasionally patients with hypersalivation, known as "water brash," literally "foam at the mouth." One such patient the authors saw produced saliva at the rate of 10 ml/min during periods of esophageal stimulation. Water brash is induced by acid reflux, wherein esophageal acid triggers an esophagosalivary reflex. Although increased salivation accompanies acid reflux in most patients with reflux esophagitis, the response is markedly exaggerated in some patients. The complaint of dysphagia in patients with reflux disease generally indicates the presence of an esophageal stricture. This symptom, however, may also be caused by abnormal esophageal motor function that may accompany reflux disease. Occasionally, the initial complaint is the sensation of a lump in the throat, referred to as globus sensation.[41] The genesis of globus, which is distinct from dysphagia, has been attributed to an increase in upper esophageal sphincter pressure, believed to be elicited by acid reflux.[42] An increase in UES pressure, however, was not confirmed in subsequent studies.[43] An unusual complaint is referred ear pain via the auricular nerve of Arnold. In adults, chronic blood loss associated with esophagitis occasionally leads to symptoms of anemia. Frank hemorrhage, however, is rare. The type and severity of reflux symptoms vary widely among patients but do not correlate well with the degree of esophageal injury.

GE reflux accompanied by regurgitation and aspiration may cause respiratory tract symptoms such as nonseasonal asthma, recurrent pneumonitis, nocturnal choking, or morning hoarseness. In some cases, these symptoms occur in the absence of any histologic abnormality of the esophageal mucosa. Findings from recent studies suggest that an esophagobronchial reflex may exist whereby acid reflux may stimulate receptors in a damaged esophageal mucosa to elicit bronchoconstriction.[44, 45, 46]

In infants and young children, symptoms of GE reflux differ considerably from those in adults. The predominant symptoms in young children is excessive regurgitation, which may be accompanied by respiratory symptoms. Significant symptoms are iron-deficiency anemia and failure to thrive. Difficulty in swallowing heralds the development of a stricture. A curious symptom in children is intermittent cervical torticollis or peculiar posturing known as Sandifer's syndrome.[47]

The clinical course of reflux symptoms varies widely, from spontaneous remission without treatment to intractable symptoms or severe complications during treatment. The substantial majority of patients have mild reflux disease, albeit their symptoms vary in frequency and intensity. In many cases, reflux disease may be situational, such as that associated with pregnancy or vomiting. In such cases the reflux disease commonly resolves without recurrence once the offending circumstance is past. In cases of spontaneous reflux disease, the reflux symptoms may resolve without therapy or with minimal therapy, only to return again at irregular intervals. In other patients, reflux symptoms subside or disappear during aggressive medical therapy, only to return as soon as the therapy is stopped or tapered. Lastly, reflux symptoms, such as heartburn, may be refractory, occur almost continuously, and require surgical therapy. Esophageal complications of reflux disease include stricture, hemorrhage, perforation, and Barrett's epithelium, whereas nonesophageal complications involve the respiratory tract or oral cavity.

Complications

Stricture

Peptic stricture of the esophagus is a serious sequela of aggressive reflux esophagitis. Repetitive, prolonged exposure to gastric refluxate may cause transmural inflammation that leads to fibrosis with loss of esophageal wall compliance or frank stricture. About 10 per cent of patients with severe reflux esophagitis develop a peptic stricture during the course of their disease. The incidence of stricture formation is increased in the presence of certain risk factors, such as Barrett's esophagus, or severe impairment of esophageal motor function, such as occurs in scleroderma.

Although peptic strictures nearly always occur in the distal esophagus, they occasionally develop at a higher level. They are usually short (e.g., 2 to 4 cm in length)

but may be extensive and involve the entire length of the thoracic esophagus. The latter situation is observed most often in the rare circumstance when fulminant reflux esophagitis ensues during a period of nasogastric intubation (Fig. 34–3) or in patients with Zollinger-Ellison syndrome. In some instances, a ring-like annular stricture may develop in the distal esophagus or at the esophagogastric junction (Fig. 34–4). The latter circumstance may simulate a tight Schatzki's ring, which is a mucosal plication covered below with columnar epithelium and above with squamous epithelium.

Esophageal peptic strictures generally develop insidiously over months; occasionally they evolve rapidly within a few weeks. For example, the authors have observed that an occlusive stricture that developed three weeks after an initial endoscopic examination demonstrated only severe erosive esophagitis. The loss of esophageal wall compliance associated with transmural inflammation and fibrosis is more variable than is generally appreciated. Most peptic strictures do not progress inexorably to marked narrowing of the esophageal lumen. The majority arrest as segments of mild to moderate narrowing, 1.5 to 2.0 cm in diameter, often unaccompanied by dysphagia.

Dysphagia is the characteristic symptom of stricture formation. Symptom onset is often insidious, and the patient may gradually alter the diet as an adaptation

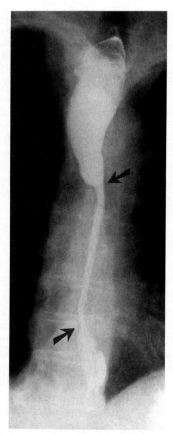

Figure 34–3. Long esophageal stricture caused by nasogastric intubation following cholecystectomy. The stricture *(arrows)* involves the distal half of the esophagus.

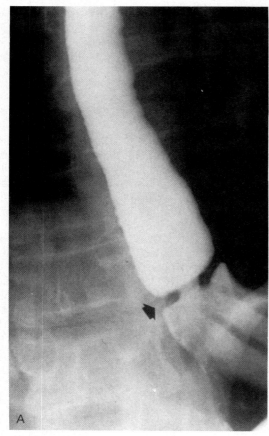

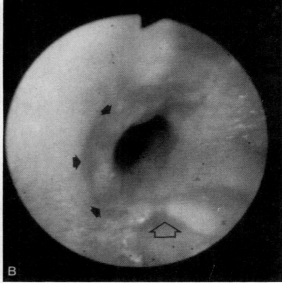

Figure 34–4. Annular stricture at the esophagogastric junction. *A*, Esophagram shows a tight ring *(arrow)* at the esophagogastric junction that simulates the appearance of a Schatzki's ring. The irregularity of the luminal contour in the distal esophagus is caused by esophagitis. *B*, Endoscopic examination shows a fixed inflammatory ring *(small arrows)* with proximal scarring *(open arrow)* from peptic esophagitis.

to progressive narrowing of the esophageal lumen. Initially, the dysphagia is limited to solids, but it may involve liquids as well if the stricturing becomes severe. Occasional patients with peptic stricture present at the emergency room with acute esophageal obstruction caused by impacted food proximal to the stricture. A more typical clinical history is that of frequent heartburn that begins to wane or disappears as the stricture develops. Some patients with peptic stricture may not have any clinical history of heartburn.

Hemorrhage or Perforation

Hemorrhage is an uncommon complication of reflux peptic esophagitis and is more likely to be related to an accompanying inflamed hiatus hernia or Barrett's esophagus than to peptic esophagitis. Hemorrhage may occur as the presenting symptom or against a background of known reflux esophagitis. Episodes of hemorrhage may be caused either by diffuse ulcerative esophagitis, or, more commonly, by a discrete, penetrating esophageal ulcer. Insidious blood loss from chronic reflux esophagitis occurs more commonly than from frank hemorrhage. The patients may present with Hemoccult-positive stool or symptoms from iron-deficiency anemia. These features are more common in children than in adults. Acute esophageal perforation occurs rarely in reflux esophagitis. It has been reported in occasional patients with severe peptic esophagitis

associated with the Zollinger-Ellison syndrome or complicating a Barrett's ulcer.

Barrett's Esophagus

In some patients, peptic esophagitis may be complicated by a unique reparative process wherein the original squamous epithelial cell lining of the esophagus is replaced by a metaplastic columnar-type epithelium. This condition is termed columnar-lined, or Barrett's esophagus. The clinical significance of Barrett's esophagus lies in its malignant potential. Although the actual incidence of esophageal adenocarcinoma arising from a Barrett's esophagus is not known, a risk of about 10 per cent is widely quoted.[48]

Although areas of columnar epithelium may persist within the esophagus from birth, the vast majority of cases of Barrett's esophagus are caused by an epithelial regenerative process associated with reflux esophagitis. The prime role of gastroesophageal reflux in the pathogenesis of Barrett's esophagus is supported by clinical, radiologic, endoscopic, manometric, and pH esophageal studies.[49]

An anatomic aberration that confuses the issue of Barrett's esophagus is the fact that islands of columnar epithelium are found frequently in an otherwise normal esophagus. This phenomenon might be expected because the human esophagus is lined entirely with columnar epithelium during early fetal development.

Later, squamous epithelium replaces the columnar cell lining, beginning initially in the middle of the esophagus and then spreading proximally and distally.[50] Isolated islands and patches of ectopic columnar epithelium found in the human esophagus could result from the arrest of the re-epithelialization process. Ectopic columnar epithelial islands are found most commonly in the proximal esophagus at, or immediately below, the upper esophageal sphincter in about 4 per cent of adult patients who have upper GI endoscopy[51] and in young children. Proximal esophageal islets of columnar epithelium are usually an incidental finding observed at endoscopic examination. Occasionally, however, dysphagia has been noted in association with these proximal "inlet patches" of heterotopic gastric mucosa. In one series of 244 patients who had esophageal columnar epithelium, 20 per cent had islets of columnar cells located immediately above the Z line. These islets were not accompanied by mucosal inflammation and, like other patches or focal areas of columnar epithelium, usually are not of clinical importance.[52] To avoid conflicts of interpretation that occur when tissue biopsies are obtained in the distal esophagus near the Z line, it has been recommended that mucosal samples should be obtained at distances of 3 cm or more above the Z line.

Barrett's esophagus is found in 12 per cent of endoscoped patients with persistent symptoms of gastroesophageal reflux.[53] When endoscopy is done to assess the severity of esophagitis, an 8- to 20-per cent incidence of Barrett's esophagus has been reported.[54] Additionally, Barrett's epithelium is detected in about 40 per cent of patients with chronic peptic stricture of the esophagus.[55] Although Barrett's esophagus is usually found in patients older than 40 years of age, it also occurs in children and young adults, suggesting a bimodal age distribution.

Generally, clinical symptoms of patients with a Barrett's esophagus are those associated with underlying reflux esophagitis. Often, pyrosis is severe early in the patient's clinical course. However, heartburn may diminish or disappear later as columnar cell epithelialization of the distal esophagus becomes more extensive. Dysphagia commonly is the presenting complaint of the patient with Barrett's esophagus because of the high incidence of stricture formation with this disease. The patient may deny any past history of heartburn symptoms prior to an initial episode of obstruction for solids caused by development of an esophageal adenocarcinoma.

The development of a Barrett's ulcer may be heralded clinically by the onset of odynophagia and chronic substernal chest pain. Development of a severe, boring-type pain may occur rarely when a Barrett's ulcer perforates into adjacent tissues or structures. Occasionally, significant bleeding may result from either a Barrett's ulcer or a zone of sponge-like, papillomatous mucosa that is associated with a columnar epithelial lining.

Stricture formation in Barrett's esophagus can develop anywhere in the esophageal body. Generally,

however, a Barrett's stricture causes less severe stenosis than its squamous epithelial counterpart. The Barrett's stricture usually occurs at or within 1 cm of the neosquamocolumnar junction. Commonly, esophagitis exists proximal to the stricture, with little or no inflammation within or distal to the stenosis. As a rule, esophageal narrowing involves a longer esophageal segment in Barrett's stricture than in peptic reflux disease.

It has been suggested that in Barrett's esophagus, benign strictures occur at the neosquamocolumnar junction, whereas malignant strictures occur below this junctional area. However, in a recent study of 28 patients, 5 of 11 benign strictures were located below the squamocolumnar line.[56] Nonetheless, all Barrett's strictures (Fig. 34–5) should be viewed with suspicion and biopsied to ascertain their underlying histology.

A Barrett's ulcer is a solitary lesion found exclusively within the region of columnar epithelium. Occasionally, it may have a focus of squamous mucosa at the rim of its crater. Barrett's ulcer exhibits the classic morphology of a gastric ulcer (i.e., rounded contour, sharp margins, and deep excavations). It occurs, most often, on the posterior or posterolateral esophageal

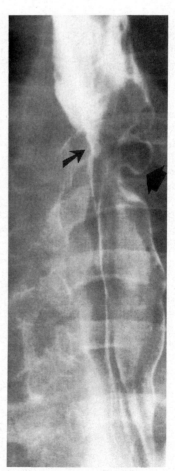

Figure 34–5. Proximal stricture associated with Barrett's esophagus. An accompanying pseudodiverticulum *(large arrow)* is present. The long arrow indicates the proximal margin of the columnar epithelium, as determined at endoscopy.

wall above the esophageal vestibule. These ulcers may hemorrhage severely or, in rare instances, perforate the esophageal wall. They may heal with subsequent stricture formation.

In Barrett's esophagus associated with chronic peptic esophagitis, the columnar epithelium can assume hyperplastic characteristics that may be either focal or widespread. This phenomenon has been called "papillomatous neotransformation."[52] The columnar mucosal surface appears spongy or porous and can be mistaken for a zone of malignant degeneration. Such areas are friable and may be the source of spontaneous, often repetitive bleeding.

The increased risk of esophageal adenocarcinoma in patients with Barrett's esophagus has recently been estimated to be about 30 to 40 times that of the general population.[57, 58] Although this is an impressive figure, it nonetheless represents a smaller risk than the previous estimate of 10 per cent of Barrett's patients.[54] Primary adenocarcinoma, arising in an otherwise normal esophagus and surrounded by normal squamous epithelium, is relatively rare. However, adenocarcinoma occurring in Barrett's columnar-lined esophagus may account for 5 to 10 per cent of all esophageal malignancies. Adenocarcinoma that is found in the distal portion of a Barrett's esophagus may be difficult to differentiate from adenocarcinoma arising from the gastric cardia that has spread upward into the gullet. The finding of dysplastic changes within the adjacent Barrett's epithelium and the position of the tumor mass (e.g., more than 50 per cent above the gastroesophageal junction) may be helpful in establishing the origin of the cancer. When adenocarcinoma develops within a Barrett's esophagus, it may be multifocal in origin and often is far advanced at the time of clinical recognition.[59]

Pharynx and Mouth Disturbances

Occasional patients with gastroesophageal reflux have recurrent or persistent complaints referable to the throat. These complaints consist of sore throat, globus, or cervical dysphagia.[60] On direct examination, the hypopharynx may be injected and edematous. In rare cases, recurrent GE reflux and regurgitation may cause severe gingivitis or gradual destruction of the teeth.

Pulmonary Symptoms

The potential for GE reflux to produce hoarseness, coughing, wheezing, or pneumonia often is not fully appreciated. However, pulmonary symptoms attributed to gastroesophageal reflux have been reported to occur in about 10 per cent of adult patients with GE reflux disease.[61] Better appreciated is the relationship between GE reflux and chronic respiratory symptoms in the pediatric population.[62] GE reflux may be an important cause of intrinsic asthma, although it is not known how often this association occurs.

Some reports suggest that aspiration of gastric fluid may cause laryngeal problems manifested by morning hoarseness, vocal cord ulceration, laryngospasm, transient apnea, or even respiratory arrest.[63] Aspiration is believed to account for some cases of infant death syndrome.[64]

Two mechanisms have been suggested to explain respiratory complications of GE reflux disease: (1) direct laryngeal and pulmonary aspiration of regurgitated refluxed gastric contents and (2) neurally mediated reflex bronchoconstriction caused by refluxate irritation of the esophageal lining. Pulmonary aspiration of refluxed gastric material is not easy to document, and clinical studies seldom demonstrate this association conclusively. In a study of patients with GE reflux or a history of aspiration, 24-hour pH monitoring showed a drop in intraluminal pH concurrent with symptoms of wheezing, coughing, and pyrosis in 20 per cent of the patients.[65] However, about half the patients developed pulmonary symptoms unassociated with any acid reflux. Recent findings indicate that upper sphincter pressure virtually disappears during sleep.[66] This finding suggests that considerable potential exists for pharyngoesophageal reflux and aspiration at night. Several reports present evidence to suggest a vagally mediated bronchoconstrictor mechanism that is activated by acid stimulation of esophageal receptors in some asthmatic patients and experimental animals. This response is ablated in the dog following high cervical vagotomy.[67] Nothwithstanding, the authors have never precipitated an episode of clinical asthma or dyspnea in any patient, a number of whom were asthmatics, in the 15 years they have been doing esophageal acid infusion studies.

Esophageal Cancer

The association between columnar esophageal epithelium and the development of esophageal adenocarcinoma is well recognized. The possibility exists, however, that chronic peptic esophagitis may contribute to the pathogenesis of squamous esophageal carcinoma. This association has often been suspected, but a definite connection is unproved. In a recent study, 25 per cent of patients with squamous cell carcinoma of the distal esophagus exhibited an associated reflux peptic esophagitis.[68] In the authors' practice, however, the association of esophageal carcinoma and non-Barrett's peptic esophagitis has been rare.

DIAGNOSTIC EVALUATION

The diagnostic evaluation of GE reflux disease depends on a careful clinical history and a discriminating selection of diagnostic clinical tests. Findings from physical examination or blood tests are seldom helpful other than in the evaluation of an associated anemia.

Clinical History

In most patients with reflux disease, the history is sufficiently typical to permit a clinical trial of therapy without obtaining comprehensive diagnostic tests. In patients with an atypical history, refractory symptoms, or complications of esophagitis, specific diagnostic tests are warranted. Tests that may be useful in individual patients with known or suspected reflux disease include esophagography, endoscopy with or without biopsy, acid infusion (Bernstein test), esophageal manometry, esophageal scintigraphy, and 24-hour pH monitoring.

X-ray Examination

Overall, esophagography has a low sensitivity for detecting GE reflux disease because the substantial majority of cases have mild reflux changes that do not show any morphologic abnormality on radiographs and are often difficult to diagnose at endoscopy without the benefit of biopsy. The diagnostic sensitivity is improved, albeit only slightly, by double-contrast examination. However, in cases of moderate to severe macroscopic esophagitis that is readily seen on endoscopy, esophagography has a sensitivity of 80 to 90 per cent.[69, 70] Morphologic findings of esophagitis include thickened esophageal folds, contour irregularity, thickening of the esophageal wall, and luminal narrowing.[71, 72] The finding of transverse, or feline type, esophageal folds (Fig. 34–6 A) is suggestive but not diagnostic of

the presence of reflux disease. In the authors' opinion, radiography is the best method available for evaluating esophageal compliance, (i.e., distensibility) or for demonstrating subtle esophageal strictures, rings, or webs. For this purpose, the esophagus must be dilated maximally by having the patient drink a barium solution rapidly and using an abdominal bolster that retards esophageal emptying of barium. Use of a barium-coated marshmallow (Fig. 34–6 B) represents an effective ancillary method for demonstrating esophageal rings and subtle strictures. The presence of stricture in the proximal esophagus or a discrete penetrating esophageal ulcer suggests the presence of an underlying columnar-lined esophagus.

When done properly, the X-ray method also provides excellent information about esophageal motor function that compares favorably with information obtained by esophageal manometry.[73, 74] The X-ray examination also demonstrates abnormal esophageal volume clearance as well as free or stress-induced GE reflux of barium in a substantial subset of the patients, mainly in those patients with low basal LES pressure. Therefore, the finding of reproducible GE reflux strongly suggests low LES tone. Lastly, the X-ray examination documents the presence and size of a hiatus hernia and serves as a screening examination for the esophagus, stomach, and duodenum.

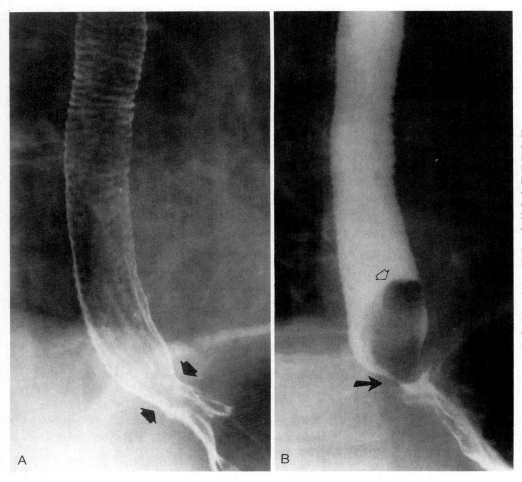

Figure 34–6. Transverse ridging, or "felinization," of the esophagus in a patient with complaints of heartburn and dysphagia. *A,* Double-contrast examination shows compacted transverse folds in the distal half of the esophagus. Some narrowing *(arrows)* is seen at the esophagogastric junction. *B,* Single-contrast examination following the swallowing of a marshmallow. The marshmallow *(open arrow)* is impacted proximal to a short segmental stricture *(closed arrow)* located at the esophagogastric junction. The serrations of the esophageal luminal contour are caused by closely spaced transverse mucosal folds.

Endoscopy

Esophageal endoscopy provides a direct view of the esophageal mucosa and allows directed biopsy when needed. Visual inspection yields a gross anatomic examination of the esophageal interior. Without endoscopy or esophageal biopsy, only a presumptive diagnosis of reflux disease can be made from other diagnostic tests or the clinical history.

The macroscopic features of esophagitis include mucosal erosion, ulceration, pseudomembrane formation, and scarring.[75] In some cases the mucosa is hemorrhagic. When the mucosal changes are moderate to severe, tissue biopsy generally is not needed for diagnosis. Moderate to severe esophageal narrowing or stricture generally is detected readily at endoscopy, but mild narrowing, which may be detected on X-ray examination, commonly goes undetected at endoscopy when using endoscopes of standard diameter. Mild superficial esophagitis or reflux changes may escape detection unless biopsy material is obtained.[5] Therefore, when the macroscopic findings are equivocal or the esophagus appears normal in an individual with suspected reflux disease or Barrett's esophagus, biopsy is warranted.

The diagnosis of Barrett's esophagus requires endoscopic examination supported by tissue biopsy. Macroscopically, Barrett's esophagus is easiest to identify when the lower esophagus is lined circumferentially over several centimeters by columnar epithelium. The displaced neosquamocolumnar junction is the most significant clue to the presence of Barrett's columnar lining. The columnar epithelium is often redder in appearance than normal gastric tissue. A delicate "villoid pattern" may be appreciated, and a submucosal venous pattern is visible beneath the surface.

Barrett's esophagus generally occurs in association with a hiatus hernia and active reflux esophagitis.[49] In many instances, severe inflammation or stricture formation may obscure anatomic detail at or immediately above the anatomic gastroesophageal junction. A thin, arc-like ridge, which occasionally is completely circumferential, is often observed at the distal esophagus. This structure marks the site of the original squamocolumnar junction and often identifies proximal displacement of the Z line. If doubt exists concerning the exact site or presence of columnar epithelium, Lugol's solution may be used to stain the glycogen in the squamous epithelium black, but it does not stain the columnar epithelium. Lugol's solution (3 to 5 ml) is applied to the esophageal mucosa through an irrigation tube passed down the biopsy channel of the endoscope.

Linear, finger-like, flame-like, or spiked projections of Barrett's columnar epithelium may extend orad from the distal esophagus, the GE junction may appear "star-like," or the lower esophagus may be lined circumferentially by columnar epithelium, either completely or partially with intervening islets of preserved squamous epithelium (Fig. 34–7).

Histology

Esophageal biopsy should be done with jumbo biopsy forceps because small pinch biopsies often are not of any diagnostic value. Biopsies done during direct

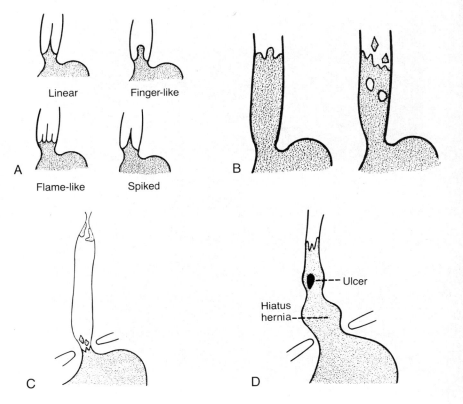

Figure 34–7. Examples of esophageal distribution of Barrett's columnar epithelium. *A,* Solitary projection. *B,* Complete or partially circumferential distribution. *C,* Patches of heterotopic columnar epithelium at both ends of esophagus. *D,* Barrett's ulcer. (Adapted from Savary M., and Miller G. (eds.): The Esophagus: Handbook and Atlas of Endoscopy. Solothurn, Switzerland, Gassmann AG, 1978.)

Linear Finger-like

Flame-like Spiked

Ulcer

Hiatus hernia

viewing may be taken from designated areas of the esophagus or from specific areas of suspicion. Biopsy material may also be obtained by blind endoscopic technique using a suction biopsy instrument. In some cases the suction probe may be passed adjacent to the endoscope to allow a directed suction biopsy. In practice, however, suction biopsies of the esophagus are seldom done.

The classic histologic features of esophagitis are epithelial erosion or ulceration accompanied by inflammatory infiltrate.[1] The infiltrate may contain acute or acute and chronic inflammatory cells. Necrosis, pseudomembrane, or fibrosis may also be present. These criteria, however, generally identify only patients with moderate or severe esophagitis. Mild esophagitis may feature only spotty epithelial erosions and some mixed cellular infiltrate. More subtle histologic changes (Fig. 34–8) that suggest reflux disease consist of epithelial basal cell hyperplasia and prominent papillae.[4, 5, 6] Intraepithelial polymorphologic neutrophils or eosinophils may be present. The histologic finding of basal cell hyperplasia is believed to be caused by increased cell turnover as a response to epithelial injury.[76]

Endoscopically directed biopsy permits correlation of the biopsy information with the endoscopist's visual assessment of the esophageal surface topography. Targeted biopsies are particularly important when focal lesions, such as an ulcer, surface irregularities, and strictures, are present. Difficulty in diagnosis occurs when columnar-lined epithelium is not obvious or

widely distributed within the esophagus. In this situation, serial biopsies are taken, beginning in the gastric cardiac region, continuing proximally at 1- to 2-cm intervals through the site of possible Barrett's epithelium, and into the squamous epithelium above.

In the Barrett's esophagus, the normal squamous cell lining may be replaced by one type or a combination of three types[77] of columnar epithelium: a distinctive, specialized columnar epithelium, a junctional-type epithelium, and a gastric fundus-type epithelium (Fig. 34–9, A–C). These types of epithelium may be intermixed but more frequently are present in a stratified, zonal arrangement.

Specialized columnar epithelium is characterized by mucous cells, goblet cells, and a villous structure. The columnar cells lack intestinal absorptive capabilities or ultrastructural characteristics of true intestinal cells and appear to be an example of "incomplete" intestinal metaplasia.[78] Specialized columnar epithelium is frequently the most proximal cell type encountered within the Barrett's esophagus. Junctional-type epithelium has a predominantly foveolar surface pattern, contains mucous glands, and resembles the epithelium of normal gastric cardia. It is usually present in the Barrett's esophagus between the specialized columnar-type and the more distally located gastric fundus-type epithelium. Fundus-type epithelium is the only variety of Barrett's columnar epithelium that contains both parietal and chief cells. These cells may secrete hydrochloric acid and pepsin. The glandular structures of

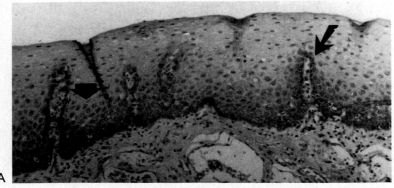

A

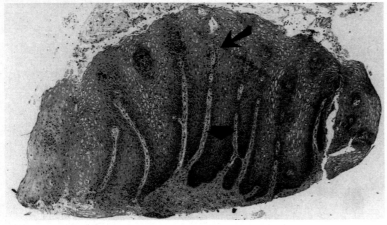

B

Figure 34–8. Micrographs of esophageal mucosa. *A,* Asymptomatic patient, large-forceps biopsy. Normal appearance of a relatively thin basal zone layer *(broad arrow)* and normal papilla *(thin arrow).* Normal basal zone height is less than 15 per cent of the total epithelial thickness, and normal papillary extension is less than 66 per cent of the length of the epithelial layer. Hematoxylin and eosin stain, ×80. *B,* Patient with symptomatic reflux. Marked hyperplasia of the basal zone layer *(broad arrow)* is present and the papillae *(thin arrow)* are substantially elongated. Hematoxylin and eosin stain, ×40. (Courtesy of R. Komorowski, M.D.)

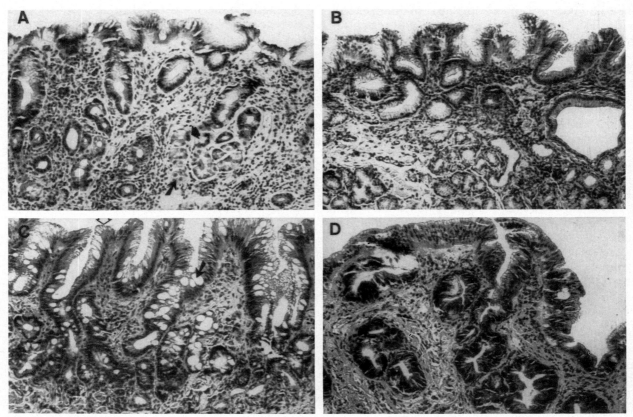

Figure 34–9. Types of Barrett's esophagus. Morphologic features of three types of Barrett's epithelia *(A–C)* and severe dysplasia *(D)*. *A*, Gastric fundic-type epithelium, which resembles atrophic lining of fundus and body of stomach. The surface is foveolar, and glandular zones contain chief cells *(broad arrow)* and parietal cells *(long arrow)*. *B*, Junctional-type epithelium, which resembles epithelium of normal gastric cardia. This type has a foveolar surface pattern. Mucus-secreting cells are prominent. Chief cells and parietal cells are absent. *C*, Specialized columnar epithelium which resembles intestinal mucosa with villiform surface and crypts. The villi are lined by secretory columnar cells with poorly defined brush borders *(open arrow)* and goblet cells *(closed arrow)*. This type of epithelium appears to be an incomplete form of intestinal metaplasia. *D*, High-grade dysplasia in an area of Barrett's specialized columnar epithelium shows cellular stratification, glandular distortion, and crowded, hyperchromatic cell nuclei. Classically these nuclei are pleomorphic and elongated and extend into the upper pole, away from the basal location. (Hematoxylin and eosin stain, × 100.) (Courtesy of J. Trier, M.D.)

the fundic epithelium, however, are sparse and foreshortened, causing it to appear atrophic compared to normal gastric mucosa. Enzyme characteristics of these Barrett's columnar epithelial cells are sufficiently dissimilar from those of true gastric fundic and intestinal mucosal cells to suggest a metaplastic origin.

Barrett's columnar epithelium is prone to cell dysplasia or neoplastic change that may be a precursor to malignancy (Fig. 34–9, *D*). Dysplasia has been found in all three types of Barrett's epithelia, particularly the specialized columnar type. Positive dysplastic alterations in Barrett's columnar cells have recently been classified as low-grade or high-grade, depending on the degree of nuclear pleomorphism, hyperchromatism, and alteration of polarity.[79] High-grade cellular dysplasia represents an ominous occurrence in the neoplastic spectrum that includes adenocarcinoma in situ.

Bernstein Test

The acid infusion, or Bernstein, test is a useful method for determining whether the patient's symp-

toms are of esophageal origin.[80] For this test, 0.1 N HCl is infused into the distal esophagus at a minimum rate of 1 ml/min using a saline infusion as a control. Although the test was done originally with the subject upright, the supine position is used currently by many workers. Findings from numerous studies show excellent correlation between esophagitis symptoms and provocation of heartburn by esophageal acid infusion. The test has a sensitivity of about 80 to 90 per cent.[81] However, false positive as well as false negative results do occur. For example, acid-induced symptoms may be caused by gastritis or peptic ulcer disease as well as by esophagitis. Findings from earlier studies suggested that intraluminal acid provoked heartburn by inducing nonperistaltic esophageal activity.[82] Although this circumstance may occur, the substantial majority of positive responses are not associated with abnormal esophageal motor activity. A consensus exists that acid-induced heartburn results from a direct action of acid on damaged esophageal epithelium.[1]

Although the Bernstein test may be performed as an isolated test, it is generally done as part of a manometric examination of esophageal motor function. Additional tests often combined with manometry include pH testing for acid reflux and measurement of esophageal acid clearance.

Esophageal Manometry

In the past, esophageal manometry was done in patients with reflux disease mainly to assess LES pressure. This practice was based on the notion that resting LES pressure correlated directly with sphincter competency. Although sample values of LES pressure, obtained by station or rapid pull-through technique, do not generally discriminate patients with reflux disease from control subjects,[83, 84] manometric assessment of LES pressure is warranted in selected patients, mainly those considered for surgical therapy. Depending on patient selection, only about 25 to 50 per cent of patients with GE reflux disease have hypotensive sample values of resting LES pressure, (e.g., less than 10 mm Hg). Furthermore, an even smaller percentage have markedly low values of less than 6 mm Hg, which allow distinct separation from control values.[81] Notwithstanding, discrimination of patients with markedly low LES pressure identifies those individuals who are unlikely to respond satisfactorily to conventional medical therapy. Many of the patients with substantial LES hypotension are identified initially on barium studies that show copious GE reflux.

Manometry also yields a quantitative assessment of esophageal body motor function in response to swallowing and esophageal acid infusion. Swallowing should include wet swallows, 5-ml water boluses, and dry swallows. Current evidence suggests that a subset of patients with reflux disease have abnormal esophageal peristalsis with either a decreased incidence of complete peristaltic sequences after swallowing, hypotensive peristaltic waves, or impaired responses to esophageal distention.[36, 85] The prevalence of impaired peristaltic function increases with the more severe forms of esophagitis. About 50 per cent of patients with moderate or severe esophagitis exhibit some degree of impaired esophageal peristaltic function.[36] Demonstration of impaired esophageal peristalsis implies that such individuals will have abnormal esophageal acid clearance.

Acid Reflux

Two ancillary tests commonly included with esophageal manometry are the acid reflux, or Tuttle, test and determination of esophageal acid clearance.[34, 35] Both of these tests require that a pH electrode be positioned in the distal esophagus, conventionally 5 cm above the LES. Testing for acid reflux is generally done during basal conditions and after the stomach has been loaded with 200 ml of 0.1 N HCl. When standard stress maneuvers are included, a minimum of two reflux episodes are required for an abnormal positive response. The test is referred to as standard acid reflux

testing, or SART.[86] Acid GE reflux is observed as an abrupt drop in esophageal pH to less than 4.0 that lasts for more than 5 sec. Such reflux episodes are generally associated with a common-cavity phenomenon wherein an abrupt increase in intraluminal esophageal pressure occurs that equilibrates with intragastric pressure.[16] Findings from earlier studies suggest that the acid reflux test yields good separation of esophagitis patients from individuals without reflux disease.[65, 87] False negative findings, however, are encountered, and acid reflux may be recorded in individuals without reflux disease.[15, 88] The rationale behind the test tends to regard GE reflux as an all-or-none phenomenon, rather than stressing quantitative differences in reflux rate between symptomatic patients and normal subjects.

Acid Clearance

The other acute test featuring esophageal pH monitoring is the acid-stripping, or acid-clearing, test.[34] For this test, 15 ml of 0.1 N HCl is injected into the esophagus in the supine subject, and the subject is asked to swallow every 30 sec. Normally, esophageal pH is returned to a value of greater than 4.0 in about 15 swallows or less. An abnormal acid clearance time, or an increased number of swallows for acid clearance, is encountered in a substantial percentage of patients with reflux disease.[35, 89] The test measures simply esophageal acid clearance and does not reliably discriminate patients with reflux disease from other individuals. The test results may be abnormal in any patient with abnormal esophageal motor function or impaired salivation.

Isotope Studies

An isotope method of quantitative scintigraphy has been used to evaluate GE reflux.[90, 91] Initially the method was proposed to quantitate GE reflux, but in reality only a qualitative evaluation of reflux is obtained. A nonabsorbable isotope such as technetium-99m sulfur colloid is placed in the stomach and counts are monitored over the chest. Episodes of GE reflux are heralded by an abrupt increase in counts over an esophageal region of interest. The test is done with the subject supine while incremental pressure is applied to the abdomen. Although initial findings suggested that the isotope method had a high sensitivity for detecting patients with reflux disease, this expectation has not been substantiated.[92] Currently the test seems most useful for determining reflux episodes in children.[93, 94]

The isotope method has also been used to quantitate esophageal transit.[95] For this test, the subject swallows a radioactive bolus, and the disappearance rate of maximal counts over the esophageal region of interest is taken as a measurement of transit. A modified method enables the counts to be transposed to bolus volume so that the test becomes a measurement of esophageal volume clearance.[30] Limitations of the method are that some isotope adheres to the esophageal mucosa and generally only a few swallows are recorded to minimize radiation exposure.

Although the diagnosis of reflux-related respiratory disease can be inferred from a detailed clinical history and the results of endoscopy or esophageal pH monitoring, convincing proof is difficult to obtain. In some instances, radionuclide testing may provide objective evidence to substantiate the occurrence of pulmonary aspiration of refluxed gastric material. For such testing, ^{99m}Tc-sulfur colloid is placed in the stomach at bedtime, and scans are obtained over the lung in the morning.[96] The appearance of activity over the lungs substantiates the occurrence of regurgitation and aspiration.

Long-Interval pH Monitoring

A major diagnostic test of increasing importance is long-interval esophageal pH monitoring (Fig. 34–10). Such testing can be done for 12- to 24-hour intervals in inpatients or as an abbreviated 4-hour study utilizing a standardized meal. Recently, suitable instrumentation has become available to obtain 24-hour ambulatory studies of patients in their daily environment. Additionally, newer instruments allow the possibility of recording esophageal motor activity concurrently

with esophageal pH. A substantial benefit of continuous esophageal pH monitoring is that the method yields a temporal profile of acid reflux events and acid clearance. Variables for measurement include the number of reflux episodes, acid clearance times, and esophageal exposure to acid. These values can be determined while the subject is upright as well as recumbent. In general, subjects with reflux disease exhibit a higher rate of acid reflux and increased esophageal exposure to acid than do normal subjects,[97, 98] but about 20 per cent of symptomatic patients yield values within the upper range of normal.[15] Additionally, pH monitoring gives important information relevant to relating patient symptoms to the occurrence or nonoccurrence of reflux events. Thus, in some cases the test results clearly establish that the patient's clinical complaint is not related to acid reflux or to abnormal esophageal motility (when motor function is recorded). In selected cases, long-interval pH monitoring provides an objective method for documenting the efficacy of medical or surgical therapy.

Measurement of Salivation

Quantitation of salivation may be desirable in occasional patients who are suspected of having impaired salivation as a significant determinant in the pathogen-

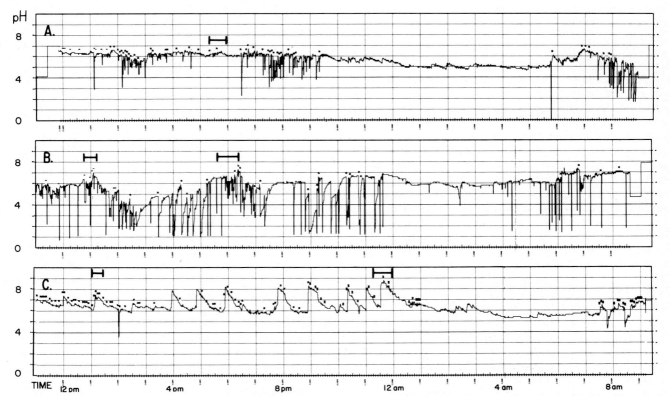

Figure 34–10. Examples of ambulatory 24-hour esophageal pH recordings from three patients. The pH is given on the vertical scale, whereas time of day is indicated on the horizontal scale. The heavy horizontal bars within each tracing represent meals. *A*, Normal 24-hour pH recording. Brief reflux episodes occur mainly during the day. *B*, Abnormal acid reflux test (total time during which pH < 4.0 equals 19 per cent). *C*, Alkaline reflux recording. This patient has pyrosis refractory to medical treatment. Clearly demarcated episodes of alkaline reflux are present.

esis of their reflux disease. Normal awake subjects exhibit a basal salivary flow of about 0.3 to 0.5 ml/min that is stimulated fourfold to sixfold by the sucking of a peppermint lozenge.[29] Measurement of salivation is done simply by collecting saliva by expectoration for a 15-minute basal period and for a 15-minute period during lozenge stimulation.

Test Selection

When evaluating an individual patient, the clinician is confronted with making a judicious selection of diagnostic tests. As a general rule, clinical symptoms are best evaluated by a careful clinical history. Evaluation of clinical symptoms is supplemented by the Bernstein test, or, in some cases, by long-interval esophageal pH monitoring. Objective evidence of reflux disease is best established by endoscopy, with or without biopsy, and less commonly by radiography. An abnormal prevalence of GE reflux is determined by esophageal pH monitoring, or, in some cases, by radiography or scintigraphy. Esophageal body motor function is evaluated equally well by radiography or manometry, whereas only manometry quantitates resting LES pressure. Esophageal pH monitoring is the only suitable method for evaluating esophageal acid clearance. Optimal selection of a given test depends on the issue under consideration: source of symptoms, prevalence of reflux, morphologic evidence of reflux disease, strength of LES tone, or efficacy of esophageal clearance. For this reason, a clear formulation of specific questions is essential before ordering any diagnostic tests.

The authors rely heavily on the clinical history for patient evaluation. When symptoms typical of GE reflux seem to be present in untreated patients, the authors are content to make a presumptive diagnosis of reflux disease and prescribe medical treatment without recourse to diagnostic tests. In most cases, the patients respond favorably, on one or more occasions, thereby obviating any additional work-up. However, some patients present with refractory symptoms unresponsive to treatment or do not respond satisfactorily to aggressive medical therapy. In other cases, symptoms suggesting complications of reflux disease, such as stricture or a respiratory problem, may be present that warrant additional diagnostic work-up. Once additional work-up is judged necessary, the authors generally obtain an esophagram and an esophageal endoscopy. The endoscopy determines the presence or absence of mucosal abnormalities, whereas the esophagram evaluates for esophageal stricture, esophageal motor function, volume clearance, and reproducible reflux related to hypotensive LES pressure. When doubt exists about clinical symptoms, a Bernstein test or ambulatory pH monitoring is commonly performed. Ambulatory pH monitoring is useful for evaluating patients with pulmonary symptoms, chest pain suspected to be related to GE reflux, or intractable heartburn without macroscopic esophagitis. Presently,

the authors utilize esophageal manometry less than previously. Manometry is performed as a method of optimizing the treatment rationale for using prokinetic agents in patients with severe symptoms who are not surgical candidates, or in patients who are serious candidates for surgery. In nearly all cases, the authors combine the Bernstein, reflux, and acid clearance tests with manometry and use isotope studies only for investigational purposes.

DIFFERENTIAL DIAGNOSIS

Although generally they are quite characteristic, symptoms from GE reflux need to be distinguished from symptoms related to gastritis, peptic ulcer disease, dyspepsia, biliary tract disease, coronary artery disease, and esophageal motor disorders. Often certain details of the clinical history suggest that reflux-like symptoms are non-esophageal in origin. For example, a history of peptic ulcer disease, cholelithiasis, pain radiation to the back, or symptoms exacerbated by exercise raises the possibility of non-esophageal origin of symptoms. Endoscopy and an upper gastrointestinal series offer a means of not only examining the esophagus but also of evaluating the remainder of the upper gastrointestinal tract for symptom-producing lesions. The biliary tract is evaluated most efficiently by sonography. The evaluation of unexplained chest pain may include a stress electrocardiogram and coronary arteriogram. Potential esophageal motor disorders may be evaluated by radiography, manometry, or, in some cases, ambulatory recording using intraluminal strain gauges. To evaluate acid regurgitation as a cause of respiratory tract symptoms, pH monitoring may be done with the electrode positioned in the proximal esophagus or pharynx. In some cases, symptoms related to dyspepsia may be reproduced by loading the stomach with gas during fluoroscopy, using CO_2-releasing granules, and observing for symptomatic gas reflux or belching.

MANAGEMENT AND TREATMENT

General Principles

A clear rationale for the therapy of GE reflux disease depends on a careful definition of specific aims. In many cases, the goal of therapy is simply to alleviate or eliminate symptoms, whereas, in other cases, the major goal is to minimize or eliminate GE reflux. These goals are set against the background that reflux disease is generally a chronic condition characterized by recurrent symptoms. Effective therapy often minimizes symptoms while having no long-term effect on the underlying mechanism(s) that contributes to the development of reflux disease. In a minority of cases, such as patients with a stricture, Barrett's esophagus, or respiratory tract symptoms, the minimization or elimination of GE reflux is the desirable therapeutic goal.

Options for treating GE reflux disease include both medical and surgical therapy. Ideally, therapy should be based on a knowledge of the mechanisms involved in the pathogenesis of reflux disease in the individual patient. In many cases, however, the details of the pathogenesis may not be known, and general therapeutic measures are prescribed presumptively. Specific therapeutic measures may be directed toward accomplishing any or all of the following: (1) decrease GE reflux, (2) increase resting LES pressure, (3) enhance gastric emptying, (4) make esophageal refluxate innocuous, (5) improve esophageal motor function, (6) enhance esophageal acid clearance, (7) stimulate salivation, (8) improve esophageal protection, and (9) promote esophageal healing. Additionally, some potential exists in the future for therapeutic depression of transient LES relaxations using drug therapy or other measures.

Four broad goals of therapy are to decrease GE reflux, neutralize refluxate, enhance esophageal clearance, and protect the esophageal mucosa. Therapy directed toward decreasing GE reflux includes measures designed to decrease gastric volume, increase resting LES pressure, or decrease the rate of transient LES relaxations. Gastric volume may be kept at a minimum by instructing the patient to avoid large meals and to refrain from a snack before going to bed. Dietary fat should be kept to a minimum because fat slows gastric emptying and also decreases LES pressure. Prokinetic agents may be useful if gastric emptying is abnormal. Instructions designed to prevent reduction of basal LES pressure include minimizing the dietary intake of fat, chocolate, alcohol, and coffee and avoiding smoking.[99] Low basal LES pressure can generally be increased by oral prokinetic agents such as bethanechol, metaclopromide, or cisapride.[100] Additionally, many potent new prokinetics that appear to have minimal side effects are in the offing. The rate of transient LES relaxations is diminished by minimizing gastric volume and distention. The potential exists for new pharmacologic agents that might retard the occurrence of nondeglutitive LES relaxations. Algenic acid is believed to retard GE reflux by creating a barrier of foam at the cardia. The predominant effect of surgical therapy is to reduce or eliminate GE reflux.

Measures designed to decrease the potency of refluxate to cause esophageal injury are directed mainly toward increasing the pH of the refluxate toward neutrality. Such an increase in pH not only prevents esophageal injury from acid but also, perhaps even more importantly, places the pH in a range in which pepsin is inactive and the damaging effects of some types of bile acids are diminished. The pH of esophageal refluxate may be increased using liberal amounts of antacid to neutralize gastric acid or by suppressing gastric secretion of acid. Agents that decrease gastric secretions include histamine (H_2) blockers; selective anticholinergics, such as pirenzepine, which does not affect motor function; and, more recently, omeprazole, an agent that antagonizes the parietal cell proton pump and is undergoing field testing at present. H_2 blocking agents, such as cimetidine, ranitidine, and newer long-acting agents, are currently the major pharmacologic agents used to reduce gastric acid secretion. These agents substantially reduce, but do not abolish, gastric acid production. At present such agents are a mainstay in the medical therapy of reflux disease.[101, 102] However, healing of esophagitis following treatment with H_2 blocking agents appears to be inversely related to the extent of esophageal erosions, and low-dose maintenance therapy does not prevent relapse.[103]

Nonspecific anticholinergics, such as probanthine and belladonna, cause an appreciable reduction in gastric acid secretion but have a depressant effect on gastric and esophageal motor function. Therefore, such agents are contraindicated for the treatment of reflux disease. Recently, selective muscarinic antagonists, such as pirenzepine, have been developed that selectively depress gastric acid secretion while having negligible effect on gastroesophageal motor function. Such agents are not potent depressors of gastric acid secretion but may have some clinical value when combined with H_2 blockers, particularly in patients with gastric hypersecretion.

Whereas H_2 blockers and anticholinergics block gastric acid secretion stimulated by histamine and acetylcholine, respectively, omeprazole blocks an enzyme, hydrogen potassium ATPase, that is involved in the final common pathway of acid secretion by the parietal cell. This new potent agent can virtually abolish acid production. Early clinical trials suggest that omeprazole is extremely effective in abolishing reflux symptoms and healing esophagitis,[104] but ruling on its safety awaits further clinical trials.

Therapy directed toward improvement of esophageal clearance includes tilting up the head of the bed with blocks, prokinetic agents, and increasing salivation. Findings from several studies confirm that the use of bed blocks improves acid clearance time and reduces esophageal exposure to acid while having negligible effect on the number of reflux episodes. In some cases, prokinetic agents, such as bethanechol, may improve impaired esophageal acid clearance. Increased salivation may be stimulated by chewing gum as well as by sucking on lozenges or antacid tablets. Such therapy may ameliorate heartburn symptoms.

Lastly, efforts may be made to protect the esophageal mucosa. Agents such as sucralfate[105] seem to bind to the esophageal mucosa and act as a physical barrier that prevents mucosal injury.

Peptic Reflux Disease

When treating garden-variety peptic reflux disease, either of two general strategies may be adopted for a given patient. The most common, or conservative, approach is to follow a course of incremental therapy, starting with simple forms of medical therapy and using progressively more aggressive forms of therapy if symptoms do not subside. A second tactic that can be adopted profitably in some patients is to "pull all the stops'' and overshoot the mark by pursuing maximally aggressive medical therapy initially and then backing off as appropriate. These two treatment strategies are not mutually exclusive and can be used to advantage in different types of patients. For example, in patients with severe symptoms, severe esophagitis, substantial LES hypotension, or markedly impaired esophageal clearance, aggressive initial therapy is warranted in an attempt to control symptoms and tissue injury rapidly. Initial aggressive therapy may define refractory patients quickly and thereby avoid a prolonged interval of medical therapy before surgical therapy is considered.

A cornerstone of medical therapy is the institution of lifestyle changes that include dieting toward an ideal body weight, decreasing the size of meals, avoidance of eating between meals, using bed blocks, and minimizing the ingestion of fat, chocolate, and coffee. Smoking should be discontinued or kept to a minimum. The next level of therapy beyond lifestyle changes is therapy designed to make esophageal reflux less acid either by neutralization or by depression of gastric acid secretion. These treatments, therefore, include the use of antacids, H$_2$ blockers, or pirenzepine, either alone or in combination. Ancillary therapy may also include the use of sucralfate in an attempt to protect the esophageal mucosa as well as recommendations of gum, lozenges, or antacid tablets to increase salivary flow as a means of increasing endogenous antacid.[29, 106] In general, lifestyle changes, making refluxate less acid, and protecting the esophageal mucosa represent universal forms of therapy that are of potential benefit in peptic reflux disease regardless of the specific mechanisms that contribute to the pathogenesis of clinical disease in the individual patient. Therefore, these methods can be used empirically with the confidence that they represent an implicitly sound rationale. The one exception is in "alkaline esophagitis," for which attempts to neutralize gastric juice or decrease gastric acid secretions have no rationale. Unlike agents that make refluxate less acid and potentially act as universal therapy in all patients with peptic reflux disease, prokinetic agents are potentially useful only in those patients with impaired motor function of the esophageal or gastric smooth muscle. Although prokinetic agents can be used empirically, a clear rationale for their aggressive use depends on the demonstration of abnormal gastroesophageal motor function. For example, it makes no sense to press on with agents to increase basal LES pressure or enhance esophageal motor function if these variables are already normal.

The authors make a presumptive diagnosis of reflux disease in new patients with reflux-like symptoms. If symptoms suggestive of complications, such as stricture, are absent, these patients are treated initially with a combination of lifestyle changes, elevation of the head of the bed, and antacids or antacids plus H$_2$ blockers, without recourse to diagnostic tests. The majority of patients respond satisfactorily. Such treatments are simply repeated if recurrent symptoms are not unduly frequent or severe. If the therapeutic response is suboptimal after using an H$_2$ blocker or the patient has symptoms suggestive of complications from reflux disease, endoscopic and radiographic examinations of the esophagus are performed routinely. If these tests show objective evidence of reflux disease or if the X-ray findings suggest hypotensive LES tone or impaired esophageal peristalsis, a prokinetic drug, such as bethanechol, metaclopramide, or cisapride, is added to the therapeutic regimen. Thus, the authors' practice is to use prokinetic agents not as single-drug therapy but rather as part of a full medical regimen that includes antacids and an H$_2$ blocker.[107] A modest percentage of patients treated in this manner exhibit a favorable response to the addition of a prokinetic agent. If the response remains suboptimal, esophageal manometry with pH testing is done to better evaluate LES function, esophageal peristalsis, and esophageal acid clearance. When doubt exists about whether the patient's symptoms are esophageal, a Bernstein test is done at some point. Ambulatory pH monitoring is also useful to evaluate ambiguous symptoms or to evaluate for the potential of reflux-associated respiratory disease.

Surgical therapy is considered when the patient has established reflux disease associated with persistent clinical symptoms, which are refractory to medical therapy or associated with significant respiratory tract complications. In some cases, surgical therapy to control GE reflux is considered in patients who have reflux-related pulmonary disease in the presence of normal esophageal mucosa.[108] Overall, surgical therapy is actively considered in about 5 per cent of the authors' patients with reflux disease. After the pros and cons of surgical therapy are fully discussed with the patient, about half of these patients elect surgery.

Surgical therapy consists mainly of different types of fundoplication, of which the Nissen and the Belsey Mark IV are the most common (Fig. 34–11). A new procedure has been introduced recently that consists of placing a Silastic ring (Angelchik prosthesis) around the distal esophagus. Overall, a substantial majority of patients who undergo fundoplication experience considerable improvement or even cessation of their reflux symptoms. In many cases, peptic esophagitis heals following effective surgery. Findings from one study suggest that after surgery, both symptoms and mucosal changes are improved at a one- to two-year follow-up, whereas only the symptoms are improved at five years after surgery.

The mechanism whereby fundoplication reduces or abolishes GE reflux is not fully established. Available evidence, however, suggests strongly that fundoplication creates a mechanical compression that causes a mild to modest high-pressure zone at the cardia. On manometry this effect is generally manifested as an increase in LES pressure. Any intrinsic LES tone may augment the passive pressure. However, experimental studies show that the fundoplication may act as a mechanical valve mechanism to prevent GE reflux, even in resected specimens. Even a small amount of passive pressure may be sufficient to prevent GE reflux. This fact is suggested by recent findings that indicate

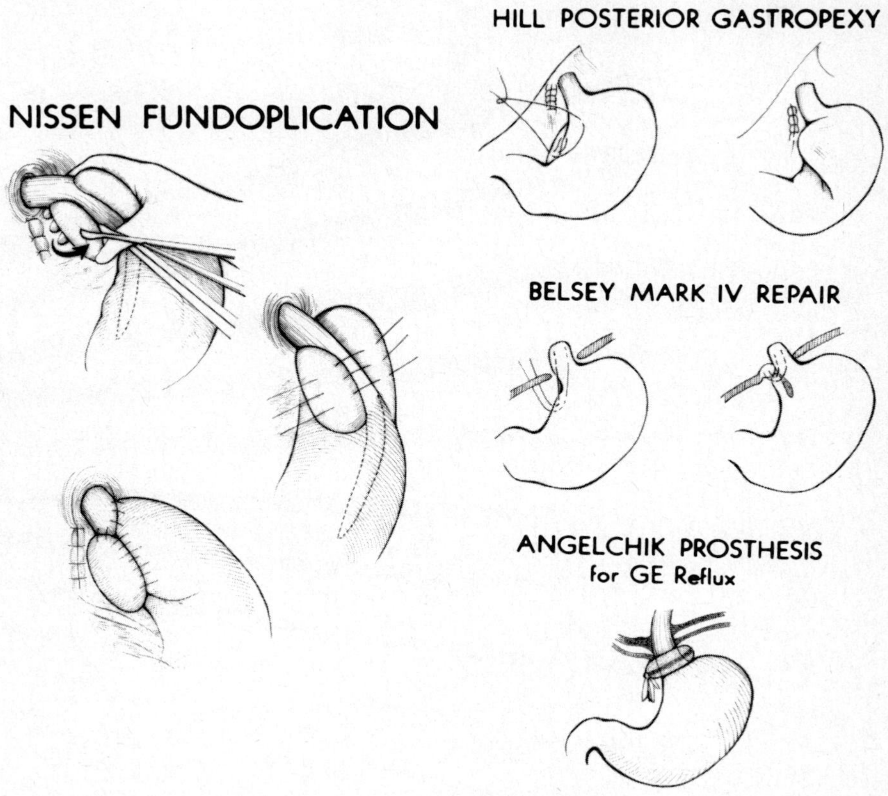

Figure 34–11. Antireflux operations. Operative techniques used in constructing an antireflux barrier are shown for four antireflux surgical procedures.

that a high rate of transient LES relaxations may continue after fundoplication, but the transient sphincter relaxations are no longer associated with GE reflux owing to a small residual LES pressure.

Alkaline Reflux Disease

Alkaline reflux esophagitis is treated medically by a trial of lifestyle changes and a prokinetic agent. As discussed earlier, antacids and H_2 blockers have little to offer. If the symptoms are particularly severe or refractory, or if stricture develops, surgical therapy is warranted. Revision of a gastroenterostomy is often done because alkaline esophagitis generally occurs in the setting of a postoperative stomach wherein excessive bile refluxes into the stomach. In occasional instances, alkaline esophagitis is treated by fundoplication.

Complications of Reflux Disease

Esophageal Stricture

Mechanical dilation of the esophagus is an important therapeutic method for treating the complication of peptic stricture. A variety of mercury-filled, rounded or tapered dilators are available for bougienage and remain the mainstay of treatment for uncomplicated peptic stricture. These dilators are of little benefit, however, when the stricture is unyielding, is angulated,

or causes severe luminal narrowing. In 1950, Puestow introduced a dilation technique whereby a series of metal olives mounted onto a semiflexible rod are passed over a guide wire inserted across the stenotic esophageal segment. A recent introduction is a semiflexible, tapered, polyvinyl bougie with a hollow center. This bougie is threaded onto an endoscopically inserted steel guide wire for directed passage through the stricture. Savary-Gilliard dilators consist of a series of 10 dilators, ranging in size from 5 to 18 mm (No. 15 to 54 Fr) that fit over a stainless steel guide wire 182 cm long and 0.8 mm in diameter (Fig. 34–12). The wire has a graduated flexible spring tip that reduces the tendency to penetrate tissue or retroflex upon itself. A radiopaque marker is incorporated into the dilator to aid in fluoroscopic monitoring.[109] The American dilation system, an adaptation of the Savary dilator, offers several different features. The distal central lumen of the American dilator does not impact on the guide wire tip, as can occur with the Savary. The distal tapered end of the bougie shaft is shorter, and the bougies are completely radiopaque. These dilators are calibrated with two sets of markings, one for identifying the shaft tip, the other to mark the point of maximal bougie diameter. There are 12 dilators (No. 15 to 54 Fr) in this system. Both the Savary and the American plastic dilators are easily passed through the mouth, and the flexible tip traverses the pharynx readily. The polyvinyl material is less apt to injure the patient's teeth than is the metal, and the supine position is not required for the patient during the dilation procedure.

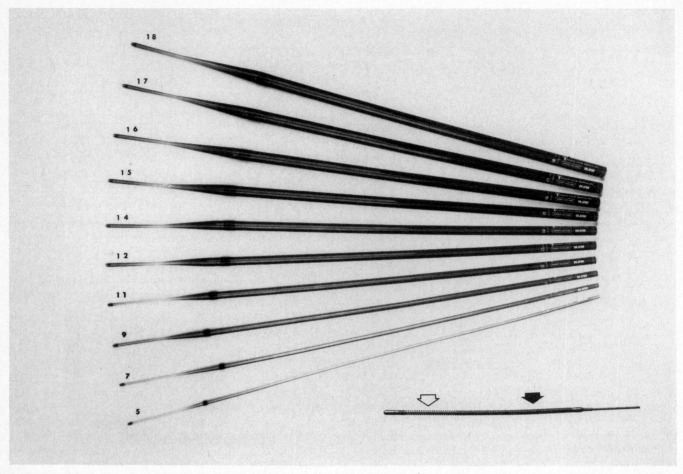

Figure 34–12. Savary-Gilliard dilators, which consist of a series of 10 semi-flexible, tapered, polyvinyl bougies with hollow centers. Sizes range from 5 to 18 mm in diameter. These dilators can be threaded over an endoscopically inserted guide wire. The tip of the guide wire *(black arrow, lower right)* is progressively flexible to its end *(white arrow)* to decrease the risk of perforation during insertion. (Courtesy of Wilson-Cook, Inc., Winston-Salem, NC.)

Pneumatic balloon dilators, such as those used to treat vascular stenosis, have been adapted for use in treating gastrointestinal tract strictures.[110] This new type of dilator can be inflated with air, fluid, or dilute radiopaque contrast medium (Fig. 34–13). When fully inflated, the balloons range in diameter from 4 to 30 mm. The collapsed balloon is threaded over an endoscopically placed guide wire and positioned across the stricture. Balloon pressure generated during inflation is monitored by a pressure gauge. This method has a mechanical advantage over conventional dilation because the distending force is applied only at right angles to the long axis of the stricture without the shear forces required to push a conventional dilator across a stricture.

Dilation of esophageal strictures can be done with the patient either recumbent or sitting. Fluoroscopic monitoring may be necessary, particularly when wire-guided dilators are used.

Although esophageal dilation is usually performed without premedicating the patient, dilation is often best accomplished following intravenous premedication with meperidine hydrochloride (Demerol) (25 to 40 mg) or midazolam hydrocloride (Versed) (2 to 3 mg). Saliva should be aspirated during the dilation procedure.

When using hollow, tapered plastic dilators or Maloney mercury-filled rubber bougies, the general rule is to pass no more than three dilators that meet moderate or more resistance during any single session. This approach has been associated with a low incidence of esophageal perforation. The introduction of Gruntzig-type balloon dilators has altered the traditional, stepwise approach to stretching a stricture. With the use of three progressively larger inflatable balloons, esophageal peptic strictures can be dilated dramatically during one session. For example, strictures in one report were dilated from an initial mean stricture diameter of 7.8 mm to 15 mm in one setting. Patient discomfort was used for determining the final diameter of dilatation.[111] Complications seem to be negligible using this approach, but caution is urged until more experience is accrued.[112, 113]

Successful dilation of peptic strictures to a lumen size of greater than 14 mm (No. 42 Fr) generally provides relief from dysphagia. The schedule for serial

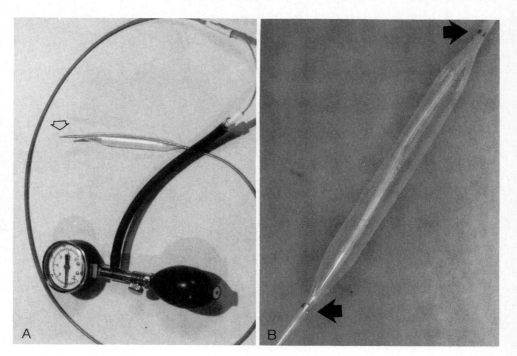

Figure 34–13. Gruntzig-type pneumatic balloon (Rigiflex TTS) used for dilating esophageal strictures. When fully inflated, balloons of different sizes range from 4 to 30 mm in diameter. *A,* A pressure-monitoring gauge. Arrow points to the hollow, tapered tip which fits over a guide wire. *B,* Close-up view of inflated balloon. Arrows point to radiopaque markers. (Courtesy of Micro-Vasive Co., Milford, ME.)

dilations is based on the type of stricture, its response to initial and subsequent dilation, and the patient's tolerance to the procedure. Each stricture is unique and requires an individually tailored approach to the initial dilation and subsequent follow-up dilations. Controversy continues as to the best method for treating peptic strictures (i.e., medical management with dilation alone or operative treatment). Many published reports confirm the benefit of conservative, long-term medical management of esophageal peptic strictures.[114, 115, 116] On the other hand, a review of the postoperative results in 160 patients who underwent an antireflux operation and dilation for esophageal peptic stricture suggests that the results of early operation are comparable to, or better than, those for conservative treatment by dilation alone.[117]

Barrett's Esophagus

At present, there is no effective treatment, medical or surgical, for Barrett's esophagus per se. Management of the reflux esophagitis that accompanies Barrett's esophagus, however, is an attainable goal. Healing of Barrett's ulcers with long-term H_2 receptor blocker medication and antacids may occur.[118] Barrett's strictures frequently require esophageal dilatation. Operative therapy may be needed to control intractable gastroesophageal reflux symptoms or mucosal damage. Neither intensive medical therapy nor antireflux surgery, however, has been shown conclusively to cause regression of Barrett's epithelium. Although postfundoplication regression of Barrett's epithelium (and, presumably, a reduced risk of cancer development) has been cited in several reports,[119, 120] the validity of these observations is controversial.

Because of the frequent association of cellular dysplasia and adenocarcinoma in Barrett's esophagus (Fig. 34–14), it is presumed that malignancy evolves from a sequential progression of epithelial neoplastic changes. This dysplasia-cancer sequence is the basis for proposed clinical surveillance programs for the Barrett's esophagus patients, albeit definitive information about the frequency with which dysplasia progresses to cancer is unavailable. Several practical issues plague a meaningful cancer-surveillance program of Barrett's esophagus patients. For example, dysplasia is found in only about 5 to 10 per cent of Barrett's esophagus patients who have no detectable adenocarcinoma. High-grade dysplasia does not always mean that invasive cancer is present. Invasive cancer may already be present when high-grade dysplasia is the only endoscopic finding. Lastly, multifocal areas of dysplasia and cancer may coexist.

Although some type of endoscopic surveillance program for Barrett's esophagus patients seems appropriate for early detection of dysplastic alterations in the columnar-lined esophagus, the efficacy and cost-effectiveness of endoscopic surveillance programs is a hotly debated issue. Presently, a validated, well-accepted program is not established for endoscopic surveillance of premalignant changes in patients with Barrett's esophagus.

Because multifocal sites of dysplasia may exist in the Barrett's esophagus, tissue sampling should be taken from as many areas of involvement as possible. The authors biopsy specimens at the same axial level, beginning at the anatomic GE junction and continuing at 2-cm increments to a level about 2 cm above the highest projection of recognizable columnar epithelium (Fig. 34–15). Biopsy specimens are also obtained of any discrete areas of mucosal irregularities, ulcers, or

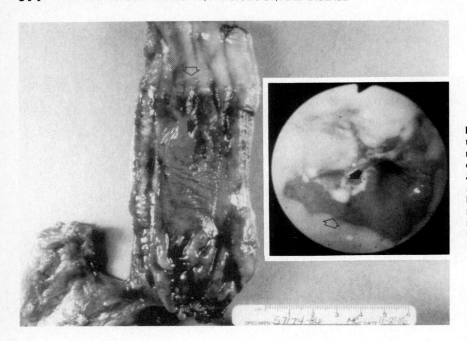

Figure 34–14. Barrett's esophagus with stricture, high-grade dysplasia, and transmural adenocarcinoma. Inset at right was taken during endoscopy at 28 cm from incisor teeth. Shown are the squamocolumnar junctional interphase *(open arrow)*, strictured lumen, and surface irregularity caused by underlying adenocarcinoma *(closed arrow)*. The resected esophageal specimen shows the same anatomic features identified by similar arrows.

strictures. A diagrammatic record of the columnar epithelial distribution and the specific sites of tissue biopsy or brushings is essential for subsequent location of dysplastic changes.

Depending on the histologic findings from the esophageal biopsies or cytology brushings, the authors' endoscopic surveillance program is as follows: When there is no epithelial dysplasia, repeat endoscopic examination is done at one-year intervals. If low-grade dysplasia is detected, endoscopy and tissue biopsy are repeated in three to six months. If low-grade dysplasia persists on biopsy, this shorter surveillance interval is maintained. When high-grade dysplasia is demonstrated on the initial examination, endoscopy and tissue

biopsy are repeated within six weeks. If repeat biopsy shows the presence of high-grade dysplasia, this diagnosis should be confirmed by a second experienced pathologist.

If the diagnosis is confirmed, consideration is given to a primary esophagectomy with esophagogastrectomy or intestinal interposition operation. These possibilities are discussed thoroughly with the patient. The mortality rate for esophagectomy is on the order of 5 to 10 per cent. Some authorities believe the surgical mortality is too high a risk unless there is established evidence that invasive carcinoma is present. Others think the esophagus should be removed. At this writing, the jury is still out.

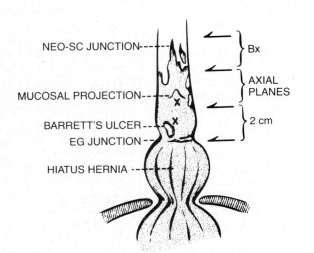

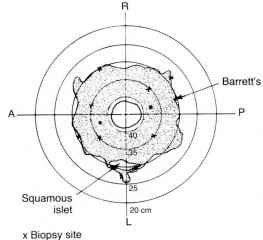

x Biopsy site
• Cytology site

Figure 34–15. Endoscopic method for surveillance of Barrett's esophagus. Biopsy-recording technique. *A*, Designated levels, increments, and structures within the Barrett's esophagus are detailed for tissue biopsy. *B*, The grid represents a view into the esophagus, giving distances from incisor teeth and orientation points. In this example, the extent of Barrett's distribution within the distal esophagus has been plotted *(shaded area)*. An area of preserved squamous islet is noted, and the sites of tissue biopsy and cytology have been marked.

Pulmonary Complications

Regurgitation accompanied by pulmonary aspiration is a potentially serious complication of reflux disease in adults as well as children. Vigorous medical management often is required, but frequently medical treatment does not control the problem.

Infants with GE reflux and suspected associated pulmonary disease are treated initially by "thickening" the diet, feeding them in the upright position, and maintaining them upright for 30 to 60 minutes after eating. Other effective measures are harness restraint in the prone, head-up position during sleep and bethanechol treatment.[121]

Young children with reflux-related pulmonary complications initially are treated conservatively by altering their nighttime posture, avoiding food and fluid intake for several hours before their bedtime, and giving them antacids. An antireflux surgical procedure is often beneficial in those children who are refractive to intensive medical management.[122] Retarded pediatric patients are particularly prone to GE reflux and its complications and generally respond poorly to conservative treatment. Both a Nissen fundoplication and an Angelchik prosthesis have been shown to be effective in this special pediatric group.[123] Long-term evaluation, however, of the continued effectiveness and possible complications of antireflux procedures is not yet available.

The medical management of the adult patient with pulmonary complications secondary to GE reflux includes all those measures outlined previously for treating aggressive peptic esophagitis. Particular attention must be paid to having an empty stomach at bedtime. Elevation of the patient's trunk at night and judicious use of H_2 blockers have been reported to decrease GE reflux and nocturnal asthma significantly in some patients.[124]

In those patients with persistent pulmonary symptoms from regurgitation and aspiration who are refractive to a trial of intensive medical management, an antireflux operation should be performed. Before surgery, however, the occurrence of undue GE reflux or pulmonary aspiration should be verified by objective testing. In some instances, surgical therapy for pulmonary complications is warranted even though the esophageal mucosa is normal.

Complications of Operative Therapy

Failure of a surgical antireflux procedure implies a recurrence of untoward GE reflux owing to improper construction of the antireflux barrier at the time of operation or to disruption of the repair. Reports of complications and failure rates for antireflux operations vary considerably. For example, despite refinements in

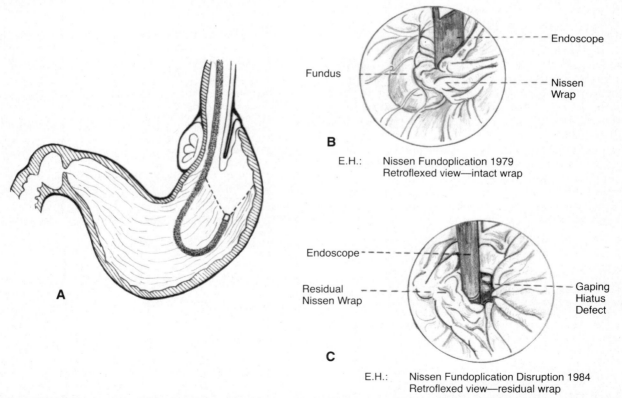

Figure 34–16. Endoscopic evaluation of a fundoplication wrap. *A,* With the endoscope flexed upon itself in the stomach, the fundoplication wrap can be inspected around its entire circumference. *B,* Retroflexed view of an intact Nissen wrap. The cone of tissue created by the fundoplication is seen surrounding the shaft of the endoscope for 270 degrees. One border is contiguous with the lesser curvature of the esophagus and stomach. *C,* View of disrupted fundoplication seen from below. The hiatus is gaping; the wrap has loosened and flattened.

the Nissen fundoplication and Belsey Mark IV operations, these procedures still have a 10 to 20 per cent rate of failure.[125, 126] Such failures may be evaluated by endoscopy (Fig. 34–16) as well as by radiography. A five-year follow-up of patients who had a Hill posterior gastropexy showed that 18 per cent developed a return of clinically significant gastroesophageal reflux.[127] The Angelchik prosthetic device has a reported failure rate ranging from 3 to 10 per cent.[128]

Patients with a "failed" fundoplication operation may develop heartburn, esophagitis, dysphagia, and peptic stricture. When a fundoplication, especially a Nissen, is made too tight, dysphagia or the gas-bloat syndrome can occur.[129] Other complications reported with the Nissen fundoplication include peritonitis and the development of an esophagogastric or gastropericardial fistula.

Gastric ulceration has been reported after fundoplication in several series.[130] The majority of these gastric ulcers occur high on the lesser curvature of the stomach, close to the fundoplication, and the majority of patients have a recurrent hiatus hernia. Anatomic distortion caused by the fundoplication wrap is the most likely cause of the ulcer, although gastric distention, reflux bile gastritis, and ischemia may play some role.

The Angelchik prosthesis has been associated with a number of dramatic complications. Prior to the inclusion of a completely circumferential Teflon strap, the prothesis was reported to migrate from the chest to the pelvis.[131] With the addition of the 360-degree Teflon strap, major migration no longer seems to be a problem. Local tissue disruption, however, may still occur (e.g., erosion into the stomach).

The only effective treatment for patients with a failed antireflux operation is another operation. In most instances, the esophagus can be preserved at first reoperation and a standard antireflux procedure done. A first reoperation morbidity rate of 3 per cent and good to excellent long-term results have been reported in 86 per cent of patients.[132] With multiple repeat operations, there is an increasing surgical mortality, morbidity, and poor results. In this circumstance, consideration should be given to definitive resection of the esophagus and replacement with a tubular structure from another segment of the gut.

References

1. Dodds, W. J., Hogan, W. J., and Miller, W. N. A report on reflux esophagitis. Am. J. Dig. Dis. 21:49, 1976.
2. Nebel, O. T., Formes, M. F., and Castell, D. O. Symptomatic gastro-esophageal reflux: incidence and precipitating factors. Am. J. Dig. Dis. 21:953, 1976.
3. Johanessen, T. Symptoms of esophagitis in general practice. In Sanberg, N., and Walan, A. (eds.). Function and Disease of the Oesophagus. Philadelphia, Smith, Kline and French, 1985, pp. 77–78.
4. Ismail-Beigi, F., Horton, P. F., and Pope, C. E., II. Histological consequences of gastroesophageal reflux in man. Gastroenterology, 58:163, 1970.
5. Ismail-Beigi, F., and Pope, C. E., II. Distribution of the histological changes of gastroesophageal reflux in the distal esophagus of man. Gastroenterology 66:1109, 1974.
6. Behar, J., and Sheahan, D. C. Histologic abnormalities in reflux esophagitis. Arch. Pathol. 99:387, 1975.
7. Weinstein, W. M., Bogoch, E. R., and Bowes, K. L. The normal human esophageal mucosa: a histological reappraisal. Gastroenterology 68:40, 1975.
8. Winkelstein, A. Peptic esophagitis. A new clinical entity. JAMA 104:906, 1935.
9. Winans, C. S., and Harris, L. D. Quantitation of lower esophageal sphincter competence. Gastroenterology 52:773, 1967.
10. Pope, C. E., II. A dynamic test of sphincter strength: its application to the lower esophageal sphincter. Gastroenterology 52:779, 1967.
11. Cohen, S., and Harris, L. D. The lower esophageal sphincter. Gastroenterology 63:1066, 1972.
12. Dodds, W. J., Hogan, W. J., Helm, J. F., and Dent, J. Pathogenesis of reflux esophagitis. Gastroenterology 81:376, 1981.
13. Dodds, W. J., Dent, J., Hogan, W. J., Helm, J. F., Hauser, R., Patel, G. K., and Egide, M. S. Mechanisms of gastroesophageal reflux in patients with reflux esophagitis. N. Engl. J. Med. 308:1547, 1982.
14. DeMeester, T. R., Johnson, L. F., Joseph, G. J., Toscano, M. S., Hall, A. W., and Skinner, D. B. Patterns of gastroesophageal reflux in health and disease. Ann. Surg. 184:459, 1976.
15. Schlesinger, P. K., Donahue, P. E., Schmid, B., and Layden, T. J. Limitations of 24-hour intraesophageal pH monitoring in the hospital setting. Gastroenterology 89:797, 1985.
16. Dent, J., Dodds, W. J., Friedman, R. H., Sekiguchi, T., Hogan, W. J., and Arndorfer, R. C. Mechanism of gastroesophageal reflux in recumbent asymptomatic human subjects. J. Clin. Invest. 65:256, 1980.
17. Werlin, S. L., Dodds, W. J., Hogan, W. J., and Arndorfer, R. C. Mechanisms of gastroesophageal reflux in children. J. Pediatr. 97:244, 1980.
18. Benz, L. J., Hootkin, L. A., Margulies, S., Donner, M. W., Cauthorne, R. T., and Wendrix, T. R. A comparison of clinical measurements of gastroesophageal reflux. Gastroenterology 62:1, 1972.
19. Eastwood, G. L., Castell, D. O., and Higgs, R. H. Experimental esophagitis in cats impairs lower esophageal sphincter pressure. Gastroenterology 69:146, 1975.
20. Wesdorp, E., Bartelsman, J., Pape, K., Dekker, W., and Tytgat, G. N. Oral cimetidine in reflux esophagitis: a double blind controlled trial. Gastroenterology 74:821, 1978.
21. Bright-Asare, P., and El-Bassoussi, M. Cimitidine, metoclopramide, or placebo in the treatment of symptomatic gastroesophageal reflux. J. Clin. Gastroenterol. 2:149, 1980.
22. Goyal, R. K., and Rattan, S. Nature of the vagal inhibitory innervation to the lower esophageal sphincter. J. Clin. Invest. 55:119, 1975.
23. Holloway, R. H., Hongo, M., Berger, K., and McCallum, R. W. Gastric distention: a mechanism for postprandial gastroesophageal reflux. Gastroenterology 89:779, 1985.
24. McCallum, R. W., Berkowitz, D. M., and Lerner, E. Gastric emptying in patients with gastroesophageal reflux. Gastroenterology 80:285, 1981.
25. Goldberg, H. I., Dodds, W. J., Gee, S., Montgomery, C., and Zboralske, F. F. Role of acid and pepsin in acute experimental esophagitis. Gastroenterology 56:223, 1969.
26. Gillison, E. W., De Castro, V. A. M., Nyhus, L. M., Kusakari, K., and Bombeck, C. T. The significance of bile in reflux esophagitis. Surg. Gynecol. Obstet. 134:419, 1972.
27. Harmon, J. W., Johnson, L. F., and Maydonovitch, C. L. Effects of acid and bile salts on the rabbit esophageal mucosa. Dig. Dis. Sci. 26:65, 1981.
28. Schweitzer, E. J., Harmon, J. W., Bass, B. L., and Batzri, S. Bile acid efflux precedes mucosal barrier disruption in the rabbit esophagus. Am. J. Physiol. 247:G480, 1984.
29. Helm, J. F., Dodds, W. J., Hogan, W. J., Soergel, K. H., Egide, M. S., and Wood, C. M. Acid neutralizing capacity of human saliva. Gastroenterology 83:69, 1982.
30. Helm, J. F., Dodds, W. J., Pelc, L. R., Palmer, D. W., Hogan, W. J., and Teeter, B. C. Effect of esophageal emptying and saliva on clearance of acid from the esophagus. N. Engl. J. Med. 310:284, 1984.

31. Kapila, Y. V., Dodds, W. J., Helm, J. F., and Hogan, W. J. Relationship between swallow rate and salivary flow. Dig. Dis. Sci. *29*:528, 1984.

32. Helm, J. F., Dodds, W. J., Riedel, D. R., Teeter, B. C., Hogan, W. J., and Arndorfer, R. C. Determinants of esophageal acid clearance in normal subjects. Gastroenterology *85*:607, 1983.

33. Teeter, B. C., Helm, J. F., Dodds, W. J., Linehan, J. H., Hogan, W. J., Pelc, L. R., and Egide, M. S. Computerized model of the mechanisms governing esophageal acid clearance. (Abstract.) Dig. Dis. Sci. *27*:664, 1982.

34. Booth, D. J., Kemmerer, W. T., and Skinner, D. B. Acid clearing from the distal esophagus. Arch. Surg. *96*:731, 1968.

35. Stanciu, C., and Bennett, J. R. Studies of esophageal acid clearing. The function of the esophagus. *In* Sorenson, H. R., Jepsen, O., and Pedersen, S. A. (eds.). The Function of the Esophagus. Odense, Odense University Press, 1973, pp. 22–26.

36. Kahrilas, P. J., Dodds, W. J., Hogan, W. J., Kern, M., Arndorfer, R. C., and Reece, A. Esophageal peristaltic dysfunction in peptic esophagitis. Gastroenterology *91*:897, 1986.

37. Orlando, R. C. Esophageal epithelial resistance. J. Clin. Gastroenterol. *8*:12, 1986.

38. Mittal, R. K., Lange, R. C., and McCallum, R. W. Identification and mechanism of delayed esophageal acid clearance in subjects with hiatus hernia. Gastroenterology *92*:130, 1987.

39. Dodds, W. J., Dent, J., and Hogan, W. J. Pregnancy and the lower esophageal sphincter. Gastroenterology *74*:1334, 1978.

40. Price, S. F., Smithson, K. W., and Castell, D. O. Food sensitivity in reflux esophagitis. Gastroenterology *75*:240, 1978.

41. Chodosh, P. L. Gastro-esophago-pharyngeal reflux. Laryngoscope *87*:1418, 1977.

42. Hunt, P. S., Connell, A. M., and Smiley, T. B. The cricopharyngeal sphincter in gastric reflux. Gut *11*:303, 1970.

43. Stanciu, C., and Bennett, J. R. Upper esophageal sphincter yield pressure in normal subjects and in patients with gastro-oesophageal reflux. Thorax *29*:459, 1974.

44. Tuchman, D. N., Boyle, J. T., Pack, A. I., Scwartz, J., Kokonos, M., Spitzer, A. R., and Cohen, S. Comparison of airway responses following tracheal or esophageal acidification in the cat. Gastroenterology *87*:872, 1984.

45. Mansfield, L. E., Hameister, H. H., Spaulding, H. S., Smith, N. J., and Glab, N. The role of the vagus nerve in airway narrowing caused by intraesophageal hydrochloric acid provocation and esophageal distention. Ann. Allergy *47*:431, 1981.

46. Spaulding, H. S., Mansfield, L. E., Stein, M. R., Sellner, J. C., and Gremillion, D. E. Further investigation of the association between gastroesophageal reflux and bronchoconstriction. J. Allergy Clin. Immunol. *69*:516, 1982.

47. Werlin, S. L., D'Souza, B. J., Hogan, W. J., Dodds, W. J., and Arndorfer, R. C. Sandifer syndrome. An unappreciated clinical entity. Dev. Med. Child Neurol. *22*:374, 1980.

48. Haggitt, R. C., and Dean, P. J. Adenocarcinoma in Barrett's epithelium. *In* Spechler, S. J., and Goyal, R. K. (eds.). Barrett's Esophagus: Pathophysiology, Diagnosis, and Management. New York, Elsevier Science Publishing Company, 1985, pp. 153–166.

49. Hamilton, S. R. Pathogenesis of columnar lined (Barrett's) esophagus. *In* Spechler, S. J., and Goyal, R. K., (eds.). Barrett's Esophagus: Pathophysiology, Diagnosis, and Management. New York, Elsevier Science Publishing Company, 1985, pp. 29–37.

50. Johns, B. A. E. Developmental changes in the oesophageal epithelium in man. J. Anat. *86*:431, 1952.

51. Jabbari, M., Goresky, C. A., Lough, J., Yaffe, C., Daly, D., and Côté, C. The inlet patch: heterotopic gastric mucosa in the upper esophagus. Gastroenterology *89*:352, 1985.

52. Savary, M., and Miller, G. (eds.). The Esophagus. Handbook and Atlas of Endoscopy. Solothurn, Switzerland, Gassmann, AG, 1978.

53. Winters, C., Jr., Spurling, T. J., Chobanian, S. J., Curtis, D. J., Esposito, R. L., Hacker, J. F., III, Johnson, D. A., Cruess, D. F., Cotelingam, J. D., Gurney, M. S., and Cattau, E. L., Jr. Barrett's esophagus. A prevalent, occult complication of gastroesohageal reflux disease. Gastroenterology *92*:118, 1987.

54. Spechler, S. J., and Goyal, R. K. Barrett's esophagus. N. Engl. J. Med. *315*:362, 1986.

55. Spechler, S. J., Sperber, H., Doos, W. G., and Schimmel, E. M. The prevalence of Barrett's esophagus in patients with chronic peptic esophageal strictures. Dig. Dis. Sci. *28*:769, 1983.

56. Lackey, C., Rankin, R. A., and Welsh, J. D. Stricture location in Barrett's esophagus. Gastrointest. Endosc. *30*:331, 1984.

57. Cameron, A. J., Ott, B. J., and Payne, W. S. The incidence of adenocarcinoma in columnar-lined (Barrett's) esophagus. N. Engl. J. Med. *313*:857, 1985.

58. Spechler, S. J., Robbins, A. H., Rubins, H. B., Vincent, M. E., Heeren, T., Doos, W. G., Colton, T., and Schimmel, E. M. Adenocarcinoma and Barrett's esophagus: an overrated risk? Gastroenterology *87*:927, 1984.

59. Banner, B. F., Memoli, V. A., Warren, W. J., and Gould, V. E. Carcinoma with multidirectional differentiation arising in Barrett's esophagus. Ultrastruc. Pathol. *4*:205, 1983.

60. Nostrant, T. T., Ossakow, S., and Straho, K. Esophageal reflux and dysmotility as a basis for persistent cervical symptomatology. (Abstract.) Gastroenterology *88*:1519, 1985.

61. Dairs, M. V. Relationship between pulmonary disease, hiatal hernia and gastroesophageal reflux. N.Y. State J. Med. *72*:935, 1972.

62. Eiler, A. P., Byrne, W. J., Ament, M. E., Fonkalsrud, E. W., Strobel, C. T., Siegel, S. C., Katz, R. M., Rachelefsky, G. S.: Recurrent pulmonary disease in children: a complication of gastroesophageal reflux. Pediatrics *63*:47, 1979.

63. Foglia, R. P., Fonkalsrud, E. W., Ament, M. E., Byrne, W. J., Berquist, W., Siegel, S. C., Katz, R. M., and Rachelefsky, G. S. Gastroesophageal fundoplication for the management of chronic pulmonary disease in children. Am. J. Surg. *140*:72, 1980.

64. Herbst, J. J., Minton, S. D., and Books, L. S. Gastroesophageal reflux causing respiratory distress and apnea in newborn infants. J. Pediatr. *95*:763, 1979.

65. Mansfield, L. E., and Stein, M. R. Gastroesophageal reflux and asthma: a possible reflux mechanism. Ann. Allergy *41*:224, 1978.

66. Kahrilas, P. J., Dodds, W. J., Dent, J., Haeberle, B., Hogan, W. J., and Arndorfer, R. C. The effect of sleep, spontaneous gastroesophageal reflux and a meal on UES pressure in normal human volunteers. Gastroenterology. *92*:466, 1987.

67. Mansfield, L. E., Hameister, H. H., Spaulding, H. S., Smith, N. J., and Glab, N. The role of the vagus nerve in airway narrowing caused by intraesophageal hydrochloric acid provocation and esophageal distention. Ann. Allergy *47*:431, 1981.

68. Kuylenstierna, R., and Munch-Wikland, E. Esophagitis and cancer of the esophagus. Cancer *56*:837, 1985.

69. Ott, D. J., Dodds, W. J., Wu, W. C., Gelfand, D. W., Hogan, W. J., and Stewart, E. T. Current status of radiology in evaluating for gastroesophageal reflux disease. Clin. Gastroenterol. *4*:365, 1982.

70. Ott, D. J., Chen, Y. M., Gelfand, D. W., Munitz, A., and Wu, W. C. Analysis of a multiphasic radiographic examination for detecting reflux esophagitis. Gastrointest. Radiol. *11*:1, 1986.

71. Dodds, W. J., Goldberg, H. I., Montgomery, C., Ludemann, W. B., and Zboralske, F. F. Sequential gross microscopic and roentgenographic features of acute feline esophagitis. Invest. Radiol. *5*:209, 1970.

72. Ott, D. J., Wu, W. C., and Gelfand, D. W. Reflux esophagitis revisited: prospective analysis of radiologic accuracy. Gastrointest. Radiol. *6*:1, 1981.

73. Dodds, W. J. Cannon Lecture: Current concepts of esophageal motor function. Clinical implications for radiology. AJR *128*:549, 1977.

74. Dodds, W. J. Radiology of the esophagus. *In* Margulis, A. R., and Burhenne, H. J. (eds.). Alimentary Tract Radiology, Vol. I. Ed. 3. St. Louis, C. V. Mosby Company, 1983, pp. 529–603.

75. Monnier, P. H., and Savary, M. Contribution of endoscopy to gastro-oesophageal reflux disease. Scand. J. Gastroenterol. *106*:26, 1984.

76. Livstone, E. M., Sheahan, D. G., and Behar, J. Studies of esophageal epithelial cell proliferation in patients with reflux esophagitis. Gastroenterology *73*:1315, 1977.

77. Paull, A. P., Trier, J. S., Dalton, M. D., Camp, R. C., Loeb, P., and Goyal, R. K. The histologic spectrum of Barrett's esophagus. N. Engl. J. Med. 295:476, 1976.
78. Rothery, C. A., Patterson, J. E., Stoddard, C. J., and Day, D. W. Histological and histochemical changes in the columnar lined (Barrett's) esophagus. Gut 27:1062, 1986.
79. Riddell, R. H., Goldman, H., and Ransohoff, D. F. Dysplasia in inflammatory bowel disease: standard classification with provisional clinical applications. Hum. Pathol. 14:931, 1983.
80. Bernstein, L. M., and Baker, L. A. A clinical test for esophagitis. Gastroenterology 34:760, 1958.
81. Behar, J., Biancani, P., and Sheahan, D. G. Evaluation of esophageal tests in the diagnosis of reflux esophagitis. Gastroenterology 71:9, 1976.
82. Siegel, C. I., and Hendrix, T. R. Esophageal motor abnormalities induced by acid perfusion in patients with heartburn. J. Clin. Invest. 42:686, 1963.
83. Dilawari, J. B., Edwards, D. A. W., and Girmes, D. H. The probability of symptoms or of radiographic evidence of reflux predicted by lower oesophageal sphincter pressure. Proceedings of the Fourth International Symposium on Gastrointestinal Motility, Banff, Alberta, Canada, Sept. 6–8, 1973, Vancouver, Mitchell Press, 1974, pp. 441–448.
84. Stanciu, C., and Bennett, J. R. Correlation between a physiological test of gastrooesophageal reflux and sphincter squeeze. Proceedings of the Fourth International Symposium on Gastrointestinal Motility, Banff, Alberta, Canada, Sept. 6–8, 1973, Vancouver, Mitchell Press, 1974, pp. 131–138.
85. Gill, R. C., Bowes, K. L., Murphy, P. D., and Kingma, Y. J. Esophageal motor abnormalities in gastroesophageal reflux and the effects of fundoplication. Gastroenterology 91:364, 1986.
86. Skinner, B. D., and Booth, D. J. Assessment of distal esophageal function in patients with hiatal hernia and/or gastroesophageal reflux. Ann. Surg. 172:627, 1970.
87. Bombeck, C. T., Helfrich, G. B., and Nyhus, L. M. Planning surgery for reflux esophagitis and hiatus hernia. Surg. Clin. North Am. 50:29, 1970.
88. Venkatachalam, B., Da Costa, L. R., and Beck, I. T. What is a normal esophagogastric junction? Gastroenterology 62:521, 1972.
89. Miller, W. N., Ganeshappa, K. P., Dodds, W. J., Hogan, W. J., Barreras, R. F., and Arndorfer, R. C. Effect of bethanechol on gastroesophageal reflux. Am. J. Dig. Dis. 22:230, 1977.
90. Fisher, R. S., Malmud, L. S., Roberts, G. S., and Lobis, I. F. Gastroesophageal (GE) scintiscanning to detect and quantitate GE reflux. Gastroenterology 70:301, 1976.
91. Chernow, B., Johnson, L. F., Janowitz, W. R., and Castell, D. O. Pulmonary aspiration as a consequence of gastroesophageal reflux. Dig. Dis. Sci. 24:839, 1979.
92. Jenkins, A. F., Cowan, R. J., and Richter, J. E. Gastroesophageal scintigraphy: is it a sensitive screening test for gastroesophageal reflux disease? J. Clin. Gastroenterol. 7:127, 1985.
93. Rudd, T. G., and Christie, D. L. Demonstration of gastroesophageal reflux in children by radionuclide gastroesophagography. Radiology 131:483, 1979.
94. Heyman, S. Esophageal scintigraphy (milk scans) in infants and children with gastroesophageal reflux. Radiology 144:891, 1982.
95. Tolin, R. D., Malmud, L. S., Reilley, J., and Fisher, R. S. Esophageal scintigraphy to quantitate esophageal transit (quantitation of esophageal transit). Gastroenterology 76:1402, 1979.
96. Ghaed, N., and Stein, M. R. Assessment of a technique for scintigraphic monitoring of pulmonary aspiration of gastric contents in asthmatics with gastroesophageal reflux. Ann. Allergy 42:306, 1979.
97. Johnson, L. F., and DeMeester, T. R. Advantage of distal esophageal 24 hour pH monitoring over other tests for gastroesophageal reflux (GER). (Abstract.) Gastroenterology 66:716, 1974.
98. Johnson, L. F. 24-hour pH monitoring in the study of gastroesophageal reflux. J. Clin. Gastroenterol. 2:387, 1980.
99. Castell, D. O. Medical therapy for reflux esophagitis: 1986 and beyond. Ann. Intern. Med. 104:112, 1986.
100. McCallum, R. W., Fink, S. M., Winnam, G. R., Avella, J., and Callachari, C. Metoclopramide in gastroesophageal reflux

101. Hine, K. R., Holmes, G. K. T., Melikian, V., Lucey, M., and Fairclough, P. D. Ranitidine in reflux oesophagitis. Digestion 29:119, 1984.
102. Sherbanuik, R., Wensel, R., Bailey, R., Trantuan, A., Grace, M., Kirdeikis, P., Jewell, L., Pare, P., Levesque, D., Farley, A., et al. Ranitidine in the treatment of symptomatic gastroesophageal reflux disease. J. Clin. Gastroenterol. 6:9, 1984.
103. Koeltz, N. R., Birchler, R., Bretholz, A., et al. Healing and relapse of reflux esophagitis during treatment with ranitidine. Gastroenterology 91:1198, 1986.
104. Dammonn, H. G., Blum, A. L., Lux, G., and Krankenhaus, B. Differences in healing tendency of reflux oesophagitis with omeprazole and ranitidine. Results of an Austrian-German-Swiss multi-center trial. Dtsch. Med. Wochenschr. 111:123, 1986.
105. Elsborg, L., Bech, B., and Stubgaard, M. Effect of sucralfate on gastroesophageal reflux in esophagitis. Hepatogastroenterology 32:181, 1985.
106. Graham, D. Y., Smith, J. L., and Patterson, D. J. Why do apparently healthy people use antacid tablets? Am. J. Gastroenterol. 78:257, 1983.
107. Lieberman, D. A., and Keeffe, E. B. Treatment of severe reflux esophagitis with cimetidine and metoclopramide. Ann. Intern. Med. 104:21, 1986.
108. Editorial: Management of gastroesophageal reflux. Lancet 1:1054, 1984.
109. Dumon, J., Meric, B., Sivak, M. V., and Fleischer, D. A new method of esophageal dilatation using Savary-Gilliard bougies. Gastrointest. Endosc. 31:379, 1985.
110. Kozarek, R. Endoscopic Gruntzig balloon dilatation of gastrointestinal stenosis. J. Clin. Gastroenterol. 30:359, 1984.
111. Graham, D. Y., and Smith, J. L. Balloon dilatation of benign and malignant esophageal strictures. Blind retrograde balloon dilatation. Gastrointest. Endosc. 31:171, 1985.
112. Lindor, K. D., Ott, B. J., and Hughes, R. W., Jr. Balloon dilatation of upper digestive tract strictures. Gastroenterology 89:545, 1985.
113. Taub, S., Rodan, B. A., Bean, W. J., Koerner, R. S., Mullin, D. M., and Feng, T. S. Balloon dilatation of esophageal strictures. Am. J. Gastroenterol. 81:14, 1986.
114. Starlurger, M., Appel, W. H., Schemper, M., and Schiessel, R. Long-term treatment of peptic esophageal stenosis with dilatation and cimetidine. Factors influencing clinical results. Eur. Surg. Res. 17:207, 1985.
115. Wesdorp, I. C., Bartelsman, J. F., den Hartog Jager, F. C., Huibregtse, K., and Tytgat, G. N. Results of conservative treatment of benign esophageal strictures. A followup study in 100 patients. Gastroenterology 82:487, 1982.
116. Patterson, D. J., Graham, D. Y., Smith, J. L., Schwartz, J. T., Alpert, E., Lanza, F. L., and Cain, G. D. Natural history of benign esophageal stricture treated by dilatation. Gastroenterology 85:346, 1983.
117. Mercer, C. D., and Hill, L. D. Surgical management of peptic esophageal stricture: twenty-year experience. J. Thorac. Cardiovasc. Surg. 91:371, 1986.
118. Wesdorp, I. C. E., Bartelsman, J., Schipper, M. E. I., and Tytgat, G. N. Effect of long-term treatment with cimetidine and antacids in Barrett's oesophagus. Gut 22:724, 1981.
119. Skinner, D. B., Walther, B. C., and Little, A. C. Surgical treatment of Barrett's esophagus. In Spechler, S. J., and Goyal, R. K. (eds.). Barrett's Esophagus: Pathophysiology, Diagnosis, and Management. New York, Elsevier Science Publishing Company, 1985, pp. 211–221.
120. Brand, D. L., Ylvisaker, J. T., Gelfance, M., and Pope, C. E., II. Regression of columnar esophageal (Barrett's) epithelium after anti-reflux surgery. N. Engl. J. Med. 32:844, 1980.
121. Strickland, A. D., and Chang, J. H. T. Results of treatment of gastroesophageal reflux with bethanechol. J. Pediatr. 103:311, 1983.
122. Pennell, R. C., Lewis, E. L., Cradock, T. V., Danis, R. K., and Kaminsky, D. L. Management of severe gastroesophageal reflux in children. Arch. Surg. 119:553, 1984.

123. Gourley, G. R., Pellett, J. R., Li, B. U., and Adkins, W. N., Jr. A prospective randomized double-blind study of gastro-esophageal reflux surgery in pediatric-sized developmentally disabled patients: Nissen fundoplication versus Angelchik prosthesis. J. Pediatric Gastroenterol. Nutr. 5:52, 1986.
124. Goodall, R. J. R., Earis, J. E., Cooper, D. N., Bernstein, A., and Temple, J. G. Relationship between asthma and gastro-oesophageal reflux. Thorax 36:116, 1981.
125. Bushkin, F. L., Neustein, C. L., Parker, T. H., and Woodward, E. R. Nissen fundoplication for reflux peptic esophagitis. Ann. Surg. 185:672, 1977.
126. Belsey, R. H. R. Mark IV repairs of hiatal hernia by the transthoracic approach. World J. Surg. 1:475, 1977.
127. Hill, L. D. Progress in the surgical management of hiatus hernia. World J. Surg. 1:425, 1977.

128. Condon, R. E. More misadventures with the esophageal collar. Surgery 93:477, 1983.
129. Brand, D. L., Eastwood, I. R., Martin, D., Carter, W. B., and Pope, C. E., II. Esophageal symptoms, manometry, and histology before and after antireflux surgery. Gastroenterology 76:1393, 1979.
130. Bremmer, C. G. Gastric ulceration after a fundoplication operation for gastroesophageal reflux. Surg. Gynecol. Obstet. 148:62, 1979.
131. Durans, D., Armstrong, C. P., and Taylor, T. V. The Angel-chik antireflux prosthesis—some reservations. Br. J. Surg. 72:525, 1985.
132. Little, A. G., Ferguson, M. K., and Skinner, D. B. Reoperation for failed antireflux operations. J. Thorac. Cardiovasc. Surg. 91:511, 1986.

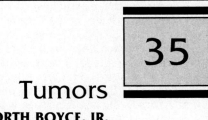

Tumors

H. WORTH BOYCE, JR.

Esophageal cancer is one of the most lethal of all malignancies. For clinical purposes, cancer of the esophagus means squamous cell carinoma as this lesion accounts for about 98 per cent of primary esophageal malignancies. Adenocarcinoma originating in the esophagus accounts for no more than 2 per cent of all malignancies in this organ. When it does occur, adenocarcinoma usually is associated with a columnar cell–lined esophagus.[1]

The natural history and delayed onset of symptoms of esophageal cancer result in late diagnosis and incurability. The answer to this problem depends on the development of more effective and safe systemic therapeutic agents or methods of earlier diagnosis, perhaps possible only by screening high-risk individuals. Benign esophageal tumors are sufficiently rare that they often are discovered as a surprise finding with somewhat atypical symptoms and signs.

CANCER OF THE ESOPHAGUS

Squamous Cell Carcinoma

Etiology. The cause of esophageal squamous cell carcinoma is unknown, but epidemiologic studies from several areas of the world strongly suggest a relationship to ingested substances found in soil and food, water, tobacco, alcohol, nitrosamines, *Candida* infec-

tions, aflatoxin, and riboflavin and vitamin A deficiencies.

The risk of esophageal cancer increases by a factor of 18 in alcoholics who drink more than 80 gm of ethanol per day and by a factor of 44 in those who also have a daily consumption of 20 gm of tobacco.[2] A high prevalence of esophageal cancer in France has been related to alcohol consumption, in both prospective and retrospective studies. In the United States alcohol alone does not appear to increase the risk of esophageal cancer but it is associated with a significant risk increase in persons who also use tobacco.[3] In high-incidence areas of Iran and China, little, if any, alcohol is ever consumed. In Australia there is a high consumption of alcohol and tobacco but a low prevalence of squamous cell carcinoma. In Italy the tar content of cigarettes is reported to be related to the risk of developing esophageal carcinoma and to be greater for esophageal cancer than for carcinoma of the lung.[4]

Both men and women in the Bantu population of South Africa have a high incidence that has been attributed to a beer ("cidiviki") that is now made from maize.[5] In Linxian County, China, where the prevalence of esophageal cancer is as high as any area in the world, a high incidence of pharyngoesophageal cancer has been found in domestic fowl, suggesting a common carcinogen from the soil.[6]

There appears to be a definite relationship between esophageal cancer and other medical conditions such as achalasia,[7] corrosive injury (lye) of the esophagus,[8] iron deficiency and the Paterson-Kelly or Plummer-Vinson syndrome,[3, 5] tylosis,[9] and thyroid disease.[10] Tylosis (hyperkeratosis of palms and soles) is a rare genetic disorder with autosomal dominant inheritance and full penetrance. Persons with this condition have a 100 per cent chance of developing esophageal cancer during their lifetime and at a much younger age than the usual.[9]

An unusual form of chronic esophagitis was found in 80 per cent of 430 men and women in northern Iran studied by esophagoscopy and biopsy. Dysplasia of the esophageal mucosa was found in 16 cases and invasive carcinoma in 11. Further study of 20 patients one year after the initial diagnosis of precancerous mucosal dysplasia revealed 4 with invasive cancer and 1 with carcinoma in situ.[11]

Incidence and Epidemiology. Although relatively infrequent in most of western Europe and North America, cancer of the esophagus is, overall, one of the most common cancers in the world.[12] Current estimates are that about 8000 new cases of esophageal cancer are diagnosed each year in the United States and that this disease accounts for 4 per cent of all cancer deaths.[3] The disease is more common in males than in females, with a ratio of 3:1. In Curacao and the Transkei in South Africa,[13] the sex incidence is about equal. Black males in this country are at highest risk. Incidence per 100,000 adjusted to the 1950 United States population has been reported as 1.2 for white females, 3.6 for black females, 4.1 for white males, and 15.6 for black males.[14] The patient usually is over 60 years old, but women seem to be affected at a younger age by several years.

Squamous cell carcinoma of the esophagus has a variation in incidence of up to 500 times from one area of a country to another, from one country to another, and from one ethnic group to another in the same country. However, there is no evidence that the natural history of this disease varies in different parts of the world. The incidence between the sexes favors males, but the male-female ratio does vary in areas of high prevalence from 20:1 (France) to 1:1 in areas of low prevalence (Finland).[2] There is a reversal of the usual male sex predominance in Iran and Ceylon. Also, in Ceylon, this neoplasm is the most common carcinoma of the gastrointestinal tract.

Prevalence rates vary widely around the world. The current rate in the United States is said to be 5 to 7 new cases per 100,000 male population per year.[5] Much higher prevalence rates are reported from southern African countries, Iran, China, India, Ceylon, and Puerto Rico. For example, in the Iranian province of Mazandaran, the prevalence is reported up to 110 per 100,000 males and 184 per 100,000 among females. In this area, a 20-fold variation in prevalence has been observed within a 300-mile span. A belt from the Caspian littoral in Iran to the northern provinces of China is known as the "Asian esophageal cancer belt."[3, 13] In the United States, the areas of highest incidence are around Charleston, South Carolina, Washington, D.C., and Alaska.

Pathology. Preneoplastic lesions in the esophagus are associated with conditions that result in chronic irritation and involve inflammation, hyperplasia, atypia, dysplasia, and carcinoma in situ. There appears to be a common association and a progressive relationship between dysplasia and frank carcinoma.[15]

Squamous cell carcinoma most often develops in the midthoracic segment and regularly invades the submucosa extensively before producing dysphagia or other symptoms. The histologic features of squamous cell carcinoma vary widely. Some are well differentiated with typical epidermoid features of keratinization, pearl formation, and intracellular bridges. Others are so poorly differentiated that they are difficult or impossible to classify. There are no clinical clues that correlate with the degree of differentiation; neither does there appear to be any relation between histopathology and the uniformly dismal prognosis except for the recently recognized superficially invasive variety.[16–18] Most lesions are greater than 4 cm in linear extent before diagnosis, but on occasion relatively massive involvement, up to 10 cm long, is found at initial diagnosis. The malignant cells spread readily via submucosal lymphatics to often extend in both directions, but especially in a cephalad direction, well beyond the macroscopic margin of the tumor. This feature has resulted in a need for the surgeon to establish a resection line well beyond both margins of the visible carcinoma. Even so, residual cancer cells are found in as many as 35 per cent of patients after the optimum gross extent of esophageal resection.[19]

The lymphatic drainage of the esophagus is disconcerting in that the first relay nodes already belong to the common mediastinal system. The anatomy of the long lymphatic channels that drain both the lungs and the lower esophagus and transport the lymph to either the right or left lateral tracheal chain explains the multicentric nature of the metastases.

The size of the intramural neoplasm is related to lymph node metastases. When the primary lesion exceeds 5 cm in size, over 90 per cent will have regional lymph node metastases. The growth pattern of this tumor in its earlier stages favors longitudinal and extramural extension over circumferential spread. Consequently, lumen stenosis occurs relatively late, as does the resulting dysphagia. The combination of this growth pattern plus patient delay in seeking medical help after onset of dysphagia regularly leads to a poor prognosis.

Once the cancer spreads through the muscle layers, it easily extends into the periesophageal tissues as there is no esophageal serosa to retard its migration. All mediastinal structures are vulnerable to metastasis, but the most common sites of involvement are the trachea, bronchi, lungs, pleura, major vessels, and diaphragm, depending on the site of origin of the cancer.

Esophagopulmonary fistula occurs in 6 to 12 per cent of persons with squamous cancer. The consensus is that these fistulas are primarily the result of local growth of the carcinoma as they appear at various times during the course of the disease, both before and after treatment. It is unfair to blame a fistula on the radiation therapist or the method used, because the therapy has done its job by destroying the cancer that involves both structures.

Distant, blood-borne metastases are less common as a clinical problem late in this disease than in many other visceral carcinomas. Autopsy findings in squamous cell carcinoma reveal that about 85 per cent of cadavers have metastases. The average number of metastatic sites per patient is 3.3. The most common metastatic sites are lymph nodes (73 per cent), lungs (52 per cent), and liver (47 per cent). The liver is the most common site of clinically apparent distant metastases, whereas the lung is the site of metastases most often detectable by radiography.[12] During life, bone metastases are reported in 5.2 per cent of cases, but 14 per cent have bone metastases on autopsy.[13, 20]

Superficially invasive or "early" squamous cell carcinomas have been recognized with increasing frequency in Japan, Europe, and the United States as a result of the increasing use of endoscopy. This type of lesion represents about 4 per cent of all esophageal cancers and from 7 to 13 per cent of all resected carcinomas in some reports.[18, 21] The European experience with this cancer is reported from a survey of 902,207 endoscopies in which there were 6719 (0.7 per cent) instances of esophageal cancer, of which 51 (0.75 per cent) were considered early or limited to the mucosa and submucosa. Twenty-five (49 per cent) of these patients were alive without evidence of cancer an average of 30 months after surgery.[17] Early esophageal cancer detection rates are as high as 70 per cent of all esophageal cancer in Northern China owing to mass screening by exfoliative balloon cytology. The reported five-year survival rate for these patients after surgery is over 85 per cent.[22, 23]

The pathology of squamous esophageal cancer is unique in another respect because there is an unusually high incidence (10 to 16.4 per cent) of associated carcinomas in the head and neck regions. Additional primary cancers may be found in 2.4 per cent. Thorough clinical investigation and surveillance is necessary in patients with upper aerodigestive tract carcinoma to rule out associated malignancy, which may greatly influence therapy and prognosis.[24, 25]

Clinical Manifestations. Dysphagia is the classic symptom of esophageal obstruction owing to esophageal carcinoma. Unfortunately, it also indicates extensive involvement of the esophagus and surrounding structures by malignancy in at least 90 per cent of cases. For practical purposes, the disease must be considered incurable in the majority of patients when dysphagia begins. The exceptions to this extremely poor prognosis are some patients who have superficial invasive squamous cell carcinoma. Although dysphagia is reported to be a complaint in some patients who have minimal involvement of the esophageal wall, all indications are that malignancy is present months, and probably years, before there is sufficient esophageal stenosis to produce dysphagia. It has been estimated that when dysphagia appears, about two thirds of the circumference of the esophageal wall is involved.[26]

The patient who develops dysphagia probably has had numerous early clues but is unable to interpret sensations that are transient and unfamiliar. In one series, 10 per cent of 300 patients with squamous cell carcinoma of the esophagus were forewarned by an unusual sensation of substernal oppression, discomfort, or fullness that usually was transient.[27] Although unable to recognize the significance of subtle early symptoms of esophageal stenosis, the patient begins subconsciously to alter eating habits. A definite but subtle hang-up or "dragging" sensation first occurs with solids. There is a tendency to drink more fluids and to chew solids more thoroughly. It takes longer to eat a meal. Next comes the practice of altering the consistency of the diet by avoiding those foods most likely to cause these mild, uncomfortable "predysphagia" sensations. A large bolus of any solid material can cause problems, but the most common items involved have been beef, especially if charcoal-broiled with a firm outer consistency, apples, and fresh breads. Fresh bread causes plugging of the stenosis because it is modified by mixing with saliva during chewing to form a miniature dough ball with a putty-like consistency. These three items of solid food, and others of similar form, provide a bolus challenge to the developing malignant stenosis and usually cause the patient sufficient discomfort to make him or her remember the precise date of onset. After onset, the patient tolerates or denies the significance of the dysphagia for three to six months before seeking medical attention. By the time of the first medical evaluation, most have altered dietary intake to soft and liquid foods and have lost weight.

Dysphagia is never psychogenic or "functional." True dysphagia is sensed by the patient within 10 sec of the act of swallowing and is indicative of a mechanical obstruction or a neuromotor disorder. Consequently, it is imperative that the diagnostic evaluation of this symptom be continued until the cause is determined.

Dysphagia is most commonly perceived as a blockage in the midesophagus or high epigastrium. In some cases, the patient will complain of food sticking or hang-up in the cervical region, although the stenosing lesion is located more distally in the esophagus. This fact requires total examination of hypopharynx, esophagus, and proximal stomach even if one lesion is found that explains that complaint as more than one lesion may occur in the same patient.[24, 25]

Excessive salivation (sialorrhea) may be noted early after esophageal stenosis develops but usually becomes a significant problem later on.

As the degree of esophageal obstruction progresses, regurgitation occurs, swallowing becomes uncomfortable, and the patient has less desire to tolerate the problem. He or she then consumes fewer calories than needed, and weight loss begins. Most patients will have lost between 10 and 20 pounds of body weight when first seen. Nutritional assessment reveals protein and total calorie malnutrition. In addition to dysphagia, anorexia and odynophagia (painful swallowing) will further aggravate the undernutrition.

Anemia of mild degree is common but rarely presents a significant problem initially. It usually is of the hypochromic, microcytic type owing to low oral intake of dietary iron and, to a lesser extent, blood loss. Dehydration may mask the degree of anemia.

Pain associated with malignant esophageal stenosis occurs in several forms. First is the pressure or aching sensation associated with delay of passage or impaction of a solid bolus against an unyielding, narrow lumen. This pain can be perceived at any level from the cervical esophagus to the gastroesphageal junction. It may be noted in the neck, jaws, or retrosternal or intercapsular areas. It can simulate the pain of coronary insufficiency. Because of this impact pain or discomfort, the patient quickly learns to alter the foods eaten and to drink more liquids to minimize its occurrence.

Another pain noted by some patients during swallowing is that due to a topical effect of the substances swallowed. Such things as alcohol, citrus juices, and certain medications (potassium chloride and ferrous sulfate among others) may cause burning pain. Radiation, candidal, or viral esophagitis also may be the cause of odynophagia in patients with esophageal cancer. Esophagoscopy should be done to evaluate for the presence of infectious esophagitis as specific therapy will help in most cases. This type pain and the impact pain described previously are the main causes of odynophagia. They can be controlled by alteration of oral intake or therapy for esophagitis.

A third type of pain associated with esophageal cancer is the most ominous of all related symptoms and indicates extensive mediastinal metastasis. It is a steady, aching pain in the midchest, back, or epigastrium and is indicative of the late stage of this disease. Narcotics, often in large doses, are needed for adequate relief. When dysphagia is relieved by palliative therapy, this pain often assumes prominence as the patient's main complaint.

Pulmonary sequelae, either from regurgitation and transadital aspiration or via an esophagopulmonary fistula, usually develop later in the course of this disease. The patient may be prone to pulmonary complications because of aspiration and fistula drainage but also is at great risk because of immunologic incompetence resulting from visceral protein deficiency. Pulmonary infection often is the immediate cause of death. Unexplained cough may be an early manifestation of mediastinal invasion and tracheal or bronchial involvement. Cough should always lead the clinician to suspect the possibility of a developing fistula.

Less common clinical manifestations include hiccup, hoarseness owing to laryngeal nerve paralysis or aspiration, bleeding, hypercalcemia, hypokalemic alkalosis, and focal bone pain from metastasis. Bleeding from the carcinoma typically is manifested only as occult blood in the stool. Bleeding noted before or soon after initial diagnosis usually is mild but can be severe from the tumor itself without major vessel involvement. Late in the disease, bleeding (hematemesis) is an ominous sign that may indicate erosion into a major vessel.

Hypercalcemia can produce a confusing clinical syndrome in esophageal cancer patients. It is manifested by the rapid onset of progressive weakness, vague gastrointestinal complaints, drowsiness, or stupor. It is important to consider this possibility and not to attribute deterioration only to the effects of carcinoma. In one series of 149 patients with esophageal cancer, 73 had a serum calcium determination and 12 (16 per cent) had a value greater than 11 mg/dl.[28] Severe hypokalemic alkalosis has been reported related to ACTH-producing metastases from carcinoma of the esophagus.[29] Metastasis to the adrenals may result in adrenal insufficiency as the presenting syndrome.

Squamous cell carcinoma of the cervical esophagus is relatively rare, accounting for less than 10 per cent of all cases, but it produces some different symptoms than those located in the thoracic esophagus. The cervical esophagus is located in a relatively confined space in close proximity to the spine posteriorly, the trachea anteriorly, and the carotid arteries, thyroid gland, and neck muscles. Because of these relationships, symptoms and signs might be expected that would lead to earlier diagnosis. Sadly, these patients have no better prognosis than those with cancer of the thoracic esophagus with two to eight months of symptoms elapsing before they seek medical attention and another two to six months of delay before diagnosis. Symptoms and signs to be expected include dysphagia, weight loss, hoarseness, aspiration, and pain.[30]

Diagnosis. Until recently there was no evidence that a clinically recognizable stage exists that will permit a true "early" diagnosis of this disease. True early carcinoma in the form of the superficial invasive type that often is found by accident is the exception to the usual clinical reality. "Early" in the typical case of advanced disease refers to a time soon after onset of symptoms, but it can not be equated with an "early" stage of neoplastic growth. In this disease, the onset of its major symptom (i.e. dysphagia) is, in the majority of patients, a sign of incurability. The clinician has little or no chance to successfully apply curative surgical or irradiation therapy. Unfortunately, many physicians and surgeons have not yet accepted this and continue to recommend radical "curative" surgical procedures that rarely have a chance of success. It appears that the only opportunity for effecting cure in this disease is to develop screening procedures for patients who have been identified as at highest risk and who may have localized disease. Good surgical technique and irradiation therapy can cure if the patient is referred when the carcinoma is localized to the esophagus, an extremely rare finding nowadays.

The presumptive diagnosis and even the level of the lesion can be determined readily in most patients by taking a good history. It is important to emphasize again that the symptom of dysphagia never is psychogenic and that its presence in the history makes complete radiographic, endoscopic, and, in a few cases, manometric study imperative.

Physical Examination. The physical examination

usually reveals some degree of undernutrition, ranging from mild weight loss to classic marasmus. About half of the patients will lose over 20 pounds of weight by the time of diagnosis. About 10 per cent will report no weight loss. Rarely is there physical evidence of metastasis of squamous cell carcinoma at the time of initial diagnosis. Carcinoma of the cervical esophagus may present with a syndrome that mimics acute suppurative thyroiditis with tenderness and a mass or with hoarseness. This lesion more often produces abnormal physical findings than thoracic esophageal cancer. A careful examination of the neck may reveal a palpable neck mass, loss of laryngeal crepitus, or unilateral vocal cord paralysis, indicative of incurable disease.[30]

Radiographic Studies. Standard chest radiographs assist primarily by revealing evidence of pulmonary complications of esophageal carcinoma, such as pneumonia and metastasis into mediastinum or lung parenchyma. Subtle changes such as mediastinal widening, posterior tracheal indentation, and abnormality of the azygoesophageal line also may be seen.[31]

Barium contrast radiography is the preferred initial study, which will provide strong evidence for the diagnosis in nearly all patients if it is properly performed. Double-contrast technique is best for study of mucosal detail. It is imperative that the radiologist examine the hypopharyngeal and proximal gastric areas as well as the esophagus regularly during this examination. Unexpected second primary carcinoma in the pharynx or the rare metastasis to the stomach may be detected by a thorough examination.

The common features of malignant change in the esophageal wall include nodularity, rigidity, abrupt luminal angulation or "shelving," ulceration, and stenosis of the lumen. The stenosis typically has asymmetric margins, distinctively different from the usual smooth, tapered stenosis of a benign lesion. The lumen proximal to a malignant stenosis usually is only mildly to moderately dilated as the patient rarely will challenge the stenosis by ingesting sufficient volumes of fluid and solids to cause severe dilatation (Fig. 35–1).

Esophageal carcinoma classically presents in one or a combination of three forms: infiltrative, polypoid, or ulcerative. The infiltrative form causes only minimal changes in the surface contour of the mucosa. Polypoid lesions appear as irregular, nodular filling defects in the barium column, often combined with infiltrative or ulcerative features or both. The ulcerative type rarely, if ever, occurs in primary form but instead is a change more often seen in combination with the infiltrative and polypoid lesions.

The differential diagnosis occasionally may be difficult when lesions such as candidal esophagitis, ulcerative reflux-related esophagitis, or adenocarcinoma of the gastric cardia invading the distal esophagus are present. In those instances in which a standard barium contrast study fails to clearly define the level or the cause of dysphagia, it is imperative that a bolus challenge study be performed. Challenging the luminal patency and motility of the esophagus with a solid bolus of adequate size (13 mm barium pill or a marsh-

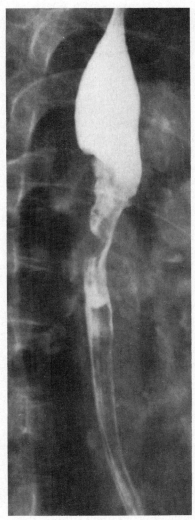

Figure 35–1. Carcinoma of the esophagus. A circumferential lesion with marked luminal narrowing is seen high in the esophagus. Mucosal irregularity suggests that this is not a benign tumor. (Courtesy of C. A. Rohrmann, M.D.)

mallow) will make it unlikely that any type of symptomatic esophageal stenosis will be missed.

Endoscopy. Squamous cell carcinoma that has grown to produce esophageal stenosis and dysphagia will produce abnormalities of the mucosal surface. Usually there is inflammation, nodularity, erosion, and ulceration present to provide ample evidence of disease. Subtle surface changes in the mucosa will be missed if there is any residual food, barium, or tissue debris present. Therefore, it is essential to be certain that the area is cleared before endoscopy, either by a clear liquid diet for one to two days or lavage just before the examination. When the lumen is stenosed, peroral dilation may be necessary to permit endoscopic examination and tissue sampling from the narrowed segment and beyond.

Suspicion of early cancer is based on endoscopic findings that will appear unremarkable to the casual observer. The following signs should create suspicion and are sufficient justification for cytologic and biopsy study: mucosal discoloration, slight or subtle reddening, shallow depression, uneven grainy surface appearance of the mucosa, and plateau-like elevations. The morphology of superficial invasive carcinoma has been classified as (1) white, elevated; (2) red, depressed or flat; (3) mixed, and (4) normal-appearing mucosa.[16] Superficial invasive carcinoma may have relatively gross changes indicative of malignancy or very minimal changes mimicking reflux esophagitis or normal-appearing mucosa. These observations and the importance of accurate diagnosis of this lesion justify a more vigorous use of biopsy and cytologic study of minor mucosal changes with a benign appearance.

Fiberoptic esophagoscopy with biopsy and cytology is the favored method for confirming a diagnosis of esophageal carcinoma. Endoscopic visualization plus biopsy and brush cytology will provide an accurate diagnosis in nearly 100 per cent of cases.[32] *Brush cytology* permits sampling of large areas of mucosa. *Biopsy* alone is 98 per cent accurate when at least seven biopsy specimens are taken. Seventeen per cent of all lesions subsequently proved to be malignant were thought to be benign on endoscopic inspection.[33]

Biopsy touch cytology has been recommended as the most accurate method. This is performed by carefully transferring the biopsy specimen from forceps to a glass slide and rotating the specimen gently over the slide using a 21 gauge needle. A total of six to eight slides is recommended. A 100 per cent positive rate is reported for the biopsy touch smear, compared with 82 per cent for brush cytology and 89 per cent for biopsy.[34]

Salvage cytology is performed by aspirating the content of the endoscope biopsy channel into a mucus trap in the suction line. This method collects residual cellular debris left in the channel from the biopsy forceps that proves diagnostic of malignancy in 88 per cent of cases.[35]

Staining of the mucosa with Lugol's iodine solution may aid in tissue sampling because neoplastic cells do not stain.[36, 37] The normal squamous cells around the tumor margin stain a dark brown color, so the clinician can precisely direct forceps or cytology brush to the nonstained area of neoplasm. Nonstaining alone is not diagnostic of neoplasm, however, as areas of severe inflammation also may fail to stain with iodine.

The *Nabeya capsule* has been developed in Japan and *mesh-covered balloons* are used in China for screening high risk populations for esophageal cancer. The crevices in the sponge or mesh trap cellular material by an abrading action on withdrawal. The material captured is then examined after cytologic preparation and staining.

A tiny *Geiger counter* that is pulled through the esophagus has been used to measure radioactivity concentrated in malignant tissue following a dose of 500 microcuries of radioactive phosphorous (^{32}P) given 18 hours earlier.[38] The method proved 95 per cent accurate in differentiating benign and malignant lesions. It has been found useful in the diagnosis of some "early" carcinomas.[39]

Staging. The proper extent of staging or preoperative evaluation has not been determined. Chest radiography, esophagoscopy, computed tomography, bronchoscopy, biopsy of any accessible lymph nodes, and laparoscopy are acceptable procedures. Mediastinoscopy, azygos venography, and transtracheal mediastinal lymphography are rarely used. Bronchoscopy should be done prior to thoracotomy because of the frequency of airway invasion.[40] Laparoscopy has proved to be the most sensitive method for detecting small hepatic and peritoneal metastases.[41] Endoscopic ultrasonography currently is under investigation and appears to have merit for preoperative staging.[42]

Esophagogastroscopy originally done for diagnosis will provide helpful information on the extent of gross esophageal wall involvement. Peroral dilation should be done to open the lumen adequately to permit evaluation of the distal extent of the lesion as well as the condition of the stomach. At least 90 per cent of persons with evidence of more than 5 cm involvement of the length of the esophageal wall already have metastasis to the mediastinal nodes.

Computer-assisted tomography has been reported to be of value for staging the extent of esophageal mural and extraesophageal mediastinal and upper abdominal involvement by carcinoma. Initial reports offer impressive evidence that CT is remarkably precise in demonstrating wall thickness, intraluminal masses, and periesophageal invasion.[43, 44] It appeared that this technique could provide sufficient data for staging to permit a more accurate preoperative determination of resectability and thereby help reduce the hazards of exploratory surgery currently in use for this purpose. There are reports of over 90 per cent accuracy for CT in local tumor staging, but recently it has been pointed out that mediastinal and celiac lymph node metastases are not identified reliably in many cases.[45, 46] The role of CT has not been completely defined.

Laparoscopy is a safe and efficient method for staging esophageal carcinoma and can obviate the need for laparotomy in inoperable cases.[46] This method has proved more accurate than scintography and ultrasonography and should be considered as a valuable method for preoperative staging in patients with esophageal carcinoma. Metastatic lesions of liver and peritoneum under 1 cm in diameter often are undetected by CT but can be diagnosed at laparoscopy in over 85 per cent of cases.[41]

Therapy. Physicians who accept responsibility for medical care of patients with esophageal cancer must accept the fact that overall five-year "cure" rates for this neoplasm have not changed significantly during the past 40 years. This is despite the excellent progress made in supportive care, surgical technique, and irradiation therapy. The reason for the persistently poor results is that rarely is diagnosis ever made early enough to permit either surgery or irradiation therapy to be curative.

Management options that are available for palliation for most of these patients include surgical removal of the primary lesion with esophagogastric anastomosis or colon interposition, a combination of irradiation and surgery, external irradiation, internal irradiation, peroral dilation, placement of a peroral esophageal prosthesis, and intraluminal tumor ablation by laser vaporization or coagulation probes. It is safe to say that chemotherapy to date has not been shown to have a role in treating this disease, but research presently under way using combinations of several agents may prove beneficial.

General supportive care, restoration of adequate nutritional status, and treatment of specific sequelae of the carcinoma all are essential to proper therapy. No single method likely will be adequate for treating esophageal carcinoma.

The author's philosophy agrees completely with that of Lawrence, who has stated that the treatment plan should effectively deal with the major symptom of dysphagia as palliation is the primary accomplishment that can be hoped for at this time.[47] Other authors emphasize that surgery should be attempted only in those patients without clinical evidence of metastatic disease.[48] The role of resection intended only for palliation has been properly emphasized by an increasing number of surgeons.[49, 50]

Surgery. Preoperative assessment of the patient's general status as well as of the extent of malignancy or staging is the first step in decision making. While this is being done, therapy must be directed toward treating the sequelae of esophageal cancer, usually obstruction, mediastinal pain, malnutrition, and pulmonary infection secondary to aspiration and often immune incompetence. Most patients with this disease have been cigarette smokers for many years and as a consequence suffer the risks of chronic obstructive pulmonary disease. Peroral dilation may be started promptly and, in nearly all cases, a lumen adequate for taking liquid and soft foods safely can be established within a few days.[51] The risk of continued aspiration is reduced, the patient can swallow saliva and food, and nutritional deficits can begin to be restored. Most patients are significantly underweight, debilitated, and obviously poor surgical risks. Therefore, even in those few cases for which surgery seems appropriate, there should be no rush until improved total body nutrition and restoration of optimum pulmonary function have been achieved.

Surgical classification of patients into subgroups has made the reports more understandable, but it has created confusion about survival statistics. Even by the most liberal standards, no more than 50 per cent of all patients should be considered "operable," (i.e., are considered able to survive the operation and live at least four weeks). Operable also is defined as the situation in which the patient may be offered operation with a reasonable risk and expectation of resection of the cancer.

Unfortunately, the criteria for operability appear to be somewhat loose in many reports, with a wide discrepancy in the final staging criteria for operability and resectability. The surgeon who recognizes that nearly all surgery merely is palliative should have results for operability and resectability that are quite close.

"Resectable" indicates that the tumor can be resected. At best, about 30 to 40 per cent of all squamous cell carcinomas are considered resectable.[52, 53] Further refinements in staging should permit the unfortunate discrepancy between operability and resectability to be minimized. In a review of over 83,000 cases reported in the literature, 54 per cent were deemed operable and only 39 per cent were resectable.[53] The most common cause of inoperability is tracheobronchial invasion, a finding that provides clear indication for bronchoscopy in the staging process.[40] A very small number will be labeled "resectable for cure" (i.e., extraesophageal involvement is minimal and all suspiciously involved tissue can be removed safely). Unfortunately, accurate assignment to the categories of resectable and resectable for cure is possible only after surgical exploration. The price for this determination is general anesthesia, a thoracotomy, and the risks inherent with these procedures.

Survival statistics usually are reported for the resectable-for-cure group, from which five-year cure rates as high as 25 per cent may be seen. This 25 per cent actually may represent 6 of 24 patients whose tumors were considered resectable for cure from a total of 100 patients, giving an overall five-year survival rate of only 6 per cent. The primary physician should keep these classifications and reporting procedures, as well as the track record of surgical colleagues, in mind when developing a realistic therapeutic plan.

Distal esophageal carcinomas are considered operable more often because they are technically more easily resected. Adenocarcinoma of the gastric cardia involving the distal esophagus should not be included with statistics on surgery for squamous cell carcinoma of the esophagus.

The surgical procedure of choice for most patients is esophagogastrectomy with primary esophagogastrostomy.[54] The best results indicate an operative mortality rate between 2.8 and 17 per cent with significant complications in 5.3 to 12 per cent. Survival rates will vary depending on the way they are calculated. The overall five-year survival rate averages less than 10 per cent but may be reported to be as high as 25 per cent depending on type of cancer, location, staging, and extent of surgical resection. Mean survival times after esophagogastrectomy vary from 7.7 to 25 months.[19, 54-56]

The surgical reports just mentioned are among the best available and cannot be considered indicative of what can be expected in the average hospital. A review of 4109 patients from major centers reports an overall postoperative mortality rate of 22 per cent (range of 6 to 41 per cent) and a cumulative five-year survival rate of 9.6 per cent.[57] A report from the Cleveland Clinic reveals a drop in operative mortality from 20 per cent to 7.1 per cent over the past 15 years with an increase in two-year survival from 10.9 to 31.5 per cent. Their overall five-year survival rate remained low at 6 per cent.[19]

The conclusion of Earlam and Cunha-Melo is the best available for giving an overview of the results of surgery for squamous cell cancer and is quoted as follows: "After trying to standardize the data, it appears that of 100 patients with the condition, 58 will be explored and 39 have the tumour resected, of whom 13 will die in the hospital. Of the 26 patients leaving hospital with the tumour excised, 18 will survive for 1 year, 9 for 2 years and 4 for 5 years. Oesophageal resection for squamous cell carcinoma has the highest operative mortality of any routinely performed surgical procedure today."[53] This review reflects statistics more representative of the average hospital, but it will be contested by those who specialize in esophageal surgery. Most patients with operable cancers will not have the good fortune to be operated on by an esophageal surgeon with an operative mortality rate under 10 per cent.

As yet there is no evidence from properly controlled studies that the combination of surgical resection with preoperative or postoperative radiation has enhanced the degree of palliation or cure of squamous cell cancer of the esophagus.[58] The relative merits of various combinations of surgery, irradiation, and chemotherapy will not be known until properly controlled, randomized studies are performed.[59]

The most common fatal complications of surgery are pulmonary, cardiovascular, and septic complications usually related to anastomotic leak. The major risk of surgery for esophageal cancer is such an anastomotic leak, which previously has occurred in at least 10 per cent of cases. Since the introduction of parenteral nutrition and use of the end-to-end stapler the incidence of anastomotic leak has decreased to about 2 per cent in some reports.

Radiation. The practice in most centers has been to refer those patients with the greatest chance of cure for surgery and to refer all others for palliative or "curative" radiation. There is at present no proof that surgery alone is better than radiation therapy alone as no study randomizing patients with similar staging of disease has been undertaken. Three reports of patients who received radiation therapy at a stage when their disease would have been classed as operable have been published. The one-year survival rates were 42, 44, and 46 per cent; the two year survival rates were 8, 15, and 27 per cent; and the three year survival rates were 6, 6, and 20 per cent, respectively all being equal to or better than surgical results in patients at a similar stage of disease reported by other authors.[60] Other reports indicate that radiation therapy can give five-year survival rates equal to or better than surgical resection.[19, 61] It should be pointed out that both the occasional operator and the occasional irradiator are at a considerable disadvantage and cannot expect the same results as can be achieved in specialized treatment centers.

A critical review of the literature on radiotherapy in 49 reports of a total of 8489 patients over the period of 1954 through 1979 has been published by Earlam and Cunha-Melo.[60] Although most reports include patients who have more disseminated disease (i.e., have been evaluated and considered inoperable), the one-year survival rate is 18 per cent and the five-year survival rate after radiotherapy is 6 per cent. These rates are similar to those for surgery; there is no operative mortality and the stomach and voice remain intact. If the patient has an adverse reaction during the course of irradiation, treatment can be modified or discontinued.

It has been stated that radiation therapy transiently may worsen dysphagia, and evidence indicates this worsening is likely to peak about five days into a course of treatment. Dysphagia may recur or slowly worsen any time after radiation therapy and 50 per cent or more may need continued peroral dilation. Peroral esophageal dilation properly performed during and after radiation therapy carries no significant risk.[51]

Radiation esophagitis occasionally is a problem and may be managed symptomatically in most patients. Both dysphagia and odynophagia may occur but rarely are persistent. The clinician must be aware that these patients are prone to develop candidal or viral esophagitis, which causes a syndrome similar to radiation esophagitis. These conditions are readily diagnosed by endoscopy with biopsy and usually respond to specific therapy.

Mortality from radiation therapy is nonexistent in most series. This is ascribed to the fact that if the patient becomes ill, the therapeutic regimen is altered to suit patient tolerance. This lack of therapy-related mortality gives radiation a distinct edge as the treatment of choice over surgery in most patients with squamous cell carcinoma of the esophagus.[62]

The latest approach for either high-dose or low-dose palliative irradiation is via an intraluminal after-loading delivery system using cobalt-60 or iridium-192 seeds, respectively. This therapy has the advantage that it can be used as primary therapy or as an adjunct to external irradiation.[63]

Chemotherapy. Unfortunately, little progress has been made in the chemotherapy of esophageal cancer over the past decade. Eleven chemotherapy combination regimens have been reported to date. Cisplatin has been used in most of these in varying dosages and schedules, but its toxicity has far exceeded its efficacy. Complete remissions of this carcinoma are very rare and when they do occur are short in duration. Most clinicians will agree with Kelsen and associates that for now the use of systemic chemotherapy in esophageal carcinoma should still be considered investigational.[64]

Peroral Dilation. The first order of therapeutic business should be to restore the stenotic esophageal lumen to a diameter sufficient to allow the patient to ingest fluid and food as well as the significant volume of saliva produced every day. Peroral dilation should begin as soon as possible in patients with dysphagia.[65, 66] When proper instruments and technique are used there is no increased risk to dilating a malignant stenosis either before, during, or after radiation therapy.[51]

Peroral dilation can restore esophageal lumen patency to a diameter adequate to permit adequate swallowing in over 90 per cent of patients.[51] Either flexible, tapered dilators (Savary), metal olives on a flexible shaft (Eder-Puestow), or rubber dilators (Maloney) are used in progressive sizes under fluoroscopic control. Most malignant stenoses can be dilated to a size of No. 48 to 51 French (16 to 17 mm). Lumen diameter must be greater than No. 39 French (13 mm) if solid food dysphagia is to be relieved. A maintenance program for frequency of dilation is an individual matter based on each patient's response.[66, 67]

Peroral Esophageal Prosthesis. When dilation is unsuccessful, a peroral polyvinyl prosthesis may be inserted by pulsion technique through the stenosis using only mild sedative-analgesic medication and anesthetic gargle.[65, 66, 68, 69] This palliative method is necessary in about 15 per cent of all patients who fail to respond adequately to peroral dilation. The prosthesis remains in position for the rest of the patient's life and permits adequate swallowing in most cases (Fig. 35–2). Complications are uncommon, and the method is recognized as having less risk than surgical placement of a traction-type prostheses.[70]

The prosthesis also is useful to block leakage and stop the pulmonary soilage via an esophagopulmonary fistula. Esophagopulmonary fistula can be treated in most patients adequately in a palliative fashion only by an esophageal prosthesis that is best positioned by the peroral route.[66]

Laser. Transendoscopic ablation of obstructing intraluminal cancer by laser photocoagulation offers another relatively safe but often temporary palliation for dysphagia. The value of this method relative to other treatments currently is being evaluated, but preliminary results are encouraging.[71, 72]

Pain Therapy. Pain from the region of the carcinoma may be a major problem. Typically, it becomes serious enough to require regular drug therapy relatively late in the course but may occur as the first symptom, preceding dysphagia in 10 per cent of patients. It ordinarily is a constant, deep, aching or boring pain noted in the retrosternal area, back, or epigastrium and may be referred to neck, jaws, or shoulders. Typically, it responds incompletely to medications containing combinations of aspirin or acetaminophen plus codeine. Dilaudid, morphine sulfate, methadone, or other potent narcotics usually are required and should be prescribed at a dose and frequency adequate to provide relief.[73] Liquid morphine preparation is useful in patients with dysphagia. A sedative at bedtime may help by enhancing the analgesic effect of a narcotic drug.

Nutritional Support. During the initial physical and laboratory examination, an assessment of the patient's nutritional status should be made. Dysphagia and pain can be managed adequately within several days so the patient can swallow food and medications. The treatment of the protein and calorie malnutrition so common in these patients should be initiated early. In some patients, it may be appropriate to begin this restoration by central venous alimentation, by surgical placement of a feeding tube via jejunostomy under local anesthesia, or by placement of a nasoenteric Silastic feeding tube. Percutaneous endoscopic gastrostomy is currently favored as the ideal method for providing enteral nutritional supplementation. For those depleted patients who are considered surgical candidates, it is best to delay the operation for several weeks and attempt to restore nitrogen balance and immune competence by either enteral or central venous nutrition.[74] Oral feeding is encouraged as tolerated at the same time. It is essential to make every effort to deliver adequate calories, replace nitrogen deficits, and thereby restore the patient's immune competence. Early postoperative deaths often result as much from the consequences of malnutrition and infection, especially pneumonia, as from spread of the carcinoma.

Other important aspects of supportive care include maintenance of good oral hygiene, restoration of adequate dentition, and pulmonary toilet. Needless to say, the care, compassion, and ready availability of a knowledgeable physician to provide psychologic support, for both the patient and concerned family members, is of major importance to the quality of the patient's remaining life.

Selection of Therapy. In 1931, Turner indicated that the attitude of most doctors toward esophageal carcinoma was one of studied neglect or benevolent despair.[75] Although there are enthusiasts for each form

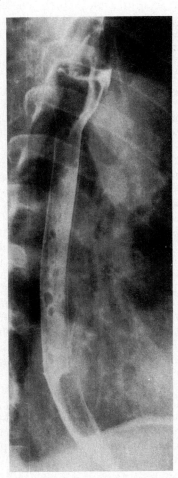

Figure 35–2. A peroral esophageal prosthesis is shown in the midesophagus for palliation of obstruction by a squamous cell carcinoma that failed to respond adequately to radiation and later dilation therapy.

of therapy who report better results for highly selected subgroups, the overall results nearly 60 years later give reason for despair. There is, by present standards, no available method for making an "early" diagnosis of this disease except by screening methods in high-risk populations. In 1957, Palmer pointed out the fallacy of the "early" diagnosis. In 16 patients, either esophageal cancer was found before symptoms developed or symptoms suggestive of the diagnosis were recognized while the patient was under active medical surveillance for conditions unrelated to the esophagus. Those with symptoms found before diagnosis were examined within nine days of onset. Only four patients survived one year and just two were alive at two years.[76]

Whatever the treatment happens to be, the overall survival can be expected to be higher in females, patients with distal esophageal lesions, those with more localized disease, those with the best nutritional status, and those without other significant disease. These factors must be considered in selection of therapy and in interpretation of treatment results. Untreated, the average patient will survive about eight months from the onset of symptoms or four to five months after diagnosis.

Most treatment must be considered primarily palliative because of the natural history of this disease. All patients should be evaluated thoughtfully by staging methods before decisions on therapy are made. The goal of therapy will remain to cure, but perceptive clinicians know that this is impossible in 95 per cent of cases because patients regularly come to medical attention after the chance for cure has passed. If clinicians can be convinced that each patient should be evaluated carefully with the reality of the situation in mind, they will begin to see better palliation, improved quality of life, and therapy properly directed toward all of the sequelae of the carcinoma rather than fruitless, high-risk attempts to remove the primary lesion and its metastases. Lawrence properly states that the main benefits of surgery are palliative even in cases that initially appear favorable.[47]

Adenocarcinoma

Incidence. Adenocarcinoma primary in the esophagus has been estimated to account for 0.76 to 10 per cent of all esophageal cancer.[77, 78] Adenocarcinomas arising in a columnar cell–lined esophagus appear to constitute the majority.[1] Evidence is accumulating to indicate that adenocarcinoma and squamous cell carcinoma of the esophagus primarily affect different racial groups (i.e., most adenocarcinomas occur in white males with a columnar-lined esophagus, whereas black males are at by far a greater risk for squamous cell cancer.[78]

The risk that adenocarcinoma will develop in the columnar-lined esophagus recently has been re-evaluated and found to be far less than originally reported. The prevalence ratio of adenocarcinoma was 7 per cent and the incidence was one case per 175 person-

years. That incidence is more than 40-fold greater than would be expected in a group of men of similar ages in the general population.[79]

Etiology. The common association between a columnar-lined esophagus and the development of adenocarcinoma is attributed to the malignant potential of the metaplastic and later dysplastic epithelium that occurs in this condition. An association between primary esophageal adenocarcinoma and a columnar-lined esophagus has been reported in 86 per cent of cases.[1] Most reports of adenocarcinoma in patients with a columnar-lined esophagus emphasize the histories of heavy alcohol and smoking as possible major contributors to this malignant potential.[78, 79] Adenocarcinoma in the absence of columnar-lined esophagus arises from columnar epithelium in the esophageal mucous glands.

Clinical Picture. Adenocarcinoma may present as an infiltrating, stenosing lesion but most often it is first manifested as an ulceration or as polypoid, relatively soft masses that are easy to dilate but are poorly responsive to dilation. Some patients have large, bulky tumors that appear to occlude the lumen totally but cause little dysphagia. This rarely occurs with squamous cell cancer. The typical patient, a white male who smokes cigarettes and drinks alcohol, presents with dysphagia and some weight loss and usually has evidence of extraesophageal metastasis on staging evaluation. Metastases are present more often with adenocarcinoma and distal esophageal malignancies. Symptoms of gastroesophageal reflux related to the columnar-lined esophagus often are mild or absent despite the fact that esophagitis appears responsible for the squamous epithelial destruction that precedes the cephalad migration of metaplastic columnar epithelium.

Diagnosis. A proper history suggests distal malignant esophageal obstruction. Barium contrast radiography nearly always suggests the diagnosis. If no lesion is apparent, a bolus challenge with barium pill or marshmallow will identify the level of the stenosis accurately. Fiberoptic endoscopy with biopsy and cytology will provide the histologic diagnosis in virtually all cases. An initial negative report by either radiography or endoscopy should never be accepted as accurate in a patient with dysphagia and weight loss. Computed tomography may provide evidence of mural thickening or periesophageal metastasis, but this method is considered primarily to assist in staging rather than initial diagnosis. Endoscopic ultrasonography provides a means to more precisely evaluate the esophageal wall and periesophageal region for lesions not apparent on endoscopic inspection.[42]

Therapy. Adenocarcinoma accounts for the majority of malignant lesions reported in the distal esophagus.[19] However, many of the distal lesions actually originate in the cardia and invade the distal esophagus. Esophagogastrectomy is the surgical procedure of choice for cancers that are considered resectable for cure or for palliative resection after careful staging procedure.[19, 54, 56] Interpretation of surgical reports is difficult because most include adenocarcinomas originating in the gastric cardia along with those primary in the esophagus. Good palliation may be obtained by palliative resection with relief of dysphagia in most patients, although periodic dilation of the anastomosis often is needed. Postoperative complications occur early in up to 72 per cent and late in 38 per cent, most of the latter being anastomotic strictures. The best operative mortality rates reported for esophagogastrectomy are between 2.1 and 7.1 per cent.[19, 54]

Radiation therapy is less effective for this lesion than for squamous cell cancer and does not appear to enhance survival when combined with surgery. Chemotherapy as yet has no proved role in therapy of this malignancy.

Peroral esophageal dilation and prosthesis can effectively palliate dysphagia, but only prosthesis offers relief for a significant period of time.

Other Malignant Primary Tumors

Adenoid Cystic Carcinoma. Adenoid cystic carcinoma of the esophagus occurs most commonly in elderly men, is located most often in the middle third of the esophagus, has a high rate of distant metastases before diagnosis, and has a poor prognosis.[80] This cancer is considered clinically and morphologically distinct from the more common adenoid cystic carcinoma of salivary gland origin.

Malignant Melanoma. Malignant melanoma primary in the esophagus is an exceedingly rare and highly malignant lesion accounting for only 0.1 per cent of primary esophageal malignancies. These tumors usually are polypoid, large, focally ulcerated, and mostly covered by intact squamous mucosa. Survival after surgery averages about eight months.[81]

Pseudosarcoma. Pseudosarcoma is a rare malignant neoplasm that consists of two separate cellular components. An intraluminal polypoid mass contains sarcomatous tissue, and squamous cell carcinoma is present in or adjacent to the base of the sarcomatous polyp. Either of the tissue elements may metastasize. Initial biopsy of the primary lesion may sample only one of the tissue types and create confusion. Esophagectomy is considered the best therapy, but the prognosis for cure is poor.[82] This lesion is different from the carcinosarcoma that has the two tissue elements intermingled rather than side by side. The sarcoma component seems to metastasize more often and hence has a poorer prognosis.[83]

Primary Esophageal Lymphoma, Oat Cell Carcinoma, and Malignant Carcinoid. These are extremely rare malignancies that have a variety of clinical features that mimic more common lesions.[84–86] Their presence is confirmed only by histopathologic study and they usually are a surprise to the clinician.

Leiomyosarcoma. Leiomyosarcoma has been reported rarely, with only 45 cases found in a recent review. This malignancy may be polypoid or infiltrating in its gross morphology. The presenting symptom is dysphagia that may date back over several years related to slow growth of the obstructing tumor. Usually there is no ulceration of the overlying mucosa. Diagnosis is suspected by radiography and endoscopy, but differentiation between leiomyosarcoma and leiomyoma depends on histologic examination after resection. Current opinion is that the less radical resection procedures may be as effective as radical resection as long as all gross tumor is removed.[87]

BENIGN TUMORS OF THE ESOPHAGUS

Leiomyoma. Leiomyomas arise primarily from the circular smooth muscle layer and are the most common benign tumor of the esophagus, being reported in up to 5 per cent of autopsy specimens.[88] About 7.5 per cent of leiomyomas of the intestinal tract are found in the esophagus.

They occur as oval or round, intramural masses usually from 3 to 8 cm in largest dimension but may rarely be very large, be pedunculated, have bizarre configurations, or be multiple. These tumors are covered by normal squamous epithelium and rarely are associated with mucosal ulceration unless they extend into the stomach. Consequently, bleeding is a rare manifestation.

Most leiomyomas are asymptomatic and are found incidentally during radiographic examination (Fig. 35–3). When they are symptomatic, either dysphagia or pain may be the presenting complaint. Asphyxia can result from retrograde prolapse of a pedunculated tumor into the oropharynx. Diagnosis usually is suspected by barium radiography and endoscopic features. Biopsy through normal overlying mucosa should not be done.

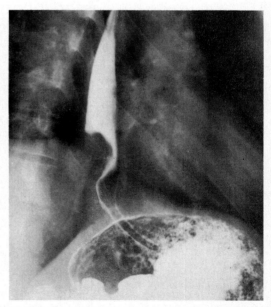

Figure 35–3. Leiomyoma of the esophagus. This large filling defect was found in a patient with no esophageal symptoms. A soft tissue density seen in the mediastinum adjacent to the defect in the barium column reveals the extent of this tumor. (Courtesy of C. A. Rohrmann, M.D.)

When leiomyomas of large size are associated with symptoms, surgical removal should be considered. It has been estimated that about 10 per cent of reported leiomyomas will require surgical removal. Enucleation is associated with a 1.8 per cent mortality rate and resection with a 10.5 per cent mortality rate.[88]

Lipoma. Lipomas of the esophagus are exceedingly rare, are more common in men, and present as pliable and pedunculated, with changing shape on radiographs. Symptoms usually are mild, with dysphagia being predominant. Lipomas on long pedicles have first become manifest as a mass in the oropharynx without significant prior symptoms.[89] Other mesenchymal tumors, such as fibrolipoma, fibromyxoma, and hamartoma, may present as pedunculated polyps.

Granular Cell Tumor. Granular cell tumor (granular myoblastoma, Abrikossoff tumor) is a lesion that currently is believed to originate from neural elements (Schwann cells). It is most often reported in tongue and skin, but with increased use of fiberoptic endoscopy the esophagus is being recognized as a relatively common site. This tumor usually is submucosal, slightly elevated, grayish-white to yellow with a smooth, intact mucosal covering. Size varies from several millimeters to 2 cm for benign lesions and up to 10 cm in the rarer malignant variety. Granular cell tumors rarely cause symptoms. Removal of small tumors has been done transendoscopically, but biopsy is all that is usually needed. Symptomatic lesions should be removed surgically.[90]

Squamous Cell Papilloma. Squamous cell papilloma is a benign esophageal tumor that usually is asymptomatic and found incidentally during endoscopy. This lesion may be mimicked by polypoid squamous cancer. It is best treated by resection with a diathermy snare during endoscopy.[91]

References

1. Haggitt, R. C., Tryzelaar, J., Ellis, H., and Colcher, H. Adenocarcinoma complicating columnar epithelium-lined (Barrett's) esophagus. Am. J. Clin. Pathol. 70:1, 1978.
2. Wienbeck, M., and Berges, W. Oesophageal lesions in the alcoholic. Clin. Gastroenterol. 10:375, 1981.
3. Wynder, E. L., Reddy, B. S., McCoy, G. D., Weisberger, J. H., and Williams, G. M. Diet and gastrointestinal cancer. Gastroenterology 5:463, 1976.
4. La Vecchia, C. L., Liati, P., Decarli, A., Negrello, I., and Franceschi, S. Tar yields of cigarettes and the risk of oesophageal cancer. Int. J. Cancer 38:381, 1986.
5. Levin, B., Riddell, A., and Kirsner, J. B. Management of precancerous lesions of the gastrointestinal tract. Clin. Gastroenterol. 5:827, 1976.
6. McConnell, R. B. Genetic aspects of gastrointestinal cancer. Clin. Gastroenterol. 5:483, 1976.
7. Carter, R., and Brewer, L. A. Achalasia and esophageal carcinoma: studies in early diagnosis for improved surgical management. Am. J. Surg. 130:114, 1975.
8. Appelqvist, P., and Salmo, M. Lye corrosion carcinoma of the esophagus. Cancer 45:2655, 1980.
9. Schwindt, W. D., Berhardt, L. C., and Johnson, S. A. M. Tylosis and intrathoracic neoplasms. Chest 57:590, 1970.
10. Arnott, S. J., Pearson, J. G., Finlayson, N. D. C., and Shearman, D. J. C. The association of squamous esophageal cancer and thyroid disease. Br. J. Cancer 25:33, 1971.
11. Crespi, M., Grassi, A., Amiri, G., Munoz, N., Aramesh, B., and Mojtabai, A. Oesophageal lesions in Northern Iran: a premalignant condition? Lancet 2:217, 1979.
12. Day, N. E. The geographic pathology of cancer of the oesophagus. Br. Med. Bull. 40:329, 1984.
13. Silber, W. Carcinoma of the oesophagus: aspects of epidemiology and aetiology. Proc. Nutr. Soc. 44:101, 1985.
14. Maram, E. S., Kurland, L. T., Ludwig, J., and Brian, D. D. Esophageal carcinoma in Olmsted County, Minnesota, 1935–1971. Mayo Clin. Proc. 52:24, 1977.
15. Ohta, H., Nakazawa, S., Segawa, K., and Yoshino, J. Distribution of epithelial dysplasia in the cancerous esophagus. Scand. J. Gastroenterol. 21:392, 1986.
16. Monnier, P. H., Savary, M., Pasche, R., and Anani, P. Intraepithelial carcinoma of the oesophagus: endoscopic morphology. Endoscopy 13:185, 1981.
17. Froelicher, P., and Miller, G. The European experience with esophageal cancer limited to the mucosa and submucosa. Gastrointest. Endosc. 32:88, 1986.
18. Schmidt, L. W., Dean, P. J., and Wilson, R. T. Superficially invasive squamous cell carcinoma of the esophagus. A study of seven cases in Memphis, Tennessee. Gastroenterology 91:1456, 1986.
19. Galandiuk, S., Hermann, R. E., Gassman, J. J., and Cosgrove, D. M. Cancer of the esophagus. The Cleveland Clinic experience. Ann. Surg. 203:101, 1986.
20. Anderson, L. L., and Lad, T. E. Autopsy findings in squamous-cell carcinoma of the esophagus. Cancer 50:1587, 1982.
21. Barge, J., Molas, G., Maillard, J. N., Fekete, F., Bogomoletz, W. V., and Potet, F. Superficial esophageal carcinoma: an esophageal counterpart of early gastric cancer. Histopathology 5:499, 1981.
22. Coordinating group for research in esophageal cancer, Linhsien County, Honan. Early diagnosis and surgical treatment of esophageal cancer under rural conditions. Chin. Med. J. (Engl.) 2:113, 1976.
23. Guojun, H., Lingfang, S., Dawei, Z., Zhangcai, L., Guoqing, W., Shuxian, L., and Fubao, C. Diagnosis and surgical treatment of early esophageal carcinoma. Chin. Med. J. (Engl.) 94:229, 1981.
24. Grossman, T. W., Toohill, R. J., Duncavage, J. A., Lehman, R. H., and Malin, T. C. Role of esophagoscopy in the evaluation of patients with head and neck carcinoma. Ann. Otol. Rhinol. Laryngol. 92:369, 1983.
25. Fogel, T. D., Harrison, L. B., and Son, Y. H. Subsequent upper aerodigestive malignancies following treatment of esophageal cancer. Cancer 55:1882, 1985.
26. Edwards, D. A. W. Carcinoma of the esophagus and fundus. Postgrad. Med. J. 50:223, 1974.
27. Watson, W. L., and Goodner, J. T. Carcinoma of the esophagus. Am. J. Surg. 93:259, 1957.
28. Benrey, J., Graham, D. Y., and Goyal, R. K. Hypercalcemia and carcinoma of the esophagus. Ann. Intern. Med. 80:415, 1974.
29. Lohrenz, F. N., and Custer, G. S. ACTH producing metastases from carcinoma of the esophagus. Ann. Intern. Med. 62:1017, 1965.
30. Lee, D. J., Harris, A., Gillete, A., Munoz, L., and Kashima, H. Carcinoma of the cervical esophagus: diagnosis, management and results. South. Med. J. 77:1365, 1984.
31. Lindell, M. M., Jr., Hill, C. A., and Libshitz, H. I. Esophageal cancer: radiographic chest findings and their significance. AJR 133:461, 1979.
32. Winawer, S. J., Sherlock, P., Belladonna, J. A., Melamed, M., and Beattie, E. J., Jr. Endoscopic brush cytology in esophageal cancer. JAMA 232:1358, 1975.
33. Graham, D. Y., Schwartz, J. T., Cain, C. D., and Gyorkey, F. Prospective evaluation of biopsy number in the diagnosis of esophageal and gastric carcinoma. Gastroenterology 82:228, 1982.
34. Young, J. A., Hughes, H. E., and Lee, F. D. Evaluation of endoscopic brush and biopsy touch smear cytology and biopsy histology in the diagnosis of carcinoma of the lower oesophagus and cardia. J. Clin. Pathol. 33:811, 1980.

35. Graham, D. Y., and Spjut, H. J. Salvage cytology. A new alternative fiberoptic technique. Gastrointest. Endosc. 25:137, 1979.
36. Mandard, A. M., Tourneux, J., Gignoux, M., Blanc, L., Segol, P., and Mandard, J. C. In situ carcinoma of the esophagus. Macroscopic study with particular reference to the Lugol test. Endoscopy 12:51, 1980.
37. Nishizawa, M., Okada, T., Hosoi, T., and Makino, T. Detecting early esophageal cancers, with special reference to the intraepithelial stage. Endoscopy 16:92, 1984.
38. Nelson, R. S., Dewey, W. C., and Rose, R. G. The use of radioactive phosphorus P^{32} and a miniature Geiger tube to detect malignant neoplasia of the gastrointestinal tract. Gastroenterology 46:8, 1964.
39. Endo, M., Kobayashi, S., Suzuki, H., Takemato, T., and Nakayama, K. Diagnosis of early esophageal cancer. Endoscopy 3:61, 1971.
40. Melissas, J., Minnaar, R., and Mannell, A. Bronchoscopic findings in patients with oesophageal carcinoma. S. Afr. J. Surg. 24:24, 1986.
41. Shandall, A., and Johnson, C. Laparoscopy or scanning in oesophageal and gastric carcinoma? Br. J. Surg. 72:449, 1985.
42. Takemoto, T., Aibe, T., Fuji, T., and Okita, K. Endoscopic ultrasonography. Clin. Gastroenterol. 15:305, 1986.
43. Daffner, R. H., Halber, M. D., Postlethwait, R. W., Korobkin, M., and Thompson, W. M. CT of the esophagus: II. Carcinoma. AJR 133:1051, 1979.
44. Moss, A. A., Schnyder, P., Thoeni, R. F., and Margulis, A. R. Esophageal carcinoma: Pretherapy staging by computed tomography. AJR 136:1051, 1981.
45. Taylor, C. R. Carcinoma of the esophagus—current imaging options. Am. J. Gastroenterol. 81:1013, 1986.
46. Becker, C. D., Barbier, P., and Porcellini, B. CT evaluation of patients undergoing transhiatal esophagectomy for cancer. J. Comput. Assist. Tomogr. 10:607, 1986.
47. Lawrence, W. L., Jr. Surgical management of gastrointestinal cancer. Clin. Gastroenterol. 5:703, 1976.
48. Adelstein, D. J., Forman, W. B., and Beavers, B. Esophageal carcinoma. Cancer 54:918, 1984.
49. Cooper, J. D., Jamieson, W. R. E., Blair, N., Todd, T. R. J., Ilves, R., and Pearson, F. G. The palliative value of surgical resection for carcinoma of the esophagus. Can. J. Surg. 24:145, 1981.
50. Payne, W. S. Palliation of esophageal carcinoma. Ann. Thorac. Surg. 28:208, 1979.
51. Heit, H. A., Johnson, L. F., Siegel, S. R., and Boyce, H. W., Jr. Palliative dilatation for dysphagia in esophageal carcinoma. Ann. Intern. Med. 89:629, 1978.
52. Postlethwait, R. W. Carcinoma of the thoracic esophagus. Surg. Clin. North Am. 63:933, 1983.
53. Earlam, R., and Cunha-Melo, J. R. Oesophageal squamous cell carcinoma: I. A critical review of surgery. Br. J. Surg. 67:381, 1980.
54. Ellis, F. H., Jr., Gibb, S. P., and Watkins, E., Jr. Overview of the current management of carcinoma of the esophagus and cardia. Can. J. Surg. 28:493, 1985.
55. Griffith, J. L., and Davis, J. T. A twenty-year experience with surgical management of carcinoma of the esophagus and gastric cardia. J. Thorac. Cardiovasc. Surg. 79:447, 1980.
56. Payne, W. S., Trastek, V. F., Piehler, J. M., Pairolero, P. C., and Bernatz, P. E. Current techniques for the surgical management of malignant lesions of the thoracic esophagus and cardia. Mayo Clin. Proc. 61:564, 1986.
57. Moertel, C. G. The esophagus. In Holland, F. J., and Frei, E. (eds.). Cancer Medicine XXV. Alimentary Tract Cancer. Philadelphia, Lea & Febiger, 1982, pp. 1753–1760.
58. Launois, B., Delarue, D., Campion, J. P., and Kerbaol, M. Preoperative radiotherapy for carcinoma of the esophagus. Surg. Gynecol. Obstet. 153:690, 1981.
59. Steiger, Z., Franklin, R., Wilson, R. F., Leichman, L., Seydel, H., Loh, J. J., Vaishamapayan, G., Knechtges, T., Astaw, I., Dindogru, A., Rosenberg, J. C., Buroker, T., Torres, A., Hoschner, D., Miller, P., Pietruk, T., and Vaitkevicius, V. Eradication and palliation of squamous cell carcinoma of the esophagus with chemotherapy, radiotherapy and surgical therapy. J. Thorac. Cardiovasc. Surg. 82:713, 1981.
60. Earlam, R., and Cunha-Melo, J. R. Oesophageal squamous cell carcinoma: II. A critical review of radiotherapy. Br. J. Surg. 67:457, 1980.
61. Pearson, J. G. The present status and future potential of radiotherapy in the management of esophageal cancer. Cancer 39:882, 1977.
62. Hancock, S. L., and Glatstein, E. Radiation therapy of esophageal cancer. Semin. Oncol. 11:114, 1984.
63. Rowland, C. G., and Pagliero, K. M. Intracavitary irradiation in palliation of carcinoma of oesophagus and cardia. Lancet 2:981, 1985.
64. Kelsen, D. P., Fein, R., Coonley, C., Heelan, R., and Bains, M. Cisplatin, vindesine, and mitoguazone in the treatment of esophageal cancer. Cancer Treat. Rep. 70:255, 1986.
65. Boyce, H. W., Jr., and Palmer, E. D. Techniques of clinical gastroenterology. Springfield, Illinois, Charles C Thomas, 1975, pp. 237–251.
66. Boyce, H. W., Jr. Palliation of advanced esophageal cancer. Semin. Oncol. 11:186, 1984.
67. Tulman, A. B., and Boyce, H. W., Jr. Complications of esophageal dilation and guidelines for their prevention. Gastrointest. Endosc. 27:229, 1981.
68. Tytgat, G. N. J., den Hartog Jager, F. C. A., and Bartelsman, J. F. W. M. Endoscopic prosthesis for advanced esophageal cancer. Endoscopy 18:32, 1986.
69. Earlam, R., and Cunha-Melo, J. R. Malignant oesophageal strictures: a review of techniques for palliative intubation. Br. J. Surg. 69:61, 1982.
70. Unruh, H. W., and Pagliero, K. M. Pulsion intubation versus traction intubation for obstructing carcinomas of the esophagus. Ann. Thorac. Surg. 40:337, 1985.
71. Fleischer, D., and Kessler, F. Endoscopic Nd:YAG laser therapy for carcinoma of the esophagus: a new form of palliative treatment. Gastroenterology 85:600, 1983.
72. Lightdale, C. J., Zimbalist, E., and Winawer, S. J. Outpatient management of esophageal cancer with endoscopic Nd:YAG laser. Am. J. Gastroenterol. 82:46, 1987.
73. Oster, M. W., Vizel, M., and Turgeon, L. R. Pain of terminal cancer patients. Arch. Intern. Med. 138:1801, 1978.
74. Haffejee, A. A., and Angorn, I. B. Nutritional status and the nonspecific cellular and humoral immune response in esophageal carcinoma. Ann. Surg. 189:475, 1979.
75. Turner, G. G. Some experience in the surgery of the esophagus. N. Engl. J. Med. 205:657, 1931.
76. Palmer, E. D. Carcinoma of the esophagus—survival and the fallacy of "early diagnosis." Armed Forces Med. J. 8:1317, 1957.
77. Bosch, A., Frias, Z., and Caldwell, W. L. Adenocarcinoma of the esophagus. Cancer 43:1557, 1979.
78. Rogers, E. L., Goldkind, S. F., Iseri, O. A., Bustin, M., Goldkind, L., Hamilton, S. R., and Smith, R. R. L. Adenocarcinoma of the lower esophagus. J. Clin. Gastroenterol. 8:613, 1986.
79. Spechler, S. J., Robbins, A. H., Rubins, H. B., Vincent, M. E., Heeren, J., Doos, W. G., Colton, T., and Schimmel, E. M. Adenocarcinoma and Barrett's esophagus. An overrated risk? Gastroenterology 87:927, 1984.
80. Petursson, S. R. Adenoid cystic carcinoma of the esophagus. Cancer 57:1464, 1986.
81. Boulafendis, D., Damiani, M., Sie, E., Bastounis, E., and Samaan, H. A. Primary malignant melanoma of the esophagus in a young adult. Am. J. Gastroenterol. 80:417, 1985.
82. Halvorsen, R. A., Foster, W. L., Williford, M. E., Roberts, L., Jr., Postlethwait, R. W., and Thompson, W. M. Pseudosarcoma of the esophagus: barium swallow and CT findings. J. Can. Assoc. Radiol. 34:278, 1983.
83. Xu, L., Sun, C., Wu, L. -H., Chang, Z. -R., and Liu, T. Clinical and pathological characteristics of carcinosarcoma of the esophagus: report of four cases. Ann. Thorac. Surg. 37:197, 1984.
84. Matsuura, H., Saito, R., Nakajima, S., Yoshihara, W., and Enomoto, T. Non-Hodgkin's lymphoma of the esophagus. Am. J. Gastroenterol. 80:941, 1985.

85. Sabanthan, S., Graham, G. P., and Salama, F. D. Primary oat cell carcinoma of the oesophagus. Thorax *41*:318, 1986.
86. Siegal, A., and Swartz, A. Malignant carcinoid of oesophagus. Histopathology *10*:761, 1986.
87. Choh, J. H., Khazei, A. H., and Ihm, H. J. Leiomyosarcoma of the esophagus: report of a case and review of the literature. J. Surg. Oncol. *32*:223, 1986.
88. Postlethwait, R. W. Benign tumors and cysts of the esophagus. Surg. Clin. North Am. *63*:925, 1983.
89. Zonderland, H. M., and Ginai, A. Z. Lipoma of the esophagus. Diagn. Imaging Clin. Med. *53*:265, 1984.
90. Coutinho, D. S. S., Soga, J., Yoshikawa, T., Miyashita, K., Tanaka, O., Sasaki, K., Muto, T., and Shimizu, T. Granular cell tumors of the esophagus: a report of two cases and review of the literature. Am. J. Gastroenterol. *80*:758, 1985.
91. Toet, A. E., Dekker, W., Orth, J. O., and Blok, P. Squamous cell papilloma of the esophagus: report of four cases. Gastrointest. Endosc. *31*:77, 1985.

36

Rings and Webs

CHARLES E. POPE, II

DEFINITION

Although the terms "ring" and "web" have been used interchangeably in the medical literature, it would seem preferable to restrict the term *esophageal web* to a thin (2 to 3 mm) structure consisting of mucosa and submucosa alone. Such webs can occur anywhere along the length of the esophagus. *Ring* might be used to refer to a thicker structure composed of both mucosa and muscle. This classification immediately falls afoul of the most famous of all esophageal rings, the lower esophageal ring (Schatzki's ring), which is, in fact, a web as defined here. Short concentric strictures occurring at the lower end of the esophagus have also been dignified with the term "lower esophageal ring." There is no common usage in the medical literature; careful attention to the definition of the individual author is necessary. Another classification is by site of origin[1]; this will be followed in the present chapter.

UPPER ESOPHAGEAL WEBS

Webs occurring in the upper 2 to 4 cm of the esophagus usually consist of squamous epithelium, possess eccentric lumens, and are associated with iron-deficiency anemia. When associated with dysphagia, the term Paterson-Brown-Kelly or Plummer-Vinson syndrome is given.[2] In most patients presenting with this syndrome, iron-deficiency anemia can be demonstrated and other physical signs of iron deficiency, such as spooning of the nails, are present.[3, 4] Dysphagia, often associated with aspiration symptoms, is the usual clinical presentation. The web is associated with the occurrence of postcricoid carcinoma, often after symptoms of the web have been present for many years.[5]

Diagnosis is made by barium swallow, which shows a thin web, usually best seen in the lateral projection (Fig. 36–1). As barium passes through the upper esophagus rapidly, it is sometimes necessary to obtain a cine study. Some workers would also include a longer, tube-like stricture under the term Plummer-Vinson syndrome.[2] Esophagoscopy is not easy in such patients; occasionally the web is ruptured in an attempt to visualize it. Treatment is by dilation, either endoscopically or by bougienage. Replacement of iron stores is recommended to prevent recurrence and possibly to decrease the likelihood of postcricoid carcinoma.

An unusual cause for an upper esophageal web, which might be confused with the Plummer-Vinson syndrome, is the formation of a web between a patch of ectopic gastric mucosa and squamous epithelium above and below.[6] The patient was not anemic and responded well to dilation.

A recent report draws attention to the association between a cervical web and a Zenker's diverticulum.[7] Such webs are not appreciated during radiologic study, even retrospectively. The webs can be felt during surgery with an intraesophageal exploring finger; they can be excised.

A third cause for the formation of an upper esophageal web is involvement of the esophagus by graft-versus-host disease following bone marrow transplantation.[8] Three patients with chronic graft-versus-host disease developed dysphagia; high cervical webs were found by radiography or endoscopy. In two patients the webs were easily ruptured by the endoscope or a bougie; the third patient suffered a perforation and a protracted period of morbidity.

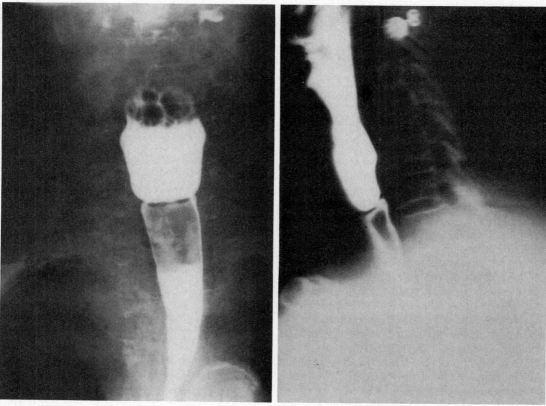

Figure 36–1. Esophageal web. Anteroposterior and lateral views of an upper esophageal web in a 62-year-old woman with iron deficiency anemia and dysphagia. It is unusual to obtain this clear a definition in the anteroposterior plane; the lateral view is usually more productive. (Courtesy of F. E. Templeton, M.D.)

ESOPHAGEAL BODY WEBS

Webs consisting of squamous epithelium can infrequently obstruct the body of the esophagus anywhere along its length. These webs can be single[9], double,[10] or multiple.[11] They do not seem to arise in patients suffering from reflux and may well represent a remnant of embryologic development in which the esophagus fails to recanalize completely. Some authors believe that such webs can result from ongoing reflux.[12] Treatment is usually by bougienage. A web occurring in the terminal esophagus may well become confused with the lower esophageal ring (Schatzki's ring).

RINGS AND WEBS IN THE TERMINAL ESOPHAGUS

In 1953, Schatzki and Gary described a thin luminal narrowing in the terminal esophagus associated with dysphagia, which they called the "lower esophageal ring."[13] They subsequently followed one of their patients to autopsy and demonstrated that the ring projected into the lumen and marked the junction of esophageal and columnar epithelium. There was no sign of fibrosis or inflammation. A similar squamocolumnar junction was described in 15 patients with the clinical and X-ray manifestations of a lower esophageal ring who went to surgery for relief of dysphagia.[14] A ring marking the squamocolumnar junction was found in 9 of 100 esophagi examined at autopsy,[15] a prevalence similar to that found in radiologic examination of asymptomatic individuals. Not all authorities are happy with the idea that the lower esophageal ring marks the boundary between esophageal and columnar epithelium[16]; this unhappiness is based on studies attempting to correlate ring position as seen by X-ray and localization by manometric or biopsy methods. Such studies are indeed difficult as the esophageal muscle and the epithelium both move during swallowing, the only time that the ring can be demonstrated. Another study shows that the mucosal junction in patients with rings, as measured by potential difference changes, and the lower esophageal sphincter, as measured simultaneously manometrically, are extremely close to one another.[17]

In addition to the mucosal ring, a muscular ring can occasionally be demonstrated just proximal to the squamocolumnar junctional ring. This is not a fixed structure, and will only be demonstrated on some swallows. There is very little surgical or autopsy material on such muscular rings; some authorities do not even recognize them as a separate entity.

The clinical presentation of a lower esophageal ring is often sufficiently distinctive to make the diagnosis. Classically, the patient suffers from *intermittent dysphagia*. During meals a bolus of meat or bread may become impacted; the patient will regurgitate the offending bolus and then will be able to continue eating without further dysphagia. This event usually happens intermittently and often increases slowly in frequency over a number of years. Dysphagia is the rule if luminal diameter is under 13 mm but unlikely if ring diameter is over 20 mm. Dysphagia that occurs every day is very unlikely to be caused by a lower esophageal ring. These patients do not often suffer from symptoms of esophageal reflux and have no other manifestations of systemic illness.

Another classic presentation of a lower esophageal ring is sudden, total esophageal obstruction caused by meat impaction. A barium swallow taken at this time will often show a foreign body lodged in the lower portion of the esophagus. The patient then undergoes esophagoscopy and the piece of meat is removed; the endoscopist usually comments that the esophagus appears normal. A follow-up barium swallow is interpreted as normal and the patient is discharged with the diagnosis of hysterical dysphagia. This sequence is often repeated two or three times before the correct diagnosis is made. Of course, physical examination provides no clues to the diagnosis; it usually reveals only normal-appearing patients who are usually in the fifth to seventh decades of life at the onset of their symptoms. Frequently, however, a history of intermittent dysphagia of a more transitory nature for several decades can be elicited. The clinical history of the muscular ring at the lower end of the esophagus is identical to that of the lower esophageal ring, with intermittent dysphagia being the main presenting symptom.

The lower esophageal ring is best demonstrated when the lower segment of the esophagus is distended. The patient takes a deep breath and holds it as the peristaltic wave approaches the area of the diaphragm. This maneuver causes the lower esophageal segment to balloon out and makes the ring visible (Fig. 36–2). It should be noted that the lower esophageal ring is usually symmetric and quite thin. If asymmetry is seen, a web in the lower esophagus should be suspected. Of more importance is the finding of a relatively thick (0.5 to 1.0 cm) ring. This is probably not a lower esophageal ring but might represent a localized ring stricture caused by peptic digestion of the esophagus. This is an important diagnosis to consider, as its therapy is quite different. If the segment is not filled adequately, no statement can be made as to whether or not a ring is present. An ancillary measure is the administration of a bolus that can be arrested in the area of the ring, thus calling special attention to this particular area. Bread or marshmallows soaked in barium are the most easily available bolus materials. Theoretically, it is possible to calibrate the lumen of the ring by giving barium tablets of known size. Practically, however, as the ring produces only intermittent dysphagia, arrest of the bolus cannot always be demonstrated unless the ring diameter is very small. Radiography is more efficient in demonstrating rings than is endoscopy; single-contrast prone examination is more efficient than double-contrast examination.[18]

Endoscopy can help to differentiate whether the ring

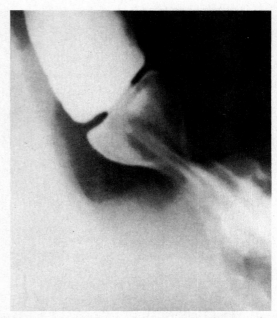

Figure 36–2. Close-up view of a lower esophageal ring. Note the impression of the ring on the column of barium as well as the notches formed by seeing the ring from the side.

seen on X-ray represents true lower esophageal ring or whether it is an annular stricture. A stricture will usually resist passage of the endoscope and will often be associated with mucosal changes of reflux esophagitis, such as ulceration and bleeding.

Therapy directed toward the lower esophageal ring depends in part on the frequency and intensity of the patient's complaints. Demonstration and explanation of the problem often will convince the patient to eat more slowly and to chew food more thoroughly. This advice may give complete relief. If symptoms are more troublesome, mechanical methods of alleviating the obstruction must be found. Bougienage with large dilators has been recommended.[19] If this form of therapy is to be used, it is wise to use a large dilator, such as a No. 50 French, without progressively stretching the ring with dilators of smaller caliber. If relief is not obtained after one dilation, it might be repeated under fluoroscopic control to make sure that the dilator has indeed passed through the ring. Occasionally this form of therapy will not produce good results. It is then necessary to use a pneumatic dilator, preferably a 4-inch bag. The technique is similar to that used in the dilation of a patient with achalasia, and fluoroscopic localization of the dilating bag is essential. It also seems likely that the new rigid balloons that can be placed endoscopically will be utilized for such dilations. One dilation should cure the condition permanently. Although the ring may still be demonstrated radiographically after this procedure, the patient will not complain of recurring bouts of dysphagia.

Surgical attempts to remove this lesion have also been recommended.[20] These include fracture of the ring digitally through a gastrostomy opening or actual segmental removal of portions of the ring. Repair of associated hiatus hernias has also been employed in treatment of symptomatic rings, but occasionally the patient will still complain of intermittent dysphagia even though the ring structure has been reduced to a position below the diaphragm. It would seem that surgical therapy for this lesion alone would not be warranted, because intraluminal therapy with a dilator will frequently give good relief in these patients, for whom instruction about the nature of the condition is inadequate.

References

1. Rinaldo, J. A. Esophageal webs and rings. *In* Vantrappen, G., and Hellemans, J. (eds.). Diseases of the Esophagus. Berlin, Springer-Verlag, 1974, p. 571.
2. Logan, J. S. The Plummer-Vinson stricture. Ulster Med. J. *47*(Suppl 2):1, 1978.
3. Chisholm, M., Ardran, G. M., Callender, S. T., and Wright, R. Iron deficiency and autoimmunity in post-cricoid webs. Q. J. Med. *40*:421, 1971.
4. Chisholm, M., Ardran, G. M., Callender, S. T., and Wright, R. A follow-up study of patients with post-cricoid webs. Q. J. Med. *40*:409, 1971.
5. Chisholm, M. The association between webs, iron, and post-cricoid carcinoma. Postgrad. Med. J. *50*:215, 1974.
6. Weaver, G. A. Upper esophageal web due to a ring formed by a squamocolumnar junction with ectopic gastric mucosa (another explanation of the Patterson-Kelly, Plummer-Vinson syndrome). Dig. Dis. Sci. *24*:959, 1979.
7. Mercer, C. D., and Hill, L. D. Esophageal web associated with Zenker's diverticulum: a possible cause of continuing dysphagia after diverticulectomy. Can. J. Surg. *28*:375, 1985.
8. McDonald, G. B., Sullivan, K. M., Schuffler, M. D., Shulman, H. M., and Thomas, E. D. Esophageal abnormalities in chronic graft-vs-host disease in humans. Gastroenterology *80*:914, 1981.
9. Ikard, R. W., and Rosen, H. E. Midesophageal web in adults. Ann. Thor. Surg. *24*:355, 1977.
10. Longstreth, G. F., Wolochow, D. A., and Tu, R. T. Double congenital midesophageal webs in adults. Dig. Dis. Sci. *24*:162, 1979.
11. Shiflett, D. W., Gilliam, J. H., Wu, W. C., Austin, W. E., and Ott, D. J. Multiple esophageal webs. Gastroenterology *77*:556, 1979.
12. Weaver, J. W., Kaude, J. V., and Hamlin, D. J. Webs of the lower esophagus: a complication of gastroesophageal reflux? AJR *142*:289, 1984.
13. Schatzki, R., and Gary, J. E. Dysphagia due to a diaphragm-like localized narrowing in the lower esophagus ("lower esophageal ring"). AJR *70*:911, 1953.
14. Wilkins, E. W., Jr., and Bartlett, M. K. Surgical treatment of the lower esophageal ring. N. Engl. J. Med. *268*:461, 1963.
15. Goyal, R. K., Bauer, J. L., and Spiro, H. M. The nature and location of lower esophageal ring. N. Engl. J. Med. *284*:1775, 1971.
16. Hendrix, T. R. Schatzki ring, epithelial junction, and hiatal hernia—an unresolved controversy. Gastroenterology *79*:584, 1980.
17. Eckardt, V. F., Adami, B., Hücker, H., and Leeder, H. The esophagogastric junction in patients with asymptomatic lower esophageal mucosal rings. Gastroenterology *79*:426, 1980.
18. Ott, D. J., Chen, Y. M., Wu, W. C., Gelfand, D. W., and Munitz, H. A. Radiographic and endoscopic sensitivity in detecting lower esophageal mucosal ring. AJR *147*:261, 1986.
19. Eastridge, C. E., Pate, J. W., and Mann, J. A. Lower esophageal ring: experiences in treatment of 88 patients. Ann. Thorac. Surg. *37*:103, 1984.
20. Eastridge, C. E., Salazar, J., Pate, J. W., and Farrell, G. Symptomatic lower esophageal ring: treatment of 24 patients. South. Med. J. *72*:919, 1979.

37

Diverticula
CHARLES E. POPE II

DEFINITION

Esophageal diverticula are outpouchings of one or more layers of the esophageal wall. These outpouchings occur in three main areas: (1) immediately above the upper esophageal sphincter (*Zenker's diverticulum*), (2) near the midpoint of the esophagus (*traction diverticulum*), and (3) immediately above the lower esophageal sphincter (*epiphrenic diverticulum*).

ETIOLOGY AND PATHOGENESIS

Although esophageal diverticula have been described in infants and children,[1] they are usually discovered in later life. This late appearance is undoubtedly dictated by the factors that produce diverticula. It is commonly stated that *Zenker's diverticula* and *epiphrenic diverticula* may result from motor abnormalities of the esophagus, and that the midesophageal or traction diverticulum is a response to scarring and traction on the walls of the esophagus by external inflammatory processes. This latter explanation is probably incorrect, as the midesophageal diverticulum may well represent an expression of abnormal motor activity of the esophagus.

There has been speculation that Zenker's diverticulum represents an expression of motor incoordination at the cricopharyngeus. Cine-esophagrams have been reported to show premature contraction of the cricopharyngeus,[2] and manometric evidence of such incoordination has also been presented.[3–6] However, using infused catheters and noncompliant tubing, two different laboratories found no evidence of incoordination.[7, 8] In a personal study employing intraluminal strain gauge transducers, no incoordination was observed in any of five patients with moderate- to large-sized Zenker's diverticula.

The pathogenesis of the midesophageal diverticulum remains uncertain. Although fibrous adhesions from tuberculous mediastinal nodes are thought to produce diverticula, the actual demonstration of such adhesions is rare in autopsy material. A congenital origin for midesophageal diverticula has been suggested,[9] but abnormalities in motor function seem more likely to play a causal role. Manometric changes consisting of high-amplitude, prolonged contractions in upper and lower esophagus have been described,[10] and have been confirmed by a study in which manometric abnormalities were shown in 10 of 12 consecutive patients investigated. The manometric findings were not uniform: five patients were thought to have diffuse spasm, one had vigorous achalasia, and four others showed prolongation of the peristaltic wave.[11] In addition to a prolonged wave, extremely high amplitude waves have been described in two of six patients with midesophageal diverticula.[12]

A motility disturbance can be implicated by other observations. A midesophageal diverticulum with a bolus of meat stuck well below the diverticulum is shown in Figure 37–1. Subsequent esophagoscopy and repeated barium swallow revealed no organic obstruction in this area. At autopsy seven years later no evidence of luminal compromise or adhesion of fibrous bands was found. However, the esophageal muscular wall was thickened. These findings are certainly consistent with a disturbance in motor function, although they do not prove it.

Epiphrenic diverticula (Fig. 37–2) can also be shown to be associated with motor abnormalities of the esophagus. As with Zenker's diverticulum, incoordination of sphincteric relaxation and esophageal peristalsis might occur. The lower esophageal segment would then be subject to increasing amounts of pressure. A high incidence of motor abnormalities of the esophagus has been reported when the esophagus was evaluated radiologically.[13] Investigation of 65 patients with lower esophageal diverticula revealed abnormalities of peristalsis in 50.[14] The manometric patterns were varied; *diffuse spasm, achalasia,* and *nonspecific patterns* were seen. In another study, failure of sphincteric relaxation

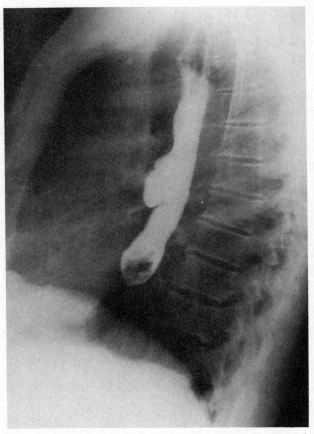

Figure 37–1. A large midesophageal diverticulum is seen in the midthoracic area. Below this is an impacted bolus of meat, causing esophageal obstruction. Subsequent films after the bolus was removed showed no narrowing at the site where the bolus was arrested.

associated with high-amplitude, prolonged peristaltic waves was described.[15]

Scleroderma may be associated with wide-mouthed multiple diverticula of the esophagus.[16] These esophageal diverticula resemble those found in the colons of patients with scleroderma.

An even more unusual diverticulum is one that remains in an intraluminal location rather than protruding outside the muscular wall, as is the usual case.[17] This intraluminal location allows the diverticulum to prolapse down into the stomach. The cause of this type of diverticulum is not known; both reported patients had undergone repeated instrumentation with bougies or endoscopes.

SYMPTOMS

Zenker's diverticulum presents the most classic group of symptoms. Transient dysphagia may be noted early in the course. However, when the pharyngeal sac becomes large enough to retain contents, the patient may complain of pulmonary *aspiration, gurgling* in the throat, appearance of a *mass* in the neck, or *regurgitation* of food into the mouth. Some patients develop

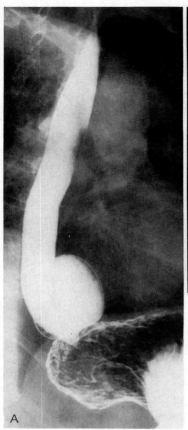

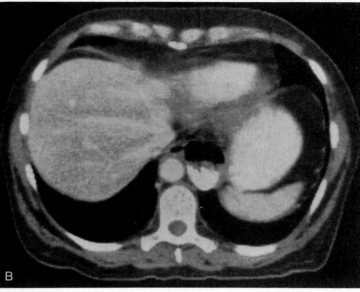

Figure 37–2. Epiphrenic diverticulum. *A,* An epiphrenic diverticulum is seen immediately above the stomach. In this projection, it might be confused with a hiatus hernia. *B,* A CT scan shows the air-filled diverticulum and its connection to the esophagus, which also contains air. (Courtesy of C. A. Rohrmann, M.D.)

a series of maneuvers used to empty the pouch consisting of pressure on the neck and repeated coughing and clearing of the throat. The sac may become so large that its retained contents may push anteriorly on the esophagus and completely obstruct it.

The midesophageal diverticula are much more likely to be found in a totally asymptomatic patient. However, occasional patients with such diverticula will complain of dysphagia or, rarely, of esophageal obstruction owing to a retained bolus.

It is difficult to tell whether the symptoms of an epiphrenic diverticulum are caused by the presence of the diverticulum itself or by the associated motor abnormalities in the esophagus. One symptom seems to be unique to the presence of the diverticulum: the *regurgitation* of massive amounts of fluid, usually occurring at night. Presumably, this fluid has been stored in the diverticulum during waking hours and is regurgitated during periods of recumbency.

DIAGNOSIS AND DIFFERENTIAL DIAGNOSIS

Zenker's diverticula are most often discovered during X-ray examination (Fig. 37–3). Occasionally, the entire first glass of barium taken will disappear into the capacious confines of an especially large divertic-

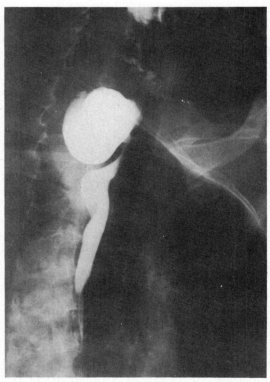

Figure 37–3. Zenker's diverticulum. This diverticulum is large enough to cause esophageal obstruction when it fills with contents.

ulum. It is better to find such diverticula radiographically than to perforate a hitherto unknown diverticulum during the passage of an endoscope or other tube! Traumatic diverticula in the cervical region have occasionally been produced by vigorous suction during birth[18] or, in one instance, by tripping while running with a carrot held in the mouth.[19]

Small diverticula can be missed if they are superimposed on the main column of barium in the esophagus. This can be avoided by rotating the patient during the examination. Another possible source of confusion might be an esophagus with many tertiary contractions. This may give a temporary appearance of numerous diverticula in the lower esophagus. However, the changing patterns on subsequent swallows will eliminate this source of confusion.

It is not necessary to perform endoscopy to investigate esophageal diverticula. In fact, the procedure may represent a hazard to the patient, as it is difficult to avoid entering the pharyngeal esophageal diverticulum with the tip of the instrument. Therefore, when it is known that a Zenker's diverticulum exists, an endoscopic procedure necessary for other reasons should always be performed under direct vision. Manometric examination will not be helpful clinically, although it may throw light on the pathogenesis of these structures.

COMPLICATIONS

As mentioned previously, esophageal diverticula can produce symptoms by compression of the esophagus when full of material (Zenker's diverticulum) or by serving as a reservoir for fluid, which is then available for reflux into the pharynx (Zenker's diverticulum) or esophagus (epiphrenic diverticulum). A very rare complication is the formation of a fistula between a Zenker's diverticulum and the trachea, leading to constant aspiration.[20]

Another uncommon complication is the occurrence of carcinoma in a diverticulum. Four of 1249 patients with Zenker's diverticulum were found to have cancer.[21] Although most of these cancers had spread to regional structures by the time of discovery, a few are still localized within the diverticulum and excision of the diverticulum is adequate therapy. Epiphrenic diverticula can also be the locus for squamous cell carcinoma.[22]

TREATMENT

The main method of treatment is surgical. There are three methods of surgical correction of a Zenker's diverticulum: (1) a two-stage operation involving mobilization of the diverticulum and excision subsequently when granulation tissue has formed around the diverticulum; (2) excision of the diverticulum in one step; and (3) a cricopharyngeal myotomy, leaving the diverticulum undisturbed. The most common method currently employed is the one-stage diverticulectomy. In

a large series reported from the Mayo Clinic, quite satisfactory results were obtained, with a symptomatic and X-ray recurrence of approximately 4 per cent.[23] However, the symptomatic and radiographic recurrence may be higher after one-stage diverticulectomy.[24] Reoperation after surgery for a Zenker's diverticulum is associated with much higher perioperative morbidity, although good long-term results can be expected.[23]

If the diverticulum is small, it can be treated with cricopharyngeal myotomy.[3] This can actually be done under local anesthesia so that the patient can assist the surgeon by swallowing on command.[25] When cricopharyngeal myotomy is done, the diverticulum can be ignored if it is small, suspended by diverticulopexy, or resected. Long-term results of cricopharyngeal myotomy are not yet available. An alternative method of treatment is the endoscopic division of the septum between the diverticulum and the mouth of the esophagus.[7] In a series of 107 patients, good clinical relief of symptoms with a very low mortality and morbidity rate was obtained. This procedure does require a fair amount of endoscopic skill.

Midesophageal diverticula usually do not require any form of therapy. The diverticula tend to be small and not to retain material. It is conceivable that if an associated motor abnormality becomes too troublesome, a long myotomy might be offered to the individual.

Simple excision of epiphrenic diverticula would seem to have an unacceptably high mortality and morbidity rate.[10] However, when attention is directed to the associated motor condition, be it achalasia or diffuse spasm, and a myotomy is performed in the lower esophageal wall, better results have been reported.[10, 14] The need for surgical therapy is dictated by the clinical manifestations of the epiphrenic diverticulum.

INTRAMURAL DIVERTICULOSIS

A condition exists in which many small diverticula of the esophagus are seen, so-called intramural diverticulosis.[26] Presenting usually with *dysphagia,* these patients are found to have numerous small (1 to 3 mm), flask-shaped outpouchings, usually associated with a smooth stricture in the upper esophagus[27] (Fig. 37–4). *Candida* has been found in some cases on biopsy and recovered in culture in other patients. However, the majority of reported cases are not associated with presence of *Candida.*[28]

The pathology of this condition would suggest that the diverticula represent dilated ducts coming from submucosal glands.[28, 29] The glands themselves do not take part in this process. The term pseudodiverticulosis might be more appropriate, as no true diverticulum of the muscular esophageal wall exists. High-amplitude peristaltic contractions have been recorded from one patient with this disease[30]; more patients will need to be investigated before high intraluminal pressures can be accepted as a causal factor.

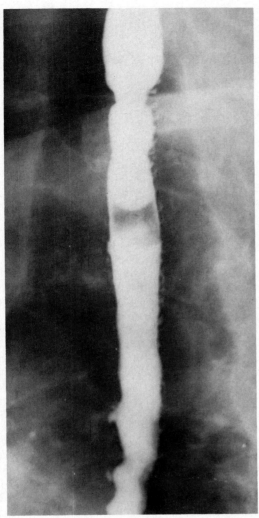

Figure 37–4. Intramural diverticulosis. A short stricture is seen at the upper end of the esophagus. In this area and below are seen numerous small outpouchings. (Courtesy of C. A. Rohrmann, M.D.)

Treatment consists of dilation of the associated stricture. Following dilation, the pseudodiverticula still remain, but may be less prominent.

References

1. Meadows, J. A., Jr. Esophageal diverticula in infants and children. South. Med. J. *63*:691, 1970.
2. Lund, W. S. The cricopharyngeal sphincter: its relationship to the relief of pharyngeal paralysis and the surgical treatment of the early pharyngeal pouch. J. Laryngol. *82*:353, 1968.
3. Ellis, F. H., Jr., Schlegel, J. F., Lynch, V. P., and Payne, W. S. Cricopharyngeal myotomy for pharyngo-esophageal diverticulum. Ann. Surg. *170*:340, 1969.
4. Lichter, I. Motor disorder in pharyngo-esophageal pouch. J. Thorac. Cardiovasc. Surg. *76*:272, 1978.
5. Duranceau, A., Rheault, M. J., and Jamieson, G. G. Physiologic response to cricopharyngeal myotomy and diverticulum suspension. Surgery *94*:655, 1983.
6. Bonavina, L., Khan, N. A., and DeMeester, T. R. Pharyngoesophageal dysfunctions. Arch. Surg. *120*:541, 1985.
7. van Overbeek, J. J. M. The Hypopharyngeal Diverticulum. Amsterdam, Van Goruum Assen, 1977, p. 92.
8. Knuff, T. E., Benjamin, S. B., and Castell, D. O. Pharyngoesophageal (Zenker's) diverticulum: a reappraisal. Gastroenterology *82*:734, 1982.
9. Duda, M., Serý, Z., Vojáček, K., Roček, V., and Rehulka, M. Etiopathogenesis and classification of esophageal diverticula. Int. Surg. *291*, 1985.
10. Allen, T. H., and Clagett, O. T. Changing concepts in the surgical treatment of pulsion diverticula of the lower esophagus. J. Thorac. Cardiovasc. Surg. *50*:455, 1965.
11. Kaye, M. D. Oesophageal motor dysfunction in patients with diverticula of the mid-thoracic oesophagus. Thorax *29*:666, 1974.
12. Dodds, W. J., Stef, J. J., Hogan, W. J., Hoke, S. E., Stewart, E. T., and Arndorfer, R. C. Radial distribution of esophageal peristaltic pressure in normal subjects and patients with esophageal diverticulum. Gastroenterology *69*:584, 1975.
13. Bruggeman, L. L., and Seaman, W. B. Epiphrenic diverticula. AJR *119*:266, 1973.
14. Debas, H. T., Payne, W. S., Cameron, A. J., and Carlson, H. C. Physiopathology of lower esophageal diverticulum and its implications for treatment. Surg. Gynecol. Obstet. *151*:593, 1980.
15. Hurwitz, A. L., Way, L. W., and Haddad, J. K. Epiphrenic diverticulum in association with an unusual motility disturbance: report of surgical correction. Gastroenterology *68*:795, 1975.
16. Clements, J. L., Abernathy, J., and Weens, H. S. Atypical esophageal diverticula associated with progressive systemic sclerosis. Gastrointest. Radiol. *3*:383, 1978.
17. Schreiber, M. H., and Davis, M. Intraluminal diverticulum of the esophagus. AJR *129*:595, 1977.
18. Girdany, B. R., Sieber, W. K., and Osman, M. Z. Traumatic pseudodiverticulums of the pharynx in newborn infants. N. Engl. J. Med. *280*:237, 1969.
19. Scarpa, F. J., Skudlarick, J. L., and Sawyers, J. L. Pharyngeal pseudodiverticulum in an adult. JAMA *234*:740, 1975.
20. Stanford, W., Barloon, T. J., and Lu, C. C. Esophagotracheal fistula from a pharyngoesophageal diverticulum. Chest *84*:229, 1983.
21. Huang, B., Unni, K. K., and Payne, W. S. Long-term survival following diverticulectomy for cancer in pharyngoesophageal (Zenker's) diverticulum. Ann. Thorac. Surg. *38*:207, 1984.
22. Saldana, J. A., Cone, R. O., Hopens, T. A., and Bannayan, G. A. Carcinoma arising in an epiphrenic esophageal diverticulum. Gastrointest. Radiol. *7*:15, 1982.
23. Huang, B., Payne, W. S., and Cameron, A. J. Surgical management for recurrent pharyngoesophageal (Zenker's) diverticulum. Ann. Thorac. Surg. *37*:189, 1984.
24. Einarsson, S., and Hallen, O. On the treatment of esophageal diverticula. Acta Otol. Laryngol. *64*:30, 1967.
25. Hiebert, C. A. Surgery for cricopharyngeal dysfunction under local anesthesia. Am. J. Surg. *131*:408, 1976.
26. Mendl, K., McKay, J. M., and Tanner, C. H. Intramural diverticulosis of the esophagus and Rokitansky-Aschoff sinuses in the gallbladder. Br. J. Radiol. *33*:496, 1960.
27. Castillo, S., Aburashed, A., Kimmelman, J., and Alexander, L. C. Diffuse intramural esophageal pseudodiverticulosis. Gastroenterology *72*:541, 1977.
28. Fromkes, J., Thomas, F. B., Mekhjian, H., Caldwell, J. H., and Johnson, J. C. Esophageal intramural pseudodiverticulosis. Am. J. Dig. Dis. *22*:690, 1977.
29. Umlas, J., and Sakhuja, R. The pathology of esophageal intramural pseudodiverticulosis. Am. J. Clin. Pathol. *65*:314, 1976.
30. Murney, R. G., Linne, J. H., and Curtis, J. High-amplitude peristaltic contractions in a patient with esophageal intramural pseudodiverticulosis. Dig. Dis. Sci. *28*:843, 1983.

38

Esophageal Diseases Caused by Infection, Systemic Illness, and Trauma

GEORGE B. McDONALD

INFECTIONS

The physician's approach to the patient who might have an esophageal infection depends on how immunosuppressed the patient is. Those with more normal immune defenses may be infected with *Candida albicans* or rarely *herpes simplex virus* (HSV) but are unlikely to harbor unusual fungi, viruses, or parasites. These patients usually present with persistent heartburn or dysphagia. When patients with these symptoms come to endoscopy, brushings and biopsies should be obtained for fungal stains. Expensive tests looking for other organisms are not warranted.

On the other hand, when severely immunosuppressed patients have an esophageal infection, the presentation can be deceptive and the range of infecting organisms broad. Dysphagia and esophageal pain are common, but fever, nausea, and bleeding may be the only manifestations. Occasionally the presence of oral thrush or nasolabial herpetic lesions in a patient with acutely painful swallowing is enough to make a diagnosis, but there are usually compelling reasons to carry out endoscopic brushings and biopsies. The endoscopist should be prepared to sample the surface, edges, and base of esophageal lesions. The pathologist should use not only routine histologic stains but also more specific stains for bacteria and viruses. Specimens should be placed in transport media for viral and fungal culture. Treatment of specific esophageal infection is dependent on the organisms discovered by these techniques.

Fungal Infections

Incidence and Predisposing Factors

Fungal infection occurs not only in immunocompromised patients but also in those with less obvious immune defects (diabetic, malnourished elderly, postoperative, and antiobiotic- and steroid-treated patients, for example).[1-5] Esophageal stasis also predisposes patients to infection.[6] In addition, fungal elements can be found in brushings and biopsies of esophageal abnormalities in about 5 per cent of apparently normal patients presenting for endoscopy.[7, 8] Many of these patients had no esophageal symptoms, and fungal infection was often not suspected on the basis of either clinical history or endoscopic appearance.

Clinical Presentation

The sudden development of painful swallowing and retrosternal pain is common in acute fungal infection.[7, 9] Melena and hematemesis may occur, especially if platelet counts are low.[10, 11] Untreated patients may show sloughing of the epithelium, perforation, formation of large tumor-like masses, or intramural bleeding. Fever can be seen with *Candida* esophagitis, but because this organism can traverse the normal small intestinal mucosa, diffuse visceral candidiasis may be present as well.[12] Oral thrush may accompany esophageal infection, particularly in patients with acquired immunodeficiency syndrome (AIDS).[13]

Fungal esophagitis may also be asymptomatic, as shown by its high prevalence at autopsy in immunosuppressed patients and by its chance discovery during routine endoscopy.[7-10, 14] Dysphagia resulting from strictures and bleeding from ulcerative esophagitis are the usual manifestations of infection in chronic mucocutaneous candidiasis as well as in some apparently normal people.[5, 7, 8, 15] In chronic mucocutaneous candidiasis, infection of the mouth, larynx, skin, and nails may also be present.[5, 15] Dysphagia is the presenting complaint in intramural pseudodiverticulosis of the upper esophagus, a disorder associated with chronic *Candida* infection.[5, 16, 17]

Rarely, *Histoplasma capsulatum* may erode from mediastinal nodes into the esophageal wall, presenting either as an extrinsic compression, or as a stricture, or as a mass.[18, 19, 19a]

Diagnosis

Endoscopic brushings and biopsy specimens, properly stained, are the most accurate diagnostic method (Fig. 38–1). Although contrast X-rays show abnormalities in many cases, the changes are not always specific for fungal infection and cannot identify unusual fungi, viruses, and bacteria, which may also be present in immunosuppressed patients.[6, 11] Nonetheless, X-rays are useful in patients with chronic symptoms and in some patients with acute infection, especially when low platelet counts preclude biopsy or when a perforation is suspected.

X-ray changes in acute fungal esophagitis are best seen with double-contrast studies, which typically show longitudinally oriented plaques and pseudomembranes and impaired motility[6, 20, 21] (Fig. 38–2A). With more

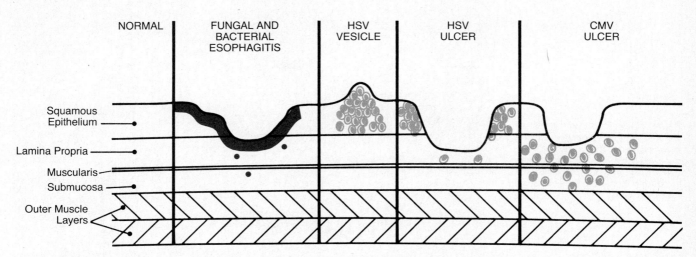

NORMAL   FUNGAL AND   HSV   HSV   CMV
         BACTERIAL   VESICLE   ULCER   ULCER
         ESOPHAGITIS

Squamous Epithelium

Lamina Propria

Muscularis

Submucosa

Outer Muscle Layers

Figure 38–1. Microscopic location of common organisms causing esophageal infection. Fungi and bacteria can usually be recovered from the surface layers of esophageal erosions and ulcers. Herpes simplex virus (HSV) is seen within epithelial cells but rarely may be found at the ulcer base. Cytomegalovirus (CMV) usually is found in subepithelial cells, such as fibroblasts and endothelium. Detection of herpesvirus in biopsy specimens may require immunohistology and *in situ* hybridization methods.

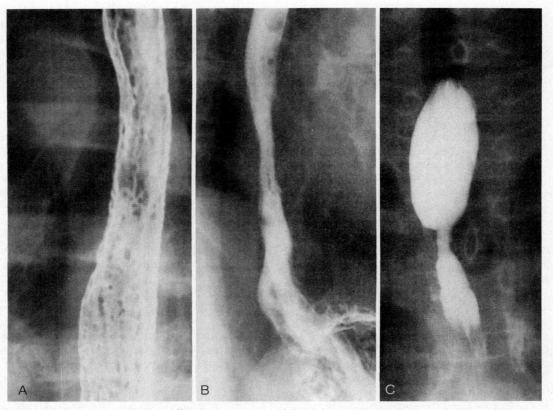

Figure 38–2. Barium contrast X-rays showing different appearances of *Candida* esophagitis. *A,* Acute *Candida* infection in a patient with acquired immunodeficiency syndrome (AIDS). Symptoms were nausea, vomiting, and painful swallowing. X-ray shows multiple small plaques aligned vertically. *B,* Long *Candida* stricture in a patient with chronic mucocutaneous candidiasis. X-ray shows irregular narrowing of the distal esophagus. *C,* Focal stenosis in the thoracic esophagus caused by *Candida* infection in a patient with mucocutaneous candidiasis. (Courtesy of Charles A. Rohrmann, M.D.)

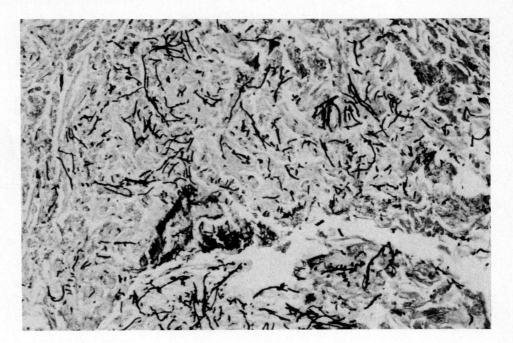

Figure 38–3. Photomicrograph of an esophageal biopsy showing yeast and mycelial forms of *Candida albicans,* stained darkly with silver. Fungi may be difficult to see in routine hematoxylin and eosin stains. (× 480).

extensive inflammation, submucosal edema leads to irregular thickening of folds and a cobblestone appearance.[20, 21] Later, the esophageal wall has a shaggy outline due to coalescing plaques and ulcers.[20–22] Polypoid masses, intramural hematomas, adherent clots, and perforation may also be seen.[6, 20, 23–25] Rarely, the entire mucosa will slough, leaving a smooth radiographic appearance.[23] Dense, fibrotic strictures occur in some patients.[24]

In chronic esophageal candidiasis, constriction of the lumen is the most prominent X-ray abnormality.[5, 7] The narrowing may be focal or involve long segments (Fig. 38–2, *B* and *C*). Intramural pseudodiverticulosis may also be seen[5] (see Fig. 37–4, p. 639).

Esophagoscopy reveals the same spectrum of lesions, including patchy white plaques, confluent pseudomembranes, ulcerations, friable mucosa, polypoid lesions, adherent clots, and diffuse mucosal bleeding.[1, 2, 7, 9] The completely denuded esophagus has a smooth, gray, friable appearance. Plaques and exudate overlying ulcerations should be brushed with a sheathed cytology brush, smeared onto slides, and stained with Gram's and periodic acid–Schiff (PAS) or silver stains.[1, 2, 9, 26] Mycelial forms and large numbers of yeast are abnormal. Biopsy specimens showing fungal elements are also diagnostic (Fig. 38–3) but may be less sensitive than brushings, even when properly stained[26] (Fig. 38–1).

Cultures of biopsy or brush material are not useful in telling whether a fungal infection is present or absent, as *Candida albicans* is a normal commensal organism.[1] As most fungal infections are due to *Candida* species, a presumptive diagnosis can be based on just brushings or biopsies.[26, 27] However, in some patients, unusual fungi may cause esophagitis resistant to conventional antifungal drugs, including ketoconazole.

Other *Candida* species (especially *C. tropicalis* and *C. glabrata*), *Aspergillus, Mucor, Blastomyces,* and *Cryptococcus* may be recognized by fungal culture.[27–31a] Serologic tests have no current role in the diagnosis of either acute or chronic fungal esophagitis.

Treatment

There are no controlled trials comparing antifungal agents for established *Candida* esophagitis, but, in general, severely immunosuppressed patients should be treated with either oral ketoconazole or intravenous amphotericin (Table 38–1).[1, 13, 32] Ketoconazole may rarely cause liver damage and may lead to the increased growth of other fungi, such as *Aspergillus.* Amphotericin causes renal and systemic toxicity and may not eradicate oral lesions because of low salivary levels. Miconazole and oral amphotericin (not available in the United States) are reserved for patients unable to tolerate ketoconazole or intravenous amphotericin. Treatment duration is 7 to 10 days, followed by prophylactic antifungal agents for as long as host resistance is low.[33, 34] When fungal esophagitis is found in normal or minimally immunocompromised patients, less toxic oral therapy with nystatin or clotrimazole is often successful (Table 38–1).[1, 7, 8] Ketoconazole is the drug of choice in patients with AIDS and when nystatin and clotrimazole have failed to eradicate fungi. Coexisting viral or unusual fungal infections should also be considered when symptoms persist.[11, 35]

Treatment of esophageal involvement with histoplasmosis has traditionally been surgical.[18] Several cases, including these with esophageal abscess and fistula, have been successfully treated with amphotericin.[19, 19a]

Table 38–1. TREATMENT OF COMMON ESOPHAGEAL INFECTIONS

Organism	Patient's Immune Status	Prophylaxis	Treatment of Esophagitis
Candida*	N or ↓	Not usually indicated	Nystatin suspension, 1 to 3 million units orally, every 6 hours or Clotrimazole, 100 mg tablets, to be sucked every 6 hours or Ketoconazole tablets, 200–400 mg orally, once daily
	↓ ↓ ↓	Nystatin suspension, 1–3 million units orally, every 4–6 hours or Clotrimazole, 100 mg tablets, to be sucked every 6 hours or Ketoconazole tablets, 200–400 mg orally, once daily	Amphotericin, 0.3–0.5 mg/kg/day, intravenously or Ketoconazole tablets, 400 mg orally, once daily or Miconazole, 200–600 mg every 8 hours, intravenously or Amphotericin, 10 mg lozenges, to be sucked 4–8 times daily
Herpes simplex virus (HSV)†	N or ↓	Not usually indicated	Acyclovir, 200 mg capsules orally, 5 times daily
	↓ ↓ ↓	Acyclovir, 200–400 mg tablets orally, 4–5 times daily or Acyclovir, 800 mg orally, twice daily or Acyclovir, 250 mg/m^2 every 12 hours, intravenously	Acyclovir, 250 mg/m^2 every 8 hours, intravenously or Acyclovir, 400 mg orally, 5 times daily
Cytomegalovirus (CMV)	↓ ↓ ↓	*For seronegative patients:* Transfusion of only seronegative blood products. CMV immune globulin is under study. *For seropositive patients:* Acyclovir and ganciclovir are under current study	Ganciclovir (DHPG), 5 mg/kg every 12 hours, intravenously‡ or Foscarnet‡
Varicella-zoster virus (VZV)	N or ↓	Not usually indicated	Acyclovir, 500 mg/m^2 every 8 hours, intravenously or Orally administered acyclovir (under study)
	↓ ↓ ↓	*If prior infection:* Acyclovir, 400 mg orally, 3 times daily *If no prior infection:* Postexposure VZ immune globulin. VZV vaccine is under study	Acyclovir, 500 mg/m^2 every 8 hours, intravenously

*Some *Candida* species are resistant to amphotericin.
†HSV strains resistant to acyclovir have been reported.
‡Ganciclovir (DHPG) and Foscarnet are investigational drugs active against CMV. Optimal dosages for enteric CMV infections are not yet established.

Viral Infections

Three herpesviruses, herpes simplex virus (HSV), cytomegalovirus (CMV), and varicella-zoster virus (VZV), cause ulcerative esophagitis. Most of these infections occur in immunosuppressed patients, although HSV esophagitis may occur in the normal host. The pathogenesis of ulceration differs among these viruses, HSV and VZV causing epithelial necrosis, and CMV affecting submucosal tissue.

Herpes Simplex Virus (HSV)

The earliest esophageal lesions are vesicles, the centers of which slough to form discrete, circumscribed ulcers with raised edges. When adjacent ulcers coalesce, there may be denudation of wide areas of epithelium, leading to large ulcers.[11, 36, 37] Patients usually present with painful swallowing, retrosternal pain, and heartburn but may have only nausea, vomiting, or hematemesis.[11, 37–41] Diagnosis requires endoscopic brushing and biopsies, but a presumptive diagnosis can be made in patients with esophageal symptoms and HSV infections of the mouth or nares. X-rays of the esophagus may show abnormalities highly suggestive of HSV infection (Fig. 38–4) but are too insensitive to

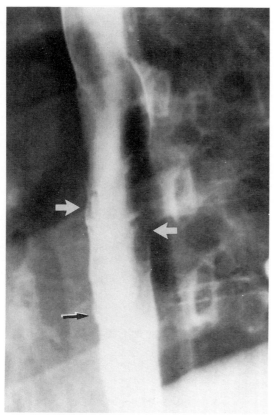

Figure 38–4. Barium contrast X-ray showing multiple herpes simplex virus ulcers in the esophagus of a marrow transplant patient with dysphagia. Small ulcers surrounded by edema give the appearance of targets *(large arrows)* or shallow irregularities when viewed in profile *(small arrow)*. (Courtesy of Charles A. Rohrmann, M.D.)

detect small erosions and cannot reliably indicate the cause, especially in patients with multiple esophageal infections.[11, 21, 35, 42, 43] Endoscopic diagnosis of herpesvirus infection requires extensive brushing and biopsies. Platelet counts should be greater than 50,000 cells per cubic millimeter before biopsy of the edge and center of ulcers is undertaken. HSV can be detected in exfoliated epithelial cells and in tissue sections by several methods. Routine histologic stains may show characteristic epithelial cells with occasional multinucleation, "ground glass" nuclear staining, and intranuclear (Cowdry type A) inclusions. There is little HSV in the granulation tissue bed of an HSV ulcer[11, 36] (Fig. 38–1). More specific and sensitive techniques include immunohistologic identification of infected cells with monoclonal antibodies to HSV antigens and *in situ* hybridization for HSV nucleic acid.[41] Both brushings and biopsy specimens should be placed in viral transport media for viral culture. Cultures can be read in 24 to 36 hours using immunologic staining of centrifugation cultures.[43a]

In patients with intact immune responses, esophageal HSV infection runs a course parallel to nasolabial infection, with spontaneous healing.[44, 45] In immunodeficient patients, symptoms may not resolve until immune function returns.[11, 41] Bleeding from large ulcers and HSV pneumonia are consequences of untreated HSV esophagitis; another complication is superinfection of the denuded esophagus with fungi and bacteria.[9, 11, 35, 39, 40, 46] Rarely, HSV may cause gastritis, ulcerative enteritis, and fulminant hepatitis. HSV infections can be treated effectively (and prevented) with acyclovir (Table 38–1).[47–50] Symptoms usually resolve within one week, but large ulcerations may take longer to re-epithelialize.[11, 36, 41] Reflux of acid peptic juice causes intense pain even when virus is no longer present; antireflux therapy is useful in treating these symptoms. Submucosal fibrosis may lead to stricture formation.

Cytomegalovirus (CMV)

Cytomegalovirus infection occurs only in immunosuppressed patients and differs from HSV esophagitis in several respects. CMV may be activated from latency or acquired from blood-product transfusions.[51, 52] Esophageal infection occurs within submucosal fibroblasts and endothelial cells, not in the epithelium, and is usually part of a widespread visceral infection.[11, 41, 53–56] CMV lesions first appear as serpiginous ulcers in otherwise normal mucosa but coalesce to form giant ulcers, particularly in the distal esophagus.[11, 41, 53] Patients present with nausea, vomiting, painful swallowing, heartburn, and hematemesis, in addition to involvement of other organs with CMV.[11, 41, 53, 56] Esophageal X-rays may be nonspecifically abnormal or show large ulcers.[21, 57] Diagnosis requires endoscopic biopsies of the center of the ulcer; brushings of overlying exudate are seldom useful[11, 41] (Fig. 38–1). Routine histologic stains show large cells in the submucosa bearing amphophilic intranuclear inclusions as well as small intracytoplasmic inclusions. Immunohistology with monoclonal antibodies to CMV antigens and *in situ* hybridization for CMV DNA are useful in finding infected cells that are neither large nor inclusion-bearing.[41, 58] Culturing biopsy specimens for CMV can be useful if newer methods are used[43a]; otherwise days to weeks may pass before cultures become positive. In contrast to HSV infections, CMV can frequently be found in the mucosa and submucosa of the stomach and intestine in patients with CMV esophagitis.[11, 41, 54, 56, 57] HSV, fungi, and bacteria may coexist with CMV in esophageal ulcers in patients with profound, prolonged immunosuppression.[11, 41]

Treatment of established CMV esophagitis or enteritis is dependent on immune reconstitution. Antiviral drugs (Table 38–1) active against CMV *in vitro* appear to be effective in immunosuppressed patients and are under current study.[59–60a] Untreated CMV esophagitis is associated with protracted nausea and vomiting in marrow transplant patients, many of whom have persistent esophageal pain related to acid peptic reflux.[41] Re-epithelialization may not occur unless CMV infection disappears, and even then healing takes weeks to months.

Varicella-Zoster Virus (VZV)

Varicella-zoster virus may rarely involve the esophagus in children with chicken pox and adults with herpes zoster, often with spontaneous resolution.[37, 61] However, VZV can cause necrotizing esophagitis in severely immunosuppressed patients with herpes zoster.[11, 37, 61] Both vesicles and confluent necrosis can be seen in the esophagus. Routine histologic stains of brushings and biopsy specimens show epithelial cell changes similar to those of HSV infection. Immunohistology can differentiate these two viruses. Esophageal VZV may also be a harbinger of disseminated visceral VZV in the absence of skin involvement.[11] VZV is sensitive to acyclovir, but there is little experience with treatment of visceral VZV with this drug (Table 38–1).

Bacterial Infections

Bacterial infections of the esophagus are unusual, occurring either in profoundly granulocytopenic patients or as part of an infection involving contiguous organs (tuberculosis, for example). In the immunocompromised patient, gram-positive cocci and gram-negative bacilli from the oropharnyx can cause esophageal ulcers, pseudomembranes, and bacteremia[11, 62] (Fig. 38–1). These infections are usually missed because other organisms (viruses, fungi) are commonly present and because bacteria are difficult to see on routine histologic stains.[11, 62] In one autopsy series, bacterial esophagitis accounted for 16 per cent of 123 cases of infective esophagitis.[62] In two cancer-center populations, the prevalence of bacterial esophagitis among patients being endoscoped was 11 and 12 per cent,

respectively.[11, 62] Although most patients with these infections are symptomatic, fever and bacteremia may be the only manifestation of esophageal infection.[11, 62–64] Bacterial esophagitis caused by *Lactobacillus* and beta-hemolytic streptococci has also been described in immunocompetent patients.[65, 66]

Tuberculosis of the esophagus is a rare disease, usually seen in patients with obvious tuberculosis elsewhere (lungs, lymph nodes, spine).[67] Dysphagia and retrosternal pain point to esophageal involvement with ulcerations just above the tracheal bifurcation. Tumor-like masses on X-ray can be confused with carcinoma, but endoscopic biopsies of ulcerated tissue show epitheloid granulomas.[68–69a] Computed tomography of the mediastinum gives a clear picture of the pathology involved.[69a, 70] A rare "granular" form of esophageal tuberculosis occurs after miliary spread of primary infection.

Syphilis involving the esophagus is rare. Earlier literature described gummas, diffuse ulceration, and strictures of the esophagus in tertiary syphilis. Dysphagia occurs rarely in secondary syphilis.[71] Histology shows perivascular lymphocytic infiltration; specific immunostaining should be done if this diagnosis is a possibility.

Diphtherial membranes may extend from the oropharynx into the esophagus. Dysphagia due to neuromuscular abnormalities can be seen in tetanus.[72]

Parasitic Infections

Chagas' disease is due to infection with *Trypanosoma cruzi,* a South American parasite that destroys ganglion cells throughout the body. Chronic Chagas' syndrome develops 10 to 30 years after the acute disease, with heart, esophageal, and intestinal abnormalities.[73–75] In the esophagus, the clinical picture is similar to that of achalasia, and manometric findings may be identical. Diagnosis depends on finding other organs involved and on serologic tests.[75]

Infection with *Cryptosporidium* and with *Pneumocystis carinii* have been reported in patients with AIDS, both causing nonspecific inflammation in the distal esophagus.[76, 76a] Esophageal involvement with amebic liver abscess, echinococcal cyst, and nematode infestation has been described.[77]

SYSTEMIC ILLNESSES

Skin Disorders

Rare cases of esophageal involvement occur with most skin diseases that affect the oral cavity, especially the bullous skin disorders.[78]

Dystrophic Epidermolysis Bullosa

Dystrophic epidermolysis bullosa is an inherited disorder in which trauma to the skin and mucous membranes causes bullae and scarring. Esophageal involvement is common with the recessive form of the disease, most patients presenting with dysphagia and aspiration in childhood.[79-81] Esophageal bullae occur at sites of trauma by ingested material at the proximal and distal esophagus and at the level of the carina.[81, 82] These bullae may resolve, ulcerate, or heal by scar formation, leaving webs and strictures.[80-82] Medical management includes soft foods, steroids, phenytoin, and careful balloon dilation of strictures.[81] Some patients require esophageal resection and reconstruction with colon or gastric tubes.[79, 83, 84]

Pemphigus Vulgaris

Pemphigus vulgaris affects skin, mouth, and other mucous membranes with weeping bullous lesions. Patients are usually 40 to 60 years old. Rare cases of esophageal involvement have been reported, usually in patients with obvious skin and mouth lesions.[85-87] Isolated esophageal bullae have been seen.[88] The diagnosis is established by histology showing acantholysis and intraepithelial bullae and by specific immunohistology.[85, 88] Steroid treatment is effective, but esophageal bleeding, strictures, and formation of epithelial casts may occur.[85, 86]

Bullous Pemphigoid

Bullous pemphigoid is a chronic disease of the elderly, in whom tense, pruritic skin bullae arise. Oral bullae occur in about 20 per cent of cases, but scarring is unusual. Esophageal bullae occur rarely; sloughing of the epithelium as a cast has been described.[89-91] The diagnosis is by histology showing subepithelial bullae, circulating antibodies to basement membrane, and immunohistology. Steroid treatment is effective.

Benign Mucous Membrane Pemphigoid

Benign mucous membrane pemphigoid (also known as cicatricial pemphigoid) is a chronic blistering disease of the mucous membranes of the eyes, mouth, genitalia, and adjacent areas of skin.[92] These lesions are most common in middle and older age and have a tendency for scar formation. Esophageal involvement includes bullae, webs, and dense strictures.[93, 94] Frequent dilations may be needed for chronic strictures.

Drug-induced Skin Diseases

Drug-induced skin diseases (Stevens-Johnson syndrome, toxic epidermal necrolysis) may rarely affect the esophagus with a blistering process and desquamation of large areas of epithelium.[95-99] Both focal and long strictures and webs may result, requiring dilation.

Other Skin Diseases

An erosive type of *lichen planus* may affect both oral cavity and esophagus, causing pain and dysphagia.[100, 101] *Acanthosis nigricans* appears as granular nodules in the esophagus in patients with carcinoma elsewhere.[102, 103] *Leukoplakia* and similar lesions of the oral cavity can be seen in the esophagus.[78] Hyperkeratotic papules may stud the esophagus in *Darier's disease*.[78] Squamous papillomas of the esophagus have been described in patients with focal dermal hypoplasia.[103a] *Tylosis* (diffuse palmoplantar keratoderma) is a hereditary skin disease that rarely predisposes to bronchial, laryngeal, and esophageal cancer.[78, 104-106]

Behçet's Disease

Behçet's disease is a multisystem inflammatory process characterized by oral and genital ulcers, ocular inflammation, skin lesions, and vasculitis. It is most common in Japan and the Middle East, but cases have been reported from many countries. Ileum and colon are commonly involved, but the esophagus is affected only rarely.[107] Esophageal lesions include ulcerations that can tunnel under the mucosa, strictures, and perforation.[107-109] Strictures may be localized to the upper esophagus or involve long segments of the midesophagus. Biopsies show nonspecific inflammation, and rarely vasculitis. Esophageal inflammation may respond to steroid therapy.

Graft-Versus-Host Disease (GVHD)

Patients who have received an allogeneic bone marrow transplant may develop GVHD, an immunologic reaction against host tissues by donor lymphoid cells.[110] Histologic changes of acute GVHD can be found in the esophagus, but more extensive damage occurs in chronic GVHD, a multisystem disorder that involves the skin, eyes, mucous membranes, liver, and esophagus.[110-112] Esophageal symptoms include dysphagia, retrosternal pain, and aspiration. Barium contrast X-rays may reveal webs, rings, and tight strictures in the upper esophagus and midesophagus but often fail to show the generalized desquamation apparent on endoscopy.[112] There may be poor acid clearing because of salivary gland involvement as well as motor abnormalities. Dilations, antireflux measures, and immunosuppressive therapy are usually successful, but there is an increased risk of esophageal perforation during dilation.[110, 111]

Crohn's Disease

Esophageal involvement in patients with extensive Crohn's disease has been described in some 50 patients. Rarely, the esophagus is the only organ affected. Painful dysphagia is a common presenting symptom.[113] X-ray and endoscopy show small aphthous ulcers, inflammatory strictures, sinus tracts, filiform polyps, and fistulas to adjacent viscera.[113-117] Granulomas can occasionally be found in endoscopic biopsy specimens.[113, 117, 118] Inflammatory lesions respond to steroid therapy, but strictures and fistulas may require surgery.[113, 118]

Ulcerative Colitis

Earlier literature described an association between ulcerative colitis and inflammatory esophagitis,[119] but infectious causes were not excluded in these cases. Aphthous ulcers of the mouth occur in 8 per cent of patients with ulcerative colitis[120] and may rarely be seen in the esophagus.[121] However, herpes simplex virus can produce similar lesions in patients with colitis.[122]

Sarcoidosis

Several well-documented cases of sarcoidosis involving the esophagus have been reported, most with accompanying dysphagia.[123] Esophageal strictures are due to transmural granulomatous involvement, which may also affect muscle and vagal nerves.[123-125] It may be difficult to differentiate esophageal Crohn's disease from sarcoidosis.[126]

Metastatic Cancer

Cancers originating near the esophagus may cause dysphagia by external compression, invasion, or intramural metastases. This is most common with lung, breast, and gastric cancers, but more remote tumors (prostate, pancreas, thyroid) can involve the esophagus.[127-130] The diagnosis is best made by barium contrast X-ray and CT.[128, 129, 131, 132] Endoscopy can exclude primary esophageal lesions but often fails to obtain a tissue diagnosis of cancer unless there is transmural infiltration.[132, 133] Treatment with radiation therapy and placement of an endoprosthesis may provide palliation.[134]

Esophageal involvement with lymphoma and Kaposi's sarcoma, formerly a rarity, has been recognized in AIDS patients.[135-137] These tumors may coexist with viral and fungal infections of the esophagus.[135] Radiation therapy may provide palliation.

Collagen Vascular Diseases

Motility disorders of the esophagus can be seen with progressive systemic sclerosis, mixed connective tissue disease, polymyositis-dermatomyositis, Sjögren's syndrome, systemic lupus erythematosus, and Raynaud's phenomenon (see pp. 559–593). Epithelial damage occurs when there is poor clearing of acid (salivary disease, poor peristalsis, and lower esophageal sphincter involvement), immune suppression leading to esophageal infection, or retention of pills causing esophagitis (see later discussion).

TRAUMA

Perforation

Causes

The most common causes of esophageal perforation are medical tubes and instruments, forceful vomiting, and foreign bodies.[138-140] Less frequent (and often missed) are perforations caused by trauma to the cervical spine, gunshot wounds, caustic ingestion, anastomotic leaks, necrotizing infection, necrosis of tumors during chemoradiation therapy, extension of a Barrett's ulcer, and the introduction of gases under high pressure.

Any medical instrument that enters the esophagus can perforate the esophagus, but the frequency is highest when some form of therapy is undertaken. Rigid esophagoscopy (usually for stricture dilation) has a risk of perforation of 1 in 100.[141] Diagnostic fiberoptic upper endoscopy carries a risk of perforating the normal esophagus of less than 1 in 1000, but the risk rises when biopsy, sclerotherapy, balloon dilation of strictures, and electrocautery are done through the endoscope.[142] Perforation is also more likely after dilation of tight peptic strictures, forceful balloon dilation for achalasia, placement of an endoprosthesis for esophageal cancer, and esophageal balloon tamponade of varices. An increasingly frequent cause is attempted endotracheal intubation, especially when done out of hospital during resuscitation.[143] Both nasogastric and endotracheal tubes may readily perforate the neonatal esophagus.[144] Surgical instruments can perforate during mediastinoscopy, vagotomy, hiatus hernia repair, or any periesophageal procedure.[140]

Both foreign bodies and the procedures used to extract them may perforate. Bones and coins were formerly the leading offenders, but these have recently been joined by bottle tops, toys, and small batteries.[139, 140] Perforation may result from either a sharp edge or pressure necrosis, and the foreign body may itself migrate into adjacent structures.[140]

Diagnosis

Perforations are recognized by symptoms (odynophagia; chest, neck, abdominal, upper neck pain; respiratory distress), signs (subcutaneous crepitation, mediastinal crunching sound with the heart beat, fever, shock), leukocytosis, and X-ray abnormalities.[138-140, 145-147] However, when X-rays are done routinely after medical instrumentation, some asymptomatic patients are found to have been perforated.[148] Perforation may be apparent only at autopsy in some patients.[145] The most important determinants of survival are the size and location of the perforation and whether gross contamination outside the esophagus has occurred. Delay in recognition usually leads to more contamination and a much higher early mortality rate, and it also complicates long-term management. Perforations discovered early can usually be closed primarily or, in some cases, treated without operation. Perforations diagnosed late may require an esophageal exclusion procedure and one or more operations months later to restore esophageal continuity.

Plain films are abnormal in over 80 per cent of esophageal perforations, but some changes (pleural effusion and mediastinal widening) develop over hours to days.[149, 150] Plain films of the neck usually show air in the soft tissues and prevertebral space after perforation of the cervical esophagus.[149, 150] Projections with the neck hyperextended allow better views of the esophageal inlet.[138] Later changes of air-fluid collections and abscesses can be seen on plain film but are better appreciated by CT.[151] Perforations of the posterior wall of the cervical esophagus may reach the retropharyngeal space and extend into the mediastinum. Anterolateral and piriform sinus perforations enter the pretracheal space and may also reach the mediastinum. A surgical approach may involve both neck and mediastinum if so directed by CT.[151]

The thoracic esophagus lies just beneath the right pleura. Perforations here lead to air, fluid, and pus collections in the mediastinum and right pleural space.[138, 150, 151] CT can be useful in defining mediastinal abnormalities, especially when the perforation site has sealed over.[152] In contrast, perforations of the distal esophagus usually lead to air and fluid reaching the left pleural space, mediastinum, or abdomen.[138, 150] Perforation into the abdomen can also involve the retroperitoneal space and lesser sac.[153, 154] A combined thoracoabdominal approach may be required in the surgical treatment of such cases.

Contrast studies and CT are usually needed to better define the site of perforation and anatomic extent of damage. Contrast X-ray studies should be done immediately after procedures that carry a high risk of perforation (balloon dilation for achalasia, stent placement for palliation of carcinoma).[148, 155] Water-soluble contrast medium should be used in small boluses at first, avoiding aspiration because of this agent's pulmonary toxicity[156] (Fig. 38–5). Although barium contrast material clearly is superior in demonstrating small perforations,[149, 157] it causes an inflammatory response in the mediastinal, pleural, and peritoneal cavities.[156] However, when examination with water-soluble contrast material fails to show a perforation, barium should be used for better definition.[156, 157]

Treatment

Nonoperative Management. Esophageal perforation is a highly lethal complication that demands early surgical consultation. Nonoperative approaches apply only to very specific situations. Some cases of esophageal perforation caused by medical instruments can be managed without operation, provided that the diagnosis is made early, the perforation is confined to a small space, and there is no obvious contamination of the perforation site with gastric contents, saliva, and food.[155, 158, 159] Exceptions are perforations into the

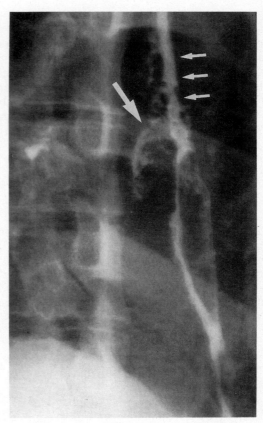

Figure 38–5. Water-soluble contrast X-ray of the distal esophagus, showing a perforation *(large arrow)*. This perforation occurred during rubber bougie dilatation of a lye stricture *(small arrows)*. (Courtesy of Charles A. Rohrmann, M.D.)

abdominal or pleural cavities, which require immediate surgical repair.[155, 159] It is less clear whether perforations caused by foreign bodies, nasogastric and endotracheal tubes, blunt trauma, and the like can be managed safely without surgery as these cases are usually not recognized promptly. Most authors recommend operation in cases of spontaneous perforation.[140, 160]

Nineteen consecutive instrumental perforations in patients without malignancy have been reported from Amsterdam.[155] Most had been perforated during dilation of strictures, but the perforations were recognized within two hours. Fourteen patients recovered after a week's treatment with antibiotics, parenteral or enteral nutrition, and protection of the perforation site by a nasoesophageal tube whose side holes straddled the leak. Five patients were treated surgically by primary closure and drainage because of either intra-abdominal perforation or suspected gross contamination. All patients recovered.[155]

Recent surgical literature supports nonoperative management for highly selected cases, including some whose perforations are not recognized until later.[140, 146, 158, 159, 161, 162] Perforations in the hypopharynx and cervical esophagus contained within the soft tissues can occasionally be managed without surgery unless there is mediastinal involvement.[140, 148, 163] However, when these perforations are caused by retained foreign bodies rather than medical instruments, the amount of contamination can be high, and they are better approached with surgical drainage.[139] In newborn infants, endotracheal and nasogastric tubes are the cause of most cervical perforations, which usually can be managed without surgical repair.[144] Reports of endotracheal tube perforation in adults, however, emphasize the need for early surgery to avoid death or a prolonged recovery.[143] With perforation of the thoracic esophagus, deciding between operative and nonoperative management is not easy, as even small perforations can lead to sepsis, mediastinitis, and pleural contamination.[145] Nonoperative treatment can be considered for patients with minimal signs and symptoms and drainage of the leak back into the esophagus.[158, 159] These "contained" perforations are more likely to occur in patients with esophageal cancer or previous inflammation or irradiation than in those with normal mediastinal anatomy. All patients managed conservatively should be watched closely for abscess formation, continued leak, and mediastinal extension.

Perforation of esophageal cancer during endoscopy, dilation, or placement of an endoprosthesis is a difficult problem. Most of these perforations occur in patients whose cancer is inoperable, during attempts at palliative treatment.[155, 164] The Amsterdam group has reported 35 consecutive perforations in such patients, all treated without operation, with antibiotics, nutritional support, and protection of the perforation site.[155] In 10 patients, the site was sealed off by immediate placement of an endoprosthesis; only one patient developed mediastinitis. In 24 patients, nonoperative treatment was followed by placement of an endoprosthesis within one week, with no deaths related to perforation.[155] Similar results have been reported in 34 patients undergoing placement of an endoprosthesis for cancer in Nottingham.[148] Eight patients had perforations in the hypopharynx, away from the tumor; all recovered after nasopharyngeal suction and antibiotics. Twenty-four patients had perforation through the tumor. All had received prophylactic antibiotic (cephalosporin) and had the endoprosthesis placed to seal off the perforation. Twenty patients recovered after medical therapy without developing mediastinitis, but four died as a result of perforations that had entered the pleural cavity.[148] Attempts at resection of the cancer or esophagus after the cancer has been perforated have usually been in vain.[140, 160]

Perforations can also be sealed effectively with a Celestin-type endoprosthesis, and success with this approach has been reported in a small number of patients with nonmalignant conditions, including spontaneous rupture.[165, 166] These prostheses are pulled into position through a gastrostomy at laparotomy and may obviate major thoracic surgery in high-risk patients.[165]

Surgical Management. Surgery is necessary when there is suspected contamination of a perforation site, obvious infection, sepsis, pleural or peritoneal perforation, or respiratory failure, and when nonoperative treatment has failed (abscess formation, failure of perforation site to close).[140, 146, 159, 167] Some surgeons,

however, believe that all patients with a hole in the esophagus should be operated on.[160] For cervical perforations, primary closure and drainage of surrounding tissue is optimal, but with small leaks, drainage alone may suffice.[145, 159] For perforations in the thoracic esophagus, the defect should be closed if possible and supported with a local tissue flap when the defect cannot be closed primarily.[145, 159, 160] When a large perforation leads to continued leakage, the only options are major operations that resect the esophagus, exclude the lumen from above and below, or place an endoprosthesis in the lumen. Although these operations may be the only way to control persistent mediastinal and pleural infection, mortality in this group of patients is high.[159, 160, 162, 167] Several reviews supply details of current surgical approaches to this difficult problem.[140, 159]

Intramural Hematoma

Bleeding into the wall of the esophagus can be seen with any of the conditions that cause perforation, including vomiting, foreign body ingestion, and medical instrumentation.[168–173] Another form of incomplete perforation is the double-barreled esophagus, in which the mucosa is dissected off the muscular layer to form two channels.[173a] Hematomas also occur spontaneously, particularly in patients with platelet and clotting factor abnormalities.[169, 174] Presenting symptoms include retrosternal or epigastric pain, dysphagia, and bleeding.[168–170, 173a] The diagnosis is made by barium contrast X-ray showing double columns of contrast separated by a radiolucent stripe and large, tumor-like intramural masses.[169, 173–175] CT can provide accurate information about the extent of intramural dissection and whether or not a perforation has occurred.[176] Most hematomas resolve spontaneously.[168, 169]

Nasogastric Tube Strictures

Occasionally patients who have had nasogastric tubes in place for a long time will develop strictures owing to local irritation and persistent reflux.[177, 178] These strictures, usually discovered only after the tube is pulled, may involve the length of the esophagus and prove difficult to dilate.[179] New Silastic tubes may cause less damage.[180]

Pill Esophagitis

Pills that have been reported to cause esophageal mucosal injury are listed in Table 38–2.[181, 181a] Tetracycline, potassium chloride, quinidine and emepronium account for most of the reported cases.[181a] Although patients with pre-existing esophageal narrowings are at risk, most reported cases have occurred in patients without prior swallowing problems.[181] In normal subjects, swallowed pills remain in the esophagus for 5

Table 38–2. PILLS CAUSING ESOPHAGEAL
MUCOSAL INJURY

Antibiotics (tetracycline, doxycycline, clindamycin, others)
Potassium chloride (especially slow-release forms)
Iron preparations
Quinidine
Alprenolol (beta-blocker)
Analgesics (aspirin, nonsteroidal anti-inflammatory drugs)
Emepronium (anticholinergic)
Clinitest (and similar chemicals in tablet form)

minutes or longer, lodging either just above the lower esophageal sphincter or in the upper esophagus.[182–184] Large pills coated with gelatinous material will stick, especially when too little water is taken.[183–185] Bedtime pill taking may contribute to this problem, as the supine position and decreased salivation and swallowing during sleep may lead to pill retention in the esophagus.[184] Some tablets not intended for oral use (Clinitest, for example) cause esophageal injury by thermal and chemical effects.[186] When papain solutions are placed in the esophagus to dissolve meat boluses, esophagitis may result, particularly if mucosal damage was present beforehand.[186a]

The most common symptom is retrosternal pain on swallowing, which usually develops after days to weeks of pill taking.[181] Some patients have slowly progressive dysphagia caused by strictures and inflammatory masses in the esophagus.[181, 187, 188] Bleeding, perforation, stricture formation, and death have been reported more commonly with pills containing potassium chloride, iron, quinidine, and alprenolol than with antibiotic pills, perhaps because antibiotics are usually taken for shorter periods of time.[181]

The diagnosis is suggested by the history or by a barium esophagogram showing an ulcer, stricture, or mass.[181, 187–190] These lesions may resemble peptic strictures and carcinomas, particularly when they occur in the mid- and upper esophagus.[181, 187, 188] Endoscopy reveals either discrete ulcers or heaped up, inflamed mucosa, often with profuse exudate.[181, 187] Lesions may resemble carcinoma as well as peptic strictures. Pill fragments may be seen. Biopsies show inflammatory changes, but cytology should be interpreted cautiously, as hyperplastic cells resulting from inflammation can be confused for carcinoma.[181, 187]

In uncomplicated cases, symptoms and epithelial inflammation resolve one to six weeks after pills are stopped.[181, 181a] Continuation of offending pills, especially potassium chloride, may lead to complications such as stricture formation and perforation. Strictures may require dilation but generally resolve if injury to the epithelium ceases.[181, 187, 189] Patients with known esophageal abnormalities should receive certain chronic medications as liquids or pulverized material, and bedridden patients especially should wash down pills with 6 ounces of water.[183, 184]

Radiation and Chemotherapy

Treatment for cancer may cause esophageal symptoms either directly (thoracic radiation) or indirectly (decreased salivary flow leading to peptic esophagitis or immunosuppression leading to infection). Radiation therapy of over 30 Gy (3000 rad) to the mediastinum commonly causes retrosternal burning and painful swallowing, usually mild and limited to the duration of therapy.[191–194] Incidence and severity rise with increasing doses of radiation, more severe esophagitis occurring after 50 Gy (5000 rad).[192, 194, 195] In one series, esophagitis was the most common toxic effect of 50-Gy radiation therapy for lung cancer, affecting 24 per cent of patients; 9 per cent had moderate or severe esophagitis.[193] Strictures, perforations, and fistulas have been described, usually after 60-Gy radiation.[195–199] Histologically, acute radiation esophagitis is characterized by basal cell necrosis, submucosal edema, capillary dilatation, and swollen endothelial cells. After several weeks, superficial erosions occur, owing to failure of regeneration and to blood vessel damage.[197, 200] Several months after high-dose radiation therapy, there is regeneration of epithelium and submucosal healing by fibrosis but also striking abnormalities of esophageal smooth muscle in some patients.[191, 195, 197, 200] Dysphagia during radiation therapy is probably attributable to both epithelial damage and disordered motility, which in turn may predispose to peptic esophagitis.[198, 200] If radiation ports include the neck, salivary flow may be markedly diminished, removing another barrier to acid damage.[197, 201]

Animal studies suggest that prostaglandin metabolites are involved in radiation damage to the esophagus, and that inhibitors of cyclo-oxygenase enzymes (indomethacin, aspirin, and meclofenamic acid) protect the animal esophagus from damage.[202–204] A randomized, double-blind study in lung cancer patients receiving thoracic radiation showed modest therapeutic benefit with indomethacin prophylaxis.[205]

Much more serious esophageal damage occurs in patients who receive certain chemotherapeutic drugs along with mediastinal radiation.[198, 206, 207] As occurs elsewhere in the body, chemotherapy potentiates radiation injury in the esophagus, which may show damage with radiation doses under 25 Gy (2500 rad).[208] This effect is particularly common with doxorubicin (Adriamycin) but has also been described with bleomycin, dactinomycin, cyclophosphamide, fluorouracil, etoposide, methotrexate, and cisplatin.[206–212] Severe esophagitis, stricture formation, and rarely fistulas occur in 25 to 40 per cent of patients treated with both chemotherapy and radiation therapy. These patients may also have recurrences of symptoms with subsequent courses of chemotherapy alone.[206–208] Severe esophageal toxicity can be lessened by separating chemotherapy and radiation doses by a week.[207]

Chemotherapy alone may cause severe dysphagia because of oropharyngeal "mucositis," but esophageal involvement is unusual. Agents that commonly cause mucositis include dactinomycin, bleomycin, cytarabine, daunorubicin, fluorouracil, methotrexate, and vincristine.[213] Vinca alkaloid drugs are neurotoxic; reversible dysphagia without esophagitis has been described with vincristine.[214] Chemotherapy-induced vomiting may lead to Mallory-Weiss tear, intramural hematoma, and esophageal perforation, all potentially lethal in patients with low platelet counts and immunodeficiency. Perforations and fistulas may also develop when cancer therapy results in necrosis of tumors involving the esophageal wall.

Sclerotherapy for Varices

Recent literature on endoscopic sclerotherapy for varices has been paralleled by case reports and small series of complications from this procedure. These include esophageal ulcers, strictures, intramural hematoma, perforation, abscess, and sepsis. Ulceration at the site of injection is very common, persisting for 1 to 3 weeks, then usually healing.[215, 216] However, as many as 25 per cent of patients have persistent ulceration, and some fail to heal after months of aggressive medical therapy.[217, 218] The published incidence of persistent ulceration and stricture formation varies widely, suggesting that technique, type of sclerosant, volume injected, and frequency of sclerosis are important factors.[219–221] Injection of sclerosant results in mural necrosis followed by fibrosis; the bases of these chronic ulcers are relatively avascular.[222]

Transient dysphagia and retrosternal pain occur after sclerotherapy because of edema, inflammation, and disordered motility.[223, 224] Strictures may develop two weeks afterward in up to 50 per cent of patients.[221, 225, 226] Poor acid clearing may be a factor in stricture formation, but intensity of submucosal fibrosis is probably more important.[224, 227, 228] Most authors suggest H$_2$-blocker medication, antireflux measures, and perhaps sucralfate to prevent ulceration and stricturing, but there is little evidence of efficacy. Dilation of strictures is usually effective,[224, 226] but refractory strictures have been reported.[229]

Aorto-esophageal Fistula

Foreign bodies, especially those with sharp projections such as bones and pins, may erode into the aorta over the course of a week. In most cases, there is sentinel arterial bleeding, followed later by more massive hemorrhage.[230–232] Similar fistulas can occur with lung and esophageal cancer, an aneurysm of the aorta and after penetration of an esophageal ulcer.[231–235] As with many aortoenteric fistulas, the diagnosis can be difficult, even with endoscopy and angiography. Bleeding is usually fatal, but a small number of patients have survived after emergency thoracotomy.[232–235]

References

1. Mathieson, R., and Dutta, S. K. Candida esophagitis. Dig. Dis. Sci. 28:365, 1983.
2. Trier, J. S., and Bjorkman, D. J. Esophageal, gastric, and intestinal candidiasis. Am. J. Med. 77:39, 1984.
3. Gundry, S. R., Borkon, A. M., McIntosh, C. L., and Morrow, A. G. Candida esophagitis following cardiac operation and short-term antibiotic prophylaxis. J. Thorac. Cardiovasc. Surg. 80:661, 1980.
4. Dutta, S. K., and Al-Ibrahim, M. S. Immunological studies in acute pseudomembranous esophageal candidiasis. Gastroenterology 75:292, 1978.
5. Rohrmann, C. A., and Kidd, R. Chronic mucocutaneous candidiasis: radiologic abnormalities in the esophagus. AJR 130:473, 1978.
6. Levine, M. S., Macones, A. J., and Laufer, I. Candida esophagitis: accuracy of radiographic diagnosis. Radiology 154:581, 1985.
7. Kodsi, B. E., Wickremesinghe, C., Kozinn, P. J., Iswara, K., and Goldberg, P. K. Candida esophagitis: a prospective study of 27 cases. Gastroenterology 71:715, 1976.
8. Scott, B. B., and Jenkins, D. Gastro-oesophageal candidiasis. Gut 23:137, 1982.
9. Wheeler, R. R., Peacock, J. E., Cruz, J. M., and Richter, J. E. Esophagitis in the immunocompromised host: role of esophagoscopy in diagnosis. Rev. Infect. Dis. 9:88, 1987.
10. Eras, P., Goldstein, M., and Sherlock, P. Candida infections of the gastrointestinal tract. Medicine 51:367, 1972.
11. McDonald, G. B., Sharma, P., Hackman, R. C., Meyers, J., and Thomas, E. D. Esophageal infections in immunosuppressed patients after marrow transplantation. Gastroenterology 88:1111, 1985.
12. Krause, W., Matheis, H., and Wulf, K. Fungaemia and funguria after oral administration of Candida albicans. Lancet 1:598, 1969.
13. Tavitian, A., Raufman, J. P., and Rosenthal, L. E. Oral candidiasis as a marker for esophageal candidiasis in the acquired immunodeficiency syndrome. Ann. Intern. Med. 104:54, 1986.
14. Clotet, B., Grifor, M., Parra, O., Boix, J., Junca, J., Tor, J., and Foz, M. Asymptomatic esophageal candidiasis in the acquired immunodeficiency syndrome-related complex. Ann. Intern. Med. 105:145, 1986.
15. Kobayashi, R. H., Rosenblatt, H. M., Carney, J. M., Byrne, W. J. Ament, M. E., Mendoza, G. R., Dudley, J. P., and Stiehm, E. R. Candida esophagitis and laryngitis in chronic mucocutaneous candidiasis. Pediatrics 66:380, 1980.
16. Troupin, R. H. Intramural esophageal diverticulosis and moniliasis: a possible association. AJR 104:613, 1968.
17. Castillo, S., Aburashed, A., Kimmelman, J., and Alexander, L. C. Diffuse intramural esophageal pseudodiverticulosis. Gastroenterology 72:541, 1977.
18. Gilliland, M. D., Scott, L. D., and Walker, W. E. Esophageal obstruction caused by mediastinal histoplasmosis: beneficial effects of operation. Surgery 95:59, 1984.
19. Jenkins, D. W., Fisk, D. E., and Byrd, R. B. Mediastinal histoplasmosis with esophageal abscess. Two case reports. Gastroenterology 70:109, 1976.
19a. Coss, K. C., Wheat, L. J., Conces, D. J., Brashear, R. E., and Hull, M. T. Esophageal fistula complicating mediastinal histoplasmosis. Response to amphotericin B. Am. J. Med. 83:343, 1987.
20. Lewicki, A. M., and Moore, J. P. Esophageal moniliasis: a review of common and less frequent characteristics. AJR 125:218, 1975.
21. Frager, D. H., Frager, J. D., Brandt, L. J., Wolf, E. L., Rand, L. G., Klein R. S., and Beneventano, T. C. Gastrointestinal complications of AIDS: radiologic features. Radiology 158:597, 1986.
22. Athey, P. A., Goldstein, H. M., and Dodd, G. D. Radiologic spectrum of opportunistic infections of the upper gastrointestinal tract. AJR 129:419, 1977.
23. Jones, J. M. Necrotizing candida esophagitis: failure of symptoms and roentgenographic findings to reflect severity. JAMA 244:2190, 1980.
24. Farman, J., Tavitian, A., Rosenthal, L. E., Schwartz, G. E., and Raufman, J. P. Focal esophageal candidiasis in acquired immunodeficiency syndrome (AIDS). Gastrointest. Radiol. 11:213, 1986.
25. Ho, C. S., Cullen, J. B., and Gray, R. R. An unusual manifestation of esophageal moniliasis. Report of two cases. Radiology 123:287, 1977.
26. Young, J. A., and Elias, E. Gastro-oesophageal candidiasis: diagnosis by brush cytology. J. Clin. Pathol. 38:293, 1985.

27. Knoke, M., and Bernhardt, H. Endoscopic aspects of mycosis in the upper digestive tract. Endoscopy 12:295, 1980.
28. Bentlif, P. S., and Wiedermann, B. Esophagitis caused by Torulopsis glabrata. Case report. Am. J. Gastroenterol. 71:395, 1979.
29. McKenzie, R., and Khakoo, R. Blastomycosis of the esophagus presenting with gastrointestinal bleeding. Gastroenterology 88:1271, 1985.
30. Jacobs, D. H., Macher, A. M., Handler, R., Bennett, J. E., Collen, M. J., and Gallin, J. I. Esophageal cryptococcosis in a patient with the hyperimmune immunoglobulin E–recurrent infection (Job's) syndrome. Gastroenterology 87:201, 1984.
31. Young, R. C., Bennett, J. E., Vogel, C. L., Carbone, D. P., and DeVita, V. T. Aspergillosis. The spectrum of the disease in 98 patients. Medicine 49:147, 1970.
31a. Tom, W., and Aaron, J. S. Esophageal ulcers caused by Torulopsis glabrata in a patient with acquired immune deficiency syndrome. Am. J. Gastroenterol. 82:766, 1987.
32. Fazio, R. A., Wickremesinghe, P. C., and Arsura, E. L. Ketoconazole treatment of Candida esophagitis—a prospective study of 12 cases. Am. J. Gastroenterol. 78:261, 1983.
33. Hann, I. M., Prentice, H. G., and Corringham, R. Ketoconazole versus nystatin plus amphotericin B for fungal prophylaxis in severely immunocompromised patients. Lancet 1:826, 1982.
34. Quintiliani, R., Owens, N. J., Quercia, R. A., Klimek, J. J., and Nightingale, C. H. Treatment and prevention of oropharyngeal candidiasis. Am. J. Med. 77:44, 1984.
35. Agha, F. P., Lee, H. H., and Nostrant, T. T. Herpetic esophagitis: a diagnostic challenge in immunocompromised patients. Am. J. Gastroenterol. 81:246, 1986.
36. Nash, G., and Ross, J. S. Herpetic esophagitis. A common cause of esophageal ulceration. Hum. Pathol. 5:339, 1974.
37. Buss, D. H., and Scharyj, M. Herpesvirus infection of the esophagus and other visceral organs in adults. Incidence and clinical significance. Am. J. Med. 66:457, 1979.
38. Berg, J. W. Esophageal herpes: a complication of cancer therapy. Cancer 8:731, 1955.
39. Fishbein, P. G., Tuthill, R., Kressel, H., Friedman, H., and Snape, W. J. Herpes simplex esophagitis. A cause of upper-gastrointestinal bleeding. Dig. Dis. Sci. 24:540, 1979.
40. Rattner, H. M., Cooper, D. J., and Zaman, M. B. Severe bleeding from herpes esophagitis. Am. J. Gastroenterol. 80:523, 1985.
41. Spencer, G. D., Hackman, R. C., McDonald, G. B., Amos, D. E., Cunningham, B. A., Meyers, J. D., and Thomas, E. D. A prospective study of unexplained nausea and vomiting after marrow transplantation. Transplantation 42:602, 1986.
42. Levine, M. S., Laufer, I., Kressel, H. Y., and Friedman, H. M. Herpes esophagitis. AJR 136:863, 1981.
43. Shortsleeve, M. J., Gauvin, G. P., Gardner, R. C., and Greenberg, M. S. Herpetic esophagitis. Radiology 141:611, 1981.
43a. Gleaves, C. A., Reed, E. C., Hackman, R. C., and Meyers, J. C. Rapid diagnosis of invasive cytomegalovirus infection by examination of tissue specimens in centrifugation culture. Am. J. Clin. Pathol. 88:354, 1987.
44. Springer, D. J., DaCosta, L. R., and Beck, I. T. A syndrome of acute self-limited ulcerative esophagitis in young adults, probably due to herpes simplex virus. Dig. Dis. Sci. 24:535, 1979.
45. Deshmukh, M., Shah, R., and McCallum, R. W. Experience with herpes esophagitis in otherwise healthy patients. Am. J. Gastroenterol. 79:173, 1984.
46. Ramsey, P. G., Fife, K. H., Hackman, R. C., Meyers, J. D., and Corey, L. Herpes simplex virus pneumonia. Clinical, virologic, and pathologic features in 20 patients. Ann. Intern. Med. 97:813, 1982.
47. Hirsch, M. S., and Schooley, R. T. Treatment of herpesvirus infections. N. Engl. J. Med. 309:963, 1034, 1983.
48. Meyers, J. D., Wade, J. C., Mitchell, C. D., Saral, R., Lietman, P. S., Durack, D. T., Levin, M. J., Segreti, A. C., and Balfour, H. H., Jr. Multicenter collaborative trial of intravenous acyclovir for the treatment of mucocutaneous herpes simplex virus infection in the immunocompromised host. Am. J. Med. 73:229, 1982.
49. Shepp, D. H., Newton, B. A., Dandliker, P. S., Flournoy, N., and Meyers, J. D. Oral acyclovir therapy for mucocutaneous herpes simplex virus infections in immunocompromised marrow transplant recipients. Ann. Intern. Med. 102:783, 1985.
50. Wade, J. C., Newton, B., Flournoy, N., and Meyers, J. D. Oral acyclovir for prevention of herpes simplex virus reactivation after marrow transplantation. Ann. Intern. Med. 100:823, 1984.
51. Meyers, J. D., Flournoy, N., and Thomas, E. D. Cytomegalovirus infections and specific cell-mediated immunity after marrow transplant. J. Infect. Dis. 142:816, 1980.
52. Villar, L. A., Massanari, R. M., and Mitros, F. A. Cytomegalovirus infection with acute erosive esophagitis. Am. J. Med. 76:924, 1984.
53. St. Onge, G., and Bezahler, G. H. Giant esophageal ulcer associated with cytomegalovirus. Gastroenterology 83:127, 1982.
54. Gertler, S. L., Pressman, J., Price, P., Brozinsky, S., and Miyai, K. Gastrointestinal cytomegalovirus infection in a homosexual man with severe acquired immunodeficiency syndrome. Gastroenterology 85:1403, 1983.
55. Toghill, P. J., and McGaughey, M. Cytomegalovirus oesophagitis. Br. Med. J. 2:294, 1972.
56. Freedman, P. G., Weiner, B. C., and Balthazar, E. J. Cytomegalovirus esophagogastritis in a patient with acquired immunodeficiency syndrome. Am. J. Gastroenterol. 80:434, 1985.
57. Balthazar, E. J., Megibow, A. J., Hulnick, D., Cho, K. C., and Beranbaum, E. Cytomegalovirus esophagitis in AIDS: radiographic features in 16 patients. AJR 149:919, 1987.
58. Myerson, D., Hackman, R. C., Nelson, R. A., Ward, D. C., and McDougall, J. K. Widespread presence of histologically occult cytomegalovirus. Hum. Pathol. 15:430, 1984.
59. Erice, A., Jordan, M. C., Chace, B. A., Fletcher, C., Chinnock, B. J., and Balfour, H. H. Ganciclovir treatment of cytomegalovirus disease in transplant recipients and other immunocompromised hosts. JAMA 257:3082, 1987.
59a. Chachoua, A., Dieterich, D., Krasinski, K., Greene, J., Laubenstein, L., Wernz, J., Buhles, W., Koretz, S. 9-(1,3-dihydroxy-2-propoxymethyl)guanine (Ganciclovir) in the treatment of cytomegalovirus gastrointestinal disease with the acquired immunodeficiency syndrome. Ann. Intern. Med. 107:133, 1987.
60. Ringden, O., Lonnqvist, B., Paulin, T., Ahlmen, J., Kluitmalm, G., Wahren, B., and Lernestedt, J. O. Pharmacokinetics, safety, and preliminary clinical experiences using foscarnet in the treatment of cytomegalovirus infections in bone marrow and renal transplant recipients. J. Antimicrob. Chemother. 17:373, 1986.
60a. Weber, J. N., Thom, S., Barrison, I., Unwin, R., Forster, S., Jeffries, D. J., Boylston, A., and Pinching, A. J. Cytomegalovirus colitis and oesophageal ulceration in the context of AIDS: clinical manifestations and preliminary report of treatment with Foscarnet (phosphonoformate). Gut 28:482, 1987.
61. Rosen, P., and Hadju, S. Visceral herpesvirus infections in patients with cancer. Am. J. Clin. Pathol. 56:459, 1971.
62. Walsh, T. J., Belitsos, N. J., and Hamilton, S. R. Bacterial esophagitis in immunocompromised patients. Arch. Intern. Med. 146:1345, 1986.
63. Gilver, R. L. Esophageal lesions in leukemia and lymphoma. Dig. Dis. Sci. 15:31, 1970.
64. McDonald, G. B., and Vracko, R. Systemic absorption of oral cholestyramine. Gastroenterology 87:213, 1984.
65. McManus, J. P. A., and Webb, J. N. A yeast-like infection of the esophagus caused by Lactobacillus acidophilus. Gastroenterology 68:583, 1975.
66. Howlett, S. A. Acute streptococcal esophagitis. Gastrointest. Endosc. 25:150, 1979.
67. Pelemans, W., and Hellemans, J. Tuberculosis of the esophagus. In Vantrappen, G., and Hellemans, J. (eds.). Diseases of the Esophagus. New York, Springer-Verlag, 1974, pp. 553–555.
68. de Mas, R., Lombeck, G., and Riemann, J. F. Tuberculosis of the oesophagus masquerading as ulcerated tumor. Endoscopy 18:153, 1986.

69. Seivewright, N., Feehally, J., and Wicks, A. C. B. Primary tuberculosis of the esophagus. Am. J. Gastroenterol. *79*:842, 1984.

69a. Damtew, B., Frengley, D., Wolinksy, E., and Spagnuolo, P. J. Esophageal tuberculosis: mimicry of gastrointestinal malignancy. Rev. Infect. Dis. *9*:140, 1987.

70. Williford, M. E., Thompson, W. M., Hamilton, J. D., and Postlethwait, R. W. Esophageal tuberculosis: findings on barium swallow and computed tomography. Gastrointest. Radiol. *8*:119, 1983.

71. Pelemans, W., and Vantrappen, G. Syphilis of the esophagus. *In* Vantrappen, G., and Hellermans, J. (eds.). Diseases of the Esophagus. New York, Springer-Verlag, 1974, pp. 556–557.

72. Wang, L., and Karmody, C. S. Dysphagia as the presenting symptom of tetanus. Arch. Otolaryngol. *111*:342, 1985.

73. Koberle, F. Chagas' disease and Chagas' syndrome: the pathology of American trypanosomiasis. Advanc. Parasitol. *6*:63, 1968.

74. Earlham, R. J. Gastrointestinal aspects of Chagas' disease. Am. J. Dig. Dis. *17*:559, 1972.

75. Mota, E., Todd, C. W., Maguire, J. H., Portugal, D., Santana, O., Ribeiro Filho, R., and Sherlock, I. A. Megoesophagus and seroreactivity to *Trypanosoma cruzi* in a rural community in northeast Brazil. Am. J. Trop. Med. Hyg. *33*:820, 1984.

76. Kazlow, P. G., Shah, K., Benkov, K. J., Dische, R., and LeLeiko, N. S. Esophageal cryptosporidiosis in a child with acquired immune deficiency syndrome. Gastroenterology *91*:1301, 1986.

76a. Grimes, M. M., LaPook, J. D., Bar, M. H., Wasserman, H. S., and Dwork, A. Disseminated *Pneumocystis carinii* infection in a patient with acquired immunodeficiency syndrome. Hum. Pathol. *18*:307, 1987.

77. Geboes, K., and Pelemans, W. Miscellaneous and rare diseases. *In* Vantrappen, G., and Hellemans, J. (eds.). Diseases of the Esophagus. New York, Springer-Verlag, 1974, p. 839.

78. Geboes, K., and Janssens, J. The esophagus in cutaneous diseases. *In* Vantrappen, G., and Hellemans, J. (eds.). Diseases of the Esophagus. New York, Springer-Verlag, 1974, pp.823–833.

79. Schuman, B. M., and Arciniegas, E. The management of esophageal complications of epidermolysis bullosa. Am. J. Dig. Dis. *17*:875, 1972.

80. Agha, F. P., Francis, I. R., and Ellis, C. N. Esophageal involvement in epidermolysis bullosa dystrophica: clinical and roentgenographic manifestations. Gastrointest. Radiol. *8*:111, 1983.

81. Feurle, G. E., Weidauer, H., Baldauf, G., Schulte-Braucks, T., and Anton-Lamprecht, I. Management of esophageal stenosis in recessive epidermolysis bullosa. Gastroenterology *87*:1376, 1984.

82. Tishler, J. M., Han, S. Y., and Helman, C. A. Esophageal involvement in epidermolysis bullosa dystrophica. AJR *141*:1283, 1983.

83. Harmel, R. P. Esophageal replacement in two siblings with epidermolysis bullosa. J. Pediatr. Surg. *21*:175, 1986.

84. Fonkalsrud, E. W., and Ament, M. E. Surgical management of esophageal stricture due to recessive dystrophic epidermolysis bullosa. J. Pediatr. Surg. *12*:221, 1977.

85. Kaplan, R. P., Touloukian, J., Ahmed, A. R., and Newcomer, V. D. Esophagitis dissecans superficialis associated with pemphigus vulgaris. J. Am. Acad. Dermatol. *4*:682, 1981.

86. Kaneko, F., Mori, M., Tsukinaga, I., and Miura, Y. Pemphigus vulgaris of esophageal mucosa. Arch. Dermatol. *121*:272, 1985.

87. Yamamoto, H., Kozawa, Y., Otake, S., and Shimokawa, R. Pemphigus vulgaris involving the mouth and esophagus. Report of a case and review of the literature. Int. J. Oral Surg. *12*:194, 1983.

88. Barnes, L. M., Clark, M. L., Estes, S. A., and Bongiovanni, G. L. Pemphigus vulgaris involving the esophagus. A case report and review of the literature. Dig. Dis. Sci. *32*:655, 1987.

89. Foroozan, P., Enta, T., Winship, D. H., and Trier, J. S. Loss and regurgitation of the esophageal mucosa in pemphigoid. Gastroenterology *53*:548, 1967.

90. Eng, T. Y., Hogan, W. J., and Jordon, R. G. Oesophageal involvement in bullous pemphigoid. A possible cause of gastrointestinal haemorrhage. Br. J. Dermatol. *99*:207, 1978.

91. Sharon, P., Greene, M. L., and Rachmilewitz, D. Esophageal involvement in bullous pemphigoid. Gastrointest. Endosc. *24*:122, 1978.

92. Person, J. R., and Rogers, R. Bullous and ciratricial pemphigoid. Mayo Clin. Proc. *52*:54, 1977.

93. Benedict, E. B., and Lever, W. F. Stenosis of the esophagus in benign mucous membrane pemphigus. Ann. Otol. Rhinol. *61*:1120, 1952.

94. Agha, F. P., and Ragi, M. R. Esophageal involvement in pemphigoid: clinical and roentgen manifestations. Gastrointest. Radiol. *7*:109, 1982.

95. Calcaterra, T. C., and Strahan, R. W. Stevens-Johnson syndrome. Oropharyngeal manifestations. Arch. Otolaryngol. *93*:37, 1971.

96. Stein, M. R., Thompson, C. K., Sawicki, J. E., and Martel, A. J. Esophageal stricture complicating Stevens-Johnson syndrome. A case report. Am. J. Gastroenterol. *62*:435, 1974.

97. Peters, M. E., Gourley, G., and Mann, F. A. Esophageal strictures and web secondary to Stevens-Johnson syndrome. Pediatr. Radiol. *13*:290, 1983.

98. Herman, T. G., Kushner, D. C., and Cleveland, R. H. Esophageal stricture secondary to drug-induced toxic epidermal necrolysis. Pediatr. Radiol. *14*:439, 1984.

99. Heer, M., Altorfer, J., Burger, H. R., and Walti, M. Bullous esophageal lesions due to cotrimoxazole: an immune-mediated process? Gastroenterology *88*:1954, 1985.

100. Lefer, L. G., Lichen planus of the esophagus. Am. J. Dermatopathol. *4*:267, 1982.

101. Al-Shihabi, B. M., and Jackson, J. M. Dysphagia due to pharyngeal and oesophageal lichen planus. J. Laryngol. Otol. *96*:567, 1982.

102. Krebs, A. Acanthosis nigricans mit Befall des Oesophagus und Mangel an vitamin A. Schweiz. Med. Wschr. *92*:545, 1962.

103. Itai, Y., Kogure, T., Okuyama, Y., and Akiyama, H. Radiological manifestations of oesophageal involvement in acanthosis nigricans. Br. J. Radiol. *49*:592, 1976.

103a. Brinson, R. R., Schuman, B. M., Mills, L. R., Thigpen, S., and Freedman, S. Multiple squamous papillomas of the esophagus associated with Goltz syndrome. Am. J. Gastroenterol. *82*:1177, 1987.

104. Harper, P. S., Harper, R. M. J., and Howel-Evans, A. W. Carcinoma of the oesophagus with tylosis. Q. J. Med. *49*:317, 1970.

105. Tyldesley, W. R., and Kempson, S. A. Ultrastructure of the oral epithelium in leukoplakia associated with tylosis and esophageal carcinoma. J. Oral Pathol. *4*:49, 1975.

106. Ritter, S. B., and Peterson, G. Esophageal cancer, hyperkeratosis, and oral leukoplakia. Occurrence in a 25-year old woman. JAMA *235*:1723, 1976.

107. Mori, S., Yoshihira, A., Kawamura, H., Takeuchi, A., Hashimoto, T., and Inaba, G. Esophageal involvement in Behçet's disease. Am. J. Gastroenterol. *78*:548, 1983.

108. Anti, M., Marra, G., Rapaccini, G. L., Barone, C., Manna, R., Bochicchio, G. B., Fedeli, G. Esophageal involvement in Behçet's syndrome. J. Clin. Gastroenterol. *8*:514, 1986.

109. Yashiro, K., Nagasako, N., Hasegawa, K., Maruyama, M., Suzuki, S., and Obata, H. Esophageal lesions in intestinal Behçet's disease. Endoscopy *18*:57, 1986.

110. McDonald, G. B., Shulman, H. M., Sullivan, K. M., and Spencer, G. D. Intestinal and hepatic complications of human bone marrow transplantation. Gastroenterology *90*:460, 770, 1986.

111. McDonald, G. B., Sullivan, K. M., Schuffler, M. D., Shulman, H. M., and Thomas, E. D. Esophageal abnormalities in chronic graft-versus-host disease in humans. Gastroenterology *80*:914, 1981.

112. McDonald, G. B., Sullivan, K. M., and Plumley, T. F. Radiographic features of esophageal involvement in chronic graft-versus-host disease. AJR *142*:501, 1984.

113. Geboes, K., Janssens, J., Rutgeerts, P., and Vantrappen, G.

Crohn's disease of the esophagus. J. Clin. Gastroenterol. *8*:31, 1986.

114. Degryse, H. R., and De Schepper, A. M. Aphthoid esophageal ulcers in Crohn's disease of ileum and colon. Gastrointest. Radiol. *9*:197, 1984.

115. Levine, M. S. Crohn's disease of the upper gastrointestinal tract. Radiol. Clin. North Am. *25*:79, 1987.

116. Cockey, B. M., Jones, B., Bayless, T. M., and Shauer, A. B. Filiform polyps of the esophagus with inflammatory bowel disease. AJR *144*:1207, 1985.

117. Huchzermeyer, H., Paul, F., Seifert, E., Frohlich, H., and Rasmussen, C. W. Endoscopic results in five patients with Crohn's disease of the esophagus. Endoscopy *8*:75, 1977.

118. Davidson, J. T., and Sawyers, J. L. Crohn's disease of the esophagus. Am. Surg. *49*:168, 1983.

119. Christopher, N. L., Watson, D. W., and Farber, E. R. Relationship of chronic ulcerative esophagitis to ulcerative colitis. Ann. Intern. Med. *70*:971, 1969.

120. Greenstein, A. J., Janowitz, M. D., and Sachar, D. M. The extraintestinal complications of Crohn's disease and ulcerative colitis. A study of 700 patients. Medicine *55*:401, 1976.

121. Zimmerman, H. M., Rosenblum, G., and Bank, S. Aphthous ulcers of the esophagus in a patient with ulcerative colitis. Gastrointest. Endosc. *30*:298, 1984.

122. Wormann, B., Sommer, A., and Ottenjann, R. Association of herpes virus infection of the esophagus and idiopathic inflammatory bowel disease. Endoscopy *17*:36, 1985.

123. Pelemans, W., and Vantrappen, G. Granulomatous esophagitis. *In* Vantrappen, G., and Hellemans, J. (eds.). Diseases of the Esophagus. New York, Springer-Verlag, 1974, p. 568.

124. Wiesner, P. J., Kleinman, M. S., Condemi, J. J., Resnicoff, S. A., and Schwartz, S. I. Sarcoidosis of the esophagus. Am. J. Dig. Dis. *16*:943, 1971.

125. Davies, R. J. Dysphagia, abdominal pain, and sarcoid granulomata. Br. Med. J. *3*:564, 1972.

126. Oakley, J. R., Lawrence, D. A., and Fiddian, R. V. Sarcoidosis associated with Crohn's disease of the ileum, mouth, and oesophagus. J. R. Soc. Med. *76*:1068, 1983.

127. Antler, A. S., Ough, Y., Pitchamoni, C. S., Davidian, M., and Thelmo, W. Gastrointestinal metastases from malignant tumors of the lung. Cancer *49*:170, 1982.

128. Steiner, H., Lammer, J., and Hackl, A. Lymphatic metastases to the esophagus. Gastrointest. Radiol. *9*:1, 1984.

129. Caramella, E., Bruneton, J. N., Roux, P., Aubanel, D., and Le Comte, P. Metastasis of the digestive tract. Report of 77 cases and review of the literature. Eur. J. Radiol. *3*:331, 1983.

130. Boccardo, F., Merlano, M., Canobbio, L., Rosso, R., and Aste, H. Esophageal involvement in breast cancer. Report of six cases. Tumori *68*:149, 1982.

131. Gale, M. E., Birmbaum, S. B., Gale, D. R., and Vincent, M. E. Esophageal invasion by lung cancer: CT diagnosis. J. Comput. Assist. Tomogr. *8*:694, 1984.

132. Anderson, M. F., and Harell, G. S. Secondary esophageal tumors. AJR *135*:1243, 1980.

133. Roark, G. D., and Schoppe, L. E. Painful dysphagia from infiltrating oat cell carcinoma. J. Clin. Gastroenterol. *5*:331, 1983.

134. den Hartog Jager, F. C., Bartelsman, J. F., and Tytgat, G. N. Palliative treatment of obstructing esophagogastric malignancy by endoscopic positioning of a plastic prosthesis. Gastroenterology *77*:1008, 1979.

135. Pass, H. I., Potter, D. A., Macher, A. M., Reichert, C., Shelhammer, J. H., Masur, H., Ognibene, F., Grelmann, E., Lane, H. C., Fauci, A., and Roth, J. A. Thoracic manifestations of the acquired immune deficiency syndrome. J. Thorac. Cardiovasc. Surg. *88*:654, 1984.

136. Patow, C. A., Stark, T. W., Findlay, P. A., Steis, R., Longo, D. L., Masur, H., and Macher, A. M. Pharyngeal obstruction by Kaposi's sarcoma in a homosexual male with acquired immune deficiency syndrome. Otolaryngol. Head Neck Surg. *92*:713, 1984.

137. Bernal, A., and del Junco, G. W. Endoscopic and pathologic features of esophageal lymphoma: a report of four cases in patients with acquired immune deficiency syndrome. Gastrointest. Endosc. *32*:96, 1986.

138. Phillips, L. G., and Cunningham, J. Esophageal perforation. Radiol. Clin. North Am. *22*:607, 1984.

139. Berry, B. E., and Ochsner, J. L. Perforation of the esophagus: a 30 year review. J. Cardiovasc. Thorac. Surg. *65*:1, 1973.

140. Michel, L., Grillo, H. C., and Malt, R. A. Esophageal perforation. Ann. Thorac. Surg. *33*:203, 1982.

141. Radmark, T., Sandberg, N., and Pettersson, G. Instrumental perforation of the oesophagus. A ten year study from two ENT clinics. J. Larygol. Otol. *100*:461, 1986.

142. Silvis, S. E., Nebel, O., Rogers, G., Sugawa, C., and Mandelstam, P. Endoscopic complications: results of the 1974 American Society for Gastrointestinal Endoscopy survey. JAMA *235*:928, 1976.

143. Dubost, C., Kaswin, D., Duranteau, A., Jehanno, C., and Kaswin, R. Esophageal perforation during attempted endotracheal intubation. J. Thorac. Cardiovasc. Surg. *78*:44, 1979.

144. Johnson, D. E., Foker, J., Munson, D. P., Nelson, A., Athinarayanan, P., and Thompson, T. R. Management of esophageal and pharyngeal perforation in the newborn infant. Pediatrics *70*:592, 1982.

145. Michel, L., Grillo, H. C., and Malt, R. A. Operative and nonoperative management of esophageal perforations. Ann. Surg. *194*:57, 1981.

146. Goldstein, L. A., and Thompson, W. R. Esophageal perforations: a 15 year experience. Am. J. Surg. *143*:495, 1982.

147. Love, L., and Berkow, A. E. Trauma to the esophagus. Gastrointest. Radiol. *2*:305, 1978.

148. Hine, K. R., and Atkinson, M. The diagnosis and management of perforations of esophagus and pharynx sustained during intubation of neoplastic esophageal strictures. Dig. Dis. Sci. *31*:571, 1986.

149. Appleton, D. S., Sandrasagra, F. A., and Flower, C. D. Perforated oesophagus: review of twenty-eight consecutive cases. Clin. Radiol. *30*:493, 1979.

150. Han, S. Y., McElvein, R. B., Aldrete, J. S., and Tishler, J. M. Perforation of the esophagus: correlation of site and cause with plain film findings. AJR *145*:537, 1985.

151. Endicott, J. N., Molony, T. B., Campbell, G., and Bartels, L. J. Esophageal perforations: the role of computerized tomography in diagnosis and management decisions. Laryngoscope *96*:751, 1986.

152. Brown, B. M. Computed tomography of mediastinal abscess secondary to post-traumatic esophageal laceration. J. Comput. Assist. Tomogr. *8*:765, 1984.

153. Han, S. Y., and Tishler, J. M. Perforations of the abdominal segment of the esophagus. AJR *143*:751, 1984.

154. Allen, K. S., Siskind, B. N., and Burrell, M. I. Perforation of distal esophagus with lesser sac extension: CT demonstration. J. Comput. Assist. Tomogr. *10*:612, 1986.

155. Wesdorp, I. C., Bartelsman, J. F., Huibregtse, K., den Hartog Jager, F. C., and Tytgat, G. N. Treatment of instrumental oesophageal perforation. Gut *25*:398, 1984.

156. Dodds, W. J., Stewart, E. T., and Vlymen, W. J. Appropriate contrast media for evaluation of esophageal disruption. Radiology *144*:439, 1982.

157. Foley, M. J., Ghahremani, G. G., and Rogers, L. F. Reappraisal of contrast media used to detect upper gastrointestinal perforations: comparison of ionic water-soluble media with barium sulfate. Radiology *144*:231, 1982.

158. Cameron, J. L., Kieffer, R. F., Hendrix, T. R., Mehigan, D. G., and Baker, R. R. Selective nonoperative management of contained intrathoracic esophageal disruptions. Ann. Thorac. Surg. *27*:404, 1979.

159. Brewer, L. A., Carter, R., Mulder, G. A., and Stiles, Q. R. Options in the management of perforations of the esophagus. Am. J. Surg. *152*:62, 1986.

160. Richardson, J. D., Martin, L. F., Borzotta, A. P., and Polk, H. C. Unifying concepts in treatment of esophageal leaks. Am. J. Surg. *149*:157, 1985.

161. Erwall, C., Ejerblad, S. A., Lindholm, C. L., and Aberg, T. Perforation of the oesophagus. A comparison between surgical and conservative treatment. Acta Otolaryngol. (Stockh.) *97*:185, 1984.

162. Lyons, W. S., Seremetis, M. G., de Guzman, V. C., and Peabody, J. W. Ruptures and perforations of the esophagus:

the case for conservative supportive management. Ann. Thorac. Surg. 25:346, 1978.

163. Shockley, W. W., Tate, J. L., and Stucker, F. J. Management of perforations of the hypopharynx and cervical esophagus. Laryngoscope 95:939, 1985.

164. Ogilvie, A. L., Dronfield, M. W., Ferguson, R., and Atkinson, M. Palliative intubation of oesophagogastric neoplasms at fibreoptic endoscopy. Gut 23:1060, 1982.

165. Quale, A. R., Moore, P. J., Jacob, G., Griffith, C. D., and Rogers, K. Treatment of oesophageal perforation by intubation. Ann. R. Coll. Surg. Engl. 67:101, 1985.

166. Asplund, C. M., and Hill, L. D. Delayed lower esophageal perforation: management with Celestin tube. Ann. Otol. Rhinol. Laryngol. 94:114, 1985.

167. Sarr, M. G., Pemberton, J. H., and Payne, W. S. Management of instrumental perforations of the esophagus. J. Thorac. Cardiovasc. Surg. 84:211, 1982.

168. Kerr, W. F. Spontaneous intramural rupture and intramural haematoma of the oesaphagus. Thorax 35:890, 1980.

169. Shay, S. S., Berendson, R. A., and Johnson, L. F. Esophageal hematoma: four new cases, a review, and proposed etiology. Dig. Dis. Sci. 26:1019, 1981.

170. Spiller, R. C., Catto, J. V., and Kane, S. P. Spontaneous dissecting intramural haematoma of the oesophagus: a rare cause of haematemesis and dysphagia. Endoscopy 13:128, 1981.

171. Watts, H. D. Postemetic hematomas: a variant of the Mallory-Weiss syndrome. Am. J. Surg. 132:320, 1976.

172. Heceta, W. G., Wruble, L. D., and Pate, J. W. Esophageal obstruction due to intermuscular hematoma following pneumatic dilation. Chest 69:115, 1976.

173. Van Steenbergen, W., Fevery, J., Broeckaert, L., Ponette, E., Baert, A., and DeGroote, J. Intramural hematoma of the esophagus: unusual complication of variceal sclerotherapy. Gastrointest. Radiol. 9:293, 1984.

173a. Pellicano, A., Watier, A., and Gentile, J. Spontaneous double-barrelled esophagus. Report of two cases and review of the literature. J. Clin. Gastroenterol. 9:149, 1987.

174. Ashman, F. C., Hill, M. C., Saba, G. P., and Diaconis, J. N. Esophageal hematoma associated with thrombocytopenia. Gastrointest. Radiol. 3:115, 1978.

175. Bradley, J. L., and Han, S. Y. Intramural hematoma (incomplete perforation) of the esophagus associated with esophageal dilation. Radiology 130:59, 1979.

176. Demos, T. C., Okrent, D. M., Studlo, J. D., and Flisak, M. E. Spontaneous esophageal hematoma diagnosed by computed tomography. J. Comput. Assist. Tomogr. 10:133, 1986.

177. Douglas, W. K. Oesophageal stricture associated with gastro-duodenal intubation. Br. J. Surg. 43:404, 1956.

178. Nagler, R., and Spiro, H. M. Persistent gastroesophageal reflux during prolonged gastric intubation. N. Engl. J. Med. 269:495, 1965.

179. Viard, H., Favre, J. P., and Petiot, A. Les oesophagites sténosantes post-opératoires. A propos de 11 cas observés après interventions n'intéressant pas l'hiatus oesophagien. Chirurgie (Paris) 101:577, 1975.

180. Balkang, T. J., Baker, B. B., Bloustein, P. A., and Jafek, B. W. Cervical esophagostomy in the dog. Endoscopic, radiographic, and histopathologic evaluation of esophagitis induced by feeding tubes. Ann. Otol. Rhinol. Laryngol. 86:588, 1977.

181. Kikendall, J. W., Friedman, A. C., Oyewole, M. A., Fleischer, D., and Johnson, L. F. Pill-induced esophageal injury. Case reports and review of the medical literature. Dig. Dis. Sci. 28:174, 1983.

181a. Bott, S., Prakash, C., and McCallum, R. W. Medication-induced esophageal injury: survey of the literature. Am. J. Gastroenterol. 82:758, 1987.

182. Evans, K. T., and Roberts, G. M. Where do all the tablets go? Lancet 2:1237, 1976.

183. Hey, H., Jorgensen, F., Sorensen, K., Hasselbalch, H., and Wamberg, T. Oesophageal transit of six commonly used tablets and capsules. Br. Med. J. 285:1717, 1982.

184. Channer, K. S., and Virjee, J. P. The effect of size and shape of tablets on their esophageal transit. J. Clin. Pharmacol. 26:141, 1986.

185. Marvola, M., Rajaniemi, M., Marttila, E., Vahervuo, K., and Sothman, A. Effect of dosage form and formulation factors on the adherence of drugs to the esophagus. J. Pharm. Sci. 72:1034, 1983.

186. Burrington, J. D. Clinitest burns of the esophagus. Ann. Thorac. Surg. 20:400, 1975.

186a. Davis, R., Thomas, L. C., and Guice, K. S. Esophagitis after papain. J. Clin. Gastroenterol. 9:127, 1987.

187. Ravich, W. J., Kashima, M., and Donner, M. W. Drug-induced esophagitis simulating esophageal carcinoma. Dysphagia 1:13, 1986.

188. Wong, R. K., Kikendall, J. W., and Dachman, A. H. Quinaglute-induced esophagitis mimicking an esophageal mass. Ann. Intern. Med. 105:62, 1986.

189. Creteur, V., Laufer, I., Kressel, H. Y., Caroline, D. F., Goren, R. A., Evers, K. A., Glick, S. N., and Gatenby, R. A. Drug-induced esophagitis detected by double-contrast radiography. Radiology 147:365, 1983.

190. Agha, F. P., Wilson, J. A. P., and Nostrand, T. T. Medication-induced esophagitis. Gastrointest. Radiol. 11:7, 1986.

191. Phillips, T. L., and Margolis, L. Radiation pathology and the clinical response of lung and esophagus. Front. Radiat. Ther. Oncol. 6:254, 1972.

192. Hellman, S., Kligerman, M. M., von Essen, C. F., and Scibetta, M. P. Sequelae of radical radiotherapy of carcinoma of the lung. Radiology 82:1055, 1964.

193. The Lung Cancer Study Group. Effects of postoperative mediastinal radiation on completely resected stage II and stage III epidermoid cancer of the lung. N. Engl. J. Med. 315:1377, 1986.

194. Cox, J. D., Byhardt, R. W., Wilson, J. F., Haas, J. S., Komaki, R., and Olson, L. E. Complications of radiation therapy and factors in their prevention. World J. Surg. 10:171, 1986.

195. Seaman, E. B., and Ackerman, L. V. The effect of radiation on the esophagus. A clinical and histologic study of the effects produced by the betatron. Radiology 68:534, 1957.

196. Novak, J. M., Collins, J. T., Donowitz, M., Farman, J., Sheahan, D. G., and Spiro, H. M. Effects of radiation on the human gastrointestinal tract. J. Clin. Gastroenterol. 1:9, 1979.

197. Berthrong, M., and Fajardo, L. F. Radiation injury in surgical pathology. Part II. Alimentary tract. Am. J. Surg. Pathol. 5:153, 1981.

198. Lepke, R. A., and Libshitz, H. I. Radiation injury of the esophagus. Radiology 148:375, 1983.

199. Papazian, A., Capron, J. P., Ducroix, J. P., Dupas, J. L., Quenum, C., and Besson, P. Mucosal bridges of the upper esophagus after radiotherapy for Hodgkin's disease. Gastroenterology 84:1028, 1983.

200. Berthrong, M. Pathologic changes secondary to radiation. World J. Surg. 10:155, 1986.

201. Kuten, A., Ben-Aryeh, H., Berdicevsky, I., Ore, L., Szargel, R., Gutman, D., and Robinson, E. Oral side effects of head and neck irradiation: correlation between clinical manifestations and laboratory data. Int. J. Radiat. Oncol. Biol. Phys. 12:401, 1986.

202. Northway, M. G., Libshitz, H. I., Osborne, B. M., Feldman, M. S., Mamel, J. J., West, J. H., and Szwarc, I. A. Radiation esophagitis in the opossum: radioprotection with indomethacin. Gastroenterology 78:883, 1980.

203. Northway, M. G., Eastwood, G. L., Libshitz, H. I., Feldman, M. S., Mamel, J. J., and Szwarc, I. A. Antiinflammatory agents protect opossum esophagus during radiotherapy. Dig. Dis. Sci. 27:923, 1982.

204. Ambrus, J. L., Ambrus, C. M., Lillie, D. B., Johnson, R. J., Gastpar, H., and Kishel, S. Effect of sodium meclofenamate on radiation-induced esophagitis and cystitis. J. Med. 15:81, 1984.

205. Nicolopoulos, N., Mantidis, A., Stathopoulos, E., Papaodyssees, S., Kouvaris, J., Varveris, H., and Papavasiliou, C. Prophylactic administration of indomethacin for irradiation esophagitis. Radiother. Oncol. 3:23, 1985.

206. Feld, R. Complications in the treatment of small cell carcinoma of the lung. Cancer Treat. Rev. 8:5, 1981.

207. Umsawasdi, T., Valdivieso, M., Barkley, H. T., Booser, D.

J., Chiuten, D. F., Murphy, W. K., Dhingra, H. M., Dixon, C. L., Farha, P., and Spitzer, G. Esophageal complications from combined chemoradiotherapy (cyclophosphamide + Adriamycin + cisplatin + XRT) in the treatment of non-small cell lung cancer. Int. J. Radiat. Oncol. Biol. Phys. *11*:511, 1985.

208. Newburger, P. E., Cassady, J. R., and Jaffe, N. Esophagitis due to Adriamycin and radiation therapy for childhood malignancy. Cancer *42*:417, 1978.

209. Greco, F. A., Brereton, M. D., Kent, H., Zimbler, H., Merrill, J., and Johnson, R. E. Adriamycin and enhanced radiation reaction in normal esophagus and skin. Ann. Intern. Med. *85*:294, 1978.

210. Horwich, A., Lokich, J. J., and Bloomer, W. D. Doxorubicin, radiotherapy and oesophageal stricture. Lancet *2*:561, 1975.

211. Boal, D. K., Newburger, P. E., and Teele, R. L. Esophagitis induced by combination radiation and Adriamycin. AJR *132*:567, 1979.

212. Eagan, R. T., Fleming, T. R., Lee, R. E., Ingle, J. N., Frytak, S., and Creagen, E. T. Chemotherapy response as a prognosticator for survival in patients with limited squamous cell lung cancer treated with combined chemotherapy and radiotherapy. Int. J. Radiat. Oncol. Biol. Phys. *6*:879, 1980.

213. McDonald, G. B., and Tirumali, N. Intestinal and liver toxicity of antineoplastic drugs. West. J. Med. *140*:250, 1984.

214. Chisholm, R. C., and Curry, S. B. Vincristine-induced dysphagia. South. Med. J. *71*:1364, 1978.

215. Westaby, D., Melia, W. M., MacDougall, B. R. D., Hegarty, J. E., and Williams, R. Injection sclerotherapy for oesophageal varices: a prospective, randomized trial of different treatment schedules. Gut *25*:129, 1984.

216. Soehendra, N., de Heer, K., Kempeneers, I., and Frommelt, L. Morphologic alterations of the esophagus after endoscopic sclerotherapy of varices. Endoscopy *15*:291, 1983.

217. Evans, D. M. D., Jones, D. B., Cleary, B. K., and Smith, P. M. Oesophageal varices treated by sclerotherapy, a histopathological study. Gut *23*:615, 1982.

218. Subramanyam, K., and Patterson, M. Chronic esophageal ulceration after endoscopic sclerotherapy. J. Clin. Gastroenterol. *8*:58, 1986.

219. Barsoum, M. S., Abdel-Wahab Mooro, H., Bolous, F. I., Ramzy, A. F., Rizk-Allah, M. A., and Mahmoud, F. I. The complications of injection sclerotherapy of bleeding oesophageal varices. Br. J. Surg. *69*:79, 1982.

220. Paquet, K. T. Endoscopic paravariceal injection sclerotherapy of the esophagus—indications, technique, complications: re-

sults of a period of 14 years. Gastrointest. Endosc. *29*:310, 1983.

221. Sorensen, T., Burcharth, F., Pedersen, M. L., and Findahl, F. Oesophageal stricture and dysphagia after endoscopic sclerotherapy for bleeding varices. Gut *25*:473, 1984.

222. Ayres, S. J., Goff, J. S., and Warren, G. H. Endoscopic sclerotherapy for bleeding esophageal varices: effects and complications. Ann. Intern. Med. *98*:900, 1983.

223. Agha, A. P. The esophagus after endoscopic injection sclerotherapy: acute and chronic changes. Radiology *153*:37, 1984.

224. Sauerbruch, T., Wirsching, R., Leisner, B., Weinzierl, M., Pfahler, M., and Paumgartner, G. Esophageal function after sclerotherapy of bleeding varices. Scand. J. Gastroenterol. *17*:745, 1982.

225. Helpap, B., and Bollweg, L. Morphologic changes in the terminal oesophagus with varices following sclerosis of the wall. Endoscopy *13*:229, 1981.

226. Haynes, W. C., Sanowski, R. A., Foutch, P. G., and Bellapravalu, S. Esophageal strictures following endoscopic variceal sclerotherapy: clinical course and response to dilation therapy. Gastrointest. Endosc. *32*:202, 1986.

227. Reilly, J. J., Schade, R. R., and Van Thiel, D. S. Esophageal function after injection sclerotherapy: pathogenesis of esophageal stricture. Am. J. Surg. *147*:85, 1984.

228. Sauerbruch, T., Wirsching, R., Holl, J., Grobl, J., and Weinzierl, M. Effects of repeated injection sclerotherapy on acid gastroesophageal reflux. Gastrointest. Endosc. *32*:81, 1986.

229. Tabibian, N., and Alpert, E. Refractory sclerotherapy-induced esophageal strictures. Ann. Intern. Med. *106*:59, 1987.

230. Sloop, R. D., and Thompson, J. C. Aorto-esophageal fistula: report of a case and review of the literature. Gastroenterology *53*:768, 1967.

231. Carter, R., Mulder, G. A., and Snyder, E. N. Aortoesophageal fistula. Am. J. Surg. *136*:26, 1978.

232. Wilson, R. T., Dean, P. J., and Lewis, M. Aortoesophageal fistula due to a foreign body. Gastrointest. Endosc. *33*:448, 1987.

233. Ctercteko, G., and Mok, C. K. Aorto-esophageal fistula induced by a foreign body. J. Thorac. Cardiovasc. Surg. *80*:233, 1980.

234. Snyder, D. M., and Crawford, E. S. Successful treatment of primary aorto-esophageal fistula resulting from aortic aneurysm. J. Thorac. Cardiovasc. Surg. *85*:457, 1983.

235. Lambert, D. R., Llaneza, P. R., Gaglani, R. D., Lach, R. D., and Beaver, W. L. Esophageal-atrial fistula. J. Clin. Gastroenterol. *9*:345, 1987.

IV

THE STOMACH AND DUODENUM: ANATOMY, PHYSIOLOGY, AND DISEASE

Anatomy, Embryology, and Developmental Anomalies

JAMES E. McGUIGAN
MARVIN E. AMENT

39

ANATOMY OF THE STOMACH

General Anatomic Considerations

The stomach is a capacious, saccular organ that is connected superiorly with the inferior termination of the esophagus and inferiorly with the first portion of the duodenum. It is the most dilated region of the gastrointestinal tract, although its shape and capacity may vary substantially with age, body habitus, and degree of distention. The stomach is J-shaped in most normal individuals. Its capacity in the adult approximates 1500 ml. The stomach is located in the superior part of the abdomen, extending from the left hypochondrium into the epigastrium and reaching the umbilicus. It is relatively fixed at its upper and lower connections with the esophagus and duodenum but quite mobile between these sites of fixation.

The stomach has two curvatures, which have been designated the lesser and greater curvatures. The greater curvature, which extends to the left from the gastroesophageal junction, is four to six times as long as the opposing lesser curvature. The stomach and proximal duodenum are attached to the lesser omentum (hepatoduodenal ligament) and to the greater omentum. The long axis of the stomach first passes downward, then forward, to the right, and finally slightly upward and posteriorly. Much of the anterior surface of the stomach is shielded by the right and left lobes of the liver. Downward and to the left, the anterior surface of the stomach rests against the inner surface of the anterior abdominal wall. The left lateral portion of the stomach in the hypochondrium is covered by the ribs, pleural cavity, and diaphragm. The posterior surface of the stomach comprises a large portion of the anterior wall of the lesser peritoneal sac (omental bursa). The greater curvature of the stomach is located immediately above and anterior to the transverse colon. The greater curvature of the stomach is more freely movable than is the lesser curvature and is altered with position, contraction, relaxation, and distention.

The posterior surface of the stomach rests on the transverse mesocolon and the anterior surface of the pancreas. The fundus of the stomach is nestled within the cavity of the left diaphragm and laterally is in contact with the spleen. Peritoneum clothes all of the gastric surfaces. The two layers of the visceral peritoneum extend from the inferior portion of the greater curvature of the stomach as the greater omentum; on the left, they attach to the spleen as the gastrosplenic ligament.

Anatomic Regions of the Stomach

The stomach has been separated into various anatomic regions (Fig. 39–1). That portion of the stomach which immediately adjoins the esophagus has been termed the *cardia (cardiac portion)* of the stomach. The cardia is located approximately 2.5 cm to the left of the midline at the level of the ninth thoracic vertebra. The gastric *fundus* is the dome-shaped portion of the stomach that extends to the left and superiorly from the cardia. The gastric *body,* or *corpus*, is the major portion of the stomach and extends inferiorly from the fundus and the cardia to the general region of the *incisura angularis,* which is a notchlike indentation located in the lower part of the lesser curvature (Fig. 39–2).

The *antrum* of the stomach has been defined in several ways. The gross anatomic description of the antrum is usually that of the distal portion of the stomach which extends from the incisura angularis to

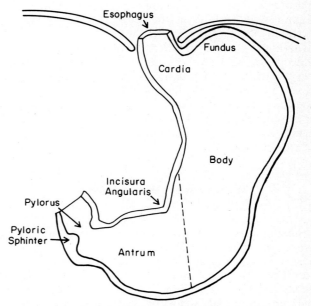

Figure 39–1. Anatomic regions of the stomach.

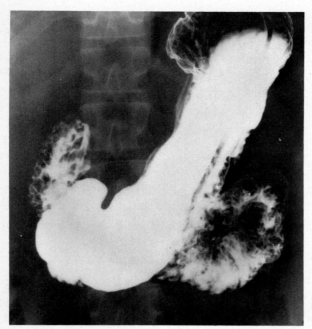

Figure 39–2. Upper gastrointestinal radiograph demonstrating incisura angularis located on distal lesser curvature. (Courtesy of James W. Weaver, M.D.)

the proximal limit of the pylorus. When the extent of the antrum is delineated functionally or by histologic features of its mucosa it includes the pylorus, and the demarcation between the antrum and the corpus is variably higher on the lesser curvature of the stomach and may extend up to two thirds of the length of the lesser curvature.

The *pylorus* is the most distal and narrowly tubular part of the stomach, with a thick muscular wall forming the *pyloric sphincter.* The lumen passing through the pyloric sphincter is termed the *pyloric canal* or *pyloric channel,* and is approximately 2.5 cm in length. The pylorus is usually located approximately 2.5 cm to the right of the midline at the level of the first lumbar vertebra and is posterior to the quadrate lobe of the liver and anterior to the neck of the pancreas. The mucosa of the gastric antrum is relatively free of parietal cells and contains the pyloric glands and the cells that contain the hormone gastrin. The oxyntic (parietal) portion of the stomach, which contains acid-secreting parietal cells and the major portion of the zymogen (chief) cells, comprises the body and fundus of the stomach.

Tissue Layers of the Stomach

The stomach, like most other portions of the gastrointestinal tract, is composed of four tissue layers: *mucosa, submucosa, muscularis propria,* and *serosa.* The mucous membrane lining of the lumen of the stomach is thick and vascular, with a smooth, soft, and velvety surface. The lining of the stomach is grayish pink in color and is thrown into numerous folds, or rugae, which, for the most part, are longitudinally directed. The mucosa of the cardia, antrum, and pylorus is paler than that of the rest of the stomach. In the filled or distended stomach, the folds flatten out and may be stretched evenly and smoothly. Numerous, barely visible gastric pits (*foveolae gastricae*) may be seen to invaginate the gastric mucosa.[1]

The major muscular component (muscularis propria) of the gastric wall, separated from the gastric mucosa by the intervening submucosa, is composed of three muscle layers: outer longitudinal, middle circular, and inner oblique. The outer longitudinal fibers, adjacent to the serosa, are most concentrated along the greater and lesser curvatures of the stomach. The middle circular fibers encircle the body of the stomach and are thickened at the pylorus to form the pyloric sphincter. The innermost oblique muscle fibers loop over the fundus and pass down over the anterior and posterior walls of the stomach. Recently a transverse gastric band has been described in normal human subjects using imaging techniques. The band is located in a position corresponding to the junction of the oblique and circular muscle layers of the stomach and separates a major portion of the gastric antrum from the gastric corpus. The anatomic basis for the band and its potential role in regulation of gastric emptying remain to be established.[1a] The serosa envelops the muscle layers of the stomach as the visceral peritoneum.

Arterial Blood Supply and Venous and Lymphatic Drainage of the Stomach

The arterial blood supply of the stomach is derived from branches of the celiac artery. The left gastric artery arises from the celiac artery, passes upward and to the left to reach the distal esophagus, then descends along the lesser curvature of the stomach to supply blood to the lower third of the esophagus and the upper right portion of the stomach. The right gastric artery, arising from the hepatic branch of the celiac artery, runs to the left along the lesser gastric curvature, supplying blood to the lower right portion of stomach. Blood supply to the gastric fundus is provided by short gastric arteries that arise from the splenic artery at the hilus of the spleen. The upper part of the greater curvature of the stomach is supplied by blood from the left gastroepiploic artery, which arises from the splenic artery at the splenic hilus. The lower portion of the greater curvature receives its blood supply from the right gastroepiploic artery, which originates from the gastroduodenal branch of the hepatic artery.

The left and right gastric veins, draining the lesser curvature of the stomach, enter directly into the portal vein. The short gastric veins, draining the fundus, and the left gastroepiploic veins, draining the upper portion of the greater curvature, join the splenic vein. Blood from the lower portion of the greater curvature is drained by the right gastroepiploic vein, which enters the superior mesenteric vein. The lymphatic drainage of the stomach parallels its arterial supply.[2]

Innervation of the Stomach

The stomach is innervated by both sympathetic and parasympathetic components of the autonomic nervous system. The sympathetic innervation of the stomach is supplied by postganglionic fibers arising from the celiac plexus through nerve plexuses located adjacent to the gastric and gastroepiploic arteries; the preganglionic sympathetic fibers arise from the sixth through the eighth (principally seventh and eighth) thoracic segments of the spinal cord. The sympathetic nerves to the stomach contain afferent pain-transmitting nerve fibers,[3] as well as motor fibers to the pyloric sphincter. The parasympathetic nerve supply to the stomach is derived from the right and left vagus nerves and their branches. The left vagus nerve, usually in the form of one or two vagal trunks, enters the abdomen on the anterior surface of the stomach. It then gives off several nerve filaments to the region of the cardia, an occasional celiac branch, and a longer major branch that runs anterior and to the right of the lesser curvature as the *anterior nerve of Latarjet*. This nerve supplies anterior gastric branches to the anterior surface of the stomach and terminates in a "crow's-foot" distribution in the region of the pylorus and distal antrum. The right vagus nerve, also usually as one or two trunks, enters the abdomen on the posterior surface of the gastroesophageal junction and supplies branches to both surfaces of the stomach and *posterior nerve of Latarjet,* which has a distribution to the posterior surface of the stomach similar to that of the anterior nerve. Both nerves of Latarjet travel in the lesser omentum 1 to 2 cm from the lesser curvature of the stomach. Vagal nerve fibers connect with gastric ganglion cells in the submucosa (Meissner's plexus) or with ganglion cells in the muscularis propria (Auerbach's plexus). Postganglionic fibers from these plexuses innervate both secretory components (glands and secretory cells) and motor components (muscle) of the stomach. Acid-secreting parietal cells, zymogen cells, and gastrin-secreting cells are innervated by postganglionic vagal fibers.

Microscopic Anatomy of the Gastric Mucosa

The innermost lining of the human stomach is composed of simple columnar epithelium that is punctuated generously by numerous pits (foveolae), approximately 3.5 million in number, which serve approximately 15 million branched, tubular glands. The epithelium, which lines the foveolae gastricae and the intervening mucosal surface, is uniform; however, differences in the gastric glands permit histologic identification of three principal gastric regions. The first region, which is 1.5 to 3 cm in length, contains the *cardiac glands* and corresponds with the gastric cardia (Fig. 39–1). The second region (the oxyntic, or acid-secreting, portion of the stomach) constitutes the fundus and body—the proximal two thirds of the stomach—and contains the *oxyntic (fundic,* or *parietal,* cell) *glands.*

The third region of the stomach contains the *pyloric,* or *antral, glands,* corresponds principally with the antrum of the stomach, and comprises the distal portions of the stomach, including the pylorus, and extends farther superiorly along the lesser than the greater curvature of the stomach (Fig. 39–1).

Surface Epithelium. The mucosa of the stomach is lined principally by a single epithelial layer of tall columnar cells, 20 to 40 μ in height. These *surface mucous cells* cover the surface of the gastric folds and ridges and extend into the gastric pits. This columnar epithelium commences abruptly at the cardia with the termination of the stratified squamous epithelium of the esophagus. The surface mucous cells have basally located nuclei with large supranuclear cytoplasmic regions densely packed with ovoid, spherical, or discoid granules within membranes of well-developed Golgi complexes (Fig. 39–3). These granules contain neutral polysaccharide protein mucin that can be stained readily by mucicarmine and periodic acid–Schiff reagents. When discharged into the lumen of the stomach, these granules produce a layer of mucus that lubricates the gastric mucosa. These cells appear to originate in the deeper portions of the foveolae and in the necks of the glands and then migrate upward, replacing those lost at the surface by desquamation. Surface mucous cells are completely renewed every one to three days.[4-6]

Oxyntic Glands. The oxyntic glands, also designated *parietal* or *gastric glands,* are relatively straight, branched epithelial tubular glands, approximately 50 μ in outer diameter (Fig. 39–4 and 39–5). They are closely packed and oriented perpendicularly to the gastric mucosal surface. The superficial portions of these tubular glands are nearly straight; their deepest portions are tortuous. The oxyntic glands average approximately 1.2 mm in length. One or more gastric glands pierce the deepest portion of each foveola. The constricted entrance of the gland from the gastric lumen has been called the *neck* of the gland. The average foveola is approximately 70 μ wide and 200 μ deep.

At least four types of cells have been identified as constituents of the oxyntic glands: (1) mucous neck cells, (2) zymogen or chief cells, (3) oxyntic or parietal cells, and (4) endocrine or endocrine-like cells. The *mucous neck cells,* located immediately below the base of the pit of the proximal constriction of the oxyntic glands, are interspersed, singly or in groups of two or three cells, among parietal cells. Mucous neck cells, which are relatively few in number, have basal nuclei and cytoplasm that is packed with granules containing an acidic mucus (glycosaminoglycan); it differs from the neutral mucus contained in and secreted by surface mucous cells. Mucous neck cells exhibit more cytoplasmic basophilia by light microscopy and more rough endoplasmic reticulum by electron microscopy than do surface mucous cells. The Golgi apparatus is extremely well developed in these cells. The cytoplasmic mucus-containing granules are more spherical and larger than those of surface mucous cells, and the granules often lie deep in the cell adjacent to the nucleus, as well as near the apex.

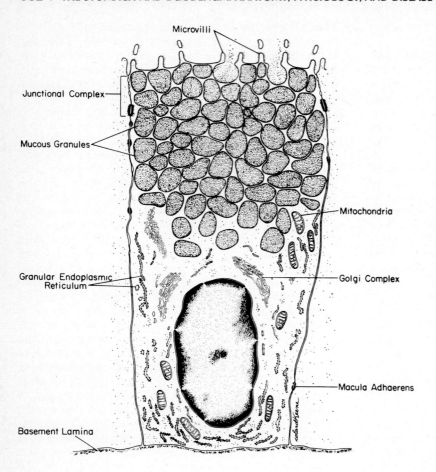

Figure 39–3. Surface mucous cell, illustrating some of its salient features. (From Ito, S. Functional gastric morphology. *In* Johnson, L. R., et al. [eds.]. Physiology of the Gastrointestinal Tract, Vol. 1. 2nd ed. New York, Raven Press, 1987. Used with permission.)

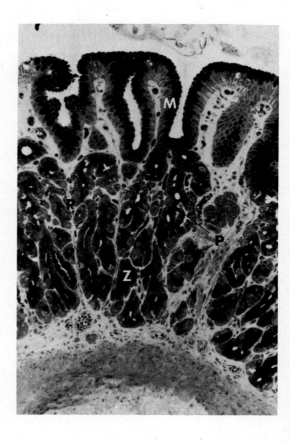

Figure 39–4. Photomicrograph of normal human gastric oxyntic gland mucosa (parietal cell region). Mucous cells (M) line the foveolae. Large, oval, light-staining parietal cells (P) are seen in the midportion of the glands. In the base of the glands, dark-staining zymogen cells (Z) may be seen. × 250. (Courtesy of Clinton B. Lillibridge, M. D.)

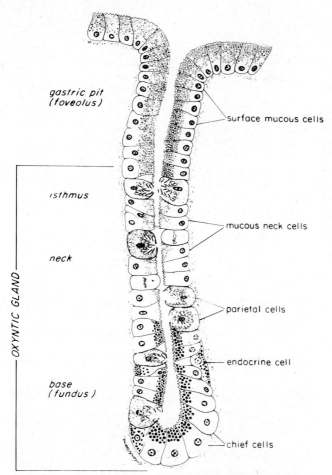

gastric pit
(foveolus)

surface mucous cells

OXYNTIC GLAND

isthmus

mucous neck cells

neck

parietal cells

endocrine cell

base
(fundus)

chief cells

Figure 39–5. Diagrammatically simplified tubular oxyntic gland from the corpus of a mammalian stomach. (From Ito, S. Functional gastric morphology. *In* Johnson, L. R., et al. [eds.]. Physiology of the Gastrointestinal Tract, Vol. 1. 2nd ed. New York, Raven Press, 1987. Used with permission.)

The *parietal (oxyntic) cells* are located principally in the upper (luminal) half of the oxyntic glands, but are also interspersed among the chief (zymogen) cells in the lower half of the gastric glands (Fig. 39–4). Parietal cells are present in much fewer numbers (almost absent) in the antral glands. The parietal cells are large (20 to 35 μ) and are usually either spherical or pyramidal in shape. Their tapered apical ends usually face the tubular glandular lumen, with their broader basal surfaces placed against the basement membrane of the

glands. The nucleus of the parietal cell is large and round, and cytoplasm is strongly eosinophilic. Parietal cells contain numerous rod-shaped or oval mitochondria with little rough endoplasmic reticulum.[7] The Golgi complex is small and basal in location. The most conspicuous morphologic feature of the parietal cell is an extensive tubulovesicular canalicular system (Fig. 39–6).

The apical luminal cell surfaces of parietal cells are deeply invaginated by intracellular (secretory) canaliculi, which represent virtual intracellular extensions of the glandular lumen. These canaliculi, which are lined by microvilli, extend in continuity with an abundance of smooth membranes in the cytoplasm as the tubulovesicular system. Transport of hydrochloric acid across this vast internalized surface occurs during its secretion. With stimulation of acid secretion, the microvilli become more abundant and the tubulovesicular system diminishes (Fig. 39–5). With inhibition of acid secretion, the reverse occurs. Human parietal cells also contain and secrete intrinsic factor.[8]

The *chief (zymogen) cells* are present in greatest numbers in the deepest portions of the oxyntic glands, lining the glandular lumen in the lower one half or one third of the glandular tubule. Zymogen cells appear as irregularly truncated pyramids approximately 7 by 16 μ. The apical cytoplasm of these cells contains numerous large, highly refractile zymogen granules, which range from 1 to 3 μ in diameter. The granules contain pepsinogens (groups I and II), the zymogen precursors of pepsins. The fine structure of the zymogen cells is similar to that of other cell types involved in synthesis and secretion of proteolytic enzymes, such as the pancreatic acinar cells. Large oval or round granules of relatively low density are found in the apical cytoplasm. The supranuclear region contains a well-developed Golgi apparatus. Granular endoplasmic reticulum is found throughout the cytoplasm but is especially concentrated in the basal portions of the cells. Basophilic staining of these cells is accounted for by the presence of abundant ribosomes, both free in the cytoplasm and attached to reticulum membranes.

A variety of *endocrine cells* are present in the epithelial lining of the gastric glands. These cells are scattered, usually singly, among parietal and zymogen cells. These endocrine cells are rounded or pyramidal in shape and rest on the basal membrane. Their cytoplasm is filled with small granules which, in many instances, may be stained with silver or chromium

Figure 39–6. Gastric parietal cell of mouse, resting (left) and after stimulation with pilocarpine (right). The cell contains a prominent nucleus (N), abundant mitochondria (M), smooth endoplasmic reticulum (R), vacuoles (V), and canaliculi (C) that swell conspicuously in response to stimulation. (Reproduced with permission from Davenport, H. W.: Physiology of the Digestive Tract. 3rd ed. Copyright 1971 by Year Book Medical Publishers, Inc., Chicago. Courtesy of A. D. Hally.)

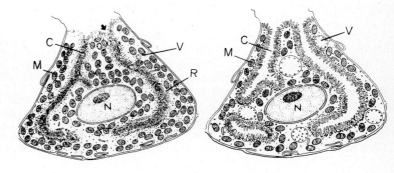

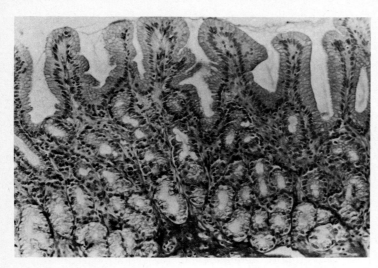

Figure 39–7. Human gastric antrum. Hematoxylin and eosin stain, × 300. (Courtesy of Clinton B. Lillibridge, M. D.)

salts. One group of these endocrine cells contains granules that reduce silver salt without pretreatment (argentaffin cells).[9–11] These cells have been shown to contain 5-hydroxytryptamine (5-HT, or serotonin).[12] Other populations of endocrine cells require exposure to a reducing substance before their granules will react with silver (argyrophil cells). Explanations for the affinity for metallic salts exhibited by these cells and for differences in the staining properties of these two populations of cells have not been elucidated.

Antral Glands. In the antral mucosal portion of the stomach, the foveolae gastricae (gastric pits) are much deeper than in other regions of the stomach (Fig. 39–7). The glands, usually referred to as antral or pyloric glands, are branched and extensively coiled tubular glands. Most of the mucosal epithelial cells lining the gland lumens have pale cytoplasm, with their nuclei located adjacent to basement membranes, and appear similar to mucous neck cells and to the cells lining duodenal Brunner's glands.

Argentaffin and argyrophil cells are also interspersed singly or in small clusters along the course of the antral glands. Some of the antral gland endocrine cells contain biogenic monoamines, such as 5-HT, and yield positive argentaffin and chromaffin reactions and also display a characteristic formaldehyde-induced yellow fluorescence. These cells are referred to as enterochromaffin cells (EC cells). Gastrin is contained in cytoplasmic granules of a population of endocrine cells designated as *gastrin cells* (or *G cells*) (Fig. 39–8).[13] These cells are located principally in the middle and deeper portions of the antral glands. Gastrin cells contain vesicular to fairly dense cytoplasmic secretory granules of variable size (200 to 400 nm), which are located principally in the basal portion of the cell (Fig. 39–9). The gastrin cells, like many but not all of the gut endocrine cells, possess an apical surface, covered with microvilli, that is in contact with the gastric lumen. Apical contact with the lumen may represent the cell's receptor pole for interaction with luminal contents. Endocrine cells of the gut that have apical contact with the gut lumen have been referred to as *open* cells, whereas those cells

that do not possess a surface exposed to the lumen have been called *closed* cells. Evidence has been provided that gastrin cells may also contain an ACTH-like peptide as well as enkephalin-endorphin related peptides.[14, 15]

Somatostatin has been demonstrated in cytoplasmic

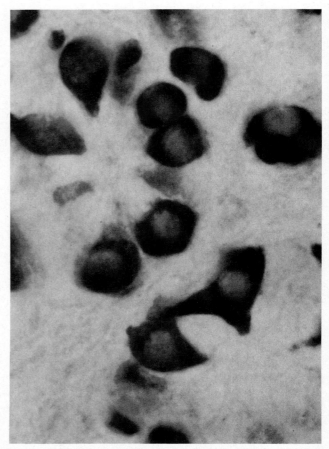

Figure 39–8. Human antral mucosa gastrin cells (G cells), with dark-staining cytoplasm, identified by immunocytochemistry using indirect immune peroxidase technique with antibodies to human gastrin I (G17). × 1200.

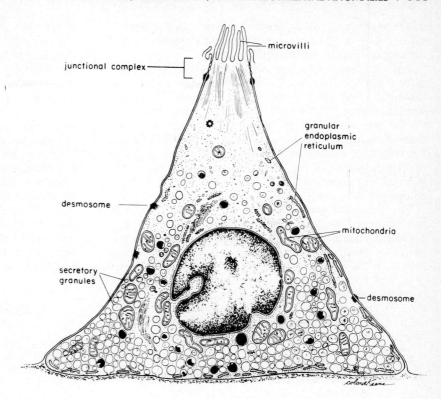

Figure 39–9. Diagram of a G cell from the pyloric gland. Gastrin endocrine cells have infranuclear secretory granules and a wide basal cytoplasm on the lamina propria. Of the many types of endocrine cells in the stomach, only the G cell and EC cell have a luminal border with microvilli. (From Ito, S. Functional gastric morphology. *In* Johnson, L. R., et al. [eds.]. Physiology of the Gastrointestinal Tract, Vol. 1. 2nd ed. New York, Raven Press, 1987. Used with permission.)

granules in endocrine cells (D cells) in the walls of both antral and oxyntic glands.[16] These cells give off cytoplasmic extensions, rich in somatostatin, which terminate on or in near proximity to potential effector cells, including gastrin cells, chief cells, and parietal cells. In the oxyntic gland region, some of these extensions appear to terminate on enterochromaffin-like (ECL) endocrine cells and in the antral glands on 5-HT–storing enterochromaffin cells. It has been proposed that somatostatin may exert local (paracrine) effects by direct communication with putative effector cells. Somatostatin cells are most frequent in the middle and lower zones of the glands and are often in close approximation to gastrin cells. It has been estimated that the ratio of somatostatin-containing cells to gastrin cells is approximately 1:3. Somatostatin-containing cells in the fundus of the stomach, unlike those of the antrum, rarely possess an apical surface in contact with the gastric lumen. Vasoactive intestinal peptide (VIP) is present in a small number of nerves and nerve cell bodies in the gastric mucosa, but not in discrete endocrine-type mucosal cells. Numerous VIP neurons can be demonstrated in the submucosa. VIP-containing nerve terminals are associated chiefly with small blood vessels, smooth muscle, and ganglion cells of the submucosal and myenteric plexuses.

Cardiac Glands. The glands in the cardia of the stomach are lined by cells similar to mucous neck cells and the mucosal epithelial cells of the pyloric glands. There is a gradual transition between the cardiac glands and the oxyntic glands containing zymogen and parietal cells.

The *lamina propria* is the connective tissue component of the gastric mucosa and lies beneath and adja-

cent to the gastric mucosa epithelium. The *muscularis mucosae,* a delicate smooth muscle layer, constitutes the deepest layer of the mucosa. Immediately deep to the mucosa is the submucosa, a connective tissue layer containing small arteries and veins; lymphoid elements, including lymphocytes and plasma cells; and the submucosal neural plexuses.

ANATOMY OF THE DUODENUM

The duodenum is a tubular organ, approximately 30 cm in length, which is in continuity with the stomach and, for the most part, is located retroperitoneally. It is shaped approximately in the form of the letter C, with its cavity toward the left and the head of the pancreas resting in this concavity. The first portion of the duodenum is approximately 5 cm in length, begins at the pylorus, and runs upward, backward, and to the right at the level of the first lumbar vertebra. The first 2.5 cm of the duodenum are freely movable and clothed by the same layers of peritoneum that envelop the stomach. The distal 2.5 cm are covered only anteriorly by peritoneum and thus are retroperitoneal. The second, or descending, portion of the duodenum is approximately 8 cm in length. Just inferior to the mid-portion of the descending duodenum is the ampulla of Vater, at which the major pancreatic and common bile ducts gain entry into the intestinal lumen. The accessory pancreatic duct may enter 2 cm superior (proximal) to the ampulla of Vater. The third, or horizontal, portion of the duodenum is approximately 10 cm long and crosses transversely anterior to the inferior vena cava and aorta. The fourth portion of the duodenum, which is about 5 cm in length, ascends along the left side of the aorta and then descends abruptly at the ligament of Treitz as the jejunum.

The duodenum is a muscular tube with outer longitudinal and inner circular smooth muscle layers. Its lumen is lined by mucosa, which in many respects is similar to that of other portions of the small intestine, which are described in detail elsewhere. Although there are minor gross and microscopic differences between the duodenum, jejunum, and ileum, each of the three parts of the small intestine has the same general organization, and transitions between these components are gradual.

The duodenal glands, or Brunner's glands, begin in the vicinity of the gastric pyloric mucosa and are usually present, in gradually diminishing numbers, in the proximal two thirds of the duodenum. They are not usually found in the jejunum or ileum. They are generously branched and coiled tubular glands arranged in lobules approximately 0.5 and 1.0 mm in diameter, penetrating the mucosa and located for the most part in the submucosa. Brunner's gland secretion is clear in appearance, viscous, and alkaline (pH 8.2 to 9.3).[17]

EMBRYOLOGIC DEVELOPMENT OF THE STOMACH AND DUODENUM

During the fifth week of intrauterine development, the primitive stomach develops as a dilatation in the foregut, caudal to the developing lung buds. During the following weeks, differential rates of growth occur in the wall of this expanded area, which result in an asymmetric shape. Rotation occurs along both a longitudinal axis and an anterior-posterior axis; the left border becomes the anterior wall, the right border becomes the posterior wall, and the stomach comes to lie more horizontally. The longitudinal rotation also results in the left and right vagus nerves predominantly innervating the anterior and posterior stomach walls, respectively. The cephalic and caudal ends of the stomach, which originated as midline structures, finally lie on an axis that runs from above left to below right. The greater curvature of the stomach, which develops from the original posterior wall, faces downward and to the left. The pyloric portion of the stomach migrates upward and to the right, and the cardiac portion migrates downward and to the left.

The duodenum is formed from the most distal portion of the embryonic foregut and the most proximal portion of the midgut. These two embryonic portions of the primitive foregut meet and fuse distal to what will become the ampulla of Vater. The duodenum also rotates to the right during gastric rotation and forms the C loop in its retroperitoneal position. During organogenesis, the intestinal lumen is temporarily obliterated; failure of recanalization results in stenosis or atresia. The dorsal mesentery in the 8-mm embryo extends from the terminal esophagus to the cloaca. The ventral mesentery is present only in the distal esophagus, stomach, and upper duodenum. During gastric rotation, the liver extends into the ventral mesentery. Eventually, the ventral mesentery extends from the lesser curvature of the stomach to the lesser omentum, to and encasing the liver, and then further extends as the falciform ligament to the ventral abdominal wall. That portion of the dorsal mesentery that suspends the primitive foregut is called the dorsal mesogastrium and extends to the left in the form of a large sac, the omental bursa. That which originally was the right peritoneal surface of the dorsal mesogastrium becomes the lining of the interior of this sac. That which was the left surface of the dorsal mesogastrium constitutes the exterior of the omental bursa. The anterior wall of this sac envelops the spleen and attaches to the greater gastric curvature. The posterior surface of this sac is pressed against the dorsal body wall and covers the pancreas.

CONGENITAL ABNORMALITIES OF THE STOMACH AND DUODENUM

Atresia

Gastric, antral, and pyloric *atresias* are conditions in which the stomach is totally occluded by a blindly ending stomach or by two apparent membranes connected by an atretic strand of mucosa and submucosa while the seromuscular layer remains normal.[18] Rarely, the stomach ends blindly, and the pylorus is replaced by a fibrous band that links the stomach to the duodenum.

Etiology and Pathogenesis. The pathogenesis of the condition is unknown, but local vascular factors may play a part. Complete atresia is an autosomal recessive disorder.[19] In those who have partial obstruction, the cause is unknown. The pathogenesis is secondary to failure of recanalization of the gastric lumen. The reported male-to-female ratio has been approximately 11:15, and the incidence of these abnormalities is 1 per cent of all gastrointestinal atresias. In the autosomal recessive variety of this condition, there is little chance that the patient's child would have this condition unless the mate is heterozygous or also is affected. The condition has been reported in those with chromosome 21 trisomy. Junctional epidermolysis bullosa has been associated with complete pyloric atresia in a number of reported cases.

Clinical Features and Diagnosis. Nonbilious vomiting in a newborn infant with a scaphoid lower abdomen and distended stomach is a typical feature of the condition. The mothers usually have hydramnios. Radiographic examination discloses only a large, air-filled stomach with no second "bubble." These patients develop hypokalemic alkalosis, dehydration, and starvation if they are not managed appropriately.

Treatment. Laparotomy, gastroduodenostomy, gastrojejunostomy, or incision of the membrane of atretic segment is the appropriate therapy for the condition.

Membranes

Congenital pyloric and antral membranes are conditions in which the stomach fails fully to recanalize. The cause of pyloric and antral membranes has not been determined. The conditions are congenital in nature, but the majority are not detected during infancy and childhood. The number of reported cases is small.[20] The antral and pyloric membranes usually contain either squamous or columnar epithelium and usually have a central ring of variable diameter.

Clinical Features and Diagnosis. The membranes may produce no obstructive symptoms until adult life. Patients with this condition have been described as late as the sixth decade. Less commonly, infants may have projectile vomiting in the neonatal period.[21] Symptoms may be precipitated by inflammation and edema around the central orifice of the membrane. At times, the condition may not be detected by upper gastrointestinal series and may require endoscopy in order to define it. Ultrasonographic study of the antrum shows a partitioning of the antrum by the membrane and narrowing of the gastric channel. Upper gastrointestinal series shows the pyloric region to be rounded and blunted, and no muscular indentation of the antrum or duodenal cap is visualized. Emptying of the stomach is greatly delayed, and, when it occurs, barium passes in a thin stream from the center of the obstruction.

Treatment. Surgical treatment is simple and consists of incision or excision of the membrane combined with pyloroplasty and antroplasty. Nonoperative treatment through an endoscope has been described in which the membranes have been cut endoscopically.

Microgastria

Congenital *microgastria* or *hypoplasia* is a condition in which the stomach fails to become differentiated from the primitive foregut. The number of recognized cases is small and, therefore, a male-to-female sex ratio has not been established. The incidence of this condition also has not been established. Its prevalence is extremely rare.[22] This congenital condition has not been described in families but has been found in association with other congenital malformations.[23] Typically, the stomach remains tiny and simple and persists in the midline without development of the curvature or rotation into the normal oblique position. The cause of congenital microgastria has not been identified.

Clinical Features and Diagnosis. This condition is diagnosed by upper gastrointestinal examination and is always associated with failure of rotation of the stomach without differentiation into fundus, body, and pyloric areas. The esophagus is usually dilated and takes over some storage function. Vomiting, hematemesis, malnutrition, and secondary anemia are noted at birth and intensify if the condition is not corrected.

Treatment and Prognosis. Surgical correction is impossible; nursing or feeding in the upright position is the only treatment possible. This condition has been found primarily in infants with serious cardiac abnormalities and appears to be the principal limiting factor in their life expectancy.[24] These patients generally have poor health and most die early. Two patients followed for long periods slowly developed functional stomachs.

Gastric Duplication

Gastric *duplication* or triplication is a rare condition in which a mass or mass lesions develop in the stomach that are distinct from it and that contain all layers of the gastric wall.[25] Synonyms for gastric duplication are gastric enterocystoma, cardioduodenal duct, and reduplication of the stomach.

Etiology and Pathogenesis. Gastric duplications are very rare,[26] and triplications are even rarer. The male-to-female ratio was 1:8 in one series of duplications. The risk of recurrence for a patient's sibling or a patient's child is unknown in either condition. True gastric duplications have a distinctive wall of three layers of smooth muscle and the lining of the gastric epithelium. They vary in size and shape and may be tubular, fusiform, or spherical. They rarely communicate with the lumen of the stomach. Gastric duplications are found most commonly along the greater curvature of the stomach,[27] as are triplications. They also may occur at the pylorus or as an extragastric pouch communicating with the pancreas.

Clinical Features and Diagnosis. These conditions may present as an asymptomatic upper abdominal mass or a mass with vomiting or gastrointestinal bleeding; they may simulate pyloric stenosis. They may also present as diffuse peritonitis caused by rupture of the duplication or triplication. An abdominal mass is almost always palpable. Radiographic studies with contrast material sometimes verify the diagnosis but usually demonstrate only pressure effects along the greater curvature of the stomach and obstruction. These features, with depression of the splenic flexure, are suggestive of gastric duplication or triplication. Communication between the duplication and the stomach occurs in 20 per cent of cases. Bleeding may present as hematemesis, melena, or unexplained anemia.[28] Perforation of the cyst into the abdomen is a serious complication, resulting in peritonitis. Rarely, carcinoma develops in the duplication.

Pathogenesis of this condition is probably the persistence of a solid stage, with failure of coalescence of vacuoles forming a lumen.

Treatment. Complete surgical excision of the duplication or triplication is the treatment of choice and is the most common therapy. In the case of complete duplication, gastrogastrostomy allows free drainage of secretions.

Neonatal Gastric Perforations

Perforation of the stomach in the neonatal period is a rare and dramatic occurrence. Eighty to 90 per cent of cases occur in the first five days of life.[29, 30]

Etiology and Pathogenesis. Patients who are predisposed to the condition are premature infants who have been hypoxic or have had nasogastric tubes placed in the stomach.[31] Neonatal peptic ulceration and distal small intestinal obstruction are other associated conditions.[32] The greater curvature of the stomach is the most frequent point of rupture. Pathologically, the perforations appear as linear breaks in the gastric wall. Diffuse hemorrhage is often present in the submucosa, accompanied by mucosal edema and thrombosis of blood vessels.

Clinical Features and Diagnosis. Symptoms occur rapidly after birth, in most cases with an acute onset. The infant refuses to feed and may vomit blood. The infant rapidly develops respiratory distress, with increasing abdominal distention. The abdomen is tympanitic and tender. Shock follows if the condition is not diagnosed rapidly. Abdominal radiographs in the upright and supine positions will show free air under the diaphragm.[33] A laparotomy is required to establish the diagnosis.

Treatment and Prognosis. A nasogastric tube should be placed for decompression, and fluid and electrolyte deficits should be corrected. The gastric defect is usually obvious. Affected areas should be sutured. Plication may be necessary to reinforce the closure. Careful search must be made for a distal intestinal obstruction. A gastrostomy should be made to ensure postoperative decompression. Emergency surgical repair is requisite. Prognosis largely depends on promptness of surgery.[30]

Infantile Hypertrophic Pyloric Stenosis

Hypertrophic pyloric stenosis is a congenital obstructing lesion involving the gastric outlet at the level of the pylorus. It is the most common disorder requiring abdominal surgery during the first six months of life.[34, 35] It occurs in one of 250 births. Its frequency is highest in Caucasians,[36] less common in non-Caucasians, and rare in Asiatics, especially the Chinese.

Etiology and Pathogenesis. The cause and pathogenesis of pyloric stenosis are subject to speculation. There have been several theories about its cause. One particularly interesting observation was made by Dodge, who showed that administration of pentagastrin to pregnant dogs induced pyloric hypertrophy in some offspring, presumably by enhancing antral contractions of the fetus.[37] The condition is rare outside early infancy, suggesting that stomachs of newborn infants are particularly susceptible to the pathophysiologic influences involved.

Genetics. It is believed that pyloric stenosis is a polygenic and sex-modified condition in its mode of inheritance. Familial aggregations of pyloric stenosis occur frequently, but they do not obey mendelian principles. Males are affected three or four times as frequently as females.[38] Identical twins usually show concordance for the condition.[39] Male relatives of female patients are especially likely to be affected.[40] If a patient and the mother both had pyloric stenosis, a brother would have a risk of one in five and a sister a risk of one in 14. If the patient alone were affected, there is a chance of one in 20 that a brother would also be affected and one in 40 for a sister. If a woman has pyloric stenosis, there is a one in five chance that her sons will have the condition and a one in 14 chance that her daughters will. If the patient is male and had pyloric stenosis as an infant, there is a one in 20 chance for his sons to have it and a one in 40 chance for his daughters. Patients with pyloric stenosis are most likely to belong to blood group B, O, or AB.[41]

Other factors that predispose to pyloric stenosis are being a first-born male, having a high birth weight, and being born to professional parents.[42] Pyloric stenosis has been seen in association with trisomy 18, long arm deletion 21, Turner's syndrome (XO), Smith-Lemli-Opitz syndrome, Cornelia deLange Amsterdam dwarf syndrome, esophageal atresia, partial thoracic stomach, phenylketonuria, maternal myasthenia gravis, rubella embryopathy, and Hirschsprung's disease.[41]

Pathology. Histologically, these individuals have pyloric muscular hypertrophy and mucosal edema. Some lymphocyte infiltration is often seen in the submucosal muscular layers. There are no significant changes in the autonomic ganglia. Following successful surgery, the tumor mass disappears, and operation at a later date reveals only a small scar; however, in some instances the muscular hypertrophy may not disappear for many years, although the patient can be completely free of symptoms.

Clinical Features and Diagnosis. The typical infant with hypertrophic pyloric stenosis begins to vomit at three to four weeks of age. However, 20 per cent have onset of symptoms in the first week of life.[43] Rarely, symptoms may not begin until the third month of life. Initially, there may be only regurgitation, but soon the characteristic projectile nonbilious vomiting occurs. Regurgitation through the nostrils is common. Typically, the vomitus is free of bile; however, red blood or "coffee grounds" may be present in one fifth of cases.[44] Vomiting may occur immediately after feeding, but may be delayed until a sufficient volume accumulates. Following vomiting, the infant still has a voracious appetite and wants to feed again. Only when the infant becomes severely wasted may he or she become weak and lose interest in feeding. Constipation develops because the infants do not retain a sufficient volume of feeding. Stools become hard and irregular. Urinary output is gradually reduced, and the urine becomes concentrated.

Typically, parents, physicians, and nurses attribute the vomiting to improper feeding habits or to formula intolerance. Several formula changes may take place before the diagnosis is established.

Physical examination typically demonstrates a wasted and at times dehydrated infant, the degree related to the duration of symptoms. *Visible peristalsis* and a *palpable pyloric tumor* are the characteristic diagnostic features of pyloric stenosis. The infant is best examined during a test meal while feeding. The abdomen is exposed and the child is held in the mother's left arm when the infant feeds from the breast or bottle. The examiner sits at the same level facing the mother and watches the infant's peristalsis. Even when peristalsis is not seen, epigastric distention may be observed.

The site of the tumor varies according to the position and degree of dilatation of the stomach; it may be found from the level of the umbilicus to high up in the angle between the liver and the stomach. The latter position is the most frequent. Hypertrophy of the pylorus is felt as an olive-like lump, which contracts and relaxes as the baby feeds. The tumor may be impossible to feel when located behind the dilated antrum. For this reason it is best to palpate the abdomen immediately after the child has vomited or after aspiration of the gastric contents.

Jaundice occurs in less than 3 per cent of patients with pyloric stenosis.[45] It is caused by elevated serum levels of the unconjugated bilirubin. Pathogenesis of the jaundice is not known, but it appears to be secondary to inhibition of glucuronyl transferase activity caused by deficiency of glucose.

A plain film of the abdomen should be obtained in the erect posture in patients in whom a definite mass is not palpated after an adequate test meal. A plain film should demonstrate a distended stomach and relative lack of intestinal gas. Ultrasonography has become the commonest method to diagnose hypertrophic pyloric stenosis. Of the three pyloric measurements made (pyloric muscle diameter, pyloric muscle thickness, and pyloric muscle length) the last was the most accurate (97.8 per cent). Upper gastrointestinal series should be done only if the pylorus cannot be identified by ultrasonography (Fig. 39–10). If an upper gastrointestinal series is done, the stomach should be aspirated beforehand. Following ingestion of small amounts of barium mixture, the baby should be made to lie semiprone. The diagnostic radiographic abnormalities that are seen include elongation and narrowing of the pyloric channel, indentation of the duodenal cap and pyloric antrum by the tumor, and a double track produced by partial blockage of the canal by thickened mucosa (Fig. 39–10).[46]

Treatment. The first step in the management of pyloric stenosis is replacement of fluid and electrolytes when dehydration is present. Hypochloremic alkalosis will be corrected when adequate sodium, chloride, and potassium have been given. Only when the child's condition is stable is he or she ready for surgical treatment. The preferred surgical procedure is the Ramstedt pyloromyotomy, in which a longitudinal incision is made on the anterior surface of the pylorus through the serosa down to the submucosa, resulting in a division of the ring of pyloric muscle.[47] Some vomiting is expected during the first few postoperative days, especially when the preoperative history is a long one.[48]

Medical therapy for pyloric stenosis is used in Europe, particularly in the Scandinavian countries.[49] This therapy involves the use of either atropine, methyl nitrate, or scopolamine methyl nitrate. Because of its high failure rate surgery becomes necessary in one third of cases. For this reason it is not used in the United States.

The prognosis is excellent. After pyloromyotomy, symptoms gradually vanish, and pyloric hypertrophy eventually disappears. Following surgery, the growth and development of affected infants are within the expected range. Long-term follow-up studies indicate liquid emptying is significantly faster following pyloromyotomy than in normal controls, and duodenal reflux is greater.[50]

Adult Hypertrophic Pyloric Stenosis

Symptoms of congenital hypertrophic pyloric stenosis may on rare occasion be seen in adults.[51]

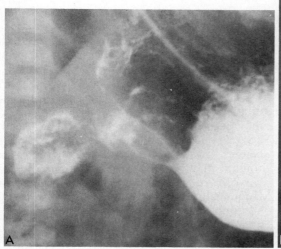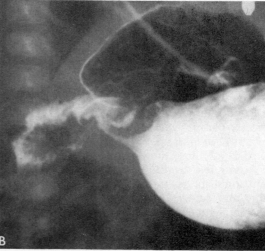

Figure 39–10. *A,* Upper gastrointestinal series in a three-month-old infant with hypertrophic pyloric stenosis. The pyloric channel is elongated and shows a thin column of barium. More barium is moving through the channel in *B* than in *A.*

Etiology and Pathogenesis. The incidence of adult hypertrophic pyloric stenosis is unknown. Many physicians believe this condition is secondary to local disease such as pyloric ulcer disease, cancer, gastritis, and prolonged pyloric spasm, leading to hypertrophy of the circular pyloric muscle bundle. Others believe the condition in adults is the same entity observed in infants and children, but is milder and later in its clinical appearance.

The histologic and anatomic abnormalities in adult hypertrophic pyloric stenosis are indistinguishable from those in the infantile form. The absence of documented associated local disease and demonstration of the familial interoccurrence of infantile congenital hypertrophic pyloric stenosis with the adult form support, at least in some instances, a genetic predisposition for development of the adult form of hypertrophic pyloric stenosis.[52]

Clinical Features and Diagnosis. Symptoms in some patients may extend from infancy. Nausea and vomiting, with epigastric pain, weight loss, and anorexia, are the most common symptoms. They may be either persistent or episodic. Ultrasonography should be considered the method of choice for screening adults with this condition. Findings should be comparable to those in infants. The lesion may be demonstrated by upper gastrointestinal series. In contrast to congenital pyloric stenosis in the infant, there is no palpable abdominal mass in adult hypertrophic pyloric stenosis, because the mass is small. The pyloric channel is substantially elongated and narrowed. Emptying of barium from the stomach is usually delayed.[53] The condition must be differentiated from pyloric channel peptic ulcer disease and gastric carcinoma involving this portion of the stomach.

Treatment. Surgical treatment is required for alleviation of symptoms associated with adult hypertrophic pyloric stenosis. Pyloromyotomy or local resection of the involved region of the pylorus is the surgical procedure of choice. The need for a certain diagnosis and, in particular, the need to exclude localized carcinoma in the region of the pylorus are important reasons to resect the involved area.[54]

Volvulus of the Stomach

Volvulus of the stomach is a very rare disorder. Fewer than 50 cases have been reported. This disorder may occur around either of two axes: *organoaxial* (cardiopyloric line) or *mesenteroaxial* (a line connecting the center of both curvatures).[54a]

In organoaxial volvulus, the gastric antrum rotates upward and from left to right. In mesenteroaxial volvulus, the antrum rotates upward and from right to left, producing an "upside down" stomach. In either case, the gastric ligaments, particularly the gastrosplenic, are normally long or relaxed.[55]

Clinical Features and Diagnosis. Recurrent crying and vomiting and refusal of feedings are occasional symptoms. The epigastrium is distended, and giant peristaltic waves may be visible. Vomiting after meals suggests the diagnosis. The radiologic features may be diagnostic. Plain films reveal gastric distention, often with a double fluid level. Upper gastrointestinal series demonstrate the volvulus, unless gastric filling is impossible because of gastroesophageal obstruction.

Treatment. Emergency medical treatment may be provided by passage of a gastric tube to relieve symptoms. Surgery is required to cure the condition and consists of reduction of the volvulus and anterior gastropexy.

Congenital Duodenal Obstruction

Several different congenital abnormalities may result in partial or complete obstruction of the gastrointestinal tract at the level of the duodenum. These include *duodenal stenosis, duodenal atresia,* and *annular pancreas.*

Duodenal atresia means complete obliteration of the lumen of the duodenum. Duodenal stenosis indicates partial obstruction. Both atresia and stenosis may affect the duodenum proximal to (20 per cent) or distal from (80 per cent) the ampulla of Vater.[56] Both conditions are rare and occur in one of 16,000 to 20,000 births. Duodenal obstruction may be present in any one of several forms: the lumen may be entirely discontinuous, with no evidence of a remnant of the intestinal channel; a membranous ring or web may be present in the duodenum; the duodenum may terminate in a dilated blind end with a fibrous cord running to the distal undilated bowel; or diaphragmatic obstruction of the duodenum may be relatively complete, with only a tiny lumen.

Etiology and Pathogenesis. The cause of the duodenal atresia and stenosis has not been defined. Two hypotheses have been proposed. In the sixth or seventh week of embryonic development, epithelial proliferation in the duodenum occludes its lumen. In normal embryologic development, this transient obstruction is shortly relieved by recanalization secondary to vacuolization; it has been suggested that this fails to occur in patients with duodenal atresia or stenosis. Alternatively, others have proposed that duodenal stenosis and atresia result from ischemia caused by vascular defects in the embryo.

Clinical Features and Diagnosis

Complete Obstruction. In the newborn infant, vomiting begins within a few hours after birth or following the first feedings.[57] The vomiting is usually bilious, because most atresias involve the postampullary duodenum. Distention is limited to the epigastrium. Meconium may be passed. Polyhydramnios occurs in 50 per cent of the patients and jaundice in one third.[58] Duodenal atresia may be recognized in the fetus when a "double bubble" is recognized on real time ultrasonography.[59]

Partial Obstruction (Stenosis of Diaphragm). When duodenal obstruction is partial, symptoms of obstruction are intermittent and may fail to appear for weeks,

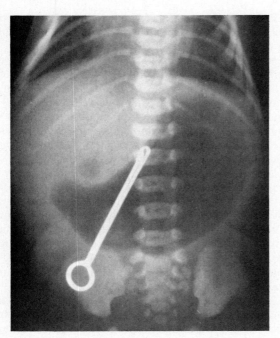

Figure 39–11. Flat plate of the abdomen in a patient with duodenal atresia, showing the "double bubble" sign.

months, or years. The clinical and radiographic findings indicate either partial or complete duodenal obstruction. Plain films of the abdomen usually show gastric and duodenal gaseous distention proximal to the "double bubble" sign (Fig. 39–11). Protracted vomiting and dehydration may occur with little in the stomach. Total absence of gas from the intestinal tract distal to the obstruction suggests atresia or extrinsic obstruction severe enough to completely occlude the lumen. Air scattered in the lower bowel may indicate partial duodenal obstruction.

In less than 2 per cent of patients with duodenal atresia or stenosis, the intestine is shorter than normal. Approximately 54 per cent of the patients are premature by birth weight. Vomiting is the first symptom in over 80 per cent of patients and is bile stained in three fourths of them. Abdominal distention, usually localized to the upper abdomen, is seen in over one third of patients. Meconium is passed in more than 52 per cent of patients prior to surgery. Jaundice occurs in approximately one third of patients and occasionally requires exchange transfusion.

Approximately 30 per cent have chromosome 21 trisomy syndrome. Malrotation of the colon with incomplete intestinal fixation occurs in approximately 22 per cent, and congenital heart disease occurs in 20 per cent of the patients. Annular pancreas is the commonest anomaly associated with duodenal atresia and stenosis.[60] Tracheoesophageal fistula and renal malformations are slightly less common. A male-to-female ratio for the condition is 1:1. The condition occurs in one of 10,000 live births, and there is no racial predilection. The risk of recurrence for a patient's sibling is one in 10,000 and for the patient's own child one in 10,000.

Treatment. The usual surgical treatment is duodenojejunostomy; gastrojejunostomy may be an alternative for those with atresia of the first part of the duodenum. During surgery, the remaining portions of the small intestine and colon should be examined to look for other sites of atresia and for malrotation, which sometimes accompanies duodenal atresia or stenosis. It is usually not possible to resect localized duodenal diaphragms or stenotic atretic segments. For patients with these, a bypass procedure is preferable.

Prognosis and Complications. The mortality rate associated with surgical correction of duodenal stenosis or atresia is related to early diagnosis and correction before perforation and peritonitis occur. Survival rate is 91 per cent for duodenal defects. This represents a major improvement over past decades.

Congenital Extrinsic Duodenal Obstruction

The extrinsic variety of duodenal obstruction occurs more commonly in males. It is usually secondary to congenital Ladd's bands, with or without associated malrotation. It may also occur with an *annular pancreas, preduodenal portal vein,* or *duplication* of the *duodenum. Incomplete rotation* of the duodenojejunal loop can result in redundancy and kinking of the jejunum, with partial intestinal obstruction noted in the presence of normal rotation of the colon.[61]

Clinical Signs. When obstruction is complete, the symptoms and signs are the same as for intrinsic duodenal obstruction. The diagnosis is more difficult when obstruction is only partial; persistent regurgitation may be the only sign. Bilious vomiting is one of the most common signs.

Diagnosis. The upper gastrointestinal series demonstrates site, severity, and cause of most partial obstructions of the duodenum.

Treatment. Gastrojejunostomy or duodenojejunostomy is used as a corrective measure for proximal duodenal obstruction.[60]

Annular Pancreas

Annular pancreas is a rare condition, in which obstruction occurs at the level of the second portion of the duodenum and is produced by an anomalous ring of pancreatic tissue.

Etiology and Pathogenesis. There are several forms of incomplete rotation of the dorsal and ventral anlagen of the pancreas, which result in portions of the pancreas remaining on both sides of the second part of the duodenum. The exact mode of formation of the defect is not known; perhaps several different variations in rotation may result in annular rings of the pancreas producing various grades of obstruction. Several investigators believe that obstruction, when present, is due to a stenosis of the duodenum, and that there is no true constriction by the surrounding pancreas.

There is an equal male-to-female sex ratio in this

condition, which occurs in one of 10,000 live births. Chromosome 21 trisomy is found in 20 to 30 per cent of patients. Anomalies of other organs are detected in 40 to 50 per cent of patients. The risk of occurrence in siblings or children of the patient is unknown.

Clinical Features and Diagnosis. All grades of obstruction are found, ranging from complete duodenal obstruction in the neonate associated with maternal hydramnios and bile-stained vomitus to intermittent vomiting and failure to thrive in the older infant and child.[62, 63] Nonobstructing, symptomless forms may be found at operation or autopsy.

Major diagnostic criteria for this condition are intestinal obstruction with a "double bubble" gas pattern by plain films of the abdomen, and the demonstration of a collar of pancreas surrounding the duodenum at laparotomy (Fig. 39–12). Both CT scan and ultrasonography may also be used to establish the diagnosis.[62]

Complications. Defective pancreatic drainage with pancreatitis later in life is a potential problem. Occasional stasis ulcer of the duodenum with perforation into the annular pancreas is another. Failure to thrive secondary to occasional vomiting is a third complication in cases that are diagnosed late in infancy and childhood.

Treatment. The operation of choice is either duodenostomy or duodenojejunostomy. Operative dissection or division of the pancreatic annulus should not be attempted.

Prognosis. Following surgical correction of the obstruction, patients are usually asymptomatic.

Malrotation with Duodenal Obstruction

The most common cause of duodenal obstruction in childhood is *intestinal malrotation.*

Etiology and Pathogenesis. The failure of attachment of the mesentery to the posterior abdominal wall results in an incompletely rotated or highly mobile cecum. The second portion of the duodenum may be obstructed by peritoneal bands when the cecum is not completely rotated. These bands extend from the cecum to the right posterior lateral abdominal wall.

In a second type of malrotation, the colon has rotated normally, but the hepatic flexure of the colon is higher than normal and lies medial to the duodenum, which is compressed by bands originating from the hepatic flexure. When the duodenojejunal loop has failed to complete its rotation while the cecocolic loop assumes its normal position in fixation, the duodenum and ligament of Treitz remain to the right of the midline.[64] Bands commonly obstruct the distal portion of the third part of the duodenum. This anomaly of rotation may also lead to kinking of the duodenum.

In the fourth variety, bands occur in the absence of any error of rotation in either the duodenum or the colon. This condition is considered to represent hypertrophy of hepatoduodenal ligaments that obstruct the duodenum at the junction of its first and second portions.

Clinical Features. Seventy per cent of the symptomatic patients have evidence of *high intestinal obstruction* within the first three weeks of life.[65] Typically, the newborn infant retains food for the first 24 to 48 hours, then begins vomiting, which becomes bilious. Abdominal distention, localized at the upper abdomen, is frequent, and visible peristaltic waves can occur. *Volvulus* also may lead to vascular obstruction of the midgut, which may be manifested by melena, currant jelly stools, and, eventually, sepsis, perforation, and peritonitis.

Malrotation is associated with *annular pancreas, congenital atresia,* or *stenosis* of the duodenum in 25 per cent of patients. Nonrotation is also associated with midgut volvulus found in patients with omphaloceles, gastroschisis, and hernias through the foramen of Bochdalek. The dorsal mesentery supports the entire intestine in these latter cases. Congenital heart disease is the most common extraintestinal abnormality associated with malrotation.

Less than 5 per cent of patients become symptomatic later than the first few months of life.[66] They have intermittent symptoms of obstruction, recurring at frequent intervals after meals. Rarely they have a malabsorption syndrome.[67] Even rarer is a watery diarrhea syndrome associated with chylous ascites, which occurs secondary to chronic lymphatic and venous obstruction. Many patients with anomalies of intestinal rotation are asymptomatic throughout life.

Diagnosis. The flat film of the abdomen may be normal or demonstrate dilatation of the proximal duodenum and the stomach. In the small infant with severe obstruction, air may be absent from the intestine. Upper gastrointestinal series delineates the sites of obstruction and reveals the malrotation by demonstrating the cecum in the right upper abdomen (Fig. 39–13). Ultrasonography may be used to diagnose intestinal obstruction and volvulus in utero.[68]

Treatment. Surgery is the only treatment for midgut volvulus with duodenal obstruction. Infarction of the intestine requires resection of the involved intestine. The surgical procedure required consists of division of

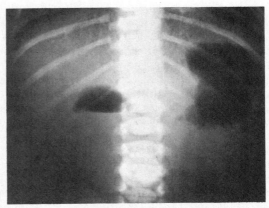

Figure 39–12. Upright film of the abdomen in a patient with annular pancreas shows the "double bubble" sign. Duodenal atresia cannot at times be separated from annular pancreas until exploratory laparotomy.

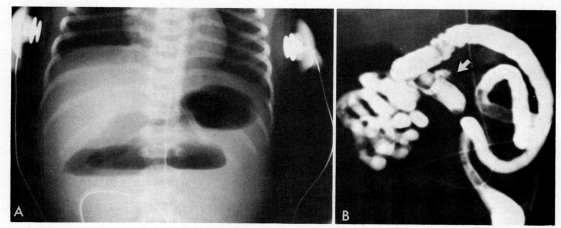

Figure 39–13. *A*, Upright film of the abdomen in a patient with malrotation and complete high bowel obstruction. The limited numbers of air-fluid levels indicate the obstruction is high. *B*, The cecum is located in the midline and high in the abdomen. The small intestine is entirely displaced in the right side of the abdomen and twisted around the superior mesenteric artery.

obstructing bands and relief of the volvulus; stabilization of the cecum may be necessary to avoid recurrent episodes of volvulus.

Prognosis and Complications. Fifteen to 20 per cent of the infants and children operated on for malrotation die. This occurs because of extensive ischemia of the small intestine, which may have to be removed, and may result in severe malabsorption. Total parenteral nutrition now provides many of these patients with massive small intestinal resection the opportunity for intestinal adaptation and in some instances for life support for those whose intestines cannot adapt (see pp. 2007–2023).

There is an equal male-to-female ratio in this condition. The frequency is unknown. The risk of occurrence for a patient's sibling or a patient's own child is also unknown. Over one half the patients become symptomatic within the first ten days of life and three fourths within the first month of life. Hydrops fetalis may be a clinical sign of volvulus in the newborn.[69] The remainder of the patients can continue to be asymptomatic or can develop symptoms at any age.

Gastric Diverticulum

Gastric diverticulum is a rare abnormality and, in general, does not produce symptoms. There are no characteristic symptoms or signs; the diagnosis is made usually by radiographic studies. The sex ratio of this phenomenon is unknown. Its incidence is very rare. Its risk in the patient's sibling or patient's child is small.

Clinical Findings. No characteristic clinical findings are present. The abnormality is usually identified radiographically as an outpouching extending from the juxtacardiac posterior gastric wall. The diverticulum involves all layers of the gastric wall. Gastric diverticula may occur near the pylorus, in association with high, small intestinal obstruction; in these instances, they represent acquired lesions.

Complications. Patients occasionally may present

with severe vomiting, which is produced by pressure effects of the diverticulum causing pyloric or duodenal obstruction.

Specific treatment for this condition is rarely indicated.

Gastric Teratoma

This is an exceedingly rare congenital abnormality. The cause of the gastric teratoma and its pathogenesis are unknown.

This condition usually presents as a large, upper abdominal mass, with calcification as shown on radiographs suggesting the diagnosis. Confirmation requires demonstration of gross and microscopic pathology.

Clinical Findings. In one fifth of patients, the condition presents with an upper abdominal mass or gastrointestinal bleeding. Respiratory difficulties associated with intestinal obstruction may be produced by pressure from the large abdominal mass. There are no usual associated congenital anomalies.

This condition has been found primarily in males. It is extremely rare. The risk for the patient's siblings and children is small.

Treatment. Surgical resection of the tumor, by either partial or total gastrectomy, is indicated. It has been stated that patients with this condition nearly always survive surgery without difficulty.

References

1. Bloom, W., and Fawcett, D. W. A Textbook of Histology. Ed. 10. Philadelphia, W. B. Saunders Co., 1975, pp. 644, 647.
1a. Moore, J. G., Dubois, A., Christian, P. E., Elgin, D., and Alazraki, N. Evidence for a midgastric transverse band in humans. Gastroenterology *91*:540, 1986.
2. Coller, F. A., Kay, E. B., and McIntyre, R. S. Regional lymphatic metastases of carcinoma of the stomach. Arch. Surg. *43*:748, 1941.
3. Kimura, C. Visceral sensation. Acta Neuroveg. *28*:405, 1966.
4. Baker, B. L. Cell replacement in the stomach. Gastroenterology *46*:202, 1964.

5. Lipkin, M. P., Sherlock, P., and Bell, B. Cell proliferation kinetics in the gastrointestinal tract of man. II. Cell renewal in stomach, ileum, colon, and rectum. Gastroenterology 45:721, 1963.

6. MacDonald, W. C., Trier, J. S., and Everett, N. B. Cell proliferation in the stomach, duodenum, and rectum of man. Gastroenterology 46:405, 1964.

7. Lillibridge, C. B. The fine structure of normal human gastric mucosa. Gastroenterology 47:269, 1964.

8. Hoedemaeker, P. J., Abels, J., Wachters, J. J., Arends, A., and Niewig, N. O. Investigations about the site of production of Castle's gastric intrinsic factor. Lab. Invest. 13:1394, 1964.

9. Dawson, A. B. Argentophile and argentaffin cells in the gastric mucosa of the rat. Anat. Rec. 100:319, 1948.

10. Holcenberg, J., and Benditt, E. P. A new histochemical technique for demonstration of enterochromaffin cells. J. Histochem. Cytochem. 7:303, 1959.

11. Holcenberg, J., and Benditt, E. P. A new color reaction for tryptamine derivatives. Histochemical applications to enterochromaffin cells. Lab. Invest. 10:144, 1961.

12. Pentilla, A. Histochemical reactions of the enterochromaffin cells and the 5-hydroxytryptamine content of the mammalian duodenum. Acta Physiol. Scand. 69, Suppl. 281:7, 1966.

13. McGuigan, J. E. Gastric mucosal intracellular localization of gastrin by immunofluorescence. Gastroenterology 55:315, 1968.

14. Larsson, L.-I. Adrenocorticotropin-like and melanotropin-like peptides in a subpopulation of human gastrin cell granules: Bioassay, immunoassay, and immunocytochemical evidence. Proc. Natl. Acad. Sci. 78:2990, 1981.

15. Larsson, L.-I., and Stengaard-Pedersen, K. Enkephalin/endorphin-related peptides in antropyloric gastrin cells. J. Histochem. Cytochem. 29:1088, 1981.

16. Larsson, L.-I., Goltermann, N., DeMagistris, L., Rehfeld, J. F., and Schwartz, T. W. Somatostatin cell processes as pathways for paracrine secretion. Science 205:1393, 1979.

17. Grossman, M. I. The glands of Brunner. Physiol. Rev. 38:675, 1958.

18. Brandon, F. M., and Weidner, W. A. Antral mucosal membrane, a congenital obstructing lesion of the stomach. AJR 411:386, 1972.

19. Bar-Maor, J. A., Nissan, S., and Nevo, S. Pyloric atresia: a hereditary congenital anomaly with autosomal recessive transmission. J. Med. Genet. 9:70, 1972.

20. Liechtl, R. E., Mikkelson, W. P., and Snyder, W. H. Prepyloric stenosis caused by congenital squamous epithelial diaphragm—resultant infantilism. Surgery 53:670, 1963.

21. Dodge, J. A. The stomach. In Anderson, C. M., and Burke, V. (eds.). Paediatric Gastroenterology. Oxford, Blackwell Scientific Publications, 1976, p. 93.

22. Schultz, R. D. Microgastrie congénitale. Ann. Radiol. 14:285, 1971.

23. Rubinstein, B., Bloom, H., Fluck, R., and Grand, M. J. H. Anomalous position of the foregut. AJR 86:582, 1961.

24. Young, G. B. Duplication of the stomach. Br. J. Radiol. 38:853, 1965.

25. Gray, D. H. Total reduplication of the stomach: A rare anomaly. Aust. N.Z. J. Surg. 41:130, 1971.

26. Grosfeld, J. L., Boles, E. T., and Reiner, C. Duplication of the pylorus in the newborn: a rare cause of gastric outlet obstruction. J. Pediatr. Surg. 5:365, 1970.

27. Parker, B. C., Guthrie, J., France, N. E., and Atwell, J. D. Gastric duplications in infancy. J. Pediatr. Surg. 7:294, 1972.

28. Cloutier, R. Pseudocyst of the pancreas secondary to gastric duplication. J. Pediatr. Surg. 8:67, 1973.

29. Holgersen, L. O. The etiology of spontaneous gastric perforation of the newborn: a re-evaluation. J. Pediatr. Surg. 16:608, 1981.

30. Dubos, J. P., Hanesse, M., Ricout, M., Bouchez, M. C., Hadrzynski, C., Lequien, P., and Ponte, C. Les perforations gastriques néonatales. Ann. Pediatr. 31:641, 1985.

31. Bayatpour, M., Bernard, L., McCune, F., and Barill, W.: Spontaneous gastric rupture in the newborn. Am. J. Surg. 137:267, 1979.

32. Houch, W. S., and Griffon, J. A.: Spontaneous linear tears of the stomach in the newborn infant. Ann. Surg. 193:763, 1981.

33. Jones, T. B., Kirchen, S. G., Lee, F. A., and Heller, R. M.: Stomach rupture associated with esophageal atresia, tracheo-esophageal fistula and ventilatory assistance. AJR 134:675, 1980.

34. Benson, D. C. Infantile pyloric stenosis. Prog. Pediatr. Surg. 1:63, 1970.

35. Bell, M. J. Infantile pyloric stenosis: experience with 305 cases at Louisville Children's Hospital. Surgery 64:983, 1968.

36. Shim, W. K. T., Campbell, A., and Wright, S. W. Pyloric stenosis in the racial groups of Hawaii. J. Pediatr. 70:89, 1970.

37. Dodge, J. A. Production of duodenal ulcers and hypertrophic pyloric stenosis by administration of pentagastrin to pregnant and newborn dogs. Nature 225:284, 1970.

38. Dodge, J. A. Infantile pyloric stenosis. A multifactorial condition. Birth Defects 8:15, 1972.

39. Dodge, J. A. Genetics of hypertrophic pyloric stenosis. Clin. Gastroenterol. 2:523, 1973.

40. Dodge, J. A. Abnormal distribution of ABO blood groups in infantile pyloric stenosis. J. Med. Genet. 8:468, 1971.

41. Whalen, J. V., and Asch, M. J. Report of two patients with hypertrophic pyloric stenosis and Hirschsprung's disease. Am. Surg. 51:480, 1985.

42. Franklin, E. A., and Saldino, R. N. Hypertrophic pyloric stenosis complicating esophageal atresia with tracheo-esophageal fistula. Am. J. Surg. 117:647, 1969.

43. Geer, L. L., Gaisie, G., Mandell, V. S., Scatliff, J. H., and Thullen, J. D.: Evolution of pyloric stenosis in the first week of life. Pediatr. Radiol. 15:205, 1985.

44. Scharli, A., Sieber, W. K., and Kiesewetter, W. B. Hypertrophic pyloric stenosis at the Children's Hospital of Pittsburgh from 1912 to 1967. J. Pediatr. Surg. 4:108, 1969.

45. Arias, I. M., Schorr, J. B., and Eraad, C. M. Clinic Conference: congenital hypertrophic pyloric stenosis with jaundice. Pediatrics 24:338, 1959.

46. Cremin, B. J., Cywes, S., and Louw, J. H. The Radiological Diagnosis of Digestive Tract Disorders in the Newborn. London, Butterworth, 1973.

47. Prosser, R. Infantile hypertrophic pyloric stenosis. Surgery 58:881, 1965.

48. Benson, C. D., and Lloyd, J. R. Infantile pyloric stenosis. A review of 1,120 cases. Am. J. Surg. 107:429, 1964.

49. Day, L. R: Medical management of pyloric stenosis. JAMA 207:949, 1969.

50. Berglund, G., and Rabo, E. A long-term followup investigation of patients with hypertrophic pyloric stenosis—with special reference to heredity and later morbidity. Acta Paediatr. Scand. 62:130, 1963.

51. Zavala, C., Bolio, A., Montalvo, R., and Lisuer, R. Hypertrophic pyloric stenosis: adult and congenital types occurring in the same family. J. Med. Genet. 6:126, 1969.

52. Woo-Ming, M. Familial relationship between adult and infantile hypertrophic pyloric stenosis. Br. Med. J. 1:476, 1961.

53. Wellman, K. F., Kagan, A., and Fang, H. Hypertrophic pyloric stenosis in adults. Survey of the literature and report of a case of the localized form. Gastroenterology 46:601, 1964.

54. Skoryna, S. C., Dolan, H. S., and Gley, A. Development of primary pyloric hypertrophy in adults in relation to the structure and function of the pyloric canal. Surg. Gynecol. Obstet. 108:83, 1959.

54a. Gean, A. D., and Deluca, S. A. Acute gastric volvulus. Am. Fam. Pract. 34:99, 1986.

55. Campbell, J. B., Rappaport, L. N., and Sherker, L. B. Acute mesentero-axial volvulus of the stomach. Radiology 103:153, 1972.

56. Sheridan, R. L., Shay, S. S., and d'Avis, J. C. Adult duodenal web associated with reflex esophagitis. Am. J. Gastroenterol. 81:718, 1986.

57. Fonkalsrud, E. W., DeLorimier, A. A., and Hays, D. M. Congenital atresia and stenosis of duodenum: a review compiled from the members of the surgical section of the American Academy of Pediatrics. Pediatrics 43:79, 1969.

58. Girvan, D. P., and Stephens, C. A. Congenital duodenal obstruction: A 20-year review of its surgical management and consequences. J. Pediatr. Surg. 9:833, 1974.

59. Brown, W. Case history: Diagnosis of fetal duodenal atresia. Radiography 50:30, 1984.

60. Rescorla, F. J., and Grosfeld, J. L. Intestinal atresia and stenosis: analysis of survival in 120 cases. Surgery *98*:668, 1985.
61. Wayne, E. R., and Burrington, J. D. Extrinsic duodenal obstruction in children. Surg. Gynecol. Obstet. *136*:87, 1973.
62. Novetsky, G. J., Berlin, L., Smith, C., and Epstein, A. J.: CT diagnosis of annular pancreas. J. Comput. Assist. Tomogr. *8*:1031, 1984.
63. Feuchtwanger, M. M., and Weiss, Y. Side to side duodeno-duodenostomy for obstructing annular pancreas in the newborn. J. Pediatr. Surg. *3*:398, 1968.
64. Berdon, W. E., Baker, D. H., Bull, S., and Santulli, T. V. Midgut malrotation and volvulus. Radiology *96*:375, 1970.
65. Firor, H. V., and Harris, V. J. Rotational abnormalities of the gut. AJR *120*:315, 1974.
66. Ellenberg, D. J., and del Castillo, J. Duodenal obstruction from peritoneal (Ladd's) bands in a ten-year-old child. Ann. Emerg. Med. *13*:56, 1984.
67. Rees, J. R., and Redo, S. F. Anomalies of intestinal rotation and fixation. Am. J. Surg. *116*:834, 1968.
68. Samuel, N., Dicker, D., Feldberg, D., and Goldman, J. A. Ultrasound diagnosis and management of fetal intestinal obstruction and volvulus in utero. J. Perinat. Med. *12*:333, 1984.
69. Nogami, W., Weber, T., and Lemons, J. A. Hydrops fetalis associated with midgut volvulus. J. Pediatr. Surg. *20*:177, 1985.

Motor Function of the Stomach in Health and Disease

RICHARD W. McCALLUM

Advances in our knowledge of gastrointestinal motility have progressed geometrically. Recognition of gastric emptying abnormalities as clinicopathologic entities has spurred an abundance of research and pharmaceutical trials, paving the way for an accumulation of information on the diagnosis and management of disorders of delayed gastric emptying. Gastric stasis has now been appreciated as part of the clinical expression of a number of medical conditions, and new clinical entities such as "idiopathic" gastric stasis and gastrointestinal pseudo-obstruction are accepted. Pioneering diagnostic techniques are opening the way to more sophisticated technologic advances capable of defining and quantitating delayed gastric emptying. New therapeutic methods have arisen from the concepts of gastrointestinal electrophysiology and radionuclide measurements of gastrointestinal transit. A new pharmacologic division of "prokinetic" agents capable of regularizing and coordinating gastrointestinal transit has arrived, with promising agents on the horizon.

PHYSIOLOGY OF GASTRIC EMPTYING

Gastric Emptying of Liquids and Solids

Gastric emptying of solids and liquids occurs separately, as different anatomic areas of the stomach are involved in each. Historically this concept can be dated to the beginning of the twentieth century. Most of the early theories of how the stomach functioned as a reservoir and an emptier derived from fluoroscopic observations, starting with those of Cannon.[1] The general idea was that the distal portion of the stomach, or the antrum, could be seen to undergo orderly peristaltic contractions and worked as a pump, whereas the proximal aspect of the stomach, which did not appear to contract very much, functioned as a storage area. This idea of the antrum as a pump was further advanced in the early part of the present century by observations in animals with duodenal fistulas, in which material emptying from the stomach into the duodenum came out in spurts, resembling bursts of antral contractions. In the 1950s, Thomas[2] and others, using balloon kymographs, showed that certain materials in foods, such as fat in the intestine, were powerful inhibitors of antral contractions, and they also slowed gastric emptying. In the 1960s, there was an explosive growth in all areas of gastrointestinal physiology, but particularly in motility. Contributing factors were better instrumentation for both electrical and manometric recordings, the ability to label and track foods, and developments in related areas such as gastrointestinal hormones. Among the most important developments, in terms of understanding the physiology of the stomach, was the penchant in the early 1960s for surgeons to invent new operations for gastric and duodenal ulcers. These operations had profound effects on gastric motility, focusing further interest on the stomach. Most importantly, electrophysiologic studies reinforced the earlier radiographic ideas that the stomach really

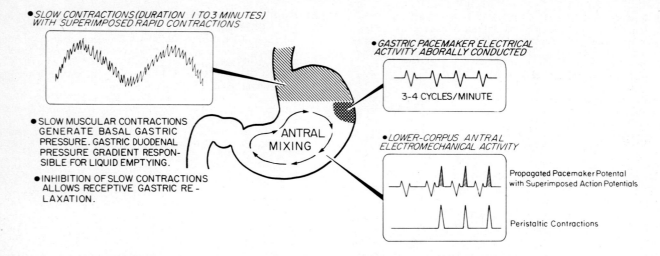

PERISTALIC CONTRACTIONS TRITURATE DIGESTIBLE SOLIDS TO NEAR LIQUIFIED FORM

Figure 40–1. Motor activity of proximal stomach and electrical and motor activity of distal stomach, summarizing their contributions to gastric emptying of liquids and digestible solids, respectively.

is two organs in one—the distal portion of the stomach, which is electrically active, and the proximal portion, which is electrically silent and thought to be a reservoir.

Gastric Emptying of Liquids

Liquid emptying is controlled by the fundus and proximal body of the stomach directly related to the gastroduodenal pressure gradient generated by two types of gastric contractions: rapid phasic contractions superimposed on slow, sustained, or tonic contractions[3] (Fig. 40–1). These sustained contractions result in the development of the basal gastric pressure within the stomach and a gastric-duodenal pressure gradient responsible for liquid emptying.

Deglutition and gastric distention will result in prompt relaxation of the proximal gastric wall by inhibition of the sustained contractions.[4] This so-called receptive or adaptive relaxation permits the fundus and upper body of the stomach to act as a reservoir for a large volume of food while maintaining low intragastric pressures. Abolition of adaptive relaxation after vagotomy indicates that this reflex is mediated by inhibitory vagal neurons,[5] which are noncholinergic, nonadrenergic, and partially dopaminergic.[6, 7] It was this concept that any change in the amplitude of the slow, sustained contractions of the proximal stomach will change the gastric emptying of liquids that led to the postulate that the proximal portion of the stomach controls liquid emptying.[8] By use of a gastric barostat to alter intragastric pressure, it was further demonstrated that the rate of liquid emptying from the stomach increases linearly with increasing intragastric pressure.[9] A vagotomy, even a parietal cell vagotomy, which vagally denervates the proximal portion of the stomach, is followed by increased pressure after gastric distention and a more rapid gastric emptying of liquids,[6, 10] which can result in loose stools and even the full picture of the dumping syndrome.

Pattern of Gastric Electrical Activity

The stomach can also be divided into two regions on the basis of its electrical activity[10, 11] (Fig. 40–1). The proximal portion of the stomach, which encompasses the fundus and the orad third of the gastric corpus, is thought to be electrically silent. The rest of the stomach (the distal portion) demonstrates a well-defined, phasic electrical activity. In this part of the stomach, the membrane potential of smooth muscle cells is not maintained at a stable level but is interrupted by an omnipresent, recurring variation in electrical potential. These potentials have been labeled "slow waves," "basic electrical rhythm," "control potentials," or "pacesetter potentials," all such terms referring to the same phenomenon.

Gastric slow waves are generated from an area in the midcorpus along the greater curvature.[11, 12] This area behaves as a gastric pacemaker. There is some similarity to the atrium of the heart in that this pacemaker site has the highest rate of slow-wave production and sets the pace for the entire stomach. From their site of origin, the slow waves propagate circumferentially and longitudinally to the pylorus at a rate of 3 cycles per minute in humans and 5 to 6 cycles per minute in dogs.[10] In the duodenum the rate increases to 11 to 12 cycles/min in humans. The slow waves apparently do not propagate retrogradely to the proximal part of the stomach. However, most observations regarding fundic electrical status were in dogs. More recently, in studies in humans using intraoperatively placed electrodes, myoelectrical activity has been identified in the human fundus.[12a]

Gastric slow waves propagate myogenically and do not depend on special conduction fibers, as do cardiac potentials. In fact, no such conduction system is found in the stomach. The gastric smooth muscle cells communicate with one another—electrically, that is—through gap junctions.[13] Gap junctions are areas in which the outer lamellae of the muscle cells are fused or are closely apposed, and they provide a low-resistance pathway between cells. Therefore, changes in the membrane potential in any cell are shared by the adjacent cells through the gap junctions.

Electrical Basis of Gastric Motility

Gastric contraction is a mechanical manifestation of an electrical event that occurs at the surface membrane of smooth muscle cells. As an aid in understanding the mechanism of electromechanical coupling, let us first review the shape of gastric slow waves, which depends on the method of recording. Intracellular recordings show that each slow wave is characterized by an initial upstroke potential and a subsequent plateau potential.[14] On extracellular recordings, each slow wave appears as a composite of a triphasic (positive-negative-positive) potential complex and an isopotential segment (Fig. 40–2). This triphasic potential complex is sometimes referred to as the initial potential.

Gastric action potentials produce contraction, but gastric slow waves do not. In the stomach, the term action potential refers to a potential change that causes the smooth muscle to contract. Using the technique of simultaneous mechanical and intracellular microelectrode recordings, Morgan and Szurszewski[15] demonstrated that a gastric action potential triggers a mechanical response by increasing the size of the plateau potential above a certain threshold. The plateau potential of an action potential looks like a depression on the extracellular electromyogram, and it is referred to as the second potential (Fig. 40–2). In the distal antrum, one or more depolarizing potentials, called spikes, can be superimposed on the plateau potential. These electrical undulations, also called pacesetter potentials or electrical control activity, change the

permeability of the membrane and make the cells susceptible to calcium fluxes, which are the basis for muscle contraction. Therefore, muscle contractions tend to follow these pacesetter potentials. Not every pacesetter potential results in a contraction. Whether the cell is highly sensitive or insensitive to contraction in response to one of these pacesetter potentials depends on the physiologic status of the stomach related to eating or fasting and the hormonal milieu and messengers at the cell receptor level. Certain neural transmitters or hormones may increase or decrease the sensitivity of the cell to contract on the tail of one of these pacesetter potentials. The maximal rate of contraction is three contractions per minute, but not every pacesetter potential results in contractions, nor do all contractions necessarily sweep the entire distal two thirds of the stomach. They may start somewhere along the stomach or they may start at the beginning of this pacesetter and fade out before they reach the terminal antrum.

Excitatory agents of gastric contraction such as acetylcholine and pentagastrin increase the magnitude of contraction by increasing the amplitude of the plateau potential above the mechanical threshold.[11] Conversely, inhibitory agents such as norepinephrine and prostaglandin E_2 reduce the force of contraction by decreasing the amplitude of the plateau potential.[16] Therefore, the force of gastric contraction is directly related to the duration and the amplitude of the plateau potential.

Gastric Emptying of Solids

The contractions of the distal portion of the stomach are the peristaltic waves. These circular rings of muscular contraction increase in amplitude and velocity as they move distally. During the postprandial state,

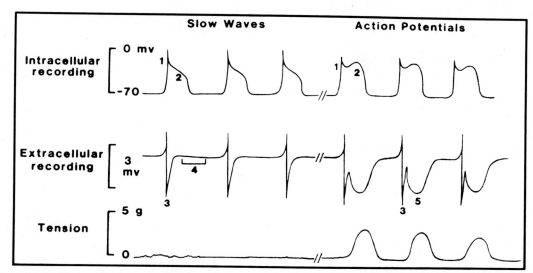

Figure 40–2. Schematic diagram of the electromechanical activity of the stomach. In intracellular recording, each slow wave is composed of initial upstroke potential *(1)* followed by a plateau potential *(2)* and a subsequent return to baseline. Their extracellular counterparts are the initial potential *(3)* and the isopotential segment *(4)*. The shape of action potentials differs from that of slow waves in that the amplitude of the plateau potential is greater in the intracellular recording and in that the isopotential segment is replaced by a downward potential deflection known as the second potential *(5)* in the extracellular recording. Note that peaks of contractions coincide with peaks of plateau potentials and second potentials.

rhythmic sets of peristaltic waves occur that constitute the digestive or fed pattern of the distal part of the stomach. The amount and type of food needed to initiate a posprandial pattern in humans have not yet been determined. Besides their obvious transport function, these contractions have an important mixing and grinding effect on solid foods. As the peristaltic wave approaches the distal antrum, the terminal antrum and pylorus close. The classic Code and Carlson radiographs[17] showed peristaltic contraction coming into the terminal antrum and barium beginning to flow. Some barium is pushed forward down through the duodenum. However, at this point the pylorus appears to close while the wave progresses into the terminal antrum, radiographically obliterating the antrum. At the same time, the barium that remains in the terminal antrum is retropelled back into the proximal stomach. It has been estimated that particles greater than 1 mm in size will not pass out of the stomach during this digestive phase.[18] Thus, large solid particles retained in the stomach by the antropyloric closure are retropelled and in turn propelled back down towards the pylorus. This "antral mill" effect involves pressures of up to 60 mm Hg being generated by the gastric contractions. Through this grinding action, along with mixing with acid and pepsin, most solid particles are reduced to chyme-like consistency (process of trituration), allowing outflow into the duodenum. This chymous consistency minimizes damage to the duodenal mucosa and maximizes absorption.

Neural and Hormonal Regulation. Both the proximal and distal portions of the stomach are controlled by neural and hormonal mechanisms. Neural influences involve input from vagal and sympathetic fibers. For example, gastric distention, which produces a vagal reflex, tends to relax the proximal part of the stomach while it contracts the antrum,[19] again reinforcing the idea that manometrically at least the stomach really has two regions that often act in opposite ways. Dopaminergic pathways, found to be inhibitory, are involved in control of gastric emptying.[7] Levodopa delays gastric emptying in humans as measured by radioisotope techniques.[20] Dopamine receptors of the classification of D_2 (found in pituitary cells) are also present in the gastrointestinal tract, and dopamine is an inhibitor of smooth muscle function in the gastrointestinal tract. Serotonergic pathways mediated by 5-hydroxytryptamine may elicit direct effects on smooth muscle

or act indirectly by the stimulation of intramural neurons to release acetylcholine and perhaps substance P.[21] A variety of hormones affect antral contractions, including secretin, gastrin gastric inhibitory peptide, motilin, vasoactive intestinal peptide, glucagon, neurotensin, somatostatin, and cholecystokinin.[22–25] Only motilin, which enhances intragastric pressure, may have a potential physiologic influence on actually enhancing gastric emptying.[26] Recently it has been demonstrated that pharmacologic doses of histamine can delay gastric emptying in normal humans,[27] implying that H_1 receptor activity may play a role in modulating postprandial gastric emptying.[28] While most of the hormones mentioned above delay gastric emptying at pharmacologic doses, cholecystokinin and gastrin may do so at physiologic doses. Gastrin and cholecystokinin have different effects on the two regions of the stomach. They relax the proximal third of the stomach, increase the contractility of the antrum, and increase pyloric and duodenal contractility and pressure resulting in impedance to emptying. Opiate-induced effects on gastric motility are similar and may even result in nausea and vomiting.[26] Whether gastrointestinal hormones change the basic electrical rhythm and, by inducing a tachygastria on a bradygastria, result in altered gastric emptying—specifically slow emptying—has not been clearly established in humans. Animal studies indicate that glucagon and possibly opiates result in nausea and vomiting in dogs with associated gastric dysrhythmias.[29, 30] Although in humans thyroid disease may alter the pacesetter, variations in thyroid function do not change gastric emptying.

Theories of Solid Food Digestion. A hypothesis proposed in 1980 tried to extend the observations related to Code and Carlson radiographs. The idea was that as a peristaltic contraction sweeps into the terminal antrum an acceleration of liquid in a parabolic fashion occurs (Fig. 40–3). Small particles with less inertia would tend to accelerate more rapidly than large particles and hence make their way into the center, or faster-moving stream; whereas the larger particles would tend to stick to the sides, or slower-moving streams. As the wave continues, some material would empty into the duodenum, but ultimately the pylorus could close. Because the small particles are in the faster-moving portions, they would arrive first and could be successfully swept through the pylorus into the duodenum, whereas the larger particles would be

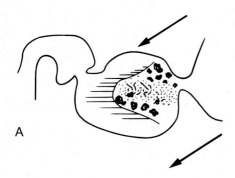

A

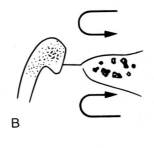

B

Figure 40–3. Keller's 1980 hydrodynamic hypothesis of sieving. *A*, Larger particles tend to remain at sides while smaller particles are propelled more quickly in the center of the stream; contractions cause acceleration of liquid in a parabolic fashion. *B*, Small particles are swept out just before pyloric closure, whereas larger particles are retained and retropulsed.

trapped in the distal antrum and retropelled; in being retropelled they would be tumbled and broken apart by sheer forces. If this entire hypothesis had been correct, pyloroplasty itself would greatly alter grinding and sieving, but it does not seem to do so.[31, 32] It may be that the intermittent to-and-fro fluid flows created do rely on a complex coordination between antral and duodenal contractions rather than pyloric closure.[33] An alternative or complementary hypothesis proposes that particle movement depends on how fast or how slowly the particles sink or float away from the central-moving stream.[34] Such factors as density, sphere diameter, and velocity are the determinants. In this hypothesis, particle transit varies inversely with particle diameter and density but directly with fluid viscosity and fluid velocity. By combining both these theories, antroduodenal coordination is facilitated by hydrodynamic sieving, and resection of the terminal antrum destroys these actions and prevents the sieving process from discriminating between solids and liquids.

Role of the Pylorus and Duodenum. Under certain circumstances it can be demonstrated that the pylorus can have an important regulatory influence. Schulze-Delrieu and Wall[35] implicated the pylorus as an important regulator initially after the ingestion of a liquid meal, consistent with the observation that if pyloroplasty is added to a proximal gastric vagotomy, emptying of liquids is greatly accelerated.[36] Bortolotti and colleagues[37] showed that circular muscle myectomy of the duodenal muscle increased the rate of gastric emptying of liquid. All of these experiments support the idea that the antrum, pylorus, and duodenum work in a coordinated fashion and also receive input from the fundus.

Determinants and Control Mechanisms of Gastric Emptying. Several factors affect the rate of gastric emptying (Fig. 40–4). The primary determinant of the emptying of liquids from the stomach is volume. The elimination of liquids is an exponential (first-order) process in relation to volume; that is, the volume of liquid emptied per unit of time is directly proportional to the volume present in the stomach.[38] If the stomach is filled with saline, saline is rapidly emptied, and the larger the volume, the faster the saline empties; it is an exponential or logarithmic relationship. Emptying of neutral, isosmolar, and calorically inert solutions is rapid; for example, half of a 500-ml load of isotonic saline is emptied from a human stomach in 12 minutes.[39] If, instead, the stomach is filled with a nutrient solution, the nutrients are emptied much more slowly and the logarithmic relationship (that is, the proportionality of speed of emptying to volume) no longer holds. A series of control mechanisms are stimulated by the composition of the gastric nutrients—their osmolarity, acidity, fat, and amino acid content, and presence of some sugars. Other nutrients, such as alcohol (a highly caloric substance) and lysine or short-chained fatty acids, do not seem to have much effect. Solutions that are hypertonic or contain acid, fat, or certain amino acids all retard gastric emptying by the action of specific small bowel receptors on the poorly characterized neural or hormonal pathways mentioned previously (Fig. 40–4).

Acidic solutions slow gastric emptying, with higher acid concentrations causing more profound inhibition of emptying than lower acid concentrations.[40] The inhibitory effect of an acid may be related to its anion, in that acids with high molecular weight cause less retardation of emptying than acids with low molecular weight. In general, increasing osmolarity of a solution results in slower gastric emptying, although some hyposmolar solutions may also inhibit elimination.[41] Fatty acids, monoglycerides, and diglycerides all delay gastric emptying. The fatty acid chain length determines the degree of inhibition, with chain lengths of 10 to 14 carbons causing the greatest delay.[42] The emptying of

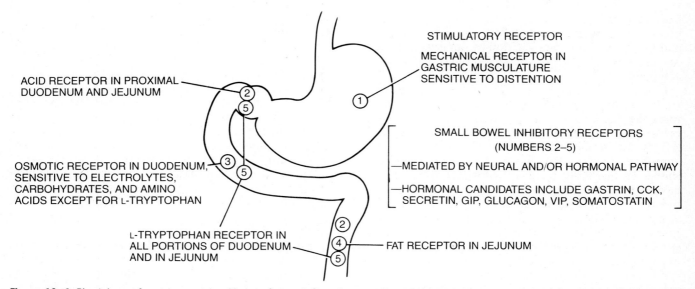

Figure 40–4. Physiology of gastric emptying. Various factors influencing gastric emptying are depicted. Location of mechanical and osmotic receptors *(1 and 3)* are from studies performed in humans. The other receptors were localized from studies in dogs. CCK, Cholecystokinin; GIP, gastric inhibitory polypeptide; VIP, vasoactive intestinal polypeptide.

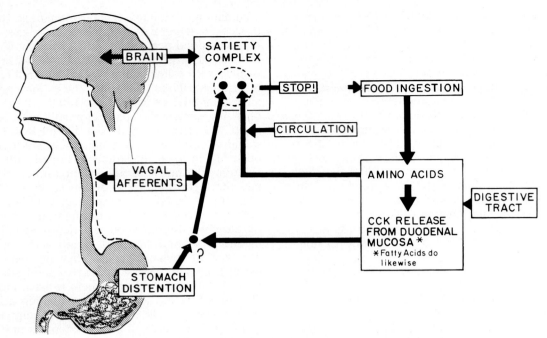

Figure 40–5. Hypothesis of factors contributing to recognition of satiety.

amino acids, except for L-tryptophan, is determined by the osmolality of the solution. Only L-tryptophan delays gastric emptying in concentrations that are considered possible under physiologic conditions of protein digestion.[43]

Hunt and Stubbs[44] demonstrated that the rate of gastric emptying of a meal could be predicted by its nutritive density (that is, the number of kilocalories present per unit volume). Isocaloric concentrations of fat, carbohydrates, and protein (4 gm of fat/100 ml = 9 gm of carbohydrate/100 ml = 9 gm of protein/100 ml = 36 kcal/100 ml) leave the stomach at similar rates. Nutritive density probably exerts its influence via the previously mentioned small bowel receptors. Carbohydrates and amino acids, except for L-tryptophan, retard gastric emptying via the osmoreceptors, and fats slow emptying by action of putative fatty acid receptors, which are as yet unidentified and uncharacterized.

Fat is the most powerful of all the substances controlling gastric emptying. Fat in the intestine tends to relax the fundus with lower intragastric pressure and increases the reservoir function of the proximal stomach. It also inhibits antral contractility, slowing gastric emptying on that basis. Fat in the intestine has been shown to markedly increase pyloric contraction and narrow the pyloric lumen in a tonic way, so that if the pylorus can act as a resistance to outflow, fat might work at that site as well.[45] Finally, fat has been shown to change intestinal peristalsis, particularly duodenal peristalsis, from a propagated series of waves to segmenting activity. Propagation of contractions is associated with transit whereas segmenting activities are not. The idea would be that, by converting the intestinal activity to segmenting activity, the duodenum would act as a brake.[46] Hence, a powerful inhibitor

such as fat may act at multiple sites, increasing the reservoir function, decreasing the pumping action, and increasing the resistance of the pylorus and the duodenum.

The concept that satiety and a decision to stop eating at a certain point in a meal are related to signals from gastric distention and postprandial hormone release has been proposed. It is proposed that gastrointestinal hormones, specifically cholecystokinin (CCK),[47–51] feedback on the satiety center, inhibiting smooth muscle and augmenting a feeling of fullness and gastric distention with afferent input to the central nervous system. In addition, the concentration of the absorbed nutrients (fat and protein) could influence the satiety center (Fig. 40–5). This background allows questions to be asked relating to the status of gastric emptying in conditions of profound satiety and decreased food intake, such as anorexia nervosa. There are no data on CCK levels in this entity, but gastric emptying of solids is definitely delayed (see pp. 697–698). Similarly, CCK and other gastrointestinal hormone levels in other gastric stasis settings have not been studied. Could obesity be in part attributable to rapid gastric emptying and increased capacity for food intake? This rapid gastric emptying could result from impaired release of CCK (and other hormones, as, for example, somatostatin) or deficient CCK receptor binding at the satiety center level. CCK levels have not been measured in morbid obesity, but gastric emptying has been shown to be more rapid in some reports.[52]

Emptying of Nondigestible Solids. Solids that cannot be broken down to sufficiently small size (less than 1.0 mm) are eliminated from the stomach by a different mechanism. A distinct cycle of electromechanical activity during the fasting state that begins in the proximal stomach and migrates aborally through the small bowel has been described.[53] This cycle, which recurs approximately every 1½ hours, is called the migrating motor complex or the interdigestive myoelectric complex (Fig. 40–6A and B). The complex is composed of four phases. Phase 1 is a period of motor inactivity with only rare action potentials or contractions, lasting 45 to 60 minutes. During phase 2 there are intermittent peristaltic contractions that increase in frequency and amplitude over an approximately 30-minute period. In the 5- to 15-minute period designated as phase 3, there is a salvo of peristaltic contractions generated by action potentials occurring with every pacesetter potential (i.e., three contractions per minute). In the fasting state, as opposed to the fed state, the pylorus remains open as a phase 3 interdigestive contraction approaches and the contraction, having no "hole" in its center through which retropulsion can occur, sweeps indigestible solids out of the stomach. It is this effect that gives phase 3 of the interdigestive cycle the name of "housekeeper" of the gastrointestinal tract.[53] Phase 4

is a short transition period between the electromechanical surge of phase 3 and the inactivity of phase 1.

The periodicity of the interdigestive myoelectric complex is thought to be determined by signals from the central nervous system. Caloric intake of adequate amounts can return the cycle to a digestive pattern at any time. It has been postulated that the gastrointestinal hormone motilin plays some yet to be clarified role.[26] These interdigestive cycles are switched off by neural and hormonal mediators. Truncal vagotomy is known to delay the onset of a pattern of gastric contraction.[54] Gastrin has been shown to inhibit fasting elecromechanical cycles.[55] Recent data in dogs suggest that central nervous system input is required for initiation of migrating myoelectrical complexes (MMC) in the stomach and that central vagal input, but not central sympathetic input, is essential for cycling of plasma motilin.[56]

Simultaneous increments in gastric, biliary, and pancreatic secretion promote this housekeeper effect and

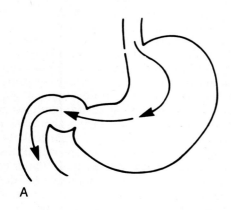

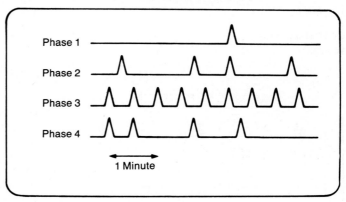

MOTOR ACTIVITY DURING FASTING
(INTERDIGESTIVE PHASES)

Phase 1

Phase 2

Phase 3

Phase 4

1 Minute

Figure 40–6. An example of a normal migrating motor complex in man during the fasting state. A motility catheter is positioned with a transducer recording antral motility and transducers located 10 (A + 10 cm), 20 (A + 20 cm) and 30 cm (A + 30 cm) beyond the pylorus to measure small bowel motility. A salvo of motor activity is signaled by a contraction front appearing in the antrum with a maximal frequency of 3 per minute and amplitudes in excess of 50 mm Hg. There is propagation of this activity into the proximal and distal small bowel as illustrated. Small bowel contractions are seen at a maximal rate of 11/min. Note the propagative (peristaltic) nature of the motor activity front as it sequentially traverses the antrum, duodenum, and small bowel at an average velocity of 7 cm/min.

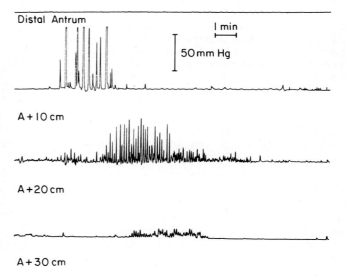

Distal Antrum

1 min

50 mm Hg

A + 10 cm

A + 20 cm

A + 30 cm

B

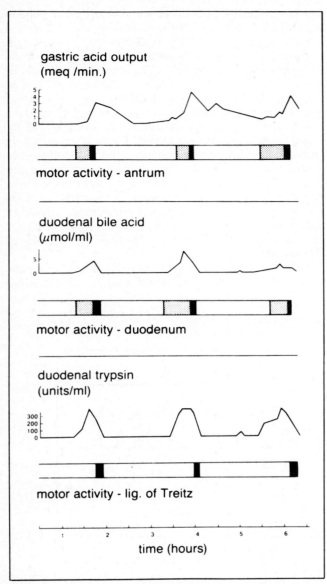

Figure 40–7. Schematic depiction of the interrelationships between the migrating motor complex (MMC) and the associated physiologic secretory functions of the stomach as depicted by gastric acid output, and of the duodenum as evidenced by the duodenal bile concentrations and duodenal trypsin levels.

together provide a deterrent for bacterial colonization and bezoar development as well as aiding digestion of remaining chyme (Fig. 40–7).

The motility cycle during fasting has a number of implications. The variation in the peaking of glucose in glucose-tolerance testing has been correlated with the phase of the fasting cycle when the glucose load is administered. Variations in plasma levels of drugs could relate to unpredictable gastric emptying and hence absorption if they are given to the patient in the fasting state; hence the instructions to take some medications before or with meals. During clinical motility testing it is important to differentiate any expected drug-induced increase in motility from the phase 2 and particularly phase 3 parts of the MMC cycle. Therefore drugs must be administered only after the duration of the subject's MMC cycle has been studied.

CLINICAL PRESENTATION OF DISORDERED GASTRIC MOTOR FUNCTION

The clinical manifestations of delayed gastric emptying usually form a constellation of symptoms. Occasionally, the patient may experience only one or two "uncomfortable" symptoms. Nausea and vomiting are the most disquieting of all the symptoms. Some patients with gastric emptying disorders may complain only of postprandial bloating or fullness, which is probably due to the accumulation of solids or liquids leading to gastric distention. Anorexia and early satiety, although of possible constitutional origin, in the framework of the appropriate signs and symptoms may indicate gastric stasis. Although abdominal pain is present in gastric retention states, also probably owing to distention, its presence as a dominant part of a patient's presentation should arouse suspicion to at least consider other clinical entities, either anatomically independent from the stomach or mechanically related, that could result in delayed gastric emptying. Such possibilities would include gastric ulcer, posterior penetrating duodenal ulcer, gastric cancer, relapsing pancreatitis, biliary tract disease, "upset stomach" possibly related to gastritis or a viral insult, and pancreatic cancer. Important clues relate to the aggravation and provocation of symptoms with meals, particularly large volume ones. Vomiting and significant weight loss can vary and need not always be elicited. Patients may have learned that weight can be maintained with liquid caloric intake with less chance of vomiting if small and frequent liquid-soft meals are the major form of nutrition. It should be remembered, however, that disordered motility of the duodenum and small bowel can present with a symptom complex similar to that of gastric stasis. Here there may be more emphasis on abdominal pain and sometimes suspicion of biliary dyskinesia and sphincter of Oddi dysfunction and at times a past history of cholecystectomy. Alternatively, there may be a history of pain medication requirements reaching addictive proportions.

Patients with symptoms suggestive of rapid emptying will complain of anxiety, weakness, dizziness, tachycardia, sweating, flushing, and decreased consciousness, all occurring in the postprandial setting, either immediately or within 2 hours.

Physical findings may be entirely normal or remarkable only for epigastric distention or fullness. A succussion splash, although more characteistic or a mechanical gastric outlet obstruction, may be found in gastric stasis patients, especially those with significant liquid retention. Epigastric tenderness may be elicited but is an uncommon finding.

Table 40–1. CONDITIONS PRODUCING SYMPTOMATIC GASTRIC MOTOR DYSFUNCTION

ACUTE CONDITIONS

Abdominal pain, trauma, inflammation
Postoperative state
Acute infections, gastroenteritis
Acute metabolic disorders:
 Acidosis, hypokalemia,
  hypercalcemia or hypocalcemia,
  hepatic coma, myxedema
Immobilization
Hyperglycemia (glucose >200 mg/dl)
Pharmaceutical Agents and Hormones
Opiates, including endorphins and narcotics (e.g., morphine)
Anticholinergics
Tricyclic antidepressants
Beta-adrenergic agonists
Levodopa
Aluminum hydroxide antacids
Gastrin
Cholecystokinin
Somatostatin

CHRONIC CONDITIONS

Mechanical
 Gastric ulcer
 Duodenal ulcer
 Idiopathic hypertrophic pyloric stenosis
 Superior mesenteric artery syndrome
Acid-peptic disease
 Gastroesophageal reflux
 Gastric ulcer disease, nonulcer dyspepsia
Gastritis
 Atrophic gastritis ± pernicious anemia
 Viral gastroenteritis (acute, ?chronic gastritis)
Metabolic and endocrine
 Diabetic ketoacidosis (acute)
 Diabetic gastroparesis (chronic)
 Addison's disease
 Hypothyroidism
 Pregnancy?
 Uremia?
Collagen vascular diseases
 Scleroderma
 Dermatomyositis
 Polymyositis
 Lupus?
Pseudo-obstruction
 Idiopathic, hollow visceral myopathy
 Secondary (e.g., amyloidosis, Chagas' disease, muscular dystrophies, cancer-associated syndrome)
Postgastric surgery
 Postvagotomy or postgastric resections
Medications
 Anticholinergics, narcotic analgesics, levodopa, tricyclic antidepressants
Hormones (pharmacologic studies)
 Gastrin, cholecystokinin, somatostatin
Anorexia nervosa: bulimia
Idiopathic
 Gastric dysrhythmias: tachygastria
 Gastroduodenal dyssynchrony
 Central nervous system: tabes dorsalis depression

Clinical Syndromes

Patients with suspected gastric motor disorders need to be questioned specifically about some of the aspects summarized in Tables 40–1 and 40–2. Evidence of a more diffuse neuropathy or myopathy of the gastrointestinal tract should evoke a number of possibilities.

Systemic sclerosis, in which dysphagia and degrees of constipation may be elicited, Raynaud's phenomenon, collagen vascular disorders, amyloidosis, and vasculitis have to be considered. Another entity with a diffuse GI involvement is hollow viscus myopathy or neuropathy, which may present as either a rare familial disorder or with sporadic nonfamily history. The neuropathic form results from a degeneration of Auerbach's myenteric plexus and may be grouped under the heading of "chronic idiopathic intestinal pseudo-obstruction."[57] In addition to gastrointestinal tract symptoms, there may be evidence of bladder dysfunction and lens problems of the eye. Such patients as these and persons with the other entities summarized earlier, with diffuse involvement of smooth muscle, may have histories of previous laparotomies and also can have severe episodes of diarrhea punctuating prolonged periods of constipation. Diarrhea is caused by bacterial overgrowth, and with the accompanying malabsorption, this can make the weight loss more profound.

Physical examination will also include evaluation for orthostatic hypotension, raising the question of autonomic neuropathy. Further symptoms, such as urinary dysfunction and gustatory sweating, would suggest a

Table 40–2. HISTORICAL FINDINGS AND THEIR IMPLICATIONS IN PATIENTS WITH SUSPECTED GASTRIC MOTOR DYSFUNCTION

Finding	Implication
Timing of Symptoms	
Minutes after meals	Psychoneurotic vomiting, bulimic vomiting, vomiting due to gastric outlet obstruction (channel ulcer), early dumping syndrome
Hours after meals	Mechanical obstruction, gastroparesis
Before breakfast	Pregnancy, uremia, alcoholism, increased intracranial pressure, after gastric surgery
Duration of Symptoms	
Hours to days	Acute infections, drugs, toxins or poisons, acute inflammatory conditions, pregnancy
Weeks to months	Mechanical obstruction, gastroparesis, brain tumors, psychogenic vomiting
Quality of Vomitus	
Partially digested old food	Gastroparesis, obstruction
Undigested food	Esophageal obstruction or diverticulum
Bile present	Gastric outlet patent
Feculent odor	Gastroparesis with stasis, intestinal obstruction, gastrocolonic fistula
Blood present	Cancer or inflammation
Amenorrhea	Pregnancy, anorexia nervosa
Headache	Brain tumor
Previous surgery	Postvagotomy gastroparesis, dumping syndrome, other postgastrectomy syndromes, mechanical obstruction

From Schiller, L. R. Practical Gastroenterology 7(4):309, 1982. Used by permission.

search for symptoms and signs relevant to diabetes, dysproteinemias, and collagen vascular disorders, as well as porphyria. In relationship to the autonomic neuropathy, evidence of metabolic imbalance related to past histories of ketoacidosis could be pursued. Standard blood counts and chemistries would provide supportive evidence, but a blood glucose test may need to be accompanied by a glucose tolerance study to identify the severity of the problem. In the chemistry profile, the role of hypokalemia or hypocalcemia, or both, also has to be considered. Addison's disease can present as an abdominal crisis involving abdominal pain and, in some cases, unexplained nausea and vomiting.[58]

A careful history of the psychologic profile and personality of the individual, as well as current lifestyle and background psychiatric overtones, must be obtained. Acute stress can elicit nausea and vomiting, but it is not known whether chronic stress can really lead to recurrent nausea and vomiting. Certainly overtones of anorexia nervosa and bulimia may be associated with disturbances in gastric emptying. Some patients may be taking anticholinergic medications, particularly antidepressants or other medications (Table 40–3) that could impair the interpretation of the gastric emptying test.

Any surgical procedure involving either a vagotomy or a gastric resection raises the spectrum of "dumping syndrome" (particularly for liquids) on one hand or of chronic postgastric surgery stasis (particularly for solids) on the other hand. In the same patient a dumping or rapid emptying of liquids can be present concomitantly with vomiting and slow emptying of solids. It is possible that even a fundoplication for gastroesophageal reflux disease and reduction of a hiatus hernia can result in dumping of liquids and delayed gastric emptying of solids owing to inadvertent vagotomy or vagal nerve damage.

Some patients present with a picture of an acute onset of gastroenteritis. The diarrhea resolves, but the upper gastrointestinal symptoms persist. Viral infections have often been suspected of causing alterations in gut myenteric plexus or smooth muscle function, or both. Acute viral gastroenteritis involving the parvovirus-like agents termed Norwalk or Hawaii virus have been reported to result in significant gastric retention of liquids, but this seems to resolve or improve after the acute illness.[59] There have been some recent reports relating to cytomegalovirus in an Italian series,[60] hence the past history of family illness or travel is extremely important. Whether patients presenting with gastroenteritis may have underlying bacterial overgrowth of the upper gastrointestinal tract owing to hypochlorhydria and achlorhydria or jejunal diverticula has been speculated upon. There is evidence that antibiotic treatment of bacterial overgrowth has resulted in improved small bowel motility.[61]

Finally, in view of the often profound weight loss that occurs, the question of malignancy may arise. A past history of abdominal radiation, no matter how distant, could be implicated. Infiltrative disorders such as lymphoma must be considered, as well as the possibility of paraneoplastic syndromes. Although it has been suspected that metastatic malignancy may result in celiac node involvement or mechanical compression of the stomach, as in pancreatic cancer, other settings can be cited in which the malignancy is distant from the gastric area and yet unexplained retention and vomiting occur.[62] Here the role of a humoral agent inhibiting neural function has been invoked but not further explored. One should not overlook the need for brain CT scanning to exclude cerebellar tumors, meningiomas, and other space-occupying lesions, particularly in younger patients with unexplained vomiting.

Table 40–3. FACTORS AFFECTING INTERPRETATION OF A GASTRIC EMPTYING TEST

Metabolic States
Hyperglycemia ± acidosis
Hypokalemia
? Parenteral nutrition
Metastatic malignancy
   Malignant cachexia
   Chemotherapy
   Radiation therapy

Drugs or Medications
A. Delay Emptying:
   Opiates—narcotic analgesics
   Anticholinergics (including antidepressants)
   Levodopa
   Beta-adrenergic agonists
   Progesterone (? role of menstrual cycle)
   Cigarette smoking
   Aluminum hydroxide antacids
   ? Carafate
   Alcohol (exceeding social doses)
B. Increase Emptying:
   Beta-adrenergic antagonists
   Metoclopramide
   Domperidone
   Cisapride

Diagnostic Tests

Upper Gastrointestinal X-Rays and Endoscopy

Some patients need no further diagnostic testing at this point. Such a clinical setting would usually relate to acute metabolic or septic events, administration of chemotherapy or other medications, or recent surgery that can chronologically be linked to the onset of symptoms. It is crucial, however, that all women of childbearing age have a pregnancy test so as to avoid proceeding with further tests that may involve hazardous exposure.

Most other patients, especially those with symptoms related to delayed gastric emptying, need to have mechanical obstruction and other related conditions excluded. The first step is often a carefully performed barium contrast study (upper GI series). Although barium is a non-nutritive liquid, and it is not emptied by the same mechanism as food, valuable information can be gained from this study, including identification of carcinoma or peptic ulcer disease. A diagnosis of gastric retention is supported by poor emptying of barium from the stomach, gastric dilatation, and the presence of retained food or gastric bezoar. Mechanical obstruction may produce the same picture, and endoscopic inspection of the gastric outlet, stomach, and duodenum is essential to exclude obstruction. On the other hand, if barium passes out of the stomach freely, such a result does not indicate that no disease is present, but merely that there is no mechanical obstruction. A considerable defect in the emptying of solids or of nutritive liquids may still be present. Even the development of the barium "burger" meal has not helped in addressing solid food gastric emptying.[63] The barium burger is difficult to quantitate objectively, as the burger quickly dissociates from the barium, and in addition, significant radiation exposure limits its role for following the therapeutic attempts planned for patients.

Endoscopy is necessary in all patients to establish the anatomic status of the upper gastrointestinal tract. In addition, biopsy specimens of any observed lesions can be obtained. This is specifically indicated when atrophic gastritis, and consequently achlorhydria, is suspected or when endoscopic evidence of antral gastritis raises the question of whether or not a bacterial gastritis may be present related to the organism *Campylobacter pylori*.[64] Postoperatively, endoscopy is the procedure of choice to evaluate the role of bile reflux and also the ease of passage of the instrument into the efferent limb or the Roux-en-Y loop of bowel, as the case may be. In systemic diseases such as scleroderma and amyloidosis, evidence of impaired esophageal motility or strictures, or both, may be present. Culture of the duodenum through endoscopic aspiration should be routinely performed in these patients. Duodenal dilatation may be seen, particularly in diabetic neuropathy, scleroderma, and a myopathic form of chronic idiopathic intestinal pseudo-obstruction. Unfortunately, biopsies in these patients with chronic intestinal pseudo-obstruction will not be in any way diagnostic of the underlying disorder, as only a full-thickness biopsy with specimens several centimeters long would be adequate to show neural disease. Such specimens are usually obtained only at laparotomy and hence cannot be advocated routinely. However, if any surgery is being contemplated in such patients, it is crucial that tissue be obtained for full histologic study and special stains.

Categorization of Patients and Additional Diagnostic Tests

At this point in their investigation, patients will fall into two categories—those presenting with a clear clinical picture and those in whom the clinical picture is still confusing. An example of the first category is a patient with long-standing diabetes mellitus who has nausea and vomiting of old food, a dilated stomach

Table 40–4. LABORATORY DIAGNOSIS OF MOTILITY DISORDERS

Two General Methods
1. Manometry: Fasting and fed patterns of phasic pressure activity in the antrum and upper small bowel, as well as responses to pharmacologic provocation.
2. Radioscintigraphy: Gastric emptying and intestinal transit of radiolabeled solid and liquid components of a meal.

with residual food present on upper gastrointestinal X-rays, and poor emptying of barium from the stomach. Such a patient should undergo endoscopy to exclude gastric outlet obstruction, but further investigation would not be indicated. A diagnosis of diabetic gastroparesis could be made and therapy started. On the other hand, another patient might be just as symptomatic but have normal barium study findings and no abnormalities on endoscopy. Diagnosis in such a patient requires additional studies (Tables 40–4 and 40–5).

Assessment of Gastric Emptying

Intubation techniques all have important clinical relevance and have revealed much about the role of liquids.[38, 65] The saline load test of Boyle and Goldstein[66] can still contribute to decision-making during nasogastric tube aspiration for gastric outlet obstruction and may have some predictive role regarding the potential for surgical intervention. More recently, extensive work with the fractional test meal and intubation techniques have disclosed much about the contributions of gastric acid and other gastric constituents to the final emptied material[67] (Fig. 40–8). Phenol red and other nonabsorbable markers can identify constituents of the pyloric effluent. In general, the invasive aspect of the test makes demands on patient tolerance and so repetition is limited. Such tests, quite popular at one time, are not used in clinical practice, primarily because they are less standardized and because they may be normal even when an emptying problem (for example, poor solid emptying) is present. Modification to include a solid food aspect (homogenized meal) is very complex and clinically impractical.[68] Intubation tests continue to be useful in a research setting.

Radionuclide Measurements of Gastric Emptying. The need to quantitate gastric emptying with greater reliability and fidelity to the physiologic process than

Table 40–5. ADDITIONAL STUDIES IN GASTRIC MOTILITY DISORDERS

Ancilliary Tests:
1. Electrogastrogram: Fasting and fed patterns.
2. Endoscopy with antral biopsies for routine and special histologic studies; specimens for bacterial overgrowth in the small intestine and also studies for *Campylobacter pylori*
3. Esophageal function testing, including motility, pH monitoring and Bernstein test.
4. Gastric analysis (looking for hypersecretory or achlorhydric settings).
5. Psychologic evaluation

METHOD

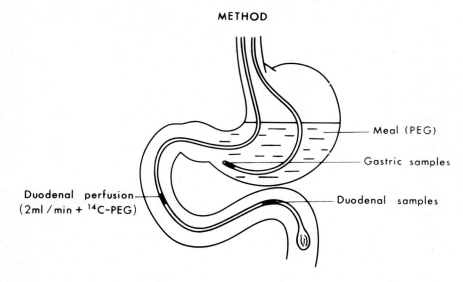

Figure 40–8. Diagram depicting duodenal and gastric intubations for using both gastric and duodenal markers. Recovery of the gastric marker from the duodenum permits evaluation of gastric emptying, and recovery of the duodenal marker from a distal duodenal sampling port allows measurement of pancreatic and biliary contributions. PEG, polyethylene glycol.

was possible using the methods discussed earlier has been spurred in part by the advent of drugs effective in treating gastric stasis syndromes. Radioisotopes, or radionuclides, have gone far in recent years toward meeting this need. Being noninvasive, radionuclide testing is more physiologic than are intubation methods, and the ability of radionuclides to "tag" a solid test meal offers quantitative results not possible with barium radiography.

The current status of radionuclide applications to the study of gastroparesis may be more appreciated in light of the previous decade's experience with isotope "tagging" of tests meals. Radioactive technetium or chromium in some form was in general use and was presumed to remain steadfastly bonded to the test meal, even well into the final phase of digestion, whether the meal was meat, cornflakes, or porridge. However, in actuality isotopes easily strayed from the meals to which they were "affixed," becoming bound to random liquids such as mucus and bile and even attaching to gastric mucosa, creating serious doubts about what was being measured.[69]

These early studies on gastric emptying led to a new era ushered in by Meyer and colleagues,[69] that may be designated "the chicken liver era." Technetium-99m (^{99m}Tc) bound to sulfur colloid is injected into the wing of a live chicken; most of the ^{99m}Tc becomes bound to cytoplasmic protein in the chicken's Kupffer cells, which holds the isotope until late in the digestive process. The chicken is killed 30 minutes later and its liver is resected, diced into 1-cm cubes, mixed with beef stew, heated, and offered to the patient along with crackers and liquids. The patient then usually lies supine under a gamma camera interfaced with a computer to help in interpreting the data. A series of scintiscans over the abdomen can be acquired, showing the movement of isotope into the antrum and the subsequent arrival of the test meal in the small bowel (Fig. 40–9A). The interfaced computer may be used to outline the stomach as the defined area of interest, and gamma counts are monitored (if necessary by continuous 1-minute frames) over the stomach for as

long as necessary, at least 2 hours, or to 50 per cent emptying from stomach. In the next phase of development, a double-isotope technique provided a means to quantitate the gastric emptying of solids and liquids simultaneously. Indium-111 diethylene triamine pentracetic acid (^{111}In DTPA) was selected for the liquid, or water, phase of the meal because of its distinctive gamma spectrum[70, 71] (Fig. 40–9B and C). The gamma camera needs to sense two gamma peaks sufficiently separate to minimize overlapping, and ^{111}In has a gamma peak of 247 KEV (kilo electron volts) that is well removed from the 140 KEV gamma ray of ^{99m}Tc. Estimates of radiation dose to various organs from 500 microcuries of ^{99m}Tc and 100 microcuries of ^{111}In are no more than that received from two abdominal flat plate X-rays.

Methodologic Questions with Radionuclide Meals. One of the problems of applying radionuclide techniques to gastric emptying tests is the decay rate of the isotope being used. It is necessary to have a gamma camera that carefully distinguishes the gamma peaks of ^{111}In and ^{99m}Tc and makes corrections for any slight overlap. Another difficulty is that ^{111}In dissociates from water and becomes nonspecifically adsorbed to chicken liver and beef stew at about the rate of 10 per cent every 30 minutes.[70] Still another problem requiring vigilance in the interpretation of individual test meal results is the removal of small amounts of ^{99m}Tc from the Kupffer cells (less than 5 per cent).[69]

A word about the avoidance of scanning-related artifactual errors is in order. Reliable gamma counts from a patient undergoing a gastric emptying study depend on a carefully defined anatomic region of interest, and this can be difficult in patients who may have had surgery that has altered the architecture of the region under study. Because radionuclide techniques constitute a two-dimensional representation of a three-dimensional process, erroneous gamma counts may arise as a consequence of the changing depth of radioactivity. This situation is more aptly illustrated in the anterior migration of food that was initially located posteriorly in the proximal stomach during gastric

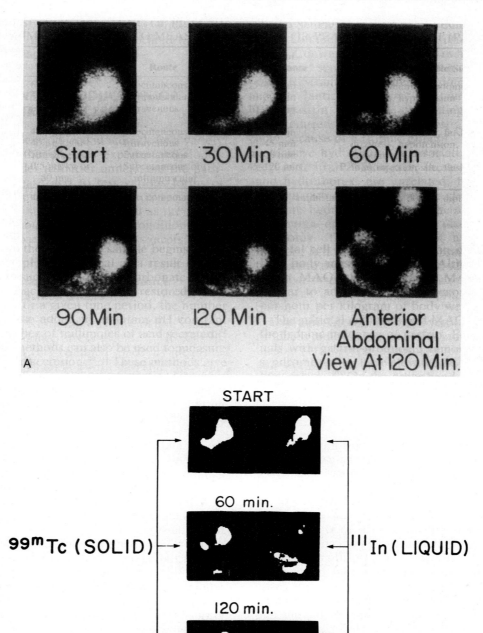

Figure 40–9. *A,* A series of scintiscans illustrating gastric emptying of an isotope-labeled solid meal (chicken liver). Isotope can be appreciated moving from the proximal stomach to the antrum over the first 60 minutes. By 2 hours there is less isotope present in the stomach as well as decreasing density. At 2 hours a full abdominal anterior imaging shows at least half of the isotope present in the duodenum and small bowel, confirming that gastric emptying has occurred. *B,* Scintigraphic display of isotope transit with the dual isotope method in a normal subject. In the top frame, all of the nuclide markers for both the solid and liquid phases are in the gastric outline. At 60 minutes, most of the solid marker (approximately 75 per cent) remains in the gastric region whereas only a small amount (approximately 20 per cent) of the liquid marker is retained in the stomach. By 120 minutes, although a significant amount of technetium (solid marker) is in the small bowel, some remains in the gastric confines. All the indium (liquid marker) has emptied from the stomach at 120 minutes.

Illustration continued on following page

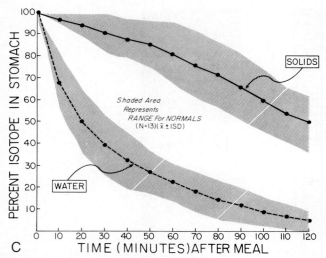

Figure 40–9 *Continued C,* Gastric emptying of a group of normal subjects, using the dual isotope method. The mean and 1SD (1 standard deviation) of the fraction of isotope remaining in the stomach are depicted at various time intervals after ingestion of the meal. Note the exponential nature of liquid emptying and the linear process of solid food emptying. Also note that for the first 50 minutes or so, there is very little emptying of the solid food marker, and this part of the gastric emptying curve is referred to as the "lag phase." Linear emptying of the solid food marker then commences and continues. At this point, the solid food component is homogenized and triturated and is emptying in a similar fashion to liquid components.

emptying.[72] If only a posteriorly positioned gamma camera is used, it will underestimate the gamma radiation emanating from the food as it moves away from it; that is, the gastric emptying rate appears to be faster than is the case with the exclusive use of an anteriorly positioned camera, which conversely overestimates the gamma radiation as the food approaches it. Practically, the approximately 15 per cent difference in counts between the two camera positions is acceptable, as it is assumed to be constant within the spectrum of nonobese normal subjects and patients with gastric emptying disorders. The same holds true in research, in which the same subject is compared basally and after pharmacologic manipulation. However, in obese patients, because the anterior gamma camera will be a considerable distance from the stomach, the error may become significant.

In the presence of duodenal gastric reflux, the quantitation of isotope that is actually emptied is complicated by refluxed isotope that adds to the quantity of counts being estimated in the stomach. Fortunately, this problem is seen in relatively few patients, usually in the postgastric resection setting.

For radionuclide gastric emptying methodology to find favor with nuclear medicine sections in community hospitals, a way was found to eliminate the need to house live chickens. A more adaptable test meal can be made using commercial chicken liver, diced into cubes and injected with ^{99m}Tc-sulfur colloid. When ^{111}In is added to the water, this version of the dual isotope method yields gastric emptying results comparable to those obtained using the *in vivo* labeled technique.[73] Moreover, the affinity of ^{99m}Tc-sulfur colloid for commercial chicken liver is reasonably good, with approximately 10 per cent leaching of the isotope per hour after it is injected with diced liver and cooked before placing it in human gastric juice. ^{99m}Tc-sulfur-colloid labeling of omelette preparation is another meal used to study gastric emptying of solids. It results in very little isotope loss by *in vitro* evaluation, and the gastric emptying rate in humans is only slightly faster than after a chicken liver meal.[74]

Vegetarians can be given an isotope-labeled egg salad sandwich, which, despite its nonspecificity, is an adequate clinical if not research test of solid food emptying. Although this meal gives a composite measure of both solid and liquid emptying, the results are reproducible and sensitive enough for clinical application.[75] Alternatively, labeling of nutrient liquids such as Ensure may be required for different clinical settings (personal data).

In the future, counts may not be acquired as they are now, by maintaining patients lying in a fixed position for a period of time. Routine counts may be obtained at intermittent but regular intervals, such as every 10 or 15 minutes. The former method allows for the same gastric region of interest to be used for the whole study, thus simplifying analysis. Taking intermittent counts allows the patient to move between scans, which may be important in studying disabled or elderly patients. It may be more practical to take initial counts and then sample for 5 minutes at hourly intervals. This could provide accurate data while freeing gamma camera time in busy hospital settings. The only concern with these interval scanning approaches is movement in the stomach's location and hence variation in the area of interest assumed by the computer to be the stomach.

Gastric emptying is influenced by a number of factors, including the size, consistency, and caloric content of the meal,[76] body position, and concurrent drug administration. Therefore, whatever radionuclide technique is used, the principle of uniformity of method is critically important. Furthermore, the numerical results obtained will vary according to the method of analysis. Before establishing measurement of gastric emptying as a clinical test, a method must be decided on, a normal range established for a particular laboratory, and the technique kept consistent. Any substantial changes in method must be taken into account in the analysis of the data.

Interpretation of Radionuclide Gastric Emptying. How should gastric emptying tests be analyzed? The recent literature abounds with ways of presenting data on gastric emptying, a summary of which, along with this author's personal preference, follows. Percentage of gastric emptying as a function of time is one way of expressing the data, in terms of either isotope retained in the stomach (Fig. 40–9C) or isotope leaving the stomach. Another method acknowledges a lag phase or a lag period. A lag period occurs upon ingestion of a meal and is due to receptive relaxation and the time it takes the antrum to begin actively functioning as a grinding and mixing organ. This interval before active emptying occurs is often called the lag period and can range from 0 to 50 minutes. At its conclusion, gastric emptying of the solid component begins to occur in a linear fashion (Fig. 40–9C). At this point there is similarity noted between the emptying rates of the solid and liquid markers. Since the solid is triturated and homogenized, its emptying characteristics approach that of a liquid. Thus, two distinct phases, the lag period and the linear gastric emptying period, provide two components of the gastric emptying curve. The time it takes for 50 per cent gastric emptying of the stomach is a useful indicator for liquids, which empty rapidly. However, for measuring solid food emptying in severe gastric stasis settings, this approach is not meaningful. The area under the curve is very useful and this method combines a lot of information into one calculation. There is a developing interest in the generation of mathematical curves and the exponential function to describe the emptying process. Gastric emptying data can be analyzed by linear regression calculation and power exponential. The power exponential addresses some of the questions concerning analysis of emptying data by fitting nonlinear curves with nonlinear least squares.[77] These concepts may be more applicable to research centers than to the community hospital clinical setting. For day-to-day clinical tests, percentage emptied over a set time period, integrated changes, and area under the curve are adequate indices.

What other factors may influence the test meal result? Gastric emptying of a chicken liver meal in different study positions, supine or standing, was found to be similar. The supine position may emphasize the early lag phase to a greater extent, but the net result is not significantly different. Reproducibility of results on a day-to-day basis is also found to be quite satisfactory with about a 10 to 15% variation in the results analyzed at 2 hours after completing the test meal (personal data).

A physician may be asked to comment on the results of a gastric emptying test (Table 40–3).[78] It is important that the patient be in a stable metabolic state when undergoing a gastric emptying test. Metabolic imbalance associated with sepsis, hyperglycemia, electrolyte disarray, the immediate postsurgery period, acidosis, parenteral nutrition, and hyperosmolar states must be corrected. Interpretation of test results may be difficult in patients with metastatic malignancy because of malignant cachexia or the effects of chemotherapy or radiation therapy. Total parenteral nutrition has been demonstrated to cause significant gastric stasis by an unknown mechanism.[79] Elemental diets, probably owing to their high concentration of amino acid and hyperosmolality, take longer to empty from the stomach than does blenderized "whole" food of comparable caloric composition.[80] Medications that influence motility must be withdrawn at least 12 hours before a gastric emptying test, particularly opiates, anticholinergics, levo-dopa, and beta-adrenergic agonists. Cigarette smoking and aluminum hydroxide antacids also

influence motility to a slight degree.[81] Cigarette smoking has been shown to delay emptying of solids,[82] although it may accelerate emptying of liquids.[83] Alcohol (in social doses) does not affect gastric emptying.[84, 85] Gastrointestinal transit has been shown to vary during a woman's menstrual cycle, with prolongation occurring during the luteal phase, when progesterone levels are high.[86] Whether or not gastric emptying contributes to these changes in gastrointestinal transit has not been determined. Although progesterone or estrogen may conceivably alter gastric motility, pregnant women (at least from 16 weeks of pregnancy until term) are reported to have normal gastric emptying as demonstrated by the dye dilution method.[87] However, no studies have been reported of gastric emptying in women between the fifth and sixteenth week, the period in which vomiting of pregnancy most often occurs. It is recommended that gastric emptying studies in premenopausal women be performed during the first 14 days of the menstrual cycle to minimize progesterone input. Some drugs may stimulate gastric emptying—metoclopramide, domperidone, cisapride, and possibly beta blockers, among others.[88]

A final consideration in the assessment of gastric emptying is whether patients who are nauseated at the time should be studied. The delayed gastric emptying attributed to lack of antral motility may be explained by contributions from the central nervous system. The use of an antiemetic is indicated before or during the test meal study to minimize the central contributions from nausea. Antiemetics in small single doses do not alter gastric emptying.

Another important use of the radiolabeled test meal technique is as a marker for therapeutic trials. Do putative therapeutic agents for gastric stasis objectively change gastric emptying? The results of the dual-isotope gastric emptying in Figure 40–10 indicate that metoclopramide accelerated liquid and solid food emptying back to the normal rate. This would imply that a therapeutic trial of this agent (or future putative agents) would be indicated. Alternatively, the patient could be studied while receiving chronic oral medication to see if a gastric emptying improvement is present or sustained, or both.

Nonradionuclide Assessment of Gastric Emptying. A new attempt at quantifying gastric emptying rates has recently been proposed.[89] Liquid gastric emptying was assessed by real time ultrasonography and compared with scintiscanning. Although some correlation was made, interpretation was hampered by low numbers and the presence of air in the stomach. The method also limits assessment to liquids.

A radiographic emptying test that uses radiopaque markers and fluoroscopic equipment available at virtually every hospital has been reported.[90] Ten pieces of nasogastric tubing are ingested, and abdominal X-rays are taken over 6 hours. A good correlation was found for gastric emptying of solids between radionuclide meal techniques. This method promises to be a noninvasive test of disturbances in gastric emptying, particularly those involving the interdigestive migrating motor complex (MMC), which is important in the

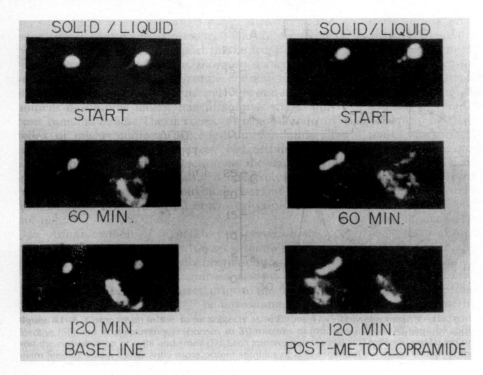

SOLID / LIQUID SOLID / LIQUID

START START

60 MIN. 60 MIN.

120 MIN. 120 MIN.
BASELINE POST-METOCLOPRAMIDE

Figure 40–10. Example of a dual gastric emptying technique where the solid food marker is chicken liver labeled ^{99m}Tc-sulfur colloid and the liquid marker is water labeled with ^{111}In-DTPA. Note that in the baseline state, there is no appearance of the solid food marker in the duodenum and small intestine and, for the liquid component, isotope is clearly visible in the stomach after 2 hours. Following the administration of metoclopramide, significant acceleration in gastric emptying can be appreciated for both the solid and the liquid meal components. After 2 hours there is substantial isotope appreciated in the small bowel in the case of the solid food component, and for liquids no isotope is appreciated in the stomach in 2 hours.

emptying of nondigestible solids from the stomach. These studies may unmask an abnormality in the MMC before a gastric emptying problem for solids is recognizable clinically.

Techniques of Measuring Gastric Motility
(Table 40–4)

Catheter perfusion techniques and also probes containing transducers are available. A comparison of perfusion and catheters with transducers is valuable. Perfusion catheters are cheap and easy to build or buy; however, they are thicker than the usual transducer tube, making them harder to pass through the nose and sometimes less acceptable to the patient. Another disadvantage of perfusion is that infusing a constant rate of water over time may perturb motility and hence change the physiological environment. Transducers, on the other hand, are more expensive. They tend to be thinner probes and, because they do not disturb the luminal environment, they accurately record the physiologic setting. Both methods have limitations: both attach subjects to machinery, although more recently telemetry techniques allow recordings outside the hospital setting. The most recent advance in the transducer recording area is the ultraminiature silicone pressure sensor device[91] (Fig. 40–11). This is a very small, 2.7-mm tube. The transducers are arranged spacially to sense the antrum, duodenum, and small bowel and are encased in a flexible polyurethane sheath that easily passes through the nose and can be tolerated for long periods of time. Measurements can be made for up to 24 hours to sample a number of MMCs and provide more opportunity to observe disturbed or disrupted complex (Fig. 40–12). (A shorter study period of 2 to 6 hours may not contain more than one or two such

complexes.) Figure 40–12 is an example of a disrupted MMC showing impaired propagation into the duodenum with some higher amplitude contractions. This manometric finding could occur in the following di-

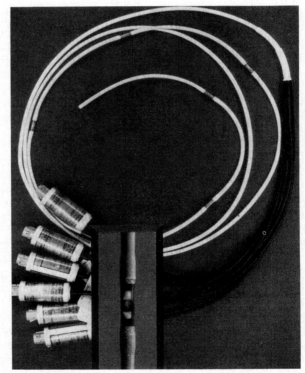

Figure 40–11. The improved recording probe showing six pressure transducers, 10 cm apart and a rubber tubex tip. The probe is 2.7 mm in diameter (8 French). A magnified inset of a transducer is shown upper right, indicating that it is encased in a flexible polyurethane sheath.

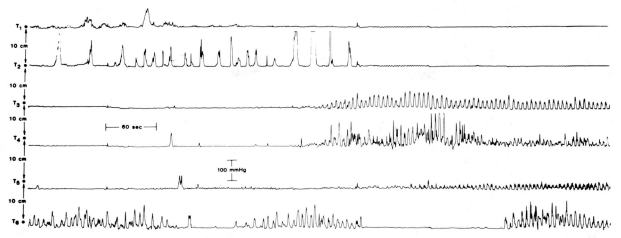

Figure 40–12. Example of an abnormal migrating motor complex in a patient in the fasting state. Pressure sensor placement is illustrated schematically on the left, and time and pressure calibrations are also shown. In this subject T1 and T2 are in the body and antrum of the stomach, respectively. T3 to T5 are in the duodenum, and T6 is in the proximal jejunum. Note that in the antrum the migrating motor complex propagation is already disturbed with rather rapid contraction frequencies at the T2 site, with small contraction amplitudes on many occasions. Propagation is disrupted and abnormal in the duodenum and, in turn, in the small intestine. There is no sequential propagation observed; in the duodenum many contraction amplitudes are abnormally high and, if anything, there may be retrograde propagation illustrated at the level of T6. These findings are consistent with the diagnosis of gastroduodenal motor disorder (or gastroduodenal dyssynchrony) and also could be seen as part of the spectrum of suspected gastric-duodenal dysrhythmias or under the umbrella term of nonulcer dyspepsia.

agnostic settings: *gastroduodenal dyssynchrony* or *gastroduodenal motor dysfunction* (synonymous terms), *nonulcer dyspepsia,* or a *gastric* (or *duodenal*) *dysrhythmia*, all entities which are more frequently observed in symptomatic female patients.

Correlations of Emptying and Motility Studies. In healthy individuals there is a positive correlation between postcibal antral contractile activity and the rate of emptying of a radiolabeled meal measured radioscintigraphically.[92] Whether there is also a quantitative relationship between impairment of postcibal gastrointestinal motility and gastric stasis is not completely known. A motility index or area under the curve estimates total activity based on contraction amplitudes and duration, and the calculation can be applied to the antral and duodenal response to a meal, usually over a 2-hour period.[92] Whether such measurements should be derived from a sample of two or three meals rather than one is debated. Although the observation of a hypomotility response (Fig. 40–13) does not allow for a specific diagnosis or for the distinction of a myopathy from a neuropathy, it does indicate that normal propagation of solid food from the antrum into the duodenum is unlikely. The finding of postprandial hypomotility in patients in whom delayed gastric emptying has been established using a radionuclide method could help identify a problem with antral motility as the etiology of the slow emptying rather than other causes such as increased duodenal impedance and motor resistance (e.g., duodenal dyscoordination).

Patients with clinically suspected gastrointestinal dysmotility who are undergoing manometric and a radioscintigraphic studies fall into two main motility categories: patients with postcibal antral hypomotility and normal small bowel motility, and patients with normal antral motility but with abnormal intestinal motility. Those with postcibal antral hypomotility have delayed gastric emptying of solids but usually not of liquids. Patients with intestinal dysmotility, on the other hand, have a normal lag period for solid emptying but a reduced slope of solid emptying from the stomach once emptying begins. This variation in the emptying phase can be easily overlooked by single indices of gastric emptying such as t½ (50 per cent). Liquid emptying could also be slow with intestinal disturbances.

One contribution of recording motility of the antrum and duodenum is in predicting responses to a potential therapeutic agent. For example (Fig. 40–14), the atonic antrum in the diabetic patient with gastroparesis can be transformed after administration of metoclopramide, with appearance of frequent (three contractions per minute) good amplitude contractions in the antrum and at the antropyloric junction. Such responses assist the physician in prescribing this therapy. Contractile responses due to agents such as metoclopramide, bethanechol, domperidone, or cisapride indicate the problem is a neuropathy of the enteric nervous system, not a myopathy.

Ancillary Tests. Ancillary testing (Table 40–5) that might be useful include endoscopy and antral biopsies to unmask *severe gastritis*, particularly *atrophic gastritis*. Patients with achlorhydria can have delayed gastric emptying, and those with hypersecretion can have rapid emptying. *Bacterial overgrowth* is an important aspect when evaluating the antrum and duodenum. Whether *Campylobacter pylori* and its associated gastritis underlie the antral hypomotility in patients with idiopathic gastric stasis of apparent sudden onset is a serious question. Also of interest are reports of increased titers of cytomegalovirus in Italian patients and the possibility that Norwalk agent and other viruses

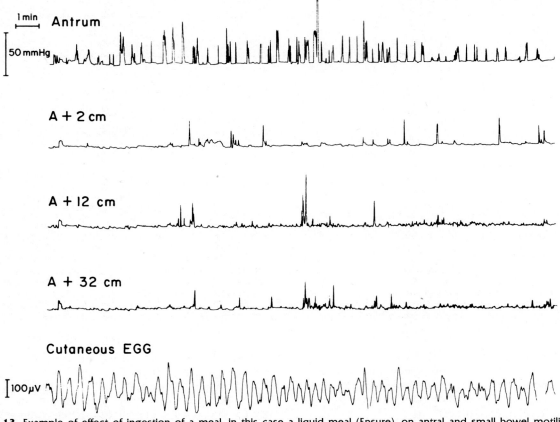

Figure 40–13. Example of effect of ingestion of a meal, in this case a liquid meal (Ensure), on antral and small bowel motility. This "fed pattern," as it is generally termed, is illustrated here by a motility catheter positioned with a transducer recording antral motility, and transducers located 2 (A + 2 cm), 12 (A + 12 cm), and 32 (A + 32 cm) beyond the pylorus, to measure small bowel motility. There is a simultaneous recording of the electrical activity of the stomach through a continuous electrogastrogram (EGG). Within 30 minutes of eating, the antral motility increases in amplitude (up to 50 mm Hg or greater) and frequency, here attaining maximal frequency of 3 contractions per minute. Small bowel motility can also be observed to increase in amplitude and frequency. The amplitude of the EGG increases compared with that occurring in the fasting state, while the frequency remains the same (3 cycles/minute).

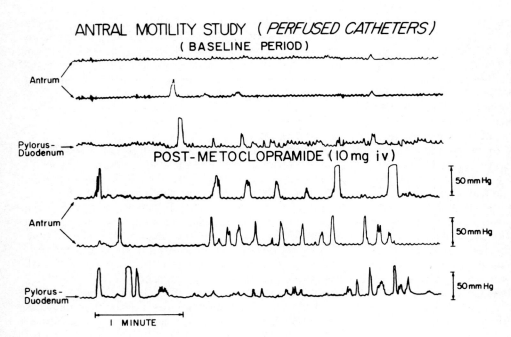

Figure 40–14. A continuously profused catheter system in the antrum of the stomach measures contractions in millimeters of mercury at 3-cm intervals extending into the pylorus and proximal duodenum. Recordings are made in the basal state and then beginning 10 minutes after the intravenous administration of 10 mg metoclopramide. In the basal state, there was relative atony in this insulin-dependent diabetic patient and symptoms consistent with gastric stasis, as well as objective evidence of delayed gastric emptying on a radionuclide scan. Metoclopramide increased the amplitude and frequency (contractions per minute) of antral and duodenal contractions, and there is evidence of coordination between antral and duodenal motility. The activity level induced by the intravenous metoclopramide may resemble the activity pattern of a phase 2 period of a migrating motor complex (MMC).

may play a pathologic role. Testing of esophageal function should be considered because of the overlap of gastroesophageal reflux disease with delayed gastric emptying. Also spastic esophageal motor disorders can be identified in some of the patients with idiopathic motor disorders of the stomach, small bowel, and colon—so-called pseudo-obstruction (particularly those patients with familial visceral myopathy syndromes).[93] As the latter disease also involves the bladder with urinary retention, cystometrograms may be indicated. Sphincter of Oddi dysfunction, dyskinesia, and hypertension may also be present in this patient population, which is particularly consistent with the impression of the coincidence, predominantly in females, of the postcholecystectomy syndrome and gastric stasis. Psychologic evaluations are very important in understanding the patient's personality profile, pain thresholds, adaptation to chronic disease, and potential coping mechanisms regarding treatment and should be performed routinely as part of a "team" approach to the care of these patients.

Electrogastrography. The electrogastrogram (EGG) is the recording of the basal electrical rhythm or the gastric slow wave. Cutaneous recordings are now being performed in more laboratories and this study is slowly evolving from a research tool to a diagnostic method. Silver–silver chloride electrodes are commonly used. Electrical stability of electrodes, not size, is important. The optimal electrode location will depend on the nature of the signal desired; for example, largest possible amplitude; lowest artifacts from ECG, respiration, and subject movement; and the position of the subject's internal organs, particularly the antrum of the stomach and the diaphragm.[94] For most subjects, the EGG with the greatest signal-to-noise ratio is obtained with bipolar electrodes: Electrodes are placed in the epigastrium between the naval and xiphoid,[95] with a limb lead as a reference electrode.

The subject typically lies supine. Prior to the attachment of electrodes, the subject's skin is prepared by shaving if necessary, cleaning with alcohol, and either rubbing with electrode jelly or lightly abrading with fine sandpaper or the equivalent. The skin resistance should be lowered to approximately 5000 ohms to avoid skin potential responses that will otherwise confound the EGG. A thin coating of electrode jelly is applied to the electrodes before they are attached to the subject's skin with tape. EGGs may be made simultaneously from multiple locations using a single reference electrode.[96]

Recording of the EGG can be accomplished with commercial polygraphs if sufficient amplification and appropriate filtering are available. Commercial polygraphs also provide an internal voltage needed to neutralize the relatively constant DC potential between the two electrodes. When the voltage and polarity are adjusted properly, the constant potential between the electrodes is reduced, leaving the desired cyclic potential, the EGG. It is recommended that the output of the amplifiers go to both an ink-writer and either an FM tape recorder for later analysis or directly to a

computer for on-line analysis. Fast Fourier transform to develop a power spectrum of the signal frequency for given time periods is the most commonly agreed upon method for analysis of data.

To validate this cutaneous technique, consenting patients at surgery have had serosal electrodes implanted on their stomachs, and postoperatively their responses were recorded simultaneously from the cutaneous site as well as from the surgically implanted electrodes[97] (Fig. 40–15). Excellent correlations were obtained. Therefore, the cutaneous EGG recordings now available in a number of laboratories can be regarded as becoming more reliable and reproducible. Some of these laboratories also record from the antral mucosa by an intragastric electrode on a probe, and the electrode is sucked against the mucosa or held by a magnet technique.[98, 99]

For now, the main role for EGG in humans is monitoring for dysrhythmias. A possible future role for the EGG could be to assess postprandial antral motility. Antral activity, reflected by pressure measurements in the stomach, is associated with a marked

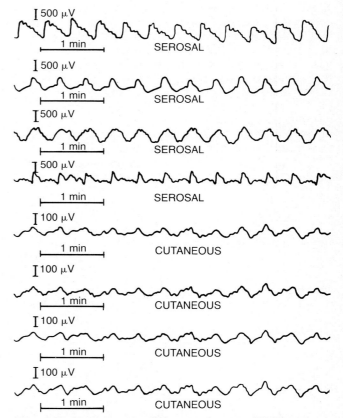

Figure 40–15. Depiction of electrogastrogram (EGG) simultaneously recorded from electrodes implanted intraoperatively on the gastric serosa compared with recordings from cutaneous electrodes placed on the abdomen between the navel and xiphoid. The basal electrical rhythm of approximately 3 cycles per minute is displayed by both techniques. Note the fivefold attenuation of the signal from the cutaneous electrodes related to the depth of fat between the skin and underlying stomach. This study verifies the accuracy of recording the EGG from a cutaneous and, thus, noninvasive site.

increase in the amplitude of the electrical slow wave signal (Fig. 40–16). If it is assumed to be a reflection of electromechanical coupling, the augmented electrical signal postprandially represents the antral motility index. Responses with prokinetic agents could similarly be expected, and hence cutaneous EGG could potentially provide a noninvasive means for assessing antral motility and responses to physiologic and pharmacologic provocation.

Disturbances in Normal Gastric Electrical Activity

Disturbances in the normal gastric electrical activity were first reported in dogs.[100] Two types of abnormalities were described: slow waves that are unusually fast in rate and slow waves that are normal in rate but highly irregular in rhythm. These abnormalities were designated as tachygastria and arrhythmia, respectively. Subsequently, bradygastria was added to the list of gastric dysrhythmias; it refers to slow waves that are abnormally slow in rate.

Tachygastria and bradygastria have distinct electrical characteristics. tachygastria usually originates from an ectopic focus in the distal antrum, and its slow waves may also propagate in a retrograde fashion, contrary to the usual antegrade manner. Each episode of tachygastria ($\geq$ 6 cycles per minute) is followed by a pause that appears as an electrically silent period on the extracellular electromyogram. In contrast, bradygastria ($\leq$ 1 cycle per minute) usually does not arise from a discrete area in the stomach; rather, it appears in both the corpus and the antrum simultaneously, and its slow waves usually propagate antegradely.

Although the etiologic mechanism of gastric dysrhythmias is currently unknown, they can be induced

pharmacologically both in humans and in animals under experimental conditions. Agents such as epinephrine, glucagon, met-enkephalin, beta-endorphin, prostaglandin E_2, secretin, and insulin have all been demonstrated to cause gastric dysrhythmia.[101, 102] The characteristics of tachygastria and bradygastria induced by these agents are similar to the corresponding spontaneous varieties.[101, 102] The fact that so many substances with diverse chemical structures can cause similar electrical disturbances in the stomach raises the possibility that they may act through a common paracrine pathway. One candidate as the mediator for the mechanism is the intramural synthesis and release of endogenous postaglandins.[16]

Clinical Implications of Gastric Dysrhythmia

Gastric dysrhythmias have been described in a variety of clinical conditions (Table 40–6). Most of the studies, however, have been isolated case reports, and the role of gastric dysrhythmia in human disease has yet to be examined with careful scientific scrutiny. The first well-documented report of tachygastria in humans was published in 1978.[103] The patient was a 5-month-old male infant who was debilitated from severe gastric retention and had symptoms of intractable nausea, vomiting, and weight loss. The symptoms were attributed to impaired motor function of the stomach, and were unrelieved by conventional medical therapy and surgical procedures such as pyloroplasty or gastrojejunostomy. Subsequently, the patient underwent resection of the distal three fourths of the stomach and gastrojejunostomy, after which the symptoms dramatically subsided. When the surgical tissue was carefully studied *in vitro* by means of intracellular microelectrode techniques, an abnormally fast electrical rhythm (occurring at a rate of 5 to 20 cycles per minute), was detected. Furthermore, addition of excitatory stimulants to the gastric smooth muscle failed to generate plateau potentials, and no contractions were noted. This detailed account of abnormal electrophysiologic findings at the cellular levels provided a rational explanation for the clinical problem of gastric atony in this patient.

The association between tachygastria and abnormal gastric motor function was described in a 26-year-old woman with persistent nausea, vomiting, and abdominal pain who was found to have antral tachygastria and severe impairment of antral motor function.[104] This patient also required a subtotal gastrectomy for relief of her symptoms. Subsequent studies revealed gastric dysrhythmias in 9 to 14 patients with unexplained nausea, vomiting, and epigastric bloating for periods

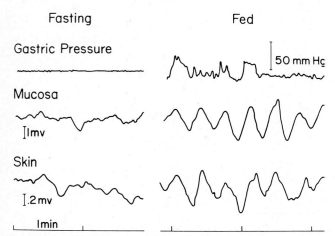

Figure 40–16. Change in the gastric slow wave signal recorded by both an invasive technique relying on an electrode suctioned to the antral mucosa of the stomach and a noninvasive cutaneous technique with electrodes placed on the abdominal skin. Following a meal there is evidence of an increase in gastric pressure indicated by amplitudes of up to 25 mm Hg, and at the same time an increase in the activity and amplitude of the slow wave recorded by both techniques—the intragastric mucosa recordings and the cutaneous skin recordings of the EGG.

Table 40–6. CLINICAL CONDITIONS ASSOCIATED WITH GASTRIC DYSRHYTHMIAS

Idiopathic gastroparesis	Post-vagotomy state
Secondary gastroparesis	Miscellaneous
Diabetes mellitus	Asymptomatic persons
Anorexia nervosa	Postoperative period
Gastric ulcer	

that ranged from 5 months to 10 years.[98] The role of gastric dysrhythmia in human disease was further suggested by its high prevalence in patients who suffer from gastroparesis in association with diabetes mellitus[105] or anorexia nervosa.[99]

Gastric dysrhythmias are not exclusive to stomachs with impaired motor function. They are also present in asymptomatic persons,[102] during the immediate postoperative period,[106–108] and in a variety of unrelated clinical conditions.[104] In such circumstances, however, gastric dysrhythmias tend to be transient. Whether gastric dysrhythmias are directly responsible for abnormal motor function of the stomach and dyspeptic symptoms is unclear. Their normal frequency (that is, how many minutes per day asymptomatic subjects have dysrhythmias) has not been established. It could be postulated that teleologically nauseated patients have dysrhythmias as a protective mechanism against eating. Or is the dysrhythmia primarily responsible for abnormal motility, nausea, and vomiting related to gastric stasis? The finding of a gastric dysrhythmia in a patient with dyspeptic symptoms, however, may indicate an underlying motor dysfunction of the stomach and may warrant further investigation with use of such techniques as gastrointestinal manometry and radioscintigraphy.

Causes of Delayed Gastric Emptying States

Organic obstructing lesions of the duodenum or antropyloric region will produce gastric retention whether due to *peptic ulcer disease, pyloric hypertrophy* (infantile or adult), *antral carcinoma, pancreatic carcinoma* invading the duodenum, or the radiologic identification of superior mesenteric artery syndrome. If the radionuclide-labeled test meal documents delayed gastric emptying and these lesions have been ruled out by the appropriate diagnostic techniques, the diagnosis is a gastric disorder of hypomotility, and a search should begin for the specific cause and the various clinical states associated with delayed gastric emptying. Some are well known, whereas others have only recently been described, often overshadowed by the symptom complex or severity of the primary disease (see Table 40–1).

Diabetic Gastroparesis

This entity is a well-described phenomenon originally suspected 50 years ago and defined in 1958 as gastroparesis diabeticorum.[109] Wide variations in the reported incidence of this disorder are largely attributed to different methods of measuring gastric emptying and to patient selection. Accurate quantitation of gastric emptying can now be performed by means of radionuclide test meals.

Diabetic gastroparesis was originally thought to be a vagal neuropathy, in part because of its association with a peripheral neuropathy; however, such neuropathy should cause more rapid liquid emptying, an

uncharacteristic finding. An inverse correlation has been noted between the gastric emptying rate and elevated blood glucose levels.[110] Furthermore, a metabolic cause associated with hyperglycemia has been postulated on the basis of elevated urinary levels of myoinositol in poorly controlled diabetes; the significance of this finding is based on the fact that inositol is an integral part of the nerve unit.[111] Abnormal neural control of gastric muscular action may be a significant component in the pathogenesis of gastroparesis diabeticorum. Clinical correlation of this electrophysiologic phenomenon is observed in two thirds of diabetic patients who are unable to eliminate 1.0-cm radiopaque markers at 6 hours from ingestion.[90] The duration and the rate of antral contractions are decreased, and normal aboral propagation of phase 3 interdigestive myoelectric activity is disturbed or absent in the antrum of such symptomatic diabetic patients.[112, 113] The prokinetic agent metoclopramide can restore normal motility. The antral smooth muscle is normal by light and electron microscopic parameters.

That asymptomatic diabetic patients suffer from gastroparesis suggests that this unrecognized delay in gastric emptying may be in part responsible for poor diabetic control. Timing of carbohydrate absorption and insulin administration are critical in control of brittle diabetes. In patients with less difficult control, other causes, such as infection or insulin antibody formation, may be responsible for episodic decompensations. Because elevated blood glucose levels can delay gastric emptying,[110] a vicious cycle may arise. Long-standing diabetes and peripheral neuropathy in an insulin-dependent diabetic patient should arouse suspicion of delayed gastric emptying as a possible cause of poor control of blood glucose levels.

Abnormal gastric emptying of solids is the most sensitive initial finding in gastroparesis diabeticorum, with additional impairment of liquid emptying in more advanced settings (Fig. 40–17). In addition to diminished antral motor activity, pyloric dysmotility may contribute to delayed gastric emptying,[114] because duration of pyloric activity was greater in diabetic patients with nausea or vomiting than in control subjects, and prolonged or intense tonic contraction or pylorospasm was noted in these same patients.

Effect of Gastric Surgery on Emptying

Superselective or proximal gastric vagotomy alters gastric receptive relaxation, augmenting the gastroduodenal pressure gradient and causing rapid emptying of liquids.[115] Truncal vagotomy decreases antral motility and slows solid food emptying. The degree and frequency of impaired gastric emptying with vagotomy as tested by radionuclide-labeled meals varies widely. The decreased acid secretion following truncal vagotomy may also retard gastric emptying.

The effects of truncal vagotomy and pyloroplasty on gastric emptying are transient; gastric emptying usually returns to normal within three years.[116, 117] After truncal vagotomy, liquid emptying time is prolonged, but when

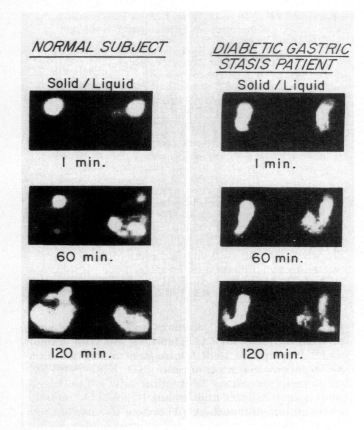

Figure 40–17. A series of gastric scintiscans illustrating comparison of dual emptying of solids and liquids for a normal subject and a diabetic patient with gastric stasis. The solids marker is chicken liver labeled with ^{99m}Tc-sulfur colloid, and the liquid component is water labled with ^{111}In-DTPA. The diabetic patient has no evidence of solid food leaving the stomach after 2 hours and has a well-outlined stomach. This may be the only abnormality in diabetic gastroparesis, with normal emptying of liquids often present. In the example presented here, this is an advanced form of diabetic gastroparesis in which liquid emptying is also impaired, as illustrated by significant retention at 60 minutes and 2 hours.

a pyloroplasty is performed, liquid emptying is normal, hence the use of the drainage procedure. After antrectomy a slight increase in liquid emptying rates is noted. Up to one month after antrectomy and truncal vagotomy, increased gastric emptying of solids is observed, with normalization usually occurring by the sixth month postoperatively, indicating adaptation to the lack of the antral pulverizing effect. In the absence of gastric outlet obstruction, gastric retention for more than one month after antrectomy and vagotomy heralds a chronic process. This complication is recognized in 3 to 9 per cent of patients,[118] and these chronic symptoms can reach disabling proportions, often necessitating surgical revisions.

A predisposing condition to chronic postoperative gastric retention is preoperative gastric outlet obstruction.[119] The probable cause of such a circumstance is a chronically distended stomach with the resultant excessively stretched and poorly responsive gastric smooth muscle. Patients with chronic postgastric surgery retention usually have a history of preoperative

vomiting. Vagotomy also increases the risk of postoperative gastric stasis.[118] Only 3 per cent of patients with subtotal gastrectomy without vagotomy have gastric atony, as opposed to 9 per cent of those with a vagotomy and hemigastrectomy. Thus, the combination of preoperative gastric outlet obstruction and vagotomy with either a pyloroplasty or a gastroenterostomy adversely affects the results of surgery. After vagotomy and drainage, 27 per cent of patients with preoperative gastric outlet obstruction in one series had prolonged postoperative stasis, compared with only 5 per cent of those who had no obstruction before surgery.[120]

The implication here is that if patients have duodenal ulcer disease and gastric outlet obstruction and do not rapidly improve, they should undergo surgery in a timely fashion. Preoperatively, a period of gastric aspiration to decompress the stomach and return tone should be included.

In patients undergoing truncal vagotomy and hemigastrectomy, an interesting phenomenon is observed. Unlike asymptomatic patients, those with postoperative gastric stasis were found to have absent phase 3 interdigestive motor activity, which was re-established after the administration of metoclopramide, a gastrointestinal prokinetic agent.[121] High gastric resection may also interfere with the gastric pacemaker, and this may contribute to the delayed emptying.

Gastroesophageal Reflux

Gastric retention with accumulation of acid and gastric contents logically may be postulated as a contributory factor in the production of gastroesophageal reflux. Approximately 60 per cent of patients with reflux have delayed gastric emptying of solids[122, 123]; liquid emptying is normal or delayed, depending on the test meal.[122–124] Regardless, rates of emptying do not correlate with lower esophageal sphincter pressure.[122] That patients with gastroesophageal reflux may have subjective and objective findings of impaired gastric emptying is clear, and it may be the harbinger of subsequent reflux. The delay in gastric emptying produces gastric distention, which in turn promotes more transient relaxations of the lower esophageal sphincter.[125]

The gastric motility disturbance may be primary (idiopathic) or secondary to an identifiable disease. Because fat delays gastric emptying as well as lowering LES pressure, it is appropriate to recommend small, soft, and semi-solid low-fat meals for reflux patients.

In the pediatric age group, gastric retention of liquids, as determined by radionuclide-labeled formula, has been documented and contributes to the failure to thrive or pulmonary aspiration observed in this population.[126, 127]

An antireflux operation, fundoplication, is often successful in patients with reflux esophagitis. When gastric emptying studies are performed, surgical failures appear to correlate with slower solid emptying,[128] whereas increased liquid emptying occurred more often, probably attributable to impaired receptive relaxation related to surgical trauma or entrapment, or both, of the vagus nerve. This author has also observed that a population of postfundoplication patients presenting with increasing symptoms of gastroesophageal reflux (and therefore termed relative or absolute failures) have an accompanying delay in gastric emptying. The cause of the delayed gastric emptying in this failed operative group may reflect that the patient had the delay in gastric emptying from the onset, as has been summarized earlier, and there would be no reason to believe that a fundoplication would really improve the rate of gastric emptying of solids. It is interesting that the literature would indicate that symptoms tend to recur over a period of three to five years, such that by five years there is significant documentation of reflux by esophageal pH studies. It may be indicative that the continued delay in gastric emptying slowly weakens the efficacy of the antireflux procedure.

Fink and colleagues[129] have reported that the slow gastric emptying of solids in the population of patients with gastroesophageal reflex can be correlated with the degree and severity of antral gastritis. Presumably this antral gastritis continues after surgery. The cause of the gastritis is not clear. Could gastric stasis itself promote gastritis, or could gastritis induce a smooth muscle impairment? The cause of the latter gastritis could be bile reflux (some comparisons with the gastritis of gastric ulcer) and raises questions about the competence of the pylorus and the status of duodenal motility in gastroesophageal reflux disease.

Another possibility is that at the time of fundoplication, there is vagal damage in the form of an accidental vagotomy or perhaps entrapment of the vagus nerve in the fundoplication wrap. There are estimates implying that accidental vagotomies or vagal nerve damage could occur in as many as 30 per cent of patients undergoing fundoplication, particularly in the setting of a second antireflux operation. Such vagal damage would certainly explain both the more rapid gastric emptying of liquids found in such postoperative settings,[6] and the possibility that impaired antral innervation could result in delayed gastric emptying of solids.

Achlorhydria, Atrophic Gastritis, and Pernicious Anemia

Patients with atrophic gastritis have delayed gastric emptying as determined by a chromium-labeled meal.[130] A study with the dual-isotope technique in 17 patients with achlorhydria—8 with atrophic gastritis and 9 with pernicious anemia treated with vitamin B_{12} and without neurologic involvement—showed that gastric emptying of solids was delayed, but liquid emptying was normal.[131] Instillation of acid and pepsin into the stomach increased solid emptying by 20 per cent, while metoclopramide sped up gastric emptying by 40 per cent.[131] Thus, restoration of the gastric secretory contents influenced gastric emptying, but reversing delayed gastric emptying with metoclopramide implies re-estab-

lishment of perturbed gastric motility, through an effect on gastric smooth muscle.

Clinically it could be speculated that delayed gastric emptying may be causally related to the occurrence of cancer in pernicious anemia. Higher concentrations of nitrosamines resulting from higher bacterial counts and delayed gastric emptying may represent a risk factor for gastric cancer. In postantrectomy patients, achlorhydria develops, possibly partly explaining the gastric stasis occurring in some of these patients.

There is paucity of information on gastric acid production, histamine receptors, and gastric emptying. In the only known human study evaluating histamine receptor activity and gastric emptying, histamine given intravenously at a dosage of 40 mg/kg/hr, for maximal acid output, combined with cimetidine (300 mg) produced a dramatic delay in gastric emptying in five normal volunteers.[27] The same test at 20 mg/kg/hr of histamine plus 300 mg of cimetidine intravenously and cimetidine alone did not significantly delay gastric emptying. Thus, histamine, through an H_1 receptor mechanism, may be one of the factors modulating gastric emptying in humans. The extremes of acid production, not intermediate levels, appear to accelerate gastric emptying in humans, which, at first glance, may fit into the physiologic scheme of digestion. That is, patients with Zollinger-Ellison syndrome (and to some degree routine duodenal ulcer disease) have more rapid emptying, whereas achlorhydric, atrophic gastritis patients have slow emptying.

Intestinal Pseudo-obstruction

Primary chronic pseudo-obstruction most notably affects the small and large intestine and occasionally the esophagus and stomach.[57, 132] A myopathic form called hereditary hollow viscus myopathy (familial visceral myopathy) is characterized by degeneration of smooth muscle. This entity may exist without familial involvement. A neuropathic form (familial visceral neuropathy) displays a diffusely abnormal myenteric plexus with normal smooth muscle histologically. Secondary intestinal pseudo-obstruction is associated with a variety of systemic disorders, such as myotonic dystrophy and progressive muscular dystrophy.[133, 134, 134a] In the Riley-Day syndrome of familial dysautonomia, gastric stasis may occur, accompanying the more obvious signs of neurologic dysfunction, such as labile hypertension, vasomotor instability, and peripheral neuropathy.[135] The autonomic neuropathy of variegate and acute intermittent porphyria has been implicated. Amyloidosis and dysproteinemias may influence gastric function as well as intestinal transit.[135–137] A diffuse smooth muscle impairment can develop in patients with advanced malignancy outside the GI tract.[62]

Anorexia Nervosa

Anorexia nervosa is a psychiatric disorder predominantly affecting young women. Profound anorexia, epigastric pain, bloating, and distention, as well as

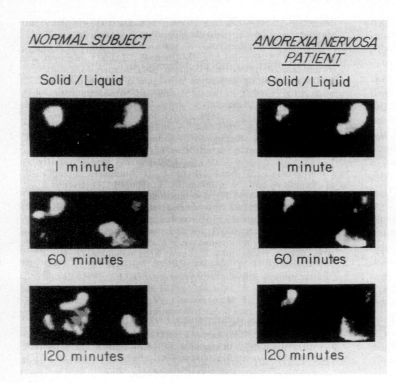

Figure 40–18. A series of scintiscans taken over a span of 2 hours contrasting the gastric emptying of solids and liquids in a patient with anorexia nervosa compared to a normal subject, using the dual isotope technique. Here the solid meal component is chicken liver labeled with ^{99m}Tc-sulfur colloid and the liquid marker is water labeled with ^{111}In-DTPA. Gastric emptying of the solid food component is dramatically slow in the patient with anorexia nervosa, whereas liquid emptying is preserved and normal.

nausea and vomiting, are common components of the symptom complex. Delayed gastric emptying of solids with preservation of normal liquid emptying has been documented in affected patients, possibly contributing to the production or perpetuation of the syndrome[138] (Fig. 40–18). The mechanism of the gastric emptying abnormality has not been discovered, but gastric neuromuscular involvement has been suggested by the reversal of delayed gastric emptying by metoclopramide[138] and domperidone,[139] a more selective dopamine antagonist. Likewise, the neuroendocrine and psychiatric components that initiate or aggravate the condition have not been elucidated. Delayed gastric emptying in these patients should prompt consideration of a caloric liquid diet and pharmacologic manipulation of gastric emptying, together with psychiatric counseling as part of the initial therapeutic approach.

Gastric Ulcer

The reported variability concerning gastric emptying in gastric ulcer patients may be attributed to different techniques of assessing gastric motor function. To date, studies have indicated a transient delay in gastric emptying, especially if the active ulcer is in the proximal stomach. Abnormalities of the interdigestive migrating motility complex and increased duodenogastric reflux have been noted in gastric ulcer patients irrespective of the location of the gastric ulcer.[140] Antral motility is also significantly diminished during phase 3 activity, which generally originated in the duodenum in two thirds of these patients. Of interest, bile salt concentration in the gastric aspirate is significantly increased, indicating the possibility of an additional

motor abnormality; however, the pathogenetic importance of this finding is not clear. Whether delayed gastric emptying is primary or results from the ulcer (secondary) remains a question. One hypothesis is that chronic antral gastritis may cause dysmotility and a chronic motor dysfunction may underlie recurrence of gastric ulcer. A long-term therapeutic approach with a prokinetic agent would seem to have good rationale.

Connective Tissue Diseases

Of all the connective tissue diseases, progressive systemic sclerosis (PSS) is best known for causing motility disturbance in the esophagus and, to some extent, in the small and large bowel. Prolonged patency of the lower esophageal sphincter and diminution or absence of peristalsis in the body of the esophagus characterize its esophageal involvement. Gastric involvement, on the other hand, has not been demonstrated to be a major feature of PSS. Of 10 patients with gastrointestinal symptoms of PSS, five had evidence suggestive of delayed gastric emptying.[141] On barium radiography, these five patients showed prolonged retention of small amounts of barium, although the earlier phases of gastric emptying appeared normal. Of these five patients, three had no upper abdominal symptoms. Using radionuclide methodology, delayed emptying of solids and liquids was documented[142] in patients with esophageal involvement, suggesting that slow emptying could augment the damage caused by the frequent gastroesophageal reflux with its attendant severe esophagitis and stricture formation. Additional gastric emptying studies should be performed in patients with Raynaud's phenomenon or cutaneous findings of scleroderma to categorize the pathophysiologic

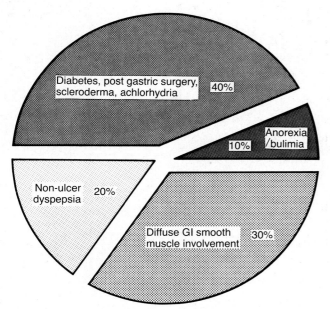

Figure 40–19. Breakdown of the patients presenting for a gastric emptying study at the University of Virginia.

state and to tailor appropriate treatment to the individual patient.

To date, reports of delayed gastric emptying in other connective tissue disorders have been patchy. A minority of patients with systemic lupus erythematosus, attributable to either vasculitis or an autonomic neuropathy, were found to have gastric involvement.[143] Delay of both esophageal and gastric emptying of solids and liquids has been documented in polymyositis and dermatomyositis, which correlated with the severity of skeletal muscle weakness.[144] Smooth muscle dysfunc-

tion may be neurologic in origin or result from muscular fibrosis or atrophy.

Summary of Clinical Classifications of Gastric Motor Disorders

Forty to 50 per cent of patients with the symptoms of gastric stasis who undergo a radionuclide study for diagnosis have diabetes mellitus, postgastric surgery problems, scleroderma, anorexia nervosa, or atrophic gastritis (Fig. 40–19). The remaining 50 per cent are said to have idiopathic gastric stasis[145] (Fig. 40–20), and the abnormality is invariably delayed gastric emptying of solids only, indicating impaired antral motility or abnormal duodenal motility affecting duodenal impedence and increasing resistance. One of the important clinical areas under the umbrella term of idiopathic gastric stasis is *nonulcer dyspepsia* (Table 40–7). In fact, up to 60 per cent of patients with *nonulcer dyspepsia* may have an underlying antral motility problem (Fig. 40–21). They complain of postprandial distress, of which profound satiety is a major component. These symptoms include epigastric discomfort, burning (often evolving into heartburn), bloating, belching, fullness, and nausea. Vomiting is infrequent. Many of these patients indeed have gastroesophageal reflux disease, some may have gastritis with and without *Campylobacter pylori*, and others have duodenal-gastric (bile) reflux related to disturbances of duodenal motility.

The other major subgroup of idiopathic gastric stasis is the group with *diffuse dysfunction of smooth muscle* throughout the gastroentestinal tract (Table 40–8). Fifty per cent of patients who have gastric stasis also

Figure 40–20. A series of scintigrams to highlight the gastric emptying abnormality present in patients with idiopathic gastric stasis. Here the gastric emptying of solids and liquids is evaluated using the dual isotope technique, in which the solid component is chicken liver labeled with ^{99m}Tc-sulfur colloid and the liquid component is water labeled with ^{111}In-DTPA. The patient with idiopathic gastric stasis will invariably have a normal liquid emptying component (fundic motility), whereas solid food emptying is always abnormal, consistent with the concept of impaired antral motility.

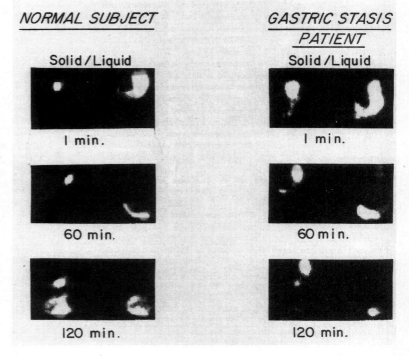

Table 40–7. PATIENTS WITH THE DIAGNOSIS OF NONULCER DYSPEPSIA

1. Up to 60 per cent will actually have delayed gastric emptying with impaired antral motility.
2. *Subgroups*
   A. Gastroesophageal reflux patients
   B. Gastritis patients:
      ?Viral, ?Campylobacter pylori as causative agent
      ?Duodenogastric (bile) reflux
   C. "Idiopathic" Role of duodenal and small bowel motility factors
3. Overall, less vomiting, more postprandial discomfort, nausea, heartburn, belching, indigestion

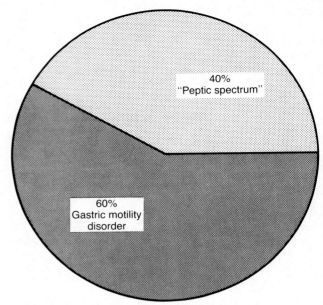

Figure 40–21. Breakdown of patients presenting to the University of Virginia, Gastroenterology Division, under the umbrella term of nonulcer dyspepsia.

have other gastrointestinal abnormalities, such as gastroduodenal motor dysfunction, and small and large bowel motor dysfunction, including atony and constipation. The author applies the term *irritable gut* (Fig. 40–22) or "unhappy" smooth muscle to some of these cases, with the recognition that each component of the *irritable gut* is a symptom arising from an organ-specific site. These patients have different severities of neuropathy from the esophagus to rectum, with gastric symptoms triggering the initial physician contact.

Particularly impressive is the female predominance (90 per cent), especially of white, professional women younger than 45 years old. Although symptoms may influence the timing of a visit to a physician, psychologic assessment has not been useful in determining a predictable patient profile. Nevertheless, psychologic stress, independent of any identifiable psychopathology, correlates with exacerbations of symptoms. Although it is tempting to link this female predominance to the hormonal influences of the menstrual cycle, no studies support this concept. There is information obtained from a breath testing technique that small bowel transit is slow in pregnant women.[73] Also, the abdominal pain is not always cyclic. Perhaps this female population has a supersensitive dose response to normal circulating levels of progesterone. Another hypothesis is that males also have degrees of this problem, but females present at a lower symptomatic threshold or are more openly concerned and inquisitive about their health status.

TREATMENT OF PATIENTS WITH GASTRIC MOTOR DISORDERS

Table 40–9 summarizes an approach to the treatment of patients with gastric motor dysfunction. If an un-

derlying disease has been identified, such as diabetes mellitus or any of the acute processes listed in Table 40–1, it should be treated and the gastric motor problem may resolve. This result is particularly likely for acute gastric retention, but it may also be true to some extent for diabetic gastroparesis. There are several anecdotal reports of spontaneous improvement in gastric motor function in diabetic patients with gastroparesis with strict control of blood sugar concentrations. In addition, in history taking, note should be made of any relationship between motion and symptoms because experimentally induced motion sickness was found to be associated with tachygastria.[146]

Diet. Dietary advice and nutritional support are also important. Many patients with gastric motor disorders will have lost weight and will be catabolic. Efforts should be made to increase nutrient intake via the oral

Table 40–8. SUBGROUPS IN CATEGORY OF "IDIOPATHIC"

Irritable bowel or constipation or both
1. Patients who may present with a gastric motility disturbance, but have a more diffuse impairment of gastrointestinal smooth muscle (e.g., duodenal-gastric dyssynchrony, intestinal pseudo-obstruction, or colonic involvement
2. Abdominal pain is often a very prominent and difficult management problem
3. Predominance of white females under age 45 years

Table 40–9. TREATMENT OF GASTRIC MOTOR DYSFUNCTION

1. Treat underlying disease process, if possible.
2. Dietary advice and nutritional support
   a. Malnutrition: Enteral supplements; intubation feeding techniques; parenteral alimentation
   b. Rapid emptying: Dry foods; avoid hypertonic, glucose-rich beverages; small, frequent feedings
   c. Slow emptying: Increase nutritive liquids; avoid hypertonic beverages; decrease undigestible material (fiber-rich foods)
3. Drug therapy
   a. Traditional antiemetic drugs
   b. Bethanechol (Urecholine)
   c. Metoclopramide (Reglan)
   d. Domperidone
   e. Cisapride
   f. Investigational drugs
4. Long-term nutritional support by feeding jejunostomy or parenteral nutrition
5. Surgery

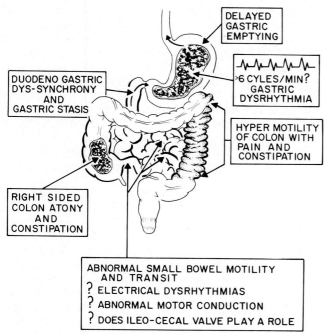

Figure 40–22. A working hypothesis to facilitate understanding of the concept of a diffuse "irritable gut" syndrome. Rather than use the term irritable bowel syndrome, which seems to be indicative of an alteration in bowel habits and accompanying lower abdominal pain, this concept suggests that each specific organ segment of the gastrointestinal tract has its own symptomatic manifestations of irritability, based on pathophysiology of its smooth muscle.

route (liquid feedings are always better tolerated than regular foods) or, if necessary, by enteric tube feeding or parenteral alimentation. Re-establishment of adequate nutrient intake removes much of the urgency about correcting gastric motor dysfunction and permits an orderly evaluation.

In individuals taking food by mouth who have gastric motor dysfunction, adjustment of the type of food ingested may ameliorate symptoms. Patients with the rapid gastric emptying, or dumping, syndromes should be advised to eat more dry foods and to avoid hypertonic, glucose-rich beverages, as precipitous emptying of hypertonic liquids is thought to be responsible for the production of symptoms in these patients. Small, frequent feedings without milk products are also advised in patients with rapid emptying in an attempt to smooth out the caloric load presented to the intestine.

In patients with slow gastric emptying, it is sensible to increase nutritive liquids in the diet because emptying of liquids may be less affected than the emptying of solids. It is important to use liquids that are isotonic, however, as interdigestive motor activity that clears the stomach of such material is often absent in these patients. Because fiber can slow emptying, a high-fiber diet in patients with slow emptying may exacerbate retention.[147] This limits a high-fiber approach for any associated constipation in this patient group.

Pharmacologic Therapy. "Kinetic," as defined in *Dorland's Medical Dictionary*, means "pertaining to or producing motion." "Prokinetic" implies favoring

"forward motion." Prokinetic (or promotility or pro-transit) agents attempt to return abnormally slow gastric emptying states to normal. They attempt to regularize the impaired setting but are thought to affect the normal emptying stomach only minimally. Therefore, appropriate studies to evaluate putative prokinetic agents are best performed in gastric stasis patients.

Developmental Background. The background of the development of these agents is very interesting and worth reviewing briefly. It is recognized that there is a vomiting center in the lateral reticular formation and that there is also a chemoreceptor trigger zone (CTZ) located on the floor of the fourth ventricle. Nausea and vomiting can result from a number of factors, ranging from visceral pain to pregnancy to cytotoxic drug therapy. Emesis can also be induced by dopamine agonists such as apomorphine, bromocriptine, and levodopa. Changes in gastrointestinal motility were observed in nausea and vomiting induced by apomorphine, radiation sickness, and motion sickness in animal models.[146] These changes in gastrointestinal activity are likely to be induced by central mechanisms involving the vagal nuclei, which are located in the immediate vicinity of the CTZ and vomiting center. Therefore, an agent that would have a central anti-emetic action as well as peripheral actions on gastrointestinal motility would be very attractive therapeutically.

The development of the dopamine antagonist metoclopramide (Reglan) relied on integrating previous knowledge that dopamine is a centrally acting emetic agent with the concepts of dopamine receptors located throughout the smooth muscle of the gastrointestinal tract. Dopamine has been known to mediate receptive relaxation of the stomach in dogs.[7] Receptive relaxation is defined as the normal physiologic relaxation of the proximal portion of the stomach in response to ingestion of a bolus, a function that is crucial to the reservoir and accommodative functions of the proximal half of the stomach. As receptive relaxation is mediated through the vagus nerve, vagotomy abolishes it. Rapid emptying of liquids results, producing symptoms of dumping and, in some, diarrhea. Hence, pharmacologic inhibition of dopamine-induced receptive relaxation should enhance gastric emptying because there would be a lower reservoir or storage capacity. This theoretical possibility is substantiated by the action on gastric emptying of such agents as metoclopramide and domperidone. These agents act on dopamine receptors.

Recently, both pharmacologic and receptor-binding experiments have shown that dopamine receptors can be classified into at least three broad categories. Dopamine 1 receptors are coupled to adenyl cyclase. Dopamine 2 receptors are pituitary cells that lack a dopamine-sensitive adenyl cyclase. Dopamine 3 receptors may be synthesized in the corpus striatum. Dopamine 2 receptors are the predominant subgroup in the gut, except for the lower esophageal sphincter,[148] and act to inhibit neurotransmitters, except perhaps in the colon, where dopamine 2 receptors help to stimulate motility.[149] As expected, agents that block dopamine 2 receptors eliminate the dopamine-mediated inhibition of gastrointestinal smooth muscle.

Dopamine-receptor antagonists all have a centrally acting antiemetic effect and elevate prolactin concentrations, but only metoclopramide and domperidone are thought to be true prokinetic agents in that they stimulate gastrointestinal motility. It is important to note that the property of being a centrally acting antiemetic does not guarantee a prokinetic effect on gastrointestinal motility. An example is the effect of tetrahydrocannabinol, an active ingredient of marijuana, which is also used as an antiemetic in patients receiving cancer chemotherapy. This agent, when ingested orally, actually delays gastric emptying in normal subjects.[150]

Metoclopramide

Metoclopramide (methoxy-2-chloro-5-procainamide) (Reglan in United States, Maxolon in United Kingdom, and Primperan in France and Europe) was first described by Justin-Besancon and associates[150a] in France as an antiemetic in pregnancy in the early 1960s. The drug, developed by the Delargrange Company in the early 1960s in Europe, is a procainamide derivative that differs from procainamide in lacking the 5-chloro and 2-methoxy aryl substituents, and as a result lacks both the local anesthetic and the antiarrhythmic properties of procainamide.

Mechanism of Action. Metoclopramide's mechanisms of action are several: (1) it is cholinergic in that it is dependent on intramural cholinergic neurons; (2) it appears to antagonize the inhibitory neurotransmitter dopamine in gastrointestinal smooth muscle; and (3) it may possibly have a direct effect on smooth muscle, an action not blocked by neural toxins.[151]

Although metoclopramide has a cholinergic action that is unlike conventional cholinergic compounds, it needs intrinsic stores of acetylcholine to achieve its effects on gastrointestinal smooth muscle. Postsynaptic activity results from the drug's ability to augment acetylcholine release from postganglionic nerve terminals and to sensitize the muscarinic receptors of gastrointestinal smooth muscle.[152, 153] Metoclopramide's effect on gastric emptying may be observed after vagotomy,[154] although this agent's actions on upper gastrointestinal smooth muscle are reduced or abolished by atropine.[155] Metoclopramide is not a cholinomimetic agent in the usual sense, however, as it does not increase gastric acid secretion or stimulate endogenous gastrin release.

Levodopa inhibits gastric emptying of a mixed solid-liquid meal in normal persons. Metoclopramide antagonizes this effect, returning gastric emptying to normal.[20] It also blocks the effect of subemetic doses of apomorphine (a dopamine agonist), which causes gastric stasis and spasm of the pylorus and duodenum. By neutralizing this effect, it accelerates gastric emptying by increasing gastric tone and amplitude of the antral contractions while decreasing relaxation of the proximal stomach. It also relaxes the pylorus and duodenum

while increasing peristalsis of the jejunum and accelerating intestinal transit time from the duodenum to the ileocecal valve.[156] The ability of metoclopramide to orchestrate upper gastrointestinal motility seems to be unique to this agent, consisting of an action that coordinates gastric, pyloric, and duodenal motor functions to produce net aboral movement. This coordinating effect of metoclopramide, although not completely understood, clearly separates this agent's effects from the nonspecific cholinergic stimulation associated with an agent like bethanechol, which does not result in net aboral movement or an increased rate of gastric emptying.[144]

Bethanechol is a cholinomimetic drug that increases gastric acid and salivary secretion; although previously it was thought to be so, it is *not prokinetic*. Bethanechol increases lower esophageal sphincter pressure (LESP) to a degree similar to that caused by metoclopramide and augments gastric contractions.[121, 157] Unlike metoclopramide, it does not accelerate gastric emptying in patients with stasis.[158] The limitations of this agent are that it produces significant abdominal cramping pain and urinary frequency, and it lacks an antiemetic component. There may be a role, however, for bethanechol in augmenting metoclopramide's therapeutic efficacy. Theoretically, presence of an agent akin to acetylcholine, particularly in diabetes, could potentiate the effects of metoclopramide.[159] Therefore, combination therapy with metoclopramide is worth a trial in patients not responding to metoclopramide alone.

The anticholinesterase agent *edrophonium (Tensilon)* may have actions and side effects similar to those of bethanechol, but is neither antiemetic nor prokinetic.

Pharmacokinetics. Metoclopramide is rapidly and almost completely absorbed by the gastrointestinal tract after oral administration. However, considerable variations (up to fivefold) in peak plasma concentration among individual recipients have been reported with the same oral dose. Sulfate conjugation in the gut or during first pass through the liver is the principal determinant of bioavailability of orally administered metoclopramide.[152] There is only partial metabolism, and 80 per cent of an oral dose is excreted in the urine within 24 hours, either as unchanged drug (20 per cent) or sulfate and glucuronide conjugates of metoclopramide. Because absorption may be delayed in patients with gastroparesis, "loading" by parenteral administration may initiate gastric and small intestinal motility, an effect that can be sustained by subsequent oral dosing. The onset of pharmacologic action of metoclopramide is 1 to 30 minutes after intravenous administration, 10 to 15 minutes after intramuscular administration, and 30 to 60 minutes after oral administration. Pharmacologic effects persist for 1 to 2 hours after administration of a single dose.

Although the exact metabolic fate of metoclopramide is not clearly established, it appears to be only minimally metabolized. Metoclopramide and its metabolites are excreted mainly in the urine. Elimination half-life has been reported as 2.6 to 5 hours in healthy subjects and about 14 hours in patients with moderate to severe renal impairment.

Therapeutic Effects. Metoclopramide's action as a prokinetic agent begins in the esophagus and extends to small bowel. It has been studied in the United States for 15 years and has been available in Europe for over 20 years. A good recent review of its pharmacology and clinical application is available.[152] In 1981, parenteral metoclopramide was approved in the United States to facilitate tube placement in the stomach and small bowel and also to accelerate small bowel transit and minimize fluoroscopic examination time in patients having small bowel series. Oral metoclopramide was subsequently approved for treating patients with diabetic gastric stasis. In 1984, the agent was approved for the oral treatment of gastroesophageal reflux disease. The injectable form of metoclopramide has also been approved for treating the nausea and vomiting associated with cancer chemotherapy. Its prokinetic effects are less pronounced in the distal than in the proximal small bowel and are only minimal in the colon.[159, 159a] In the stomach, the drug increases both the frequency of antral contractions, up to the maximum of three per minute, and the amplitude of these contractions in both normal subjects and patients with gastric stasis syndromes.[138, 149] In the small bowel, metoclopramide induces the equivalent of a migrating motor complex, inasmuch as the increase in gastric motility that it induces extends into the duodenum and small bowel.[152]

Diabetic Gastroparesis. Controlled trials[160–163] have shown that metoclopramide gives symptomatic relief while accelerating gastric emptying of solids and liquids in diabetic gastroparesis. A period of time (days) may elapse before it is clinically effective because of delayed absorption due to the gastroparesis. In patients who have been helped symptomatically but in whom gastric emptying is unaffected, metoclopramide's efficacy is explained by its centrally acting antiemetic properties.

Postgastric Surgery. In postgastric resection gastroparesis, subjective and objective improvements achieved in controlled trials attest to metoclopramide's efficacy in antrectomized patients.[121, 152]

Idiopathic Gastric Stasis. A full understanding of the pathophysiology of gastric stasis is not possible in some patients; such cases are termed idiopathic. In these patients and including those with anorexia nervosa or gastric ulcer disease, metoclopramide has also been shown to enhance gastric emptying.[138, 152]

However, the long-term therapeutic value of metoclopramide in these patients has not been established. In patients with chronic idiopathic intestinal pseudo-obstruction, metoclopramide has been shown to be less effective, possibly because some of these patients have a primary smooth muscle disorder, whereas others have a myenteric nerve lesion.

Dosage and Administration. The usual dose of metoclopramide is 10 mg fifteen to thirty minutes before meals and at bedtime. In older patients, the initial dose should be 5 mg three to four times a day, which is then slowly increased to a therapeutic level as tolerated. A syrup preparation is available for children. Maintenance doses of metoclopramide may also be used in the long-term management of gastric stasis; for example, 20 mg may be indicated before a large evening meal or before retiring to maximize gastric emptying and minimize side effects.

Metoclopramide may also be administered subcutaneously. This can be a valuable route for treating patients who are severely nauseated and frequently vomit up the oral form before it can be absorbed. No suppository form is available. The subcutaneous route guarantees sustained plasma levels and allows patients to treat themselves at home during periods of severe symptoms. It is well tolerated in a dose of 1 ml, or 5 mg, at each subcutaneous site. The author recommends a trial of this route of therapy in all patients with "refractory" gastric stasis. Side effects, of course, must be closely monitored.

Side Effects

The incidence of side effects of metoclopramide is approximately 20 per cent.[152] The main side effects are *drowsiness* or *restlessness,* and *anxiety* (akathisia). There are also mild effects, such as dry mouth, light-headedness, constipation, diarrhea, and rash. *Extrapyramidal reactions,* such as oculogyric crises, opisthotonos, trismus, and torticollis, affect about 1 per cent of patients. These effects can be reversed immediately with diphenhydramine (Benadryl) and also are more slowly reversible by discontinuing the drug.

At therapeutic levels of metoclopramide, parkinsonian motor disorders, such as *tremor, rigidity,* and *akinesia,* have only rarely been reported and have been reversible on stopping the drug. However, dosages in children, the elderly, and patients with renal failure must be monitored carefully. Tardive dyskinesia is a very rare but reported possibility. Some of the patients had underlying Parkinson's disease. Metoclopramide elevates serum prolactin levels in all patients, some of whom may have associated breast enlargement, nipple tenderness, galactorrhea, or menstrual irregularity. Contraindications to the use of metoclopramide include evidence of significant *mechanical obstruction,* simultaneous use of *other dopamine antagonists,* such as phenothiazines (a relative contraindication; augments side effects), *anticholinergic agents* (antagonism of metoclopramide's effects), *pheochromocytoma,* and *parkinsonism.* Although metoclopramide may alleviate nausea and vomiting in parkinsonism, the drug may also negate the effects of dopamine agonists used in treatment of the disease.

Domperidone

Domperidone (Motilium) a benzimidazole derivative (Fig. 40–23), is a specific dopamine antagonist that stimulates the gastrointestinal tract and has antiemetic properties, but it does not readily cross the blood-brain barrier and rarely causes extrapyramidal side

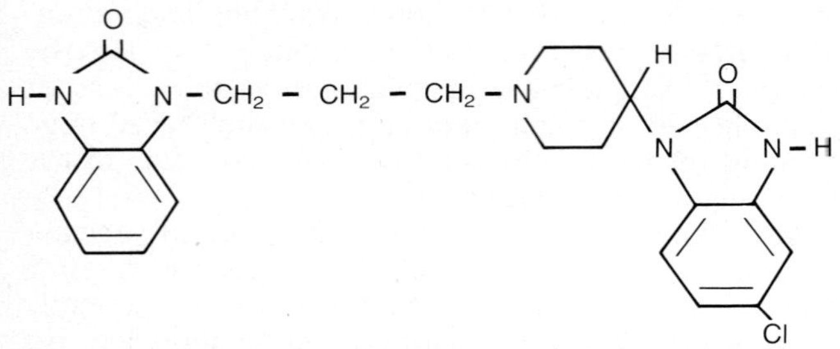

Figure 40–23. Molecular structure of domperidone.

effects. Recent reviews of this experimental agent are available.[164, 165] The wide dissociation between the peripheral and central effects of domperidone has been demonstrated in animal studies by the low brain concentration after systemic administration, the marked differences in the effect of intracerebral and systemic domperidone in antagonizing the behavioral effects of dopamine, and the wide difference in the intravenous dosage needed to counteract the peripheral (emetic) and central effects of apomorphine.[164] These observations indicate that the CTZ is outside the blood-brain barrier, clearly indicating that it is on the CTZ that domperidone exercises its antiemetic action, and side effects related to dopamine depletion in the central nervous system, (e.g., basal ganglion) are not seen. Domperidone does not seem to have any cholinergic activity, as its actions are not blocked by atropine.

Pharmacokinetics. Peak plasma concentrations of domperidone occur from 10 to 30 minutes after intramuscular and oral administration, and from 1 to 3 hours after rectal administration of suppositories. This suppository form is available in Europe. Bioavailability of intramuscular domperidone is about 90 per cent, whereas that of oral domperidone is 13 to 17 per cent. The low oral bioavailability is probably due to metabolism in gut wall and liver during "first-pass." The detection of drug in the wall of the stomach and small bowel suggests that part of its mechanism of action is through this pathway. This would suggest local effects on smooth muscle, so plasma levels of domperidone may not reflect or necessarily correlate with smooth muscle actions. After oral administration, 31 per cent of the drug is excreted in the urine and 60 per cent in the feces over a period of four days. The elimination half-life of domperidone is 7.5 hours in healthy subjects and can be prolonged up to 20.8 hours in patients with very severe renal dysfunction, but accumulation does not occur in mild renal dysfunction.[164]

Mechanism of Gastrointestinal Effects. Domperidone has a high affinity for gastrointestinal tissue, and high concentrations of the drug are found in the esophagus, stomach, and small intestine. Currently, the entire effect of domperidone on gastrointestinal smooth muscle is explained by its antagonism of dopamine receptors. This commences with partial inhibition of receptive relaxation in the stomach, augmentation of antral motility, and, in addition, improved antroduodenal coordination of peristaltic waves and acceleration of small intestinal transit. Domperidone probably has a minimal effect on colonic motility.

Gastric Stasis. The effect of domperidone on gastric motility involves increased peristaltic activity of the antrum and duodenum as well as increased amplitude. Data on domperidone's effect on gastric emptying of solids and liquids in patients with gastric retention states, as well as on dose-response effects of parenteral domperidone in patients with diabetes, postsurgical stasis, gastroesophageal reflux, scleroderma, and idiopathic gastric stasis are available.[166] Ten milligrams of domperidone does not accelerate gastric emptying significantly, whereas doses of 20, 30, and 40 mg orally will[166, 167] (Fig. 40–24). In a recent double-blind crossover trial, domperidone, in oral doses of 20 to 30 mg four times a day, was shown to be significantly better than placebo in improving the symptoms of gastric retention in patients with *idiopathic gastric stasis*.[168] An open-labeled trial indicates that a dose of 20 mg significantly improves the symptoms in patients with diabetic gastroparesis.[167] Daily dose regimens have ranged from 40 to 120 mg in the United States, and the duration of treatment experience for any one patient has ranged up to 2 years.

Side Effects. Domperidone is particularly well tolerated and seldom causes important side effects. However, it has a potent effect on prolactin secretion, which results in side effects that are more inconvenient than disabling. *Breast enlargement, nipple tenderness,* and *galactorrhea* are particularly notable in women. The accompanying hyperprolactinemia can result in *amenorrhea*. Amenorrhea as well as more significant prolactin side effects are more frequent with domperidone than metoclopramide, probably because domperidone is given in larger doses. Other side effects occasionally reported include *dry mouth, transient skin rash* or *itching, headache, diarrhea,* and *nervousness*.

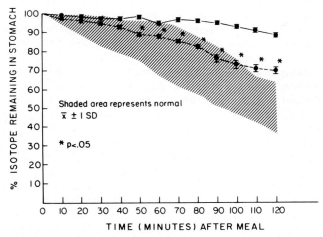

Figure 40–24. The effect of 20 mg domperidone administered intravenously to 13 patients with gastric stasis either secondary to diabetes mellitus or postgastric surgery or idiopathic. The delayed gastric emptying of the solid meal (isotope-labeled chicken liver) is accelerated in a statistically significant fashion, so that the emptying rate returns to the normal range (shaded area) over the 2-hour observation period of the study.

Extrapyramidal and true acute dystonic reactions are rare. Central nervous system side effects have not been reported. Thus, domperidone is potentially useful in treating children and patients with parkinsonism.

The author has used this agent in more than 100 patients being treated in double-blind or open-labeled trials for periods of up to 3 years. The drug has been well tolerated, with side effects related to hyperprolactinemia observed in 10 to 15 per cent of patients. A New Drug Application is being submitted to FDA for the treatment of diabetic gastroparesis and idiopathic gastric stasis syndromes. One important observation from Japan is that parenteral and even oral administration of domperidone to patients with chemotherapy-induced nausea and vomiting was associated with cardiac arrhythmias, which has led to discontinuation of parenteral domperidone in that country. Although no cardiac arrhythmias have been reported with this drug in the United States or Europe, all studies with parenteral domperidone in the United States have also been suspended at this time.

In summary, although direct comparative studies of the two drugs are lacking, domperidone seems to be as efficacious as metoclopramide as a prokinetic agent, but generally it requires larger doses. Its minimal side effects give it an attractive potential for long-term maintenance use, which is often required in diabetic and other patients with gastric retention. Another attractive aspect is that domperidone is available in a rectal (suppository) preparation, a feature that could be valuable in maintenance of high blood levels of the drug during nausea and vomiting. Information is lacking as to whether domperidone has any corrective role in gastric dysrhythmic states.

Cisapride

Cisapride, a benzamide derivative, is a new prokinetic agent under investigation in the United States and Europe by Janssen Pharmaceutica. Devoid of antidopaminergic properties of cholinomimetic effects (Fig. 40–25), cisapride is thought to facilitate acetylcholine release at the myenteric plexus without effects at the secretory gland level.[169] In vitro, it stimulates ileal contractility, increases gastric tonic and phasic motility, and furthers antroduodenal coordination.[170] In vivo, it stimulates digestive and interdigestive antroduodenal motility and improves gastric emptying.[171] There are animal data on the esophagus, stomach, small bowel, and colon to support a prokinetic effect.

Cisapride also appears to be an effective antagonist of serotonin in the guinea pig intestinal mucosa.[172]

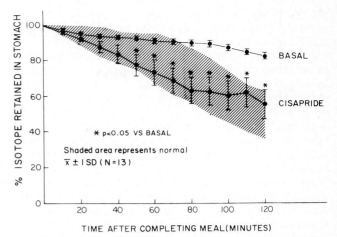

Figure 40–26. The effect of cisapride administered in a dose of 10 mg intravenously on gastric emptying of an isotope-labeled solid meal (chicken liver) in 19 patients with delayed gastric emptying that was attributed to diabetes mellitus, followed gastric surgery, or was considered idiopathic. Compared to the very slow baseline emptying state, cisapride significantly accelerated gastric emptying and returned it to the normal range (see shaded area) during the 120 minutes of the study.

Such an agent may regulate intestinal ion transport and hence may have a role in diarrheal states or abnormal motility of the colon and small intestine. On the other hand, this drug may be the first agent that promises a prokinetic approach to idiopathic constipation.

Pharmacokinetics. In humans, the plasma level of cisapride decays triexponentially, with a half-life of 19.4 hours after intravenous administration. The bioavailability after oral administration is in the range of 35 to 40 per cent. Plasma levels after administration of a 10 mg tablet peaked at 1.5 to 2.0 hours.

Therapeutics. In humans, cisapride, in doses of 2, 4, and 8 mg intravenously and 4 and 16 mg orally, increases gastric emptying, antral peristalsis, and small bowel transit[173] without affecting gastric secretion and serum prolactin levels. The incidence of side effects in the subjects receiving the agent was negligible. However, the one side effect reported was loose stool, suggesting an effect on the colon in humans. Cisapride, in a 10-mg intravenous dose, significantly accelerated gastric emptying of solids (Fig. 40–26) and liquids in patients with diabetic, postgastric surgery, and idiopathic gastric stasis syndromes.[174]

The drug remains experimental in the United States, although approval in some European countries will begin in 1988.

Naloxone

The role of the opiate peptides as neurotransmitters of gastrointestinal motility and secretion is being pursued extensively. Morphine has an inhibitory effect on gastric emptying, which can be demonstrated by systemic or intracerebroventricular administration of the opiate. Studies have demonstrated that naloxone is a potent μ receptor opiate antagonist. In a dose of 5 mg

Figure 40–25. Molecular structure of cisapride. This compound is devoid of both antidopaminergic and cholinomimetic effects. It facilitates acetylcholine release at the myenteric plexus without having effect at the secretory gland level.

intravenously, naloxone accelerated gastric emptying of both solids and liquids but not to a statistically significant degree over a 2-hour period for which data are available.[175] One study[176] has addressed the effect of naloxone on abnormally slow gastric emptying rates. In a daily dose of 1.6-mg subcutaneously, it accelerates gastric emptying of solids and transit time to the cecum in patients with small intestinal pseudo-obstruction. Such evidence raises the question whether naloxone may indeed have a role in patients with delayed gastric emptying or impaired small bowel motility, or both. A body of information is already available on irritable bowel syndrome suggesting that naloxone may be useful in decreasing pain and improving bowel habits. An oral equivalent to naloxone, naltrexone, may have therapeutic benefits for patients who do not require parenteral administration.

Antiemetics

The response to prokinetic agents can be augmented and supplemented by traditional antiemetic drugs, such as prochlorperazine (Compazine), tremethobenzamide (Tigan), and chlorpromazine (Phenergan) orally, parenterally, or by suppository.[177] These agents may be helpful in reducing nausea and vomiting, making patients more able to tolerate diagnostic studies, and, in particular, able to ingest meals. The acute use of antiemetics will not interfere with interpretation of the gastric emptying results. In sustained high doses there is concern that the small anticholinergic component related to these agents may interfere with gastric prokinetic drug use and interpretation of tests.

Patients receiving dexamethasone for chemotherapy-induced vomiting notice less suppression of appetite with dexamethasone than with other antiemetics, raising the question of whether this agent has some accompanying beneficial effect on gastrointestinal motility. Similar observations regarding appetite improvements have, of course, been noted in many patients receiving prednisone for different reasons. Only one report suggests that prednisolone was effective in patients with idiopathic nausea and vomiting or that accompanying endoscopic antral gastritis.[178] Prednisone does dramatically improve the nausea and vomiting related to Addison's disease.[58]

Surgical Treatment of Gastric Stasis

Surgical therapy for patients with continuing symptoms, malnutrition, and inability to function may be necessary in certain selected cases of idiopathic gastric stasis and rarely in diabetic gastroparesis. A case in point refers to a female patient with severe nausea, vomiting, and weight loss, diagnosed as having tachygastria and tachydysrhythmia with pacesetter potentials in the orad direction arising from an antral ectopic focus, and asynchrony between duodenum and jejunum.[104] Distal hemigastrectomy and resection of the jejunal segment produced weight gain and relieved

symptoms. Subtotal gastrectomy was required for a definitive result in the case of an infant with unexplained gastric stasis tachygastria that was unresolved by pyloroplasty or gastrojejunostomy.[103] These drastic measures came after exhaustive attempts at pharmacologic and dietary control failed. At present, any consideration for operation can only be condoned after such patients have been referred to special centers to undergo full investigations related to motility and electrophysiology, as well as psychiatric assessment. Other options would include a trial of home hyperalimentation or feeding jejunostomy to see if time may play some role in helping motility return.

Any patient undergoing or being considered for an antrectomy because of refractory gastric stasis should have the operation at a center with special interest in gastrointestinal motility research. Special electron microscopy and stains of smooth muscle tissue and nerve ganglia are indicated. In the case of idiopathic gastric stasis there have been antrectomies performed in the hope that suspected antral ectopic pacemakers inducing dysrhythmias would be resected. Follow-up in these settings indicated <50 per cent sustained improvement after antrectomy. It is hoped that more refined EGG studies preoperatively will allow better documentation of which patients have evidence of a dysrhythmia. If antrectomy is contemplated when medical therapy fails, electrodes should be placed on the gastric remnant or the serosa at the time of surgery for postoperative recordings to detect a possible dysrhythmia. This then makes possible the option of gastric pacing. The author and colleagues have demonstrated that electrical stimulation of serosal electrodes from an external source can significantly improve gastric emptying of a solid meal,[179] and there may be a further role for "gastric pacing" using portable stimulation. However, this is purely experimental at present. No vagotomy should be performed in the idiopathic setting for fear of disturbing remaining motility in the small bowel.

Antrectomy and hemigastrectomy may have a role in treatment of a patient whose condition is termed "idiopathic," in whom prolonged medical treatment, including experimental agents has failed, and who has no apparent dysrhythmia. In addition, this operation should be considered in severe diabetic gastric stasis, particularly in a young patient whose other diabetic complications are minimal or well tolerated. The goal here is to remove a nonfunctioning antrum, performing a wide gastroduodenal anastomosis in the hope that food will empty by gravity. A truncal vagomoty is not recommended, although possibly a selective parietal cell vagotomy may be done in the hope of increasing liquid emptying. Also, a Billroth II antrectomy is not recommended because severe bile reflux can result. The author has documented 50 per cent improvement in gastric emptying of a radionuclide meal and a much improved course in two diabetic patients and in one patient with idiopathic stasis for whom he has recommended this procedure. Based on the total patient experience of the author's group, this would indicate that less than 5 per cent of all gastric stasis patients may warrant such consideration.

Postoperative gastric stasis occurs in patients who have undergone an antrectomy and vagotomy for chronic peptic ulcer disease, usually in the setting of complicated gastric outlet obstruction. These are the patients who in turn go on to have revision of their Billroth I anastomosis to a Billroth II, and later on have an additional Roux-en-Y procedure. Pharmacologic approaches with prokinetic agents in this subgroup of patients is worth trying but has a very low success rate. There is limited gastric smooth muscle, and it has lost its length-tension relationship. New evidence has been found that the Roux limb itself may be the site of dysmotility and that it is possible that this Roux limb is actually an obstructive element for emptying from the gastric remnant. The incidence of this Roux-en-Y syndrome at the Mayo Clinic is 25 to 30 per cent.[180] Such a Roux limb has been used successfully for years in the operation performed for Zollinger-Ellison syndrome. It seems that in the clinical setting of the antrectomized patient who has delayed gastric emptying already present before the addition of the Roux-en-Y procedure, a "double jeopardy" situation develops. Mathias and colleagues[181] have shown abnormal motor patterns in Roux limbs in these patients and hypothesize that loss of electrical synchrony in the implanted jejunal limb may be a contributing factor. This is consistent with observations in the animal setting in which ectopic pacemakers can appear in Roux limbs and drive the limb in a reverse or orad direction.[182] Vogel and colleagues[183, 184] and Hocking and associates,[185] in studying dogs undergoing gastric resections and Roux procedures, have stressed how the addition of a vagotomy seemed to correlate with the finding of delayed gastric emptying. There has been a call for reassessment of the Roux-en-Y procedure, and at the time of this writing, the author believes that this procedure cannot be condoned when there is evidence that delayed gastric emptying is present initially. There may be selective situations in which bile reflux gastritis is so overwhelming that there is a defensible indication for diversion of bile to be achieved by a Roux-en-Y procedure. However, if done in a setting of gastric stasis documented for solids, it will not result in improved gastric emptying and symptoms will remain.

It is the conclusion of the author, based on experiences with two recent cases of extreme malnutrition and debilitation following gastric operations and Roux-en-Y procedures, that total gastrectomy and esophagojejunal anastomosis may possibly be of help in improving nutrition and overcoming vomiting. In these cases, vomiting did stop and nutrition was stable. Other clinicians at the Mayo Clinic also find that total gastrectomy can be effective (K. Kelly, personal communication). However, when a long history of abdominal pain is also present, this symptom is usually not helped by total gastrectomy. This is particularly so when the abdominal pain dates back to the initial peptic ulcer experience and has persisted during surgical revisions. Here attempts at addressing the pain needs of the patient are a different and difficult problem but should not be used as an indication for such surgery as total gastric resection.

Summary of Therapeutic Approaches for Gastric Stasis

This review has addressed the rapidly evolving field of prokinetic agents in the gastrointestinal tract. The gold standard at the current time—the "digoxin," if you will (based on a cardiology analogy) of gastrointestinal smooth muscle—is metoclopramide, the drug about which the most data have been accumulated and currently the only approved prokinetic agent in the United States. Domperidone, the selective peripheral dopamine antagonist available in Europe and in many other countries, has a better safety profile and long-term maintenance treatment potential. Cisapride may be the first agent with total esophagus-to-colon propulsive properties and with an excellent safety profile. Future developments in the prokinetic approaches will take place in four areas: (1) defining dysrhythmias of gastrointestinal smooth muscle and finding antiarrhythmic agents; (2) developing drugs that perturb myenteric plexus mechanisms (e.g., suppress inhibition or augment stimulation); assessing the role of serotonin and serotonin receptor antagonists, which are currently very topical in regard to this site of modulation[186]; (3) evaluating the role of peptides, particularly CCK, and the development of both antagonists (in the case of CCK) or perhaps peptide agonists in other settings; and (4) pursuing the concept of electrical stimulation pacing of the gastrointestinal tract, including the stomach.

RAPID GASTRIC EMPTYING

Rapid gastric emptying has been associated with duodenal ulcer. Duodenal ulcer patients are observed to empty solids more quickly than normal persons.[187] Other reports, however, have shown that liquid emptying is normal in patients with duodenal ulcers.[188, 189] The cause and effect relationship between rapid gastric emptying of solids and duodenal ulcer have not yet been determined. It was demonstrated in a family with a duodenal ulcer diathesis that gastric emptying of liquids was rapid.[190] Such studies support the concept that gastric emptying is a factor in the pathogenesis of certain subgroups of duodenal ulcer by accelerating emptying of unbuffered acid into the duodenum. A study using mixed liquid-solid scintigraphy noted in duodenal ulcer patients the existence of a subgroup with normal emptying and another with rapid gastric emptying.[191] Gastric emptying studies after ulcers are healed are necessary to clarify this association. Although rapid gastric emptying may be important in the pathogenesis of duodenal ulcer, it should be stated that this motility abnormality is relatively asymptomatic. Interestingly, aluminum hydroxid, antacids, and

Carafate (an aluminum salt) do act to slow rapid gastric emptying[81] and it could be speculated that the decreased acid load to the duodenal bulb may assist healing.

Zollinger-Ellison syndrome is associated with rapid gastric emptying of both liquids[67] and solids.[192] The mechanism is unclear, but it may involve defective inhibitory receptor processes due to extensive duodenal and proximal jejunal inflammation. Cimetidine does not normalize gastric emptying, indicating that acid hypersecretion per se is not the cause of the accelerated emptying.[192] Although the diarrhea that Zollinger-Ellison patients usually experience is multifactorial, rapid gastric emptying may well be a contributing factor.

Postgastric Surgery

Some patients with gastroenterostomy, partial gastrectomy, vagotomy with pyloroplasty or antrectomy, or proximal gastric vagotomy experience a postprandial symptom complex known as the *dumping syndrome*. The early dumping symptoms are those of epigastric fullness and pain, nausea, vomiting, diarrhea, and weakness occurring 10 to 30 minutes after meals. Palpitations, sweating, and weakness occurring 1 to 3 hours after meals are labeled late dumping symptoms and are ascribed to hypoglycemia. The incidence of the dumping symdrome is difficult to ascertain because of the varying criteria used in its diagnosis. After proximal gastric vagotomy, the incidence may be as low as 0.9 per cent,[193] whereas after truncal vagotomy and antrectomy, it may be as high as 22 per cent.[194] After truncal or selective vagotomy with drainage, symptoms of dumping can be elicited in 10 to 30 per cent of patients, but severe symptoms are present in less than 5 per cent.[195]

Rapid gastric emptying is a major factor in the pathogenesis of the dumping syndrome (Fig. 40–27). As stated earlier, vagotomies or subtotal gastrectomies as a group result in an initial phase of rapid liquid emptying. With regard to solid emptying, subgroups of patients with vagotomy and pyloroplasty can be identified, one with rapid gastric emptying of solids.[196] It is clear that patients with the dumping syndrome have an increased initial emptying rate for liquids compared with asymptomatic patients after similar gastric operative procedures.[197] In this study, rapid gastric emptying also correlated with decreases in plasma volume. The intraluminal hyperosmolarity caused by the rapid gastric emptying may be responsible for the shift in plasma fluid

Malabsorptive states, such as pancreatic exocrine insufficiency and celiac sprue, may conceivably cause rapid gastric emptying. Inasmuch as small bowel inhibitory receptors are more sensitive to fatty acids than to whole fat, maldigestion of fat should theoretically decrease the inhibition of gastric emptying. However, normal gastric emptying of liquids has been noted in patients with pancreatic exocrine insufficiency.[198]

In the past, *hyperthyroidism* was often listed as a

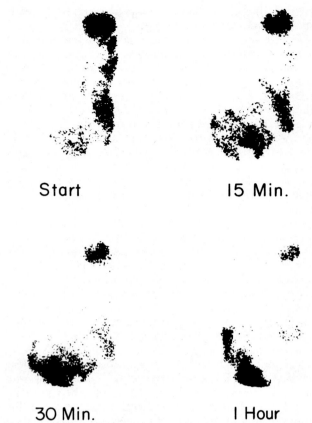

Start   15 Min.

30 Min.   1 Hour

Figure 40–27. Representative scintiscans of the abdomen demonstrating rapid gastric and intestinal transit of an isotope-labeled chicken liver meal in a patient with symptoms of "dumping syndrome" following a Billroth II gastric resection. Note that by 30 minutes the isotope is appreciated in the cecal area with only a small residual in the gastric remnant. By 1 hour the isotope is entering the ascending colon.

cause of rapid gastric emptying. A recent study, however, has shown that the emptying rates of liquids and solids are normal in hyperthyroidism.[199]

Therapy of Rapid Gastric Emptying Disorders

The dumping syndrome is the only disorder of rapid gastric emptying that warrants therapy directed specifically at the emptying problem. Dietary manipulations, such as frequent small feedings, temporarily separating solid from liquid intake, and decreasing carbohydrate intake, may reduce but rarely eliminates the symptoms of dumping. Anticholinergic drugs can slow gastric emptying, as can levodopa, codeine, and other opiates, and can alleviate some of the dumping manifestations. Pectin, a type of dietary fiber, causes some symptomatic improvement in addition to delayed liquid emptying in dumping syndrome patients.[200] The mechanism of pectin action is not clear. Acarbose,[201] a disaccharidase inhibitor, may also be efficacious in the dumping syndrome and is currently undergoing therapeutic trials. Remedial surgery for the dumping syndrome has unpredictable results,[202] although several operative techniques have been tried.

When patients have a pyloroplasty or a gastroenterostomy, the pyloroplasty can be overcome by reconstructing the pylorus, or the gastroenterostomy can be taken down and the defects in the stomach and small intestine closed. The procedures will increase resistance to outflow of chyme and slow the rate of gastric emptying, thus combatting the symptoms produced by rapid emptying. The danger is that the rate of emptying after the reconstruction will be so slow that symptoms of gastric stasis will then ensue.[202] Another alternative is to convert an operative result to a Roux gastrectomy. The rate of emptying from the gastric remnant into a Roux limb is approximately that found in healthy persons. Thus, the symptoms of rapid emptying may abate after conversion to a Roux gastrectomy.

Recent investigation in an animal model for dumping have focused on the role of electrical pacing of a segment of proximal small bowel to reverse or hinder the aboral flow of contents.[203]

References

1. Cannon, W. B. The movements of the stomach studied by means of Roentgenrays. Am. J. Physiol. *1*:359, 1898.
2. Thomas, J. E. Mechanics and regulation of gastric emptying. Physiol. Rev. *37*:453, 1957.
3. Wilbur, B. G., and Kelly, K. A. Effect of proximal, complete gastric and truncal vagotomy on canine gastric electrical activity, motility and emptying. Ann. Surg. *178*:295, 1973.
4. Jahnberg, T. Gastric adaptive relaxation. Effects of vagal inactivation and vagotomy. An experimental study in dogs and in man. Scand. J. Gastroent. *12*(Suppl.):1, 1977.
5. Abrahamsson, H. Studies on inhibitory nervous control of gastric motility. Acta Physiol. Scand. *390*(Suppl.):1, 1973.
6. Brandsborg, O., Bransborg, M., Loygreen, N. A., Mikkelsen, K., Moller, B., Rokkjaer, M., and Andrup, E. Influence of parietal cell vagotomy and selective gastric vagotomy on gastric emptying rate and serum gastrin concentrations. Gastroenterology *72*:212, 1977.
7. Valenzuela, J. E. Dopamine as a possible nerve transmitter in gastric relaxation. Gastroenterology *71*:1019, 1976.
8. Wilbur, B. G., and Kelly, K. S. Effect of proximal gastric, complete gastric and truncal vagotomy on canine gastric electric activity, motility and emptying. Ann. Surg. *178*:295, 1973.
9. Strunz, U. T., and Grossman, M. I. Effect of intragastric pressure on gastric emptying and secretion. Am. J. Physiol. *234*:E552, 1978.
10. Kelly, K. A., Code, C. F., and Elveback, L. R. Patterns of canine gastric electrical activity. Am. J. Physiol. *217*:461, 1969.
11. Hinder, R. A., and Kelly, K. A. Human gastric pacesetter potential: site of origin, spread, and response to gastric transection and proximal gastric vagotomy. Am. J. Surg. *133*:29, 1977.
12. Kelly, K. A., and Code, C. F. Canine gastric pacemaker. Am. J. Physiol. *220*:112, 1971.
12a. Schirmer, B. D., Shaffrey, B. E., Bellahsene, B. E., and McCallum, R. W. Identification of myoelectric activity in the fundus of the human stomach. Gastroenterology *92*:1621, 1987.
13. Gabella, G. Structure of muscles and nerves in the gastrointestinal tract., *In* Johnson, L. R. (ed.). Physiology of the Gastrointestinal Tract, Vol. 1. New York, Raven Press, 1981, pp. 197–241.
14. Szurszewski, J. H. Electrical basis for gastrointestinal motility. *In* Johnson, L .R. (ed.). Physiology of the Gastrointestinal Tract, Vol. 2. New York, Raven Press, 1981, pp. 1435–1466.
15. Morgan, K. G., and Szurszewski, J. H. Mechanisms of phasic

and tonic actions of pentagastrin of canine gastric smooth muscle. J. Physiol. (Lond.) *301*:229, 1981.
16. Sanders, K., Menguy, R., Chey, W., You, C., Lee, K., Morgan, K., Kreulen, D., Schmalz, P., Muir, T., and Szurszewski, J. One explanation for human antral tachygastria (Abstract). Gastroenterology *76*:1234, 1979.
17. Code, C. F., and Carlson, H. C. Motor activity of the stomach. *In* Code, C. F., and Heidel, H. (eds.). Handbook of Physiology, Section 6, Volume 4: Alimentary Canal. Baltimore, Williams & Wilkins, 1968, pp. 1903–1916.
18. Meyer, J. H., Thomson, J. B., Cohen, M. B., et al. Sieving of solid food by the canine stomach and sieving after gastric surgery. Gastroenterology *76*:804, 1979.
19. Scratcherd, T., and Grundy, D. Nervous afferents from the upper gastrointestinal tract which influence gastrointestinal motility. *In* Weinbeck, M. (ed.). Motility of the Digestive Tract. New York, Raven Press, 1982, pp. 7–17.
20. Berkowitz, D. M., and McCallum, R. W. Interaction of levodopa and metoclopramide on gastric emptying. Clin. Pharmacol. Ther. *27*:414, 1980.
21. Fernandez, A. G., and Massingham, R. Peripheral receptor populations involved in the regulation of gastrointestinal motility and the pharmacologic actions of metoclopramide-like drugs. Life Sciences *36*:1, 1985.
22. Kelly, K. A. Effect of gastrin on gastric myoelectric activity. Am. J. Dig. Dis. *15*:399, 1970.
23. Valenzuela, J. E. Effect of intestinal hormones and peptides on intragastric pressure in dogs. Gastroenterology, *71*:766, 1976.
24. Valenzuela, J. E., and Defilippi, C. Inhibition of gastric emptying in humans by secretin, the octapeptide of cholecystokinin, and intraduodenal fat. Gastroenterology *81*:898, 1981.
25. Valenzuela, J. E., and Grossman, M. I. Effect of pentagastrin and caerulein on intragastric pressure in dogs. Gastroenterology *69*:1383, 1975.
26. Itoh, Z., Takeuchi, S., Aizawa, I., Mori, K., Taminato, T., Seino, Y., Imura, H., and Yanihara, N. Changes in plasma motilin concentration and gastrointestinal contractile activity in conscious dogs. Am. J. Dig. Dis. *23*:929, 1978.
27. Ricci, D., Lange, R., Magyar, L., and McCallum, R. W. Effect of histamine receptor stimulation on gastric emptying in man. Clin. Res. *13*:682A, 1983.
28. Corinaldes, R., Scarpignato, C., Galassi, A., Stanghellini, V., Callamelli, R., Bertaccini, G., and Barbara, L. Effect of cimetidine and ranitidine on gastric emptying of a mixed meal in man. Int. J. Clin. Pharmacol. Ther. Toxicol. *22*:498, 1984.
29. Monges, H., Salduca, J., and Nandy, B. Electrical activity of the gastrointestinal tract in dogs during vomiting. *In* Daniel, E. E. (ed.). Proceedings of the Fourth International Symposium on Gastrointestinal Motility. Vancouver, Mitchell Press, 1976, pp. 479–488.
30. Kim, C. H., and Malagelada, J. R. Electrical activity of the stomach: clinical implications. Mayo Clin. Proc. *61*:205, 1986.
31. Meyer, J. H., Thompson, J. B., Cohen, M. B., et al. Sieving of solid food by the normal and ulcer operated canine stomach. Gastroenterology *76*:804, 1979.
32. Hinder, R. A., and San-garde, B. A. Individual and combined roles of the pylorus and antrum in the canine gastric emptying of a liquid and digestible solid. Gastroenterology *84*:281, 1983.
33. Schuurks, J. A. J., and VanNeuten, J. M. Gastroduodenal coordination. *In* Akkermans, L. M. A., Johnson, A. G., and Read, N. N. (eds.). Gastric and Gastroduodenal Motility. New York, Praeger Scientific, 1984.
34. Amidon, G. L. Fluid mechanics and intestinal transit. Gastroenterology *88*:858, 1985.
35. Schulze-Delrieu, K., and Wall, J. P. Determinants of flow across isolated gastroduodenal functions in cats and rabbits. Am. J. Physiol. *245*:259, 1983.
36. Clarke, R. J., and Alexander-Williams, J. The effect of preserving antral innervation and of a pyloroplasty on gastric emptying in man. Gut *14*:300, 1973.
37. Bortolotti, M., Pandolfo, N., and Nebiacolombo, C., Labo, G., and Mattioli, F. Modifications in gastroduodenal motility induced by the extramucosal section of circular duodenal musculature in dogs. Gastroenterology *81*:910, 1981.

38. Hunt, J. N., and Spurrell, W. R. The pattern of emptying of the human stomach. J. Physiol. (Lond.) *113*:157, 1957.

39. Hunt, J. N. Some properties of an alimentary osmoreceptor mechanism. J. Physiol. (Lond.) *132*:267, 1956.

40. Hunt, J. N., and Knox, M. T. The slowing of gastric emptying by four strong acids and three weak acids. J. Physiol. (Lond) 22:187, 1972.

41. Hunt, J. N., and Pathak, J. D. The osmotic effects of some simple molecules and ions on gastric emptying. J. Physiol. (Lond.) *154*:254, 1960.

42. Hunt, J. N., and Knox, M. T. A relation between the chain length of fatty acids and the slowing of gastric emptying. J. Physiol. (Lond.) *194*:327, 1968.

43. Stephens, J. R., Woolson, R. F., and Cooke, A. R. Effects of essential and non-essential amino acids on gastric emptying in the dog. Gastroenterology *69*:920, 1975.

44. Hunt, J. N., and Stubbs, D. F. The volume and energy content of meals as determinants of gastric emptying. J. Physiol. (Lond.) *245*:209, 1975.

45. Keinke, O., and Ehrein, J. J. Effect of oleic acid on canine gastroduodenal motility, pyloric diameter and gastric emptying. Q. J. Exp. Physiol. *68*:675, 1983.

46. Brink, B. M., Schlegel, J. F., and Code, C. F. The pressure profile of the gastroduodenal junction zone in dogs. Gut *6*:163, 1965.

47. Gibbs, J., Young, R. C., Smith, G. P. Cholecystokinin decreases food intake in rats. J. Comp. Physiol. Psychol. *84*:888, 1973.

48. Della-Fera, M. A., and Baile, C. A. Cholecystokinin octapeptide continuous picomole injections into the cerebral ventricles of sheep suppress feeding. Science *206*:471, 1979.

49. Straus, E., Ryder, S. W., Eng, J., and Yalow, R. S. Immunochemical studies relating to cholecystokinin in brain and gut. Recent Prog. Hormone Res. *37*:447, 1981.

50. Crawley, J. N., and Kiss, J. Z. Paraventricular nucleus lesions abolish the inhibition of feeding induced by systemic cholecystokinin. Peptides *6*:927, 1985.

51. Shillabeer, G, and Davison, J. S. The effect of vagotomy on the increase in food intake induced by the cholecystokinin antagonist, proglumide. Regul. Peptides *12*:91, 1985.

52. Pambianco, D., Plankey, M., and McCallum, R. W. Effects of the Garren gastric bubble in marked obesity. Am. J. Gastroenterol. (Abstract.) Vol. *82*, 1987.

53. Code, C. F., and Marlett, J. A. The interdigestive myoelectric complex of the stomach and small bowel of dogs. J. Physiol. (Lond.) *246*:387, 1975.

54. Marik, F., and Code, C. F. Control of the interdigestive myoelectric activity in dogs by the vagus nerves and pentagastrin. Gastroenterology *69*:387, 1975.

55. Thomas, P. A., Schang, J. C., Kelly, K. A., and Co, V. L. W. Can endogenous gastrin inhibit canine interdigestive gastric motility? Gastroenterology *78*:716, 1980.

56. Hashmonai, M., Go, V. L. W., and Szurszewski, J. H. Effect of total sympathectomy and of decentralization on migrating complexes in dogs. Gastroenterology *92*:978, 1987.

57. Schuffler, M. D., Rohrmann, C. A., Chaffee, R. G., Brand, D.L., Delaney, J. H., and Young, J. H. Chronic intestinal pseudo-obstruction: a report of 27 cases and review of the literature. Medicine (Baltimore) *60*:173, 1981.

58. Smalley, W. E., Valenzuela, G., and McCallum, R. W. Nausea and vomiting with adrenocortical insufficiency: is it central in origin or a gastrointestinal motility disturbance? Am. J. Gastroenterol. (in press).

59. Meeroff, J. C., Schreiber, D. S., Trier, J. S., and Blacklow, N. R. Abnormal gastric motor function in viral gastroenteritis. Ann. Intern. Med. *92*:370, 1980.

60. Bortoloth, M., Bersain, G., and Labo, G. Association between chronic idiopathic gastroparesis and cytomegalovirus infection (Abstract). Gastroenterology *92*:1324, 1987.

61. Vantrappen, G., Janssens, J., and Ghoos, Y. The interdigestive motor complex of normal subjects and patients with bacterial overgrowth of the small intestine. J. Clin. Invest. *59*:1158, 1977.

62. Shivshanker, K., Bennett, R. W., Jr., and Haynie, T. P.

63. Perkel, M. S., Fajman, W. A., Hersh, T., Moore, C., Davidson, E. D., and Hann, C. Comparison of the barium test meal and the gamma camera scanning technique in measuring gastric emptying. South. Med. J. *74*:1065, 1981.

64. Marshall, B. J. *Campylobacter pyloridis* and gastritis. J. Infect. Dis. *153*:650, 1986.

65. George, J. D. A new clinical method for measuring the role of gastric emptying: the double sampling test meal. Gut *9*:237, 1968.

66. Goldstein, H., and Boyle, J. The saline load test—a bedside evaluation of gastric retention. Gastroenterology *49*:375, 1965.

67. Dubois, A., VanEerdewegh, P., and Gardner, J. D. Gastric emptying and secretin in Zollinger-Ellison syndrome. J. Clin. Invest. *59*:255, 1977.

68. Malagelada, J. R., Longstreth, G. F., Summerskill, W. H. J., et al. Measurement of gastric function during digestion of ordinary solid meals in man. Gastroenterology *70*:203, 1976.

69. Meyer, J. H., MacGregor, M. B., Gueller, R. ^{99m}Tc-tagged chicken liver as a marker of solid food in the human stomach. Am. J. Dig. Dis. *21*:296, 1976.

70. McCallum, R. W., Grill, B. B., Lange, R. C., Plankey, M., Glass, E., and Greenfeld, D. G. Definition of a gastric emptying abnormality in patients with anorexia nervosa. Dig. Dis. Sci. *30*:713, 1985.

71. Collins, P. J., Horowitz, M., Cook, D. J., Harding, P. E., and Shearman, D.J. Gastric emptying in normal subjects—a reproducible technique using a single scintillation camera and a computer system. Gut *24*:1117, 1983.

72. Tothill, P., McLoughlin, G.P., and Heading, R. C. Techniques and errors in scintigraphic measurements of gastric emptying. J. Nucl. Med. *19*:256, 1978.

73. Christian, P. E., Moore, J. G., and Dante, F. L. Comparison of Tc-labeled liver and liver pate as markers for solid phase gastric emptying. J. Nucl. Med. *25*:364, 1984.

74. Knight, L. C., DeVegvar, M. L., Fisher, R. S., et al. Tc-sulfur-colloid scrambled eggs versus in vivo chicken liver in normal subjects. J. Nucl. Med. *23*:21, 1983.

75. McCallum, R. W., Berkowitz, D. M., and Lerner, E. Gastric emptying in patients with gastroesophageal reflux. Gastroenterology *80*:285, 1981.

76. Moore, J. G., Christian, P. E., and Coleman, R. E. Gastric emptying of varying meal weights and composition in man. Evaluation by dual liquid and solid phase isotopic method. Dig. Dis. Sci. *26*:16, 1981.

77. Elashoff, J. E., Reedy, T. J., and Meyer, J. H. Analysis of gastric emptying data. Gastroenterology *83*:1306, 1982.

78. Minami, H., and McCallum, R. W. The physiology and pathophysiology of gastric emptying in humans. Gastroenterology *86*:1592, 1984.

79. MacGregor, I.L., Wiley, Z. D., Lavigne, M. E., and Way, L. W. Total parenteral nutrition slows gastric emptying of solid foods (Abstract). Gastroenterology *74*:1059, 1978.

80. Bury, K. D., and Jambunathan, G. Effects of elemental diets on gastric emptying and gastric secretion in man. Am. J. Surg. *127*:59, 1974.

81. McCallum, R. W., Caride, V. J., Prokop, E. K., and Troncale, F. J. Effect of sucralfate and an aluminum hydroxide gel on gastric emptying of solids and liquids. Clin. Pharmacol. Ther. *37*:629, 1985.

82. Harrison, A., and Ippoliti, A. Effect of smoking on gastric emptying (Abstract). Gastroenterology *76*:1152, 1979.

83. Buckler, K. G. Effects of gastric surgery upon gastric emptying in cases of peptic ulceration. Gut *8*:137, 1967.

84. Moore, J. G., Christian, P. E., and Datz, F. L. Effect of creme on gastric emptying in humans. Gastroenterology *81*:1072, 1981.

85. Barboriak, J. J., and Meade, R. C. Effect of alcohol on gastric emptying in man. Am. J. Clin. Nutr. *23*:1151, 1970.

86. Wald, A., Van Thiel, D. H., Hoechstetter, L., Gavaler, J. S., Egler, K. M., Verm, R., Scott, L., and Lester, R. Gastrointestinal transit: the effect of the menstrual cycle. Gastroenterology *80*:1497, 1981.

Tumor-associated gastroparesis: correction with metoclopramide. Am. J. Surg. *145*:221, 1983.

87. Hunt, J. N., and Murray, F. A. Gastric function in pregnancy. J. Obstet. Gynaecol. Br. Commonw. *65*:78, 1978.
88. Rees, M. R., Clark, R. A., and Holdsworth, C. D. The effect of beta-adrenoreceptor agonists and antagonists on gastric emptying in man. Br. J. Clin. Pharmacol. *10*:551, 1980.
89. Holt, S., Cervantes, J., Wilkinson, A., and Wallace, J. H. Measurement of gastric emptying rate in humans by real-time ultrasound. Gastroenterology *90*:918, 1986.
90. Feldman, M., Smith, H. J., and Simon, T. R. Gastric emptying of solid radiopaque markers: studies in healthy subjects and diabetic patients. Gastroenterology *87*:895, 1984.
91. Mathias, J. R., Sninsky, C. A., Millar, H. D., Clench, M. H., and Davis, R. H. Development of an improved multi-pressure-sensor probe for recording muscle contraction in human intestine. Dig. Dis. Sci. *30*:119, 1985.
92. Malagelada, J. R., and Stanghellini, V. Manometric evaluation of functional upper gut symptoms. Gastroenterology *88*:1223, 1985.
93. Faulk, D. L., Anuris, S., and Christensen, J. Chronic intestinal pseudo-obstruction. Gastroenterology *74*:1922, 1978.
94. Mirizzi, N., and Scafoglieri, V. Optimal direction of the electrogastrographic signal in man. Med. Biol. Eng. Comput. *21*:385, 1983.
95. Rabov, V. G. Diagnostic possibilities of electrogastrography from parts of the body distant from the stomach. Klin. Med. *52*:115, 1974.
96. Bellahsene, B. E., Hamilton, J. N., and Reichelderfer, M. An improved method for recording and analyzing the electrical activity of the human stomach. IEEE Trans. Biomed. Eng. *BME-32*:911, 1985.
97. Bellahsene, B. E., Schirmer, B., and McCallum, R. W. Validation of cutaneous EGG recordings by comparing with recordings from intragastric surgically implanted electrodes (Abstract). Gastroenterology *92*:1313, 1987.
98. You, C. H., Lee, K. Y., Chey, W. Y., et al. Electrogastrographic study of patients with unexplained nausea, bloating and vomiting. Gastroenterology *79*:311, 1980.
99. Abell, T. L., Lucas, A. R., Brown, M. L., et al. Gastric electrical dysrhythmias in anorexia nervosa (Abstract). Gastroenterology *88*:1300, 1985.
100. Code, C. F., and Marlett, J. A. Canine tachygastria. Mayo Clin. Proc. *49*:325, 1974.
101. Kim, C. H., Azpiroz, F., and Malagelada, J. R. Characteristics of spontaneous and drug-induced gastric dysrhythmias in a chronic canine model. Gastroenterology (in press).
102. Stoddard, C. J., Smallwood, R. H., and Duthie, H. L. Electrical arrhythmias in the human stomach. Gut *22*:705, 1981.
103. Telander, R. L., Morgan, K. G., Kreulen, D. L., Schmalz, P. F., Kelly, K. A., and Szurszewski, J. H. Human gastric atony with tachygastria and gastric retention. Gastroenterology *75*:497, 1978.
104. You, C. H., Chey, W. Y., Lee, K. Y., Menguy, R., and Bortoff, A. Gastric and small intestinal myoelectric dysrhythmia associated with chronic intractable nausea and vomiting. Ann. Intern. Med. *95*:449, 1981.
105. Abell, T. L., Camilleri, M., Malagelada, J. R. High prevalence of gastric electrical dysrhythmias in diabetic gastroparesis (Abstract). Gastroenterology *88*:1299, 1985.
106. Sarna, S. K., Bowes, K. L., and Daniel, E. E. Post-operative gastric electrical control activity (ECA) in man. *In* Daniel, E. E. (ed.). Proceedings of the Fourth International Symposium on Gastrointestinal Motility. Vancouver, Mitchell Press, 1973, pp. 73–83.
107. Bertrand, J., Dorval, E. D., Metman, E. H., de Calan, L., and Ozoux, J. P. Electrogastrography and serosal electrical recording of the antrum after proximal vagotomy in man (Abstract). Gastroenterology *86*:1026, 1984.
108. Geldof, H., van der Schee, E. J., van Blankenstein, M., and Grashuis, J. L. Gastric dysrhythmia: an electrogastrographic study (Abstract). Gastroenterology *84*:1163, 1983.
109. Kassander, P. Asymptomatic gastric retention in diabetes (gastroparesis diabeticorum). Ann. Intern. Med. *48*:797, 1958.
110. MacGregor, I. L., Deveney, C., Way, L. W., and Meyer, J. H. The effect of acute hyperglycemia on meal-stimulated gastric, biliary, and pancreatic secretion and serum gastrin. Gastroenterology *70*:197, 1976.
111. Greene, D. A., DeJesus, P. F., Jr., and Winegrad, A. I. Effects of insulin and dietary myoinositol on impaired motor nerve conduction velocity in acute streptozotocin diabetes. J. Clin. Invest. *55*:1326, 1975.
112. Fox, S., and Behar, J. Pathogenesis of diabetic gastroparesis: a pharmacologic study. Gastroenterology *78*:757, 1980.
113. Achem-Karam, S. R., Funakosa, A., Vinik, A. I., and Ouyang, C. Plasma motilin concentration and interdigestive migrating motor complex in diabetic gastroparesis: effect of metoclopramide. Gastroenterology *88*:492, 1985.
114. Mearin, F., Camillan, M., and Malagelada, J. R. Pyloric dysfunction in diabetes with recurrent nausea and vomiting. Gastroenterology *90*:1919, 1986.
115. Gleystien, J. J., and Kalbfleisch, J. H. Progression of changes in gastric emptying of hypertonic liquids after proximal gastric vagotomy. Dig. Dis. Sci. *26*:119, 1981.
116. Kalbasi, H., Hudson, F. R., Herring, A., Moss, S., Glass, H. I., and Spencer, J. Gastric emptying following vagotomy and antrectomy and proximal gastric vagotomy. Gut *16*:509, 1975.
117. MacGregor, M. G., Martin, P., and Meyer, J. H. Gastric emptying of solid food in normal man and after subtotal gastrectomy and truncal vagotomy with pyloroplasty. Gastroenterology *72*:206, 1977.
118. Kraft, R. O., Fry, W. J., and DeWeese, M. S. Post-vagotomy gastric atony. Arch. Surg. *88*:865, 1964.
119. Bergin, W. F., and Jordan, P. H., Jr. Gastric atonia and delayed gastric emptying after vagotomy for obstructing ulcer. Am. J. Surg. *98*:612, 1959.
120. Harper, F. B. Gastric dysfunction after vagectomy. Am. J. Surg. *112*:194, 1966.
121. Malagelada, J. R., Rees, W. D., Mazzotta, L. J., et al. Gastric motor abnormalities in diabetic and post vagotomy gastroparesis: effect of metoclopramide and bethanechol. Gastroenterology *78*:186, 1980.
122. McCallum, R. W., Mensh, R., and Lange, R. Definition of gastric emptying abnormalities present in gastroesophageal reflux patients (Abstract). Gastroenterology *80*:1226, 1981.
123. Maddern, G. J., Chatterton, B. E., Collins, P. J., Horowitz, M., Shearman, D. J., and Jamieson, G. G. Solid and liquid gastric emptying in patients with gastro-esophageal reflux. Br. J. Surg. *72*:344, 1985.
124. Behar, J., and Ramsly, G. Gastric emptying and antral motility in reflux esophagitis. Gastroenterology *74*:253, 1978.
125. Holloway, R. H., Hongo, M., and McCallum, R. W. Gastric distension. A mechanism for postprandial gastroesophageal reflux. Gastroenterology *89*:779, 1985.
126. Hillemeier, A. C., Lange, R., McCallum, R. W., Seashore, J., and Gryboski, J. Delayed gastric emptying in infants with gastroesophageal reflux. J. Pediatr. *98*:190, 1981.
127. Hillemeier, A. C., Grill, B. B., McCallum, R. W., and Gryboski, J. Esophageal and gastric motor abnormalities in gastroesophageal reflux during infancy. Gastroenterology *84*:741, 1983.
128. Maddern, G. J., Jamieson, G. G., Chatterton, B. E., et al. Is there an association between failed antireflux procedures and delayed gastric emptying? Ann. Surg. *202*:162, 1985.
129. Fink, S. M., Barwick, K., DeLuca, V., Sanders, F. J., Kandathil, M., and McCallum, R. W. The association of histologic gastritis with gastroesophageal reflux and delayed gastric emptying. J. Clin. Gastroenterol. *6*:301, 1984.
130. Davies, W. T., Kirkpatrick, J. R., Owen, G. M., and Shields, R. Gastric emptying in atrophic gastritis and carcinoma of the stomach. Scand. J. Gastroenterol. *6*:297, 1971.
131. Frank, E. B., Lange, R. C., and McCallum, R. W. Abnormal gastric emptying in patients with atrophic gastritis with or without pernicious anemia. Gastroenterology *80*:551, 1981.
132. Schuffler, M. D. Chronic intestinal pseudo-obstruction syndromes. Med. Clin. North Am. *65*:1331, 1981.
133. Schuffler, M. D., Rohrmann, C. A., Chaffee, R. G., Brand, D. L., Delaney, J. H., and Young, J. H. Chronic intestinal pseudo-obstruction: a report of 27 cases and review of the literature. Medicine (Baltimore) *60*:173, 1981.

134. Goldberg, H. I., and Sheft, O. J. Esophageal and colon changes in myotonia dystrophica. Gastroenterology 63:134, 1972.

134a. Bevans, M. Changes in musculature of gastrointestinal tract and myocardium in progressive muscular dystrophy. Arch. Pathol. 40:225, 1945.

135. Linde, L. M., and Westover, J. L. Esophageal and gastric abnormalities in dysautonomia. Pediatrics 29:303, 1962.

136. Gilat, T., and Spiro, H. M. Amyloidosis and the gut. Am. J. Dig. Dis. 13:619, 1968.

137. Intriere, A. D., and Brown, C. H. Primary amyloidosis: report of a case of gastric involvement only. Gastroenterology 30:833, 1956.

138. McCallum, R. W., Grill, B. B., Lange, R., Planky, M., Glass, E., and Greenfeld, D. G. Definition of gastric emptying abnormality in patients with anorexia nervosa. Dig. Dis. Sci. 30:713, 1985.

139. Russell, D. M., Freedman, M. L., Feiglin, D. H., Jeejeeboy, K. N., Swinson, R. P., and Garfinkel, P. E. Delayed gastric emptying and improvement with domperidone in a patient with anorexia nervosa. Am. J. Psychiatry 140:1235, 1983.

140. Miranda, M., DeFilippi, C., and Valenzuela, J. E. Abnormalities of the interdigestive motility complex and increased duodenogastric reflux in gastric ulcer patients. Dig. Dis. Sci. 30:16, 1985.

141. Peachey, R. D., Creamer, B., and Pierce, J. N. Sclerodermatous involvement of the stomach and small and large bowel. Gut 10:285, 1969.

142. Maddern, G. J., Horowitz, M., Jamieson, G. G., Chatterdon, B. E., Collins, P. J., and Roberts-Thomson, P. Abnormalities of esophageal and gastric emptying in progressive systemic sclerosis. Gastroenterology 87:922, 1984.

143. Brown, C. H., Shirey, E. K., and Haserick, J. R. Gastrointestinal manifestations of systemic lupus erythematosis. Gastroenterology 31:649, 1956.

144. Horowitz, M., McNeil, J. D., Maddern, G., et al. Abnormalities of gastric and esophageal emptying in polymyositis and dermatomyositis. Gastroenterology 90:234, 1986.

145. Ricci, D. A., and McCallum, R. W. Idiopathic gastric stasis, survey of. Dig. Dis. 1:79, 1983.

146. Stern, R. M., Stewart, W. R., Lindblad, I., et al. Tachygastria and motion sickness. Dig. Dis. Sci. 29:566A, 1984.

147. Russell, J., and Bass, P. Canine gastric emptying of polycarbophil: an indigestible, particulate substance. Gastroenterology 89:307, 1985.

148. Ke, M. Y., Oertel, R., and McCallum, R. W. The effects of Dazopride, a new prokinetic agent, on esophageal motor function in the cat: comparison with metoclopramide. Clin. Res. 32:691, 1984.

149. Wiley, J., and Owyany, C. Dopaminergic modulation of colonic myoelectric and motor activities (Abstract). Gastroenterology 86:1299, 1984.

150. Sridhar, K., Ricci, D., Lange, R., et al. Effects of tetrahydrocannabinol on gastric emptying of solids in humans (Abstract). Gastroenterology 86:1265, 1984.

150a. Justin-Besancon, L., Laville, C., and Thominet, M. Le Métoclopramide et ses homologues. Introduction à leur étude biologique. C. R. Acad. Sci. (Paris) 258:4384, 1964.

151. Cohen, S., and DiMarino, A. J. Mechanisms of metoclopramide on opossum lower esophageal sphincter muscle. Gastroenterology 71:996, 1976.

152. McCallum, R. W., and Albibi, R. Metoclopramide: pharmacology and clinical application. Ann. Intern. Med. 98:86, 1983.

153. Beani, L., Bianchi, C., and Cremer, C. Effects of metoclopramide on isolated guinea pig colon. 1. Peripheral sensitization to acetylcholine. Eur. J. Pharmacol. 12:220, 1970.

154. Conell, A. M., and George, J. D. Effect of metoclopramide on gastric function in man. Gut 10:678, 1969.

155. Eisner, M. Gastrointestinal effects of metoclopramide in man: in vitro experiments with human smooth muscle preparations. Br. Med. J. 4:649, 1968.

156. Johnson, A. G. Gastroduodenal motility and synchronization. Postgrad. Med. J. 49:29, 1973.

157. McCallum, R. W., Kline, M. M., Curry, N., et al. Comparative effects of metoclopramide and bethanechol on lower exophageal sphincter pressure in reflux patients. Gastroenterology 68:1114, 1975.

158. McCallum, R. W., Fink, S. M., Lerner, E., and Berkowitz, D. M. Effects of metoclopramide and bethanechol on delayed gastric emptying present in gastroesophageal reflux patients. Gastroenterology 84:1573, 1983.

159. Malagelada, J. R., Rees, W. D., Mazzotta, L. J., et al. Gastric motor abnormalities in diabetic and post-vagotomy gastroparesis: effect of metoclopramide and bethanechol. Gastroenterology 78:286, 1980.

159a. Battel, W. M., Snape, W., et al. Abnormal colonic motility in progressive systemic sclerosis. Ann. Intern. Med. 94:749, 1981.

160. Ricci, D. A., Saltzman, M. B., Meyer, C., Callachan, C., and McCallum, R. W. Effects of metoclopramide in diabetic gastroparesis. J. Clin. Gastroenterol. 7:25, 1985.

161. Snape, W. J., Battle, W. M., Schwartz, S. S., Braunstein, S. N., Goldstein, H. A., and Alavi, A. Metoclopramide to treat gastroparesis due to diabetes mellitus. Ann. Intern. Med. 96:444, 1982.

162. McCallum, R. W., Ricci, D. A., Rakatansky, H., et al. A multicenter placebo controlled clinical trial of oral metoclopramide in diabetic gastroparesis. Diabet. Care 6:643, 1983.

163. Saltzman, M. B., and McCallum, R. W. Diabetes and the stomach—symposium on gastrointestinal manifestations of diabetes mellitus. Yale J. Biol. Med. 56:179, 1983.

164. Brogden, R. N., Carmine, A. A., Heel, R. C., Speight, T. M., and Avery, G. S. Domperidone: a review. Drugs 24:360, 1982.

165. Friedman, G. The GI Drug Column: Domperidone. Am. J. Gastroenterol. 78:47, 1983.

166. Albibi, R., DuBovic, S., Lange, R. C., and McCallum, R. W. A dose response study of the effects of domperidone on gastric retention states in man. Am. J. Gastroenterol. 78:679, 1983.

167. Horowitz, M., Harding, P. E., Chatterton, B. E., Collins, P. J., and Shearman, D. J. Acute and chronic effects of domperidone on gastric emptying in diabetes autonomic neuropathy. Dig. Dis. Sci. 30:1, 1985.

168. McCallum, R. W., Ricci, D., DuBovic, S., et al. Effect of domperidone on gastric emptying and symptoms in patients with idiopathic gastric stasis (Abstract). Gastroenterology 86:1179, 1984.

169. Van Neuten, J. M., Reyntjens, A., Schurkes, J. A. J. Gastrointestinal motility stimulating properties of the non-antidopaminergic and non-cholinergic compound R 41 619. Gastroenterol. Clin. Biol. 7:706, 1983.

170. Schuurkes, J. A. J., Verlinden, M., Kermans, L .M. A., et al. Stimulation effects of R 51 619 on antroduodenal motility in the conscious dog. Gastroenterol. Clin. Biol. 7:707, 1983.

171. Corazziari, E., Scopmaro, F., Bontempo, I., et al. Effect of R 41 519 on distal esophageal motor activity and gastric emptying. Ital. J. Gastroenterol. 15:185, 1983.

172. Cooke, H. J., and Carey, H. V. The effects of cisapride on serotonin-evoked mucosal responses in guinea pig ileum. Eur. J. Pharmacol. 98:148, 1984.

173. Reboa, G., Arnulfo, G., and DiSomma, C. Prokinetic effects of cisapride on normal and reduced antro-duodenal reflexes. Curr. Ther. Res. 36:18, 1984.

174. McCallum, R. W., Petersen, J., Lange, R., et al. Cisapride accelerates gastric emptying of solid and liquid meal components in patients with gastric stasis (Abstract). Gastroenterology 90:1541, 1986.

175. Mittal, R., Frank, E. B., Lange, R., et al. Effect of morphine and naloxone on lower esophageal sphincter pressure and gastric emptying in man. Dig. Dis. Sci. 31:936, 1986.

176. Schang, J. C., Devroede, G., Perrault, R. Naloxone therapy in small intestinal pseudo-obstruction. Preliminary results about two cases. Am. J. Gastroenterol. 79:828, 1984.

177. McCallum, R. W., Newman, G. A. Functional disorders of the upper gastroenestinal tract. In Bayless, T. M., Brain, M C., and Chernick, R. M. (eds.). Current Therapy in Internal Medicine. Ed. 2. Philadelphia/Toronto, B. C. Decker, 1987, pp. 637–643.

178. Farthing, M. J. G., Fairchlough, P. D., Hegarty, J. E.,

Swarbrick, E. T., and Dawson, A. M. Treatment of chronic erosive gastritis with prednisolone. Gut *22*:759, 1981.

179. Bellahsene, B., Schirmer, B., and McCallum, R. W. Effect of electrical stimulation on gastric emptying (Abstract). Am. J. Gastroenterol. (in press).

180. Gustavsson, G., Ilstrup, D. M., Morrison, P., and Kelly, K. A. The Roux-stasis syndrome after gastrectomy. Am. J. Surg. (in press).

181. Mathias, J. R., Fernandez, A., Sinitsky, C. A., Clench, M. H., and Davis, R. H. Nausea, vomiting and abdominal pain after Roux-en-Y anastomosis: motility of the jejunal limb. Gastroenterology *88*:101, 1985.

182. Morrison, P., Kelly, K. A., and Hocking, M. Electrical dysrhythmias in the Roux-en-Y jejunal limb and their correction by pacing. Gastroenterology *88*:1508, 198⁵.

183. Vogel, S. B., Vair, D. B., and Woodward, E. R. Alterations in gastrointestinal emptying of 99m-technetium-labelled solids following sequential antrectomy, truncal vagotomy, and Roux-Y gastroenterostomy. Ann. Surg. *198*:506, 1983.

184. Vogel, S. B., Hocking, M. P., and Woodward, E. R. Radionuclide evaluation of gastric emptying in patients undergoing Roux-Y biliary diversion for reflux gastritis and postgastrectomy dumping. Surg. Forum *34*:173, 1983.

185. Hocking, M. P., Vogel, S. B., Falasca, C. A., and Woodward, E. R. Delayed gastric emptying of liquids and solids following Roux-en-Y biliary diversion. Ann. Surg. *194*:494, 1981.

186. Bucheit, K. H., Engel, G., Mutschler, E., et al. Study of contractile effect on 5-hydroxytryptamine (5-HT) in the isolated longitudinal muscle strip from guinea pig ileum. Arch. Pharmacol. *329*:36, 1985.

187. Fordtran, J. S., and Walsh, J. H. Gastric acid secretion rate and buffer content of the stomach after eating: Results in normal subjects and in patients with duodenal ulcer. J. Clin. Invest. *52*:645, 1973.

188. George, J. D. Gastric acidity and motility. Am. J. Dig. Dis. *13*:376, 1968.

189. Cobb, J. S., Bank, S., Marks, I. N., et al. Gastric emptying after vagotomy and pyloroplasty: relation to some postoperative sequelae. Am. J. Dig. Dis. *16*:207, 1971.

190. Rotter, J. I., Rubin, R., Meyer, J. H., et al. Rapid gastric emptying—an inherited pathophysiologic defect in duodenal ulcer (Abstract). Gastroenterology *76*:1229, 1979.

191. Howlett, P. J., Sheiner, J. H., Barber, D. C., et al. Gastric emptying in control subjects and patients with duodenal ulcer before and after vagotomy. Gut *17*:542, 1976.

192. Harrison, A., Ippoliti, A., and Cullison, R. Rapid gastric emptying in Zollinger-Ellison syndrome (Abstract). Gastroenterology *78*:1180, 1980.

193. Goligher, J. C., Hill, G. L., Kenny, T. E., et al. Proximal gastric vagotomy without drainage for duodenal ulcer: results after 5 to 8 years. Br. J. Surg. *65*:145, 1978.

194. Sawyer, J. C., Herrington, J. L., and Burney, D. P. Proximal gastric vagotomy compared with vagotomy and antrectomy and selective gastric vagotomy and pyloroplasty. Ann. Surg. *186*:510, 1977.

195. Koelz, H. R., and Gewertz, B. L. The stomach, part 1: vagotomy. Clin. Gastroenterol. *8*:305, 1979.

196. MacGregor, I. L., Martin, P., and Meyer, J. H. Gastric emptying of solid food in normal man and after subtotal gastrectomy and truncal vagotomy with pyloroplasty. Gastroenterology *72*:206, 1977.

197. Ralphs, D. N. L., Thomson, J. P. S., Haynes, S., et al. The relationship between the rate of gastric emptying and the dumping syndrome. Br. J. Surg. *65*:637, 1978.

198. Regan, P. T., Malagelada, J. R., Dimagno, E. P., et al. Postprandial gastric function in pancratic insufficiency. Gut *20*:249, 1979.

199. Wiley, Z. D., Lavigne, M. E., Liu, K. M., et al. The effect of hyperthyroidism on gastric emptying rates and pancreatic exocrine and biliary secretion in man. Dig. Dis. Sci. *23*:1003, 1978.

200. Leeds, A. R., Ralphs, D. N. L., Ebied, F., Metz, G., and Dilawari, J. B. Pectin in the dumping syndrome: reduction of symptom and plasma volume changes. Lancet *1*:1075, 1981.

201. McLoughlin, J. C., Buchanan, K. D., and Alam, M. J. A glycoside-hydrolase inhibitor in treatment of dumping syndrome. Lancet *2*:603, 1979.

202. Brooke-Cowden, G. L., Broosch, J. W., Giff, S. P., et al. Postgastrectomy syndromes. Am. J. Surg. *131*:464, 1976.

203. Gladen, H. E., and Kelly, K. A. Electrical pacing for short bowel syndrome. Surg. Gynecol. Obstet. *153*:697, 1981.

41

Gastric Secretion in Health and Disease

MARK FELDMAN

The purpose of this chapter is to review current concepts of regulation of gastric secretion and methods of measuring gastric secretion. The emphasis will be largely clinical, and, wherever possible, data obtained from studies in humans are cited. However, recent studies in animals have led to important insights into the mechanisms of gastric secretion at the cellular level; accordingly, these data are also reviewed.

FUNCTIONAL GASTRIC ANATOMY

The anatomy of the human stomach is discussed in detail on pages 659–665 and elsewhere.[1, 2] The gastric mucosa is bordered by the apical plasma membrane of surface epithelial cells at the luminal surface and by the muscularis mucosae beneath the gastric glands. The gastric mucosal epithelium includes cells that line the surface, cells that line the gastric pits, and cells composing the gastric glands beneath the pits. Cells that line the surface and the pits are the same throughout the stomach; they are columnar in type and secrete mucus and bicarbonate. It has been speculated by Heatley that gastric mucus and bicarbonate secretion by these cells protects the surface of the gastric mucosa from damage by luminal acid-pepsin.[3] Surface cells may have other functions, including maintenance of a lumen-negative potential difference in the gastric mucosa and disposal of H^+ ions.[4, 5]

In contrast to surface cells and cells that line gastric pits, cells composing gastric glands differ from one region of the stomach to another. The stomach can be divided into three glandular areas on the basis of these differences (Table 41–1). The cardiac gland area is a thin rim of glands just distal to the esophagogastric squamocolumnar junction. The glands secrete mucus and certain pepsinogens (group II pepsinogens). The oxyntic gland area corresponds anatomically to the gastric fundus and body, occupying around 75 per cent of the total glandular area. Oxyntic glands contain many different kinds of cells, including parietal (oxyntic) cells, chief cells, and mucous neck cells. Both chief cells and mucous neck cells of oxyntic glands secrete pepsinogen I and pepsinogen II. It is believed that mucous neck cells or closely related undifferentiated cells are responsible for constantly replacing the gastric epithelium by proliferation and differentiation. The pyloric gland area, which corresponds anatomically to the gastric antrum and the pylorus, constitutes 20 to 25 per cent of the gastric mucosal area and contains mucous cells and G (gastrin) cells.

Oxyntic and pyloric glands also contain enterochromaffin cells, which contain serotonin, and several types of endocrine cells (for example, somatostatin cells and gut glucagon cells). Some of these peptides may be secreted into the tissue (paracrine secretion) rather than into the circulation (endocrine secretion). Certain peptides that may affect gastric secretion (for example, vasoactive intestinal polypeptide, somatostatin, gastrin-releasing peptide, enkephalins) are also present within nerves in the stomach (neurocrine secretion). There is evidence that certain hormonal peptides, such as gastrin and somatostatin, are secreted into gastric juice (exocrine secretion), although this may not be of physiologic importance,[6, 7] probably because receptors for regulatory peptides are present on the basolateral cell membrane and not on the luminal cell membrane.

Nonepithelial cells within the lamina propria are also of importance in the physiology and pathophysiology of gastric secretion. For example, mast cells contain histamine,[8] which plays a central role in stimulation of gastric acid secretion. Moreover, plasma cells within lamina propria synthesize immunoglobulin A, which is secreted into gastric mucus and gastric juice. Certain immunoglobulin G molecules synthesized by plasma cells under pathologic conditions, such as atrophic gastritis, may be directed against parietal cell antigens, such as the gastrin receptor, thus reducing acid secretion in a potentially reversible manner.[9, 10]

Table 41–1. CELLS WITHIN GASTRIC GLANDS AND THEIR SECRETORY PRODUCT(S)

Gland Area (% of total)	Cell Within Glands	Secretory Product(s)
Cardiac (<5%)	Mucous	Mucous, pepsinogens (group II)
	Endocrine	See footnote*
Oxyntic (75%)	Parietal (oxyntic)	HCl, intrinsic factor
	Chief	Pepsinogens (groups I and II)
	Mucous Neck	Mucous, pepsinogens (groups I and II)
	Enterochromaffin	Serotonin
	Endocrine	See footnote*
Pyloric (20–25%)	Mucous	Mucus, pepsinogens (group II)
	G-cell	Gastrin
	Enterochromaffin	Serotonin
	Endocrine (besides gastrin)	See footnote*

*Cardiac, oxyntic, and pyloric glandular mucosae contain at least nine different types of endocrine cells. In some of these cells the hormonal product has been identified. Examples include D cells (somatostatin) and A cells (gut glucagon). See page 996 for further description of gastric endocrine cells.

This chapter deals with regulation of gastric secretion of hydrochloric acid (HCl), intrinsic factor, mucus, and bicarbonate ion (HCO_3^-). Regulation of the functions of enterochromaffin cells and of gastric endocrine cells (besides gastrin cells) is discussed elsewhere (see p. 996).

ACID (HCl) SECRETION

One function of gastric acid is to facilitate peptic digestion of dietary protein. The integral relationship between acid and pepsinogen secretion is most apparent in nonmammalian vertebrates in whom acid and pepsinogen are secreted by the same cell (oxyntopeptic cell). In general, a stimulant or inhibitor of acid secretion will have the same effect on pepsinogen secretion. However, there is no evidence that acid secretion regulates pepsinogen secretion, or vice versa.[11] A second function of gastric acid is to inactivate microorganisms such as bacteria, which are ingested with food or fluids.[12] Agents that reduce gastric acidity result in bacterial overgrowth of the stomach and small intestine.[13] There is also some evidence that gastric acid facilitates the intestinal absorption of iron[14] and calcium,[15] although the importance of gastric acid in calcium absorption has been questioned.[16]

Under basal (fasting) conditions in normal humans, acid is usually secreted at low rates relative to the maximal capacity for acid secretion. Basal acid output averages 7 to 10 per cent of maximum. A physiologic event (e.g., a meal) or pathologic condition (e.g., a gastrin-producing tumor) increases gastric HCl secretion above basal rates by increasing the concentration of chemical mediators near parietal cells. These mediators, after binding to a specific cellular receptor on the parietal cell, initiate a series of intracellular chemical reactions that result in increased HCl secretion.

The intracellular chemical reactions resulting in HCl secretion are reviewed first, followed by the chemical mediators that interact with parietal cells to initiate these chemical reactions via the release of "second" intracellular messengers.

Intracellular Chemical Reactions

Hydrogen ions (protons) are secreted by parietal cells into gastric juice against a concentration gradient 2,000,000:1 or greater. Chloride ions, which accompany hydrogen ions when acid is secreted, are secreted against both a concentration gradient and an electrical gradient (the gastric lumen is negatively charged compared with the interstitial fluid, with a potential difference of approximately 44 mV). Thus, HCl secretion by parietal cells must be an active, energy-dependent process.

Studies by various groups of investigators demonstrated that ATP provides the energy necessary for active pumping of protons out of the parietal cell into gastric juice.[17-20] These workers have characterized an enzyme H^+,K^+-ATPase, that catalyzes a one-to-one exchange of hydrogen for potassium ions.[21] This enzyme, which is magnesium dependent, has been found only on secretory surfaces of parietal cells (apical plasma membrane, tubulovesicular membrane) and not on the basolateral surface of parietal cells or on other gastric epithelial cells. H^+,K^+-ATPase has been found in several species, including rabbits, pigs, and humans. Unlike Na^+,K^+-ATPase, H^+, K^+-ATPase is not inhibited by ouabain. There is a close relationship between the activity of H^+,K^+-ATPase and gastric acid secretion.[22, 23]

The mechanism of HCl secretion by the parietal cell is shown schematically in Figure 41–1. Protons (hydrogen ions) are generated within the parietal cell from H_2O; the corresponding hydroxyl ions are combined with CO_2 under the action of carbonic anhydrase to form HCO_3^- ions, which are then exchanged for Cl^- ions at the basolateral membrane of the parietal cell. At high rates of acid secretion, such as occur after a meal, large amounts of HCO_3^- enter the blood stream from the parietal cell, the so-called "alkaline tide." However, one recent study showed that alkalosis occurs after a meal even when gastric H^+ secretion is blocked by cimetidine.[24] This suggests that postprandial alkalosis may not be a result of gastric H^+ secretion. Chloride ions entering the parietal cell in exchange for HCO_3^- are transported into the secretory canaliculus along with K^+ ions via Cl^- and K^+ conductance pathways closely associated with the H^+,K^+-ATPase. H^+ ions are exchanged for the K^+ ions on a 1:1 basis, a transport process catalyzed by H^+,K^+-ATPase and involving a phosphorylated intermediate protein. Thus, the net result is secretion of H^+ and Cl^- at concentrations of 160 mM, whereas K^+ ions are primarily recycled rather than secreted. As the apical membrane of the parietal cell and other gastric epithelial cells is very impermeable to H^+, most acid secreted by parietal cells remains in the gastric lumen rather than diffusing back into the tissue.

When acid secretion is stimulated (for example, by histamine or pentagastrin), there is a dramatic morphologic transformation of the membrane of the parietal cell.[1, 2] Tubulovesicular membranes, quite prominent in the cytoplasm of the resting cell, diminish or disappear in concert with a six- to tenfold increase in an apical plasma membrane and the appearance of long apical microvilli.[1, 25] There is evidence that the H^+,K^+-ATPase and the K^+ and Cl^- conductances (also called symporters) are transported from the tubulovesicles to the secretory canaliculus just prior to initiation of acid secretion.[26]

Although it is not yet known exactly how the activity

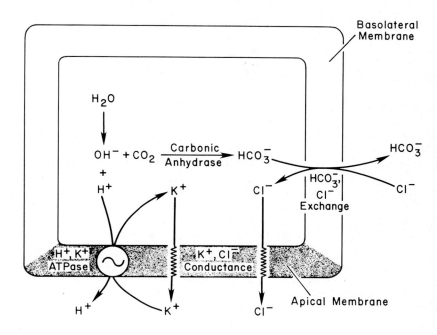

Figure 41–1. Model of HCl secretion by the parietal cell. Hydrogen ions are secreted in exchange for K^+ ions by the activity of a H^+,K^+-ATPase, the proton pump. Closely associated with this ATPase are conductance pathways for K^+ and Cl^-. K^+ ions are largely recycled by the cell, whereas Cl^- ions are secreted with H^+. Intracellular pH would rise as a result of accumulation of OH^- ions left over after H^+ is pumped out of the cell. OH^- ions are thus converted to HCO_3^- by carbonic anhydrase; HCO_3^- is then exchanged for Cl^- ions at the basolateral membrane of the cell. The net result is secretion of HCl by the cell and utilization of CO_2, H_2O, and energy (ATP). The author gratefully acknowledges Dr. G. Sachs for his advice in the preparation of this model.

of the H^+,K^+-ATPase and the K^+ and Cl^- conductance pathways are regulated, compounds that inhibit the ATPase have been developed. One group of compounds, the substituted benzimidazoles (e.g., omeprazole), markedly inhibit gastric HCl secretion *in vitro* and *in vivo*.[22, 23, 26–28] For example, a single oral dose of omeprazole inhibits acid secretion for more than 48 hours in humans.[28] Omeprazole is taken up into the parietal cell, and, in the presence of acid within the secretory canaliculus, is converted to an active metabolite that binds irreversibly to a site on the H^+,K^+-ATPase, inactivating this transporting enzyme.[26, 27] H^+ secretion is inhibited by the drug until new proton pump units can be synthesized and inserted into the apical membrane of the parietal cell, a renewal process that requires more than 24 hours. Substituted benzimidazoles inhibit HCl secretion stimulated by intracellular mediators *in vitro*, such as cyclic AMP and K^+, whereas cimetidine and atropine have no effect under similar conditions. These findings have been interpreted to indicate that activation of H^+,K^+-ATPase is the terminal step in the acid secretory process. Substituted benzimidazoles do not block the morphologic transformation of parietal cells from a "resting" to a "stimulated" appearance, even though these agents block H^+ secretion. In contrast, cimetidine and atropine block both the morphologic transformation of parietal cells and H^+ secretion.[29]

Chemical Mediators, Receptors, and Intracellular Second Messengers

At least four endogenous substances increase gastric acid secretion when infused exogenously: histamine, gastrin, acetylcholine or its stable derivatives, and calcium. Receptors for three of these substances—histamine (H_2 receptor), gastrin (gastrin receptor), and acetylcholine (muscarinic receptor)—are present on the basolateral membrane of canine,[30, 31] and presumably also human, parietal cells (Fig. 41–2). These three agonists interact with their respective receptors on the outer membrane of the parietal cell and then initiate intracellular biochemical reactions which ultimately activate the proton pump.* The parietal cell is somewhat permeable to calcium ions; thus, calcium, when administered exogenously, may enter the parietal cell and, presumably by a calmodulin-dependent step, activate the proton pump. Exogenous calcium administration also increases circulating gastrin concentrations, thus increasing the amount of gastrin reaching gastrin receptors on the parietal cells.[32] As gastrin does not enter the parietal cell, it must act via a second, intracellular messenger, and mounting evidence suggests that the second messenger for gastrin may be intracellular calcium.[26, 33–36] The source of this intracellular

calcium may be the microtubular-microfilamentous system,[36] a system of structural actin-like proteins that appear to play an important role in acid secretion by the parietal cell.[37] There is evidence[33, 34] that acetylcholine, released by postganglionic nerves near the muscarinic receptor on the parietal cell, increases HCl secretion by increasing the permeability of the parietal cell to extracellular calcium (Fig. 41–2). It has been suggested[38] that acetylcholine (and perhaps gastrin[26]) activates phospholipase C to release inositol phosphates from membrane phospholipids, such as phosphatidylinositol bisphosphate, with the inositol phosphates then releasing intracellular calcium. Thus, stimulation of HCl secretion by acetylcholine and by gastrin may both be mediated by increases in intracellular calcium, although there is controversy regarding the source of calcium (extracellular or intracellular).[33, 36, 39]

Unlike gastrin, which reaches its receptor on the parietal cell via the blood (endocrine effect), and acetylcholine, which reaches the muscarinic receptor on the parietal cell after diffusion across a synapse (neurocrine effect), histamine diffuses to the H_2 receptor on the parietal cell after local release from mast cells in the lamina propria of the oxyntic mucosa (paracrine effect).[8] In some species, gastrin increases histamine release from mast cells or mast-like cells,[35] but not in other species.[40] Little is known about regulation of histamine release and histamine degradation in the gastric mucosa of humans. Thus, it is unknown whether histamine is released continuously from mast cells at a constant rate or whether histamine release is regulated (e.g., after a meal).

When histamine binds to the H_2 receptor on the parietal cell, it increases the affinity of a guanosine triphosphate (GTP)-regulatory protein for cytosolic GTP. Once the GTP-regulatory protein has bound GTP, adenylate cyclase is activated, converting cytosolic ATP to cyclic AMP (cAMP, Fig. 41–2).[41] Through one or more intermediate steps involving phosphorylated protein kinases, cAMP accumulation in parietal cells activates the proton pump. Agents that delay degradation of intracellular cAMP, such as the phosphodiesterase inhibitor theophylline, will augment the stimulatory effect of histamine on HCl secretion.[41] One study suggested that histamine, in addition to increasing cAMP within the parietal cell, may also increase intracellular calcium concentrations,[34] although this could not be confirmed in another laboratory.[33]

In addition to a histamine-activated stimulatory GTP-regulatory protein (Gs), which activates adenylate cyclase in the parietal cell, there is also a closely related inhibitory GTP-regulatory protein (Gi), which prevents activation of adenylate cyclase. Soll and colleagues have demonstrated that Gi can be activated by prostaglandin E_2.[42] Their data suggest that prostaglandin E_2 acts on a membrane receptor (near the H_2 receptor), which activates Gi and prevents histamine from activating adenylate cyclase via Gs. Thus, prostaglandins can inhibit histamine-stimulated parietal cell function *in vitro*[43] and acid secretion induced by a

---

*In canine parietal cells, the gastrin receptor interacts equally with gastrin and cholecystokinin (CCK), even though CCK is a much weaker stimulant of acid secretion than gastrin *in vivo* in the dog.[3] The explanation for this paradox is uncertain.

variety of stimulants, including histamine, *in vivo*.[44] Agents that reduce prostaglandin synthesis *in vivo*, such as indomethacin, augment basal and histamine-stimulated acid secretion,[45, 46] suggesting that endogenous prostaglandins may normally play a physiologic, inhibitory role in acid secretion at the parietal cell level.

Besides the endogenous stimulants of acid secretion discussed earlier (histamine, gastrin, acetylcholine, and calcium), two additional neuropeptides, enkephalin (an opiate-like peptide) and bombesin (or its mammalian equivalent, gastrin-releasing peptide) have been reported to increase acid secretion in humans when given parenterally.[47, 48]* However, increases in acid secretion during parenteral infusion of these peptides does not necessarily prove that the substance causes an increase in acid secretion under physiologic conditions. Nevertheless, studies using specific antagonists suggest that endogenous opiates play a physiologic role in acid secretion. Naloxone and nalmefene (opiate receptor antagonists) reduce acid secretion in response to food, sham feeding, and gastrin in humans.[52–54] Furthermore, stimulatory opiate receptors have been demonstrated on isolated parietal cells of guinea pigs.[55] Bombesin is a potent gastrin-releaser and presumably stimulates

---

*Of interest, endogenous opiate-like peptides and bombesin, as well as several other peptides, including calcitonin gene-related peptide, inhibit acid secretion when administered into the central nervous system of dogs or rats.[49, 50] On the other hand, intracerebral administration of thyrotropin-releasing hormone, oxytocin, and other peptides increases acid secretion.[51] The physiologic significance of these interesting observations is as yet unknown and the observed effects vary with site of central nervous system application, species, and dose of peptide.

acid secretion via gastrin.[48] Until a specific antagonist is discovered, it will be difficult to assess the physiologic role of bombesin in gastric acid secretion.

Several endogenous substances are capable of reducing gastric acid secretion when infused intravenously. These include prostaglandin E_2 (see earlier discussion), several peptides (e.g., secretin,[56] somatostatin,[57] glucagon,[58] gastric inhibitory peptide,[59] neurotensin,[60] calcitonin gene-related peptide,[61] corticotropin-releasing factor,[62] thyrotropin-releasing hormone,[63] and peptide YY[64]), dopamine,[65] and magnesium and zinc ions.[66, 67] It is uncertain which of these plays a physiologic role in suppressing acid secretion in humans, although current evidence favors such a role for prostaglandins,[45, 46] somatostatin[68–70] and secretin.[71] Hydrogen ions within the gastric lumen also inhibit acid secretion in response to physiologic stimuli—for example, food, sham feeding, and distention.[72–74] The inhibitory effect of luminal acid on gastric acid secretion is mediated by inhibitory effects on gastrin release (discussed later in this chapter) and perhaps by stimulatory effects on secretin release. Inhibition is not due to a topical effect of acid on the parietal cell.[75]

Under certain pathologic conditions, increased amounts of stimulatory chemical mediators can lead to gastric acid hypersecretion. Thus, gastrin-producing tumors (gastrinoma, Zollinger-Ellison syndrome) and systemic mastocytosis with hyperhistaminemia can lead to massive acid hypersecretion and peptic ulcer disease. It has been speculated that duodenal ulcer patients with idiopathic basal acid hypersecretion have increased basal acetylcholinergic activity.[76, 77] Elevating serum calcium concentrations acutely above normal increases acid secretion and serum gastrin concentration.[66] On the other hand, individuals with severe

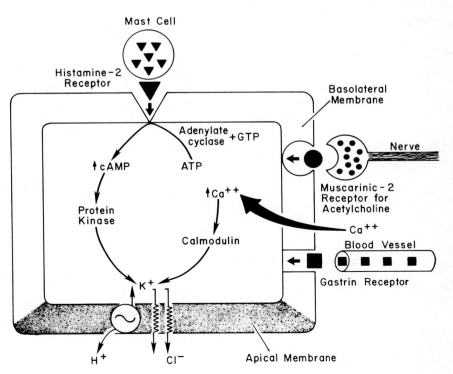

Figure 41–2. Model for receptors on the basolateral membrane of the parietal cell and their intracellular mediators. Histamine from mast cells activates the proton pump (shown on the apical membrane of the cell) by increasing intracellular cyclic AMP (cAMP), whereas acetylcholine from nerves and gastrin from the blood act by increasing intracellular calcium. Although the increase in intracellular calcium is shown to arise from extracellular calcium, there is evidence that gastrin and perhaps acetylcholine release calcium from intracellular stores (see text).

hypocalcemia are often achlorhydric.[78, 79] When serum calcium concentrations are restored to normal, parietal cells again secrete acid.

With this background describing chemical mediators, cellular receptors, and intracellular second messengers (Fig. 41–2), it is easier to understand how acid-antisecretory drugs and ulcer operations reduce acid secretion. Any factor that reduces the concentration of secretagogues near the parietal cell will reduce HCl secretion. Thus, factors that lower serum gastrin concentrations (e.g., somatostatin, certain prostaglandins, antrectomy) will lower HCl secretion. Vagotomy may reduce release of acetylcholine near muscarinic receptors on the parietal cell, although this has not yet been demonstrated. Agents that stabilize mast cells and prevent histamine release reduce acid secretion under certain conditions.[80] Chemical compounds that block stimulatory receptors on parietal cells also inhibit HCl secretion by interfering with agonist-receptor interactions and the subsequent generation of intracellular second messengers. Although gastrin receptor antagonists such as proglumide have been used experimentally, they are only weak inhibitors of acid secretion *in vivo*.[81] On the other hand, histamine$_2$ receptor antagonists (e.g., cimetidine, ranitidine, famotidine) and muscarinic receptor antagonists (e.g., atropine) are strong inhibitors of HCl secretion. It is now known that there are two types of muscarinic receptors, M_1 and M_2, and that the muscarinic receptor on the parietal cell is of the M_2 type.[82] Atropine and related nonselective muscarinic antagonists reduce HCl secretion by acting on M_2 receptors on parietal cells and on M_1 receptors on other cells (e.g., postganglionic neurons), whereas M_1-selective anticholinergic agents such as pirenzepine may act primarily on cells other than parietal cells (e.g., postganglionic neurons).[83, 84] Pirenzepine may reduce acid secretion by blocking acetylcholine release from these neurons, acting in some ways like a medical vagotomy.[84]

As mentioned earlier, prostaglandin compounds prevent histamine-induced activation of adenylate cyclase by activating a Gi protein. Theoretically, calcium channel antagonists might block HCl secretion, and some of these agents will modestly inhibit acid secretion *in vitro*[85] and *in vivo*,[86] although the effects are not great or consistent.[87, 88] Finally, agents that act on the proton pump interfere with the terminal steps of the HCl secretory process. These agents include the substituted benzimidazoles (e.g., omeprazole, see earlier discussion).[26] Acid antisecretory agents are discussed in more detail on pages 845 to 854 and 894 to 898.

Gastric Acid Secretion in Humans

Methods of Measuring Acid Secretion. Acid secretion in humans is usually expressed as the amount of acid secreted under maximal stimulation (MAO, or maximal acid output), as the amount of acid secreted under basal conditions (BAO, or basal acid output), or as the amount of acid secreted in response to a particular stimulus, such as a meal. Before reviewing factors that influence MAO, BAO, and acid secretion stimulated by meals, it is necessary to review methods of measuring acid secretion.

Gastric Aspiration Method. Aspiration of gastric juice using a nasogastric tube is the simplest and most widely used method of measuring acid secretion. It is important that the aspirating ports of the tube be positioned, usually by fluoroscopy, in the most dependent portion of the stomach. Even when the tube has been positioned correctly, approximately 10 per cent of gastric juice escapes aspiration and empties into the duodenum.[89] These losses are even greater after pyloroplasty or gastroenterostomy. Besides emptying from the stomach, a secreted hydrogen ion may be neutralized by bicarbonate-containing alkaline secretions (such as duodenal fluid that has refluxed into the stomach, nonparietal gastric secretion, or saliva) or may diffuse back across the gastric mucosa. All three mechanisms (pyloric losses of H^+, neutralization of H^+, and H^+ back diffusion) result in an underestimation of the true rate of gastric acid secretion. Despite these limitations, gastric aspiration is a useful technique for measuring acid secretion because losses of acid are usually small relative to the rate of acid secretion. BAO, MAO, or peak acid output (PAO) and the cephalic phase of acid secretion are usually measured with this method (see later discussion). Also, tests to evaluate completeness of vagotomy (e.g., sham feeding test) employ this aspiration method (see pp. 757–758). Gastric aspiration cannot accurately measure acid secretion while food is in the stomach.

The H^+ concentration in a sample of aspirated gastric juice (C_{H+}) can be determined by one of two methods.* First, the specimen can be titrated *in vitro* with a base (e.g., NaOH). The number of millimoles of base needed to titrate a volume of gastric juice to a pH endpoint (e.g., 7.0) represents the "titratable" acidity (in millimoles per liter) of the sample. Which pH endpoint to use is somewhat arbitrary and controversial.[91] A second method of determining c_{H+} is to measure pH of gastric juice with a glass electrode. Because the glass electrode measures H^+ activity (a_{H+}), not concentration (c_{H+}), it is necessary to convert a_{H+} to c_{H+} by the following equation: $c_{H+} = a_{H+}/\gamma_{H+}$, where γ_{H+} is the activity coefficient for H^+ in gastric juice. Tables of activity coefficients for gastric juice have been developed by Moore and Scarlata.[91]

In Vivo Intragastric Titration Method. This technique is used to measure acid secretion after a meal. A nasogastric tube is inserted into the stomach. Then, either a meal is eaten in a normal manner or a homogenized meal is infused into the stomach through the tube. A sample of gastric contents (meal plus secreted fluid) is obtained at frequent intervals and the

---

*The H^+ concentration or pH of a sample of aspirated gastric juice does not necessarily equal the H^+ concentration or pH of gastric contents *in vivo*. Using two intragastric pH electrodes, Krawiec and associates showed that the intraluminal pH in the antrum is significantly higher than the pH in the body of the same stomach.[90]

Table 41–2. DOSE, ROUTE, TIMING OF PEAK RESPONSE, AND POSSIBLE SIDE EFFECTS OF VARIOUS STIMULANTS USED TO MEASURE MAXIMAL OR PEAK ACID OUTPUT (PAO)

Stimulant	Dose	Route	Timing of Peak Response	Possible Side Effects
Pentagastrin	6 μg/kg	Subcutaneous	15–45 min	Nausea, sweating, abdominal or chest pain, faintness, hypotension
	6 μg/kg	Intramuscular	10–30 min	
	6 μg/kg/hr	Intravenous	10–30 min	
Histamine*				
Acid phosphate	40 μg/kg	Subcutaneous	20–60 min	Pain at injection site, flushing, headache,
Acid phosphate	40 μg/kg/hr	Intravenous	30–45 min	dizziness, hypotension, nausea, abdominal pain,
Dihydrochloride	50 μg/kg	Subcutaneous	30–45 min	palpitations
Betazole	0.5 mg/kg or 50 mg	Subcutaneous or intramuscular	45–120 min	Pain at injection site, flushing

*Prior to admistering any of these histamine compounds, administer an H_1-antihistamine, such as 50 mg diphenhydramine (Benadryl) intramuscularly.

pH is measured. If the pH of the sample begins to fall below the original pH of the meal as a result of acid secretion, a base, such as sodium bicarbonate, is infused into the stomach until the pH is restored to the original meal pH. For a given time period, the number of millimoles of base added to maintain pH constant is equal to the number of millimoles of acid secreted.[92] Indicator-dilution methods can also be used to measure food-stimulated acid secretion.[93, 94] These methods give results similar to *in vivo* intragastric titration.[95]

Maximal Secretory Capacity (MAO or PAO). The maximal secretory capacity can be estimated by the MAO or PAO following administration of a maximally effective dose of pentagastrin, histamine, or the histamine analogue betazole (3-beta-aminoethylpyrazole). Doses of these agents, possible routes of administration, time until peak responses, and possible side effects are given in Table 41–2.

MAO represents the sum of the four 15-minute acid outputs following pentagastrin or histamine administration (acid output = volume × H^+ concentration). PAO is defined as the sum of the two highest consecutive 15-minute acid outputs following stimulation, multiplied by 2 to express results in millimoles per hour. MAO and PAO are indirect estimates of the total population of functional parietal cells.[96, 97] The lower panels of Figure 41–3 display MAO and PAO in 100 healthy men and 50 healthy women. MAO in the 150 subjects ranged from 4.7 to 58.4 mmol/hr, corresponding to a range of 0.25 to 3.0 billion parietal cells.[96] On the average, women have lower maximal secretory capacities than men, and histologic studies confirm that women have fewer parietal cells.[98] Women are also less responsive than men to stimulants of acid secretion, such as gastrin, even when differences in MAO are taken into consideration. For example, the serum gastrin concentration required to produce half of MAO is two to three times higher in women than in men.[99] The reason for this is unknown, although a study in rats has suggested that estradiol may directly inhibit H^+,K^+-ATPase activity.[100]

Figure 41–4 indicates that the MAO and PAO are fairly constant from one day to another in the same person; MAO usually but not always remains relatively constant over long periods of time.[101] MAO (and hence

parietal cell mass) is a function of sex, body weight, lean body mass, and age.[102] Although children have lower MAOs than do adults, MAOs in children are similar to adult values when expressed as millimoles per hour per kilogram of body weight.[103]

The parietal cell mass and MAO can increase under the trophic influence of gastrin. For example, individuals with gastrin-producing tumors (Zollinger-Ellison syndrome) often have elevated MAOs and parietal cell hyperplasia.[104] On the other hand, antrectomy leads to a decrease in serum gastrin concentrations, parietal cell atrophy, and a decrease in MAO.[105] The parietal cell atrophy and fall in MAO after antrectomy can to some extent be prevented experimentally with exogenous gastrin.[105, 106] The gastrin antagonist proglumide

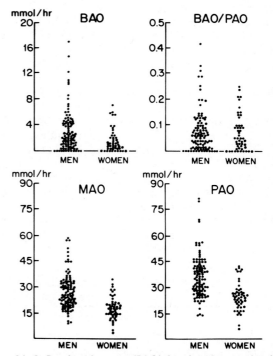

Figure 41–3. Basal acid output (BAO), basal acid output/peak acid output (BAO/PAO), maximal acid output (MAO) and peak acid output (PAO) in 100 healthy men and 50 healthy women. Upper and lower limits of normal, derived from these data, are shown in Table 41–3.

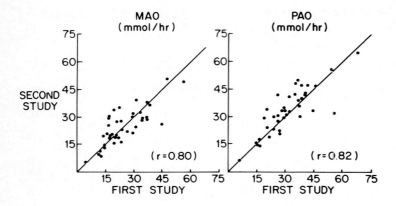

Figure 41–4. Reproducibility of maximal acid output (MAO) and peak acid output (PAO) in 40 healthy subjects studied on two separate days. Either 6 μg/kg pentagastrin or 40 μg/kg histamine phosphate was given subcutaneously on both studies. There was a significant ($P < 0.001$) correlation between MAO and PAO. Line represents the line of identity rather than the linear regression plot of the data.

can inhibit the trophic effect of gastrin.[107] Experimental evidence suggests that histamine, chronic hypercalcemia (perhaps mediated through gastrin), and chronic vagal stimulation also can increase parietal cell mass.[108–110] Because patients with duodenal ulcer have, on the average, larger parietal cell populations and MAO than nonulcer controls,[98] it is possible that some trophic factor (perhaps gastrin or increased vagal activity) leads to an increase in parietal cell mass and MAO in these patients.

MAO decreases by 50 to 60 per cent after truncal or proximal gastric vagotomy.[111, 112] Vagotomy does not lead to atrophy of parietal cells,[113] possibly because vagotomy also increases serum gastrin concentrations.[114] Thus, MAO cannot be used to estimate parietal cell mass after vagotomy. Some studies have reported that MAO after histamine stimulation can sometimes be restored by administering cholinergic agents after vagotomy, suggesting that MAO had decreased because of loss of the permissive effect of acetylcholine.[115, 116] However, this could not be confirmed by other workers.[117, 118] Moreover, the effect of vagotomy on MAO cannot be simulated by giving large intravenous doses of atropine.[119, 120] Thus, the explanation for the large and rapid decrease in maximal secretory capacity after vagotomy is uncertain. A recent *in vitro* study of human oxyntic glands obtained endoscopically from vagotomized patients indicated that the maximal response of these glands to histamine was reduced by 60 per cent, and this reduction was not overcome by adding dibutyrl cAMP, suggesting an intracellular defect induced by the vagotomy.[121]

Basal Acid Secretion (BAO). Gastric acid secreted in the absence of all intentional and avoidable stimulation is called basal acid secretion. BAO varies from

hour to hour in the same individual and tends to follow a circadian pattern.[122] The lowest secretory rates occur between 5 and 11 A.M., whereas the highest rates occur between 2 and 11 P.M. The cause of these cyclic variations in basal acid secretion is not known. The rate of basal acid secretion can also be influenced by the emotional state of the individual.[123]

It is apparent from Figure 41–3 that BAO varies considerably among healthy individuals. BAO is higher in men than in women. However, this is probably because men have a larger maximal acid secretory capacity, for, as shown in Figure 41–3, the ratio of BAO to PAO was very similar in men and women (averaging 0.08 in men and 0.07 in women). The fact that BAO/PAO varied from 0 to 0.42 in healthy individuals suggests that factors other than parietal cell mass are responsible for differences in basal acid secretion among subjects.

When basal serum gastrin concentrations and basal acid secretion are measured simultaneously, there is either no correlation[124] or a negative correlation.[125] Moreover, there is no correlation between serum gastrin levels and circadian changes in BAO.[122] At present, then, there is no evidence that differences in basal acid secretion between subjects or in the same subject are attributable to differences in circulating gastrin levels.

Upper limits of normal BAO and BAO/PAO, derived from data in the 150 healthy men and women in Figure 41–3, are listed in Table 41–3. Upper and lower limits of MAO and PAO are also shown. These 95 per cent confidence limits provide guidelines for diagnosis of acid hypersecretory and hyposecretory states.

Meal-Stimulated Acid Secretion. When an appetizing meal is eaten, gastric acid secretion promptly increases above basal rates so that within 90 minutes

Table 41–3. UPPER AND LOWER LIMITS OF NORMAL ACID OUTPUTS
IN HEALTHY ADULT MEN AND WOMEN*

	BAO (mmol/hr)		MAO (mmol/hr)		PAO (mmol/hr)		BAO/PAO	
	Men	*Women*	*Men*	*Women*	*Men*	*Women*	*Men*	*Women*
Upper limit of normal	10.5	5.6	47.8	30.2	60.6	40.1	0.29	0.23
Lower limit of normal	—	—	6.9	5.0	11.6	8.0	—	—

*Upper and lower limits of normal (95 per cent confidence limits) were derived from data in Figure 41–3 from 100 healthy men and 50 healthy women. There are no lower limits of normal for BAO or for the ratio of BAO to PAO because many normal subjects have a BAO of zero. BAO, Basal acid output; MAO, maximal acid output; PAO, peak acid output.

or so acid secretion rates approach the maximal secretory capacity (Fig. 41–5, top). This acid secretory response to a meal does not appear to be affected significantly by the temperature of the meal[126] or by the level of physical activity of the individual after the meal (e.g., rest versus exercise).[127] Although acid secretion increases rapidly after a meal, the hydrogen ion concentration actually decreases temporarily (i.e., the pH increases). Intragastric pH remains above 3.0 for more than 60 minutes because food protein in the stomach buffers most of the acid that has been secreted (Fig. 41–5, bottom). By 120 minutes after the meal, postprandial intragastric pH decreases below basal levels because food buffers have either been utilized or have been emptied from the stomach, while at the same time gastric acid secretion continues at a relatively high rate (Fig. 41–5).

Three mechanisms contribute to stimulation of acid secretion after a meal: (1) cephalic-vagal stimulation; (2) gastric distention; and (3) chemical reactions of food with gastrointestinal mucosa.

Cephalic-Vagal Stimulation. The thought, sight, smell, and taste of appetizing food sends afferent signals to various centers within the brain. Efferent messages then travel downward from the hypothalamus through the midbrain and brainstem to the dorsal motor nuclei of the vagus nerves in the medulla. The vagi contribute long preganglionic neurons that travel to the stomach, where axons terminate near short, postganglionic neurons that innervate target cells (e.g., parietal cells in oxyntic glands, gastrin cells in pyloric glands). The central and peripheral neurotransmitters involved in the cephalic phase of acid secretion are uncertain. The findings that atropine[128] and naloxone[52, 54] reduce the cephalic phase of acid secretion suggest that central or peripheral cholinergic and opiate pathways could be involved. Furthermore, antiserum to bombesin blocks gastrin release induced by nerve stimulation,[129] suggesting that gastrin-releasing peptide may be the neurotransmitter that releases gastrin from antral G cells during vagal stimulation.[130]

The cephalic phase of acid secretion in humans is usually studied by employing a sham-feeding technique in which subjects see, smell, taste, and chew appetizing food without swallowing it. Sham feeding causes a large increase in gastric acid output, although the peak response is only 50 to 60 per cent of that achievable with maximal exogenous doses of pentagastrin or histamine. During sham feeding, several investigators have documented significant increases in serum gastrin concentrations.[73, 77, 131–133] Gastrin release could contribute to the acid secretory response to sham feeding.[73] Whether vagal stimulation also potentiates the acid secretory response to circulating gastrin is unknown, although such potentiation has been demonstrated between cholinergic agonists and gastrin in humans.[134] In contrast, vagotomy reduces the responsiveness of parietal cells to circulating gastrin.[135]

The relative importance of thought, sight, smell, and taste of appetizing food in the cephalic phase of gastric acid secretion has recently been studied systemati-

cally.[136] Discussing appetizing food for 30 minutes (without sight, smell, or taste) increased acid secretion in healthy subjects and also increased serum gastrin concentrations significantly. Discussing food resulted in an acid secretory response that averaged 66 per cent of the response to modified sham feeding, which activates thought, sight, smell, and taste. Discussing topics other than food (e.g., current events, sports) did not increase acid secretion or serum gastrin significantly. The sight of appetizing food (without smell or taste), the smell of appetizing food (without sight or taste), or the combination of sight and smell (without taste) also increased acid secretion and serum gastrin concentration significantly. Compared with food discussion, however, sight and smell were less potent stimulants of acid secretion (Fig. 41–6). These studies indicate that thinking about food is a potent stimulant of gastric acid secretion in healthy humans. Moreover, the sight and smell of food increase gastric acid secretion and serum gastrin concentrations, probably by provoking thoughts related to food. Thus, thought, sight, and smell can increase acid secretion in the absence of food intake. Taste also appears to play a relatively important role in eliciting gastric acid secretion as a component of the cephalic phase, as the major difference between the combined sight and smell experiment and the sham

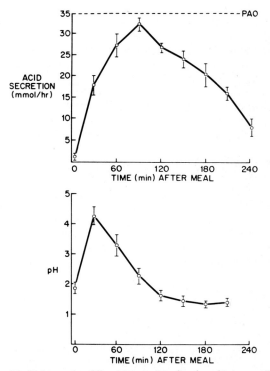

Figure 41–5. Mean (± SE) acid secretion (top) and intragastric pH (bottom) following an eaten sirloin steak meal. On one day (top), acid secretion was measured by *in vivo* intragastric titration to pH 5.5 in six subjects. On a second day (bottom), intragastric pH was allowed to seek its natural level in ten subjects. The mean (± SE) basal acid secretion rate (top) and basal pH (bottom) prior to the meal are shown at 0 minute. Peak acid output (PAO) is also indicated.

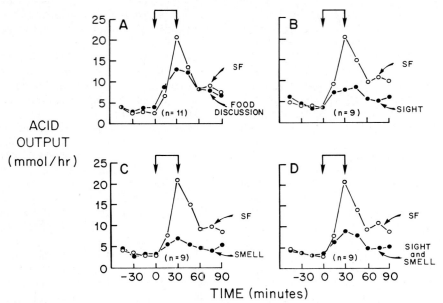

ACID OUTPUT (mmol/hr)

TIME (minutes)

Figure 41–6. Comparison in the same subjects as in Figure 41–5 between mean gastric acid secretory responses to 30 minutes of sham feeding (SF) and acid secretory responses to 30 minutes of food discussion *(A)*, sight of appetizing food *(B)*, smell of appetizing food *(C)*, and the combination of sight and smell *(D)*. Each intervention started at 0 minutes and lasted until 30 minutes *(arrows)*. For each comparison, sham feeding was a significantly more potent stimulus of acid secretion. As a percentage of the response to sham feeding, mean responses were 66 per cent with food discussion, 28 per cent with sight, 23 per cent with smell, and 33 per cent with sight and smell. PAO to pentagastrin averaged approximately 38 mM/hr in these subjects. (Reprinted with permission from: Role of thought, sight, smell, and taste of food in the cephalic phase of gastric acid secretion in man, by Feldman, M., and Richardson, C. T., Gastroenterology *90*(2):428–433. Copyright 1986 by The American Gastroenterological Association.)

feeding experiment was that subjects could taste food in the latter (see Fig. 41–6D).

Gastric Distention. Distention of the stomach stimulates acid secretion by activating both long vagovagal reflexes[137] and short intragastric reflexes.[138] The observation that proximal gastric vagotomy reduces distention-induced acid secretion by 80 to 95 per cent suggests that the vagus plays a major role in this type of acid secretion,[139] much as it does in the cephalic phase of acid secretion.

Two methods have been used to measure acid secretory responses to gastric distention in humans. Either a balloon is used selectively to distend the fundus[139] or antrum[140] and acid secretion is measured by aspiration, or a liquid test meal is used to distend the entire stomach and acid secretion is measured by indicator dilution[141] or *in vivo* intragastric titration.[74] The peak acid secretion rate in response to distention with a fundic balloon or a liquid meal amounts to 20 to 50 per cent of pentagastrin-stimulated PAO. Studies using liquid meals indicate that even small distending volumes (50 to 100 ml) can stimulate acid secretion.[89]

Studies using balloons to distend the fundus or antrum separately have shown that fundic distention is a good stimulus for acid secretion in humans, whereas antral distention does not elicit acid secretion. In fact, when the antrum was distended with a balloon during intravenous pentagastrin infusion, acid output decreased, suggesting that antral distention activates a neural or humoral mechanism that inhibits gastric acid secretion.[142] Antral distention did not inhibit acid secretion in dogs after proximal gastric vagotomy,[143]

suggesting that antral inhibition of acid secretion is mediated via a vagal pathway.

The observations that muscarinic and histamine$_2$ receptor antagonists reduce distention-induced acid secretion in humans suggest that acetylcholine and histamine play at least a permissive role in this response.[139, 144] However, there is no evidence that distention actually causes the release of acetylcholine or histamine in the vicinity of parietal cells. With respect to distention and gastrin release, studies in dogs with antral pouches have demonstrated repeatedly that antral distention releases gastrin into the circulation. In humans, studies with balloons or liquid meals have often, but not always, demonstrated that gastric distention releases gastrin. It is unclear to what extent, if at all, the acid secretory response to distention is due to gastrin release. The finding that gastric distention still significantly stimulated acid secretion even when the gastrin response to distention was blocked by the beta-adrenergic antagonist propranolol suggests that the acid secretory response to distention is, at least in part, independent of gastrin.[145]

Chemical Reactions of Food with Gastrointestinal Mucosa. The acid secretory response to intragastrically administered homogenized food (containing protein, carbohydrate, and fat) is much greater than the acid response to distention with a similar volume of intragastric saline, reaching 60 to 70 per cent of PAO (Fig. 41–7).[146] The acid secretory response to food is a net result of both gastric and intestinal mechanisms, some stimulatory and others inhibitory. In general, the stomach and possibly the upper small intestine have a net

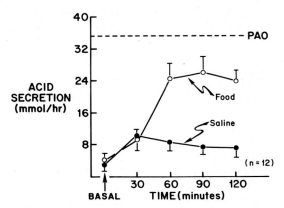

Figure 41–7. Mean (± SE) acid secretion in response to gastric distention with 600 or 700 ml intragastric saline (pH 5) or in response to 600 ml intragastric food (pH 5) in 12 subjects. Basal acid secretion is shown, as is peak acid output (PAO).

stimulatory role in acid secretion, whereas the jejunum and ileum[147] and possibly the colon[148] play an inhibitory role. Following small intestinal resection,[149] acid secretion increases, suggesting that the predominant effect of the small intestine on acid secretion is inhibitory.

Protein is the major constituent of food that stimulates acid secretion. Undigested proteins, such as albumin, are weak stimulants of acid secretion if peptic digestion is prohibited.[146] In contrast, peptic digests of protein, such as polypeptides, peptones, and amino acids, are more potent stimulants of acid secretion. Not all amino acids are equally effective in stimulating acid secretion, however.[150] Amino acids and peptides stimulate gastric acid secretion mainly by releasing gastrin. The rises in plasma gastrin 17 (G17) concentrations in response to a mixed amino acid meal is sufficient to account for the entire acid secretory response to the meal.[151] Thus, G17 appears to be the major physiologic mediator of the acid secretory response to dietary protein. Amino acids and peptides also release big gastrins (G34I and G34II) into the circulation. Evidence from studies in animals *in vivo* and *in vitro* suggests that amino acids in the gastric lumen are converted to amines, which are then taken up by antral gastrin cells and which stimulate the gastrin cells to secrete gastrin into the circulation.[152]

There are other, nongastrin mechanisms by which meals containing amino acids and peptides could stimulate gastric acid secretion. First, amino acids within the gastric lumen might stimulate parietal cells directly.[153] Such a mechanism has been shown in dogs but not yet in humans. Second, amino acids could stimulate acid secretion via release of a nongastrin circulating secretogogue from the small intestine, an entero-oxyntin.[154] A third mechanism by which amino acids could stimulate acid secretion is via the circulation following absorption. In one study, intravenously administered amino acids were as potent a stimulant of acid secretion as an equal amount of intraduodenal amino acids, leading to a secretion rate that was 30 to 35 per cent of PAO.[155] This suggests that the stimulatory "intestinal" phase of acid secretion may be largely due to absorbed amino acids.

Carbohydrates infused into the small intestine or intravenously inhibit gastric acid secretion in response to food or sham feeding.[156, 157] Although dietary glucose releases gastric inhibitory polypeptide (GIP) from the small intestine, the amount of GIP released is insufficient to explain the acid secretory inhibition observed.[59] The mechanism by which carbohydrates reduce acid secretion is uncertain.

Fat is an inhibitor of acid secretion whether it is infused into the stomach,[94] intestine,[158] or veins.[159] The mechanism by which fat inhibits acid secretion is unknown. Several gut peptides, including GIP, neurotensin, glucagon, vasoactive intestinal polypeptide (VIP), peptide YY, and cholecystokinin (CCK), are released into the circulation by meals containing fat. It has not been shown, however, that rises in the circulating concentrations of any of these peptides are sufficient to account for the acid secretory inhibition observed.[158] The inhibition of acid secretion by fat is not due to suppression of gastrin release.[94, 146, 158] One study has shown that intraduodenal fat inhibited pentagastrin-stimulated acid secretion before, but not after, proximal gastric vagotomy.[160] These investigators suggested that inhibition of gastric acid secretion by fat might depend on intact vagus nerves and be mediated by the gut peptide neurotensin. Some studies have provided evidence that inhibition of gastric acid secretion by glucagon and peptide YY is dependent on intact vagal function.[161, 162]

Coffee and many other beverages (milk, beer, wine, soft drinks) increase gastric acid secretion and serum gastrin concentrations.[163, 164] Decaffeinated coffee stimulates about as much acid secretion as does regular coffee, indicating that coffee contains stimulants of acid secretion and gastrin release other than caffeine.[165]

Total, 24-Hour Acid Secretion. Recently, by combining gastric aspiration and *in vivo* intragastric titration methods, it has been possible to measure gastric acid secretion over an entire 24-hour period in humans.[166] As shown in Figure 41–8, acid secretion in seven normal men increased several-fold following breakfast, lunch, and dinner meals and then returned to basal rates within 4 to 5 hours. For the entire 24-hour period, acid secretion averaged a little more than 200 mmol, with just over two thirds of this acid secreted during the day (9 A.M. to 9 P.M.) and just under one third during the night (9 P.M. to 9 A.M.). Men with chronic duodenal ulcer secreted a little over 400 mmol acid/day.

GASTRIN RELEASE

The physiology of gastrin release is discussed on pages 716 to 718. In this section, regulation of gastrin release as it relates to meal-stimulated gastric acid secretion will be reviewed.

As mentioned previously, cephalic-vagal stimulation, gastric distention, and chemical reactions of food constituents (mainly amino acids and peptides) all contribute to the gastrin response to a meal. There is evidence

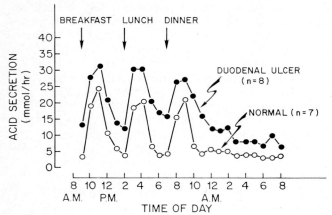

Figure 41–8. Mean (± SE) acid secretion throughout an entire 24-hour period in seven healthy men and eight patients with chronic duodenal ulcer disease. Breakfast, lunch, and dinner meals were given at 9 A.M., 2 P.M., and 7 P.M., respectively, and acid secretion was measured for the next 2 hours by *in vivo* intragastric titration. For the rest of the study, acid secretion was measured by gastric aspiration. Total 24-hour acid secretion averaged 208.3 mM in normal subjects and 408.3 mM in duodenal ulcer patients (*p* <0.02). (Reprinted with permission from: Total 24-hour gastric acid secretion in patients with duodenal ulcer: comparison with normal subjects and effects of cimetidine and parietal cell vagotomy, by Feldman, M., and Richardson, C. T. Gastroenterology 90[3]:540–544. Copyright 1986 by The American Gastroenterological Association.)

that the cephalic vagal stimulation activates not only pathways that release gastrin but also pathways that inhibit gastrin release. When atropine is administered prior to sham feeding, the ensuing gastrin response to sham feeding is markedly enhanced.[128] Blockade of an inhibitory cholinergic pathway by atropine leads to unopposed stimulation of gastrin release by a separate, atropine-insensitive (and therefore probably noncholinergic) vagal pathway. The nature of the neurotransmitter that releases gastrin during vagal stimulation is speculative, although one candidate is gastrin-releasing peptide, the mammalian counterpart of bombesin.[129, 130] Another candidate is gamma-aminobutyric acid (GABA).[167] Gastric distention also activates both a cholinergic reflex that inhibits gastrin release and a separate stimulatory reflex for gastrin release.[74] Atropine, given prior to distention, markedly enhances distention-induced gastrin release, presumably by blocking the inhibitory, cholinergic reflex that normally suppresses gastrin release after distention. On the other hand, distention-induced gastrin release can be blocked by giving propranolol prior to gastric distention, suggesting that stimulation of gastrin release by distention involves adrenergic nerves and a beta receptor mechanism.[145]

The gastrin response to an eaten meal is due mainly to the amino acid component of the meal. Women release considerably more gastrin in response to a protein meal than men (for unclear reasons), but this does not result in increased acid secretion because women's parietal cells are less responsive to gastrin.[99] There is evidence that food does not stimulate gastrin

release maximally in humans because the gastrin response to intravenous bombesin infusion is much larger than the gastrin response to a protein meal.[48, 168]

Luminal acid is the major mechanism that regulates meal-stimulated gastrin release by a negative feedback mechanism. Thus, eating food releases gastrin, which stimulates acid secretion; as a result, intragastric pH eventually decreases (Fig. 41–5). When antral pH decreases below 2.5 to 3.0, antral gastrin release is suppressed (negative feedback). The mechanism by which a low intragastric pH suppresses gastrin release is uncertain. The presence of microvilli on the luminal surface of antral gastrin cells suggests that acid may suppress these cells directly. Acid may also protonate amines derived from dietary amino acids, preventing passive uptake of these protonated, positively charged amines by gastrin cells and stimulation of gastrin release.[169] In the case of cephalic-vagal stimulation (e.g., during sham feeding), luminal acid suppresses gastrin release, and this suppression can be prevented by atropine[73] and possibly by indomethacin,[170] suggesting that inhibition may be mediated via a cholinergically dependent pathway or by endogenous prostaglandins.

INTRINSIC FACTOR (IF) SECRETION

Intrinsic factor (IF) is an approximately 45,000-molecular-weight glycoprotein, which, in humans, is secreted by parietal cells.[171] In other species, such as rodents, IF is secreted by chief cells. The role of IF in vitamin B_{12} absorption is discussed on pages 1048 to 1050, but can be summarized briefly as follows.[172] Vitamin B_{12} is released from dietary protein by the action of gastric acid and pepsin. Two vitamin B_{12}–binding proteins are present in gastric juice: IF and R proteins (also called cobolophilin[173] or haptocorrin[174]). R proteins are so named because of their rapid migration during electrophoresis; they are secreted into saliva, gastric juice, and bile.[175, 176] R proteins are more efficient at binding vitamin B_{12} in the stomach than is IF, especially at a low pH, and therefore most vitamin B_{12} initially becomes bound to R proteins. In the upper small intestine, R protein–vitamin B_{12} complexes are cleaved by pancreatic proteolytic enzymes, and the freed vitamin B_{12} then becomes bound to IF. The IF-B_{12} complex (which is resistant to pancreatic proteolysis[177]) eventually attaches to a specific receptor on ileal mucosa. Vitamin B_{12} is then absorbed into portal venous blood and transported to tissues by another vitamin B_{12}-binding protein, transcobalamin II.

When radioactive vitamin B_{12} is administered orally to patients with IF deficiency, low amounts of radioactive vitamin B_{12} are excreted in the urine (abnormal part I Schilling test). If exogenous IF is administered to IF-deficient patients, together with radioactively labeled vitamin B_{12}, urinary excretion of the vitamin should become normal (part II Schilling test). In addition to IF deficiency, vitamin B_{12} malabsorption may be due to bacterial overgrowth of the small intestine (vitamin B_{12} competed for by bacteria), pancreatic insufficiency[178] (impaired proteolytic cleavage of R–B_{12} complex), or ileal disease or resection (absent absorptive site).

Normally, IF secretion far exceeds the amount necessary for vitamin B_{12} absorption. All stimulants of gastric acid secretion discussed earlier in this chapter also stimulate IF secretion, although the duration of the IF secretory response to these stimulants tends to be much briefer than the duration of the acid secretory response. Patients with low or absent acid secretion often have reduced IF secretion. However, continued IF secretion in low amounts may be sufficient to prevent vitamin B_{12} deficiency and pernicious anemia. Agents that reduce H^+ secretion by parietal cells by blocking the H^+, K^+-ATPase (e.g., omeprazole) do not reduce IF secretion by these cells,[179] whereas agents that reduce acid secretion by blocking receptors on the parietal cell membrane, such as histamine$_2$ receptor antagonists, reduce IF secretion.[180] In rare patients, IF secretion is absent despite normal acid secretion. This usually occurs in children (juvenile pernicious anemia[181]), although cases in adults have been reported.[182] In even rarer cases, juvenile pernicious anemia may result from secretion of an abnormal IF molecule or from an intracellular block in IF secretion.[183, 184]

Circulating antibodies to parietal cells and IF are found in many patients with pernicious anemia, atrophic gastritis, achlorhydria, or hypochlorhydria. Whether these antibodies play a role in the pathogenesis of these disorders is uncertain, although some evidence suggests that they may.[9, 10] In these patients, antral mucosa may be spared (type A gastritis) or involved (type B gastritis). When the antral mucosa is spared, markedly elevated serum gastrin concentrations develop,[185] probably as a result of prolonged achlorhydria.[186]

PEPSINOGEN SECRETION

As shown in Table 41–1, pepsinogens are present in mucous cells of cardiac glands, in chief and mucous neck cells of oxyntic glands, and in mucous cells of pyloric glands. In addition, pepsinogens are present in mucous cells of duodenal Brunner's glands. These proenzymes, when secreted, are activated by acid to an active form, pepsin. Once this reaction begins, pepsin can activate additional pepsinogen autocatalytically. Pepsinogens belong to a family of enzymes called aspartic proteases (EC 3.4.23); renin also belongs to this family.[187]

Using electrophoresis, Samloff has detected at least eight proteolytic enzymes in extracts from gastric mucosa.[188] Five fractions (1 to 5), which migrate toward the anode most rapidly, are identical immunologically and have been referred to as group I pepsinogens (also called PGI or PGA). The DNA sequence for PGA in humans is located on chromosome 11[189, 190] and the complete amino acid sequence of PGI in several spe-

cies, including humans, has been reported.[187, 191] PGIs appear to be expressed and secreted only in oxyntic mucosa. Migrating slightly behind the group I pepsinogens are two fractions, 6 and 7, which are immunologically similar to each other and distinct from group I pepsinogens. These latter group II pepsinogens (also called PGII or PGC) are secreted not only from oxyntic mucosa but also from cardiac and pyloric glands and duodenal Brunner's glands. Both group I and group II pepsinogens are active at acid pH, inactivated reversibly at around pH 5.0, and irreversibly destroyed at pH 7 to 8. The pH optimal for peptic activity varies from about 1.8 to 3.5, depending on the species of pepsin, the ionic strength (osmolality), and the type and concentration of substrate.

Another protease, which is immunologically distinct from group I and II pepsinogens, is an electrophoretically slow-moving protease (SMP). This protease, which accounts for less than 5 per cent of the total proteolytic activity of gastric mucosal extracts, is probably a tissue cathepsin (i.e., an acid protease not destroyed by alkalinization and present in several tissues). This protease appears to be produced in superficial epithelial cells rather than in gastric glands.[192] SMP is the predominant protease found in fetal stomachs and is also the major protease found in gastric adenocarcinoma cells, especially in poorly differentiated tumors.[192]

Both group I and group II pepsinogens can be detected in the blood by radioimmunoassay.[188] It is unclear whether pepsinogens are secreted into the blood from intact cells or from degenerating cells. There is a modest correlation between serum group I pepsinogen concentrations and maximal acid secretion.[193] Group I (but not group II) pepsinogens are also present in urine, whereas group II (but not group I) pepsinogens are present in semen. Recent studies suggest that there may be several other proteolytic fractions in gastric mucosal extracts besides the eight fractions described here.

It is generally believed that agents that increase or decrease gastric acid secretion have a similar effect on gastric pepsinogen secretion, and this statement is for the most part true. *In vitro* studies of pepsinogen secretion using chief cells or oxyntic glands obtained from animals have shed additional light on factors that regulate pepsinogen secretion.[194–202] Certain agents that activate adenylate cyclase and increase intracellular cAMP, such as secretin, VIP, forskolin, prostaglandins, and isoproterenol, increase pepsinogen secretion *in vitro*. Furthermore, calcium ions and agents that increase intracellular calcium (carbachol, cholecystokinin, the calcium ionophore A23187) also increase pepsinogen secretion. On the other hand, histamine has no effect on pepsinogen secretion *in vitro* and gastrin has only a variable effect. This contrasts with *in vivo* studies in humans in which histamine and gastrin each stimulate pepsinogen secretion.[203] Thus, like the parietal cell, the chief cell seems to respond to two different intracellular mediators (cAMP and calcium), although the chemical agents that increase the intracellular concentrations of these mediators differ to some extent in the two types of cells. Furthermore, *in vitro* and *in vivo* results do not always coincide, whether studying pepsinogen or H^+ secretion.

In addition to proteolytic enzymes, a lipolytic enzyme is secreted into gastric juice.[204] This gastric lipase has properties that are distinct from pancreatic lipase. Stimulation of gastric lipase secretion occurs under similar conditions as stimulation of gastric pepsinogen secretion discussed earlier.[204, 205] Thus, gastric (and lingual) lipase, gastric pepsin, and salivary amylase initiate intragastric digestion of dietary fat, protein, and carbohydrate, respectively, prior to pancreatic enzymatic digestion of ingested nutrients in the upper small intestine.

MUCUS SECRETION

Mucus is secreted by superficial epithelial cells and by mucous cells in glands throughout the stomach. Gastric mucus is a viscous gel that adheres to and blankets the entire surface of the gastric mucosa, keeping it lubricated and protected from mechanical and abrasive injury.

The physicochemical properties of gastric mucus have been reviewed by Bell and colleagues.[206] Much of the research in this field has utilized mucus obtained from pigs, which is similar in structure to human mucus. The mucus gel is approximately 95 per cent water and 5 per cent glycoprotein. The intact, undegraded glycoprotein has a molecular weight of about 2 million and is a polymer consisting of four identical subunits, each with a molecular weight of 500,000. Each subunit consists of a protein core with many carbohydrate side chains attached to serine and threonine residues of the protein core. Carbohydrate side chains are approximately 15 sugars long, the major sugars being galactose, fucose, N-acetylgalactosamine, and N-acetylglucosamine. Sialic acids are also present but in lesser amounts than in mucous glycoproteins from other parts of the gut. Differences in the terminal sugar sequences of the side chains impart antigenic differences among gastric mucus glycoproteins secreted into gastric juice. Individuals secrete mucus with antigenic determinants for blood group A, B, or H (O) substance activity.

The four subunits of the intact mucus glycoprotein are joined by disulfide bridges connecting the nonglycosylated parts of the protein core. If disulfide bridges are broken—for example, by treatment with N-acetyl-L-cysteine (Mucomist) or by proteolysis with pepsin, the glycoprotein is degraded into its four subunits, loses its gel-forming and viscous properties, and becomes solubilized. Under normal conditions *in vivo*, the mucus gel is continuously being secreted by surface epithelial cells and continuously being solubilized by luminal peptic activity.

Gastric mucus may have other functions besides surface lubrication. For example, *in vitro* studies indicate that gastric mucus retards the rate of H^+ diffusion.[207, 208] The mucus gel thus provides an unstirred water layer, which slows inward diffusion of H^+ toward the mucosa. It has been speculated[3, 209] that the mucus barrier to H^+, in combination with secretion of HCO_3^- into the gel by surface epithelial cells, serves to protect the surface epithelium against injury from luminal acid and pepsin (Fig. 41–9).

Different methods are used to measure gel thickness.[210, 211] Mean thickness adjacent to human antral mucosa ranges from 0.2 to 0.6 mm. Gel thickness increases under certain conditions (e.g., following gastric distention[210] or after administration of 16,16-dimethyl prostaglandin E_2 or carbenoxolone[210, 211]). It is uncertain whether this increased thickness is attributable to increased mucus secretion, reduced mucus degradation, or both. The thickness of the mucus gel is reduced by N-acetyl-L-cysteine (Mucomist),[210] by certain nonsteroidal anti-inflammatory agents, including aspirin,[209] and by pepsin.[211]

Studies of physiologic events that regulate the secretion of mucus have been few and are difficult to interpret. Several agents, including prostaglandins, increase the amount of degraded glycoprotein subunits in luminal gastric contents.[212] However, this finding does not necessarily imply that mucus secretion has been stimulated. In fact, if mucus secretion were to remain constant and peptic degradation of the mucus gel were to increase (prostaglandins may increase pepsinogen secretion[200] *in vitro*), an increased output of degraded, soluble glycoprotein into gastric juice would occur. Under these conditions, the thickness of the

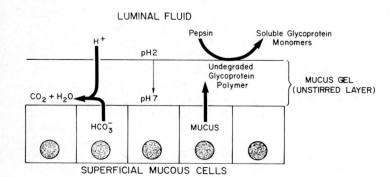

Figure 41–9. Model for surface neutralization of H^+ by HCO_3^- within unstirred layer of gastric mucus gel. HCO_3^- secretion into gel by superficial mucous cells would keep the pH near the mucosal surface alkaline. Undegraded mucus glycoprotein polymer is secreted continuously into mucus gel by superficial mucous cells, and gel is solubilized continuously by luminal pepsin. (Modified from Allen, A., and Garner, A. Gut *21*:249, 1980.)

gastric gel would actually decrease. Thus, studies reporting an increase or decrease in gastric juice glycoprotein output must be interpreted cautiously.

BICARBONATE (HCO_3^-) SECRETION

HCO_3^- is secreted throughout the stomach. Evidence suggests that HCO_3^- is secreted by surface epithelial cells; these cells contain large amounts of carbonic anhydrase.[213] As these cells also secrete mucus, a high pH mucus-bicarbonate blanket covers the gastric epithelium.[3, 209] As luminal H^+ diffuses inward toward this blanket, H^+ is converted to CO_2 and H_2O by HCO_3^-. Furthermore, as pepsin diffuses toward the mucosa, its activity declines as the pH in the microenvironment near the surrface of the mucosa approaches 7.0 (Fig. 41–9).

Under most conditions, luminal gastric HCO_3^- is overwhelmed by luminal gastric H^+. Therefore, HCO_3^- is not present in aspirated gastric juice, as it is converted to CO_2. Thus, measurement of gastric HCO_3^- secretion is difficult and indirect. One method that has been used is to measure gastric juice pCO_2 and pH and then to use the Henderson-Hasselbalch equation to calculate HCO_3^- concentration.[214] If it is assumed that all CO_2 in gastric juice arises from HCO_3^-, that the gastric mucosa is impermeable to CO_2 formed in the lumen from HCO_3^-, and that CO_2 is not lost into gastric gas or by belching, it is possible to calculate HCO_3^- secretion rates. Unfortunately, the assumptions on which these calculations are made have not been proved, especially in humans. Most investigators who use the pH-pCO_2 method also employ an H_2 receptor antagonist such as cimetidine or ranitidine to block H^+ secretion, reducing intraluminal conversion of HCO_3^- to CO_2.[214] Unfortunately, it is uncertain whether H_2 blockers themselves affect gastric HCO_3^- secretion *in vivo*, although one preliminary study suggests that they do not.[215]

A second indirect method to measure gastric HCO_3^- secretion is based on the observation that HCO_3^- neutralizes an equimolar amount of H^+ with a resultant disappearance of HCO_3^- and H^+ (as CO_2 and H_2O are formed) and a decrease in gastric juice osmolality. Using a two-component model of gastric secretion (parietal component containing HCl, nonparietal component containing HCO_3^-), this author has developed and validated *in vitro* and *in vivo* a method for measuring H^+ and HCO_3^- secretion simultaneously, as well as parietal and nonparietal volume secretion.[216] The assumptions of the method are: (1) the H^+ concentration and osmolality of the parietal component are 160 mM and 1.10 times plasma osmolality (or approximately 320 mosmol/kg), respectively*; and (2) the osmolality of the nonparietal component is equal to plasma osmolality, or approximately 290 mosmol/kg.

---

*In the original reports,[216] it was assumed that the osmolality of pure parietal secretion was 1.06 times plasma osmolality, but more recent studies have suggested that 1.10 is a more accurate figure.

Both of these assumptions have experimental support.[216]

Using the two-component model–osmolality method, it is possible to calculate the concentration of HCO_3^- in nonparietal secretions. Such calculations indicate that the HCO_3^- concentration of nonparietal secretions (60 to 90 mM) is much higher than the plasma HCO_3^- of 24 mM.[216] Thus, HCO_3^- appears to be secreted into gastric juice against both a concentration gradient and an electrical gradient, implying an active, energy-dependent process. Studies *in vitro* using metabolic inhibitors or anoxic conditions also indicate that gastric HCO_3^- secretion is largely an energy-dependent, metabolic process.[217]

The exact mechanism by which gastric HCO_3^- is secreted is unclear. The fact that there is virtually no change in gastric electrical potential difference (PD) during stimulation of HCO_3^- secretion suggests that HCO_3^- transport may take place via an electroneutral ion exchange mechanism, possibly an exchange of HCO_3^- for Cl^- at the luminal surface.[217] In support of this hypothesis is the observation in amphibian gastric mucosa *in vitro* that HCO_3^- secretion into luminal fluid ceases when the chloride in the luminal solution is replaced by another anion.[217, 218]

Using either the pH-pCO_2 method or the two-component model–osmolality method to measure gastric HCO_3^- secretion, recent studies have elucidated factors that regulate gastric HCO_3^- secretion in humans. Vagal stimulation, induced by sham feeding, for example, increases both gastric H^+ and, to a lesser extent, gastric HCO_3^- secretion.[214, 219] An example using the two-component model–osmolality method is shown in Figure 41–10. Stimulation of gastric HCO_3^- and nonparietal volume secretion by the vagus is probably cholinergically mediated because both can be inhibited by atropine and stimulated by the cholinergic agonist bethanechol.[214, 216, 219, 220] It has been known for several years that cholinergic agents like bethanechol have little effect on net gastric acid output in humans (net acid output = acid secretion − bicarbonate secretion).[221] This is probably because bethanechol stimulates H^+ and HCO_3^- secretion to approximately similar extents.[216]

Prostaglandin E_2 analogues (e.g., enprostil, trimoprostil) also stimulate gastric HCO_3^- secretion in humans.[216, 222] However, blockade of endogenous prostaglandin synthesis by indomethacin does not affect gastric HCO_3^- secretion in humans.[45] Thus, stimulation of gastric HCO_3^- secretion by prostaglandins is probably a pharmacologic rather than a physiologic action.

Although gastrin does not affect gastric HCO_3^- secretion *in vitro* in amphibians,[223] the author and colleagues have found in humans that G17 infusion inhibits basal gastric HCO_3^- secretion by approximately 50 per cent. Interestingly, G17 did not inhibit gastric HCO_3^- secretion in humans after proximal gastric vagotomy, suggesting that gastrin's inhibitory effect on gastric HCO_3^- secretion is mediated via the vagi.

Current evidence suggests that different factors may regulate gastric HCO_3^- secretion and nonparietal vol-

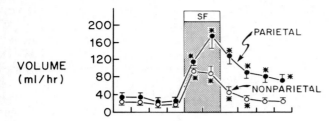

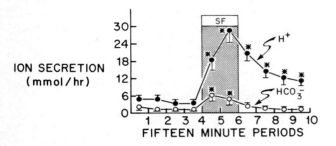

VOLUME (ml/hr)

ION SECRETION (mmol/hr)

FIFTEEN MINUTE PERIODS

Figure 41–10. Effect of sham feeding (SF) on mean parietal and nonparietal volume secretion (top) and on mean gastric H^+ and HCO_3^- secretion (bottom) in ten subjects. Significant ($P < 0.05$) increases above mean control values during four 15-minute periods before SF are shown by asterisks. (From Feldman, M. Am. J. Physiol. *248*:G188, 1985. Used with permission.)

ume secretion. For example, prostaglandin E_2 analogues increase gastric HCO_3^- secretion without increasing gastric nonparietal fluid secretion.[216, 222] On the other hand, G17 infusion decreases gastric HCO_3^- secretion, at the same time increasing nonparietal volume secretion. Patients with duodenal ulcer have normal rates of gastric HCO_3^- secretion and increased nonparietal volume secretion,[221, 224] whereas proximal gastric vagotomy has no effect on gastric HCO_3^- secretion but reduces gastric nonparietal volume secretion. It seems reasonable to propose, on the basis of current knowledge, that gastric HCO_3^- secretion is a function of surface cells via a volume-independent HCO_3^-/Cl^- exchange mechanism, whereas nonparietal volume secretion arises primarily from nonparietal cells within oxyntic and pyloric glands. This refinement of conventional two-component models of gastric secretion is still overly simplified, as surface cells must secrete at least some fluid and nonparietal glandular cells probably secrete some bicarbonate.

Little is known about the effect of food on gastric bicarbonate secretion. The observation that the pH of gastric juice decreases to 1 to 2 after a meal (Fig. 41–5) indicates that secreted HCO_3^- is easily overwhelmed by secreted H^+. However, as mentioned previously, the pH in the vicinity of the surface epithelial cells may be considerably higher than the pH in the luminal fluid because of the presence of an unstirred mucus gel on top of these cells and because of the secretion of HCO_3^- into this gel by superficial cells (Fig. 41–9).

GASTRIC SECRETION IN DISEASE

In general, measurement of gastric acid-pepsin secretion is rarely indicated clinically. Major indications include diagnosis of Zollinger-Ellison syndrome (see pp. 909–925) and evaluation of patients after peptic ulcer surgery (see pp. 962–963). However, there are

a number of diseases associated with increased or decreased acid-pepsin secretion.

Diseases Associated with Increased Acid-Pepsin Secretion

Duodenal Ulcer Disease. Chronic duodenal ulcer disease is the most common disorder associated with increased gastric acid secretion. Duodenal ulcer patients as a group have a significantly higher MAO or PAO, BAO, BAO/PAO, and total 24-hour acid secretion (Fig. 41–8) than normal subjects, although there is overlap among the two groups. There are several reasons for increased gastric acid secretion in duodenal ulcer patients; these are discussed on pages 823 to 831.

Zollinger-Ellison Syndrome (Gastrinoma). Patients with Zollinger-Ellison syndrome have elevated serum gastrin concentrations as a result of a gastrin-producing islet cell tumor, usually located in the pancreas. Increased serum gastrin concentration leads to increased basal acid secretion. Basal acid secretion is usually greater than 15 mmol/hr, and in some patients it may be as high as 150 mmol/hr. The BAO/PAO ratio is usually 0.6 or greater. This syndrome is sometimes associated with other endocrine tumors as part of multiple endocrine neoplasia, type I (MEN-I) syndrome (see p. 911).

Retained Antrum Syndrome. This rare syndrome can develop after antrectomy and Billroth II gastrojejunostomy if the most distal antral and pyloric tissue is not resected (see pp. 939–945). Because of its new location at the end of the afferent loop, the retained pyloric glands are continually bathed in alkaline secretions. Under these conditions, gastrin is released continuously into the circulation from the antral and pyloric G cells, which may lead to increased gastric acid secretion from remaining parietal cells and to recurrent peptic ulceration in some patients.

Other Causes. In some patients with hyperparathyroidism, increased acid secretion and peptic ulcer disease may result from a coexisting gastrinoma (MEN-I syndrome) (see p. 490). There is no definite evidence of increased acid secretion in patients with hyperparathyroidism without gastrinoma. Less common causes of acid hypersecretion include extensive small bowel resection, head trauma with increased intracranial pressure,[225, 226] antral gastrin cell hyperplasia (see p. 821) and foregut carcinoid tumors (see p. 1549). Carcinoid tumors may lead to acid hypersecretion by producing histamine. Histamine overproduction is also the mechanism for acid hypersecretion in some patients with systemic mastocytosis and basophilic leukemia.

Diseases Associated with Decreased Acid-Pepsin Secretion

Decreased acid and pepsin secretion is commonly observed in patients with gastric ulcer, gastritis, gastric polyps, and gastric carcinoma (see pp. 755–756 and 884–885). Patients with gastric atrophy and histamine-fast or pentagastrin-fast achlorhydria often have reduced or absent intrinsic factor secretion and are therefore at risk for developing vitamin B_{12} deficiency (see pp. 265 and 1048–1050). It has long been recognized that gastric acid–pepsin secretion declines with age.[227] Ths is probably owing to an associated atrophic gastritis. Using a low ratio of serum PGI to PGII (less than 2.9) as an indicator of atrophic gastritis, Krasinski and colleagues studied 359 free-living, institutionalized older people 60 to 99 years old and found an increasing incidence of atrophic gastritis of 24 per cent, 32 per cent, and 37 per cent for age groups 60 to 69, 70 to 79, and 80 to 99 years old, respectively.[228]

Other causes of reduced acid secretion include previous partial gastric resection or vagotomy and, on rare occasions, islet cell tumors that produce hormones that inhibit acid secretion (somatostatin, for example).[229]

Abnormalities in Gastric Mucus–Bicarbonate Secretion

Now that better techniques are available for measuring gastric mucus and HCO_3^- secretion, these methods are being applied to study of patients with diseases. Patients with duodenal ulcer have qualitatively normal gastric mucus[230] and normal gastric HCO_3^- secretion.[224, 230] Patients with gastric ulcer, on the other hand, may have a poor quality of gastric mucus and also reduced gastric HCO_3^- secretion,[230] although more studies are needed to confirm these observations. Several agents that damage the gastric mucosa (e.g., alcohol and aspirin) may act, at least partly, by decreasing gastric mucus or HCO_3^- secretion.[209] This will be a fruitful area for further investigation.

References

1. Ito, S. Functional gastric morphology. *In* Johnson, L. R. (ed.). Physiology of the Gastrointestinal Tract, New York, Raven Press, 1981.
2. Helander, H. F. The stomach. Cellular aspects. *In* Desnuelle, P., Sjostrom, H., and Noren, O. (eds.). Molecular and Cellular Basis of Digestion. New York, Elsevier, 1986, pp. 475.
3. Heatley, N. G. Mucosubstance as a barrier to diffusion. Gastroenterology 37:313, 1959.
4. McGreevy, J. M. Gastric surface cell function: potential difference and mucosal barrier. Am. J. Physiol. 247:G79, 1984.
5. Olender, E. J., Fromm, D., Furukawa, T., and Kolis, M. H$^+$ disposal by rabbit gastric mucosal surface cells. Gastroenterology 86:698, 1984.
6. Uvnas-Wallensten, K. Luminal secretion of gut peptides. Clin. Gastroenterol. 9:545, 1980.
7. Morz, R., Prager-Petz, J., and Pointner, H. Effect of luminal somatostatin on pentagastrin-stimulated gastric acid secretion in the rat. Am. J. Physiol. 245:G297, 1983.
8. Mohri, K., Reimann, H.-J., Lorenz, W., Troidl, H., and Weber, D. Histamine content and mast cells in human gastric and duodenal mucosa. Agents Actions 8:372, 1978.
9. De Aizpurua, H. J., Ungar, B., and Toh, B.-H. Serum from patients with pernicious anaemia blocks gastrin stimulation of acid secretion by parietal cells. Clin. Exp. Immunol. 61:315, 1985.
10. Loveridge, N., Bitensky, L., Chayen, J., Hausamen, T. U., Fisher, J. M., Taylor, K. B., Gardner, J. D., Bottazzo, G. F., and Doniach, D. Inhibition of parietal cell function by human gammaglobulin containing gastric parietal cell antibodies. Clin. Exp. Immunol. 41:264, 1980.
11. Hersey, S. J., Miller, M., May, D., and Norris, S. H. Lack of interaction between acid and pepsinogen secretion in isolated gastric glands. Am. J. Physiol. 245:G775, 1983.
12. Gianella, R. A., Broitman, S. A., and Zamcheck, N. Gastric acid barrier to ingested microorganisms in man: studies in vivo and in vitro. Gut 13:251, 1972.
13. Long, J., DeSantis, S., State, D., White, R. A., and Klein, S. R. The effect of antisecretagogues on gastric microflora. Arch. Surg. 118:1413, 1983.
14. Skikne, B. S., Lynch, S. R., and Cook, J. D. Role of gastric acid in food iron absorption. Gastroenterology 81:1068, 1981.
15. Hunt, J. N., and Johnson, C. Relation between gastric secretion of acid and urinary excretion of calcium after oral supplements of calcium. Dig. Dis. Sci. 28:417, 1983.
16. Bo-Linn, G. W., Davis, G. R., Buddrus, D. J., Morawski, S. G., Santa Ana, C., and Fordtran, J. S. An evaluation of the importance of gastric acid secretion in the absorption of dietary calcium. J. Clin. Invest. 73:640, 1984.
17. Forte, J. G., and Lee, H. C. Gastric adenosine triphosphatases: a review of their possible role in HCl secretion. Gastroenterology 73:921, 1977.
18. DiBona, D. R., Ito, S., Berglindh, T., and Sachs, G. Cellular site of gastric acid secretion. Proc. Natl. Acad. Sci., USA 76:6689, 1979.
19. Forte, J. G., Machen, T. E., and Obrink, K. J. Mechanisms of gastric H$^+$ and Cl$^-$ transport. Ann. Rev. Physiol. 42:111, 1980.
20. Fellenius, E., Berglindh, T., Sachs, G., Olbe, L., Elander, B., Sjostrand, S.-E., and Wallmark, B. Substituted benzimidazoles inhibit gastric acid secretion by blocking (H$^+$ + K$^+$)-ATPase. Nature 290:159, 1981.
21. Sachs, G., Berglindh, T., Cuppoletti, J., Fowler, L., Gunther, R. D., Malinowska, D., Rabon, E., Smolka, A. The gastric (H$^+$ + K$^+$)-ATPase. *In* Forte, J. G., Warnoch, D. G., and Rector, F. C., Jr. (eds.). Hydrogen Ion Transport in Epithelia. New York, John Wiley and Sons, 1984, p. 57.
22. Wallmark, B., Jaresten, B.-M., Larsson, H., Ryberg, B., Brandstrom, A., and Fellenius, E. Differentiation among inhibitory actions of omeprazole, cimetidine, and SCN$^-$ on gastric acid secretion. Am. J. Physiol. 245:G64, 1983.
23. Wallmark, B., Larsson, H., and Humble, L. The relationship between gastric acid secretion and gastric H$^+$, K$^+$-ATPase activity. J. Biol. Chem. 260:13681, 1985.

24. Vaziri, N. D., Byrne, C., Ryan, G., and Wilson, A. Preservation of urinary postprandial alkaline tide despite inhibition of gastric acid secretion. Am. J. Gastroenterol. *74*:328, 1980.

25. Aase, S., Dahl, E., Roland, M., and Hars, R. Morphometric studies of parietal cells during basal conditions and during stimulation with pentagastrin in healthy subjects. Scand. J. Gastroenterol. *18*:913, 1983.

26. Sachs, G. The parietal cell as a therapeutic target. Scand. J Gastroenterol. *21*(Suppl. 118):1, 1986.

27. Wallmark, B., Brandstrom, A., and Larsson, H. Evidence for acid-induced transformation of omeprazole into an active inhibitor of (H$^+$ + K$^+$)-ATPase within the parietal cell. Biochim. Biophys. Acta *778*:549, 1984.

28. Olbe, L., Haglund, U., Leth, R., Lind, T., Cederberg, C., Ekenved, G., Elander, E., Lundburg, P., and Wallmark, B. Effects of substituted benzimidazole (H 149/94) on gastric acid secretion in humans. Gastroenterology *83*:193, 1982.

29. Helander, H. F. Parietal cell structure during inhibition of acid secretion. Scand. J. Gastroenterol. *19*(Suppl. 101):21, 1984.

30. Soll, A. H. The actions of secretagogues on oxygen uptake by isolated mammalian parietal cells. J. Clin. Invest. *61*:370, 1978.

31. Soll, A. H., Amirian, D. A., Thomas, L. P., Reedy, T. J., and Elashoff, J. D. Gastrin receptors on isolated canine parietal cells. J. Clin. Invest. *73*:1434, 1984.

32. Barclay, G., Maxwell, V., Grossman, M. I., and Solomon, T. E. Effects of graded amounts of intragastric calcium on acid secretion, gastrin release, and gastric emptying in normal and duodenal ulcer subjects. Dig. Dis. Sci. *28*:385, 1983.

33. Muallem, S., and Sachs, G. Changes in cytosolic free Ca^{2+} in isolated parietal cells. Differential effects of secretagogues. Biochim. Biophys. Acta *805*:181, 1984.

34. Chew, C. S. Cholecystokinin, carbachol, gastrin, histamine, and forskolin increase [Ca^{2+}]$_i$ in gastric glands. Am. J. Physiol. *250*:G814, 1986.

35. Ruiz, M. C., and Michelangeli, F. Stimulation of oxyntic and histaminergic cells in gastric mucosa by gastrin C-terminal tetrapeptide. Am. J. Physiol. *251*:G529, 1986.

36. Tsunoda, Y. Gastrin induces intracellular Ca^{2+} release and acid secretion regulation by the microtubular-microfilamentous system. Biochim. Biophys. Acta *855*:186, 1986.

37. Black, J. A., Forte, T. M., and Forte, J. G. The effects of microfilament disrupting agents on HCl secretion and ultrastructure of piglet gastric oxyntic cells. Gastroenterology *83*:595, 1982.

38. Baudiere, B., Guillon, G., Bali, J.-P., and Jard, S. Muscarinic stimulation of inositol phosphate accumulation and acid secretion in gastric fundic mucosal cells. FEBS Lett. *198*:321, 1986.

39. Chew, C. S. Differential effects of extracellular calcium removal and nonspecific effects of Ca^{2+} antagonists on acid secretory activity in isolated gastric glands. Biochim. Biophys. Acta *846*:370, 1985.

40. Redfern, J. S., Thirlby, R., Feldman, M., and Richardson, C. T. Effect of pentagastrin on gastric mucosal histamine in dogs. Am. J. Physiol. *284*:G369, 1985.

41. Soll, A. H., and Wollin, A. Histamine and cylic AMP in isolated canine parietal cells. Am. J. Physiol. *237*:E444, 1979.

42. Chen, M. C. Y., Soll, A. H., Amirian, D. A., Toomey, M., and Sanders, M. J. Prostanoid inhibition of canine parietal cells: mediation by the inhibitory GTP-binding protein of adenylate cyclase. Gastroenterology, in press.

43. Soll, A. H. Specific inhibition by prostaglandins E$_2$ and I$_2$ of histamine-stimulated [^{14}C]aminopyrine accumulation and cyclic adenosine monophosphate generation by isolated canine parietal cells. J. Clin. Invest. *65*:1222, 1978.

44. Robert, A. Prostaglandins and the gastrointestinal tract. In Johnson, L. R. (ed.). Physiology of the Gastrointestinal Tract. New York, Raven Press, 1981, p. 1407.

45. Feldman, M., and Colturi, T. J. Effect of indomethacin on gastric acid and bicarbonate secretion in humans. Gastroenterology *87*:1339, 1984.

46. Levine, R. A., and Schwartzel, E. H. Effect of indomethacin on basal and histamine stimulated human gastric acid secretion. Gut *25*:718, 1984.

47. Olsen, P. S., Kirkegaard, P., Petersen, B., Lendorf, A., and Christiansen, J. The effect of a synthetic met-enkephalin analog

48. Fave, G. D., Kohn, A., de Magistris, L., Mancuso, M., and Sparvoli, C. Effect of bombesin-stimulated gastrin on gastric acid secretion in man. Life Sci. *27*:993, 1980.

(FK 33-824) on gastric acid secretion and serum gastrin in man. Scand. J. Gastroenterol. *16*:531, 1981.

49. Lenz, H. J., Klapdor, R., Hester, S. E., Webb, V. J., Galyean, R. F., Rivier, J. E., and Brown, M. R. Inhibition of gastric acid secretion by brain peptides in the dog. Role of the autonomic nervous system and gastrin. Gastroenterology *91*:905, 1986.

50. Pappas, T., Hamel, D., Debas, H., Walsh, J. H., and Tache, Y. Cerebroventricular bombesin inhibits gastric acid secretion in dogs. Gastroenterology *89*:43, 1985.

51. Rogers, R. C., and Hermann, G. E. Dorsal medullary oxytocin, vasopressin, oxytocin antagonist, and TRH effects on gastric acid secretion and heart rate. Peptides *6*:1143, 1985.

52. Feldman, M., and Cowley, Y. Effect of an opiate antagonist (naloxone) on the gastric acid secretory response to sham feeding, pentagastrin and histamine in man. Dig. Dis. Sci. *27*:308, 1982.

53. Feldman, M., Moore, L., and Walsh, J. H. Effect of oral nalmefene, an opiate-receptor antagonist, on meal-stimulated gastric acid secretion and serum gastrin concentration in man. Regul. Peptides *11*:245, 1985.

54. Konturek, S. J., Kwiecien, N., Obtulowicz, W., Swierczek, J., Bielanski, W., Oleksy, J., and Coy, D. H. Effect of enkephalin and naloxone on gastric acid and serum gastrin and pancreatic polypeptide concentrations in humans. Gut *24*:740, 1983.

55. Kromer, W., Skowronek, B., Stark, H., and Netz, S. Modulation of acid secretion from enriched guinea pig parietal cells by opioid receptors. Pharmacology *27*:298, 1983.

56. Dalton, M. D., Eisenstein, A. M., Walsh, J. H., and Fordtran, J. S. Effect of secretin on gastric function in normal subjects and in patients with duodenal ulcer. Gastroenterology *71*:24, 1976.

57. Limberg, B., and Kommerell, B. Influence of a continuous intragastric and intravenous infusion of somatostatin on stimulated gastric secretion. Res. Exp. Med. *183*:153, 1983.

58. Christiansen, J., Holst. J. J., and Kalaja, E. Inhibition of gastric acid secretion in man by exogenous and endogenous pancreatic glucagon. Gastroenterology *70*:688, 1976.

59. Maxwell, V., Shulkes, A., Brown, J. C., Solomon, T. E., Walsh, J. H., and Grossman, M. I. Effect of gastric inhibitory polypeptide on pentagastrin-stimulated acid secretion in man. Dig. Dis. Sci. *25*:113, 1980.

60. Olsen, P. S., Pedersen, J. H., Kirkegaard, P., Stadil, F., Fahrenkrug, J., and Christiansen, J. Neurotensin inhibits meal-stimulated gastric acid secretion in man. Scand. J. Gastroenterol. *18*:1073, 1983.

61. Pappas, T., Debas, H. T., Walsh, J. H., Rivier, J., and Tache, Y. Calcitonin gene-related peptide-induced selective inhibition of gastric acid secretion in dogs. Am. J. Physiol. *250*:G127, 1986.

62. Tache, Y., Goto, Y., Gunion, M., Rivier, J., and Debas, H. Inhibition of gastric acid secretion in rats and in dogs by corticotropin-releasing factor. Gastroenterology *86*:281, 1984.

63. Dolva, L. O., Hanssen, K. F., Flaten, O., Skare, S., and Schrumpf, E. Effect of thyrotropin-releasing hormone on gastric acid secretion in man. Scand. J. Gastroenterol. *17*:775, 1982.

64. Adrian, T. E., Savage, A. P., Sagor, G. R., Allen, J. M., Bacarese-Hamilton, A. J., Tatemoto, K., Polak, J. M., and Bloom, S. R. Effect of peptide YY on gastric, pancreatic, and biliary function in humans. Gastroenterology *89*:494, 1985.

65. Valenzuela, J. E., Defilippi, C., Diaz, G., Navia, E., and Merino, Y. Effect of dopamine on human gastric and pancreatic secretion. Gastroenterology *76*:323, 1979.

66. Christiansen, J., Rehfeld, J. F., and Stadil, F. Interaction of calcium and magnesium on gastric acid secretion and serum gastrin concentration in man. Gastroenterology *68*:1140, 1975.

67. Puscas, I., Sturzu, L., and Buzas, G. Effect of ZnSO$_4$ upon gastric acid secretion and carbonic anhydrase. Int. J. Clin. Pharmacol. Therap. Toxicol. *23*:609, 1985.

68. Colturi, T. J., Unger, R. H., and Feldman, M. Role of circulating somatostatin in regulation of gastric acid secretion,

gastrin release, and islet cell function: studies in healthy subjects and duodenal ulcer patients. J. Clin. Invest. *74*:417, 1984.

69. Loud, F. B., Holst, J. J., Egense, E., Petersen, B., and Christiansen, J. Is somatostatin a humoral regulator of the endocrine pancreas and gastric acid secretion in man? Gut *26*:445, 1985.

70. Short, G. M., Doyle, J. W., and Wolfe, M. M. Effect of antibodies to somatostatin on acid secretion and gastrin release by the isolated perfused rat stomach. Gastroenterology, *88*:984, 1985.

71. Chey, W. Y., Kim, M. S., Lee, K. Y., and Chang, T. M. Secretin is an enterogastrone in the dog. Am. J. Physiol. *240*:G239, 1981.

72. Walsh, J. H., Richardson, C. T., and Fordtran, J. S. pH dependence of acid secretion and gastrin release in normal and ulcer subjects. J. Clin. Invest. *55*:462, 1975.

73. Feldman, M., and Walsh, J. H. Acid inhibition of sham feeding-stimulated gastrin release and gastric acid secretion: effect of atropine. Gastroenterology *78*:772, 1980.

74. Schiller, L. R., Walsh, J. H., and Feldman, M. Distention-induced gastrin release and gastric acid secretion: effects of luminal acidification and intravenous atropine. Gastroenterology *78*:912, 1980.

75. Carter, D. C., and Grossman, M. I. Effect of luminal pH on acid secretion from Heidenhain pouches evoked by topical and parenteral stimulants. J. Physiol. *281*:227, 1978.

76. Kirkpatrick, P. M., Jr., and Hirschowitz, B. I. Duodenal ulcer with unexplained marked basal gastric acid hypersecretion. Gastroenterology *79*:4, 1980.

77. Feldman, M., Richardson, C. T., and Fordtran, J. S. Effect of sham feeding on gastric acid secretion in healthy subjects and duodenal ulcer patients: evidence for increased basal vagal tone in some ulcer patients. Gastroenterology *79*:796, 1980.

78. Babbott, F. L., Johnston, J. A., and Haskins, C. H. Gastric acidity in infantile tetany. Arch. Dis. Child. *26*:486, 1923.

79. Donegan, W. L., and Spiro, H. M. Parathyroids and gastric secretion. Gastroenterology *38*:750, 1960.

80. Boyd, E. J. S., Wilson, J. A., Wormsley, K. G., Richards, M. H., and Langman, M. J. S. Effects of a mast cell stabiliser (FPL 52694) on human gastric secretion. Agents Actions *16*:462, 1985.

81. Loewe, C. J., Grider, J. R., Gardiner, J., and Vlahcevic, Z. R. Selective inhibition of pentagastrin- and cholecystokinin-stimulated exocrine secretion by proglumide. Gastroenterology *89*:746, 1985.

82. Rosenfeld, G. C. Pirenzepine (LS519): a weak inhibitor of acid secretion by isolated rat parietal cells. Eur. J. Pharmacol. *86*:99, 1983.

83. Hammer, R., and Giachetti, A. Muscarinic receptor subtypes: M_1 and M_2 biochemical and functional characterization. Life Sci. *31*:2991, 1982.

84. Feldman, M. Inhibition of gastric acid secretion by selective and nonselective anticholinergics. Gastroenterology *86*:361, 1984.

85. Sewing, K.-F., and Hannemann, H. Calcium channel antagonists verapamil and gallopamil are powerful inhibitors of acid secretion in isolated and enriched guinea pig parietal cells. Pharmacology *27*:9, 1983.

86. Sonnenberg, A., Meckel, F., Eckhardt, U., and Scholten, T. The effect of the calcium antagonist verapamil on gastric acid secretion in humans. Hepato-gastroenterology *31*:80, 1984.

87. Levine, R. A., Petokas, S., Starr, A., and Eich, R. H. Effect of verapamil on basal and pentagastrin-stimulated gastric acid secretion. Clin. Pharmacol. Ther. *34*:401, 1983.

88. Aadland, E., and Berstad, A. Effect of verapamil on gastric secretion in man. Scand. J. Gastroenterol. *18*:969, 1983.

89. Feldman, M. Comparison of acid secretion rates measured by gastric aspiration and by in vivo intragastric titration in healthy human subjects. Gastroenterology *76*:954, 1979.

90. Krawiec, J., Odes, H. S., Schwartz, B., and Lamprecht, S. A. Regional difference in ambient intraluminal gastric acidity after cimetidine monitored by intragastric pH-metry. Am. J. Gastroenterol. *78*:272, 1983.

91. Moore, E. W., and Scarlata, R. W. The determination of

92. Fordtran, J. S., and Walsh, J. H. Gastric acid secretion rate and buffer content of the stomach after eating. Results in normal subjects and in patients with duodenal ulcer. J. Clin. Invest. *52*:645, 1973.

93. Malagelada, J.-R., Longstreth, G. F., Summerskill, W. H. J., and Go, V. L. W. Measurement of gastric functions during digestion of ordinary solid meals in man. Gastroenterology *70*:203, 1976.

94. Gross, R. A., Isenberg, J. I., Hogan, D., and Samloff, I. M. Effect of fat on meal-stimulated duodenal acid load, duodenal pepsin load, and serum gastrin in duodenal ulcer and normal subjects. Gastroenterology *75*:357, 1978.

95. Hogan, D. L., Turken, D., Stern, A. I., and Isenberg, J. I. Comparison of the serial dilution indicator and intragastric titration methods for measurement of meal-stimulated gastric acid secretion in man. Dig. Dis. Sci. *28*:1001, 1983.

96. Card, W. I., and Marks, I. N. The relationship between the acid output of the stomach following "maximal" histamine stimulation and the parietal cell mass. Clin. Sci. *19*:147, 1960.

97. Marks, I. N., Komarov, S. A., and Shay, H. Maximal acid secretory response to histamine and its relation to parietal cell mass in the dog. Am. J. Physiol. *199*:579, 1960.

98. Cox, A. J. Stomach size and its relation to chronic peptic ulcer. JAMA *54*:407, 1952.

99. Feldman, M., Richardson, C. T., and Walsh, J. H. Sex-related differences in gastrin release and parietal cell sensitivity to gastrin in healthy human beings. J. Clin. Invest. *71*:751, 1983.

100. Limlomwongse, L., and Piyachaturawat, P. Inhibition of gastric H^+ secretion, K^+-ATPase and K^+-phosphatase by estradiol in vivo and in vitro. Can. J. Physiol. *60*:680, 1982.

101. White, W. D., and Juniper, K. Repeatability of gastric analysis. Dig. Dis. *18*:7–13, 1973.

102. Baron, J. H. Lean body mass, gastric acid, and peptic ulcer. Gut *10*:637, 1969.

103. Christie, D. L., and Ament, M. E. Gastric acid hypersecretion in children with duodenal ulcer. Gastroenterology *71*:242, 1976.

104. Neuburger, P., Lewin, M., Recherche, C., and Bonfils, S. Parietal and chief cell populations in four cases of the Zollinger-Ellison syndrome. Gastroenterology *63*:937, 1972.

105. Bergegardh, S., and Olbe, L. The effect of long-term postoperative pentagastrin infusion on the maximal acid responses to pentagastrin in patients subjected to antrectomy. Scand. J. Gastroenterol. *11*:347, 1976.

106. Johnson, L. R., and Chandler, L. R. RNA and DNA of gastric and duodenal mucosa in antrectomized and gastrin-treated rats. Am. J. Physiol. *274*:937, 1973.

107. Johnson, L. R., and Guthrie, P. D. Proglumide inhibition of trophic action of pentagastrin. Am. J. Physiol. *246*:G62, 1984.

108. Marks, I. N. The effect of prolonged histamine stimulation on the parietal cell population and the secretory function of the guinea-pig stomach. Q. J. Exp. Physiol. *42*:180, 1957.

109. Neely, J. C., and Goldman, L. Effect of calciferol-induced chronic hypercalcemia on the gastric secretion from Heidenhain pouch. Ann. Surg. *155*:406, 1962.

110. Thirlby, R. C., and Feldman, M. Effect of chronic sham feeding on maximal gastric acid secretion in the dog. J. Clin. Invest. *73*:566, 1984.

111. Payne, R. A., and Kay, A. W. The effect of vagotomy on the maximal acid secretory response to histamine in man. Clin. Sci. *22*:373, 1962.

112. Feldman, M., Dickerman, R. M., McClelland, R. N., Cooper, K. A., Walsh, J. H., and Richardson, C. T. Effect of selective proximal vagotomy on food-stimulated gastric acid secretion and gastrin release in patients with duodenal ulcer. Gastroenterology *76*:926, 1979.

113. Melrose, A. G., Russell, R. I., and Dick, A. Gastric mucosal structure and function after vagotomy. Gut *5*:546, 1964.

114. Hakanson, R., Vallgren, S., Ekelund, M., Rehfeld, J. F., and Sundler, F. The vagus exerts trophic control of the stomach in the rat. Gastroenterology *88*:28, 1984.

115. Broome, A. Mechanism of the vagotomy-induced suppression

of the maximal acid response to histamine in antrectomized duodenal ulcer patients. Scand. J. Gastroenterol. 2:275, 1967.

116. Hirschowitz, B. I., and Helman, C. A. Effects of fundic vagotomy and cholinergic replacement on pentagastrin dose responsive gastric acid and pepsin secretion in man. Gut 23:675, 1982.

117. Roland, M., Berstad, A., and Liavag, I. Acid and pepsin secretion in duodenal ulcer patients in response to graded doses of pentagastrin or pentagastrin and carbacholine before and after proximal gastric vagotomy. Scand. J. Gastroenterol. 9:511, 1974.

118. Feldman, M., and Walsh, J. H. Effect of bethanechol on gastric acid secretion and serum gastrin concentration after parietal cell vagotomy. Ann. Surg. 196:14, 1982.

119. Konturek, S. J., Wysocki, A., and Oleksy, J. Effect of medical and surgical vagotomy on gastric response to graded doses of pentagastrin and histamine. Gastroenterology 51:392, 1968.

120. Rowlands, C., Temperley, J. M., and Wyllie, J. H. Pentagastrin-infusion test after atropine or vagotomy. Lancet 2:348, 1969.

121. Leth, R., Elander, B., Fellenius, E., Olbe, L., and Haglund, U. Effects of proximal gastric vagotomy and antrectomy on parietal cell function in humans. Gastroenterology 87:1277, 1984.

122. Moore, J. G., and Wolfe, M. The relation of plasma gastrin to the circadian rhythm of gastric acid secretion in man. Digestion 9:97, 1973.

123. Mittelmann, B., and Wolff, H. G. Emotions and gastroduodenal function. Experimental studies on patients with gastritis, duodenitis and peptic ulcer. Psychosom. Med., 4:5, 1942.

124. Gedde-dahl, D. Radioimmunoassay of gastrin. Fasting serum levels in humans with normal and high gastric acid secretion. Scand. J. Gastroenterol. 9:41, 1974.

125. Trudeau, W. L., and McGuigan, J. E. Relations between serum gastrin levels and rates of gastric hydrochloric acid secretion. N. Engl. J. Med. 284:408, 1971.

126. McArthur, K. E., and Feldman, M. Intragastric temperature, gastric acid secretion, and gastrin release, and gastric emptying following ingestion of hot, warm, or cold coffee in humans. Gastroenterology 90:1540, 1986.

127. Feldman, M., and Nixon, J. V. Effect of exercise on postprandial gastric secretion and emptying in humans. J. Appl. Physiol. 53:851, 1982.

128. Feldman, M., Richardson, C. T., Taylor, I. L., and Walsh, J. H. Effect of atropine on vagal release of gastrin and pancreatic polypeptide. J. Clin. Invest. 63:294, 1979.

129. Schubert, M. L., Saffouri, B., Walsh, J. H., and Makhlouf, G. M. Inhibition of neurally mediated gastrin secretion by bombesin antiserum. Am. J. Physiol. 248:G456, 1985.

130. Knuhtsen, S., Holst, J. J., Knigge, U. Olesen, M., and Nielsen, O. V. Radioimmunoassay, pharmacokinetics, and neuronal release of gastrin-releasing peptide in anesthetized pigs. Gastroenterology 87:372, 1984.

131. Mayer, G., Arnold, R., Feurle, G. Fuchs, K., Ketterer, H., Track, N. S., and Creutzfeldt, W. Influence of feeding and sham feeding on serum gastrin and gastric acid secretion in control subjects and duodenal ulcer patients. Scand. J. Gastroenterol. 9:703, 1974.

132. Knutson, U., Olbe, L., and Ganguli, P. C. Gastric acid and plasma gastrin responses to sham feeding in duodenal ulcer patients before and after resection of antrum and duodenal bulb. Scand. J. Gastroenterol. 9:351, 1974.

133. Forichon, J., Minaire, Y., Vagne, M., Sicallac, P., and Chayvialle, J. A. Effects of proximal vagotomy on gastric secretory and plasma hormonal responses to sham feeding in patients with duodenal ulcers. Hepato-gastroenterology 33:115, 1986.

134. Roland, M., Berstad, A., and Liavag, I. Effect of carbocholine and urecholine on pentagastrin-stimulated gastric secretion in healthy subjects. Scand. J. Gastroenterol. 10:357, 1975.

135. Blair, A. J., Richardson, C. T., Walsh, J. H., and Feldman, M. Effect of parietal cell vagotomy on acid secretory responsiveness to circulating gastrin in humans: relationship to postprandial serum gastrin concentration. Gastroenterology 90:1001, 1986.

136. Feldman, M., and Richardson, C. T. Role of thought, sight, smell, and taste of food in the cephalic phase of gastric acid secretion in man. Gastroenterology 90:428, 1986.

137. Barber, W. D., and Burks, T. F. Brain stem response to phasic gastric distension. Am. J. Physiol. 245:G242, 1983.

138. Grossman, M. I. Stimulation of secretion of acid by distention of denervated fundic pouches in dogs. Gastroenterology 41:385, 1961.

139. Grotzinger, U., Bergegardh, S., and Olbe, L. Effect of atropine and proximal gastric vagotomy on the acid response to fundic distention in man. Gut 18:303, 1977.

140. Bergegardh, S., and Olbe, L. Gastric acid response to antrum distention in man. Scand. J. Gastroenterol. 10:171, 1975.

141. Cooke, A. R. Potentiation of acid output in man by a distention stimulus. Gastroenterology 58:633, 1970.

142. Schoon, I. M., Bergegardh, S., Grotzinger, U., and Olbe, L. Evidence for a defective inhibition of pentagastrin-stimulated gastric acid secretion by antral distention in the duodenal ulcer patient. Gastroenterology 75:363, 1978.

143. Soon-Shiong, P., and Debas, H. T. Pyloro-oxyntic neurohumoral inhibitory reflex of acid secretion. J. Surg. Research 28:198, 1980.

144. Schoon, I.M., and Olbe, L. Inhibitory effect of cimetidine on gastric acid secretion vagally activated by physiological means in duodenal ulcer patients. Gut 19:27, 1978.

145. Peters, M. N., Walsh, J. H., and Feldman, M. Adrenergic regulation of gastrin release in man. Clin. Res. 29:310A, 1981.

146. Richardson, C. T., Walsh, J. H., Hicks, M. I., and Fordtran, J. S. Studies on the mechanisms of food-stimulated gastric acid secretion in normal human subjects. J. Clin. Invest. 58:623, 1976.

147. Miller, L. J., Malagelada, J.-R., Taylor, W. F., and Go, V. L. W. Intestinal control of human postprandial gastric function: the role of components of jejunoileal chyme in regulating gastric secretion and gastric emptying. Gastroenterology 80:763, 1981.

148. Jian, R., Besterman, H. S., Sarson, D. L., Aymes, C., Hostein, J., Bloom, S. R., and Rambaud, J. C. Colonic inhibition of gastric secretion in man. Dig. Dis. Sci. 26:195, 1981.

149. Meyers, W. C., and Jones, R. S. Hyperacidity and hypergastrinemia following extensive intestinal resection. World J. Surg. 3:539, 1979.

150. Taylor, I. L., Byrne, W. J., Christie, D. L., Ament, M. E., and Walsh, J. H. Effect of individual L-amino acids on gastric acid secretion and serum gastrin and pancreatic polypeptide release in humans. Gastroenterology 83:273, 1982.

151. Feldman, M., Walsh, J. H., Wong, H. C., and Richardson, C. T. Role of gastrin hepatadecapeptide in the acid secretory response to amino acids in man. J. Clin. Invest. 61:308, 1978.

152. Lichtenberger, L. M., Graziani, L. A., and Dubinsky, W. P. Importance of dietary amines in meal-induced gastrin release. Am. J. Physiol. 243:G341, 1982.

153. Konturek, S. J., Tasler, J., Obtulowicz, W., and Cieszkowski, M. Comparison of amino acids bathing the oxyntic gland area in the stimulation of gastric secretion. Gastroenterology 70:66, 1976.

154. Vagne, M., and Mutt, V. Entero-oxyntin: a stimulant of gastric acid secretion extracted from porcine intestine. Scand. J. Gastroenterol. 15:17, 1980.

155. Isenberg, J. I., and Maxwell, V. Intravenous infusion of amino acids stimulates gastric acid secretion in man. N. Engl. J. Med. 298:27, 1978.

156. MacGregor, I. L., Deveney, C., Way, L. W., and Meyer, J. H. The effect of acute hyperglycemia on meal-stimulated gastric, biliary, and pancreatic secretion, and serum gastrin. Gastroenterology 70:197, 1976.

157. Moore, J. G., and Crespin, F. Influence of glucose on cephalic-vagal-stimulated gastric acid secretion in man. Dig. Dis. Sci. 25:117, 1980.

158. Christiansen, J., Bech, A., Fahrenkrug, J., Holst, J. J., Lauritsen, K., Moody, A. J., and Schaffalitzky de Muckadell, O. Fat-induced jejunal inhibition of gastric acid secretion and release of pancreatic glucagon, enteroglucagon, gastric inhibitory polypeptide, and vasoactive intestinal polypeptide in man. Scand. J. Gastroenterol. 14:161, 1979.

159. Varner, A. A., Isenberg, J. I., Elashoff, J. D., Lamers, C. B.

H. W., Maxwell, V., and Shulkes, A. A. Effect of intravenous lipid on gastric acid secretion by intravenous amino acids. Gastroenterology 79:873, 1980.

160. Kihl, B., and Olbe, L. Fat inhibition of gastric acid secretion in duodenal ulcer patients before and after proximal gastric vagotomy. Gut 21:1056, 1980.

161. Loud, F. B., Christiansen, J., Holst, J. J., Petersen, B., and Kirkegaard, P. Effect of endogenous pancreatic glucagon on gastric acid secretion in patients with duodenal ulcer before and after parietal cell vagotomy. Gut 22:359, 1981.

162. Pappas, T. N., Debas, H. T., and Taylor, I. L. Enterogastrone-like effect of peptide YY is vagally mediated in the dog. J. Clin. Invest. 77:49, 1986.

163. McArthur, K., Hogan, D., and Isenberg, J. I. Relative stimulatory effects of commonly ingested beverages on gastric acid secretion in humans. Gastroenterology 83:199, 1982.

164. Peterson, W. L., Barnett, C. C., and Walsh, J. H. Effect of intragastric infusion of ethanol and wine on serum gastrin concentration and gastric acid secretion. Gastroenterology 91:1390, 1986.

165. Feldman, E. J., Isenberg, J. I., and Grossman, M. I. Gastric acid and gastrin response to decaffeinated coffee and a peptone meal. JAMA 246:248, 1981.

166. Feldman, M., and Richardson, C. T. Total 24-hour gastric acid secretion in patients with duodenal ulcer: comparison with normal subjects and effects of cimetidine and parietal cell vagotomy. Gastroenterology 90:540, 1986.

167. Harty, R. F., and Franklin, P. A. GABA affects the release of gastrin and somatostatin from rat antral mucosa. Nature 303:623, 1983.

168. Hirschowitz, B. I., Ou Tim, L., Helman, C. A., and Molina, E. Bombesin and G-17 dose response in duodenal ulcer and controls. Dig. Dis. Sci. 30:1092, 1985.

169. Lichtenberger, L. M., Nelson, A. A., and Graziani, L. A. Amine trapping: physical explanation for the inhibitory effect of gastric acidity on the postprandial release of gastrin. Studies on rats and dogs. Gastroenterology 90:1223, 1986.

170. Befrits, R., Samuelsson, K., and Johansson, C. Gastric acid inhibition by antral acidification mediated by endogenous prostaglandins. Scand. J. Gastroenterol. 19:899, 1984.

171. Levine, J. S., Nakane, P. K., and Allen, R. H. Immunocytochemical localization of human intrinsic factor: the nonstimulated stomach. Gastroenterology 79:493, 1980.

172. Donaldson, R. M. Intrinsic factor and the transport of cobalamin. In Johnson, L. R. (ed.). Physiology of the Gastrointestinal Tract. New York, Raven Press, 1981, p. 641.

173. Herzlich, B., and Herbert, V. Rapid collection of human intrinsic factor uncontaminated with cobalophilin (R binder). Am. J. Gastroenterol. 81:678, 1986.

174. Gueant, J. L., Djalali, M., Aouadj, R., Gaucher, P., Monin, B., and Nicolas, J. P. In vitro and in vivo evidences that the malabsorption of cobalamin is related to its binding on haptocorrin (R binder) in chronic pancreatitis. Am. J. Clin. Nutr. 44:265, 1986.

175. Seetharam, B., Jimenez, M., and Alpers, D. H. Effect of bile and bile acids on binding of intrinsic factor to cobalamin and intrinsic factor–cobalamin complex to ileal receptor. Am. J. Physiol. 245:G72, 1983.

176. Kanazawa, S., and Herbert, V. Mechanism of enterohepatic circulation of vitamin B_{12}: movement of vitamin B_{12} from bile R-binder to intrinsic factor due to the action of pancreatic trypsin. Trans. Assoc. Am. Physicians 96:336, 1983.

177. Nicolas, J.-P., Jimenez, M., Marcoullis, G., and Parmentier, Y. In vivo evidence that intrinsic factor-cobalamin complex traverses the human intestine intact. Biochim. Biophys. Acta 675:328, 1981.

178. Marcoullis, G., Parmentier, Y., Nicolas, J.-P., Jimenez, M., and Gerard, P. Cobalamin malabsorption due to nondegradation of R proteins in the human intestine. J. Clin. Invest. 66:430, 1980.

179. Kittang, E., Aadland, E., and Schjonsby, H. Effect of omeprazole on the secretion of intrinsic factor, gastric acid and pepsin in man. Gut 26:594, 1985.

180. Binder, H. J., and Donaldson, R. M. Effect of cimetidine on

181. Carmel, R. Gastric juice in congenital pernicious anemia contains no immunoreactive intrinsic factor molecule: study of three kindreds with variable ages at presentation, including a patient first diagnosed in adulthood. Am. J. Hum. Genet. 35:67, 1983.

182. Meeroff, J. C., Zagalsky, D., and Meeroff, M. Intrinsic factor deficiency in adults with normal hydrochloric acid production. Gastroenterology 80:575, 1981.

183. Yang, Y., Ducos, R., Rosenberg, A. J., Catrou, P. G., Levine, J. S., Podell, E. R., and Allen, R. H. Cobalamin malabsorption in three siblings due to an abnormal intrinsic factor that is markedly susceptible to acid and proteolysis. J. Clin. Invest. 76:2057, 1985.

184. Levine, J. S., and Allen, R. H. Intrinsic factor within parietal cells of patients with juvenile pernicious anemia. A retrospective immunohistochemical study. Gastroenterology 88:1132, 1985.

185. Brandsborg, M., Elsborg, L., Anderson, D., Brandsborg, O., and Bastrup-Madsen, P. Gastrin concentrations in serum and gastric mucosa in patients with pernicious anemia. Scand. J. Gastroenterol. 12:537, 1977.

186. Bins, M., Burgers, P. I. C. J., Selbach, S. G. M., van Wettum, Th.B., Lamers, C. B. H. W., and van Tongeren, J. H. M. The relation between basal gastric pH and serum gastrin. Digestion 23:271, 1982.

187. Foltmann, B. Pepsin, chymosin and their zymogens. In Desnuelle, P., Sjostrom, H., and Noren, O. (eds.). Molecular and Cellular Basis of Digestion. New York, Elsevier Science Publishers, 1986, p. 491.

188. Samloff, I. M., Pepsinogens I and II: Purification from gastric mucosa and radioimmunoassay in serum. Gastroenterology 82:26, 1982.

189. Zelle, B., van Kessel, A. G., de Wit, J., Evers, P., Arwert, F., Pronk, J. C., Mager, W. H., Planta, R. J., Eriksson, A. W., and Frants, R. R. Assignment of human pepsinogen A locus to the q12-pter region of chromosome 11. Hum. Genet. 70:337, 1985.

190. Taggart, R. T., Mohandas, T. K., Shows, T. B., and Bell, G. I. Variable numbers of pepsinogen genes are located in the centromeric region of human chromosome 11 and determine the high-frequency electrophoretic polymorphism. Proc. Natl. Acad. Sci. USA 82:6240, 1985.

191. Kageyama, T., and Takahashi, K. The complete amino acid sequence of monkey pepsinogen A. J. Biol. Chem. 261:4395, 1986.

192. Hirsch-Marien, H., Louisillier, F., Touboul, J. P., and Burtin, P. Immunochemical study and cellular localization of human pepsinogens during ontogenesis and in gastric cancers. Lab. Invest. 34:623, 1976.

193. Samloff, I. M., Secrist, D. M., and Passaro, E. A study of the relationship between serum group I pepsinogen levels and gastric acid secretion. Gastroenterology 69:1196, 1975.

194. Sanders, M.J., Amirian, D.A., Ayalon, A., and Soll, A. H. Regulation of pepsinogen release from canine chief cells in primary monolayer culture. Am. J. Physiol. 245:G641, 1983.

195. Norris, S. H., and Hersey, S. J. pH dependence of pepsinogen and acid secretion in isolated gastric glands. Am. J. Physiol. 245:G730, 1983.

196. Raufman, J.-P., Kasbekar, D. K., Jensen, R. T., and Gardner, J. D. Potentiation of pepsinogen secretion from dispersed glands from rat stomach. Am. J. Physiol. 245:G525, 1983.

197. Kasbekar, D. K., Jensen, R. T., and Gardner, J. D. Pepsinogen secretion from dispersed glands from rabbit stomach. Am. J. Physiol. 244:G392, 1983.

198. Hersey, S. J., May, D., and Schyberg, D. Stimulation of pepsinogen release from isolated gastric glands by cholecystokininlike peptides. Am. J. Physiol. 244:G192, 1983.

199. Raufman, J.-P., Sutliff, V. E., Kasbekar, D. K., Jensen, R. T., and Gardner, J. D. Pepsinogen secretion from dispersed chief cells from guinea pig stomach. Am. J. Physiol. 247:G95, 1984.

200. Berger, S., and Rauffman, J.-P. Prostaglandin-induced pepsi-

nogen secretion from dispersed gastric glands from guinea pig stomach. Am. J. Physiol. *249*:G592, 1985.

201. Norris, S. H., and Hersey, S. J. Stimulation of pepsinogen secretion in permeable isolated gastric glands. Am. J. Physiol. *249*:G408, 1985.

202. Sutliff, V. E., Raufman, J.-P., Jensen, R. T., and Gardner, J. D. Actions of vasoactive intestinal peptide and secretin on chief cells prepared from guinea pig stomach. Am. J. Physiol. *251*:G96, 1986.

203. Hirschowitz, B. I. Pepsinogen. Postgrad. Med. J. *60*:743, 1984.

204. Szafran, Z., Szafran, H., Popiela, T., and Trompeter, G. Coupled secretion of gastric lipase and pepsin in man following pentagastrin stimulation. Digestion *18*:310, 1978.

205. Fink, C. S., Hamosh, M., Hamosh, P., DeNigris, S. J., and Kasbekar, D. K. Lipase secretion from dispersed rabbit gastric glands. Am. J. Physiol. *248*:G68, 1985.

206. Bell, A. E., Sellers, L. A., Allen, A., Cunliffe, W. J., Morris, E. R., and Ross-Murphy, S. B. Properties of gastric and duodenal mucus: effect of proteolysis, disulfide reduction, bile, acid, ethanol, and hypertonicity on mucus gel structure. Gastroenterology *88*:269, 1985.

207. Williams, S. E., and Turnberg, L. A. Retardation of acid diffusion by pig gastric mucus: a potential role in mucosal protection. Gastroenterology *79*:299, 1980.

208. Pfeiffer, C. J. Experimental analysis of hydrogen ion diffusion in gastrointestinal mucus glycoprotein. Am. J. Physiol. *240*:G176, 1981.

209. Allen, A., and Garner, A. Mucus and bicarbonate secretion in the stomach and their possible role in mcosal protection. Gut *21*:249, 1980.

210. Bickel, M., and Kauffman, G. L. Gastric gel mucus thickness: effect of distention, 16,16-dimethyl prostaglandin E$_2$, and carbenoxolone. Gastroenterology *80*:770, 1981.

211. Kerss, S., Allen, A., and Garner, A. A simple method for measuring thickness of the mucus gel layer adherent to rat, frog and human gastric mucosa: influence of feeding, prostaglandin, N-acetylcysteine and other agents. Clin. Sci. *63*:187, 1982.

212. Johansson, C., and Kollberg, B. Stimulation by intragastrically administered E$_2$ prostaglandins of human gastric mucus output. Eur. J. Clin. Invest. *9*:229, 1979.

213. O'Brien, P., Rosen, S., Trencis-Buck, L., and Silen, W. Distribution of carbonic anhydrase within the gastric mucosa. Gastroenterology *72*:870, 1977.

214. Forssell, H., Stenquist, B., and Olbe, L. Vagal stimulation of human gastric bicarbonate secretion. Gastroenterology *89*:581, 1985.

215. Guslandi, M. Alkali secretion by the human stomach: effect of H$_2$ blockers. Am. J. Physiol. 248:G649, 1985.

216. Feldman, M. Gastric bicarbonate secretion in humans. Effect of pentagastrin, bethanechol, and 11,16,16-trimethyl prostaglandin E$_2$. J. Clin. Invest. *72*:295, 1983.

217. Flemstrom, G. Gastric secretion of bicarbonate. *In* Johnson, L. R. (ed..). Physiology of the Gastrointestinal Tract. New York, Raven Press, 1981, p. 603.

218. Forte, J. G. Three components of Cl$^-$ flux across the isolated bullfrog gastric mucosa. Am. J. Physiol. *216*:167, 1969.

219. Feldman, M. Gastric H$^+$ and HCO$_3^-$ secretion in response to sham feeding in humans. Am. J. Physiol. *248*:G188, 1985.

220. Feldman, M., Unger, R. H., and Walsh, J. H. Effect of atropine on plasma gastrin and somatostatin concentrations during sham feeding in man. Regul. Peptides *12*:345, 1985.

221. Feldman, M., and Schiller, L. Effect of bethanechol (urecholine) on gastric acid and nonparietal secretion in normal subjects and duodenal ulcer patients. Comparison with atropine, pentagastrin, and histamine. Gastroenterology *83*:262, 1982.

222. Heylings, J. R., and Feldman, M. Stimulation of HCO$_3^-$ secretion by the prostaglandin E$_2$ analog enprostil: studies in human stomach and rat duodenum. Prostaglandins *32*:907, 1986.

223. Flemstrom, G., Heylings, J. R., and Garner, A. Gastric and duodenal HCO$_3^-$ transport in vitro: effects of hormones and local transmitters. Am. J. Physiol. *242*:G100, 1982.

224. Feldman, M., and Barnett, C. C. Gastric bicarbonate secretion in patients with duodenal ulcer. Gastroenterology *88*:1205, 1985.

225. Mulvihill, S. J., Pappas, T. N., and Debas, H. T. Effect of increased intracranial pressure on gastric acid secretion. Am. J. Surg. *151*:110, 1986.

226. Larson, G. M., Koch, S., O'Dorisio, T. M., Osadchey, B., McGraw, P., and Richardson, J. D. Gastric response to severe head injury. Am. J. Surg. *147*:97, 1984.

227. Vanzant, F. R., Alvarez, W. C., Eusterman, G. B., Dunn, H. L., and Berkson, J. The normal range of gastric acidity from youth to old age. Arch. Intern. Med. *49*:345, 1932.

228. Krasinski, S. D., Russell, R. M., Samloff, I. M., Jacob, R. A., Dallal, G. E., McGandy, R. B., and Hartz, S. C. Fundic atrophic gastritis in an elderly population. Effects on hemoglobin and several serum nutritional indicators. J. Am. Geriatr. Soc. *34*:800, 1986.

229. Krejs, G. J., Orci, L., Conlon, J. M., Ravazzola, M., Davis, G. R., Raskin, P., Collins, S. M., McCarthy, D. M., Baetens, D., Rubenstein, A., Aldor, T. A. M., and Unger, R. H. Somatostatinoma syndrome. Biochemical, morphologic and clinical features. N. Engl. J. Med. *301*:285, 1979.

230. Guslandi, M., and Ballarin, E. Assessment of the "mucusbicarbonate" barrier in the stomach of patients with chronic gastric disorders. Clin. Chim. Acta *144*:133, 1984.

42

Diverticula, Rupture, and Volvulus

STEVEN B. RAFFIN

GASTRIC DIVERTICULA

As contrasted with the spectrum of disease emanating from colonic diverticulosis, the solitary gastric diverticulum barely warrants consideration. It is a rare radiographic discovery, with an incidence ranging from 0.03 to 0.1 per cent of upper gastrointestinal series, 0.03 to 0.30 per cent of endoscopic studies, and 0.01 to 0.11 per cent of autopsies.[1–3] First described by Baille in 1793,[4] gastric diverticula have now been reported in well over 500 patients.[5] Most are discovered in persons between the fourth and sixth decades of life, with equal sexual and racial prevalence.[6]

The Latin word *diverticulum*, meaning bypath, is descriptive of the gross anatomy. Seventy-six per cent of gastric diverticula occur high on the posterior wall of the stomach, approximately 2 cm below the esophagogastric junction and 3 cm from the lesser curvature. These pouches are almost never associated with peptic, granulomatous, or neoplastic processes[1, 5–7] and are presumed to be "congenital." Fifteen per cent of diverticula are prepyloric and are usually the result of antecedent peptic, granulomatous, or neoplastic disease or surgery; these pouches are categorized as being "acquired."[8] The remaining 8 to 10 per cent of pouches are located along the intervening mucosa.[2, 9]

A smoldering controversy exists in the literature as to the nomenclature of gastric diverticula. The original dichotomy states that "true," congenital or juxtacardiac, diverticula contain all layers of the stomach, whereas "false," acquired or juxtapyloric, diverticula contain only mucosa.[1, 6] Confusing this definition, a recent study reporting seven cases of juxtacardiac diverticula found that none had an outer muscular coat, and hence all would be labeled false despite their classic locations and lack of association with either intra- or perigastric inflammation.[5] It seems reasonable to conclude that the hoary classification of these rare pouches perpetuates misconceptions and that notation of location plus the presence or absence of associated pathologic processes serves the clinician best.[1, 5, 10]

Pathogenesis

The pathophysiology of the acquired juxtapyloric or traction diverticulum is obvious. The pouch develops from the addition of abnormal stresses to the gastric wall from *surgery, neoplasm, healing ulcer*, or *periantral inflammation*.[8] Differentiation from ulcer or malignancy may be very difficult without endoscopic visualization, cytology, and biopsy.[10]

The juxtacardiac diverticulum has been thought to arise from a weakness or pressure change high on the posterior gastric wall.[1, 2] A new hypothesis, however, suggests that these uncommon pouches develop from traction by Grassi's nerve during embryologic rotation of the stomach.[11]

Diagnosis

All positive defects of the barium-filled stomach must be diagnosed. The juxtapyloric pouch is more difficult to distinguish from a peptic or malignant process than is the juxtacardiac diverticulum. The criteria for diagnosis of the former are a pliable contour on multiple spot films and the presence of grossly normal mucosa on endoscopy. The latter has a characteristic radiographic appearance of a solitary pouch, 2 to 4 cm in diameter, with a smooth, rounded, pliable contour on barium study (Fig. 42–1).[1, 6] Both X-ray and endoscopy may reveal rugal folds entering the pouch through a narrow neck.[1] The gastroscopic view of the mouth of a juxtacardiac diverticulum is usually diagnostic (i.e., a small round stoma with sharp margins that may change size in synchrony with peristalsis). The histology of such a diverticulum obtained at surgery in symptomatic patients always shows some chronic inflammatory change.[5]

Atypical gastric diverticula are extremely unusual and find their way into case reports.[2, 9] In fact the tenth greater curvature diverticulum was described as a radiologic curiosity; it contained all layers of the normal stomach wall.[2] Other reports emphasize the value of compression films in the upper gastrointestinal series to demonstrate a pliable wall in the rare case of partial or intramural antral diverticula.[9] Additional radiologic criteria useful for differentiating intramural diverticula from an aberrant pancreas or antral leiomyoma include demonstrating an intramural rounded outpouching of barium with smooth margins, a typical location along the greater curvature of the antrum, a maximum size of approximately 10 mm, and a smooth ostium without evidence of mass or edema in the surrounding gastric mucosa.[12] Careful radiographic technique is required for both small and large pouches. A giant 10-cm diverticulum was missed totally during a barium study until the examiner positioned the patient so that the small stoma was dependent.[7] Finally, one report de-

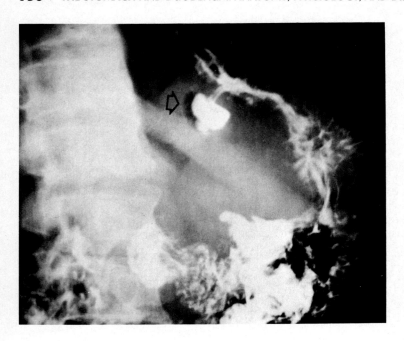

Figure 42–1. This solitary juxtacardiac gastric diverticulum *(arrow)* is easily seen on upper gastrointestinal series.

scribed a 3-cm fundal diverticulum simulating an adrenal mass on abdominal CT scan.[13]

Clinical Picture

The clinical importance of gastric diverticula has been a controversial subject for years, because more than 50 per cent of patients are asymptomatic.[1, 8] Typical ulcer-like pain or vomiting is rare in some reports[6] but common in others.[5] One study concluded that this lesion was a "potent source" of "entirely nonspecific" symptoms such as vague high abdominal pressure or fullness usually precipitated by a meal, with postprandial relief upon lying down.[14] Other reports describe exactly the opposite picture, with pain in the fasting state and upon lying down and relief with meals.[1, 5] The larger lesions with mucosal inflammation most probably account for this spectrum of complex, nonspecific dyspepsia. Based solely on history and physical examination, clinical differentiation of a juxtacardiac gastric diverticulum from an atypical peptic ulcer, pancreaticobiliary disease, or even functional complaints may be difficult.

Complications and associations of gastric diverticula are few in number. Unanticipated hemorrhage and perforation are the two catastrophic events that rarely occur.[1, 6, 15, 16] There is no obvious tendency toward carcinogenesis in these pouches, but occasionally incidental mucosal or submucosal tumors may be found inside, with aberrant pancreas heading the list. Finally, there is no correlation between gastric diverticula and other gastrointestinal diseases, including small and large bowel diverticula.[6]

Treatment

Treatment of a very rare lesion that is predominantly asymptomatic and that has few complications is impos-

sible to evaluate statistically. Medical therapy encompasses such diverse maneuvers as postural drainage, bland diet, antacids, and water-induced emesis. It is usually unsuccessful in affording more than temporary relief.[1, 5] Many physicians claim total relief of dyspeptic upper abdominal pain with surgical ablation of the pouch.[5, 7, 14] Surgical therapy may be aided by intraoperative gastroscopy to facilitate localization of fundal diverticula.[17] The clinician must be concerned, however, about the false positive effects of sham surgery in a patient with nonspecific gastrointestinal complaints.[18]

GASTRIC RUPTURE

A very rare, devastating, and poorly understood catastrophe involving the upper gut is *rupture* of the stomach,[19] which by definition excludes those cases associated with penetrating abdominal wounds or those resulting from involvement of the stomach by adjacent inflammatory processes or by ulcer or carcinoma. These obvious causes will not be discussed further; rather, spontaneous gastric perforation and rupture following blunt abdominal trauma will be examined.

Etiology

Traumatic. Up to the late 1930s, approximately 800 cases of abdominal contusion had been reported, with only 60 or so cases of rupture of the stomach.[19] A series of 200 nonpenetrating abdominal injuries contained only two cases of gastric rupture, but damage to liver, spleen, and bowel was frequent.[20] Today, motor vehicle accidents remain the most frequent cause of traumatic gastric rupture. A review of 52 cases of *gastric rupture* following blunt abdominal trauma in the English-language literature since 1930 serves to re-emphasize the rarity of this phenomenon.[21] The explanation for this apparent sparing of the stomach lies in an understanding of its anatomic position. It is well protected, lying snugly against the spine, and is partially covered by ribs, diaphragm, lung, liver, and transverse colon.[19, 22] It is also very mobile and tolerates distortion well, requiring more than 4 liters of fluid in its lumen before rupturing.[23, 24] Finally, the cardio-esophageal junction and pylorus act as escape valves for excessive gastric contents.[22, 25, 26] Further attesting to the resistance of the stomach to rupture from blunt trauma, an early investigator "directed a blow with a knobbed stick against the abdominal wall . . . but never produced rupture; . . . [and] filled the stomachs of animals and then struck them over this area with a club . . . but [produced] no complete rupture."[27] Hence the stomach appears to be the least vulnerable of the abdominal viscera to blunt trauma.

On the other hand, the gastric lumen is one of the most accessible areas of the gut to direct visualization and subsequent internal contusion. Iatrogenic perforation during fiberoptic endoscopy has been evaluated. Perforation of the esophagus or stomach occurs in 0.33 to 1 case per 1000 endoscopic procedures. Perforation of the stomach constitutes more than one half of all perforations.[28] Rarely, pneumoperitoneum may follow endoscopy without evidence of perforation. This event is benign, resolving spontaneously with nasogastric suction. Air dissecting along intramural vessels into the peritoneal cavity is the postulated mechanism, as no rents in the gastric wall are found at laparotomy.[29] Finally, gastric rupture has occurred during external cardiac compression immediately following upper gastrointestinal endoscopy complicated by cardiac arrest.[30] In this uncommon setting, prompt decompression of the distended stomach with a gastric tube following endotracheal intubation might prevent this catastrophe.

Nontraumatic. Nontraumatic, *spontaneous gastric perforation* was first described in 1845 by Carson,[31] 16 years after Cruveilhier showed that prior reported perforations were the result of peptic disease.[22] Spontaneous perforation, exclusive of the newborn period, is more common in females in the fifth decade,[22] in contrast to a peak incidence of young males sustaining rupture following blunt trauma.[19]

Several conceptual notions help explain the pathogenesis in most of the reported cases. The "magenstrasse" is firmly bound by the gastrohepatic ligament[22, 31] and is less distensible than the greater curvature, which is composed of pliable rugal folds. Seventy-three per cent of spontaneous ruptures in cases of gastric overdistention in adults occur on the lesser curvature.[22, 26, 32] In contrast, the few reported cases of gastric rupture following vomiting have occurred along the proximal greater curvature.[33]

Other factors contributing to nontraumatic gastric rupture include barium administration during upper gastrointestinal radiography,[34] cardiopulmonary resuscitation,[35, 36] nasal oxygen administration,[32] labor,[37] the postpartum period,[38] and anorexia nervosa.[39] One report[40] described the fifth case of spontaneous gastric

rupture ascribed to sodium bicarbonate ingestion. A healthy 31-year-old man used only one-half teaspoon of baking soda in one-half glass of water to treat dyspepsia after drinking margueritas and eating a spicy Mexican dinner. The patient suffered severe pain and collapse within several minutes and, at laparotomy, displayed a 5-cm linear lesser curvature tear. Fordtran and colleagues[41] have demonstrated experimentally that only small amounts of carbon dioxide (208 ml) might have been produced in the foregoing clinical setting. However, these authors warn that large amounts of gas could be generated with doses larger than one half of a level teaspoon of baking soda.

A patient with an inguinal hernia containing a ptotic stomach suffered fatal gastric rupture and serves well to summarize the pathophysiology of spontaneous gastric perforation.[25] The prerequisite anatomy was present in this patient, including obstruction of the distal stomach in the hernia sac and distention of the stomach with air and beer. The additional stress of periodic increases in abdominal pressure brought about by repeated attempts at vomiting completed the necessary sequence of events.

Clinical Picture and Treatment

The diagnosis of spontaneous gastric rupture must be considered in a setting of *abdominal distention, shock*, diffuse *peritoneal irritation*, gastrointestinal *hemorrhage*, and *cervical subcutaneous emphysema*.[19, 22] High serum amylase values may be confusing, pointing toward the false diagnosis of acute pancreatitis.[26] Some physicians suggest that a trocar be passed into the abdomen to relieve the taut distention.[22] Laparotomy and repair of the rent must follow swiftly if the patient is to survive. Unfortunately, this diagnosis is rarely made before operation or autopsy.[26] Mortality had been reported to range from 40 to 70 per cent; however, the most recent review of the literature since 1930 reports a figure of 11 per cent.[21]

GASTRIC VOLVULUS

Gastric volvulus is an uncommon, acquired twist of the stomach upon itself. Torsion of one part of the upper gut around another without vascular compromise may be asymptomatic. On the other hand, patient complaints may range from a mild dragging in the epigastrium with bloating and early satiety to intense upper abdominal pain and shock. The subtleties of the former and the urgency of the latter presentation must be kept in mind if this purely structural lesion is to be diagnosed and repaired.

Gastric volvulus was first recognized by Berti in 1886[42] during a postmortem examination. Since that inauspicious description, volvulus has been reported in about 325 adults and is more than a mere medical curiosity.[43, 44] Males are involved as frequently as females, and the peak incidence occurs during the fifth decade of life.[44]

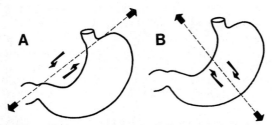

Figure 42–2. Types of gastric volvulus. The dashed line represents the axis about which the stomach twists. *A*, Organoaxial volvulus; *B*, mesenteroaxial volvulus. (Modified from Wastell, C., and Ellis, H. Br. J. Surg. *58*:557, 1971.)

Types of Volvulus

The anatomic classification of gastric volvulus is superficially straightforward, but much confusion arises from attempts at its clinical application. Basically three types of volvulus exist.[45] The *organoaxial* volvulus occurs when the stomach twists along its long axis, the cardiopyloric line, in a manner analogous to the wringing out of a wet rag (Fig. 42–2*A*). The fixed cardioesophageal junction and second part of the duodenum act as anchor points, creating a closed loop obstruction. This type of volvulus often presents acutely and has been documented to be the most common type.[43, 46] It is classically seen as the "upside-down stomach" in the patient with a large paraesophageal hiatus hernia.[47] The twist in *mesenteroaxial* volvulus occurs along an imaginary line from the middle of the lesser curvature to the middle of the greater curvature (Fig. 42–2*B*), and is at approximately right angles to the cardiopyloric axis of the organoaxial volvulus. The consensus is that this type is least common and usually causes chronic or intermittent abdominal symptoms.[43, 46] In addition, the cardioesophageal junction usually is incompletely obstructed and often allows passage of a nasogastric tube.[43] It is possible that the third type, or *mixed* gastric volvulus, is the most frequent form and is the source for the confusion over incidence statistics. Further discussion will deal with the clinically important recognition of acute and chronic situations resulting from obstruction or ischemia and lesser degrees of torsion, respectively.

Pathogenesis

The pathophysiology is not obscure. The normal stomach is well restrained by the retroperitoneal duodenum and by the gastrosplenic, gastrocolic, and gastrohepatic ligaments.[48, 49] According to cadaver studies, the stomach cannot be rotated 180 degrees unless one of these fibrous attachments is severed. If displaced with intact ligaments, the stomach will glide back into its anatomic position. Hence, *in vivo*, ligamentous laxity is the major factor permitting volvulus to occur. Rarely, supernumerary ligaments in the form of adhesions to the peritoneum or adjacent viscera will provoke abnormal torsion of the stomach.[47] Extrinsic pressure from enlarged adjoining organs or masses, or

intrinsic tumor, may distort the normal anatomy and allow the stomach to twist. Abnormally active peristalsis after a heavy meal and a low insertion of the esophagus have also been incriminated in the pathogenesis of gastric volvulus.[49]

A major pathophysiologic event incriminated in volvulus formation is the pushing or drawing of the twisted stomach into coelomic extensions, either as a paraesophageal hiatus hernia or as a hernia associated with eventration of the diaphragm.[47] For example, the presence of a paraesophageal hiatus hernia draws up the dependent greater curvature via push from organs below and negative pressure in the thoracic hernia pouch. In addition, any condition that causes elevation of the left diaphragm such as phrenic nerve paralysis or left lung resection facilitates the development of gastric volvulus.[43]

Clinical Picture

Acute volvulus, usually organoaxial, with either luminal obstruction or vascular strangulation of the stomach is a dramatic clinical event, because the patient often presents in frank shock.[43, 44, 46] A clinical triad was set forth in 1904[50] describing this acute abdominal catastrophe: (1) *violent retching* with production of little vomitus, (2) *constant, severe epigastric pain*, and (3) great *difficulty* in *advancing a nasogastric tube* past the distal esophagus. The upper abdomen may be greatly distended, with the lower quadrants retaining surprisingly soft and flat contours.[49] Rarely hematemesis may accompany mucosal ischemic necrosis resulting from gastric volvulus.[51] Reported mortality figures have ranged from 42 to 56 per cent[44]; however, recent aggressive therapy has reduced mortality rate to 16 per cent.[43, 46]

In contrast, *chronic volvulus* or *torsion* may go undetected for years, the major symptoms being low-grade pain, bloating, eructation, and pyrosis.[48, 52] Postcibal borborygmi may result from chyme passing through the entrapped gas and may be quite embarrassing at the dinner table. Patients with diaphragmatic defects may even complain of breathlessness,[47] whereas others with mild torsion may be totally asymptomatic. Without radiologic assistance the clinician may not be able to distinguish the syndrome of chronic or intermittent torsion from chronic gallbladder disease, peptic ulcer, "gastritis," or functional complaints.[47] A case of asymptomatic, intrathoracic organoaxial volvulus causing a subacute cholestatic syndrome has been reported. The common bile duct was compressed by the diaphragm as it stretched from liver to displaced duodenum.[53] Mortality in chronic volvulus has been reported to vary from 0 to 13 per cent.[44, 46]

Diagnosis

An elderly patient with known paraesophageal hiatus hernia and protracted vomiting should bring to mind the consideration of gastric volvulus.[54] Definitive di-

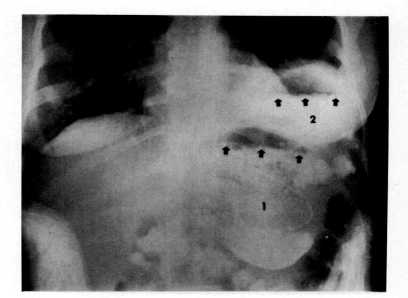

Figure 42–3. Mesenteroaxial volvulus in a patient with eventration of the diaphragm. Two air-fluid levels *(arrows)* are seen in this upright plain film of the abdomen. Numbers 1 and 2 indicate proximal and distal stomach, respectively.

agnosis resides with the radiologist. An erect film of the abdomen may rarely show two air-fluid levels in the left upper quadrant and hence be diagnostic of mesenteroaxial volvulus (Fig. 42–3).[49] The barium examination shows a tapering of the distal esophagus in acute strangulation. Actual visualization of the twisted viscus in intermittent or partially obstructed cases is also diagnostic of this condition (Fig. 42–4).[48] The

physician must be suspicious of intermittent torsion when, in a symptom-free interval, the barium examination shows only a paraesophageal hernia or eventration of the diaphragm. Fiberoptic endoscopy plays a small role in the diagnosis of acute organoaxial volvulus because the twist precludes passage of the instrument.

Treatment

A conservative approach to the treatment of volvulus has been that of gastric decompression alone. It has been suggested that if the volvulus can be corrected by nasogastric aspiration, it will not recur. Evidence to the contrary exists, recommending that nasogastric decompression be considered only as a preoperative measure.[48]

The treatment of the acute strangulating twist causing vascular insufficiency is emergency laparotomy; however, fiberoptic endoscopic derotation of mesenteroaxial and organoaxial volvulus has been reported.[55, 56] Gastric decompression via nasogastric tube or trocar and restoration of the normal anatomy with an anterior gastropexy constitute the repair in either the acute or the recurrent case. One surgeon insists that the subphrenic space be partially and permanently occupied with transpositioned colon to ensure success of the repair.[47] If any obvious anatomic defects are present, such as a rent or bulge in the diaphragm, adhesions, or a paraesophageal hiatus hernia, they, too, should be repaired.[44, 48, 49]

An innovative endoscopic approach to permanent volvulus repair has been described.[57] The gastric antrum and body were independently fixed to their adjacent ligaments by the construction of two percutaneous endoscopic gastrostomies. The patient was discharged within 48 hours and the gastrostomy tubes were removed four weeks later.

Figure 42–4. Mesenteroaxial volvulus in a patient with eventration of the diaphragm. The barium examination reveals the location of the cardioesophageal junction *(closed arrow)*. Colon accompanies stomach above the diaphragm *(open arrow)*. Numbers 1 and 2 indicate proximal and distal stomach, respectively.

References

1. Localio, S., and Stahl, W. Diverticular Disease of the alimentary tract. II. The esophagus, stomach, duodenum, and small intestine. Curr. Prob. Surg. 21, 1968.
2. Dodd, G., and Sheft, D. Diverticulum of the greater curvature of the stomach. AJR 107:102, 1969.
3. Honda, T., Mizuno, T., Takasaki, I., Kurosu, Y., and Morita, K. Gastric diverticulum: report of a case and brief review of the literature. Nihon Univ. J. Med. 20:31, 1978.
4. Baille, T. The Morbid Anatomy of Some of the Most Important Parts of the Human Body. London, 1793, Chap. vii: 92.
5. Tillander, H., and Hesselsjö, R. Juxtacardial gastric diverticula and their surgery. Acta Chir. Scand. 134:255, 1968.
6. Palmer, E. Gastric diverticula, a collective review. Int. Abstr. Surg. 92:417, 1951.
7. Seltzer, M. A huge gastric diverticulum. Am. J. Dig. Dis. 16:167, 1971.
8. Eras, P. The development of a false antral gastric diverticulum. Gastrointest. Endosc. 15:118, 1968.
9. Rabushka, S., Melamed, M., and Melamed, J. Unusual gastric diverticula. Radiology 90:1006, 1968.
10. Eras, P., and Beranbaum, S. Gastric diverticula: congenital and acquired. Am. J. Gastroenterol. 57:120, 1972.
11. Kurgan, A., and Hoffmann, J. Aetiology of gastric diverticula. An hypothesis. Med. Hypotheses 7:1471, 1981.
12. Cockrell, C. H., Cho, S. R., Messmer, J. M., Shaw, C. I., and Liv, C. I. Intramural gastric diverticula: a report of three cases. Br. J. Radiol. 57:285, 1984.
13. Schwartz, A. N., Goiney, R. C., and Graney, D. O. Gastric diverticulum simulating an adrenal mass: CT appearance and embryogenesis. AJR 146:553, 1986.
14. Palmer, E. Gastric diverticula, with special reference to subjective manifestations. Gastroenterology 35:406, 1958.
15. Graham, D., Kimbrough, R., and Fagan, T. Congenital gastric diverticulum as a cause of massive hemorrhage. Am. J. Dig. Dis. 19:174, 1974.
16. Gibbons, C., and Harvey, L. An ulcerated gastric diverticulum— a rare cause of haematemesis and melaena. Postgrad. Med. J. 60:693, 1984.
17. Anaise, D., Brand, D. L., Smith, N. L., and Soroff, H. S. Pitfalls in the diagnosis and treatment of a symptomatic gastric diverticulum. Gastrointest. Endosc. 30:28, 1984.
18. Palmer, E. Gastric diverticulosis. Am. Fam. Phys. 7:114, 1973.
19. Wolf, N. Subcutaneous rupture of the stomach. Review of the literature and report of a case. N.Y. State J. Med. 36:1539, 1936.
20. Fitzgerald, J., Crawford, E., and DeBakey, M. Surgical considerations of non-penetrating abdominal injuries. Am. J. Surg. 100:22, 1960.
21. Semel, L., and Frittelli, G. Gastric rupture from blunt abdominal trauma. N.Y. State J. Med. 81:938, 1981.
22. Albo, R., de Lorimier, A., and Silen, W. Spontaneous rupture of the stomach in the adult. Surgery 53:797, 1963.
23. Revilliod, E. Rupture de l'estomac. Rev. Méd. Suisse Rom. 5:5, 1885.
24. Morris, C., Ivy, A., and Maddock, W. Mechanism of acute abdominal distention. Arch. Surg. 55:101, 1947.
25. Gue, S. Spontaneous rupture of the stomach, a rare complication of inguinal hernia. Br. J. Surg. 57:154, 1970.
26. Mirsky, S., and Garlock, J. Spontaneous rupture of the stomach. Ann. Surg. 161:466, 1965.
27. Ritter and Vanni: as cited by Rehn: Arch., Klin. Chir. 53:383, 1896.
28. Shahmir, M., and Schuman, B. Complications of fiberoptic endoscopy. Gastrointest. Endosc. 26:86, 1980.
29. Brandborg, L. Upper gastrointestinal endoscopy. In Harkins, H., and Nyhus, L. (eds.): Surgery of the Stomach and Duodenum. Ed. 2. Boston, Little, Brown and Co., 1969, p. 173.
30. Schein, M., Falkov, A., and Decker, G. A. Gastric rupture due to external cardiac massage following gastroscopy. Gastrointest. Endos. 31:291, 1985.
31. Zer, M., Chaimoff, C., and Dintsman, M. Spontaneous rupture of the stomach following ingestion of sodium bicarbonate. Arch. Surg. 101:532, 1970.
32. Walstad, P., and Conklin, W. Rupture of the normal stomach after therapeutic oxygen administration. N. Engl. J. Med. 264:1201, 1961.
33. Watts, D. Lesions brought on by vomiting: the effect of hiatus hernia on the site of injury. Gastroenterology 71:683, 1976.
34. Sung, J., O'Hara, V., and Lee, C.-Y. Barium peritonitis. West. J. Med. 127:172, 1977.
35. Demos, N., and Poticha, S. Gastric rupture occurring during external cardiac resuscitation. Surgery 55:364, 1964.
36. Krause, S. Gastric rupture during cardiopulmonary resuscitation. Can. Anaesth. Soc. J. 31:319, 1984.
37. Miller, J. Spontaneous rupture of the stomach during labor. N. Engl. J. Med. 209:1085, 1933.
38. Christoph, R., and Pirkham, E. Unexpected rupture of the stomach in the postpartum period, a case report. Ann. Surg. 154:100, 1961.
39. Saul, S. H., Dekker, A., and Watson, C. G. Acute gastric dilatation with infarction and perforation. Report of fatal outcome in patient with anorexia nervosa. Gut 22:978, 1981.
40. Mastrangelo, M., and Moore, E. Spontaneous rupture of the stomach in a healthy adult man after sodium bicarbonate ingestion. Ann. Intern. Med. 101:649, 1984.
41. Fordtran, J., Morawski, S. G., Santa Ana, C. A., and Rector, F. C., Jr. Gas production after reaction of sodium bicarbonate and hydrochloric acid. Gastroenterology 87:1014, 1984.
42. Berti, A. Sigolare attortiglamento dell'esofago col duodeno sequito da rapida morte. Gazz. Med. Ital. Prov. Ver. 9:139, 1886.
43. Carter, R., Brewer, L., and Hinshaw, D. Acute gastric volvulus. Am. J. Surg. 140:99, 1980.
44. Wastell, C., and Ellis, H. Volvulus of the stomach. Br. J. Surg. 58:557, 1971.
45. Buchanan, J. Volvulus of stomach. Br. J. Surg. 18:99, 1930.
46. Pillay, S., Angorn, I., and Baker, L. Gastric volvulus unassociated with hiatal hernia. S. Afr. Med. J. 52:880, 1977.
47. Tanner, N. Chronic and recurrent volvulus of the stomach. Am. J. Surg. 115:505, 1968.
48. Gosin, S., and Gallinger, W. Recurrent volvulus of the stomach. Am. J. Surg. 109:642, 1965.
49. Camblos, J. Acute volvulus of the stomach. Am. Surgeon 35:505, 1969.
50. Borchardt, L. Pathology and therapy of volvulus of stomach. Arch. Klin. Chir. 74:243, 1904.
51. Metcalfe-Gibson, C. A case of haemorrhage from volvulus of the gastric fundus. Br. J. Surg. 62:224, 1975.
52. Deitel, M. Chronic or recurring organoaxial rotation of the stomach. Can. J. Surg. 16:195, 1973.
53. Llaneza, P. P., Salt, W. B., II, and Partyka, E. K. Extrahepatic biliary obstruction complicating a diaphragmatic hiatal hernia with intrathoracic gastric volvulus. Am. J. Gastroenterol. 81:292, 1986.
54. Babb, R., Peck, O., and Jamplis, R. Gastric volvulus and obstruction in paraesophageal hiatus hernia. Am. J. Dig. Dis. 17:119, 1972.
55. Haddad, J., Doherty, C., and Clark, R. Acute gastric volvulus— endoscopic derotation. West. J. Med. 127:341, 1977.
56. Lowenthal, M. N., Odes, H. S., and Fritsch, E. Endoscopic reduction of acute gastric volvulus complicating motor neuron disease. Israel J. Med. Sci. 21:552, 1985.
57. Eckhauser, M., and Ferron, J. The use of dual percutaneous endoscopic gastrostomy (DPEG) in the management of chronic intermittent gastric volvulus. Gastrointest. Endosc. 31:340, 1985.

Bezoars

STEVEN B. RAFFIN

43

There are few topics in the history of medicine that are more steeped in a bizarre and mystical lore than the subject of bezoars. The term refers to food or foreign matter that has undergone digestive change in the gut of either animals or man. The word arose from attempts at transliteration of the Arabic "badzehr," Persian "padzahr," or Turkish "panzehir," all meaning "anti-poison" or antidote.[1] From antiquity to the eighteenth century, oriental bezoars from the stomachs of goats and gazelles and occidental bezoars from the South American vicuña were highly praised for their magical medicinal properties against such diverse ailments as old age, snakebite, plagues, and evil spirits.[2] So precious were they that a gold-framed bezoar was included in the inventory of Queen Elizabeth's crown jewels in 1622.[3] Proper dosage of these animal concretions was as much a problem as was the establishment of clinical indications: ". . . for one bitten, poisoned, or stung, is the weight of twelve barley grains; the dose for weakness of the heart and loss of sexual power is one grain."[4]

More than a mere medical curiosity when found in the gut of man, bezoars present serious, current medical problems, including upper gastrointestinal ulceration with bleeding and small bowel obstruction. Bezoars have been classified into two groups: hair or trichobezoars, and plant or phytobezoars.[1, 5, 6] A third group of miscellaneous intragastric materials includes fungal agglomerations,[7] food boluses,[6, 8, 9] chemical concretions,[1, 10] and foreign bodies.[11]

CLINICAL PICTURE

Bezoars may produce symptoms ranging from a dragging or fullness in the upper quadrants to epigastric pain, which is the most frequent symptom (70 per cent). Periodic attacks of nausea and vomiting (64 per cent) are also common. A mass can be palpated in 57 per cent of phytobezoars, as contrasted with 88 per cent of trichobezoars. Gastric outlet and intestinal obstruction are also common.[1, 12, 13] The incidence of associated peptic ulceration with the more abrasive phytobezoars (14 to 24 per cent) is greater than with trichobezoars (10 per cent).[5, 14] The incidence of perforation and peritonitis is about 7 and 10 per cent, respectively—less frequent but obviously more catastrophic events.[5] Recently, three cases of gastric carcinoma accompanying bezoars have been reported.[15, 16]

DIAGNOSIS

The laboratory is of little help in diagnosis, except that an associated hypochromic, microcytic anemia and modest leukocytosis may be present. Uncommonly, patients may present with hypoproteinemia and trichobezoar.[17, 18] Erect plain films of the abdomen may show a mass invading the gastric air bubble (Fig. 43–1). The upper gastrointestinal series usually reveals a freely movable mass in the barium field.[19] There is less permeation of barium into the bulk of the phytobezoar than into the trichobezoar,[6] which may aid in differentiation. The postgastric emptying films should show the mass with a thin barium shell in either case (Fig. 43–2).

Recently, a case of postgastrectomy bezoar was diagnosed by abdominal ultrasound.[20] In this case, a complex mass with internal mobile echoes was noted. In addition, the cystic component of the lesion enlarged as the patient drank water during real-time scanning.

Gastroscopy, however, remains the best technique to diagnose and classify bezoars. Trichobezoars are black and tarry (Color Fig. 43–3, p. xxxix), whereas most phytobezoars vary in color from yellow to green. Endoscopic biopsy yielding hair or vegetable fibers is pathognomonic.[6, 21]

TYPES

Phytobezoar

The most common bezoar in current adult medicine is the phytobezoar. Plant bezoars may be composed of the digested fibers, leaves, roots, and skins of almost any plant matter and are usually smaller, more compact, and hence more abrasive than hair bezoars. They are most often found in females over the age of 40,[14] and have a prevalence in the population that now seems to parallel the number of partial gastrectomies.[10, 12, 13, 19, 22, 23]

Hypochlorhydria, diminished antral motility, and incomplete mastication are the main predisposing factors in phytobezoar formation. Diseases illustrating this pathophysiology include myotonic muscular dystrophy[24] and gastroparesis diabeticorum.[25, 26] Recently, an H_2-receptor antagonist, cimetidine, has been causally linked to phytobezoar formation.[27]

Postgastrectomy Bezoar. In the late 1930s, none of the reported patients with bezoar had had prior gastric

741

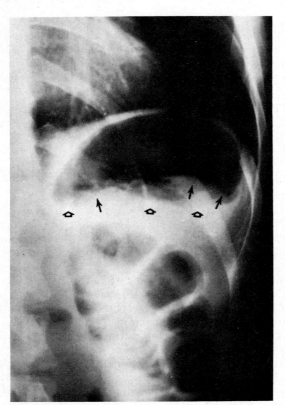

Figure 43–1. Upright plain film of the abdomen. The open arrows point to an air-fluid level in the stomach bubble. The solid arrows point to a bezoar floating in the air-fluid interface.

surgery.[1, 5] The literature of the last 20 years contains many reports that describe phytobezoars complicating the postoperative management of patients with gastric stasis and hypochlorhydria following Billroth I and Billroth II partial gastrectomies, especially when accompanied by vagotomy.[10, 12, 13, 19, 22, 23] Attesting to the

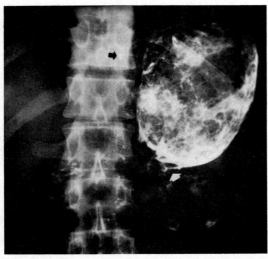

Figure 43–2. This late film in an upper gastrointestinal series of a patient following Billroth II partial gastrectomy and vagotomy demonstrates a barium-coated gastric bezoar. The white arrow points to the surgical stoma, and the solid arrows point to the vagotomy clips.

role of vagotomy in predisposing to bezoars, an interesting report described a large gastric bezoar in an autovagotomized patient, the neurolysis being secondary to encasement of the vagi by esophageal carcinoma.[29] Numerous reports exist documenting transient or complete small intestinal obstruction by wandering phytobezoars six to eight years following gastric surgery.[9, 12, 13, 23] Factors that presumably are causally related to bezoar impaction in the small bowel include the amount of undigestible material in the bezoar (pulpy, fibrous fruit or vegetables, especially oranges), the condition of the chewing mechanism, the caliber of the small bowel (diameter is smallest at a site 50 to 75 cm proximal to the ileocecal valve), and the loss of pyloric function limiting the size of food particles entering the duodenum.[12]

The standard treatment of postgastrectomy phytobezoar includes manual attempts at external disruption, a liquid diet, suction and lavage, and endoscopic internal fragmentation using biopsy forceps and polypectomy snares.[21, 26, 28] Madsen and coworkers successfully used the Teledyne Water Pik to disrupt phytobezoars rapidly in five patients. They recommend this method as a first-line approach.[30]

In addition to physical disruption, chemical attack has also proved to be very successful in treating phytobezoars. Papain and acetylcysteine, both proteolytic enzymes, have been tried with moderate success.[22, 31] However, cellulase, an enzyme specific for the resistant fibrous substrate of the bezoar, has been most successful in dissolving postgastrectomy phytobezoars.[15, 32–34] Two recent reports[35, 36] used pure cellulase in water, rather than Gastroenterase, Celluzyme, or Kanulase, with excellent results. In one regimen, patients consumed up to 1.2 liters of cellulase solution (0.5 gm/dl water) over a 24-hour period for two days. Delpre[16] successfully treated six of seven patients with postoperative phytobezoar by allowing copious clear liquids and infusing metoclopramide intravenously at a rate of 40 mg per 24 hours for three days. Perhaps combination therapy with oral cellulase and intravenous metoclopramide is the optimum therapy?

If medical treatment fails, a gastrotomy must be performed (Fig. 43–4). The surgical mortality is minimal; however, the mortality of untreated bezoar is significant but much less than the often quoted 60 per cent.[5, 14] Although there is no urgency to remove surgically symptomatic intragastric bezoars, there is great advantage to prompt laparotomy in the case of phytobezoar impaction in the small intestine. Prophylactic measures to prevent postgastrectomy bezoar formation include improving dentition; avoiding pulpy, fibrous fruit and vegetables (especially oranges); and perhaps, in cases of delayed gastric emptying without gastric outlet obstruction, using metoclopramide.[25–27, 37]

Persimmon Bezoar (Diospyrobezoar). A major subgroup of phytobezoar not related to gastric surgery is the diospyrobezoar, named for a native American tree of the ebony family, *Diospyros virginiana*, the persimmon. Its fruit, a true berry, possesses little fiber but has a luxuriant pulp. In unripe and, to a lesser degree, in ripe fruit, the well-known astringent properties are

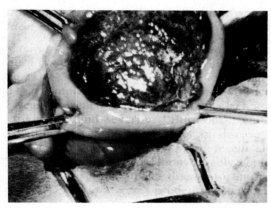

Figure 43–4. This photograph, taken during gastrotomy, demonstrates the lengthy incision needed to retrieve a large, black phytobezoar.

attributed to a substance called shiboul or phlobatannin, which coagulates on contact with dilute acid.[38] This substance is present under the skin in ripe persimmons, making the mature fruit potentially dangerous. Thus, the pathophysiology is obvious. Unripe pulp or ripe skin is ingested by a patient with free acid, and a coagulum results. Symptoms begin soon after excess ingestion of persimmons and are potentiated by drinking copious amounts of water. The unfortunate consequence in extreme instances is severe distress which may suggest an acute abdominal catastrophe to the physician. Seventy-one per cent of patients in a recent report[39] had hematemesis or melena caused by an associated gastric ulcer. Enzymatic therapy usually fails, and gastrotomy is required to remove these rock-hard bezoars.[39]

Moriel and colleagues[40] described 77 postgastrectomy ulcer patients in Israel who presented with bowel obstruction due to diospyrobezoar impaction. Seventy-one patients required laparotomy, and two died. Clearly persimmons, along with citrus pith, must be avoided by patients with loss of pyloric function.

"Cotton Bezoar." An even more bizarre phytobezoar was reported in an ex-heroin addict on methadone. This patient continued intravenous injections despite counseling, using cotton pledgets to filter the crushed tablet-water mixture. Afterward, he swallowed the cotton, thus avoiding the bitter taste of methadone. A "cotton-picking stomach syndrome" resulted.[41]

Trichobezoar

Hairballs are contained within a glairy, mucoid coat and are composed of decaying foodstuff enmeshed among enormous amounts of hair. They are always black and have a fetid odor emanating mainly from undigested dietary fat and bacterial colonization. A large ball may be present for years in an asymptomatic phase, growing slowly by accretion to eventually become a J-shaped cast of the stomach (Fig. 43–5). For unknown reasons hair strands are not usually passed through the pylorus, and hair is rarely found in the

stool of patients with trichobezoar.[42] Occasionally, a trichobezoar may attain a wet weight of over 6 pounds. Several reports exist documenting the association of protein-losing gastropathy with massive trichobezoars.[17, 18] Recently three cases of acute appendicitis have been associated with hair bezoars.[43]

Trichobezoars are most often found in females under the age of 30 years. In the past they were more common than phytobezoars, but today the relative incidence has been reversed.[1, 5, 12] Hair ingestion or trichophagia, which is the cause of the disorder, is only infrequently associated with blatant neuropsychiatric disturbances, in contrast to the ingestion of inorganic foreign bodies; however, some feel that the trait represents a personality maladjustment analogous to fingernail biting.[1]

A clue to diagnosis is the finding of deep crepitus when palpating over these large intragastric masses.[44] The treatment is surgical, because there is no way to dissolve matted hair in vivo. Soilage of the peritoneum and subsequent peritonitis at laparotomy can be a grave consequence, because the stomach contains both bacteria and putrefied material enmeshed in the hairballs.[5]

Food Bolus

The composition of a food bolus may vary from undigested pits, seeds, or citrus pith to minimally digested food in a loose aggregation.[1, 6, 8, 9] Surprisingly, boluses of meat have not been reported within either the stomach or the small bowel.[23] Food boluses differ from bezoars in that they are neither compact nor hard and show no effects of prolonged gastric retention. Food boluses as well as phytobezoars may cause gastric outlet obstruction or may become impacted in the small intestine.[8, 9, 12, 23] Careful mastication and elimi-

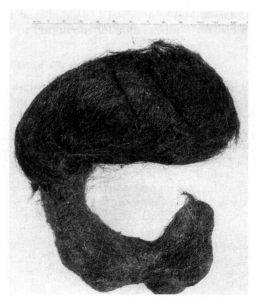

Figure 43–5. Trichobezoar surgically excised from the stomach of a 17-year-old girl with secondary gastric ulcer and profound iron-deficiency anemia. (Courtesy of Emmet B. Keeffe, M.D.)

nation of oranges from the diet of all postgastrectomy patients would probably abolish this entity.[6, 12]

Concretion

Concretions range from the mundane to the bizarre. Occasionally, agglomerated antacid tablets, aluminum hydroxide gel, or Kayexalate may cause small bowel obstruction in partially gastrectomized patients.[45, 46] Sucralfate has the potential to form an especially durable concretion.[47] Youngsters ingesting rather than sniffing glue have occasionally presented in distress with insoluble gastroliths (L. L. Brandborg, personal communication). Classically, the gastric concretion is unique to furniture finishers who drink a mixture of shellac and alcohol for the stimulating effects of the latter component. Upon subsequent ingestion of water as a chaser, the resinous contents agglutinate into a solid mass in the stomach. This lesion grows by laminar accretion, with the rate paralleling the bouts of imbibition and the gross appearance similar to growth rings on the wood furniture for which the mixture was solely concocted. These masses may exceed 4 pounds[1] and must be surgically removed.

A potentially deadly intragastric concretion consisting of shoe polish and "sleep-aid" pill fragments resulted in bromide intoxication in an alcoholic patient.[48] Endoscopic fragmentation of the mass and saline gastric lavage resulted in prompt normalization of serum bromide levels. One must be aware that concretions or bezoars are able to entrap pills and may produce prolonged toxic levels of orally administered drugs.

Foreign Bodies

True foreign body ingestion, including such diverse items as pins, nails, razor blades, buttons, and coins, is usually seen in children or psychotic individuals. Not infrequently polybezoars, consisting of metallic, plastic, or wooden trinkets enmeshed in a trichobezoar, are seen in these patients.[11] In one instance an esophageal dilator guide string "bezoar" was removed from the stomach of a woman who had last used the dilator 26 years previously.[49] Nonspecific upper quadrant pain may be the only clue to diagnosis, although laceration of the gut wall with hemorrhage or peritonitis sometimes occurs. The stomach and intestines may be literally brimful of articles, and the only therapy is laparotomy with removal of the collection.[11]

Gastrointestinal Fungal Balls

The presence of large, spongy intragastric yeast balls has been described in Scandinavian patients, predominantly following vagotomy and Billroth I gastroduodenostomy.[7, 50] These patients were not taking antibiotics, steroids, or immunosuppressive agents and had no systemic disease to account for the proliferation of *Candida* in their stomachs. It appears that postgastrectomy fungal collections are more frequent than postgastrectomy phytobezoars in Finland and Sweden. Diagnosis requires endoscopy, as it is impossible to distinguish between phytobezoars and yeast balls roentgenologically. Neither ulcer nor hemorrhage occurs in association with these foreign bodies. Although most postgastrectomy yeast balls disintegrate following gastric lavage and antimycotic therapy, they often recur months to years later.[7, 50]

References

1. DeBakey, M., and Ochsner, A. Bezoars and concretions. Surgery 4:934, 1938.
2. Dechambre, A. Dictionnaire encyclopédique des sciences médicales. Vol. 9. Paris, Victor Masson et Fils, 1868, p. 221.
3. Murdock, H. Persimmon bezoars occurring around Tulsa, Oklahoma. J. Okla. Med. Assoc. 27:442, 1934.
4. Elgood, C. A treatise of the bezoar stone. By the late Mahmud Bin Masud the Imad-ul-din, the Physician of Ispahan. Ann. Med. Hist. 7:73, 1935.
5. DeBakey, M., and Ochsner, A. Bezoars and concretions. Surgery 5:132, 1939.
6. Sanowski, R., and DiDianco, J. Pseudotumors of the stomach. Am. J. Dig. Dis. 11:607, 1966.
7. Borg, I., Heijkenskjold, F., Nilehn, B., and Wehlin, L. Massive growth of yeasts in resected stomach. Gut 7:244, 1966.
8. McCabe, R., and Knox, W. Phytobezoar in gastrectomized patients. Arch. Surg. 86:264, 1963.
9. Koh, I., Urca, I., and Tikva, P. Intestinal obstruction after partial gastrectomy due to orange pith. Arch. Surg. 100:79, 1970.
10. Cain, G., Moore, P., and Patterson, M. Bezoars—a complication of the postgastrectomy state. Am. J. Dig. Dis. 13:801, 1968.
11. Bitar, D., and Holmes, R., Jr. Polybezoar and gastrointestinal foreign bodies in the mentally retarded. Am. Surg. 41:497, 1975.
12. Buchholz, R., and Haisten, A. Phytobezoars following gastric surgery for duodenal ulcer. Surg. Clin. North Am. 52:341, 1972.
13. Shapiro, P., Babbin, G., and Matolo, N. Phytobezoar and obstruction of the small intestine following gastrectomy. West. J. Med. 124:506, 1976.,
14. Zarling, E., and Thompson, L. Nonpersimmon gastric phytobezoar. Arch. Intern. Med. 144:959, 1984.
15. Van Thiel, D., DeBelle, R., Painter, T., McMillan, W., and Haradin, A. Phytobezoar occurring as a complication of gastric carcinoma. Gastroenterology 68:1292, 1975.
16. Delpre, G., Glanz, I., Neeman, A., Avidor, I., and Kadish, V. New therapeutic approach in postoperative phytobezoars. J. Clin. Gastroenterol. 6:231, 1984.
17. Bernstein, L., Gutstein, S., Efron, G., Wagle, M., and Graham, E. Trichobezoar—an unusual cause of megaloblastic anemia and hypoproteinemia in childhood. Am. J. Dig. Dis. 18:67, 1973.
18. Hossenbocus, A., and Colin-Jones, D. Trichobezoar, gastric polyposis, protein-losing gastroenteropathy and steatorrhea. Gut 14:730, 1973.
19. Rigler, R., and Grininger, D. Phytobezoars following partial gastrectomy. Surg. Clin. North Am. 50:381, 1970.
20. Bidula, M. M., Rifkin, M. D., and McCoy, R. I. Ultrasonography of gastric phytobezoar. J. Clin. Ultrasound 14:49, 1986.
21. McKechnie, J. Gastroscopic removal of a phytobezoar. Gastroenterology 62:1047, 1972.
22. Sparberg, M., Nielsen, A., and Andruczak, R. Bezoar following gastrectomy. Am. J. Dig. Dis. 13:579, 1968.
23. Rogers, L., Davis, E., and Harle, T. Phytobezoar formation and food boli following gastric surgery. AJR 119:280, 1973.
24. Kuiper, D. Gastric bezoar in a patient with myotonic dystrophy. Am. J. Dig. Dis. 16:529, 1971.
25. Brady, P., and Richardson, R. Gastric bezoar formation secondary to gastroparesis diabeticorum. Arch. Intern. Med. 137:1729, 1977.
26. Brady, P. Gastric phytobezoars consequent to delayed gastric emptying. Gastrointest. Endosc. 24:159, 1978.

27. Nichols, T., Jr. Phytobezoar formation: A new complication of cimetidine therapy. Ann. Intern. Med. *95*:70, 1981.
28. Diettrich, N., and Gau, F. Postgastrectomy phytobezoars—endoscopic diagnosis and treatment. Arch. Surg. *120*:432, 1985.
29. Kirks, D., and Szemes, G. Autovagotomy and gastric bezoar. Gastroenterology *61*:96, 1971.
30. Madsen, R., Skibba, R., Galvan, A., Striplin, C., and Scott, P. Gastric bezoars. A technique of endoscopic removal. Dig. Dis. *23*:717, 1978.
31. Schlang, H. Acetylcysteine in removal of bezoar. JAMA *214*:1329, 1970.
32. Pollard, H., and Block, G. Rapid dissolution of phytobezoar by cellulase enzyme. Am. J. Surg. *116*:933, 1968.
33. Deal, D. Vitale, P., and Raffin, S. Dissolution of a post-gastrectomy bezoar by cellulase. Gastroenterology *64*:467, 1973.
34. Stanten, A., and Peters, H., Jr. Enzymatic dissolution of phytobezoars. Am. J. Surg. *130*:259, 1975.
35. Holloway, W., Lee, S., and Nicholson, G. The composition and dissolution of phytobezoars. Arch. Pathol. Lab. Med. *104*:159, 1980.
36. Smith, B., Mollot, M., and Berk, J. E. Use of cellulase for phytobezoar dissolution. Am. J. Gastroenterol. *73*:257, 1980.
37. Winkler, W., and Saleh, J. Metoclopramide in the treatment of gastric bezoar. Am. J. Gastroenterol. *78*:403, 1983.
38. Izumi, S., Isida, K., and Iwamoto, M. Mechanism of formation of phytobezoars with special reference to persimmon ball. Jap. J. Med. Sc. Tr., II Biochem. *2*:21, 1933.
39. Dolan, P., and Thompson, B. Management of persimmon bezoars (diospyrobezoars). South. Med. J. *72*:1527, 1979.
40. Moriel, E. Z., Ayalon, A., Eid, A., Rachmilewitz, D., Krausz, M. M., and Durst, A. L. An unusually high incidence of gastrointestinal obstruction by persimmon bezoar in Israeli patients after ulcer surgery. Gastroenterology *84*:752, 1983.
41. Kaden, W. Phytobezoar in an addict: The cottonpicking stomach syndrome. JAMA *209*:1367, 1969.
42. Davies, I. Hairballs or hair casts of stomach and gastrointestinal tract. Lancet *2*:791, 1921.
43. Kochar, A. Acute appendicitis associated with a trichobezoar. (Letter.) JAMA *252*:1681, 1984.
44. Dasgupta, H., Chandra, S., Gupta, M., Sanwal, B., Bhargawa, S., and Vaid, R. Trichobezoar—clinical diagnosis. J. Postgrad. Med. *25*:181, 1979.
45. Townsend, C., Jr., Remmers, A., Jr., Sarles, H., and Fish, J. Intestinal obstruction from medication bezoar in patients with renal failure. N. Engl. J. Med. *288*:1058, 1973.
46. Korenman, M., Stubbs, M., and Fish, J. Intestinal obstruction from medication bezoars. JAMA *240*:54, 1978.
47. Algozzine, G. Sucralfate bezoar. (Letter.) N. Engl. J. Med. *309*:1387, 1983.
48. Iberti, T., Patterson, B. K., and Fisher, C. J., Jr. Prolonged bromide intoxication resulting from a gastric bezoar. Arch. Intern. Med. *144*:402, 1984.
49. Norfleet, R, Bickford, R., and Eckberg, R. Gastric bezoars from swallowed string. JAMA *240*:855, 1978.
50. Perttala, Y., Peltokallio, P., Leiviskä, T., and Sipponen, J. Yeast bezoar formation following gastric surgery. AJR *125*:365, 1975.

44

Neoplasms of the Stomach

GLENN R. DAVIS

PATHOLOGY OF GASTRIC CANCER

The majority of malignant neoplasms of the stomach are adenocarcinomas which arise from mucous cells, and special studies indicate that the cell of origin is probably the mucous neck cell.[1] Recently, though, three cases of gastric cancer originating from the parietal cell have been identified.[2]

Microscopically, carcinoma of the stomach has been divided into a variety of groups based on cellular and extracellular characteristics. Depending upon the degree of gland formation and ability to secrete mucus, a gastric cancer may be well, moderately, or poorly differentiated. The ability to secrete mucus has, also, given way to other classifying terms, such as signet ring carcinoma, which is a tumor with large amounts of intracellular mucinous material compressing the nucleus to an eccentric location. When there is exces-sive mucus secretion, forming extracellular aggregates that may be visible macroscopically, this is referred to as colloid or mucinous carcinoma. Carcinomas are called medullary when there are solid bands or masses of cancer cells or papillary if the glandular structures are in a papillary form. The nature of the inflammatory infiltrate in the stroma has also been used to classify adenocarcinomas of the stomach.

With all these names and modifying terminology, a relatively simple pathologic entity can become very confusing. These various cellular characteristics and degrees of differentiation have been reported to exist within the same tumor and even change with time, so attempts to correlate these descriptive features with prognosis have been predictably unrewarding.

The histologic study of gastric carcinoma has been useful, though, in the epidemiologic study of gastric carcinoma. It has been observed that gastric cancers

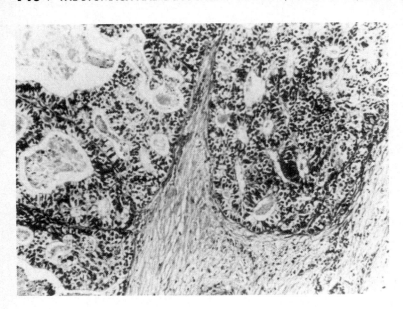

Figure 44–1. Intestinal (expanding) type of gastric cancer. (From Correa, P. Semin. Oncol. *12*:4, 1985. Used by permission.)

often display features of intestinal mucosa. After analyzing 1344 surgically removed specimens, Lauren divided gastric cancer into diffuse or intestinal type.[3] The intestinal type resembles colon cancer and has distinct large glands; in the diffuse type of gastric carcinoma the glandular structure was rarely present, and the cells were scattered either as a solitary cell or small clusters of cells. The cells which lined the glands of the intestinal type carcinoma were usually well-polarized columnar cells with a well-developed brush border identified in many (Figs. 44–1 and 44–2).

Because 14 per cent of tumors could not be classified by this method, Ming proposed dividing gastric carcinoma into expanding and infiltrative types.[4] This classification also reflects the growth pattern of the cancers. The expanding type is characterized by a group of cells which maintain a coherent relationship and grow by pushing aside other cells, that is, by expansion. The infiltrative type, on the other hand, is characterized by deep and wide infiltration of isolated individual tumor cells. Ming's expanding and infiltrative types, in general, correspond to Lauren's intestinal and diffuse types, respectively.

These observations have led to the speculation that gastric cancer encompasses two diseases with the key differentiating factor being cell cohesion.[5] When it is present, the cells "stick" to each other and form glandular-like structures (intestinal or expanding type). When there is the lack of cell cohesion, this results in independent cells which infiltrate without forming a definite mass (diffuse or infiltrating type).

Intestinal metaplasia which represents the replacement of normal gastric tissue by mucosa that resembles that of the intestine has been associated with the intestinal or expanding type of gastric cancer but not the diffuse or infiltrative type. Intestinal metaplasia

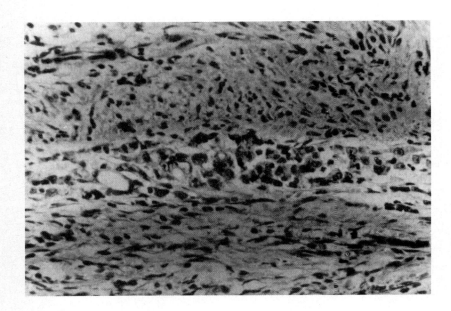

Figure 44–2. Diffuse (infiltrative) type of gastric cancer. (From Correa, P. Semin. Oncol. *12*:4, 1985. Used by permission.)

has been classified as complete (type I), in which metaplastic epithelium has characteristics of intestinal mucosa resembling biochemically and pathologically the small intestinal mucosa; or incomplete (type II), in which the immature mucosa does not have these characteristics and may resemble colon mucosa.[6] It is this latter type of intestinal metaplasia that is thought to be associated with gastric cancer, but the complete or mature type metaplasia is not (see p. 752).

Early Gastric Cancer

Saeki in 1938 identified a subgroup of patients with gastric cancer in which the depth of invasion was limited. In view of the major health problem gastric cancer represents in Japan, the Japanese Endoscopic Society in 1962 defined this phenomenon as early gastric cancer. It would be this lesion that mass screening programs would attempt to identify in order to reduce the mortality rate of gastric cancer in Japan.

Early gastric cancer (EGC) is defined as a disease in which the depth of invasion is limited to the mucosa or submucosa, regardless of lymph node involvement. Early gastric cancer is, therefore, a pathologic diagnosis, and although this term clinically suggests a lesion that is not late, not advanced, not symptomatic, not large, and therefore curable, these are not necessarily synonymous because in some cases EGC may have lymph node involvement, may be associated with non-specific symptoms, or may be fairly large.[8, 9]

Microscopically, EGC shows a wide range of histologic appearances, including varying degrees of differentiation and different patterns of mucous secretion. Both expanding and infiltrative types of carcinoma are seen in early gastric cancer. Macroscopically, EGC has been divided into three types (Fig. 44–3): protruded (type I), superficial (type II), and excavative (type III). Type II (specifically type IIc) is the most common lesion. This macroscopic classification was derived by examining resected specimens histologically and grossly. It has been suggested that types I and IIa consist almost entirely of well-differentiated adenocarcinoma, types IIb and IIc show varying degrees of differentiation, and type III includes a higher percentage of poorly differentiated and undifferentiated carcinomas.[9, 10] Figures 44–4 to 44–6 are examples of early gastric cancer.

The majority of cases of EGC occur in the distal stomach. Multicentric lesions are present in approximately 10 per cent of patients when the stomach is examined following resection. Initially it was felt that EGC was a disease peculiar to the Japanese, but early gastric cancer has been found with increasing prevalence in other parts of the world. Surveys of endoscopists in Europe and North America show that EGC represented 4 to 7 per cent of gastric cancer in the late 1970s.[11] Recent reports indicate that it still only represents 5 to 16 per cent of those who have undergone resection for gastric cancer.[12, 13] Despite this intercountry variation in incidence of EGC, histologic comparisons of EGC from Japan and Western countries have shown that they have similar features, and therefore it appears that everyone is describing the same disease.[14, 15]

Advanced Gastric Cancer

Advanced gastric cancer (AGC) denotes disease that has penetrated the muscular layer (Fig. 44–7) and usually is associated with distant or contiguous spread of tumor and, therefore, a poor chance of being cured. Advanced gastric cancer is identified by the pathologist, radiologist, and endoscopist in patterns that correspond to Borrmann's classification. These include: I, polypoid; II, ulcerative lesion in which there are discrete, sharply defined borders; III, ulcerating-infiltrating in which the ulceration does not have discrete borders; and IV, diffuse infiltrating lesions or linitis plastica (Fig. 44–8).

Classically, type I includes only the rarely seen polypoid carcinoma. In some series, Borrmann's type I includes large fungating carcinomas, though this type of lesion is more appropriately assigned to Borrmann's type III, which represents the most common gross appearance of gastric carcinoma. Greater than 50 per cent of advanced gastric cancers are located in the antrum. Tumors of the cardia and more proximal stomach accounted for approximately 10 per cent of carcinomas in older series, but more recently some authors have found a higher incidence of proximally (cardia) located carcinomas.[16] Whether this is a true increase in this location or a reflection of a decrease in distal lesions is uncertain. The lesser curvature is more often the site of gastric cancer than the greater curvature.

Is Early Gastric Cancer an "Early" Stage of Advanced Gastric Cancer?

From the concept of early gastric cancer naturally comes the assumption that EGC with time would

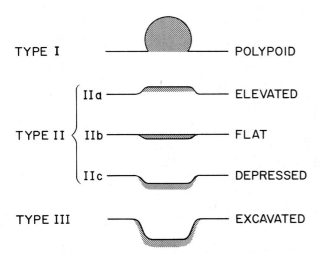

Figure 44–3. Early gastric cancer is macroscopically divided into three types. Type II is further subdivided into three subtypes.

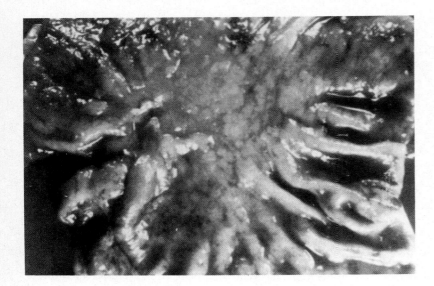

Figure 44–4. Gastrectomy specimen demonstrating type IIb early gastric cancer. (From Bogomoletz, W. Early gastric cancer. Am J. Surg. Pathol. 8:384, 1984. Used by permission.)

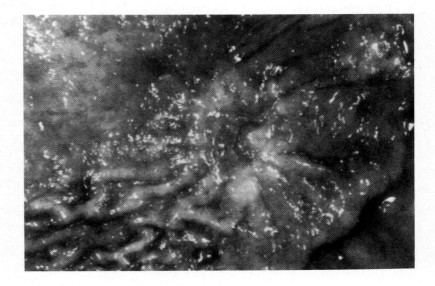

Figure 44–5. Gastrectomy specimen demonstrating type IIc early gastric cancer. (From Bogomoletz., W. Early gastric cancer. Am. J. Surg. Pathol. 8:384, 1984. Used by permission.)

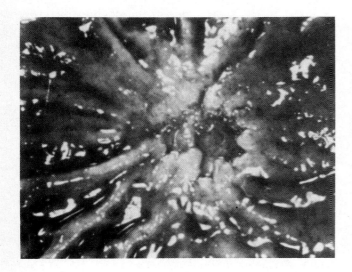

Figure 44–6. Gastrectomy specimen demonstrating type IIc-III early gastric cancer. (From Bogomoletz, W. Early gastric cancer. Am. J. Surg. Pathol. 8:385, 1984.)

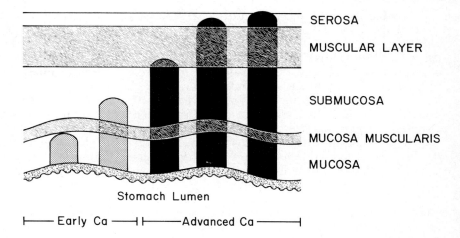

Figure 44–7. In early gastric cancer the disease is limited to the mucosa and submucosa, whereas the tumor penetrates beyond the submucosa in advanced gastric cancer. (From Dupont, G. J., and Conn, I. Curr. Probl. Cancer 4(1):15. Copyright 1980, Year Book Medical Publishers. Reproduced with permission.)

invariably become advanced gastric cancer (AGC). Some have suggested, though, that EGC may be a different disease than AGC, and because of an inability to invade, it may have an indolent course and select itself out for cure.[17] Advanced gastric cancer, on the other hand, may be a more aggressive, invasive lesion, rarely being diagnosed at a curable stage. Such a concept seems possible when one considers that it is indeed difficult to explain why in some studies, even

with lymph involvement, EGC maintains its good prognosis, why the mean age of onset with EGC is not uniformly younger than that with AGC, and why EGC is more common in some countries than others. Also, to conclusively prove that this sequence (EGC becomes AGC) occurs in humans would be difficult, perhaps impossible. Early gastric cancer is a pathologic diagnosis, and therefore the lesion has to be removed surgically and examined to determine the depth of invasion. This, in turn, would interrupt the sequence.

The evidence that supports the concept that EGC becomes AGC includes the observation that there are persons with AGC who retrospectively had what appeared to be macroscopic lesions of EGC when gastro-camera film was reviewed.[18] Also, there have been persons with macroscopic-appearing EGC who have refused surgery and have subsequently developed AGC on follow-up.[19] Animal studies have demonstrated the progression of EGC to AGC when the neoplastic process was induced by the administration of nitroso compounds.[20] It can be argued that one cannot be absolutely sure the lesion observed to be EGC macroscopically was EGC pathologically in any of these situations. However, there are cases in which EGC was diagnosed from surgical specimens, but the margins of resection still had cancer (EGC); and these persons have gone on to develop AGC.[21]

Is Early Gastric Cancer the Same as Superficial Spreading or Surface Carcinoma of the Stomach?

By definition, many carcinomas of the superficial spreading variety are EGC, i.e., confined to the mucosa and the submucosa, and therefore share the same good prognosis. It has been argued that these terms should not be used interchangeably because, even if confined to the submucosa, superficial spreading cancer is a more extensive (spread out) lesion, and EGC is a smaller lesion. This is not a uniform finding, though, and it is not unreasonable to classify the clinical entity of superficial spreading carcinoma into EGC or AGC, depending on the depth of invasion.

Figure 44–8. Borrmann classification of gastric cancer: I, polypoid; II, ulcerating; III, ulcerating-infiltrating; IV, infiltrating. (From Douglass, H. O., Jr., and Nava, H. R. Semin. Oncol. 12:33, 1985. Used by permission.)

Squamous Cell Carcinoma of the Stomach

Rarely, squamous cell carcinoma of the stomach can occur.[22, 23] In this lesion, areas of adenocarcinomatous changes usually will be detected if looked for closely, so these are also referred to as adenosquamous. Several pathogenic mechanisms have been postulated as to the origin, including (1) local extension or metastasis from esophageal squamous cell carcinoma, (2) heterotopic squamous cell epithelium, (3) squamous cell metaplasia, (4) multipotential stem cell, and (5) overgrowth of squamous components in an existing adenocarcinoma.

There are cases reported which are examples of squamous cell carcinoma occurring in each of these situations, but it has been shown that close inspection of the stomach will always identify adenocarcinoma in association with the squamous cell carcinoma. Therefore, it is felt that the origin is probably from a multipotential stem cell or that it arises from squamous metaplasia in an existing adenocarcinoma. The latter hypothesis is supported by the fact that squamous cell carcinoma has not been reported in early gastric cancer.

Hepatoid Adenocarcinoma

This rare carcinoma contains distinctive foci of hepatic differentiation.[24] In addition to the morphologic similarities to liver cells, these tumors secrete substances produced by normal liver cells, such as alpha-fetoprotein. Because the stomach and liver are both derived from the primitive foregut, it has been postulated that a disturbance of differentiation in gastric cancer might be responsible for this rare occurrence.

EPIDEMIOLOGY

Gastric cancer was the most common malignant disease in the United States as recently as the 1940s.[25] Since then, there has been a dramatic and unexplained decrease in the death rate from this disease. Because the fatality rate from gastric cancer remains high, death rates represent a good index of incidence in many countries and are perhaps the most accurate statistic to collect.[25] The age-adjusted death rate from stomach cancer in the United States was 22.5 deaths per 100,000 persons in 1940, but now it is less than 7 per 100,000 persons (8.2 and 3.9 per 100,000 males and females, respectively).[26] In the United States, this decrease has been observed regardless of sex, race, or age.

Intercountry Variation

There is a marked variation in the incidence of gastric cancer throughout the world.[26–28] Japan, Costa Rica, Chile, Hungary, and Poland are among the countries with the highest rates.

As in the United States, a similar decrease in gastric cancer has been observed in most countries, although the rate of decline has varied. Japan, which has the highest mortality rate from gastric cancer—63.1 and 30.3 deaths per 100,000 males and females, respectively—was still reporting an increase in the 1960s, but now there appears to be a trend toward decline. Whether this is the result of their mass screening effort or the same unknown factors responsible for the decrease in other countries remains uncertain. The fact that the incidence rate in Japan has surpassed the mortality rate suggests that the mass screening program has had some impact.[29]

When there is a high incidence of gastric cancer, there appears to be a predominance of the expanding type of gastric cancer; therefore, this has been termed by some the "epidemic type." When a decrease in gastric cancer is noted, it is a decrease in the expanding type with a relatively consistent incidence of the infiltrative or "endemic type."[5]

Intracountry Variation

Just as outstanding as the marked intercountry incidence variation is an intracountry variation. This is more readily demonstrated in countries such as Japan and Colombia, where there is a high incidence of gastric cancer, but has also been shown to exist in the United States in the past.[30, 31] Increased mortality rate was demonstrated in major cities and areas characterized by low socioeconomic class. Other areas of increased mortality rate had higher concentrations of first and second generation immigrants from other countries with higher incidence of gastric cancer.

Migration Studies

The intercountry variation has provided epidemiologists the opportunity to study the effect of migration from high-risk to low-risk areas. It has been noted that first generation Japanese (Issei) who migrated to Hawaii in the late 1800s and early 1900s had a similar or possibly a slightly lower incidence of gastric cancer when compared with the same generation in Japan.[32] More important, though, second generation Japanese in Hawaii (Nisei) had a lower incidence than the Issei, but still higher than that noted for the United States population. The third generation (Sansei), although still young, appear to have a lower incidence of lesions, such as atrophic gastritis and intestinal metaplasia, which are believed to be precancerous lesions. The incidence of gastric cancer in the Hawaiian Japanese now appears to be as low as that observed in the native Hawaiians.

In addition to this observed decrease of gastric cancer in migrants from high-risk areas, there are some preliminary data suggesting that persons moving from a low-risk area to a high-risk area may develop the increased risk for gastric cancer.

ETIOLOGY

Environmental Factors

The influence of migration on gastric cancer incidence suggests that exposure to an etiologic agent early in life is responsible for this disease. What this agent might be remains uncertain but since the stomach is the first point of prolonged contact with food, dietary substances have been incriminated. Attempts to identify the responsible substance through diet studies present problems beause they represent retrospective analysis of long periods of time and require that the patient recall early life dietary habits.[33] Nevertheless, from these extensive investigations of eating patterns, including case control studies from several countries, some general conclusions have been drawn.[34-37]

There appears to be an increased association of gastric cancer with starch, pickled vegetables, salted fish and meat, and smoked foods. On the other hand, whole milk, fresh vegetables, citrus fruits, vitamin C, and refrigeration are inversely associated with gastric cancer. One of the most consistent features in the dietary studies of persons with gastric cancer is an increase in salt consumption. The recent decrease in mortality rate from gastric cancer coincides with a decrease in mortality rate from cerebrovascular accidents, both of which have been attributed to a decrease in salt consumption.[38]

Other substances which may be involved in the development of gastric cancer are nitrates and nitrites.[39, 40] A decrease in salt intake usually will be associated with a decrease in nitrate and nitrite consumption also. Nitrates are a common constituent of our diet and are primarily found in vegetables, in cured meat, and to some extent in drinking water. Nitrites are also ingested, but their main source is the conversion of nitrates to nitrites. Nitrites then can be nitrosated, that is, combined with amines and amides to form nitrosamines and nitrosamides (nitroso compounds). These latter substances have been shown to be gastric carcinogens in animals.[41] Although nitroso compounds have not been definitely shown to be the cause of gastric cancer in humans, circumstantial evidence is available which helps to advance this hypothesis. High nitrate concentrations in the soil and drinking water in areas with high death rates from gastric cancer have been observed[42] (though recently a negative association with gastric cancer and nitrates in drinking water was identified in the United Kingdom[43]). There is an increased number of nitrite-forming bacteria in the upper gastrointestinal tract in persons with hypo- or achlorhydria, which is not an infrequent occurrence in persons with gastric cancer as well as in persons with possible predisposition to gastric cancer (such as pernicious anemia and atrophic gastritis).[44]

The reduced acid supposedly allows the colonization of the stomach by nitrite-forming bacteria. Increased nitrite and nitrosamine concentrations have also been found in persons who have undergone gastric surgery, another situation possibly associated with gastric can-

cer.[45] Ruddell has demonstrated higher concentrations of nitrites in gastric juice from persons with gastric cancer than in that from gastric ulcer patients or control subjects.[46]

Obviously, because these patients were not followed prospectively, it is impossible to know if these findings are causally related or an incidental effect. Recently, Hall confirmed the finding of bacterial colonization and increased nitrite concentrations in the stomach but found a negative corelation between nitroso compounds and gastric pH.[47]

Because cold temperatures inhibit the conversion of nitrate to nitrite, the general use of refrigeration and the use of less nitrate as food preservative could be an explanation for the recent decrease in gastric cancer in the United States. Likewise, it has been shown that vitamin C can inhibit nitrosation, and substances that are high in vitamin C, such as citrus fruits, have been shown to be inversely correlated with the incidence of gastric cancer.[48]

Some studies have found a decreased risk with increased dietary fiber intake and an increased risk with chocolate.[33] Coffee intake has been shown not to be associated with gastric cancer, as is alcohol, except for studies in which intake was very high or on an "empty stomach before breakfast."[34, 36, 37, 49] A consistent, strong relationship between smoking and gastric cancer has not been observed.

Genetic Factors

In 1953, Aird made the observation that blood group A was more frequent in patients with gastric cancer.[50] This was later confirmed by other studies.[28] The meaning of this association remains uncertain, and although the studies have been criticized because of the control groups used, the relationship appears real. No relationship of gastric cancer to a specific HLA antigen has been detected.[51]

Several families have been described in which there are clusters of persons with gastric carcinoma, and relatives of persons with this disease are believed to have at least two to three times greater incidence of gastric cancer. Gastric cancer has been reported in monozygous twins.[52] These latter obserations are interesting, but because environmental exposure is usually similar in these groups, it is impossible to separate out the role of genetic factors. It appears that environmental factors are most important in the etiology of gastric cancer but may be superimposed on an inherited susceptibility.

POPULATION AT RISK

A summary of possible risk factors for gastric cancer is shown in Figure 44-9.

The incidence and mortality rate of gastric cancer increase with age, relatively few cases being reported prior to 30 years of age, with a sharp increase after age 50.[53-55] In the United States, the incidence of gastric

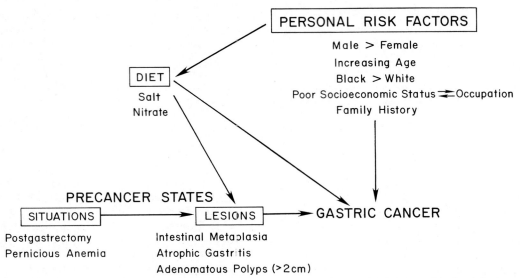

Figure 44–9. Major personal risk factors, dietary substances, and possible precancer states (situations and lesions) that are associated with gastric cancer.

cancer is higher in males than in females, although this ratio is less obvious in the young and elderly. Some series have shown that the male-to-female ratio is as high as 2:1.

The risk of gastric cancer is greatest among the lower socioeconomic groups.[28, 29] This may be the cause or the effect of the observation that this lesion is more frequent in blacks, regardless of sex. The decline in gastric cancer mortality rate has been less pronounced in the black than in the white population. Because of the numerous factors involved (occupation, socioeconomic class, diet), it is impossible to determine the importance of the racial factors.

POSSIBLE PRECANCEROUS LESIONS AND SITUATIONS

Chronic Atrophic Gastritis and Intestinal Metaplasia

In chronic atrophic gastritis, normal gastric glands are decreased or absent, there is a variable degree of inflammation, and intestinal metaplasia frequently develops. Intestinal metaplasia represents replacement of gastric mucosa by mucosa that by many standards (histologic, histochemical, and physiologic) resembles that of the intestine. Occasionally, chronic atrophic gastritis does not have intestinal metaplasia; and areas of intestinal metaplasia have been identified in the stomach of normal persons and those with only superficial gastritis. Most often, though, these two entities are found together.

Chronic atrophic gastritis and intestinal metaplasia have frequently been considered a precancerous lesion. This is based on the observation that atrophic gastritis with intestinal metaplasia is frequently found in persons with gastric cancer. Also, chronic atrophic gastritis is

much more frequent in autopsy specimens from Japanese than from Americans, a finding which is similar to the difference in gastric cancer incidence.[56] Likewise, in Colombia, persons from high-risk areas of gastric cancer had a greater incidence of intstinal metaplasia than those from low-risk areas.[30] Siurala followed 116 patients with atrophic gastritis for at least 20 years, and 10 per cent developed gastric cancer, as compared with 0.6 per cent of subjects with normal gastric mucosa or superficial gastritis.[57] In experimental carcinogenesis, atrophic gastritis and intestinal metaplasia developed in many of the animal models prior to overt cancer, suggesting that it is a part of a continuum of gastric cancer.[58]

On the other hand, chronic atrophic gastritis and intestinal metaplasia are found with increasing frequency in older but normal individuals who do not have gastric carcinoma.[59] In addition, this lesion was found in many of the patients who died from extragastric carcinoma, and an increased incidence of intestinal metaplasia in patients with peptic ulcer disease has been observed.[60]

Though it appears that there is a relationship between chronic atrophic gastritis with intestinal metaplasia and gastric cancer, intestinal metaplasia is too prevalent to be a sensitive indicator of cancer or a precancerous lesion. Therefore, it has been proposed that perhaps not all intestinal metaplasia is precancerous. Using various morphologic and histochemical analyses, intestinal metaplasia has been subdivided into two groups.[6, 7, 61] Type I, or complete type, resembles small intestinal mucosa with intestinal brush border enzymes fully represented and though there are no villi, the crypt cells are lined with goblet cells secreting nonsulfated acid mucins, mainly sialomucin. Type II intestinal metaplasia is defined as incomplete and may be divided into two subgroups. In type IIa, referred to as goblet cell metaplasia, there appear to be goblet cells secreting a nonsulfated acid mucin from normal appearing gastric glands. In type IIb, cell differentiation is more marked and the predominant mucin produced is a sulfated acid mucin or sulfomucin. This latter type IIb is felt to be associated with gastric cancer. In a prospective study involving three centers, type IIb was more commonly associated with gastric cancer than benign conditions.[62] This suggests that although intestinal metaplasia in general is not precancerous, certain subtypes of this histologic phenomenon may be more closely associated with gastric cancer and more likely to be a precancerous lesion.

It is also to be noted that studies indicate intestinal metaplasia is primarily associated with the expanding type gastric cancer, while no definite relationship can be demonstrated with the infiltrating type of gastric cancer.[63]

Gastric Ulcer

One of the more controversial issues is the relationship of gastric ulcer and gastric carcinoma. Despite the fact that these two processes share many features (such as the population affected and the high incidence of gastritis and intestinal metaplasia), chronic benign gastric ulcer rarely progresses to gastric cancer. It is accepted that gastric cancer may present as an ulcer and in those instances in which gastric cancer is found in a chronic ulcer, it was probably missed on first diagnostic studies. If an ulcer heals on therapy but is proved to be cancer at time of recurrence, this does not necessarily indicate previous benignity and subsequently degeneration, for malignant gastric ulcers occasionally may heal on intense medical therapy,[64-66]

On the other hand, recent animal studies have suggested that the presence of chronic antral ulcer in rats shortens cancer induction time,[69] and benign-appearing gastric ulcers with a small focus of cancer at a margin have been described.

Pernicious Anemia

An increased incidence of gastric cancer in patients with pernicious anemia was first suggested many years ago by autopsy studies in which 10 per cent of the patients with pernicious anemia were found to have gastric cancer.[70] Subsequent clinical studies appear to confirm this association with a prevalence of gastric cancer being 1 to 12 per cent,[71] but many of these studies were done at times when the incidence of gastric cancer was much higher. In addition, other neoplastic lesions, including gastric polyps and carcinoids, are more common in patients with pernicious anemia, and some authors have suggested that many of these lesions were actually misinterpreted as adenocarcinomas.[72] Hoffman followed 48 patients with pernicious anemia for a mean time period of greater than 11 years, and no cases of gastric cancer were found.[73]

Though this evidence may indicate an overestimation of the problem, more recent studies support the earlier observation of an increased incidence of gastric cancer in pernicious anemia.[71, 74] Borch reported an 8.1 per cent prevalence of gastric neoplastic lesions (including four gastric cancers and five carcinoids) at a primary endoscopic screening of 123 patients.[71] It has also been suggested that some patients with carcinoma are in a "prepernicious anemia stage" without overt PA.[75]

Postgastrectomy

Several reports have suggested an increased incidence of gastric cancer following gastric resection for benign disease. This was particularly noticeable because the cancer occurred even though the most common site for this problem (antrum) had been resected. In larger series, persons having undergone gastric resection had an incidence of gastric cancer of 5 to 16 per cent.[76] Subsequently, prospective "studies" (that is, endoscopic examinations, regardless of symptoms, starting approximately 20 years after the surgery) reported an incidence of approximately 2 to 5 per cent.[77-82] In other studies, it has been noticed that patients with previous gastric surgery were overrepresented in patient populations with gastric cancer.[83, 84] There is also circumstantial evidence supporting this concept, including the observation that intestinal metaplasia is more common in the gastric remnant after resection and that the higher pH in the stomach following surgery could allow for the overgrowth of nitrite-producing bacteria.

Because these studies usually compare the incidence of gastric cancer in patients with gastrectomies who are undergoing endoscopy with patients who have not had resections and are undergoing endoscopy or with the incidence in the general population, it has been felt that the problem may be overestimated. A recent case control study examined the frequency of gastric surgery in 521 patients with gastric cancer as compared with a control group which was race, sex, and age matched. Gastric surgery was not found to be more frequent in those patients with gastric cancer.[85]

Likewise, recent studies from the United States,[86] Great Britain,[87] and Japan[88] evaluated patients who had had previous gastrectomies and determined that the incidence of gastric cancer in those having undergone surgery did not differ from the expected value for the general population.

Although these more recent studies are convincing, the numerous case reports and studies supporting a predilection for gastric cancer in individuals who have had gastric surgery cannot be ignored. Routine screening cannot be unconditionally recommended, but an individual who has had previous gastric surgery and develops symptoms should be evaluated endoscopically; and any suspicious lesion and possibly even normal-appearing stomal mucosa should be biopsied, particularly if it has been greater than 10 years since the surgery.

Most patients who have developed gastric cancer following surgery have undergone antrectomy with Billroth II anastomosis and gastrojejunostomy. It has been suggested that the cancer is more common if the initial surgery was for gastric ulcer rather than duodenal ulcer,[89] but not all studies confirm this. The incidence of gastric cancer appears to be directly related to the length of time following the initial surgery. Only rare cases are reported prior to 10 years, and most cases occur 20 years after the surgical procedure. There is a prominent male-to-female ratio in this situation, and it has been reported to be as high as 36:1. In persons who develop gastric cancer following surgery, the prognosis in most studies is poor, with very few five-year survivals.

Hypertrophic Gastropathy

Cases of gastric cancer occurring in persons with hypertrophic gastropathy (Menetrier's disease) have been reported.[90] Because of the rarity of this disease, the frequency of this complication is difficult to estimate, but prospective follow-up of patients with hypertrophic gastropathy suggests that it may be as high as 10 per cent.[91, 92]

Gastric Polyps

Gastric polyps are discussed elsewhere in this chapter (pp. 763 to 765).

Gastric Dysplasia

Much attention has been given to dysplasia arising in the colon and esophagus. Dysplasia has not arrived at the same status in the stomach, where it is occasionally seen, but it has the same significance.

Dysplasia is abnormal mucosa with the potential for undergoing malignant transformation. It is characterized by cellular atypia, abnormal differentiation, and disorganized mucosal architecture.[93–95] Some have proposed that in the presence of precancerous conditions (atrophic gastritis, intestinal metaplasia, adenomatous polyps, etc.), the addition of excessive cell proliferation and cellular dedifferentiation leads to a precancerous change (dysplasia).

The precancerous condition is probably reversible, as is the precancerous change, until a critical point is reached. This critical point depends on time, genetic and environmental factors, and possibly general and local immunity.

Dysplasia can vary from mild to severe, and at times it is very difficult to distinguish between dysplasia and malignancy. When dysplasia is encountered, follow-up biopsies are recommended at frequent intervals, and if the condition persists, resection should be considered.

CLINICAL PRESENTATION

Symptoms and Signs

As has been noticed from mass screening surveys, early gastric cancer in many instances is asymptomatic. When there are symptoms with EGC, these include pain, vague discomfort, or a sense of fullness in the epigastrium and nausea.[8, 9] Whether or not these symptoms are related to the cancer is uncertain because in many instances even large mass lesions do not become symptomatic until late. Physician examination in patients with early gastric cancer usually will detect no findings referable to that lesion.

With advanced gastric cancer, abdominal discomfort and weight loss are the most common presenting complaints. Though abdominal pain is usually the first symptom, weight loss is also present in many patients at the time of presentation.[96] Some have suggested that pain is more common when the tumor is in the body or on the lesser curve but the lesions on the greater curvature are silent. The abdominal pain may be an acute or chronic pain, resembling peptic ulcer disease, or may consist of a vague upper abdominal discomfort, burning, or fullness.

Depending upon the location of the cancer, obstructive symptoms may predominate (e.g., dysphagia from tumor in the cardia, or vomiting from tumor in the antrum). A clinical picture identical to achalasia has been described with submucosal infiltration of gastric carcinoma into the esophagus.[97, 98] Overt gastrointestinal bleeding, either hematemesis or more frequently melena, may occur. Nonspecific symptoms such as anorexia, weakness, change in bowel habits, and bloating may occur.

Gastric cancer may present with the manifestations secondary to metastasis. Patients may complain of abdominal swelling from ascites secondary to liver or peritoneal metastasis. Shortness of breath secondary to anemia or pleural effusions from lung metastasis may occur. Direct extension of gastric cancer into the colon (gastrocolic fistula) may be associated with foul-smelling emesis or the finding of recently ingested material in the stool.[99] Gastric carcinoma has been reported to present with nephrotic syndrome,[100] with thrombophlebitis (Trousseau's sign), and with a neuromyopathy.[101]

Physical examination in patients with advanced gastric cancer may likewise be unrevealing, or there may be an epigastric mass (in 30 per cent of patients), hepatomegaly from hepatic metastasis, cachexia, or ascites. Evidence of distant metastasis such as the so-called sentinel node or signal node of Virchow (supraclavicular node, particularly on the left), or left anterior axillary node (Irish's node), or mass in cul-de-sac (rectal shelf of Blumer), or infiltration of the umbilicus (Sister Joseph node) may be additional or the only manifestation. These should be conscientiously looked for if the diagnosis of gastric cancer is being considered, because these findings establish unresectability of the tumor.

Pelvic examination may reveal an enlarged ovary secondary to metastasis (Krukenberg tumor), which is usually bilateral on pathologic examination. Associated skin manifestations are rare and include nodules secondary to metastasis, acanthosis nigricans (hyperpigmentation, particularly in the axilla,[102] or sign of Leser-Trélat (sudden appearance of warty keratoses and pruritus).[103] Gastric cancer has also been associated with dermatomyositis.

Laboratory Tests

In early gastric cancer, routine laboratory studies are usually normal. With advanced disease, laboratory studies may also be normal, though hematologic evaluation may reveal an anemia secondary to acute blood loss, iron deficiency from chronic blood loss, or rarely macrocytic anemia secondary to pernicious anemia. Abnormal liver tests from hepatic metastasis may be seen. Chest X-ray may reveal metastatic disease to the lung or less likely to the bone. Distortion of fundic air bubble and increased distance between the base of the left lung and gastric bubble have been described in cancers of the fundus.[104]

ESTABLISHING THE DIAGNOSIS

Radiology and Endoscopy

When the patient presents with symptoms or signs which are believed to be referable to the upper gastrointestinal tract, the usual first diagnostic procedure is radiographic or endoscopic examination of the esophagus, stomach, and duodenum. Identification of early gastric cancer by X-ray requires that special compression techniques be used and double contrast medium examination be done (procedures that are not routine in all hospitals). Likewise, detection of early gastric cancer by endoscopy demands a thorough and systematic evaluation of the stomach by an endoscopist who is trained to detect subtle changes of texture and color and is willing to take multiple biopsies. In Japan much screening is by gastrocamera, and the film can then be reviewed and discussed, and the appropriate follow-up can be taken.

Advanced gastric cancer, on the other hand, usually presents grossly in one of several ways which are identified by radiologic or endoscopic techniques. As previously mentioned, these roughly correspond to Borrmann's classification of pathologic lesions which include polypoid (I), ulcerating with sharpy demarcated edges (II), ulcerating-infiltrating (III), and diffusely infiltrating (IV) (Fig. 44–8).

Classic radiologic criteria of benign gastric ulceration include smooth margins, abrupt projection from gastric wall, and penetration beyond expected course of the gastric wall.[105] Occasionally, there can be a radiolucent band between ulcer niche and lumen which is best seen on profile and is referred to as Hampton's line. This is felt to be typical of a benign ulcer but is not always present. The most reliable sign of benignity is the presence of radiating folds and areae gastricae (normal-appearing stomach surface) around the ulcer crater.

X-ray is usually very capable of demonstrating the presence of gastric cancer when it presents as a mass lesion or nondistensible stomach secondary to a diffuse infiltrating cancer. Further evaluation by endoscopy with biopsy is indicated in all these situations to attempt to make a definite diagnosis.

Histologic diagnosis of gastric cancer can be obtained at endoscopy by biopsy, cytologic examination, or a combination of these. The reported accuracy of biopsy varies, but more recent studies indicate that biopsies alone provide the diagnosis in 79 to 85 per cent of cases.[106-108] The diagnosis is more likely to be made with exophytic lesions than infiltrative or ulcer-like lesions. When cytologic examination is added to biopsy, the diagnostic rate is reported to be greater than 95 per cent. When biopsy alone is to be used, it has been demonstrated that diagnostic accuracy increases as more biopsies are taken. Graham found that the first biopsy yielded the correct diagnosis is 70 per cent of gastric cancer cases, and four biopsies increased the yield to 95 per cent; and with seven biopsies, the yield was 100 per cent.[109] Likewise, another study demonstrated a greater than 99 per cent chance of diagnosing gastric cancer with eight biopsies.[110]

It is recommended, therefore, that multiple biopsies (seven or eight) be taken from the lesion of concern. If fewer biopsies are taken, then cytologic examination should be added. Cytologic examination should be considered strongly in infiltrative and ulcer-like lesions. Biopsies from ulcer-like lesions should be taken from both the edge and base for greatest accuracy.[111]

The most commonly used method for obtaining cytologic specimens involves the use of small brushes which are passed through the endoscope in protective plastic sheaths. The brush is extended from the sheath and placed directly on the lesion and twisted. When brushing is completed, the brush is retracted into the sheath and withdrawn. It probably does not matter whether biopsy or brushing is done first. Brushing lesions first may irritate the lesion and cause bleeding which might obscure the area and interfere with accurate biopsy.

Special Studies

Gastric Secretory Studies. Approximately 65 per cent of patients with gastric cancer have fasting achlorhydria, as compared with 15 to 25 per cent of normal persons in the cancer age range.[112] Less than 20 to 25 per cent of persons with gastric cancer have achlorhydria following maximal stimulation. The presence of achlorhydria in a patient with a gastric ulcer who does not use ulcerogenic drugs increases the likelihood of malignancy.

Pepsinogen. Persons with extensive atrophic gastritis and intestinal metaplasia have low serum pepsinogen levels. It has been suggested that a low level might identify a high-risk group of individuals who deserve intermittent evaluation for gastric cancer. In one study, a low serum pepsinogen level was found in 31 per cent of patients with gastric cancer and 6 per cent of matched control subjects.[76]

Carcinoembryonic Antigen (CEA). Serum CEA levels are less frequently elevated in gastric carcinoma than in colon carcinoma. Only 19 to 35 per cent of patients with advanced gastric cancer and 4.5 per cent of patients with EGC have elevated serum levels (> 5 ng/ml).[113, 114] Approximately 54 per cent of patients with gastric cancer had levels above 2.5 ng/ml, but so did 10 per cent of the normal population. Elevated concentrations of CEA in gastric juice have been found in 50 per cent of patients with early and advanced gastric cancer. Recent attempts to use CEA in gastric juice to separate patients revealed much overlap. Though CEA concentration greater than 100 ng/ml was seen in 88 per cent of gastric cancer cases, a similar concentration was observed in 54 per cent of patients with gastric ulcer and 89 per cent of patients with moderate to severe chronic atrophic gastritis.[115] Serum CEA levels have no role in the diagnosis of gastric cancer, but as in colon cancer, postoperative follow-up of elevated preoperative levels might be helpful.

Fetal Sulfoglycoprotein Antigen (FSA). FSA has been detected in the gastric juice of 96 per cent of patients with gastric cancer and 14 per cent of patients with benign gastric diseases.[113]

PREOPERATIVE STAGING

After identification of the gastric lesion by X-ray or endoscopy and confirmation of diagnosis with biopsy, computed tomography (CT scan) should be considered. This not only helps identify liver metastasis but may provide information about extragastric extension of stomach cancer and nodal involvement. Initially it was reported that computed tomography correlated closely with surgical findings and was useful in staging gastric adenocarcinoma by demonstrating distant metastasis, extragastric extension, and lymph node involvement.[117] Recent studies have shown that CT scan is not always reliable.[118, 119] Cook found that CT scan underestimated disease in 51 per cent of patients, and in three out of six patients predicted to have extensive disease the gastric cancer was confined to the stomach or regional nodes. Despite these latter reports, CT scanning does provide information which may be of assistance in determining type of therapy.

TREATMENT

The therapeutic stages of gastric cancer have been identified. First is local disease in which the primary therapy is surgery. Adjuvant chemotherapy may be considered in this situation. The second stage concerns disseminated disease, that is, disease in which the presence of distant metastasis has been established. Surgery is undertaken for palliation, and chemotherapy

may be the primary therapy. The third stage is locally advanced, nonresectable disease. Resection may have been attempted but was unsuccessful, and when additional therapy is undertaken, it consists of chemotherapy or irradiation therapy.

Local Disease

If there is no evidence of distant metastasis in an operable patient, surgical resection for cure should be attempted. The choice of procedure depends upon location of the tumor but usually consists of a subtotal resection for proximal and distal lesions. At times, location or size of tumor requires that total gastrectomy be done. Because wide resections might be necessary to ensure microscopically tumor-free margins[120] and because gastric cancer may have a multicentric origin, it has been suggested by some that total gastrectomy be done routinely, particularly for cancer of the proximal stomach. Because of the high mortality and morbidity rates with total gastrectomy for gastric cancer and because randomized studies showing a definite advantage of this operation over limited resection are not available, it is not possible to make this a uniform recommendation, though at times it will be necessary.[121] It is important that extensive lymphadenectomies be done when resecting for cure in patients with gastric cancer.[122, 123]

The Japanese Research Society for Gastric Cancer published their general rules in 1962 to help classify the extent of disease and determine the type of resection to be done.[124] Lymph nodes draining the stomach were divided into four groups. Group 1 nodes are strictly perigastric lymph nodes, including right and left cardiac, lesser and greater curvature, and supra- and infrapyloric nodes. Group 2 nodes are more distant than those in group 1 and include the lymph node located along the left gastric, common hepatic, and splenic arteries as well as around the celiac artery and splenic hilus. Group 3 nodes are more distant than those in group 2 and include those located in hepatoduodenal ligament, on the posterior aspect of the pancreas, at the root of the mesentery, and at the diaphragm and periesophageal nodes. Group 4 includes all lymph nodes further away than group 3. These have been designated N_1 through N_4, respectively.

An absolute curative resection can be defined as follows: (1) no evidence of distant metastasis, (2) no residual cancer at the margin of the excised stomach, (3) resection of adjacent structures if involved, and (4) adequate lymph node dissection. To achieve the latter, the most distant group of lymph nodes resected (R_1 to R_4) is at least one group farther away than where nodal involvement with cancer was found. (The "R" number is greater than the "N" number.[125])

In a curative resection, the omentum and spleen are often included in the resection to ensure removal of the splenic hilus nodes. Regardless of the type of surgery, if a curative resection has been performed, the patient might be considered for adjuvant chemotherapy or irradiation (see p. 757).

Disseminated Disease or Evidence of Distant Metastasis

When physical examination and subsequent special studies (such as lymph node or liver biopsy) confirm the presence of distant metastasis, surgery should not be undertaken unless there are symptoms that require palliation, such as obstruction or bleeding. Severe pain is not a frequent problem with gastric cancer, and when pain is present surgery is not uniformly effective in relieving it.

For distal obstruction of the stomach, palliation usually consists of simple gastrojejunostomy if there is sufficient uninvolved stomach. In some patients, in order to obtain palliation from obstruction or bleeding, partial gastric resection is necessary. Laser therapy has been used to recanalize proximal obstructing lesions,[126] and prosthetic stents have been placed for proximal lesions.[127] Total gastrectomy for palliation should be discouraged.

Some have suggested that even in the presence of distant metastasis, patients are more comfortable and even live longer with radical resection.[121] These studies have to be interpreted carefully because no randomized control group is used in these analyses, most of which are retrospective. There is no evidence that extensive debulking of the primary tumor improves response to chemotherapy in persons with distant metastasis.

Locally Advanced, Nonresectable Disease

When preoperative evaluation reveals no evidence of distant metastasis but physical examination or special studies (such as CT scan) reveal extragastric extension of the tumor, the course to pursue is not always clear. Incurability cannot be assumed in this situation, and exploratory laparotomy should be considered to evaluate the extent of the disease and attempted resection. By en bloc resection of involved adjacent organs, a curative resection sometimes can be accomplished. When this cannot be done, essentially locally advanced nonresectable disease remains. In these patients, chemotherapy and irradiation can be offered.

Chemotherapy

Gastrointestinal cancers respond poorly to chemotherapy; however, gastric cancer is considered the most responsive.[129]

Single Agent. Several drugs have been used alone in the treatment of gastric cancer. Responses (i.e., 50 per cent reduction in size of a measurable lesion) with the active agents are seen in approximately 20 to 25 per cent of patients, but the response duration is brief and adds little to the patient's survival.[130, 131] The most extensively studied agent is 5-fluorouracil (5-FU). Though oral 5-FU has been used, the usual method of administration is intravenous. Despite years of use, the dose and schedule of administration are not uniform. Daily or weekly bolus injections are the most common

route of administration, but continuous infusions for several days is an alternative.[132] 5-FU has an objective response rate of approximately 20 per cent.

Mitomycin C is another drug which has been widely used. Initially, high response rates were reported in Japan, but cumulative bone marrow toxicity was a major problem. Less frequent dosing has made this drug better tolerated, and response rates in the United States have been approximately 25 per cent.[133] Unlike colon cancer, gastric cancer has been found to be responsive to doxorubicin (Adriamycin) and nitrosoureas (approximately 25 per cent and 19 per cent response rate, respectively). The folate antagonists, triazinate and cisplatin, have recently been shown to demonstrate some activity.[134–136]

Combination Chemotherapy. 5-FU with a nitrosurea (BCNU or methyl-CCNU) was the first combination used. Not only was a greater response rate demonstrated with the combination, but an increased survival time at 18 months was observed when compared with the single agent 5-FU alone.[137] Other studies were not consistently able to confirm these results.

After the Japanese demonstrated a response with mitomycin C, this was incorporated in the combination of programs with 5-FU. No significant improvement in survival was noted, so a regimen incorporating doxorubicin (Adriamycin) with these two drugs was developed. This regimen, FAM, was associated with a response rate of 42 per cent. The median duration and survival in responding patients was 12.5 months as compared with 3.5 months in the nonresponders.[138]

Substituting the mitomycin C in the FAM regimen with methyl-CCNU (FAMe) has also been shown to have activity against gastric cancer. This combination of 5-FU, Adriamycin, and methyl-CCNU (FAMe) has been compared with FAM, and no significant difference between the two regimens was observed by the Gastrointestinal Tumor Study Group.[139] The Eastern Cooperative Oncology Group found a 39 per cent response with FAM, 29 per cent with FAMe, 29 per cent with Adriamycin and mitomycin C, and 14 per cent response rate with 5-FU and methyl-CCNU (FUMe).[140] The combination of platinum with 5-FU and Adriamycin (FAP) was shown to have a 29 per cent response rate by Wooley,[141] and more recently, Wagener reported a 50 per cent response rate suggesting that cisplatin was as effective as mitomycin in combination with 5-FU and Adriamycin.[142] This 50 per cent response rate was confirmed by Moertel.[143] Other combinations being evaluated include 5-FU, Adriamycin, and methotrexate (FAMeth).

Radiotherapy. Radiotherapy has been used in patients with locally unresectable and recurrent disease. There are reports of improved survival with external radiotherapy alone in these situations, but others have failed to confirm this. It is believed that the definitive irradiation dose (6000 to 6600 rad) cannot be delivered because of adjacent radiosensitive organs. Intraoperative radiotherapy might overcome this by allowing directed radiation therapy.[131]

Early studies have suggested that radiation treatment might be potentiated by the addition of 5-FU. Studies in patients with unresectable cancer have shown a 55 per cent response rate with radiation and 5-FU, but there was only a 17 per cent response rate with 5-FU alone and no response with the radiation alone.[144] This was confirmed in a study from the Mayo Clinic in which patients with unresectable cancer receiving irradiation and 5-FU had 13 months survival compared with approximately six months survival for patients with placebo and irradiation.[145] In subsequent studies, irradiation and combination chemotherapy have been compared with combination chemotherapy alone.

The Gastrointestinal Tumor Study Group (GITSG) compared 5-FU and methyl-CCNU versus irradiation and 5-FU in 96 patients.[146] At the end of the first year, the chemotherapy group had a 68 per cent survival rate, while the combined chemotherapy and irradiation therapy group had a survival rate of 44 per cent. At three years, though, the survival lines crossed, and there was an 18 per cent survival rate with the combined modality and a 7 per cent survival rate for the chemotherapy groups alone. The most recent follow-up has indicated eight persons are still alive from this study—six from the combined modality group and two from the chemotherapy group alone.[131] Protocol and pilot studies have been introduced using combination chemotherapy consisting of FAM with irradiation.[147]

Adjuvant Therapy. With the high rate of recurrence in gastric cancer following a curative resection, adjuvant therapy would seem reasonable to consider. Some studies using 5-FU alone have demonstrated a prolongation of time to recurrence without a definite influence on survival. Other reports using 5-FU have failed to show an advantage. There are several adjuvant chemotherapy studies under way at this time, including one by GITSG consisting of 5-FU and methyl-CCNU (FUMe).[148] For those undergoing surgery who were not receiving adjuvant chemotherapy, the median survival time was approximately 33 months, and the median time to recurrence was 30 months. In patients who had received adjuvant chemotherapy following surgery, the median survival was 48 months. The probability of five-year survival was 27 per cent in the control group and 43 per cent in the treatment group, while seven-year survival was 18 per cent and 37 per cent, respectively. ECOG found no difference in survival with adjuvant therapy with FUMe when compared with a control group, but patients with microscopic residual tumor were included. (E. Livstone, personal communication). Because of the possibility of developing leukemia following long-term methyl-CCNU use, it is no longer available. Other adjuvant protocols using FAM are under way.

If one examines the pattern of recurrence in patients who have had curative resections for gastric cancer, the majority occur locally. Gunderson and Sosin reported the results of reoperation in this group of patients.[49] In 88 per cent of their patients, the recurrence was local or regional, and 46 per cent of the patients had no evidence of distant metastasis. This raises the possibility that radiotherapy with or without chemotherapy may be useful as adjuvant therapy. Studies to evaluate this are under way.

Table 44–1. PROGNOSIS ACCORDING TO DEPTH OF INVASION AND LYMPH NODE INVOLVEMENT*

Feature	Five-Year Survival (%)
Depth of Invasion	
Mucosa	100
Submucosa	90
Muscularis propria	70
Subserosa	50
Serosa 1	40
Serosa 2	22
Serosa 3	7
Nodal involvement	
N (−)	80
N_1 (+)	39
N_2 (+)	23
N_3 (+)	11
N_4 (+)	8

*From Miwa, K. Cancer of the stomach in Japan. Gann Monograph on Cancer Research 22:61, 1979.

PROGNOSIS OF GASTRIC CANCER

Many factors have been evaluated with regard to prognosis of gastric cancer. The only factor which is consistently related to prognosis is the extent of the disease; that is, the degree of invasion of the gastric wall, the presence or absence of lymph node involvement, and peritoneal and distant metastasis. Table 44–1 presents data from Miwa as an example to demonstrate prognosis based on depth of invasion and lymph node involvement.[124]

Since it has been demonstrated that the presence or absence of lymph node involvement and distant metastasis is directly related to the degree of invasion of the gastric wall (Fig. 44–10), this latter factor appears to be the primary prognostic indicator; but the factors that influence cancer invasion in the stomach are uncertain.

Other factors may also influence prognosis, and these will be reviewed. Perhaps one or more of these is the unknown factor(s) which governs the degree of invasion.

Age and Sex

Very young and older patients with gastric cancer do not do as well as middle-aged patients. No difference in survival rates between men and women has been identified except in one study in which females had a greater seven-year survival rate.[150]

Histology

In some studies, undifferentiated adenocarcinoma is more likely to have metastasized at the time of presentation.[151] Gastric carcinoma with a nondesmoplastic stroma infiltrated with lymphocytes has been associated with a good prognosis,[152] as has a cancer cell–free dense submucosal fibrosis.[153] Lauren's intestinal type of gastric carcinoma has been associated with a better

	DEPTH OF INVASION	% WITH LYMPH NODE INVOLVEMENT		FIVE YEAR SURVIVAL	
EARLY GASTRIC CANCER	MUCOSA	7%	24%	91%	78%
	SUBMUCOSA	14%		81%	
ADVANCED GASTRIC CANCER	MUSCULARIS	45%	68%	36%	21%
	SEROSA	66%		4%	

Figure 44–10. The percentage of patients with gastric cancer who have lymph node involvement increases as the depth of invasion progresses from mucosa to serosa. The five-year survival decreases as depth of invasion increases. (In some reports, represented in the second and fourth columns, the patients were classified only as having early or advanced gastric cancer.)

prognosis than the diffuse type. Since carcinoids have a better survival and a more indolent course, gastric cancers have been stained for the number of endocrine cells, but it has been found that the presence or absence of endocrine cells in an adenocarcinoma did not affect survival.[154]

Location, Gross Appearance, and Size

Gastric neoplasms located in the distal stomach appear to have a better prognosis than those in the proximal stomach. Sharply demarcated lesions do better than diffuse disease. Polypoid (Borrmann's I) and ulcerating (II) are less likely to have nodal involvement than ulcerating-infiltrating (III) and infiltrating (IV) types. It has been noted that gastric cancers presenting as benign ulcers do better because there is less extensive invasion at the time they are discovered.[155]

In general, smaller lesions have a better prognosis than larger lesions, as the depth of invasion is usually not as great.[153]

Immunocompetence

Positive PPD and DNCB (dinitrochlorbenzene) skin tests have been shown to be less frequent in persons with gastric cancer when compared with patients with other gastrointestinal diseases and control subjects.[113] Furthermore, persons with gastric cancer and positive tests generally have less advanced disease and are more frequently able to undergo curative resection than those with negative skin tests. Whether this is the reason for or the effect of less extensive disease is uncertain. Studies of peripheral T and B cells have failed to identify any abnormality.

HLA Type

Although no specific HLA type has been identified with gastric cancer, Hayashi reported a high frequency of HLA-DR4 antigen in long-term survivors.[156]

CEA

Serum CEA concentrations have not been consistently correlated with extent of disease or survival, but recently it has been demonstrated that gastric cancer tissue itself which stained negative or weakly positive for CEA had better survival than those staining strongly positive,[157] perhaps because they respond better to chemotherapy.[158]

Other

Recent studies have shown that gastric cancers with human epidermal growth factors present on histochemical analysis have a poor prognosis.[159] Estrogen and progesterone receptors have been identified in gastric cancer.[160] The significance of this finding with regard to prognosis and response to therapy is being evaluated.

Prognosis Depending on the Type of Therapy

In this section, prognosis is evaluated on the basis of the type of therapy a patient received. Though it is understood that the type of therapy is usually dictated by extent of disease, this may not always be the situation. In addition, many series do not report details about extent of disease, and survival is reported only on the basis of type of surgical therapy.

Prognosis in Untreated Cases. Patients with gastric cancer who receive no therapy, regardless of the reason, have a mean survival time of approximately 11 months from time of diagnosis.[112] While many of these patients are not treated because they are unlikely to be cured by surgery, some with less extensive disease are not surgical candidates because they refuse surgery. If only those who are inoperable owing to cancer are considered, the prognosis is very poor. In one study, 84 per cent were dead by six months and 96 per cent by one year.

Prognosis for Patients Who Have Undergone Diagnostic Exploratory Laparotomy Alone. The mean survival time in this group of patients is consistently reported to be four to five months.[112, 161–164] This is less than the untreated group, but in those patients undergoing exploratory laparotomy alone, extensive disease and unresectability are confirmed, not just suspected. With the additional morbidity of surgery, this group has a worse prognosis.

Prognosis for Patients Who Have Undergone Palliative Surgical Procedure. Those patients who undergo palliative bypass procedure also have a mean survival period of four to five months.[112, 161–164] These patients probably are actually the same group as mentioned in the previous section but in addition to confirming extensive disease at laparotomy, a simple bypass procedure was performed. On the other hand, if the surgical procedure for palliation is noncurative resection, a mean survival time of 9 to 14 months has been reported. Five-year survivals in this group are rarely reported.[112, 162]

Prognosis for Patients Who Have Undergone Curative Resections. If at the time of laparotomy and pathologic examination it appears that a curative resection has been performed, the mean survival for such a patient is 28 months.[161] Five-year survivals of approximately 40 per cent are reported.[162]

Overall Prognosis. The overall five-year survival in patients with gastric cancer is less than 10 per cent in most series from the United States. As previously mentioned, this figure will vary with the number of cases of early gastric cancer. For instance, in Japan, where survival rates are higher than in the United States, as much as one third of all gastric cancer is EGC.

Prognosis According to Stage (TMN)

The TMN classification for gastric cancer was initially proposed in 1970[165] and revised in 1977[166] as a method of staging gastric cancer (Table 44–2). The "T" indicates the depth of tumor infiltration; mucosal and submucosal involvement is designated as T_1, muscularis invasion as T_2, and serosal invasion as T_3. In the original classification, T_4 indicated diffuse involvement of the stomach but now indicates invasion of contiguous organs. The "N" indicates the presence or absence of lymph node involvement and the extent as designated by subscripts 0 to 3. M_0 designates no metastasis, while M_1 is used if metastases are present. In 1977, the "R" classification was introduced in which R_0 is no residual tumor following surgery, R_1 is microscopic residual tumor, and R_2 is macroscopic residual tumor. From these, stages I through IV are defined as in Figure 44–11. The five-year survival rate is greater than 90 per cent in stage I, approximately 50 per cent in stage II, 10 per cent in stage III, and rarely ever seen in stage IV of the disease. Most patients in the United States are stage III or IV at the time of diagnosis.

Table 44–2. TNM CLASSIFICATION

Primary Tumor (T)

T1   Tumor limited to mucosa and submucosa regardless of its extent or location

T2   Tumor involves the mucosa and the submucosa (including the muscularis proprial), and extends to or into the serosa but does not penetrate through the serosa

T3   Tumor penetrates through the serosa without invading contiguous structures

T4   Tumor penetrates through the serosa and invades the contiguous structures

Nodal Involvement (N)

N0   No metastases to regional lymph nodes

N1   Involvement of perigastric lymph nodes within 3 cm of the primary tumor along the lesser or greater curvature

N2   Involvement of the regional lymph nodes, more than 3 cm from the primary tumor, which are removable at operation, including splenic, celiac, and common hepatic arteries

N3   Involvement of other intra-abdominal lymph nodes which are not removable to operation, such as the para-aortic, hepatoduodenal, retropancreatic, and mesenteric nodes

Distant Metastasis (M)

M0   No (known) distant metastasis

M1   Distant metastasis present

WHAT HAPPENS TO PATIENTS WITH GASTRIC CANCER?

After review of large series of patients with gastric cancer, one can predict what will happen to patients with this problem. Out of each 100 patients with gastric cancer, approximately 86 underwent surgical exploration. The other 14 were considered inoperable because of distant metastasis, had medical contraindication to surgery, or refused surgery. Of the 86 operated on, curative resection was performed in 45 (approximately half the patients), while palliative or diagnostic procedures were done in the remaining. Even though these were palliative, many were extensive resections. Postoperative mortality rate varies from series to series but averages 11 per cent in the patients undergoing curative resection and 24 per cent in those undergoing a palliative procedure. It is not unusual to see a higher

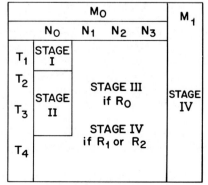

Figure 44–11. The TNM classification provides for stages as defined in this figure.

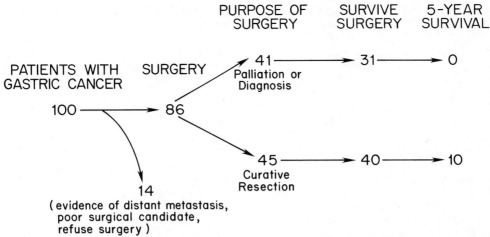

PURPOSE OF   SURVIVE   5-YEAR
SURGERY   SURGERY   SURVIVAL

Figure 44–12. This scheme, which summarizes the survival results of several large series, suggests what happens to 100 patients with the diagnosis of gastric cancer.

mortality rate in this latter group which usually consists of sicker patients with more extensive disease. The five-year survival rate in those undergoing and surviving curative resection is approximately 25 per cent, while in those undergoing palliative or diagnostic procedures, five-year survivors are unusual. The overall five-year survival rate in the United States is, therefore, approximately 10 per cent (Fig. 44–12). Obviously the survival rate will vary among institutions, depending on how many early gastric cancers are included.

GASTRIC LYMPHOMA

Primary lymphoma of the stomach is much less common than adenocarcinoma of the stomach, and in most reviews it represents less than 5 per cent of all gastric neoplasms. At larger referral centers, it may account for a higher percentage of neoplasms of the stomach because patients with lymphoma are more readily referred for irradiation and chemotherapy.

This disease represents 2 to 3 per cent of all non-Hodgkin's lymphomas and, therefore, is the most common (~ 15 to 20 per cent) of all extranodal non-Hodgkin's lymphomas.[167] Hodgkin's disease of the stomach occurs but is uncommon.

Clinical Features

The usual presenting symptoms of patients with gastric lymphoma, which include abdominal pain, nausea, vomiting, and weight loss, are not different from those seen with gastric adenocarcinoma.[168–170]

By barium examination, lymphomas may appear as polypoid, ulcerating, or infiltrative lesions. They, therefore, cannot be distinguished from gastric cancer in many instances. Some of the patterns more suggestive of lymphoma are thickening of gastric folds without luminal narrowing, extension into the duodenum

(while esophageal extension is more common with adenocarcinoma), and multiple masses and areas of ulceration.

Similarly, examination by endoscopy may confirm the presence of a neoplastic-appearing process, but on gross examination, it may be difficult to distinguish accurately between lymphoma and adenocarcinoma. When the lesion is polypoid or ulcerative, endoscopic biopsy may provide the diagnosis, but just as with adenocarcinoma, the infiltrative type of lymphoma will frequently defy diagnosis by usual endoscopic biopsy techniques. In this situation, a lift and cut technique using a snare has been suggested as a safe method of obtaining adequate tissue for histologic examination.[171] In many instances, adequate tissue for diagnosis can be obtained only at laparotomy.

Pathology

Gastric lymphomas arise from the lymphoid tissue in the submucosa and may extend into the mucosa or beyond the lamina propria through the serosa to involve adjacent regional nodes. Histologic classification of non-Hodgkin's lymphoma of the stomach is usually according to the system developed by Rappaport.[172] This classification divides lymphoma into nodular or diffuse types on the basis of architecture, and further refinement depends upon cell characteristics, i.e., well differentiated or poorly differentiated lymphocytes, histiocytes, or mixed. The most common is histiocytic of the diffuse type.

The Rappaport classification may not be perfect, and in fact, the term histiocytic may be incorrect. The large cells found in the neoplasm are not true histiocytes but transformed lymphocytes.[173] Therefore, newer classifications have been developed based on morphologic and immunologic features. All of these systems were evaluated by the National Cancer Institute recently.[174]

Table 44–3. STAGING SYSTEM FOR PRIMARY GASTRIC LYMPHOMA

I_E	Involvement of single extranodal site
II_E	Localized involvement of an extranodal site and its lymph node chain
III_E	Involvement of lymph node region on both sides of the diaphragm and localized involvement of an extranodal site
IV	Diffuse or disseminated involvement

Staging

Although staging systems for extranodal non-Hodgkin's lymphomas are difficult to use, it is important that some standard method for identifying and relaying information about disease activity and extent be available. The TNM classification developed for gastric cancer (Table 44–2) has been used by some,[175] but the most common method for staging gastric lymphoma is the Ann Arbor system or a modification of it (Table 44–3).[176] Stage I_E indicates involvement of the stomach alone without lymph node involvement. (Penetration into an adjacent structure would not change the stage.) In stage II_E, in addition to the stomach, lymph nodes are involved. Some have further separated this category into II_{1E} (involvement of contiguous nodes) and II_{2E} (involvement of noncontiguous nodes but on the same side of the diaphragm).[176] Stage III_E is lymph node involvement on both sides of the diaphragm, and stage IV is disseminated disease. In the latter two stages, it may be impossible to distinguish primary from secondary lymphoma of the stomach because a significant percentage of patients with what is considered nodal non-Hodgkin's lymphoma will have gastric involvement on pathologic evaluation. Extensive involvement of the stomach suggests that the disease started at this point and spread to nodal sites.

Treatment

With stage I_E disease, resection of the involved stomach and contiguous organs should be attempted. Radiation therapy has been the primary modality of therapy in special situations, such as poor operative candidates, and in patients who refuse surgery. Whether the addition of radiation postoperatively in I_E disease is better than resection alone has not been established.[177] Adjuvant chemotherapy in this situation has also been suggested but is not standard procedure.

Approach to stage II_E disease is not as clear. Because the disease is more extensive, combination chemotherapy and irradiation have been recommended as the best approach.[178] Others believe that because of potential problems with perforation or bleeding with rapid tumor resolution following chemotherapy or irradiation, surgery should be first performed in stage II (and perhaps in stages III and IV where large, bulky tumors are present), followed by chemotherapy and irradiation.[179, 180] Besides, exploration provides a more precise staging.

Others feel that separating II_E into II_{1E} and II_{2E} may help determine therapy. Stage II_{1E} would be disease confined to the stomach and contiguous nodes, so radical resection followed by radiotherapy or chemotherapy would be a more reasonable approach. Stage II_{2E}, with more extensive nodal involvement, would be treated with chemotherapy and irradiation primarily. In stages III_E and IV the primary therapy would be combination chemotherapy. Palliative surgical procedures or irradiation in stages III_E and IV occasionally would be necessary for obstruction or bleeding, but in many instances it is hoped that these symptoms may resolve with chemotherapy if the patient can be temporarily supported.[178]

The chemotherapeutic agents most commonly used are CAOP (cyclophosphamide, Adriamycin, vincristine, and prednisone) or C-MOPP (cyclophosphamide, vincristine, procarbazine, and prednisone).

Out of each 100 patients with gastric lymphoma, about 95 will undergo surgery. Approximately 86 will have a curative resection (i.e., no residual tumor at the conclusion of surgery). The average mortality rate is 7 per cent, leaving 80 postoperative survivors, approximately 50 per cent of whom will survive five years. In the series reviewed, at least half of these latter patients were also treated with irradiation, but these patients were not randomly assigned to different therapies, so it is difficult to assess this factor. This can be compared to the course of adenocarcinoma in Figure 44–12.

Prognosis

When Lim staged gastric lymphoma using the 1970 TNM classification, he found that, like gastric cancer, survival with lymphoma was correlated with depth of invasion and involvement of perigastric lymph nodes.[175] The T_1 lesions were associated with an 82 per cent five-year survival rate, T_2 with a 65 per cent five-year survival rate, and T_3 with a 24 per cent five-year survival. N_0 lesions had a five-year survival rate of 88 per cent, while N_1 lesions had a five-year survival rate of 32 per cent.

The N_0 lesions would correspond to the stage I_E (of the Ann Arbor Staging System), which has been shown to have a similar 75 to 80 per cent five-year survival rate, while in stage II_E there is approximately a 40 per cent five-year survival. There are seldom five-year survivors with stages III_E or IV. Approximately 50 per cent of patients with gastric lymphoma will be stage I (TNM) or stage I_E (Ann Arbor). As a comparison, approximately 5 per cent of adenocarcinoma will be detected at these early stages. The overall five-year survival rate in patients with gastric lymphoma is approximately 47 to 57 per cent.[170, 177]

Besides depth of invasion and lymph node involvement, several other factors have been evaluated as prognostic factors. Though gastric lymphomas are rare and only small groups are reported, it appears that histologic characteristics can be a prognostic indicator (which is unlike the experience with gastric cancer) with the nodular form of lymphoma doing better. Some studies have found that the larger-sized tumors (> 8 to 10 cm) are associated with a worse prognosis than smaller tumors, and lesions in the distal stomach appear to be associated with a better prognosis than proximal disease.

Pseudolymphoma

Pseudolymphoma is caused by an intense or exaggerated lymphocyte infiltration usually in the presence of benign diseases, such as peptic ulcer.[181–183] With small endoscopic biopsies it is difficult to distinguish this entity from lymphoma, and because lymphoma may present as an ulcer-like lesion, it is also difficult to distinguish the lesions clinically. Histologic examination of a surgically resected specimen is required in many cases. Pseudolymphoma has a polymorphous cellular infiltrate, follicle formation with true germinal centers, and lack of nodal involvement. It is usually a smaller lesion than lymphomas. On the other hand, presence of regional node involvement, invasion through the serosa, or invasion of vessels suggests malignant lymphoma. The regional lymph nodes in pseudolymphoma may show reactive changes, and although pseudolymphoma may infiltrate the muscular wall, it does not destroy it.

Immunologic studies are also helpful in distinguishing between the two lesions. The finding of a monoclonal pattern of immunoglobulin in cells is evidence for lymphoma.

The reasons to resect pseudolymphomatous lesions are to establish a definitive tissue diagnosis and to manage symptoms. Because the lesion is confined to the distal stomach in most cases, limited resections are usually sufficient. Recently, it has been suggested that pseudolymphoma may be a precursor lesion with malignant potential.[184]

GASTRIC POLYPS

Though any discrete protrusion into the lumen of the stomach detected by X-ray or endoscopy has been referred to as a gastric polyp, more discriminate use of the term should be considered. Many of these luminal protrusions are nonepithelial, being derived from the mesenchymal tissue of the submucosa (such as a leiomyoma), and are separate pathologic entities. In this chapter, the term "polyp" will refer only to epithelial lesions that are adenomatous (including the infrequently seen villous adenoma of the stomach) or hyperplastic. It is recommended that discrete protrusions identified on X-ray or endoscopy be referred to as a polypoid or elevated lesion until histologic diagnosis is made. Using these terms in a more discriminate manner would facilitate a more accurate assessment of incidence, malignant potential, and other clinical features of gastric polyps.

Incidence

Gastric polyps are uncommon. Review of several autopsy series revealed a 0.4 per cent incidence of gastric "polyps,"[185] and a similar incidence has been reported in routine radiographic examinations of patients whose symptoms are not given.[186] Radiographic and endoscopic survey in symptomatic patients usually reveals a higher incidence of polyps. Once again, histologic diagnosis may not always be available in these studies in which a polyp refers to any luminal protrusion.

Blackstone reported 103 epithelial polyps in 5000 examinations (endoscopic) of the upper gastrointestinal tract for an incidence of 2 per cent.[187] As a comparison, autopsy series have suggested that 7 to 51 per cent of colons examined have adenomatous polyps, albeit many of them are very small; and it is estimated that 5 to 10 per cent of asymptomatic persons undergoing barium enema examinations will have a polypoid lesion eventually proving to be an adenomatous polyp.[186, 188]

Clinical Features

Though most polyps are discovered in radiographic and endoscopic examinations in patients complaining of nausea, abdominal pain, and other gastrointestinal complaints, it is doubtful these lesions are responsible for those nonspecific symptoms in most cases. Upper gastrointestinal bleeding from an ulcerated polyp or obstructive symptoms from a pedunculated antral polyp prolapsing through the pylorus may be the only symptoms which can be definitely ascribed to a gastric polyp. Approximately 85 per cent of patients with gastric polyps have achlorhydria. An increased incidence of polyps is found in persons with atrophic gastritis, pernicious anemia, and gastric cancer, and more recently, hyperplastic polyps have been described adjacent to the gastroenterostomy site following gastric resection.

Pathology

Hyperplastic polyps, also referred to as regenerative polyps, are the most common polyp seen in the stomach, representing over 75 to 90 per cent of such lesions.[189] Some authors have referred to this as hyperplasiogenic.[190] Grossly, these polyps are usually solitary, small (< 2 cm),[191] either sessile or pedunculated, smooth lesions with no predilection for site, occurring as frequently in the antrum as in the proximal stomach. A diffuse hyperplastic gastric polyposis can be seen and may represent a form of Menetrier's disease.[192] Microscopically, these polyps consist of branching or elongated and hyperplastic glands which may be markedly dilated or cystic. Bundles of smooth muscle fibers from invaginated muscularis mucosa are often observed in the polyp. The glandular changes merge with the normal epithelium, and it may be difficult to distinguish a sharp margin for the polyp. The interstitium of the polyp usually contains a lymphocytic infiltrate of varying degree. Because hyperplastic polyps are a reactionary change of normal mucosa, they are not true neoplasms, and therefore they are not felt to be capable of malignant degeneration. Despite this, malignant change in a hyperplastic polyp has rarely been reported.[189, 193–195] Hyperplastic polyps are also frequently found in a stomach harboring a carcinoma at a different site.[189]

Adenomatous polyps represent the second most common type of polyp. These can be sessile or pedunculated and are more likely to be found in the antrum. These adenomas usually adopt a tubulovillous (villoglandular) pattern. Villous adenomas of the stomach have been reported rarely.[196] This is unlike the colon, where the majority of adenomas are tubular adenomas. Microscopically, abrupt changes between the adenomatous epithelium and the normal gastric epithelium can be seen. This polyp appears to be a true neoplasm, with glands composed of poorly differentiated cells with large hyperchromatic nuclei, scant or absent mucus, and frequent mitotic figures.

Because the adenoma is a true neoplasm, there is concern that malignant degeneration may occur. Though the relationship cannot be conclusively proved, the evidence strongly suggests that adenomatous polyps have the potential to become malignant. The incidence of malignant change in adenomatous polyps has been reported to be from 6 to 75 per cent.[189, 197] The malignant potential appears to be related to the size of the polyp, with larger adenomas (particularly > 2 cm) having a greater potential for malignant change. Other suggestive evidence includes the observation that areas of benign adenomatous polyps are occasionally found in the margin of gastric cancer.[198] In addition, adenomatous polyps are frequently found coincidentally with gastric carcinoma.[189] These findings support the malignant potential of adenomatous polyps of the stomach, and as Ming concluded, an adenomatous polyp is not a frequent precursor of gastric cancer but an important one.[189]

Polyposis Syndromes

Polypoid lesions of the stomach have been reported in many of the polyposis syndromes. Gastric polyps of the adenomatous type have been described in persons with familial polyposis coli (FPC).[189, 199, 200] As many as 50 per cent of patients with FPC who underwent esophagogastroduodenoscopy had "polyps" of the upper gastrointestinal tract in one study. Histologic findings were not provided, and some of these polyps were in the duodenum. Recently "fundic gland polyps" have been reported in patients with FPC. This consists of multiple small polypoid lesions that may be hyperplastic polyps or hamartomas.[201–203]

In Gardner's syndrome, an autosomal dominant disease, adenomatous polyps and polypoid hamartomas have been encountered in the stomach. Although no report of instances of adenocarcinoma of the stom-

ach developing from such polyps is available, because of the high malignant potential of colorectal polyps in Gardner's syndrome, if an adenoma of the stomach is found, it should be removed by whatever means necessary.

In the Peutz-Jeghers syndrome, hamartomas of the stomach have been reported in as high as 25 per cent of cases. Gastric carcinoma has been observed in persons with this syndrome, but it is unlikely that this develops from hamartomas; more likely it reflects the unexplained increase in cancer at multiple sites in patients with this syndrome. Cronkhite-Canada syndrome and Cowden's disease have also been described to have hamartomas of the stomach.[189]

APPROACH TO POLYPOID LESIONS OF THE STOMACH

A polypoid lesion is defined as a rounded, translucent "filling" defect in a barium-filled stomach. This is seen as an "elevated" lesion if double contrast medium technique is utilized. A lesion less than 0.5 cm is difficult to detect unless it is situated in a location where it is seen in profile. When 23 such filling defects on X-ray of < 3 cm were evaluated histologically by Bonfill, seven adenomas, seven hyperplastic polyps, four hamartomas, two cancers, and one each of leiomyoma, carcinoid, and "retention polyps" were found.[204] Huppler found 80 per cent of polypoid lesions were benign, and 75 per cent of these (60 per cent of total) were polyps. The 20 per cent malignant lesions included several adenomatous polyps with adenocarcinoma. These studies suggest that most polypoid lesions on X-ray are polyps.[205]

If an elevated or polypoid lesion is first encountered during upper gastrointestinal X-ray study, as is the usual situation, the lesion should be evaluated by endoscopy. The purpose of endoscopy is to search for synchronous lesions (polyps or cancer) and obtain tissue from any abnormalities found. If the lesion is amenable to endoscopic polypectomy, this should be done because this has been established as a safe diagnostic and therapeutic procedure.[206] If this cannot be accomplished (because of size, location, or shape), then the lesion(s) should be biopsied and brushed for cytologic examination. It must be remembered that there can be a discrepancy between histologic diagnosis from endoscopic biopsies of such lesions and examination of the entire lesion.[207] Yamada's classification of elevated lesions may help formulate some idea about management of certain lesions.[208] He divided elevated lesions into four types (Fig. 44–13). Type I configuration lesions are usually benign submucosal lesions. These should be biopsied several times in the same place (well biopsy).[209] Normal mucosa will be obtained usually, but in some instances, adipose tissue will be seen, confirming a submucosal lesion. If, on the other hand, adenomatous tissue is obtained, the lesions should be removed by endoscopic polypectomy or surgically, which might be safer with this type of lesion.

Type IV configuration, a pedunculated lesion, can

TYPE \ SIZE mm	I	II	III	IV	TOTAL
≤ 4	○ 2	○ 8			10
5–9	○ 2	○ 13 ◐ 2	○ 24	○ 12	53
10–19	○ 7	◐ 2	○ 8 ◐ 4	○ 31	52
20–29	○ 1	○ 2	◐ 1 ● 1	○ 4 ◐ 2	11
≥ 30	○ 1	◐ 5 ● 1	◐ 8 ● 9	◐ 1 ● 1	26
TOTAL	13	33	55	51	152

○ BENIGN
◐ EARLY GASTRIC CANCER
● ADVANCED GASTRIC CANCER

Figure 44–13. Diagnosis of polypoid or elevated lesion of the stomach based on shape and size. Type I configuration lesions, regardless of size, were benign. Most type IV lesions were benign polyps, although some contained a focus of cancer. Type II and III configurations were usually benign lesions when less than 1 cm in diameter, but when larger than 2 cm were early or advanced gastric cancer. (From Yamada, T., and Ichikawa, H. X-ray diagnosis of elevated lesions of the stomach. Radiology *110*:79–83, 1976. Used by permission.)

be removed by endoscopic polypectomy at the time it is discovered. The type II and type III lesions are sessile and less amenable to endoscopic polypectomy. These configurations are associated with many of the adenomatous polyps, and the majority of early and advanced gastric cancer. If the endoscopist does not feel polypectomy can be attempted safely, biopsies should be done. If no definitive diagnosis is made, surgical excision should be contemplated in the patients in whom there are no contraindications. In general, surgery should be done for (1) adenomatous lesions > 2 cm which are not amenable to endoscopic polypectomy; (2) sessile lesions (types II and III) in which no definitive diagnosis can be made by endoscopic biopsy; and (3) any polypoid lesion that is believed to be responsible for symptoms which warranted the investigation in the first place (and cannot be removed by endoscopic polypectomy).

The surgical procedure of choice for a single polyp is excision of the polyp with a rim of normal mucosa. Frozen sections should be obtained for immediate pathologic diagnosis. With large sessile polyps or multiple polyposis of the stomach, more extensive resection may be necessary. A particularly difficult question is how to approach a diffuse gastric polyposis when all the polyps appear to be hyperplastic. Larger polyps should be removed, but it is impossible to sample or remove all polyps to ensure that there are not any adenomas. Because the malignant potential of hyperplastic polyps is low, it is not unreasonable to let other criteria (such as symptoms) be used to determine the need for surgery, as it would probably be necessary to do a total gastrectomy to remove all polyps in this situation.

Complications from endoscopic polypectomy include hemorrhage and perforation. Symptomatic ulcers can be seen also. An antiulcer regimen for two weeks following polypectomy has been recommended.[210, 211] Disappearance or reduction in size of polypoid lesions has been observed on endoscopic follow-up, but because no histologic diagnosis was available, it is uncertain what this means. Recurrence of polyps following removal may be seen but this is uncommon.

GASTRIC CARCINOIDS

Gastric carcinoids are uncommon in the United States, accounting for approximately 3 per cent of all gastrointestinal carcinoids and only 0.3 per cent of gastric neoplasms.[212] This tumor appears to be more common in Japan and may represent as high as 41 per cent of all gastrointestinal carcinoids.[213]

Carcinoid tumors arise from the enterochromaffin cells of the gastrointestinal tract. Hyperplasia and subsequent neoplasia of these cells may be the sequence in the development of a carcinoid tumor. The factors responsible for the sequence of events are uncertain, but because gastric carcinoids are more common in persons with atrophic gastritis and, therefore, pernicious anemia, one theory suggests that achlorhydria and the resulting hypergastrinemia is responsible.[212, 214–216] Gastrin may exert a trophic effect on the endocrine cells inducing the hyperplasia, which can progress to neoplastic change with time. In accord with this concept gastric carcinoids have been reported in persons with Zollinger-Ellison syndrome and more recently in patients using omperazole, a potent inhibitor of gastric acid secretion.

Pathology

Microscopically, carcinoids arising from the foregut, such as a gastric carcinoid, are composed of uniform, round, or polygonal cells with monotonous-appearing round and centrally located nuclei. Like other carcinoid tumors, the gastric carcinoid stains with silver stains which are specific for endocrine cells storing amines or peptide hormones. The argyrophil reaction, which requires the addition of an external reducing agent, is a nondiscriminating stain and nearly all the endocrine cells of the gastrointestinal tract stain with this method. The argentaffin reaction, which produces a dark stain without the addition of the reducing agent, is not seen typically in foregut carcinoid tumors, such as in the stomach.[217, 218]

Macroscopically, the majority of gastric carcinoids are located in the body and fundus, and there may be single or multiple lesions. The carcinoid tumors are typically found in the submucosa, so endoscopic biopsies may not provide the diagnosis. Multiple biopsies from the same site and specifically in areas of ulceration are important. Many of these are polypoid and amenable to polypectomy, making the histologic diagnosis much more likely.[219]

Clinical Symptoms

Usually the patient with a gastric carcinoid has nonspecific symptoms, such as abdominal pain or dyspepsia. Gastrointestinal bleeding is not uncommonly reported. Gastric carcinoids are usually endocrinologically silent, but occasionally metastasis does occur and produces the malignant carcinoid sydrome. The syndrome with gastric carcinoids may be atypical in that instead of the classic cyanotic skin flush, there may be a splotchy bright red geographic blush. This has been attributed to release of 5-hydroxytryptophan and histamine rather than 5-hydroxytryptamine (serotonin).

Treatment and Prognosis

Gastric carcinoids like other carcinoids typically have an indolent course, and conservative therapy may be recommended for small tumors. Despite this, all carcinoids are potentially malignant and may metastasize. In fact, nearly 20 per cent have metastasized at the time surgery is performed. In small carcinoids, endoscopic removal or limited excision at surgery can be performed. More extensive resections are recommended for larger lesions, particularly those greater than 2 cm. If regional metastasis to the nodes is found, attempts at resecting as much disease as possible are advised. In those few patients who have distant metastasis, surgical excision of the primary tumor and attempts to resect metastasis are not unreasonable in view of the course of these tumors.

In those patients not suitable for surgery who have distant metastasis or malignant carcinoid syndrome, chemotherapy has been used. Doxorubicin has been most widely used and probably is the first line of treatment. 5-FU and imidazole carboxamide are two other agents used. Streptozotocin does not appear to be as effective in malignant carcinoid syndrome as it is in islet cell tumors, and in addition, it may be very toxic. Some combination chemotherapy programs have been used with perhaps slightly higher but not significantly different response rates than single agents.[220]

Leiomyoma and Leiomyosarcoma

The most common benign tumor of the stomach is the leiomyoma, which arises from smooth muscle tissue. This neoplasm is most commonly found incidentally at surgery or autopsy. In fact, one autopsy series demonstrated its presence in 50 per cent of persons over 50 years of age.[221] This observation supports the common notion that most leiomyomas are clinically silent. The asymptomatic leiomyoma is usually small (< 2 cm), while the symptomatic leiomyoma is usually larger (> 2 cm), averaging 4.5 cm. When a leiomyoma is symptomatic, it most commonly presents with gas-

trointestinal bleeding or abdominal pain. When evaluating a patient with symptoms due to a leiomyoma, an upper GI series will identify a lesion in most cases. This can be confirmed at endoscopy, but unless the lesion is ulcerated, biopsies are usually nondiagnostic. Local surgical excision for the symptomatic lesion is curative, and no recurrences have been reported.

Unless there is evidence of local extension or metastasis, it may be difficult to distinguish leiomyoma from its malignant counterpart, leiomyosarcoma. This neoplasm accounts for approximately 1 per cent of gastric malignancies. The presenting symptoms of leiomyosarcoma are similar to symptoms due to leiomyoma, but in addition, these patients are more likely to complain of weight loss. Although leiomyosarcomas are usually larger than leiomyomas at the time of discovery, there is much overlap in size. A palpable abdominal mass is seen in approximately 30 to 50 per cent of patients with leiomyosarcoma and, when present, is highly suggestive of malignancy. Still, in some cases it is only after recurrence following resection that the diagnosis of leiomyosarcoma is made.[222]

Though tumor size cannot be definitely correlated with the extent of disease, it appears that leiomyosarcomas greater than 8 cm are more likely to be associated with disseminated disease.[223] Treatment of choice is surgical extirpation. Sixty-seven per cent of persons with leiomyosarcoma will have extragastric extension when explored. Curative resection can generally be attempted in one half to one third of patients. However, local recurrence after resection remains a problem. Radiotherapy is usually not successful, and although chemotherapy has been attempted, it too is not usually helpful. Leiomyosarcomas are associated with a 25 to 30 per cent five-year survival rate.[223]

Another entity is gastric leiomyoblastoma, which, though clinically similar, is pathologically distinct from leiomyoma or leiomyosarcoma.[224] This interesting tumor has the malignant potential to invade and metastasize but even in the presence of metastases, these patients have a relatively benign course, and long survival is common when resection is performed.

Lipoma and Liposarcoma

Lipoma of the stomach is rare, arising from submucosal fat tissue. Lipomas are usually solitary and located in the distal stomach (75 per cent are located in the antrum). The most common symptom is gastrointestinal bleeding.[225]

The corresponding malignant lesion is the liposarcoma, which is also very unusual. In one series, there was one case in 1192 gastric malignancies over a 30-year period.[226] The most common presenting symptom of the liposarcoma is gastrointestinal bleeding.

Pancreatic Rests

Pancreatic rests are rare and represent the presence of ectopic pancreatic tissue in the stomach. These are usually incidental findings on upper GI series or gastroscopy, though they may produce obstruction, ulcerate and bleed, or be associated with clinical pancreatitis. These are usually submucosal lesions located on the greater curvature in the antrum. The bull's eye or target lesion is one presentation, though not always present. If a secretory duct is seen associated with the lesion, then the diagnosis is certain. The treatment of symptomatic lesions is simple excision.[227]

Metastatic Tumors to the Stomach

When a person presents with upper gastrointestinal symptoms and a history of a primary extragastric neoplasm, metastatic involvement of the stomach should be considered as a possible, though not necessarily the most likely, explanation for the symptoms. The symptoms may be nausea, vomiting, pain, or gastrointestinal bleeding. Cancer of the breast was reported to metastasize to the stomach in 12 per cent of patients at autopsy.[228]

Malignant melanoma is one of the more frequently observed metastatic lesions, and although the bull's eye or target lesion associated with a submucosal lesion is well known, it usually presents as a slightly elevated black nodule when observed at endoscopy.[229] Cancer of the lung, ovary, testes, liver, colon, and parotid gland has been demonstrated to metastasize to the stomach.[228, 230]

References

1. Chen, C. K., and Parsa, I. Cells of origin in human gastric neoplasms. Cancer Letters *21*:195, 1983.
2. Capella, C., Frigerio B., Cornaggia, M., Solcia, E., Pinzon-Trujillo, Y., and Chejfec, G. Gastric parietal cell carcinoma—a newly recognized entity: light microscopic and ultrastructural features. Histopathology *8*:813, 1984.
3. Lauren, P. The two histologic main types of gastric carcinoma: Diffuse and so-called intestinal type carcinoma. An attempt at a histo-clinical classification. Acta Pathol. Microbiol. Scand. *64*:31, 1965.
4. Ming, S. C. Gastric carcinoma—a pathobiological classification. Cancer *39*:2475, 1971.
5. Correa, P. Clinical implications of recent developments in gastric cancer, pathology and epidemiology. Semin. Oncol. *12*:2, 1985.
6. Jass, J. R. Role of intestinal metaplasia in the histogenesis of gastric carcinoma. J. Clin. Pathol. *33*:801, 1980.
7. Sipporen, P. Intestinal metaplasia and gastric carcinoma. Ann. Clin. Res. *13*:139, 1987.
8. Qizilbash, A. H., and Stevenson, G. W. Early gastric cancer. Pathol. Ann. *14*:317, 1979.
9. Bogomoletz, W. V. Early gastric cancer. Am. J. Surg. Pathol. *8*:381, 1984.
10. Morson, B. C. Pathology, staging and prognostic implications of gastrointestinal cancer. *In* Stroehlein, J. R., and Romsdahl, M. M. (eds.). Gastrointestinal Cancer. New York, Raven Press, 1981, p. 99.
11. Kawai, K., Fernandez, J. M. B., Seifert, E., Murakami, T. Proceedings of the symposium: Early gastric cancer, held at the IV World Congress of Digestive Endoscopy. Gastroenterol. Japon. *14*:266, 1979.
12. Chappius, C. W., Cohn, I., and Correa, P. Early gastric cancer. Ann. Surg. *204*:103, 1986.
13. Carter, K. J., Schaffer, H. A., and Ritchie W. P. Early gastric cancer. Ann. Surg. *199*:604, 1984.
14. Evan, D. M. D., Craven, J. L., Murphy, F., and Cleary, B. K. Comparison of "early gastric cancer" in Britain and Japan. Gut *19*:1, 1978.
15. O'Brien, M. J., Burakoff, R., Robbins, E. A., Golding, R. M., Zamcheck, N., and Gottlieb, L. S. Early gastric cancer. Clinicopathologic Study. Am. J. Med. *78*:195, 1985.
16. Antonioli, D. A., and Goldman, H. Changes in location and type of gastric adenocarcinoma. Cancer *50*:775, 1982.
17. Eckardt, V. F., Williams, D., Kanzler, G., Remmele, W., Bettendorf, V., and Paulus, W. Eighty months persistence of poorly differentiated early gastric cancer. Gastroenterology *87*:719, 1984.
18. Yoshimori, M., Yoshida, S., Nakamura, K., and Oguro, Y. Relationship between early and advanced gastric cancers. Retrospective follow-up study of gastic cancer. Jap. J. Clin. Oncol. *8*:3, 1978.
19. Oshima, A., Fujimoto, I., Hiraoka, T., Mishima, T., and Okuda, S. Evaluation of intervention trials in stomach cancer. Presented at U.S.-Japan Cooperative Cancer Research Program. Integrated seminar of epidemiology and chemical radiation carcinogenesis. Colon Cancer and Stomach Cancer: Initiator and promoter in Honolulu, Hawaii, March, 1980.
20. Saito, T., Sasaki, O., Matsukuchi, T. Iwamatsu, M., and Inokucki, K. Experimental gastric cancer: Pathogenesis and clinico-histopathologic correlation. *In* Herfarth, C. H., and Schlag, P. (eds.): Gastric Cancer. New York, Springer Verlag, 1979, pp. 22–31.
21. Matsusaka, T., Kodama, Y., Soejima, K., Miyazaki, M., Yoshimura, K., Sugimachi, K., and Inokucki, K. Recurrence in early gastric cancer. A pathologic evaluation. Cancer *46*:168, 1980.
22. Mori, M., Iwashita, A., and Enjoji, M. Adenosquamous carcinoma of stomach: A clinicopathologic analysis of 28 cases. Cancer *57*:333, 1986.
23. Mori, M., Iwashita, A., and Enjoji, M. Squamous cell carcinoma of the stomach: Report of three cases. Am. J. Gastroenterol. *8*:339, 1986.
24. Ishikura, H., Kirimoto, K., Shamoto, M., Miyamoto, Y., Yamagiwa, H., Itoh, T., and Aizawa, M. Hepatoid adenocarcinomas of the stomach: An analysis of seven cases. Cancer *58*:119, 1986.
25. Wangensteen, O. H. The problem of gastric cancer. JAMA *134*:1161, 1947.
26. Silverberg, E., and Lubera, J. Cancer Statistics, 1986. CA *36*:9, 1986.
27. Coggon, D., and Acheson, E. D. The geography of cancer of the stomach. Br. Med. Bull. *40*:335, 1984.
28. Haas, J. F., and Schottenfeld, D. Epidemiology of gastric cancer. *In* Lipkin, M., and Good, R. (eds.): Gastrointestinal Tract Cancer. New York, Plenum Medical Book Company, 1978, pp. 173–206.
29. Kawai, K., Kizu, M., and Miyaoka, T. Epidemiology and pathogenesis of gastric cancer. Frontiers Gastrointest. Res. *6*:71, 1980.
30. Munoz, N., Correa, P., Cuello, C., and Duque, E. Histologic types of gastric carcinoma in high and low risk areas. Int. J. Cancer *3*:809, 1968.
31. Hoover, R., Mason, T. J., McKay, F. W., and Frameni, J. F. Cancer by county: New resources for etiologic clues. Science *189*:1005, 1975.
32. Haenzel, W., Kurihara, M., Segi, M., and Lee, R. K. C. Stomach cancer among Japanese in Hawaii. J. Natl. Cancer Inst. *49*:969, 1972.
33. Lyon, J. L., Gardener, J. W., West, D. W., and Mahoney, K. M. Methodological issues in epidemiological studies of diet and cancer. Cancer Res. (suppl.) *43*:2392, 1983.
34. Risch, H. A., Jain, M., Choi, N. W., Fodor, J. G., Pfeiffer, C. J., Howe, G. R., Harrison, L. W., Craib, K. J. P., and Miller, A. B. Dietary factors and the incidence of cancer of the stomach. Am. J. Epidemiol. *122*:947, 1985.
35. Correa, P., Fontham, E., Pickle, L. W., Chen, V., Lin, Y., and Haenszel, W. Dietary determinants of gastric cancer in south Louisiana inhabitants. J. Natl. Cancer Inst. *75*:645, 1985.
36. Trichopoulos, D., Ouranos, G., Day, N. E., Tzonou, A., Manousos, O., Papadimitriou, C., and Trichopoulos, A. Diet

and cancer of the stomach: A case-control study in Greece. Int. J. Cancer *36*:291, 1985.

37. Jedrychowski, W., Wahrendorf, J., Popiela, T., and Rachtan, J. A case-control study of dietary factors and stomach cancer risk in Poland. Int. J. Cancer *37*:837, 1986.
38. Joossens, J. V., and Geboers, J. Nutrition and gastric cancer. Proc. Nutr. Soc. *40*:37, 1981.
39. Pocock, S. J. Nitrates and gastric cancer. Human Toxicol. *4*:471, 1985.
40. Mirvish, S. S. The etiology of gastric cancer. Intragastric nitrosamide formation and other theories. J. Nat. Cancer Inst. *71*:631, 1983.
41. Sugimura, T., and Kawachi, T. Experimental stomach carcinogenesis. *In* Lipkin, M. and Good, R. (eds.): Gastrointestinal Tract Cancer. New York, Plenum Medical Book Company, 1978, pp. 327–341.
42. Cuello, C., Correa, P., Haenszel W., Gordillo, G., Brown, C., Archer, M., and Tannenbaum, S. Gastric cancer in Colombia: Cancer risk and suspect environmental agents. J. Natl. Cancer Inst. *57*:1015, 1976.
43. Beresford, S. A. A. Is nitrate in the drinking water associated with the risk of cancer in the urban UK? Int. J. Epidemiol. *14*:57, 1985.
44. Ruddell, W. S. J., Bone, E. S., Hill, M. J., and Walters, C. L. Pathogenesis of gastric cancer in pernicious anemia. Lancet *1*:521, 1978.
45. Schlag, P., Ulrich, H., Merkle, P., Bockler, R., Peter, M., and Herfarth, C. H. Are nitrate and N-nitroso compounds in gastric juice risk factors for carcinoma in the operated stomach? Lancet *1*:727, 1980.
46. Ruddell, W. S. J., Bone, E. S., Hill M. J., Blendis, L. M., and Walters, C. L. Gastric juice nitrite: A risk factor for gastric cancer in the hypochlorhydric stomach? Lancet *2*:1037, 1976.
47. Hall, C. N., Darkin, D., Brimblecombe, R., Cook, A. J., Kirkham, J. S., and Northfield, T. C. Evaluation of nitrosamine hypothesis of gastric carcinogenesis in precancerous conditions. Gut *27*:491, 1986.
48. Mirvish, S. S., Karlowski, K., Sams, J. P., and Arnold, S. D. Studies related to nitrosamide formation: nitrosation in solvents: water and solvent systems, nitrosomethylurea formation in the rat stomach and analysis of a fish product for ureas. IARC. Sci. Publ. *19*:161, 1978.
49. Hoey, J., Montvernay, C., and Lambert, R. Wine and tobacco: Risk factors for gastric cancer in France? Am. J. Epidemiol. *113*:668, 1981.
50. Aird, I., Bentall, H. H., and Roberts, J. A. F. A relationship between cancer of the stomach and the ABO blood groups. Br. Med. J. *1*:799, 1953.
51. Nomura, A., Glober, G., Terasaki, P., and Stemmermann, G. G. HLA antigens in stomach cancer. Int. J. Cancer *25*:195, 1980.
52. Cwern, M., Garcia, R. L., Davidson, M. I., and Friedman, I. H. Simultaneous occurrence of gastric carcinoma in identical twins. Am. J. Gastroenterol. *75*:41, 1981.
53. Bloss, R. S., Miller, T. A., and Copeland, E. M., III. Carcinoma of the stomach in the young adult. Surg. Gynecol. Obstet. *150*:883, 1980.
54. Hansen, R. M., and Hanson, G. A. Gastric carcinoma in young people. Am. J. Gastroenterol. *74*:497, 1980.
55. Dixon, W. L., and Fazzari, P. J. Carcinoma of the stomach in a child. JAMA *235*:2414, 1976.
56. Imai, T., Kubo, T., and Watanabe, H. Chronic gastritis in Japanese with reference to high incidence of gastric carcinoma. J. Natl. Cancer Inst. *47*:179, 1971.
57. Siurala, M. Gastritis, its fate and sequelae. Ann. Clin. Res. *13*:111, 1981.
58. Saito, T., Sasaki, O., Matsukuchi, T., Iwamatsu, M., and Inokucki, K. Experimental gastric cancer: Pathogenesis and clinico-histopathologic correlation. *In* Herfarth, C., and Schlag, P. (eds.): Gastric Cancer. New York, Springer Verlag, 1979, pp. 22–31.
59. Stout, A. P. Gastric mucosal atrophy and carcinoma of the stomach. N. Y. State J. Med. *45*:973, 1945.
60. Guiss, L. W., and Stewart, F. W. Chronic atrophic gastritis and cancer of the stomach. Arch. Surg. *46*:823, 1943.
61. Turani, H., Lurie, B., Chaimoff, C., and Kessler, E. The

diagnostic significance of sulphated mucin content in gastric intestinal metaplasia with early gastric cancer. Am. J. Gastroenterol. *81*:343, 1986.
62. Filipe, M. I., Potet, F., Bogomoletz, W. V., Dawson, P. A., Fabiani, B., Chauveinc, P., Fenzy, A., Gazzard, B., Goldfain, D., and Zeegan, R. Incomplete sulphomucin-secreting intestinal metaplasia for gastric cancer. Preliminary data from a prospective study from three centers. Gut *26*:1319, 1985.
63. Sipponen, P., Kekki, M., and Siurala, M. Age-related trends of gastritis and intestinal metaplasia in gastric carcinoma patients and in controls representing the population at large. Br. J. Cancer *49*:521, 1984.
64. Elder, J. B., Ganguli, P. C., and Gillespie, I. E. Cimetidine and gastric cancer. Lancet *1*:1005, 1979.
65. Taylor, R. H., Menzies-Gow, N., and Lovell, D. Misleading response of malignant gastric ulcer to cimetidine. Lancet *1*:686, 1978.
66. Isenberg, J. I., Peterson, W. L., and Elashoff, J. D. Healing of benign gastric ulcer with low-dose antacid or cimetidine. N. Engl. J. Med. *308*:1319, 1983.
67. Kaneko, E., Nakamura, T., Fujino, M., Umeda, N., and Niwa, H. Endoscopic analysis in the growth of early gastric cancer. Gastroenterol. Japon. *14*:103, 1979.
68. Rollag, A., and Jacobsen, C. D. Gastric ulcer and risk of cancer. A five-year follow-up study. Acta Med. Scand. *216*:105, 1984.
69. Ohara, T. Experimental production of ulcer—carcinoma in rat glandular stomach. Jap. J. Cancer Clin. *17*:534, 1971.
70. Zamcheck, N., Grable, E., Ley, A., and Norman L. Occurrence of gastric cancer among patients with pernicious anemia at the Boston City Hospital. N. Engl. J. Med. *252*:1103, 1955.
71. Borch, K. Epidemiologic, clinicopathologic and economic aspects of gastroscopic screening of patients with pernicious anemia. Scand. J. Gastroenterol. *21*:21, 1986.
72. Rogers, L. W., and Murphy, R. C. Gastric carcinoid and gastric carcinoma. Am. J. Surg. Pathol. *3*:195, 1979.
73. Hoffman, N. R. The relationship between pernicious anemia and cancer of the stomach. Geriatrics *25*:90, 1970.
74. Stockbrugger, R. W., Menon, G. G., Beilby, J. O. W., Mason, R. R., and Cotton, P. B. Gastroscopic screening in 80 patients with pernicious anemia. Gut *24*:1141, 1983.
75. Shearman, D. J. C., Finlayson, N. D. C., Wilson, R., and Samson, R. R. Carcinoma of the stomach and early pernicious anemia. Lancet *2*:403, 1966.
76. Cleimencon, G. Risk of carcinoma in the gastric remnant after gastric resection for benign condition. *In* Herfarth, C., and Schlag, P. (eds.): Gastric Cancer. New York, Springer Verlag, 1979, pp. 129–136.
77. Peitsch, W. Remarks on the frequency and pathogenesis of primary gastric stump cancer. *In* Herfarth, C., and Schlag, P. (eds.): Gastric Cancer. New York, Springer Verlag, 1979, pp. 137–144.
78. Rosch, W. Prospective studies in patients with resected stomach and stump carcinoma. *In* Herfarth, C., and Schlag, P. (eds.): Gastric Cancer. New York, Springer Verlag, 1979, pp. 145–146.
79. Domellof, L., Eriksson, S., and Janunger, K. G. Carcinoma and possible precancerous changes of the gastric stump after Billroth II resection. Gastroenterology *73*:462, 1977.
80. Schrumpf, E., Stadaas, J., Myren, J., Serck-Hanssen, A., Aune, S., and Osnes, M. Mucosal changes in the gastric stump 20–25 years after partial gastrectomy. Lancet *2*:467, 1977.
81. Offerhaus, G. J. A., Huibregtse, K., DeBoer, J., Verhoeven, T., Van Olffen, G. H., Von De Stadt, J., and Tytgat, G. N. J. The operated stomach: A premalignant condition. Scand. J. Gastroenterol. *19*:521, 1984.
82. Farrands, P. A., Blake, J. R. S., Ansell, I. D., Cotton, R. E., and Hardcastle, J. D. Endoscopic review of patients who have had gastric surgery. Br. Med. J. *286*:755, 1983.
83. Ovaska, J. T., Havia, T. V., and Kujari, H. P. Retrospective analysis of gastric stump carcinoma—patients treated during 1946–1981. Acta Chir. Scand. *152*:199, 1986.
84. Perez, D., Narayanan, N. C., Russell, J. C., and Becker, D. R. Gastric carcinoma after peptic ulcer surgery. Am. Surgeon *50*:538, 1984.
85. Sandler, R. S., Johnson, M. D., and Holland, K. L. Risk of

stomach cancer after gastric surgery for benign conditions. A case-control study. Dig. Dis. Sci. *29*:703, 1984.

86. Schafer, L. W., Larson, D. E., Melton, J., Higgins, J. A., and Ilstrep, D. M. The risk of gastric carcinoma after surgical treatment for benign ulcer disease. N. Engl. J. Med. *309*:1210, 1983.

87. Fischer, A. B., Graem, N., and Jensen, O. M. Risk of gastric cancer after Billroth-II resection for duodenal ulcer. Br. J. Surg. *70*:552, 1983.

88. Tokudome, S., Kono, S., Ikeda, M., Kuratsune, M., Sano, C., Inokuchi, K., Kodama, Y., Ichimiya, H., Nakayama, F., Kaibara, N., Koga, S., Yamada, H., Ikejiri, T., Oka, N., and Tsurumaru, H. A prospective study on primary gastric stump cancer following partial gastrectomy for benign gastroduodenal disease. Cancer Res. *44*:2208, 1984.

89. Pickford, I. E., Craven, J. L., Hall, R., Thomas, G., and Stone, W. D. Endoscopic examination of the gastric remnant 31–39 years after subtotal gastrectomy for peptic ulcer. Gut *25*:393, 1984.

90. Wood, G. M., Bates, C., Brown, R. C., and Losowky, M. S. Intramucosal carcinoma of the gastric antrum complicating Menetrier's disease. J. Clin. Pathol. *36*:1071, 1983.

91. Scharschmidt, B. F. The national history of hypertrophic gastropathy (Menetrier's disease). Am. J. Med. *63*:644, 1977.

92. Case records of the Massachusetts General Hospital. N. Engl. J. Med. *303*:744, 1980.

93. Murson, B. C., Sobin, L. H., Grundman, E., Johansen, A., Nagayo, T., and Serck-Hanssen, A. Precancerous condition and epithelial dysplasia in the stomach. J. Clin. Pathol. *33*:711, 1980.

94. Jass, J. R. Precancerous lesions of the stomach. Gann Monograph on Cancer Research *31*:19, 1986.

95. Oehlert, W. Biological significance of dysplasias of the epithelium and of atrophic gastritis. *In* Herfarth, C., and Schlag, P. (eds.): Gastric Cancer. New York, Springer Verlag, 1979, pp. 91–104.

96. LaDue, J. S. The clinical diagnosis of gastric cancer. *In* McNeer, G., and Pack, T. T. (eds.): Neoplasms of the Stomach. Philadelphia, J. B. Lippincott Company, 1967, pp. 102–125.

97. Kolodny, M., Schrader, Z. R., Rubin, W., Hochman, R., and Sleisenger, M. Esophageal achalasia probably due to gastric carcinoma. Ann. Intern. Med. *69*:569, 1968.

98. Tucker, H. J., Snape, W. J., and Cohen, S. Achalasia secondary to carcinoma: Manometric and clinical features. Ann. Intern. Med. *89*:315, 1978.

99. Mallaiah, L., Fruchter, G., Brozinski, S., and Uddin, M. S. Malignant gastrocolic fistula. Case report and review of the literature. Am. J. Proctol. Gastroenterol. Colon Rectal Surg. *31*:12, 1980.

100. Wakashin, M., Wakashin, Y., Iesato, K., Ueda, S., Mori, Y., Tsuchida, H., Shigematsu, H., and Okuda, K. Association of gastric cancer and nephrotic syndrome. An immunologic study in three patients. Gastroenterology *78*:749, 1980.

101. Croft, P. B., and Wilkinson, M. The incidence of carcinomatous neuromyopathy in patients with various types of carcinoma. Brain *88*:427, 1965.

102. Brown, J., and Winkelmann, R. K. Acanthosis nigricans: A study of 90 cases. Medicine *47*:33, 1968.

103. Dantzig, P. I. Sign of Leser-Trelat. Arch. Dermatol. *108*:700, 1973.

104. Ballesta-Lopez, C., Cabre-Martinez, C. A., and Arcusa-Gavalda, R. Value of roentenograms in the diagnosis and prognosis of carcinoma of the stomach. Surg. Gynecol. Obstet. *152*:63, 1981.

105. Federic, M. P., and Goldberg, H. I. Conventional radiography of the alimentary tract. *In* Sleisenger, M. H., and Fordtran, J. S. (eds.): Gastrointestinal Disease. Philadelphia, W. B. Saunders Company, 1983, pp. 1634–1667.

106. Moreno-Ortero, R., Martinez-Raposo, A., Cantero, J., and Pajares, J. M. Exfoliative cytodiagnosis of gastric adenocarcinoma. Comparison with biopsy and endoscopy. Acta Cytol. *27*:485, 1983.

107. Hanson, J. T., Thoreson, C., and Morrissey, J. F. Brush cytology in the diagnosis of upper gastrointestinal malignancy. Gastrointest. Endosc. *26*:33, 1980.

108. Bemvenuti, G. A., Hattori, K., Levin, B., Kirsner, J. B., and Reilly, R. W. Endoscopic sampling for tissue diagnosis in gastrointestinal malignancy. Gastrointest. Endosc. *21*:159, 1975.

109. Graham, D. Y., Schwartz, J. T., Cain, G. D., and Gyorkey, F. Prospective evaluation of biopsy number in the diagnosis of esophageal and gastric carcinoma. Gastroenterology *82*:228, 1982.

110. Sancho-Pock, F. J., Balanzo, J., Ocana, J., Presa, E., Sala-Cladera, E., Cusso, X., and Vilardell, F. An evaluation of gastric biopsy in the diagnosis of gastric cancer. Gastrointest. Endosc. *24*:281, 1978.

111. Hatfield, A. R. W., Slavin, G., and Segal, A. W. Importance of the site of endoscopic gastric biopsy in ulcerating lesions of the stomach. Gut *16*:884, 1975.

112. Everson, T. C. Carcinoma of the stomach. *In* Everson, T. C., and Cole, W. H. (eds.): Cancer of the Digestive Tract, Clinical Management. New York, Appleton-Century-Crofts, 1969, pp. 11–73.

113. Heymer, B., and Quentmeier, A. Biological markers for staging of gastric cancer. *In* Herfarth, C., and Schlag, P. (eds.): Gastric Cancer. New York, Springer Verlag, 1979, pp. 157–162.

114. Tatsuta, M., Itoh, T., Okuda, S., Yamamura, H., Baba, M., and Tamura, H. Carcinoembryonic antigen in gastric juice as an aid in diagnosis of early gastric cancer. Cancer *46*:2686, 1980.

115. Nitti, D., Farini, R., Grassi, F., Cardin, F., Di Mario, F., Piccoli, T., Vianello, F., Farinati, F., Favretti, F., Lise, M., and Naccarato, R. Carcinoembryonic antigen in gastric juice collected during endoscopy. Cancer *52*:2334, 1983.

116. Nomura, A. M. Y., Stemmermann, G. N., and Samloff, I. M. Serum pepsinogen I as a predictor of stomach cancer. Ann. Intern. Med. *93*:537, 1980.

117. Moss, A. A., Schnyder, P., Marks, W., and Margulis, A. R. Gastric adenocarcinoma: A comparison of the accuracy and economics of staging by computed tomography and surgery. Gastroenterology *80*:45, 1981.

118. Komaki, S., and Toyoshima, S. CT's capability in detecting advanced gastric cancer. Gastrointest. Radiol. *8*:307, 1983.

119. Cook, A. O., Levine, B. A., Sirinek, K. R., and Gaskill, H. V. Evaluation of gastric adenocarcinoma. Abdominal computed tomography does not replace cellotomy. Arch. Surg. *121*:603, 1986.

120. Schrock, T. R., and Way, L. W. Total gastrectomy. Am. J. Surg. *135*:348, 1978.

121. Pichlmayr, R., and Meyer, H. J. Value of gastrectomy "de principe." *In* Herfarth, C., and Schlag, P. (eds.): Gastric Cancer. New York, Springer Verlag, 1979, pp. 196–204.

122. Soga, J., Kobayashi, K., Saito, J., Fujimaki, M., and Muto, T. The role of lymphadenectomy in curative surgery for gastric cancer. World J. Surg. *3*:701, 1979.

123. Kodama, Y., Sugimachi, K., Soejima, K., Matsusaka, T., and Inokuchi, K. Evaluation of extensive lymph node dissection for carcinoma of the stomach. World J. Surg. *5*:241, 1981.

124. Miwa, K. Cancer of the stomach in Japan. Gann Monograph on Cancer Research *22*:61, 1979.

125. Crave, J. L. Stomach cancer. *In* Fielding, J. W. L., and Priestman, T. J. (eds.): Gastrointestinal Oncology. Philadelphia, Lea & Febiger, 1986, pp. 125–138.

126. Swain, C. P., Brown, S. G., Edwards, D. A. W., Kirkham, J. S. Salmon, P. R., and Clark, C. G. Laser recanalization of obstructing foregut cancer. Br. J. Surg. *71*:112, 1984.

127. Turnbull, A., Kussin, S., Kurtz, R. C., and Bains, M. Palliative prosthetic intubation in gastric cancer. J. Surg. Oncol. *15*:37, 1980.

128. Koga, S., Kawaguchi, H., Kishimoto, H., Tanaka, K., Miyano, Y., Kimwa, O., Takeda, R., and Nishidoi, H. Therapeutic significance of noncurative gastrectomy for gastric cancer with liver metastasis. Am. J. Surg. *140*:356, 1980.

129. Smith, F. P., Byne, P. J., Cambareri, R. C., and Schein, P. S. Gastrointestinal cancer. *In* Pinedo, H. M. (ed.): Cancer Chemotherapy. New York, Elsevier, 1980, pp. 284–298.

130. O'Connell, M. J. Current status of chemotherapy for advanced pancreatic and gastric cancer. J. Clin. Oncol. *3*:1032, 1985.

131. Le Chevalier, T., Smith, F. P., Harter, W. K., and Schein, P.

S. Chemotherapy and combined modality therapy for locally advanced and metastatic gastric carcinoma. Semin. Oncol 12:46, 1985.

132. Shah, A., and MacDonald, W. C. Chemotherapy for advanced gastric cancer with 72-hour continuous intravenous 5-fluorouracil infusion at 2 week intervals. Med. Pediatr. Oncol. 11:358, 1983.

133. Schein, P. S., MacDonald, J. S., and Hoth, D. Mitomycin-C: Experience in the United States with emphasis on gastric cancer. Cancer Chemother. Pharmacol. 1:73, 1978.

134. Eare, H. M., Coombes, R. C., and Schein, P. S. Cytotoxic chemotherapy for cancer of the stomach. Clin. Oncol. 3:351, 1984.

135. Bruckner, H. W., Lokich, J. J., and Stablein, D. M. Studies of Baker's antifol, methotrexate and razoxane in advanced gastric cancer. A Gastrointestinal Tumor Study Group report. Cancer Treat. Rep. 66:1713, 1982.

136. La Cave, A. J., Izarzugara, I., and Aparicio, L. M. A. Phase II: Clinical trial of cis-dichlorodiammine platinum in gastric cancer. Am. J. Clin. Oncol. 6:35, 1983.

137. Kovach, J. S., Moertel, C. G., Schutt, A. J., Hahn, R. G., and Reitemeier, R. J. A controlled study of combined 1,3-bis (2-chlorethyl)-1-nitrosourea and 5-fluorouracil for advanced gastric and pancreatic cancer. Cancer 33:563, 1974.

138. MacDonald, J. S., Schein, P. S., Wooley, P. V., Smythe, T., Ueno, W., Hotch, D., Smith, F., Boiron, M., Gisselbrecht, C., Brunet, R., and LaGarde, C. 5-fluorouracil, doxorubicin and mitomycin (FAM) combination chemotherapy for advanced gastric cancer. Ann. Intern. Med. 93:533, 1980.

139. Gastrointestinal Tumor Study Group. A comparative clinical assessment of combination chemotherapy in the management of advanced gastric cancer. Cancer 49:1362, 1982.

140. Douglas, H. O., Lavin, P. T., and Groudsmith, A. Phase II–III: Evaluation of combinations of methyl-CCNU, Mitomycin-C, Adriamycin and 5-fluorouracil in advanced measurable gastric cancer. J. Clin. Oncol. 2:1372, 1984.

141. Wooley, P., Smith, F., Estevez, R., Gisselbrecht, C., Alvarez, C., Boiron, M., Machado, C., LaGarde, C., and Schein, P. A Phase II trial of 5-FU, Adriamycin and cisplatin (FAP) in advanced gastric cancer. Proc. Am. Soc. Clin. Oncol. 481:455, 1981.

142. Wagener, D. J. T., Yap, S. H. Wobbes, T., Burghouts, J. T. M., Van Dam, F. E., Hillen, H. F. P., Hoogendoorn, G. J., Scheerder, H., and van der Vegt, S. G. L. Phase II trial of 5-fluorouracil, Adriamycin and cisplatin (FAP) in advanced gastric cancer. Cancer Chemother. Pharmacol. 15:86, 1985.

143. Moertel, C. G., Rubin, J., O'Connell, H. J., Schutt, A. J., and Wieand, H. S. A phase II study of combined 5-fluorouracil, doxorubicin and cisplatin in the treatment of upper gastrointestinal adenocarcinoma. J. Clin. Oncol. 4:1053, 1986.

144. Falkson, G., and Falkson, H. C. Fluorouracil and radiotherapy in gastrointestinal cancer. Lancet 2:1252, 1969.

145. Moertel, C. G., Childs, D. S., Reitemeier, R. J., Colby, M. Y., and Holbrook, M. A. Combined 5-fluorouracil and super-voltage radiation therapy for locally unresectable gastrointestinal cancers. Lancet 2:865, 1969.

146. Gastrointestinal Tumor Study Group. A comparison of combination chemotherapy and combined modality therapy for locally advanced gastric carcinoma. Cancer 49:1771, 1982.

147. Weissberg, J. B. Role of radiation therapy in gastrointestinal cancer. Arch. Surg. 118:96, 1983.

148. Livstone, E. M., and Stablein, D. M. Adjuvant chemotherapy with 5-FU and methyl CCNU prolongs recurrence-free interval and survival following curative resection for gastric adenocarcinoma. Gastroenterology 80:1215, 1981.

149. Gunderson, L. L., and Sosin, H. Adenocarcinoma of the stomach: Areas of failure in a reoperation series (second or symptomatic look). Clinicopathologic correlation and implications for adjuvant therapy. Int. J. Rad. Oncol. Biol. Phys. 8:1, 1982.

150. Armstrong, C. P., and Dent, D. M. Factors influencing prognosis in carcinoma of the stomach. Surg. Gynecol. Obstet. 162:343, 1986.

151. Schmitz-Moorman, P., Heider, H. A., and Thomas, C. Cancer of the stomach—prognosis, independent of therapy in gastric cancer. In Herfarth, C., and Schlag, P. (eds.): Gastric Cancer. New York, Springer Verlag, 1979, pp. 172–181.

152. Watanabe, H., Enjoji, M., and Imai, T. Gastric carcinoma with lymphoid stroma. Its morphologic characteristics and prognostic correlations. Cancer 38:232, 1976.

153. Okada, M., Kojima, S., Murakami, M., Fuchigami, T., Yao, T., Omae, T., and Iwashita, A. Human gastric carcinoma: prognosis in relation to macroscopic and microscopic features of the primary tumor. J. Nat. Cancer Inst. 71:275, 1983.

154. Bonar, S. F., and Sweeney, E. C. The prevalence, prognostic significance and hormonal content of endocrine cells in gastric cancer. Histopathology 10:53, 1986.

155. Larson, N. E., Cain, T. C., and Bartholomew, L. G. Prognosis of the medically treated small gastric ulcer. A ten year to nineteen year follow-up study of 391 patients. N. Engl. J. Med. 264:330, 1961.

156. Hayashi, R., and Ochiai, T. HLA Type and survival in gastric cancer. Cancer Res. 46:3701, 1986.

157. Kojima, O., Ikeda, E., Uehara, Y., Majima, T., Fijita, Y., and Majima, S. Correlation between carcinoembryonic antigen in gastric cancer tissue and survival of patients with gastric cancer. Gann 75:230, 1984.

158. Smith, S. R., Howell, A., Minawa, A., and Morrison, J. M. The clinical value of immunohistochemically demonstrable CEA in breast cancer: A possible method of selecting patients for adjuvant chemotherapy. Br. J. Cancer 46:757, 1982.

159. Tahara, E., Smuiyoshi, H., Hata, J., Yasui, W., Taniyama, K., Hayashi, T., Nagae, S., and Sakamoto, S. Human epidermal growth factor in gastric carcinoma as a biologic marker of high malignancy. Jpn. J. Cancer Res. (Gann) 77:145, 1986.

160. Tokunaga, A., Nishi, K., Matsukura, N., Tanaku, N., Onda, M., Shiroto, A., Asano, G., and Hayashi, K. Estrogen and progesterone receptors in gastric cancer. Cancer 57:1376, 1986.

161. Lumpkin, W. M., Crow, R. L., Hernandez, C. M., and Cohn, I. Carcinoma of the stomach: Review of 1,035 cases. Ann. Surg. 159:919, 1964.

162. Yamada, E., Miyaishi, S., Nakazato, H., Kato, K., Kito, T., Takagi, H., Yasue, M., Kato, T., Morimoto, T., and Yamauchi, M. The surgical treatment of cancer of the stomach. Int. Surg. 65:387, 1980.

163. Clark, G. C., Boulos, P. B., and Ward, N. W. N. Cost effectiveness in the treatment of gastric cancer. Clin. Oncol. 6:303, 1980.

164. Dupont, J. B., Lee, J. R., Burton, G. R., and Cohn, I. Adenocarcinoma of the stomach: Review of 1,497 cases. Cancer 41:941, 1978.

165. Kennedy, B. J. TNM classification for stomach cancer. Cancer 26:971, 1970.

166. American Joint Committee for Cancer Staging and End-Results Reporting. Manual for Staging of Cancer. Chicago, American Joint Committee, 1977.

167. Freeman, C., Berg, J. N., and Cutler, S. J. Occurrence and prognosis of extranodal lymphomas. Cancer 29:252, 1972.

168. Levin, K. J., Ranchod, M., and Dorfman, R. F. Lymphomas of the gastrointestinal tract: A study of 117 cases presenting with gastrointestinal disease. Cancer 42:693, 1978.

169. Bedikian, A. Y., Khankhanian, N., Heilbrun, L. K., and Valdivieso, M. Primary lymphomas and sarcomas of the stomach. South. Med. J. 73:21, 1980.

170. Brooks, J. J., and Enterline, H. T. Primary gastric lymphomas. A clinicopathogic study of 58 cases with long-term follow-up and literature review. Cancer 51:701, 1983.

171. Martin, T. R., Onstad, G. R., Silvis, S. E., and Vennes, J. A. Lift and cut biopsy technique for submucosal sampling. Gastrointest. Endosc. 23:29, 1976.

172. Rappaport, H. Tumors of the hematopoietic system. In Armed Forces Institutes of Pathology. Atlas of Tumor Pathology, Section 3, Fasc. 8. Washington, D. C., 1966, pp. 97–161.

173. Perren, T. J., and Blackledge, G. Gastrointestinal lymphomas. In Fielding, J. W. L., and Priestman, T. J. (eds.): Gastrointestinal Oncology. Philadelphia, Lea & Febiger, 1986, pp. 237–255.

174. The non-Hodgkin's lymphoma pathologic classification report.

National Cancer Institute sponsored study of classification of non-Hodgkin's lymphomas. Summary and description of a working formulation for clinical usage. Cancer 49:2112, 1982.

175. Lim, F. E., Hartman, A. S., Tan, E. G. C., Cady, B., and Meissner, W. A. Factors in the prognosis of gastric lymphoma. Cancer 39:1715, 1977.

176. Carbone, P. P., Kaplan, H. S., Musshoff, K., Smithers, D. W., and Tubiana, M. Report of committee of Hodgkin's disease staging classification. Cancer Res. 31:1860, 1971.

177. Dworkin, B., Lightdale, C. J., Weingrad, D. N., DeCosse, J. J., Lieberman, P., Filippa, D. A., Sherlock, P., and Straus, D. Primary gastric lymphoma. A review of fifty cases. Dig. Dis. Sci. 27:986, 1982.

178. Gray, G. M., Rosenberg, S. A., Cooper, A. D., Gregory, P. B. and Stein, D. T. Lymphoma involving the gastrointestinal tract. Gastroenterology 82:143, 1981.

179. Fleming, I. D., Mitchell, S., and Ali Dilawari, R. The role of surgery in the management of gastric lymphoma. Cancer 49:1135, 1982.

180. Shendan, W. P., Medley, G., and Brodie, G. N. Non-Hodgkin's lymphoma of the stomach: A prospective pilot study of surgery plus chemotherapy in early and advanced disease. J. Clin. Oncol. 3:495, 1985.

181. Watson, R. J., and O'Brien, M. T. Gastric pseudolymphoma (lymphofollicular gastritis). Ann. Surg. 171:98, 1970.

182. Saraga, P., Hurlimann, J., and Ozzello, L. Lymphomas and pseudolymphomas of the alimentary tract. An immunohisto-chemical study with clinicopathologic correlations. Human Pathol. 12:713, 1981.

183. Mattingly, S., Cibull, M. L., Ram, M. D., Hagihara, P. F., and Griffin, W. O. Pseudolymphoma of the stomach. Arch. Surg. 116:25, 1981.

184. Brooks, J. J., and Enterline, H. T. Gastric pseudolymphoma: Its three subtypes and relation to lymphoma. Cancer 51:476, 1983.

185. Bentivenga, S., and Panagopoulos, P. G. Adenomatous gastric polyps. Am. J. Gastroenterol. 44:135, 1965.

186. Marshak, R. H., and Feldman, F. Gastric polyps. Am. J. Dig. Dis. 10:909, 1965.

187. Blackstone, M. O. Gastric polyps. In Blackstone, M. O. (ed.): Endoscopic Interpretation—Normal and Pathologic Appearances of the Gastrointestinal Tract. New York, Raven Press, 1984, pp. 158–169.

188. Morson, B. C., and Dawson, I. M. P. Adenomas and the adeno-carcinoma sequence. Gastrointestinal Pathology. Oxford, St. Louis, Blackwell Scientific Publications, 1979, pp. 615–647.

189. Ming, S. The classification and significance of gastric polyps. In International Academy of Pathology Monograph: The Gastrointestinal Tract, 1977, p. 149.

190. Elster, K., Carson, W., Eidt, H., and Thomasko, A. Significance of gastric polypectomy (histological aspect). Endoscopy 15:148, 1983.

191. Smith, H. J., and Lee, E. L. Large hyperplastic polyps of the stomach. Gastrointest. Radiol. 8:19, 1983.

192. Palmer, E. D. What Menetrier really said. Gastrointest. Endosc. 15:83, 1968.

193. Papp, J. J., and Joseph, J. I. Adenocarcinoma occurring in a hyperplastic polyp. Gastrointest. Endosc. 23:38, 1976.

194. Remmele, W., and Kolb, E. F. Malignant transformation of hyperplasiogenic polyps of the stomach. Endoscopy 10:63, 1978.

195. Bosseckert, H., and Rabbe, G. Multiple polyps in the stomach—how many polyps should be ectomized. Endoscopy 15:150, 1983.

196. Herrington, J. L., Powell, S., and Granda, A. Villous adenoma of the stomach. World J. Surg. 7:295, 1983.

197. Nakamura, T., and Nakano, G. Histopathological classification and malignant change in gastric polyps. J. Clin. Pathol. 38:754, 1985.

198. Tomasulo, J. Gastric polyps. Histologic types and their relationship to gastric carcinoma. Cancer 27:1346, 1971.

199. Watanabe, H., Enjoji, M., Yao, T., and Ohsato, K. Gastric lesions in familial adenomatosis coli. Hum. Pathol. 9:269, 1978.

200. Ranzi, T., Castagnone, D., and Veko, P. Gastric and duodenal polyps in familial polyposis coli. Gut 22:363, 1981.

201. Iida, M., Yao, T., Watanabe, H., Itoh, H., and Iwashita, A. Fundi gland polyposis in patients without familial adenomatosis coli: Its incidence and clinical features. Gastroenterology 86:1437, 1984.

202. Nishiura, M., Hirota, T., Itabashi, M., Ushio, K., Yamada, T., and Oguro, Y. A clinical and histopathological study of gastric polyps in familial polyposis coli. Am. J. Gastroenterol. 79:98, 1984.

203. Jarrinem, H., Nyberg, M., and Peltokallio, P. Upper gastrointestinal tract polyps in familial adenomatosis coli. Gut 24:333, 1983.

204. Bonfield, R. E., Martel, W., and Batsakis, J. G. The significance of small gastric filling defects. Surg. Gynecol. Obstet. 127:1231, 1968.

205. Huppler, E. G., Priestley, J. T., Marlock, C. G., and Gage, R. P. Diagnosis and results of treatment in gastric polyps. Surg. Gynecol. Obstet. 110:309, 1960.

206. ReMine, S. G., Hughes, R. W., and Weiland, L. H. Endoscopic gastric polypectomies. Mayo Clin. Proc. 56:371, 1981.

207. Seifert, E., and Elstr, K. Endoskopische Polypektomie am Magen: Indikation, Technik und Ergebnisse. Dtsh. Med. Wochenschr. 97:1199, 1972.

208. Yamada, T., and Ichikawa, H. X-ray diagnosis of elevated lesions of the stomach. Radiology 110:79, 1976.

209. Bjork, J. T. Nonepithelial neoplasms of the stomach. Gastrointest. Endosc. 30:107, 1984.

210. Lanza, F. L., Graham, D. Y., Nelson, R. S., Godiness, R., and McKechnie, J. C. Endoscopic upper gastrointestinal polypectomy. Am. J. Gastroenterol. 75:345, 1981.

211. Hughes, R. W. Gastric polyps and polypectomy: Rationale, technique and complications. Gastrointest. Endosc. 30:101, 1984.

212. Morgan, J. E., Kaiser, C. W., Johnson, W., Doos, W. G., Dayal, Y., Berman, L., and Nabseth, D. Gastric carcinoid (gastrinoma) associated with achlorhydria (pernicious anemia). Cancer 51:2332, 1983.

213. Mizuma, K., Shibuya, H., Totsuka, M., and Hayasaka, H. Carcinoid of the stomach: A case report and review of 100 cases reported in Japan. Ann. Chir. Gynaecol. 72:23, 1983.

214. Carney, J. A., Go, V. L. W., Fairbanks, V. F., Breanndan, S., Moore, M. B., Alport, E. C., and Nora, F. E. The syndrome of gastric argyrophil carcinoid tumors and nonantral gastric atrophy. Ann. Intern. Med. 99:761, 1983.

215. Borch, K., Renvall, H., and Leidberg, G. V. Gastric endocrine cell hyperplasia and carcinoid tumors in pernicious anemia. Gastroenterology 88:638, 1985.

216. Helling, T. S., and Wood, W. G. Gastric carcinoid and atrophic gastritis. Arch. Surg. 118:765, 1983.

217. Wilander, E., El-Salhy, M., and Pitkanen, P. Histopathology of gastric carcinoids: A survey of 42 cases. Histopathology 8:183, 1984.

218. Lewin, K. J., Ulich, T., Yang, K., and Layfield, L. The endocrine cells of the gastrointestinal tract. Tumors. Part II. Pathol. Annu. 21:185, 1986.

219. Caletti, G. C., Guizzardi, G., Brocchi, E., Grigioni, W. F., D'Errico, A., and Labo, G. Gastric carcinoid: A clinical and endoscopic assessment of four cases. Endoscopy 18:101, 1986.

220. Harris, A. L. Carcinoid tumors. In Fielding, J. W. L., and Priestman, T. J. (eds.): Gastrointestinal Oncology. Philadelphia, Lea & Febiger, 1986, pp. 256–274.

221. Morson, B. C., and Dawson, I. M. P. Nonepithelial tumors. In Gastrointestinal Pathology. Oxford, Blackwell Scientific Publications, 1979, pp. 187–199.

222. Delikaras, P., Golematis, B., Missitzis, J., Bang, L., Nakopoulou, L., and Paulsen, J. Smooth muscle neoplasms of the stomach. South. Med. J. 76:440, 1983.

223. Bedikian, A. Y., Khankhanian, N., Valdivieso, M., Heilbrun, L. K., Benjamin, R. S., Yap, B. S., Nelson, R. S., and Bodey, G. P. Sarcoma of the stomach: Clinicopathologic study of 43 cases. J. Surg. Oncol. 13:121, 1980.

224. Plantinga, E. R. M., Mravunac, M., and Joosten, H. J. M. Gastric leiomyoblastoma: Three interesting cases. Acta Chir. Scand. 145:571, 1979.

225. Johnson, D. C. I., DeGennaro, V. A., Pizzi, W. F., and Nealan, T. F. Gastric lipomas. A rare cause of massive upper gastrointestinal bleeding. Am. J. Gastroenterol. 75:299, 1981.
226. Bedikian, A. Y., Khankhanian, N., Heilbrun, L. K., and Valdivieso, M. Primary lymphomas and sarcomas of the stomach. South Med. J. 73:21, 1980.
227. Kilman, W. J., and Berk, R. N. The spectrum of radiographic features of aberrant pancreatic rests involving the stomach. Radiology 123:291, 1977.

228. Lightdale, C. J., and Sherlock, P. The diagnosis and treatment of gastrointestinal malignancies. Front. Gastrointest. Res. 6:138, 1980.
229. Nelson, R. S., and Lanza, F. Malignant melanoma metastatic to the upper gastrointestinal tract. Gastrointest. Endosc. 24:156, 1978.
230. Burbige, E. J., Radigan, J. J., and Belber, J. P. Metastatic lung carcinoma involving the gastrointestinal tract. Am. J. Gastroenterol. 74:504, 1980.

45 Stress Ulcers, Erosions, and Gastric Mucosal Injury

ANDRÉ ROBERT
GORDON L. KAUFFMAN, JR.

Gastric mucosal stress erosions are a common occurrence among patients placed in intensive care units after a variety of acute conditions, such as severe trauma and septic shock. We will review here the clinical setting, course, and treatment of stress erosions, and their experimental production in animals.

STRESS EROSIONS: CLINICAL ASPECTS

Although there is some variation in the histology of acute gastric mucosal erosions of various etiologies, these lesions usually occur in several clinical situations: first, in patients who have sustained severe trauma, who have ongoing sepsis, or who are being treated for serious medical illnesses; second, in patients who have significant thermal burn injury, referred to as Curling's ulcer; third, in patients with intra- or extracranial central nervous system disease, following craniotomy or traumatic cerebral or spinal cord injuries; and fourth, in patients who chronically ingest drugs that have adverse effects on the gastric mucosa. Massive upper gastrointestinal bleeding, which usually occurs three to seven days after the insult, is the most common presentation of acute gastric mucosal ulceration and has been termed acute hemorrhagic gastritis. Rarely are there prodromal signs, such as abdominal pain, which may alert the physician to the potential occurrence of massive upper gastrointestinal bleeding. Rarely does perforation complicate acute gastric mucosal ulceration. With the exception of certain patients with central nervous system injury, gastric acid hypersecretion is not present in patients who develop these acute erosions. This entity, then, is distinct from chronic gastric or duodenal ulcer or the exacerbation of a pre-existing quiescent gastric or duodenal ulcer. The histologic features of stress ulcer, as contrasted with chronic gastric ulcer, are shown in Figure 45–1. Once hemorrhage becomes manifest, the seriousness of the condition is reflected in the mortality rate, which approaches 50 per cent.

Underlying Conditions Associated with Acute Gastric Mucosal Erosions

Association with Trauma, Sepsis, Significant Underlying Disease, or Serious Illness. Severe trauma, including major surgical procedures, ongoing sepsis, and underlying diseases, such as pulmonary and renal insufficiency, predisposes patients to develop acute gastric mucosal erosions.[1, 2] Nearly all such patients have been shown endoscopically to develop these lesions.[1] They initially appear in the proximal portion of the gastric mucosa and may progress to involve the entire body mucosa. Under conditions of severe trauma and stress, the gastric antral mucosa may also develop acute ulcerations which tend to regress as the patient's condition improves. A small percentage of patients will develop life-threatening hemorrhage from these acute gastric mucosal lesions. Exactly what percentage of patients at risk this represents is not known, but it has been reported that only one patient of 64 bled from acute gastric mucosal erosions within 10 days of trauma,[3] and out of 2300 general surgical admissions to an intensive care unit, 1.8 per cent bled and 0.4 per cent required surgery to control upper gastrointestinal bleeding that was considered to be stress related.[4] The majority of patients who bleed from acute gastric mucosal erosions do so three to seven days following the traumatic event, but some patients may not bleed until 14 to 21 days after the injury.

In a series of 300 patients admitted to an intensive care unit, prospectively studied to determine significant factors predisposing to upper gastrointestinal bleeding, an illness severity score was defined.[5] The nine categories were (1) ventilatory assistance for more than 24 hours, (2) shock (systolic pressure $\leq$90 mm Hg), (3) sepsis, (4) congestive heart failure or myocardial infarction, (5) acute renal failure (serum creatinine $\geq$3.0 mg/100 ml), (6) central nervous system injury, (7) steroid administration, (8) coagulopathy (platelets $\leq$50,000 per cu mm or prothrombin time <30 per cent of control), and (9) serum bilirubin >5.0 mg/100 ml. Bleeding was the end point, that is, a 4+ guaiac nasogastric aspirate continuous for more than 16 hours, bright red blood per nasogastric tube, or fall in hematocrit. One hundred patients were randomized to not receive prophylactic therapy. In this group, there was a direct relationship between severity of illness and likelihood of upper gastrointestinal hemorrhage; those with 0 to 2 risk factors had an 11 per cent incidence of bleeding, those with 3 to 6 risk factors had a 34 per cent incidence of bleeding, and those with 7 or more risk factors had a 50 per cent incidence of bleeding. Overall, this "control" group had a 20 per

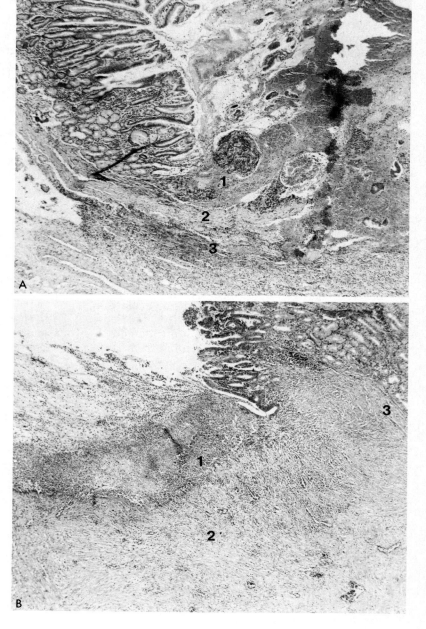

Figure 45–1. *A,* Acute gastric ulcer. The mucosa is disrupted with prominent hemorrhage (1). The muscularis mucosae (2) extends into the ulcer, where it too is disrupted. The ulcer extends to the submucosa, where there is some inflammation but no fibrosis (3). *B,* Chronic gastric ulcer. The base of the ulcer contains inflammatory exudate, necrotic tissue, and granulation tissue (1). Beneath this there is extensive fibrosis (2). The muscularis mucosae on the extreme right merges with the scar (3). (Courtesy of W. C. MacDonald, M.D., Head, Division of Gastroenterology, University of British Columbia, Vancouver, Canada.)

cent incidence of upper gastrointestinal bleeding, which was associated with a 17 per cent mortality rate.

Recently, 174 patients were prospectively evaluated for subsequent occurrence of "stress" bleeding after admission to a medical or respiratory intensive care unit.[6] Occult bleeding was defined as multiple, at least three, positive results of occult blood testing; overt bleeding was defined as any episode of coffee-ground emesis requiring lavage, hematemesis, or melena. Evidence of overt or occult gastrointestinal bleeding developed in 14 per cent. Diagnoses of malignancy, sepsis, or chronic obstructive pulmonary disease were common among those who bled; however, only a coagulopathy and the need for mechanical ventilation for more than five days were those factors with which "stress" bleeding was most closely associated. The set of patients who bled, when compared to those who did not bleed, had a higher mortality rate (64 versus 9 per cent), longer duration of intensive care stay (median of 14.2 versus 4.2 days), greater number of patients who required ventilatory support (84 versus 26 per cent), and longer ventilatory support (median 14.2 versus 4.2 days). The three (12 per cent) patients in this report who died of gastrointestinal bleeding each required ventilatory support, and none appear to have been treated prophylactically. Endoscopic evaluation of 18 patients admitted to an intensive care unit in the placebo arm of a randomized prospective trial demonstrated that only five (28 per cent) had normal-appearing mucosa.[7] Endoscopic signs of bleeding cleared or did not develop in 11 patients. There was one death from bleeding in a placebo-treated patient.

Measurement of intramural pH in stomachs of patients in an intensive care unit has been suggested as a method of identifying patients who will bleed massively.[8] Intramural pCO_2 is in equilibrium with that of the gastric juice which, when measured with intra-arterial $[HCO_3^-]$, allows calculation of the intramural pH using the Henderson-Hasselbalch equation. Seven of 103 patients studied developed massive bleeding from stress erosions, six of whom died. Predictive factors for gastrointestinal bleeding were number of risk factors and intramural pH. Bleeding from stress erosions was seen only in patients whose intramural pH had fallen below the lower limit of normal (pH 7.24). A relationship between arterial blood $[HCO_3^-]$, as in systemic acidosis, and probability of massive bleeding was identified.

From these observations of patients in the intensive care unit setting, it is reasonable to conclude that 10 to 20 per cent will have evidence of upper gastrointestinal bleeding if no prophylactic therapy is given, that the risk of bleeding is proportional to the severity of the illness, and that the mortality rate doubles or triples once overt bleeding has begun. Measuring intramural pH may allow the identification of certain patients who are prone to bleed.

Acute gastric mucosal erosions are multiple, shallow, and well demarcated but are not associated with a fibrous base or intense inflammatory reaction, a fact that distinguishes them from chronic peptic ulcer.

Acute gastric erosions usually extend to but not through the submucosa. Deeper penetration with perforation of the gastric wall has been reported to occur in only 13 per cent of patients.[9] Bleeding is usually from multiple shallow ulcers rather than deeper penetration through the submucosa and muscularis. Acute mucosal lesions may grossly assume any geometric shape and vary in length from 2 to 25 mm.

Unlike patients with chronic peptic ulcer, epigastric pain is rarely associated with acute gastric mucosal ulceration.[9] Painless gastrointestinal bleeding, manifested as hematemesis or melena or both, is usually the first and often the only clinical manifestation.

Association with Burns. Acute gastric mucosal ulceration associated with severe burns is referred to as "Curling's ulcer." Curling, in 1842, described acute duodenal ulceration in 10 extensively burned patients.[10] An endoscopic evaluation of 32 adult patients who sustained significant burn injury identified an 86 per cent incidence of acute gastric mucosal ulceration.[11] Patients with burns of 35 per cent or more of the body have a greater tendency to develop these lesions. The most common presenting sign is bleeding, hematemesis being at least twice as frequent as melena. Pain may precede or accompany bleeding in 4 per cent, and perforation has been reported to occur in 12 per cent of patients with burn-induced gastroduodenal mucosal ulceration.[12] In 15 per cent of patients with burns, both gastric and duodenal ulcers may be present.

The acute gastric mucosal ulcers are predominantly multiple and less than 2 cm in greatest diameter. They are shallow lesions that may penetrate through the gastric mucosa but rarely penetrate the muscularis. Sharply demarcated, they are not associated with surrounding inflammation or edema. The duodenal ulcers associated with burns tend to be single, histologically exhibiting evidence of chronic inflammation with deeper penetration, and as such, they more frequently perforate.[13]

Association with Central Nervous System Trauma. Injury to the central nervous system, due to either trauma or surgery, is associated with acute gastric mucosal ulceration. Since his description, this lesion has borne Harvey Cushing's name.[14] Cushing's ulcers may be found in the esophagus, stomach, or duodenum and histologically tend to be deep and often full thickness.[15] For this reason, perforated ulcers are more frequently found with Cushing's ulcers than with trauma- or sepsis-induced gastric mucosal ulcerations. The incidence of endoscopic mucosal lesions is 50 to 75 per cent in patients with head injuries, and bleeding may occur in 40 to 80 per cent of these patients.[16, 17] Injury to the spinal cord has also been associated with acute gastric mucosal ulceration.[3] Fifty-two of 2000 patients with spinal cord injuries developed gastrointestinal bleeding, most frequently observed in patients with complete cervical cord injuries.[18] In this study, the administration of anticoagulants and steroids increased the risk of bleeding.

Increased gastric acid secretion is associated with central nervous system lesions,[19] a fact that may account for some of the histologic differences between Cushing's ulcers and other forms of stress-induced acute gastric mucosal ulceration. In particular, the decerebrate state has been associated with increased rates of gastric acid secretion and upper gastrointestinal bleeding.[20] Certain patients with injuries of the central nervous system have significantly higher levels of serum gastrin than trauma patients without central nervous system injury; this may, in part, account for the observed hypersecretory state.[15]

Association with Drug Ingestion. A number of agents, such as nonsteroidal anti-inflammatory compounds and ethanol, are toxic to the gastric mucosa and may cause dyspepsia as well as acute gastric mucosal ulceration. These drug-induced acute gastric mucosal ulcers are often distributed in the proximal portion of the stomach and both grossly and histologically may be indistinguishable from stress-induced acute gastric mucosal ulcers. It is not known whether there is a common mechanism of mucosal injury between drug-induced and stress-induced ulceration. Massive bleeding from drug-induced lesions is rare, as is perforation. Epigastric discomfort, nausea, or anorexia may occur at any dose of nonsteroidal anti-inflammatory compounds in susceptible individuals; however, these effects are more common at higher doses. Dyspepsia, with or without peptic ulceration, is likely to worsen with ingestion of these compounds. Each of these compounds is a cyclo-oxygenase inhibitor and is an effective anti-inflammatory compound. Why there should be a difference in mucosal toxicity is unknown. There is no randomized, prospective study in arthritic patients comparing the efficacy of a series of these compounds against joint symptoms and gastric mucosal toxicity. Endoscopic evidence of injury is poorly correlated with gastrointestinal complaints. Each patient with arthritis should be treated with a drug that is effective, and gastrointestinal complaints should be minimized by coadministering antacid, antisecretory agents, or sucralfate. No one regimen should be considered the standard as individual variability of response is great.

Patients with drug-induced mucosal injury may present with chronic hypochromic, microcytic anemia due to chronic bleeding. Two studies[21, 22] using ^{51}Cr-labeled erythrocytes have demonstrated that 900 mg of aspirin four times per day for two weeks produces an average fecal blood loss of 3.6 ml per sample compared to 1.1 ml per sample after naproxen, 375 mg twice per day, and that 650 mg of aspirin four times per day for seven days produces fecal blood loss of about 5 ml per day compared to etodolac, 600 mg twice per day, which was associated with fecal blood loss of about 0.75 ml per day.

Endoscopic evidence of mucosal injury was found to be lower in patients taking corticosteroids (14 per cent) than in those taking aspirin (50 per cent),[23] and in the former group, only patients taking more than 10 mg of prednisone (or equivalent) for longer than six months had lesions. In another endoscopically controlled study of rheumatoid arthritis patients taking aspirin, at least eight 300 mg tablets per day for three months, 6 per cent taking enteric-coated aspirin alone and 23 per cent taking regular aspirin were found to have gastric mucosal damage.[24] In another study in healthy volunteers, regular aspirin (three tablets four times a day for four weeks) caused antral erosions in all subjects.[25] When the same subjects were switched to enteric-coated aspirin, only two of nine developed lesions. Duodenal erosions also developed in five of nine subjects on regular aspirin, but in none of those taking enteric-coated aspirin.

It may well be asked, is one nonsteroidal anti-inflammatory compound less toxic to the gastric mucosa than another? Any of these agents can cause gastric mucosal injury; however, aspirin appears to be the most toxic, followed by indomethacin, phenylbutazone, and ibuprofen, as evaluated endoscopically.[26] Further endoscopic evaluation of the gastric mucosa following several days of various nonsteroidal anti-inflammatory compounds in normal volunteers has demonstrated a similar gradation of propensity to cause mucosal injury. In one such study, aspirin, 3600 mg per day for seven days, caused the most severe injury, followed by indomethacin, 150 mg per day, and naproxen, 750 mg per day. Lesser injury was seen with naproxen, 500 mg per day, and ibuprofen, 1600 to 2400 mg per day.[27] A comparison of aspirin, 2600 to 3900 mg per day, sulindac, 300 to 400 mg per day, and naproxen, 500 to 750 mg per day, for seven days in a single-blind crossover study again identified aspirin as the most toxic to the gastric mucosa with a mean endoscopic score of 3.53 to 3.80, followed by naproxen, 1.07 to 2.27, and sulindac, 0.93. Flurbiprofen,[28] 100 to 200 mg per day, compared favorably to aspirin, 2600 mg per day for seven days, in terms of causing gastric mucosal injury evaluated endoscopically. A newer compound, etodolac,[29] 400 to 1200 mg per day, produced significantly less injury, with a 0.2 to 0.7 score, than aspirin, 3900 mg per day for seven days, which was associated with a mean score of 3.8.

Diagnosis of Acute Gastric Mucosal Ulceration

Familiarity with the conditions that predispose to development of acute gastric mucosal ulceration, such as severe trauma, sepsis, respiratory failure, renal failure, hypotension, jaundice, thermal burns, central nervous system injury, and chronic illness (particularly in the elderly), should provide the physician with a high index of suspicion that upper gastrointestinal bleeding may occur. Unfortunately, very few symptoms other than hematemesis and melena usually precede significant upper gastrointestinal hemorrhage.

Routine upper gastrointestinal barium series are virtually of no diagnostic value. These patients are seriously ill, confined to bed with tubes, at times uncooperative and, as such, limit the radiologist's ability to obtain an optimal study. In addition, the lesions of acute gastric mucosal ulceration are too superficial to visualize adequately. Should visceral angiography be a necessary diagnostic procedure, the presence of barium in the bowel may reduce its diagnostic accuracy.

Upper gastrointestinal endoscopy should be the first test performed to identify the bleeding source. The value of routine early endoscopy in all patients seen with acute upper gastrointestinal bleeding has been questioned in terms of reducing overall morbidity and mortality, but in patients in whom there is a high index of suspicion that the bleeding is due to acute gastric mucosal erosions not controlled by routine medical measures, endoscopy should be undertaken. A diagnosis will be made in nearly 90 per cent of these patients.[30] In a series of 183 patients with acute hemorrhage of the upper gastrointestinal tract, the primary cause of bleeding, as judged endoscopically, was acute gastric erosion, but in 43 per cent of these patients, more than one source of bleeding was identified.[31] The relative ease and diagnostic accuracy of upper gastrointestinal endoscopy makes it the primary diagnostic procedure in patients suspected of bleeding from acute gastric mucosal erosions.

In those patients who continue to bleed and in whom endoscopy has not provided a diagnosis, visceral angiography should be performed. A bleeding rate of 0.5 ml per minute appears to be the major requirement for visualization of a dye blush at the bleeding site.[32] A blush is usually visualized on a selective left gastric artery injection in patients with bleeding from acute gastric mucosal ulceration. If angiography reveals the location of bleeding, the catheter should be left in place for potential therapeutic use of vasoconstrictor drugs.

Nonsurgical Therapy of Bleeding Acute Gastric Mucosal Ulcers

Medical Therapy. Of prime importance in the treatment of bleeding from acute gastric mucosal ulcers is correction of the underlying predisposing condition. If that is hypovolemic shock, adequate intravascular volume must be established. The incidence of stress bleeding in injured patients correlates directly with the number of units of transfused blood required during resuscitation. Patients requiring less than four units rarely develop these lesions, whereas those requiring more than ten units often do.[33] If the underlying condition is sepsis, a thorough evaluation of possible sources must be undertaken. In a recent report[34] comparing the efficacy of antacids and cimetidine as prophylactic medications in 77 critically ill patients, there were five episodes of major gastrointestinal bleeding. Each of these patients was refractory to both medications in that intragastric pH could not be kept ≥ 4, with ongoing sepsis or respiratory failure being the major stressors. Inability to maintain the gastric luminal fluid at pH ≥ 4 with any single or combination medical prophylactic regimen suggests an untreated septic focus; whether this is due to higher rates of acid secretion or more rapid gastric emptying is not known.

The likelihood of bleeding is greater if the infectious process is intraperitoneal or pulmonary than if it is peripheral. Sepsis must be managed by surgical drainage, appropriate antibiotic therapy, or both. If the underlying condition is respiratory insufficiency, adequate respiratory function must be maintained. Artificial ventilation and occasionally tracheostomy may be required.

Nasogastric intubation with a large-bore tube allows gastric decompression and reduces the risk of vomiting and aspiration, providing access to the gastric mucosa for saline irrigation and information about the rate of bleeding. The Ewald tube is the best tube for this purpose, since the stomach often contains large clots that cannot be aspirated through a conventional nasogastric tube. With iced saline lavage, nearly 80 per cent of patients will stop bleeding.[1] Some consideration has been given to the use of intragastric levarterenol,[35] but its advantage over saline has not been proved clinically. If the bleeding is controlled with iced saline lavage, the tube is left in place for antacid instillation. Keeping the gastric luminal contents at pH ≥ 7 by instillation of antacids appears to be effective in reducing the incidence of rebleeding once it is initially controlled in stress- and burn-induced acute gastric mucosal erosions.[36, 37] Although there are a few published studies of the efficacy of the histamine H_2-receptor antagonist cimetidine in controlling established upper gastrointestinal bleeding, these have not been blind or controlled. To date, there are no prospective randomized endoscopically controlled studies that indicate that cimetidine is effective in controlling established bleeding from acute gastric mucosal erosions.[38] The effectiveness of antacids and cimetidine in prophylaxis will be discussed later in this chapter.

Somatostatin has been reported to control established bleeding from peptic ulcer.[39, 40] This peptide inhibits stimulated gastric acid and pepsin secretion[41] and reduces splanchnic blood flow.[42] In one report,[43] in patients who were bleeding from chronic peptic ulcer and considered too high a risk for surgical intervention, somatostatin given intravenously was significantly more effective in stopping the bleeding (80 per cent) than was cimetidine (10 per cent). It is yet to be determined if somatostatin is effective in reducing hemorrhage from acute gastric mucosal erosions.

The use of prostaglandin for established bleeding from acute gastric mucosal erosions is theoretically attractive, but there are no reported clinical trials using any of the prostaglandin analogues for this specific purpose. Anecdotal reports suggest that 15(R)-15-methyl PGE_2 may be effective in arresting bleeding in seriously ill patients refractory to other medical forms of therapy.[44, 45]

In patients with drug-induced acute gastric mucosal ulceration, discontinuation of the offending drug, in conjunction with acid neutralization, will in most cases eliminate the need for other forms of therapy.

Angiographic Therapeutic Techniques. Angiographic methods for the control of upper gastrointestinal hemorrhage include intra-arterial infusion of vasopressin and transcatheter arterial embolization.[46]

Consideration of these modalities may be made when therapy has failed. Intraceliac or left gastric artery vasopressin is administered as a continuous infusion at a rate of 0.2 to 0.4 units per minute for 48 to 72 hours with tapering of the dose before the infusion is discontinued.[47] Vasopressin is metabolized by the liver, so major side effects are infrequent. This form of therapy should be undertaken with extreme caution in patients with cardiac ischemia. Other complications may occur locally at the arterial catheter site. The infusion of vasopressin is usually associated with prompt reduction in blood loss. In one randomized study, initial control of bleeding occurred in 80 per cent of patients and complete control in 67 per cent.[48] In another randomized study, vasopressin reduced massive upper gastrointestinal bleeding, but no improvement in survival rate was observed, even in noncirrhotic patients.[49]

The second angiographic technique for control of bleeding is occlusion of the bleeding artery by transcatheter embolization. Autologous clot with additives such as oxidized cellulose, aminocaproic acid, thrombin, or surgical gelatin has been used.[43] For this technique, one major artery should be supplying the area of bleeding, but in the stomach this is rarely the case. The submucosal plexus is so extensive that no gastric artery is an end vessel. Although it has been reported to be a successful technique for control of upper gastrointestinal bleeding,[50] very few patients with acute gastric mucosal ulceration bleeding have been studied. Collateralization and recannulation predispose to rebleeding. Occasionally, end-organ necrosis has resulted from this technique.

Endoscopic Therapeutic Techniques. Techniques for control of upper gastrointestinal bleeding via the gastroscope include mono- and bipolar electrocauterization, argon laser photocoagulation, and neodymium-YAG laser photocoagulation.[50–54] Presently, each of these techniques is being investigated with respect to its efficacy in controlling hemorrhage in experimental bleeding ulcer models in animals and its safety in terms of depth of tissue injury.[55] These techniques have been used to treat upper gastrointestinal bleeding from a variety of lesions in randomized but uncontrolled studies. Reports on monopolar electrocauterization therapy indicate about 95 per cent hemostatic efficacy and no complications.[56, 57] Argon laser photocoagulation has been reported to be 96 per cent effective with no complications.[58] YAG laser photocoagulation has been reported to be 90 to 94 per cent effective with a 1 to 2 per cent incidence of perforation.[55–59] The true efficacy of each technique, and its safety, must be more completely evaluated in order to place this modality in proper perspective for use in patients with acute gastric mucosal erosion hemorrhage.

Surgical Therapy of Bleeding Acute Gastric Mucosal Ulcers

In 75 to 85 per cent of patients, bleeding from acute gastric mucosal erosions will be controlled with saline lavage, antacids, or vasoconstrictor therapy.

Surgical intervention should be considered when patients require in excess of four to six units of blood per 24 to 48 hours, particularly if attempts at therapeutic endoscopy have failed. In general, the consensus of opinion favors early rather than late surgical intervention once all available nonsurgical modalities have been exhausted.

No randomized controlled studies comparing different types of surgical procedures in the treatment of acute gastric mucosal ulceration have been conducted. Therefore, a variety of operations have been proposed, ranging from vagotomy and pyloroplasty with oversewing of bleeding lesions to gastric devascularization or total gastrectomy. No one approach has emerged as the treatment of choice. The only observation that is uniform is that the mortality rate for all forms of surgical therapy is 30 to 40 per cent.

The effects of a variety of surgical approaches on mortality and rebleeding rates are indicated in Table 45–1. Vagotomy and drainage procedure, usually pyloroplasty, with oversewing has been advocated by some as the primary operative procedure. The cumulative rebleeding rate following vagotomy and pyloroplasty is 41 per cent and the mortality rate is 47 per cent. Recognizing a significant rebleeding rate following vagotomy and pyloroplasty, proponents of this operation consider total gastrectomy as a second procedure if recurrent bleeding is not again controlled by medical means.[60] The results for vagotomy and hemigastrectomy are not different from those for vagotomy and pyloroplasty for rates of rebleeding (30 versus 41 per cent) or mortality (47 versus 47 per cent). These data have influenced some[61] to recommend the most simple, rapid, and atraumatic procedure, vagotomy and pyloroplasty, as the treatment of choice.

Total gastrectomy for the surgical treatment of bleeding acute gastric mucosal ulcers has been considered to be the treatment of choice by others because of the virtual lack of postoperative rebleeding.[62, 63] Although the mortality rate in one series was 100 per cent following total gastrectomy, this procedure has not been uniformly fatal. The authors suggest that the number of stress factors, recurrent bleeding, respiratory failure, and reoperation were positively correlated

Table 45–1. RESULTS OF SURGICAL THERAPY FOR BLEEDING ACUTE GASTRIC MUCOSAL ULCERATION

Procedure	Mortality (%)	Rebleeding (%)	Reference No.
Vagotomy and pyloroplasty (oversewing lesions)	55	61	50
	38	25	47
	32	36	47
	62	43	49
Vagotomy and hemigastrectomy	63	37	50
	57	28	47
	33	11	47
	33	44	49
Total gastrectomy	18	0	47
	100	0	49
Gastric devascularization	38	9	50

with the mortality rate, and on this basis recommend rapid intervention and generous extirpative surgery once intensive medical measures fail to control hemorrhage.

The gastric devascularization procedure[64] is the newest addition to the surgical alternatives for control of bleeding. In this procedure, right gastric arteries and the left and right gastroepiploic arteries are ligated near their respective origins, the entire blood supply to the stomach being via the short gastric vessels. Although low rates of rebleeding were reported for this procedure, the mortality rate remains high, 38 per cent. On that count, gastric devascularization offers no advantage over alternative procedures.

Prophylaxis Against Bleeding from Acute Gastric Mucosal Ulceration

In view of the mortality rate (80 per cent) associated with significant hemorrhage from acute gastric mucosal ulceration and the relatively ineffective means to control bleeding once it occurs, much attention and research have been aimed at preventing this complication. Reduction of intraluminal gastric acidity is a very important prophylactic aspect. Critically ill patients do not hypersecrete hydrochloric acid, but the endogenous mechanisms that maintain the physiologic proton gradient across the gastric epithelium without causing damage seem to be less effective than normal.

Antacids. The effectiveness of antacids in the prevention of bleeding was studied in a prospective randomized controlled trial in 100 critically ill patients.[65] One group of 51 patients received antacid (Mylanta II), 30 ml initially and 30 ml at hourly intervals, provided that the pH of the gastric luminal contents was greater than 3.5; 60 ml was given if the pH of the contents was less than 3.5. The nasogastric tube was clamped for the hour between antacid administration. In the randomized group of patients who were not to receive antacid titration, the nasogastric tube was connected to intermittent suction. Patients who had frank blood in the nasogastric aspirate or had 4+ guaiac test results for the aspirate were considered to have upper gastrointestinal bleeding. Only two of the 51 patients (4 per cent) who received antacids bled. Twelve of the 49 patients (25 per cent) who did not receive antacids bled. Risk factors such as respiratory failure, sepsis, peritonitis, jaundice, renal failure, and hypotension were analyzed, and a positive correlation was found between the number of risk factors and the incidence of gastrointestinal bleeding.

The efficacy of antacids in the prevention of gastrointestinal bleeding in patients with burns of greater than 35 per cent of the total body surface area has also been established.[37] Twenty-four patients were selected to receive antacid therapy, which was administered as 60 ml aliquots to keep the gastric luminal contents at pH 7. The luminal contents were evaluated for pH at hourly intervals, and antacids were administered accordingly to keep the pH at 7. No antacids were given to 24 patients who had burns of equal severity. Significant gastrointestinal hemorrhage was defined as requiring three or more units of blood over 24 hours to maintain vital signs and hematocrit. Only one of 24 patients (4 per cent) who received antacids developed significant upper gastrointestinal hemorrhage. In contrast, seven of 24 patients (29 per cent) receiving no antacid therapy developed significant gastrointestinal complications, six developed hemorrhage, and one suffered perforation.

Histamine H$_2$ Receptor Antagonists. Two studies have suggested that ranitidine may be more effective than cimetidine in preventing the gastric luminal fluid pH from falling. In the first study,[66] 100 patients admitted to a surgical intensive care unit were randomized to receive either cimetidine (300 mg IV followed by 50 mg per hour) or ranitidine (50 mg IV followed by 12.5 mg per hour) for the duration of their stay in the unit. Intragastric pH was measured every four hours. Antacids were administered when the intragastric pH dropped below 5.0. The number of pH readings <5 and total number of pH readings were recorded for each patient. There was no difference overall in the number of patients who had at least one gastric pH reading <5; however, there was a larger proportion of patients with >10 to 25 per cent of gastric pH determinations <5 in the cimetidine-treated group than in the ranitidine-treated group. Similarly, in a second study,[67] 48 patients admitted to an intensive care unit were randomized to receive cimetidine (200 mg every six hours, 200 mg every four hours, or 400 mg every four hours) or ranitidine (50 mg every six hours, 50 mg every four hours, or 100 mg every four hours) intravenously over 15 minutes. The drugs were administered in dose increments as needed to maintain the intragastric pH >4. Intragastric pH was measured every two hours. Cimetidine was successful in maintaining the pH above 4 in five of 28 patients, and ranitidine succeeded in ten of 20 patients, a statistically significant difference, suggesting that ranitidine may be more effective than cimetidine, at these dose levels, in maintaining the intragastric pH above 4. No patient in either study was reported to have had significant gastrointestinal bleeding. Neither drug provided adequate maintenance of intragastric pH at 4 to 5 in all the patients, suggesting that intragastric pH must be monitored in patients receiving either drug to identify those patients whose dose may require a change or for whom antacids must be added to the prophylactic regimen.

A pharmacodynamic study[68] of intravenous cimetidine administration demonstrates that an infusion (300 mg followed by 37.5 to 100 mg per hour) provided better control of intragastric pH ($\geq$4) than a bolus regimen (300 mg every eight hours to 400 mg every four hours). The difference in ability to maintain intragastric pH above 4 was entirely due to less than adequate serum cimetidine levels (0.5 to 1.2 mg/100 ml) with the bolus regimen. A nonrandomized study suggested that the histamine H$_2$ receptor antagonists were also effective in preventing bleeding from acute gastric mucosal ulceration in critically ill patients.[69]

Subsequently, several prospective randomized studies were performed to evaluate the efficacy of the histamine H_2 receptor antagonist cimetidine in the prevention of bleeding in patients admitted to an intensive care unit with fulminant hepatic failure, with renal transplantation, and with central nervous system injury. Cimetidine may be more effective than placebo treatment in prophylaxis against acute gastric mucosal erosion bleeding in certain clinical settings. One endoscopically controlled, randomized double-blind prospective study of 39 patients admitted to an intensive care unit had a cimetidine (300 mg every six hours) and placebo control arm.[7] Fourteen of 21 patients treated with cimetidine and five of 18 patients in the placebo-treated group had normal-appearing mucosa 18 hours after being admitted to the unit. Endoscopic signs of bleeding cleared or did not develop in 20 (95 per cent) patients treated with cimetidine and in 11 (61 per cent) patients in the placebo-treated group. Significantly fewer blood transfusions were given to patients treated with cimetidine than with placebo. There was one death from upper gastrointestinal bleeding in a placebo-treated patient. Another study of the effectiveness of cimetidine in prophylaxis against upper gastrointestinal bleeding following renal transplantation was conducted comparing the incidence of gastrointestinal hemorrhage in 35 consecutive patients treated with cimetidine (200 mg intravenously every 12 hours followed by 200 mg three times per day and 400 mg orally at bedtime) with the incidence in 33 transplant recipients who had not received cimetidine.[70] The 35 patients treated with cimetidine had no episodes of upper gastrointestinal hemorrhage, compared with six of 33 patients (18 per cent) who did not receive cimetidine. Likewise, in a study of 50 patients with severe head injury, patients were randomized to receive cimetidine therapy (300 mg intravenously every four hours) or to have no cimetidine therapy.[17] Patients with bright red blood per nasogastric tube or gastric contents with 4+ guaiac test results for three consecutive eight-hour periods were considered to have significant upper gastrointestinal bleeding. Five of 26 patients (19 per cent) in the cimetidine group developed gastrointestinal bleeding compared with 18 of 24 patients (75 per cent) in the control group.

These observations are to be balanced against others which have not demonstrated cimetidine to be more effective than placebo in prophylaxis against these lesions. Two hundred twenty-one patients admitted to an intensive care unit were randomized to receive cimetidine (300 mg every six hours) or placebo.[71] Criteria for bleeding were hematemesis or gastric aspirate of more than 50 ml fresh blood, melena, drop in hematocrit > 2 gm/dl associated with melena or coffee-ground gastric drainage of at least 100 ml. No antacids were given. Intragastric pH was not measured. Six of 114 (5.3 per cent) patients given cimetidine and 11 of 107 (10.2 per cent) patients given placebo bled. This difference did not reach statistical significance. The same number of patients, 13, died in each group. Another randomized double-blind study of the efficacy of cimetidine (20 mg/kg per 24 hours) in preventing upper gastrointestinal hemorrhage utilized the appearance of ^{51}Cr-labeled erythrocytes in gastric contents to determine blood loss.[72] This was a double-blind controlled study. Intragastric pH was measured in each 24-hour gastric juice sample. Although cimetidine-treated patients had fewer days in which intragastric pH was below 3.5 (17.5 per cent) compared to placebo-treated patients (72.2 per cent), blood loss in the cimetidine-treated patients was 5.24 ml, nearly twice the blood loss in placebo-treated patients, 2.18 ml per 24 hours. Five patients treated with cimetidine bled significantly, whereas only one placebo-treated patient bled. Finally, a double-blind, randomized, endoscopically controlled study of the efficacy of cimetidine versus placebo treatment in the prevention of stress bleeding in patients with acute spinal injury has also failed to demonstrate a prophylactic effect of cimetidine (1.2 to 2.4 gm per 24 hours).[73] One hundred five patients were entered into the study. Antacids were given but intragastric pH was not measured. Endoscopic evaluation demonstrated that 12 of 43 (28 per cent) cimetidine-treated patients and 11 of 41 (27 per cent) placebo-treated patients had visible gastroduodenal ulcerations or erosions.

Cimetidine versus Antacids. A comparison[74] of cimetidine (300 mg every six hours intravenously) and antacids (30 ml every hour to keep gastric content at pH $\geq$ 3.5) in a randomized prospective trial of 75 critically ill patients in whom significant gastrointestinal bleeding was indicated by frank blood via the nasogastric tube or 4+ guaiac examination of gastric contents on three consecutive readings showed that none of the patients given antacids, but seven of the 38 given cimetidine (18 per cent), developed significant gastrointestinal bleeding during the study period. A number of studies have been conducted to address the question of whether cimetidine is as effective as antacid prophylaxis. Few studies demonstrate cimetidine to be superior to antacids, and the majority of investigators conclude that either cimetidine is equally effective when compared to antacids or antacids are more effective.

Seventy-five patients with fulminant hepatic failure were included in two trials,[75] which, however, were not designed properly. The authors concluded that the histamine H_2 receptor antagonists were more effective in the prophylaxis against hepatic failure–induced gastric mucosal bleeding than were antacids. It has been suggested that the antacid dose schedule used in these studies, every four hours, was inadequate and might account for the lesser effect of antacids compared with histamine H_2 receptor antagonists.[76]

Equal prophylactic efficacy of cimetidine and antacids, however, has been concluded in the following studies. First, 44 patients admitted to an intensive care unit were randomized to receive cimetidine (300 mg every six hours to 400 mg every four hours) or antacid (Mylanta II, 30 to 90 ml per hour), keeping the intragastric pH $\geq$ 4.[77] Endoscopy was performed at 74 hours. Erosions occurred in five of 21 (24 per cent) cimetidine-treated patients and eight of 16 (50 per cent) antacid-treated patients. Intragastric pH $\geq$ 4 was maintained in 79 per cent of cimetidine-treated patients and 98 per cent of antacid-treated patients; there was no significant bleeding in any patient enrolled in this study. Second, a double-blind randomized study of the comparative efficacy of cimetidine or antacids versus placebo was reported in patients requiring mechanical ventilation.[78] Fourteen patients were randomized to the control group, 11 to the cimetidine group (300 mg every six hours), and 11 to the antacid group (Mylanta II, 30 ml per hour). Intragastric pH was not measured. Gastrointestinal bleeding occurred in nine patients; it was occult in two, and overt in seven. Bleeding did not occur in any patient in the antacid group, whereas in one patient of the cimetidine group and in five of the control group, bleeding did occur. Third, a double-blind endoscopically controlled study compared cimetidine (400 mg every four hours), antacids (30 ml every two hours), and placebo as prophylactic therapy against stress-induced bleeding in patients with thermal injury.[79] Intragastric pH was measured hourly. Endoscopically normal gastric and duodenal mucosa was seen in 23 per cent of the cimetidine group and 14 per cent of the antacid treatment group. Gastric erythema and ulcer were seen in 77 and 23 per cent of the cimetidine and in 71 and 14 per cent of the antacid-treated groups, respectively. No catastrophic gastrointestinal bleeding occurred in any patient in this study.

Other investigators claim that antacids are more effective than cimetidine as a prophylactic measure in patients at risk of developing these lesions. First, a randomized prospective study of 300 patients in an intensive care unit setting was reported, in which the bleeding end point was persistent 4 + positive guaiac nasogastric aspirate for > 16 hours, bright red bleeding through the nasogastric tube, guaiac positive stools, or a fall in hematocrit.[5] One hundred patients were randomized to receive cimetidine (300 mg every six hours), antacids to maintain intragastric pH $\geq$ 4, or nothing. Patients were stratified for a number of risk factors, which were correlated with the incidence of gastrointestinal bleeding. Cimetidine at this fixed dose was not as effective as antacids in maintaining intragastric pH $\geq$ 4. Because the effect of antacids was significantly more dramatic than that of cimetidine (7 per cent compared to 32 per cent bled, in the group of patients with the 3 to 6 severity index score), the authors concluded that antacids may be more effective than cimetidine in this setting. Second, 144 patients admitted to an intensive care unit were randomly assigned to receive either cimetidine (300 to 600 mg every six hours) or antacids (Mylanta II, 30 ml every hour) to maintain intragastric pH.[80] Prophylaxis failure was considered to be an intragastric pH $\leq$ 4 on three of six consecutive hourly determinations or development of significant upper gastrointestinal bleeding requiring blood transfusion. No patient given antacids failed this form of therapy, whereas 26 per cent of patients given cimetidine failed by the above criteria. Significant upper gastrointestinal bleeding, requiring transfusion, occurred in only one patient who had been randomized to receive cimetidine. Third, cimetidine treatment (300 to 400 mg every four to six hours) was associated with

adequate intragastric fluid pH maintenance in 23 per cent of patients and an upper gastrointestinal bleeding incidence of 5 per cent, compared to antacid treatment (Maalox, 30 to 60 ml every hour), in which no bleeding occurred in a randomized prospective study of 77 critically ill patients.[81] The authors concluded that antacids were the preferred agent for gastric neutralization in this setting.

Complications of both antacids and cimetidine must be kept in mind when determining the appropriate prophylactic medical regimen. Antacids have been associated with diarrhea, ileus, hypophosphatemia, hypermagnesemia, and metabolic alkalosis. Cimetidine has been associated with mental changes, stimulation or depression, thrombocytopenia, and drug-drug interactions. These complications are reversible following discontinuation of the offending medication.

Sucralfate. Sucralfate is a basic aluminum salt of sucrose octasulfate which has been demonstrated in randomized prospective studies to be as effective as antacids and histamine H_2 receptor antagonists in the acute healing of duodenal ulcers. The mechanism by which this compound works is not well established. Although originally purported to work via an endogenous prostaglandin-mediated mechanism, other mechanisms are also probably involved. Several clinical trials have compared sucralfate to placebo, antacids, and cimetidine as prophylactic therapeutic agents against acute gastric mucosal erosion bleeding in severely ill patients.

First, 100 critically ill patients were randomized, 52 receiving antacids (30 to 60 ml Mylanta II to maintain intragastric pH $\geq$ 3.5) and 48 receiving sucralfate (1 gm suspended in 30 ml saline every six hours).[82] Any patient who had frank blood in the nasogastric aspirate or three consecutive strongly positive guaiac nasogastric aspirates was considered a failure. No life-threatening hemorrhage occurred in any patient. Three of 48 (6 per cent) sucralfate and two of 52 (4 per cent) antacid-treated patients were failures. The authors concluded that sucralfate therapy is as effective as antacids in the prevention of bleeding from these lesions.

Second, a randomized prospective study of 50 patients who had abdominal aortic aneurysmectomy compared the efficacy of antacids (30 ml Mylanta II each hour to maintain intragastric pH $\geq$ 3.5) or sucralfate (1 gm in 30 ml normal saline every six hours) in preventing stress-induced gastrointestinal bleeding.[83] Any patient who had frank bleeding or strongly guaiac positive nasogastric aspirate on three consecutive readings was considered a failure. Intragastric pH was measured hourly. No patient in the antacid-treated group and only one in the sucralfate-treated group were failures of therapy, and no patient died of gastrointestinal bleeding.

Third, prophylaxis with the combination therapy pirenzepine, a μ_1 antagonist, plus sucralfate was as effective as pirenzepine plus cimetidine or antacids in 100 intensive care unit patients.[84] In this randomized prospective study, all patients received pirenzepine (50 mg each day), while in the various arms, patients received sucralfate (1 gm every four hours), antacids (10 ml every two hours), or cimetidine (2 gm every 24 hours). Intragastric pH was measured every eight hours. Bloody nasogastric aspirate, hematemesis, and melena were used as the criteria for acute upper gastrointestinal hemorrhage. Five (15 per cent) patients who received cimetidine, four (12 per cent) who received antacids, and four (12 per cent) who received sucralfate died owing to underlying disease. Hemorrhage contributed to death in one patient who received cimetidine.

Finally, a recent abstract, again comparing sucralfate to antacids in preventing acute gastrointestinal bleeding in 62 ventilator-dependent patients, indicates that 52 per cent of patients (11 of 21) given cimetidine, 39 per cent of patients (7 of 18) given antacids, and 21 per cent (4 of 19) given sucralfate developed coffee-ground nasogastric aspirates.[85] Eight per cent of patients had bright red blood per nasogastric tube, four in the antacid-treated group, one in the cimetidine-treated group, and none in the sucralfate group. These observations support the hypothesis that sucralfate, which has no effect on gastric acid secretion, is as effective as antacids or histamine H_2 receptor antagonists as a prophylactic agent against acute gastric mucosal erosion bleeding in critically ill patients. This compound is not absorbed and consequently is associated with few side effects. Caution should be exercised in patients who recently have had an upper gastrointestinal anastomosis, as with the use of antacids.

The potential adverse effect of neutralizing gastric acid or blocking its production in terms of the development of pneumonia in critically ill patients on ventilators has recently been addressed in two randomized, prospective studies in which prophylaxis with sucralfate was compared to antacids or histamine H_2 receptor antagonists. Gastric bleeding was monitored; however, the development of pneumonia, length of stay in the intensive care unit, and mortality were additionally addressed. The hypothesis being tested in these two studies is that a more neutral intragastric pH allows greater bacterial colonization than one which is acidic and that this colonization leads to a greater frequency of pneumonia due to chronic aspiration of gastric contents. In the first study,[86] 95 patients were randomized to prophylactically receive either sucralfate (1 gm every four hours) or a histamine H_2 receptor antagonist. These patients were in an intensive care unit, had been intubated for 24 hours, and were mechanically ventilated. Each patient had a nasogastric tube in place, and intragastric pH was monitored. Bleeding was assessed by examination of nasogastric aspirates for presence of occult blood with guaiac testing, hemolyzed blood, or active bleeding. The diagnosis of ventilator-associated pneumonia required a new and persistent infiltrate on chest X-ray that was consistent with pneumonia and at least three of the following: (1) purulent sputum with > 25 leukocytes per high power field, (2) a significant respiratory or nosocomial pathogen isolated from a tracheal aspirate culture, (3)

peripheral leukocytosis > 10,000 per cu mm, or (4) temperature > 38°C. Comparing the sucralfate to antacid-treated patients, 79 versus 64 per cent had no bleeding, 12 versus 32 per cent had occult blood, 5 versus 2 per cent had coffee-ground aspirate, and 5 versus 2 per cent had bright red blood per nasogastric tube, respectively. Twelve per cent of patients treated with sucralfate developed pneumonia, whereas 26 per cent treated with antacid or H_2 antagonists did, a trend which did not reach statistical significance. The mean number of ventilator days was 7.8 for patients treated with sucralfate, compared to 14.5 days for patients treated with antacids or H_2 receptor antagonists, a statistically significant difference. Similarly, the number of ICU days was greater in the antacid or H_2 receptor antagonist–treated group compared to the sucralfate-treated group, a statistically significant difference. Aerobic bacterial isolates of the numerous organisms—*S. aureus, E. coli*, mixed gram-negative bacilli, *H. influenzae*, β-hemolytic streptococci, mixed *S. aureus*, gram-negative bacilli, *S. pneumoniae*, and *Serratia* species—were greater in the H_2 receptor antagonist–treated patients than in the sucralfate-treated patients. The author concluded from these data that rates of ventilator-associated pneumonia, morbidity, and mortality are lower in patients receiving prophylactic sucralfate compared with those receiving antacids or histamine H_2 receptor antagonists, and that perhaps agents which do not elevate intragastric pH should be used as prophylactic agents to prevent acute gastric mucosal erosion bleeding.

Another study which lends support to this hypothesis also prospectively studied not only the prophylactic efficacy of sucralfate (1 gm every four hours) versus antacids (10 ml every two hours) against gastrointestinal bleeding but also the rate of nosocomial pneumonia in 100 ventilated patients in an intensive care unit.[87] Intragastric pH was measured every eight hours. Bleeding was defined as macroscopically visible hematemesis, bloody nasogastric aspirate, or melena. The diagnosis of pneumonia was made by an unbiased physician using all the following criteria: pulmonary changes on chest X-ray, temperature $\geq$ 38.5°C, leukocytosis, and bacteria in a tracheal smear. One in 50 patients in each prophylactic group showed signs of acute upper gastrointestinal hemorrhage. In 4 per cent of antacid-treated patients and in 54 per cent of sucralfate-treated patients the intragastric pH was < 4.0. In terms of nosocomial pneumonia, 10 per cent of patients receiving sucralfate and 34 per cent of patients receiving antacids developed signs sufficient to fulfill the criteria. The authors concluded that sucralfate provided adequate protection against stress bleeding while also minimizing the risk of nosocomial pneumonia. It has also been suggested that, in addition to not interfering with the intragastric pH, sucralfate may have some antibacterial activity which results in a lesser degree of bacterial overgrowth than in the antacid-treated patient.[88] In this study, the rate of overgrowth in human gastric juice at various controlled pH values to which either antacids or sucralfate was added was significantly retarded for *Pseudomonas aeruginosa* and *E. coli*.

Further confirmatory studies are in order before embracing the concept that in the ventilator-dependent patient, allowing the intragastric pH to fall to 4 or below with sucralfate prophylaxis may be more appropriate than maintaining the pH $\geq$ 4 when taking into account the morbidity and mortality rates associated with nosocomial pneumonitis.

Prostaglandins. Considering the experimental work which has demonstrated that many prostanoids, natural or synthetic, at nonantisecretory doses confer gross and histologic protection of the gastric mucosa against a multiplicity of ulcerogens, it is surprising that few studies have addressed the efficacy of prostanoids in prophylaxis against stress-induced acute gastric mucosal erosion bleeding. Several studies using synthetic prostanoids in this setting are ongoing and have yet to be reported. There are anecdotal reports in which 15(R)-15-methyl prostaglandin E$_2$ (50 μg every six hours), given orally, was associated with cessation of upper gastrointestinal bleeding that was refractory to other medical forms of therapy.[44, 45] To date, only one study, randomized and prospective, comparing the efficacy of 15(R)-15-methyl prostaglandin E$_2$ to antacids in the prevention of upper gastrointestinal bleeding in patients in an intensive care unit has been published.[89] Forty-six patients were randomized to receive either 15(R)-15-methyl prostaglandin E$_2$ (100 μg every four hours) or antacids (30 to 60 ml every hour to maintain intragastric pH $\geq$ 3.5). Intragastric pH was measured hourly. Nasogastric aspirate was examined every four hours for frank or occult blood. Any patient who had frank blood in the aspirate or positive occult blood test on three consecutive readings over a 12-hour period was considered to have gastrointestinal bleeding and prophylaxis was considered a failure. Three of 22 (14 per cent) patients in the antacid-treated group bled, compared to 12 of 24 (50 per cent) patients in the prostaglandin-treated group. There were no deaths in the antacid-treated patients, whereas one patient in the prostaglandin-treated group died of hypoxic brain injury, not related to gastrointestinal bleeding. Upper gastrointestinal bleeding was not a major clinical problem in any of these patients. This study, standing alone, cannot be considered to be definitive because ongoing studies using other synthetic prostanoids will soon be reported. It does, however, suggest that it is unlikely that the prostanoids will prove to be prophylactically superior to those compounds which are presently being used.

Elemental Diets. In 1980, an article appeared which was a retrospective study in 146 severely burned patients, comparing the nutritional efficacy of regular diet compared to an "elemental" diet.[90] Major upper gastrointestinal bleeding occurred in 30 per cent of patients taking a regular diet, whereas only 3 per cent of patients on the elemental diet developed this complication of severe burn injury. These authors concluded that the elemental diet was associated with a decrease in major upper gastrointestinal bleeding while still contributing to calorie intake. A second retrospective

study appeared in 1983 in which the incidence of upper gastrointestinal bleeding in mechanically ventilated patients receiving enteral alimentation was compared to that in patients receiving prophylactic antacids or cimetidine.[91] Fourteen of 20 (70 per cent) patients receiving antacids, seven of nine (78 per cent) receiving cimetidine, and none of 14 patients receiving an elemental diet developed gastrointestinal bleeding. More recently, a prospective randomized study[92] suggested that continuous intragastric feeding with an elemental diet provides sufficient proton neutralization to maintain intragastric pH $\geq$ 3.5, which may account for the potential beneficial effect of continuous intragastric infusion of an elemental diet against stress-induced acute gastric mucosal erosion bleeding.

Conclusions. It is reasonable to conclude from these studies that prophylactic therapy is better than none for the prevention of upper gastrointestinal bleeding in patients at risk to develop acute gastric mucosal erosions. These studies use somewhat artificial bleeding end points, because the clinician really wants to know about the effect of these drugs on life-threatening massive gastric mucosal bleeding. Whether guaiac positive nasogastric aspirates or endoscopically visualized gastric mucosal erosions are predictors of massive bleeding is not clear. Because the incidence of bleeding is very low, it is unlikely that we will be able to answer the question to our satisfaction, and what data are published will have to serve as the basis for recommendations. A case for using antacids as the standard prophylactic medication can easily be made. Hourly gastric pH monitoring and antacid titration are the mainstay of stress ulcer prophylaxis, with high-potency antacids being the preferred agents. Histamine H$_2$ receptor antagonists may serve as adjunctive therapy in patients requiring large doses of antacids, having acid-base abnormalities from high gastric output states, or in whom a recent gastrointestinal anastomosis was performed. Parenteral histamine H$_2$ receptor antagonists should be used prophylactically when antacids are either contraindicated or the response is unreliable, and rarely should they be used alone.

Sucralfate, as a prophylactic agent, appears to be as effective as antacids or histamine H$_2$ receptor antagonists insofar as studies have been reported on its use in patients predisposed to develop stress bleeding. Advantages of its use include twice or three times per day dosing, lack of side effects, and perhaps cost, when consideration is given to the relative ease of administration, which does not require pH monitoring at one- or two-hour intervals.

Additional experience with the use of various synthetic prostaglandins in this clinical setting is required before a more definitive statement can be made regarding their use. Particular attention to side effects will be important in this evaluation. Anecdotal reports, however, seem sufficiently encouraging to suggest that 15(R)-15-methyl PGE$_2$ may be given intragastrically to patients, refractory to all forms of medical therapy and support, who continue to bleed from the gastric mucosa.

In those patients who continue to bleed, attempts at

therapeutic endoscopy may stem the tide; however, if they are ineffective, gastrectomy is indicated for life-threatening hemorrhage.

EXPERIMENTAL PRODUCTION OF STRESS ULCERS

Stress ulcers can be produced in animals by a variety of methods. As for other diseases, experimental models are important in order to better understand the pathogenesis of the disease and to test various forms of treatment. We will review some of the most recognized methods to produce stress ulcers as well as the results obtained under various experimental conditions, and we will discuss the pathogenesis of stress ulcers.

Experimental Methods to Produce Stress Ulcers

Restraint Ulcers. Restraint was one of the earliest methods used to produce stress ulcers.[93–95] It consists of placing rats into a very confined space, by means of either rods, plaster, metal box with movable sides and ends, surgical tape, or window screen. The animals are usually fasted overnight prior to restraint, although this may not be essential. The duration of restraint varies from two to 24 hours, depending on whether the ambient temperature is normal or very cold. Restrained animals placed in a room at 4°C develop ulcers within two to four hours.

These ulcers are located in the gastric corpus, i.e., the portion of the glandular stomach secreting acid and pepsin. The gastric antrum and the forestomach are not affected. The mucosal erosions are superficial and do not penetrate the muscularis mucosae. After release from confinement, the ulcers usually heal within a week. Contrary to the sex ratio in humans, female rats are more sensitive to restraint ulcers than are male rats. Restraint ulcers are prevented by antisecretory agents (anticholinergics,[94] certain prostaglandins[96]). Pentagastrin, although stimulating gastric secretion, also reduced the severity of restraint ulcers, presumably because of a trophic effect.[97]

Massive hydrothorax is associated with restraint ulcers in fed rats.[94] However, these two changes, ulcers and hydrothorax, are unrelated, for it is possible to prevent one and not the other. For instance, fasting prevents hydrothorax but not the ulcers, whereas anticholinergic agents prevent the ulcers but not the hydrothorax. The mechanism of hydrothorax due to restraint is not known. The pleural fluid is a yellowish transudate that coagulates on standing, and is probably identical to plasma. Because the development of hydrothorax is abundant and rapid, the hematocrit increases.[94]

Exertion Ulcers. Forced exertion in rotating cages produces multiple gastric ulcers in rats.[98] As in restraint ulcers, (1) exertion ulcers are located in the corpus and are smaller and more numerous than restraint ulcers (Fig. 45–2), (2) female rats are more sensitive to their formation than are male rats, and (3) these ulcers are prevented by antisecretory agents,[98] certain prostaglandins,[99] and prednisolone.[98] The first demonstration of exertion ulcers was by Selye,[100] who found that a variety of stress conditions, including forced muscular exercise, produced a nonspecific alarm reaction, of which gastric ulcers were a constant feature. In dogs, forced exertion leads to gastric ulcers when gastric acid secretion is stimulated by histamine.[101]

Activity Stress Ulcers. Rats placed in running-wheel

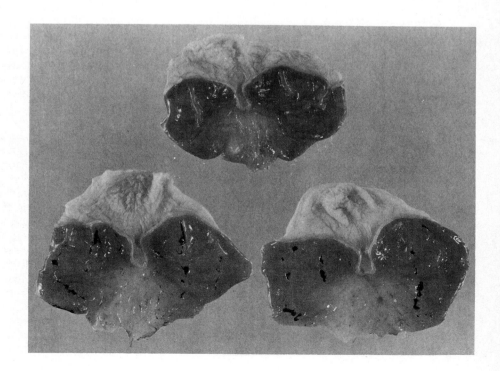

Figure 45–2. Exertion ulcers in rats. *Top,* Normal stomach, open along the lesser curvature. The upper portion (forestomach) is lined with squamous epithelium. The lower portion is glandular and is divided into corpus (darker area on each side of midline) and antrum (triangular central area). *Bottom,* Stomachs after forced exertion for two hours and 45 minutes. Note multiple bleeding ulcers in the corpus.

activity cages and given food for only one hour a day develop gastric ulcers in the corpus within four to 12 days.[102] In some cases, the crater penetrates through the muscularis mucosae. Several other species are also susceptible to activity stress ulcers (hamsters, gerbils, guinea pigs, chipmunks). Gastric secretion is reduced by the procedure. Female rats are more susceptible to activity stress ulcers than are male rats. Activity stress ulcers penetrate deeper than do exertion ulcers, probably because they are more chronic; they progress for several days, whereas exertion ulcers are produced within three hours.

Shock-Induced Ulcers. Traumatic shock produced in rats and guinea pigs by tumbling in a rotating drum produces gastric ulcers as well as intense mesenteric congestion.[103] Hemorrhagic shock also causes gastric ulcers in rats and rabbits.[104, 105] Septic shock elicited in dogs by intraperitoneal injection of mixed bacteria and bile is followed by development of bleeding gastric erosions within two days, as well as by increased basal, food-stimulated, and pentagastrin-stimulated acid secretion.[106] These ulcers are prevented by a histamine H_2 blocker, cimetidine, at doses that totally block basal secretion and inhibit stimulated acid output by more than 80 per cent. On the other hand, 16,16-dimethyl prostaglandin E_2 prevents these acute gastric erosions even at doses that do not affect gastric secretion. The authors concluded that cimetidine prevents the development of sepsis-induced gastric erosions by inhibiting acid secretion, whereas 16,16-dimethyl PGE_2 acts through cytoprotection, that is, by a mechanism yet unknown but other than inhibition of gastric secretion.

Curling's Ulcers. Extensive skin burns have been known to produce gastroduodenal ulcers in humans ever since Curling's original observation.[10] Such ulcers can be produced in rats[107] and dogs.[108] In dogs, hemorrhage, sepsis, and injection of histamine increase the incidence and severity of such ulcers. However, Curling's ulcers were also produced in germ-free mice, a fact indicating that concomitant infection is not essential.[109]

Neurologically Induced Ulcers. Cushing was the first to recognize that gastroduodenal ulcers were particularly frequent in patients with neurologic trauma.[4] Similar ulcers are produced experimentally by electrical stimulation of various areas of the hypothalamus in monkeys and cats.[110–112] In two of these studies,[111, 112] the site of ulceration was not mentioned; in the third one,[110] ulcers were found in the stomach (fundus and antrum) and the duodenum. In most cases, increased acid secretion accompanied ulcer formation, although a cause-and-effect relationship has not been established.

The Executive Monkey. In 1958, interest was stimulated by reports that monkeys placed in a situation in which they had to "decide," by pressing a lever, whether a nearby monkey would receive electric shocks, developed gastroduodenal ulcers which sometimes perforated and were lethal.[113] The experiment was called "the executive monkey." Although subsequent studies in other laboratories could not reproduce these results, a similar method proved successful in monkeys subjected to multiple psychologic stress procedures.[114] Gastroduodenal lesions ranging from discoloration of the mucosa to disruption of mucosal integrity were produced in 88 per cent of the animals after four to ten weeks.

Drug-Induced Gastric Ulcers and Erosive Gastritis. Although stress ulcers and drug-induced ulcers are separate entities, they have several features in common, such as rapid onset, rapid healing once the stress condition or the drug is discontinued, multiplicity within a single stomach, and the fact that they usually are confined to the mucosa and do not penetrate the deeper layers of the gastric wall. We will consider here only the drugs known to produce gastroduodenal damage in humans. These agents are the nonsteroidal anti-inflammatory compounds, corticosteroids, and reserpine.

Nonsteroidal Anti-Inflammatory Compounds (NOSAC). Nonsteroidal anti-inflammatory compounds, such as aspirin, indomethacin, and phenylbutazone, are ulcerogenic in experimental animals. In humans, aspirin is the most important among these, in large part because, being an over-the-counter drug, it is used by many more patients than prescription drugs and is self-administered for a variety of ailments. The usual experimental procedure in rats consists of administering the drug orally after fasting the animals for 24 hours. Ulcers develop in the corpus two to five hours after administration, provided that acid is present in the stomach.[115, 116] Exposure to cold temperature markedly aggravates aspirin-induced ulcers.[117, 118]

Parenteral (subcutaneous, intraperitoneal, intravenous) administration of NOSAC (aspirin, indomethacin) can also produce gastric erosions in animals if the gastric contents are highly acid.[115, 116, 119] This shows that direct contact of the drug with the luminal side of the gastric mucosa is not required for ulcer formation, although in animals, aspirin is more ulcerogenic when given orally. This is also the case in humans: enteric-coated aspirin, which releases the drug only in the intestine, causes less gastric damage than regular aspirin tablets that disintegrate in the stomach.[22, 23]

Because acid is necessary for formation of NOSAC-induced ulcers, these are prevented by antisecretory drugs such as anticholinergics, histamine H_2 blockers, and antisecretory prostaglandins as well as by antacids. However, cytoprotective prostaglandins that do not affect gastric secretion prevent formation of NOSAC-induced gastric lesions even in the presence of acid, by an as-yet-unknown mechanism. This cytoprotective property of certain prostaglandins was also demonstrated in humans. Fecal occult blood was measured daily in human volunteers receiving high doses of aspirin (two tablets four times a day) and in arthritic patients treated with indomethacin (50 mg three times a day).[120–122] Such treatment increased the amount of occult blood originating from the gastric mucosa. The increase in fecal blood loss was prevented by concurrent treatment with prostaglandin E_2 given orally; by this route, this prostaglandin does not affect acid secretion.

Steroid-Induced Ulcers. Although the incidence of

chronic peptic ulcer in humans due to corticoid treatment does not appear to be high, many cases have been reported. Multiple, bleeding gastric ulcers can readily be produced in rats by cortisol or prednisolone.[123] These ulcers appear after two to three days and are localized in the corpus. Again, antisecretory drugs and antacids prevent their formation. It is interesting that pregnancy and lactation in rats markedly reduce their incidence,[124] an observation in accord with the known fact that peptic ulcer in women usually disappears during pregnancy and lactation.

Reserpine-Induced Ulcers. One of the side effects of reserpine treatment in humans is the development of gastric intolerance and sometimes gastroduodenal ulcer. Gastric ulcers are readily produced in rats by reserpine. Although the mechanism is not clear, these ulcers are associated with a sustained increase in gastric acid secretion.[125]

Pathogenesis of Stress Ulcers

Several factors contribute to the formation of stress ulcers. They are discussed below and are summarized in Table 45–2.

Acid Hypersecretion. Stress ulcers in animals usually are not associated with acid hypersecretion. In fact, acid secretion is markedly decreased during restraint[126–128] and exertion.[98–100] Nevertheless, at least small amounts of luminal acid must be present for the formation of stress ulcers as well as of aspirin-induced ulcers,[116] since they are prevented by administration of antisecretory drugs.[98, 129] In certain forms of stress ulcer, however, increase in acid secretion occurs. This is the case for ulcers following certain neurologic lesions,[110] sepsis,[106] and the combination of cold plus restraint.[128, 130, 131] Whether the observed hyperacidity contributes to ulcer formation is unknown.

Gastric Anoxia. Ulcers due to severe stress may result from a combination of cardiovascular shock and the presence of injurious agents (e.g., acid and pepsin, irritants) in the gastric lumen. Stress-induced cardio-

vascular shock may impair vascular perfusion of the stomach to the extent that mucosal cells become anoxic and malnourished and, as a consequence, cannot adequately resist the irritating properties of luminal contents. Sepsis was found to induce hypoxia of the canine gastric mucosa with consequent impairment of microcirculatory blood flow and formation of gastric mucosal edema. These changes were prevented by methylprednisolone.[132] Corticoids (prednisolone), given as single treatment at a dose that by itself is not ulcerogenic, also inhibited restraint and exertion ulcers, presumably by preventing vascular collapse.[93, 95] Prednisone and isoproterenol, a β-adrenergic agent, prevented formation of cold-restraint ulcers in rats; prior treatment with indomethacin abolished the protection, a finding suggesting that the protective effect of these two agents requires an intact prostaglandin synthetic pathway.[133] Stress ulcers (produced by cold and restraint) are accompanied by a decrease in gastric mucosal blood flow.[130, 131, 134] These ulcers, however, developed only in animals who in addition exhibited high-amplitude contractions of the stomach for more than one hour.[134] It was concluded that increased gastric motility and reduced blood flow may play a role in the development of stress ulcers.

Alteration of Natural Defense Mechanisms. When one considers the composition of gastrointestinal contents, it is surprising that the mucosa, with which they are in continuous contact, does not become inflamed and necrotic. If these contents (consisting of acid and pepsin, food particles, spices, microorganisms and their toxins, bile acids, and sometimes alcohol and drugs) were introduced into any other cavity (peritoneum, lung, bladder, uterus) or beneath the skin, the tissues would die. Yet, the gastrointestinal mucosa resists. Some natural defense mechanisms must account for this protection. The following mechanisms can be considered.

Role of Mucus. Mucus normally covers the gastrointestinal mucosa. It has long been regarded as a substance affording natural protection against potentially damaging agents present in the lumen of hollow or-

Table 45–2. ETIOLOGY OF STRESS ULCERS

Ulcerogenic Conditions		Antiulcer Conditions	
Sensitizing Factors	*Immediate Causes*	*Counteracting the Immediate Causes*	*Counteracting the Sensitizing Factors*
Prostaglandin deficiency Spontaneous Drug-induced (NOSAC,* steroids)	Luminal contents Acid-pepsin Bile acids Alcohol Drugs Microorganisms Toxins	Antisecretory agents, antacids	Prostaglandins Mucus stimulation Prostaglandins Carbenoxolone
Mucus deficiency Spontaneous Drug-induced (NOSAC,* steroids)			
Reduced cell turnover			Trophic agents Gastrin Epidermal growth factor Growth hormone
Stress-shock	Ischemia-anoxia	Antishock measures (intravenous solutions, transfusions, antibiotics)	

*NOSAC = *Nonsteroidal anti-inflammatory compounds.*

gans.[135] Mucus could provide a physical shield to the penetration of noxious substances. The following experimental observations support this concept.

1. *Stress (prolonged fasting, restraint) reduces mucus secretion in rats.* The hexosamine content of gastric juice and gastric mucosa was much lower in fasted animals developing ulcers than in animals whose mucosa remains intact. The decrease in hexosamine (an index of mucus content) preceded the formation of ulcers.[136] Gastric ulcers produced by restraint stress were associated with a reduction in the amount of mucus adherent to the mucosa.[137] Conversely, secretin prevented bleeding from cold and restraint–induced gastric ulcers while restoring mucus (glycoprotein) to normal.[138]

2. *Administration of high doses of prednisolone to rats and dogs produces gastric ulcers within a few days.* In rats, prednisolone markedly decreased the levels of hexosamines in the gastric mucosa (corpus and antrum), but the decrease occurred prior to the formation of ulcers (steroid ulcers).[139, 140] The hexosamine content of gastric juice was also lowered by prednisolone. Histologic examination of the stomach with special mucus stains revealed the disappearance of mucus granules from the surface epithelium and the mucus neck cells within 24 hours of prednisolone administration—that is, before ulcers had developed.[123]

3. *Aspirin, an ulcerogenic agent, reduces the mucus content of rat and dog gastric juice and mucosa.*[141] These studies suggest that mucus reduction in gastric juice and gastric mucosa may predispose to ulcer formation. This has been ascribed to the inhibition of prostaglandin formation by aspirin because certain prostaglandins were shown to stimulate mucus secretion in rats and dogs[142, 143] and to double the thickness of the gastric gel mucus in rats, under certain conditions.[144, 145]

4. *If mucus is indeed a natural protective substance for the gastric mucosa, the mechanism by which it exerts such an effect is not clear.* It could act as a physical as well as a chemical barrier to irritants present in the gastric lumen.[146] Mucus could also provide a physical barrier to the penetration of noxious substances. *In vitro* studies showed that gastric mucus retards the diffusion of hydrogen ions and can maintain a pH gradient of 2.31 on the luminal side and 7.26 on the epithelial side of the mucus layer.[145, 147]

Epithelial Renewal. The rate of epithelial renewal may affect mucosal resistance. Gastrin, epidermal growth factor, and growth hormone are trophic agents; they stimulate protein and DNA synthesis as well as cell division in gastric mucosal cells. These three agents were found to inhibit formation of restraint ulcers (pentagastrin,[97] growth hormone[148]) and aspirin ulcers (epidermal growth factor[149]).

Tissue Mediators. Three types of substances released by the gastric mucosa have been studied for their ability to either prevent or aggravate tissue injury. These are arachidonic acid metabolites, PAF (platelet activating factor), and free radicals.

Arachidonic Acid Metabolites. Arachidonic acid is the common precursor for prostaglandins, thromboxanes, and leukotrienes.

Prostaglandins. Several prostaglandins have been isolated in relatively large amounts from the gastric mucosa.[150] When administered to animals and humans, certain prostaglandins of the E series inhibited gastric secretion[151] and were cytoprotective.[152]

Aspirin-like drugs, by inhibiting cyclo-oxygenase activity, block the biosynthesis of prostaglandins in tissues.[153] Most properties of NOSAC (anti-inflammatory, analgesic, antipyretic) are believed to be due chiefly to the prostaglandin depletion they elicit. Similarly, NOSAC-induced ulcers may be caused by a local (gastric, duodenal) depletion of prostaglandins. The sequence of events would be as follows: NOSAC (e.g., aspirin, indomethacin) → prostaglandin deficiency in the stomach and duodenum → decreased mucosal resistance to the gastric contents (e.g., acid, pepsin, food debris, bile salts) due to lack of prostaglandin cytoprotection → mucosal damage (gastritis, bleeding, sometimes frank ulcer). Certain prostaglandins are believed to be cytoprotective by preventing this deficiency; the prostaglandins would maintain cellular integrity despite treatment with aspirin-like drugs and despite the hostile environment provided by the gastrointestinal contents.

The protective role of endogenous prostaglandins for the stomach was demonstrated in animal studies using models of gastric mucosal injury. Intragastric administration of a variety of mild irritants 15 minutes before giving necrotizing agents (absolute ethanol, 0.6 M HCl, 0.2 M NaOH) protected the gastric mucosa from necrosis.[154, 155] These mild irritants were shown to stimulate prostaglandin formation by the gastric mucosa, and their protective effect was blocked by prior treatment with indomethacin.[154, 155] Similarly, mild physical stress (restraint) applied for ten days markedly reduced the severity of gastric mucosal lesions produced by 40 per cent ethanol; again, indomethacin abolished the protection.[156]

Although aspirin or stress can produce gastric ulcerations, the combination of aspirin plus stress, such as restraint or exposure to cold, leads to ulcerogenic synergism. For instance, the combination of aspirin in doses that are not ulcerogenic along with a stressful condition which alone is also not ulcerogenic produces within 30 minutes multiple, deep, and bleeding ulcers.[117, 118] Figure 45–3 illustrates such synergism. The mechanism of this potentiation has not been explained. It could be due to several factors: (a) a decrease in prostaglandin formation by the stomach, caused by aspirin; (b) an increase in gastric acid secretion; (c) a reduction in gastric mucosal blood flow. These possibilities were explored with the following findings: (a) aspirin decreased prostaglandin formation, but the reduction was the same whether the animals were exposed to cold or not; (b) cold and restraint tripled the acid output, but aspirin did not; (c) gastric mucosal blood flow was decreased by aspirin and by stress, but the reduction was not enhanced when both conditions were applied. It was concluded that the potentiation

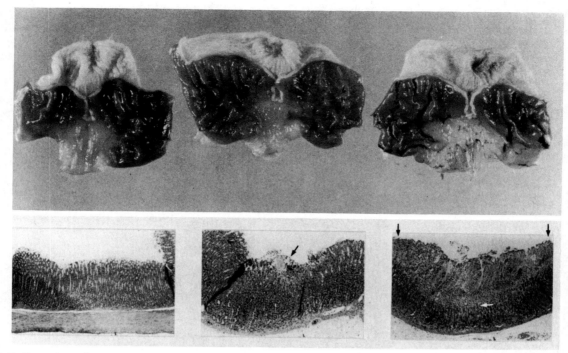

Figure 45–3. Synergism of stress and aspirin on ulcer formation. *Top,* Rat stomachs opened to show the mucosa. *Bottom,* Histologic sections of the corresponding stomachs. (Hematoxylin-eosin, × 25.) *Left,* Stomach of animal exposed to restraint and cold (4°C) for one hour. No lesion. *Middle,* Stomach of animal given 50 mg/kg of aspirin in 0.1 M HCl, orally, one hour earlier. A few small erosions (black spots, top), corresponding to shallow erosions (arrow, bottom) in the mucosa. *Right,* Stomach of animal given aspirin and exposed to restraint and cold. Multiple, severe, and extensive erosions throughout the corpus mucosa (top), corresponding to necrotic ulcerations (bottom) occupying a large area of the mucosa (between the two vertical arrows) and extending to two-thirds deep in the mucosa (horizontal arrow).

of ulcer formation by aspirin plus stress was most likely due to two factors acting jointly: acid hypersecretion and a decrease in gastric prostaglandins.[131] The lack of cytoprotective prostaglandins caused by aspirin would reduce the mucosal resistance and allow the excess acid to cause ulcers.

Thromboxanes and leukotrienes. Conversely, thromboxane A_2 and thromboxane mimetic agents are potent gastric vasoconstrictors and can cause severe gastric lesions.[157–159] Leukotriene C_4 is also a vasoconstrictor.[157, 160] The development of gastric necrotic lesions by absolute ethanol was associated with a sevenfold increase in LTC_4 production by the gastric mucosa. Oral pretreatment with nordihydroguaiaretic acid, a 5-lipoxygenase inhibitor that blocks the synthesis of LTC_4, protected the mucosa against injury produced by ethanol.[161] These findings suggest that both thromboxanes and leukotrienes may play a role in ulcer formation.

Platelet Activating Factor (PAF). PAF is a phospholipid synthesized and released by leukocytes, macrophages, and endothelial cells.[162] It is believed to play a role in inflammatory processes and in the development of endotoxic shock.[163] When infused intravenously to rats, it caused gastric vascular congestion, subepithelial edema, and neutrophil accumulation. It also aggravated gastric damage produced by topical administration of 20 per cent ethanol and 2 mM acidified taurocholate.[164] PAF may therefore contribute to the pathogenesis of gastric ulceration.

Oxygen-Derived Free Radicals. Oxygen-derived free radicals, often generated in organs rendered ischemic and later resupplied with blood, can lead to severe tissue damage, including gastric mucosal lesions. Gastric ulcerations were produced by oral administration of HCl to rats rendered hypotensive by bleeding and then retransfused with their own blood. These ulcers were prevented either by allopurinol (which inhibits xanthine oxidase, the enzyme responsible for the formation of superoxide radicals) or by superoxide dismutase (a scavenger of superoxide radicals).[165] In other studies, the degree of lipid peroxidation by the gastric mucosa was markedly increased when lesions were produced by ethanol; treatment with PGE_2 or $PGF_2\alpha$ prevented both the lesions and the increase in peroxide formation.[166] These studies suggest that free radicals may be mediators of acute gastric injury produced by various conditions, including severe stress.

Lowered Intramucosal pH. The intramural pH of the gastric mucosa during hemorrhagic shock was studied in rabbits and dogs and was correlated with the presence of mucosal ulcerations.[167–169] In rabbits, the pH fell from 7.35 to 6.62 during hemorrhagic shock when fundic pouches were irrigated with HCl. This was associated with severe ulcerations. When the fundic pouches were irrigated with neutral buffer, the fall in intramural pH caused by hemorrhage was much less, and gastric lesions were minimal. Similar results were obtained in dog gastric pouches, especially when the irrigating fluid contained acid and sodium taurocholate. These results suggest that a substantial portion of the decrease in intramural pH is caused by back diffusion of luminal H^+. The capacity of the gastric mucosa to dispose of influxing H^+ may be compromised during hemorrhagic shock, a factor that may be critical in the pathogenesis of acute gastric ulceration.

Energy Deficit. It was postulated that a deficit in gastric mucosal energy during stress might lead to ulcer formation. This was substantiated by the observation that in rats and rabbits the ATP levels in the corpus decrease markedly during hemorrhagic shock, although such decrease does not take place in the antrum. Under these conditions, only the corpus becomes ulcerated.[104, 105]

SUMMARY

Many clinical studies have been cited in this chapter, and the specifics of each will provide the reader with reasonable information on which to base a decision regarding all appropriate prophylactic regimens. The incidence of life-threatening bleeding due to acute gastric mucosal erosion is very low, perhaps due to better critical care monitoring, diagnosis, and therapy, such as the standard use of some of the prophylactic modalities presented in this chapter. Based on information available, no one form of prophylaxis can be recommended above all others. Several principles, however, can be identified. A high index of suspicion that acute gastric mucosal erosion bleeding may occur must attend the care of any patient with ongoing sepsis or respiratory failure or who sustained severe trauma, thermal burns, or central nervous system injury. Antacids should be administered on an hourly basis, with intragastric pH maintained ≥ 4. In those patients who have a recent upper gastrointestinal anastomosis or a complication of antacid therapy, a histamine H_2 receptor antagonist should be administered, again, maintaining the intragastric pH ≥ 4. Patients who are ventilated present more of a dilemma based on available information. If subsequent studies support the hypothesis that neutral intragastric pH is inadvisable because it predisposes to bacterial overgrowth, increasing the risk of pneumonia, with which is associated greater morbidity and mortality than with upper gastrointestinal bleeding, then the use of sucralfate prophylactically may be more appropriate than antacids or histamine H_2 receptor antagonists. Intragastric infusion of elemental formulas not only provides nutrition to the critically ill patient but also may provide sufficient proton neutralization to assist in the maintenance of intragastric pH at levels ≥ 4.

Stress ulcers can be produced experimentally, the animal of choice being the rat. The methods include restraint, especially combined with exposure to cold, forced exercise, and administration of aspirin. The pathogenesis of such ulcers involves various factors, some common to all models, others not. Some gastric acid, not necessarily in increased amounts, must be present for stress ulcers to develop. Gastric anoxia

may also play a role, as may a decrease in intramucosal pH. Alterations in certain natural defense mechanisms are also important, particularly a decrease in gastric mucus. Certain tissue mediators appear to favor ulcer formation; among these are thromboxanes, leukotrienes, platelet activating factor (PAF), and free radicals. Other mediators, such as prostaglandins, are beneficial, and their depletion (such as after treatment with aspirin) may lead to ulcer formation.

References

1. Lucas, C. E., Sugawa, C., Riddle, J., Rector, F., Rosenburg, B., and Walt, A. J. Natural history and surgical dilemma of "stress" gastric bleeding. Arch. Surg. *102*:266, 1971.
2. Skillman, J. J., Bushnell, L. S., Goldman, H., and Silen, W. Respiratory failure, hypotension, sepsis and jaundice: A clinical syndrome associated with lethal hemorrhage from acute stress ulceration of the stomach. Am. J. Surg. *123*:25, 1971.
3. Stremple, J. F., Mori, H., Lev, R., and Glass, G. B. J. The stress ulcer syndrome. Curr. Probl. Surg. February, 1973, pp 3–4.
4. Greenburg, A. G. Invited commentary. World J. Surg. *5*:148, 1981.
5. Zinner, M. J., Zuidema, G. D., Smith, P. L., and Mignosa, M. The prevention of upper gastrointestinal tract bleeding in patients in an intensive care unit. Surg. Gynecol. Obstet. *153*:214, 1981.
6. Schuster, D. P., Rowley, H., Feinstein, S., McGue, M. K., and Zucherman, G. R. Prospective evaluation of the risk of upper gastrointestinal bleeding after admission to a medical intensive care unit. Am. J. Med. *76*:623, 1984.
7. Peura, D. A., and Johnson, L. F. Cimetidine for prevention and treatment of gastroduodenal mucosal lesions in patients in an intensive care unit. Ann. Intern. Med. *103*:173, 1985.
8. Fiddian-Green, R. G., McGough, E., Pittenger, G., and Rothman, E. Predictive value of intramural pH and other risk factors for massive bleeding from stress ulceration. Gastroenterology *85*:613, 1983.
9. David, E. McIlrath, D. C., and Higgins, J. A. Clinical experience with acute peptic gastrointestinal ulcers. Mayo Clin. Proc. *46*:15, 1971.
10. Curling, T. B. On acute ulceration of the duodenum in cases of burns. Med. Surg. Trans. (London) *25*:260, 1842.
11. Czaja, A. J., McAlhany, J. C., and Pruitt, B. A. Acute gastroduodenal disease after thermal injury: An endoscopic evaluation of incidence and natural history. N. Engl. J. Med. *291*:925, 1974.
12. Pruitt, B. A., and Goodwin, C. W. Stress ulcer disease in the burned patient. World J. Surg. *5*:209, 1981.
13. Sevitt, S. Duodenal and gastric ulceration after burning. Br. J. Surg. *54*:32, 1967.
14. Cushing, H. Peptic ulcers and the interbrain. Surg. Gynecol. Obstet. *55*:1, 1932.
15. Bowen, J. C., Fleming, W. H., and Thompson, J. C. Increased gastrin release following penetrating central nervous system injury. Surgery *75*:720, 1974.
16. Kamada, T., Fusamoto, H., Kawano, S., Hoguchi, M., Hiramatsu, K., Masazawa, M., Abe, H., Fuggi, C., and Sugimoto, T. Gastrointestinal bleeding following head injury, a clinical study of 433 cases. J. Trauma *17*:44, 1977.
17. Haloran, L. G., Zfass, A. M., Gayle, W. E., Wheeler, C. B., and Miller, J. D. Prevention of acute gastrointestinal complications after severe head injury: A controlled trial of cimetidine prophylaxis. Am. J. Surg. *139*:44, 1980.
18. Kiwerski, J. Bleeding from the alimentary canal during the management of spinal cord injury patients. Paraplegia *24*:92, 1986.
19. Gordon, M. J., Skillman, J. J., Zervas, W. T., and Silen, W. Divergent nature of gastric mucosal permeability in gastric acid secretion in sick patients with general and neurosurgical disease. Ann. Surg. *178*:285, 1973.

20. Watts, C., and Clark, K. Gastric acidity in the comatose patient. J. Neurosurg. 30:107, 1969.
21. Lussier, A., Arsenault, A., and Varady, J. Gastrointestinal microbleeding after aspirin and naproxen. Clin. Pharmacol. Ther. 23:402, 1978.
22. Arnold, J. D., Mullane, J. F., Hayden, D. M., March, L., Hart, K., Perdomo, C. A., Fencik, M., and Berger, A. E. Etodolac, aspirin, and gastrointestinal microbleeding. Clin. Pharmacol. Ther. 35:716, 1984.
23. Caruso, I., and Porro, G. B. Gastroscopic evaluation of anti-inflammatory agents. Br. Med. J. 1:75, 1980.
24. Silvoso, G. R., Ivey, K. J., Butt, J. H., Lockard, O. O., Holt, S. D., Sisk, C., Baskin, W. N., Makercher, P. A., and Hewett, J. Incidence of gastric lesions in patients with rheumatic disease on chronic aspirin therapy. Ann. Intern. Med. 91:517, 1979.
25. Hoftiezer, J. W., Silvoso, G. R., Burks, M., and Ivey, K. J. Comparison of the effects of regular and enteric coated aspirin on gastroduodenal mucosa of man. Lancet 2:609, 1980.
26. Lanza, F. L., Royer, G. L., Jr., Nelson, R. S., Chen, T. T., Seckman, C. E., and Rack, M. F. The effects of ibuprofen, indomethacin, aspirin, naproxen, and placebo on the gastric mucosa of normal volunteers. Dig. Dis. Sci. 24:823, 1979.
27. Lanza, F. L., Nelson, R. S., and Rack, M. F. A controlled endoscopic study comparing the toxic effects of sulindac, naproxen, aspirin, and placebo on the gastric mucosa of healthy volunteers. J. Clin. Pharmacol. 24:89, 1984.
28. Lanza, F. L., Royer, G. L., Nelson, R. S., Seckman, C. E., Schwartz, J. H., Rack, M. F., and Gernaat, C. M. Effects of flurbiprofen and aspirin on the gastric and duodenal mucosa: An endoscopic comparison. Am. J. Med. 80(suppl. 3A):31, 1986.
29. Lanza, F. L., Panagides, J., and Salom, I. L. Etodolac compared with aspirin: An endoscopic study of the gastrointestinal tract of normal volunteers. J. Rheumatol. 13:299, 1986.
30. Peterson, W. L., Barnett, C. C., Smith, J. H., Allen, M. H., and Corbett, D. B. Routine early endoscopy in upper gastrointestinal tract bleeding: A randomized controlled trial. N. Engl. J. Med. 304:925, 1981.
31. Sugawa, C., Werner, M. H., Hayes, D. F., Lucas, C. E., and Walt, A. J. Early endoscopy: A guide to therapy for acute hemorrhage in the upper gastrointestinal tract. Arch. Surg. 107:133, 1973.
32. Baum, S., Nusbaum, M., Blakemore, W. S., and Finkelstein, A. K. The preoperative radiographic demonstration of intra-abdominal bleeding from undetermined sites by percutaneous selective celiac and superior mesenteric arteriography. Surgery 58:797, 1965.
33. Lucas, C. F. Stress ulceration: The clinical problem. World J. Surg. 5:139, 1981.
34. Martin, L. F., Max, M. M., and Polk, H. C., Jr. Failure of gastric pH controlled antacids or cimetidine in the critically ill: A valid sign of sepsis. Surgery 88:59, 1980.
35. Kislow, M. L., and Wagner, M. Intragastric instillation of levarterenol: A method for control of upper gastrointestinal tract hemorrhage. Arch. Surg. 107:387, 1973.
36. Simonian, S. J., and Curtis, L. E. Treatment of hemorrhagic gastritis by antacid. Ann. Surg. 184:429, 1976.
37. McAlhany, J. C., Czaja, A. J., and Pruitt, B. A. Antacid control of complications from acute gastroduodenal disease after burns. J. Trauma 16:645, 1976.
38. Eden, K., and Korn, F. Current status of cimetidine in upper gastrointestinal bleeding. Gastroenterology 74:466, 1978.
39. Reichlin, S. Somatostatin. N. Engl. J. Med. 309:1556, 1983.
40. Mulvihill, S., Pappas, T. N., Passaro, E., and Debas, H. T. The use of somatostatin and its analogs in the treatment of surgical disorders. Surgery 100:467, 1987.
41. Gomez-Pan, A., Reed, J. D., Albinus, M., Reed, J. D., Shaw, S., and Hall, R. Direct inhibition of gastric acid and pepsin secretion by growth-hormone release-inhibiting hormone in the cat. Lancet 1:888, 1975.
42. Keller, U., Perruchoud, A., Kayasseh, L., and Gyr, N. Effect of therapeutic somatostatin on splanchnic blood flow in man. Eur. J. Clin. Invest. 8:335, 1978.
43. Kayasseh, L., Keller, U., Gyr, K., and Stadler, G. A. Soma-tostatin and cimetidine in peptic ulcer hemorrhage: A randomized controlled trial. Lancet 1:844, 1980.
44. Groeger, J. S., Dazza, S. J., Carlon, G. C., Turnbull, A. D., Pierri, M. K., and Howland, W. S. Prostaglandin therapy in a case of refractory stress ulcer bleeding. Crit. Care Med. 10:486, 1982.
45. Weiss, J. B., Peskin, G. W., and Isenberg, J. I. Treatment of hemorrhagic gastritis with 15(R)-15-methyl prostaglandin E_2: Report of a case. Gastroenterology 82:558, 1982.
46. Eckstein, M. R., and Athanasoulis, C. A. Gastrointestinal bleeding: An angiographic perspective. Surg. Clin. North Am. 64:37, 1984.
47. Athanasoulis, C. A., Wallman, A. C., Novelline, R. A., Krudy, A. G., and Sniderman, K. W. Angiography: Its contribution to the emergency management of gastrointestinal hemorrhage. Radiol. Clin. North Am. 14:265, 1976.
48. Athanasoulis, C. A. Medical progress: Therapeutic application of angiography. N. Engl. J. Med. 302:1117, 1980.
49. Conn, H. O., Ramsby, G. R., Storer, E. H., Machnick, M. G., Joshi, P. M., Phillips, M. M., Cohen, G. A., Fields, G. W., and Petroski, D. Intraarterial vasopressin in the treatment of upper gastrointestinal hemorrhage: A prospective controlled clinical trial. Gastroenterology 68:211, 1975.
50. Goldman, N. L., Land, W. C., Bradley, E. L., and Anderson, J. Transcatheter therapeutic embolization in the management of massive upper gastrointestinal bleeding. Radiology 120:513, 1976.
51. Papp, J. P. Endoscopic electrocoagulation in the management of upper gastrointestinal tract bleeding. Surg. Clin. North Am. 62:797, 1982.
52. Johnston, J. H., Sones, J. Q., Long, B. W., and Posey, E. L. Comparison of heater probe and YAG laser in endoscopic treatment of major bleeding from peptic ulcers. Gastrointest. Endosc. 31:175, 1985.
53. Overholt, B. F. Laser treatment of upper gastrointestinal hemorrhage. Am. J. Gastroenterol. 80:721, 1985.
54. Himal, H. S. Endoscopic control of upper gastrointestinal bleeding. Can. J. Surg. 28:305, 1985.
55. Jensen, D. M. Endoscopic control of gastrointestinal bleeding. In Berk, J. E. (ed.). Developments in Digestive Diseases. Vol. 3. Philadelphia, Lea & Febiger, 1980.
56. Gaisford, W. D. Endoscopic electrohemostasis of acute upper gastrointestinal bleeding. Am. J. Surg. 137:47, 1979.
57. Papp, J. P. Endoscopic electrocoagulation of actively bleeding arterial upper gastrointestinal lesions. Am. J. Gastroenterol. 71:516, 1979.
58. Fruhmorgan, P., Bodem, F., Reidenbach, H. D., Kaduk, B., and Demling, L. Endoscopic photocoagulation by laser irradiation in the gastrointestinal tract in man. Acta Hepatogastroenterol. 25:1, 1978.
59. Kiefhaber, P., Nath, P., and Moritz, K. Endoscopic control of massive gastrointestinal hemorrhage by irradiation with a high power Neodymium-YAG laser. Progr. Surg. 15:140, 1977.
60. Cheung, L. Y. Treatment of established stress ulcer disease. World J. Surg. 5:235, 1981.
61. Cody, H. S., and Wichem, W. A. Choice of operation for acute gastric mucosal hemorrhage. Report of 36 cases and literature review. Am. J. Surg. 135:322, 1971.
62. Menguy, R., Gadacz, T., and Zajtchuk, R. The surgical management of acute gastric mucosal bleeding. Arch. Surg. 99:198, 1969.
63. Hubert, J. P., Kernan, P. D., Welch, J. S., ReMine, W. H., and Beahrs, O. H. The surgical management of bleeding stress ulcers. Ann. Surg. 191:672, 1980.
64. Richardson, J. D., and Aust, J. B. Gastric devascularization: A useful salvage procedure for massive hemorrhagic gastritis. Ann. Surg. 185:649, 1977.
65. Hastings, P. R., Skillman, J. J., Bushnell, L. S., and Silen, W. Antacid titration in the prevention of acute gastrointestinal bleeding. A controlled randomized trial of 100 critically ill patients. N. Engl. J. Med. 298:1041, 1978.
66. Reid, S. R., and Barjliff, C. D. The comparative efficacy of cimetidine and ranitidine in controlling gastric pH in critically ill patients. Can. Anesth. Soc. J. 33:287, 1986.

67. More, D. G., Raper, R. F., Munro, I. A., Walston, C. J., Bowtagy, J. S., and Shenfield, G. M. Randomized, prospective trial of cimetidine and ranitidine for control of intragastric pH in the critically ill. Surgery 97:215, 1985.

68. Ostro, M. J. Russell, J. A., Soldin, S. J., Mahon, W. A., and Jeejeebhoy, K. N. Control of gastric pH with cimetidine: Boluses versus primed infusion. Gastroenterology 89:532, 1985.

69. MacDonald, A. S., Steele, J. B., and Bottomly, M. G. Treatment of stress-induced upper gastrointestinal hemorrhage with metiamide. Lancet 1:68, 1976.

70. Jones, R. H., Rudge, C. J., Bewick, M., Parsons, V., and Weston, M. J. Cimetidine: Prophylaxis against upper gastrointestinal haemorrhage after renal transplantation. Br. Med. J. 1:398, 1978.

71. Groll, A., Simon, J. B., Wigle, R. D., Tagichi, K., Todd, R. J., and Depew, W. T. Cimetidine prophylaxis for gastrointestinal bleeding in an intensive care unit. Gut 27:135, 1986.

72. Van Denberg, B., and van Blankenstein, M. Prevention of stress-induced upper gastrointestinal bleeding by cimetidine in patients on assisted ventilation. Digestion 31:1, 1985.

73. Zach, G. A., Gyr, K. E., von Alvensleben, E., Mills, J. G., Slatder, G. A., Dunn, S. L., and Bloom, S. A double-blind randomized, controlled study to investigate the efficacy of cimetidine, given in addition to conventional therapy in the prevention of stress ulceration and haemorrhage in patients with acute spinal injury. Digestion 29:214, 1984.

74. Priebe, H. J., Skillman, J. J., Bushnell, L. S., Long, P. C., and Silen, W. Antacids versus cimetidine in preventing acute gastrointestinal bleeding: A randomized trial of 75 critically ill patients. N. Engl. J. Med. 302:426, 1980.

75. MacDougall, B. R. D., Bailey, R. J., and Williams, R. H2 receptor antagonists and antacids in the prevention of acute gastrointestinal hemorrhage in fulminant hepatic failure. Lancet 1:617, 1977.

76. Priebe, H. J., and Skillman, J. J. Methods of prophylaxis in stress ulcer disease. World J. Surg. 5:223, 1981.

77. Poleski, M. H., and Spanier, A. H. Cimetidine versus antacids in the prevention of stress erosions in critically ill patients. Am. J. Gastroenterol. 81:107, 1986.

78. Friedman, C. J., Oblinger, M. J., Suratt, P. M., Bowers, J., Goldberg, S. K., Sperling, M. H., and Blitzer, A. H. Prophylaxis of upper gastrointestinal hemorrhage in patients requiring mechanical ventilation. Crit. Care Med. 10:316, 1982.

79. McElwee, H. P., Sirinek, K. R., and Levine, B. A. Cimetidine affords protection of stress ulceration following thermal injury. Surgery 86:620, 1979.

80. Stothert, J. C., Simonowitz, D. A., Dellinger, E. P., Farley, M., Edwards, W. A., Blair, A. D., Culter, R., and Carrico, C. J. Gastric pH monitoring as a prognostic indicator for the prophylaxis of stress ulceration in the critically ill. Am. J. Surg. 140:761, 1980.

81. Weigelt, J. A., Aurbakken, C. M., Gwertz, B. L., and Synder, W. H. Cimetidine vs. antacid in prophylaxis for stress ulceration. Arch. Surg. 116:597, 1981.

82. Borrero, E., Margolis, I. B., and Bank, S. A randomized trial of sucralfate vs. antacid in preventing acute gastrointestinal bleeding in 100 critically ill patients. Am. J. Surg. 148:809, 1984.

83. Borrero, E., Ciervo, J., and Chang, J. B. Antacids vs. sucralfate in preventing acute gastrointestinal tract bleeding in abdominal aortic surgery. Arch. Surg. 121:810, 1986.

84. Tryba, M., Zevourow, F., Torok, M., and Zeng, M. Prevention of acute stress bleeding with sucralfate, antacids, or cimetidine: A controlled study with pirenzepine as a basic medication. Am. J. Med. 79(suppl. 2C):55, 1985.

85. Cannon, L. A., Heiselman, D. E., Gardner, W. G., and Jons, J. Sucralfate versus antacids and cimetidine in preventing acute gastrointestinal bleeding in the ventilator patient. Crit. Care Med. 14:388, 1986 (abstract).

86. Driks, M. R., Craven, D. E., Celli, B. R., Manning, M., Burke, R. A., Garvin, G. M., Kunches, L. M., Farber, H. W., Wedel, S. A., and McCabe, W. R. Nosocomial pneumonia in intubated patients given sucralfate as compared with antacids or histamine type 2 blockers: The role of gastric colonization. N. Engl. J. Med. 317:1376, 1987.

87. Tryba, M. The risk of acute stress bleeding and nosocomial pneumonia in ventilated ICU patients: Sucralfate vs antacids. Am. J. Med 83(3B):117, 1987.

88. Tryba, M., and Manthey-Stiers, R. Antibacterial activity of sucralfate in human gastric juice. Am. J. Med. 83(3B):125, 1987.

89. Skillman, J. J., Lisbon, A., Long, P. C., and Silen, W. 15(R)-15-methyl prostaglandin E2 does not prevent gastrointestinal bleeding in seriously ill patients. Am. J. Surg. 147:451, 1984.

90. Choctaw, W. T., Fujita, C., and Zawacki, B. E. Prevention of upper gastrointestinal bleeding in burn patients: A role of "elemental" diet. Arch. Surg. 115:1073, 1980.

91. Pingleton, S. K., and Hadzimar, S. K. Enteral alimentation and gastrointestinal bleeding in mechanically ventilated patients. Crit. Care Med. 11:13, 1983.

92. Valentine, R. J., Turner, W. W., Borman, K. R., and Weigelt, J. A. Does nasoenteral feeding afford adequate gastroduodenal stress prophylaxis? Crit. Care Med. 14:599, 1986.

93. Rossi, G., Bonfils, S., Lieffogh, F., and Lambling, A. Technique nouvelle pour produire des ulcérations gastriques chez le rat blanc: L'ulcère de contrainte. C. R. Soc. Biol. 150:2124, 1956.

94. Brodie, D. A., and Hanson, H. M. A study of the factors involved in the production of gastric ulcers by the restraint technique. Gastroenterology 38:353, 1960.

95. Robert, A., Phillips, J. P., and Nezamis, J. E. Production, by restraint, of gastric ulcers and of hydrothorax in the rat. Gastroenterology 51:75, 1966.

96. Kawarada, Y., Lambeck, J., and Matsumoto, T. Pathophysiology of stress ulcer and its prevention. II. Prostaglandin E1 and microcirculatory responses in stress ulcer. Am. J. Surg. 129:217, 1975.

97. Takeuchi, K., and Johnson, L. R. Pentagastrin protects against stress ulceration in rats. Gastroenterology 76:327, 1979.

98. Robert, A., Northam, J. I., and Nezamis, J. E. Exertion ulcers in the rat. Am. J. Dig. Dis. 15:497, 1970.

99. Dajani, E. Z., Driskill, D. R., Bianchi, R. G., and Collins, P. W. Comparative gastric antisecretory and antiulcer effects of prostaglandin E1 and its methyl ester in animals. Prostaglandins 10:205, 1975.

100. Selye, H. A syndrome produced by diverse noxious agents. Nature 138:32, 1936.

101. Lillehei, C. W., and Wangensteen, O. H. Effect of muscular fatigue on histamine-provoked ulcer with observations on gastric secretion. Proc. Soc. Exp. Biol. Med. 67:49, 1948.

102. Paré, W. P. Psychological studies of stress ulcer in the rat. Brain Res. Bull. 5(suppl. 1):73, 1980.

103. Noble, R. L., and Collip, J. B. Quantitative method for the production of experimental traumatic shock without hemorrhage in unanesthetized animals. Q. J. Exp. Physiol. 31:187, 1942.

104. Menguy, R., Desbaillets, L., and Masters, Y. F. Mechanisms of stress ulcer: Influence of hypovolemic shock on energy metabolism in the gastric mucosa. Gastroenterology 66:46, 1974.

105. Menguy, R., and Masters, Y. F. Mechanism of stress ulcer. III. Effects of hemorrhagic shock on energy metabolism in the mucosa of the antrum, corpus, and fundus of the rabbit stomach. Gastroenterology 66:1168, 1974.

106. Odonkor, P., Mowat, C., and Himal, H. S. Prevention of sepsis-induced gastric lesions in dogs by cimetidine via inhibition of gastric secretion and by prostaglandin via cytoprotection. Gastroenterology 80:375, 1981.

107. Foss, D. L., Stavney, L. S., Haraguchi, T., Harkins, N., and Nyhus, L. M. Pathophysiologic and therapeutic considerations of Curling's ulcer in the rat. JAMA 187:592, 1964.

108. Friesen, S. R. The genesis of gastroduodenal ulcer following burns. An experimental study. Surgery 28:123, 1950.

109. Einheber, A., Wren, R. E., Porro, R. F., and Dobeck, A. S. Curling's ulcer in the germ-free mouse. Nature 214:298, 1967.

110. French, J. D., Porter, R. W., von Amerongen, F. K., and Raney, R. B. Gastrointestinal hemorrhage and ulceration associated with intracranial lesions. Surgery 32:395, 1952.

111. Longmire, R. L. Experimental observations on "psychoso-

matic" mechanisms. I. Gastrointestinal disturbances. Arch. Neurol. Psychiatry 72:267, 1954.

112. Feldman, S., Behar, A. J., and Birnbaum, D. Gastric lesions following hypothalamic stimulation. Arch. Neurol. 4:308, 1961.

113. Porter, R. W., Brady, J. K., Conrad, D., Mason, J. W., Galambos, R., and Rioch, D. M. Some experimental observations on gastrointestinal lesions in behaviorally conditioned monkeys. Psychosom. Med. 20:379, 1958.

114. Natelson, B. H., Dubois, A., and Sodetz, F. J. Effect of multiple-stress procedures on monkey gastroduodenal mucosa, serum gastrin and hydrogen ion kinetics. Am. J. Dig. Dis. 22:888, 1977.

115. Brodie, D. A., and Hooke, K. F. Effects of route of administration on the production of gastric hemorrhage in the rat by aspirin and sodium salicylate. Am. J. Dig. Dis. 16:985, 1971.

116. Cooke, A. R. The role of acid in the pathogenesis of aspirin-induced gastrointestinal erosions and hemorrhage. Am. J. Dig. Dis. 18:225, 1973.

117. Rainsford, K. D. A synergistic interaction between aspirin, or other nonsteroidal anti-inflammatory drugs, and stress which produces severe gastric mucosal damage in rats and pigs. Agents Actions 5:553, 1975.

118. Meeroff, J. C., Paulsen, G., and Guth, P. H. Parenteral aspirin produces and enhances gastric mucosal lesions and bleeding in rats. Dig. Dis. 20:847, 1975.

119. Bugat, R., Thompson, M. R., Aures, D., and Grossman, M. I. Gastric mucosal lesions produced by intravenous infusion of aspirin in cats. Gastroenterology 71:754, 1976.

120. Cohen, M. M. Mucosal cytoprotection by prostaglandin E_2. Lancet 2:1253, 1978.

121. Yik, K. Y., Dreidger, A. A., and Watson, W. C. Prostaglandin E_2 tablets prevent aspirin-induced blood loss in man. Dig. Dis. Sci. 11:972, 1982.

122. Johansson, C., Kollberg, B., Nordeman, R., Samuelsson, K., and Bergstrom, S. Protective effect of prostaglandin E_2 in the gastrointestinal tract during indomethacin treatment of rheumatic disease. Gastroenterology 78:479, 1980.

123. Robert, A., and Nezamis, J. E. Histopathology of steroid-induced ulcers. An experimental study in the rat. Arch. Pathol. 77:407, 1964.

124. Kelly, P., and Robert, A. Inhibition by pregnancy and lactation of steroid-induced ulcers in the rat. Gastroenterology 56:24, 1969.

125. La Barre, J., and Desmarez, J. A propos des phénomènes hypersécrétoires et des manifestations ulcéreuses gastriques apparaissant chez le rat traité par la réserpine. C. R. Soc. Biol. 151:1451, 1957.

126. Menguy, R. Effects of restraint stress on gastric secretion in the rat. Am. J. Dig. Dis. 5:911, 1960.

127. Brodie, D. A., Marshall, R. W., and Moreno, O. N. Effect of restraint on gastric acidity in the rat. Am. J. Physiol. 202:812, 1962.

128. Hayase, M., and Takeuchi, K. Gastric acid secretion and lesion formation in rats under water-immersion stress. Dig. Dis. Sci. 31:166, 1986.

129. Beattie, D. Effect of drugs on rats exposed to cold-restraint stress. J. Pharm. Pharmacol. 29:748, 1977.

130. Murakami, M., Lam, S. K., Inada, M., and Miyake, T. Pathophysiology and pathogenesis of acute gastric mucosal lesions after hypothermic restraint stress in rats. Gastroenterology 88:660, 1985.

131. Robert, A., Leung, F. W., and Guth, P. H. Ulcer potentiation by stress and aspirin: Role of acid, mucosal blood flow and prostaglandins. Gastroenterology 1988 (in press).

132. Payne, J. G., and Bowen, J. C. Hypoxia of canine gastric mucosa caused by Escherichia coli sepsis and prevented with methylprednisolone therapy. Gastroenterology 80:84, 1981.

133. Hernandez, D. E., Adcock, J. W., Nemeroff, C. B., and Prange, A. J., Jr. The role of the adrenal gland in cytoprotection against stress-induced gastric ulcers in rats. J. Neurosci. Res. 11:193, 1984.

134. Garrick, T., Leung, F. W., Buack, S., Hirabayashi, K., and Guth, P. H. Gastric motility is stimulated but overall blood flow is unaffected during cold restraint in the rat. Gastroenterology 91:141, 1986.

135. Hollander, F. The mucous barrier in the stomach. In Sandweiss, D. J. (ed.). Peptic Ulcer. Philadelphia, W. B. Saunders Co., 1951, p. 65.

136. Robert, A., Bayer, R. B., and Nezamis, J. E. Gastric mucus content during development of ulcers in fasting rats. Gastroenterology 45:740, 1963.

137. Somasundaram, K., and Ganguly, A. K. Gastric mucosal protection during restraint stress in rats: Alteration in gastric adherent mucus and dissolved mucus in gastric secretion. Hepato-gastroenterol. 32:24, 1985.

138. Murakami, M., Fujisaki, H., Oketani, K., and Wakabayashi, T. Effect of secretin on stress-induced gastric bleeding in rats. Dig. Dis. Sci. 30:346, 1985.

139. Robert, A., and Nezamis, J. E. Effect of prednisolone on gastric mucus content and on ulcer formation. Proc. Soc. Exp. Biol. Med. 114:545, 1963.

140. Menguy, R., and Masters, Y. F. Effect of cortisone on muco-protein secretion by gastric antrum of dogs: Pathogenesis of steroid ulcer. Surgery 54:19, 1963.

141. Menguy, R., and Masters, Y. F. Effects of aspirin on gastric mucous secretion. Surg. Gynecol. Obstet. 120:92, 1965.

142. Bolton, J. P., Palmer, D., and Cohen, M. M. Stimulation of mucus and nonparietal cell secretion by the E_2 prostaglandins. Am. J. Dig. Dis. 23:359, 1978.

143. Bolton, J. P., Palmer, D., and Cohen, M. M. Effect of the E_2 prostaglandins on gastric mucus production in rats. Surg. Forum. 27:402, 1976.

144. Bickel, M., and Kauffman, G. L., Jr. Gastric gel mucus thickness: Effect of distention, 16,16-dimethyl prostaglandin E_2, and carbenoxolone. Gastroenterology 80:770, 1981.

145. Kerss, S., Allen, A., and Garner, A. A simple method for measuring thickness of the mucus gel layer adherent to rat, frog and human gastric mucosa: Influence of feeding, prostaglandin, N-acetylcysteine and other agents. Clin. Sci. 63:187, 1982.

146. Williams, S. E., and Turnberg, L. A. Retardation of acid diffusion by pig gastric mucus: A potential role in mucosal protection. Gastroenterology 79:299, 1980.

147. Williams, S. E., and Turnberg, L. A. Demonstration of a pH gradient across mucus adherent to rabbit gastric mucosa: Evidence for a "mucus-bicarbonate" barrier. Gut 22:94, 1981.

148. Vanamee, P., Winawer, S. J., Sherlock, P., Sonnenberg, M., and Lipkin, M. Decreased incidence of restraint-stress induced gastric erosions in rats treated with bovine growth hormone. Proc. Soc. Exp. Biol. Med. 135:259, 1970.

149. Konturek, S. J., Brzozowski, T., Piastucki, I., Radecki, T., and Dembiska-Kiec, A. Epidermal growth factor (EGF) and gastric cytoprotection. Role of endogenous prostaglandins (PGs) and DNA synthesis. Gastroenterology 80:1196, 1981.

150. Bennett, A., Stamford, I. F., and Stockley, H. L. Estimation and characterization of prostaglandins in the human gastrointestinal tract. Br. J. Pharmacol. 61:579, 1977.

151. Robert, A. The inhibitory effects of prostaglandins on gastric secretion: Their possible role in the treatment of gastric hypersecretion and peptic ulcer. In Glass, G. B. J. (ed.). Progress in Gastroenterology. New York, Grune & Stratton, Inc., 1977, pp. 777–801.

152. Robert, A. Cytoprotection by prostaglandins. Gastroenterology 77:761, 1979.

153. Vane, J. R. Inhibition of prostaglandin synthesis as a mechanism of action for aspirin-like drugs. Nature (New Biol.) 231:232, 1971.

154. Robert, A., Nezamis, J. E., Lancaster, C., Davis, J. P., Field, S. O., and Hanchar, A. J. Mild irritants prevent gastric necrosis through "adaptive cytoprotection" mediated by prostaglandins. Am. J. Physiol. 245:G113, 1983.

155. Konturek, S. J., Brzozowski, T., Piastucki, I., Radecki, T., Dembinski, A., and Dembinska-Kiec, A. Role of locally generated prostaglandins in adaptive gastric cytoprotection. Dig. Dis. Sci. 27:967, 1982.

156. Wallace, J. L., and Cohen, M. M. Gastric mucosal protection with chronic mild restraint: Role of endogenous prostaglandins. Am. J. Physiol. 247:G127, 1984.

157. Whittle, B. J. R., Oren-Wolman, N., and Guth, P. H. Gastric vasoconstrictor actions of leukotriene C_4, $PGF_{2\alpha}$, and throm-

boxane mimetic U-46619 on rat submucosal microcirculation *in vivo*. Am. J. Physiol. *248*:G580, 1985.

158. Whittle, B. J. R., Kauffman, G. L., and Moncada, S. Vaso-constriction with thromboxane A₂ induces ulceration of the gastric mucosa. Nature *292*:472, 1981.

159. Kauffman, G. L., Jr., and Whittle, B. J. R. Gastric vascular actions of prostanoids and the dual effect of arachidonic acid. Am. J. Physiol. *242*:G582, 1982.

160. Gulati, N., Philpot, M. E., Gulati, O. P., Mahnsten, C., and Huggel, H. Effects of leukotriene C₄ and prostaglandin E₂ on the rat mesentery *in vitro* and *in vivo*. Prostaglandins, Leuko-trienes Med. *10*:257, 1983.

161. Peskar, B. M., Lange, K., Hoppe, U., and Peskar, B. A. Ethanol stimulates formation of leukotriene C₄ in rat gastric mucosa. Prostaglandins *31*:283, 1986.

162. Vargaftig, B. B., Chignard, M., Benveniste, J., Lefort, J., and Wal, F. Background and present status of research on platelet-activating factor (PAF-acether). Ann. N. Y. Acad. Sci. *370*:119, 1981.

163. Doebber, T. W., Wu, M. S., Robbins, J. C., Choy, B. M., Chang, M. N., and Shen, T. Y. Platelet activating factor (PAF)

involvement in endotoxin-induced hypotension in rats. Studies with PAF-receptor antagonist kadsurenone. Biochem. Biophys. Res. Comm. *123*:799, 1985.

164. Wallace, J. L., and Whittle, B. J. R. Picomole doses of platelet-activating factor predispose the gastric mucosa to damage by topical irritants. Prostaglandins *31*:989, 1986.

165. Itoh, M., and Guth, P. H. Role of oxygen-derived free radicals in hemorrhagic shock-induced gastric lesions in the rat. Gastro-enterology *88*:1162, 1985.

166. Mizui, T., and Doteuchi, M. Lipid peroxidation: A possible role in gastric damage induced by ethanol in rats. Life Sci. *38*:2163, 1986.

167. Kivilaakso, E., Fromm, D., and Silen, W. Relationship be-tween ulceration and intramural pH of gastric mucosa during hemorrhagic shock. Surgery *84*:70, 1978.

168. Kivilaakso, E., Barzilai, A., Schiessel, R., Fromm, D., and Silen, W. Experimental ulceration of rabbit antral mucosa. Gastroenterology *80*:77, 1981.

169. Kivilaakso, E. Pathogenetic mechanisms in experimental gastric stress ulceration. Scand. J. Gastroenterol. *20*(suppl. 110):57, 1985.

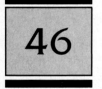

46

Gastritis

WILFRED M. WEINSTEIN

Gastritis is diagnosed frequently in clinical practice and is the subject of numerous publications. In both arenas there is often uncertainty regarding what is being described. This is often because of loosely used terminology or because the same terms (e.g., acute, chronic) mean different things to individuals who work in different fields.

When biopsies are taken, the endoscopist provides the macroscopic findings for the pathologist. There-fore, effective dialogue between them is essential. Such dialogue is enhanced if the endoscopist uses descriptive rather than dynamic terms to describe mucosal ap-pearances, and also employs accurate descriptions for the locations of lesions that are biopsied.

CLASSIFICATION AND NOMENCLATURE

Table 46–1 gives the classification of gastritis and its associations. The starting point in the classification is based on the gross appearance, namely, whether the gastritis is *erosive/hemorrhagic* or *nonerosive*. Erosive/ hemorrhagic patterns refer to endoscopically visible abnormalities. Only rarely are erosions or diffuse mu-cosal hemorrhages detected histologically in the ab-sence of gross (endoscopic) abnormalities. Nonerosive gastritis is a diagnosis that can only be made histolog-ically. The endoscopic appearance of the gastric mu-cosa does not, in the vast majority of instances, predict the presence, absence, or type of mucosal inflamma-tion.[1] Within each major category of gastritis the associated histologic appearance may be *nonspecific* or *specific*. Specific refers to more distinctive histologic features, which markedly narrow the differential di-agnosis even if they are not pathognomonic.

Gastritis will be considered in three groups. These groups and their associated disorders or clinical settings are shown in Table 46–1. The first two will be the nonspecific types of erosive/hemorrhagic and nonero-sive gastritis. The third group will be the *specific* types of gastritis combining the erosive/hemorrhagic (where applicable) and nonerosive types. Specific types of gastritis are uncommon. They include Menetrier's dis-ease, eosinophilic gastritis, and certain infections.

Table 46–1. TYPES OF GASTRITIS AND THEIR ASSOCIATED DISORDERS OR CLINICAL SETTINGS

I. Erosive/hemorrhagic gastritis: nonspecific types
  Stress lesions; seriously ill patients
  Drugs
    Nonsteroidal anti-inflammatory drugs
    Others: Potassium chloride, iron
  Alcohol
  Localized gastric trauma
    Mechanical and interventional
    Caustic
    Radiation
  Postgastrectomy
  Ischemia
  Idiopathic
    Incidental
    Chronic erosive gastritis
II. Nonerosive nonspecific gastritis
  Healthy aging
  Campylobacter pylori
  Peptic ulcer
    Gastric ulcer
    Duodenal ulcer
  Postgastrectomy
  Pernicious anemia
  Gastric adenocarcinoma
  Possible associations
    Gastroesophageal reflux
    Dermatitis herpetiformis
III. Specific types of gastritis
  Confined to the stomach
    Menetrier's disease
    Lymphoid hyperplasia
    Isolated unexplained granulomas
  In gastrointestinal tract
    Crohn's disease
    Eosinophilic gastritis
  In systemic disease
    Sarcoidosis
    Infections and infestations

EROSIVE/HEMORRHAGIC GASTRITIS: NONSPECIFIC TYPES

Table 46–1 gives the settings in which these lesions may be encountered. The most important are those that occur in seriously ill patients, in alcoholics, and in patients on nonsteroidal anti-inflammatory drugs. These are considered in Chapter 45. Other drugs, notably potassium chloride[2] and iron,[3] have been reported to cause erosions and/or hemorrhages over the short-term in human volunteers.

Caustic injury is discussed in Chapter 11. *Postgastrectomy gastritis* is discussed later in this chapter.

Definitions

An erosion classically refers to a defect in the mucosa that does not traverse the muscularis mucosae. The distinction between erosion and ulcer at endoscopy is of necessity often arbitrary. Erosions are flat or minimally depressed breaks in the mucosa with white bases and surrounding erythema. When a black-based erosion is present, it implies recent hemorrhage. A subepithelial hemorrhage refers to the appearance of discrete petechiae or bright-red areas of what appear to be "blood under a clear plastic wrap." Although some endoscopists describe these lesions as submucosal hemorrhages, this implies a degree of clairvoyance that is not verifiable. The term *subepithelial hemorrhage* is preferred because it leaves open the possiblity that the lesion is located in either the mucosa or submucosa.

It is not possible to determine on gross appearance alone whether a zone of subepithelial hemorrhage might be due to an underlying vascular abnormality.[4] Not infrequently, the findings of erythema and friability (petechiae or bleeding after contact with the endoscope) are designated as erosions.[5] This designation should be avoided. Whereas there is good interobserver agreement for erosions and subepithelial hemorrhages,[1] there is not for erythema,[1] nor is there any standardized test for friability.

The diagnosis of nonspecific erosive or hemorrhagic gastritis is made on the basis of the endoscopic appearance. Biopsies are not usually required, or they may be contraindicated because of the associated serious illness. These lesions are often unaccompanied by any significant inflammatory reaction either within the lesion itself or in the adjacent intact mucosa.[6, 7]

Mechanical and Interventional Trauma

Nasogastric tube suction is a well-recognized source of gastric erosions or subepithelial hemorrhages.

Prolapse gastropathy refers to the finding of a demarcated area of subepithelial hemorrhage just distal to the region of the gastroesophageal junction.[8] Typically, there is a history of retching followed by hematemesis or abdominal pain. At endoscopy one may see a "knuckle" of gastric mucosa prolapsing into the distal esophagus.[8] It is likely that some subepithelial hemorrhages incidentally discovered in the fundus at endoscopy are similarly induced by retching associated with endoscopic intubation. The linear gastric erosions in the proximal stomach of patients with large diaphragmatic hernias may also be due to trauma to mucosal folds in the course of respiratory excursions.[9]

By their very nature, techniques to control bleeding in the stomach (laser, electrocoagulation, and heater probe) may induce erosions or ulcers in and adjacent to the treated areas.[10] Their time course has not been studied in humans.[11]

Radiation Injury

Primary radiation therapy to the stomach for peptic ulcer[12] is no longer employed. It was reported to produce both hemorrhagic and nonerosive injury.[13]

Secondary irradiation injury as a result of large doses (exceeding 4500 rad) to the abdomen is uncommon because this form of radiotherapy is not often employed. The acute response to massive irradiation occurs largely in the antrum and prepyloric region. Ulcers may progress quickly to perforation or gastric outlet obstruction.[14] A more delayed change may be pyloroduodenal narrowing, with symptoms of gastric outlet obstruction.

Patients who have received abdominal radiation and are on chemotherapy for malignancy may develop abdominal pain and gastrointestinal bleeding. If erosive gastritis or discrete ulcers are found, it is important to consider opportunistic-associated disease.

Ischemia

Discrete ischemic injury to the stomach is rarely recognized. Erosive gastritis has been reported in association with atheromatous embolization of cholesterol[15] and with vasculitis.[16] Small numbers of patients with chronic gastric ulcers and erosions have been reported to heal their lesions after intestinal revascularization.[17, 18]

Idiopathic Erosive/Hemorrhagic Gastritis

Incidental. Occasionally, gastric erosions or subepithelial hemorrhages are encountered unexpectedly. The true prevalence of this phenomenon is impossible to gauge from existing data. In a Finnish study of 358 control subjects for a gastric carcinoma study, erosions were reported in 2.5 per cent.[19] In a U.S. study of paid, largely unemployed individuals, a surprisingly large number, 12 per cent, were found to have erosive gastritis.[20] In neither of these studies was it possible to exclude mechanical (prolapse) injury or prior alcohol or nonsteroidal anti-inflammatory drug ingestion as contributing factors.

In the evaluation of patients with dyspepsia it is often impossible to know if a few erosions or hemorrhages seen in the stomach represent a purely incidental finding or are the cause of the patient's symptoms. It is well recognized that there is a poor correlation between the presence of erosions and symptoms of pain in patients on anti-inflammatory drugs or with "stress" lesions (see Chapter 45). In a Norwegian study[5] of patients with "nonulcer dyspepsia," 14 per cent had gastric erosions, primarily in the antrum. It is not known how many of those individuals were habitual users of nonsteroidal anti-inflammatory drugs or alcohol. Given the unavailability of any provocative tests to determine whether erosions in a given patient are causing their dyspepsia, it seems logical to treat these individuals as for dyspepsia in general.[21]

Chronic Erosive Gastritis. This rare condition has also been termed *diffuse varioliform gastritis*.[22] It is characterized by the persistence or recurrence of multiple gastric erosions in the absence of any known risk factors for their development (Table 46–1).

The pathogenesis is unknown. An earlier study suggested a hypersensitivity mechanism because of the observation of increased numbers of IgE-containing cells in the mucosa.[22] Subsequently it has been shown that increased numbers of these cells may also be seen in biopsies from the edges of duodenal and gastric

ulcers.[23] It is not known what proportion of these IgE-staining cells are plasma cells and what proportion are mast cells.

The spectrum of reported symptoms is broad and includes nondescript abdominal pain, ulcer-type symptoms, nausea, and vomiting. Uncommon features include occult gastrointestinal bleeding, hematemesis, profound anorexia, and weight loss.[24–27] There may be laboratory evidence of anemia or hypoalbuminemia. Symptoms often wax and wane and do not necessarily bear a strict relationship to the number of erosions seen endoscopically at any given time. In all these cases a nonsteroidal drug and alcohol ingestion should be excluded in order to consider the condition truly idiopathic.

Double constrast barium x-ray of the stomach may be highly suggestive.[27] Typically there are nodules at the crests of thickened folds in the body, antrum or both. Some of the nodular defects may contain central barium-filled craters.[27] Endoscopic examination is required to establish the diagnosis with certainty, primarily by excluding other conditions. The small (usually less than 1 cm in diameter) nodules are generally positioned at the crests of rugal folds. Many or all contain central umbilications, some with a white base suggesting exudate. The role of endoscopic biopsy is largely to rule out other more *specific* forms of erosive gastritis and malignancy. Biopsies in the vicinity of the erosions usually show a nonerosive nonspecific gastritis of variable severity, with accompanying foveolar hyperplasia.[27, 28] The erosion itself may contain a volcano-like pseudomembrane at the surface.[28] In some patients there are more usual-appearing erosions without the associated tiny mounds.

When the lesions are circumscribed, endoscopic biopsies should be taken to rule out the possibility of underlying lymphoma or diffuse carcinoma. Deep snare biopsies should be taken only if underlying malignancy is a serious consideration. Depending upon the clinical setting, biopsies may also aid in the differential diagnosis of specific forms of erosive gastritis, such as Crohn's disease, or infections in the immunocompromised host.

No therapy has been found to be uniformly effective. In large part this is a reflection of the waxing and waning nature of the condition, and it may also be because so few cases have been studied systematically. Clinical and endoscopic responses have been reported with a variety of therapies: therapy for peptic ulcer, sodium cromoglycate, and corticosteroids.[25–27] A reasonable initial approach is to begin with conventional peptic ulcer treatment before resorting to other types of empiric therapy.[25, 26]

The natural history of the disorder is highly variable. Some patients have apparent remissions within months, whereas in others the condition persists for years.

NONEROSIVE NONSPECIFIC GASTRITIS

This form is commonly referred to as chronic gastritis. It is a histologic entity that is very common in the general population. Nonerosive, nonspecific gastritis appears to be a final common pathway of injury in response to diverse causes. It has attracted attention because of its possible pathogenic relationship to disorders such as peptic ulcer and gastric cancer and most recently because of the link with *Campylobacter pylori*. In Japan chromoendoscopy with Congo red and methylene blue dyes has been used for large surveys of nonerosive nonspecific gastritis.[29] However, mucosal biopsy is required to definitively characterize the presence and severity of nonerosive gastritis.

Histologic Patterns

In order to understand the histologic patterns and distribution of nonerosive nonspecific gastritis it is important to recall that the stomach has two major gland zones from a histologic point of view. The fundic gland mucosa occupies both the fundus and the body of the stomach. The antral (pyloric) gland mucosa occupies the anatomic antrum. Between these zones are transition areas that combine features of adjacent gland types. The antral-fundic gland transition zone is often more extensive along the lesser curvature of the stomach.

The terms *type A* and *type B gastritis* were originally coined to refer to nonerosive fundic gland and antral gland gastritis, respectively.[30] However, commonly both gland zones are involved simultaneously, but with severity and extent predominating in one zone more than in the other.

The histologic patterns of nonerosive, nonspecific gastritis are outlined in Table 46–2. The designation of *superficial* or *atrophic* provides a general picture of

Table 46–2. OVERALL HISTOLOGIC CLASSIFICATION OF NONEROSIVE, NONSPECIFIC GASTRITIS

Type of Gastritis*	Inflammatory Cells	Glands
Superficial	Confined to pit regions	Intact
Atrophic	Extension into gland zones	Variable gland loss

*The affected gland zone (fundic or antral gland) is given and then the designation, superficial or atrophic. Special features (e.g., neutrophils, intestinal metaplasia) may be highlighted in the description or final diagnosis (see text).

the severity and mucosal depth of the inflammatory response. Changes are often patchily distributed and of variable severity in a given patient. *Superficial gastritis* is characterized by the presence of increased numbers of inflammatory cells in the pit or foveolar regions (Fig. 46–1). Glands are preserved. *Atrophic gastritis* is characterized by a variable gland loss and encroachment of inflammatory cells into the gland zones (Fig. 46–2). It is not uncommon to see a spectrum of mild to severe atrophic gastritis in the same stomach or even in the same biopsy specimen. Some biopsies with severe gland atrophy have only minimal inflammatory change (Fig. 46–3).

Special Histologic Features. In addition to grading the gastritis as superficial or atrophic, special features when present are noted. In some disease models these features may be the actual focus for study.[31, 32] There are three major categories of special features: (1) prominent neutrophil infiltrates; (2) epithelial changes; (3) intestinal or pseudopyloric metaplasia.

Normally the predominant inflammatory cells in

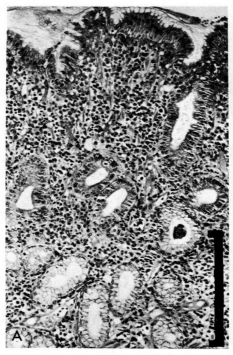
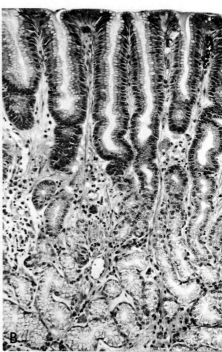

Figure 46–1. *A,* Superficial antral gland gastritis. The lamina propria inflammatory cells are concentrated in the upper half of the mucosa. The antral glands (bracketed zone) are intact. Compare with *B,* normal antral gland mucosa. (Hematoxylin and eosin stain, × 120.)

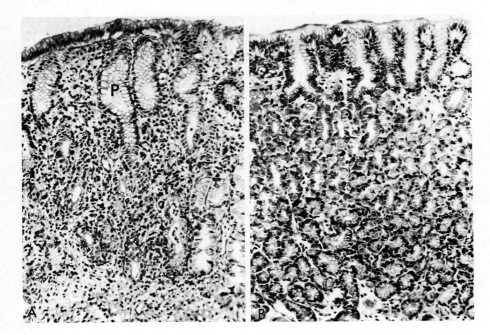

Figure 46–2. *A,* Severe atrophic fundic gland gastritis in a biopsy from the midbody, greater curvature. Most of the fundic glands are absent, and there is a dense inflammatory cell infiltrate. The pit epithelium (P) is preserved. Compare with *B,* normal fundic gland mucosa. (Hematoxylin and eosin stain, × 120.)

nonerosive nonspecific gastritis are mononuclear, i.e., lymphocytes and plasma cells. Not uncommonly there are prominent collections of neutrophils or eosinophils free in the lamina propria and in the lining epithelium.

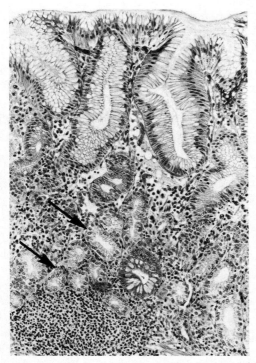

Figure 46–3. Atrophic fundic gland gastritis with minimal inflammation. Biopsy from the midbody greater curvature in an achlorhydric patient. The surface epithelium and the pits are normal. The normal fundic gland elements (parietal and chief cells) are absent. There is pseudopyloric metaplasia as evidenced by the clear-staining mucus type glands *(arrows)*. A lymphoid aggregate lies deep in the mucosa (lower left). (Hematoxylin and eosin stain, × 120.)

The terms "*active*" and "*chronic active*" can be used to highlight the presence of neutrophils.

The surface epithelium in all forms of nonerosive nonspecific gastritis is often normal or only minimally affected. If the epithelium is abnormal, it is usually the pit (foveolar) zone more so than the surface. The epithelial changes are characterized by mucin-depleted cells with disturbed nuclear polarity, enlarged nuclei, and an apparent increase in mitotic figures.[31] Even more atypical epithelial changes may be observed in certain circumstances, as in hepatic arterial infusion chemotherapy.[33]

Two types of metaplasia may be present in nonerosive nonspecific gastritis. One is *intestinal metaplasia* (Fig. 46–4). The typical feature is the intestinal type goblet cell. The metaplasia may be patchy, with isolated collections of goblet cells in the surface epithelium or pits. In general, extensive intestinal metaplasia accompanies more severe forms of atrophic gastritis. Sometimes the intestinal metaplasia is so extensive that the appearance is indistinguishable from that of small intestinal mucosa, with full-blown villus formation, complete with a brush border and Paneth cells.

A second type of metaplasia, namely, *pseudopyloric metaplasia,* occurs in the fundic gland zone when there is moderate or severe atrophic gastritis. The normal fundic glands are replaced in part or totally by mucus glands that are indistinguishable from those of the antral gland or cardiac gland mucosa (Fig. 46–3). Thus, a biopsy from the fundic gland zone that exhibits severe atrophic gastritis or atrophy with pseudopyloric metaplasia may appear indistinguishable ("antralized") from an antral gland gastritis. For this reason it is essential for the pathologist to know the precise site where a given biopsy was taken. Pseudopyloric metaplasia is more frequent along the lesser curvature of the body of the stomach as a proximal extension of antral gland gastritis.[34] Therefore, biopsy samples

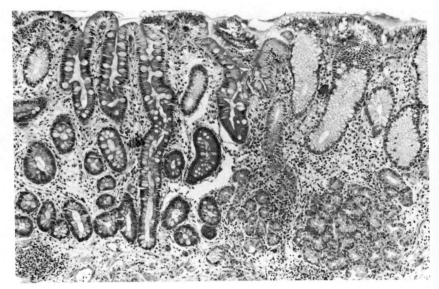

Figure 46—4. Intestinal metaplasia of the fundic gland zone. Biopsy from the same patient and near the same area as the biopsy illustrated in Figure 46—3. The left half of the biopsy shows full-thickness mucosal intestinal metaplasia with rudimentary villi and numerous goblet cells. (Hematoxylin and eosin stain, × 75.)

taken to assess the maximal degree of fundic gland atrophy should be obtained from the proximal or mid body on the greater curvature, where the fundic gland mucosa is normally thicker.

Other Histologic Features. A variety of *endocrine cells* may be demonstrated with silver stains or with specific antisera in areas of intestinal metaplasia of the stomach.[35] In severe atrophic fundic gland gastritis, especially in the presence of hypergastrinemia there may also be endocrine cell hyperplasia (Fig. 46–5) in zones of pseudopyloric metaplasia.[36–38]

Both *lipid islands* (*gastric xanthelasma*) and *intramucosal cysts* appear to be more common in the postoperative stomach.[31, 39–41]

Clinical Features

As indicated previously, the presence (friability, erythema, etc.) or absence of apparent endoscopic abnormalities generally bears little relationship to the presence or absence of nonerosive nonspecific gastritis.[1]

In clinical practice there is rarely any need to determine whether a patient has nonerosive nonspecific gastritis. The only exception to this might be to document gastric atrophy of the fundic gland mucosa in a case of otherwise atypical pernicious anemia.

The capacity to secrete acid is progressively reduced as atrophic fundic gland gastritis develops. Serum gastrin levels are elevated in approximately 75 per cent of individuals with severe atrophic fundic gland gastritis.[36] The hypergastrinemia results from the loss of the normal acid inhibition of gastrin release. In addition there may be gastrin cell hyperplasia.[42] However, when there is concomitant severe atrophic antral gland gastritis, fasting serum gastrin levels may not be elevated.[36, 43]

A small proportion of patients with nonerosive antral gland gastritis have autoantibodies that react with antral gastrin cells.[44] It is not known whether these autoantibodies have any biologic capacity to compromise gastrin cell function or to cause gastrin cell atrophy.

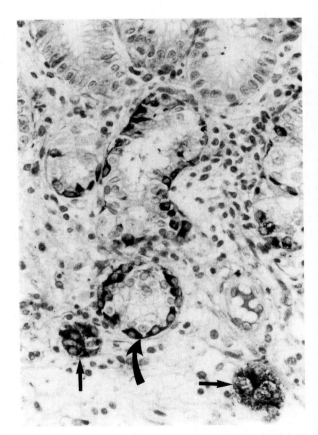

Figure 46—5. Endocrine cell hyperplasia in atrophic fundic gland gastritis. There is a ringlet of black-staining endocrine cells in a zone of pseudopyloric metaplasia *(curved arrow).* There are also isolated buds of black-staining endocrine cells deeper in the mucosa *(straight arrows).* (Grimelius silver stain, × 160.)

In a large Finnish population study it was shown that a low ratio of pepsinogen I to pepsinogen II was predictive of moderate to severe fundic gland gastritis.[45] This ratio was also found to decrease progressively with advancing age in a group of elderly U.S. patients who did not undergo mucosal biopsy.[46] Serum pepsinogen determinations appear to be useful for epidemiologic survey studies of moderate to severe nonerosive fundic gland gastritis.

Parietal cell antibodies and intrinsic factor antibodies will be discussed in the section on pernicious anemia.

Nonerosive Gastritis and Dyspepsia. It is logical to suppose that a subset of patients with nonerosive nonspecific gastritis might have abdominal symptoms based upon the presence of the inflammatory change or upon its consequences such as motor abnormalities. At the present time there is no reliable way to identify this subset. As discussed subsequently, nonerosive gastritis is so common in the general population that it is difficult to attribute symptoms to it without some additional "marker(s)." Another form of proof would be to demonstrate in sufficient numbers of patients (with an appropriate control group) that symptoms and inflammatory changes receded in parallel.

Conditions Associated with Nonerosive Nonspecific Gastritis

Healthy Aging. Earlier population biopsy surveys outside North America indicated that nonerosive nonspecific gastritis was common.[47-50] After the fourth decade approximately 50 per cent of the population was found to have superficial antral and fundic gland gastritis, which developed into more atrophic patterns with advancing age. In most studies the antral gland gastritis was more severe than the fundic gland gastritis, especially along the lesser curvature. There was age-dependent proximal extension of the antral gland zone into the fundic zone with both pseudopyloric metaplasia and intestinal metaplasia.[34] In some populations the severity of the nonerosive gastritis and its rate of progression may be related to genetic factors. There is also preliminary data in asymptomatic individuals that Campylobacter pylori infection (discussed below) has an increased prevalence with age, but it is not known whether it is responsible for the age-related gastritis.

More recent studies indicate that the trends may be changing, with a "slowing" of the progression in both the body and antrum, more marked in the latter.[51-53] These apparent trends may reflect environmental factors that are also responsible for the decrease in gastric ulcer and gastric cancer that has been observed in certain countries.

There are no large-scale biopsy studies of a normal population in North America. The absolute prevalence of antral and fundic gland gastritis may be lower or less severe in North America compared with countries that have higher prevalence rates for gastric ulcer and adenocarcinoma. Nevertheless, the same general pattern of age dependency most likely exists in North America.[46]

Campylobacter pylori. There has been enormous investigative enthusiasm in this area ever since 1983 when Warren and Marshall described "curved bacilli" in the gastric mucosa.[54] The intense interest centers around the nature of the relationship between *Campylobacter pylori,* nonerosive gastritis, and peptic ulcer.[55-57]

The intent in this section is to focus on the relationship between *C. pylori* and nonerosive nonspecific gastritis. Other aspects, specifically the historical perspectives, and the relationship with peptic ulcers[55-57] will not be discussed in detail.

C. pylori is a gram-negative microaerophilic organism that requires special culture conditions.[58] It is a small (3×0.5 μm) rod and appears bent or spiral (Fig. 46–6). The organism is probably not a true *Campylobacter.*[59] It is likely that there are various strains of this organism which may differ in pathogenicity.[60] *C. pylori* is sensitive to a variety of antibiotics *in vitro* and to bismuth compounds.[32, 61]

Diagnosis of **C. pylori.** When biopsies are obtained for culture they must be ground or minced and incubated promptly.[62] The relationship between the actual number of organisms per unit of tissue ("colony count") and the severity of the associated mucosal inflammation has not been defined.

With conventional hematoxylin and eosin stained slides the organisms can often be appreciated at ordinary high-power magnification, but visualization is facilitated with oil immersion. The organisms cluster on the luminal aspect of the surface and pit mucus

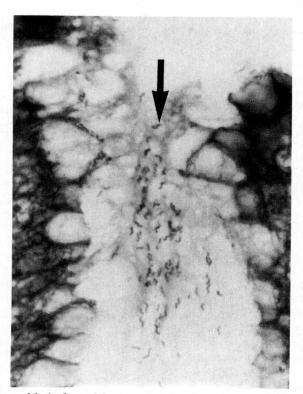

Figure 46–6. *Campylobacter pylori.* A group of organisms at the opening *(arrow)* of a gastric pit. The organisms have a bent or spiral appearance. (Giemsa stain, × 600.)

cells (Fig. 46–6). Within a given biopsy there is often considerable variation in the numbers of organisms. With electron microscopy the organisms are seen to concentrate over intercellular junctions.[63] Studies are required to address the question of the frequency of invasion of epithelial or glandular cells.

Visualization at light microscopy is facilitated with special stains using either silver techniques (Warthin-Starry) or Giemsa stains. Other techniques have included monoclonal antibody staining,[64] acridine orange with fluorescence, and phase contrast. There appears to be a good correlation between the finding of *C. pylori*–type organisms on biopsy and culture positivity.[32]

An adjunct to the examination of biopsies is to prepare smears from brushings of gastric mucosa.[65] This has the theoretical advantage of being able to sample a larger area of mucosa.

Other Diagnostic Techniques. *C. pylori* has a high endogenous urease activity. A rapid "bedside" *urease test* that can be done with a single gastric biopsy has been described.[66] A breath test has been employed in survey studies; ^{13}C-urea is administered orally and urea-derived $^{13}CO_2$ is measured in the breath.[67]

Systemic and local antibody production to *C. pylori* can be demonstrated.[68–71] The use of *serologic tests*, especially with more sensitive techniques such as ELISA, may prove useful in prevalence and in natural history studies. It will be important to know how the organism load, as determined by culture, and the severity of inflammatory response will correlate with the serologic titers.

C. pylori *and Nonerosive Nonspecific Gastritis.* Based primarily on morphologic studies and to a lesser extent on gastric biopsy cultures it has been demonstrated that *C. pylori* occurs in from 70 to more than 90 per cent of patients with nonerosive antral gland gastritis.[58, 69, 72–74] It has also been reported in children with nonerosive gastritis.[75] Many of the subjects with nonerosive antral gastritis have been asymptomatic. There appears to be a lesser frequency of finding organisms in the fundic gland mucosa, but this is not a uniform finding.[76] In individuals without nonerosive antral gland gastritis less than 10 per cent are found to have *C. pylori*. Preliminary prevalence data using the ^{13}C-urea breath test indicate that 75 per cent of asymptomatic individuals over the age of 65 may have *C. pylori* infection.[77]

How *C. pylori* acts as a variable in the link between peptic ulcer, gastritis, and gastric carcinoma remains to be defined. The severity of the inflammatory change associated with *C. pylori* may be very mild, and many investigators have focused on neutrophilic infiltrates which seem to correlate best with the presence or absence of the organisms.[55, 56, 74, 78] Because *C. pylori* is so commonly found in nonerosive gastritis, it is not being designated as a *specific* type of gastritis histologically.

Does this ubiquitous organism cause gastritis or does it colonize areas of pre-existing gastritis? The ultimate answer may be that it can do both, namely, a pathogen

sometimes, and commensal often. Drs. Marshall and Morris ingested *C. pylori* and developed mild upper gastrointestinal tract symptoms.[60, 79] In both cases a nonerosive superficial antral gland gastritis developed, with neutrophils as part of the inflammatory response. In Dr. Morris' case a superficial fundic gland gastritis was also documented.[60]

It has also been speculated that *C. pylori* may have been responsible for two miniepidemics of nonerosive, nonspecific gastritis.[80, 81] These were reported in volunteers for secretory studies and the individuals developed self-limited upper abdominal complaints, but with hypochlorhydria that persisted in some for months. Endoscopy in one of these studies[81] was reported to be normal. Spontaneous hypochlorhydria has also been reported in the Zollinger-Ellison syndrome.[80, 82] In "*epidemic gastritis*" or spontaneous hypochlorhydria the published histology reveals that the inflammatory change is largely confined to the pit regions and to the superficial gland zones. Thus, the condition appears to be due to severe functional impairment of parietal cells rather than obliteration of the fundic gland zone.

A preliminary controlled trial dealing with eradication of the *C. pylori* in antral gastritis was reported.[32] This was a mixed group of patients with erosive and nonerosive gastritis, some symptomatic and some asymptomatic. Bismuth salicylate was superior to erythromycin in clearing *C. pylori*, and this clearance was associated with a significant improvement in both neutrophil and mononuclear scores. In these small groups there was no correlation with symptom improvement.[32] Uncontrolled preliminary observations[83] suggest that *C. pylori* may recur fairly promptly after its apparent eradication with either colloidal bismuth or amoxicillin. The efficacy of antibiotics in the temporary or more prolonged clearance of the organisms may not parallel *in vitro* sensitivities.[32]

C. pylori *and Other Conditions.* The association between the finding of *C. pylori* and peptic ulcer disease has also been reported in numerous studies.[56] Approximately two-thirds of patients with gastric ulcer and more than 80 per cent with duodenal ulcer have been found to have *C. pylori* in the stomach. The organism has also been found in the duodenum, especially in association with areas of gastric surface cell metaplasia.[73] It remains to be seen whether eradication of *C. pylori* is itself an important factor in the healing rate or relapse rate of peptic ulcers.

There are preliminary indications that, compared with the prevalence in antral gland gastritis, *C. pylori* is a less frequent occurrence in the stomach of patients with pernicious anemia[84] and in the gastric remnant mucosa after gastrectomy.[85, 86] There are conflicting preliminary results concerning whether *C. pylori* may normally reside in histologically normal fundic gland mucosa.[76, 85]

Does *C. pylori* cause chronic dyspepsia? To answer this is a major challenge because dyspepsia is difficult to define for studies and because the organism is so commonly found in asymptomatic individuals with nonerosive antral gastritis. It might be tempting for some physicians who encounter patients with chronic dyspepsia to advocate that they have endoscopy with biopsies for culture and histologic testing to determine whether there is infection with *C. pylori*. Until there is an infinitely larger body of evidence in relation to dyspepsia and *C. pylori*, this temptation should be resisted. One rational alternative is to treat short-term with some form of bismuth compound as a second line of empiric therapy that the physician normally uses in the general approach to dyspepsia.[21]

Peptic Ulcer

Gastric Ulcer. It has been conventional wisdom for many years that chronic gastric ulcers in the body of the stomach are invariably associated with a diffuse antral gland gastritis.[87, 88] This diffuse antral gland gastritis appears to be independent of age and has been shown to be more severe in gastric ulcer than in duodenal ulcer.[89, 90] The fundic gland zone is often inflamed as well, but initially less severely than the antrum. In recent reports from Japan and Finland it has been shown that the nonerosive gastritis in the gastric body of patients with previous gastric ulcers progresses more rapidly with time (three to seven years average follow-up) than in control subjects.[51, 91] Additionally, in the Finnish study it was estimated that the antral gastritis, unlike the fundic gland gastritis, did not progress more rapidly in the ulcer patients than in the control subjects.[91] As discussed earlier, these changing patterns may reflect environmental changes in relation to diet and habits, and may not just represent a phenomenon peculiar to the gastric ulcer diathesis.

The association between antral gastritis and gastric ulcer led to the notion that the basic defect in gastric ulcer is actually the diffuse nonerosive gastritis. The pathogenesis of this mucosal change is basically the same as that proposed for gastric ulcer in general (see pp. 880–887). More recent studies also indicate some link between nonerosive antral gastritis and delayed gastric emptying,[92, 93] but their cause and effect relationships are not clear.

One exception to the antral gastritis–gastric ulcer link was reported in patients who habitually took aspirin.[94] Approximately half the patients did not have antral gastritis, suggesting a novel nongastritis pathway for the formation of some aspirin-associated gastric ulcers. Prospective studies of gastric ulcers associated with other nonsteroidal anti-inflammatory drugs have not been reported. Nevertheless, in a clinical setting one might suspect that ingestion of these drugs may have been overlooked as a factor in pathogenesis if biopsies from the edge of a gastric ulcer fail to show any inflammatory changes.

Duodenal Ulcer. In patients with duodenal ulcer there is a greater prevalence of antral gastritis than in control subjects and a better preserved or more "juvenile" fundic gland mucosa.[95, 96] In a provocative study from Hong Kong it was found that the inflammatory cell activity in the gastric antrum was significantly reduced when there was duodenal ulcer healing, even on placebo![97] This relationship between antral gastritis

and duodenal ulcer will undoubtedly receive more attention especially with regard to a possible contribution from *Campylobacter pylori*.

Postgastrectomy. The syndrome of alkaline reflux gastritis is discussed on page 980. This section focuses on the nature of the mucosal inflammatory changes.

After partial gastrectomy for duodenal ulcer, fundic gland gastritis develops or worsens more rapidly than in control subjects within the first two years after surgery and thereafter appears to progress at the same rate as in the general population.[98] The changes appear to be more marked after Billroth II anastomoses[31] and also might be expected to be more severe in those who have had surgery for gastric ulcers. It is not known whether highly selective vagotomy is associated with an accelerated development of nonerosive gastritis compared with control populations.

There is a common perception that there is severe nonerosive gastritis in these patients, especially those labeled as having the syndrome of "alkaline reflux gastritis." In actual fact, half or more may have only minimal or no evidence of inflammatory change.[31, 99, 100] The major abnormality in many patients is the epithelium at the stoma where there are epithelial abnormalities and prominent foveolar cell hyperplasia.[31] The inflammatory cell density at the stoma may actually be less than in the remainder of the stomach.[31, 100] Other mucosal abnormalities that occur more commonly in the postoperative stomach are stomal erosions,[99] intramucosal cysts,[31, 41] and lipid islands.[39, 40]

The well-recognized[101] lack of correlation between the histologic features of the postoperative stomach, symptoms, endoscopic appearances, and tests of duodenal-gastric reflux is discussed on pages 962 to 969. For many years it has been suggested that increased duodenal-gastric reflux may cause gastritis and symptoms in patients with intact stomachs. There is no concrete evidence that this is true.

Pernicious Anemia. It merits re-emphasis that the finding of diffuse atrophic fundic gland gastritis and hypo- or achlorhydria is not uncommon in the elderly population.[46] Only a small subset of these individuals have classic pernicious anemia.

Addisonian pernicious anemia is a megaloblastic anemia with absolute achlorhydria. Vitamin B_{12} malabsorption (documented by Schilling's test) is due to severe fundic gland gastritis with a diminished ability to secrete intrinsic factor. Therapy consists of monthly injections of vitamin B_{12}.

Immunologic abnormalities and associations with autoimmune diseases figure prominently in pernicious anemia.[102, 103] For many of the immunologic abnormalities it is unclear whether they are important in pathogenesis or merely represent epiphenomena. Serum antibodies to parietal cells are found in up to 90 per cent of patients with pernicious anemia. Cytotoxic antibodies to parietal cells have been demonstrated.[104] The serum intrinsic factor antibodies which occur are of two types.[102] Type I is a blocking antibody that combines with intrinsic factor and is found in about 70 per cent of patients. Type II is a binding antibody which prevents uptake of the intrinsic factor–vitamin B_{12} complex and is present in about 40 per cent of patients, and only in those with type I antibodies. It has been shown that corticosteroids can improve vitamin B_{12} absorption in pernicious anemia.[105] It was also claimed, using fluoroscopically placed suction biopsy instruments, that parietal cells returned on corticosteroid therapy.[105] This observation might have been due to a sampling phenomenon because small numbers of parietal cells may normally be found in some biopsies of patients with pernicious anemia.[43]

Familial patterns in first-degree relatives of patients with pernicious anemia have been documented. These are reflected by an increased frequency of the finding of parietal cell and intrinsic factor antibodies, absolute achlorhydria, and more severe fundic gland gastritis.[106, 107] It is not known how many of these relatives develop overt pernicious anemia within their lifetimes.

The severe fundic gland atrophy in pernicious anemia may be associated with only a minimal inflammatory cell infiltrate (Fig. 46–3). Extensive pseudopyloric metaplasia and variable amounts of intestinal metaplasia are common. The pseudopyloric metaplasia may be so extensive that the biopsy specimen may seem to be antral in origin. The surface epithelium is often remarkably well preserved. Even in the presence of absolute achlorhydria, residual tiny nests of parietal and chief cells may be present.[43] In some cases the antral gland mucosa exhibits nonerosive gastritis as well. It is usually less severe than that of the fundic gland zone but sometimes is very severe and extensive. In antral gland mucosae spared of severe change, increased numbers of gastrin cells can be demonstrated with immunocytochemical techniques.[42] This increase in gastrin cell number is part of the reason for the elevated serum gastrin levels that occur in 75 per cent or more of patients with pernicious anemia.[36]

There may also be impressive endocrine cell hyperplasia in the fundic gland mucosa (Fig. 46–5).[36–38, 108] This hyperplasia can be demonstrated with the use of silver stains and is roughly correlated with the magnitude of serum gastrin elevation.[36] Frank gastric carcinoids, although uncommon, have been increasingly recognized in pernicious anemia.[108–110] It is believed that they have the potential to metastasize when they exceed 2 cm, and they should be removed when they occur as isolated lesions.[110] When they are multifocal and smaller, one has to make an individualized choice between a major gastric resection and periodic endoscopic surveillance.

In endoscopic surveys of pernicious anemia, the most common lesions encountered are hyperplastic or inflammatory polyps, found in 10 to 40 per cent of patients.[109, 111] These innocuous non-neoplastic lesions may occur either in the body or in the antrum.

The risk of gastric adenocarcinoma in pernicious anemia has been estimated to be three times that of the general population.[111] However, this increased risk is not borne out in countries that have lower prevalence rates in general for gastric cancer.[109, 112] The relationship between the nonerosive gastritis of pernicious anemia and gastric carcinoma will be discussed in the next section.

Should endoscopic screening be done in patients with pernicious anemia? The recommendations from Stockbrugger et al. seem reasonable.[109] They suggest that all patients with pernicious anemia should undergo endoscopy with biopsies once, at or after the time of diagnosis. There are no guidelines for how many biopsies to take. My approach is to take four from the antrum and at least six from the body and fundus; these sites are spaced equidistant along lesser and greater curvatures. If carcinoids, adenomatous neoplasms, or high-grade dysplasias are not discovered, then repeated surveillance endoscopy is not indicated.[111]

If a patient is found to have high-grade dysplasia, more biopsies should be taken immediately to rule out coexisting carcinoma. Thereafter, I recommend periodic endoscopy and biopsy surveillance at one- to two-year intervals only for those who were initially found to have high-grade dysplasia or small isolated carcinoids. High-grade dysplasia is considered to be a potential precursor lesion for invasive carcinoma. Fortunately, it is a rare, chance occurrence. Surgical resection would need to be considered if intramucosal carcinoma were found in follow-up.

It should be recognized that crucial data are not available to support these recommendations. *First*, the natural history of high-grade dysplasia is unknown, in terms of how often and over what period of time it has the capacity to develop into carcinoma with the capability to metastasize.[113] *Second*, the cure rate for cancers detected in a long-term surveillance program in this setting is unknown. *Third*, one has to take into account the potential morbidity and mortality from extensive gastric resections.

Gastric Adenocarcinoma. Adenocarcinoma of the gastric antrum and body are commonly associated with a more extensive (than in control populations) antral gland and fundic gland gastritis with prominent intestinal metaplasia.[114–116] Adenocarcinomas of the gastric cardia differ in that nonerosive gastritis of adjacent fundic gland mucosa is minimal or absent.[117, 118] There appears to be an increase in the incidence of cancers of the cardia, despite an overall decline in gastric adenocarcinoma in North America.[118]

It is suspected that severe nonerosive gastritis with extensive intestinal metaplasia may be a precursor lesion for some types of gastric cancer. However, this finding is very common in the same general populations in which gastric adenocarcinoma has a high prevalence.[119, 120] Therefore, there has been considerable interest in trying to find more specific markers for heightened cancer risk in intestinal metaplasia. None have been documented convincingly, and some results have been conflicting.[119–121] The same environmental and genetic factors proposed in the pathogenesis of gastric cancer have also been proposed for the severe nonerosive gastritis that accompanies some of these neoplasms.[122] As indicated earlier, whatever is accounting for the changing patterns of nonerosive gastritis in the general population[51-53] may also be part of the reason for the decline in the incidence of gastric adenocarcinoma.

The risk of gastric stump cancer 15 to 25 years after gastrectomy (especially Billroth II) is established in some countries but not in others.[123-126] It has been speculated but not proved that this risk may be related to the development of a more severe form of postoperative nonerosive gastritis in the gastric remnant.

Endoscopy and Biopsy Screening for Malignancy. Should physicians do repeated surveillance endoscopy in patients with severe nonerosive gastritis who might statistically have a greater than normal risk for the development of gastric adenocarcinoma? This question especially applies to patients with severe atrophic gastritis with achlorhydria, whether or not they have pernicious anemia,[127] and postgastrectomy patients, especially 20 years after Billroth II operations for gastric ulcer.[126] Screening would be for grossly visible tumors and for microscopic changes such as high-grade dysplasia and intramucosal carcinoma. For most North American populations in which the endemic gastric rates are low, repeated endoscopic biopsy surveillance of such patients is not justified. Even in countries where there is a greater endemic gastric cancer rate, the benefits in terms of case detection and prolongation of life are not strikingly apparent.[125]

A more desirable alternative to repeated endoscopic biopsy screening of the statistically higher risk patient is to caution the patient to report the development of any symptoms that might suggest gastric carcinoma and to screen these individuals regularly for signs of occult gastrointestinal bleeding.

Associations That Require Corroboration. There are two reports of antral gastritis and symptomatic gastroesophageal reflux.[92, 128] One study had dyspeptic control subjects[128] and the 20 normal control subjects in the second study[92] were 25 years younger than the patient group.

In a study of more than 100 patients with dermatitis herpetiformis it was found that 26 per cent were achlorhydric, significantly greater than a smaller number of patients with celiac sprue.[129] Normal control subjects were not studied.

SPECIFIC TYPES OF GASTRITIS

Table 46–1 gives the disorders that will be considered in this section. Most of these disorders are uncommon or rare. The designation *specific gastritis* refers to distinctive histologic features which markedly narrow the differential diagnosis or occasionally are pathognomonic. Some of these disorders, for example, Crohn's disease of the stomach, may be characterized by both erosive and nonerosive gastritis. The gross (endoscopic) appearances are usually not distinctive, except in certain rare circumstances, as in Menetrier's disease.

Menetrier's Disease

Menetrier's disease is a rare condition of unknown etiology. The definition in earlier reviews and reports has often been fuzzy. Therefore, the definition used here is one modified from that proposed in the excellent review by Appelman.[130] Namely, authentic cases of Menetrier's disease are those that have (1) giant folds, especially in the fundus and body of the stomach; (2) hypoalbuminemia; and (3) histologic features of foveolar hyperplasia, atrophy of glands, and a marked overall increase in mucosal thickness. Hypochlorhydria, e.g., with a peak acid output less than 10 mM per hour, can be expected when the process involves most of the fundic gland mucosa.

Pathology. The thickened folds are most prominent in the body of the stomach along the greater curvature (Fig. 46–7). At the crests of these folds there may be erosions, ulcerations, or a confluent polypoid appearance.

The histologic hallmark is that of marked elongation and tortuosity of the foveolae (pits), often associated with prominent cystic dilatations (Fig. 46–8). These cysts may penetrate the muscularis mucosae and extend into the submucosa. The lamina propria round cell content is increased in the pit regions. As expected, in the face of the marked foveolar hyperplasia there is an accompanying extensive reduction in the numbers of parietal and chief cells, with replacement by mucus glands (pseudopyloric metaplasia). In some cases there may be residual pockets of relatively intact fundic glands. When the process involves the antrum, then antral gland atrophy may also be present.

Gastric protein loss through this abnormal mucosa has been demonstrated often. It has been postulated that the protein loss occurs in a paracellular fashion via tight junctions.[131] Submucosal lymphangiectasia may also be associated and thus may contribute to the protein-losing gastropathy.[132]

Clinical Features and Diagnosis. As indicated by Appelman,[130] clinical reports of the disorder are often incomplete in relation to a full definition of the disease.[133, 134]

Menetrier's disease is usually diagnosed after the age of 50 and is more common in men. The spectrum of symptoms is broad; among the most common are epigastric pain, weight loss, diarrhea, and edema. The latter may sometimes be the first manifestation of the disease. The physical examination is nonspecific. There may be epigastric tenderness, edema, and signs of anemia, with stools positive for occult blood. The most characteristic laboratory abnormalities are low serum albumin and total serum proteins. The average peak acid output is in the range of 10 mM per hour, but hypochlorhydria is not a universal finding.[134] Patients with Menetrier's disease may have an increased risk of vascular or thromboembolic phenomena.[134]

Menetrier's disease has also been reported in children. This is not likely the same disorder as in adults. In children the thick folds (commonly without histo-

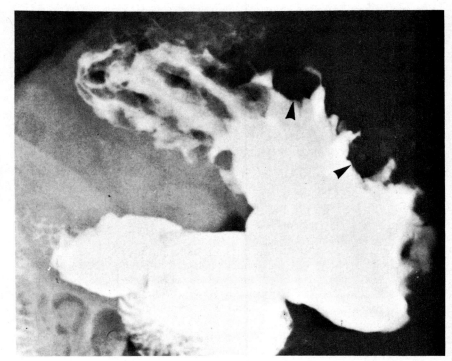

Figure 46–7. Menetrier's disease. The barium X-ray shows markedly thickened folds of the gastric fundus and body. These thick folds create a "thumbprint" effect *(arrowheads).* (Courtesy of Marvin Weiner, M.D.)

logic documentation) and hypoproteinemia are reversible.[135] These reversible cases are probably due to various infections. One prominent candidate appears to be *Cytomegalovirus.*[136, 137]

Barium X-ray reveals enlarged gastric folds in the fundus and body, with frequent sparing of the antrum (Fig. 46–7). The folds may be so enlarged, nodular, and tortuous that there is an appearance of barium-filled craters between the folds. Endoscopy confirms the X-ray findings and may also reveal associated superficial mucosal erosions or ulcers. The mucosal folds are pliable but they do not flatten fully with air insufflation at endoscopy. Endoscopic biopsies, even

with the "jumbo" pinch forceps, may not sample the full thickness of the mucosa and thus may be suggestive of the diagnosis but do not prove it. In these biopsies there may be foveolar hyperplasia, a nonspecific finding, but sampling is commonly not deep enough to document the gland atrophy and accompanying cystic changes.

Most patients thought to have Menetrier's disease are no longer subjected to open biopsy at laparotomy.[134] A full-thickness mucosal biopsy ("large particle biopsy") can be obtained with an electrocautery snare device. However, in many circumstances even this diagnostic approach may not be used. For example,

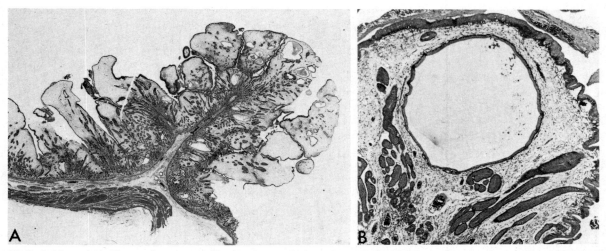

Figure 46–8. *A,* Menetrier's disease. Low-power view to show a thickened mucosa with a polypoid configuration. (Hematoxylin and eosin stain, × 5.) *B,* Higher power view to show a large mucosal cyst near the surface. (Hematoxylin and eosin stain, × 30.) (Courtesy of Klaus Lewin, M.D.)

patients already known to have the characteristic radiologic and laboratory findings over a period of years need not have a tissue diagnosis established with a full-thickness mucosal biopsy. Even in other clinical circumstances, when ominous disorders such as infiltrating carcinoma are excluded, patients may simply be followed, without documentation by full-thickness mucosal biopsy, and the diagnosis is established with time on the basis of its chronicity.[134]

Differential Diagnosis. The differential diagnosis of a symptomatic patient with thick gastric folds has long been a fashionable topic for discussion. The real concern is to exclude an infiltrating neoplasm, such as a diffuse carcinoma or lymphoma. In many cases, apparently thick folds on barium x-ray are found at endoscopy not to be thickened. Thick folds in the fundus and body of the stomach may be observed in the Zollinger-Ellison syndrome and in some patients with duodenal ulcer, but the clinical pictures are not those of Menetrier's disease. Some degree of foveolar hyperplasia may occasionally be seen in the Zollinger-Ellison syndrome and may result in transient confusion with Menetrier's disease.[138]

An even rarer condition than Menetrier's disease is *hypertrophic, hypersecretory gastropathy*.[130, 139] In this condition, there is acid hypersecretion and gastric protein loss. However, parietal and chief cell numbers are not markedly reduced, as they are in Menetrier's disease. The histologic appearance of the gastric lesions of the Cronkhite-Canada syndrome may be identical to that seen in Menetrier's disease,[140] but differential diagnosis on clinical grounds should be easy.

Perhaps the major question is what to call those cases that are not typical. In our experience they outnumber *bona fide* cases of Menetrier's disease. Examples include those with typical histologic features but without apparent protein loss and hypochlorhydria.[130] Other examples include those that have undergone spontaneous remission or progression to atrophic gastritis.[130, 141] It is recommended that these cases not be designated as Menetrier's disease until they are proved to be chronic and typical, recognizing in the meantime that they may represent part of the evolution of or natural progression of this disease.[130] The term I prefer for these variant cases is *idiopathic hypertrophic gastropathy*.

Finally, more localized examples of thick folds may be seen, especially in the gastric antrum. The histologic findings may mimic those of Menetrier's disease or hyperplastic polyps,[142] and again the main issue in differential diagnosis is to rule out underlying malignancy.

Therapy and Outcome. Some patients with associated gastric ulcers or erosions may benefit symptomatically from peptic ulcer therapy. Patients with few symptoms and minimal hypoalbuminemia require no specific therapy. Isolated successes in terms of abatement of symptoms and reversal of hypoalbuminemia have been associated with a variety of therapies including anticholinergics, H_2 receptor antagonist therapy, parietal cell vagotomy,[134] and oral tranexamic acid.[143]

It seems that fewer patients are now having partial gastric resections for persistent abdominal symptoms and hypoalbuminemia.[134] The results of surgery have generally been reported to be favorable.[133] Radical or total gastrectomy should be reserved for desperate situations. A few cases of carcinoma have been reported either coincidentally at the time of diagnosis or later in the course of the disease.[133, 144] The recommendation to perform annual endoscopic biopsy surveillance[144] of both the involved and uninvolved stomach seems premature. Endoscopic biopsy surveillance also represents a formidable challenge in a stomach that is occupied by massively thickened folds with numerous nooks and crannies.

Lymphoid Hyperplasia ("Pseudolymphoma")

This very uncommon condition represents a localized lymphoid hyperplasia of the stomach.[145, 146] The term "gastric pseudolymphoma" has been used widely because it may mimic lymphoma. Other conditions that less commonly enter into the differential diagnosis are small cell adenocarcinoma of the stomach and the very rare multisystem disease lymphomatoid granulomatosis.[147]

Localized lymphoid hyperplasia is usually detected in the evaluation of a patient with symptoms of peptic ulcer or incidentally in the follow-up biopsy of the edges of gastric ulcers. The most common gross appearance is that of a gastric ulcer, either surrounded by benign-appearing margins or by raised thickened folds that suggest malignancy. A second less common pattern is that of a plaque-like deformity with thickened, indurated gastric folds. Histologically there is massive hyperplasia of lymphoid follicles that usually contain germinal centers. The infiltrates most commonly occupy the mucosa and upper submucosa, but occasionally they are transmural.

The pathogenesis of localized lymphoid hyperplasia of the stomach is unknown. In many instances the lesions probably represent an idiosyncratic inflammatory reaction to gastric ulcer.

A presumptive diagnosis can be made in some cases using some combination of "jumbo" pinch biopsy forceps, large particle snare biopsy, endoscopically directed fine needle aspirates, and immunocytochemistry. Sometimes, even with large particle biopsy it may be impossible to exclude a lymphoma, and surgical resection must be performed. A tiny number of patients with localized lymphoid hyperplasia either have had associated gastric lymphoma or have progressed to lymphoma.[146, 148] Pathologists commonly perform immunocytochemistry for cytoplasmic immunoglobulins to differentiate between lymphoma (monotypic staining pattern) and benign localized lymphoid hyperplasia of the stomach (polytypic staining pattern). However, some cases that appear benign may actually have a monotypic staining pattern.[149] These patients, as well as all those who do not have total resections of the lesions, should have periodic endoscopic biopsy surveillance for the development of lymphoma.

Isolated Idiopathic Granulomatous Gastritis

This is a diagnosis of exclusion which refers to the histologic finding of isolated mucosal granulomas in the absence of a specific disease (Fig. 46–9).

When granulomas are found incidentally in gastric biopsies some are those of the *foreign body type*. These granulomas contain various types of foreign debris and are considered to represent a reaction to some form of prior mucosal injury, such as ulceration or erosion.

Isolated idiopathic granulomatous gastritis is sometimes associated with marked gross structural changes, especially in the gastric antrum. There may be narrowings or masses that simulate carcinoma[151] and ulcerative lesions which may perforate.[152, 153] Apparent resolution has been documented rarely.[151]

When multiple granulomas are encountered, with or without associated gross structural changes, a variety of other (usually rare) conditions of the stomach must be considered. These are displayed in Table 46–3, and most are discussed in this section on specific types of gastritis.

Crohn's Disease

Gastric involvement in Crohn's disease is usually confined to the antrum and pylorus and most commonly coexists with disease in the proximal duodenum. It had been traditionally stated that gastric involvement in Crohn's disease was very uncommon. This may hold for stenotic transmural disease. However, more recent

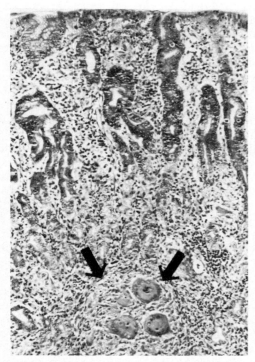

Figure 46–9. Isolated unexplained granuloma with three discrete giant cells deep in the mucosa *(arrows)*. (Hematoxylin and eosin stain, × 120.)

Table 46–3. CONDITIONS WHICH MAY BE ASSOCIATED WITH THE FINDINGS OF GASTRIC GRANULOMAS

Isolated idiopathic granulomas
  Foreign-body type
  As mass, ulcer, or in normal-appearing mucosa
Noninfectious
  Crohn's disease
  Sarcoidosis
  Chronic granulomatous disease (childhood)[209]
  Allergic granulomatosis[167]
Infectious
  Tuberculosis
  Histoplasmosis
  Parasitic

studies indicate that mucosal lesions similar to those observed elsewhere in the gastrointestinal tract are more common than was formerly appreciated.[154–157]

The gastroduodenal involvement is almost invariably accompanied by evidence of Crohn's disease elsewhere in the small intestine or colon or both. Only rarely is it the initial presentation of the disease, and one should be very cautious about making the diagnosis of Crohn's disease isolated to the stomach alone, without involvement of the more conventional sites.

Gastric involvement by Crohn's disease may be clinically silent and may be detected in the course of a general radiologic investigation of the disease. Symptoms attributed specifically to gastroduodenal involvement are peptic ulcer-like pain and symptoms of delayed gastric emptying, with early satiety, nausea, and postprandial vomiting.

Air contrast barium X-ray may suggest evidence of the mucosal changes of Crohn's disease with shallow erosions and nodularity.[156] If there is transmural disease, then the antral lumen is narrowed, often extending to the postbulbar duodenum.[156] Gastric fistulas are rare.[158] Endoscopy is less useful in defining degrees of luminal narrowing but is more sensitive in detecting the aphthoid and serpiginous erosions, ulcerations, and mucosal irregularities.[154, 157] Of course, the presence of erosions or ulcers in a patient with Crohn's disease may be due to other causes. Similarly, in patients who have gastric antral narrowing, underlying infiltrative malignancy may need to be considered.

In reported studies, biopsies of involved and immediately adjacent areas may yield the finding of mucosal granulomas in two thirds or more of patients.[154, 155, 157] In practice, when meticulous screening of multiple sections is not performed the yield is probably considerably less. Under these circumstances one has to decide whether to *suggest* Crohn's disease of the stomach based on how typical the gross findings are.

In the presence of active peptic ulcer–like symptoms and gastroduodenal Crohn's disease, an empirical trial of peptic ulcer therapy may be warranted. When there is gastroduodenal narrowing due to Crohn's disease, medical therapy, including corticosteroids, may improve the symptoms of delayed gastric emptying, but operative bypass may ultimately be required.[159] The outcome after gastrojejunostomy bypass is generally favorable.[159, 160]

Eosinophilic Gastritis

This refers to gastric involvement in the rare disorder, eosinophilic gastroenteritis, which is discussed on pages 1123 to 1131. The stomach, especially the antrum, is often involved.[150, 161, 162] All layers of the gastric wall may be involved, but there may be selective predominance of eosinophilic infiltrates in the mucosa, the muscle layers, or the subserosa.[161, 162] The clinical features that can be attributed to gastric involvement include early satiety, nausea, vomiting due to relative or absolute pyloric obstruction and signs or symptoms of anemia from chronic blood loss due to associated ulceration when there is extensive mucosal involvement.

Barium X-ray may reveal antral abnormalities with thick mucosal folds, nonspecific narrowing, or nodular defects. Biopsies of target lesions in the mucosal form of the disease will reveal evidence of eosinophilic infiltrates. In children with this disease random biopsies, even from a normal-appearing antral mucosa, may reveal eosinophilic infiltrates and thus may be useful in diagnosis.[150]

Therapy with corticosteroids is used to control symptoms in eosinophilic gastroenteritis (see pp. 1130–1131). Some patients require surgery because of persistent pyloric outlet obstruction.

In patients with peripheral eosinophilia, abdominal pain, and eosinophilic gastritis, the main condition to rule out is a parasitic infestation, especially with nematodes. The entity of *eosinophilic granuloma* is sometimes a confusing misnomer. It actually refers to *inflammatory fibroid polyps*.[163] These isolated polypoid lesions are similar to those that occur in the ileum. In the stomach they most commonly occur in the antrum.[163, 164] They originate in the submucosa and consist of variable numbers of eosinophils in a stroma of fibrous and vascular tissue.[163, 164] If they cause symptoms, it is either because of pyloric outlet obstruction or because of surface ulceration (pain and bleeding). They are *not* associated with peripheral eosinophilia and do not recur after resection. Prominent but not massive eosinophilic infiltrates in the stomach may occasionally be detected in other settings, but either they are not associated with peripheral eosinophilia or they are not chronic. These include milk-sensitive enteropathy of infancy[165] and certain connective tissue disorders.[166] The rare disorder, *allergic granulomatosis*, appears to be distinct from eosinophilic gastroenteritis.[167]

Sarcoidosis

Involvement of the gastrointestinal tract in sarcoidosis is rare, but the stomach is the most commonly affected site.[168, 169] "Silent" granulomas were found in suction biopsies from fundic gland mucosa in 6 of 60 patients with disseminated sarcoidosis.[170] Symptoms attributable to gastric involvement by sarcoidosis are variable, ranging from those of gastric outlet obstruc-

tion to upper gastrointestinal tract bleeding. Reported changes in the stomach have included a linitus plastica appearance, ulceration or erosions, and thick gastric folds. Granulomas are found in and adjacent to these lesions. However, when a granulomatous type of inflammation is detected in gastric lesions in a patient with disseminated sarcoidosis, it is essential to rule out other conditions, especially infections, before attributing the changes to sarcoidosis.

Infections

When an infectious gastritis is suspected, biopsy tissue for conventional morphologic examination alone is often insufficient. Establishment of a specific diagnosis usually requires special stains of tissue sections, culture of gastric biopsy material (especially for fungi and viruses), and mucosal smears.

The apparent increase in the numbers of cases of infectious gastritis is largely seen in immunocompromised patients, with AIDS (see pp. 1233–1257), transplantation, or cancer chemotherapy as the basis of the impaired host defense.

Phlegmonous and Emphysematous Gastritis. Fortunately, these life-threatening illnesses are rare. Most reports describe one or two cases and review the previous literature.[171–174]

Phlegmonous gastritis is a purulent bacterial inflammation of the submucosa of the stomach. Classically it results in sloughing of the overlying mucosa and extension through to the serosa. In order to accept a case as representing phlegmonous gastritis, bacteria should be seen (and possibly also cultured) in the submucosal exudate. There may be small vessel thrombosis associated with the purulent infection. At laparotomy the stomach appears dark red and distended. Pus may actually be expressed from the serosal surface. Depending upon the severity of the condition and the timing of laparotomy, perforation may have occurred, with resultant diffuse peritonitis and purulent ascites. In more than half the cases, alpha-hemolytic streptococci have been isolated, but a variety of other organisms have been detected, including anthrax.[175]

Emphysematous gastritis is even more rare and may be a variant of phlegmonous gastritis.[172, 176] It is associated with gas-forming organisms (e.g., coliform bacteria or *Clostridium welchii*), which form gas blebs in the submucosa. Emphysematous gastritis is distinct from benign collections of air in the gastric wall, so-called *gastric emphysema* and *pneumatosis cystoides intestinalis*.[177] Gas in the gastric wall might also be found as a result of an abscess associated with the extremely rare condition of *gastric actinomycosis*.[178]

A variety of predisposing clinical factors have been reported for the development of phlegmonous and emphysematous gastritis—even endoscopic polypectomy![179] There is no common thread, with the possible exception of underlying debility[173, 174] and concomitant infections elsewhere in the body. Ischemia may be important in the pathogenesis in some cases but is difficult to prove. In emphysematous gastritis the prior ingestion of corrosives or the presence of gastric malignancy may trigger the process.[177]

The typical patient presents with an acute abdomen, sometimes accompanied by hematemesis. More dramatic clues are the vomiting of frank pus or a cast of the stomach. Plain films of the abdomen, ultrasound, or CT scans may suggest a localized or diffuse thickening of the gastric wall. In the emphysematous variant, gas may be seen in the gastric wall.

Therapy should consist of vigorous antibiotic coverage for sepsis of unknown etiology, and prompt laparotomy. If only the antrum is involved, then a localized resection may suffice; otherwise total gastrectomy may be required. Death is almost inevitable with medical therapy alone. The mortality rate, even with prompt surgical therapy, is in the range of 20 per cent.

Tuberculosis. The stomach is rarely involved by tuberculosis and modern reviews of abdominal tuberculosis hardly mention it.[180] Not surprisingly, gastric tuberculosis has now been reported in AIDS.[181] The clinical manifestations attributable to gastric tuberculosis are similar to those of Crohn's disease, and the radiologic appearances may be identical, including the pyloroduodenal involvement. The specific diagnosis rests on the demonstration of caseating granulomas in biopsy tissue and on positive cultures. Acid-fast bacilli are seen only rarely in tissue sections. A positive gastric washing by itself has little significance if there is coexisting pulmonary tuberculosis. If the diagnosis of gastric or gastroduodenal tuberculosis is suspected but cannot be proved, a course of empirical antituberculous therapy may be required. Irreversible pyloroduodenal obstruction at the time of diagnosis or later in the course of healing may dictate a need for surgery.

Syphilis. Gastric syphilis is rare. The gummatous reaction of tertiary syphilis in the stomach is of historical interest. However, there are scattered case reports of gastric involvement in secondary syphilis.[182–184] The gastric involvement is characterized by thick gastric folds, commonly associated with erosions. The picture may resemble a gastric malignancy.

The proof that syphilis causes gastric lesions and symptoms rests with the demonstration of the organism in the gastric mucosa, appropriate serologic testing, and evidence that the lesions regress after therapy. *Treponema pallidum* spirochetes can be demonstrated in gastroscopic biopsy material by silver impregnation and fluorescent antibody techniques. The histologic appearance of the gastric mucosa in secondary syphilis is nonspecific, although the inflammatory infiltrate with mononuclear cells (plasma cells and lymphocytes) is more dense than one usually sees in other types of gastritis.

Fungal Infections

Candida albicans. If searched for, *Candida albicans* and to a lesser extent *Torulopsis glabrata* are commonly found in gastric ulcer or erosion beds in immunocompromised hosts.[185–188] It is somewhat surprising that, despite the great prevalence of esophageal candidiasis in AIDS, there is so little apparent gastric candidiasis in this disease (see pp. 1250 and 1256).

Candida albicans can be cultured more often than it can be found in tissue sections.[188] In the immunocompetent host with *Candida*-associated gastric ulcers or erosions it is assumed that the fungus is simply colonizing, because healing rates are not affected by the presence or absence of the organism.[187, 188]

Smears of exudates combined with cultures, and examination of biopsy specimens from ulcer edges for the presence of mycelia, establish the diagnosis. If gastric erosions or ulcers are seen in an immunocompromised host, it is worth while to look for associated fungal infection and to treat it, if present, in conjunction with therapy for peptic ulcer. The rationale would be to theoretically minimize the risk of dissemination[185] or of vascular invasion in the bed of the ulcer.[186]

Histoplasmosis. Disseminated histoplasmosis involves the stomach rarely, and when it does, the usual feature is bleeding from gastric ulcers or from erosions on giant gastric folds that are infiltrated with the granulomas of *Histoplasma capsulatum*.[189, 190] However, histologic demonstration of the organisms in tissue does not necessarily imply that the organisms are viable or that infection is active. Active infection must be proved by culture of the organism from gastric biopsy tissue.[190] The time course of the gastric lesion's response to amphotericin therapy is not clearly documented.

Mucormycosis. Mucormycosis is a disease that is produced by a member of the Phycomycetes class.[191] These fungi are widely distributed, and they become pathogenic in debilitated patients. Many of the reports of gastric involvement originate from Africa, and in some of these patients there is no underlying debility. The stomach is the most frequently affected part of the gastrointestinal tract in mucormycosis and may be unassociated with rhinocerebral involvement. The typical lesion is a perforated or deep bleeding ulcer with black indurated edges. The vessels at the ulcer base are thrombosed and contain broad nonseptate hyphae. Most cases are lethal; if the disease is recognized, partial gastrectomy offers the best hope for survival.

Viral Infections

Cytomegalovirus. Cytomegalovirus may be found in the stomach in a variety of settings: after renal and bone marrow transplantation,[192–195] in cytomegalovirus mononucleosis,[196] in childhood,[136, 137] and in AIDS.[197, 198] The diagnosis is established by finding the typical cytomegalic cells with their intranuclear inclusions (see Fig. 46–10*B*) in tissue sections and in a positive viral culture.

Cytomegalovirus infection is so common in the immunosuppressed patient that it is difficult to know in an individual patient whether an area of erosive or nonerosive gastric inflammation is due to the virus or whether the virus is simply colonizing. For example, in bone marrow transplantation the finding of cytomegalovirus in association with inflammatory change or erosions does not exclude the possibility that the inflammatory change is actually caused by *graft-versus-host disease,* chemotherapy, or the "stress state."[195] Once there is proven and rapid therapy available for cytomegalovirus, it might be possible to define the

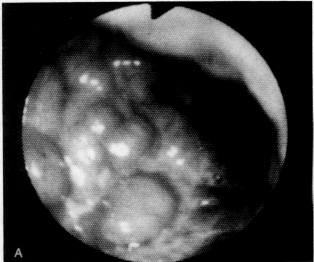

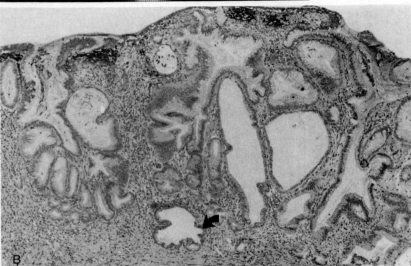

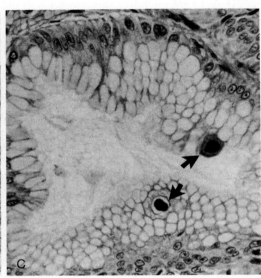

Figure 46–10. *A,* Endoscopic photo of the midbody greater curvature of a patient with AIDS and culture proven cytomegalovirus-associated gastritis. The mucosa has a thickened bumpy appearance. (From Weinstein, W. M. *In* Sivak, M. V. (ed.): Gastroenterological Endoscopy. Philadelphia, W. B. Saunders Co., 1987.) *B,* Endoscopic biopsy from the abnormal area shown in *A.* There is massive foveolar hyperplasia with tortuous cystic change and absence of fundic gland elements. The arrow points to a cystic area that is shown in higher power in *C.* (Hematoxylin and eosin stain, × 60.) *C,* High-power view of the cystic area deep in the mucosa in *B.* There are two cytomegalic cells with the typical intranuclear inclusions of cytomegalovirus *(arrows).* (Hematoxylin and eosin stain, × 300.)

potential role of cytomegalovirus as an actual cause of gastric mucosal injury versus its role as a colonizer.

There are a few reports of cytomegalovirus infection associated with striking thickening of gastric mucosal folds, in patients with AIDS, and in apparently immunocompetent children.[136, 137, 197, 198] The process seems to affect the gastric fundus and body more commonly (see Fig. 46–10). In the childhood cases the process may be reversible.[136, 137] It is reasonable to attribute such cases to cytomegalovirus infection because the pattern of inflammation is so unusual and is otherwise not explainable.

Herpes Simplex Virus. Gastric erosions associated with presumed herpesvirus in the immunocompromised host have been recognized only rarely.[195, 199]

Parasites and Nematodes. *Cryptosporidium* is hardly ever described in the stomach, and it is unclear whether its presence here accounts for any symptoms in patients with AIDS who have chronic cryptosporidiosis.[200]

Anisakiasis of the stomach is increasingly recognized, especially in Japan,[201] but there are now some cases appearing in the United States.[202] The ascaris-like larvae, which measure 2 to 3.5 cm, are acquired by eating raw or poorly cooked fish. They embed themselves in the gastric mucosa and produce severe abdominal pain which subsides within a few days. The worms can be demonstrated in the gastric mucosa with double contrast barium X-rays[203] or at endoscopy.[201] It is claimed that pain subsides within hours of endoscopic removal of the worms.[201] Otherwise, the patient will ache for a few days until the larvae die.

Strongyloides stercoralis is common in many parts of the world, including parts of the United States. In immunocompromised patients it may lead to overwhelming dissemination if it goes unrecognized.[204] It predominates in the small bowel, and the diagnosis is made by the examination of stools and duodenal aspirates. Occasionally strongyloides is found in the gastric mucosa or elsewhere in the gastric wall of immunosuppressed patients.[172, 205]

If one searches the world's literature diligently enough, it is possible to uncover isolated reports of a variety of other infestations of the stomach. These include *schistosomiasis*,[206] *Necator americanus*,[207] and even *amebiasis*.[208]

References

1. Sauerbruch, T., Schreiber, M. A., Schussler, P., and Permanetter, W. Endoscopy in the diagnosis of gastritis. Diagnostic value of endoscopic criteria in relation to histological diagnosis of gastritis. Endoscopy 16:101, 1984.
2. Moore, J. G., Alsop, W. R., Freston, J. W., and Tolman, K. G. The effect of oral potassium chloride on upper gastrointestinal mucosa in healthy subjects: Healing of lesions despite continuing treatment. Gastrointest. Endosc. 32:210, 1986.
3. Laine, L., Bentley, E., and Chandrasoma, P. The effect of oral iron therapy on the upper gastrointestinal tract: A prospective evaluation. Dig. Dis. Sci. 1988 (in press).
4. Jabbari, M., Cherry, R., Lough , J. O., Daly, D. S., Kinnear, D. G., and Goresky, C. A. Gastric antral vascular ectasia: The watermelon stomach. Gastroenterology 87:1165, 1984.
5. Nesland, A. A., and Berstad, A. Erosive prepyloric changes in persons with and without dyspepsia. Scand. J. Gastroenterol. 20:222, 1985.
6. Laine, L., and Weinstein, W. M. The histology of erosive "gastritis" in alcoholic patients: A prospective study (abstract). Gastroenterology 92:1488, 1987.
7. Redfern, J. S., Lee, E., and Feldman, M. Effects of indomethacin on gastric mucosal prostaglandins in humans. Correlation with mucosal damage. Gastroenterology 92:969, 1987.
8. Shepherd, H. A., Harvey, J., Jackson, A., and Colin-Jones, D. G. Recurrent retching with gastric mucosal prolapse: A proposed prolapse gastropathy syndrome. Dig. Dis. Sci. 29:121, 1984.
9. Cameron, A. J., and Higgins, J. A. Linear gastric erosion. A lesion associated with large diaphragmatic hernia and chronic blood loss anemia. Gastroenterology 91:338, 1986.
10. Bown, S. G., Swain, C. P., Storey, D. W., Collins, C., Matthewson, K., Salmon, P. R., and Clark, C. G. Endoscopic laser treatment of vascular anomalies of the upper gastrointestinal tract. Gut 26:1338, 1985.
11. Fleischer, D. Endoscopic therapy of upper gastrointestinal bleeding in humans. Gastroenterology 90:217, 1986.
12. Clayman, C. B., Palmer, W. L., and Kirsner, J. B. Gastric irradiation in the treatment of peptic ulcer. Gastroenterology 55:403, 1968.
13. Goldgraber, M. B., Rubin, C. E., Palmer, W. L., Dobson, R. L., and Massey, B. W. The early gastric response to irradiation, a serial biopsy study. Gastroenterology 27:1, 1954.
14. Berthrong, M., and Fajardo, L. F. Radiation injury in surgical pathology. Part II. Alimentary tract. Am. J. Surg. Pathol. 5:153, 1981.
15. Bourdages, R., Prentice, R. S. A., Beck, I. T., Dacosta, L. R., and Paloschi, G. B. Atheromatous embolization to the stomach: An unusual cause of gastrointestinal bleeding. Am. J. Dig. Dis. 21:889, 1976.
16. Shepherd, H. A., Patel, C., Bamforth, J., and Isaacson, P. Upper gastrointestinal endoscopy in systemic vasculitis presenting as an acute abdomen. Endoscopy 15:307, 1983.
17. Cherry, R. D., Jabbari, M., Goresky, C. A., Herba, M., Reich, D., and Blundell, P. E. Chronic mesenteric vascular insufficiency with gastric ulceration. Gastroenterology 91:1548, 1986.
18. Hojgaard, L., and Krag, E. Chronic ischemic gastritis reversed after revascularization operation. Gastroenterology 92:226, 1987.
19. Ihamaki, T., Varis, K., and Siurala, M. Morphological, functional and immunological state of the gastric mucosa in gastric carcinoma families: Comparison with a computer-matched family sample. Scand. J. Gastroenterol. 14:801, 1979.
20. Akdamar, K., Ertan, A., Agrawal, N. M., McMahon, F. G., and Ryan, J. Upper gastrointestinal endoscopy in normal asymptomatic volunteers. Gastrointest. Endosc. 32:78, 1986.
21. Kahn, K. L., and Greenfield, S. The efficacy of endoscopy in the evaluation of dyspepsia. A review of the literature and development of a sound strategy. J. Clin. Gastroenterol. 8:346, 1986.
22. Lambert, R., Andre, C., Moulinier, B., and Bugnon, B. Diffuse varioliform gastritis. Digestion 17:159, 1978.
23. Andre, C., Bruno, H. B. D., Moulinier, B., Andre, F., and Daniere, S. Evidence for anaphylactic reactions in peptic ulcer and varioliform gastritis. Ann. Allergy 51:325, 1983.
24. O'Brien, T. K., Saunders, D. R., and Templeton, F. E. Chronic gastric erosions and oral aphthae. Am. J. Dig. Dis. 17:447, 1972.
25. Andre, C., Gillon, J., Moulinier, B., Martin, A., and Fargier, M. C. Randomised placebo-controlled double-blind trial of two doses of sodium cromoglycate in treatment of varioliform gastritis: Comparison with cimetidine. Gut 23:348, 1982.
26. Farthing, M. J. G., Fairclough, P. D., Hegarty, J. E., Swarbrick, E. T., and Dawson, A. M. Treatment of chronic erosive gastritis with prednisolone. Gut 22:759, 1981.
27. Elta, G. H., Fawaz, K. A., Dayal, Y., McLean, A. M., Phillips, E., Bloom, S. M., Paul, R. E., and Kaplan, M. M. Chronic erosive gastritis—a recently recognized disorder. Dig. Dis. Sci. 28:7, 1983.
28. Franzin, G., Manfrini, C., Musola, R., Rodella, S., and Fratton, A. Chronic erosions of the stomach—a clinical, endoscopic and histological evaluation. Endoscopy 16:1, 1984.
29. Tatsuta, M., and Shigeru, O. Location, healing and recurrence of gastric ulcers in relation to fundal gastritis. Gastroenterology 69:897, 1975.
30. Strickland, R. G., and Mackay, I. R. A reappraisal of the nature and significance of chronic atrophic gastritis. Am. J. Dig. Dis. 18:426, 1973.
31. Weinstein, W. M., Buch, K. L., Elashoff, J., Reedy, T., Tedesco, F. J., Samloff, I. M., and Ippoliti, A. F. The histology of the stomach in symptomatic patients after gastric surgery: A model to assess selective patterns of gastric mucosal injury. Scand. J. Gastroenterol. 20(Suppl. 109):77, 1985.
32. McNulty, C. A. M., Gearty, J. C., Crump, B., Davis, M., Donovan, I. A., Melikian, V., Lister, D. M., and Wise, R. Campylobacter pyloridis and associated gastritis: Investigator blind, placebo controlled trial of bismuth salicylate and erythromycin ethylsuccinate. Br. Med. J. 293:645, 1986.
33. Weidner, N., Smith, J. G., and LaVanway, J. M. Peptic ulceration with marked epithelial atypia following hepatic arterial infusion chemotherapy. A lesion initially misinterpreted as carcinoma. Am. J. Surg. Pathol. 7:261, 1983.
34. Kimura, K. Chronological transition of the fundic-pyloric border determined by stepwise biopsy of the lesser and greater curvatures of the stomach. Gastroenterology 63:584, 1972.
35. Mingazzini, P., Carlei, F., Malchiodi-Albedi, F., Lezoche, E., Covotta, A., Speranza, V., and Polak, J. M. Endocrine cells in intestinal metaplasia of the stomach. J. Pathol. 144:171, 1984.
36. Borch, K., Renvall, H., Liedberg, G., and Andersen, B. N. Relations between circulating gastrin and endocrine cell proliferation in the atrophic gastric fundic mucosa. Scand. J. Gastroenterol. 21:357, 1986.
37. Rode, J., Dhillon, A. P., Papadaki, L., Stockbrugger, R., Thompson, R. J., Moss, E., and Cotton, P. B. Pernicious anaemia and mucosal endocrine cell proliferation of the nonantral stomach. Gut 27:789, 1986.
38. Bordi, C., Ferrari, C., D'Adda, T., Pilato, F., Carfagna, G., Bertele, A., and Missale, G. Ultrastructural characterization of fundic endocrine cell hyperplasia associated with atrophic gastritis and hypergastrinaemia. Virchows Arch. [Pathol. Anat.] 409:335, 1986.
39. Domellof, L., Eriksson, S., Helander, H. F., and Janunger, K. G. Lipid islands in the gastric mucosa after resection for benign ulcer disease. Gastroenterology 72:14, 1977.
40. Terruzzi, V., Minoli, G., Butti, G. C., and Rossini, A. Gastric lipid islands in the gastric stump and in non-operated stomach. Endoscopy 12:58, 1980.
41. Kato, Y., Sugano, H., and Rubio, C. A. Classification of intramucosal cysts of the stomach. Histopathology 7:931, 1983.
42. Arnold, R., Hulst, M. V., Neuhof, C. H., Schwarting, H., Becker, H. D., and Creutzfeldt, W. Antral gastrin-producing G-cells and somatostatin-producing D cells in different states of gastric acid secretion. Gut 23:285, 1982.
43. Lewin, K. J., Dowling, F., Wright, J. P., and Taylor, K. B. Gastric morphology and serum gastrin levels in pernicious anaemia. Gut 17:551, 1976.
44. Uibo, R. M., and Krohn, K. J. E. Demonstration of gastrin

cell autoantibodies in antral gastritis with avidin-biotin complex antibody technique. Clin. Exp. Immunol. 58:341, 1984.

45. Samloff, I. M., Varis, K., Ihamaki, T., Siurala, M., and Rotter, J. I. Relationships among serum pepsinogen I, serum pepsinogen II and gastric mucosal histology. A study in relatives of patients with pernicious anemia. Gastroenterology 83:204, 1982.
46. Krasinski, S. D., Russell, R. M., Samloff, I. M., Jacob, R. A., Dallal, G. E., McGandy, R. B., and Hartz, S. C. Fundic atrophic gastritis in an elderly population. Effect on hemoglobin and several serum nutritional indicators. J. Am. Geriatr. Soc. 34:800, 1986.
47. Haenszel, W., Correa, P., Cuello, C., Guzman, N., Burbano, L. C., Lores, H., and Munoz, J. Gastric cancer in Colombia. II. Case-control epidemiologic study of precursor lesions. J. Natl. Cancer Inst. 57:1021, 1976.
48. Kreuning, J., Bosman, F. T., Kuiper, G., Wall, A. M., and Lindeman, J. Gastric and duodenal mucosa in "healthy" individuals. J. Clin. Pathol. 31:69, 1978.
49. Cheli, R., Simon, L., Aste, H., Figus, I. A., Nicolo, G., Bajtai, A., and Puntoni, R. Atrophic gastritis and intestinal metaplasia in asymptomatic Hungarian and Italian populations. Endoscopy 12:105, 1980.
50. Siurala, M., Varis, K., and Kekki, M. New aspects of epidemiology, genetics, and dynamics of chronic gastritis. In van der Reis, L., (ed.): Frontiers in Gastrointestinal Research. Vol. 6. Basel, S. Karger, 1980, p. 148.
51. Tatsuta, M., Iishi, H., Ichii, M., Noguchi, S., Okuda, S., and Taniguchi, H. Chromoendoscopic observations on extension and development of fundal gastritis and intestinal metaplasia. Gastroenterology 88:70, 1985.
52. Ihamaki, T., Kekki, M., Sipponen, P., and Siurala, M. The sequelae and course of chronic gastritis during a 30- to 34-year bioptic follow-up study. Scand. J. Gastroenterol. 20:485, 1985.
53. Imai, T., and Murayama, H. Time trend in the prevalence of intestinal metaplasia in Japan. Cancer 52:353, 1983.
54. Warren, J. R., and Marshall, B. Unidentified curved bacilli on gastric epithelium in active chronic gastritis. Lancet 1:1273, 1983.
55. McNulty, C. A. M. Campylobacter pyloridis–associated gastritis. J. Infect. 13:107, 1986.
56. Rathbone, B. J., Wyatt, J. I., and Heatley, R. V. Campylobacter pyloridis—a new factor in peptic ulcer disease? Gut 27:635, 1986.
57. Blaser, M. J. Gastric campylobacter-like organisms, gastritis, and peptic ulcer disease. Gastroenterology 93:371, 1987.
58. Buck, G. E., Gourley, W. K., Lee, W. K., Subramanyam, K., Latimer, J. M., and DiNuzzo, A. R. Relation of Campylobacter pyloridis to gastritis and peptic ulcer. J. Infect. Dis. 153:664, 1986.
59. Romaniuk, P. J., Zoltowska, B., Trust, T. J., Lane, D. J., Olsen, G. J., Pace, N. R., and Stahl, D. A. Campylobacter pylori, the spiral bacterium associated with human gastritis, is not a true Campylobacter sp. J. Bacteriol. 169:2137, 1987.
60. Morris, A., and Nicholson, G. Ingestion of Campylobacter pyloridis causes gastritis and raised fasting gastric pH. Am J. Gastroenterol. 82:192, 1987.
61. Marshall, B. J., McGechie, D. B., Rogers, P. A., and Glancy, R. J. Pyloric Campylobacter infection and gastroduodenal disease. Med. J. Aust. 142:439, 1985.
62. Goodwin, C. S., Blincow, E. D., Warren, J. R., Waters, T. E., Sanderson, C. R., and Easton, L. Evaluation of cultural techniques for isolating Campylobacter pyloridis from endoscopic biopsies of gastric mucosa. J. Clin. Pathol. 38:1127, 1985.
63. Hazell, S. L., Lee, A., Brady, L., and Hennessy, W. Campylobacter pyloridis and gastritis: Association with intercellular spaces and adaptation to an environment of mucus as important factors in colonization of the gastric epithelium. J. Infect. Dis. 153:658, 1986.
64. Engstrand, L., Pahlson, C., Gustavsson, S., and Schwan, A. Monoclonal antibodies for rapid identification of Campylobacter pyloridis. Lancet 2:1402, 1986.
65. The Gastrointestinal Physiology Working Group. Rapid identification of pyloric Campylobacter in Peruvians with gastritis. Dig. Dis. Sci. 31:1089, 1986.
66. Morris, A., McIntyre, D., Rose, T., and Nicholson, G. Rapid diagnosis of Campylobacter pyloridis infection. Lancet 1:149, 1986.
67. Graham, D. Y., Klein, P. D., Evans, D. J., Jr., Evans, D. G., Alpert, L. C., Opekun, A. R., and Boutton, T. W. Campylobacter pylori detected noninvasively by the 13C-urea breath test. Lancet 1:1174, 1987.
68. Rathbone, B. J., Wyatt, J. I., Worsley, B. W., Shires, S. E., Trejdosiewicz, L. K., Heatley, R. V., and Losowsky, M. S. Systemic and local antibody responses to gastric Campylobacter pyloridis in non-ulcer dyspepsia. Gut 27:642, 1986.
69. Booth, L., Holdstock, G., MacBride, H., Hawtin, P., Gibson, J. R., Ireland, A., Bamforth, J., DuBoulay, C. E., Lloyd, R. S., and Pearson, A. D. Clinical importance of Campylobacter pyloridis and associated serum IgG and IgA antibody responses in patients undergoing upper gastrointestinal endoscopy. J. Clin. Pathol. 39:215, 1986.
70. Von Wulffen, H., Heesemann, J., Butzow, G. H., Loning, T., and Laufs, R. Detection of Campylobacter pyloridis in patients with antrum gastritis and peptic ulcers by culture, complement fixation test, and immunoblot. J. Clin. Microbiol. 24:716, 1986.
71. Goodwin, C. S., Blincow, E., Peterson, G., Sanderson, C., Cheng, W., Marshall, B., Warren, J. R., and McCulloch, R. Enzyme-linked immunosorbent assay for Campylobacter pyloridis: Correlation with presence of C. pyloridis in the gastric mucosa. J. Infect. Dis. 155(3):488, 1987.
72. Goodwin, C. S., Armstrong, J. A., and Marshall, B. J. Campylobacter pyloridis, gastritis, and peptic ulceration. J. Clin. Pathol. 39:353, 1986.
73. Johnston, B. J., Reed, P. I., and Ali, M. H. Campylobacter-like organisms in duodenal and antral endoscopic biopsies: Relationship to inflammation. Gut 27:1132, 1986.
74. Wyatt, J. I., Rathbone, B. J., and Heatley, R. V. Local immune response to gastric Campylobacter in non-ulcer dyspepsia. J. Clin. Pathol. 39:863, 1986.
75. Drumm, B., Sherman, P., Cutz, E., and Karmali, M. Association of Campylobacter pylori on the gastric mucosa with antral gastritis in children. N. Engl. J. Med. 316:1557, 1987.
76. Peterson, W. L., Lee, E. L., and Feldman, M. Gastric campylobacter-like organisms in healthy humans: Correlation with endoscopic appearance and mucosal histology. (Abstract.) Gastroenterology 90:1585, 1986.
77. Graham, D. Y., Klein, P. D., Opekun, A. R., Alpert, L. C., Klish, W. J., Evans, D. J., Evans, D. G., Michalaetz, P. A., Yoshimura, H. H., Adam, E., and Boutton, T. W. Epidemiology of Campylobacter pyloridis infection. Gastroenterology 92:1411(abstract), 1987.
78. Marshall, B. J. Campylobacter pyloridis and gastritis. J. Infect. Dis. 153:650, 1986.
79. Marshall, B. J., Armstrong, J. A., McGechie, D. B., and Glancy, R. J. Attempt to fulfil Koch's postulates for pyloric campylobacter. Med. J. Aust. 142:436, 1985.
80. Ramsey, E. J., Carey, K. V., Peterson, W. L., Jackson, J. J., Murphy, F. K., Read, N. W., Taylor, K. B., Trier, J. S., and Fordtran, J. S. Epidemic gastritis with hypochlorhydria. Gastroenterology 76:1449, 1979.
81. Gledhill, T., Leicester, R. J., Addis, B., Lightfoot, N., Barnard, J., Viney, N., Darkin, D., and Hunt, R. H. Epidemic hypochlorhydria. Br. Med. J. 290:1383, 1985.
82. Wiersinga, W. M., and Tytgat, G. N. Clinical recovery due to target parietal cell failure in a patient with Zollinger-Ellison syndrome. Gastroenterology 73:1413, 1977.
83. Tytgat, G. N. J., Rauws, E., and Langenberg, W. The role of colloidal bismuth subcitrate in gastric ulcer and gastritis. Scand. J. Gastroenterol. 21(suppl. 122):22, 1986.
84. O'Connor, H. J., Axon, A. T. R., and Dixon, M. F. Campylobacter-like organisms unusual in type A (pernicious anaemia) gastritis. Lancet 2:1091, 1984.
85. Gustavsson, S., Phillips, S. F., Malagelada, J.-R., and Rosenblatt, J. E. Assessment of Campylobacter-like organisms in the postoperative stomach, iatrogenic gastritis, and chronic gastroduodenal diseases: preliminary observations. Mayo Clin. Proc. 62:265, 1987.
86. O'Connor, H. J., Wyatt, J. I., Dixon, M. F., and Axon, A. T. R. Campylobacter-like organisms and reflux gastritis. J. Clin. Pathol. 39:531, 1986.

87. Oi, M., Oshida, K., and Sugimura, S. The location of gastric ulcer. Gastroenterology *36*:45, 1959.

88. Gear, M. W. L., Truelove, S. C., and Whitehead, R. Gastric ulcer and gastritis. Gut *12*:639, 1971.

89. Aukee, S. Gastritis and acid secretion in patients with gastric ulcers and duodenal ulcers. Scand. J. Gastroenterol. 7:567, 1972.

90. Zaterka, S., Vieira, F. E., Neves, D. P., daSilva, E. P., Carneiro-Leao, G., and Bettarello, A. Chronic gastritis and peptic ulcer. Acta Hepato-gastroenterol. *24*:381, 1977.

91. Maaroos, H. I., Salupere, V., Uibo, R., Kekki, M., and Sipponen, P. Seven-year follow-up study of chronic gastritis in gastric ulcer patients. Scand. J. Gastroenterol. *20*:198, 1985.

92. Fink, S. M., Barwick, K. W., DeLuca, V., Sanders, F. J., Kandathil, M., and McCallum, R. W. The association of histologic gastritis with gastroesophageal reflex and delayed gastric emptying. J. Clin. Gastroenterol. *6*:301, 1984.

93. Moore, S. C., Malagelada, J.-R., Shorter, R. G., and Zinsmeister, A. R. Interrelationships among gastric mucosal morphology, secretion, and motility in peptic ulcer disease. Dig. Dis. Sci. *31*:673, 1986.

94. MacDonald, W. C. Correlation of mucosal histology and aspirin intake in chronic gastric ulcer. Gastroenterology *65*:381, 1973.

95. Kekki, M., Sipponen, P., and Siurala, M. Progression of antral and body gastritis in active and healed duodenal ulcer and duodenitis. Scand. J. Gastroenterol. *19*:382, 1984.

96. Cheli, R, and Giacosa, A. Duodenal ulcer and chronic gastritis. Endoscopy *18*:125, 1986.

97. Hui, W.-M., Lam, S.-K., Ho, J., Ng, M.M.-T, Lui, I., Lai, C.-L., Lok, A.S.-F., Lau, W.-Y., Poon, G.-P., Choi, S., and Choi, T.-K. Chronic antral gastritis in duodenal ulcer. Natural history and treatment with prostaglandin E$_1$. Gastroenterology *91*:1095, 1986.

98. Kekki, M., Saukkonen, M., Sipponen, P., Varis, K., and Siurala, M. Dynamics of chronic gastritis in the remnant after partial gastrectomy for duodenal ulcer. Scand. J. Gastroenterol. *15*:509, 1980.

99. Hoare, A. M., Jones, E. L., Alexander-Williams, J., and Hawkins, C. F. Symptomatic significance of gastric mucosal changes after surgery for peptic ulcer. Gut *18*:295, 1977.

100. Saukkonen, M., Sipponen, P., Varis, K., and Siurala, M. Morphologic and dynamic behavior of the gastric mucosa after partial gastrectomy with special reference to the gastroenterostomy area. Hepatogastroenterology *27*:48, 1980.

101. Ritchie, W. P. Alkaline reflux gastritis: A critical reappraisal. Gut *25*:975, 1984.

102. Field, S. P., and Sachar, D. B. The immunology of pernicious anemia. *In* Shorter, R. G., and Kirsner, J. B. (eds.): Gastrointestinal Immunity for the Clinician. Orlando, Grune & Stratton, Inc., 1985, p. 61.

103. Leshin, M. Southwestern internal medicine conference; polyglandular autoimmune syndromes. Am. J. Med. Sci. *290*:77, 1985.

104. DeAizpurua, H. J., Coscrove, L. J., Ungar, B., and Toh, B.-H. Autoantibodies cytotoxic to gastric parietal cells in serum of patients with pernicious anemia. N. Engl. J. Med. *309*:625, 1983.

105. Jeffries, G. H., Todd, J. E., and Sleisenger, M. H. The effect of prednisolone on gastric mucosal histology, gastric secretion, and vitamin B$_{12}$ absorption in patients with pernicious anemia. J. Clin. Invest. *45*:803, 1966.

106. Varis, K., Ihamaki, T., Harkonen, M., Samloff, I. M., and Siurala, M. Gastric morphology, function and immunology in first-degree relatives of probands with pernicious anemia and controls. Scand. J. Gastroenterol. *14*:129, 1979.

107. Kekki, M., Varis, K., Pohjanpalo, H., Isokoski, M., Ihamaki, T., and Siurala, M. Course of antrum and body gastritis in pernicious anemia families. Dig. Dis. Sci. *28*:698, 1983.

108. Borch, K., Renvall, H., and Liedberg, G. Gastric endocrine cell hyperplasia and carcinoid tumors in pernicious anemia. Gastroenterology *88*:638, 1985.

109. Stockbrugger, R. W., Menon, G. G., Beilby, J. O. W., Mason, R. R., and Cotton, P. B. Gastroscopic screening in 80 patients with pernicious anaemia. Gut *24*:1141, 1983.

110. Moses, R. E., Frank, B. B., Leavitt, M., and Miller, R. The syndrome of type A chronic atrophic gastritis, pernicious anemia, and multiple gastric carcinoids. J. Clin. Gastroenterol. *8*:61, 1986.

111. Borch, K. Epidemiologic, clinicopathologic, and economic aspects of gastroscopic screening of patients with pernicious anemia. Scand. J. Gastroenterol. *21*:21, 1986.

112. Schafer, L. W., Larson, D. E., Melton, L. J., III, Higgins, J. A., and Zinsmeister, A. R. Risk of development of gastric carcinoma in patients with pernicious anemia: A population-based study in Rochester, Minnesota. Mayo Clin. Proc. *60*:444, 1985.

113. Ming, S.-C., Bajtai, A., Correa, P., Elster, K., Jarvi, O. H., Munoz, N., Negayo, T., and Stemmerman, G. N. Gastric Dysplasia. Significance and pathologic criteria. Cancer *54*:1794, 1984.

114. Imai, T., Kubo, T., and Watanabe, H. Chronic gastritis in Japanese with reference to high incidence of gastric carcinoma. J. Natl. Cancer Inst. *47*:179, 1971.

115. Stemmermann, G., Haenszel, W., and Locke, F. Epidemiologic pathology of gastric ulcer and gastric carcinoma among Japanese in Hawaii. J. Natl. Cancer Inst. *58*:13, 1977.

116. Sipponen, P., Kekki, M., Haapakoski, J., Ihamaki, T., and Siurala, M. Gastric cancer risk in chronic atrophic gastritis: Statistical calculations of cross-sectional data. Int. J. Cancer *35*:173, 1985.

117. MacDonald, W. C. Clinical and pathologic features of adenocarcinoma of the gastric cardia. Cancer *29*:724, 1972.

118. Antonioli, D. A., and Goldman, H. Changes in the location and type of gastric adenocarcinoma. Cancer *50*:775, 1982.

119. Sipponen, P., Kekki, M., and Siurala, M. Atrophic chronic gastritis and intestinal metaplasia in gastric carcinoma. Comparison with a representative population sample. Cancer *52*:1062, 1983.

120. Ectors, N., and Dixon, M. F. The prognostic value of sulphomucin positive intestinal metaplasia in the development of gastric cancer. Histopathology *10*:1271, 1986.

121. Silva, SA., and Filipe, M. I. Intestinal metaplasia and its variants in the gastric mucosa of Portuguese subjects: A comparative analysis of biopsy and gastrectomy material. Hum. Pathol. *17*:988,1986.

122. Bonney, G. E., Elston, R. C., Correa, P., Haenszel, W., Zavala, D. E., Zarama, G., Collazos, T., and Cuello, C. Genetic etiology of gastric carcinoma: I. Chronic atrophic gastritis. Genet. Epidemiol. *3*:213, 1986.

123. Schafer, L. W., Larson, D. E., Melton, L. J., Higgins, J. A., and Ilstrup, D. M. The risk of gastric carcinoma after surgical treatment for benign ulcer disease. A population-based study in Olmsted County, Minnesota. N. Engl. J. Med. *309*:1210, 1983.

124. Offerhaus, G. J. A., Huibregtse, K., DeBoer, J., Verhoeven, T., Van Olffen, G. H., van de Stadt, J., and Tytgat, G. N. The operated stomach: A premalignant condition. A prospective endoscopic follow-up study. Scand. J. Gastroenterol. *19*:521, 1984.

125. Sonnenberg, A. Endoscopic screening for gastric stump cancer—Would it be beneficial? A hypothetical cohort study. Gastroenterology *87*:489, 1984.

126. Caygill, C. P. J., Hill, M. J., Kirkham, J. S., and Northfield, T. C. Mortality from gastric cancer following gastric surgery for peptic ulcer. Lancet *1*:929, 1986.

127. Svendsen, J. H., Dahl, C., Svendsen, L. B., and Christiansen, P. M. Gastric cancer risk in achlorhydric patients. A long-term follow-up study. Scand. J. Gastroenterol. *21*:16, 1986.

128. Volpicelli, N. A., Yardley, J. H., and Hendrix, T. R. The association of heartburn with gastritis. Dig. Dis. Sci. *22*:333, 1977.

129. Gillberg, R., Kastrup, W., Mobacken, H., Stockbrugger, R., and Ahren, C. Gastric morphology and function in dermatitis herpetiformis and in coeliac disease. Scand. J. Gastroenterol. *20*:133, 1985.

130. Appelman, H. D. Localized and extensive expansions of the gastric mucosa: Mucosal polyps and giant folds. *In* Appelman, H. D. (ed.): Pathology of the Esophagus, Stomach, and Duodenum. Contemporary Issues in Surgical Pathology. 4th ed. New York, Churchill Livingstone, 1984, p. 79.

131. Kelly, D. G., Miller, L. J., Malagelada, J.-R., Huizenga, K. A., and Markowitz, H. Giant hypertrophic gastropathy (Menetrier's disease): Pharmacologic effects on protein leakage and mucosal ultrastructure. Gastroenterology 83:581, 1982.

132. Miura, S., Asakura, H., and Tsuchiya, M. Lymphatic abnormalities in protein-losing gastrophy, especially in Menetrier's disease. Angiology 32:345, 1981.

133. Scharschmidt, B. F. The natural history of hypertropic gastropathy (Menetrier's disease). Report of a case with 16 year follow-up and review of 120 cases from the literature. Am. J. Med. 63: 644, 1977.

134. Searcy, R. M., and Malagelada, J.-R. Menetrier's disease and idiopathic hypertrophic gastropathy. Ann. Intern. Med. 100:565, 1984.

135. Knight, J. A., Matlak, M. E., and Condon, V. R. Menetrier's disease in children: Report of a case and review of the pediatric literature. Pediat. Pathol. 1:179, 1983.

136. Coad, N. A. G., and Shah, K. J. Menetrier's disease in childhood associated with cytomegalovirus infection: A case report and review of the literature. Br. J. Radiol. 59:615, 1986.

137. Marks, M. P., Lanza, M. V., Kahlstrom, E. J., Mikity, V., Marks, S. C., and Kvalstad, R. P. Pediatric hypertrophic gastropathy. Am. J. Roentgenol. 147:1031, 1986.

138. Fegan, C., Sunter, J. P., and Miller, I. A. Menetrier's disease complicated by development of the Zollinger-Ellison syndrome. Br. J. Surg. 72:929, 1985.

139. Overholt, B. F., and Jeffries, G. H. Hypertrophic, hypersecretory protein-losing gastropathy. Gastroenterology 58:80, 1970.

140. Daniel, E. S., Ludwig, S. L., Lewin, K. J., Ruprecht, R. M., Rajacich, G. M., and Schawbe, A. D. The Cronkhite-Canada syndrome. An analysis of clinical and pathologic features and therapy. Medicine 61:293, 1982.

141. Berenson, M. M., Sannella, J., and Freston, J. W. Menetrier's disease. Serial morphological, secretory and serological observations. Gastroenterology 70:257, 1976.

142. Stamp, G. W. H., Palmer, K., and Misiewicz, J. J. Antral hypertrophic gastritis: A rare cause of iron deficiency. J. Clin. Pathol. 38:390, 1985.

143. Kondo, M., Ikezaki, M., Kato, H., and Masuda, M. Antifibrinolytic therapy of giant hypertrophic gastritis (Menetrier's disease). Scand. J. Gastroenterol. 13:851, 1978.

144. Wood, G. M., Bates, C., Brown, R. C., and Losowsky, M. S. Intramucosal carcinoma of the gastric antrum complicating Menetrier's disease. J. Clin. Pathol. 36:1071, 1983.

145. Ranchod, M., Lewin, K. J., and Dorfman, R. F. Lymphoid hyperplasia of the gastrointestinal tract. A study of 26 cases and review of the literature. Am. J. Surg. Pathol. 2:383, 1978.

146. Orr, R. K., Lininger, J. R., and Lawrence, W. Gastric pseudolymphoma. A challenging clinical problem. Ann. Surg. 200:185, 1984.

147. Rubin, L. A., Little, A. H., Kolin, A., and Keystone, E. C. Lymphomatoid granulomatosis involving the gastrointestinal tract. Two case reports and a review of the literature. Gastroenterology 84:829, 1983.

148. Brooks, J. J., and Enterline, H. T. Gastric pseudolymphoma. Its three subtypes and relation to lymphoma. Cancer 51:476, 1983.

149. Eimoto, T., Futami, K., Naito, H., Takeshita, M., and Kikuchi, M. Gastric pseudolymphoma with monotypic cytoplasmic immunoglobulin. Cancer 55:788, 1985.

150. Katz, A. J., Goldman, H., and Grand, R. J. Gastric mucosal biopsy in eosinophilic (allergic) gastroenteritis. Gastroenterology 73:705, 1977.

151. Weinstock, J. V. Idiopathic isolated granulomatous gastritis. Spontaneous resolution without surgical intervention. Dig. Dis. Sci. 25:233, 1980.

152. Compton, C. C., and Von Lichtenberg, F. Necrotizing granulomatous gastritis and gastric perforation of unknown etiology: A first case report. J. Clin. Gastroenterol. 5:59, 1983.

153. Hanada, M., Takami, M., Hirata, K., and Nakajima, T. Hyalinoid giant cell gastritis. A unique gastric lesion associated with eosinophilic hyalinoid degeneration of smooth muscle. Acta Pathol. Jpn. 35:749, 1985.

154. Rutgeerts, P., Onette, E., Vantrappen, G., Geboes, K., Broeckaert, L., and Talloen, L. Crohn's disease of the stomach and duodenum: A clinical study with emphasis on the value of the endoscopy and endoscopic biopsies. Endoscopy 12:288, 1980.

155. Schmitz-Moormann, P., Malchow, H., and Pittner, P. M. Endoscopic and bioptic study of the upper gastrointestinal tract in Crohn's disease patients. Pathol. Res. Pract. 179:377, 1985.

156. Gore, R. M., and Ghahremani, G. G. Crohn's disease of the upper gastrointestinal tract. CRC Crit. Rev. Diagn. Imag. 25:305, 1985.

157. Tanaka, M., Kimura, K., Sakai, H., Yoshida, Y., and Saito, K. Long-term follow-up for minute gastroduodenal lesions in Crohn's disease. Gastrointest. Endosc. 32:206, 1986.

158. Jacobson, I. M., Schapiro, R. H., and Warshaw, A. L. Gastric and duodenal fistulas in Crohn's disease. Gastroenterology 89:1347, 1985.

159. Priebe, W. M., and Simon, J. B. Crohn's disease of the stomach with outlet obstruction: A case report and review of therapy. J. Clin. Gastroenterol. 5:441, 1983.

160. Fielding, J. F., Toye, D. K. M., Beton, D. C., and Cooke, W. T. Crohn's disease of the stomach and duodenum. Gut 11:1001, 1970.

161. Klein, N. C., Hargrove, R. L., Sleisenger, M. H., and Jeffries, G. H. Eosinophilic gastroenteritis. Medicine 49:299, 1970.

162. Cello, J. P. Eosinophilic gastroenteritis—a complex disease entity. Am. J. Med. 67:1097, 1979.

163. Johnstone, J. M., and Morson, B. C. Inflammatory fibroid polyp of the gastrointestinal tract. Histopathology 2:349, 1978.

164. Ishikura, H., Sato, F., Naka, A., Kodama, T., and Aizawa, M. Inflammatory fibroid polyp of the stomach. Acta Pathol. Jpn. 36:327, 1986.

165. Katz, A. J., Twarog, F. J., Zeiger, R. S., and Falchuk, Z. M. Milk-sensitive and eosinophilic gastroenteropathy: Similar clinical features with contrasting mechanisms and clinical course. J. Allergy Clin. Immunol. 74:72, 1984.

166. DeSchryver-Kecskemeti, K., and Clouse, R. E. A previously unrecognized subgroup of "eosinophilic gastroenteritis." Association with connective tissue disease. Am. J. Surg. Pathol. 8:171, 1984.

167. Abell, M. R., Limond, R. V., Blamey, W. E., and Martel, W. Allergic granulomatosis with massive gastric involvement. N. Engl. J. Med. 282:665, 1970.

168. Sprague, R., Harper, P., McClain, S., Trainer, T., and Beeken, W. Disseminated gastrointestinal sarcoidosis. Case report and review of the literature. Gastroenterology 87:421, 1984.

169. Chinitz, M. A., Brandt, L. J., Frank, M. S., Frager, D., and Sablay, L. Symptomatic sarcoidosis of the stomach. Dig. Dis. Sci. 30:682, 1985.

170. Palmer, E. D. Note on silent sarcoidosis of the gastric mucosa. J. Lab. Clin. Med. 52:231, 1958.

171. Miller, A. I., Smith, B., and Rogers, A. I. Phlegmonous gastritis. Gastroenterology 68:231, 1975.

172. Williford, M. E., Foster, W. L., Halvorsen, R. A., and Thompson, W. M. Emphysematous gastritis secondary to disseminated strongyloidiasis. Gastrointest. Radiol. 7:123, 1982.

173. Mittleman, R. E., and Suarez, R. V. Phlegmonous gastritis associated with the acquired immunodeficiency syndrome/pre-acquired immunodeficiency syndrome. Arch. Pathol. Lab. Med. 109:765, 1985.

174. Blei, E. D., and Abrahams, C. Diffuse phlegmonous gastroenterocolitis in a patient with an infected peritoneojugular venous shunt. Gastroenterology 84:636, 1983.

175. Dutz, W., Saidi, F., and Kohout, E. Gastric anthrax with massive ascites. Gut 11:352, 1970.

176. Gonzalez, L. L., Schowengerdt, C., Skinner, H. H., and Lynch, P. Emphysematous gastritis. Surg. Gynecol. Obstet. 116:79, 1963.

177. Kussin, S. Z., Henry, C., Navarro, C., Stenson, W., and Clain, D. J. Gas within the wall of the stomach. Report of a case and review of the literature. Dig. Dis. Sci. 27:949, 1982.

178. VanOlmen, G., Larmuseau, M. F., Geboes, K., Rutgeerts, P., Penninckx, F., and Vantrappen, G. Primary gastric actinomycosis: A case report and review of the literature. Am. J. Gastroenterol. 79:512, 1984.

179. Lifton, L. J., and Schlossberg, D. Phlegmonous gastritis after endoscopic polypectomy. Ann. Intern. Med. 97:373, 1982.

180. Palmer, K. R., Patil, D. H., Basran, G. S., Riordan, J. F., and Silk, D. B. A. Abdominal tuberculosis in urban Britain— a common disease. Gut 26:1296, 1985.

181. Brody, J. M., Deborah, K. M., Zeman, R. K., Klappenbach, R. S., Jaffe, M. H., Clark, L. R., Benjamin, S. B., and Choyke, P. L. Gastric tuberculosis: A manifestation of acquired immunodeficiency syndrome. Radiology 159:347, 1986.

182. Sachar, D. B., Klein, R. S., Swerdlow, F., Bottone, E., Khilnani, M. T., Waye, J. D., and Wisniewski, M. Erosive syphilitic gastritis: Dark-field and immunofluorescent diagnosis from biopsy specimen. Ann. Intern. Med. 80:512, 1974.

183. Butz, W. C., Watts, J. C., Rosales-Quintana, S., and Hicklin, M. D. Erosive gastritis as a manifestation of secondary syphilis. Am. J. Clin. Pathol. 63:895, 1975.

184. Morin, M. E., and Tan, A. Diffuse enlargement of gastric folds as a manifestation of secondary syphilis. Am. J. Gastroenterol. 74:170, 1980.

185. Eras, P., Goldstein, M. J., and Sherlock, P. Candida infection of the gastrointestinal tract. Medicine 51:367, 1972.

186. Peters, M., Weiner, J., and Whelan, G. Fungal infection associated with gastroduodenal ulceration: Endoscopic and pathologic appearances. Gastroenterology 78:350, 1980.

187. Gotlieb-Jensen, K., and Andersen, J. Occurrence of Candida in gastric ulcers. Significance for the healing process. Gastroenterology 85:535, 1983.

188. DiFebo, G., Miglioli, M., Calo, G., Biasco, G., Luzza, P., Gizzi, G., Cipollini, F., Rossi, A., and Barbara, L. Candida albicans infection of gastric ulcer. Frequency and correlation with medical treatment. Results of a multicenter study. Dig. Dis. Sci. 30:178, 1985.

189. Fisher, J. R., and Sanowski, R. A. Disseminated histoplasmosis producing hypertrophic gastric folds. Dig. Dis. Sci. 23:282, 1978.

190. Orchard, J. L., Luparello, F., and Brunskill, D. Malabsorption syndrome occurring in the course of disseminated histoplasmosis. Case report and review of gastrointestinal histoplasmosis. Am. J. Med. 66:331, 1979.

191. Lyon, D. T., Schubert, T. T., Mantia, A. G., and Kaplan, M. H. Phycomycosis of the gastrointestinal tract. Am. J. Gastroenterol. 72:379, 1979.

192. Strayer, D. S., Phillips, G. B., Barker, K. H., Winokur, T., and DeSchryver-Kecskemeti, K. Gastric cytomegalovirus infection in bone marrow transplant patients: An indication of generalized disease. Cancer 48:1478, 1981.

193. Franzin, G., Musola, R., and Mencarelli, R. Changes in the mucosa of the stomach and duodenum during immunosuppressive therapy after renal transplantation. Histopathology 6:439, 1982.

194. Komorowski, R. A., Cohen, E. B., Kauffman, H. M., and Adams, M. B. Gastrointestinal complications in renal transplant recipients. Am. J. Clin. Pathol. 86:161, 1986.

195. McDonald, G. B., Shulman, H. M., Sullivan, K. M., and Spencer, G. D. Intestinal and hepatic complications of human bone marrow transplantation. Part II. Gastroenterology 90:770, 1986.

196. Campbell, D. A., Piercy, J. R. A., Shnitka, T. K., Goldsand, G., Devine, R. D. O., and Weinstein, W. M. Cytomegalovirus-associated gastric ulcer. Gastroenterology 72:533, 1977.

197. Balthazar, E. J., Megibow, A. J., and Hulnick, D. H. Cytomegalovirus esophagitis and gastritis in AIDS. Am. J. Roentgenol. 114:1201, 1985.

198. Elta, G., Turnage, R., Eckhauser, F. E., Agha, F., and Ross, S. A submucosal antral mass caused by cytomegalovirus infection in a patient with acquired immunodeficiency syndrome. Am. J. Gastroenterol. 81:714, 1986.

199. Howiler, W., and Goldberg, H. I. Gastroesophageal involvement in herpes simplex. Gastroenterology 70:775, 1976.

200. Garone, M. A., Winston, B. J., and Lewis, J. H. Cryptosporidiosis of the stomach. Am. J. Gastroenterol. 81:465, 1986.

201. Sugimachi, K., Inokuchi, K., Ooiwa, T., Fujino, T., and Ishii, Y. Acute gastric anisakiasis. Analysis of 178 cases. JAMA 253:1012, 1985.

202. Kliks, M. M. Anisakiasis in the western United States: Four new case reports from California. Am. J. Trop. Med. Hyg. 32:526, 1983.

203. Kusuhara, T., Watanabe, K., and Fukuda, M. Radiographic study of acute gastric anisakiasis. Gastrointest. Radiol. 9:305,1984.

204. Scowden, E. B., Schaffner, W., and Stone, W. J. Overwhelming strongyloidiasis. An unappreciated opportunistic infection. Medicine 57:527, 1978.

205. Ainley, C. C., Clark, D. G., Timothy, A. R., and Thompson, R. P. H. Strongyloides stercoralis hyperinfection associated with cimetidine in an immunosuppressed patient: Diagnosis by endoscopic biopsy. Gut 27:337, 1986.

206. Capdevielle, P., Coignard, A., LeGal, E., Boudon, A., and Delprat, J. Ulcere pre-pylorique et bilharziose gastrique. Gastroenterol. Clin. Biol. 3:153, 1979.

207. Dumont, A., Seferian, V., and Barbier, P. Endoscopic discovery and capture of Necator americanus in the stomach. Endoscopy 15:65, 1983.

208. Wongpaitoon, V., Kanjanapanjapol, S., Nithiyanant, P., and Nirapathpongporn, S. Gastric ameboma, a complication of amebic liver abscess: A case report. J. Med. Ass. Thai. 68:378, 1985.

209. Varma, V. A., Kahn, L. B., Sessions, J. T., and Lipper, S. Chronic granulomatous disease of childhood presenting as gastric outlet obstruction. Am. J. Surg. Pathol. 6:673, 1982.

210. Weinstein, W. Gastritis and inflammatory disorders of the stomach. In Sivak, M. V. (ed.): Gastroenterologic Endoscopy. Philadelphia, W. B. Saunders Co., 1987.

47

Duodenal Ulcer and Drug Therapy

ANDREW H. SOLL

Duodenal ulcer is a break in the mucosa of the duodenum extending through the muscularis mucosae,[1] with an ulcer crater surrounded by an acute and chronic inflammatory cell infiltrate, a picture similar to that of gastric ulcer (see p. 880). Duodenal ulcer (DU) is a common disease. For 1975 it was estimated that approximately 4 million people in the United States suffered from either gastric or duodenal ulcer, with a direct cost (i.e., hospital care, physician costs, drug costs) of about 1.5 billion dollars and indirect costs (i.e., time loss from work plus loss of lifetime earnings in the event of ulcer death) of 1.7 billion dollars.[2] Therefore, peptic ulcer accounted for 10 per cent of the total medical costs for digestive diseases, which were estimated for 1975 to be 25 billion dollars.[3]

This chapter could be entitled Duodenal Ulcer Diseases, the plural reflecting the likelihood that duodenal ulcer is involved in a heterogeneous set of disorders, each resulting in a hole in the duodenal mucosa. At present, understanding of these subsets goes little beyond the recognition that they exist, but understanding remains limited about their genetics, pathophysiology, clinical presentation, and therapy. Other differences, such as apparent pathophysiologic subsets, may be more apparent than real.

EPIDEMIOLOGY

Epidemiologic studies intend to elucidate patterns of disease incidence and prevalence that may highlight causal or protective factors. Epidemiologic studies of duodenal ulcer are difficult because estimates of the occurrence of the disease depend upon the mode of detection (symptoms, X-ray, endoscopy, or autopsy), the period assessed (the disease is intermittent), and the care used to differentiate duodenal from gastric ulcer (their epidemiology differs). In the literature, incidence and prevalence often are not clearly distinguished.

Prevalence

Prevalence may be defined as the proportion of the population with a given disease at a single point in time, over a period of time, or over a lifetime. In Finland, an endoscopic survey of 358 normal subjects found a point prevalence of active duodenal ulcers of 1.4 per cent.[4] The data in the National Health Interview Survey provide an estimate for the 12-month prevalence of peptic ulcers in the United States of 1.8 per cent for males and 1.7 per cent for females in 1981[5] and 1.9 per cent for males and 2.0 per cent for females for 1984 (Dr. John Kurata, personal communication).

Several lines of evidence indicate that the lifetime prevalence of duodenal ulcer is about 10 per cent for American males and about 4 per cent for American females.[6, 7] A mail survey of Massachusetts physicians found a lifetime prevalence in males of 7.7 per cent for duodenal ulcers.[8] Lifetime prevalence in the Finnish study, estimated from the presence of either an active duodenal ulcer (1.4 per cent), a scarred duodenum, or history of ulcer surgery (4.2 per cent), was 5.9 per cent.[4] This latter figure may be an underestimation to the extent that many ulcers heal without leaving a scar or requiring an operation and because the mean patient age in this study was only 46 years old. In addition, no breakdown was provided by sex, and half the subjects in the Finnish study were females, who have a lower prevalence of duodenal ulcer than males. Although 10 per cent of the population may be affected by duodenal ulcer during their lifetime, the prevalence of active disease at a given point in time is probably in the range of 1 to 2 per cent.

Incidence

Incidence is the occurrence of new cases per population base is a given period of time. Bonnevie estimated the incidence of duodenal ulcer from the compilation of all new cases of ulcer disease occurring among 500,000 residents of Copenhagen County, Denmark, between 1963 and 1968.[9] Cases were indexed by radiographic or operative findings of an ulcer crater or a constantly deformed duodenal bulb. The yearly incidence of duodenal ulcers was 0.15 per cent in males and 0.03 per cent in females. The age-specific incidence increased almost linearly with age, reaching 0.3 per cent in males aged 75 to 79 years old. Gastric ulcers were much less frequent, with an incidence in both males and females of 0.03 per cent. These figures for duodenal ulcer are similar to an estimated annual incidence in York County, England, of 0.21 per cent in males and 0.06 per cent in females.[10] The estimated annual incidence rate of duodenal ulcers in male Massachusetts physicians over age 25 was 0.29 per cent.[8] Interview data from the National Center for Health Statistics for 1975 provide an annual incidence of peptic ulcers in the United States of 0.29 per cent.[11] The incidence of duodenal ulcer in the population attending a large Health Maintenance Organization (HMO) in the United States is much lower: 0.08 per cent for males and 0.04 per cent for females.[12] The smaller magnitude of these latter estimates may reflect factors such as the younger age and lower risk of this population attending a HMO, or a different threshold for evaluating symptoms and diagnosing duodenal ulcer. Taken together, these figures allow an estimate for the United States of 200,000 to 400,000 new cases of duodenal ulcer per year.

Trends in Incidence

Duodenal ulcer was infrequently recognized before the beginning of this century, and its occurrence increased steadily until about 1960.[7] Over the last 20 years several indirect indicators, such as rates of hospitalization, operation, and death, suggest a marked decrease in duodenal ulcer incidence in England, Eu-

rope, and the United States.[7, 13, 14] One survey in the United States, based upon a sample of hospital discharge records, showed a decline of 43 per cent in the rate of hospitalization for duodenal ulcer over the period from 1970 to 1978.[15] Since 1978, estimated rates of hospitalization for uncomplicated duodenal ulcer have continued to fall in the United States, but at an apparently reduced rate (Fig. 47–1A).[16] In England and Wales, a decline in hospital admissions for duodenal ulcer was evident in a study of discharges and death records obtained by the Hospital Inpatient Enquiry (HIPE).[17] Analysis of data from the National Disease and Therapeutic Index, a sample of office-based physicians regarding visits for different diseases, indicated a decline in visits for DU between 1958 and 1984, reflecting a probable decline in incidence.[18]

The most dramatic changes thus appear in hospitalization rates for uncomplicated duodenal ulcer, whereas hospitalization rates for DU complicated by hemorrhage or perforation has declined very little (Fig. 47–1A). While there has been a decline in hospitalization for DU, hospitalizations for both gastric and

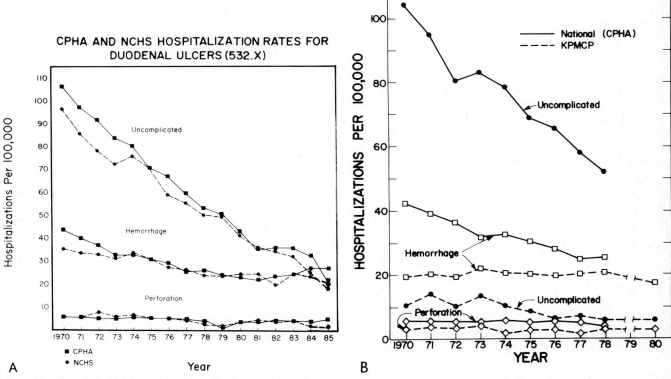

Figure 47–1. Hospitalization discharge rates for duodenal ulcer (DU). *A,* Hospitalization discharge rates for duodenal ulcer are broken down into those for uncomplicated duodenal ulcer and those for duodenal ulcer complicated by hemorrhage and perforation. Data are collected by the Commission on Professional and Hospital Activities (CPHA, closed squares) and the National Center for Health Sciences (NCHS, closed circles), as indicated. Both data bases indicate a marked decline in hospitalizations for uncomplicated DU. In contrast, hospitalizations due to perforation remained stable, and those due to hemorrhage decreased slightly until 1979 and subsequently remained stable. (From Kurata, J. H., and Corboy, E. D. Current peptic ulcer time trends: an epidemiological profile. J. Clin. Gastroenterol., in press, 1988. Used by permission.) *B,* Hospitalization discharge rates for duodenal ulcer are compared for the data from the Kaiser-Permanente Medical Care Program (KPMCP), a large health maintenance organization, and the CPHA for the years 1970 to 1980. Note the marked decline in the discharge rates for uncomplicated DU for the CPHA data, but not for KPMCP. Rates for hemorrhage and perforation for the KPMCP data remained constant over this period. (Reprinted by permission of the publisher from: Hospitalization and mortality rates for peptic ulcers: A comparison of a large health maintenance organization and United States data, by Kurata, J. H., Honda, G. D., and Frankl, H. Gastroenterology *83*[5]:1008–1016. Copyright 1982 by The American Gastroenterological Association.)

unspecified peptic ulcer have increased. The increase in gastric ulcer hospitalization is largely due to an increase in cases with hemorrhage, with both rates almost doubling.[16]

In other studies the decrease in the incidence of duodenal ulcer is less dramatic. Analysis of hospital discharge records from a large HMO in California for 1970 to 1980 revealed a rate of hospitalization for uncomplicated duodenal ulcer that was one third of the national rate, with an insignificant decline of only 19 per cent over the period surveyed (Fig. 47–1B).[19] Following age adjustment these latter rates were comparable to the data obtained from the Commission on Professional and Hospital Activities,[15] suggesting that the HMO population had a similar risk of peptic ulcer disease, as did the national population. Of interest, during this same period the rate of hospitalization for a diagnosis of gastritis and duodenitis significantly increased for the HMO population. Data based upon all hospital admissions in Hong Kong from 1970 to 1980[20] indicated an increase in peptic ulcer disease of 21 per cent over this period, with an increase in perforations of 71 per cent. The increase in perforations was largely accounted for by duodenal ulcers and increased with age in both males and females. Because the patterns differ in different studies, the trends in DU incidence remain controversial.[21–23]

Some of the variability in the data regarding trends in DU incidence reflects the age of the population under consideration. In general, the incidence of duodenal ulcer increases with age until an age of about 60 years. The declining trend in the incidence of duodenal ulcer evident in the HIPE data from England and Wales primarily reflected a decline in rates for younger men and women. In contrast, rates were stable for elderly men and increased for elderly women, a trend reflected in the rates of duodenal ulcer perforation.

There are multiple genetic and environmental factors that may influence duodenal ulcer. Susser proposed that the initial emergence of DU reflected a susceptible cohort of individuals born in the later nineteenth century; this possibility seems unlikely to explain complex current trends. Other environmental factors are probably active, with two likely candidates being cigarette smoking and NSAID (nonsteroidal anti-inflammatory drugs) consumption. Smoking is a clear risk factor for duodenal ulcer (see discussion under Risk Factors), but the increase in DU perforation rates in elderly females does not correspond to smoking trends, but rather seems to parallel an increase in prescription rates for NSAIDs. NSAID prescriptions increased from 7.6 million in 1967 to 22 million in 1985, with the greatest rates noted in elderly females.[17] Other environmental variables include changing dietary habits and stress resulting from urbanization since the turn of the century.[7, 24] The epidemiology of DU is itself complex, with patterns dependent upon the specific subpopulation being assessed and upon several environmental and genetic variables.

The controversy regarding the incidence trends for DU is partly due to difficulty encountered when conclusions are based upon indirect markers of incidence, such as hospitalization rates or mortality rates. Apparent incidence will be influenced by refinement in the diagnosis of duodenal ulcer resulting from the increasing availability of endoscopy and double contrast radiography; these techniques better discriminate duodenal ulcer from ulcer-negative dyspepsia, duodenitis, and gastric ulcer. Diagnostic and hospitalization practices have changed; increasing outpatient evaluation and treatment has an obvious impact on hospitalization rates. The efficacy of treatment may also influence hospitalization rates, as will decisions to defer surgery in favor of prolonged medical therapy. An additional factor influencing trends are the changes in the criteria and coding system for mortality and hospitalization data over the last two decades.[21] For example, the coding system for cause of death was revised in 1964 and 1965, after which ulcer disease was no longer listed as the underlying cause of death when the death certificate indicated that the ulcer was associated with a vascular, neurogenic, or other chronic condition. Another important change occurred in 1970, when a new category, "Peptic Ulcer, Unspecified," was created. Current trends in duodenal ulcer incidence are not clear; duodenal ulcer appears to be decreasing in some populations, stable in others, and increasing in some. Prospective studies will be necessary to further define these trends and provide insight into causal factors underlying the changes.

Regional Differences

There appears to be real variation in the prevalence of duodenal ulcer among certain geographic regions, although reliable data are difficult to collect. The overall prevalence of duodenal ulcers and the occurrence of perforation is higher in Scotland and, to a lesser extent, in the north of England than in the south of England.[7] The incidence in the city of York was greater than the incidence in the surrounding countryside, consistent with the view that urbanization might be an exacerbating factor.[10] In Australia, the occurrence of both duodenal and gastric ulcer was much greater in New South Wales than in Victoria, Queensland, or Western Australia.[25] Duodenal ulcer appears more common in South India than in North India and in selected regions of Africa compared to surrounding areas.[7, 26] Of interest, the ulcer disease found in India tends to occur in younger patients, with a very high male-to-female ratio (18:1) and is frequently complicated by a stenosing involvement of the duodenum but rarely by perforation and hemorrhage, suggesting different pathogenic mechanisms from those characteristic of duodenal ulcer in the Western world.[26, 27] The genetic and environmental factors underlying these possible regional differences remain unknown, although dietary factors have been hypothesized to be important in India (see below). Defining the mechanisms accounting for regional variation may greatly increase our understanding of ulcer pathogenesis.

Occupational and Social Class

Despite the belief that duodenal ulcer affects highly stressed professional and executive individuals, the available evidence suggests, if anything, that duodenal ulcer is slightly more common among unskilled laborers.[7, 10] In the United States, interview data from the National Health Survey suggest an inverse relationship between peptic ulcer and family income.[11] Duodenal ulcer has been observed more frequently among persons with a low level of educational achievement, an effect partly accounted for by a higher frequency of cigarette smoking.[28] None of these patterns are strong predictors of risk.

Racial Factors

Data from the National Center for Health Statistics indicate that crude rates for duodenal ulcer prevalence, hospitalization, and mortality are higher for whites than for nonwhites.[29] However, these crude rates oversimplify a complex situation because age-adjusted mortality rates from all causes are higher for nonwhites, leaving age adjustment inadequate to clarify the picture. Age-specific mortality rates indicate a somewhat higher mortality rate from ulcer disease in nonwhites than in whites up to the age of 65, with the reverse true at more advanced ages.[29] Even with the limitations of these data, there is little reason to suspect that race is a major risk factor for duodenal ulcer.

Sex

Duodenal ulcer is estimated to be 1.5 to 3 times more common in males than in females.[6, 9, 10] The male-to-female ratios for duodenal ulcer hospitalization and mortality rates were respectively 1.8:1 and 2.4:1 in 1970, with both ratios decreasing in 1983 to 1.3:1.[30] Whether this apparent change reflects more than the decline in the rates for men remains to be established. A true increase in incidence rates for women has been hypothesized because of changing smoking and social patterns. A recent study did find a correlation between the proportion of women who smoked and ulcer mortality rates in women (see discussion of smoking, under Risk Factors).[31]

RISK FACTORS FOR DUODENAL ULCER

Diet

Folklore has incriminated dietary indiscretion as a cause of ulcers. Although certain foods, beverages, and spices may cause dyspepsia, there are no convincing data that dietary factors cause, perpetuate, or reactivate duodenal ulcers. However, diet, particularly the content of unrefined wheat, has been hypothesized to influence the regional distribution of duodenal ulcer,

accounting for the higher incidence in the rice-eating belt in the South of India, compared with the wheat-eating areas in the North.[7, 26, 32, 33] This hypothesis was bolstered by a clinical trial in which patients with X-ray documented duodenal ulcers from the rice-eating belt in India were randomized to either a diet of unrefined wheat in the form of chapattis or to their usual rice diet. The recurrence rate on the wheat diet was 14 per cent over a five-year period, compared with 81 per cent on the rice diet.[32] In a Norwegian study duodenal ulcer recurrence rates during a six-month period were also found to be higher in patients on a low-fiber diet compared to patients on a normal or high-fiber diet.[34] The mechanisms accounting for these effects remain speculative.

Coffee is a strong stimulant of acid secretion and produces dyspepsia in many individuals. The dyspepsia may result from other actions, such as enhanced esophageal reflux.[35] Caffeine is not the important variable, for decaffeination does not reduce either effect of coffee.[36] There is little evidence that coffee is a significant risk factor for duodenal ulcer. Coffee consumption during college has been associated with a slightly increased risk of duodenal ulcers in later years,[37] whereas coffee consumption at the time of presentation was not an obvious risk factor.[28] Others found coffee consumption to be lower in duodenal ulcer patients than in control subjects,[38] probably reflecting a voluntary decrease in coffee consumption once duodenal ulcer symptoms develop. Other caffeine- and non-caffeine-containing beverages (Coca Cola, Tab, acid-neutralized coffee, 7 UP, and beer) are also potent stimulants of acid secretion, producing more than 50 per cent of the maximal acid secretory response to pentagastrin.[39] Tea is also a strong stimulant of gastric acid secretion.[40] Although some foods and beverages may be unexpectedly effective stimuli of acid secretion, there are no data to indicate that consumption of specific foods imparts an increased risk for duodenal ulcer. Although one report suggested that male college students who drank milk subsequently developed fewer peptic ulcers than their non-milk-drinking counterparts,[37] a causal relationship between either a bland diet or milk consumption and ulcer incidence is doubtful.

Alcohol

Alcohol in high concentrations damages the gastric mucosal barrier to hydrogen ion and is associated with acute gastric mucosal lesions and upper gastrointestinal bleeding. However, these acute effects do not appear to cause chronic duodenal ulcer. Previous studies have not found ethanol to be a risk factor for duodenal ulcer,[28, 37] although an association not accounted for by smoking habits has been recently reported.[41] The stimulatory effects of alcohol *per se* on acid secretion in humans are controversial, but there is no question that wine, beer, and other alcoholic beverages are acid secretagogues.[42, 43] The stimulation of acid secretion often reflects constituents other than ethanol and, in the case of wine, may involve induction of gastrin release.[43] In some studies duodenal ulcer patients consumed less ethanol than their asymptomatic counterparts, probably for the same reasons that coffee consumption is reduced.[38] In a multivariant analysis of factors predicting healing of duodenal ulcers, a moderate consumption of alcohol was found to favor healing.[44] Despite a questionable association between alcohol consumption and duodenal ulcer, cirrhosis regardless of cause appears associated with an increased risk of duodenal ulcers (see p. 832).

Drugs

Aspirin and other nonsteroidal anti-inflammatory drugs (NSAID) cause acute gastric mucosal damage (see p. 775), produce chronic gastric ulcers (see p. 885), and precipitate upper gastrointestinal bleeding (see p. 397). Determining the impact of drugs on the incidence of ulcers and bleeding is difficult, and no studies have adequately ascertained the incidence of drug-related ulcer disease.[45] With the data presently available, NSAID use has been firmly linked to the development of gastric ulcers, but the association with duodenal ulcer remains controversial.[46, 47] However, ingestion of 3.9 gm of aspirin by normal subjects for eight days did produce duodenal, as well as gastric, injury.[48] The damage was less with enteric-coated aspirin and was present only in the first portion of the duodenum, suggesting a requirement for an acidic environment. In therapeutic doses for one week, tolmetin, naproxen, and indomethacin also produced hemorrhagic lesions in the duodenum.[49] In an endoscopic study of arthritic patients taking 2.4 gm of aspirin daily, 4 per cent had duodenal ulcers and 13 per cent had duodenal erosions,[50] but these estimates may be low because individuals with symptoms or a history of peptic disease were excluded. In contrast, gastric ulcers were found in 25 per cent of a similar group of arthritis clinic patients.[51] In subjects over 65 years old, prior NSAID consumption was a relative risk factor for perforation of both gastric and duodenal ulcers.[52] Especially in elderly females, a time trend links NSAID consumption and perforation of duodenal ulcers.[17] Examining patients over 60 years old, NSAID consumption was a relative risk factor for bleeding from both duodenal and gastric ulcers.[53] Damage from NSAIDs in the duodenum is probably dose dependent, as it is in the stomach where ulcers were clearly associated with aspirin consumption on four or more days per week.[46] In addition, mucosal damage on the first day of NSAID consumption is more pronounced than after seven days of treatment, suggesting that adaptation to injury occurs in some subjects,[54] and therefore, acute damage may not predict the clinically significant sequelae of chronic ulceration. In conclusion, NSAIDs can induce acute injury to the duodenal mucosa and probably cause or exacerbate ulcers,

bleeding, and perforation, but with a relatively lower risk than that for the gastric mucosa.

The effect of corticosteroids on the risk of peptic ulcer is controversial. Although an earlier assessment of pooled data from randomized trials of steroid treatment for a variety of underlying conditions suggested an increased risk with the administration of steroids for more than 30 days or at a total dose in excess of 1 gm of prednisone,[55] this difference was not evident in a survey of more recent trials.[56] The low risk for ulcer associated with steroid treatment does not justify concomitant prophylactic therapy with antiulcer agents unless there are other specific indications.[57]

Cigarette Smoking

Several lines of evidence support an association between smoking and duodenal ulcer: (1) The available epidemiologic studies indicate that smokers are at increased risk for both duodenal and gastric ulcers and that this risk may be proportional to the amount smoked.[28, 58, 59] (2) Data from several clinical trials indicate that smoking impairs ulcer healing, promotes recurrences, and increases the risks of complications (see discussion under Therapy). (3) The death rates from ulcer disease also appear greater in patients who smoke, although it is unclear whether this apparent increase in mortality rate reflects more severe ulcer disease or the cardiac and pulmonary consequences from smoking.[58] Subsequent to gastric surgery, peptic ulcer patients who smoke experience increased mortality rates associated with smoking-related disorders.[60] (4) In both males and females, there is also a positive correlation in the time trends from 1920 to 1980 between cigarette smoking and duodenal ulcer death, further supporting a causal association between smoking and death from duodenal ulcer.[31] Although the mechanisms remain uncertain, the link between smoking and duodenal ulcer is convincing.

THE GENETICS OF DUODENAL ULCER DISEASES

An important recent advance in understanding duodenal ulcer has been the realization that it is not a single disease, but a group of disorders. Earlier workers recognized the familial aggregation of duodenal ulcer, but the patterns of inheritance were complex and interpreted as polygenic. More recently, the concept of genetic heterogeneity,[61] i.e., the existence of several discrete genetic syndromes underlying "common" duodenal ulcer, was proposed to account for the familial aggregation and the lack of a simple Mendelian pattern of inheritance. The elucidation of several rare genetic syndromes accompanied by ulcer disease, plus the recognition in family studies that several physiologic and biochemical abnormalities associated with duodenal ulcer are inherited traits, has allowed tentative discrimination of discrete subtypes of duodenal ulcer.

The elucidation of specific genetic abnormalities in duodenal ulcer may aid in sorting out pathophysiologic mechanisms: environmental, psychologic, and physiologic variables may interact differently within these separate subgroups. There may be important prognostic or therapeutic consequences of genetic or pathophysiologic heterogeneity, especially if therapy can be adapted for a specific subtype of duodenal ulcer. For example, if an operation is planned for a patient with antral G cell hyperfunction, antrectomy is a logical choice. Alternatively, in a patient with familial duodenal ulcer with rapid gastric emptying, an operation that would predispose to dumping, such as antrectomy with truncal vagotomy, should be avoided. The appropriate therapies for any subtype of duodenal ulcer will require evaluation in a controlled clinical setting.

Evidence for the Existence of Genetic Factors in Duodenal Ulcer Disease

Familial Aggregation. Twenty to 50 per cent of duodenal ulcer patients have a positive family history of duodenal ulcer, compared to 5 to 15 per cent of nonulcer subjects.[62, 63] The familial aggregation of both duodenal and gastric ulcers is distinct; the first-degree relatives of patients with duodenal ulcers had a threefold increase in the prevalence of duodenal ulcer but not of gastric ulcer. In contrast, relatives of patients with gastric ulcer had a threefold increase in the prevalence of gastric ulcer but not of duodenal ulcer.[64]

Twin Studies. The finding that concordance of peptic ulcer is more common in monozygotic than dizygotic twins indicates the existence of a genetic factor.[62, 63] Because the concordance for ulcer in monozygotic twins was less than 100 per cent, factors other than genetic must also be operative. These studies also indicated that twins shared either duodenal or gastric ulcer, further supporting the separate genetic transmission of ulcers in these two locations.[62]

Association with Blood Groups, HLA Antigens, and Secretor Status. Indirect evidence for heritable factors in ulcer disease has been sought by determining association with various genetic traits.[62, 63] Individuals with blood group O have about a 30 per cent increase in risk of duodenal ulcer, compared with individuals with blood groups A, B, or AB. Blood group O does not appear with greater frequency in patients with solitary gastric ulcers. When the presence of ABO blood group antigens in body fluids, such as saliva, is determined, individuals who are not secretors have a 50 per cent increase in risk of duodenal ulcer. Individuals with both blood group O and nonsecretor status have 150 per cent increase in risk of developing duodenal ulcers. Therefore, the risk with both genetic markers is more than additive. The association with blood group O is more of a risk factor in late- than early-onset duodenal ulcer, as noted subsequently. The pathophysiologic basis for these associations is not clear.

HLA antigens have been examined in DU patients. In one study, HLA-B5 phenotype was increased in Caucasian duodenal ucler patients compared with control subjects,[62] whereas others found an increased frequency of HLA-B12 in DU subjects.[65] It is possible that HLA antigens will be associated with DU only in selected subgroups of patients. For example, Bw35 was found in 12 of 49 duodenal ulcer patients whose onset of disease occurred above age 30, whereas none of 22 patients with onset before age 30 had this marker.[66] This type of finding further supports the hypothesis that duodenal ulcer is a heterogeneous set of disorders.

Genetic Subtypes of "Common" Duodenal Ulcer

Certain biochemical and physiologic markers have allowed discrimination of discrete genetic subtypes in "common" DU occurring in otherwise phenotypically normal individuals (Table 47–1). Duodenal ulcer may also be associated with rare, multisystem syndromes having a genetic basis, as will be discussed subsequently.

The Association of Duodenal Ulcer with Increased Serum Pepsinogen I. Two immunochemically distinct types of pepsinogen are produced by the human stomach. Pepsinogen I (PG I) is found only in chief cells and mucous neck cells in the acid-secreting fundic mucosa and has been shown to consist of five electrophoretically distinct, but immunologically indistinguishable, isoenzymes.[67] Pepsinogen II (PG II), which consists of two electrophoretically distinct isoenzymes, is present in the gastric fundus and antrum. These pepsinogens are the source of the acid protease activity of gastric juice, a potentially important aggressive factor in the pathogenesis of duodenal ulcer.[68] Pepsinogen concentrations in serum can be measured by radioimmunoassay; PG I values correlate with the maximal acid secretory capacity, indicating that there is an association between the secretory mass of parietal and chief cells. However, this correlation between serum PG I and acid secretory capacity is evident only in subjects with histologically normal gastric mucosa; with the development of gastritis, serum PG levels are altered and this relationship breaks down.[69]

Serum PG I concentrations are elevated in 30 to 50 per cent of DU patients (Fig. 47–2),[70] thus confirming earlier observations utilizing a proteolytic assay for pepsinogen.[71] Increased serum PG I is a highly signifi-

Table 47–1. SUBTYPES OF FAMILIAL DUODENAL ULCER DISEASE*

Hyperpepsinogenemia I
Antral G cell hyperfunction
Normopepsinogenemia I
Rapid gastric emp"ying
Childhood or early-onset duodenal ulcer
With postprandial hypergastrinemia
With elevated acid secretion
Combined duodenal and gastric ulcers (?)
Immunologic forms of duodenal ulcer (??)

*Adapted from Rotter.[62]

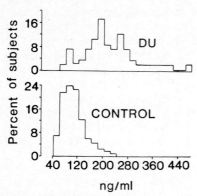

Figure 47–2. Serum pepsinogen I concentrations in normal control subjects and patients with duodenal ulcer (DU). About half of patients with DU have pepsinogen I concentrations above normal. (From Grossman, M. I. (ed.). Peptic Ulcer. A Guide for the Practicing Physician. Copyright 1981, Year Book Medical Publishers, Chicago. Reproduced with permission. Data from Samloff et al.[70])

cant risk factor for DU; a serum level of PG I above 130 μg/L imparts a threefold increase in risk for DU.[69]

Samloff and coworkers, noting a bimodal distribution of serum PG I in duodenal ulcer patients, suggested that hyperpepsinogenemia I was present in a discrete subgroup of DU patients.[70] In two large kindreds, each identified by a proband with duodenal ulcer and hyperpepsinogenemia I, hyperpepsinogenemia I was found to be inherited as an autosomal dominant trait (Fig. 47–3).[72] Hyperpepsinogenemia I was present in half of the offspring of hyperpepsinogenemic family members and in none of the offspring of normopepsinogenemic members.[72] Further evidence for autosomal dominant inheritance of hyperpepsinogenemia I in DU was provided by a study of 123 sibships of duodenal ulcer patients[73] and in another study from India.[74]

Hyperpepsinogenemia I is a marker for the ulcer diathesis. In the kindred study mentioned above, DU occurred in about 40 per cent of the family members with hyperpepsinogenemia I and in none of the nor-

mopepsinogenemic family members.[72] In the sibship study also about 40 per cent of the siblings with hyperpepsinogenemia had duodenal ulcer, whereas only seven of 57 normopepsinogenemic siblings had duodenal ulcer and three of these siblings had serum PG I values at the upper range of normal.[73] Thus, the risk of DU is increased only in the hyperpepsinogenemic I siblings. The genetic factor predisposing to ulcer disease may be acting through an increase in the parietal and chief cell mass. Acid secretion, studied in eight members of one kindred, was elevated only in the hyperpepsinogenemic siblings,[72] thus supporting a link between hyperpepsinogenemia I and elevated acid secretory capacity. The additional factors accounting for disease expression in only 40 per cent of subjects with the genetic predisposition (hyperpepsinogenemia I) remain to be defined.

Normopepsinogenemic Familial Duodenal Ulcer. Familial aggregation of duodenal ulcer also occurs in normopepsinogenemic I families. Sixteen of 85 siblings of normopepsinogenemic probands with duodenal ulcer also had ulcers.[73] PG I levels were normal in these 85 siblings, including the subgroup with DU. No pathophysiologic abnormalities nor other markers of disease predisposition were identified and thus the pattern of inheritance could not be discerned.

Familial Duodenal Ulcer Associated with Rapid Gastric Emptying. A family has been reported in which eight of 16 members in three generations had DU and rapid gastric emptying, which appeared to be related to the ulcer diathesis.[75] Several family members had symptoms consistent with postprandial hypoglycemia, and furthermore, dumping syndrome was a major problem in five family members who underwent ulcer surgery. Gastric emptying, studied using external scintigraphy following a glucose meal, was found to be rapid in three nonoperated family members with duodenal ulcers and in one of two clinically normal members. The abnormal gastric emptying pattern in this family appears to be distinct from the impaired slowing of gastric emptying by food found in ordinary duodenal

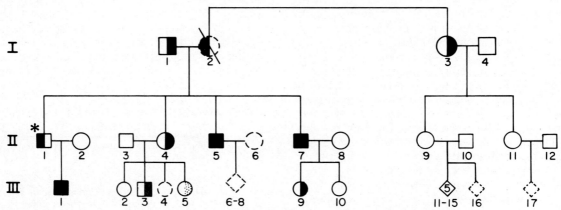

Figure 47–3. Genealogic chart for a family with hyperpepsinogenic I duodenal ulcer. Genetic transmission of hyperpepsinogenemia I is consistent with an autosomal dominant trait, with variable penetrance of duodenal ulcer. *Key:* ◐ = duodenal ulcer; ◑ = PGI (> 100 ng/ml); ○ = borderline PG I (> 90 ng/ml); □ = tested and normal; ⟨ ⟩ = not tested; * = subtotal gastrectomy; ⊠ = deceased. The numeral within the symbol denotes the number of offspring. (From Rotter, J. I., Sones, J. Q., Samloff, I. M., et al. Reprinted by permission of the New England Journal of Medicine 300:63, 1979.)

ulcer patients. Therefore, DU associated with rapid gastric emptying appears to be an unusual inherited form of the disorder.

Familial Hypergastrinemic Duodenal Ulcer. In addition to gastrinoma, hypergastrinemia in duodenal ulcer may be related to hyperfunction of antral gastrin (G) cells, a condition that may be associated with hyperplasia of antral G cells.[76, 77] Two families have been described in which antral G cell hyperfunction appeared to be an inherited basis for DU.[78] The two probands had aggressive duodenal ulcer disease, basal and postprandial hypergastrinemia, hyperpepsinogenemia I, an increased basal and maximal gastric acid output, and a normal serum gastrin response to secretin. Four of their ten first-degree relatives also had postprandial hypergastrinemia and hyperpepsinogenemia I. The pattern of inheritance of inappropriate hypergastrinemia of antral origin is variable and controversial.[77]

Childhood Duodenal Ulcer. Duodenal ulcer with the onset within the first two decades of life appears to represent another distinct familial subtype. A positive family history for duodenal ulcer occurs in about 50 per cent of early-onset DU patients, compared to about 20 per cent of patients with an onset beginning with the fourth decade.[62, 79] Further evidence for the genetic separation of early-onset duodenal ulcer is that this group has more hypersecretory subjects than does the late-onset group. In contrast, blood group O is associated with late- but not early-onset DU.[79] It is not known whether the relatives of childhood duodenal ulcer patients also have an early onset of their disease, which, if observed, would support the independent segregation and distinct genetic nature of childhood duodenal ulcer.

Combined Gastric and Duodenal Ulcer. The interrelationship between gastric and duodenal ulcers is complex. Gastric ulcers (GU) can be divided into three types: ulcers occurring in the body of the stomach (corpus or primary proximal gastric ulcers), ulcers occurring in the prepyloric region (within 3 cm of the pylorus), and ulcers occurring in a patient with duodenal ulcer.[80] Primary proximal gastric ulcers are genetically and pathophysiologically distinct from duodenal ulcers, with one clear difference being gastric hyposecretion in GU.[80, 81] In contrast, prepyloric ulcers are associated with normal or even increased acid secretion and are genetically and pathophysiologically distinct from primary proximal GU. Patients with prepyloric ulcers and with duodenal ulcers appear indistinguishable.

The occurrence of duodenal and gastric ulcers in the same patient may represent an entity distinct from either primary proximal gastric ulcer or duodenal ulcer. Acid secretion is not decreased in combined duodenal and gastric ulcer, as it is with primary proximal gastric ulcers.[81] Combined gastric and duodenal ulcer is segregated in families separately from either duodenal or gastric ulcer.[64] Furthermore, duodenal and gastric ulcers occur in the same patient at rates twentyfold greater than expected from their incidence as single

entities.[32] One additional distinguishing feature is that gastric ulcers occurring in combination with duodenal ulcer are more frequently located in the prepyloric region of the stomach than are gastric ulcers not associated with duodenal ulcers.[81, 82]

Immunologic Form of Duodenal Ulcer. Circumstantial evidence suggests the existence of immunologic forms of duodenal ulcer, possibly with a genetic basis. Evidence for this association is based upon reports of a high incidence of allergic disorders in children with DU, a tentative association of duodenal ulcer with certain HLA subtypes, and the finding of high titers of antibodies to IgA in some patients with duodenal ulcer.[83] Parietal cell antibodies have been detected in DU patients, and the suggestion has been made that these antibodies may activate parietal cell function, thus producing hypersecretion. A serum IgG component has been reported to be present in some hypersecretory duodenal ulcer patients, causing a delayed stimulation of acid secretion in rats.

Duodenal Ulcer Linked to Rare Genetic Syndromes (Table 47–2)

Multiple Endocrine Neoplasm Syndrome (MEN), Type I. The well-recognized MEN type I syndrome is characterized by an autosomal dominant inheritance with a high but somewhat variable penetrance expressed as pituitary, parathyroid, and pancreatic islet cell adenomas. The association with DU results from gastrin-producing islet cell tumors (see p. 909). Gastrinomas also occur sporadically, with a frequency roughly equal to that of the familial form associated with MEN type I. There is no evidence for a familial aggregation for gastrinoma other than in type I MEN.

Systemic Mastocytosis. Systemic mastocytosis is characterized by mast cell infiltration of many tissues and symptoms of flushing, maculopapular rash, pruritus, abdominal pain, and diarrhea. Duodenal ulcers occur in 30 to 40 per cent of these patients and may be associated with hypertrophy of the gastric mucosa and basal acid hypersecretion; the presentation can be reminiscent of the Zollinger-Ellison syndrome.[84] A number of families have been reported with this entity, with both dominant and recessive inheritance patterns described.[85, 86] Dominant inheritance with variable pen-

Table 47–2. RARE GENETIC SYNDROMES ASSOCIATED WITH DUODENAL ULCERS*

Multiple endocrine adenomatosis, type I†
Systemic mastocytosis†
Ulcer-tremor-nystagmus
Amyloidosis, type IV
Stiff-skin syndrome‡
Pachydermoperiostosis‡
Multiple lentigines—ulcer syndrome‡
Leukonychia-gallstone-ulcer syndrome

*Adapted from Rotter.[62]
†The sporadic forms are also likely to be associated with duodenal ulcers.
‡Association with duodenal ulcer is likely but is not firmly established.

etrance may best explain these pedigrees.[62] Histamine appears to be the chemical transmitter involved. Serum histamine levels may or may not be elevated in the setting of ulcer disease.[84] The measurement of histamine in serum is difficult, so significant elevations may not be detected. However, the histamine content of gastric mucosa in these patients is generally increased, underlining the importance to parietal cell function of histamine released within the gastric mucosa.

Tremor-Nystagmus-Ulcer Syndrome. A family has been reported with an autosomal dominant syndrome characterized by essential tremor, congenital nystagmus, a narcolepsy-like sleep disorder, and DU.[87] Seventeen family members were affected, 12 with tremor, 12 with nystagmus, and eight with duodenal ulcer, with neurologic features dominating the clinical picture. The pathophysiologic mechanisms involved in the ulcer disease are not clear; acid secretion was comparable to that generally found in duodenal ulcer patients.

Amyloidosis, Type IV. Amyloidosis may occur with a variety of genetic syndromes, in addition to its common association with plasma cell dyscrasias and chronic inflammatory and infectious disorders. Duodenal ulcer can be a feature of the genetic syndrome. In one large family nine of twelve affected members had DU.[88] The pattern of inheritance suggested an autosomal dominant trait, and the predominant clinical features were neuropathy and nephropathy due to amyloid infiltration. The ulcer disease did not appear to be a simple reflection of amyloid infiltration of the duodenal mucosa.

Other Rare Genetic Syndromes Linked to DU. Several other rare genetic syndromes also appear to be associated with DU (Table 47–2).[62] A multisystem stiff-skin syndrome, inherited on an autosomal dominant basis, is characterized by renal stones, joint enlargement, diabetes, and DU.[89] A Chinese family has been reported with four male members in two generations having pachydermoperiostosis and DU.[90] Pachydermoperiostosis is a rare autosomal dominant syndrome characterized by periosteal new bone formation, digital clubbing, thickened oily skin, and coarse facial features. DU has also been linked to an autosomal dominant syndrome characterized by multiple lentigines, café-au-lait spots, hypertelorism, myopia, and non-insulin-dependent diabetes mellitus.[91] In two families, DU appeared associated with hereditary white nails (hereditary leukonychia totalis) and gallstones in an autosomal dominant pattern.[92]

PSYCHOLOGIC ASPECTS OF DUODENAL ULCER

The importance of psychodynamic factors in the genesis of duodenal ulcer remains controversial despite decades of investigation.[93, 94] Study of the psychodynamic aspects of ulcer disease is hampered by several factors, including difficulty in defining the incidence of ulcer disease and its recurrences. Adequate blinding is difficult because many patients and investigators have started with the notion that ulcers are related to psychologic factors. Adequate sampling of ulcer populations and control groups generally has not been done. Furthermore, because many distinct pathogenetic mechanisms appear operative, it is possible that psychodynamic factors are of major importance only in a subset of DU patients. An early hypothesis was that duodenal ulcer reflected pure behavioral patterns or psychologic conflict. However, the associated psychologic variables in DU are more complex, and delineation requires factoring in the patient's individual defense mechanisms, anxieties, and responses to extrinsic stress.

Psychologic Conflict and Personality Type

Alexander[95] championed the classic psychosomatic theory that there exists a specific "ulcer" personality, characterized by an exaggerated dependency-independency conflict. The conflict remains unconscious and the dependency needs, which are deep-seated wishes to be loved and cared for, induce in the adult a sense of shame and lessened self-confidence. As a defense against an awareness of this dependency, ulcer patients may display exaggerated self-sufficiency, driving ambition, or aggressiveness. A prospective study by Weiner and coworkers[96] provided evidence that personality conflicts predispose to DU. Two thousand army recruits were screened for serum pepsinogen and two groups were selected: 63 "hypersecretors" with values greater than 1 SD from the mean and 57 "hyposecretors" with values more than 1 SD below the mean. Upper gastrointestinal X-rays were performed before the start of basic training, along with a prospective psychologic examination by three investigators who had no knowledge of the medical status of the recruits. The degree of dependency and the conflicts surrounding this dependency need were assessed. Predictions regarding the likelihood of duodenal ulcer were made on the basis of a high degree of dependency need, and ten recruits were selected. Nine of these ten recruits selected by their dependency profile were pepsinogen hypersecretors; four of these subjects had duodenal ulcers at the outset of the study, and three others developed active ulcers during basic training. These studies suggest that the hypersecretion of acid or pepsin combined with abnormal psychodynamic factors may predispose to duodenal ulcer in some patients.

Others reject the view that a dependent personality has specificity for ulcer disease, proposing instead the association of DU with other personality traits or conflicts.[94, 97] Certain traits more commonly describe peptic ulcer patients than control subjects, including hypochondriasis, lowered ego strength, and excessive dependency.[98] Multivariate analysis assessing dependency, anxiety, and neurotic tendencies discriminated three subgroups among 79 DU patients, with 32 patients predominantly anxious and dependent, 31 patients anxious and neurotic, and 16 patients displaying a balanced personality with good ego strength.[99] Independently validating such subgroups is difficult, but deserves further effort.

The Role of Stress in the Genesis of Duodenal Ulcer

Rats subjected to cold and restraint conditions develop acute gastric erosions but not duodenal lesions. Monkeys obligated to avoid electric shock have been reported to develop duodenal ulcers, although not consistently.[94] In experimental models stress is difficult to define as a causal factor for duodenal ulcer.

Both patients and physicians believe that peptic ulcer disease can exacerbate during or after stressful life events. Occupational, educational, or financial problems or family illness may precede the development or recurrence of duodenal ulcer, suggesting a causal association.[100] During the blitz of London in the fall of 1941, an increased number of perforated peptic ulcers occurred.[101] Such observations suggest that stress is causally related to ulcer disease, but establishing this point has been difficult because the definition and quantification of stress itself is problematic.[102] A survey of air traffic controllers, who work in an environment with obvious stress, revealed a frequent complaint of dyspepsia, but the incidence of duodenal ulcers was not obviously increased.[103] The number of stressful life events and their associated distress scores failed to differentiate 74 duodenal ulcer patients from age-matched control subjects.[104] The important variable is probably not the intensity of external stress, but rather the individual's interpretations and reactions to the stress, and few studies have adequately assessed the individual's cognitive appraisal and response to the stressful events in relation to personality patterns and defenses.[103] Although rigorous studies are lacking, some duodenal ulcer patients appear markedly affected by stressful life events, reacting with excess anxiety, frustration, and hostility and perceiving life events more negatively than control subjects.[93, 94, 98] It is likely that these psychologic factors impact negatively on ulcer disease, at least in a subset of patients.

Mechanisms Potentially Linking Psychologic Factors to Ulcer Disease

Emotional factors influence gastric function, as Beaumont observed through the gastric fistula of his patient Alexis St. Martin. Anxiety, resentment, guilt, and feelings of humiliation may alter acid secretion, although there is disagreement whether specific emotions produce selected changes.[94] Vagotomy blocks these effects. Both healthy individuals and patients with duodenal ulcer show these responses, so they are not specific for ulcer disease. A patient's psychic state may not only alter basal acid secretion, but also may alter the sensitivity of parietal cells to exogenous stimulation. In an 18-month-old child with gastric fistula,[105] histamine increased acid secretion when the patient was active and interacting with others, but not when she was depressed and withdrawn. Variation in

both basal and maximal acid secretion has been found in a few subjects that appears associated with stressful life events.[100]

Although most attention has been focused on the study of acid secretion, emotional factors may also affect pepsin and mucus secretion and alter mucosal blood flow and gastric motility.[94] Psychodynamic factors have been hypothesized to produce erosions and ulceration not only through increases in acid secretion, but also through impairment of mucosal defense,[93, 94] but these speculations remain untested. Although no firm conclusions can be reached, psychodynamic predisposition and psychic conflict (Fig. 47–4*A*), coupled with enhanced susceptibility to stressful life events (Fig. 47–4*C*), may underlie or exacerbate duodenal ulcer in some patients. These factors may act through an increase in acid secretion or an impairment in mucosal defense (Fig. 47–4*B*); however, duodenal ulcers will only occur in those patients with an adequate parietal cell mass to support an acid-peptic process (Fig. 47–4*D*). As distinct genetic and pathophysiologic mechanisms are characterized for subsets of DU patients, blinded and objective clinical studies may begin to sort out basic questions regarding the psychophysiologic aspects of duodenal ulcer.

PATHOGENESIS AND PATHOPHYSIOLOGY OF DUODENAL ULCER

Duodenal ulcers are dependent upon acid and peptic activity; occurrence is rare in persons who secrete less than 10 mEq of acid per hour, and healing of duodenal

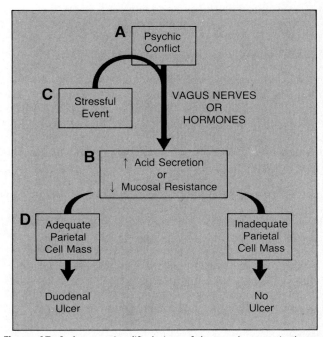

Figure 47–4. An oversimplified view of the psychosomatic theory of duodenal ulcer. The psychic conflict (*A*), amplified by a stressful life event (*C*), mediates an alteration of acid secretion or mucosal resistance (*B*) to produce duodenal ulcer in patients who have an adequate parietal cell mass (*D*). (From Fordtran, J. S. Pract. Gastroenterol. 3:24, 1979. Used by permission.)

ulcers is enhanced by agents that inhibit acid secretion. Thus, acid is an essential permissive factor for duodenal ulcer. However, hypersecretion of acid occurs in only a small proportion of DU patients. Mucosal resistance to injury is also a major variable, as underlined by the occasional gastrinoma patient who remains ulcer-free despite extreme hypersecretion of acid and pepsin. On the other hand, duodenal ulcers can develop in the setting of normal acid secretion or persist during effective therapeutic inhibition of acid secretion; their occurrence may thus also reflect a breakdown in the resistance of the mucosa to normal concentrations of acid and pepsin or a breakdown in the mechanisms that are continually called upon to repair superficial injury.

Attempts to establish a single pathophysiologic mechanism in duodenal ulcer have been unsuccessful because the pathogenesis does not reflect a single process; rather, duodenal ulcer appears to be a set of diseases, all expressed by a hole in the duodenal mucosa. Many abnormalities have been found in DU patients, but none has reliably discriminated duodenal ulcer patients from normal persons. In family studies, it has been possible to associate markers, such as hyperpepsinogenemia I, with a predisposition to duodenal ulcer. However, only 40 per cent of family members with this dominant trait develop ulcers, and 60 per cent remain ulcer-free.[72, 73] The factors that cause the expression of ulcer disease in some hyperpepsinogenemic family members, but not in others, are unknown, but may include environmental risks such as smoking or drugs, mucosal inflammation or infection, or psychodynamic factors. Male sex confers an increased risk in the hyperpepsinogenemic I families, as in duodenal ulcer in general.

Despite the fact that duodenal ulcer is an intermittent, recurring disease, the pathophysiology is often approached as if a constant abnormality will be present. However, acid secretion or mucosal resistance to injury may vary over time and may be abnormal only at times when the patient is predisposed to ulcer formation. In one study acid secretory rates were found to be higher in patients with active ulcers than in patients with ulcers inactive for three months;[106] however, individual patients were not evaluated longitudinally so that the findings are difficult to interpret. In another study basal acid secretion was measured periodically in DU patients. Basal secretion was variable but was found to be greater during the first episode of duodenal ulcer than subsequently and showed no correlation with ulcer recurrence.[107]

The pathophysiologic abnormalities hypothesized to cause duodenal ulcer are complex and inadequately defined to allow a simple discussion. The following arbitrary division (Table 47–3) has been offered in the absence of any firm basis for formulating subgroups.

Increased Acid and Peptic Secretory Mass

Gastric acid secretion in response to stimulation with pentagastrin, gastrin, histamine, betazole, or caffeine

Table 47–3. PROPOSED PATHOPHYSIOLOGIC ABNORMALITIES IN DUODENAL ULCER

Pathophysiologic Abnormality	Manifestation or Marker	Proposed mechanisms or Subsets[a]

↑ Parietal cell and chief cell mass	↑ MAO[ab]
	 ↑ Serum pepsinogen I[b]
		Gastrinoma
		   Sporadic
		   MEN, type I
		 Antral G cell hyperfunction[c]
		 Systemic mastocytosis
		   Sporadic
		   Familial
		 Basophilic leukemia
		 Familial hyperpepsinogenemia I DU[d]
		 Familial, early-onset, hypersecretory DU[d]

↑ Basal secretory drive	↑ BAO/ MAO	Gastrinoma Antral G cell hyperfunction with basal hypergastrinemia Systemic mastocytosis Short bowel syndrome Retained antrum ↑ Vagal tone (?) ↓ Inhibitory pathway (??)
↑ Postprandial secretory drive	Postprandial hypergastrenemia ↓ Acid inhibition of postprandial gastrin response ↑ Parietal cell sensitivity to gastrin ↑ Vagal responsiveness to food	Antral G cell hyperfunction
Rapid gastric emptying	↑ Duodenal acidification	Familial Sporadic
Impaired mucosal defense	*C. pylori* infection or duodenitis ↓ or altered mucus secretion ↓ Bicarbonate secretion ↓ Prostaglandin synthesis ↓ Blood flow ↓ Mucosal cell turnover or restitution	Associated gastroduodenitis Alpha₂-antitrypsin deficiency (??) Familial normopepsinogenemic duodenal ulcer (??) Nonsteroidal anti-inflammatory agents or cigarette smoking

[a]Many other subsets probably exist, such as deranged stimulatory or inhibitory pathways influencing basal or postprandial acid secretion, although these remain to be identified.
[b]These abnormalities are generally associated, but in an undefined fashion.
[c]Most cases of antral G cell hyperfunction do not have an increase in secretory mass, which appears more likely when serum gastrin level is elevated in the basal state.
[d]These may represent the same or very similar disorders.

is on the average greater in DU patients than in normal subjects, but considerable overlap exists (Fig. 47–5).[108–110] Basal and nocturnal acid secretion are also increased in a proportion of DU patients.[111, 112] Twenty-four-hour acid secretion can also be increased in DU (Fig. 47–6), probably more as a result of increased interdigestive

Figure 47–5. Maximal acid output in response to intravenous infusion of histamine acid phosphate at a dose of 40 μg per kg of body weight per hour in 54 normal men and 237 men with duodenal ulcer. Median value in millimoles per hour is significantly greater in duodenal ulcer patients (40) than in normal subjects (25). However, the overlap is considerable, and about 70 per cent of duodenal ulcer patients fall within the normal range. (Data have been redrawn from Kirkpatrick, J. R., Lawrie, J. H., Forrest, A. P. M., et al. Gut *10*:760, 1969. Used by permission.)

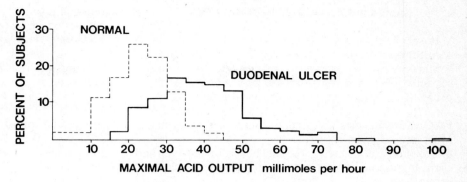

and nocturnal secretion than of increased food-stimulated secretion.[112]

The maximal capacity of the stomach to secrete acid (maximal acid output, or MAO; see p. 718) is a function of total parietal cell mass,[109, 113] and this mass is 1.5 to 2 times greater in DU patients than in control subjects (Fig. 47–7). However, the values for normal subjects and DU patients overlap, and only between 20 and 50 per cent of DU patients hypersecrete acid.[114] Some of this variation may be accounted for by the specific population that is being studied.[109] Roughly one third of DU patients also have hyperpepsinogenemia I (Fig. 47–2),[70] and the patients with acid hypersecretion and hyperpepsinogenemia I probably represent the same overall group. Some DU patients with hypersecretion have inherited the abnormality as part of familial hyperpepsinogenemia I,[72, 73] but the proportion accounted for by such patients has not been established. In both Chinese and Scottish patients, acid hypersecretion was more common when the onset of DU occurred before age 30, but no clear familial basis was identified in these early-onset patients.[79]

Little is known about the potential humoral, neural, or mucosal trophic factors that maintain the fundic mucosal mass in normal subjects or that increase it in some patients with DU. Gastrin does have a trophic effect on the fundic mucosa under certain experimental conditions.[115] In patients with the Zollinger-Ellison syndrome the sustained increase in circulating gastrin is probably the trophic factor accounting for the increase in the secretory mass. Histamine has not been demonstrated to have a trophic effect on the fundic mucosa. However, hypersecretion of acid and a presumed increased secretory mass occur in two diseases linked to proliferation of histamine-containing cells: systemic mastocytosis[84] and myeloproliferative disorders such as chronic granulocytic leukemia.[116, 117]

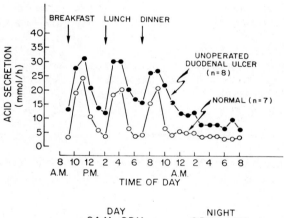

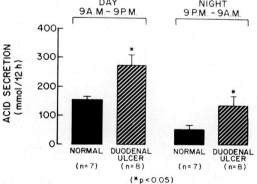

Figure 47–6. Mean hourly gastric acid secretion during a 24-hour period in eight unoperated DU patients and in seven normal subjects. *Top,* Meals were infused into the stomach as indicated. In these subjects duodenal ulcer patients had a higher basal output and higher nocturnal output, but the relative response to a meal was not markedly increased. *Bottom,* Mean acid secretion during the day and night hours is illustrated, with statistical differences shown by the asterisks (p < 0.05). (From Feldman, M., and Richardson, C. T. Gastroenterology *90*:540, 1986. Used with permission.) (Reprinted by permission of the publisher from: Gastric secretion and emptying after ordinary meals in duodenal ulcer, by Malagelada, J-R., Longstreth, G. F., Deering, T. B., et al. Gastroenterology *73*(5):989–994. Copyright 1977 by The American Gastroenterological Association.)

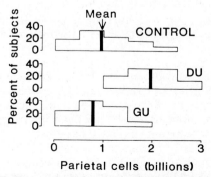

Figure 47–7. The number of parietal cells in stomachs of patients with duodenal ulcer (DU) and gastric ulcer (GU) and in normal subjects. Note that patients with DU have a higher number of parietal cells than normal, but there is marked overlap with the normal range. (Data redrawn from Cox, A. J. Arch. Pathol. *54*:407, 1952. Used by permission.)

Increased Basal Acid Secretory Drive

Basal acid output (BAO) varies with total acid secretory capacity, and therefore may be increased in subjects with an increased maximal acid secretory capacity. Determining the ratio of BAO to MAO or peak acid output (PAO) adjusts for the effect of variable parietal cell number, and an elevated BAO/PAO ratio suggests an increased basal secretory drive. Most investigators consider a BAO/PAO ratio above 0.3 to indicate an increased basal secretory drive, and such increased ratios have been found in a small proportion of DU patients.[109, 110, 118, 119] Furthermore, basal output may vary over time in the same patient,[107] so that repeat studies will be necessary to confirm a persistent abnormality.

The physiology of acid secretion is complex, and the parietal cell is regulated by input from endocrine, neural, and paracrine pathways; gastrin, acetylcholine, and histamine are the primary respective chemotransmitters delivered by these pathways (see p. 716).[120] Increased activity of any of these pathways might increase basal secretory drive in DU patients. Other hypotheses for increased basal acid secretion are an increased sensitivity of the parietal cell to endogenous secretagogues and an abnormality in one of the inhibitory pathways regulating acid secretion.

In both normal persons and duodenal ulcer patients, basal acid secretion is inhibited by anticholinergic agents, indicating that the parietal cell in the basal state is under cholinergic control. Alexander, who championed the psychosomatic basis for duodenal ulcer disease, hypothesized increased vagal tone as an important pathogenic mechanism.[95] Several recent studies have supported the view that increased vagal tone underlies an increased BAO/PAO ratio in some DU patients.[118, 119, 121] Evidence for increased vagal tone includes a finding that patients with an increased BAO/PAO ratio show little additional secretory response to sham feeding, suggesting that these subjects were already under maximal vagal tone.[119, 121] Anticholinergic agents were found to cause a 95 per cent inhibition of the increased BAO, indicating that the increase in basal acid output was largely dependent upon cholinergic input.[118] The mechanisms increasing vagal tone remain unknown; the hypothesis that psychodynamic factors are involved stands without experimental support.

Basal acid output may also be increased by hypergastrinemia, with the most dramatic example being the elevated BAO/PAO ratio found in patients with gastrinoma (see pp. 909–925). A similar mechanism may operate in those unusual patients with inappropriate G-cell hyperfunction who have basal hypergastrinemia. In ordinary DU, fasting serum gastrin levels are generally normal and therefore are an unlikely cause of an increased basal secretory drive. However, some investigators have found basal serum gastrin levels to be elevated in DU patients, proposing that this factor may contribute to the increase in BAO.[110]

Basal acid secretion is markedly inhibited by histamine H_2 receptor antagonists, indicating that the parietal cell is under histamine, as well as cholinergic, tone in the basal state. Whether or not abnormalities in histamine delivery to the parietal cell occur in DU is unknown, as will be discussed subsequently.

Dragstedt reported that nocturnal acid secretion was increased in DU,[111] a finding confirmed by others.[112] The proportion of ulcer patients with abnormal nocturnal acid secretion has not been defined. Experience in the therapy of DU has established that suppression of nocturnal acid secretion is sufficient to induce healing of most duodenal ulcers (see p. 851). Nocturnal acid secretion is under diurnal control,[122] probably mediated by vagal pathways, but whether the diurnal pattern is disturbed in DU remains unknown.

Increased Postprandial Acid Secretory Response

Alterations in meal-stimulated gastric acid secretion in DU are controversial.[109, 110] Although an increase in meal-stimulated acid secretion has been found in DU subjects, these increases may be largely accounted for by the observed increased secretory mass and maximal acid output in DU.[110] A potentially important finding, if confirmed, is that the acid secretory response to a meal is prolonged in DU subjects (Fig. 47–8), with the acid secretory response thus outlasting the buffering effects of food.[110, 123]

Hypergastrinemia

The status of the gastrin and the antral gastrin cell in duodenal ulcer remains unclear, with varying reports

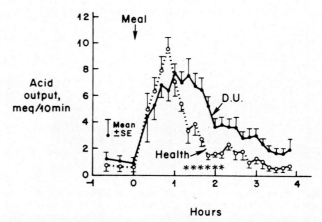

Figure 47–8. Gastric acid output after meals in patients with duodenal ulcer (DU) and normal subjects (Health). Significant differences ($p < 0.05$) are noted for 10-minute intervals (*). Hourly outputs for the second, third, and fourth hours were significantly greater in DU patients than in normal subjects ($p < 0.05$). In contrast to other studies, this figure illustrates an increased duration and total acid output in response to a meal in DU patients, rather than an increase in peak acid output (see text). (Reprinted by permission of the publisher from: Gastric secretion and emptying after ordinary meals in duodenal ulcer, by Malagelada, J-R., Longstreth, G. F., Deering, T. B., et al. Gastroenterology 73[5]:989–994. Copyright 1977 by The American Gastroenterological Association.)

of abnormalities in the number of G cells, the content and heterogeneity of gastrin, and the density of the G-cell granules, which may reflect secretory activity (see p. 94). Abnormalities in both basal- and meal-stimulated gastrin release have been found in some but not all studies,[76, 110, 124] underlining the possibility that abnormal gastrin release occurs in only a proportion of DU patients. Apart from the obvious hypergastrinemia found with gastrinomas, patients may present with increased release of antral gastrin, a syndrome labeled antral G-cell hyperfunction.[76, 77, 124] Abnormalities may vary from enhanced meal-stimulated gastrin release to basal and meal-stimulated hypergastrinemia and an increased fundic secretory mass. The hypersecretion of acid in the latter instances may resemble that found in gastrinoma patients. In some patients with G cell hyperfunction, there is an increased number of G cells in the antral mucosa.[125] As discussed previously, two families have been reported with DU associated with hypergastrinemia and increased acid secretion, indicating that G-cell hyperfunction may occur as a distinct genetic syndrome.[78] An exaggerated postprandial gastrin response has also been described in patients with early-onset duodenal ulcer and a normal maximal acid secretory capacity: a familial basis has been suggested, but not established, for this presumed subset.[126] The prevalence of G-cell hyperfunction in ordinary duodenal ulcer remains unknown; postprandial hypergastrinemia was found in about 10 per cent of DU patients in one clinic.[124] The pathophysiologic significance of this abnormality is unclear; a relation of hypergastrinemia to the magnitude and duration of the acid secretory response to a meal has not been established.

The relationship between parietal cell mass and G cell function is of particular interest because of the evidence suggesting that gastrin has a trophic effect on the fundic mucosa.[115] In patients with basal hypergastrinemia due to either gastrinoma or antral G cell hyperfunction, an increased secretory mass is often found, suggesting that the continuous increase in serum gastrin concentration is a causal factor. However, maximal acid output is generally normal in patients with postprandial hypergastrinemia and normal basal gastrin levels,[126] indicating that a transient increase in serum gastrin is not sufficient to increase the parietal cell mass beyond the normal range. However, in this same study a correlation was found between the magnitude of the meal-stimulated gastrin release and the maximal acid output,[126] suggesting that the postprandial gastrin response may be a determinant of the secretory mass but that an increase in secretory mass above the normal range is uncommon without sustained hypergastrinemia.

Increased Sensitivity to Secretagogues

An additional factor that may underlie basal or postprandial hypersecretion of acid is an enhanced sensitivity of the parietal cell to secretagogues. DU patients, or at least some DU patients, appear more sensitive to both exogenous gastrin infusion and to endogenously released gastrin than are control subjects.[127, 128] Suggested mechanisms for this greater sensitivity to gastrin in duodenal ulcer patients include enhanced vagal tone (which may influence parietal cell sensitivity to gastrin), an altered affinity of the parietal cell receptor for gastrin, and impairment of an inhibitory pathway, such as that mediated by somatostatin. These findings have been disputed by a large study of DU patients which indicated that the difference was only apparent and resulted from the relatively high basal acid output in DU male patients.[129]

Another potential mechanism underlying an acid hypersecretion in DU is an enhanced amplitude of the response to vagal stimulation. This proposed abnormality differs from the increased vagal tone that may underlie the increase in BAO found in some DU patients. An increased secretory response to sham feeding has been reported in duodenal ulcer,[130–132] although in only one of these studies was the difference not associated with an increased maximal secretory capacity.[132] An increased acid secretory response to insulin-induced hypoglycemia was also reported in a subgroup of DU patients with normal maximal acid output.[133] Abnormalities in vagal regulation of acid secretion remain theoretical, awaiting methodology to quantitate the physiologic impact of the inhibitory and stimulatory pathways. Circulating pancreatic polypeptide has been proposed as an index of vagal tone and responsiveness, but no clear pattern has emerged to clarify pathophysiologic mechanisms (see p. 88).

Impaired Inhibitory Mechanisms

A variety of stimulatory and inhibitory mechanisms utilizing paracrine, endocrine, and neurocrine pathways are undoubtedly important in modulating secretion of acid, pepsin, and gastrin (see pp. 713–734). Excessive activity of a stimulatory pathway or impaired function of an inhibitory pathway could explain the secretory abnormalities observed in DU patients. The existence of such abnormalities in DU remains largely speculative.

Impaired Acid Inhibition of Gastrin Release. It has been proposed that the enhanced gastrin release found in some DU patients may reflect impaired feedback inhibition of gastrin release by acid. Using the technique of intragastric titration, acidification of a protein meal inhibited the acid secretory and serum gastrin responses less in DU patients than in control subjects,[134] although others have not confirmed this finding.[123, 124] In one study, the serum gastrin response to intragastric amino acids was greater in DU patients than in control subjects at both pH 2.5 and 5.5. The DU group showed good inhibition at the acidic pH, and the authors concluded that these DU patients had gastrin cells with increased sensitivity to amino acids, rather than impaired acid inhibition.[124] However, the patients in this latter study were selected for marked G-cell hyperfunction, so that they may represent a distinct subgroup.

Other Inhibitory Mechanisms. There are several lines of evidence indicating that gastric distention, gastric or duodenal acidification, and infusion of fat can each activate mechanisms that inhibit acid secretion. Whether defects in such inhibitory mechanisms explain acid hypersecretion in DU remains uncertain. In the study by Cooper and coworkers, acidification of the gastric contents from pH 5.5 to 2.5 in normal subjects reduced both the gastrin and acid secretory responses to intragastric amino acids.[124] In contrast, in DU patients the gastrin—but not the acid secretory—response was inhibited as the stomach was acidified. These studies suggest a possible impairment in acid feedback inhibition of secretory function independent of gastrin release. Somatostatin is a major candidate for mediating acid feedback inhibition of gastrin release; somatostatin inhibits acid secretion both by effects on gastrin release and on the fundic mucosa. Although there is no experimental support for abnormalities in somatostatin or other inhibitory mechanisms in DU, these mechanisms deserve further investigation.

Fat inhibits acid secretion by mechanisms that remain undefined. The inhibitory effects of fat have been reported to be reduced in DU patients, but the reproducibility of this abnormality remains unknown.[135]

Depending upon the conditions, gastric distention produces both stimulatory and inhibitory effects on acid secretion. Antral distention has been reported to have reduced inhibitory effects on pentagastrin-stimulated acid secretion in DU patients, as compared to control subjects.[136]

Rapid Gastric Emptying

The rate of emptying of gastric contents both in the fasting and in the postprandial state determines the rate of delivery of acid and pepsin to the duodenum and therefore will influence duodenal pH. Rapid gastric emptying, particularly of liquid meals, has been found in DU patients,[123, 137, 138] although emptying rates overlap with the normal range and negative studies have been reported.[139] Accelerated gastric emptying may also be an inherited abnormality in rare cases of duodenal ulcer (see pp. 820–821).

In normal subjects gastric emptying is delayed by glucose, acid, and fat. Impaired acid inhibition of gastric emptying has been reported in DU patients.[137, 138] Inhibition of gastric emptying by fat and glucose may be also impaired.[138] Impaired inhibition of gastric emptying with fat, glucose, or acid in DU patients was dose-dependent, rendering differentiation with normal subjects a difficult problem.[138] The role of rapid gastric emptying in the pathogenesis of duodenal ulcer remains speculative, but decreased reservoir function of the stomach, with rapid emptying of the buffer provided by food, may increase the effective free hydrogen ion load delivered to the duodenum, especially during the late postprandial period.[123]

Peptic Activity

Despite the fact that ulcers of the stomach and duodenum are referred to as "peptic," emphasis in investigation and consideration of pathophysiology and therapy is generally focused on acid, rather than on pepsin and peptic activity. Peptic activity is closely linked to gastric pH because pepsinogen is converted to the active protease pepsin by high concentrations of hydrochloric acid, and pepsin is inactivated when the pH is increased above 4.0. The role of peptic activity in duodenal ulceration has been difficult to study because of the many isoenzymes of pepsin and because of a lack of correlation between pepsin assays *in vitro* and the ulcerogenic potential of the protease activity present in gastric juice *in vivo*.[68, 140] Acid alone is less ulcerogenic than an acid plus pepsin.[141, 142] However, secretagogue-stimulated gastric juice is more ulcerogenic than its measurable acid and pepsin components.[140, 142] Thus, either endogenous pepsins are more ulcerogenic than reflected in a comparable level of acid protease activity *in vitro*, or gastric juice contains ulcerogenic factors in addition to acid and pepsin, such as bile acids. Although there is a correlation between hyperpepsinogenemia and duodenal ulcer, this relationship also includes the hypersecretion of acid. Pepsins in DU patients have been reported to have increased activity over a wider than normal pH range.[68] The pathogenic importance of primary derangements in pepsinogen secretion or in the protease activity of the pepsin family remain to be established.

Histamine and Duodenal Ulcer

The ability of histamine H_2 receptor antagonists to markedly inhibit the acid secretory response to food, gastrin, and vagal stimuli has established the central role of histamine in the physiology of acid secretion. But, despite the obvious importance of histamine, knowledge remains limited regarding the cells that store histamine within the fundic mucosa and factors regulating histamine formation and release. One of the complicating factors in this area is the fact that histamine in the fundic mucosa is potentially stored in two cell types; mast cells and histamine-containing endocrine-like cells, the latter being called enterochromaffin-like (ECL) cells because of their silver staining properties. The proportion of these two histamine cells in the fundic mucosa appears to be highly variable among species.[120] Mast cells are prominent in the fundic mucosa of humans, but the exact make-up of the fundic mucosal histamine cell population remains uncertain. Histamine is rapidly degraded in the gastric mucosa, probably by the parietal cell and capillary endothelial cells. Especially in light of this rapid degradation, studies of histamine release into gastric juice or blood or studies inferring the pattern of histamine release from decreases in mucosal histamine content are difficult to interpret. Thus, little information exists regarding the physiology or pathophysiology of histamine release in duodenal ulcer. Several studies have found the histamine content of the fundic mucosa of duodenal ulcer patients to be about 30 per cent less than in control subjects, suggesting an abnormality in histamine release or metabolism,[143–145] which remains undefined. Some patients with systemic mastocytosis may have an increased acid secretion, and this is consistent with increased delivery of histamine to the parietal cell. Whether abnormalities in histamine release account for hypersecretion of acid in other patients with duodenal ulcer remains to be established.

Impaired Mucosal Defense

Several mechanisms are involved in the maintenance of mucosal integrity in an acid-peptic environment, including mucosal barrier function,[146] cell restitution and renewal, mucus and mucosal bicarbonate secretion, and mucosal blood flow (see pp. 772–792). The possibility of impairment of these defensive mechanisms remains largely uncharted territory in the pathophysiology of duodenal ulcer. Because many patients with DU have normal acid secretion, their predisposition to ulcer disease probably rests with defective mucosal resistance to the acid-peptic environment of the duodenum. However, despite the probable existence of defects in mucosal resistance to injury, acid-peptic activity remains an essential permissive factor in the pathogenesis of "peptic" ulcers.

Bicarbonate Secretion and Duodenal pH. Development of ulcers requires the delivery to the duodenum of acid in excess of the neutralizing capacity of bicarbonate-rich secretions from the pancreas, biliary tree, and duodenal mucosa.[147] In the duodenum, the free H^+ concentration and total acid content (including buffered H^+) in the fasting state and in response to a meal have been difficult to determine. The available evidence suggests that postprandial duodenal pH is

lower and remains lower for more prolonged periods in duodenal ulcer patients than in normal subjects, although these distributions overlap.[123] The low duodenal pH in DU patients may reflect an increase in the delivered H^+ load as a result of acid hypersecretion or an increased rate of gastric emptying. Until recently, there was no evidence for defective duodenal neutralization mechanisms; however, Isenberg and coworkers have recently developed methodology for isolating the duodenum in humans, allowing measurement of duodenal bicarbonate secretion.[147, 148] Basal and acid-stimulated duodenal bicarbonate secretion was found to be depressed in 11 of 12 DU patients compared to control subjects (Fig. 47–9), with the difference evident in the proximal but not distal duodenum.[148] These differences were of sufficient magnitude to nearly separate the ranges for normal subjects and DU patients; few of the proposed abnormalities in DU are this marked. The magnitude of this defect would be expected to alter the mucosal pH gradient, and recent studies have examined the juxtamucosal pH using a microelectrode under endoscopic guidance. Under conditions of luminal acidification to a pH of 1.5, juxtamucosal pH in the gastric fundus and body and in the duodenum remained near neutral, whereas pH values in the esophagus and antrum fell sharply at luminal pH values below 3. With this luminal acidification, DU patients were unable to maintain as high a pH value as were normal subjects.[149] These two recent studies indicate that DU patients have an impaired mucosal/bicarbonate barrier against luminal acid, in part due to impaired duodenal bicarbonate secretion. This impaired barrier, especially when coupled with the hypersecretion of gastric acid, might result in markedly increased acidification at the mucosal surface in DU patients. However, the pathophysiologic implications of these findings must be interpreted with caution.[150] In the study of duodenal bicarbonate secretion, the ulcers were inactive and all duodenal endoscopic examinations were grossly normal; thus, despite the defects in bicarbonate secretion, patients were ulcer-free. It is possible

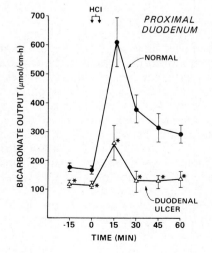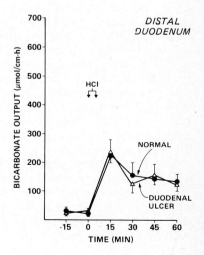

Figure 47–9. Duodenal bicarbonate output in normal subjects and duodenal ulcer patients. Data are the mean (± SE) for duodenal bicarbonate output from the proximal and distal duodenum. After basal bicarbonate secretion was measured, 100 mM hydrochloric acid was infused for five minutes and bicarbonate production was measured. The asterisks denote p < 0.01 for DU patients versus normal subjects. Proximal bicarbonate secretion was measured in 16 normal subjects and 12 DU patients, and distal bicarbonate secretion was measured in nine normal subjects and in nine DU patients. (From Isenberg, J. I., Selling, J. A., Hogan, D. L., et al. N. Engl. J. Med. *316*:374, 1987. Used with permission.)

that inflammatory changes, even in the absence of active ulcer craters, impair duodenal function. Bicarbonate secretion is stimulated by prostaglandins and inhibited by NSAIDs, which inhibit prostaglandin production,[147] thus raising the possibility that defective prostaglandin production may underlie the defect in mucosal bicarbonate secretion. However, studies of duodenal prostaglandin production in DU are controversial, as noted below. In contrast to these findings, gastric bicarbonate secretion was found to be similar in DU patients and normal subjects.[151]

Abnormal Mucus. Mucous gel in patients with gastric ulcer and to a lesser extent with duodenal ulcer has been reported to have an increased proportion of lower molecular weight glycoprotein, resulting in weaker gel formation.[152] This finding might imply that mucus would provide a less effective unstirred layer and diffusion barrier for acid and pepsin.

Prostaglandins and Duodenal Ulcer. Aspirin and other NSAIDs inhibit endogenous mucosal prostaglandin (PG) synthesis and produce mucosal injury and ulcers (see p. 775), although a causal relationship between inhibition of prostaglandin production and duodenal ulcer remains controversial. Study of the role of endogenous prostaglandins in the pathogenesis of peptic ulcer has been difficult and several studies, each using different methodologies, have yielded inconsistent findings.[153–155] Methodologic difficulties preclude firm conclusions,[156] but with the limited present data DU does not appear to be characterized by marked deficiency in duodenal prostaglandin production. This conclusion is consistent with the observations that, in general, NSAIDs, in doses that markedly inhibit endogenous prostaglandin production in the gastric mucosa,[157] impose at most a modest risk for duodenal ulcer. Therefore, it seems reasonable to assume that only a component of duodenal mucosal resistance to acid-peptic injury is prostaglandin-dependent and that prostaglandin-independent mechanisms are generally sufficient to maintain mucosal integrity. However, these data do not warrant dismissing prostaglandin deficiency in DU pathogenesis. NSAIDs can enhance basal and stimulated acid secretion,[158, 159] suggesting that endogenous prostaglandins may exert negative feedback control of acid secretion. Furthermore, these data suggest that the enhancement of acid secretion by NSAIDs may be much more pronounced in some individuals, possibly reflecting a greater dependency of acid secretory control and mucosal defense upon endogenous prostaglandin production. It is of interest that cigarette smoking, a clear risk factor in duodenal ulcer, decreases prostaglandin production, as will be discussed subsequently.

Infection and Inflammatory Change. A peptic ulcer is a hole in the mucosa surrounded by inflammatory infiltrate, but causality in the relationship between the break in the mucosa and the inflammatory change is unclear. Mucosal inflammation is frequently associated with peptic ulcer, and it is of interest that the changes observed with DU include both antral gastritis and duodenitis.

Antral Gastritis and Duodenal Ulcer. About 80 per cent of DU patients have antral gastritis.[160–162] This condition is clearly distinct from the fundic gland gastritis that is found in asymptomatic individuals as a function of increasing age and is associated with autoimmune phenomena, such as parietal cell antibodies and pernicious anemia (see p. 800). In contrast to patients with gastric ulcer who may have moderate fundic gland gastritis, DU patients have minimal fundic gland gastritis, probably less than in normal subjects.[163] Furthermore, in DU patients fundic gland gastritis may not progress with age, as it does in the normal population.[164] This preservation of a "juvenile" (uninflamed) fundic mucosa in DU patients may account for the greater acid secretory capacity found in DU patients and possibly for the low incidence of gastric carcinoma in unoperated DU patients (see p. 838).

Duodenitis and Duodenal Ulcer. The association of duodenitis with DU[165] is complex and poorly understood, possibly reflecting distinct causal factors in different patients. Duodenal inflammation is not common in the normal population; a chronic cellular infiltrate was present in 12 per cent of normal subjects, and only 4 per cent had polymorphonuclear infiltration, the latter being a cardinal feature of acute duodenitis.[166] Reports vary as to the proportion of DU patients with duodenitis,[160, 165, 167, 168] probably due to sampling problems, the activity of the ulcer disease, and true variability among DU patients. Most patients with an active DU have acute duodenitis in the vicinity of the crater, whereas other patients may have more widespread duodenitis.[168] Gastric type metaplasia is also common in the bulb of DU patients. Controlled histologic studies of healed duodenal ulcers revealed marked acute inflammation and gastric metaplasia at the site of ulceration, often covered by a single layer of epithelial cells; in most patients less inflammation was evident on the opposite duodenal wall.[169] These latter observations support an association between DU and duodenitis, but they do not clarify the causality of the relationship. In some patients, in particular those with hypersecretion, increased acid-peptic activity may itself compromise mucosal integrity, resulting in an ulcer crater with a secondary inflammatory response. Consistent with this view that the inflammatory response is a secondary process, duodenitis has been found to improve in some patients with ulcer healing.[168] In contrast, in other patients duodenitis persists after apparent healing,[168] suggesting that the inflammation is an independent factor. The persistence of an inflammatory change after ulcer healing raises the possibility that this inflammatory change also preceded the ulceration, disrupting regional mucosal structure and function, thus predisposing to ulceration in the face of normal acid-peptic activity.

Duodenitis also occurs in the absence of obvious duodenal ulcer disease,[161] as discussed subsequently. Duodenitis rarely occurs as an isolated histologic finding, but is usually associated with antral gastritis, consistent with the association of antral gastritis and duodenal ulcer.[161]

Gastroduodenitis and Campylobacter pylori. Both infectious and autoimmune mechanisms have been hypothesized to explain the inflammation associated with DU. Autoimmune mechanisms,[170] possibly with a genetic component (see pp. 819–822), remain speculative. In contrast, in the last few years a newly described organism *Campylobacter pylori* has been discovered to be a frequent resident of the human gastroduodenum (see p. 798). Although the organism is found in asymptomatic "normal subjects," it appears that the presence of this organism is much more commonly associated with active gastritis and characterized by polymorphonuclear infiltration involving the antral—but not fundic—mucosa.[171, 172, 172a] *C. pylori* was cultured from 88 per cent of subjects with "active" gastritis, but in only 5 per cent with inactive gastritis or no histologic changes.[173] In the duodenum, *C. pylori* occurs in association with both duodenitis and ulceration, but not in normal duodenum.[172, 173] *C. pylori* is found adherent to gastric type surface cells, both in the antrum and in patches of gastric metaplasia in the duodenum.[174] In sampling the antrum, *C. pylori* was isolated from the antrum of 95 per cent of 61 DU patients.[175] About 85 per cent of DU patients in another series had duodenal colonization by *C. pylori*.[176] Of 573 DU patients examined in 14 studies, *C. pylori* was isolated from the gastroduodenal mucosa in 84 per cent, compared with 57 per cent of 408 patients with ulcer-negative dyspepsia (six studies), and 21 per cent of 117 normal subjects (eight studies) (M. L. Skoglund, personal communication).

Even though adequately controlled, blinded studies are not yet available, an association between *C. pylori* and peptic disease is likely. However, the pathogenic significance of *C. pylori* rests upon establishing a causal relationship between presence of the organism and the gastroduodenitis or ulcer. Clearance of *C. pylori* following treatment with colloidal bismuth compounds occurs in some patients and has been associated with improvement of gastritis and healing of duodenal ulcers.[171, 177] Studying patients with DU and *C. pylori*, Marshall and coworkers[176] compared ulcer healing with cimetidine versus colloidal bismuth plus tinidazole, a regimen they found advantageous for clearing *C. pylori*. They found that patients with persistent *C. pylori* infection had delayed ulcer healing. Furthermore, in a one-year follow-up patients persistently positive for *C. pylori* were more likely to relapse than were patients who were cleared of the organism. These preliminary findings that persistent *C. pylori* infection may be associated with delayed healing and more frequent recurrence are very intriguing but require confirmation because of the ubiquitous nature of *C. pylori* and the challenge of establishing causal relationships in the pathophysiology of acid-peptic disease.

Viral etiologies have also been considered for duodenal ulcer.[178] Supporting evidence has included the findings that antibodies to herpes type I virus are more frequently present and in higher titer in DU patients than in control subjects.[179] Although herpesvirus has not been isolated from the gastric or duodenal mucosa,

it has been found in vagal ganglia.[178, 179] Cytomegalovirus has been isolated from the gastric mucosa of patients receiving immunosuppressants after renal transplantation,[180] a clinical setting in which duodenal ulcers are common and virulent. No further studies of this topic have been reported.

ASSOCIATED DISEASES

Duodenal ulcer may be associated with several other chronic diseases. Demonstrating a true association between DU and disease "X" requires examining a random sample of the population for both diseases, alone and in combination. A true association exists if the prevalence of both diseases in the same subject exceeds the product of the individual prevalence rates. Disease associations rarely have been studied in random samples and generally have been sought among patients ascertained by the presence of one of the two diseases. This approach risks what has been called Berkson's fallacy, which reflects bias in a hospital referral population as a result of the relative referral rates for any given disease.[181] Thus, the bias in a hospital referral population generally will indicate a greater prevalence of a given disease than actually exists in a random sample. Furthermore, not only will a patient with a given disease be more likely to be included in a referral population, but patients presenting to a hospital are more likely to be carefully examined for other medical problems. Lastly, patients with both diseases are more likely to come to medical attention.[181] Attention is needed to account for or eliminate biases in the patient population under study.

Because duodenal ulcer is common, many apparent associations are due to chance alone. Assuming that the DU prevalence rate in the male population is 10 per cent, by chance alone the DU prevalence rate may reach 34 per cent in 1 of 20 clinical trials with 50 male patients presenting with disease X. In considering a potentially biased patient sample, historical control groups are useless. Concurrent control groups matched for age, sex, smoking history, and drug consumption are essential, but rarely available. Furthermore, the study of disease associations with DU is dependent upon the mode of establishing the ulcer diagnosis (symptoms, radiography, endoscopy, surgery, or autopsy) and the care with which duodenal and gastric ulcers have been differentiated. Some of the diseases reported to be associated with duodenal ulcer are listed in Table 47–4. Other possible associations for which the data are not compelling have not been included.[182, 183] The association of DU with uncommon inherited syndromes, such as gastrinoma and systemic mastocytosis, are considered elsewhere (see pp. 821–822).

Chronic Pulmonary Diseases

An association between DU and chronic obstructive pulmonary disease has been recognized in studies as-

Table 47–4. CHRONIC DISEASES ASSOCIATED WITH DUODENAL ULCERS

Probable or Definite Associations
  Gastrinoma and multiple endocrine neoplasia, type I
  Systemic mastocytosis
  Basophilic leukemia
  Chronic pulmonary disease*
  Chronic renal failure (especially posttransplant or hemodialysis
    patients)
  Cirrhosis of the liver
  Renal stones* (in the absence of MEN I or
    hyperparathyroidism)
  Alpha antitrypsin deficiency*
Associations Claimed, but Firm Evidence Lacking
  Coronary heart disease*
  Cystic fibrosis*
  Carcinoma of the lung*
  Crohn's disease (may reflect gastroduodenal Crohn's disease)
  Hyperparathyroidism (MEN I may fully account for the
    association)
  Polycythemia vera
  Chronic pancreatitis

---

*An association may have a genetic basis.

---

certaining either pulmonary or ulcer patients. Peptic ulcers occur in up to 30 per cent of patients with chronic pulmonary disease, and the frequency of chronic lung disease in peptic ulcer patients is increased two- to threefold.[62, 183–185] Bronchial hypersecretion, airflow restriction, and peptic ulcer have been linked in a large population study.[186] In a controlled study of 29 DU and 27 GU patients, ventilatory dysfunction not accounted for by smoking was found in the GU, but not the DU, patients.[187] Chronic lung disease is responsible for five times more deaths of peptic ulcer patients than expected.[184] This association is still evident after correction for smoking,[185] and is present in both ambulatory and hospitalized patients, as well as in autopsy series. A skewed ascertainment of cases did not appear to underlie this association, since it was also evident in a survey of all autopsy cases of DU in Copenhagen County.[184] The mechanisms for the association have not been established. The observations that the occurrence of ulcers does not correlate with the clinical severity of lung disease, the degree of CO_2 retention, or the kind of therapy utilized for the pulmonary disease indicate that the association does not result from the physiologic sequelae or therapy of the pulmonary disease itself.[62] A re-evaluation of the data collected by Monson provides further evidence against the concept that pulmonary disease causes the associated duodenal ulcer; of the 27 individuals with both disorders, duodenal ulcers preceded the clinical onset of chronic pulmonary disease in 21 patients by an average of 11 years (Rotter and coworkers, unpublished observations). A genetic basis for the association has been suggested possibly as a reflection of a pleiotropic manifestation of a single gene.[62]

Two defined syndromes, alpha$_1$-antitrypsin deficiency and cystic fibrosis, are also examples of suspected associations of chronic pulmonary disease with peptic ulcers. The relative risk for peptic ulcers in

alpha$_1$-antitrypsin deficiency is estimated to be 1.5 to 3 times greater than the general population.[62] With the lack of protease inhibitors, the unopposed proteolytic activity is thought to promote breakdown of pulmonary tissue; one can speculate that a similar mechanism could produce peptic ulcers. Apart from decreased pancreatic bicarbonate secretion, specific abnormalities causing ulcers in cystic fibrosis remain undefined.

Cirrhosis

Both the incidence and prevalence of duodenal ulcer appear to be increased in cirrhosis,[183] although no series provides an age- and sex-matched control group. In 219 cirrhotic patients followed for an average of four years, the annual incidence of DU was about 2.2 per cent,[188] or about tenfold greater than overall estimates for the normal population. About 15 per cent of this series had duodenal ulcers at the outset or developed duodenal ulcers during the four-year study, a roughly two- to threefold increase in the period (not lifetime) prevalence compared with the normal population. In an endoscopic study cirrhotic patients had duodenal or prepyloric ulcers at a point prevalence rate several times higher than normal.[189] No consistent differences have been noted in the DU incidence among the different forms of cirrhosis.[189, 190] Of interest, the normal male predominance in duodenal ulcer is not evident in patients with cirrhosis.[190] The death rate from duodenal ulcer in cirrhotic patients is five times higher than in the general population.[184] Despite early suggestions that portacaval anastomosis increased the incidence of DU, no significant differences either in the incidence of new ulcers or in the exacerbation of an existing ulcer diathesis have occurred during controlled trials.[188] Decreased hepatic metabolism of GI hormones, increased acid secretion, and altered blood flow are hypothesized, but unsubstantiated, mechanisms accounting for the association between DU and cirrhosis.

Renal Failure and Transplantation

An increased incidence of DU in patients with renal failure on maintenance hemodialysis has been reported,[183, 191, 192] although other studies suggest a low prevalence of DU in this population.[193] An endoscopic survey of 249 patients under 60 years old on maintenance hemodialysis found 6.4 per cent with active DU and 4.8 per cent with evidence of a duodenal ulcer scar.[194] Although this point prevalence for DU seems somewhat high, the authors found a point prevalence of duodenal ulcer of 15 per cent in their population of 11, 219 outpatients undergoing endoscopy for a variety of indications. Of interest was the finding that 18 per cent of 142 of the uremic patients on vitamin D replacement had evidence of duodenal ulcer disease, compared to only 3 per cent of the population not taking vitamin D; this finding remains unexplained.

Studies of calcium metabolism were not reported for this population.

Data are more consistent regarding an increased risk of peptic ulceration after renal transplantation.[183, 191, 193, 195–197] In a mean follow-up period of 23 months, 12 of 95 consecutive cadaveric transplant patients developed DU.[196] After renal transplantation, ulcers frequently present with complications and high mortality rates.[193, 195, 196] Fifty-nine of 68 patients with peptic ulcers after renal transplantation presented with bleeding or perforation; the mortality rate was 43 per cent.[193] The mechanisms precipitating ulcer formation in transplant patients are unknown, although the finding of cytomegalovirus inclusion bodies in gastroduodenal mucosa of nine of 20 transplanted patients is of interest.[180] It appears that acid secretion, if anything, is normal or low in uremic patients.[198, 199] As with cirrhotic patients, serum gastrin levels are inversely related to acid secretory capacity in a similar fashion to that found in normal subjects. Secretory capacity was inversely related to the duration, but not the degree, of uremia.[197] However, in some patients an increase in acid secretion may occur after transplantation.[197, 200] The post-transplantation use of steroids, but not azathioprine, has been associated with ulcer formation, but the supporting data are weak.[45, 195] Hypercalcemia, produced by too much calcium in the dialysis bath, was related to ulcer formation in four to seven patients on hemodialysis.[201] Studies of the relation of *C. pylori* to peptic ulceration in uremic patients pre- and post-transplantation have not been reported.

Because of the high rate of complications, some authors have suggested that prophylactic surgery be performed on patients with pre-existing ulcers before they undergo transplantation.[193] Others have argued that pre-existing ulcers are inaccurate predictors of post-transplantation ulcers.[200] Transplantation and the attendent immunosuppression do not appear to prevent a response to ulcer therapy.[191, 195, 196] In an uncontrolled trial, 30 patients placed on prophylactic cimetidine from the day of transplantation experienced no bleeding, whereas six of 33 previous patients had significant bleeding episodes.[191] Some centers place all renal transplant patients on prophylactic H_2 blocker therapy in the immediate postoperative period.[194] However, H_2 blockers are present on immune cells, including suppressor T cells, and have immune modulatory effects (see p. 845). There is no clear consensus regarding the effects of H_2 antagonists on the survival of renal transplants in humans, although cimetidine has been reported to enhance transplant rejection in a canine model.[202]

Renal Stones

There is an association between duodenal ulcers and renal stones in MEN type I, reflecting the presence of both gastrinoma and hyperparathyroidism. However, renal stones may also be associated with duodenal ulcer in the absence of hyperparathyroidism. Following the exclusion of hyperparathyroidism, renal stones occurred in 7 per cent of 200 ulcer patients and in 1 per cent of control subjects.[203] Calculi preceded the ulcers in nine of these 14 patients, thus making it unlikely that this association reflected only sequelae of ulcer therapy, such as an increased milk consumption or calcium carbonate intake. Genetic factors have been associated with renal calculi and may underlie the condition in at least a subset of patients with idiopathic hypercalciuria. In three large families, an association was found between renal stones and duodenal ulcers; neither hyperparathyroidism nor gastrinoma occurred in these families (J. Rotter, personal communication).

Coronary Heart Disease

An association of ulcer and coronary artery disease has been suggested,[62, 183] possibly reflecting the high milk intake of many DU patients.[204] However, a familial basis for this apparent association has also been proposed.[62] Enhanced catecholamine secretion, as reflected in increased urinary catechols, occurred in patients with angina pectoris and myocardial infarction and in patients with duodenal ulcers;[62, 205] whether these findings reflect an association between ulcers and coronary disease remains speculative.

Other Disease Associations

An increased risk of DU has been reported in polycythemia vera,[183] although this association has not been rigorously tested. An alteration in mucosal blood flow due to increased viscosity has been proposed to underlie this association. Patients with polycythemia vera, a myeloproliferative disorder, often have elevated blood basophil counts.[206] Because basophils contain histamine, it is possible that histamine delivery to the parietal cells is increased in this disorder. Duodenal ulcers have been found more frequently in patients with reduced exocrine pancreatic function than in a control group,[207] possibly as a result of the decrease in pancreatic bicarbonate output available for neutralization of gastric acid in the duodenum. A quite variable incidence of DU has been reported for Crohn's disease;[181, 183] however, endoscopy is needed to differentiate gastroduodenal Crohn's disease and acid-peptic ulceration. An increased incidence of peptic ulcers has been reported among patients with carcinoid syndrome, myasthenia gravis, and abdominal aortic aneurysm, although supporting data are weak.[183]

Disorders Associated with a Decreased Incidence of Duodenal Ulcer

Patients with fundic gland gastritis (type A) and the associated atrophy of the fundic mucosa have a decreased incidence of DU (see p. 794). The autoimmune disorders that are associated with gastritis and are part of the polyglandular failure syndrome (i.e., Addison's disease, autoimmune thyroid disease, insulin-dependent diabetes, hypoparathyroidism),[208] may also have a decreased incidence of DU. This latter association may underlie the decreased prevalence of duodenal ulcer found in diabetes mellitus,[183] although these relationships have not been carefully studied. An inverse relationship between blood pressure and ulcer disease has also been reported but remains unexplained and unconfirmed.[209] Duodenal ulcer is rare and gastric cancer frequent in Pima Indians, findings that probably relate to the occurrence of chronic gastritis, acid hyposecretion, and a delay in gastric emptying found in this population.[210] A negative association between gastric carcinoma and duodenal ulcer has been suspected in the general population, probably because the chronic gastritis and acid hyposecretion associated with gastric carcinoma diminishes the likelihood of duodenal ulcer.[211] However, the universality of this inverse association has been challenged.[212]

CLINICAL ASPECTS

Symptoms

In the era of classic diseases, duodenal ulcer was an easy entity to recognize. The "classic" case was characterized by gnawing or burning epigastric pain occurring one to three hours after meals, frequently awakening the patient at night (about 1 or 2 A.M.), but rarely occurring before breakfast. Alkali and food produce relief, and thus "classic" patients tend to "feed their ulcers." Moynihan[215] stated that most patients with dyspepsia could be correctly diagnosed solely by their symptoms. Unfortunately, today the clinician who diagnoses duodenal ulcer when—and only when—confronted with this picture will be often misled. Some DU patients who are free of symptoms present with complications such as hemorrhage or perforation. Presentation of DU without pain has been noted more frequently in elderly patients.[214] Although the available studies support certain features of the "classic picture," symptoms are neither specific nor sensitive for separating DU from other causes of epigastric discomfort (Table 47–5).[215-219] Epigastric pain is a primary complaint in 60 to 86 per cent of duodenal ulcer patients, with the pain described as vague discomfort or cramping, as often as burning, gnawing, or hunger-like in nature. Radiation of the pain to the back occurs in about 20 per cent. Fifty to 88 per cent describe a pain that awakens them at night. In two studies about 80 per cent of DU patients described pain relief with alkali and about 60 per cent described relief with food;[215, 217] however, Horrocks and De Dombal[216] found only 39 per cent of duodenal ulcer patients with an alkali relief pattern and 20 per cent with food relief, underlining the magnitude of observer and/or patient variability. Of the patients presenting with epigastric pain who noted relief with food, only 31 per cent were subsequently found to have duodenal ulcer as the

underlying disorder,[220] so this clue lacks specificity. Clusters of pain, i.e., symptomatic periods lasting up to a few weeks, followed by symptom-free periods of often several months, are described in about 50 per cent of patients.

Many patients report symptoms that are at odds with those expected from the "classic" presentation. About one half of DU patients do not relate their pain to meals, and occasionally pain occurs with eating or within 30 minutes after eating. Only 20 per cent of DU patients have the classic increase in appetite, while 20 to 45 per cent experience anorexia or weight loss (Table 47–5). Nausea and vomiting, even in the absence of pyloric obstruction, occur in 25 to 60 per cent of cases. Other dyspeptic symptoms, such as belching, bloating distention, and fatty food intolerance, occur in 40 to 70 per cent of cases. Heartburn, characteristic of reflux esophagitis, occurs in 20 to 60 per cent of cases. Symptoms of irritable bowel syndrome have also been reported to be quite common.[219] The considerable variability among the available series probably reflects both patients selection and observer bias.

The development of a complication will often be evident by a change in symptoms. The primary DU pain is visceral and therefore is dull, aching, or gnawing and is not well localized. An increase or change in the quality of the pain, a more discrete localization, the loss of alkali relief, or the onset of radiation to the

Table 47–5. SYMPTOMATOLOGY OF DUODENAL ULCERS*

Symptom	Gastric Ulcer (%)	Duodenal Ulcer (%)	Nonulcer Dyspepsia (%)
Age	>50	30–60	20–29
Pain/discomfort†	100	100	100
Features of the pain:			
Primary pain			
Epigastric	67	61–86	52–73
Right hypochondrium	6	7–17	4
Left hypochondrium	6	3–5	5
Frequently severe	68	53	37
Within 30 minutes of food	20	5	32
Gnawing pain	13	16	6
Increased by food	24	10–40	45
Clusters (episodic)	16	56	35
Relieved by alkali	36–87	39–86	26–75
Food relief	2–48	20–63	4–32
Occurs at night	32–43	50–88	24–32
Not related to food or variable	22–53	21–49	22–65
Radiation to back	34	20–31	24–28
Increased appetite		19	
Anorexia	46–57	25–36	26–36
Weight loss	24–61	19–45	18–32
Nausea	54–70	49–59	43–60
Vomiting	38–73	25–57	26–34
Heartburn	19	27–59	28
Nondyspeptic symptoms	2	8	18
Fatty food intolerance		41–72	53
Bloating	55	49	52
Belching	48	59	60

*Data combined from three series[215-217] for gastric ulcer, duodenal ulcer, and nonulcer dyspepsia.

†Patients were ascertained for these series by dyspepsia or upper abdominal pain presenting in a hospital setting.

back may occur with posterior penetration, which may be associated with acute pancreatitis. Protracted vomiting may indicate pyloric outlet obstruction. The sudden development of severe, diffuse abdominal pain may indicate perforation; and the onset of dizziness may indicate ulcer hemorrhage.

Correlation Between Pain, Acid, and Ulcers

One would expect that acid bathing an ulcer crater underlies the pain experienced by duodenal ulcer patients. W. L. Palmer's demonstration that aspiration of gastric contents relieved pain and that reinfusion of the acidic (but not neutralized) gastric juice precipitated pain supported this concept.[221] But this study lacked control group results for the placebo effects that influence pain perception. More recent studies of the precipitation of ulcer pain by acid have been contradictory. A controlled, blinded study in which solutions of varying pH were infused into the stomach of 13 patients with active DU did not find that acidic solutions consistently produced pain.[222] However, in two double-blind studies direct duodenal infusion of acid, but not saline, induced pain in patients with endoscopic and histologic duodenitis[223] and with active duodenal ulcers.[223, 224] In the study of 40 patients with symptomatic DU confirmed by endoscopy, a five-minute endoscopic infusion into the duodenum of HCl (0.1 N, 10 ml/minute) reproduced ulcer pain in 16 patients, whereas infusion of saline produced pain in four patients.[224] The reason pain was produced in only 16 of 40 patients was not established, but the short duration and slow rate of infusion may have influenced the results. Acid bathing a DU or inflamed duodenum appears to account for a component of ulcer pain, but other factors are also likely. Duodenal dysmotility or spasm is another element hypothesized to induce pain.

Antacids relieve pain in many DU patients, suggesting that buffering of gastric acid is the responsible mechanism. However, a direct study of this question indicated that antacids and an identically appearing liquid with no buffering capacity taken orally produced comparable degrees of pain relief.[225] In two other studies infusion of antacids was somewhat superior to placebo infusion in pain relief.[226, 227] Although buffering capacity may underlie some pain relief by antacids, placebo effects also have a powerful influence on pain perception in DU patients.

A frequent dissociation between the presence of an ulcer crater and symptoms has been found in several recent clinical trials. Ulcer healing does not guarantee disappearance of symptoms; although the majority of patients who are ulcer-free by endoscopy are asymptomatic, 4 to 39 per cent of ulcer-free patients do have persistent symptoms.[228–230] Conversely, in clinical trials, ulcers may be present without producing symptoms; from 15 to 44 per cent of symptom-free patients have been found to have a duodenal ulcer crater at endoscopy.[228–230] The data from one of these series are illustrated (Fig. 47–10) to emphasize that the disappearance of symptoms by no means guarantees ulcer healing, nor does the persistence of symptoms necessarily predict a persistent ulcer crater. The pain experienced by DU patients reflects factors more complex than acid bathing an ulcer crater.

Family History

Because genetic forms of DU exist, a thorough family history may yield important information. Symptoms and diseases that may occur in addition to ulcer disease and dyspepsia are endocrine disorders, possibly suggestive of multiple endocrine adenomatosis (MEN, type I), kidney stones, or a presentation consistent

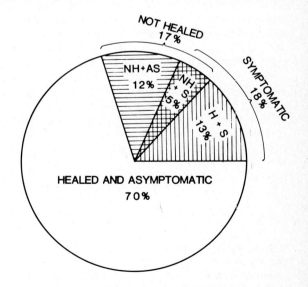

Figure 47–10. Status of healing and symptoms in patients treated for six weeks with cimetidine or antacids. Note that only about one third of the symptomatic patients had persistent ulcer craters, whereas about two thirds of the patients with persistent ulcer craters had become asymptomatic. (Redrawn by permission of the publisher from: Cimetidine versus antacid therapy for duodenal ulcer: a multicenter trial, by Ippoliti, A. F., Sturdevant, R. A. L., Isenberg, J. I., et al. Gastroenterology 74[2 pt. 2]:393–395. Copyright 1978 by The American Gastroenterological Association.)

	HEALED (H)	NOT HEALED (NH)
ASYMPTOMATIC (AS)	70%	12%
SYMPTOMATIC (S)	13%	5%

with the other rare forms of duodenal ulcer. A family history of DU is more likely when the patient developed symptoms at an early age (see p. 819).

Physical Examination

In uncomplicated cases, physical examination generally will reveal little more than epigastric tenderness, which is neither a specific nor a sensitive sign of duodenal ulcer.[231] Evidence of diseases that may be associated with DU or that may influence therapeutic decisions, such as cardiovascular and respiratory disorders, should be sought. Unusual findings may be present when DU is associated with rare genetic disorders, as discussed previously. The development of complications of ulcers, especially obstruction and perforation, may become evident on physical examination. Evidence for other processes that can cause abdominal pain should be sought, including musculoskeletal disorders.

Laboratory Studies

Routine laboratory studies generally add little to the work-up, but should include a complete blood count, creatinine, and serum calcium. A fasting serum gastrin is indicated in cases unresponsive to therapy, patients with a positive family history, or patients requiring surgery. Measurement of serum group I pepsinogen by radioimmunoassay, when available, may provide an index of the secretory mass and a clue to familial ulcer disease. In the setting of fasting hypergastrinemia, a high serum pepsinogen I level provides evidence for either gastrinoma or antral G cell hyperfunction, whereas a low serum pepsinogen I suggests atrophic (chronic) gastritis and a hyposecretory fundic mucosa.[232] Because there is a large overlap between maximal acid secretory capacity of duodenal ulcer patients and normal subjects, measurement of acid secretion is of little diagnostic or prognostic value in individual cases. However, acid secretory studies are useful as a first step following the detection of hypergastrinemia, as hypo- or achlorhydria is a surprisingly common cause of hypergastrinemia in patients initially suspected of acid peptic disease.[233] The finding of decreased acid secretion obviously eliminates a need for secretin tests or other evaluation for gastrinoma. Acid secretory studies may also be useful in cases refractory to therapy (see pp. 713–734).

Differential Diagnosis

Duodenal ulcers must be distinguished from other causes of epigastric distress. This differential diagnosis includes peptic diseases of the stomach and esophagus, gastric cancer, and a variety of less common diseases, such as Crohn's disease. However, in as many as half the patients presenting with epigastric pain, it is not possible to arrive at a specific pathologic diagnosis even after complete work-up.

Gastric Ulcer. The differences in the presentation of gastric and duodenal ulcers do not allow separation by symptoms with any precision. Gastric ulcer patients, compared to those with duodenal ulcer, tend to be older and may have more pain, which occurs sooner after meals and is less likely to be relieved by antacids or food (Table 47–5). However, clinical features do not allow differentiation, and radiography or endoscopy is necessary for firm diagnosis (see pp. 890–894).

Gastroesophageal Reflux. Heartburn or pyrosis, the symptom most commonly associated with esophageal reflux, usually originates in the epigastric area or xiphoid area and radiates retrosternally. Pyrosis often occurs when the individual is supine or bending over, especially after meals. Duodenal ulcer patients commonly complain of typical heartburn (Table 47–5), which is probably related to esophageal reflux, rather than the duodenal disease. Earlam[234] argues that the esophagus is a major source of symptoms in DU patients. Both esophageal reflux and DU commonly coexist and therefore need to be independently evaluated and treated (see pp.594–619).

Drug-Induced Dyspepsia. Many drugs cause epigastric distress with or without nausea and vomiting. Anti-inflammatory agents may cause gastric ulcers, acute hemorrhagic gastritis, and dyspepsia (see p. 775) and may be a factor in duodenal erosions and ulcer formation. Many other drugs, such as theophylline and digitalis, may cause dyspeptic symptoms. Caffeine, coffee, and smoking can also cause symptoms in many patients. A history of drug intake is important in dyspeptic patients, as a reduction in dose or discontinuation may relieve symptoms and avoid a costly work-up.

Non-Ulcer Dyspepsia (NUD). Dyspepsia is a vague and probably heterogeneous symptom complex characterized by epigastric discomfort or pain. Most dyspeptic patients have no obvious disease in the upper gastrointestinal or biliary tract, except for the possible association with gastroduodenal inflammation, as discussed below. Such patients constitute 30 to 60 per cent of cases presenting with chronic upper abdominal complaints.[215, 216, 220, 235, 236] and by their number and nature they are a challenging and frustrating group. NUD is a more frequent diagnosis in younger than older dyspeptic patients; in one series of 197 consecutive patients presenting with abdominal pain, NUD was diagnosed in 70 per cent of patients under 40, and in only 40 per cent of patients over 60.[220]

Non-ulcer dyspepsia is a poorly defined entity that may hide several disorders, each with distinct mechanisms underlying the symptoms. Some dyspeptic patients have the "classic" duodenal ulcer syndrome, characterized by an epigastric burning or gnawing pain one to three hours postprandially, with relief by food and alkali. "Ulcer" symptoms in the absence of gross ulceration has been referred to as "Moynihan's disease,"[237] even though Moynihan described this classic symptomatology in association with an ulcer crater.[213]

In other dyspeptic patients, epigastric discomfort occurs shortly after meals and is frequently associated with belching, bloating, fullness, and nausea; antacids offer little relief and eating often precipitates symptoms.[236, 238] The term "functional indigestion" aptly describes this latter group. Some dyspeptic patients complain of a combination of these symptoms. Although the symptoms of NUD are generally not associated temporally with obvious bowel dysfunction, many patients also have irritable bowel syndrome. Other complaints are also frequent (Table 47–5). The pain in NUD patients may radiate to the back and may be associated with a spinal reflex or abdominal wall syndrome, as discussed subsequently.

The symptoms in the patients with functional indigestion are typical of gastroparesis, and some of these patients have gastric dysmotility.[238] In these patients, poor gastric compliance may be present, and gastric distention produces pain at much lower volumes than in normal subjects, just as does colonic distention in patients with the irritable bowel syndrome.[239] Some patients with functional indigestion have delayed gastric emptying of a radiolabeled mixed meal and may respond to treatment with metoclopramide.[236, 238] Distinct food intolerances are often prominent complaints in patients with NUD, as well as in patients with duodenal ulcers.[215, 217, 236] Fat intolerance is common in both disorders, possibly reflecting the ability of fat to delay gastric emptying and enhance duodenal reflux.

It is important to assess the role of psychologic factors in patients both with ulcers and with NUD. In one study of 96 patients presenting with persistent or recurrent abdominal pain, 80 per cent were diagnosed as being depressed, suffering from chronic tension, or having prominent hysterical features.[240] About half of these patients responded to psychiatric management. Recognizing these psychologic elements early in the evaluation of the patient may influence decisions regarding further diagnostic studies and management. Physicians caring for patients with chronic abdominal pain need refined skills for detecting and assessing the role of psychologic factors in the genesis of symptoms. This task may be difficult, because many of these patients manifest what psychiatrists label as alexithymia, or an inability to read or describe feelings, except in terms of pain or action.[241]

Gastroduodenitis, NUD, and Ulcers. The clinical and pathogenic implications of inflammatory changes in the antral and duodenal mucosa remain problematic (see pp. 800 and 830). In particular, a causal relationship between inflammatory changes in the duodenum and dyspeptic symptoms has been difficult to establish.[166, 223, 236, 242] The visible changes of duodenitis are edema and thickened folds, erythema, petechial hemorrhages, and erosions. With the exception of clear-cut erosive duodenitis, these visible changes of duodenitis are poor predictors of symptoms; these changes may occur in asymptomatic subjects, whereas individuals with classic dyspeptic symptoms may have normal-appearing duodenal mucosa.[243] A poor correlation is also found between histologic changes and symptoms,

in that many patients with typical dyspeptic symptoms have a normal duodenal histologic appearance. One feature that seems to distinguish patients with duodenal ulcer and symptomatic duodenitis is the infiltration of the lamina propria with neutrophils, an unusual finding in normal subjects.[161, 166, 243] Although there may be several mechanisms for pain in duodenitis, some patients experience pain with acid irrigation of the duodenal bulb.[223]

The proportion of patients with NUD who have duodenitis varies among different series, probably reflecting patient selection. Dyspeptic patients selected for classic ulcer symptoms may be more likely to have duodenitis at endoscopy.[161] Others have found that duodenitis is an infrequent finding in NUD.[244]

Although the natural history of duodenitis has not been defined, patients who present with an endoscopic diagnosis of erosive duodenitis not infrequently evolve into duodenal ulcer disease.[161, 245, 246] In a series of 502 endoscopies performed for a variety of indications, symptomatic duodenitis was found in 2.8 per cent.[246] Of these 14 patients, six later developed ulcers, while six improved without documented crater formation. Several previous studies that had examined the natural history of NUD in the pre-endoscopic era yielded predictions for the development of duodenal ulcer varying from 3 to 40 per cent, a difference in part reflecting the length of the study (six to 27 years), the patient population (hospital referral or general practice), and the fact that screening was only by single contrast radiography.[247–250] In a primary care patient population, NUD will result in frank ulcer disease in only a small proportion of patients. Unfortunately, symptoms are an unreliable way of discriminating patients with NUD from those with ulcer disease.[161]

Musculoskeletal Pain. Neuromuscular mechanisms can produce chronic abdominal pain that may be confused with pain of visceral origin and may not be recognized unless specifically sought.[251] Pain of parietal origin may be impossible to differentiate by clinical history from visceral pain. Ashby[252] has described a spinal reflex syndrome in which a vicious circle of reflex pain and spasm may be initiated by a painful trigger stimulus, which itself is often transient. Excessive afferent neuronal barrage is hypothesized as perpetuating spinal reflex syndrome. Spasm of abdominal, intercostal, and paraspinous muscles may underlie these reflexes, possibly through compression of peripheral nerves or the spinal root. Clues to the existence of this syndrome are a segmental distribution of pain, intercostal, abdominal, or paraspinous tenderness, altered cutaneous sensation, and an increase of pain with tensing abdominal muscles or twisting the spine. Paraspinous tenderness and spasm may be the only evidence of a trigger point and patients may be unaware of this tenderness until precipitated by palpation. Psychologic tension may provoke pain of spinal reflex origin, presumably by enhancing muscle spasm, facilitating spinal reflexes, and causing preoccupation with the pain.[252] Ashby evaluated 73 patients consecutively referred to a general surgical practice for chronic abdominal pain and found clinical evidence supporting the diagnosis of a reflex spinal origin in 53. Forty-nine of these 53 patients had relief with the injection of a local anesthetic that produced a temporary intercostal block. Tenderness over the transverse spinal process often indicated the appropriate site for injection.[252] No evidence for visceral disease was found during the follow-up of these patients.

Peripheral nerve entrapment, which frequently occurs at the border of the rectus abdominis sheath or at the site of surgical scars, may be an important factor in some patients with chronic abdominal pain.[253, 254] Regardless of whether the origin of the pain is peripheral or spinal, interruption of the afferent reflex arc frequently promotes at least temporary relief. Injection with phenol may provide permanent relief of the pain of peripheral origin.[253] It is important to stress that although parietal pain can cause reflex visceral symptoms, visceral disease can also cause spinal root or referred parietal pain, probably through summation or visceroparietal reflexes. Thus, the existence of underlying visceral disease should be kept in mind, despite an obvious neuromuscular element in the pain. Spasm of the rectus abdominis is another cause of abdominal pain that may escape notice if not specifically sought. Clues to the presence of abdominal wall spasm are an increase in pain and/or tenderness with tensing of the abdominal musculature. Rectus muscle spasm may even be dramatic enough to mimic perforated peptic ulcer, and paradoxically it may occur shortly after administration of parenteral morphine, suggesting a causal relationship.[255]

Abdominal pain can also result from nerve root involvement secondary to diabetic radiculopathy.[256] The absence of paresthesia, the intermittent nature of symptoms, and the occasional presence of anorexia and weight loss can divert attention from the radicular origin. The presence of peripheral or autonomic neuropathy due to diabetes, which would be a clue to the neural origin of the symptoms, may not be apparent.

Carcinoma. Gastric carcinoma may present with dyspepsia, and operable gastric cancer is the most important differential diagnosis to consider. Patients with gastric carcinoma are generally older, with a shorter presenting history, and complain of a continuous pain that is increased by food and associated with anorexia. However, 10 per cent describe pain relief by food, and weight loss, early satiety, nausea, and vomiting may be absent in early cases.[257] Pain in gastric cancer patients is not clustered; symptom-free periods longer than one month are very unusual.[216] The risk of gastric carcinoma in patients with dyspepsia presenting in a primary care setting is probably less than 1 per cent.[258] However, a risk as high as 22 per cent may be found in selected patient populations, such as those presenting to specialty clinics.[216] Therefore, gastric carcinoma must be excluded, especially in patients over 50 years of age presenting with persistent symptoms. Differentiation requires air-contrast radiography or endoscopy. Other neoplastic processes, such as gastric

lymphoma or leiomyosarcoma, may also present with dyspepsia.

Crohn's Disease. Crohn's disease may involve the stomach or duodenum and produce symptoms and a radiographic appearance which mimics duodenal ulcer. Usually, radiographic abnormalities are present in other portions of the duodenum and small intestine. Endoscopy with biopsy may reveal the diagnosis.[259]

Other Gastric Lesions. Infiltrative diseases of the stomach, which may also present with dyspepsia, include eosinophilic granuloma, tuberculosis, syphilis, and sarcoidosis. Adult hypertrophic pyloric stenosis usually presents with vomiting plus epigastric pain. Hypertrophic gastritis (Menetrier's disease) also may present with dyspeptic symptoms. Atrophic gastritis, on the other hand, is generally asymptomatic.

Rare Duodenal Lesions. Lesions, such as duodenal carcinoma, polyps, webs, congenital reduplication, duodenal tuberculosis, and annular pancreas, may present with bleeding, obstruction, or pain that mimics ulcers. Duodenal carcinoma is a rare disease, but was the cause of gastrointestinal bleeding in eight of 850 endoscopies.[260] Seven duodenal carcinomas were found in 1200 consecutive duodenoscopic examinations.[261] Localized duodenal lymphoma may also mimic duodenal ulcer and even respond to therapy for a period of time.[262] Duodenal and pancreatic carcinoma may present as benign-appearing duodenal ulcers, so that follow-up endoscopy with biopsy is indicated for ulcers that fail to respond to therapy.[263] It is fascinating that duodenal biopsies in ulcer patients heal, rather than ulcerate, suggesting that ulcer formation requires local mucosal susceptibility to injury. In patients with active duodenal ulcer disease, biopsies of recently healed craters were performed without complication, but the biopsies were followed by four weeks of antisecretory therapy.[169]

Other Abdominal Lesions. Biliary tract disease is generally easily differentiated from ulcers because of the right upper quadrant location of the pain and tenderness and radiation of the pain to the right scapular region. However, 25 per cent of the patients with biliary tract disease may have epigastric pain without the typical radiation, and ulcers may occasionally present with primarily right upper quadrant pain.[216] The pain associated with peptic ulcers or ulcer-negative dyspepsia may also radiate to the back (Table 47–5).

The abrupt presentation of acute pancreatitis is usually easily differentiated from uncomplicated duodenal ulcer. Intestinal ischemia may produce a postprandial pain, usually located in the periumbilical region or lower abdomen, that is not generally relieved by alkali. Intestinal ischemia has been reported to produce gastroduodenal ulceration,[264] so that this diagnosis may require exclusion in unusual circumstances. Celiac axis compression has also been credited with causing intermittent upper abdominal pain, although the existence of the disorder is highly controversial.[265] Giardiasis may produce upper abdominal discomfort, nausea and anorexia, although these symptoms are often associated with diarrhea and occasionally evidence of malabsorption. Dyspeptic symptoms may persist over months, interspersed with periods of diarrhea lasting two to three days. Thus, especially when dyspeptic symptoms are associated with diarrhea, examining stools and duodenal aspirates for giardia may be worth while. Strongyloidiasis can also produce upper abdominal pain and nausea (see p. 1174).

Endoscopy and Upper Gastrointestinal Radiography

Radiography. A definitive radiographic diagnosis of duodenal ulcer requires demonstration of barium within an ulcer niche, which is generally round or oval and may be surrounded by a smooth mound of edema. Folds radiating to the crater may be present. Secondary signs of ulcers include deformity of the duodenal bulb secondary to spasm, edema, or scarring. This deformity may be evidenced by flattening of the superior or inferior fornicis, eccentricity of the pyloric channel, pseudodiverticuli, or exaggerated outpouching of recesses at the base of the bulb. In the presence of deformity of the duodenal bulb, edema of the folds, or postoperative deformity, ulcer craters may be very difficult to detect.[266, 267] False positive results occur when barium is trapped between folds; therefore, it is important to document that the configuration of a suspected crater is constant on multiple x-rays. Important variables in detecting ulcers are the technique, skill, and interest of the radiologist and the ability of the patient to fully cooperate.[266, 268, 269] With routine radiographic techniques 50 per cent of duodenal ulcers may be missed,[270, 271] whereas with optimal biphasic radiography, using compression and even hypotonic duodenography, 80 to 90 per cent of ulcer craters can be detected.[266, 272, 273] The sensitivity of individual examiners for detecting ulcers varies between 44 and 80 per cent,[268] with increased sensitivity obtained at the cost of an increased false positive rate. Lesion size can also be an important variable, with lesions less than 0.5 cm being difficult to detect reliably.[268] Double-contrast radiography is somewhat more sensitive than single-contrast technique,[266] although the difference in some studies is modest.[268] A combined technique including compression spot views with the bulb filled with barium can improve detection of anterior ulcers.[266, 268]

Endoscopy. Endoscopy with flexible, fiberoptic instruments provides a sensitive, specific, and safe method for diagnosing peptic ulcers.[258] Endoscopy, allowing direct inspection and biopsy, detects superficial lesions such as erosions, inflammatory conditions such as Crohn's disease, and the rare duodenal ulcer resulting from carcinoma of the duodenum or pancreas. Determining the sensitivity of endoscopy depends upon the gold standard used for comparison; experienced endoscopists probably detect 85 to 95 per cent of gastroduodenal lesions, failing to detect 5 to 10 per cent of lesions found by a second endoscopist, by radiography, or at surgery.[269, 270, 272] The specificity of endoscopy is generally greater than 90 per cent.[269, 270] Enlarged folds and spasm may obscure ulcer visualization at endoscopy. The use of glucagon or anticholinergic agents to reduce duodenal spasm may increase the endoscopic yield, as well as the radiographic yield.

The risks of upper endoscopy are low, but real.[258] In a 1974 survey of American Society for Gastrointestinal Endoscopy members, data from 211,410 procedures indicated a complication rate of 0.13 per cent. Major complications were perforation (0.03 per cent); bleeding (0.03 per cent); cardiopulmonary complications (0.06 per cent), and infection (0.008 per cent). Predisposition to cardiopulmonary complications resulted from underlying medical conditions and was often precipitated by drug reactions to topical anesthetics or sedation (laryngeal spasm, respiratory arrest, hypotension, and even postendoscopy, sedation-related automobile accidents). The complication rate will obviously vary with the nature and severity of illness in the patient population and with the experience of the endoscopic team.

Comparison of Endoscopy and Radiography. Several studies have compared the ability of endoscopy and radiography to detect ulcer craters. Routine single-contrast radiography of the duodenal bulb by resident radiologists detected from 36 to 50 per cent of the duodenal ulcers found by endoscopy.[270, 271] In another study in which faculty radiologists performed or directly supervised radiography using a biphasic technique (barium-filled and air-contrast views) plus compression, x-ray studies had a 57 per cent predictive value for detection of duodenal ulcer compared to endoscopy.[274] In dedicated hands, double-contrast radiography coupled with hypotonic duodenography detected 82 per cent of duodenal ulcers found at surgery, compared to 88 per cent detected by endoscopy.[272] The sensitivity of radiography versus endoscopy has been assessed by determining the false negative rate of radiography in patients presenting with dyspepsia; of 140 dyspeptic patients with normal double-contrast radiography, only three had gastric or duodenal ulcers at subsequent endoscopy.[273] Of patients with typical ulcer pain and a negative single-contrast x-ray, 8.7 per cent had DU on endoscopy, while another 5.4 per cent had duodenitis.[275] In optimal conditions radiography may detect nearly as many duodenal ulcers as endoscopy; however, when other gastroduodenal lesions were considered, radiography had a sensitivity of 54 per cent, compared to 92 per cent for endoscopy.[269]

Choices in Diagnosing Duodenal Ulcers

The goal in evaluating a patient with upper gastrointestinal symptoms is to expediently arrive at definitive diagnosis when significant disease exists, without exposing patients to costly and potentially risky diagnostic procedures when unnecessary. The first decision is whether and when to perform endoscopy or radiography in a patient with upper abdominal complaints. Initial clinical evaluation can often discriminate patients with heartburn suggesting esophageal reflux or symptoms suggesting biliary tract disease; endoscopy is not the first line approach in these patients. Other patients presenting with dyspepsia may have clinical features which suggest an increased risk of significant disease, such as weight loss, evidence of systemic illness, or complications such as GI bleeding or obstruction, which would justify immediate diagnostic evaluation. Other factors, such as the age of the patient (and thus the risk of carcinoma), and the length and intensity of symptoms, may also mitigate for more rapid evaluation. However, in patients with simple dyspepsia, especially those under 50 years old with a new onset of symptoms, an argument can be made to pursue an initial trial of therapy with antacids or H_2 blockers, and defer diagnostic procedures. Many of these patients will respond to therapy or to time, with resolution of symptoms. In those patients whose symptoms do not respond after a few weeks, and in patients whose symptoms recur or are improved but not resolved after a standard course of therapy, definitive evaluation is indicated.[258, 276] The yield of definitive diagnostic studies depends upon the specific case; endoscopy in patients under 40 years old has a lower yield compared to procedures performed in patients over 65, or in patients referred because of abnormal radiography, suspicion of malignancy, or upper GI bleeding.[277] Dyspepsia in a 27-year-old graduate student preparing for oral examinations may require only reassurance and follow-up, while the new onset of symptoms in a 60-year-old patient requires thorough evaluation. In some patients, initial evaluation may be deferred pending, for example, response to withdrawal of an anti-inflammatory drug or a therapeutic trial. A major risk of deferring evaluation is that some patients may be lost to follow-up, rather than returning for evaluation of persistent or recurrent symptoms.

The choice of diagnostic procedures to evaluate gastroduodenal disease depends upon several patient variables, as well as the available facilities and technical expertise. Double-contrast radiography in skilled hands will detect many of the lesions found at endoscopy. However, the overall sensitivity and specificity of endoscopy has been consistently superior to radiography in detecting ulcers (especially small ulcers or ulcers in a deformed bulb), erosions, and inflammatory lesions and in allowing biopsy. The cost of the two procedures is an important consideration, and varies considerably among localities.[256] The lesser cost makes radiography in skilled hands an acceptable screening procedure in some instances. However, endoscopy is the diagnostic procedure of choice for most suspected disorders of the upper GI tract. Patients express little preference between radiography and endoscopy.[267, 278]

In the past, it has been a common practice to perform radiography before endoscopy, with the expectation that radiography would provide valuable information for the endoscopist. In controlled studies, x-ray knowledge of radiographic findings has not enhanced the sensitivity or specificity of subsequent endoscopy.[258, 267, 279] Radiography as a second procedure infrequently reveals lesions in endoscopy-negative patients, unless technical difficulties circumvented a complete endoscopic examination. Adding endoscopy to high-quality, double-contrast radiography is indicated when symptoms remain unexplained or abnormalities are detected that required biopsy or further evaluation. Endoscopy can be expected to substantially increase the detection of ulcers in situations in which the sensitivity of radiography is compromised, such as a deformed duodenal bulb or enlarged folds or in a postoperative stomach. Performing radiography after endoscopy is unlikely to add information that will alter management, and therefore rarely warrants the added cost and patient inconvenience.

Once the diagnosis of DU has been made, endoscopy is not indicated to follow patients who become symptom-free or to routinely evaluate symptomatic recurrences that mimic the initial episode. However, if symptoms persist despite compliance with medical therapy, endoscopy may reveal the presence of another disease process (e.g., gastritis, duodenitis, or carcinoma) or the presence of a persistent ulcer crater that may warrant a change in management or consideration of surgery. With giant duodenal ulcers, or ulcers presenting with complications, endoscopy is warranted to monitor healing in response to therapy. For example, in an elderly patient with a history of duodenal ulcer complicated by hemorrhage or perforation and with contraindications to surgery, it is reasonable to repeat endoscopy to monitor ulcer status in response to initial and maintenance therapy.

It is both satisfying for the physician to make a definitive diagnosis and a relief for the patient to know the origins of symptoms, and occasionally such diagnostic successes influence therapy or eventual outcome. In one series, upper panendoscopy changed the diagnosis in 45 per cent of 84 patients and revealed two unsuspected carcinomas; management was altered in 44 per cent of patients, but not always in response to a change in diagnosis.[278] In another series, about 50 per cent of 1526 consecutive endoscopies confirmed significant abnormalities and about 30 per cent of endoscopies led to unexpected diagnostic or therapeutic consequences.[277]

Atypical Duodenal Ulcers

Giant Duodenal Ulcers. Most duodenal ulcers are less than 1 cm in diameter, but when greater than 2 cm in diameter, these giant ulcers create unique problems for the patient and for the clinician. The symptomatology of giant duodenal ulcer has not been carefully studied, but moderate to severe upper abdominal pain radiating to the back is often present. In some cases, giant duodenal ulcers present with a prolonged, typical DU history, although in some cases there may be few, if any, previous symptoms suggesting ulcer disease. Giant duodenal ulcers are usually on the posterior wall and are frequently complicated by bleeding and posterior penetration and, to a lesser extent, by pyloric obstruction. Surprisingly, the diagnosis is delayed in up to one third of the cases, largely because of difficulty making an accurate radiologic diagnosis.[280, 281] Giant duodenal ulcer may mimic a deformed bulb or diverticulum, and diagnosis requires close attention to the shape, rigidity, contractions, and mucosal pattern of the duodenal bulb. Postbulbar narrowing is frequent, and filling defects, often due to thrombi, may be noted. Endoscopy provides the diagnosis in most cases, although the extent of the ulceration may not be appreciated and the lesion may be interpreted as severe erosive duodenitis. The potential for complications is underlined by reports of mortality rates as high as 40 per cent in earlier series.[280–283] Medical management is often more difficult than with ordinary DU, although reports of response to newer treatment modalities remain limited. Therapeutic responses to H_2 blockers occur,[284, 285] but slow healing and recurrences even on maintenance therapy are common. The utility of the more potent H_2 blockers, omeprazole, and other modalities remains to be tested in a comparative fashion.

Pyloric Channel Ulcers. Ulcers located in the pyloric channel may have a unique presentation characterized by pain occurring shortly after eating, poor relief by antacids, and vomiting, the latter often reflecting pyloric obstruction.[286] In one series, patients with pyloric channel ulcers were more likely to undergo operation than were those with ulcers in the duodenal bulb,[182] suggesting that pyloric channel ulcers follow a complicated course. Underlining the potential for complications of juxtapyloric ulcers, 55 per cent of 89 patients with ulcers at or within 2 cm of the pylorus presented with either perforation or bleeding; obstructed patients were excluded from this series.[287] Juxtapyloric ulcers may also have an increased tendency for recurrence either on maintenance H_2 blocker therapy or following highly selective vagotomy.[287]

Postbulbar Ulcers. Generally, ulcers in the duodenum are located within 2 to 3 cm of the pylorus. Ulcers located more distally have been found in 10 per cent on a necropsy series, although only 15 of 4016 radiographic examinations found ulcers in more distal sites.[288] Whereas ulcers in the immediate postbulbar area have not been associated with increased acid secretion, ulcers in the more distal duodenum or even proximal jejunum are almost invariably associated with a hypersecretory state, such as gastrinoma. Symptoms of postbulbar ulcers may be severe but are generally indistinguishable from ordinary DU. The reported cases have frequent complications, although patient selection limits valid comparisons. In reported postbulbar ulcers, bleeding may occur in up to 60 per cent;[288, 289] intractability and obstruction, but not perforation, are also common. Both endoscopy and radiography may miss postbulbar ulcers; an area of narrowing or apparent spasm may be the only finding, in which case hypotonic duodenography using atropine

or glucagon, possibly with air contrast, may be needed to reveal the ulcer. Differential diagnosis should include diverticuli, adhesive bands, annular pancreas, and neoplasia of the pancreas and rarely duodenum. There are insufficient data in the literature to comment on the response of postbulbar ulcers to medical management, but ulcers occurring with gastrinomas generally respond well to vigorous medical management (see p. 917).

NATURAL HISTORY

Clinical trials performed in the last several years to test new therapeutic modalities have greatly increased our knowledge of the course of duodenal ulcer disease. However, a great deal remains to be learned before physicians will be able to predict outcome and choose the most appropriate therapy for an individual patient.

Patients who present with epigastric pain may delay weeks or years before seeking medical advice. More than 50 per cent of ulcer patients have had symptoms for more than two years before presentation, indicating the relatively mild and tolerable nature of their symptoms. As noted earlier, symptoms usually recur, appearing in clusters with intervening asymptomatic periods that may last a few months to a few years.[290] Bardhan, following patients for 12 months after documented DU healing, observed that without medical treatment 26 per cent of patients remained symptom-free, 33 per cent had one relapse, 24 per cent had two recurrences, and 17 per cent experienced three or more recurrences.[291] The placebo-treated control groups drawn from several other clinical trials of maintenance therapy also indicate that 50 to 80 per cent of patients will experience an ulcer recurrence during the six to 12 months following initial ulcer healing (Fig. 47–11).[291–294] These recurrences often produce symptoms, although asymptomatic ulcers are frequently found at surveillance endoscopy, and some patients develop symptoms without a recurrent ulcer crater. These data are largely drawn from patients studied at tertiary referral centers and thus may reflect a population with more severe duodenal ulcer disease than is found in the community in general. Patients vary considerably in their tendency to develop recurrent ulcers; patients whose ulcers healed rapidly on placebo or H_2 blocker therapy were found to have a lower recurrence rate than patients whose ulcers required longer to heal.[295, 296]

Thus, duodenal ulcers rapidly and frequently recur in many patients following initial ulcer healing. However, recurrences may not continue indefinitely, especially in a primary care patient patient population. Fry, following his general practice patients with duodenal ulcer, observed that the severity of symptoms was maximal for about eight years after presentation, whereas by ten years 60 per cent of his patients were asymptomatic and only 5 per cent had severe symptoms.[297] Fifteen years after presentation, 76 per cent were symptom-free. Another series composed of DU

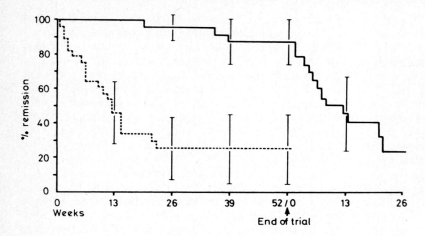

Figure 47–11. Duodenal ulcer recurrence during follow-up. The percentage of patients who remain in remission during follow-up therapy on either placebo *(dashed line)* or cimetidine therapy *(solid line)* are shown. For the 52 weeks of the trial, 12 per cent of the cimetidine-treated patients experienced symptomatic recurrence, compared with 75 per cent of the placebo-treated patients. Note that the rate of ulcer recurrence following discontinuation of cimetidine therapy at 52 weeks paralleled the initial rate found for placebo-treated patients. (From Gudmand-Høyer, E., Birger-Jensen, K., Krag, E., et al. Br. Med. J. *1:*1095, 1978. Used by permission.)

patients randomly selected from subjects with positive upper gastrointestinal radiographs also yielded data questioning the adage "once an ulcer, always an ulcer."[298] Patients were followed for 13 years, at which time 68 per cent were either asymptomatic or had mild symptoms. Only 12 per cent had moderate to severe symptoms; 20 per cent had undergone operations for duodenal ulcer.[298] In this latter study, cases diagnosed in general practice followed a milder course than those diagnosed in a hospital, although the difference was small. Thus, depending upon population selection, about two thirds of DU patients may experience disease "burnout" over a 10- to 15-year period. Data from trials with low-dose maintenance therapy to prevent recurrences also indicate that recurrences tend to be higher during the first year of the trial, with lower rates occurring during the subsequent two to three years.[296, 299] The ability to select these fortunate patients who will have their disease burnout spontaneously or be easily managed by low-dose maintenance would greatly influence decisions regarding medical or surgical therapy.

Therapeutic decisions will also rest upon the anticipated risk of major complications and the ultimate complication, death, but these risks in an unselected patient population cannot be predicted. Fourteen per cent of Fry's patients developed hemorrhage and 8 per cent developed perforation during the 15-year follow-up period,[297] indicating a yearly complication rate of about 1.5 per cent. In a series of male DU patients followed for eight years on no therapy, complication rates were about 2.7 per cent per year for those without prior complications.[300] In this series patients with duodenal and gastric ulcers had similar complication rates, with the exception that patients with combined DU and GU fared less well. Bonnevie estimates that the lifetime risk of serious complications of duodenal ulcers is about 20 per cent;[301] assuming that ulcer disease is active for eight to 15 years,[297, 298] these data also suggest that 1 to 3 per cent of DU patients develop complications during the course of a year. Of interest, patients with a prior history of complications did not demonstrate an increased risk of complications when placed on maintenance therapy.[296, 299] An optimist would interpret these latter data to suggest that maintenance therapy markedly reduces complication rates for those patients able to comply with therapy.

Bonnevie[301] found that life expectancy by actuarial analysis for duodenal ulcer patients is modestly decreased only during the first year or two after diagnosis. This decrease was limited to patients over 50 years of age who were first diagnosed in the hospital. Patients with combined duodenal and gastric ulcer disease had a somewhat increased mortality rate.[301] The benign nature of duodenal ulcer in general practice is reflected in the occurrence of only one DU-related death among the 265 patients followed by Fry for up to 15 years.[297] Duodenal ulcer mortality rates reflect the consequences of complications or of surgery. DU is a common disorder and most patients who die with duodenal ulcers have multiple diseases and die of other causes. However, ascertaining primary and secondary causes from death certificates may be misleading. Despite these considerations, statistics are unnecessary to convince a clinician that a patient presenting with a massive hematemesis or septic shock following ulcer perforation is at risk of dying from ulcer disease.

MEDICAL TREATMENT

The Data Base for Clinical Judgments Regarding Therapy

Double-blind, randomized clinical trials (RCT), utilizing fiberoptic endoscopy to document the status of an ulcer crater during the therapeutic period, have begun to provide a basis for rational decisions regarding the management of duodenal ulcer. These trials are not perfect tools and some caution is necessary in extrapolating the knowledge gained to clinical practice.[302] These RCT have been performed on selected patient populations, often collected at referral centers, and therefore these patients may not reflect those encountered in the community practice of medicine. One major variable is the length of time it takes for patients to seek medical care and to be referred to and arrive at the center conducting the RCT; many ulcers spontaneously heal in two to four weeks and those persisting long enough to arrive at tertiary centers may be a more difficult variety of ulcer.

Symptoms often provide misleading information about the ulcer status, since as many as 30 per cent of patients in symptomatic remission still harbor a persisting ulcer crater. Endoscopy has thus become the gold standard of ulcer healing, but classifying persisting erosions or duodenitis is problematic. With the focus of endoscopy on the status of the crater, many clinically significant aspects of ulcer disease often receive less attention. The goals of therapy in clinical practice are not only to heal ulcer craters but also to relieve pain, treat and prevent complications, minimize ulcer recurrences, reduce untoward consequences of diagnosis and therapy, and minimize the costs of medical care and the time lost from work. The benefit to the patient of ensuring that all duodenal ulcers have healed and remain healed is questionable. This situation contrasts with that of gastric ulcer patients, in whom the risk of carcinoma dictates monitoring healing of the ulcer crater.

Factors That Influence Ulcer Healing

As with most aspects of medicine, the natural history of the disease process may have a greater impact on outcome than the efforts expended and drugs prescribed by practitioners. The natural history of duodenal ulcers varies from spontaneous healing in a few weeks to ulcers that are refractory to months of full-dose therapy. As alluded to above, the outcome of trials will be influenced by the proportion of slow-healing and fast-healing ulcers that have been included. These factors will be reflected in the rate of placebo-induced ulcer healing that varies from 24 to 75 per cent in different trials (Fig. 47–12).[302–304] Many variables have been proposed to influence the spontaneous rate of ulcer healing. The following section will consider these variables, because eliminating factors such as NSAID use or cigarette smoking may be as effective as prescribing therapeutically active drugs.[44]

Smoking. There is no doubt that smoking impairs the healing of duodenal ulcers, promotes recurrences, and increases the risk of complications. Impaired duodenal ulcer healing in smokers compared to nonsmokers has been found in numerous studies,[44, 58, 59, 228, 305–307] although an occasional exception has been reported.[308] The differences between smokers and nonsmokers are most dramatic in placebo-treated groups. Active therapy with most drugs (H$_2$ blockers, prostaglandins, antacids, sucralfate, colloidal bismuth, etc.) generally reduces—but does not always eliminate—the deleterious effects of smoking. Lam argues that misoprostol[309] and sucralfate[307] more effectively reverse the deleterious effects of smoking on healing than do antisecretory agents. However, the data supporting a particular advantage for any specific agent in smokers are too limited to allow firm conclusions to be drawn.[310] Underlining the impact of cigarettes, nonsmoking was a

more important predictive factor in the healing of duodenal ulcers than was treatment with H$_2$ blockers.[44]

The impact of smoking on ulcer recurrence rates is also dramatic, especially in the placebo group.[44, 304, 311] Smoking, placebo-treated patients have a yearly recurrence rate of 72 per cent, compared to a rate of 21 per cent in their nonsmoking counterparts (Fig. 47–13).[312] Maintenance therapy with active drugs reduces recurrences in smokers, but even on maintenance drug therapy, recurrences are generally greater in smokers than in nonsmokers. Another convincing aspect of the association between smoking and DU is the correlation with the quantity of cigarettes smoked; a minimal risk with fewer than 10 cigarettes smoked daily has been reported, whereas in those who smoke above 30 cigarettes daily, healing is markedly impaired and recurrences in three months can reach 100 per cent.[59, 313–315]

Smoking may also be a risk factor for ulcer complications, an expected result if smoking impairs healing and promotes recurrences. Eighty-seven per cent of patients presenting with duodenal ulcer perforations were smokers. Smokers also accounted for 80 per cent of patients undergoing ulcer operations, and the reduced life expectancy after gastric surgery was strongly associated with smoking related disorders.[59, 60]

The mechanisms have been proposed for the deleterious effects of smoking on ulcer disease, including increased gastric emptying promoting duodenal acidification, increased basal and maximal acid secretion, decreased pancreatic bicarbonate secretion, altered gastroduodenal motility leading to reflux of duodenal contents, increased pepsinogen I secretion, and altered blood flow.[312, 316, 317] Decreased effectiveness of antisecretory agents has been proposed as a mechanism for the relative resistance of smokers to healing and main-

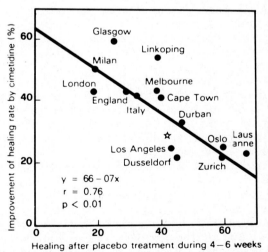

Figure 47–12. The improvement in healing with cimetidine as a function of placebo healing rates. Data from clinical trials comparing cimetidine with placebo were plotted, expressing the percentage improvement in healing above placebo rates with cimetidine treatment as a function of the placebo healing rates. There is an obvious inverse relationship between improvement with cimetidine and the placebo healing rates. (From Bianchi Porro, G., and Petrillo, M. Scand. J. Gastroenterol. *21*(suppl. 121):46, 1986. Used with permission.)

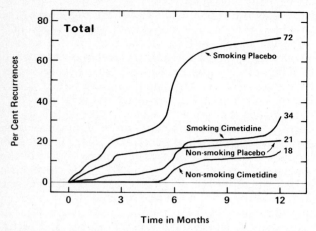

Figure 47–13. Ulcer recurrences in patients according to smoking history and treatment group. Patients with healed duodenal ulcers were entered in a 12-month trial comparing the effects of placebo and cimetidine treatment on recurrence rates. Illustrated is the percentage of patients presenting with either symptomatic or asymptomatic recurrences during the trial. Note that the highest recurrence rates occurred in smoking, placebo-treated patients. Smokers who received cimetidine maintenance recurred at a rate comparable with placebo-treated nonsmokers. (From Sontag, S., Graham, D. Y., Belsito, A., et al. N. Engl. J. Med. *311*:689, 1984. Used with permission.)

tenance therapy,[318] but these effects have not been consistently found. Smoking also decreases gastric mucosal prostaglandin production,[319, 320] possibly impairing ulcer healing and promoting ulcer recurrence.

Although no data establish that the cessation of smoking will return healing and recurrence rates to normal, this outcome is likely and provides yet another reason to encourage patients to stop smoking.

Aspirin and Other NSAIDs. Since aspirin and other NSAIDs cause gastric erosions and ulcers, promote bleeding, and appear to be a risk factor for duodenal ulcers (see discussion of risk factors, p. 818), there is sufficient reason to interdict use of NSAIDs in DU patients. Healing of duodenal ulcers can take place despite continued NSAID use,[321, 322] although the healing may be impaired.[323] A variable in healing may be the finding that 24-hour antisecretory therapy was more effective reversing the adverse effects of NSAIDs on DU healing than was inhibition of only nocturnal acid secretion.[321] Prostaglandin analogues have a theoretical advantage in treating and preventing NSAID-related ulcers,[324] but comparative trails with antisecretory agents have not been reported.

Beverage Consumption. Coffee is a strong stimulant of acid secretion and a cause of dyspepsia, but not a known risk factor for ulcer disease. Decaffeinated coffee and many other beverages are also strong acid secretagogues (see p. 817). Based upon these considerations, the physician could get trapped into recommending elimination of all beverages that are strong secretagogues, thus restricting a patient to little more than bread and water. It is more reasonable to recommend moderation in the consumption of coffee and related secretagogues, especially on an empty stomach.

Many patients are told to stop drinking alcohol, although there are no data to indicate that modest alcohol consumption retards ulcer healing. To the contrary, one study suggests that moderate alcohol intake promotes ulcer healing.[44] Alcohol abuse, on the other hand, may interfere with healing.[314]

Diet. Before the advent of specific therapy for duodenal ulcer, dietary manipulations were utilized, although support for their effect on duodenal ulcer healing was scant.[325] Frequent feedings, justified on the basis that small meals may reduce gastric distention, actually increased acid secretion. Bedtime snacks stimulate nocturnal acid secretion. A bland diet was prescribed, largely because spices and fruit juices produced dyspepsia in some subjects. However, investigators, appropriately from Texas, have found that red and black peppers cause acute gastric mucosal injury comparable to that produced by aspirin;[326] whether ingestion of pepper or other spices actually impairs ulcer healing is unknown, but avoiding substances that produce dyspepsia is safe advice to give to a duodenal ulcer patient. Milk, because of its soothing nature, was a mainstay of therapy until it was shown to be a strong secretogogue, largely because of its calcium and protein.[327] Milk thus stimulates more acid secretion than it buffers and is not an effective antacid. Recent studies have indicated that the phospsholipids in milk may have some protective properties against acute acid-induced damage in the rat.[328] Growth factors similar to epidermal growth factor have been isolated from human milk and found to protect against cysteamine-induced duodenal ulcers in mice. Despite this scientific support for the dairy industry, one controlled study compared ulcer healing in patients placed on cimetidine (1 gm daily) and then randomized to a normal diet or a diet supplemented with 2 liters of milk daily.[329] Pain relief was comparable in the two groups, but ulcers healed in 78 per cent of patients on the normal diet, compared to 53 per cent of patients on the milk-supplemented diet. Spiro[330] argues that since milk and a bland diet "often" produce subjective benefit in patients with dyspepsia, their use should not be discarded solely because of a lack of scientific validation. However, DU patients should be cautioned that milk is not an antacid nor specific therapy for their ulcer.

A resurgence of interest in dietary therapy has focused upon the dietary fiber content. Two controlled trials have indicated that recurrence rates are significantly higher on a low-fiber than on a high-fiber diet (see p. 817).[32, 34] No effects of fiber on ulcer healing were found in a trial in which patients were placed on low-dose antacid tablets four times daily and then randomized to either a high- or low-fiber diet. Healing rates in both groups were above 60 per cent in four weeks, probably reflecting the influence of the antacids (see p. 848).[331] Low-fiber diets may enhance recurrence rates, although the mechanisms involved remain unknown.

Acid Secretion. There is little doubt that acid-peptic activity is a causal factor or at least a permissive factor for ulcer formation. Therefore, one might anticipate that measuring acid output might predict ulcer healing rates; negative correlations between healing and maximal acid output have been reported.[313, 314, 332] However, this relationship is not evident in other studies, possibly because other variables are important, such as nocturnal duodenal pH or factors that influence mucosal resistance, such as concomitant *C. pylori* infection.

Most studies have allowed supplemental antacids as needed for pain, and since very low dose antacid consumption can hasten ulcer healing, antacid consumption can be an important variable in placebo healing rates.

Time Profile of the Ulcer Disease. There is controversy about whether the length of the symptomatic period prior to presentation is an important variable in predicting ulcer healing rates.[44, 305] There are conflicting data regarding whether patients with long-standing ulcer disease will have slow healing either on placebo or active drug.[44, 305 333, 334]

Characteristics of the Ulcer. As noted earlier (see p. 841), certain characteristics of the ulcer may influence healing rates. Longer healing times will obviously be necessary for larger ulcers, and some investigators have reported an overall negative correlation between healing and ulcer size.[313, 332] Prepyloric ulcers and pyloric channel ulcers appear to heal with more reluctance than do ulcers in the duodenum.[287, 335] Some studies have found this difference only in the placebo group,[332] whereas other have not found therapy to reverse the slow healing of prepyloric ulcers.[335] Stenosis of the duodenal bulb, detected at endoscopy, has also been associated with impaired healing.[305] Patients harboring both gastric and duodenal ulcers may also have delayed healing.[300]

Sex and Age. Young females may heal better than young males.[44] Overall, the effect of age is variable.[228, 336] Disease with an onset in youth and with a positive history may be associated with poor healing.[79, 314] Elderly patients with DU often fare less well; they more often present without abdominal pain, are more likely to bleed and rebleed, require more transfusions, and have a prolonged hospital stay.[337]

Psychodynamic Factors Including the Physician-Patient Relationship. Psychosocial factors and the clinical setting may influence not only perception of symptoms but also ulcer healing rates. The physician-patient relationship may be an important variable; one study found that the duration of pain during a recurrence varied significantly among patients treated by different physicians.[338] Participation in a clinical trial and administration of a placebo may influence healing, but this possibility is difficult to test. Stressful life situations, such as occupational, financial, and family problems, have been reported to be more frequent in patients with duodenal ulcers that required longer than six weeks to heal.[339]

Psychodynamic factors should be assessed in the initial evaluation of a patient with chronic abdominal pain, as insight into these factors may guide the diagnostic as well as the therapeutic approach. The impor-

tance of psychosomatic mechanisms in the pathogenesis of duodenal ulcer remains unclear, and psychotherapy has not been shown to alter the course of ulcer disease. Therefore, psychotherapeutic intervention should be reserved for those patients in whom it is indicated on independent grounds. Because psychodynamic factors are so frequently present in patients presenting with chronic abdominal pain,[240] careful psychologic evaluation is indicated for most, if not all, patients presenting with ulcer or non-ulcer dyspepsia.

Pharmacology of the Drugs Used to Treat Ulcer Disease

H$_2$ Receptor Antagonists. Three H$_2$ receptor antagonists—cimetidine (Tagamet), ranitidine (Zantac), and famotidine (Pepcid)—have been approved by the FDA for use in the United States. These agents are specific receptor antagonists that inhibit acid secretion by blocking histamine H$_2$ receptors on the parietal cell.

Cimetidine shares the imidazole ring structure of histamine itself. Cimetidine is well absorbed in the small intestine and reaches a peak blood level in 45 to 90 minutes, with a two-hour half-life. About 50 per cent of the oral dose is excreted unchanged by the kidneys with the remainder being excreted after metabolism into a sulfoxide. The renal excretion of cimetidine accounts for the recommendation that the dose be reduced by 50 per cent in the face of renal failure.[340] Postmarketing surveillance of cimetidine has indicated it to be a very safe drug,[341] although several side effects have been reported,[340, 342] as noted below.

Ranitidine is chemically quite different from cimetidine, based upon a furan ring instead of an imidazole ring structure. In contrast to cimetidine, about 50 per cent of a ranitidine dose is eliminated by hepatic metabolism, and therefore, impaired hepatic capacity to metabolize drugs will increase the half-life or ranitidine. Such effects have been found in both cirrhotic and elderly subjects;[343] dose reduction might be necessary in such patients, except that ranitidine is essentially free of dose-related adverse effects.[344]

Famotidine is chemically distinct from both ranitidine and cimetidine, being based upon a thiazole ring structure. About 70 per cent of the drug is eliminated intact in the urine.[345] With severe renal failure (creatinine clearance <10 ml/min), the daily dose of famotidine should be reduced from 40 to 20 mg. No dosage adjustment is necessary with hepatic failure. Famotidine is a long-acting but competitive H$_2$ antagonist, with an antisecretory potency of about five to eight times that of ranitidine and 50 to 80 times that of cimetidine. Peak antisecretory activity is reached one to three hours after ingestion of a 40 mg oral dose, and activity persists for 10 to 12 hours.[346] Intravenous administration produces a similar time for the antisecretory effects, but with twice the potency of oral administration.

Side Effects of H$_2$ Receptor Antagonists

Antiandrogenic Effects. Cimetidine has dose-dependent antiandrogen effects leading to gynecomastia and impotence. Gynecomastia is rare with less than eight weeks of therapy at normal doses of cimetidine and occurred in only 0.2 per cent of patients treated for 26 weeks.[347] The majority of cases of gynecomastia and impotence reported with cimetidine have been during therapy for hypersecretory disorders in which higher doses are used for prolonged time periods. Gynecomastia and impotence have been reported rarely with ranitidine therapy, and when patients with hypersecretory disorders are switched from cimetidine to ranitidine, the untoward antiandrogen effects usually resolve.[347] Hyperprolactinemia can occur with intravenous injection of 300 mg of cimetidine and with intravenous doses of ranitidine above 100 mg.[347] Neither drug given orally produces hyperprolactinemia. In general, the endocrine side effects of both drugs are probably qualitatively, but not quantitatively, similar. These endocrine effects have little clinical impact, in ordinary DU at normal doses, in that they rarely occur as side effects in clinical trials.

Drug Interactions. Cimetidine inhibits cytochrome P_{450} and therefore interferes with drugs metabolized by this pathway, including the benzodiazepines, diazepam, and chlordiazepoxide.[348] The metabolism of lorazepam and oxazepam, which are eliminated by glucuronidation, are not influenced by cimetidine. Warfarin, theophylline, propranolol, and phenytoin are also metabolized by cytochrome P_{450} and have clinically significant interactions with cimetidine. This inhibition is not due to the H_2 receptor, because ranitidine, which is more potent at the H_2 receptors, is tenfold less effective in inhibition cytochrome P_{450}-dependent mixed-function oxidases.[348, 349] Famotidine, at therapeutic doses appears free of effects on hepatic metabolism of drugs.[346, 349a] Increased toxicity of lidocaine has been reported during the initiation of infusions in patients on cimetidine;[350, 351] this latter effect may be due to reduced clearance and is probably not a result of decreased P_{450} metabolism. In light of these drug interactions, patients on drugs with a narrow therapeutic margin, such as phenytoin, warfarin, and theophylline, that are metabolized by the hepatic cytochrome P_{450} pathway should be treated with antiulcer agents other than cimetidine.

H_2 Receptor Effects on the Immune System. H_2 receptors have been identified on immune cells; interleukin-1 and -2 levels are reduced in patients on cimetidine therapy.[352] Patients on cimetidine have also been shown to have altered immunoregulation,[353] which may have an impact on rejection of kidney transplants and skin reactivity. Altered immune regulation was hypothesized as a causal factor in a case of polymyositis and nephropathy developing on cimetidine therapy.[353] During a controlled trial, the responsiveness of peripheral blood lymphocytes to mitogenic stimulation was found to be increased on cimetidine, but not ranitidine, therapy.[354] Others have reported that ranitidine altered T suppressor cell function.[355] The relative effects and the clinical significance of the various H_2 receptor antagonists on the immune system require further study.

Other Side Effects. CNS symptoms, including confusion, somnolence, and dizziness, have been reported with cimetidine. Altered mental status is noted particularly in elderly patients, in the ICU setting, and when compounded by renal or hepatic dysfunction.[356] These CNS effects are less frequent with ranitidine, although reported experience with ranitidine in the ICU setting is limited compared to cimetidine. Unusual reactions probably common to cimetidine and ranitidine include bone marrow depression, anaphylactoid reactions, interstitial nephritis, malaise, increases in serum creatinine or transaminases, and rare cases of hepatitis, all of which appear reversible. The small increases in serum creatinine probably reflect only minor changes in tubular function. Causality in the cases of hepatitis have been supported by rechallenge.[357, 358] Bradycardia, probably resulting from interaction with cardiac H_2 receptors, has occurred with the rapid infusion of H_2 blockers. Reversible headaches, which may be severe, have been reported with ranitidine therapy. Clinical experience with famotidine is limited, but based upon available data, untoward effects such as drug interactions or endocrine or CNS side effects appear to be minimal.[345, 346, 349a]

Omeprazole. Omeprazole is a substituted benzimidazole with a unique antisecretory action based upon inhibition of the parietal cell H^+/K^+-ATPase, the pump responsible for acid secretion.[359] This specific ATPase is present in the parietal cell membranes that line the apical surface and the tubulovesicles that fill the cytoplasm in the resting state. With stimulation, these tubulovesicles transform into secretory channels that drain into the lumen, thereby positioning the H^+/K^+-ATPase for the job of secreting acid. Being a weak base, omeprazole is absorbed at the alkaline pH in the small intestine and concentrated from the circulation by pH partition into the acidic tubulovesicular and canalicular compartments of the parietal cell. In an acid enviroment a sulfoxide metabolite of omeprazole is formed that irreversibly binds to the H^+/K^+-ATPase, thereby irreversibly inactivating the enzyme. Because omeprazole is acid-labile, it must be administered in an enteric-coated form. Omeprazole has a prolonged duration of antisecretory action, not because of its half-time in the circulation, but rather because of its irreversible inactivation of the parietal cell H^+/K^+-ATPase. The antisecretory action persists for between 24 and 72 hours. Probably as a result of increased absorption of the acid-labile drug after the antisecretory effect has been induced, bioavailability of omeprazole increases over five days of treatment.[360] Omeprazole inhibits acid secretion in humans over a dose range from 5 to 30 mg daily. A single 10-mg dose has little effect on acid secretion, but after five days a 93 per cent reduction in basal secretion and a 66 per cent reduction in pentagastrin-stimulated acid secretion was found.[361] After seven days of treatment with 10, 20, or 30 mg daily, 24-hour H^+ activity was decreased by 27, 90, and 97 per cent, respectively.[362] After a second week of therapy no further inhibition was observed, and no further inhibition was found at a dose of 60 mg daily, leading to the conclusion that the optimal acid secretory inhibition would be produced by a 20 to 30-mg daily dose. A 20-mg dose has been selected as the daily dose for treatment of DU. A variability in the inhibitory response is evident with doses of omeprazole below 20 mg. After seven days on the 10-mg dose, some patients have virtually no inhibition of acid secretion, while others experience greater than 90 per cent inhibition. Thus, the effects of the 10-mg dose are too variable to produce reliable clinical effects.[362, 363] The variability in response is less at omeprazole doses above 20 mg, but is still evident in the spread of gastric pH values obtained from patients after seven days on 30 mg of omeprazole daily (Fig. 47–14). Treatment of 10 DU patients with 20 mg of omeprazole daily for 8 days produced >99 per cent inhibition of 24-hour gastric acidity in 6 patients, but only about 50 per cent reduction in the other 4 patients. The patients with the reduced response to omeprazole had lower plasma concentrations of the drug, but whether this difference reflected inactivation by gastric acid, decreased absorption, or rapid degradation was not established.[363a]

Probably because the primary action of omeprazole only occurs after being concentrated and activated in the acidic compartments of the parietal cell, the drug appears free of significant side effects in short-term use, although clinical experience remains too limited to predict the spectrum of untoward effects. An elevation of liver enzymes was noted in one small, poorly controlled series. Other studies have failed to find abnormalities in liver function,[345, 346, 364] and thus far clinical hepatitis has not been reported. Altered diazepam, phenytoin, and 7-hydroxycoumarin metabolism has been found on omeprazole, suggesting interactions with the hepatic cytochrome P_{450},[346a] but the importance of drug interactions with omeprazole remains to be defined.

Omeprazole is undergoing clinical evaluation, but is not yet approved by the FDA for use in the United States.

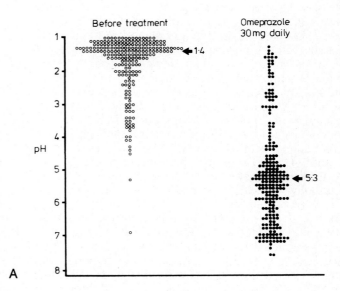

A

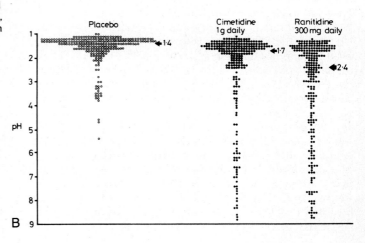

B

Figure 47–14. pH values of gastric aspirates before and during treatment with antisecretory agents. *A,* The pH of gastric juice aspirates was determined hourly in nine subjects before and after seven days of treatment with 30 mg of omeprazole daily. The arrows indicate the mean pH values. *B,* Hourly gastric aspirate pH values are shown for patients treated with placebo, cimetidine (1 gm daily), and ranitidine (300 mg daily). (From Walt, R. P., Gomes, M. F. A., Woods, E. C., et al. Br. Med. J. *287*:12, 1983. Used with permission.)

Nonselective and Selective Antimuscarinic Agents. Anticholinergics decrease basal gastric acid secretion by about 40 to 50 per cent and inhibit meal-stimulated gastric acid secretion by about 30 per cent.[365] Their use in acid peptic disorders has been limited by the well-recognized side effects, such as dry mouth, blurred vision, exacerbation of glaucoma, ileus, urinary retention, and tachycardia.

Pirenzepine is an inhibitor of acid secretion that also blocks muscarinic receptors. This compound is structurally related to the tricyclic antidepressants but is highly hydrophilic and its permeability across the blood-brain barrier is low.[366] Considerable evidence has been advanced that pirenzepine is a selective antimuscarinic agent that inhibits acid secretion with a greater relative potency than has been found for interaction with receptors on smooth muscle, heart, and salivary glands.[365, 367] Secretory inhibition by pirenzepine is of a similar magnitude to that found with nonselective anticholinergic agents. However, presumably because of presumed receptor selectivity, the usual therapeutic dosage (50 mg bid or tid) produces fewer typical cholinergic side effects (dry mouth, 14 per cent; blurred vision, 2 per cent) and few patients drop out of clinical studies as a result of side effects.[367] Pirenzepine is somewhat less effective than cimetidine in inhibiting basal and pentagastrin-stimulated acid secretion.[368, 369] Telenzepine, another selective antimuscarinic agent undergoing development, is four to twenty times more potent than pirenzepaine, but appears to have a similar relative specificity for muscarinic receptor subtypes and therefore has similar side effects at therapeutic dosages.[370] Pirenzepine and telenzepine are undergoing clinical trials; neither is yet approved for use in the United States.

Antacids. One of the few firm conclusions offered in the last edition of this textbook was that antacids healed duodenal ulcers by virtue of buffering gastric acid; even this conclusion must now be tempered with caution. Based upon the concept that optimal healing with antacids would occur with maximal buffering of gastric acid, a protocol was designed administering antacids one and three hours after meals and at bedtime, thus advantage was taken of the postprandial delay in gastric emptying, thereby extending the time antacids were present in the stomach buffering acid.[371] Because antacids are very rapidly emptied from the stomach, the nighttime dose provided essentially no reduction in nocturnal acid secretion.[372] In clinical trials antacids enhanced healing of DU to the same degree as did other active drugs, possibly indicating that decreasing acidity during daytime hours was sufficient to induce healing of most ordinary duodenal ulcers. Over the past several years, the doses of antacids have been decreased to as low as 120 mM of acid neutralizing capacity daily. With this modest capacity for acid neutralization,[373, 374] one may question whether "antacids" induce healing by mechanisms other than acid neutralization, such as binding of bile acids, or inactivation of pepsin.[375] An alternate hypothesis is that antacids enhance mucosal resistance to injury; a "cytoprotective" effect against alcohol injury has been found with two aluminum hydroxide–containing compounds, sucralfate and antacids, as well as with aluminum hydroxide and with aluminum sulfate alone.[376] Whether aluminum complexes, *per se*, influence the healing of duodenal ulcers in humans remains the subject of investigation.

Despite their apparent benignity as therapeutic agents, antacids have several side effects. Magnesium-containing antacids cause a dose-dependent diarrhea and hypermagnesemia, especially in the face of renal failure. Aluminum hydroxide blocks the intestinal absorption of phosphate, and in only two weeks of therapy with moderate doses, significant hypophosphatemia can develop, especially if the patient is on a low phosphate diet or is phosphate-depleted for other reasons.[377] Prolonged therapy with aluminum hydroxide can disrupt mineral metabolism, depleting phosphate and increasing urinary and fecal excretion of calcium, and eventually producing osteoporosis and osteomalacia.[378] Antacids may also contain considerable sodium, which can cause sodium overload in susceptible patients. Ingestion of large amounts of calcium and absorbable alkali, particularly calcium carbonate, can lead to hypercalcemia, alkalosis, and renal impairment, the milk-alkali syndrome.[379] Antacids also bind certain drugs, limiting their absorption, and this list of interacting drugs includes antibiotics, warfarin, digoxin, anticonvulsants, cimetidine, and anti-inflammatory drugs.[381]

Significant absorption of aluminum can occur even on low therapeutic doses. Patients consuming only 120 mM of antacid tablets daily show significant elevations of serum and urinary aluminum levels during four weeks of therapy (Fig. 47–15).[382] Aluminum is absorbed from several formulations.[383] Simultaneous consumption of citric acid markedly increased absorption of aluminum, with roughly tenfold elevations in serum aluminum concentration resulting from consumption of four Al-Mg tablets (120 mM neutralizing capacity).[382] Aluminum is generally excreted in the urine, but neurotoxicity can develop, especially in the setting of renal failure. It is uncertain to what extent aluminum deposition occurs in tissues with chronic use, but reports of aluminum deposits in brain tissue in Alzheimer's disease underline the need for caution and for more data. In light of the effect of citric acid on aluminum absorption, in the absence of further data, antacids should probably be taken alone or with water.

Patient compliance was a problem with the high-dose regimen, because of its cumbersome nature and because of the diarrhea that occurs in as many as 25 per cent of patients taking Al-Mg antacids. Reducing the dose of the magnesium-containing antacids[384] or alternating them with aluminum-containing antacids may reduce this problem. The incidence of diarrhea is reduced in the recent studies utilizing lower daily doses.[382, 385] The balance of aluminum and magnesium is different in different preparations, so that the choice of the specific Al-Mg antacid preparation may also influence the incidence of diarrhea.[385]

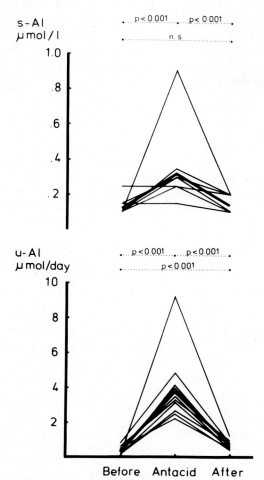

s-Al
μmol/l

p<0.001   p<0.001

n.s.

1.0

.8

.6

.4

.2

u-Al
μmol/day

p<0.001   p<0.001

p<0.001

10

8

6

4

2

Before   Antacid   After

Figure 47–15. Serum concentrations and urinary excretion of aluminium before, during, and after four weeks of antacid treatment. The dose of antacids was one tablet of aluminium-magnesium antacids four times daily. The after measurements were performed three to four days after cessation of therapy. Lines indicate values for 10 healthy subjects. Tablets were Link (1100 mg), with 30 mM buffering capacity. (From Berstad, A., and Weberg, R. Scand. J. Gastroenterol. *21*(suppl. 125):32, 1986. Used with permission.)

Prostaglandins. Prostaglandins are derived from 20-carbon oxygenated fatty acids, converted by cyclooxygenase to a five-carbon ring plus a seven-carbon and an eight-carbon side chain. Prostaglandins are produced by the gastroduodenal mucosa and play a role in mucosal resistance to injury, but their importance to the pathogenesis of duodenal ulcer remain uncertain (see p. 830). Prostaglandins particularly of the E and I group inhibit acid secretion acting directly on the parietal cell to selectively inhibit histamine-stimulated cyclic AMP production. Prostaglandin receptors appear to interact with the inhibitory GTP (guanosine triphosphate) binding protein of adenylate cyclase, thus reducing cyclic AMP production.[386] Under certain circumstances, prostaglandins also enhance gastric mucosal resistance to injury by mechanisms independent of their antisecretory properties (see p. 782).

The naturally occurring prostaglandins are unstable, being metabolized primarily by hydroxylation at the 15 position on the eight-carbon side chain. Several analogues have been synthesized with modified structure on this side chain to provide resistance to degradation. Topical action appears critical in that oral administration gives greater antisecretory efficacy and fewer side effects that does systemic administration.[387] Prostanoids that have been under study include misoprostol, enprostil, rioprostil, timoprostil, and arboprostil; none are yet approved by the FDA for clinical use for duodenal ulcer in the United States.

Misoprostol (Cytotec) is a 15-deoxy-15-hydroxy-16-methyl analogue of prostaglandin E_1. Misoprostol shares the properties of other E type prostaglandins, displaying a moderate inhibition of basal and food-stimulated acid secretion in humans.[388, 389] Enprostil is a 15-dehydro analogue of PGE_2 that has a high potency and duration of antisecretory actions compared to natural prostanoids.[387, 390] Although structurally related, there are subtle differences in the actions of these prostanoids on gastric function, such as the ability of high concentrations of PGE_2 and misoprosol, but not enprostil, to stimulate adenylate cyclase and the ability of enprostil, but not misoprostol, to inhibit gastrin release.[386, 391] These E-type prostanoids enhance mucosal resistance to injury in animal models,[387, 392] but the relevance of such actions to the therapy of acid peptic lesions in man remains unclear.[156, 393] Endoscopic studies demonstrated that both misoprostol and enprostil prevent NSAID-induced injury to gastroduodenal mucosa in humans.[394, 395] The protective effects of misoprostol against NSAID-induced endoscopic damage are dose-dependent over a range from 25 to 200 μg (F. E. Silverstein, personal communication). However, this range also produces the antisecretory actions of misoprostol, making it difficult to restablish protective effects independent of antisecretory actions. In a recent study, misoprostol was found to be significantly more effective than cimetidine in protecting gastric mucosa against NSAID(tolectin)-induced injury.[396] Of interest, the lesser degree of NSAID-induced duodenal injury was prevented equally by cimetidine and misoprostol.[396] These findings support the hypothesis that acid-independent actions are important in protecting gastric, if not duodenal, mucosa against NSAID damage.

A frequent side effect of the E type prostanoids is crampy abdominal pain and diarrhea, which are dose-dependent effects. Diarrhea occurred in 3 to 30 per cent of patients on therapeutic doses, probably depending definition of the side effect and the mode of data collecting. The diarrhea is often mild and transient and usually does not require discontinuation of the drug. Prostaglandins of the E group may also be uterotrophic. Two doses of misoprostol (400 μg) were given to 56 pregnant women the night before they were to undergo elective abortion; this dose induced partial or complete abortion in 10 per cent of these women, whereas no abortions occurred in 55 placebo-treated subjects.[397] Misoprostol is clearly contraindicated in women of childbearing potential not on contraception. All patients should be informed of this risk, to minimize the risk that the drug be inadvertently given by the patient to a pregnant woman. In a similar study of 51 pregnant women receiving two doses of enprostil (35 μg), no abortions occurred, although abdominal pain, nausea, and vomiting appeared more frequently than in the placebo group.[397] These studies indicate that actions on the uterus may differ among E-type prostaglandins, although firm conclusions are not possible with the limited doses that have been tested thus far.

Sucralfate. Sucralfate (Carafate) is a sulfated disaccharide complex with aluminum hydroxide that does not alter gastric acid or pepsin secretion and has minimal buffering effect in the stomach. Several mechanisms have been proposed for its antiulcer actions, such as binding to the base of the ulcer crater, decreasing peptic activity by impairing the pepsin-substrate interaction, and increasing mucosal prostaglandin production.[398, 399] A direct cytoprotective effect of sucralfate has been hypothesized, possibly related to the content of aluminum hydroxide.[376] The binding of this agent to the ulcer base is enhanced at a pH below 3.5, leading to the recommendation that the drug be administered 30 to 60 minutes before meals. Sucralfate has minimal untoward effects, with about 5 per cent of patients complaining of a metallic taste, nausea, or constipation.[398, 400] Sucralfate is negatively charged at low pH, and it may bind other drugs if taken simultaneously, although the clinical consequences appear minor.[400] Although the drug is assumed to act locally, without significant systemic effects, a preliminary study in humans found that 0.5 to 2.2 per cent of a radioactive label tagged to sucralfate was excreted in the urine, indicating that some absorption is occurring.[401] Following eight weeks of sucralfate therapy, there was a trend suggesting an increase in serum aluminum concentrations, but the numbers were too small for valid interpretation.[402] Urinary aluminum levels have not been reported in patients on sucralfate therapy, but such data are needed in light of the marked increases found with other aluminum-containing compounds and the potential toxicity of systemic aluminum (see p. 848). Whether citric acid or other factors influence aluminum absorption from sucralfate remains unknown. The untoward consequences of prolonged or repeated sucralfate therapy, although likely to be small, require further study.

Colloidal Bismuth Suspensions (CBS). Colloidal bismuth does not affect gastric acid, and its mechanism of ulcer healing is controversial. It decreases pepsin activity,[403] increases mucus secretion, and binds to the mucoproteins in the necrotic ulcer base.[404, 405] An abundance of macrophages surrounded the ulcer base in colloidal bismuth–treated rats, but not in the control group.[404] Tripotassium dicitrate bismuthate caused more bismuth precipitation in the ulcer base than did bismuth subnitrate, bismuth subcarbonate, or bismuth subsalicylate,[404] but potential variability among colloidal bismuth preparations has not been confirmed. The most dramatic of the actions of colloidal bismuth is the potential to clear *C. pylori* from the gastroduodenum, a property shared by several preparations, including bismuth subsalicylate.[177] In patients with active ulcers and *C. pylori* infection, ulcer healing on therapy with combinations of cimetidine, bismuth subcitrate, or the antibiotic tinidazole occurred in 92 per cent of patients who cleared the organism, but in only 60 per cent of those with persistent infection.[172a, 176] Such data suggest an association, but causality in relationship between *C. pylori* infection and ulcer crater formation remains to be defined. Bismuth combined with tinidazole eradicated *C. pylori* most effectively, but regardless of the specific therapy some patients remain with persistent infection. Recurrent infections after cessation of therapy are also common.

Colloidal bismuth is minimally absorbed from the gastrointestinal tract, but at the end of six weeks of therapy, serum bismuth concentrations are elevated; the mean in 500 patients was 7 μg/L, with only two patients in the pretoxic range of 50 to 100 μg/ml.[406] After therapy, urinary bismuth levels increased from 5 to 240 μg/L,[407] and remained elevated tenfold two weeks after therapy was stopped. There is a low risk of bismuth toxicity, particularly encephalopathy, with standard doses of colloidal preparations for a four- to six-week treatment period; however, caution is needed with prolonged use, with higher doses, or in the setting of renal failure. As a result of these considerations, colloidal bismuth is currently recommended only for intermittent therapy. Bismuth subsalicylate, the active agent in Pepto-Bismol, is not approved for use in duodenal ulcer, but is under active study and appears to share many properties of other colloidal bismuth compounds.

Tricyclic Antidepressants. The tricyclic antidepressants doxepin and trimipramine are weak inhibitors of gastric acid secretion, possibly resulting from antagonism of cholinergic or histamine H_2 receptors.[408, 409] Both agents have several side effects, although doxepin may have a reduced risk of cardiac arrhythmias compared to the other tricyclic compounds.

Carbenoxolone. Carbenoxolone, a licorice extract, effectively treats certain acid-peptic disorders, but its development as an accepted therapy has been limited by side effects which include fluid retention, congestive heart failure, hypokalemia, and hypertension.[410] The action of carbenoxolone is unknown; it is not related to alteration of gastric acid or pepsin secretion. Alteration of prostaglandin metabolism has been reported.[411] For treating duodenal ulcer a capsule preparation, Duogastrone, delivers carbenoxolone into the duodenal bulb. However, one third of patients treated with Duogastrone develop hypertension or hypokalemia. At best, carbenoxolone is equivalent to cimetidine in duodenal ulcer healing, and therefore, in light of the side effects, carbenoxolone is not likely to be approved for use in the United States. A deglycyrrhizinated licorice derivative of carbenoxolone, Caved-S, may have fewer side effects,[410] but experience with this preparation remains too limited to judge its efficacy.

Therapeutic Modalities for Healing Duodenal Ulcers

Secretory Inhibition by H₂ Antagonists and Ulcer Healing

Cimetidine and Ranitidine. Despite the observation that less than half of DU patients hypersecrete gastric acid, inhibition of acid secretion induces ulcer healing in most patients and is effective in reducing recurrences. Cimetidine was the first antisecretory agent established by double-blind, randomized trials to induce healing of duodenal ulcers more effectively than placebo. Using a regimen of 1 to 1.2 gm of cimetidine daily in four divided doses, 70 to 85 per cent of duodenal ulcers healed during a four- to six-week treatment period, compared with healing rates in placebo-treated patients, which vary from 20 to 65 per cent.[44, 292, 412] The slightly different treatment regimens used in the United States (300 mg, four times daily) and in Europe (200 mg three times daily and 400 mg before bed) resulted in equivalent healing.[413] Healing during a four-week period was roughly comparable with daily doses of cimetidine from 0.8 to 2 gm, even though inhibition of acid secretion is somewhat more pronounced at the higher doses.[230]

Extensive experience is available to indicate that ranitidine is also more effective than placebo in expediting duodenal ulcer healing, resulting in 75 to 95 per cent healing in a four- to six-week treatment period.[414] In initial trials, doses of 100 mg bid and 150 mg bid were found to be roughly comparable, with only a slight advantage for the higher dose. Ranitidine (200 or 300 mg daily) and cimetidine in the standard 1 gm qid dose were compared in seven studies; at four and eight weeks, respectively, mean ulcer healing rates with ranitidine were 73 and 92 per cent, compared to 67 and 93 per cent with cimetidine.[414] There are no data to suggest a difference between ranitidine and cimetidine in inducing initial healing of ordinary duodenal ulcer.

In initial trials with cimetidine, the drug was given before meals and at bedtime on the assumption that acid secretion needed to be inhibited throughout the day and night to induce ulcer healing. However, frequent dosage compromised both patient compliance and position in a competitive market place. A cimetidine regimen of 400 mg bid was found to be equivalent to the qid regimen both in inhibition of 24-hour acid secretion and in ulcer healing.[415]

Impact of Placebo Healing Rates. The rate of healing on placebo had a great impact on the potential benefit from active drug, and in fact, a highly significant negative correlation can be demonstrated between placebo healing rates and the degree of improvement in healing over placebo produced by active drug (Fig. 47–12). It may be a challenge to establish efficacy of a given drug when the placebo healing rates are high. Trials from the United States had higher placebo healing rates than did trials from the United Kingdom, so that in the U.S. studies it was initially more difficult to establish efficacy of cimetidine.[334]

Ulcer Healing with Only Nighttime Therapy. Man is a species that secretes considerable amounts of acid during nocturnal hours, driven by a circadian diurnal cycle. Nocturnal acid, being unbuffered by food, causes prolonged duodenal acidification. Dragstedt[111] hypothesized that nocturnal acid secretion was the most important pathophysiologic factor in duodenal ulcer. Underlying the importance of nocturnal acid secretion, inhibition of only nocturnal acid secretion markedly decreased recurrence rates (see discussion under Maintenance Therapy). Building on this data base, several investigators examined the acid secretory effects and ulcer healing efficacy of administering H₂ receptor antagonists only at night.

DU healing over four weeks was not statistically different comparing cimetidine 400 mg bid (68 per cent) and 800 mg hs (84 per cent).[416] A multicenter European trial with a total of 574 patients found healing at four weeks on 400 mg bid and 800 mg hs to be 74 and 79 per cent, respectively. Healing with these doses at eight weeks was 94 and 96 per cent, respectively.[417] Three controlled trials have found comparable ulcer healing with ranitidine at a dose of 300 mg hs versus 150 mg bid.[418–420] No significant side effects were detected in these studies with either cimetidine or ranitidine, despite the use of the higher single dose.

Acid Secretory and Ulcer Healing Correlates. The effects of various regimens on acid secretion have been studied, examining both acid output, expressed in mEq per hour, and gastric acidity, generally determined on hourly gastric aspirates and expressed either in pH units or as hydrogen ion concentration. The absolute inhibition of acid secretion varies among studies, but in one representative report an 800 mg hs dose of cimetidine reduced nocturnal acid output by 69 per cent, compared to only 27 per cent inhibition found utilizing a regimen with a 400 mg nighttime dose (Fig. 47–16).[421] The 150 mg dose of ranitidine at night reduced nocturnal acid secretion by 72 per cent, while a 300-mg dose reduced nighttime acid secretion by 85 per cent.[421] These regimens have the similar rank order of efficacy decreasing nocturnal acidity, with 400 mg cimetidine decreasing acidity by 34 per cent; 150 mg ranitidine and 800 mg cimetidine producing decreases of 54 and 56 per cent, respectively; and 300 mg of ranitidine producing an 85 per cent decrease.[421] A relatively small difference in secretory inhibition can have a large effect on nocturnal gastric acidity. For example, the 400-mg dose of cimetidine kept only 17 per cent of the overnight intragastric pH reading above 5, whereas 100 per cent of the nighttime pH values were above 5 with 150 mg of ranitidine.[422]

Overall, a strong correlation is evident between the mean four-week DU healing rates and the suppression of nocturnal gastric acidity (Fig. 47–17).[423] Of interest, this relationship was not evident comparing drug suppression of nocturnal acid output. These findings suggest that the effect of therapy on gastric or duodenal pH is an important end point to enhance healing, but the reason for this apparently critical dependence upon pH is unclear. One possibility is that peptic activity is

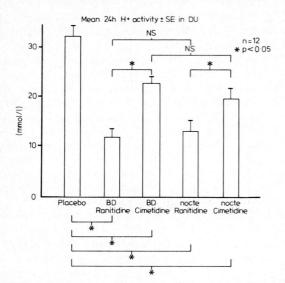

Figure 47–16. Effects of antisecretory agents on nocturnal acid output in DU patients. Nocturnal acid output was determined by continuous aspiration between 11 PM and 7 AM in patients respectively on placebo, ranitidine (150 mg bid), cimetidine (400 mg bid), ranitidine (300 mg hs), and cimetidine (800 mg hs). These treatments respectively produced 72, 27, 84, and 69 per cent decreases in acid output. The data are means from 12 patients, each treated with these five regimens. Statistical differences are indicated by the asterisks (p < 0.05). (From Gledhil T., Howard, O. M., Buck, M., et al. Gut 24:904, 1983. Use with permission.)

dependent upon the pH of gastric juice; decreased activity is evident with pH values above 4, with irreversible loss of activity at a pH of about 6.[424] The peptic activity in gastric juice of DU patients has been reported to persist at higher pH values than in normal subjects;[68] thus, near neutralization of gastric contents may be necessary to maximally inhibit peptic activity, and inactivate pepsin. It remains speculative whether therapy must maximally inhibit pepsin activity to optimally enhance duodenal ulcer healing.

A large, single evening dose (6 P.M.) of an H_2 antagonist produces more prolonged inhibition of acid secretion than does a bedtime dose; however, the nighttime dose produces a greater degree of anacidity and more inhibition of peptic activity during the nighttime hours.[424] A comparison of these regimens on ulcer healing has not been performed.

Regardless of any uncertainty regarding details, a firm conclusion can be reached that inhibition of only nighttime acid secretion is sufficient to induce healing of duodenal ulcers at a rate comparable to that found with a regimen that inhibits acid secretion throughout the day. Furthermore, a nighttime regimen not only is effective, but may have the advantage of being somewhat more physiologic.

Famotidine. The newest member of the H_2 receptor blockers approved for use in the United States is famotidine. By virtue of its antisecretory potency and long duration of action, famotidine is an obvious candidate for nighttime administration for healing DU. Famotidine, 40 mg hs, produced comparable ulcer healing as did ranitidine (300 mg hs).[425] Duodenal ulcer healing with famotidine doses of 40 mg hs, 40 mg bid, and 20 mg bid was compared to healing with placebo; after eight weeks of therapy, each dose of famotidine produced about 82 per cent ulcer healing, compared to 45 per cent healing in the placebo-treated patients.[426] These three dose regimens of famotidine also produced comparable healing to ranitidine 150 mg bid.[427] The 20-mg hs dose of famotidine increased the mean pH between 11 A.M. and 7 A.M. to 5.35, and the 40-mg dose resulted in a similar pH of 5.80.[428]

Omeprazole. Omeprazole rapidly heals duodenal ulcers. In initial trials different doses of omeprazole were evaluated. Daily doses between 20 and 40 mg produced comparable ulcer healing: 63 to 83 per cent at two weeks, and 90 to 100 per cent at four weeks.[429–432] A 10-mg dose healed DU less rapidly than a 30-mg dose, but the lower dose still induced 83 per cent healing by four weeks.[432] In a small study comparing 30 and 60 mg, at two weeks the higher dose induced

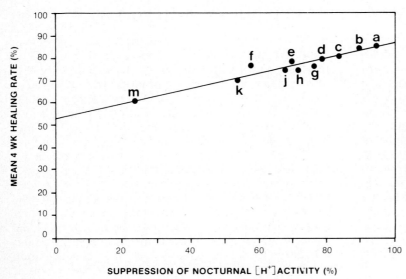

Figure 47–17. The correlation between suppression of nocturnal intragastric acidity and four-week healing rates in DU. For the several regimens indicated below, mean four-week healing rates for available clinical trials were plotted as a function of the percentage suppression of mean nocturnal gastric acidity. A significant correlation was found (r = 0.93; n = 11; p < 0.001). (From Hunt, R. H., Howden, C. W., Jones, D. B., et al. Scand. J. Gastroenterol. 21(suppl. 125):22, 1986. Used with permission.)

100 per cent healing, compared to 63 per cent with the low dose.[431] However, by four weeks the results were comparable with both doses. Compared to ranitidine, omeprazole (20 and 40 mg) induced significantly more rapid healing and pain relief at two and four weeks, but not at eight weeks.[430] In a second comparison with ranitidine, 20 mg of omeprazole induced healing more rapidly at two weeks, although both drugs produce comparable healing and pain relief after four weeks.[433] In a comparison with cimetidine (1 gm daily), omeprazole (30 mg) induced more rapid healing and pain relief at two and four weeks of therapy.[434] Thus, undoubtedly because of increased antisecretory efficacy, omeprazole heals duodenal ulcers more rapidly than H_2 blockers, but the advantage in ordinary DU after four weeks of therapy appears modest.

Antimuscarinic Agents. There is very little evidence to support the use of nonselective antimuscarinic agents for the treatment of duodenal ulcer. Although these agents probably enhance healing, recent controlled trials have studied them only in combination with low-dose antacids, which may heal ulcers at a comparable rate.[435, 436]

Several controlled trials have demonstrated that pirenzepine (100 to 150 mg daily) produced ulcer healing in the usual 70 to 87 per cent of duodenal ulcers in four to six weeks, clearly superior to the placebo healing rates of 13 to 54 per cent.[367] Pirenzepine also produced ulcer healing comparable to that found with cimetidine (1 gm daily).

Antacid Therapy. The initial controlled trial indicating that antacids healed ulcers more rapidly than placebo utilized the high-dose regimen of Al-Mg antacids taken one and three hours after meals and at bedtime, delivering a daily buffering capacity of 1000 mmol.[228] Ulcer healing occurred after four weeks in 78 per cent of patients, compared to 45 per cent treated with an identically appearing placebo. Over the past several years, trials have shown effective healing with progressively lower doses of antacids, with less frequent dosing, and with tablet antacids. In one study, liquid antacid at three doses[103, 207] and 414 mmol of buffering capacity daily was compared to placebo, and healing rates significantly greater than placebo were found with the doses of 207 and 414 mmol daily.[384] Other studies have also found liquid antacids at a daily dose under 300 mmol to be equally effective to cimetidine.[385] In a Hong Kong trial, antacid tablets delivering 175 mmol of buffering capacity daily in seven doses increased four-week ulcer healing from a placebo rate of 33 to 77 per cent.[333] The lowest antacid dose reported has been Al-Mg tablets, each with 30 mmol buffering capacity, taken one hour before meals and at bedtime; healing was 74 per cent at four weeks, compared to a placebo healing rate of 29 per cent.[375] Although antacid therapy promotes ulcer healing, there was initial uncertainty regarding whether pain relief was superior to placebo and comparable to that found with H_2 blockers.[228, 229, 333] More recent studies have found pain relief with antacids to be comparable to other modes of effective therapy.[382, 384, 385]

Direct comparisons of tablet with liquid preparations are limited. Tablets may empty from the stomach more slowly and therefore have a longer time to buffer acid[373] or alter mucosal defense mechanisms. Because of these differences, it is possible that the potency of tablet antacids is greater than that of liquid formulations. Because tablets are probably as effective as liquid preparations, their use will have the added advantage of increased patient compliance, especially on a regimen reduced to four doses daily. It is possible that acid buffering capacity is not the only variable to consider in comparing antacid regimens; aluminum content or availability may be more important, but this information is not readily available with some of the newer formulations.

Prostaglandins. Five prostanoid analogues have been shown to be more effective than placebo in healing duodenal ulcer;[393] the most extensive data are for misoprostol and enprostil. Misoprostol induces dose-dependent healing of duodenal ulcers and doses greater than 100 μg qid heal ulcers more rapidly than placebo.[393, 397] Misoprostol doses of 200 μg qid and 400 μg bid are equally effective to cimetidine in healing duodenal ulcers.[397] With the longer half-life and potency of enprostil, the dosage schedule of 35 μg bid has been used and has been found equally effective as cimetidine.[437, 438] In two studies ranitidine (150 mg bid and 300 mg hs, respectively) was found somewhat superior to enprostil (35 μg bid and 70 μg hs, respectively) in healing duodenal ulcers and relieving pain.[393, 439] However, rioprostil given in a 600-μg nighttime dose was of equivalent efficacy to ranitidine (300 mg hs) in healing DU; diarrhea was infrequent with this nighttime dose of rioprostil.[440] Experience with rioprostil is too limited to allow conclusions regarding efficacy in relation to other therapies. In all these studies it is of interest that healing of duodenal ulcers with prostanoids has only been found with antisecretory doses; doses below the threshold for inhibition of acid secretion have not been found to heal duodenal ulcers.[393, 441] These findings leave the clinical relevance of "cytoprotection" uncertain. Prostaglandins have a theoretical advantage for treatment of ulcers related to NSAID use; in a preliminary report misoprostol was more effective than placebo in healing of gastroduodenal erosions and ulcers in rheumatoid patients on high-dose aspirin.[324] A direct comparison with H_2 blockers will be necessary to determine whether healing of NSAID ulcers with prostanoids reflects more than secretory inhibition and is thus a specific indication for prostanoid therapy.

Sucralfate. Duodenal ulcer healing after four to six weeks of treatment with sucralfate (1 gm qid) was superior to placebo[442, 443] and comparable to cimetidine.[307, 444] Following the trend of decreasing dosage frequencies, comparable duodenal ulcer healing has been reported with 2 gm bid (30 minutes before breakfast and hs) and the standard 1 gm qid regimen.[445, 446]

Colloidal Bismuth. Treatment with colloidal bismuth preparations heals duodenal ulcers at a rate greater than placebo[447, 448] and comparable to other effective forms of therapy, such as cimetidine[449] and ranitidine.[311, 450] Colloidal bismuth tablets, which have been used for most of the recent studies, produce comparable duodenal ulcer healing, but avoid the unpleasant taste of liquid colloidal bismuth.[451] In a preliminary trial, bismuth subsalicylate tablets (Pepto-Bismol) were as effective as cimetidine in inducing healing of DU.[452] The most exciting aspect of treatment with colloidal bismuth is the effect on ulcer recurrence rates and *C. pylori*, as considered elsewhere.

Tricyclic Antidepressants. Trimipramine (50 mg hs) was found more effective than placebo in enhancing duodenal ulcer healing,[409] although the benefit from active therapy is not always dramatic. Limited data indicate that either trimipramine or doxepin can produce healing comparable to cimetidine.[409] More data from controlled clinical trials are needed before the comparative value of these agents for treatment of duodenal ulcers can be determined.

Carbenoxolone. Several, but not all, studies demonstrate that carbenoxolone is more effective in healing duodenal ulcers than placebo.[453, 454] Duodenal ulcer healing with carbenoxolone was also comparable to that produced by cimetidine.[455, 456] Experience with this compound is limited and will likely remain so because of the side effects.

Ulcers That Fail to Heal

About 20 per cent of duodenal ulcers fail to heal during four weeks of standard ulcer therapy. However, about half of these persisting ulcers will heal if the same therapy is continued for another four weeks.[423] It is of interest that in the clinical trials available, this trend for progressive healing over time may not hold for ulcers treated with placebo therapy.[423] Ulcers are considered refractory if healing is not evident after eight to 12 weeks of therapy; in clinical trials only about 5 per cent of ulcers fall into the resistant category.

Do Persistent Symptoms Reflect a Refractory Ulcer? It is important to determine if persistent symptoms reflect a refractory ulcer crater; symptoms may persist after the crater has healed (Fig. 47–10) or may be related to another process, such as functional dyspepsia, reflux esophagitis, or biliary tract disease. A patient who recently presented to the author underlined the point that refractory symptoms may not reflect refractory ulcers. This patient originally presented with "classic" peptic ulcer symptoms and had a duodenal ulcer at endoscopy. The initial response to therapy was excellent. However, after two weeks of therapy, symptoms recurred, this time lacking food and alkali relief, and persisted after the six-week course of therapy. At repeat endoscopy only an ulcer scar was found. Upon physical examination there was spasm of the paraspinous musculature in the lower thoracic region; pressure over this trigger point reproduced this patient's abdominal pain, and injection at the trigger point of Xylocaine

relieved the abdominal complaints. This patient had a spinal reflex syndrome,[252] probably triggered by his ulcer pain and illustrating the interplay between visceral and parietal pain mechanisms. Duodenal ulcer is common; it may often occur simultaneously with other common disorders.

Conditions Underlying Refractory Ulcers. Several conditions may underlie the failure of duodenal ulcers to heal, the most obvious of which is poor patient compliance with therapy. Other factors have been associated with refractory ulcers, such as cigarette smoking, the onset of ulcer disease at a young age, a long duration of ulcer disease, large ulcers, prepyloric ulcers, a positive family history, psychologically stressful situations or responses, and NSAID consumption. These same factors are associated with impaired initial healing and with recurrences. However, with the probable exception of smoking, these factors do not have a consistently high predictive value and are therefore not significant in many series. Some patients who initially respond well to therapy, may subsequently develop refractory ulcers for reasons that remain undefined.

Hypersecretion and/or Failure of Antisecretory Therapy. In very unusual instances the failure of an ulcer to respond to therapy may result from the presence of a definitive hypersecretory state, such as the gastrinoma (see p. 912). In cases of ordinary—but refractory—duodenal ulcer, evidence has been presented for and against a role of basal or nocturnal acid hypersecretion, an increased maximal acid output, and/or resistance to the action of antisecretory agents. Refractory ulcer patients often have acid secretion indistinguishable or insignificantly elevated above the range found for DU patients who heal normally.[457, 458] In contrast, in a recent series of patients initially treated with ranitidine, the 31 patients who healed normally had a BAO of 5.5 mEq per hour, whereas the 12 patients with refractory ulcers had a BAO of 19.6 mEq per hour.[459] It seems likely that some—but certainly not all—patients with refractory ulcers have basal acid hypersecretion. Whether nocturnal gastric acidity or duodenal pH profile would have a better predictive value for refractory ulcer patients remains unknown.

The failure of ordinary DU patients to heal on cimetidine has been credited with a failure of the standard regimen of cimetidine to adequately inhibit acid secretion, especially during nighttime hours.[458] However, the magnitude of inhibition by cimetidine varies among DU patients, and a good inhibitory response has been found in patients with ulcers that fail to heal on therapy.[457] The reason for these different outcomes is not clear; measuring drug effects on nocturnal gastric or duodenal acidity might better correlate with the success or failure of therapy than would drug effects on daytime BAO or on secretagogue or meal-stimulated acid secretion, but such data are not available from prospective studies. It is likely that in some patients refractory ulceration is linked to the magnitude of residual acid secretion on therapy, if not true resistance to antisecretory agents. This statement is based upon the findings that increasing the antisecretory efficacy of therapy induces healing in many refractory ulcers (see Therapeutic Approach to Refractory Ulcers).

Several studies have addressed possible mechanisms for insensitivity to H_2 blocker therapy. In general, the pharmacokinetics of cimetidine absorption, distribution, and serum levels are not altered in refractory patients.[457, 460] Transient, profound resistance to cimetidine was documented in a normal subject, but the mechanism was not established.[461] Following abdominal surgery or renal transplantation, and in patients with sepsis, burns, and possibly head trauma, cimetidine has been reported to poorly inhibit acid secretion and to poorly control acid-peptic complications.[462, 463] A patient with hyperparathyroidism and gastrinoma appeared resistant to cimetidine when hypercalcemic, recovering sensitivity after removal of parathyroid tissue.[464] Specific mechanisms of drug resistance that may be operative in the setting of acute illnesses remain to be defined.

Resistance to H_2 receptor antagonists may theoretically reflect acid secretion driven by histamine-*in*dependent mechanisms, such as vagal/cholinergic pathways, gastrin, or even another secretagogue. In order for this argument to be tenable, it is necessary to document impaired effects of the most potent H_2 antagonists in these patients. In such instances, combinations with antimuscarinic agents or gastrin antagonists (when available for clinical use) might be useful both for sorting out pathogenic mechanisms and for therapy.

Another possible mechanism for resistance to H_2 receptor blockers is "down regulation" of the receptor, a phenomenon that could occur following initial drug treatment. Conflicting data exist as to whether tachyphylaxis follows therapy with H_2 antagonists. After one month of therapy with cimetidine, the inhibitory response to cimetidine was diminished.[465] After nine months of maintenance therapy with ranitidine (150 mg hs), reduced inhibition of pentagastrin stimulation was found in response to intravenous ranitidine, despite normal ranitidine pharmacokinetics.[466] These findings suggesting down regulation of H_2 receptors conflict with the observation that the acid secretory response was enhanced following cessation of four or more weeks of antisecretory therapy (see Rebound Acid Secretion After Antisecretory Therapy). Further studies are required to sort out the impact of therapy on acid secretory mechanisms.

Refractory Ulcers: Acid-Independent Factors? In some instances persistent ulceration may reflect primarily a defect in mucosal resistance. Duodenitis has been noted in some of the patients with refractory ulcers;[457] duodenitis may be an independent factor underlying refractory ulcers or promoting ulcer recurrence in some patients (see Duodenitis, p. 830). *C. pylori* has been isolated from the gastroduodenal mucosa of patients with refractory ulcers; a causal relationship between the presence of *C. pylori* and slow healing is uncertain, but supported by data linking

healing with elimination of the organism (see under Therapeutic Approach to Refractory Ulcers, use of colloidal bismuth). Nonhealing ulcers may also rarely be due to duodenal or pancreatic carcinoma, or possibly *Candida* infection.[467]

Therapeutic Approach to Refractory Ulcers. Patient compliance with a therapeutic regimen should be established before an ulcer can be considered refractory and before further diagnostic testing or a change in therapy is justified. In most cases endoscopy is indicated to confirm that refractory symptoms indeed reflect a refractory ulcer and this confirmation is essential before consideration of surgery. Once a refractory ulcer has been confirmed, measurement of fasting serum gastrin is indicated. Determining basal, stimulated, or preferably nocturnal acid secretory rates and testing inhibition by antisecretory agents will certainly increase understanding of the case, but management decisions can generally be made without this information.

More of the Same Therapy. At least half of the 20 per cent of DU failing to heal during an initial four weeks of therapy are likely to heal during four to eight more weeks of the same therapy.[423, 457] Therefore, it is generally a waste of clinical energy to consider an ulcer refractory until the patient has complied with at least eight weeks of therapy. Once a patient has been confirmed to have a refractory ulcer, several options are available. With continuation of therapy with the same drug beyond eight weeks some additional ulcer healing will occur. Of 66 patients who had ulcers that were refractory after three months of cimetidine (1 gm daily), 56 per cent healed with an average additional treatment period of 7.4 months.[457] The value of increasing the dose at least of cimetidine is uncertain. In Bardhan's series, the benefit of increasing cimetidine to 2 or 3 gm daily was not dramatic, but the use of higher doses was not evaluated in a controlled fashion.[457] Others have also found that cimetidine in doses above 1.2 gm daily fails to dramatically improve healing of refractory ulcers.[460, 468, 469] Probably because cimetidine blood levels at a dose of 200 mg to 300 mg are already at the top of the dose response curve for secretory inhibition,[470] higher doses of cimetidine during the daytime offer little additional antisecretory effect.[372, 458] However, larger doses produce a more prolonged elevation of blood levels, leading to more prolonged antisecretory action, an effect of particular advantage at night (Fig. 47–16). Because inhibition of nocturnal acid secretion is an important factor for ulcer healing (see above section), increasing the nighttime dose of cimetidine to 800 mg may be a reasonable initial step in treating ulcers reluctant to heal.

Patients who develop refractory ulcers while on ranitidine at a daily dose of 300 mg may benefit from increasing the dose of ranitidine to 300 mg bid.[459] Although nighttime regimens of all three available H_2 blockers are comparable to bid dosage for treating *ordinary* duodenal ulcers, 24-hour acid suppression may be advantageous for refractory ulcers. Although untested in clinical trials, it is reasonable to treat refractory ulcers by adding a morning dose to the full-dose nighttime regimen. In patients on NSAIDs, healing seems to be enhanced by switching from an hs regimen to 24-hour suppression twice daily antisecretory dosage.[321]

The Benefits of a Switch: Swapping Antisecretory Agents. The available H_2 blockers appear comparable in their ability to induce initial healing of ordinary DU; whether increased antisecretory potency (famotidine > ranitidine > cimetidine) is beneficial for refractory ulcers remains to be established. In uncontrolled reports, ranitidine appears to heal cimetidine-resistant ulcers, but the benefits relative to continued therapy with cimetidine were not ascertained in these studies. In a controlled study, duodenal ulcers remaining unhealed after six weeks of cimetidine therapy were randomized to continued cimetidine or to ranitidine therapy. About 62 per cent of ulcers in both groups healed over the next six weeks,[471] consistent with the expected benefits from simply extending therapy. No controlled studies are available for the use of famotidine for ulcers resistant to other therapies.

Prostanoids are logical candidates for therapy of ulcers refractory to H_2 blockers because these agents inhibit acid secretion by a different mechanism and may possess other properties conducive to healing. A preliminary, controlled study did find that misoprostol was more effective than placebo in healing ulcers refractory after 10 weeks of H_2 blocker therapy.[472] However, without a comparison to continued therapy with H_2 blockers, this result cannot be interpreted.

Maximal Antisecretory Therapy with Omeprazole. Omeprazole has been evaluated in 11 patients whose duodenal ulcers failed to respond to at least three months of therapy with H_2 antagonists, alone or in combination with other antiulcer agents.[473] Nine of the patients responded to omeprazole (40 mg daily) in two weeks, and all healed by four weeks of therapy. Omeprazole has proved highly effective in gastrinoma patients,[364] further supporting its efficacy in "difficult" ulcers.

Colloidal Bismuth. In a trial from Hong Kong, patients (25 of 212) whose ulcers failed to decrease in size after four weeks of cimetidine (1 gm daily) therapy were randomized to colloidal bismuth tablets or to continued cimetidine at an increased dose (1.6 gm daily).[468] Overall, colloidal bismuth healed 85 per cent of the cimetidine failures, a rate comparable to the initial healing rates, while continued cimetidine therapy healed only 40 per cent of the initial cimetidine failures. In another series, 43 patients who had persistent ulceration after eight weeks of cimetidine or ranitidine therapy, were randomized to 1 gm of cimetidine daily, 2 gm of cimetidine daily, or to colloidal bismuth subcitrate. Although the numbers are small, after four weeks of this second round of therapy, ulcers healed in 47 per cent of patients on low-dose cimetidine, in 43 per cent on high-dose cimetidine and in 86 per cent on colloidal bismuth.[469] The efficacy of colloidal bismuth compounds in treatment failures with antisecretory agents requires further study, as does a potential role for *C. pylori* in these refractory ulcers.

Sucralfate. In a study comparing initial healing with cimetidine and sucralfate, the patients who failed to heal after four weeks of therapy were crossed over to the other therapy; during a subsequent four-week treatment period, sucralfate and cimetidine each healed about 68 per cent of the other's initial treatment failures.[307] In an uncontrolled series, 32 patients whose ulcers failed to heal on either ranitidine or cimetidine were placed on sucralfate; 82 per cent healed in six weeks of additional therapy.[474] More studies are needed to determine if sucralfate has a role in therapy of refractory ulcers.

Other Drugs. Uncontrolled studies have suggested that the tricyclic antidepressant doxepin induces healing in DU patients who failed to respond to cimetidine;[409] confirmation in controlled trials is required.

A Role for Combination Therapy? Utilizing a combination of agents is attractive because utilizing therapeutic modalities that act by different mechanisms may have complementary effects in refractory ulcers. Combination therapy is not indicated in the initial treatment of routine, uncomplicated DU.

Combinations of Antisecretory Agents. Adding antimuscarinic agents to H_2 blockers has the theoretical advantage of inhibiting acid secretion stimulated by separate pathways and might be of value, especially in patients with increased cholinergic drive, if such patients could be identified. However, variable additional antisecretory efficacy has been achieved with the combination of antimuscarinic agents and cimetidine, with the benefits in different studies being significant,[458] modest,[372] or negligible.[470] The combination of ranitidine and pirenzepine produced inhibition of food-stimulated acid secretion,[475, 476] without developing hypergastrinemia.[476] If this combination also produces profound inhibition of nocturnal acid secretion and if serum gastrin levels remain normal on sustained therapy, then this combination could be very useful when maximal antisecretory therapy is desired over a prolonged period. However, data regarding the efficacy of combination therapy in treating refractory ulcers remains limited and contradictory, with one trial supporting the efficacy of pirenzepine plus cimetidine in H_2-refractory ulcers[477] and others finding no additional benefit compared to continued therapy with H_2 antagonists.[370, 478] The combination of ranitidine or famotidine and pirenzepine remains untested in controlled trials.

Sucralfate Plus Antisecretory Agents. Sucralfate requires an acid environment to dissolve, a factor that may limit the effectiveness of combining this agent with antisecretory agents, although this theoretical disadvantage may not be clinically significant. The combination of cimetidine and sucralfate was tested on initial healing of duodenal ulcers; the combination produced a modest enhancement of healing at two, but not four, weeks,[479] leaving little justification for the cost of combination for treating ordinary DU. The value of combination therapy for healing refractory ulcers has not been reported.

Antacids Plus Antisecretory Agents. When a patient is on an antacid regimen, replacement of the nighttime antacid dose by either an H_2 antagonist or anticholinergic agent may be worthwhile, because liquid antacids are rapidly emptied and are essentially ineffective buffering nocturnal acid secretion.[372] The combination of cimetidine plus antacids has been found to be more effective than cimetidine alone in reducing gastric acidity during the daytime hours,[372] but whether this effect translates into increased therapeutic efficacy remains untested. When antacids and cimetidine are combined, taking the two medications at the same time may impair absorption of cimetidine.[380] Because both antacids and sucralfate are capable of binding many other drugs, caution should be exercised regarding drug absorption in combination therapy.

Colloidal Bismuth Plus Antisecretory Agents. Bismuth is optimally precipitated from tripotassium dicitrate bismuthate at a pH of about 3.0.[404] The combination of bismuth and antisecretory agents may be beneficial if increasing the gastric pH increases the antiulcer effectiveness of bismuth,[460] but this possibility remains untested.

Refractory Ulcers: Overview. The preliminary findings that refractory ulcers effectively heal on maximal acid inhibition with omeprazole[473] argues that acid is a necessary pathogenic factor for such ulcers. If these results with omeprazole are confirmed, one might add a corollary to Schwartz's dictum: "no acid, no refractory ulcers." This interpretation does not imply that acid is the sole pathogenic factor but rather that acid is a necessary permissive factor for most, if not all, duodenal ulcers. It should be kept in mind that simply because maximal antisecretory therapy is effective in refractory ulcers, this approach may not be the only or the optimal regimen for long-term management. It appears that refractory ulcers occur in two settings:

1. Ulcers that are associated with acid hypersecretion or resistance to antisecretory therapy. Such ulcers may require extra-effort antisecretory therapy to bring the acid secretion down into the normal therapeutic range so that healing can occur. Better understanding of the mechanisms underlying refractory ulcers may result from studies of the acid secretory response to the therapeutic regimens that fail and to those that finally succeed. A further question concerns whether pepsin activity or resistance to inactivation at higher pH values plays a role.

2. Ulcers associated with an underlying defect in mucosal resistance to a normal acid-peptic environment. Such ulcers may be associated with factors such as smoldering duodenal inflammation or infection with *C. pylori*. These ulcers may require near antacidity throughout the day to heal and may respond poorly to surgical therapy, such as highly selective vagotomy, that fails to maximally suppress acid secretion. If *C. pylori* is pathogenic, these ulcers may respond to colloidal bismuth or other therapy that clears this organism.

Recurrences Following Healing of Acute Ulcers

Although an occasional patient may experience a single episode of duodenal ulceration, frequent recurrences are part of the natural history of ulcer disease (see p. 841). The factors that underlie ulcer recurrence are the same set of factors that promote ulcer formation and since these factors are not well understood, no definitive answers can be provided for the pathogenesis of ulcer recurrences. Cigarette smoking is one variable with high predictive value for recurrences (Fig. 47–13). Basal acid hypersecretion has been associated with recurrent ulcer following highly selective vagotomy.[480, 481] Although increased basal or nocturnal acid secretion or increased maximal acid output has been proposed as underlying recurrent duodenal ulcer, such secretory abnormalities are probably of importance in only a small number of patients. It is possible that the hypersecretion of acid is not continuously present in a given patient, but may occur intermittently, therefore confounding study of its role in recurrent ulcer. Ulcer recurrence has been correlated with an increased peptic activity in gastric juice.[296]

The natural history, or tendency of ulcers to recur and complicate, is highly variable among patients. Patients who readily heal on placebo therapy appear to have a more "benign" form of ulcer disease, and are less disposed to recurrences.[295] Patients with ulcers that slowly heal or are refractory to initial therapy, are also more prone to recurrences.[296] Ulcers that were only partly healed upon entering a maintenance trial did less well than completely healed ulcers.[482] During a 24-month trial of maintenance cimetidine therapy, there was a 48 per cent recurrence rate among 61 patients who initially had refractory ulcers, but only a 20 per cent recurrence rate occurred among patients with nonrefractory ulcers.[299] Prepyloric ulcers, occurring alone or in combination with duodenal ulcers, may also be more prone to recurrence.[287]

Ulcer Recurrence: Does the Initial Therapy Matter? Despite macroscopic ulcer healing, marked inflammation is found at the site of ulceration[169] and may underlie the tendency of ulcers to recur, and to recur at the same site. Recent attention has focused on whether recurrence rates differ among the specific therapies used for treating duodenal ulcers, possibly due to promoting a better quality of healing at a histologic level. One problem encountered in comparing ulcer recurrence rates among initial therapies is compensating for the possibility that some therapies heal more recalcitrant ulcers that are therefore more prone to relapse, while less efficacious initial therapy heals more benign ulcers, which are less prone to relapse.

Recurrences after Antisecretory Therapy. Recurrences are frequent for ulcers initially healed on H$_2$ receptor antagonists, and following discontinuation of therapy recurrence rates are at least as great as those found for ulcers healed on placebos.[406, 483] The rate of recurrence does not depend upon the length of the full-dose treatment period; recurrences were comparable following initial treatment with cimetidine for between one and six months.[484] The dose and potency of the antisecretory agents used do not appear to influence the rate of recurrence; recurrence rates are probably comparable regardless of whether ulcers were healed with cimetidine, ranitidine, or famotidine, although detailed comparisons of these drugs are not available. Recurrence rates are also high for ulcers healed on omeprazole therapy, and probably are comparable to that found with H$_2$ blockers.[430, 434] Despite the efficacy of H$_2$ blockers and omeprazole for initial healing, their use does not alter the natural history of duodenal ulcer disease. Recurrence rates following initial healing with antacids have not been significantly different from H$_2$ blockers.[485, 486] Recurrence following anticholinergic agents plus antacids,[436] and following pirenzepine,[487] may be somewhat less than with H$_2$ blocker therapy, but more data are needed before firm conclusions can be reached.[406]

Data for recurrences following healing with prostaglandins are limited, but review of the data from the trials with misoprostol indicate recurrence rates somewhat lower than with cimetidine.[488] Of interest, acute antral gastritis was reduced to a greater extent in patients on misoprostol than in placebo-treated patients.[162] Extrapolating this latter finding to ulcer recurrences will require information regarding duodenal histopathology and a direct comparison with other therapies. Prostaglandins have no known effect on *C. pylori* in the gastroduodenum.

Recurrence Rates with Agents That Heal Acid-Independent Mechanisms. Five of six trials have shown lower recurrence rates following initial therapy colloidal bismuth compared to H$_2$ antagonists.[406] Combining the data from these six trials, the recurrence rate in one year following healing and cessation of bismuth therapy was 59 per cent, compared to a rate of 85 per cent following H$_2$ blocker therapy.[406] These differences were not due to differences in initial healing rates, because healing rates with colloidal bismuth were, if anything, slightly better than with H$_2$ blockers. The factors that account for the lower recurrence rate with bismuth therapy are not yet defined. Bismuth is cleared slowly and continues to be excreted for weeks after therapy is stopped,[407] possibly accounting for prolonged antiulcer effects. Elimination of *C. pylori* from the gastroduodenum is another very interesting possibility; when this organism is cleared following bismuth therapy recurrence rates appear lower than when organisms persist.[172a, 176, 488a] In a small group of DU patients, electron microscopic examination after six weeks of colloidal bismuth therapy revealed nearly normal surface morphology of the duodenal epithelial cells, whereas microvilli generally remained abnormal after cimetidine therapy.[489] Two studies have indicated that recurrence rates following healing on sucralfate therapy are less than with cimetidine,[307, 490] although confirmation with larger groups is required to support firm conclusions. Increasing evidence indicates that recurrence rates are not comparable among all therapies, with the best present evidence indicating a reduced recurrence rate with bismuth compounds.

Rebound Acid Hypersecretion after Antisecretory Therapy. A few studies have considered whether rebound acid hypersecretion occurs after stopping a course of antisecretory therapy. The postprandial acid secretory response was tested before and after four weeks of ranitidine therapy (150 mg bid); the secretory response was increased two days after stopping therapy, but returned to the initial values by four to six weeks.[491] In another study, an increase in the acid secretory response to impromidine, an H$_2$ agonist, was found after three months on maintenance treatment with ranitidine. The effectiveness of ranitidine given by intravenous bolus was unimpaired.[492] Possible mechanisms for this hypersecretory response to H$_2$ therapy might be "up-regulation" by prolonged receptor blockage of the number of H$_2$ receptors, their affinity, or their coupling to adenylate cyclase. An increase in parietal cell mass, possibly secondary to hypergastrinemia from decreased acid feedback inhibition, is a possible mechanism for posttreatment acid hypersecretion in response to all stimuli. The frequency with which changes in acid secretion occur with therapy is uncertain, and some studies find no alterations one week after cessation of therapy.[493] Changes specific for a given secretagogue (and therefore receptor) require a study focused at that question. It seems unlikely that acid rebound is of sufficient magnitude to increase the risk of ulcer recurrence; if so, then tapering antisecretory therapy, rather than abrupt cessation, would be appropriate.

Maintenance Therapy for Ulcer Recurrence

After initial healing of an acute DU, continued treatment with H$_2$ receptor antagonists reduces the very high spontaneous recurrence rate found in placebo-treated patients.[298, 494] Data from five separate one-year trials of patients on 400 mg of cimetidine nightly indicated that 60 to 85 per cent remained free of recurrences, compared to 17 to 39 per cent of the placebo-treated patients who were recurrence-free.[304] Higher doses of cimetidine were of no advantage in some studies,[294] but in others fewer recurrences were found using cimetidine at doses of 800 mg hs or 400 mg bid.[287, 296, 304]

From the above data, many patients do well on maintenance therapy with low-dose cimetidine (400 mg hs), but a proportion may require therapy with greater antisecretory efficacy. Because the efficacy of maintenance therapy probably reflects suppression of nocturnal acid secretion and because 800 mg hs cimetidine is superior the 400 mg dose for inhibiting nocturnal acid secretion (Fig. 47–16), it is not surprising that some patients respond better to this higher dose. Strom and coworkers interpreted their data to indicate that duodenal ulcers readily healing in six weeks on cimetidine (1 gm daily) responded well to maintenance therapy with 400 mg of cimetidine nightly. In contrast, DU patients who healed slowly on initial therapy and patients with prepyloric ulcers were more effectively maintained on 800 mg of cimetidine daily.[296]

For maintenance ulcer therapy, ranitidine (150 mg hs) is clearly superior to placebo, with recurrences of 16 per cent in one year on therapy compared to a placebo recurrence rate of 72 per cent.[494] Early trials indicated that ranitidine (150 mg hs) was as effective as cimetidine (400 mg hs) in preventing recurrences,[495] but in two recent trials DU recurrence rates on ranitidine (150 mg hs) were lower than on cimetidine (400 mg hs). In these latter trials using the same doses, recurrences in one year on ranitidine were 16[496] and 23 per cent,[497] compared to rates of 43 and 34 per cent on cimetidine. It is possible that this difference relates to the slightly greater suppression of nocturnal acidity with 150 mg ranitidine compared to 400 mg of cimetidine (Fig. 47–16). However, these findings[496, 497] need to be interpreted with some caution, since these recurrence rates for both drugs are not in line with several previous studies.

Famotidine is also useful for maintenance therapy in duodenal ulcer. Recurrence rates in patients treated for one year with 20 mg and 40 mg of famotidine nightly were 23 and 25 per cent, respectively, compared to a recurrence rate of 57 per cent in the placebo-treated patients.[498] The famotidine dose approved for initial maintenance is 20 mg nightly.

In summary, ulcer recurrences are reduced on antisecretory therapy, and inhibiting nocturnal acid secretion appears to underlie the efficacy of this therapeutic approach. Extrapolating from the above data, about 15 to 20 per cent of patients will require more antisecretory efficacy for successful maintenance therapy than that achieved with 400 mg of cimetidine nightly. An increased dose of cimetidine (800 mg daily) or ranitidine (150 mg hs) may be more effective in preventing recurrences. It is likely that 20 mg of famotidine will produce at least a comparable decrease in recurrence rates to that found with 150 mg of ranitidine nightly, but trials directly comparing these drugs have not been reported.

The results of long-term clinical trials with anticholinergics to prevent ulcer complications and recurrences are conflicting,[499] and because other effective forms of therapy are available, there is no rationale for the long-term use of anticholinergics in duodenal ulcer. In controlled trials, patients on pirenzepine (50 to 100 mg hs) had lower recurrence rates than placebo-treated patients, and the recurrence rate on pirenzepine was roughly comparable to cimetidine (400 mg hs).[367] It is possible that pirenzepine at 75 mg daily and cimetidine (400 mg nightly) is a combination that will be effective in ulcers refractory to low-dose cimetidine maintenance.[477]

There are only limited data regarding maintenance therapy with prostaglandins. In two trials, enprostil (35 μg hs) was found to be significantly less effective than ranitidine (150 mg hs) in preventing ulcer recurrences.[500, 501] Whether higher doses of enprostil will have a greater impact on recurrence rates remains to be established.

Because omeprazole is effective in preventing recurrences in gastrinoma patients, it undoubtedly would be effective in ordinary duodenal ulcer. However, the antisecretory response to low doses (5 to 10 mg) is quite variable among patients, possibly complicating the use of a maintenance dose less than 20 mg. Maintenance on very potent antisecretory regimens is not necessary in the majority of duodenal ulcer patients, and their prolonged use entails several theoretical risks (see Consequences of Medicinal Hypochlorhydria). Until there is more information regarding these risks in humans, prolonged use of omeprazole seems best reserved for patients who fail on other regimens.

Experience with sucralfate for maintenance therapy remains limited; both 1 and 2 gm daily doses of sucralfate were found to have reduced recurrence rates compared to placebo.[502]

Unfortunately, once maintenance treatment with antisecretory agents is stopped, duodenal ulcer recurrence is similar to that for patients placed on placebo after initial ulcer healing (Fig. 47–11), thus emphasizing that the length of antisecretory therapy does not alter the natural history of duodenal ulcer disease.

Asymptomatic Recurrences. Asymptomatic recurrences are common and occur as a function of how often endoscopy is performed. Recurrences on maintenance therapy are more likely to be asymptomatic than are recurrences on placebo.[503] In a two-year follow-up of 261 patients on 400 mg of cimetidine nightly, 25 per cent had symptomatic relapses and 49 per cent had asymptomatic relapses.[299] Although asymptomatic recurrences are of importance to the FDA and to drug companies conducting trials, their importance to the patient and physician depends upon whether they will become symptomatic or develop complications. It is well known that ulcers may initially present with complications without heralding symptoms. In contrast, asymptomatic recurrences on maintenance therapy infrequently have complications.[299, 503] These break-through ulcers occurring on maintenance therapy may heal slowly, but most remain asymptomatic.[503] Of interest, Boyd and coworkers observed that patients who complied with therapy were more likely to have mild, asymptomatic recurrences, whereas symptomatic recurrences occurred more frequently in patients who did not comply with therapy.[503] Atlhough conclusions still rest on a thin data base, ulcers that recur on maintenance therapy without associated symptoms or complications (i.e., found on surveillance or incidental endoscopy or X-ray) should not be cause for clinical distress, although an effort to induce healing with higher dose maintenance therapy, a course of full-dose therapy, or an altered regimen is appropriate.

The Efficacy of Prolonged Maintenance Therapy. Maintenance therapy continued into the second and third years appears to produce at least comparable decreases in recurrences as those found during the initial maintenance trial.[299, 504] Although the data are limited, there is an indication that recurrence rates of patients followed into second and third years of maintenance are lower than the rates occurring during the first year of therapy and this difference is not due to surgical or other dropouts.[296, 299, 304] A few series have followed patients for three to five years on maintenance therapy with cimetidine; patients entered these series often with a history of complications or an initial referral for ulcer surgery.[287, 299, 304, 505] Sixty per cent or more of the patients in these series did well on maintenance therapy; the proportion who failed or had complications varied, probably as a function of the patient population and the vigor with which medical therapy was pursued as an alternate to surgery. In series from Gray and coworkers, 60 per cent of patients who had been surgical candidates at the outset did well on low-dose cimetidine maintenance.[505] Twenty of the 50 patients underwent surgery; seven because of symptomatic recurrences on maintenance therapy, seven with complications (two with bleeding, five with pyloric stenosis), and five patients who elected surgery when maintenance therapy could not be stopped without relapse. Of those patients who failed to respond to cimetidine, their failure was evident within seven months into the trial.[505] Whether these "medical failures" would have responded to higher doses of cimetidine or to other agents is unknown. In a second series, 18 per cent failed long-term management and underwent surgery for complications or recurrences on therapy.[304] Of the remaining patients in this latter series on continuous maintenance, 24 per cent were asymptomatic and ulcer free, and 56 per cent had one or more relapses which responded to full-dose cimetidine therapy.[304] The argument has been that low-dose cimetidine maintenance therapy decreases recurrence rates, but serves to delay rather than reduce the total number of operations.[506] However, this series was drawn from a surgical clinic, and it is likely that operations were recommended rather than manipulating the medical regimen to induce healing and maintain the patient in a symptom- and complication-free status.

Overall, with continued compliance, 60 to 90+ per cent of patients on maintenance therapy will fare well for prolonged periods; recurrences may occur, but they are likely to be asymptomatic and free of complications. For recurrences on maintenance therapy, increasing the nighttime dose of antisecretory agent may be effective, but is not necessary in most patients. Once a patient is established on maintenance therapy, there is no indication that the relative success deteriorates with extended treatment periods. If anything, there may be a tendency for patients to have fewer recurrences over time,[296, 299] but more experience with such extended treatment periods is necessary to fully assess the benefits and risks.

Impact of Therapy on Complications

A major rationale for initial and maintenance medical therapy, in addition to alleviation of symptoms, is to reduce the risk of complications. Because complications can only occur when an ulcer crater is present, it is difficult to conceive that therapy which hastens ulcer healing or reduces recurrences will fail to decrease the risk of complications. The complication rate in duodenal ulcer is low, and the effect of medical therapy on that complication rate has not been firmly established; complications in most clinical trials are only noted in the methods section as the reason for patient dropouts. In the absence of direct studies of this point, Schiller and Fordtran reviewed data from 48 randomized trials of ulcer healing during four to six weeks of therapy, focusing upon the causes for patient dropouts.[507] Dropouts due to complications were very infrequent and comparable between the placebo and active drug treatment groups. However, placebo-treated patients were six times more likely to drop out for intractable pain or worsening of ulcer symptoms than were patients on active treatment. Because there was no standardization in the reporting of these complications, these findings have to be interpreted with caution.

In randomized clinical trials of maintenance therapy for six to 12 months, complications appeared to occur less frequently on than off therapy. During 659 patient months on cimetidine maintenance, no complications occurred despite an symptomatic ulcer recurrence rate of about 2 per cent per month.[299] The absence of complications was particularly notable in this series because 61 of the 261 patients studied entered with refractory ulcers. Strom and coworkers followed 43 patients, 63 per cent of whom entered the study with a history of complications of hemorrhage or perforation; despite a recurrence rate of 33 per cent, none of the patients developed complications on maintenance therapy and, of interest, the patients with a history of complications were not more liable to recurrence than were the other patients. These observations suggest that many patients, even those with a history of complications or refractory ulcers, may do well on maintenance therapy. However, complications do develop on maintenance therapy.[304, 505] Nine patients on maintenance or full-dose cimetidine were reported presenting with perforation.[508] Pyloric stenosis was a surprisingly frequent complication, occurring in five of the 50 patients followed by Gray on cimetidine maintenance.[505] Once pyloric stenosis has developed, patients often respond poorly to medical therapy, with the majority eventually requiring surgery.[509] Further studies are needed to define the short- and long-range effects of different therapeutic modalities on ulcer complication rates, so that this information can be factored into therapeutic decisions.

Consequences of Medicinal Hypochlorhydria

Hypochlorhydria, Hypergastrinemia, ECL Cells, and Histamine

Hypergastrinemia. Normally the secretion of gastrin from the antral mucosa is subjected to feedback inhibition by acid. Pernicious anemia (PA) is the extreme case; the absence of acid feedback inhibition produces profound hypergastrinemia, especially when the antrum is spared from severe gastritis. Antisecretory agents increase both postprandial and basal gastrin levels as a function of their potency and duration of inhibitory effects. Even with cimetidine, the least potent of the H[2] blockers, meal-stimulated gastrin release is enhanced after one month of therapy with 1.2 gm daily.[465] A small increase in fasting serum gastrin concentrations was observed after three months of treatment with full-dose cimetidine, but both basal and meal-stimulated gastrin levels returned to normal within five days of stopping therapy.[510] Limited data exist regarding the effects on serum gastrin levels of therapy with a single nighttime dose of an H[2] blocker or of maintenance therapy. After 12 months of therapy with 150 mg of ranitidine nightly, fasting serum gastrin levels had increased an average of 65 per cent.[510a] As expected, treatment with potent antisecretory agents produces an increase in fasting and postprandial gastrin levels and increased serum pepsinogen I levels. The effects of omeprazole on serum gastrin appear to be dose-dependent over doses from 10 to 30 or 40 mg and time-dependent, progressively increasing over a two-week treatment period.[362, 511, 512] After a 14-day treatment period with 30 mg of omeprazole daily, fasting serum gastrin levels in nine DU patients increased from a basal value of 15 pg/ml to 77 pg/ml.[362] Similar increases were seen in a group of eight normal subjects given a 40-mg dose of omeprazole for 14 days (Fig. 47–18). Of interest, in three of the eight normal subjects fasting serum gastrin increased to about 260 pg/ml (125 pmol/L, Fig. 47–18). Two of these three subjects also displayed an exaggerated serum gastrin response to a test meal, suggesting that they may have antral G cell hyperfunction.[512] In most subjects, the elevated serum gastrin levels return to normal in one week after stopping therapy, but in some subjects the decline in serum gastrin appears somewhat slower (Fig. 47–18). The effects of more prolonged omeprazole therapy on serum gastrin levels in humans have not been reported. The variability in the magnitude of gastrin response is impressive and underlines the importance of examining gastrin levels in individual patients receiving prolonged therapy with potent antisecretory agents.

In the rat and dog prolonged therapy with omeprazole leads to dose-dependent increases in serum gastrin, which can be dramatic at higher doses. Gastrin

levels return to normal within about a week after stopping therapy.[513] There is some species variability in the serum gastrin response to the same degree of acid inhibition, and the rat displays much greater increases in serum gastrin than does man.[513]

Consequences of Hypergastrinemia. Sustained hypergastrinemia is the probable cause of the profound increase in the fundic mucosal secretory mass that occurs in the Zollinger-Ellison syndrome (see p. 909). Basal hypergastrinemia appears necessary to produce trophic effects on fundic cell mass, but the threshold at which gastrin induces the secretory mass remains to be established. If the fundic secretory mass increases, then rebound hypersecretion of acid may occur upon stopping antisecretory therapy, but this possibility seems of minor clinical consequence (see discussion of rebound).

An important consequence of hypergastrinemia is a trophic effect on a specific endocrine cell, the enterochromaffin-like (ECL) cell. The most dramatic example of this phenomenon occurs in the female rat, in which the prolonged administration of potent antisecretory agents in very high doses produced hyperplasia of ECL cells and the formation of carcinoid tumors composed of these cells.[514, 515] Larsson and coworkers, studying the effects of omeprazole, provided strong evidence for a causal association with profound inhibition of acid secretion producing hypergastrinemia, which in turn caused hyperplasia of ECL cells.[516] As a function of the degree and duration of acid secretory inhibition, a similar sequence of events can be expected in the rat with other antisecretory agents, regardless

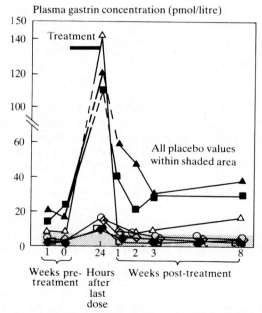

Figure 47–18. Individual fasting serum gastrin concentrations before, during, and after a two-week treatment period with a daily dose of 40 mg of omeprazole or placebo. Each point represents the mean of duplicate determinations. (From Sharma, B. K., Lundborg, P., Pounder, R. E., et al. Scand. J. Gastroenterol. *21*(suppl. 118):143, 1986. Used with permission.)

of the mechanism by which they inhibit acid secretion. In the rat, prolonged, high-dose administration of the H_2 receptor antagonists ranitidine[516] and loxtidine[515] also produced ECL cell hyperplasia. In lifelong (2-year) studies in the rat, loxtidine also induced carcinoid formation.[515] Similar studies in the mouse revealed much less hyperplasia of ECL cells and no carcinoid formation with lifelong (1-year) treatment. ECL hyperplasia is also much less prominent in the dog than in the rat. These species differences remain unexplained.

Evidence indicates that ECL cell hyperplasia also occurs in the human fundic mucosa at least with extreme, prolonged hypergastrinemia; hyperplasia of ECL cells and occasional carcinoid tumors have been found in pernicious anemia and in Zollinger-Ellison syndrome.[517-519] The duration and degree of hypergastrinemia necessary for production of ECL hyperplasia and carcinoid formation in humans remain unknown; other pathogenic factors in addition to hypergastrinemia may be involved. Although it is likely that sustained basal hypergastrinemia will be necessary to produce ECL hyperplasia, the long-term consequences of exaggerated meal-stimulated hypergastrinemia also need elucidation.

Implications of Hypergastrinemia. The degree of hypergastrinemia produced with standard therapeutic doses of even the most potent antisecretory agents is quite modest in most patients and is very unlikely to produce significant hyperplasia of ECL cells in short treatment periods. However, with the variability in the gastrin response to two weeks of antisecretory therapy (Fig. 47–18), it is possible that some patients may experience profound hypergastrinemia with prolonged therapy. Until the trophic effect of gastrin on ECL cells in humans has been fully characterized, more studies are necessary to monitor gastrin levels and ECL density on an individual basis in patients on sustained therapy with potent, long-acting antisecretory agents. Monitoring must detect this occasional patient with profound changes in gastrin levels (Fig. 47–18) or ECL cell density, rather than depending upon trends in the larger population of treated patients. Because the changes in response to gastrin may only be evident in the ECL cells, this cell compartment must be directly determined, rather than depending upon estimates of total endocrine cells. One other point of interest is that in the rat ECL cells produce and contain large amounts of histamine. In humans there was little evidence for histamine being present in ECL cells until the recent demonstration of immunoreactivity with antihistamine antibodies.[520] The amount of histamine-like immunoreactivity contained in these ECL cells in normal fundic mucosa is small, and the physiologic and pathophysiologic consequences of this histamine in ECL cells remain to be unraveled.

The mechanism of the apparent variability of gastrin response to antisecretory therapy has not been established, but two possibilities seem likely. The first is probable antral G cell hyperfunction.[512] Second, sensitivity to acid inhibitory effects of therapy varies among individuals (Fig. 47–14), and some patients experience profound hypochlorhydria with standard antisecretory therapeutic doses. To illustrate this point, bacterial overgrowth (see following section) on cimetidine therapy is an inverse function of the pretreatment acid secretory capacity.[521] It is possible that patients with relatively low initial acid secretion may be more sensitive to antisecretory agents and therefore more liable to develop bacterial overgrowth and hypergastrinemia. Such sequelae may be of particular importance in patients treated for esophagitis or gastric ulcer with the potent, prolonged-acting antisecretory agents.

Antisecretory Drugs, Bacterial Overgrowth, and Cancer. Gastric acid markedly decreases the bacterial count in the stomach and essentially sterilizes food, and as a result, bacterial counts in the small intestine remain low. Conversely, with hypochlorhydria, bacterial overgrowth occurs in the stomach. pH values below 4 are usually bactericidal, but with higher pH values mouth flora or occasionally fecal flora flourish.[521, 522] The consequences of bacterial overgrowth are several. PA patients have a tendency to develop chronic or intermittent diarrhea and malabsorption. With hypochlorhydria, there is also an increased risk of infection with enteropathogenic organisms, with the best data relating to nontyphoid salmonellosis.[521, 523] The risk for other infections, including cholera and parasitic infections (giardiasis, strongyloidiasis, and *Entamoeba histolytica*), may also be increased.[521, 523] Brucellosis and pseudomembranous enterocolitis have also been reported. Another consequence of hypochlorhydria is that the gastric bacterial flora may reduce dietary nitrate, thereby increasing nitrite concentrations, which in turn may lead to the formation of N-nitroso compounds, which are known carcinogens in animal models.[521, 524] This mechanism has been proposed to underlie the increased cancer risk in PA, but a causal association remains controversial.

A question of pertinence to a much larger population is whether these several risks are of concern to patients who acquire medicinal hypochlorhydria as a result of antisecretory therapy for peptic ulcer disease. Bacterial overgrowth occurs with antisecretory therapy as a function of the potency of the agent used.[521, 522, 525] Gastric bacterial counts also increase in patients on antacid therapy, but not with sucralfate or bismuth therapy. Postmarketing surveillance indicated some increased risk of diarrhea in patients on cimetidine therapy,[341] but whether this was due to enteric infection is not known. A few cases of cholera have been reported in patients on H_2 blockers, but whether the therapy actually predisposed to infection was not established.[522] The consequences of the occurrence of N-nitroso compounds in the stomach with antisecretory therapy remain controversial,[521, 524] and with the present limited data base there is no indication of an increased risk of gastric cancer resulting from prolonged antisecretory therapy. Of interest, postmarketing surveillance indicated that both gastric cancer and death in takers of cimetidine were considerably greater than in nontakers. However, this difference reflected the takers starting cimetidine therapy with pre-existing cancer or other diseases that increased their morbidity and mortality rates. No evidence supported a causal relationship between these risks and their antiulcer therapy.[524] As gastric pH approaches neutrality for longer periods of time as a result of therapy with potent antisecretory agents, the potential risks of medicinal hypochlorhydria require careful monitoring.

Recommendations for Treatment of Duodenal Ulcer

Initiation of Therapy. The first step in treating a duodenal ulcer is to attempt to withdraw potential offending agents, such as aspirin or other NSAIDs, cigarettes, and excess alcohol and, to the extent possible, to address stressful psychosocial situations. When does one initiate specific therapy in a patient with duodenal ulcer symptoms? In many instances, therapy will be initiated upon demonstration of an ulcer crater. However, in practice, ulcer disease may be suspected from the presence of characteristic symptoms, and therapy (e.g., H$_2$ blockers, antacids, sucralfate) may be started without endoscopic or radiographic demonstration of an ulcer crater. The validity of this approach can be debated, particularly because symptoms are not accurate predictors of the presence of a crater. However, this approach places the emphasis where it belongs—on treating patients and their symptoms—rather than on the ulcer crater *per se*. In low-risk patients, patients under 45 years old and without evidence of complications or markers of organic disease, this approach may be cost-effective.[276, 526] However, it is important to document that symptoms in fact reflect duodenal ulceration in those patients in whom the diagnosis is in doubt, especially if there is suspicion of significant organic disease, or if symptoms do not respond to a brief "therapeutic trial" or are recurrent. Establishing a specific diagnosis and a correlation between symptoms and the presence of an ulcer crater is also essential before embarking upon an expensive, "extra-effort" regimen or prolonged maintenance therapy or before surgery is considered.

At present, duodenal ulcers can be treated in the United States with H$_2$ receptor blockers (cimetidine, ranitidine, and famotidine), antacids, or sucralfate, with the expectation that in 70 to 95 per cent of patients the ulcers will heal in four to eight weeks of therapy. These approved therapies appear equally effective for initial healing and pain relief, so that healing efficacy does not provide a basis for selection among these modalities. Unfortunately, competition in the market place has not reduced the cost of antiulcer therapy, so that the cost factor is at present a minor consideration in selecting a specific therapy.

The emerging evidence that ulcer recurrence rates differ among therapies is another factor influencing the choice among specific regimens. Current evidence indicates that recurrence rates following colloidal bismuth therapy are lower than with H$_2$ antagonists.

Further data are needed to establish the relative recurrence rates among other therapies; such data would influence therapeutic decisions.

The available antiulcer agents are surprisingly free of side effects, so that a given agent would only be contraindicated under specific instances, such as renal failure contraindicating magnesium-containing antacids, or potential drug interactions contraindicating the use of cimetidine. Selecting a simple regimen with twice daily or nighttime dosing will increase patient compliance and therefore be an advantage. In the case of H$_2$ receptor antagonists, a single evening or nighttime dose is an effective and probably "physiologic" approach. With such a regimen, acid secretion during the day is unaltered, thereby allowing acid to suppress bacterial overgrowth and N-nitrosamine production while food is being ingested. The elevation in postprandial serum gastrin that normally occurs with antisecretory therapy probably will be reduced with acid suppression limited to the nighttime hours. However, both the degree to which nocturnal hypochlorhydria elevates fasting gastrin levels and the potential consequences of bacterial overgrowth need to be directly studied with both the potent, long-acting antisecretory agents, such as famotidine, as well as with higher doses of shorter acting agents, such as cimetidine. The most potent antisecretory agents, such as omeprazole, heal DU more rapidly than other therapies, but the advantages after six weeks over other therapies are minimal. Although the potential risks of such potent antisecretory agents in a short treatment period are few, the gain probably will not warrant their use as initial therapy in ordinary DU. Whether such potent agents are more effective in the treatment of acute complications, such as hemorrhage, remains to be established.

Because many ulcers heal and most patients become symptom-free on placebo, one can argue against automatic treatment of all patients with agents that are costly and carry a potential risk.[526] This point is underlined by the finding in one study that cimetidine therapy was the fifth most important determinant of healing rate, ranking behind female sex, moderate alcohol consumption, abstinence from smoking, and a young age.[44] Even though relief of symptoms is often quite rapid with placebo, in most trials treatment with active drugs produces more rapid pain relief and decreases the risk of intractability, if not other complications (see Effects of Therapy on Complications). Thus, it is difficult to justify withholding specific therapy from patients whose symptoms lead them to seek medical care.

Assuming the patient is asymptomatic, the initial round of therapy for an uncomplicated duodenal ulcer can be stopped after four weeks. Progressively more ulcers heal as therapy with standard agents is extended to eight weeks, with healing rates of 90 to 95 per cent achieved in many series,[423] but the advantages of doubling the treatment costs in patients who are asymptomatic and uncomplicated after a four-week treatment period are debatable. Prolonging therapy beyond eight weeks is not justified, because there are no data to indicate that the quality of healing, i.e., the risk of recurrences or complications, will be altered with longer treatment periods. Continued treatment is clearly indicated for patients with persistent symptoms due to refractory ulcer (see below), a history of frequent symptomatic recurrences, or complications. Two studies indicated that in uncomplicated DU, treatment with cimetidine for only the duration of persistent symptoms yielded comparable healing results to therapy for four to six weeks.[527, 528] However, experience with this approach is too limited to recommend it as a general practice.

Recommendations for Refractory Ulcers. Symptom-free patients are not always ulcer-free, but the benefit of proving that an asymptomatic patient following treatment for an uncomplicated DU is ulcer-free does not justify the costs. However, if symptoms persist after eight weeks, an endoscopic confirmation of a refractory ulcer is important. Such refractory ulcers can be treated with a continuation of the same drug, with the expectation that about half of these ulcers will heal during another six weeks of therapy. In general, the benefits of higher doses of antisecretory agents are uncertain. If confirmed, the good response of patients with refractory ulcers to either increasing the dosage of ranitidine to 300 mg bid[459] or switching to omeprazole[473] suggests that maximal suppression of acid secretion will benefit many patients with truly refractory ulcers. After eight weeks, if symptoms or a history of complications warrant the cost of stepping up therapy, the most convenient regimen would be to combine an optimal nighttime dose of cimetidine (800 mg), ranitidine (300 mg), or famotidine (40 mg) with daytime secretory inhibition achieved with the same dose (or half that dose) given in the morning.

A cost-effective alternative to these high-dose, high-cost regimens would be to add low-dose daytime antacids to the normal dose or, if necessary, to high-dose antisecretory therapy. A switch to or addition of sucralfate is another choice, but the data available at present do not lead one to anticipate a dramatic advantage over continued therapy with H$_2$ antagonists in refractory ulcer patients. When available, omeprazole will most likely occupy "cleanup position" for treating ulcers refractory to other therapies, especially if rapid healing is needed because of complications. However, as with other therapies, frequent and rapid recurrences can be expected after omeprazole is stopped in refractory patients, and high-dose maintenance therapy may be necessary for ulcers that require aggressive therapy for initial healing.[473] Present data, although limited, suggest that colloidal bismuth preparations will effectively heal many ulcers refractory to H$_2$ blockers. It will be of considerable interest to establish the recurrence rate in refractory ulcers healed by bismuth therapy.

Recommendations Regarding Therapy for Ulcer Recurrences. Duodenal ulcer is a recurrent disease that can either be approached with intermittent therapy for recurrences or with continuous low-dose maintenance therapy. Certain factors will favor the selection of continuous maintenance therapy, such as a history of complications, age > 60 years, associated serious illness, and continued treatment with NSAIDs.[291] Smoking or the history or refractory ulceration or disabling symptoms with recurrences also favor selecting maintenance therapy. Patients who have an abrupt onset of symptoms (or complications) would also fare better on maintenance therapy because they would not have sentinel dyspeptic symptoms heralding the onset of a recurrence, thus allowing an early start of full-dose therapy. Ulcers recurring after gastric surgery respond as well to therapy as do ulcers in unoperated patients,[374, 529, 530] and medical therapy has far fewer consequences, especially in the short term, than does reoperation for recurrent ulcers.

For patients who do not fall into these high-risk categories, the frequency of recurrences can be used to select the mode of therapy. Because roughly 83 per cent of patients have less than two recurrences per year,[291] intermittent therapy is cost-effective in this majority of patients. Thus, in a low-risk patient, intermittent therapy could be used initially. However, after a patient returns for a second recurrence within a year, it is reasonable to follow a full-dose treatment period with continuous maintenance therapy. The data in clinical trials often reflect a patient population drawn from tertiary referral centers, which may not reflect behavior of patients in the community. The challenge for the physician is to predict the natural history of the ulcer disease for the patient under their care.

Pounder[531] proposed a model for evaluating the outcome of intermittent versus continuous low-dose maintenance therapy. From clinical trial data, the recurrence rate per month on placebo therapy was estimated to be 8.5 per cent, compared to a recurrence rate of 2.5 per cent for patients receiving 400 mg of cimetidine nightly. If patients who recur on either regimen are treated with full-dose cimetidine, one can anticipate that 77 per cent will heal in four weeks. From these estimates, one can predict that utilizing intermittent cimetidine therapy for recurrences leaves 16.5 per cent of patients with active ulcers at any point in time, compared to 3 per cent of patients on continuous low-dose therapy with active ulcers.[531] Thus, using intermittent therapy, considerably more patients will be at risk for complications and symptomatic recurrences. Whether these risks and the attendant costs counterbalance the added cost of continuous low-dose maintenance therapy is a decision that needs to be individualized for each patient, based on the anticipated or demonstrated frequency of recurrences and the anticipated risk associated with recurrences.

Using the model proposed by Pounder, recurrence rates following initial therapy are a major determinant of the number of patients with active ulcers at any point in time. If recurrences are indeed reduced with a given therapy, as appears to be the case with colloidal bismuth compared to H$_2$ blockers, then initial therapy with bismuth would reduce the proportion of patients with active ulcers during the first year of follow-up.[406, 483] However, recurrence rates are only reduced and in at least 60 per cent of patients ulcers still recur within a year; the optimal approach to these patients remains unknown. For example, it is not known whether patients who recur following bismuth therapy will again heal better (recur more slowly) with bismuth than with other therapy. Because of reduced recurrence rates, colloidal bismuth may have an advantage as an initial therapy. Whether repeated courses of bismuth are advantageous to other approaches remains unknown. If decreased recurrence rates and the efficacy of bismuth compounds for refractory ulcers are shown to result from clearance of *C. pylori*, then when tests to detect the presence of *C. pylori* in DU patients become clinically avaiable, such testing would provide a.basis for selecting therapies.

A great deal of clinical experience supports the safety and efficacy of "low-dose," nighttime H_2 blockers (cimetidine, 400 mg; ranitidine, 150 mg; famotidine, 20 mg) for maintenance therapy. Opting for these lower doses is reasonable, especially if the patient does not have a history of complications. Failure on low-dose maintenance does not necessarily predict failure on higher doses or more potent agents; if a patient has a breakthrough recurrence while on low-dose cimetidine, then better inhibition of nocturnal acid secretion will probably be achieved with a switch to ranitidine (150 mg) or famotidine (20 mg). At current prices, these latter two options are preferable because of a lower cost than 800 mg of cimetidine. Of course, a frequent cause of failure is patient noncompliance, a possibility that should be addressed before management is changed.

There is no solid evidence to indicate that patients become resistant to repeated short courses of full-dose therapy or that recurrence rates increase over time on low-dose maintenance therapy. Data regarding side effects and risks of long-term maintenance therapy will be essential before a patient can decide upon long-term therapy with fully informed consent. Such therapy appears very safe, but little data exist on the consequences of prolonged exposure to the degree of nocturnal hypochlorhydria achieved with these agents.

Recommendations Regarding Surgery for Duodenal Ulcer

There is a general consensus that indications for emergency surgery include continuing hemorrhage, unremitting pyloric obstruction, and most instances of perforation. In other instances the decision for surgery is semi-elective, based the occurrence of complications despite compliance with medical management, symptomatic ulcer craters refractory to medical therapy, the unwillingness or inability of the patient to continue drug therapy, and the development of untoward effects that necessitate stopping drug therapy. In patients who present with intractable pain, it is essential to establish that intractable symptoms are associated with refractory duodenal ulceration, since as many as 50 per cent of symptomatic patients do not have a duodenal ulcer. Operations developed for duodenal ulcer are not effective in ulcer-negative dyspepsia.

There is great variability among physicians regarding the decision to operate electively on patients with duodenal ulcer.[532] Such decisions entail weighing unknowns: the long-term benefits and risks of medical management versus surgery (Table 47–6; see also p. 939). Although short-term mortality rates are usually less than 1 per cent, 10 to 40 per cent of patients who have undergone traditional surgical procedures (truncal vagotomy with or without resection) experience sufficient symptoms to alter their life-style, and 5 to 10 per cent of patients experience moderate to severe incapacitation. Certain psychosocial factors may have a major impact on the long-term outcome of surgery, particularly when the indication for surgery is intractable pain; such patients tend to experience greater physical and psychologic disability from their operations.[533-535] Any patient who becomes incapacitated from chronic abdominal pain is likely to be a personality type who will experience difficulty handling any physical or psychologic stress, whether secondary to ulcers or to ulcer surgery. Following gastric surgery, patients often develop new symptoms to replace their abdominal pain[534] and experience considerable psycho-

Table 47–6. BENEFIT/RISK RATIO FOR SURGERY AND LONG-TERM THERAPY OF DUODENAL ULCER

Surgery		Long-Term Medical Therapy	
Benefits	*Risks*	*Benefits*	*Risks*
Decreases ulcer recurrences and complications	Perioperative morbidity and mortality	Decreased recurrence rate Probably ↓ complication rate	Ongoing costs of medical care Long-term untoward effects of drugs
May reduce ongoing cost of medical care for ulcer	*Short-term side effects:* Dumping Disordered gastric motility	Ulcers generally continue to respond to medical therapy	Requires continued patient compliance
	Long-term side effects: Weight loss and malabsorption, Anemia and osteoporosis (?) Risk of suicide and psychologic morbidity Long-term increase in medical costs for some patients	Not permanent, i.e., can be stopped or replaced by new therapy	Risks of hypochlorhydria Enteric infection Gastric bacterial overgrowth with N-nitroso production and possible carcinogenesis Hypergastrinemia with possible ECL cell hyperplasia

logic morbidity and a high suicide rate.[536] Several factors have been associated with a poor surgical outcome, including an age less than 50 years, a broken home setting, social mobility, and the presence of personal conflicts.[533] Before embarking on elective surgical intervention, a thorough psychologic evaluation is a prudent measure to elucidate psychologic factors that might influence both the outcome and the therapeutic decision.

A concern regarding surgery, especially in a younger patient, is the long-range risk of carcinoma developing in the gastric remnant. Several series indicate that 3 to 10 per cent of operated patients develop gastric carcinoma, with the increased risk becoming evident 10 to 15 years after ulcer surgery.[537–539] This risk contrasts with the very low rate of gastric carcinoma found in unoperated duodenal ulcer patients. However, other series have not confirmed an increased risk of gastric carcinoma following surgery;[60, 540, 541] whether these differences are real, reflecting true regional or population differences, remains unclear. The risk of gastric carcinoma is at least a theoretical risk, mitigating against surgery especially in younger patients. Of interest, smoking appears the most important variable predicting late mortality rate following gastric surgery,[60] and death from lung cancer is at least as frequent as death from gastric cancer.

Parietal cell or highly selective vagotomy has the advantages of a lower long-term morbidity rate than traditional procedures but at the expense of a recurrence rate averaging about 10 per cent. This procedure is technically demanding, and the most important variable in the outcome appears to be the experience and specific technical skills of the surgeon.[481] The recurrences that follow surgery are frequently mild, without life-threatening complications, and generally respond well to medical therapy.[287, 481, 530] These are no data to indicate an increased risk of gastric carcinoma following highly selective vagotomy.

Even when a patient's ulcer history is severe enough to consider elective surgery, maintenance drug therapy offers a viable alternative. Well over half of the patients who face this choice are effectively managed on medical therapy, although many require continued drug therapy and develop recurrences when therapy is stopped. The ability to predict the natural history of the ulcer disease for a given patient would be a handy skill for the physician deciding between surgery and maintenance drug therapy. Patients with a history of complications are at greater risk for future complications when not on therapy,[300] but maintenance therapy may reverse this increased risk.[296, 299] Thus, a history of complications is no longer a definite indication for surgery. One would certainly defer operation if duodenal ulcer disease indeed tended to "burn out" over a 10- to 15-year period (see Natural History discussion), or if patients who initially respond to maintenance therapy prove to have a decreased risk of recurrences after the first year. For patients complying with maintenance therapy, the risk of complications requiring emergent surgery is very small. Patients on

medical management retain the option for elective surgery and with present knowledge, deferring surgery does not have obvious deleterious consequences.

Certain features of the ulcer may influence the responsiveness to medical therapy, because postbulbar, prepyloric, pyloric channel, and giant duodenal ulcers and possible combined duodenal and gastric ulcers tend to be more difficult to treat medically. Patients who have had pyloric outlet obstruction may also be a group who will respond poorly to medical management. However, patients refractory to medical management may also have a poor surgical outcome.[287, 457, 535, 542] although others argue that cimetidine resistance does not predict a poor surgical result.[543, 544]

Based upon estimated recurrence rates and risks with both medical and surgical therapy, Sonnenberg[22] concluded that although recurrences would be higher on maintenance medical therapy, the major threat to life is emergency surgery, a very infrequent event, especially in patients compliant with the therapeutic regimen. This risk was outweighed by the immediate morbidity and mortality associated with elective surgery, even when the operation was a highly selective vagotomy. Therefore, although surgery reduces the frequency of ulcer recurrence and complications, this decrease appears insufficient to compensate for the short and long-term consequences of the surgical procedure itself.

In summary, long-term medical therapy with several agents decreases the rate of ulcer recurrence and appears to decrease the risk of complications, but continued therapy is necessary for sustained benefit. The efficacy of maintenance drug therapy appears unaltered over a period of time as long as five years, and the risk of untoward drug effects is acceptably low, although clinical experience with the benefits and risks of such prolonged treatment remains limited. Even if further studies reveal significant risks, medical therapy can be stopped or replaced with a more effective, less hazardous modality. Because maintenance therapy has fewer untoward consequences than surgery, at least in the short term, maintenance drug therapy is a preferable initial choice over early elective surgery. Most likely, the majority of physicians and surgeons—treating their own ulcers—would not hesitate to stay on long-term medical therapy as long as they remained free of symptoms and complications. When, despite an optimal medical regimen, complications or symptomatic recurrences develop and surgery is to be undertaken, a highly selective vagotomy performed by a surgeon experienced in this technique will most likely minimize untoward surgical sequelae, with a small risk of failure. The importance of correlating ulcer-like symptoms with the presence of active ulceration cannot be overemphasized, because ulcer surgery is not appropriate for conditions other than ulcer disease.

Acknowledgments

I am indebted to my many colleagues who have shared with me their wisdom, knowledge, references, and moral support and to Rebecca Fox and Therese Sonnenfeld who have provided the secretarial support without which completion would have remained elusive.

References

1. Ivy, A. L., Grossman, M. I., and Bachrach, W. H. Peptic Ulcer. Philadelphia, The Blakiston Co., 1950, pp. 139–146.
2. Von Haunalter, G., and Chandler, V. V. Cost of Ulcer Disease in the United States. Stanford, Stanford Research Institute Project 5894, 1977.
3. Paringer, L., and Berk, A. Costs of illnesses and disease fiscal year 1975. Report number 2. Contract No. 1-OD-5-2121. Washington, D. C., Public Services Laboratory, Georgetown University, 1977.
4. Ihamaki, T., Varis, K., and Siurala, M. Morphological, functional and immunological state of the gastric mucosa in gastric carcinoma families. Comparison with a computer-matched family sample. Scand. J. Gastroenterol. *14*:801, 1979.
5. Current Estimates from the National Health Interview Survey, United States, 1979. Vital and Health Statistics. Data from the National Health Survey, series 10, No. 136. National Center for Health Statistics, United States Department of Health and Human Services Publication No. (PHS)81:1564, 1981, p. 34.
6. Grossman, M. I. Peptic Ulcer: Definition and Epidemiology. *In* Rotter, J., Samloff, I. M., and Rimoin, D. L. (eds.): The Genetics and Heterogeneity of Common Gastrointestinal Disorders. New York, Academic Press, 1980, p. 21.
7. Langman, M. J. S. Peptic Ulcer. *In* The Epidemiology of Chronic Digestive Disease. Chicago, Year Book Medical Publishers, Inc., 1979, p. 9.
8. Monson, R. R., and MacMahon, B.: Peptic ulcer in Massachusetts physicians. N. Engl. J. Med. *281*:11, 1969.
9. Bonnevie, O. The incidence of duodenal ulcer in Copenhagen County. Scand. J. Gastoenterol. *10*:385, 1975.
10. Pulvertaft, C. N. Peptic ulcer in town and country. Br. J. Prev. Soc. Med. *13*:131, 1959.
11. Prevalence of Selected Chronic Digestive Conditions, United States, 1975. Vital and Health Statistics. Data from the National Health Survey. National Center for Health Statistics, United States Department of Health and Human Services. DHEW Publication No. (PHS)79:1558, 1979, p. 14.
12. Kurata, J. H., Honda, G. D., and Frankl, H. The incidence of duodenal and gastric ulcers in a large Health Maintenance Organization. Am. J. Publ. Health *75*(6):625, 1985.
13. Brown, R. C., Langman, M. J. S., and Lambert, P. M. Hospital admissions for peptic ulcer during 1958–1972. Br. Med. J. *1*:35, 1976.
14. Coggon, D., Lambert, P., and Langman, M. J. S. Twenty years of hospital admissions for pepic ulcer in England and Wales. Lancet *1*:1302, 1981.
15. Elashoff, J. D., and Grossman, M. I. Trends in hospital admissions and death rates for peptic ulcer in the United States from 1970 to 1978. Gastroenterology *78*:280, 1980.
16. Kurata, J. H., and Corboy, E. D. Changing pattern of peptic ulcer trends. J. Clin. Gastroenterol., in press, 1988.
17. Walt, R., Katschinski, B., Logan, R., Ashley, J., and Langman, M. Occasional survey: Rising frequency of ulcer perforation in elderly people in the United Kingdom. Lancet *1*:489, 1986.
18. Sonnenberg, A. Changes in physician visits for gastric and duodenal ulcer in the United States during 1958–1984 as shown by National Disease and Therapeutic Index (NDTI). Dig. Dis. Sci. *32*(1):1, 1987.
19. Kurata, J. H., Honda, G. D., and Frankl, H. Hospitalization and mortality rates for peptic ulcers: A comparison of a large Health Maintenance Organization and United States Data. Gastroenterology *83*:1008, 1982.
20. Koo, J., Ngan, Y. K., and Lam, S. K. Trends in hospital admission, perforation, and mortality of peptic ulcer in Hong Kong from 1970 to 1980. Gastroenterology *84*:1558, 1983.
21. Kurata, J. H., Elashoff, J. D., Honda, G. D., and Haile, B. M. A reappraisal of time trends in ulcer disease: Factors related to changes in ulcer hospitalization and mortality rates. Am. J. Publ. Health *73*:1066, 1983.
22. Sonnenberg, A. Geographic and temporal variations in the occurrence of peptic ulcer disease. Scand. J. Gastroenterol. *20*(suppl. 110):11, 1985.
23. Bonnevie, O. Changing demographics of peptic ulcer disease. Dig. Dis. Sci. *30*(11)(Nov. 85 suppl.):8S, 1985.
24. Susser, M. Period effects, generation effects and age effects in peptic ulcer mortality. J. Chron. Dis. *35*:29, 1982.
25. Hugh, T. B., Coleman, M. J., McNamara, M. E., Norman, J. R., and Howell, C. Epidemiology of peptic ulcer in Australia. A study based on government statistics in four states. Med. J. Aust. *21*:81, 1984.
26. Tovey, F. I. Peptic ulcer in India and Bangladesh. Gut *20*:329, 1979.
27. Moshal, M. G., Spitaels, J. M., Robbs, J. V., MacLeod, I. N., and Good, C. J. Eight-year experience with 3392 endoscopically proven duodenal ulcers in Durban, 1972–79. Rise and fall of duodenal ulcers and a theory of changing dietary and social factors. Gut *22*:327, 1981.
28. Friedman, G. D., Siegelaub, A. B., and Seltzer, C. C. Cigarettes, alcohol, coffee and peptic ulcer. N. Engl. J. Med. *290*:469, 1974.
29. Kurata, J. H., and Haile, B. H. Racial difference in peptic ulcer disease: Fact or myth. Gastroenterology *83*:166, 1982.
30. Kurata, J. H., Haile, B. M., and Elashoff, J. D. Sex differences in peptic ulcer disease. Gastroenterology *88*:96, 1985.
31. Kurata, J. H., Elashoff, J. D., Nogawa, A. N., and Haile, B. M. Sex and smoking differences in duodenal ulcer mortality. Am. J. Publ. Health *76*(6):700, 1986.
32. Malhotra S. L. A comparison of unrefined wheat and rice diets in the management of duodenal ulcer. Postgrad. Med. J. *54*:6, 1978.
33. Rydning, A., and Berstad, A. Dietary fiber and peptic ulcer. Scand. J. Gastroenterol. *21*:1, 1986.
34. Rydning, A., Berstad, A., Aadland, E., and Odegaard, B. Prophylactic effect of dietary fibre in duodenal ulcer disease. Lancet *2*:736, 1982.
35. Cohen, S. Pathogenesis of coffee-induced gastrointestinal symptoms. N. Engl. J. Med. *303*:122, 1980.
36. Cohen, S., and Booth, G. H., Jr. Gastric acid secretion and lower-esophageal-sphincter pressure in response to coffee and caffeine. N. Engl. J. Med. *293*:897, 1975.
37. Paffenbarger, R. S., Jr., Wing, A. L., and Hyde, R. T. Chronic disease in former college students. XIII. Early precursors of peptic ulcer. Am. J. Epidemiol. *100*:307, 1974.
38. Ostensen, H., Gudmundsen, T. E., Burhol, P. G., and Bonnevie, O. Smoking, alcohol, coffee, and familial factors: Any associations with peptic ulcer disease? A clinically and radiologically prospective study. Scand. J. Gastroenterol. *20*(10):1227, 1985.
39. McArthur, K., Hogan, D., and Isenberg, J. I. Relative stimulatory effects of commonly ingested beverages on gastric acid secretion in humans. Gastroenterology *83*:199, 1982.
40. Dubey, P., Sundram, K. R., and Nundy, S. Effect of tea on gastric acid secretion. Dig. Dis. Sci. *29*(3):202, 1984.
41. Piper, D. W., Nasiry, R., McIntosh, J., Shy, C. M., Pierce, J., and Byth, K. Smoking, alcohol, analgesics, and chronic duodenal ulcer. A controlled study of habits before first symptoms and before diagnosis. Scand. J. Gastroenterol. *19*:1015, 1984.
42. Lenz, H. J., Ferrari-Taylor, J., and Isenberg, J. I. Wine and five percent ethanol are potent stimulants of gastric acid secretion in humans. Gastroenterology *85*:1082, 1983.
43. Peterson, W. L., Barnett, C., and Walsh, J. H. Effect of intragastric infusions of ethanol and wine on serum gastrin concentration and gastric acid secretion. Gastroenterology *91*(6):1390, 1986.
44. Sonnenberg, A., Muller-Lissner, S. A., Vogel, E., Schmid, P., Gonvers, J. J., Peter, P., Strohmeyer, G., and Blum, A. L.: Predictors of duodenal ulcer healng and relapse. Gastroenterology *81*:1061, 1981.

45. Kurata, J. H., Elashoff, J. D., and Grossman, M. I. Inadequacy of the literature on the relationship between drugs, ulcers, and gastrointestinal bleeding. Gastroenterology 82:373, 1982.

46. Levy, M. Aspirin use in patients with major upper gastrointestinal bleeding and peptic-ulcer disease. N. Engl. J. Med. 290(21):1158, 1974.

47. Piper, D. W., McIntosh, J. H., Ariotti, D. E., Fenton, B. H., and MacLennan, R. Analgesic ingestion and chronic peptic ulcer. Gastroenterology 80:427, 1981.

48. Lanza, F., Royer, G. L., and Nelson, R. S. Endoscopic evaluation of the effects of aspirin, buffered aspirin, and enteric-coated aspirin on gastric and duodenal mucosa. N. Engl. J. Med. 303(3):136, 1980.

49. Lanza, F. L., Royer, G. L., Nelson, R. S., Chen, T. T., Seckman, C. E., and Rach, M. F.: A comparative endoscopic evaluation of the damaging effects of nonsteroidal anti-inflammatory agents on the gastric and duodenal mucosa. Am. J. Gastroenterol. 75(1):17, 1981.

50. Lockard, O. O., Jr., Ivey, K. J., Butt, J. H., Silvoso, G. R., Sisk, C., and Holt, S. The prevalence of duodenal lesions in patients with rheumatic diseases on chronic aspirin therapy. Gastrointest. Endosc. 26(1):5, 1980.

51. Silvoso, G. R., Ivey, K. J., Butt, J. H., Lockard, O. O., Holt, S. D., Sisk, C., Baskin, W. N., Mackercher, P. A., and Hewett, J. Incidence of gastric lesions in patients with rheumatic disease on chronic aspirin therapy. Ann. Intern. Med. 91:517, 1979.

52. Collier, D. St. J., and Pain, J. A.: Non-steroidal anti-inflammatory drugs and peptic ulcer perforation. Gut 26:359–363, 1985.

53. Somerville, K., Faulker, G., and Langman, M. Non-steroidal anti-inflammatory drugs and bleeding peptic ulcer. Lancet 1:462, 1986.

54. Graham, D. Y., Smith, J. L., and Dobbs, S. M.: Gastric adaptation occurs with aspirin administration in man. Dig. Dis. Sci. 28(1):1, 1983.

55. Conn, H. O., and Blitzer, B. L. Nonassociation of adrenocorticosteroid therapy and peptic ulcer. N. Engl. J. Med. 294:473, 1976.

56. Messer, J., Reitman, D., Sacks, H. S., Smith, H., Jr., and Chalmers, T. C. Association of adrenocorticosteroid therapy and peptic-ulcer disease. N. Engl. J. Med. 309(1):21, 1983.

57. Spiro, H. M.: Is the steroid ulcer a myth (editorial)? N. Engl. J. Med. 309(1):45, 1983.

58. Harrison, A. R., Elashof, J. D., and Grossman, M. I. Peptic Ulcer Disease. In Smoking and Health, Report of the Surgeon General. Washington, D.C., U.S. Public Health Service, Office on Smoking and Health, DHEW Publication No. 79-50066, 1979, pp. 9–36.

59. McCarthy, D. M. Smoking and ulcers—time to quit (editorial). N. Engl. J. Med. 311(11):726, 1984.

60. Ross, A. H. M., Smith, M. A., Anderson, J. R., and Small, W. P. Late mortality after surgery for peptic ulcer. N. Engl. J. Med. 307(9):519, 1982.

61. Rotter, J. I., and Rimoin, D. L. Peptic ulcer disease—a heterogeneous group of disorders? Gastroenterology 73:604, 1977.

62. Rotter, J. I. Peptic ulcer. In Emery, A. E. H., and Rimoin, D. L. (eds.): The Principles and Practice of Medical Genetics. New York, Churchill Livingstone, 1983, pp. 863–878.

63. McConnell, R. B. Peptic ulcer: Early genetic evidence—families, twins, and markers. In Rotter, J. I., Samloff, I. M., and Rimoin, D. L. (eds.): The Genetics and Heterogeneity of Common Gastrointestinal Disorders. New York, Academic Press, 1980, p. 31.

64. Doll, R., and Kellock, T. D. The separate inheritance of gastric and duodenal ulcers. Ann. Eugen. 16:231, 1951.

65. Ellis, A., and Woodrow, J. C. HLA and duodenal ulcer. Gut 20:760, 1979.

66. Goedhard, J. G., Biemond, I., Pena, A. S., Kreuning, J., Schreuder, G. M., and Van Rood, J. J. HLA and duodenal ulcer in The Netherlands. Tissue Antigens 22:213–218, 1983.

67. Samloff, I. M. Pepsinogens and their relationship to peptic ulcer. In Rotter, J. I., Samloff, I. M., and Rimoin, D. L. (eds.): The Genetics and Heterogeneity of Common Gastrointestinal Disorders. New York, Academic Press, 1980, p. 43.

68. Pearson, J. P., Ward, R., Allen, A., Roberts, N. B., and Taylor, W. H. Mucus degradation by pepsin: Comparison of mucolytic activity of human pepsin 1 and pepsin 3: Implications in peptic ulceration. Gut 27:243, 1986.

69. Samloff, I. M., Stemmermann G. N., Heilbrun, L. K., and Nomura, A.: Elevated serum pepsinogen I and II levels differ as risk factors for duodenal ulcer and gastric ulcer. Gastroenterology 90:570, 1986.

70. Samloff, I. M., Liebman, W. M., and Panitch, N. M. Serum group I pepsinogens by radioimmunoassay in control subjects and patients with peptic ulcer. Gastroenterology 69:83, 1975.

71. Mirsky, I. A. Physiologic, psychologic, and social determinants in the etiology of duodenal ulcer. Am. J. Dig. Dis. 3:285, 1958.

72. Rotter, J. I., Sones, J. Q., Samloff, I. M., Richardson, C. T., Gursky, J. M., Walsh, J. H., and Rimoin, D. L. Duodenal-ulcer disease associated with elevated serum pepsinogen I. An inherited autosomal dominant disorder. N. Engl. J. Med. 300(63):53, 1979.

73. Rotter, J. I., Petersen, G., Samloff, I. M., McConnell, R. B., Ellis, A., Spence, M. A., and Rimoin, D. L. Genetic heterogeneity of hyperpepsinogenemic I and normopepsinogenemic I duodenal ulcer disease. Ann. Intern. Med. 91:372, 1979.

74. Habibullah, C. M., Mujahid, Ali, M., Ishaq, M., Prasad, R., Pratap, B., and Saleem, Y. Study of duodenal ulcer disease in 100 families using total serum pepsinogen as a genetic marker. Gut 25:1380, 1984.

75. Rotter, J. I., Rubin, R., Meyer, J. H., Samloff, M. I., and Rimoin, D. L. Rapid gastric emptying—an inherited pathophysiologic defect in duodenal ulcer (abstract)? Gastroenterology 76:1229, 1979.

76. Arnold, R., Koop, H., and Creutzfeldt, W. Hormones and their role in ulcer disease. In Holtermuller, K.-H., and Malagelada, J.-R. (eds.): Advances in Ulcer Disease, Amsterdam, Excerpta Medica, 1980, p. 207.

77. Lamers, C. B. H. W., Jansen, J. B. M. J., Rotter, J. I., and Samloff, I. M. Serum pepsinogen I in hereditary hypergastrinemic peptic ulcer syndromes. In Rotter, J. I., Samloff, I. M., and Rimoin, D. L. Pepsinogens in Man: Clinical and Genetic Advances. New York, A. R. Liss, 1985, pp. 273–281.

78. Taylor, I. L., Calam, J., Rotter, J. I., Vaillant, C., Samloff, I. M., Cook, A., Simkin, E., and Dockray, G. J. Family studies of hypergastrinemic, hyperpepsinogenemic I duodenal ulcer. Ann. Intern. Med. 95:421, 1981.

79. Lam, S. K., Koo, J., Sircus, W. Early- and late-onset duodenal ulcers in Chinese and Scots. Scand. J. Gastroenterol. 18:651, 1983.

80. Johnson, H. D. Gastric ulcer, classification, blood group characteristics, secretion patterns and pathogenesis. Ann. Surg. 162:996, 1965.

81. Lam, S. K., and Lai, C. L. Gastric ulcers with and without associated duodenal ulcer have different pathophysiology. Clin. Sci. Mol. Med. 55:97, 1978.

82. Bonnevie, O. The incidence in Copenhagen County of gastric and duodenal ulcers in the same patient. Scand. J. Gastroenterol. 10:529, 1975.

83. Rotter, J. I., and Heiner, D. C.: Are there immunologic forms of duodenal ulcer? J. Clin. Lab. Immunol. 7:1, 1982.

84. Ammann, R. W., Vetter, D., Deyhle, P., Tschen, H., Sulser, H., and Schmid, M. Gastrointestinal involvement in systemic mastocytosis. Gut 17:107, 1976.

85. Selmanowitz, V. J., Orentreich, N., Tiangco, C. C., and Demis, D. J., Uniovular twins' discordance for cutaneous mastocytosis. Arch. Dermatol. 102:34, 1970.

86. Shaw, J. M. Genetic aspects of urticaria pigmentosa. Arch. Dermatol. 97:137, 1968.

87. Neuhauser, G., Daly, R. F., Magnelli, N. C., Barreras, R. F., Donaldson, R. M., Jr., and Opitz, J. M. Essential tremor, nystagmus and duodenal ulceration. Clin. Gent. 9:81, 1976.

88. Van Allen, M. W., Frohlich, J. A., and Davis, J. R. Inherited predisposition to generalized amyloidosis. Neurology 19:10, 1969.

89. Stevenson, R. E., Lucas, T., and Martin, J. R. Stiff skin and multiple system disease in four generations (abstract). Am. J. Hum. Genet. 31:84A, 1979.

90. Lam, S. K., Hui, W. K. K., Ho, J., Wong, K. P., Rotter, J.

I., and Samloff, I. M. Pachydermoperiostosis, hypertrophic gastropathy, and peptic ulcer. Gastroenterology *84*(4):834, 1983.

91. Halal, F., Gervais, M. H., Baillargeon, J., and Lesage, R. Gastrocutaneous syndrome: Peptic ulcer, multiple letigenes/café-au-lait spots, hypertelorism and myopia. Am. J. Med. Genet. *11*:161, 1982.

92. Ingegno, A. P., and Yatto, R. P. Hereditary leukonychia, duodenal ulcer and gallstones (abstract). Gastroenterology *82*:1089, 1982.

93. Fordtran, J. S. Psychological factors in duodenal ulcer. Pract. Gastroenterol. *3*:24, 1979.

94. Weiner, H. Peptic ulcer. *In* Psychobiology and Human Disease. Amsterdam, Elsevier North Holland, 1977.

95 Alexander, F. Psychosomatic Medicine. New York, Norton, 1950.

96. Weiner, H., Thaler, M., Reiser, M. F., and Mirsky, I. A. Etiology of duodenal ulcer. I. Relation of specific psychological characteristics to rate of gastric secretion (serum pepsinogen). Psychosom. Med. *19*:1, 1957.

97. Weisman, A. D. A study of the psychodynamics of duodenal ulcer exacerbations. With special reference to treatment and the problem of "specificity." Psychosom. Med. *18*:2, 1956.

98. Feldman, M., Walker, P., Green, J. L., and Weingarden, K. Life events stress and psychosocial factors in men with peptic ulcer disease. A multidimensional case-controlled study. Gastroenterology *91*:1370, 1986.

99. Magni, G., Di Mario, F., Rizzardo, R., Pulin, S., and Naccarato, R. Personality profiles of patients with duodenal ulcer. Am. J. Psychiat. *143*(10):1297, 1986.

100. Peters, M. N., and Richardson, C. T. Stressful life events, acid hypersecretion, and ulcer disease. Gastroenterology *84*:114, 1983.

101. Stewart, D. N., and Winser, D. M. Incidence of perforated peptic ulcer: Effect of heavy air-raids. Lancet *1*:259, 1942.

102. Rabkin, J. G., and Struening, E. L. Life events, stress, and illness. Science *194*:1013, 1976.

103. Feldman, E. J., and Sabovich, K. A. Stress and peptic ulcer disease (editorial). Gastroenterology *78*:1087, 1980.

104. Piper, D. W., McIntosh, J. H., Ariotti, D. E., Calogiuri, J. V., Brown, R. W., and Shy, C. M. Life events and chronic duodenal ulcer: A case control study. Gut *22*:1011, 1981.

105. Engle, G. L., Reichsman, F., and Segal, H. L. A study of an infant with a gastric fistula. I. Behavior and the rate of total hydrochloric acid secretion. Psychosom. Med. *18*:374, 1956.

106. Achord, J. L. Gastric pepsin and acid secretion in patients with acute and healed duodenal ulcer. Gastroenterology *81*:15–18, 1981.

107. Littman, A. Basal gastric secretion in patients with duodenal ulcer: A long term study of variations in relation to ulcer activity. Gastroenterology *43*:166, 1962.

108. Johnson, D., and Jepson, K. Use of pentagastrin in a test of gastric acid secretion. Lancet *2*:585, 1967.

109. Lam, S. K., Pathogenesis and pathophysiology of duodenal ulcer. Clin. Gastroenterol. *13*:447–472, 1984.

110. Blair, A. J., III, Feldman, M., Barnett, C., Walsh, J. H., and Richardson, T. Detailed comparison of basal and food-stimulated gastric acid secretion rates and serum gastrin concentrations in duodenal ulcer patients and normal subjects. J. Clin. Invest. *79*:582–587, 1987.

111. Dragstedt, L. R. Gastric secretion tests (editorial). Gastroenterology *52*(3):587, 1967.

112. Feldman, M., and Richardson, C. T. Total 24-hour gastric acid secretion in patients with duodenal ulcer. Gastroenterology *90*:540, 1986.

113. Grossman, M. I., and Elashoff, J. Antrectomy and maximal acid output (editorial). Gastroenterology *78*:165, 1980.

114. Cox, A. J. Stomach size and its relation to chronic peptic ulcer. Arch. Pathol. *54*:407, 1952.

115. Johnson, L. R. The trophic action of gastrointestinal hormones. Gastroenterology *70*:278, 1976.

116. Hirasuna, J. D., Shelub, I., and Bolt, R. J. Hyperhistaminemia and peptic ulcer. West. J. Med. *131*:140, 1979.

117. Olinger, E. J., McCarthy, D. M., Young, R. C., and Gardner, J. D. Hyperhistaminemia and hyperchlorhydria in basophilic granulocytic leukemia. Gastroenterology *71*:667, 1976.

118. Kirkpatrick, P. M., Jr., and Hirschowitz, B. I. Duodenal ulcer with unexplained marked basal gastric acid hypersecretion. Gastroenterology *79*:4, 1980.

119. Feldman, M., Richardson, C. T., and Fordtran, J. S. Effect of sham feeding on gastric acid secretion in healthy subjects and duodenal ulcer patients. Evidence for increased vagal tone in some ulcer patients. Gastroenterology *79*:796, 1980.

120. Soll, A. H., and Berglindh, T. Physiology of isolated gastric glands and parietal cells: Receptors and effectors regulating function. *In* Johnson, L. R. (ed): Physiology of the Gastrointestinal Tract. 2nd ed. New York, Raven Press, 1987, p. 883.

121. Kohn, A., Annibale, B., Suriano, G., Severi, C., Spinella, S., and Delle Fave, G. Gastric acid and pancreatic polypeptide responses to modified sham feeding: Indication of an increased basal vagal tone in a subgroup of duodenal ulcer patients. Gut *26*:776, 1985.

122. Moore, J. G. Circadian rhythm of gastric acid secretion in man. Nature *226*:1261, 1970.

123. Malagelada, J.-R. Longstreth, G. F., Deering, T. B., Summerskill, W. H. J., and Go, V.-L. W. Gastric secretion and emptying after ordinary meals in duodenal ulcer. Gastroenterology *73*:989, 1977.

124. Cooper, R. G., Dockray, G. J., Calam, J., and Walker, R. Acid and gastrin responses during intragastric titration in normal subjects and duodenal ulcer patients with G-cell hyperfunction. Gut *26*:232, 1985.

125. Lewin, K. J., Elashoff, J. D., Yang, K., Walsh, J., and Ulich, T. Primary gastrin cell hyperplasia. Report of five cases and a review of the literature. Am. J. Surg. Pathol. *8*(11):821, 1984.

126. Lam, S. K., and Ong, G. B. Identification of two subgroups of familial early-onset duodenal ulcers. Ann. Intern. Med. *93*:540, 1980.

127. Lam, S K., Isenberg, J. I., Grossman, M. I., Lane, W. H., and Walsh, J. H. Gastric acid secretion is abnormally sensitive to exogenous gastrin released after peptone test meals in duodenal ulcer patients. J. Clin. Invest. *65*:555, 1980.

128 Lam, S. K., and Koo, J. Gastrin sensitivity in duodenal ulcer. Gut *26*:485, 1985.

129. Hirschowitz, B. I. Apparent and intrinsic sensitivity to pentagastrin of acid and pepsin secretion in peptic ulcer. Gastroenterology *86*:843, 1984.

130. Mayer, G., Arnold, R., Feurle, G. Fuchs, K., Ketterer, H., Track, N. S., and Creutzfeldt, W. Influences of feeding and sham feeding upon serum gastrin and gastric acid secretion in control subjects and duodenal ulcer patients. Scand. J. Gastroenterol. *9*:703, 1974.

131. Konturek, S. J., Kwiecien, N., Obtulowicz, W., Mikos, E., Sito, E., Oleksy, J., and Popiela, T. Cephalic phase of gastric secretion in healthy subjects and duodenal ulcer patients: Role of vagal innervation. Gut *20*:875, 1978.

132. Lam, S. K., and Sircus, W. Vagal hyperactivity in duodenal ulcer: With and without excessive acid secretion. Rendic. Gastroenterol. *7*:5, 1975.

133. Lam, S. K., and Sircus, W. A comparison of acid and gastrin secretory responses to hypoglycemia and meals in duodenal ulcer with and without acid hypersection to pentagastrin. Digestion *14*:1, 1976.

134. Walsh, J. H., Richardson, C. T., and Fordtran, J. S. pH dependence of acid secretion and gastrin release in normal and ulcer subjects. J. Clin. Invest. *55*:462, 1975.

135. Kihl, B., and Olbe, L. Fat inhibition of gastric acid secretion in duodenal ulcer patients before and after proximal gastric vagotomy. Gut *21*:1056, 1980.

136. Schoon, I. M., Bergegardh, S., Grotzinger, U., and Olbe, L. Evidence for a defective inhibition of pentagastrin-stimulated gastric acid secretion by antral distension in the duodenal ulcer patient. Gastroenterology *75*(3):363, 1978.

137. Lam, S. K., Isenberg, J. I., Grossman, M. I., Lane, W. H., and Hogan, D. L. Rapid gastric emptying in duodenal ulcer patients. Dig. Dis. Sci. *27*:598, 1982.

138. Williams, N. S., Elashoff, J., and Meyer, J. H. Gastric emp-

tying of liquids in normal subjects and patients with healed duodenal ulcer disease. Dig. Dis. Sci. *31*(9):943, 1986.

139. Holt, S., Heading, R. C., Taylor, T. V., Forrest, J. A., and Tothill, P. Is gastric emptying abnormal in duodenal ulcer? Dig. Dis. Sci. *31*(7):685, 1986.

140. Samloff, I. M. Pepsins, peptic activity, and peptic inhibitors. J. Clin. Gastroenterol. *3*(suppl. 2):91, 1981.

141. Alphin, R. S., Vokac, V. A., Gregory, R. L., Bolton, P. M., and Tawes, J. W., III. Role of intragastric pressure, pH, and pepsin in gastric ulceration in the rat. Gastroenterology *73*:495, 1977.

142. Joffe, S. N., Roberts, N. B., Taylor, W. H., and Baron, J. H. Exogenous and endogenous acid and pepsins in the pathogenesis of duodenal ulcers in the rat. Dig. Dis. Sci. *25*:837, 1980.

143. Thon, K. P., Lorenz, W., Ochmann, C. H., Weber, D., Rohde, H., and Roher, H. D. Sample taking problems in measuring actual histamine levels of human gastroduodenal mucosa: Specific and general relevance in clinical trials on peptic ulcer pathogenesis and selective proximal vagotomy. Gut *26*(11):1165, 1985.

144. Parsons, M E. Histamine and the pathogenesis of duodenal ulcer disease (editorial). Gut *26*:1159, 1985.

145. Man, W. K., Thompson, J. N., Baron, J. H., and Spencer, J. Histamine and duodenal ulcer: Effect of omeprazole on gastric histamine in patients with duodenal ulcer. Gut *27*:418, 1986

146. Sanders, M. J., Ayalon, A., Roll, M., and Soll, A. H. The apical surface of canine chief cell monolayers resists H$^+$ back-diffusion. Nature *313*(5997):52, 1985.

147. Isenberg, J. I., Hogan, D. L., Koss, M. A., and Selling, J. A. Human duodenal mucosal bicarbonate secretion. Evidence for basal secretion and stimulation by hydrochloric acid and a synthetic prostaglandin E$_1$ analogue. Gastroenterology *91*:370, 1986.

148. Isenberg, J. K., Selling, J. A., Hogan, D. L., and Koss, M. A. Impaired proximal duodenal mucosal bicarbonate secretion in patients with duodenal ulcer. N. Engl. J. Med. *361*(7):374, 1987.

149. Quigley, E. M. M., and Turnberg, L. A. pH of the microclimate lining human gastric and duodenal mucosa in vivo. Studies in control subjects and in duodenal ulcer patients. Gastroenterology *92*:1876, 1987.

150. Feldman, M. Bicarbonate, acid and duodenal ulcer. N. Engl. J. Med. *316*(7):408, 1987.

151. Feldman, M., and Barnett, C. C. Gastric bicarbonate secretion in patients with duodenal ulcer. Gastroenterology *88*:1205, 1985.

152. Younan, F., Pearson, J., Allen, A., and Venables, C. Changes in the structure of the mucous gel on the mucosal surface of the stomach in association with peptic ulcer disease. Gastroenterology *82*:827, 1982.

153. Ahlquist, D. A., Dozois, R. R., Zinsmeister, A. R., and Malagelada, J.-R. Duodenal prostaglandin synthesis and acid load in health and in duodenal ulcer disease. Gastroenterology *85*:522, 1983.

154. Hillier, K., Smith, C. L., Jewell, R., Arthur, M. J. P., and Ross, G. Duodenal mucosa synthesis of prostaglandins in duodenal ulcer disease. Gut *26*:237, 1985.

155. Rachmilewitz, D., Ligumsky, M., Fich, A., Goldin, E., Eliakim, A., and Karmeli, F. Role of endogenous gastric prostanoids in the pathogenesis and therapy of duodenal ulcer. Gastroenterology *90*:963, 1986.

156. Hawkey, C. J., and Rampton, D. S. Prostaglandins and the gastrointestinal mucosa: Are they important in its function, disease or treatment? Gastroenterology *89*:1162, 1985.

157. Ligumsky, M., Golanska, E. M., Hansen, D. G., and Kauffman, G. L. Aspirin can inhibit gastric mucosal cyclo-oxygenase without causing gastric mucosal lesions (abstract). Gastroenterology *82*:1117, 1982.

158. Feldman, M., and Colturi, T. J. Effect of indomethacin on gastric acid and bicarbonate secretion in humans. Gastroenterology *87*:1339, 1984.

159. Levine, R. A., and Schwartzel, E. H. Effect of indomethacin on basal and histamine stimulated human gastric acid secretion. Gut *25*:718, 1984.

160. Meikle, D. D., Taylor, K. B., Truelove, S. C., and Whitehead, R. Gastritis duodenitis, and circulating levels of gastrin in duodenal ulcer before and after vagotomy. Gut *17*:719, 1976.

161. Greenlaw, R., Sheahan, D. G., DeLuca, V., Miller, D., Myerson, D., and Myerson, P. Gastroduodenitis. A broader concept of peptic ulcer disease. Dig. Dis. Sci. *25*(9):660, 1980.

162. Hui, W.-M., Lam, S. K., Ho, J., Ng, M.-M., Lui, I., Lai, C.-L., Lok, A.-S., Lau, W.-Y., Poon, G.-P., Choi, S., and Choi, T.-K. Chronic antral gastritis in duodenal ulcer. Natural history and treatment with prostaglandin E$_1$. Gastroenterology *91*(5):1095, 1986.

163. Cheli, R., and Giacosa, A. Duodenal ulcer and chronic gastritis. Endoscopy *18*:125, 1986.

164. Kekki, M., Sipponen, P., and Siurala, M. Progression of antral and body gastritis in patients with active and healed duodenal ulcer and duodenitis. Scand. J. Gastroenterol. *19*:382, 1984.

165. Cheli, R. Duodenitis and duodenal ulcer. A biopsy study. Digestion *1*:175, 1968.

166. Kreuning, J., Bosman, F. T., Kuiper, G., Wal, A. M., and Lindeman, J.: Gastric and duodenal mucosa in "healthy" individuals. J. Clin. Pathol. *31*:69, 1978.

167. Earlam, R. J., Amerigo, J., Kakavoulis, T., and Pollock, D. J. Histological appearances of oesophagus, antrum and duodenum and their correlation with symptoms in patients with duodenal ulcer. Gut *26*:95, 1985.

168. Paoluzi, P., Pallone, F., Zaccardelli, E., Ripoli, F., Marcheggiano, A., and Carratu, R. Outcome of ulcer-associated duodenitis after short-term medical treatment. Dig. Dis. Sci. *30*(7):624, 1985.

169. Fullman, H., Van Deventer, G., Schneidman, D., Walsh, J., Elashoff, J., and Weinstein, W. "Healed" duodenal ulcers are histologically ill. Gastroenterology *88*(5:2):1390, 1985.

170. Kirk, R. M., Could chronic peptic ulcers be localised areas of acid susceptibility generated by autoimmunity? Lancet *1*(8484):772, 1986.

171. Goodwin, C. S., Armstrong, J. A., and Marshall, B. J. Campylobacter pyloridis, gastritis, and peptic ulceration. J. Clin. Pathol. *39*:353, 1986.

172. Rathbone, B. J., Wyatt, J. I., and Heatley, R. V. Campylobacter pyloridis—a new factor in peptic ulcer disease? Gut *27*:635, 1986.

172a. Dooley, C. P., and Cohen, H. The clinical significance of campylobacter pylori. Ann. Intern. Med. *108*:70, 1988.

173. Andersen, L. P., Holck, S., Povlsen, C. O., Elsborg, L., and Justesen, T. Campylobacter pyloridis in peptic ulcer disease. I. Gastric and duodenal infection caused by C. pyloridis: Histopathologic and microbiologic findings. Scand. J. Gastroenterol. *22*:219, 1987.

174. Steer, H. W. Surface morphology of the gastroduodenal mucosa in duodenal ulceration. Gut *25*:1203, 1984.

175. Lambert, J. R., Dunn, K. L., Eaves, E. R., Korman, M. G., and Hansky, J. Campylobacter pyloridis in diseases of the human upper gastrointestinal tract. Gastroenterology *92*:1509, 1986.

176. Marshall, B. J., Goodwin, C. S., Warren, J. R., Murray, R., Blincow, E., Blackbourn, S., Phillips, M., Waters, T., and Sanderson, C. Long term healing of gastritis and low duodenal ulcer relapse after eradication of Campylobacter pyloridis: A prospective double-blind study. Gastroenterology *92*(5:2):1518, 1987.

177. McNulty, C. A. M., Gearty, J. C., Crump, B., Davis, M., Donovan, I. A., Melikian, V., Lister, D. M., and Wise, R. Campylobacter pyloridis and associated gastritis: Investigator blind, placebo controlled trial of bismuth salicylate and erythromycin ethylsuccinate. Br. Med. J. *293*:645, 1986.

178. Viruses and duodenal ulcer (editorial). Lancet *1*(8222):705, 1981.

179. Vestergaard, B. F., and Rune, S. J. Type-specific herpes simplex virus antibodies in patients with recurrent duodenal ulcer. Lancet *1*:1273, 1980.

180. Franzin, G., Muolo, A., and Griminelli, T. Cytomegalovirus inclusions in the gastroduodenal mucosa of patients after renal transplantation. Gut *22*:698–701, 1981.

181. Donaldson, R. M., Jr. Factors complicating observed associations between peptic ulcer and other diseases. Gastroenterology *68*:1608, 1975.

182. Grossman, M. I. (ed.): Peptic Ulcer. A Guide for the Practicing Physician. Chicago, Year Book Medical Publishers, Inc., 1981, p. 179.
183. Langman, M. J. S., and Cooke, A. R. Gastric and duodenal ulcer and their associated diseases. Lancet 1:680, 1976.
184. Bonnevie, O. Causes of death in duodenal and gastric ulcer. Gastroenterology 73:1000, 1977.
185. Monson, R. R. Duodenal ulcer as a second disease. Gastroenterology 59:712, 1970.
186. Kauffmann, F., and Brille, D. Bronchial hypersecretion, chronic airflow limitation, and peptic ulcer. Am. Rev. Respir. Dis. 124:646, 1981.
187. Kellow, J. E., Tao, Z., and Piper, D. W. Ventilatory function in patients with gastric and duodenal ulcer. Gastroenterology 91:590, 1986.
188. Phillips, M. M., Ramsby, G. R., and Conn, H. O. Portacaval anastomosis and peptic ulcer: A nonassociation. Gastroenterology 68:121, 1975.
189. Kirk, A. P., Dooley, J. S., and Hunt, R. H. Peptic ulceration in patients with chronic liver disease. Dig. Dis. Sci. 25:756, 1980.
190. Tabaqchali, S., and Dawson, A. M. Peptic ulcer and gastric secretion in patients with liver disease. Gut 5:417, 1964.
191. Jones, R. H., Rudge, C. J., Bewick, M., Parsons, V., and Weston, M. J. Cimetidine: Prophylaxis against upper gastrointestinal haemorrhage after renal transplantation. Br. Med. J. 1:398, 1978.
192. Margolis, D. M., Saylor, J. L., Geisse, G., DeSchryver-Kecskemeti, K., Harter, H. R., and Zuckerman, G. R. Upper gastrointestinal disease in chronic liver failure. A prospective evaluation. Arch. Intern. Med. 138:1214, 1978.
193. Owens, M. L., Passaro, E., Jr., Wilson, S. E., and Gordon, H. E. Treatment of peptic ulcer disease in the renal transplant patient. Ann. Surg. 186:17, 1977.
194. Andriulli, A., Malfi, B., Recchia, S., Ponti, V., Triolo, G., and Segoloni, G. Patients with chronic renal failure are not at a risk of developing chronic peptic ulcers. Clin. Nephrol. 23:245–248, 1985.
195. Peptic ulcer after renal transplantation (editorial). Lancet 1:366, 1979.
196. Archibald, S. D., Jirsch, D. W., and Bear, R. A. Gastrointestinal complications of renal transplantation. 1. The upper gastrointestinal tract. Can. Med. Assoc. J. 119:1291, 1978.
197. Gingell, J. C., Burns, G. P., and Chisholm, G. D. Gastric acid secretion in chronic uraemia and after renal transplantation. Br. Med. J. 4:424, 1968.
198. Paimela, H. Persistence of gastric hyoacidity in uraemic patients after renal transplantation. Scand. J. Gastroenterol. 20:873, 1985.
199. Muto, S., Murayama, N., Asano, Y., Hosoda, S., and Miyata, M.: Hypergastrinemia and achlorhydria in chronic renal failure. Nephron 40:143, 1985.
200. Chisholm, G. D., Mee, A. D., Williams, G., Castro, J. E., and Baron, J. H. Peptic ulceration, gastric secretion, and renal transplantation. Br. Med. J. 1:1630, 1977.
201. Goldstein, H., Murphy, D., Sokol, A., and Rubini, M. E. Gastric acid secretion in patients undergoing chronic dialysis. Arch. Intern. Med. 120:645, 1967.
202. Burleson, R. L., Kronhaus, R. J., Marbarger, P. D., and Jones, D. M. Cimetidine, posttransplant peptic ulcer complications, and renal allograft survival: A clinical and investigational perspective. Arch. Surg. 117(7):933, 1982.
203. Golematis, B., Melissas, J., Hatzitheofilou, C., Dreiling, D. A., and Kambysi-Dea, S. The incidence of urolithiasis in peptic ulcer patients. Am. J. Gastroenterol. 68:367, 1977.
204. Briggs, R. D., Rubenberg, M. L., O'Neal, R. M., Thomas, W. A., and Hartroft, W. S. Myocardial infarction in patients treated with Sippy and other high-milk diets. An autopsy study of fifteen hospitals in the U.S.A. and Great Britain. Circulation 21:538, 1960.
205. Brandsborg, O., Brandsborg, M., Lovgreen, N. A., and Christensen, N. J. Increased plasma noradrenaline and serum gastrin in patients with duodenal ulcer. Eur. J. Clin. Invest. 8:11, 1978.
206. Gilbert, H. S., Warner, R. R. P., and Wasserman, L. R. A study of histamine in myeloproliferative disease. Blood 28:795, 1966.
207. Schulze, S., Pedersen, N. T., Jorgensen, M. J., Mollman, K.-M., and Rune, S. J. Association between duodenal bulb ulceration and reduced exocrine pancreatic function. Gut 24:781, 1983.
208. Eisenbarth, G. S., and Lebovitz, H. E. Minireview. Immunogenetics of the polyglandular failure syndrome. Life Sci. 22:1675, 1978.
209. Medalie, J. H., Neufeld, H. N., Goldbourt, U., Kahn, H. A., Riss, E., and Oron, D. Association between blood-pressure and peptic-ulcer incidence. Lancet 2:1225, 1970.
210. Sasaki, H. Nagulesparan, M., Samloff, I. M., Straus, E., Sievers, M. L., and Dubois, A. Low acid output in Pima Indians: A possible cause for the rarity of duodenal ulcer in this population. Dig. Dis. Sci. 29(9):785, 1984.
211. Bateson, E. M. Cancer of the stomach and duodenal ulcer: Report of two cases with a discussion of the significance of this rare association. Clin. Radiol. 23:208, 1972.
212. Goldin, E., Zimmerman, J., Okon, E., and Rachmilewitz, D. Should we worry about gastric cancer in duodenal ulcer patients? J. Clin. Gastroenterol. 7(3):227, 1985.
213. Moynihan, B. G. A. On duodenal ulcer: with notes of 52 operations. Lancet 1:340, 1905.
214. Clinch, D., Banerjee, A. K., and Ostick, G. Absence of abdominal pain in elderly patients with peptic ulcer. Age and Ageing 13:120, 1984.
215. Edwards, F. C., and Coghill, N. F. Clinical manifestations in patients with chronic atrophic gastritis, gastric ulcer, and duodenal ulcer. Quart. J. Med. 37:337, 1968.
216. Horrocks, J. C., and De Dombal, F. T. Clinical presentation of patients with "dyspepsia." Gut 19:19, 1978.
217. Earlam, R. A computerized questionnaire analysis of duodenal ulcer symptoms. Gastroenterology 71:314, 1976.
218. Rinaldo, J. A., Jr., Scheinok, P., and Rupe, C. E. Symptom diagnosis. A mathematical analysis of epigastric pain. Ann. Intern. Med. 59:145, 1963.
219. Sjodin, I., Svedlund, J., Dotevall, G., and Gillberg, R. Symptom profiles in chronic peptic ulcer disease. A detailed study of abdominal and mental symptoms. Scand. I. Gastroenterol. 20(4):419, 1985.
220. Mollmann, K. M., Bonnevie, O., Gudbrand-Hoyer, E., and Wulff, H. R. A diagnostic study of patients with upper abdominal pain. Scand. J. Gastroenterol. 10:805, 1975.
221. Palmer, W. L. The "acid test" in gastric and duodenal ulcer. Clinical value of experimental production of the typical distress. JAMA 88:1778, 1927.
222. Harrison, A., Isenberg, J. I., Schapira, M., and Hagie, L. Most patients with active symptomatic duodenal ulcers fail to develop ulcer-type pain in response to gastroduodenal acidification. J. Clin. Gastroenterol. 4:105, 1982.
223. Joffee, S. N., and Primrose, J. N. Pain provocation test in peptic duodenitis. Gastrointest. Endosc. 29:282, 1983.
224. Kang, J. Y., Yap, I., Guan, R., and Tay, H. H. Acid perfusion of duodenal ulcer craters and ulcer pain: A controlled double blind study. Gut 27:942, 1986.
225. Sturdevant, R. A. L., Isenberg, J. I., Secrist, D., and Ansfield, J. Antacid and placebo produced similar pain relief in duodenal ulcer patients. Gastroenterology 72:1, 1977.
226. Lorber, S. H., Stelzer, F. A., and Mayer, E. M. Effect of antacid and placebo on pain of duodenal ulcer (abstract). Gastroenterology 74:1058, 1978.
227. Rune, S. J., and Zachariassen, A. Acute relief of epigastric pain by antacid in duodenal ulcer patients. Scand. J. Gastroenterol. 15(suppl):41, 1980.
228. Peterson, W. L., Sturdevant, R. A. L., Frankl, H. D., Richardson, C. T., Isenberg, J. I., Elashoff, J. D., Sones, J. Q., Gross, R. A., McCallum, R. W., and Fordtran, J. S. Healing of duodenal ulcer with an antacid regimen. N. Engl. J. Med. 297:341, 1977.
229. Ippoliti, A. F., Sturdevant, R. A. L., Isenberg, J. I., Binder, M., Camacho, R., Cano, R., Cooney, C., Kline, M. M., Koretz, R. L. Meyer, J. H., Samloff, I. M., Schwabe, A. D.,

Strom, E. A., Valenzuela, J. E., and Wintroub, R. H. Cimetidine versus intensive antacid therapy for duodenal ulcer. Gastroenterology 74:393, 1978.

230. Bardhan, K. D., Saul, D. M., Edwards, J. L., Smith, P. M., Fettes, M., Forrest, J., Heading, R. C., Logan, R. F. A., Dronfield, M. W., Langman, M. J., Larkworthy, W., Haggie, S. J., Wyllie, J. H., Corbett, C., Duthie, H. L., Fussey, I. V., Holdsworth, C. D., Balmforth, G. V., and Maruyama, T. Comparison of two doses of cimetidine and placebo in the treatment of duodenal ulcer: A multicentre trial. Gut 20:68, 1979.

231. Priebe, W. M., DaCosta, L. R., and Beck, L. T. Is epigastric tenderness a sign of peptic ulcer disease? Gastroenterology 82:16, 1982.

232. Walsh, J. H. Functional and provocative tests for gastroduodenal disorders. J. Clin. Gastroenterol. 3(suppl. 2):73, 1981.

233. Spindel, E., Harty, R. F., Leibach, J. R., and McGuigan, J. E. Decision analysis in evaluation of hypergastrinemia. Am. J. Med. 80:11, 1986.

234. Earlam, R. Dogma disputed: On the origin of duodenal-ulcer pain. Lancet 1(8435):973, 1985.

235. Oddsson, E., Binder, V., Thorgeirsson, T., Jonasson, T. A., Gunnlaugsson, O., Wulff, M., Jonasson, K., Wulff, H. R., Bjarnason, O., and Riis, P. A prospective comparative study of clinical and histological characteristics in Icelandic and Danish patients with gastric ulcer, duodenal ulcer, and X-ray negative dyspepsia. I. Design and clinical features. Scand. J. Gastroenterol. 12:689, 1977.

236. Thompson, W. G. Functional dyspepsia. In The Irritable Gut. Baltimore, University Park Press, 1979.

237. Spiro, H. M. Moynihan's disease? The diagnosis of duodenal ulcer. N. Engl. J. Med. 291:567, 1974.

238. Camilleri, M., Thompson, D. G., and Malagelada, J.-R. Functional dyspepsia. Symptoms and underlying mechanism. J. Clin. Gastroenterol. 8(4):424, 1986.

239. Lasser, R. B., Bond, J. H., and Levitt, M. D. The role of intestinal gas in functional abdominal pain. N. Engl. J. Med. 293:524, 1975.

240. Gomex, J., and Dally, P. Psychologically mediated abdominal pain in surgical and medical outpatient clinics. Br. Med. J. 1:1451, 1977.

241. Nemiah, J. C., Freyberger, H., and Sifneds, P. E. Alexithymia: A view of the psychosomatic process. In Hill, O. (ed.): Modern Trends in Psychosomatic Medicine 3. London, Butterworths, 1976, p. 430.

242. Whitehead, R., and Piris, J. Morphological Aspects of Non-Ulcer Dyspepsia. In Wastell, C., and Lancet, P. (eds.): Cimetidine, The Westminister Hospital Symposium. Edinburgh, Churchill Livingstone, 1978, pp. 111–125.

243. Toukan, A. U., Kamal, M. F., Amr, S. S., Arnaout, M. A., and Abu-Romiyeh, A. S. Gastroduodenal inflammation in patients with nonulcer dyspepsia. A controlled endoscopic and morphometric study. Dig. Dis. Sci. 30(4):313, 1985.

244. Lance, P., Wastell, C., and Schiller, K. F. R. A controlled trial of cimetidine for the treatment of nonucler dyspepsia. J. Clin. Gastroenterol. 8(4):414, 1986.

245. Cotton, P. B., Price, A. B., Tighe, J. R., and Beales, J. S. M. Preliminary evaluation of "duodenitis" by endoscopy and biopsy. Br. Med. J. 3:430, 1973.

246. Thomson, W. O., Robertson, A. G., Imrie, C. W., Joffe, S. N., Lee, F. D., and Blumgart, L. H. Is duodenitis a dyspeptic myth? Lancet 1:1197, 1977.

247. Krag, E. Pseudo-ulcer and true peptic ulcer. A clinical, radiographic and statistical follow-up study. Acta Med. Scand. 178:713, 1965.

248. Barfred, A. Pseudo-ulcer and true peptic ulcer. In Proceedings of the World Congress of Gastroenterology, Vol. 1. Baltimore, Williams & Wilkins, 1959, p. 352.

249. Brummer, P., and Hakkinen, I. X ray negative dyspepsia. A follow-up study. Acta Med. Scand. 165:329, 1979.

250. Gregory, D. W., Davies, G. T., Evans, K. T., and Rhodes, J. Natural history of patients with X-ray-negative dyspepsia in general practice. Br. Med. J. 4:519, 1972.

251. Abdominal pain: Abdominal pain of spinal origin (editorial). Lancet 1:1190, 1977.

252. Ashby, E. C. Abdominal pain of spinal origin. Value of intercostal block. Ann. R. Coll. Surg. Engl. 59:242, 1977.

253. Mehta, M., and Ranger, I. Persistent abdominal pain. Treatment by nerve block. Anaesthesia 26:330, 1971.

254. Roberts, H. J. Abdominal pain of spinal origin (letter). Lancet 2:195, 1977.

255. Young, D. Rectus muscle spasm stimulating perforated peptic ulcer (letter). Lancet 1:1190, 1976.

256. Longstreth, G. F., and Newcomer, A. D. Abdominal pain caused by diabetic radiculopathy. Ann. Intern. Med. 86:166, 1977.

257. Gray, D. B., and Ward, G. E. Delay in diagnosis of carcinoma of the stomach. An analysis of 104 cases. Am. J. Surg. 83:524, 1952.

258. Kahn, K. L., and Greenfield, S. The efficacy of endoscopy in the evaluation of dyspepsia. J. Clin. Gastroenterol. 8(3):346, 1986.

259. Danzi, J. T., Farmer, R. G., Sullivan, B. H., and Rankin, G. B. Endoscopic features of gastroduodenal Crohn's disease. Gastroenterology 70:9, 1976.

260. Sharon, P., Stalnikovicz, R., and Rachmilewitz, D. Endoscopic diagnosis of duodenal neoplasms causing upper gastrointestinal bleeding. J. Clin. Gastroenterol. 4:35, 1982.

261. Wald, A., and Milligan, F. D. The role of fiberoptic endoscopy in the diagnosis and management of duodenal neoplasms. Dig. Dis. 20(6):499, 1975.

262. Grischkan, D., Brown, L., Mazansky, H., Archer, B., and Price, F. Localized duodenal lymphoma masquerading as a duodenal ulcer. Can. J. Surg. 25(2):213, 1982.

263. Greenhall, M. J., Gough, M. H., and Kettlewell, M. G. W. Duodenal ulceration—is endoscopic biopsy necessary? Br. Med. J. 282:1061, 1981.

264. Cronstedt, J., Willen, R., Balldin, G., Kalczynski, J., Berg, N. O., Bergman, G., and Offenbartl, K. Gastro-duodenal ulceration in abdominal angina. Acta Chir. Scand. 148:687, 1982.

265. Sleisenger, M. H. The celiac artery syndrome—again (editorial)? Ann. Intern. Med. 86:355, 1977.

266. Goldberg, H. I. Radiographic evaluation of peptic ulcer disease. J. Clin. Gastroenterol. 3(suppl. 2):57, 1981.

267. Tedesco, F. J. Endoscopy in the evaluation of patients with upper gastrointestinal symptoms: Indications, expectations, and interpretation. J. Clin. Gastroenterol. 3(suppl. 2):67, 1981.

268. Gelfand, D. W., Dale, W. J., Ott, D. J., Wu, W. C., and Meschan, I. The radiologic detection of duodenal ulcers: Effects of examiner variability, ulcer size and location, and technique. AJR 145:551, 1985.

269. Dooley, C. P., Larson, A. W., Stace, N. H., Renner, I. G., Valenzuela, J. E., Eliasoph, J., Colletti, P. M., Halls, J. M., and Weiner, J. M. Double-contrast barium meal and upper gastrointestinal endoscopy: A comparative study. Ann. Intern. Med. 101:538, 1984.

270. Martin, T. R., Vennes, J. A., Silvis, S. E., and Ansel, H. J. A comparison of upper gastrointestinal endoscopy and radiography. J. Clin. Gastroenterol. 2:21, 1980.

271. Tedesco, F. J., Griffin, J. W., Jr., Crisp, W. L., and Anthony, H. F., Jr. "Skinny" upper gastrointestinal endoscopy—the initial diagnostic tool: A prospective comparison of upper gastrointestinal endoscopy and radiology. J. Clin. Gastroenterol. 2:27, 1980.

272. Brown, P., Salmon, P. R., Burwood, R. J., Knox, A. J., Clendinnen, B. G., and Read, A. E. The endoscopic, radiological, and surgical findings in chronic duodenal ulceration. Scand. J. Gastroenterol. 13:557, 1978.

273. Salter, R. H. X-ray negative dyspepsia. Br. Med. J. 2:235, 1977.

274. Ott, D. J., Chen, Y. M., Gelfand, D. W., Meschan, I., Munitz, H. A., Kerr, R. M., and Wu, W. C. Positive predictive value and examiner variability in diagnosing duodenal ulcer. AJR 145:(6):1207, 1985.

275. Cameron, A. J., and Ott, B. J. The value of gastroscopy in

clinical diagnosis, a computer-assisted study. Mayo Clin. Proc. *52:*806, 1977.

276. Health and Public Policy Committee, American College of Physicians, Philadelphia, Pennsylvania. Endoscopy in the evaluation of dyspepsia. Ann. Intern. Med. *102:*266, 1985.

277. Fjosne, U., Kleveland, P. M., Waldum, H., Halvorsen, T., and Petersen, H. The clinical benefit of routine upper gastrointestinal endoscopy. Scand. J. Gastroenterol. *21:*433, 1986.

278. Lichtenstein, J. L., Feinstein, A. R., Suzio, K. D., DeLuca, V. A., and Spiro, H. M. The effectiveness of panendoscopy on diagnostic and therapeutic decisions about chronic abdominal pain. J. Clin. Gastroenterol. *2:*31, 1980.

279. Gjorup, T., Agner, E., Bording Jensen, L., Morup Jensen, A., and Mollman, K. M. The endoscopic diagnosis of duodenal ulcer disease: A randomized clinical trial of bias and of interobserver variation. Scand. J. Gastroenterol. *21:*261, 1986.

280. Mistilis, S. P., Wiot, J. F., and Nedelman, S. H. Giant duodenal ulcer. Ann. Intern. Med. *59:*155, 1963.

281. Lumsden, K., MacLarnon, J. C., and Dawson, J. Giant duodenal ulcer. Gut *11:*592, 1970.

282. Eisenberg, R. L., Margulis, A. R., and Moss, A. A. Giant duodenal ulcers. Gastrointest. Radiol. *2:*347, 1978.

283. Klamer, T. W., and Mahr, M. M. Giant duodenal ulcer: A dangerous variant of a common illness. Am. J. Surg. *135:*760, 1978.

284. Bianchi Porro, G., Lazzaroni, M., and Petrillo, M. Giant duodenal ulcers (letter). Dig. Dis. Sci. *29:*781, 1984.

285. Jaszewski, R., Crane, S. A., and Cid, A. A. Giant duodenal ulcers. Successful healing with medical therapy. Dig. Dis. Sci. *28*(6):486, 1983.

286. Texter, E. C., Jr., Baylin, G. L., Ruffin, J. M., and Legerton, C. W., Jr. Pyloric channel ulcer. Gastroenterology *24:*319, 1953.

287. Strom, M., Bodemar, G., Lindhagen, J., Sjodahl, R., and Walan, A. Cimetidine or parietal-cell vagotomy in patients with juxtapyloric ulcers. Lancet *2:*894, 1984.

288. Cooke, L., and Hutton, C. F. Postbulbar duodenal ulceration. Lancet *1:*754, 1958.

289. Swarts, J. M., and Rice, M. L., Jr. Post-bulbar duodenal ulcer with particular reference to its hemorrhagic tendency. Gastroenterology *26*(2):251, 1954.

290. Malmros, H., and Hiertonn, T. A post-investigation of 687 medically treated cases of peptic ulcer. Acta Med. Scand. *133:*229, 1949.

291. Bardhan, K. D. Intermittent treatment of duodenal ulcer for long-term medical management. A review. Postgrad. Med. J. 1987 (in press).

292. Bardhan, K. D., Saul, D. M., Edwards, J. L., Smith, P. M., Haggie, S. J., Wyllie, J. H., Duthie, H. L., and Fussey, I. V. Double-blind comparison of cimetidine and placebo in the maintenance of healing of chronic duodenal ulceration. Gut *20:*158, 1979.

293. Burland, W. L., Hawkins, B. W., and Beresford, J. Cimetidine treatment for the prevention of recurrence of duodenal ulcer: An international collaborative study. Postgrad. Med. J. *56:*173, 1980.

294. Gudmand-Hoyer, E., Birger-Jensen, K., Krag, E., Rask-Madsen, J., Rahbek, I., Rune, S. J., and Wulf, H. R. Prophylactic effect of cimetidine in duodenal ulcer disease. Br. Med. J. *1:*1095, 1978.

295. Frederiksen, H. J., Matzen, P., Madsen, P., Kragelund, E., and Krag, E. Spontaneous healing of duodenal ulcers. Scand. J. Gastroenterol. *19*(3):417, 1984.

296. Strom, M., Berstad, A., Bodemar, G., and Walan, A. Results of short- and long-term cimetidine treatment in patients with juxtapyloric ulcers, with special reference to gastric acid and pepsin secretion. Scand. J. Gastroenterol. *21:*521, 1986.

297. Fry, J. Peptic ulcer: A profile. Br. Med. J. *2:*809, 1964.

298. Greibe, J., Bugge, P., Gjorup, T., Lauritzen, T., Bonnevie, O., and Wulff, H. R. Long-term prognosis of duodenal ulcer: Follow-up study and survey of doctors' estimates. Br. Med. J. *2:*1572, 1977.

299. Bardhan, K. D., Hinchliffe, R. C. F., and Bose, K. Low dose

300. Elashoff, J. D., Van Deventer, G., Reedy, T. J., Ippoliti, A., Samloff, I. M., Kurata, J., Billings, M., and Isenberg, M. Long-term follow-up of duodenal ulcer patients. J. Clin. Gastroenterol. *5:*509, 1983.

301. Bonnevie, O. Survival in peptic ulcer. Gastroenterology *75:*1055, 1978.

302. Bonfils, S., Baron, J. H., and Blum, A. Uncontrolled factors in controlled trials of peptic ulcer. Dig. Dis. Sci. *29*(9):858, 1984.

303. Gudjonsson, B., and Spiro, H. M. Response to placebos in ulcer disease. Am. J. Med. *65:*399, 1978.

304. Bianchi Porro, G., and Petrillo, M. The natural history of peptic ulcer disease: The influence of H_2-antagonist treatment. Scand. J. Gastroenterol. *21*(suppl. 121):46, 1986.

305. Massarrat, S., and Eisenmann, A. Factors affecting the healing rate of duodenal and pyloric ulcers with low-dose antacid treatment. Gut *22:*97, 1981.

306. Korman, M. G., Shaw, R. G., Hansky, J., Schmidt, G. T., and Stern, A. I. Influence of smoking on healing rate of duodenal ulcer in response to cimetidine or high-dose antacid. Gastroenterology *80:*1451, 1981.

307. Lam, S. K., Hui, W. M., Lau, W. Y., Branicki, F. J., Lai, C. L., Lok, A. S. F., Ng, M. M. T., Fok, P. J., Poon, G. P., and Choi, T. K. Sucralfate overcomes adverse effect of cigarette smoking on duodenal ulcer healing and prolongs subsequent remission. Gastroenterology *92:*1193, 1987.

308. Barakat, M. H., Menon, K. N., and Badawi, A. R. Cigarette smoking and duodenal ulcer healing. An endoscopic study of 197 patients. Digestion *29:*85, 1984.

309. Lam, S. K., Lau, W. Y., Choi, T. K., Lai, C. L., Lok, A. S. F., Hui, W. M., Ng, M. N. T., and Choi, S. K. Y. Prostaglandin E_1 (misoprostol) overcomes the adverse effect of chronic cigarette smoking on duodenal ulcer healing. Dig. Dis. Sci. *31*(2):68S, 1986.

310. Hawkey, C. J., and Walt, R. P. Misoprostol, smoking and duodenal ulcer healing rates (letter). Lancet *1*(8529):393, 1987.

311. Lee, F. I., Samloff, I. M., and Hardman, M. Comparison of tri-potassium dicitrato bismuthate tablets with ranitidine in healing and relapse of duodenal ulcers. Lancet *1:*1299, 1985.

312. Sontag, S., Graham, D. Y., Belsito, A., Weiss, J., Farley, A., Grunt, R., Cohen, N., Kinnear, D., Davis, W., Archambault, A., Achord, J., Thayer, W. Gillies, R., Sidorov, J., Sabesin, S. M., Dyck, W., Fleshler, B., Cleator, I., Wenger, J., Opekun, A., Jr. Cimetidine, cigarette smoking, and recurrence of duodenal ulcer. N. Engl. J. Med. *311*(11):659, 1984.

313. Lam, S. K., Lai, C. L., Lee, L. N. W., Fok, K. H., Ng, M. M. T., and Siu, K. F. Factors influencing healing of duodenal ulcer. Control of nocturnal secretion by H_2 blockade and characteristics of patients who failed to heal. Dig. Dis. Sci. *30*(1):45, 1985.

314. Hasan, M., and Sircus, W. The factors determining success or failure of cimetidine treatment of peptic ulcer. J. Clin. Gastroenterol. *3:*225, 1981.

315. Piper, D. W., McIntosh, J. H., and Hudson, H. M. Factors relevant to the prognosis of chronic duodenal ulcer. Digestion *31*(1):9, 1985.

316. Muller-Lissner, S. A. Bile reflux is increased in cigarette smokers. Gastroenterology *90:*1205, 1986.

317. Massarrat, S., Enschai, F., and Pittner, P. M. Increased gastric secretory capacity in smokers without gastrointestinal lesions. Gut *27:*433, 1986.

318. Boyd, E. J. S., Wilson, J. A., and Wormsley, K. G. Smoking impairs therapeutic gastric inhibition. Lancet *1:*95–97, 1983.

319. Quimby, G. F., Bonnice, C. A., Burstein, S. H., and Eastwood, G. L. Active smoking depresses prostaglandin synthesis in human gastric mucosa. Ann. Intern. Med. *104:*616, 1986.

320. McCready, D. R., Clark, L., and Cohen, M. M. Cigarette smoking reduces human gastric luminal prostaglandin E_2. Gut *26:*1192, 1985.

321. Lam, S. K., Lai, C. L., Ng, M., Fok, K. H., and Hui, W. M. Duodenal ulcer healing by separate reduction of postprandial

and nocturnal acid secretions have different pathophysiology. Gut 26:1038, 1985.

322. O'Laughlin, J. C., Silvoso, G. R., and Ivey, K. J. Healing of aspirin-associated peptic ulcer disease despite continued salicylate ingestion. Arch. Intern. Med. 141:781, 1981.

323. Roth, S. H., Bennett, R. E., Mitchell, C. S., and Hartman, R. J. Double-blind long term evaluation of cimetidine therapy in nonsteroidal anti-inflammatory drug gastropathy. Arch. Int. Med. 147:1798, 1987.

324. Agrawal, N., Roth, S., Mahowald, M., Montoya, H., Robbins, R., Miller, S., Nutting, E., Woods, E., Crager, M., and Swabb, E. Misoprostol coadministration heals aspirin-induced gastric lesions in rheumatoid arthritis patients. Gastroenterology 92:1290, 1987.

325. Baron, H. H., and Wastell, C. Medical treatment. In Wastell, C. (ed.): Chronic Duodenal Ulcer. London, Butterworths, 1972, pp. 117–133.

326. Myers, B. M., Smith, J. L., and Graham, D. Y. Effect of red pepper and black pepper on the stomach. Am. J. Gastroenterol. 82(3):211, 1987.

327. Ippoliti, A. F., Maxwell, V., and Isenberg, J. P. The effect of various forms of milk on gastric-acid secretion. Studies in patients with duodenal ulcer and normal subjects. Ann. Intern. Med. 84:286, 1976.

328. Dial, E. J., and Lichtenberger, L. M. A role for milk phospholipids in protection against gastric acid. Studies in adult and suckling rats. Gastroenterology 87(2):379, 1984.

329. Kumar, N., Kumar, A., Broor, S. L., Vij, J. C., and Anand, B. S. Effect of milk on patients with duodenal ulcers. Br. Med. J. (Clin. Res.) 293:666, 1986.

330. Spiro, H. M. Is milk all that bad for the ulcer patient (editorial)? J. Clin. Gastroenterol. 3:219, 1981.

331. Rydning, A., and Berstad, A. Fiber diet and antacids in the short-term treatment of duodenal ulcer. Scand. J. Gastroenterol. 20:1078, 1985.

332. Lublin, H., Amiri, S., and Jensen, H. E. Antacids in the treatment of duodenal ulcer. Acta Med. Scand. 217:111, 1985.

333. Lam, S. K., Lam, K. C., Lai, C. L., Yeung, C. K., Yam, L. Y. C., and Wong, W. S. Treatment of duodenal ulcer with antacid and sulpiride. Gastroenterology 76:315, 1979.

334. Binder, H. J., Cocco, A., Crossley, R. J., Finkelstein, W., Font, R., Friedman, G., Groarke, J., Hughes, W., Johnson, A. F., McGuigan, J. E., Summers, R., Vlahcevic, R., Wilson, E. C., and Winship, D. H. Cimetidine in the treatment of duodenal ulcer. A multicenter double-blind study. Gastroenterology 74:380, 1978.

335. Lauritsen, K., Bytzer, P., Hansen, J., Bekker, C., and Rask-Madsen, J. Comparison of ranitidine and high-dose antacid in the treatment of prepyloric or duodenal ulcer. Scand. J. Gastroenterol. 20:123, 1985.

336. Hetzel, D. J., Hansky, J., Shearman, D. J. C., Korman, M. G., Hecker, R., Taggart, G. J., Jackson, R., and Gabb, B. W. Cimetidine treatment of duodenal ulceration: Short-term clinical trial and maintenance study. Gastroenterology 74:389, 1978.

337. Permutt, R. P., and Cello, J. P. Duodenal ulcer disease in the hospitalized elderly patient. Dig. Dis. Sci. 27(1):1, 1982.

338. Sarles, H., Camatte, R., and Sahel, J. A study of the variations in the response regarding duodenal ulcer when treated with placebo by different investigators. Digestion 16:289, 1977.

339. Mason, J. B., Moshal, M. G., Naidoo, V., and Schlemmer, L. The effect of stressful life situations on the healing of duodenal ulceration. S. Afr. Med. J. 60:734, 1981.

340. Somogyi, A., and Gugler, R. Clinical pharmacokinetics of cimetidine. Clin. Pharmacokinetics 8:463, 1983.

341. Humphries, T. J., Myerson, R. M., Gifford, L. M., Aeugle, M. E., Josie, M. E., Wood, S. L., and Tannenbaum, P. J. A unique postmarket outpatient surveillance program of cimetidine: report on phase II and final summary. Gastroenterology 79:593, 1984.

342. McGuigan, J. E. A consideration of the adverse effects of cimetidine. Gastroenterology 80:181, 1981.

343. Young, C. J., Daneshmend, T. K., and Roberts, C. J. C. Effects of cirrhosis and ageing on the elimination and bioavailability of ranitidine. Gut 23:819, 1982.

344. Zeldis, J. R., Friedman, L. S., and Isselbacher, K. J. Ranitidine: A new H_2-receptor antagonist. N. Engl. J. Med. 309(22):1368, 1983.

345. Friedman, G. GI drug column. Famotidine. Am. J. Gastroenterol. 82(6):504, 1987.

346. Chremos, A. N. Clinical pharmacology of famotidine: a summary. J. Clin. Gastroenterol. 9(Suppl. 2):7, 1987.

347. McCarthy, D. M. Ranitidine or cimetidine (editorial). Ann. Intern. Med. 99(4):551, 1983.

348. Powell, J. R., and Donn, K. H. The pharmacokinetic basis for H_2-antagonist drug interactions: Concepts and implications. J. Clin. Gastroenterol. 5(suppl. 1):95, 1983.

349. Abernethy, D. R., Greenblatt, D. J., Eshelman, F. N., and Shader, R. I. Ranitidine does not impair oxidative or conjugative metabolism: Noninteraction with antipyrine, diazepam, and lorazepam. Clin. Pharmacol. Ther. 35:188, 1984.

349a. Humphries, T. J. Famotidine: a notable lack of drug interactions. Scand. J. Gastroenterol. 22(Suppl. 134):55, 1987.

350. Feely, J., Wilkinson, G. R., McAllister, C. B., and Wood, A. J. J. Increased toxicity and reduced clearance of lidocaine by cimetidine. Ann. Intern. Med. 96:592, 1982.

351. Knapp, A. B., McGuire, W., Keren, G., Karmen, A., Levitt, B., Miura, D. S., and Somberg, J. C. The cimetidine-lidocaine interaction. Ann. Intern. Med. 98:174, 1983.

352. Markiewicz, K., Malec, P., and Tchorzewski, H. Changes in the interleukin-1 and interleukin-2 generation in duodenal ulcer patients during cimetidine treatment. Immunol. Lett. 10:19, 1985.

353. Watson, A. J. S., Dalbow, M. H., Stachura, I., Fragola, J. A., Rubin, M. F., Watson, R. M., and Bourke, E. Immunologic studies in cimetidine-induced nephropathy and polymyositis. N. Engl. J. Med. 308(3):142, 1983.

354. Peden, N. R., Callachan, H., Shepherd, D. M., and Wormsley, K. G. Gastric mucosal histamine and histamine methyltransferase in patients with duodenal ulcer. Gut 23:58, 1982.

355. Griswold, D. E., Alessi, S., Badger, A. M., Poste, G., and Hanna, N. Inhibition of T suppressor cell expression by histamine type 2 receptor antagonists. J. Immunol. 132:3054, 1984.

356. Cerra, F. B., Schentag, J. J., McMillen, M., Karwande, S. V., Fitzgerald, G. C., and Leising, M. Mental status, the intensive care unit, and cimetidine. Ann. Surg. 196:565, 1982.

357. Lorenzini, I., Jezequel, A. M., and Orlandi, F. Case report: Cimeditine-induced hepatitis. Electron microscopic observations and clinical pattern of liver injury. Dig. Dis. Sci. 26(3):275, 1981.

358. Van Steenbergen, W., Vanstapel, M. J., Desmet, V., Van Kerckvoorde, L., De Keyzer, R., Brijs, R., Fevery, J., and De Groote, J. Cimetidine-induced liver injury. Report of three cases. J. Hepatol. 1:359, 1985.

359. Borg, O. K., and Olbe, L. Omeprazole. A survey of preclinical data. Scand. J. Gastroenterol. 20(Suppl. 108):5, 1985.

360. Prichard, P. J., Yeomans, N. D., Mihaly, G. W., Jones, D. B., Buckle, P. J., Smallwood, R. A., and Louis, W. J. Omeprazole: A study of its inhibition of gastric pH and oral pharmacokinetics after morning or evening dosage. Gastroenterology 88:64, 1985.

361. Howden, C. W., Forrest, J. A. H., Meredith, P. A., and Reid, J. L. Antisecretory effect and oral pharmacokinetics following low dose omeprazole in man. Br. J. Pharmacol. 20:137, 1985.

362. Sharma, B. K., Walt, R. P., Pounder, R. E., Gomes, M. de F. A., Wood, E. C., and Logan, L. H. Optimal dose of oral omeprazole for maximal 24 hour decrease of intragastric acidity. Gut 25:957, 1984.

363. Howden, C. W., Derodra, J. K., Burget, D. W., and Hunt, R. H. Effects of low dose omeprazole on gastric secretion and plasma gastrin in patients with healed duodenal ulcer. Hepatogastroenterol. 33:267, 1986.

363a. Naesdal, J., Bankel, M., Bodemar, G., Gotthard, R., Lundquist, G., and Walan, A. The effect of 20 mg omeprazole daily on serum gastrin, 24-h intragastric acidity, and bile acid concentration in duodenal ulcer patients. Scand. J. Gastroenterol. 22:5, 1987.

364. McArthur, K. E., Jensen, R. T., and Gardner, J. D. Treatment of acid-peptic diseases by inhibition of gastric H^+, K^+-ATPase. Ann. Rev. Med. 37:97, 1986.

364a. Gugler, R., and Jensen, J. C. Omeprazole inhibits oxidative drug metabolism. Gastroenterology 89:1235, 1985.

365. Feldman, M. Inhibition of gastric acid secretion by selective and nonselective anticholinergics. Gastroenterology 86:361, 1984.

366. Jaup, B. H., and Blomstrand, C. H. Cerebro-spinal fluid concentrations of pirenzepine after therapeutic dosage. Scand. J. Gastroenterol. 15(suppl. 66):35, 1980.

367. Carmine, A. A., and Brogden, R. N. Pirenzipine. A review of its pharmacodynamic and pharmacokinetic properties and therapeutic efficacy in peptic ulcer disease and other allied diseases. Drugs 30(2):85, 1985.

368. Williams, J. G., Deakin, M., and Ramage, J. K. Effect of cimetidine and pirenzepine in combination on 24 hour intragastric acidity in subjects with previous duodenal ulceration. Gut 27(4):428, 1986.

369. Procacciante, F., Citone, G., Montesani, C., and Ribotta, G. Antisecretory activity of pirenzepine vs. cimetidine in man: A controlled study. Gut 25:178, 1984.

370. Londong, W. Present status and future perspectives of muscarinic receptor antagonists. Scand. J. Gastroenterol. 21(suppl. 152):55, 1986.

371. Fordtran, J. S., and Collyns, J. A. Antacid pharmacology in duodenal ulcer. Effect of antacids on postcibal gastric acidity and peptic activity. N. Engl. J. Med. 274(17):921, 1966.

372. Peterson, W. L., Barnett, C., Feldman, M., and Richardson, C. T. Reduction of twenty-four-hour gastric acidity with combination drug therapy in patients with duodenal ulcer. Gastroenterology 77:1015, 1979.

373. Barnett, C. C., and Richardson, C. T. In vivo and in vitro evaluation of magnesium-aluminum hydroxide antacid tablets and liquid. Dig. Dis. Sci. 30(11):1049, 1985.

374. Berstad, A., Aadland, E., and Bjerke, K. Cimetidine treatment of recurrent ulcer after proximal gastric vagotomy. Scand. J. Gastroenterol. 16:891, 1981.

375. Weberg, R., Berstad, A., Lange, O., Schultz, T., and Aubert, E. Duodenal ulcer healing with four antacid tablets daily. Scand. J. Gastroenterol. 20(9):1041, 1985.

376. Hollander, D., Tarnawski, A., and Gergely, H. Protection against alcohol-induced gastric mucosal injury by aluminum-containing compounds—sucralfate, antacids, and aluminum sulfate. Scand. J. Gastroenterol. 21(suppl. 125):151, 1986.

377. Shields, H. M. Rapid fall of serum phosphorus secondary to antacid therapy. Gastroenterology 75(6):1137.

378. Spencer, H., and Lender, M. Adverse effects of aluminum-containing antacids on mineral metabolism. Gastroenterology 76:603, 1979.

379. Orwoll, E. S. The milk-alkali syndrome: Current concepts. Ann. Intern. Med. 97:242, 1982.

380. Steinberg, W. M., Lewis, J. H., and Katz, D. M. Antacids inhibit absorption of cimetidine. N. Engl. J. Med. 307(7):400, 1982.

381. Hurwitz, A. Antacid therapy and drug kinetics. Clin. Pharmacokinetics 2:269, 1977.

382. Berstad, A., and Weberg, R. Antacids for peptic ulcer: Do we have anything better? Scand. J. Gastroenterol. 21(suppl. 125):32, 1986.

383. Kaehny, W. D., Hegg, A. P., and Alfrey, A. C. Gastrointestinal absorption of aluminum from aluminum-containing antacids. N. Engl. J. Med. 296:1389, 1977.

384. Kumar, N., Vij, J. C., Karol, A., and Anand, B. S. Controlled therapeutic trial to determine the optimum dose of antacids in duodenal ulcer. Gut 25:1199, 1984.

385. Lux, G., Hentschel, H., Rohner, H. G., Brunner, H., Schutze, K., Lederer, P. C., and Rosch, W. Treatment of duodenal ulcer with low-dose antacids. Scand. J. Gastroenterol. 21(9):1063, 1986.

386. Chen, M. C.-Y., Amerian, D., Toomey, M., Sanders, M., and Soll, A. H. Postanoid inhibition of canine parietal cells: Mediation by the inhibitory GTP-binding protein of adenylate cyclase. Gastroenterology, Vol. 94, 1988 (in press).

387. Roszkowski, A. P., Garay, G. L., Baker, S., Schuler, M., and Carter, H. Gastric antisecretory and antiulcer properties of enprostil, (±)-11α,15α-dihydroxy-16-phenoxy-17,18,19,20-tetranor-9-oxoprosta-4,5,13(t)-trienoic acid methyl ester. J. Pharmacol. Exp. Therap. 239(2):382, 1986.

388. Wilson, D. E. Therapeutic aspects of prostaglandins in the treatment of peptic ulcer disease. Dig. Dis. Sci. 31(2):42S, 1986.

389. Monk, J. P., and Clissold, S. P. Misoprostol. A preliminary review of its pharmacodynamic and pharmacokinetic properties, and therapeutic efficacy in the treatment of peptic ulcer disease. Drugs 33:1, 1987.

390. Deakin, M., Ramage, J., Paul, A., Gray, S. P., Billings, J., and Williams, J. G. Effect of enprostil, a synthetic prostaglandin E₂ on 24 hour intragastric acidity, nocturnal acid and pepsin secretion. Gut 27:1054, 1986.

391. Soll, A. H., Chen, M. C. Y., Amirian, D. A., Toomey, M., and Alvarez, R. Prostanoid inhibition of canine parietal cells. Am. J. Med. 81(2A):5, 1986.

392. Bauer, R. F., Bianchi, R. G., Casler, J., and Goldstin, B. Comparative mucosal protective properties of misoprostol, cimetidine, and sucralfate. Dig. Dis. Sci. 31(2):81S, 1986.

393. Hawkey, C. J., and Walt, R. P. Prostaglandins for peptic ulcer: A promise unfulfilled. Lancet 2:1084, 1986.

394. Stiel, D., Ellard, K. T., Hills, L. J., and Brooks, P. M. Protective effect of enprostil against aspirin-induced gastroduodenal mucosal injury in man. Comparison with cimetidine and sucralfate. Am. J. Med. 81(suppl. 2A):54, 1986.

395. Lanza, F. L. A double-blind study of prophylactic effect of misoprostol on lesions of gastric and duodenal mucosa induced by oral administration of tolmetin in healthy subjects. Dig. Dis. Sci. 31(2):131S, 1986.

396. Lanza, F. L., Aspinall, R. L., Swabb, E. A., Davis, R. E., Rack, M. F., and Rubin, A. A double blind placebo controlled endoscopic comparison of the cytoprotective effects of misoprostol and cimetidine on tolmetin induced gastric mucosal injury. Gastroenterology 92(no. 5, pt. 2):1491, 1987.

397. Wiqvist, N. Unpublished data, Göteborg, Sweden.

398. Richardson, C. T. Sucralfate (editorial). Ann. Intern. Med. 97(2):269, 1982.

399. Hollander, D., Tarnawski, A., Krause, W. J., and Gergely, H. Protective effect of sucralfate against alcohol-induced gastric mucosal injury in the rat. Macroscopic, histologic, ultrastructural, and functional time sequence analysis. Gastroenterology 88(no. 1, pt. 2):366, 1985.

400. Sucralfate for peptic ulcer—a reappraisal. Med. Letter Drugs Therap. 26(660):43, 1984.

401. Giesing, D., Lanman, R., and Runser, D. Absorption of sucralfate in man (abstract). Gastroenterology 82:1066, 1982.

402. Kinoshita, H., Kumaki, K., Nakano, H., Tsuyama, T., Nagashima, R., Okada, M., and McGraw, B. Plasma aluminum levels of patients on long term sucralfate therapy. Res. Commun. Chem. Pathol. Pharmacol. 35(3):515, 1982.

403. Baron, J. H., Barr, J., Batten, J., Sidebotham, R., and Spencer, J. Acid, pepsin, and mucus secretion in patients with gastric and duodenal ulcer before and after colloidal bismuth subcitrate (De-Nol). Gut 27:486, 1986.

404. Koo, J., Ho, J., Lam, S. K., Wong, J., and Ong, G. B. Selective coating of gastric ulcer by tripotassium dicitrate bismuthate in the rat. Gastroenterology 82:864, 1982.

405. Elder, J. B. Recent experimental and clinical studies on the pharmacology of colloidal bismuth subcitrate. Scand. J. Gastroenterol. 21(suppl. 122):14, 1986.

406. Miller, J. P., and Faragher, E. B. Relapse of duodenal ulcer: Does it matter which drug is used in initial treatment? Br. Med. J. 293(6555):1117, 1986.

407. Hamilton, I., Worsley, B. W., O'Connor, H. J., and Axon, A. T. R. Effects of tripotassium dicitrato bismuthate (TDB) tablets or cimetidine in the treatment of duodenal ulcer. Gut 24:1148, 1983.

408. Brown-Cartwright, D., Brater, C., Barnett, C. C., and Richardson, C. T. Effect of doxepin on basal gastric acid and salivary secretion in patients with duodenal ulcer. Ann. Intern. Med. 104:204, 1986.

409. Ries, R. K., Gilbert, D. A., and Katon, W. Tricyclic antidepressant therapy for peptic ulcer disease. Arch. Intern. Med. 144:566, 1984.

410. Davies, G. J., Rhodes, J., and Calcraft, B. J. Complications of carbenoxolone therapy. Br. J. Med. *3:*400, 1974.
411. Rask-Madsen, J., Bukhave, K., Madsen, P. E. R., and Bekker, C. Effect of carbenoxolone on gastric prostaglandin E$_2$ levels in patients with peptic ulcer disease following vagal and pentagastrin stimulation. Eur. J. Clin. Invest. *13:*351, 1983.
412. Freston, J. W. Cimetidine. I. Developments, pharmacology, and efficacy. Ann. Intern. Med. *97:*573, 1982.
413. Graham, D. Y., Schwartz, J. T., Sabesin, S. M., Mann, J. A., Davis, W. D., Jr., Font, R. G., and Cohen, N. N. Double-blind multicenter comparison of 1,200 mg. and 1,000 mg. cimetidine in hospitalized and ambulatory duodenal ulcer patients. Am. J. Gastroenterol. *76:*500, 1981.
414. Legerton, C. W., Jr. Duodenal and gastric ulcer healing rates: A review. Am. J. Med. *77*(suppl. 5B):2, 1984.
415. Kerr, G. D., Brown, P., Lennon, J., Crowe, J., McFarland, R. J., Vargese, A., Northfield, T. C., Fine, D., Findlay, J. M., Selby, B., Temple, J., Bradby, H., Gilbertson, C., Car-Locke, D. L., and McIllMurray, M. B. Cimetidine: Twice daily adminstration in duodenal ulcer. A multicentre group study. Practitioner *226:*978, 1982.
416. Capurso, L., Dal Monte, P. R., Mazzeo, F., Menardo, G., Morettini, A., Saggioro, A., and Tafner, G. Comparison of cimetidine 800 mg once daily and 400 mg twice daily in acute duodenal ulceration. Br. Med. J. *289:*1418, 1984.
417. Dickson, B. Cimetidine, 800 mg once daily: Preliminary European clinical data evaluation. Scand. J. Gastroenterol. *21*(suppl. 121):11, 1986.
418. Ireland, A., Colin-Jones, D. G., Gear, P., Golding, P. L., Ramage, J. K., Williams, J. G., Leicester, R. J., Smith, C. L., Ross, G., Bamforth, J., DeGara, C. J., Gledhill, T., and Hunt, R. H. Ranitidine 150 mg twice daily vs 300 mg nightly in treatment of duodenal ulcers. Lancet *2:*274, 1984.
419. Farley, A., L'evesque, D., Paré, P., Thomson, A. B., and Sherbaniuk, R. A comparative trial of ranitidine 300 mg at night with ranitidine 150 mg twice daily in the treatment of duodenal and gastric ulcer. Am. J. Gastroenterol. *80*(9):655, 1985.
420. Colin-Jones, D. G., Ireland, A., Gear, P., Goldring, P. L., Ramage, J. K., Williams, J. G., Leicester, R. J., Smith, C. L., Ross, G., Bamforth, J., DeGara, C. J., Gledhill, T., and Hunt, R. H. Reducing overnight secretion of acid to heal duodenal ulcers. Comparison of standard divided dose of ranitidine with a single dose administered at night. Am. J. Med. *77*(suppl. 5B):116, 1984.
421. Gledhill, T., Howard, O. M., Buck, M., Paul, A., and Hunt, R. H. Single nocturnal dose of an H$_2$ receptor antagonist for the treatment of duodenal ulcer. Gut *24:*904, 1983.
422. Chambers, J. B., Pryce, D., Bland, J. M., and Northfield, T. C. Effect of bedtime ranitidine on overnight gastric acid output and intragastric pH: Dose/response study and comparison with cimetidine. Gut *28*(3):294, 1987.
423. Jones, D. B., Howden, C. W., Burget, D. W., Kerr, G. D., and Hunt, R. H. Acid suppression in duodenal ulcer: a meta-analysis to define optimal dosing with antisecretory drugs. Gut *28:*1120, 1987.
424. Deakin, M., Glenny, H. P., Ramage, J. K., Mills, J. G., Burland, W. L., and Williams, J. G. Large single daily dose of histamine H$_2$ receptor antagonist for duodenal ulcer. How much and when? A clinical pharmacological study. Gut *28:*566, 1987.
425. Rohner, H.-G., Gugler, R. Treatment of active duodenal ulcers with famotidine. A double-blind comparison with ranitidine. Am. J. Med. *81*(suppl. 4B):8, 1986.
426. Gitlin, N., McCullough, A. J., Smith, J. L., Mantell, G., Berman, R., et al. A multicenter, double-blind, randomized, placebo-controlled comparison of nocturnal and twice-a-day famotidine in the treatment of active duodenal ulcer disease. Gastroenterology *92:*48, 1987.
427. McCullough, A. J. A multicenter, randomized, double-blind study comparing famotidine with ranitidine in the treatment of active duodenal ulcer disease. Am. J. Med. *81*(suppl. 4B):12, 1986.
428. Smith, J. L., Opekun, A. R., Antonello, A. M., and Chremos,

A. N. Ambulatory 24-hour intragastric pH and serum gastrin in duodenal ulcer patients: Comparison of famotidine with placebo. Gastroenterology *90*(5, pt. 2):1640, 1986.
429. Hutteman, W., Rohner, H. G., duBosque, G., Rehner, M., Hebbeln, H., Martens, W., Horstkotte, W., and Dammann, H. C. 20 versus 30 mg omeprazole once daily: Effect on healing rates in 115 duodenal ulcer patients. Digestion *33:*117, 1986.
430. Bardhan, K. D., Bianchi Porro, G., Bose, K., Daly, M., Hinchliffe, R. C. F., Jonsson, E., Lazzaroni, M., Naesdal, J., Rikner, L., and Walan, A. A comparison of two different doses of omeprazole versus ranitidine in treatment of duodenal ulcers. J. Clin. Gastroenterol. *8*(4):408, 1986.
431. Gustavsson, S., Adami, H.-O., Loof, L., Nyberg, A., and Nyren, O. Rapid healing of duodenal ulcers with omeprazole: Double-blind dose-comparative trial. Lancet *2:*124, 1983.
432. Prichard, P. J., Rubinstein, D., Jones, D. B., Dudley, F. J., Smallwood, R. A., Louis, W. J., and Yeomans, N. D. Double blind comparative study of omeprazole 10 mg and 30 mg daily for healing duodenal ulcers. Br. Med. J. *290:*601, 1985.
433. Classen, M., Dammann, H.-G., Domschke, W., Huttemann, W., Londong, W., Rehner, M., Simon, B., Witzel, L., and Berger, J. Omeprazole heals duodenal, but not gastric ulcers more rapidly than ranitidine. Results of two German multicentre trials. Hepatogastroenterol. *32:*243, 1985.
434. Lauritsen, K., Rune, S. J., Bytzer, P., Kelbaek, H., Jensen, K. G., Rask-Madsen, J., Bendtsen, F., Linde, J., Hojlund, M., Andersen, H. H., Mollman, K.-M., Nissen, V. R., Ovesen, L., Schlichting, P., Tage-Jensen, U., and Wulff, H. R. Effect of omeprazole and cimetidine on duodenal ulcer. A double-blind comparative trial. N. Engl. J. Med. *312*(April 11):958, 1985.
435. Adami, H.-O., Bjorklund, O., Enander, L.-K., Gustavsson, S., Loof, L., Nordahl, A., and Rosen, A. Cimetidine or propantheline combined with antacid therapy for short-term treatment of duodenal ulcer. Dig. Dis. Sci. *27*(5):388, 1982.
436. Strom, M., Gotthard, R., Bodemar, G., and Walan, A. Antacid/anticholinergic, cimetidine, and placebo in treatment of active peptic ulcers. Scand. J. Gastroenterol. *16:*593, 1981.
437. Thomson, A. B. R. Treatment of duodenal ulcer with enprostil, a synthetic prostaglandin E$_2$ analogue. Am. J. Med. *81*(suppl. 2A):59, 1986.
438. Winters, L. Comparison of enprostil and cimetidine in active duodenal ulcer disease. Summary of pooled European studies. Am. J. Med. *81*(suppl. 2A):69, 1986.
439. Lauritsen, K., Laursen, L. S., Havelund, T., Bytzer, P., Svendsen, L. B., and Rask-Madsen, J. Enprostil and ranitidine in duodenal ulcer healing: Double blind comparative trial. Br. Med. J. *292:*864, 1986.
440. Dammann, H. G., Walter, T. A., Muller, P., and Simon, B. Night-time rioprostil vs. ranitidine in duodenal ulcer healing (letter). Lancet *2:*335, 1986.
441. Euler, A. R., Tytgat, G., Berenguer, J., Brunner, H., Wood, D. R., Lookabaugh, J. L., and Phan, T. D. Failure of a cytoprotective dose of arbaprostil to heal acute duodenal ulcers. Results of a multiclinic trial. Gastroenterology *92:*604, 1987.
442. Hollander, D. Efficacy of sucralfate for duodenal ulcers: A multicenter double-blind trial. J. Clin. Gastroenterol. *3*(suppl. 2):153, 1981.
443. McHardy, G. G. A multicenter, double-blind trial of sucralfate and placebo in duodenal ulcer. J. Clin. Gastroenterol. *3*(suppl. 2):147, 1981.
444. Glise, H., Carling, L., Hallerback, B., Kagevi, I., Solhaug, J. H., Svedberg, L. E., and Wahlby, L. Short-term treatment of duodenal ulcer. A comparison of sucralfate and cimetidine. Scand. J. Gastroenterol. *21*(3):313, 1986.
445. Marks, I. N., Wright, J. P., Gilinsky, N. H., Girdwood, A. H., Tobias, R., Boyd, E., Kalvaria, I., O'Keefe, S. J., Newton, K., and Lucke, W. A comparison of sucralfate dosage schedule in duodenal ulcer healing. Two grams twice a day versus one gram four times a day. J. Clin. Gastroenterol. *8*(4):419, 1986.
446. Brandstaetter, G., and Kratochvil, P. Comparison of two sucralfate dosages (2 g twice a day versus 1 g four times a day) in duodenal ulcer healing. Am. J. Med. *79*(suppl. 2C):18, 1985.
447. Salmon, P. R., Brown, P., Williams, R., and Read, A. E.

Evaluation of colloidal bismuth (De-Nol) in the treatment of duodenal ulcer employing endoscopic selection and follow up. Gut *15*:189, 1974.

448. Moshal, M. G. The treatment of duodenal ulcers with TDB: A duodenoscopic double-blind cross-over investigation. Postgrad. Med. J. *51*(suppl. 5):36, 1975.

449. Hamilton, I., O'Connor, H. J., Wood, N. C., Bradbury, I., and Axon, A. T. R. Healing and recurrence of duodenal ulcer after treatment with tripotassium dicitrato bismuthate (TDB) tables or cimetidine. Gut *27*:106, 1986.

450. Ward, M., Halliday, C., and Cowen, A. E. A comparison of colloidal bismuth subcitrate tablets and ranitidine in the treatment of chronic duodenal ulcers. Digestion *34*(3):173, 1986.

451. Kellow, J. E., Barr, G. D., Middleton, W. R. J., and Piper, D. W. Comparison of colloidal bismuth subcitrate tablets and liquid in duodenal ulcer healing. J. Clin. Gastroenterol. *5*:417, 1983.

452. Eberhardt, R., Kasper, G., Dettmer, A., Hochter, W., and Hagena, D. Effect of oral bismuthsubsalicylate on campylobacter pyloridis and on duodenal ulcer. Gastroenterology *92*(5, pt. 2):1379, 1987.

453. Davies, W. A., and Reed, P. I. Controlled trial of duogastrone in duodenal ulcer. Gut *18*:78, 1977.

454. Sahel, J., Sarles, H., Boisson, J., Bonnet-Eymard, J., Cornet, A., Delmont, J., Dubarry, J., Dupuy, R., Gisselbrecht, R., Monges, H., Ribet, A., Roberti, A., Valla, A., Weill, J. P., and Cros, R. C. Carbenoxolone sodium capsules in the treatment of duodenal ulcer: An endoscopic controlled trial. Gut *18*:717, 1977.

455. Schenk, J., Schmack, B., Rosch, W., and Domschke, W. Controlled trial of carbenoxolone sodium vs. cimetidine in duodenal ulcer. Scand. J. Gastroenterol. *15*(suppl. 65):103, 1980.

456. Cook, P. J., Vincent-Brown, A., Lewis, S. I., Perks, S., Jewell, D. P., and Reed, P. I. Carbenoxolone (duogastrone) and cimetidine in the treatment of duodenal ulcer—a therapeutic trial. Scand. J. Gastroenterol. *15*(suppl. 65):93, 1980.

457. Bardhan, K. D. Refractory duodenal ulcer. Gut *25*:711, 1984.

458. Gledhill, T., Buck, M., and Hunt, R. H. Effect of no treatment, cimetidine 1 g/day, cimetidine 2 g/day and cimetidine combined with atropine on nocturnal gastric secretion in cimetidine non-responders. Gut *25*:1211, 1984.

459. Collen, M. J., Stanczak, C. A., and Ciarleglio, C. A. Basal acid output in patients with refractory duodenal ulcer disease. Gastroenterology *92*(5):1351, 1987.

460. Pounder, R. E. Duodenal ulcers that will not heal. Gut *25*:697, 1984.

461. Steinberg, W. M., Lewis, J. H., and Katz, D. M. Transient cimetidine resistance. J. Clin. Gastroenterol. *6*:355, 1984.

462. Danilewitz, M., Tim, L. O., and Hirschowitz, B. Ranitidine suppression of gastric hypersecretion resistant to cimetidine. N. Engl. J. Med. *306*:20, 1982.

463. Kisloff, B. Cimetidine-resistant gastric acid secretion in humans. Ann. Intern. Med. *92*:791, 1980.

464. McCarthy, D. M., Peikin, S. R., Lopatin, R. N., Long, B. W., Spiegel, A., Marx, S., and Brennan, M. Hyperparathyroidism—a reversible cause of cimetidine-resistant gastric hypersecretion. Br. Med. J. *1*:1765, 1979.

465. Sewing, K. F., Hagie, L., Ippoliti, A. F., Isenberg, J. L., Samloff, I. M., and Sturdevant, R. A. L. Effect of one-month treatment with cimetidine on gastric secretion and serum gastrin and pepsinogen levels. Gastroenterology *74*(2):376, 1978.

466. Prichard, P. J., Jones, D. B., Yeomans, N. D., Mihaly, G. W., Smallwood, R. A., and Louis, W. J. The effectiveness of ranitidine in reducing gastric acid-secretion decreases with continued therapy. Br. J. Clin. Pharmacol. *22*:663, 1986.

467. Thomas, E., and Reddy, K. R. Nonhealing duodenal ulceration due to Candida. J. Clin. Gastroenterol. *5*:55, 1983.

468. Lam, S. K., Lee, N. W., Koo, J., Hui, W. M., Fok, K. H., and Ng, M. Randomised crossover trial of tripotassium dicitrato bismuthate versus high dose cimetidine for duodenal ulcers resistant to standard dose of cimetidine. Gut *25*:703, 1984.

469. Bianchi Porro, G., Parente, F., Lazzaroni, M., and Pace, F. Colloidal bismuth subcitrate and two different dosages of cimetidine in the treatment of resistant duodenal ulcer. Preliminary results. Scand. J. Gastroenterol. *21*(suppl. 122):39, 1986.

470. Pounder, R. E., Hunt, R. H., Vincent, S. H., Milton-Thompson, G. J., and Misiewicz, J. J. 24-hour intragastric acidity and nocturnal acid secretion in patients with duodenal ulcer during oral administration of cimetidine and atropine. Gut *18*:85, 1977.

471. Quatrini, M., Basilisco, G., and Bianchi, P. A. Treatment of 'cimetidine-resistant' chronic duodenal ulcers with ranitidine or cimetidine: A randomised multicentre study. Gut *25*(10):1113, 1984.

472. Miller, S. R., Nissen, C. H., Karim, A., and Swabb, E. A. Efficacy and safety of misoprostol in the elderly. Gastroenterology *92*(5):1535, 1987.

473. Tytgat, G. N. J., Lamers, C. B. H. W., Hameeteman, W., Jansen, J. M. B. J., and Wilson, J. A. Omeprazole in peptic ulcers resistant to histamine H₂-receptor antagonists. Aliment. Pharmacol. Therap. *1*:31, 1987.

474. Guslandi, M. More about refractory duodenal ulcers (letter). Gut *25*:1433, 1984.

475. Londong, W., Londong, V., Ruthe, C., and Weizert, P. Complete inhibition of food-stimulated gastric acid secretion by combined application of pirenzepine and ranitidine. Gut *22*:542, 1981.

476. Lazzaroni, M., Sangaletti, O., Parente, F., Imbimbo, B. P., and Bianchi Porro, G. Inhibition of food stimulated acid secretion by association of pirenzepine and ranitidine in duodenal ulcer patients. Int. J. Clin. Pharm. Therap. Toxicol. *24*(12):685, 1986.

477. Dal Monte, P. R., D'Imperio, M., Ferri, M., Fratucello, F., and del Soldato, P. A combination of pirenzepine and cimetidine: A new approach to treatment of duodenal ulcer in "nonresponders." Hepatogastroenterology *32*:126, 1985.

478. Bardhan, K. D., Thompson, M., Bose, K., Hinchliffe, R. F. C., Crowe, J., Weir, D. G., McCarthy, C., Walters, J., Thomson, T. J., Thompson, M. H., Gait, J. E., King, C., and Prudham, D. Combined anti-muscarinic and H₂ receptor blockade in the healing of refractory duodenal ulcer. A double-blind study. Gut *28*:1505, 1987.

479. Van Deventer, G. M., Schneidman, D., and Walsh, J. H. Sucralfate and cimetidine as single agents and in combination for treatment of active duodenal ulcers. A double-blind, placebo-controlled trial. Am. J. Med. *79*(suppl. 2C):39, 1985.

480. Holst-Christensen, J., Hansen, O. H., Pedersen, T., and Kronborg, O. Recurrent ulcer after proximal gastric vagotomy for duodenal and pre-pyloric ulcer. Br. J. Surg. *64*:42, 1977.

481. Blackett, R. L., and Johnston, D. Recurrent ulceration after highly selective vagotomy for duodenal ulcer. Br. J. Surg. *68*:705, 1981.

482. Paoluzi, P., Ricotta, G., Ripoli, F., Proietti, F., Zaccardelli, E., Carratu, R., and Torsoli, A. Incompletely and completely healed duodenal ulcer outcome in maintenance treatment: A double-blind controlled study. Gut *26*:1080, 1985.

483. McLean, A. J., McCarthy, P., and Dudley, F. J. Cytoprotective agents and ulcer relapse. Med. J. Aust. *142*:S25-8, 1985.

484. Bardhan, K. D., Cole, D. S., Hawkins, B. W., and Franks, C. R. Does treatment with cimetidine extended beyond initial healing of duodenal ulcer reduce the subsequent relapse rate? Br. Med. J. *284*:621, 1982.

485. Ippoliti, A., Elashoff, J., Valenzuela, J., Cano, R., Frankl, H., Samloff, M., and Koretz, R. Recurrent ulcer after successful treatment with cimetidine or antacid. Gastroenterology *85*:875, 1983.

486. Bytzer, P., Lauritsen, K., and Rask-Madsen, J. Symptomatic recurrence of healed duodenal and prepyloric ulcers after treatment with ranitidine or high-dose antacid. A one-year follow-up study. Scand. J. Gastroenterol. *21*:765, 1986.

487. Eichenberger, P. M., Giger, M., Mattle, W., Pelloni, S., Muller-Lissner, S. A., Gonvers, J. J., Birchler, R., and Blum, A. L. Treatment and relapse prophylaxis of duodenal ulcer with pirenzepine and cimetidine. Scand. J. Gastroenterol. *17*(suppl. 72):197, 1982.

488. Dickson, B., Hunt, R. H., Chiverson, S. G., and Peace, K.

The impact of initial treatment on duodenal ulcer relapse. In preparation.

488a. Coghlan, J. G., Gilligan, D., Humphries, H., McKenna, D., Dooley, C., Sweeney, E., Keane, C., and O'Morain, C. Campylobacter pylori and recurrence of duodenal ulcers—a 12-month follow-up study. Lancet 2:1109, 1987.

489. Moshal, M. G., Gregory, M. A., Pilla, C., and Spitaels, J. M. Does the duodenal cell ever return to normal? A comparison between treatment with cimetidine and Denol. Scand. J. Gastroenterol. 14(suppl.):48, 1979.

490. Marks, I. N., Lucke, W., Wright, J. P., and Girdwood, A. H. Ulcer healing and relapse rates after initial treatment with cimetidine or sucralfate. J. Clin. Gastroenterol. 3(suppl. 2):163, 1981.

491. Frislid, K., Aadland, E., and Berstad, A. Augmented post-prandial gastric acid secretion due to exposure to ranitidine in healthy subjects. Scand. J. Gastroenterol. 21:119, 1986.

492. Jones, D. B., Howden, C. W., Burget, D. W., Silletti, C., and Hunt, R. H. Evidence for up-regulation of the H_2 receptor during maintenance ranitidine treatment. Gastroenterology 90(5):1480, 1986.

493. Modammed, R., Holden, R. J., Hearns, J. B., McKibben, B. M., Buchanan, K. D., and Crean, G. P. Effects of eight weeks' continuous treatment with oral ranitidine and cimetidine on gastric acid secretion, pepsin secretion, and fasting serum gastrin. Gut 24:61, 1983.

494. Strum, W. B. Prevention of duodenal ulcer recurrence. Ann. Intern. Med. 105:757, 1986.

495. Boyd, E. J. S., Peden, N. R., Browning, M. C. K., Saunders, J. H. B., and Wormsley, K. G. Clinical and endocrine aspects of treatment with ranitidine. Scand. J. Gastroenterol. 16(suppl. 69):81, 1981.

496. Silvis, S. E. Final report on the United States multicenter trial comparing ranitidine to cimetidine as maintenance therapy following healing of duodenal ulcer. J. Clin. Gastroenterol. 7(6):482, 1985.

497. Gough, K. R., Korman, M. G., Bardhan, K. D., Lee, F. I., Crowe, J. P., Reed, P. I., and Smith, R. N. Ranitidine and cimetidine in prevention of duodenal ulcer relapse. A double-blind, randomised, multicentre, comparative trial. Lancet 2:659, 1984.

498. Texter, E. C., Navab, F., Mantell, G., and Berman, R. Maintenance therapy of duodenal ulcer with famotidine A multicenter United States study. Am. J. Med. 81(suppl. 4B):20, 1986.

499. Walan, A. Anticholinergics in the treatment of peptic ulcer. Scand. J. Gastroenterol. 14(suppl. 55):84, 1979.

500. Lauritsen, K., Havelund, T., Laursen, L. S., Bytzer, P., Kjaergaard, J., and Rask-Madsen, J. Enprostil and ranitidine in the prevention of duodenal ulcer relapse: A one year double-blind comparative trial. Gastroenterology 92(no. 5, pt. 2):1494, 1987.

501. Bardhan, K. D. A comparison of maintenance treatment (MT) with enprostil (E) against ranitidine (R) in preventing duodenal ulcer (DU) relapse (preliminary results). A UK tri-center study. Gastroenterology 92(5, pt. 2):1306, 1987.

502. Marks, I. N., and Girdwood, A. H. Recurrence of duodenal ulceration in patients on maintenance sucralfate. A 12-month follow-up study. S. Afr. Med. J. 67(16):626, 1985.

503. Boyd, E. J. S., Wilson, J. A., and Wormsley, K. G. The fate of asymptomatic recurrences of duodenal ulcer. Scand. J. Gastroenterol. 19:808, 1984.

504. Korman, M. G., Hetzel, D. J., Hansky, J., Shearman, D. J. C., and Don, G. Relapse rate of duodenal ulcer after cessation of long-term cimetidine treatment. A double-blind controlled study. Dig. Dis. Sci. 25:88, 1980.

505. Gray, G. R., McWhinnie, D., Smith, I. S., and Gillespie, G. Five-year study of cimetidine or surgery for severe duodenal ulcer dyspepsia. Lancet 1:787, 1982.

506. Andersen, D., Amdrup, E., Sorensen, F. H., and Jensen, K. B. Surgery or cimetidine? II. Comparison of two plans of treatment: Operation or cimetidine given as a low maintenance dose. World J. Surg. 7:378, 1983.

507. Schiller, L. R., and Fordtran, J. S. Ulcer complications during

508. Sherlock, D. J., and Holl-Allen, R. T. J. Duodenal ulcer perforation whilst on cimetidine therapy. Br. J. Surg. 71:586, 1984.

509. Weiland, D., Dunn, D. H., Humphrey, E. W., and Schwartz, M. L. Gastric outlet obstruction in peptic ulcer disease: An indication for surgery. Am. J. Surg. 143:90, 1982.

510. Forrest, J. A. H., Fettes, M. R., McLoughlin, G. P., and Heading, R. C. Effect of long-term cimetidine on gastric acid secretion, serum gastrin, and gastric emptying. Gut 20:404, 1979.

510a. Lombardo, L., Babando, G. M., De La Pierre, M., Masoero, G., Sategna-Guidetti, C., Imarisio, P., and Di Napoli, A. Long-term treatment of duodenal ulcer with ranitidine: an endoscopic, biochemical and clinical trial. Pan. Med. 25:105, 1983.

511. Festen, H. P. M. Thijs, J. C., Lamers, C. B. H. W., Jansen, J. M. B. J., Pals, G., Frants, R. R., Defize, J., and Meuwissen, S. G. M. Effect of oral omeprazole on serum gastrin and serum pepsinogen I levels. Gastroenterology 87:1030, 1984.

512. Sharma, B., Axelson, M., Pounder, R. P., Lundborg, P., Ohman, M., Santana, A., Talbot, M., and Cederberg, C. Acid secretory capacity and plasma gastrin concentration after administration of omeprazole to normal subjects. Aliment. Pharmacol. Therap. 1:67, 1987.

513. Carlsson, E., Larsson, H., Mattsson, H., Ryberg, B., and Sundell, G. Pharmacology and toxicology of omeprazole—with special reference to the effects of the gastric mucosa. Scand. J. Gastroenterol. 21(suppl. 118):31, 1986.

514. Ekman, L., Hansson, E., Havu, N., Carlsson, E., and Lundberg, C. Toxicological studies on omeprazole. Scand. J. Gastroenterol. 20(suppl. 108):53, 1985.

515. Poynter, D., Pick, C. R., Harcourt, R. A., Selway, S. A. M., Ainge, G., Harman, I. W., Spurling, N. W., Fluck, P. A., and Cook, J. L. Association of long lasting unsurmountable histamine H_2 blockade and gastric carcinoid tumours in the rat. Gut 26:1284, 1985.

516. Larsson, H., Carlsson, E., Mattsson, H., Lundell, L., Sundler, F., Sundell, G., Wallmark, B., Watanabe, T., and Hakanson, R. Plasma gastrin and gastric enterochromaffinlike cell activation and proliferation. Studies with omeprazole and ranitidine in intact and antrectomized rats. Gastroenterology 90:391, 1986.

517. Carney, J. A., Go, V. L. W., Fairbanks, V. F., Breanndan Moore, S., Alport, E. C., and Nora, F. E. The syndrome of gastric argyrophil carcinoid tumors and nonantral gastric atrophy. Ann. Intern. Med. 99:761, 1983.

518. Elder, J. B. Inhibition of acid and gastric carcinoids. Gut 26:1279, 1985.

519. Bordi, C., Ferrari, C., D'Adda, T., Pilato, F., Carfagna, G., Bertele, A., and Missale, G. Ultrastructural characterization of fundic endocrine cell hyperplasia associated with atrophic gastritis and hypergastrinaemia. Virchows Arch. (Pathol. Anat.) 409:355, 1986.

520. Hakanson, R., Bottcher, G., Ekblad, E., Panula, P., Simonsson, M., Dohlsten, M., Hallberg, T., and Sundler, F. Histamine in endocrine cells in the stomach: A survey of several species using a panel of histamine antibodies. Histochemistry 86(1):5, 1986.

521. Stockbruegger, R. W. Bacterial overgrowth as a consequence of reduced gastric acidity. Scand. J. Gastroenterol. 111(suppl.):7, 1985.

522. Axon, A. T. R. Potential hazards of hypochlorhydria in the treatment of peptic ulcer. Scand. J. Gastroenterol. 21(suppl. 122):17, 1986.

523. Cook, G. C. Infective gastroenteritis and its relationship to reduced gastric acidity. Scand. J. Gastroenterol. 111(suppl. 122):17, 1985.

524. Langman, M. J. S. Antisecretory drugs and gastric cancer. Br. Med. J. (Clin. Res.) 290:1850, 1985.

525. Sharma, B. K., Santana, I. A., Wood, E. C., Walt, R. P., Pereira, M., Noone, P., Smith, P. L. R., Walters, C. L., and Pounder, R. E. Intragastric bacterial activity and nitrosation

short-term therapy of duodenal ulcer with active agents and placebo. Gastroenterology 90(2):478, 1986.

before, during, and after treatment with omeprazole. Br. Med. J. *289*:716, 1984.

526. Spiro, H. M. Should we take duodenal ulcer so seriously (editorial)? J. Clin. Gastroenterol. *1*:199, 1979.

527. Lance, P., and Gazzard, B. G. Controlled trial of cimetidine for symptomatic treatment of duodenal ulcers. Br. Med. J. *286*:937, March 1983.

528. Gustavsson, S., Adami, H.-O., Loof, L., Nyberg, A., and Nyren, O. Symptomatic cimetidine treatment of duodenal and prepyloric ulcers. Dig. Dis. Sci. *31*(1):2, 1986.

529. Stage, J. G., Henriksen, F. W., and Kehlet, H. Cimetidine treatment of recurrent ulcer. Scand. J. Gastroenterol. *14*:977, 1979.

530. Koo, J., Lam, S. K., and Ong, G. B. Cimetidine versus surgery for recurrent ulcer after gastric surgery. Ann. Surg. *195*:406, 1982.

531. Pounder, R. E. Model of medical treatment for duodenal ulcer. Lancet *1*:29, 1981.

532. Elashoff, J. D., Greenfield, S., Henderson, D., and Sturdevant, R. A. L. Physician recommendations of elective surgery for duodenal ulcer patients: A comparison of surgeons and medical specialists. Gastroenterology *79*:750, 1980.

533. Aagaard, J., Amdrup, E., Aminoff, C., Andersen, D., and Hanberg Sorensen, F. A clinical and socio-medical investigation of patients five years after surgical treatment for duodenal ulcer. II. Association of social and psychological factors with surgical outcome. Scand. J. Gastroenterol. *16*:369, 1981.

534. Browning, J. S., and Houseworth, J. H. Development of new symptoms following medical and surgical treatment for duodenal ulcer. Psychosom. Med. *15*:328, 1953.

535. Hansen, J. H., and Knigge, U. Failure of proximal gastric vagotomy for duodenal ulcer resistant to cimetidine. Lancet 2(8394):84, 1984.

536. Knop, J., and Fischer, A. Duodenal ulcer, suicide, psychopathology and alcoholism. Acta Psychiat. Scand. *63*:346, 1981.

537. Eberlein, T. J., Lorenzo, F. V., and Webster, M. W. Gastric carcinoma following operation for peptic ulcer disease. Ann. Surg. *187*:251, 1978.

538. Papachristou, D. N., Agnanti, N., and Fortner, J. G. Gastric carcinoma after treatment of ulcer. Am. J. Surg. *139*:193, 1980.

539. Ovaska, J. T., Havia, T. V., and Kujari, H. P. Retrospective analysis of gastric stump carcinoma patients treated during 1946–1981. Acta Chir. Scand. *152*:199, 1986.

540. Fischer, A. B., Graem, N., and Jensen, O. M. Risk of gastric cancer after Billroth II resection for duodenal ulcer. Br. J. Surg. *70*:552, 1983.

541. Tokudome, S., Kono, S., Ikeda, M., Kuratsune, M., Sano, C., Inokuchi, K., Kodama, Y., Ichimiya, H., Nakayama, F., Kaibara, N., Koga, S., Yamada, H., Ikejiri, T., Oka, N., and Tsurumaru, H. A prospective study on primary gastric stump cancer following partial gastrectomy for benign gastroduodenal diseases. Cancer. Res. *44*:2208, 1984.

542. Primrose, J. N., and Johnston, D. Is highly selective vagotomy (HSV) effective for the duodenal ulcer (DU) which fails to heal on H₂ receptor antagonists (H₂RA)? Gastroenterology 92(5, pt. 2):1580, 1987.

543. Pickard, W. R., and MacKay, C. Early results of surgery in patients considered cimetidine failures. Br. J. Surg. *71*(1):67, 1984.

544. Weaver, R. M., and Temple, J. G. Proximal gastric vagotomy in patients resistant to cimetidine. Br. J. Surg. *72*(3):177, 1985.

48

Gastric Ulcer

CHARLES T. RICHARDSON

Benign gastric ulcers have depth and penetrate the muscularis mucosae (Figs. 48–1, 48–2A [Color, p. xxxix], and 48–3). This distinguishes them from acute superficial erosions, which represent small breaks in the mucosa without depth (Color Fig. 48–2B, p. xxxix). These latter lesions may occur in patients with stress from severe medical or surgical illnesses or in patients taking nonsteroidal anti-inflammatory drugs.

Gastric ulcers can occur anywhere in the stomach, although the most frequent location is on the lesser curvature near the angularis.[1] Gastric ulcers occur occasionally in Meckel's diverticula and have been found in ectopic gastric mucosa in the gallbladder.[2]

Ulcers are usually round but may be oval, elongated, or elliptical. Most gastric ulcers vary from 1 to 2 cm in greatest dimension, but they can range from a few millimeters to several centimeters across. Most patients have a single ulcer, although a few patients have two or more ulcers (see p. 889).

INCIDENCE

The exact number of patients who have gastric ulcer disease is not known. In Japan gastric ulcers occur five to ten times more often than duodenal ulcers.[3] In the United States, about four million people have peptic ulcers (gastric or duodenal ulcers) and about 350,000 new cases are diagnosed each year. Four times as many duodenal as gastric ulcers occur in the United States.[4] Thus, approximately one million people have gastric ulcers and about 87,500 new cases of gastric ulcer

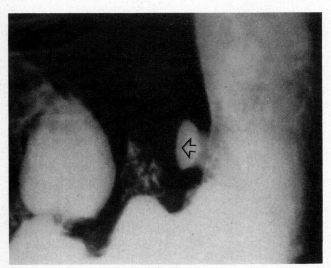

Figure 48–1. Upper gastrointestinal radiograph of the stomach and duodenum. A relatively deep gastric ulcer *(arrow)* is seen protruding from the lesser curvature of the stomach. (Courtesy of Herbert J. Smith, M.D.)

disease are diagnosed each year. Over 100,000 patients with chronic benign gastric ulcers are hospitalized yearly (Fig. 48–4), and about 3000 people die each year as a result of gastric ulcer disease.[5] Studies from Denmark[6] suggest that the incidence of new gastric ulcers occurring during a 12-month period in all persons over 15 years of age in that country is 5 per 10,000 persons. The incidence of gastric ulcers is approximately the same for men as for women. Ulcers rarely develop before age 40, and the peak incidence occurs from age 55 to 65. Results of one study demonstrated a correlation between increasing age and occurrence of ulcers.[7]

Overall, hospitalization for and deaths from peptic ulcer disease have decreased during the past 10 to 20 years.[5, 8] However, the decrease in hospitalization is due almost exclusively to a reduction in admissions for duodenal rather than for gastric ulcer. In fact, overall hospitalizations for gastric ulcer have remained stable during the past several years even though admissions for uncomplicated ulcers have decreased slightly (Fig. 48–4). Outpatient visits for gastric ulcers have de-

creased minimally in men and increased slightly in women.[9]

PATHOLOGY

Benign ulcers have elevated, firm, sometimes overhanging margins which are often indurated and hyperemic.[10] The ulcer base is covered by an adherent granular, whitish-gray exudate. Occasionally, ulcers may extend to the serosal surface and ulcers on the posterior wall may penetrate the underlying pancreas. Ulcers on the lesser curvature or anterior wall rarely penetrate through the stomach wall to the serosa.

Gastric ulcers have four microscopic zones or layers: zones of acute inflammatory exudate, fibrinoid necrosis, granulation tissue, and scar tissue (Fig. 48–3).[11] Ulcer margins are edematous and usually contain red blood cells and inflammatory cells. The muscularis mucosae surrounding ulcer craters is usually thickened, as is the submucosa. Disappearance of acute inflammatory reaction and edema in surrounding tissues is the first sign of ulcer healing.[12] Collagen fibers in the fibrous zone contract, reducing ulcer size. New epithelium grows inward from the ulcer margin and covers the layer of granulation tissue. Retraction of fibrous tissue may lead to a permanent scar.

PATHOGENESIS

The cause of gastric ulcer is poorly understood, although a number of pathophysiologic abnormalities have been described in subgroups of gastric ulcer patients. It is not known whether these defects lead to ulceration or whether some or all of them occur as a result of ulcers. In general, most of these abnormalities are thought to contribute to a breakdown in the ability of gastric mucosa to protect itself from damage by acid and pepsin or other destructive agents such as bile and pancreatic enzymes. Acid and pepsin secretion is often normal or lower than normal in patients with gastric ulcers. Therefore, it is not known whether acid and pepsin, *per se*, can damage normal mucosa and lead to ulceration (independent of a breakdown in mucosal defense) or whether acid and pepsin contribute to

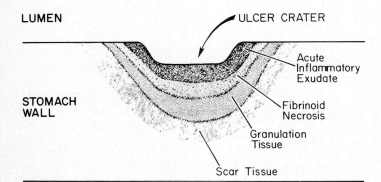

Figure 48–3. Schematic representation of an ulcer crater. The four microscopic zones and layers that compose the crater are depicted.

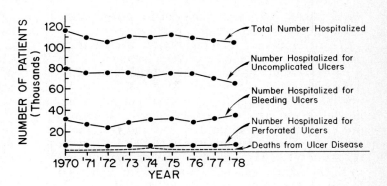

Figure 48–4. Total number of patients with gastric ulcer hospitalized each year during the period 1970 through 1978. Numbers of patients hospitalized for uncomplicated and complicated ulcer disease and deaths from ulcer disease are also shown. (Redrawn from Elashoff, J. D., and Grossman, M. I. Gastroenterology 78:280, 1980).

ulceration once mucosal damage occurs via some other mechanism.

Environmental factors, such as aspirin intake or stressful life events, may be related to ulceration in some patients. Also, most ulcers occur on the lesser curvature. Thus, this area of the stomach appears more sensitive than other areas to ulcer formation. Some studies support a role for genetic mechanisms in ulcer pathogenesis, and recently a bacterium, *Campylobacter pylori*, has been proposed as a cause of ulcer disease. How these mechanisms interact to cause ulcers in individual patients is not known. It is likely that one or several mechanisms may be important in ulcer development in some patients whereas other factors may cause ulcers in other groups of patients. The concept that different factors cause ulcers in various subgroups of patients has led to the hypothesis that gastric ulcer is not one disease but is a heterogeneous group of disorders, each with one or several causes. The ulcer crater is the clinical manifestation of one or several of these disorders.

Whether the mechanisms leading to gastric ulceration are the same as those causing duodenal ulcers is not known. It seems likely that there are a number of different causes of either disease. One author has postulated three classes of gastric ulcers.[13] According to this classification, Type 1 ulcers occur in the body of the stomach and are not associated with disease in the duodenum, pylorus, or prepyloric region. Type 2 ulcers, on the other hand, occur in the body of the stomach and are associated with an ulcer or ulcer-scar in the duodenum. This type of ulcer may occur as a result of duodenal disease. Type 3 ulcers occur in the prepyloric region and are associated with acid hypersecretion. It has been suggested that this type of ulcer may have a different pathogenesis than ulcers located in the body of the stomach. Recently, a fourth type of gastric ulcer has been hypothesized.[14] These ulcers are located in the upper portion of the stomach near the cardia. Supposedly, they have a frequent association with type O blood group, a low basal and stimulated acid output, a high incidence of upper gastrointestinal bleeding, a slower emptying of fluids, and a high percentage of deeply penetrating ulcers. These classifications and theories regarding pathogenesis of gastric ulcers remain hypothetical at the present time.

Mechanisms that may play a role in the pathogenesis of gastric ulcer disease are discussed in more detail below.

Pathophysiologic Abnormalities

Motility Defects. There are at least three methods whereby abnormal motor function might predispose to gastric ulceration. First, incompetence of the pyloric sphincter might allow duodenal contents such as bile and pancreatic enzymes to reflux into the stomach (see below). This, in turn, might produce gastritis and predispose to ulceration. Second, delayed gastric emptying, perhaps due to antral hypomotility, might lead to stasis and delayed clearing of refluxed duodenal contents, which in turn could predispose to gastritis and ulcer formation. Delayed emptying might also cause food retention in the antrum, which could lead to increased gastrin release and subsequently higher rates of acid secretion. For a number of years this latter hypothesis was thought to be a major factor in gastric ulcer pathogenesis.[15, 16] Presently, delayed gastric emptying is thought to be related to ulceration in only a minority of patients. Third, the position and movement of muscle bands in the stomach wall, especially on the lesser curvature, have been postulated as factors contributing to the vulnerability of overlying mucosa to ulceration[17] (see p. 885).

Pyloric sphincter abnormalities have been identified in small groups of gastric ulcer patients. For example, abnormally low basal pyloric sphincter pressures were found in one group of patients,[18] whereas normal basal sphincter pressures were found in another group.[19] However, when acid or fat was infused into the duodenum of patients in the second group, pressures did not increase to the same levels as occurred in normal subjects.[19] This was believed to be due to failure of the pyloric sphincter to respond to endogenously released secretin or cholecystokinin. Even after ulcers healed, the abnormality in sphincter function persisted, suggesting that the sphincter defect might have been the primary event. It was suggested that an abnormal sphincter mechanism allowed increased duodenogastric reflux of bile and pancreatic juice, which in turn led to gastritis and ulceration (see below). Additional studies are needed to confirm this abnormality and to relate it more directly to gastric ulcer pathogenesis.

Gastric motility and emptying have been evaluated in several groups of gastric ulcer patients.[19-23] Data from one study indicated that antral motility was diminished while ulcers were active but returned to normal after ulcers healed. In these patients it could not be determined whether the motility abnormality preceded the onset of gastric ulcer and thus was the primary event or whether the motor defect was secondary to ulceration. In other studies, measurements of gastric emptying have been normal[21, 22] or delayed.[23] In this latter study, gastric emptying of solids was delayed while emptying of liquids was normal.[23] Recently, an abnormality of the interdigestive, migrating motor complex was found in the stomachs of gastric ulcer patients.[24] While defects in gastric motility and/ or emptying have been described in small groups of patients, at present there is no convincing evidence that motor defects are major factors in the pathogenesis of gastric ulcers in the majority of patients.

Duodenogastric Reflux. Reflux of duodenal contents into the stomach has been postulated as a cause of gastritis, which in turn predisposes to ulceration. Reflux has been demonstrated in gastric ulcer patients by injecting barium into the duodenum and observing radiographically for regurgitation of barium into the stomach.[25] In other studies either polyethylene glycol or phenol red has been infused into the duodenum and concentrations of these markers have been measured in the stomach as an estimate of duodenogastric reflux.[26-28] More recently, reflux has been evaluated scintigraphically using technetium-labeled chemicals.[29, 30] In most instances reflux has been greater in gastric ulcer patients than in normal subjects regardless of the method used to measure reflux.

Bile acids, lysolecithin, and pancreatic secretions are thought to be the substances in duodenal juice that are most damaging to the gastric mucosa.[31-35] Of the bile acids, deoxycholic acid is believed to be the most destructive, while phospholipase A_2 also may play a role in mucosal damage.[35, 36] The exact method whereby duodenal contents harm gastric mucosa is not known. Two mechanisms have been postulated: (1) alteration of the protective mucous layer overlying epithelial cells, making it easier for acid and pepsin to reach the cells, or (2) damage to the so-called gastric mucosal barrier (see below), making it more permeable to hydrogen ion back-diffusion.

When duodenal contents have been diverted through tubes of mucosa directly into the stomachs of dogs, gastritis has occurred in the gastric mucosa near the site of entry of duodenal fluid.[37] Thus, at least in animals, there is evidence that duodenal juice can cause gastritis. Whether reflux of duodenal contents into the stomachs of ulcer patients causes gastritis is not known, although there is circumstantial evidence to suggest that it might. For example, several studies have shown that the concentration of bile acid conjugates is increased both in the fasting state and after food in gastric ulcer patients compared with normal

subjects.[38, 39] Also, there is a positive correlation between the concentration of bile acids and the severity of gastritis.[39] These studies do not prove a cause-and-effect relationship among duodenogastric reflux, bile acids, and gastritis but suggest an association. Whether gastritis, in turn, predisposes to chronic gastric ulcers also has not been established (see below).

Reflux of duodenal contents may occur with greater frequency in gastric ulcer patients than in controls; however, there are several observations that suggest that reflux of duodenal contents, *per se*, may not cause ulcers. For example, healing of ulcers does not alter bile reflux,[40] and cholestyramine, which binds bile acids, does not enhance ulcer healing.[41] Furthermore, gastritis and reflux of duodenal contents occur frequently in patients after antrectomy or subtotal gastrectomy, yet the likelihood of ulceration is low.[42] Also, there is no association between the incidence of bile reflux and ulcer morbidity.[43]

Gastritis. Chronic superficial and atrophic gastritis are frequent findings in patients with gastric ulcers.[44, 45] Gastritis usually involves the antral (pyloric) mucosa, although it may be limited only to the area immediately surrounding the ulcer or may be widespread and involve the body of the stomach as well as antral mucosa.[46, 47] Widespread gastritis is sometimes associated with ulcers in the body of the stomach.[44] A seven-year follow-up study of chronic gastritis in gastric ulcer patients indicated that antral gastritis is predominant during the early course of gastric ulcer disease but with time (4 to 7 years in this study) gastritis progresses in the body but not in the antrum.[48] Since parietal cells are located in the body, development of severe gastritis in this area might lead to parietal cell atrophy and reduced acid secretion. Theoretically, development of reduced acid secretion with time might cause gastric ulcer to be a self-limited disease.

Although gastritis is usually associated with gastric ulcers, it is not known whether gastritis is the primary event that precedes ulceration or whether gastric ulcer is the initial lesion with gastritis supervening. Results from one study indicated that the development of increasing gastritis predicted the development of gastric ulceration.[49] Furthermore, gastritis has been shown to persist during inactive ulcer disease[44, 50] and even worsen after ulcer healing.[44, 48] Results such as these suggest that gastritis may be the initial event with gastric ulcers occurring secondarily. Even with this information, however, it is still unclear whether gastritis is the precipitating event in most patients with gastric ulcers.

Gastric Mucosal Barrier. In 1954 Hollander suggested that the gastric mucosal barrier was composed of two components.[51] The anatomic integrity of the surface cells was the most important factor, while mucus covering the surface cells also played a role. Later, the term was used to describe the ability of the stomach to maintain electrical and hydrogen ion concentration gradients between lumen and blood.[52] Recent evidence indicating that the continuity of the surface epithelium can be restored within a brief period (sometimes within minutes) after injury has led investigators to return to Hollander's original proposal that the surface epithelium is an important component of the gastric mucosal barrier.[53, 54] Mucus gel or tight junctions between epithelial cells also have been postulated as factors determining barrier integrity.

A number of substances, such as aspirin, bile salts, ethyl alcohol, and acetic acid, have been shown to alter ion fluxes and potential differences across gastric mucosa and these changes have been interpreted as a reflection of damage to the "barrier."[31] How these substances disrupt the "barrier" is not known, although several mechanisms have been postulated. Studies in dogs have implicated micellar dissolution of mucosal lipids as the mechanism whereby bile salts damage the "barrier."[55] Other studies have suggested that active ion transport is inhibited or metabolic processes (such as reduction in ATP content of the gastric mucosa) are altered, leading to changes in permeability of the mucosa.

Prostaglandins. When these compounds are given orally to animals, even in small doses, the gastric mucosa is protected from damage by several noxious agents, including aspirin, bile salts, ethanol, and boiling water, to name a few.[56, 57] This ability to protect the mucosa from damage has been called "cytoprotection."[56] A number of factors likely play a role in protecting the mucosa from damage. For example, exogenous administration of prostaglandins to animals is known to increase mucosal blood flow, enhance bicarbonate and mucus secretion, and increase cell renewal and/or cell repair after injury,[56, 57] and it is now believed that one or all of these physiologic activities may play a role in so-called "cytoprotection." The "gastric mucosal barrier" discussed above may not be involved in "cytoprotection," since prostaglandins can prevent the development of gastric erosions without preventing "barrier disruption."[58]

The fact that exogenous administration of prostaglandins protects the mucosa does not mean necessarily that prostaglandins play a similar role *in vivo*, although indirect evidence suggests that they do. For example, when aspirin or other nonsteroidal anti-inflammatory drugs are given to animals or humans, gastric erosions and/or ulcerations occur.[59–61] Lesions develop presumably because these compounds inhibit endogenous prostaglandin synthesis. Studies in animals also support a role of endogenous prostaglandins in mucosal protection. In two series of experiments rabbits were immunized with prostaglandin analogs.[62–64] With the development of high-titer plasma antibodies to prostaglandins, gastric ulcers developed in a large percentage of animals. In other experiments plasma obtained from one group of immunized rabbits, which contained antibodies to prostaglandins, was transferred to another group of animals that had not been immunized.[64] The second group of animals also developed ulcers. These latter experiments demonstrated that passive transfer of sera containing antibodies to prostaglandins could cause ulcers. Results of these experiments add credence to the hypothesis that endogenous prosta-

glandins play a role in protecting the gastric mucosa from damage and, conversely, absence of certain endogenous prostaglandins may lead to mucosal damage and ulceration.

Some investigators have suggested that gastric ulcers may occur because of prostaglandin deficiency.[65–67] Measurements of prostaglandins in the mucosa from gastric ulcer patients have led to conflicting results. In 1977, Schlegel and co-workers found increased amounts of prostaglandins in the antrum of gastric ulcer patients and attributed this to inflammation.[68] In contrast, other workers have found lower levels of prostaglandins in the mucosa of gastric ulcer patients.[69, 70] In one study, prostaglandin levels were significantly lower in biopsy specimens obtained from the fundus and antrum of patients with active gastric ulcers than in tissue from healthy controls. Additionally, prostaglandin concentrations were lower in ulcer patients whose ulcers did not heal with cimetidine or antacid than in those whose ulcers did heal.[69] In another study, mucosal biopsies from fundic tissue of gastric ulcer patients generated less prostaglandins than tissue from normal subjects.[70] While results from some studies suggest that prostaglandin deficiency may play a role in gastric ulcer disease, more information is needed before the question of whether gastric ulcers in some patients are caused by decreased prostaglandin formation can be answered.

Mucosal Blood Flow. The gastric mucosa has a rich blood supply consisting of arborizing mucosal capillaries that traverse the glandular layer of the stomach (Fig. 48–5).[71] In addition, beneath the muscularis mucosae there is an extensive system of arteriovenous anastomoses that are thought to play an important role in regulating blood supply to the surface cells. This arrangement of vessels in the mucosa and submucosa is the same in all parts of the stomach. However, the blood supply to mucosal and submucosal vessels is different on the lesser curvature than on the greater curvature or in other areas of the stomach. For example, on the lesser curvature mucosal capillaries and submucosal arteries arise directly from the left gastric artery, whereas in other parts of the stomach mucosal capillaries arise from a submucous plexus of larger vessels.

Gastric mucosal ischemia is believed to be an important factor in the pathogenesis of acute mucosal injury, as occurs in patients with severe medical or surgical illnesses (stress ulceration; see pp. 772–792).[72–74] Whether similar alterations in blood flow contribute to the development of chronic gastric ulcers is not known. It is theoretically possible that the anatomic differences in blood supply to the lesser curvature compared with the remainder of the stomach may somehow contribute to chronic ulceration on the lesser curvature. Unfortunately, current methods to evaluate mucosal blood flow in humans are inadequate to detect differences in regional blood flow in normal subjects or differences in blood flow between patients with ulcer disease and normal people. Therefore, the potential role of blood flow abnormalities in the path-

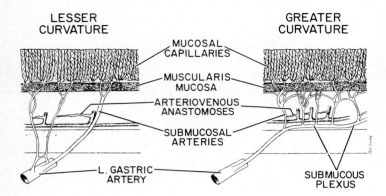

Figure 48–5. Schematic representation of blood supply to lesser and greater curvatures of the stomach. (From Barlow, T. E., Bentley, F. H., and Walden, D. N. Surg. Gynecol. Obstet. *93*:657, 1951. Used by permission.)

ogenesis of chronic gastric ulcers has not been adequately studied.

Recently, chronic mesenteric vascular insufficiency has been reported as a cause of gastric ulcers in four middle-aged women.[75] On endoscopy, ulcers in these patients appeared different from the typical chronic gastric ulcer. The ulcers were located in the antrum, were multiple, had irregular shapes with sloping edges, and had whitish, sclerotic bases. They were surrounded by mottled and erythematous mucosa that contained numerous superficial erosions. Ulcers in these patients did not heal with medical therapy but healed after balloon dilatation of the superior mesenteric artery in one patient and surgical revascularization in the others.

Mucus and Bicarbonate. A thin coat of mucus covers epithelial cells that line the gastric mucosa.[76–78] Mucus is secreted by both epithelial and mucus cells as a glycoprotein gel that adheres to the mucosal surface (Fig. 41–9, p. 726). Mucus is thought to protect underlying cells from mechanical forces of digestion, to lubricate the mucosa assisting the movement of food over the surface, and to retain water within the gel so as to provide a continuous aqueous environment for the mucosa. In addition, mucus is believed to form an unstirred layer impeding, but not blocking, diffusion of hydrogen ions from the gastric lumen to the apical membrane of epithelial cells. Although mucus gel is constantly being produced, it also is being removed continuously from the epithelial surface by mechanical forces during the mixing and grinding of food and by pepsin, which degrades mucus into glycoprotein subunits (see p. 726). The role (if any) that this process plays in causing the mucosa of gastric ulcer patients to be more vulnerable to ulceration is not known.

Nonparietal (nonacid) secretion, which is believed to consist primarily of a bicarbonate-rich fluid, also is secreted from surface epithelial cells into the mucus gel.[79] Theoretically, bicarbonate contributes to the ability of mucus to neutralize hydrogen ions that diffuse from the lumen into the mucus gel (see p. 727). Thus, in most patients, the mucosal surface is in contact with neutral fluid regardless of the amount of acid within the lumen. Mucus and bicarbonate together serve to protect the mucosa from damaging effects of hydrochloric acid, pepsin, and perhaps bile acids. Whether salivary bicarbonate, mucus that is swallowed from above, or pancreatic bicarbonate that has refluxed into the stomach from below contributes to gastric mucosal protection is not known.

How abnormalities of mucus or bicarbonate secretion might contribute to ulcer pathogenesis has not been established. Theoretically, gastric ulcer patients might secrete lower than normal amounts of mucus or bicarbonate or they may produce a qualitatively inferior mucus. So far, studies attempting to estimate the amount of mucus in gastric juice of ulcer patients compared with control subjects have led to conflicting results.[80–82] A decrease in mucus secretion has been found in patients with atrophic gastritis, a condition sometimes associated with gastric ulceration (see Gastritis, above).[77] Also, results suggest that mucus gel in gastric ulcer patients as a group (compared with normal subjects), may contain a larger quantity of lower molecular weight mucus glycoproteins, a type of glycoprotein that is associated with weaker mucus.[83] It is likely that such mucus would be less effective as a gel covering the mucosa, would be more likely to break down, and might be less able to resist the passage of larger molecules, such as pepsin, through the mucus gel.[84] More data are needed, however, before it can be determined if mucus and/or bicarbonate play a role in the pathogenesis of gastric ulcers.

Acid and Pepsin. Most patients with gastric ulcers have basal and peak acid secretory rates that are within the normal range.[85, 86] However, patients with ulcers in the body of the stomach, in general, have lower than normal acid secretory rates, whereas patients with combined gastric and duodenal ulcers or prepyloric ulcers have either normal or higher than normal acid secretion.[87] Secretion of pepsin usually parallels that of acid.

Decreased acid secretion in patients with ulcers in the body of the stomach is likely secondary to a decrease in the number of acid-secreting cells, which presumably results from gastritis. This is supported by the finding that gastritis is more widespread in patients with body ulcers than in patients with prepyloric ulcers.[44] Back-diffusion of acid through damaged mucosa also has been suggested as a possible explanation for lower rates of acid secretion in some patients. However, back-diffusion alone is not sufficient to explain low rates of acid secretion in most patients.[88]

The role of acid and pepsin in the pathogenesis of gastric ulcers is unclear. By definition, the presence of acid and pepsin is necessary for development of "peptic" ulcers and most patients with gastric ulcers secrete at least some acid and pepsin. Thus, in these patients it seems likely that acid and pepsin either contribute to the pathogenesis of ulcers, *per se*, or to the perpetuation of ulcers once they develop as a result of some other mechanism. Benign gastric ulcers have been reported in a few patients with achlorhydria.[89-91] Therefore, not all gastric ulcers result from the damaging effects of acid and pepsin, and those that do not are not true "peptic" ulcers. With regard to pepsin, it has been shown recently *in vitro* that pepsin I (a type of pepsin found in higher amounts in ulcer patients than in healthy subjects) digests mucus more effectively than another type of pepsin, pepsin III.[92] These results add further support to the belief that pepsin may lead to mucosal damage by degrading the mucus gel layer, which in turn contributes to ulceration.

Serum contains two pepsinogens (PGI and PGII) (see p. 725). PGI is synthesized mainly by the chief cells in fundic gland mucosa, whereas PGII is synthesized by chief cells in fundic glands as well as by cells in the pyloric glands and gastric antrum.[93, 94] Serum concentrations of PGI and PGII are higher in duodenal and gastric ulcer patients than in normal subjects, and the ratio of PGI to PGII is lower in gastric ulcer patients primarily because of a relatively higher PGII than PGI level.[95] This lower ratio is also seen in patients with gastritis. Whether serum pepsinogens represent a defect related to the pathogenesis of gastric ulcer disease or whether serum pepsinogens are altered in ulcer patients as a consequence of gastritis and/or ulceration is not known.

Results of a recent study demonstrated that an elevated PGII level and a low PGI/PGII ratio were risk factors for gastric ulcer at least in Japanese men.[96]

Anatomic Predisposition

Gastric ulcers can occur anywhere in the stomach although they usually occur on the lesser curvature near the angulus.[97, 98] The reason for this predilection is not known, but there are several possible contributing factors. First, histologic studies have shown that prominent muscle bundles underlie the mucosa on the lesser curvature near the angulus.[17] It has been postulated that these muscle bundles somehow cause the overlying mucosa to be more sensitive to ulceration. Second, almost all gastric ulcers occur at or near the junction of oxyntic and antral mucosa and occur on the antral side of this junctional epithelium.[99] In some patients, junctional epithelium overlies the muscle bundles on the lesser curvature. Thus, the combination of junctional epithelium above and large muscle bundles below may serve as cofactors contributing to ulceration on the lesser curvature. It is interesting that with increasing age the junction between oxyntic and antral mucosa moves proximally and this movement occurs

more rapidly on the lesser curvature.[100] Therefore, it is possible that the tendency to develop ulcers on the lesser curvature occurs when proximal movement of junctional epithelium reaches and overlies the prominent muscle bundles. The fact that the incidence of gastric ulcers increases with advancing age as does the cephalad movement of junctional epithelium supports this theory. The difference in mucosal blood supply to the lesser curvature compared with other areas of the stomach (see p. 883) may be a third factor contributing to the greater likelihood of ulcers occurring on the lesser curvature. Although these anatomic and histologic findings have been demonstrated in groups of gastric ulcer patients and groups of normal subjects, there is no proof that any or all of them actually contribute to ulcer pathogenesis in individual patients.

Environmental Factors

Nonsteroidal Anti-inflammatory Drugs. Experiments in animals indicate that aspirin causes acute mucosal erosions whether it is given orally or intravenously[101, 102] and that the severity of aspirin-induced lesions can be enhanced either by stimulating acid secretion with histamine or by infusing acid into the stomach.[101, 103] Similar lesions have been found in humans who take aspirin orally,[104] and gastrointestinal bleeding also occurs with increased frequency in patients treated with aspirin.[105] It is thought that bleeding in these latter patients originates from aspirin-induced acute mucosal lesions.

Several epidemiologic studies have demonstrated that chronic gastric ulcers occur more frequently in patients taking large doses of aspirin than in control populations.[106-109] Furthermore, there was a sixfold increase in the incidence of chronic ulcers in a group of patients taking three aspirin tablets daily in an effort to reduce recurrence of myocardial infarction compared with a control population taking placebo tablets.[110] Although these studies suggest an association between aspirin treatment and occurrence of chronic ulcers, there are no studies in animals or humans proving that aspirin actually causes chronic gastric ulcers. It seems likely, however, that aspirin contributes to chronic gastric ulceration in some patients.

The relationship between nonsteroidal anti-inflammatory drugs (other than aspirin) and the pathogenesis of chronic gastric ulcers has not been investigated adequately. Most of these drugs cause mucosal erosions in animals[111] and humans,[112] and it seems likely that many of these compounds cause chronic ulcers (see p. 784).

There are at least two mechanisms whereby aspirin and other nonsteroidal anti-inflammatory drugs might cause mucosal damage. First, aspirin alters ion transport and potential difference across gastric mucosa, changes that have been interpreted as representing damage to the "gastric mucosal barrier" (see p. 882).[113, 114] Second, nonsteroidal anti-inflammatory drugs inhibit prostaglandin synthesis (see p. 883). The second mechanism seems the more likely method whereby mucosal damage occurs.

Other Drugs. Acetaminophen also may cause mucosal damage.[115, 116] Recent epidemiologic data suggest an association between acetaminophen and development of chronic gastric ulcers,[109] but whether this is a cause-and-effect relationship has not been established.

There is no evidence that drinking caffeine-containing beverages or alcohol causes chronic gastric ulcers. Alcohol has been shown to cause gastritis,[117, 118] but there are no studies linking alcohol ingestion with chronic gastric ulceration.

Several studies indicate that ulcers do not occur more commonly in patients treated with adrenal steroids than in controls.[119, 120] However, epidemiologic data suggest that treatment with large doses of prednisone may be associated with an increased incidence of ulceration.[119] Additional information is needed to determine whether a cause-and-effect relationship exists between treatment with adrenal steroids and gastric ulcer disease.

Smoking. Smoking cigarettes has not been shown to cause gastric ulcers, although evidence suggests an association between the two.[121, 122] Ulcer patients smoke more commonly than control subjects.[120] Also, there is a positive correlation between the quantity of cigarettes smoked and the prevalence of gastric ulcer disease.[123] Other results indicate that up to 80 per cent of gastric ulcer disease might be attributable to smoking cigarettes and the daily ingestion of analgesics and nonsteroidal anti-inflammatory drugs.[124] Duodenal ulcers are less likely to heal and more likely to recur in cigarette smokers than in nonsmokers.[125, 126] This may apply also to the healing and recurrence of gastric ulcers. Epidemiologic studies have shown that death rates from peptic ulcers are higher among patients who smoke cigarettes than among those who do not.[120, 127]

If smoking cigarettes predisposes to gastric ulceration, the mechanism is not clear. Nicotine has no consistent effect on acid secretion, although it has been shown to reduce pancreatic bicarbonate secretion.[128] Theoretically, this could lead to duodenal ulceration by impairing neutralization of gastric acid in the duodenal bulb. It is difficult to understand how reduction in pancreatic bicarbonate secretion might contribute to gastric ulcer pathogenesis.

A defect in ventilatory function has been found recently in patients with chronic gastric ulcers and to a lesser extent in patients with duodenal ulcers.[129] The defect in gastric ulcer patients was more severe in smokers than in nonsmokers. Whether smoking led to the ventilatory defect, which in turn led to ulceration, or whether there was simply an association among smoking, ventilatory defects, and gastric ulcer is not known. Smoking cigarettes also has been shown to reduce pyloric sphincter pressure in gastric ulcer patients, which, as discussed above, may lead to increased duodenogastric reflux and subsequent ulceration.[130]

Dietary Salt. A statistically significant relationship has been found between salt consumption or urinary sodium chloride excretion and death rates from gastric

ulcer disease in several countries.[131] Whether this applies to patients in the United States is not known, nor is it known whether gastric ulcer patients should be advised to eat a low-salt diet.

Psychologic Stress. Studies in rats[132] have shown that "high-emotional" animals (determined by open-field tests of emotionality[133]) had a higher incidence of restraint-induced gastric ulcers than did "low-emotional" animals. However, these results may apply to development of acute superficial ulcerations as might be seen in patients with severe medical or surgical illnesses (stress-induced ulcerations) and not to chronic gastric ulcers. Prospective studies evaluating psychologic parameters in the development of acute or chronic gastric ulcers in humans have not been performed. Personality patterns and life events have been evaluated retrospectively as possible precipitating factors in gastric ulcer pathogenesis. Results from a study[134] evaluating personality traits such as neuroticism and extroversion indicated that patients with gastric ulcers as a group were no different from control subjects and there was no one personality pattern characterizing gastric ulcer patients.

Studies evaluating the relationship between stressful life events and the presence of gastric ulcers have led to conflicting results. In Australia, life stress events occurred no more frequently in ulcer patients than in control subjects, nor were they significantly different in type between the two groups.[135, 136] In contrast, data from another study indicated that 84 per cent of ulcer patients (with gastric or duodenal ulcers) experienced some stressful situation during the five- to six-day period preceding onset of dyspepsia.[137] Only 22 per cent of a control group, consisting of inguinal hernia patients, reported stressful life events prior to development of symptoms related to the hernia. The most common events reported by ulcer patients included changes in occupation, financial problems, illnesses, or some other misfortune either in their own lives or the lives of family members. An increased frequency of domestic and financial problems was found in a group of patients with chronic gastric ulcers when compared with an age- and sex-matched control group in another study.[138] Recently, a case-controlled study of multiple psychologic and social factors was carried out in the United States in men with either gastric or duodenal ulcer disease. Patients with renal stones or gallstones and a group of healthy men served as controls.[139] Both gastric and duodenal ulcer patients experienced a similar number of stressful life events, although ulcer patients perceived these events more negatively. Additional variables that differentiated ulcer patients from controls included hypochondriasis, dependency, and low ego strength.

Geographic and Socioeconomic Factors. In industrialized countries peptic ulcer disease occurs commonly and the incidence and prevalence rates of both gastric and duodenal ulcer diseases are comparable. However, in a few areas of the world ulcers occur uncommonly. For example, less than 1 per cent of black South Africans have ulcers.[140] Throughout the world duodenal ulcers tend to be more common than gastric ulcers. Exceptions (i.e., populations in which gastric ulcers are more common than duodenal ulcers) include Indian miners in Peru, inhabitants of some fishing villages in northern Norway, and Japanese men.[141] In Japan, for example, gastric ulcer accounts for 30 deaths per 100,000 men, whereas in Israel deaths have been reported in only 3 per 100,000.[142, 143] So far, these differences in the incidence and prevalence of gastric ulcer in various parts of the world have not led to the discovery of factors that either cause gastric ulcers or protect the mucosa against ulceration.

In the late 1800's and early 1900's gastric ulcer was more prevalent in people in higher social classes.[144] However, most recent studies have shown no consistent differences in ulcer incidence as related to social class,[145, 146] with one exception. In Australia, females in lower social classes have a greater incidence of gastric ulcer than those in upper classes.[147] This is thought to be secondary to the fact that women in lower social classes take large quantities of analgesics.

Infectious Agents

Bacteria and viruses have been found in gastric mucosa of many patients with gastric ulcers.[148–151] For example, Steer and Colin-Jones reported in 1975 that gram negative bacteria could be found on the surface epithelium of 80 per cent of patients with gastric ulcers.[151] The microorganism was identified as *Pseudomonas aeruginosa*. While it was believed that this bacteria might play a role in the pathogenesis of gastric ulcer disease, the hypothesis was never proved.

In 1983, Warren[152] and Marshall[153] described organisms in gastric mucosa of patients with chronic gastritis. Since by light microscopy this organism resembled *Campylobacter jejuni* but was located in the stomach, it was named *Campylobacter pyloridis*.[154] Soon after the naming of the bacterium, it was cultured by several investigators.[155–157] Later, another organism, different from *Campylobacter pyloridis*, was identified in a few patients and this organism was labeled gastric campylobacter-like organism type 2 (GCLO-2).[158] The original *Campylobacter pyloridis* organism recently has been renamed *Campylobacter pylori*.

Campylobacter pylori is found in some patients with gastritis, and the organism also has been discovered in some patients with gastric ulcers.[159, 160] One group of investigators has even developed a hypothesis in which the urease activity of the *Campylobacter* organisms leads to hydrolysis of urea at intercellular junctions, which in turn leads to back-diffusion of hydrogen ions.[161] According to this hypothesis, back-diffusion of hydrogen ions leads to ulceration. While *Campylobacter* is found in the mucosa of patients with gastric ulcers, it is not known whether the bacteria cause the disease or whether the disease, caused by some other mechanism, occurs as the initial event and the organism establishes residence in the diseased epithelium. The fact that *Campylobacter pylori* is found also in mucosa from healthy subjects has led to speculation that the organism may not cause ulcer disease but instead may occur as a secondary event. Other studies are necessary to establish the role of *Campylobacter* in the pathogenesis of gastric ulcer disease.

Cytomegalovirus (CMV) has been found in gastric ulcers of some patients, especially those who have had renal transplants.[149] As with *Campylobacter*, it is not known whether CMV actually causes ulcers or whether ulcers develop for some other reason and CMV develops in the diseased mucosa because patients are taking immunosuppressive drugs.

Heredity

Doll and Kellock[162] reported that relatives of gastric ulcer patients had a threefold increased prevalence of gastric ulcers compared with the general population, whereas duodenal ulcers occurred no more frequently than in the general population. Similarly, relatives of duodenal ulcer patients had an increased prevalence of duodenal ulcers but no increased risk of gastric ulcers. These studies suggested that, at least in some instances, the tendency to develop a gastric or duodenal ulcer was inherited and that, from the genetic standpoint, gastric and duodenal ulcer diseases were separate entities. Studies in twins have supported the concept that the tendency to develop a gastric ulcer is inherited.[163] There have been very few additional studies evaluating the genetic aspects of gastric ulcer disease. It seems likely that some inherited predisposition may be present in some gastric ulcer patients, but the exact role of heredity in the pathogenesis of gastric ulcer has not been established.

Hepatic Artery Infusion Chemotherapy

Gastric and duodenal ulcers have been reported in patients receiving chemotherapy by infusion into the hepatic artery.[164, 165] Ulceration has been associated with infusion of 5-fluorouracil alone as well as with combination chemotherapy with 5-fluorouracil, mitomycin C, doxorubicin HCl, and cisplatin. The cause of the mucosal disease is not known, but because symptoms responded to discontinuation of hepatic artery infusion and not to therapy with cimetidine, a direct toxic effect of chemotherapy has been postulated.[165]

NATURAL HISTORY

Two developments have increased our knowledge relative to the natural history of gastric ulcer disease. First, the availability of fiberoptic endoscopy has improved documentation of ulcer craters. Second, controlled clinical trials have been performed which have included groups of patients treated with placebos as well as groups treated with active medications. Evaluation of placebo-treated patients has provided information on pain relief, ulcer healing, and ulcer recurrence in the absence of active medication.

Pain disappears within 2 weeks in 30 to 40 per cent of patients treated with placebo and within 6 weeks in about 60 per cent of patients.[166] Ulcer healing, on the other hand, requires a longer period. This is illustrated in Figure 48–6. In patients treated with placebo, ulcers heal in about 45 per cent within 6 weeks, whereas by 12 weeks ulcers heal in 65 to 70 per cent.[166–168]

After ulcer healing has occurred and has been documented by endoscopy, patients in controlled clinical trials have been randomly reassigned to receive either active medication or placebo and have been followed for up to 12 months. During this period they have undergone endoscopy either at regular intervals (usually every 3 to 6 months) or when recurrent symptoms developed. In patients treated with placebos for up to 12 months, gastric ulcers recur in 55 to 89 per cent of patients.[169–171]

Most gastric ulcers recur in the same area of the stomach as the original ulcer.[172] Presumably, this occurs because the same factors predisposed the patient to both the original and recurrent ulcers. Recurrent ulcers are often smaller in size than original ulcers. This is likely due to the fact that recurrent ulcers are detected at an earlier stage of development because patients usually consult physicians sooner for evaluation of recurrent symptoms.

Whether size of the original ulcer affects the likelihood of a recurrent ulcer is controversial.[173–175] Results from one study suggested that patients with medium or large ulcers have a greater incidence of recurrence than patients with small ulcers. Likewise, ulcers recur more frequently in patients whose index ulcers were slow to heal. Complete healing of initial craters also may be important in preventing recurrent ulcers.[176] Sex of the patient or alcohol consumption does not alter the frequency of ulcer recurrences. Smoking increases

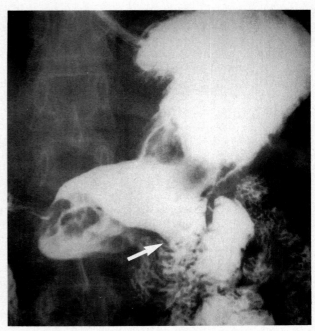

Figure 48–7. Upper gastrointestinal radiograph illustrating a gastroenteric fistula *(arrow)*. The fistula was formed when the gastric ulcer eroded into a loop of small intestine. Barium empties prematurely from the stomach into the small bowel through the fistula. (Courtesy of Herbert J. Smith, M.D.)

recurrence of duodenal ulcers[126] and may increase the incidence of gastric ulcer recurrence.

It is uncommon to see patients with more than two or three recurrences of gastric ulcers. There are at least three possible explanations for this observation. First, gastric ulcer disease may be self-limited, so that eventually the tendency to develop an ulcer disappears. Gastric atrophy and subsequent hypochlorhydria or achlorhydria that develops as a result of progressive gastritis has been postulated as a cause. Second, most patients with benign gastric ulcers may be treated surgically after two or three recurrences. Third, ulcers may recur but remain asymptomatic. In one study, 22 of 40 patients had a recurrent ulcer at endoscopy performed 4 to 8 years after documentation of the initial ulcer.[177] Of these 22 patients, 14 did not have symptoms suggestive of ulcer disease yet had an ulcer at the time of follow-up endoscopy.

Bleeding and perforation are the most frequent complications of gastric ulcers. The number of patients hospitalized each year for bleeding or perforation is shown in Figure 48–4. About 20 per cent of patients who present with a bleeding gastric ulcer develop either a recurrent bleeding ulcer or a perforated ulcer during follow-up.[178]

Occasionally, benign or malignant ulcers cause gastric outlet obstruction. When this occurs, patients usually have nausea and vomiting (especially vomiting of old food) and may present with a large stomach filled with food and fluid which can be detected on X-ray examination of the abdomen. Gastroenterocolic fistulas have occurred in a few patients as complications of benign gastric ulcers (Fig. 48–7).[179–181] Rarely, gastric

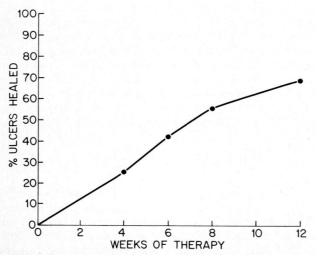

Figure 48–6. Percentage of gastric ulcers healed in patients treated with placebo. (Data from Graham, D. Y., Akdamar, K., Dyck, W., et al. Ann. Intern. Med. *102*:573, 1985; and Isenberg, J. E., Peterson, W. L., Elashoff, J., et al. N. Engl. J. Med. *308*:1319, 1983).

ulcers have penetrated into the pancreas, biliary tree, spleen, pericardium, left ventricular myocardium, and pleural space.[182–187]

It has been suggested that cancer can develop in an initially benign gastric ulcer.[188–190] This is difficult to prove because it could just as easily be said that malignant cells were present at the onset. In fact, this is a likely explanation since malignant ulcers can appear benign on X-ray and/or endoscopy and malignant cells can be missed on pathologic specimens obtained at surgery or at endoscopic biopsy or brush cytology.[191–193] Furthermore, when a small number of patients (n = 78) with benign-appearing ulcers at initial diagnosis were followed for five years, none developed gastric cancer.[194] A prospective study with endoscopic follow-up in a larger number of patients with benign-appearing gastric ulcers is needed to answer the question of whether ulcers that initially are clearly benign later become malignant.

Mortality in patients with gastric ulcers is slightly higher than in the general population.[195, 196] The total number of deaths in hospitalized patients with gastric ulcer in the United States during an eight-year period is shown in Figure 48–4. Deaths occur mostly during the first few years after initial diagnosis and occur mainly in patients over 50 years of age. There is no difference in life expectancy between men and women. Patients with combined gastric and duodenal ulcers have a greater risk of dying than those with solitary gastric ulcers.[196, 197] In the United States and most Western countries, morbidity from duodenal ulcer is more common than from gastric ulcer, although deaths from gastric ulcer occur with equal or greater frequency than those from duodenal ulcer.[4] In Japan, on the other hand, both morbidity and mortality are higher for gastric than for duodenal ulcer.

Gastric Ulcer with Coexistent Duodenal Ulcer

The incidence of coexistent duodenal ulcers in patients with gastric ulcers ranges from 7 to 64 per cent,[198–200] and in one report 42 per cent of patients with gastric ulcers had deformity of the duodenal bulb, an active duodenal ulcer, or both.[201] Whether duodenal ulcers occur first and then gastric ulcers develop as a secondary event is controversial.[197]

Gastric ulcers have been thought to be more frequently chronic and persistent in patients who also have duodenal ulcers.[200] This, however, has not been confirmed by other studies.[201, 202] There seems to be a slightly higher incidence of gastric ulcer recurrences in patients who also have duodenal ulcers.

The chances of apparently benign gastric ulcers actually being malignant are believed to be less if a coexistent duodenal ulcer or duodenal bulb deformity is present. This is supported by data from the Veterans Administration study,[201] in that there were only 1.2 per cent of patients with gastric carcinoma of 259 gastric ulcer patients who also had duodenal ulcer disease, compared with 6 per cent of the 359 gastric

ulcer patients who did not have coexistent duodenal disease. Twelve per cent of patients with malignant ulcers had concomitant duodenal ulcers, whereas 43 per cent with benign ulcers had evidence of duodenal disease. Although the presence of duodenal ulcer supports the premise that a benign-appearing gastric ulcer is actually benign, an active duodenal ulcer or a deformed duodenal bulb does not rule out gastric cancer in an individual patient.

Multiple Gastric Ulcers

Two to 8 per cent of patients with gastric ulcer disease have multiple ulcers. The age, sex, and clinical course of patients with multiple chronic gastric ulcers are no different from those of patients who have solitary ulcers.[203, 204] Furthermore, the presence of multiple ulcers at the time of initial diagnosis does not increase the likelihood of recurrent ulcer.

The finding of more than one chronic gastric ulcer in an individual patient has been used as evidence indicating that ulcers are benign.[205] This fact is not well documented, and lymphosarcoma is sometimes associated with multiple gastric ulcers.[206] Multiple refractory gastric ulcers also may be seen in patients with lymphoma complicating celiac sprue.[207]

CLINICAL MANIFESTATIONS

Most patients with chronic gastric ulcers have pain, although ulcers have been found on X-ray or endoscopy in asymptomatic patients.[177] For some reason asymptomatic ulcers occur more often in elderly than in young patients.[208] Pain resulting from an uncomplicated gastric ulcer usually is dull and localized in the midline. It can occur at any time during the day but frequently occurs within one to three hours after eating. Pain frequently is relieved by eating another meal, although in a few patients eating food may actually cause pain.[209, 210] Approximately 30 per cent of patients have pain during the night as well as during the day.[209]

The cause of pain is not known, but there are two possible explanations. First, acid bathing the ulcer crater may irritate sensory nerves in the ulcer base. Second, gastric contractions passing through the area of ulceration may cause pain. Results of two poorly controlled studies[211, 212] indicated that ulcer pain could be relieved by aspirating gastric juice from the stomach and initiated by reinfusing the fluid. In these experiments pain did not occur if acid in the gastric juice was neutralized prior to reinfusion. The hypothesis that gastric motility leads to pain in gastric ulcer patients has not been tested adequately.

Pain does not correlate with the presence or absence of gastric ulcer craters in some patients.[213] For example, a few patients continue to have pain despite endoscopic healing of ulcers, and, as mentioned above, ulcers occur in some patients who are asymptomatic.[177, 214, 215] More commonly, symptoms improve or disappear even though ulcer craters are still present.[216] The reasons for the lack of correlation in some patients between the presence of pain and ulcer craters is not known. Some may perceive pain to a greater or lesser extent than others; that is, the pain threshold may differ from one patient to another. Differences in size or depth of ulcer craters, levels of gastric acidity, or levels of endogenous antagonists of pain such as endorphins among individual patients also may contribute to the severity of ulcer pain in some patients or the ease with which pain is relieved in others.

Nausea and vomiting rarely occur in patients with uncomplicated benign gastric ulcers. On the other hand, nausea and vomiting can occur in patients who have gastric outlet obstruction resulting from an ulcer near the pylorus. Such patients frequently regurgitate food eaten several hours prior to the episode of vomiting (see Natural History, above).

The physical examination in patients with uncomplicated gastric ulcers is usually normal, although weight loss can occur in patients with either benign or malignant gastric ulcers.[209] Epigastric tenderness is occasionally present but is a nonspecific finding and has a low predictive value for gastric ulcer disease.[217]

DIFFERENTIAL DIAGNOSIS

Benign versus Malignant Gastric Ulcer

In most instances it is impossible to differentiate a benign gastric ulcer from gastric cancer on the basis of clinical presentation. Epigastric pain, anorexia, nausea, and vomiting occur in both diseases. The physical examination is rarely helpful unless an abdominal mass

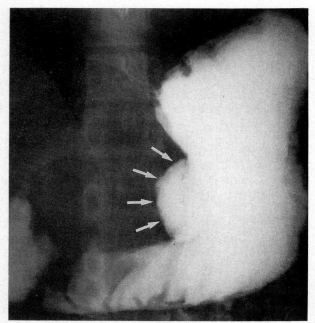

Figure 48–8. Upper gastrointestinal radiograph illustrating a large ulcer *(arrows)* on the lesser curvature of the stomach, protruding from the wall of the stomach. (Courtesy of Herbert J. Smith, M.D.)

is palpable, suggesting cancer, or there is evidence of metastatic disease. Differentiation between benign and malignant gastric ulcer is usually made by barium X-ray, endoscopy with biopsy, brush cytology, and/or response to medical therapy.

In general, location in the stomach is not helpful in differentiating benign from malignant ulcers, although ulcers in the cardia or fundus may have a greater likelihood of being malignant.[218, 219] There appears to be a higher incidence of cancer in large than in small ulcers.[191, 220] In one study 10 per cent of ulcers larger than 2 cm were malignant,[221] whereas in another report 62 per cent of ulcers 4 cm or larger were cancers.[222] From the clinical standpoint this does not mean that all patients with large gastric ulcers have cancer (Fig. 48–8) and that they should have surgery. Instead, patients with large, benign-appearing gastric ulcers should be evaluated and treated as any other patient with a gastric ulcer (see below). In fact, medical therapy of benign, giant gastric ulcers is usually effective and is not associated with a high incidence of ulcer complications.[223]

Gastric versus Duodenal Ulcers

Patients with gastric and/or duodenal ulcers present with similar symptoms and cannot be differentiated on the basis of clinical findings. The mean age of patients with gastric ulcers is approximately 10 years older than those with duodenal ulcers.[6] The highest incidence of gastric ulcers occurs in the sixth and seventh decades, whereas with duodenal ulcers the highest incidence occurs in the fifth and sixth decades. Both diseases are recurrent.

DIAGNOSIS

X-Ray

A carefully performed X-ray can detect 90 per cent of gastric ulcers,[224] although accuracy rates as low as 65 per cent have been reported.[225–229] The ability of X-ray to detect ulcers can be improved by using a double-contrast technique.[230, 231] Small ulcers (<5 mm) frequently are not found on X-ray even when a double-contrast technique is used.[232, 233]

More important than the ability of barium X-rays to locate ulcers is their ability to differentiate benign from malignant ulcers. Several studies have evaluated the frequency with which radiologically benign-appearing ulcers were found to be malignant at the time of surgery and found that 3 to 7 per cent were malignant.[221, 234, 235] The fact that some gastric ulcers are not diagnosed correctly as malignant on barium X-rays has led most physicians to recommend endoscopy in patients with radiographically diagnosed gastric ulcers even if they are benign-appearing (see Endoscopy, below).

Criteria Suggesting Benignancy. When present, probably the most reliable sign of benign gastric ulcer-

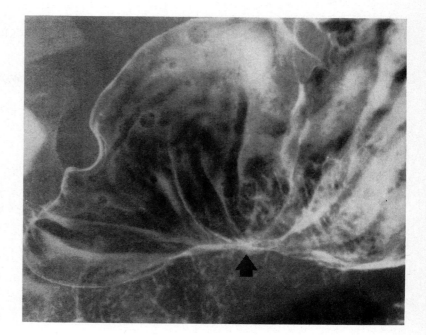

Figure 48–9. Upper gastrointestinal radiograph demonstrating folds radiating to an ulcer crater *(arrow)*. (Courtesy of Herbert J. Smith, M.D.)

ation is Hampton's sign.[224] This is characterized by a radiolucent line, usually not more than 1 mm in width, which partially or completely traverses the orifice of an ulcer. The radiolucency is due to the thin, undermined marginal mucosa of the ulcer crater.[236] The line cannot be demonstrated in most patients with benign gastric ulcers and its absence does not necessarily indicate malignancy, whereas its presence suggests benignity.[237]

Folds radiating to the edge of an ulcer crater are a second sign suggesting a benign gastric ulcer (Fig. 48–9).[238] If the folds radiate in the vicinity of the crater but are interrupted near the crater, the ulcer may be malignant rather than benign.

The ulcer collar, a translucent band that intervenes between the ulcer crater and the lumen of the stomach, is another radiologic finding indicating a benign gastric ulcer.[224] The ulcer collar most likely represents edema and inflammatory exudate surrounding the ulcer crater. An ulcer collar must be distinguished from a mass with central ulceration, which suggests malignancy.

Other criteria indicative of a benign gastric ulcer include an incisura, which is caused by spasm of circular muscle in the gastric wall opposite the ulcer[238] (Fig. 48–10), and penetration of an ulcer beyond the gastric lumen on X-ray (Fig. 48–1). The latter finding may not be a highly reliable radiologic sign of benignancy.[238]

Criteria Suggesting Malignancy. The most reliable signs of malignancy are a negative filling defect either in the ulcer crater itself or at its upper or lower margins and abnormal or effaced mucosal folds.[237, 238] Abnormal folds near the base of the crater also are a sign of malignancy. While these findings imply a malignant ulcer, they cannot be considered an absolute criterion for malignancy since they have been found also in a small percentage of patients with benign ulcers.

The best X-ray sign of a malignant lesion is the demonstration of a tumor in the vicinity of the crater.[224]

This may vary from an unmistakable ulcer within a mass (Figs. 48–11 and 48–12) to interruption or distortion of the mucosal folds on a limited segment of the periphery of the crater. A nodular or irregular base suggests cancer but is not an absolute indicator of malignancy since blood clots, granulation tissue, and

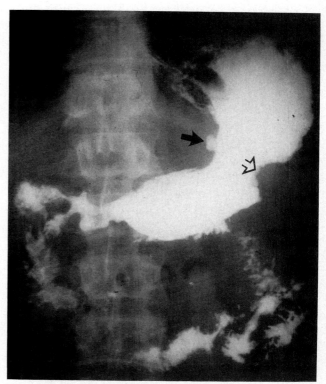

Figure 48–10. Upper gastrointestinal radiograph demonstrating an incisura *(open arrow)*, opposite the ulcer crater *(closed arrow)*. This radiograph also illustrates a markedly deformed duodenal bulb secondary to duodenal ulcer disease.

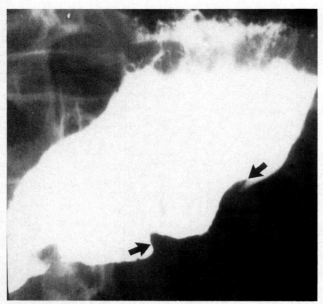

Figure 48–11. Ulcer within a mass as seen on an upper gastrointestinal radiograph. Note the sharp margins at the upper and lower edges of the ulcer crater (*arrows*). (Courtesy of Herbert J. Smith, M.D.)

food particles in a benign ulcer crater may have a similar appearance on X-ray.[239]

At one time most ulcers on the greater curvature of the stomach were believed to be malignant. However, it has been shown that many greater curvature ulcers are benign[240, 241] and are sometimes referred to as "sump-ulcers" (Fig. 48–13).[242] Greater curvature ulcers occur more frequently in elderly patients, many of whom are taking multiple oral medications including analgesics.[242]

Some patients with gastric cancer do not have a malignant-appearing ulcer on X-ray but instead have diffuse involvement of the gastric wall (*linitis plastica*).

The stomachs in these patients do not distend normally when filled with barium (Fig. 48–14).

Endoscopy

Several studies have indicated that endoscopy is more likely than X-ray to detect a gastric ulcer and that endoscopy is better at differentiating benign from malignant ulcers.[243–246] In addition, biopsy and cytologic specimens can be obtained from the ulcer crater at endoscopy.[247, 248] For these reasons, some physicians believe that endoscopy, rather than X-ray, should be performed as the initial diagnostic procedure in evaluating patients with ulcer symptoms.[249, 250] This approach, at least in the United States, is not cost effective in most patients, and therefore patients with ulcer-like symptoms usually have a barium X-ray as the initial diagnostic test.

Once an ulcer is diagnosed by X-ray, what are the indications for endoscopy? Some physicians believe that all patients with radiologically diagnosed gastric ulcers should have endoscopy regardless of whether the ulcer appears benign or malignant on X-ray. The major argument supporting this approach is that some benign-appearing ulcers on X-ray are actually malignant. As previously stated, this figure ranges from 3 to 7 per cent in most series.[221, 234, 235] The principal argument against using endoscopy in all patients with benign-appearing ulcers diagnosed by X-ray is that many gastroscopies performed in such patients will only confirm X-ray findings, increase the cost of medical care, and may misuse expensive medical resources.[251]

There is no way, based on scientific data, to settle the question of whether all patients with benign-appearing gastric ulcers on X-ray should undergo endoscopy. A subcommittee of the American Society for

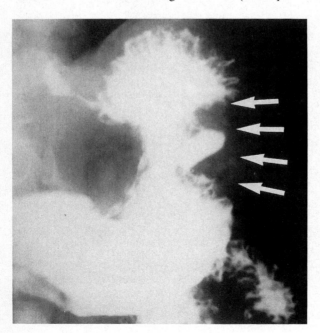

Figure 48–12. Ulcer within a relatively large mass. *Arrows* point to the serosal side of the stomach wall. (Courtesy of Herbert J. Smith, M.D.)

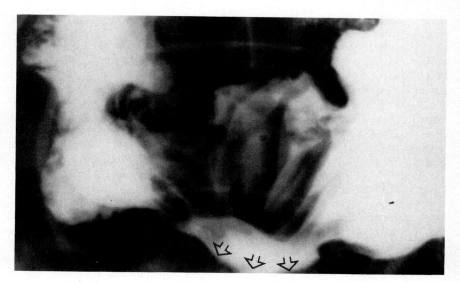

Figure 48–13. Large ulcer on the greater curvature of the stomach. Arrows are located within the crater and point to the base of the ulcer. Folds radiate to the ulcer crater. (Courtesy of Herbert J. Smith, M.D.)

Gastrointestinal Endoscopy met to design a prospective study to determine which patients with radiographically diagnosed gastric ulcers needed endoscopy.[252, 253] This group of experts concluded that such a study was not feasible for two reasons. A large number of patients would be required to carry out the study and conclusions obtained from one study might not apply to another group of patients, physicians, or economic circumstances. Furthermore, members of this subcommittee could not agree as to which patients with radiographically diagnosed ulcers needed endoscopy. Some supported the use of endoscopy in all patients with radiographically benign-appearing ulcers; a few believed gastroscopy should be performed only in patients who failed a "test of healing"; while others thought endoscopy should be performed only in patients whose ulcer on X-ray was suspicious for malignancy. The subcommittee concluded that a rigid policy regarding endoscopy in gastric ulcer patients was not justified and that the judgment of the individual physician should be used to determine which patients should undergo endoscopy.

In my opinion, all patients with benign-appearing gastric ulcers on X-ray should undergo endoscopy at some time during the course of medical treatment for an active ulcer unless there is a contraindication to endoscopy. This view is supported by recent guidelines published by the American Society for Gastrointestinal Endoscopy.[254] The timing of endoscopy during the course of ulcer therapy may vary. For example, endoscopy may be performed soon after the X-ray diagnosis is made. This is especially true in patients with ulcers that are not typically benign on X-ray or patients with large (>2.5 cm) gastric ulcers. An alternate approach is to treat patients medically for eight weeks after X-ray diagnosis and then perform endoscopy to evaluate ulcer healing (see below). Biopsy specimens can be obtained at this time if an ulcer is still present.

When endoscopy is performed, several biopsy specimens should be obtained from the ulcer margin. If the ulcer base is sampled, rather than the margin, the diagnosis of cancer may be missed. From six to ten specimens should be obtained.[246, 255, 256] Specimens should be removed in a circumferential pattern around the ulcer margin (Color Fig. 48–2C, p. xxxix). Specimens for cytology can be obtained by using a brush that is inserted through the endoscope. While this technique is not used in all laboratories, it is helpful when ulcers are located in areas of the stomach where obtaining specimens for biopsy is difficult.

It is important to remember that, if an ulcer appears benign by whichever diagnostic tests are used, the diagnosis of a benign ulcer is presumptive. All patients should be followed until ulcer healing is complete and documented by X-ray and/or endoscopy. Even though complete healing is another indicator of benignity, it is not absolute since a few malignant gastric ulcers have healed completely as visualized on X-ray and/or endoscopy.[192, 221, 257, 258]

Criteria Suggesting Benignancy. Benign gastric ul-

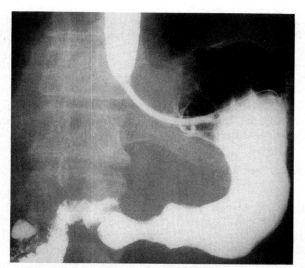

Figure 48–14. Radiograph illustrating the stomach of a patient with linitis plastica. There is minimal distention of the stomach when filled with barium.

cers penetrate the muscularis mucosae and are surrounded by an erythematous rim with smooth, regular, but slightly indurated edges (Color Fig. 48–2A and D, p. xxxix). The ulcer base is usually smooth and flat and covered by a white to gray exudate. The crater is usually round or oval but also may be somewhat linear (Color Fig. 48–2E, p. xxxix). Folds may be seen radiating to the edge of the ulcer crater (Color Fig. 48–2D, p. xxxix). If the ulcer is benign, folds usually are symmetrical and taper smoothly to the edge of the ulcer.

As mentioned previously, benign gastric ulcers have depth whereas mucosal erosions are superficial (Color Fig. 48–2A and B, p. xxxix). Depth perception of a gastric ulcer usually can be appreciated by alterations in the surrounding mucosal contour and coloration. The best method of determining ulcer depth is the "shadowing effect" provided by endoscopic light on surface irregularities.[259]

Criteria Suggesting Malignancy. Gastric cancer may appear in various forms at endoscopy. For example, an exophytic lesion is easily identifiable, whereas linitis plastica represents a more subtle finding and may be suspected only when the stomach does not distend as air is insufflated through the endoscope.

An ulcer that appears clearly to be within a mass is probably the most reliable endoscopic sign of a malignant gastric ulcer (Color Fig. 48–2E, p. xxxix). Ulcer margins, either in part or circumferentially around the crater, may appear "heaped-up" and infiltrated by tumor. Other features suggesting malignancy include ulcer margins that are irregular and overhang the ulcer crater.[259] The ulcer base also may have an uneven, nodular pattern that may represent tumor. Mucosal folds surrounding the crater often are clubbed or fused and do not extend to the edge of the ulcer.[259] This suggests that tissue surrounding the lesion is infiltrated by tumor.

As with X-ray appearance, none of the above criteria indicate necessarily that an ulcer in an individual patient is malignant. Thus, based on endoscopic visualization alone, the diagnosis of cancer is presumptive. Biopsy should be performed. If the biopsy does not reveal cancer but the endoscopic appearance suggests malignancy, endoscopy and biopsy should be repeated. In a few patients two or more endoscopic procedures with biopsy have been required to diagnose cancer. In some patients, surgery may be indicated if the index of suspicion for cancer is high yet endoscopic biopsies are normal.

Acid Secretory Studies

Most patients with gastric ulcers have acid secretory rates in the normal range. Thus, measurement of acid secretion is not useful in differentiating between normal people and patients with gastric ulcers.[85, 260] On the other hand, some patients with gastric cancer have histamine- or pentagastrin-fast achlorhydria[261] or hypochlorhydria.[262] Thus, measuring acid secretion has

been suggested as a test in gastric ulcer patients to aid in differentiating between benign and malignant ulcers. Such testing is not recommended because the incidence of achlorhydria in patients with gastric cancer is relatively small and a few patients with benign gastric ulcers also have achlorhydria.[89–91]

Measurement of acid secretion should be performed in some gastric ulcer patients to rule out Zollinger-Ellison syndrome. However, Zollinger-Ellison syndrome is rare and the occurrence of gastric ulcer alone in patients with this syndrome is unusual. Thus, acid secretory studies should be performed only in those gastric ulcer patients who for other reasons (e.g., diarrhea, postbulbar ulcers, multiple ulcers) are suspected of having Zollinger-Ellison syndrome.

Serum Gastrin Concentration

Most patients with benign-appearing gastric ulcers have serum gastrin concentrations that are higher than normal. A few patients with malignant gastric ulcers (especially those located in the body of the stomach) have markedly elevated serum gastrin concentrations.[263, 264] In general, there is an inverse relationship between serum gastrin levels and rates of acid secretion and patients with markedly elevated serum gastrin levels are usually those who also have achlorhydria. Thus, as a diagnostic test, measurement of serum gastrin concentration is of no more value than measurement of acid secretion. Serum for gastrin determination should be obtained only in those patients with gastric ulcers who because of other clinical findings (see above and pp. 912–913) are thought to have Zollinger-Ellison syndrome.

IMMEDIATE THERAPY

Medications

Results of controlled clinical trials evaluating the effectiveness of drugs used in treating patients with gastric ulcers are discussed below. Pharmacology is discussed in an abbreviated form in this chapter and on pages 845–850, but the reader is referred to Chapter 43 (pp. 708–725) in the third edition of this textbook for a detailed discussion of the pharmacology of drugs used to treat patients with peptic ulcer disease. Side effects of some of the drugs are listed in Table 48–1.

Antisecretory Drugs

Histamine H_2-receptor antagonists are the most commonly prescribed antisecretory drugs used in treating patients with benign-appearing gastric ulcers. Antimuscarinic drugs and tricyclic agents also inhibit acid secretion but are prescribed infrequently. A new class of drugs, the substituted benzimidazoles, are potent inhibitors of acid secretion and currently are being evaluated in controlled clinical trials.

Table 48–1. SIDE EFFECTS OF DRUGS USED TO TREAT PEPTIC ULCER DISEASE*†

| H₂-Receptor Antagonists | | | | |
Cimetidine	*Ranitidine*	*Famotidine*	**Antacid**	**Sucralfate**
Gynecomastia	Gynecomastia	Headache	Diarrhea‖	Constipation
Confusional states including mental confusion, agitation, and depression	Impotence	Depression	Phosphate depletion (can occur with antacids that contain aluminum hydroxide)	Diarrhea
	Decreased libido	Anxiety		Nausea
	Leukopenia	Decreased libido		Dry mouth
Impotence	Thrombocytopenia	Insomnia	Alkalosis	Rash
Decreased white blood cell count	Pancytopenia	Dizziness	Milk alkali syndrome	Dizziness
	Malaise	Constipation	Aluminum toxicity	Vertigo
Thrombocytopenia	Dizziness	Diarrhea		
Interstitial nephritis	Somnolence	Thrombocytopenia		
Pancreatitis	Depression	Palpitations		
Diarrhea	Tachycardia	Nausea		
Dizziness	Diarrhea	Vomiting		
Somnolence	Constipation	Hepatic enzyme abnormalities		
Rash	Hepatitis or hepatocellular dysfunction	Orbital edema		
Arthralgias	Rash	Arthralgia		
Drug Interactions* Warfarin-type anticoagulants Phenytoin Propranolol Chlordiazepoxide Diazepam Lidocaine Theophylline Metronidazole	Arthralgias Drug interactions§	Rash Tinnitus Taste disorder		

*See Chapter 43, pages 708–725 in the third edition of this textbook and the Physicians' Desk reference for a more detailed discussion of side effects.

†While side effects have been described in patients treated with each of these drugs, in clinical practice side effects occur rarely. This is a partial list of side effects, but in some instances a true causal relationship between the drug and the effect has not been established. In some studies in which drug side effects were described, similar side effects occurred also in patients treated with placebo.

‡Cimetidine alters microsomal enzyme systems in the liver and delays metabolism of certain drugs.

§Ranitidine has minimal effect on microsomal enzyme systems in the liver but may delay metabolism of some drugs.

‖Diarrhea usually occurs when an antacid containing magnesium hydroxide is prescribed. Diarrhea can be controlled in many patients by alternating a magnesium hydroxide–containing antacid with one that contains only aluminum hydroxide.

Histamine H₂-Receptor Antagonists. These compounds block the histamine receptor on parietal cells and thereby reduce gastric acid secretion (see p. 716). Three H₂-receptor antagonists are commercially available: cimetidine, ranitidine, and famotidine. Each of these compounds, in the doses commonly prescribed, reduces acid secretion effectively. Of the three, famotidine is the most potent, followed by ranitidine and then cimetidine. Several other H₂-receptor antagonists are undergoing clinical investigation.

Cimetidine. The effect of cimetidine (Tagamet) on the healing incidence of gastric ulcers has been evaluated in a number of controlled clinical trials and results are shown in Table 48–2.[167, 168, 265–274] Cimetidine was significantly more effective than placebo in healing gastric ulcers in most studies, although in three reports the differences between healing incidences with cimetidine and placebo were not statistically significant.[267, 269, 272]

The effect of cimetidine on gastric ulcer healing has been compared with that of antacid in two studies (Table 48–2).[168, 274] In one study,[274] patients received either 300 mg cimetidine four times daily or 15 ml Mylanta II (75 mM of neutralizing capacity) one and three hours after meals and at bedtime. The incidence of healing at 6 weeks was similar with cimetidine and antacid (59 and 61 per cent, respectively). Combining the two drugs was not significantly more effective in healing ulcers than either of the drugs given alone. Thus, in most patients it is not necessary to prescribe both cimetidine and antacid. In another study,[168] a lower daily dose of antacid, 15 ml Maalox Therapeutic Concentrate (75 mM neutralizing capacity), one hour after meals and at bedtime, was prescribed. Healing incidences were higher with cimetidine than with antacid at 4 and 8 weeks of therapy, but the differences were not statistically significant. At 12 weeks of therapy, healing was similar with cimetidine and antacid.

In most studies there is a trend for pain relief to be better with cimetidine than with placebo. However, it has been more difficult to demonstrate significant differences in pain relief with cimetidine versus placebo than differences in ulcer healing with the two forms of therapy. The explanation for this is not known. In

Table 48–2. EFFECT OF CIMETIDINE ON THE HEALING INCIDENCE OF GASTRIC ULCER

	Per Cent Ulcers Healed at Various Weeks of Therapy							
Treatment	*3*	*4*	*5*	*6*	*8*	*12*	**p**	**Reference**
CIMETIDINE VERSUS PLACEBO								
Cimetidine*				71(24)			<0.01	265
Placebo				27(22)				
Cimetidine*		71(24)					<0.02	266
Placebo		36(25)						
Cimetidine†				60(30)			NS	267
Placebo				41(29)				
Cimetidine*				95(21)			<0.05	268
Placebo				20(10)				
Cimetidine*				88(8)			NS	269
Placebo				73(11)				
Cimetidine*		69(16)					<0.001	270
Placebo		21(14)						
Cimetidine*†			84(25)				<0.05	271
Placebo			57(23)					
Cimetidine*		66(35)					NS	272
Placebo		52(25)						
Cimetidine*				86(22)			<0.05	273
Placebo				55(22)				
Cimetidine‡				66(65)			<0.05	167
Placebo				45(67)				
Cimetidine‡		56(36)			86(35)	89(35)	<0.05 at 4 and	168
Placebo		25(32)			55(31)	68(31)	8 weeks	
CIMETIDINE VERSUS ANTACID OR CIMETIDINE PLUS ANTACID								
Cimetidine‡				59(68)¶			NS	274
Antacid§				61(62)				
Cimetidine plus antacid†§				70(60)				
Cimetidine‡		56(36)			86(35)	89(35)	NS	168
Antacid‖		40(33)			69(32)	84(31)		

Numbers in parentheses represent number of patients in each group. NS, not significant.
*200 mg of cimetidine three times daily with meals and 400 mg at bedtime.
†Ulcer healing evaluated by X-ray rather than by endoscopy.
‡300 mg of cimetidine four times daily with meals and at bedtime.
§15 ml of Mylanta-II one and three hours after meals and at bedtime.
‖15 ml of Maalox Therapeutic Concentrate one hour after meals and at bedtime.
¶Data includes both inpatients and outpatients.

some studies patients in both groups were prescribed antacid as needed for pain, and this may have obscured any real differences in pain relief with cimetidine versus placebo. The other possibility is that patients actually receive pain relief to comparable degrees with placebos and active medications. Regardless of the treatment (cimetidine or placebo), pain diminishes within a few days in most patients.

The recommended dose of cimetidine in the United States is 300 mg four times daily, with meals and at bedtime. In other countries, the recommended dose is 200 mg three times daily with meals and a 400 mg dose at bedtime. Recently, 400 mg twice daily or 800 mg at bedtime has been shown to be effective in treating patients with duodenal ulcers. Whether these regimens also will be effective in treating patients with gastric ulcers remains to be established.

Patients should be treated until the ulcer heals. The percent of patients with healed ulcers at various weeks of therapy is shown in Table 48–2. In general, ulcers will heal in 60 to 90 per cent of patients treated for 6 to 8 weeks. Ulcers in a few patients will not heal even after 12 weeks of therapy. Management of these patients as well as recommendations regarding repeat X-ray or endoscopy are discussed in the section on follow-up, below.

Ranitidine. Results of several controlled clinical trials have shown that ranitidine (Zantac) is either more effective than placebo or equally as effective as cimetidine or antacid in leading to healing of gastric ulcers (Table 48–3).[275–282] Pain in most patients is relieved within a few days after beginning therapy. However, as with other forms of ulcer therapy, it is more difficult to demonstrate ranitidine's effectiveness over placebo in relieving pain than its benefit in healing ulcers.

The recommended dose of ranitidine is 150 mg twice daily, although, as shown in Table 48–3, results of several studies suggest that a single 300 mg dose at bedtime is equally as effective in healing ulcers.[278–281]

Table 48–3. EFFECT OF RANITIDINE ON THE HEALING INCIDENCE OF GASTRIC ULCER

Treatment	Per Cent Ulcers Healed at Various Weeks of Therapy					p	Reference
	2	4	6	8	12		
Ranitidine*	19(83)		68(73)			0.009	275
Placebo	12(83)		51(69)			at 6 wks	
Ranitidine*		64(17)		78(17)	88(17)	<0.05	276
Cimetidine†		55(20)		85(20)	90(20)	<0.05	
Placebo		30(20)		45(20)	55(20)		
Ranitidine*		66(96)	78(90)			NS	277
Cimetidine‡		62(101)	87(94)				
Ranitidine*		71(217)		93(204)		NS	278
Ranitidine§		65(211)		90(196)			
Ranitidine*		73(30)				NS	279
Ranitidine§		62(24)					
Ranitidine*		76(21)		100(19)		NS	280
Ranitidine§		79(19)		100(18)			
Ranitidine*		59(29)		86(29)		NS	281
Ranitidine§		73(30)		97(30)			
Ranitidine*		54(26)	69(26)			NS	282
Antacid‖		68(28)	79(28)				

Numbers in parentheses represent number of patients in each group. NS, not significant.
*150 mg of ranitidine twice daily.
†200 mg of cimetidine three times daily and 400 mg at bedtime.
‡$p < 0.05$ vs. placebo at 8 to 12 weeks.
§300 mg of ranitidine at bedtime.
‖10 ml of antacid seven times daily with a neutralizing capacity of 600 mM of acid per day.

Patients should be treated until the ulcer heals. As a general rule, patients are treated for 6 to 8 weeks. Ulcers that do not heal in this time period will occasionally heal if patients are treated for 12 weeks. Even after 12 weeks of therapy, ulcers will not heal in some patients. Management of these patients and recommendations regarding repeat X-ray or endoscopy are discussed in the section on follow-up.

Famotidine (Pepcid). This new H_2-receptor antagonist has been released recently for use in treating patients with duodenal ulcers but, as yet, has not been approved in the United States for treating patients with gastric ulcers. Results of several controlled clinical trials demonstrate that famotidine is more effective than placebo and equally effective as cimetidine in treating patients with gastric ulcers (Table 48–4).[283–286] The dose that has been used in most studies is 40 mg once daily at bedtime.

Antimuscarinics. These drugs reduce acid secretion by blocking muscarinic receptors on parietal cells and receptors on the cell body of postganglionic neurons in the wall of the stomach. The muscarinic receptors on parietal cells are M_2 receptors, whereas those on the cell body of postganglionic neurons in the wall of the stomach are M_1 receptors. M_2 receptors are located also on cells in salivary glands, on smooth muscle cells such as those in the urinary bladder, and on cardiac muscle cells. "Classic antimuscarinic" drugs, which are available currently, block both M_1 and M_2 receptors. Because these compounds block M_2 receptors, they cause side effects such as dry mouth, urinary hesitancy, and tachycardia. Clinical trials evaluating the effect of "classic antimuscarinic" drugs on healing of gastric ulcers have led to conflicting results,[287–289] and in many instances the drugs have been ineffective in healing gastric ulcers. Therefore, the compounds are not recommended for treating most patients with gastric ulcers.

One possible reason for the ineffectiveness of "classic antimuscarinic" drugs is the fact that, because of side effects, they cannot be given in doses sufficiently large enough to reduce acid secretion adequately. In an attempt to limit some of the side effects of antimuscarinic drugs, a new compound, pirenzepine, has been developed. In contrast to "classic antimuscarinic" drugs, which block both M_1 and M_2 receptors, pirenzepine is a more selective antagonist and blocks primarily M_1 receptors. Thus, reduction in acid secretion is achieved primarily by blocking M_1 receptors located on the cell bodies of postganglionic neurons in the wall of the stomach. Since pirenzepine has less effect on M_2 receptors, there is less likelihood of pirenzepine causing dry mouth, urinary hesitancy, or tachycardia. Results of clinical trials suggest that pirenzepine may be as effective as cimetidine or carbenoxolone, a licorice compound, in treating patients with gastric ulcers.[290–293] Pirenzepine has not been approved for use in treating patients in the United States.

Antimuscarinic drugs are useful when given in combination with cimetidine in treating patients who have gastric ulcers and gastric acid hypersecretion (e.g., patients with Zollinger-Ellison syndrome). In these patients a combination of an antimuscarinic drug plus an H_2-receptor antagonist is more effective in reducing acid secretion than either of the drugs given alone.[294, 295] The dose of antimuscarinic is usually one tablet (e.g., 15 mg propantheline bromide or 1 mg glycopyrrolate) given with cimetidine, ranitidine, or famotidine.

Table 48–4. EFFECT OF FAMOTIDINE ON THE HEALING INCIDENCE OF GASTRIC ULCER

Treatment	Per Cent Ulcers Healed at Various Weeks of Therapy			p	Reference
	4	6	8		
Famotidine*	42(33)	61(33)	97(33)	<0.01	283
Placebo	31(29)	45(29)	66(29)	at 8 weeks	
Famotidine*†	65(20)	95(20)	95(20)	<0.05	284
Placebo	46(24)	71(24)	79(24)	at 6 weeks	
Famotidine*‡	42(12)	69(71)	92(12)	Not given	284
Placebo	44(9)	48(73)	44(9)		
Famotidine*	48(71)		89(71)	<0.05	285
Placebo	33(73)		59(73)	at 6 weeks	
				<0.01 at	
				8 weeks	
Famotidine§	44(82)		83(84)	NS	285
Cimetidine‖	40(85)		76(91)		
Famotidine*	47¶	65	80	<0.01	286
Placebo	31	46	54	at 4, 6, and	
				8 weeks	

Numbers in parentheses represent number of patients in each group. NS, not significant.
*40 mg of famotidine once daily at bedtime.
†German trial.
‡Austrian trial.
§20 mg of famotidine twice daily.
‖200 mg of cimetidine four times daily.
¶This was a worldwide study consisting of 167 patients treated with famotidine and 169 treated with placebo. From the data presented, it was not possible to tell the number of patients in each group at each time period. Also, the number of patients entered from some countries was extremely small.

Tricyclic Antidepressants. These compounds may be useful in treating patients with gastric ulcers because of their antimuscarinic-like effects.[296] Trimipramine has been shown to be significantly (p <0.05) better than placebo in healing gastric ulcers in a small group of patients.[297] Healing incidences have ranged from 60 to 90 per cent with tricyclic agents compared with incidences of 20 to 40 per cent with placebo. These drugs are not marketed for treatment of ulcer disease in the United States.

Other Antisecretory Drugs. There are two other categories of antisecretory drugs that are being investigated. Sulpiride decreases gastric acid secretion by reducing serum gastrin concentration and by decreasing mucosal blood flow to the stomach.[298] Studies evaluating this drug in the treatment of ulcer disease have led to conflicting results.[299]

Another group of drugs, the substituted benzimidazoles, reduce acid secretion by blocking a hydrogen/potassium–adenosine triphosphatase enzyme located on the luminal surface of parietal cells.[300, 301] These compounds inactivate this enzyme, a proton pump, which is the final step in hydrogen ion secretion from parietal cells (see p. 715). Omeprazole, the drug that has undergone the most clinical testing, is a potent inhibitor of acid secretion in humans (see pp. 846 and 918). Results suggest that 20 mg of omeprazole given each morning is as effective as 150 mg of ranitidine given twice daily in treating patients with gastric ulcers.[302] While omeprazole is being tested currently in the United States, it has not been approved for clinical use. Omeprazole, given in large doses, causes carcinoid-like tumors in the stomachs of rats.[303] Additional studies are needed to determine whether this observation will have an effect on the clinical usefulness and safety of omeprazole in humans.

Antacids

Results of studies evaluating the effect of antacid or placebo in the healing of gastric ulcers are summarized in Table 48–5. One double-blind controlled study in a small number of outpatients demonstrated that the incidence of gastric ulcer healing as evaluated by barium X-ray was significantly (p <0.05) greater with antacid than with placebo.[304] Another report in hospitalized patients did not support these findings,[305] and results of still another study indicated that 15 ml of antacid given four times daily was not significantly better than placebo. After 12 weeks of antacid treatment, however, healing incidences were similar with antacid and cimetidine (Table 48–2).[168] In a recent study from Norway, the incidence of gastric ulcer healing was significantly better with one antacid tablet four times daily (neutralizing capacity, 120 mM/day) than with placebo (Table 48–5), suggesting that small doses of antacid may be effective in healing gastric ulcers.[306, 307]

Based on currently available data, the dose of antacid to be used in treating patients with gastric ulcers is not known. Since a dose of 15 ml of Maalox Therapeutic Concentrate given one hour after meals

Table 48–5. EFFECT OF ANTACID ON THE HEALING INCIDENCE OF GASTRIC ULCER

Treatment	Per Cent Ulcers Healed at Various Weeks of Therapy						p	Reference
	3	*4*	*5*	*6*	*8*	*12*		
Antacid*		100(8)					<0.05	304
Placebo		50(8)						
Antacid†	53(15)						NS	305
Placebo	62(13)							
Antacid‡		40(33)			69(32)	84(31)	NS	168
Placebo		25(32)			55(31)	68(31)		
Antacid§				67(42)			<0.001	306
Placebo				25(44)				

Numbers in parentheses represent the number of patients in each group. NS, not significant.
*2 tablets of calcium carbonate. Ulcer healing determined by X-ray rather than by endoscopy.
†Patients were hospitalized during the study. Antacid contained 200 mg of aluminum hydroxide, 200 mg of magnesium hydroxide, and 20 mg of simethicone.
‡15 ml Maalox Therapeutic Concentrate one hour after meals and at bedtime.
§Patients treated with one aluminum hydroxide plus magnesium carbonate antacid tablet four times daily (total neutralizing capacity, 120 mM acid/day).

and at bedtime was not significantly better than placebo in healing gastric ulcers, it may be reasonable to recommend a larger dose or more frequent administration of the same dose (e.g., 15 ml, 1 and 3 hours after meals and at bedtime). Antacid may be used in combination with H_2-receptor antagonists in patients whose ulcers do not heal within 8 weeks of therapy with an H_2-receptor antagonist or in patients who have pain that persists beyond 2 weeks of beginning therapy with an H_2-receptor antagonist.

Clinical pharmacology of antacids is discussed in Chapter 43 (pp. 716–719) of the third edition of this textbook. Side effects of antacids are listed in Table 48–1 and are discussed in greater detail in the above-mentioned chapter.

Coating Agents

These drugs are thought to interact with necrotic protein in the ulcer base forming a shield over the ulcer crater. Theoretically, this drug-protein complex protects the ulcer crater from acid and pepsin allowing healing to take place. There are two drugs in this category: sucralfate and colloidal bismuth. In addition to coating ulcer craters, evidence from experiments in animals suggests that sucralfate may stimulate prostaglandin synthesis and may lead to ulcer healing also by this mechanism (see p. 883).[308]

Sucralfate (Carafate). The effect of this drug in healing gastric ulcers has been tested in several clinical trials. The incidence of gastric ulcer healing was higher with sucralfate than with placebo (50 per cent versus 13 per cent in the two groups, respectively) in one study but the difference in healing between the two groups was not statistically significant.[309] In another study, the percent of ulcers healed at 6 weeks with sucralfate was slightly lower than that with cimetidine (63 per cent versus 75 per cent in the two groups, respectively) but the difference was not statistically significant.[310] In a more recent study the incidence of gastric ulcer healing was comparable with sucralfate and cimetidine,[311] and in a study performed in patients in Hong Kong, sucralfate was more effective than placebo and equally effective as cimetidine in healing gastric ulcers.[312] The dose used in most clinical trials was 1 gm four times daily. Side effects of sucralfate are listed in Table 48–1.

Sucralfate has not been approved for use in treating patients with gastric ulcers in the United States.

Colloidal Bismuth. Several controlled clinical trials have shown that colloidal bismuth is more effective than placebo in healing gastric ulcers[313–315] and is as effective as ranitidine.[316] This drug is available in a number of countries throughout the world but not in the United States.

Prostaglandin Analogs

Several prostaglandin analogs have been developed and tested in patients with gastric ulcers.[317–327] Theoretically, prostaglandin analogs might be effective in healing gastric ulcers because they reduce gastric acid secretion and/or enhance mucosal defense or both (see p. 883). Results with misoprostol or enprostil demonstrate that relatively high, antisecretory doses of these drugs (for example, 200 µg of misoprostol) are effective in healing gastric ulcers,[321–326] whereas lower, non-antisecretory doses are not.

Prostaglandin analogs are not marketed currently in the United States. If they are released for use, it seems likely that antisecretory doses will be required to adequately treat patients with active gastric ulcers. Perhaps smaller doses eventually will be shown to be effective in preventing ulcer recurrence.[327]

Other Drugs

Carbenoxolone, a licorice extract, has been shown to be more effective than placebo in healing gastric ulcers.[328–331] Two other drugs, sodium oxyferriscorbone and zinc sulfate, have also been shown to enhance healing of gastric ulcers.[332, 333] None of these compounds are available for use in the United States.

Hospitalization

Earlier studies demonstrated that hospitalization and bed rest increased the incidence of gastric ulcer healing.[334, 335] More recent results suggest the opposite.[274] Because of results from this more recent study and because it is impractical to hospitalize most patients with benign gastric ulcers, the majority should be treated as outpatients. Hospitalization should be reserved for patients with complications of ulcer disease or those with malignant ulcers who are scheduled for surgery.

Diet

Dietary restrictions do not enhance the healing incidence of gastric ulcers.[336, 337] Fiber, as a method of treating patients with gastric ulcers, has been evaluated.[306] There was no difference in ulcer healing with either a low-fiber or high-fiber diet. Patients should be advised to eat three meals a day from a diet of their own choosing. Acid secretion is stimulated equally by caffeinated and decaffeinated drinks.[338] Thus, there is no reason to substitute decaffeinated for caffeinated beverages and probably there is no reason to avoid either one. It has been postulated that ingestion of a high-fiber diet might prevent ulcers.[339] This, however, has not been tested. It also has been postulated that a diet rich in essential fatty acids may be beneficial in ulcer patients and may have contributed to the decline in the incidence and virulence of ulcer disease. This hypothesis is currently unproven.

Medical Restrictions

There is no evidence that alcohol is related to gastric ulcer pathogenesis. However, since alcohol is thought to damage gastric mucosa and may cause gastritis,[117, 118] patients with gastric ulcers should be advised to eliminate or at least decrease alcohol intake. Because salicylate-containing compounds also damage gastric mucosa (see p. 885)[340] and may delay healing of gastric ulcers,[341] these drugs should not be taken by patients with active ulcers. It is not known whether other nonsteroidal anti-inflammatory drugs also delay healing of gastric ulcers. However, it is recommended that patients avoid these compounds during the time that they have an active ulcer.

Even though patients with active gastric ulcers should refrain from taking nonsteroidal anti-inflammatory drugs, it is impossible for some patients, for example, those with rheumatoid arthritis, to stop taking these drugs. Preliminary evidence suggests that gastric ulcers may heal in patients who continue to take aspirin but are treated concomitantly with misoprostol.[342] Furthermore, chronic cimetidine therapy may prevent recurrent gastric ulcers in patients who have rheumatoid arthritis and who are taking salicylates or other nonsteroidal anti-inflammatory com-

pounds.[343] In patients with rheumatoid arthritis cessation of nonsteroidal anti-inflammatory drugs should be recommended. If it is not possible for an individual patient to stop taking these drugs, the compounds should be continued and the patient should be treated concomitantly with an H_2-receptor antagonist. Perhaps an experimental drug such as misoprostol or one of the other prostaglandin analogs might be useful in treating some patients with rheumatoid arthritis who have persistent gastric ulcers.

There is no evidence that smoking causes ulcers. However, epidemiologic studies suggest a relationship between the number of cigarettes smoked and prevalence of ulcer disease. Also, duodenal ulcers, and perhaps gastric ulcers, heal more slowly in smokers than in nonsmokers, and the recurrence of ulcers may be higher in smokers (see p. 886). Thus, patients with gastric ulcers should be advised to stop smoking cigarettes.

Immediate Therapy Summarized

1. Most patients should be treated with an H_2-receptor antagonist, although studies suggest that other drugs are equally effective. Patients should be treated until the ulcer heals as documented by either X-ray or endoscopy. The timing of the X-ray or endoscopy is discussed below in the section on follow-up.

2. Unless patients have a complication of ulcer disease, they should be treated as outpatients. Those with complications should be hospitalized.

3. Patients should be advised to eat three meals a day from a diet of their own choosing.

4. Salicylate-containing compounds and other nonsteroidal anti-inflammatory drugs should be avoided. Patients should be advised to stop smoking cigarettes.

FOLLOW-UP

Patients should be seen by their physician at least once during the initial 2 weeks of medical treatment. The purpose of this visit is to evaluate the patient's symptomatic response. If pain is not relieved by this time, another medication should be added. For example, if the patient is receiving cimetidine, addition of antacid may be beneficial. The patient should be seen again 8 weeks after initial diagnosis and a repeat barium X-ray or endoscopy performed to evaluate the extent of healing. If the ulcer was not visible on the initial X-ray and the diagnosis was made by endoscopy, then endoscopy is recommended for follow-up examinations. If the ulcer was demonstrated on the initial X-ray, some physicians advocate X-ray and not endoscopy as the method of following gastric ulcers to complete healing.[344] The 1986 guidelines on the appropriate use of gastrointestinal endoscopy published by the American Society for Gastrointestinal Endoscopy do not support or reject endoscopy in the follow-up of patients with gastric ulcers. The guidelines state sequential or periodic endoscopy may be indicated for follow-up of patients with selected large gastric ulcers to demonstrate healing.[254] In my opinion, if endoscopy is available, most patients with gastric ulcers should have repeat endoscopy with biopsy at either 6 or 8 weeks after beginning medical therapy and again at 12 weeks if the ulcer was not healed at 6 or 8 weeks. This view is supported by the observation that occasionally two or more endoscopic procedures with biopsies are required to diagnose gastric cancers in patients with endoscopically benign-appearing gastric ulcers.[192]

Most benign ulcers will heal by 12 weeks. Some large ulcers (usually >2.5 cm in width) may require 16 weeks for complete healing. This occurs because both large and small ulcers heal at the same rate, approximately 3 mm per week.[345] Thus, the larger the ulcer, the longer the period of time required for complete healing. If at any follow-up X-ray or endoscopic examination, the ulcer appears malignant or biopsies and/or cytology reveal cancer, the patient should be referred for surgery. With few exceptions, all patients whose ulcers have not healed by 12 weeks (16 weeks in patients with large ulcers) should be referred for surgery (see pp. 945–948). Exceptions to this rule include elderly patients and patients with severe medical problems other than ulcer disease in whom surgery represents an inordinately high morbidity and mortality. Whenever patients are followed with unhealed ulcers for longer than the customary 12- to 16-week period, endoscopy with biopsies and not X-ray should be performed periodically in all patients (unless there is a contraindication to endoscopy) to be as certain as possible that the ulcer is benign.

Once an ulcer has healed and this has been documented by endoscopy, endoscopic follow-up is usually not recommended even though occasionally an ulcer that appears benign and heals completely will ultimately be shown to be malignant.[346, 347] The guidelines published by the American Society for Gastrointestinal Endoscopy state that sequential or periodic endoscopy is generally not indicated for surveillance of patients with healed, benign gastric ulcers.[254]

Medical Treatment of Recurrent Ulcers

Patients with recurrent symptoms and a previous gastric ulcer should be evaluated by X-ray and/or endoscopy in the same manner as with the initial ulcer. While it is likely that recurrent symptoms represent a benign ulcer, this should not be assumed. The same rationale used to choose medication for treating patients with initial ulcers should be used in selecting a drug for treating patients with recurrent ulcers. Benign recurrent ulcers heal on medical therapy as readily as do initial ulcers[172] and may heal more quickly since recurrent ulcers are often smaller than original ulcers. Patients should be followed in the same manner as outlined for patients with initial ulcers.

Surgical Treatment of Recurrent Ulcers

Two or three recurrences of gastric ulcers have been used by some as an indication for ulcer surgery. Several reasons have been given to support this approach: (1) an increased risk of malignancy in patients with recurrent ulcers, (2) a higher incidence of complications (bleeding or perforation), and (3) a slower healing rate of recurrent ulcers. Each of these reasons has been disputed by results from clinical trials.[172, 202, 345] Thus, surgery for recurrent gastric ulcer cannot be defended on the basis of any of the reasons listed above and recurrence, *per se*, should not be used as an indication for surgery. If a recurrent benign ulcer is refractory to medical therapy and does not heal within 12 to 16 weeks, if an ulcer recurs while a patient is receiving maintenance therapy with an H_2-receptor antagonist (see below), or if there is evidence of cancer, the patient should be considered for ulcer surgery (see pp. 945–948). Otherwise, most patients with recurrent ulcers should be treated medically.

Prevention of Recurrent Ulcers

The effect of maintenance therapy with cimetidine, ranitidine, or sucralfate, but not antacid, in preventing recurrent gastric ulcers has been evaluated and compared with placebo therapy in several studies.[169–171, 348–352] Each of the drugs evaluated were significantly (p <0.05) more effective than placebo in preventing recurrent gastric ulcers for up to 12 months, the longest period studied.[169–171, 349, 350, 352] Thus, a point could be made for treating patients with healed gastric ulcers with maintenance therapy in an effort to prevent ulcer recurrence. There are several reasons for not using this approach in treating all gastric ulcer patients. First, the safety of long-term cimetidine or ranitidine treatment has not been established in large numbers of patients, although results of chronic studies in animals suggest that the drugs are safe.[353] Second, not all patients get a recurrent ulcer; therefore, it seems unjustified to treat every gastric ulcer patient with maintenance therapy to prevent ulcers in those that are ulcer-prone. Third, evidence suggests that recurrent ulcers heal on medical treatment just as readily as do initial ulcers (see above).[172] Thus, in most patients, each episode of recurrent ulcer can be treated with a separate course of medical therapy. Also, none of the currently available drugs have been approved in the United States for maintenance therapy in patients with gastric ulcers.

There are a few patients who should be treated with medication chronically. These include patients with gastric ulcer disease who are elderly and who have severe illnesses such as pulmonary, myocardial and/or renal disease; patients who have had frequent recurrent gastric ulcers (for example, three or more gastric ulcers during any one year); patients who have had a complication of ulcer disease such as bleeding or perforation, and patients who have gastric ulcer disease as a result of Zollinger-Ellison syndrome (see pp. 917–918). Since preliminary evidence suggests that chronic cimetidine therapy may prevent recurrent gastric ulcers in patients who have rheumatoid arthritis and who are taking salicylates or other nonsteroidal anti-inflammatory compounds, it seems reasonable to also treat these patients chronically with an H_2-receptor antagonist.[343] There are insufficient data to determine the dose of medication to be used in treating patients long-term. Reduced dosages such as those used in maintenance treatment of patients with duodenal ulcer disease are usually prescribed in patients with gastric ulcer disease (see pp. 858–860). Larger doses are required in patients with Zollinger-Ellison syndrome (see pp. 917–918).

References

1. Gelfand, D. W., Dale, W. J., and Ott, D. J. The location and size of gastric ulcers: radiologic and endoscopic evaluation. Am. J. Radiol. *143*:755, 1984.
2. Larsen, E. H., Diederich, P. J., and Sorensen, F. B. Peptic ulcer in the gallbladder. A case report. Acta Chir. Scand. *151*:575, 1985.
3. Sonnenberg, A. Geographic and temporal variations in the occurrence of peptic ulcer disease. Scand. J. Gastroenterol. *20*(Suppl. 110):11, 1985.
4. Kurata, J. H., and Haile, B. M. Epidemiology of peptic ulcer disease. Clin. Gastroenterol. *13*:289, 1984.
5. Elashoff, J. D., and Grossman, M. I. Trends in hospital admissions and death rates for peptic ulcer in the United States from 1970 to 1978. Gastroenterology *78*:280, 1980.
6. Bonnevie, O. The incidence of gastric ulcer in Copenhagen County. Scand. J. Gastroenterol. *10*:231, 1975.
7. Ostensen, H., Gudmundsen, T. E., Bolz, K. D., Burhol, P. G., and Bonnevie, O. The incidence of gastric ulcer and duodenal ulcer in north Norway. A prospective epidemiological study. Scand. J. Gastroenterol. *20*:189, 1985.
8. Vogt, T. M., and Johnson, R. E. Recent changes in the incidence of duodenal or gastric ulcer. Am. J. Epidemiol. *111*:713, 1980.
9. Sonnenberg, A. Changes in physician visits for gastric and duodenal ulcer in the United States during 1958–1984 as shown by National Disease and Therapeutic Index (NDTI). Dig. Dis. Sci. *32*:1, 1987.
10. Karsner, H. T. The pathology of peptic ulcer of the stomach. JAMA *85*:1376, 1925.
11. Askanazy, M. Über Bau und Entstehung des chronischen Magengeschwurs sowie Soorpilzbefunde in ihm. Virchows Arch. Pathol. *234*:111, 1921; *250*:370, 1924.
12. Magnus, H. A. The pathology of peptic ulceration. Postgrad. Med. J. *30*:131, 1954.
13. Johnson, H. D. Gastric ulcer: classification, blood group characteristics, secretion patterns and pathogenesis. Ann. Surg. *162*:996, 1964.
14. Csendes, A., Braghetto, I. and Smok, G. Type IV gastric ulcer: a new hypothesis. Surgery *101*:361, 1987.
15. Dragstedt, L. R., and Woodward, E. R. Gastric stasis: a cause of gastric ulcer. Scand. J. Gastroenterol. *5*:243, 1970.
16. Burge, H. The aetiology of benign lesser curve gastric ulcer: vagotomy and pyloroplasty in its treatment. Ann. R. Coll. Surg. Engl. *38*:349, 1966.
17. Oi, M., Ito, Y., Kumagai, F., Yoshida, K., Tanaka, Y., Yoshikawa, K., Miho, O., and Kijima, M. A possible dual control mechanism in the origin of peptic ulcer. A study on ulcer location as affected by mucosa and musculature. Gastroenterology *57*:280, 1969.
18. Valenzuela, J. E., and Defilippi, C. Pyloric sphincter studies in peptic ulcer patients. Am. J. Dig. Dis. *21*:229, 1976.
19. Fisher, R. S., and Cohen, S. Pyloric-sphincter dysfunction in patients with gastric ulcer. N. Engl. J. Med. *288*:273, 1973.
20. Garrett, J. M., Summerskill, W. H. J., and Code, C. F. Antral motility in patients with gastric ulcer. Am. J. Dig. Dis. *11*:780, 1966.
21. George, J. D. New clinical method for measuring the rate of gastric emptying: the double sampling test meal. Gut *9*:237, 1968.
22. Buckler, K. G. Effects of gastric surgery upon gastric emptying in cases of peptic ulceration. Gut *8*:137, 1967.
23. Miller, L. J., Malagelada, J. R., Longstreth, G. F., and Go, V. L. W. Dysfunctions of the stomach with gastric ulceration. Dig. Dis. Sci. *25*:857, 1980.
24. Miranda, M., Defilippi, C., and Valenzuela, J. E. Abnormalities of interdigestive motility complex and increased duodenogastric reflux in gastric ulcer patients. Dig. Dis. Sci. *30*:16, 1985.
25. Capper, W. M., Airth, G. R., and Kilby, J. O. A test for pyloric regurgitation. Lancet *2*:621, 1966.
26. Wormsley, K. G. Aspects of duodeno-gastric reflux in man. Gut *13*:243, 1972.
27. Flint, F. J., and Grech, P. Pyloric regurgitation and gastric ulcer. Gut *11*:735, 1970.
28. Fisher, R., and Cohen, S. Physiological characteristics of the human pyloric sphincter. Gastroenterology *64*:67, 1973.
29. Thomas, W. E. G. The possible role of duodenogastric reflux in the pathogenesis of both gastric and duodenal ulcers. Scand. J. Gastroenterol. *19*(Suppl. 92):151, 1984.
30. Niemela, S., Heikkila, J., and Lehtola, J. Duodenogastric bile reflux in patients with gastric ulcer. Scand. J. Gastroenterol. *19*:896, 1984.
31. Davenport, H. W. Effect of lysolecithin, digitonin and phospholipase A upon the dog's gastric mucosal barrier. Gastroenterology *59*:505, 1970.
32. Johnson, A. G., and McDermott, S. J. Lysolecithin: a factor in the pathogenesis of gastric ulceration? Gut *15*:710, 1974.
33. Silen, W., and Forte, J. G. Effects of bile salts on amphibian gastric mucosa. Am. J. Physiol. *228*:637, 1975.
34. Harmon, J. W., Lewis, C. D., and Gadacz, T. Bile salt composition and concentration as determinants of canine gastric mucosal injury. Surgery *89*:348, 1981.
35. Boyle, J. M., Neiderhiser, D. H., and Dworken, H. J. Duodenogastric reflux in patients with gastric ulcer disease. J. Lab. Clin. Med. *103*:14, 1984.
36. Ritchie, W. P., Jr., and Felger, T. S. Differing ulcerogenic potential of dehydroxy and trihydroxy bile acids in canine gastric mucosa. Surgery *89*:342, 1981.
37. Delaney, J. P., Broadie, T. A., and Robbins, P. L. Pyloric reflux gastritis: the offending agent. Surgery *77*:764, 1975.
38. Du Plessis, D. J. Pathogenesis of gastric ulceration. Lancet *1*:974, 1965.
39. Rhodes, J., Barnardo, D. E., Phillips, S. F., Rovelstad, R. A., and Hofmann, A. F. Increased reflux of bile into the stomach in patients with gastric ulcer. Gastroenterology *57*:241, 1969.
40. Black, R. B., Roberts, G., and Rhodes, J. The effect of healing on bile reflux in gastric ulcer. Gut *12*:552, 1971.
41. Black, R. B., Rhodes, J., Davies, G. T., Gravelle, H., and Sweetnam, P. A controlled clinical trial of cholestyramine in the treatment of gastric ulcer. Gastroenterology *61*:821, 1971.
42. Drapanas, T., and Bethea, M. Reflux gastritis following gastric surgery. Ann. Surg. *179*:618, 1974.
43. Stiel, D., and Piper, D. W. Duodenogastric reflux and chronic gastric ulcer. Aust. N.Z. J. Med. *11*:207, 1981.
44. Gear, M. W. L., Truelove, S. C., and Whitehead, R. Gastric ulcer and gastritis. Gut *12*:639, 1971.
45. Leading article. Gastric ulcer and gastritis. Lancet *2*:481, 1966.
46. Marks, I. N., and Shay, H. Observations on the pathogenesis of gastric ulcer. Lancet *1*:1107, 1959.
47. Capper, W. M. Factors in the pathogenesis of gastric ulcer. Hunterian Lecture delivered at the Royal College of Surgeons of England on 18 January, 1966. Ann. R. Coll. Surg. Engl. *40*:21, 1967.
48. Maaroos, H.-I., Salupere, V., Uibo, R., Kekki, M., and

Sipponen, P. Seven year follow-up study of chronic gastritis in gastric ulcer patients. Scand. J. Gastroenterol. *20*:198, 1985.

49. Tatsuta, M., Iishi, H., and Okuda, S. Location of peptic ulcers in relation to antral and fundal gastritis by chromoendoscopic follow-up examinations. Dig. Dis. Sci. *31*:7, 1986.

50. Moore, S. C., Malagelada, J.-R., Shorter, R. G., and Zinsmeister, A. R. Interrelationships among gastric mucosal morphology, secretion, and motility in peptic ulcer disease. Dig. Dis. Sci. *31*:673, 1986.

51. Hollander, F. The two component mucus barrier. Its activity in protecting the gastroduodenal mucosa against peptic ulceration. Arch. Intern. Med. *93*:107, 1954.

52. Davenport, H. W., Warner, H. A., and Code, C. F. Functional significance of gastric mucosal barrier to sodium. Gastroenterology *47*:142, 1964.

53. Lacy, E. R., and Ito, S. Ethanol-induced insult to the superficial rat epithelium. A study of damage and rapid repair. *In* Allen, A., et al. (eds.). Mechanisms of Mucosal Protection in the Upper Gastrointestinal Tract. New York, Raven Press, 1984, pp. 49–56.

54. Silen, W. Gastric mucosal defense and repair. *In* Johnson, L. R., et al. (eds.). Physiology of the Gastrointestinal Tract. 2nd ed. New York, Raven Press, 1986, pp. 1055–1069.

55. Duane, W. C., and Wiegard, D. M. Mechanism by which bile salts disrupt the gastric mucosal barrier in the dog. J. Clin. Invest. *66*:1044, 1980.

56. Robert, A. Prostaglandins and the gastrointestinal tract. *In* Johnson, L. R. (ed.). Physiology of the Gastrointestinal Tract. New York, Raven Press, 1981, pp. 1407–1434.

57. Miller, T. A. Protective effects of prostaglandins against gastric mucosal damage: current knowledge and proposed mechanisms. Am. J. Physiol. *245*:G601, 1983.

58. Larssen, K. R., Jensen, N. F., Davies, E. K., Jenson, J. C., and Moody, F. G. The cytoprotective effects of ($\pm$)-15 deoxy-16-a,b-hydroxy-16-methyl PGE$_1$ ester (SC 29333) versus aspirin-shock ulcerogenesis in the dog. Prostaglandins *21*(Suppl.):119, 1981.

59. Ligumsky, M., Grossman, M. I., and Kauffman, G. Endogenous gastric mucosal prostaglandins: their role in mucosal integrity. Am. J. Physiol. *242*:G337, 1982.

60. Whittle, B. J. R. Prostaglandin-cyclo-oxygenase inhibition and its relationship to gastric damage. *In* Harmon, J. W., (ed.). Basic Mechanisms of Gastrointestinal Mucosal Cell Injury and Protection. Baltimore, Williams and Wilkins, 1981, pp. 197–210.

61. Whittle, B. J. R. Temporal relationship between cyclooxygenase inhibition, as measured by prostacyclin biosynthesis, and the gastrointestinal damage induced by indomethacin in the rat. Gastroenterology *80*:94, 1981.

62. Olson, G. A., Leffler, C. W., Fletcher, A. M. Gastroduodenal ulceration in rabbits producing antibodies to prostaglandins. Prostaglandins *29*:475, 1985.

63. Redfern, J. S., Blair, A. J., Lee, E., and Feldman, M. Immunization with prostaglandins induces gastrointestinal (GI) ulcers in rabbits. (Abstract.) Gastroenterology *92*:1591, 1987.

64. Redfern, J. S., Blair, A. J., Lee, E., and Feldman, M. Gastrointestinal ulcer formation in rabbits immunized with prostaglandin E$_2$. Gastroenterology *93*:744, 1987.

65. Hinsdale, J. G., Engel, J. J., and Wilson, D. E. Prostaglandin E in peptic ulcer disease. Prostaglandins *6*:495, 1974.

66. Hawkey, C. J., and Rampton, D. S. Prostaglandins and the gastrointestinal mucosa: are they important in its function, disease, or treatment? Gastroenterology *89*:1162, 1985.

67. Dajani, E. Z. Is peptic ulcer a prostaglandin deficiency disease? Hum. Pathol. *17*:106, 1986.

68. Schlegel, W., Wenk, K., Dollinger, H. C., and Raptis, S. Concentrations of prostaglandin A-, E- and F-like substances in gastric mucosa of normal subjects and of patients with various gastric diseases. Clin. Sci. Mol. Med. *52*:255, 1977.

69. Wright, J. P., Young, G. O., Klaff, L. J., Weers, L. A., Price, S. K., and Marks, I. N. Gastric mucosal prostaglandin E levels in patients with gastric ulcer disease and carcinoma. Gastroenterology *82*:263, 1982.

70. Konturek, S. J., Obtulowicz, W., Kwiecien, N., and Oleksy, J. Generation of prostaglandins in gastric mucosa of patients

with peptic ulcer disease: effect of nonsteroidal antiinflammatory compounds. Scand. J. Gastroenterol. *19*(Suppl. 101):75, 1984.

71. Barlow, T. E., Bentley, F. H., and Walden, D. N. Arteries, veins and arteriovenous anastomoses in the human stomach. Surg. Gynecol. Obstet. *93*:657, 1951.

72. Guth, P. H., Pathogenesis of gastric mucosal injury. Ann. Rev. Med. *33*:183, 1982.

73. Ritchie, W. P., Jr. Acute gastric mucosal damage by bile salts, acid and ischemia. Gastroenterology *68*:699, 1975.

74. Whittle, B. J. R. Mechanisms underlying gastric mucosal damage induced by indomethacin and bile salts and the actions of prostaglandins. Br. J. Pharmacol. *60*:455, 1977.

75. Cherry, R. D., Jabbari, M., Goresky, C. A., Herba, M., Reich, D., and Blundell, P. E. Chronic mesenteric vascular insufficiency with gastric ulceration. Gastroenterology *91*:1548, 1986.

76. Hoskins, L. C., and Zamcheck, N. Studies on gastric mucus in health and disease. II. Evidence for a correlation between ABO blood group specificity, ABH(O) secretor status, and the fucose content of the glycoproteins elaborated by the gastric mucosa. Gastroenterology *48*:758, 1965.

77. Filipe, M. I. Mucins in the human gastrointestinal epithelium: a review. Invest. Cell. Pathol. *2*:195, 1979.

78. Allen, A. Structure and function of gastrointestinal mucus. *In* Johnson, L. R. (ed.). Physiology of the Gastrointestinal Tract. New York, Raven Press, 1981, pp. 617–639.

79. Flemstrom, G. Gastric secretion of bicarbonate. *In* Johnson, L. R. (ed.). Physiology of the Gastrointestinal Tract. New York, Raven Press, 1981, pp. 603–616.

80. Glass, G. B. J., and Slomiany, B. L. Derangements in gastrointestinal injury and disease. *In* Elstein, M., and Parke, D. V. (eds.). Mucus in Health and Disease. New York, Plenum Press, 1977, pp. 311–347.

81. Roberts-Thompson, J. C., Clarke, A. E., Maritz, V. M., and Denborough, M. A. Gastric glycoproteins in chronic peptic ulcer. Aust. N.Z. J. Med. *5*:507, 1975.

82. Schrager, J., and Oates. M. D. G. Human gastrointestinal mucus in disease states. Br. Med. Bull. *34*:79, 1978.

83. Younan, F., Pearson, J., Allen, A., and Venables, C. Changes in the structure of the mucous gel on the mucosal surface of the stomach in association with peptic ulcer disease. Gastroenterology *82*:827, 1982.

84. Venables, C. W. Mucus, pepsin, and peptic ulcer. Gut *27*:233, 1986.

85. Wormsley, K. G., and Grossman, M. I. Maximal Histalog test in control subjects and patients with peptic ulcer. Gut *6*:427, 1965.

86. Baron, J. H. Clinical Tests of Gastric Secretion. New York, Oxford University Press, 1979.

87. Johnson, H. D., Love, A. H. G., Rogers, N. C., and Wyatt, A. P. Gastric ulcers, blood groups and acid secretion. Gut *5*:402, 1964.

88. Thjodleifsson, B., and Wormsley, K. G. Back-diffusion—fact or fiction? Digestion *15*:53, 1977.

89. Isenberg, J. I., Spector, H., Hootkin, L. A., and Pitcher, J. L. An apparent exception to Schwarz's dictum, "no acid—no ulcer." N. Engl. J. Med. *285*:620, 1971.

90. Reid, J., Taylor, T. V., Holt, S., and Heading, R. C. Benign gastric ulceration in pernicious anemia. Dig. Dis. Sci. *25*:148, 1980.

91. Whitaker, J. A., and Cook, A. R. Achlorhydria and benign gastric ulcer. Acta Hepatogastroenterol. *26*:417, 1979.

92. Pearson, J. P., Ward, R., Allen, A., Roberts, N. B., Taylor, W. H. Mucus degradation by pepsin: comparison of mucolytic activity of human pepsin 1 and pepsin 3: implications in peptic ulceration. Gut *27*:243, 1986.

93. Samloff, I. M. Cellular localization of group I pepsinogens in human gastric mucosa by immunofluorescence. Gastroenterology *61*:185, 1971.

94. Samloff, I. M., and Liebman, W. M. Cellular localization of the group II pepsinogens in human stomach and duodenum by immunofluorescence. Gastroenterology *65*:36, 1973.

95. Ichinose, M., Miki, K., Furihata, C., Kageyama, T., Hayashi, R., Niwa, H., Oka, H., Matsushima, T., and Takahashi, K.

Radioimmunoassay of serum group I and group II pepsinogens in normal controls and patients with various disorders. Clin. Chim. Acta *126*:183, 1982.

96. Samloff, I. M., Stemmermann, G. N., Heilbrun, L. K., and Nomura, A. Elevated serum pepsinogen I and II levels differ as risk factors for duodenal ulcer and gastric ulcer. Gastroenterology *90*:570, 1986.

97. Thomas, J., Greig, M., McIntosh, J., Hunt, J., McNeil, D., and Piper, D. W. The location of chronic gastric ulcer. Digestion *20*:79, 1980.

98. Sun, D. C. H., and Stempien, S. J. Site and size of the ulcer as determinant of outcome. Gastroenterology *61*:576, 1971.

99. Oi, M., Oshida, K., and Sugimura, S. The location of gastric ulcer. Gastroenterology *36*:45, 1959.

100. Kimura, K. Chronological transition of the fundic-pyloric border determined by stepwise biopsy of the lesser and greater curvatures of the stomach. Gastroenterology *63*:584, 1972.

101. Brodie, D. A., and Chase, B. J. Role of gastric acid in aspirin-induced gastric irritation in the rat. Gastroenterology *53*:604, 1967.

102. Bugat, R., Thompson, M. R., Aures, D., and Grossman, M. I. Gastric mucosal lesions produced by intravenous infusion of aspirin in cats. Gastroenterology *71*:754, 1976.

103. Hansen, D. G., Aures, D., and Grossman, M. I. Histamine augments gastric ulceration produced by intravenous aspirin in cats. Gastroenterology *74*:540, 1978.

104. Silvoso, G. R., Ivey, K. J., Butt, J. H., Lockard, O. O., Holt, S. D., Sisk, C., Baskin, W. N., Mackercher, P. A., and Hewett, J. Incidence of gastric lesions in patients with rheumatic disease on chronic aspirin therapy. Ann. Intern. Med. *91*:517, 1979.

105. Baragar, F. D., and Duthie, J. J. R. Importance of aspirin as a cause of anaemia and peptic ulcer in rheumatoid arthritis. Br. Med. J. *1*:1106, 1960.

106. Gillies, M., and Skyring, A. P. Gastric ulcer, duodenal ulcer and gastric carcinoma. A case study of certain social and environmental factors. Med. J. Aust. *2*:1132, 1968.

107. Levy, M. Aspirin use in patients with major upper gastrointestinal bleeding and peptic-ulcer disease. N. Engl. J. Med. *290*:1158, 1974.

108. Cameron, A. J. Aspirin and gastric ulcer. Mayo Clin. Proc. *50*:565, 1975.

109. Piper, D. W., McIntosh, J. H., Ariotti, D. E., Fenton, B. H., and MacLennan, R. Analgesic ingestion and chronic peptic ulcer. Gastroenterology *80*:427, 1981.

110. Aspirin Myocardial Infarction Study Research Group of National Heart, Lung, and Blood Institute. A randomized, controlled trial of aspirin in persons recovered from myocardial infarction. JAMA *243*:661, 1980.

111. Lee, Y. H., Mollison, K. W., and Cheng, W. D. The effects of anti-ulcer agents on indomethacin-induced gastric ulcerations in the rat. Arch. Int. Pharmacodyn. Ther. *192*:370, 1971.

112. Lanza, F., Royer, G., and Nelson, R. An endoscopic evaluation of the effects of nonsteroidal anti-inflammatory agents on the gastric mucosa. Gastrointest. Endosc. *21*:103, 1975.

113. Davenport, H. W. Gastric mucosal injury by fatty and acetylsalicylic acid. Gastroenterology *46*:245, 1964.

114. Davenport, H. W. Fluid produced by the gastric mucosa during damage by acetic and salicylic acids. Gastroenterology *50*:487, 1966.

115. Ivey, K. J., Silvoso, G. R., and Krause, W. J. Effect of paracetamol on gastric mucosa. Br. Med. J. *1*:1586, 1978.

116. Hansen, D. G., and Grossman, M. I. Production of gastric ulcers in cats by intravenous acetaminophen plus histamine. (Abstract.) Clin. Res. *26*:110A, 1978.

117. Goldenberg, M. M., Honkomp, L. J., Burrous, S. E., and Castellion, A. W. Protective effect of Pepto-Bismol liquid on the gastric mucosa of rats. Gastroenterology *69*:636, 1975.

118. Lorber, S. H. Antipeptic agents, carbenoxolone and mucosal coating agents: Status report. *In* Peptic Ulcer Disease: An Update. Third International Symposium on Gastroenterology. New York, Biomedical Information Corporation, 1979, pp. 295–305.

119. Cohn, H. O., and Blitzer, B. L. Nonassociation of adrenocorticoid therapy and peptic ulcer. N. Engl. J. Med. *294*:473, 1976.

120. Piper, D. W. The treatment of chronic peptic ulcer. Front. Gastrointest. Res. *6*:109, 1980.

121. Piper, D. W., McIntosh, J. H., Greig, M., and Shy, C. M. Environmental factors and chronic gastric ulcer. A case control study of the association of smoking, alcohol, and heavy analgesic ingestion with the exacerbation of chronic gastric ulcer. Scand. J. Gastroenterol. *17*:721, 1982.

122. Ainley, C. C., Forgacs, I. C., Keeling, P. W. N., and Thompson, R. P. H. Outpatient endoscopic survey of smoking and peptic ulcer. Gut *27*:648, 1986.

123. Friedman, G. D., Siegelaub, A. B., and Seltzer, C. C. Cigarettes, alcohol, coffee and peptic ulcer. N. Engl. J. Med. *290*:469, 1974.

124. McIntosh, J. H., Byth, K., and Piper, D. W. Environmental factors in aetiology of chronic gastric ulcer: a case control study of exposure variables before the first symptoms. Gut *26*:789, 1985.

125. Korman, M. G., Shaw, R. G., Hansky, J., Schmidt, G. T., and Stern, A. I. Influence of smoking on healing rate of duodenal ulcer in response to cimetidine or high-dose antacid. Gastroenterology *80*:1451, 1981.

126. Sontag, S., Graham, D. Y., Belsito, A., Weiss, J., Farley, A., Grunt, R., Cohen, N., Kinnear, D., Davis, W., Archambault, A., et al. Cimetidine, cigarette smoking, and recurrence of duodenal ulcer. N. Engl. J. Med. *311*:689, 1984.

127. Hammond, E. G. Smoking in relation to death rates of one million men and women. Natl. Cancer Inst. Monogr. *13*:127, 1966.

128. Solomon, T. E., and Jacobson, E. D. Cigarette smoking and duodenal ulcer disease. N. Engl. J. Med. *286*:1212, 1972.

129. Kellow, J. E., Tao, Z., and Piper, D. W. Ventilatory function in chronic peptic ulcer. A controlled study of ventilatory function in patients with gastric and duodenal ulcer. Gastroenterology *91*:590, 1986.

130. Dippy, J. E., Rhodes, J., and Cross, S. Bile reflux in gastric ulcer: the effect of smoking, metoclopramide and carbenoxolone sodium. Curr. Med. Res. Opin. *1*:569, 1973.

131. Sonnenberg, A. Dietary salt and gastric ulcer. Gut *27*:1138, 1986.

132. Glavin, G. B., and Robert, E. Y. Subject emotionality and subsequent pylorus ligation–induced gastric ulcer. Pavlov J. Biol. Sci. *15*:102, 1980.

133. Pare, W. P. Relationship of various behaviors in the open-field test of emotionality. Psychol. Rep. *14*:19, 1964.

134. Piper, D. W., Greig, M., Thomas, J., and Shinners, J. Personality pattern of patients with chronic gastric ulcer. Gastroenterology *73*:444, 1977.

135. Piper, D. W., Greig, M., Shinners, J., Thomas, J., and Crawford, J. Chronic gastric ulcer and stress. Digestion *18*:303, 1978.

136. Thomas, J., Greig, M., and Piper, D. W. Chronic gastric ulcer and life events. Gastroenterology *78*:905, 1980.

137. Davies, D. T., and Wilson, A. T. M. Observations on the life-history of chronic peptic ulcer. Lancet *2*:1353, 1937.

138. Alp, M. H., Court, J. H., and Grant, A. K. Personality pattern and emotional stress in the genesis of gastric ulcer. Gut *11*:773, 1970.

139. Feldman, M., Walker, P., Green, J. L., and Weingarden, K. Life events stress and psychosocial factors in men with peptic ulcer disease. A multidimensional case-controlled study. Gastroenterology *91*:1370, 1986.

140. Palmer, E. D. The cyclic dynamism of the incidence and complications of ulcer disease. Surg. Gynecol. Obstet. *130*:709, 1970.

141. Tovey, F. I. The geographical distribution and possible factors in the etiology of peptic ulcer. Trop. Doct. *1*:17, 1974.

142. Sung, J. L., Wang, T. H., Lu, T. H., et al. Epidemiological study on peptic ulcer and gastric cancer in Chinese. Rendic. Gastroent. *6*:111, 1974.

143. Yodfat, Y. A population study of peptic ulcer; its relation to various ethnic and socioeconomic factors. Isr. J. Med. Sci. *8*:1680, 1972.

144. Susser, M. Causes of peptic ulcer: a selective epidemiologic review. J. Chron. Dis. *20*:435, 1967.

145. Pulvertaft, C. N. Comments on the incidence and natural

history of gastric and duodenal ulcer. Postgrad. Med. J. *44*:597, 1968.

146. Doll, R., Avery-Jones, F., and Buckatzsch, N. M. Occupational factors in the etiology of gastric and duodenal ulcers with an estimate of their incidence in the general population. Spec. Rep. Ser. Med. Res. Coun. No. 276:1. London, HMSO, 1951.

147. Gilles, M. A., and Skyring, A. Gastric and duodenal ulcer. The association between aspirin ingestion, smoking and family history of ulcer. Med. J. Aust. 2:280, 1969.

148. Steer, H. W. The gastro-duodenal epithelium in peptic ulceration. J. Pathol. *146*:355, 1985.

149. Cohen, E. B., Komorowski, R. A., Kauffman, H. M., and Adams, M. Unexpectedly high incidence of cytomegalovirus infection in apparent peptic ulcers in renal transplant recipients. Surgery 97:606, 1985.

150. Rathbone, B. J., Wyatt, J. I., and Heatley, R. V. *Campylobacter pyloridis*—a new factor in peptic ulcer disease? Gut 27:635, 1986.

151. Steer, H. W., and Colin-Jones, D. G. Mucosal changes in gastric ulceration and their response to carbenoxolone sodium. Gut *16*:590, 1975.

152. Warren, J. R. Unidentified curved bacilli on gastric epithelium in active chronic gastritis. (Letter.) Lancet *1*:1273, 1983.

153. Marshall, B. Unidentified curved bacilli on gastric epithelium in active chronic gastritis. (Letter.) Lancet *1*:1274, 1983.

154. Pearson, A. D., Skirrow, M. B., Rowe, B., Davies, J. R., and Jones, D. M. (eds.). Proceedings of the Second International Workshop on Campylobacter Infections. Brussels, September 6–9, 1983.

155. McNulty, C. A. M., and Watson, D. M. Spiral bacteria of the gastric antrum. (Letter.) Lancet *1*:1068, 1984.

156. Marshall, B. J., and Warren, J. R. Unidentified curved bacilli in the stomach of patients with gastritis and peptic ulceration. Lancet *1*:1311, 1984.

157. Kasper, G., and Dickgiesser, N. Isolation of campylobacter-like bacteria from gastric epithelium. Infection *12*:179, 1984.

158. Kasper, G., and Dickgiesser, N. Isolation from gastric epithelium of Campylobacter-like bacteria that are distinct from '*Campylobacter pyloridis.*' Lancet *1*:111, 1985.

159. Price, A. B., Levi, J., Dolby, J. M., Dunscombe, P. L., Smith, A., Clark, J., and Stephenson, M. L. *Campylobacter pyloridis* in peptic ulcer disease: microbiology, pathology, and scanning electron microscopy. Gut *26*:1183, 1985.

160. Goodwin, C. S., Armstrong, J. A., and Marshall, B. J. *Campylobacter pyloridis*, gastritis, and peptic ulceration. J. Clin. Pathol. *39*:353, 1986.

161. Hazell, S. L., and Lee, A. *Campylobacter pyloridis*, urease, hydrogen ion back diffusion, and gastric ulcers. Lancet *2*:15, 1986.

162. Doll, R., and Kellock, T. D. The separate inheritance of gastric and duodenal ulcers. Ann. Eugen. *16*:231, 1951.

163. Eberhard, G. Peptic ulcer in twins. A study in personality, heredity, and environment. Acta Psychiatr. Scand. *44*(Suppl. 205):1, 1968.

164. Bible, K. C., Hatfield, A. K., Lansford, C. L., and Kammer, B. A. Gastric ulceration as a complication of hepatic artery infusion chemotherapy. South. Med. J. *79*:755, 1986.

165. Shike, M., Gillin, J. S., Kemeny, N., Daly, J. M., and Kurtz, R. C. Severe gastroduodenal ulcerations complicating hepatic artery infusion chemotherapy for metastatic colon cancer. Am. J. Gastroenterol. *81*:176, 1986.

166. Freston, J. W. Cimetidine in the treatment of gastric ulcer. Gastroenterology *74*:426, 1978.

167. Graham, D. Y., Akdamar, K., Dyck, W. P., et al. Healing of benign gastric ulcer: comparison of cimetidine and placebo in the United States. Ann. Intern. Med. *102*:573, 1985.

168. Isenberg, J. I., Peterson, W. L., Elashoff, J. D., et al. Healing of benign gastric ulcer with low dose antacid or cimetidine: a double-blind, randomized, placebo-controlled trial. N. Engl. J. Med. *308*:1319, 1983.

169. Jensen, K. B., Mollmann, K.-M., Rahbek, I., Madsen, J. R., Rune, S. J., and Wulff, H. R. Prophylactic effect of cimetidine in gastric ulcer patients. Scand. J. Gastroenterol. *14*:175, 1979.

170. Machell, R. J., Ciclitira, P. J., Farthing, M. J. G., Dick, A. P., and Hunter, J. O. Cimetidine in the prevention of gastric ulcer relapse. Postgrad. Med. J. *55*:393, 1979.

171. Liedberg, G., Davies, H. J., Enskog, L., et al. Ulcer healing and relapse prevention by ranitidine in peptic ulcer disease. Scand. J. Gastroenterol. *20*:941, 1985.

172. Littman, A., and Hanscom, D. H. The course of recurrent ulcer. Gastroenterology *61*:592, 1971.

173. Smith, F. H., and Jordan, S. M. Gastric ulcer: a study of 600 cases. Gastroenterology *11*:575, 1948.

174. Hanscom, D. H., and Buchman, E. The follow-up period. Gastroenterology *61*:585, 1971.

175. Miyake, T., Ariyoshi, J., Suzaki, T., Oishi, M., Sakai, M., and Ueda, S. Endoscopic evaluation of the effect of sucralfate therapy and other clinical parameters on the recurrence rate of gastric ulcers. Dig. Dis. Sci. *25*:1, 1980.

176. Piper, D. W., Shinners, J., Greig, M., Thomas, J., and Waller, S. L. Effect of ulcer healing on the prognosis of chronic gastric ulcer. Gut *19*:419, 424, 1978.

177. Jorde, R., Bostad, L., and Burhol, P. G. Asymptomatic gastric ulcer: a follow-up study in patients with previous gastric ulcer disease. Lancet *1*:119, 1986.

178. Smart, H. L., and Langman, M. J. S. Late outcome of bleeding gastric ulcers. Gut *27*:926, 1986.

179. Lundell, L., and Svartholm, E. Gastrocolic fistula: a rare complication of benign gastric ulcer. Acta Chir. Scand. *146*:213, 1980.

180. Simpson, E. T., and White, J. A. Gastrocolic fistula complicating benign gastric ulcer. A case report and review of the literature. S. Afr. Med. J. *61*:717, 1982.

181. Krivisky, B. A., Bier, S. J., and Ostrolenk, D. G. Gastroenterocolic fistula complicating benign peptic ulcer. Mt. Sinai J. Med. *53*:299, 1986.

182. Walrond, E. R. Pancreatic-biliary fistula due to erosion by a chronic benign ulcer. West Indian Med. J. *28*:55, 1979.

183. Kumar, R. K., and Munro, V. F. Perforation of a gastric ulcer into the pericardium: A case report. Aust. N.Z. J. Surg. *50*:410, 1980.

184. Joffe, N., and Antonioli, D. A. Penetration into spleen by benign gastric ulcers. Clin. Radiol. *32*:177, 1981.

185. Ching, J. L., Owen, M. J., and Heller, C. A. Radiological gastric filling defect due to penetration into the spleen by a large gastric ulcer. Br. J. Radiol. *56*:488, 1983.

186. Porteous, C., Williams, D., Foulis, A., and Sugden, B. A. Penetration of the left ventricular myocardium by benign peptic ulceration: two cases and a review of the published work. J. Clin. Pathol. *37*:1239, 1984.

187. Brandstetter, R. D., Klass, S. C., Gutherz, P., Neglia, W., and Pinals, D. J. Pleural effusion due to communicating gastric ulcer. N.Y. State J. Med. *85*:706, 1985.

188. Finsterer, H. Ulcer-cancer of stomach. Arch. Klin. Chir. *131*:71, 1924.

189. Swynnerton, B. F., and Truelove, S. C. Simple gastric ulcer and carcinoma. Br. Med. J. *2*:1243, 1951.

190. Ekstrom, T. On the development of cancer in gastric ulcer and ulcer symptoms in gastric cancer. Acta Chir. Scand. *102*:387, 1952.

191. Comfort, M. W., Priestley, J. T., Dockerty, M. B., Weber, H. M., Gage, R. P., Solis, J., and Epperson, D. P. The small benign and malignant gastric lesion. Surg. Gynecol. Obstet. *Oct*:435, 1957.

192. Podolsky, I., Storms, P. R., Richardson, C. T., Peterson, W. L., and Fordtran, J. S. Gastric adenocarcinoma masquerading as benign gastric ulcer: a five-year experience. Dig. Dis. Sci., in press.

193. Desmond, A. M., Nicholls, J., and Brown, C. Further surgical management of gastric ulcer with unsuspected malignant change. Ann. R. Coll. Surg. Engl. *57*:101, 1975.

194. Rollag, A., and Jacobsen, C. D. Gastric ulcer and risk of cancer. A five-year follow-up study. Acta Med. Scand. *216*:105, 1984.

195. Bonnevie, O. Causes of death in duodenal and gastric ulcer. Gastroenterology *73*:1000, 1977.

196. Bonnevie, O. Survival in peptic ulcer. Gastroenterology *75*:1055, 1978.

197. Bonnevie, O. Gastric and duodenal ulcers in the same patient. Scand. J. Gastroenterol. *10*:657, 1975.

198. Wilkie, D. P. D. Coincident duodenal and gastric ulcer. Br. Med. J. *2*:469, 1926.

199. Johnson, H. D. The special significance of concomitant gastric and duodenal ulcers. Lancet *1*:266, 1955.

200. McCray, B. S., Ferris, E. J., Herskovic, T., Winawer, S. J., Shapiro, J. H., and Zamcheck, N. Clinical differences between gastric ulcers with and without duodenal deformity. Ann. Surg. *168*:821, 1968.

201. Rumball, J. M. Coexistent duodenal ulcer. Gastroenterology *61*:622, 1971.

202. Pollard, H. M., Bachrach, W. H., and Block, M. The rate of healing of gastric ulcers. Gastroenterology *8*:435, 1947.

203. Judd, E. S., and Proctor, O. Multiple gastric ulcers. Med. J. Rec. (Suppl.) *121*:93, 1925.

204. Boyle, J. D. Multiple gastric ulcers. Gastroenterology *61*:628, 1971.

205. Welch, C. E., and Allen, A. W. Gastric ulcer study of Massachusetts General Hospital cases during the ten year period 1938–1947. N. Engl. J. Med. *240*:277, 1949.

206. Snoddy, W. T. Primary lymphosarcoma of the stomach. Gastroenterology *20*:537, 1952.

207. Roehrkasse, R. L., Roberts, I. M., Wald, A., Talamo, T. S., and Mendelow, H. Celiac sprue complicated by lymphoma presenting with multiple gastric ulcers. Gastroenterology *91*:740, 1986.

208. Clinch, D., Banerjee, A. K., and Ostick, G. Absence of abdominal pain in elderly patients with peptic ulcer. Age Ageing *13*:120, 1984.

209. Horrocks, J. C., and DeDombal, F. T. Clinical presentation of patients with dyspepsia. Gut *19*:19, 1978.

210. Edwards, F. C., and Coghill, N. F. Clinical manifestations in patients with chronic atrophic gastritis, gastric ulcer, and duodenal ulcer. Q. J. Med. *37*:337, 1968.

211. Palmer, W. L. The "acid test" in gastric and duodenal ulcer. JAMA *88*:1778, 1927.

212. Bonney, G. L. W., and Pickering, G. W. Observations on the mechanism of pain in ulcer of the stomach and duodenum. I. The nature of the stimulus. Clin. Sci. *6*:63, 1946.

213. Misiewicz, J. J. Peptic ulceration and its correlation with symptoms. Clin. Gastroenterol. *7*:571, 1978.

214. Ciclitira, P. J., Machell, R. J., Farthing, M. J., Dick, A. P., and Hunter, J. A controlled trial of cimetidine in the treatment of gastric ulcer. *In* Burland, W. L., and Simpkins, M. A. (eds.). Cimetidine, Proceedings of the Second International Symposium on Histamine H_2-Receptor Antagonists. Amsterdam, Excerpta Medica, 1977, p. 283.

215. Hess, H., Wursch, T. G., Killer-Walser, R., Koelz, H.-R., Pelloni, S., Brondli, H., Sonnenberg, A., and Blum, A. L. How often does peptic ulcer produce "typical" ulcer symptoms? Hepatogastroenterology *27*:57, 1980.

216. Frost, F., Rahbek, I., Jensen, K. B., Gudmand-Hoyer, E., Krag, E., Rask-Madsen, J., Wulff, H. R., Garbol, J., Jensen, K. G., Hojlung, M., and Nissen, V. R. Cimetidine in patients with gastric ulcer: a multicentre controlled trial. Br. Med. J. *2*:795, 1977.

217. Priebe, W. M., DaCosta, L. R., and Beck, I. T. Is epigastric tenderness a sign of peptic ulcer disease? Gastroenterology *82*:16, 1982.

218. Bryk, D. Penetrated ulcer near the cardia of the stomach. Am. J. Dig. Dis. *11*:728, 1966.

219. Wohl, G. T., and Shore, L. Lesions of the cardiac end of the stomach simulating carcinoma. AJR *82*:1048, 1959.

220. Alvarez, W. C., and MacCarthy, W. C. Sizes of resected gastric ulcers and gastric carcinomas. JAMA *91*:226, 1928.

221. Wenger, J., Brandborg, L. L., and Spellman, F. A. Clinical aspects. Veterans Administration Cooperative Study on Gastric Ulcer. Gastroenterology *61*:598, 1971.

222. Robbins, S. L. Contributions of the pathologist to present-day concepts of gastric ulcer. JAMA *171*:2053, 1959.

223. Barragry, T. P., Blatchford, J. W., III, and Allen, M. O. Giant gastric ulcers. A review of 49 cases. Ann. Surg. *203*:255, 1986.

224. Dodd, G. D., and Nelson, R. S. The combined radiologic and gastroscopic evaluation of gastric ulceration. Radiology *77*:177, 1961.

225. Cotton, P. B. Fibreoptic endoscopy and the barium meal—results and implications. Br. Med. J. *2*:161, 1973.

226. Papp, J. P. Endoscopic experience in 100 consecutive cases with Olympus GIF endoscope. Am. J. Gastroenterol. *60*:466, 1973.

227. Dellipiani, A. W. Experience with duodenofibroscopes. Scott. Med. J. *19*:7, 1974.

228. Barnes, R. J., Gear, M. W. L., Nicol, A., and Dew, A. B. Study of dyspepsia in a general practice as assessed by endoscopy and radiology. Br. Med. J. *4*:214, 1974.

229. Laufer, I., Mullens, J. E., and Hamilton, J. The diagnostic accuracy of barium studies in the stomach and duodenum—correlation endoscopy. Radiology *115*:569, 1975.

230. Laufer, I. Assessment of the accuracy of double contrast gastroduodenal radiology. Gastroenterology *71*:874, 1976.

231. Goldstein, H. M. Double-contrast gastrography. Am. J. Dig. Dis. *21*:797, 1976.

232. Ott, D. J., Gelfand, D. W., and Wu, W. C. Detection of gastric ulcer: comparison of single- and double-contrast examination. AJR *139*:93, 1982.

233. Ott, D. J., Chen, Y. M., Gelfand, D. W., and Wu, W. C. Radiographic efficacy in gastric ulcer: comparison of single-contrast and multiphasic examinations. AJR *147*:697, 1986.

234. Gear, M. W. L., Truelove, S. C., Williams, D. G., Massarella, G. R., and Boddington, M. M. Gastric cancer simulating benign gastric ulcer. Br. J. Surg. *56*:739, 1969.

235. Montgomery, R. D., and Richardson, B. P. Gastric ulcer and cancer. Q. J. Med. *44*:591, 1975.

236. Shumacher, F. V., and Hampton, A. O. Radiographic differentiation of benign and malignant gastric ulcers. Ciba Clin. Symposia *8*:161, 1956.

237. Kirsh, I. E. The Veterans Administration Cooperative Study of Gastric Ulcer. 6. II. Radiological aspects of cancer after apparent healing. Gastroenterology *61*:606, 1971.

238. Kirsh, I. E. Benign and malignant gastric ulcers. Roentgen differentiation. Radiology *64*:357, 1955.

239. Sussman, M. L., and Lipsay, J. J. Roentgen differentiation of benign and malignant ulcers. Surg. Clin. N. Amer. *27*:273, 1947.

240. Findley, J. W., Jr. Ulcers of the greater curvature of the stomach. Gastroenterology *40*:183, 1961.

241. Sun, D. C. H., and Stempien, S. J. The Veterans Administration Cooperative Study on Gastric Ulcer. 3. Site and size as determinants of outcome. Gastroenterology *61*:576, 1971.

242. Kottler, R. E., and Tuft, R. J. Benign greater curve gastric ulcer: the "sump-ulcer." Br. J. Radiol. *54*:651, 1981.

243. Hermanek, P. Gastrobiopsy in cancer of the stomach. Endoscopy *5*:144, 1973.

244. Nelson, R. S., Urrea, L. H., and Lanza, F. L. Evaluation of gastric ulcerations. Am. J. Dig. Dis. *21*:389, 1976.

245. Kiil, J., and Anderson, D. X-ray examination and/or endoscopy in the diagnosis of gastroduodenal ulcer and crater. Scand. J. Gastroenterol. *15*:39, 1980.

246. Dekker, W., and Tytgat, G. N. Diagnostic accuracy of fiberendoscopy in the detection of upper intestinal malignancy. A follow-up analysis. Gastroenterology *73*:710, 1977.

247. Witzel, L., Halter, F., Gretillat, P. A., Scheurer, U., and Keller, M. Evaluation of specific value of endoscopic biopsies and brush cytology for malignancies of the esophagus and stomach. Gut *17*:375, 1976.

248. Hanson, J. T., Thoreson, C., and Morrissey, J. F. Brush cytology in the diagnosis of upper gastrointestinal malignancy. Gastrointest. Endosc. *26*:33, 1980.

249. Kiil, J., and Andersen, D. X-ray examination and/or endoscopy in the diagnosis of gastroduodenal ulcer and cancer. Scand. J. Gastroenterol. *15*:39, 1980.

250. Tedesco, F. J. Endoscopy in the evaluation of patients with upper gastrointestinal symptoms: indications, expectations, and interpretation. J. Clin. Gastroenterol. *3*(Suppl. 2):67, 1981.

251. Thompson, G., Somers, S., and Stevenson, G. W. Benign gastric ulcer: a reliable radiologic diagnosis? AJR *141*:331, 1983.

252. Tedesco, F. J., Best, W. R., Littman, A., Rubin, C. E., Sturdevant, R. A. L., and Vennes, J. A. Role of gastroscopy in gastric ulcer patients. Planning a prospective study. Gastroenterology 73:170, 1977.

253. Weinstein, W. M. Gastroscopy for gastric ulcer. Gastroenterology 73:1160, 1977.

254. Appropriate use of gastrointestinal endoscopy. A consensus statement from the American Society for Gastrointestinal Endoscopy. Prepared by the Committee on Endoscopic Utilization. Reviewed and approved by the Standards of Training and Practice Committee and by the Governing Board, June 1986.

255. Rowland, R., Durbridge, T., Hecker, R., and Fitch, R. How many endoscopic biopsy specimens? Med. J. Aust. 2:172, 1976.

256. Graham, D. Y., Schwartz, J. T., Cain, G. D., and Gyorkey, F. Prospective evaluation of biopsy number in the diagnosis of esophageal and gastric carcinoma. Gastroenterology 82:228, 1982.

257. Bachrach, W. H. Observations upon the complete roentgenographic healing of neoplastic ulceration of the stomach. Surg. Gynecol. Obstet. 114:69, 1962.

258. Novis, M. B., and Burns, D. G. Adenocarcinoma at the site of a healed gastric ulcer after 10 years of endoscopic observations. Am. J. Gastroenterol. 77:99, 1982.

259. Hogan, W. J., Bjork, J. T., Parker, H. W., Morrissey, J. F., Nelson, R. S., and Sukys, A. The gastric ulcer: a fiberendoscopic approach to detection and differential diagnosis (excerpts from the ASGE Endoscopic Teaching Syllabus). A/S/G/E Postgraduate Education Sub-Committee. Gastrointest. Endosc. 27:189, 1981.

260. Grossman, M. I., Kirsner, J. B., and Gillespie, I. E. Basal and Histalog-stimulated gastric secretion in control subjects and in patients with peptic ulcer or gastric cancer. Gastroenterology 45:14, 1963.

261. Shearman, D. J. C., Finlayson, N. D. C., and Wilson, R. Gastric function in patients with gastric carcinoma. Lancet 1:343, 1967.

262. Neeman, A., and Marks, I. N. Are acid secretory tests of diagnostic value in patients with benign-looking gastric ulcers? S. Afr. Med. J. 65:1012, 1984.

263. Trudeau, W. L., and McGuigan, J. E. Relations between serum gastrin levels and rates of gastric hydrochloric acid secretion. N. Engl. J. Med. 284:408, 1971.

264. Trudeau, W. L., and McGuigan, J. E. Serum and tissue gastrin measurements in patients with carcinoma of the stomach. (Abstract.) Gastroenterology 62:822, 1972.

265. Rahbek, I., Frost, F., Rune, S. J., et al. A controlled trial of the effect of cimetidine on the healing of gastric ulcer. In Harvegt, C. et al. (eds.). Proceedings of the National Symposium on Cimetidine ('Tagamet'). Brussels, Excerpta Medica, 1978, pp. 56–61.

266. Lambert, R. Traitement de l'ulcere gastrique par la cimetidine. Resultats de l'etude multicentrique francaise. In Harvengt, C. et al. (eds.). Proceedings of the National Symposium on Cimetidine ('Tagamet'). Brussels, Excerpta Medica, 1978, pp. 46–50.

267. Dyck, W. P., Belsito, A., Fleshler, B., Liebermann, T. R., Dickinson, P. B., and Wood, J. M. Cimetidine and placebo in the treatment of benign gastric ulcer: a multicenter double-blind study. Gastroenterology 74:410, 1978.

268. Navert, H., Larose, L., Beaudry, R., Haddad, H., Lutfi, G., Lacruz, M., and Apollon, G. Cimetidine is effective in the treatment of gastric ulcer. (Abstract.) Gastroenterology 74:1072, 1978.

269. Cremer, M., Toussaint, J., Derumier, J., and Deltenre, M. Etude en double eveugle de l'effet de la cimetidine dans l'ulcere duodenal et dans l'ulcere gastrique. In Harvengt, C. et al. (eds.). Proceedings of the National Symposium on Cimetidine ('Tagamet'). Brussels, Excerpta Medica, 1978. pp. 30–39.

270. Smith, P. M., Edwards, J. L., and Aubrey, A. A. Gastric secretory studies and cimetidine treatment in gastric ulcers. In Wastell, C., and Lance, P. (eds.). Cimetidine: The Westminster Hospital Symposium, London, Churchill Livingstone, 1978, pp. 258–272.

271. Landecker, K. D., Crawford, J., Hunt, J. H., Gillespie, P., and Piper, D. W. Cimetidine and gastric ulcer healing. Med. J. Aust. 2:43, 1979.

272. Ciclitira, P. J., Machell, R. J., Farthing, M. J. G., Dick, A. P., and Hunter, J. O. Double-blind controlled trial of cimetidine in the healing of gastric ulcer. Gut 20:730, 1979.

273. Garbol, J., Jensen, K. G., Holjlund, M., Nissen, V. R., and Olsen, P. P. A controlled trial of cimetidine ('Tagamet') in the treatment of gastric ulceration. Ugeskr. Laeger 141:3301, 1979.

274. Englert, E., Jr., Freston, J. W., Graham, D. Y., Finkelstein, W., Kruss, D. M., Priest, R. J., Raskin, J. B., Rhodes, J. B., Rogers, A. I., Wenger, J., Wilcox, L. L., and Crossley, R. J. Cimetidine, antacid and hospitalization in the treatment of benign gastric ulcer. Gastroenterology 74:416, 1978.

275. Data on file. Glaxo, Inc., Research Triangle Park, North Carolina 27709.

276. Dawson, J., Jain, S., and Cockel, R. Effect of ranitidine and cimetidine on gastric ulcer healing and recurrence. Scand. J. Gastroenterol. 19:665, 1984.

277. Single blind comparative study of ranitidine and cimetidine in patients with gastric ulcer. The Belgian Peptic Ulcer Study Group. Gut 25:999, 1984.

278. Ryan, F. P., Jorde, R., Ehsanullah, R. S. B., Summers, K., and Wood, J. R. A single night time dose of ranitidine in the acute treatment of gastric ulcer: a European multicentre trial. Gut 27:784, 1986.

279. Farley, A., Levesque, D., Pare, P., Thomson, A. B. R., Sherbaniuk, R., Archambault, A., and Mahoney, K. A comparative trial of ranitidine 300 mg at night with ranitidine 150 mg twice daily in the treatment of duodenal and gastric ulcer. Am. J. Gastroenterol. 80:665, 1985.

280. Barbara, L., Corinaldesi, R., Adamo, S., et al. A double-blind controlled trial of ranitidine 300 mg nocte and ranitidine 150 mg b.i.d. in the short-term treatment of gastric ulcer. Int. J. Clin. Pharmacol. Ther. Toxicol. 24:104, 1986.

281. Jorde, R., and Burhol, P. G. A single-centre study of gastric ulcer healing with 300 mg ranitidine at night versus 150 mg ranitidine twice daily. Scand. J. Gastroenterol. 21:833, 1986.

282. Lauritsen, K., Bytzer, P., Hansen, J., Bekker, C., and Rask-Madsen, J. Comparison of ranitidine and high-dose antacid in the treatment of prepyloric or duodenal ulcer. A double-blind controlled trial. Scand. J. Gastroenterol. 20:123, 1985.

283. Paoluzi, P., Torsoli, A., Bianchi-Porro, G., et al. Famotidine (MK-208) in the treatment of gastric ulcer. Results of a multicenter double-blind controlled study. Digestion 32(Suppl. 1):38, 1985.

284. Dammann, H. G., Walter, T. A., Hentschel, E., Muller, P., and Simon, B. Famotidine: nocturnal administration for gastric ulcer healing. Results of multicenter trials in Austria and Germany. Digestion 32(Suppl. 1):45, 1985.

285. Bianchi-Porro, G. Famotidine in the treatment of gastric and duodenal ulceration: overview of clinical experience. Digestion 32(Suppl. 1):62, 1985.

286. Lyon, D. T. Efficacy and safety of famotidine in the management of benign gastric ulcers. Am. J. Med. 81:33, 1986.

287. Baume, P. E., Hunt, J. H., and Piper, D. W. Glycopyrronium bromide in the treatment of chronic gastric ulcer. Gastroenterology 63:399, 1972.

288. Bachrach, W. H. Anticholinergic drugs. Survey of the literature and some experimental observations. Am. J. Dig. Dis. 3:743, 1958.

289. Ivey, K. J. Anticholinergics: do they work in peptic ulcer? Gastroenterology 68:154, 1975.

290. Gonvers, J. J., Realini, S., Bretholz, A., et al. Gastric ulcer: a double-blind comparison of 100 mg pirenzepine plus antacid versus 800 mg cimetidine plus antacid. Scand. J. Gastroenterol. 21:806, 1986.

291. Bianchi-Porro, G., Petrillo, M., Lazzaroni, M., et al. Comparison of pirenzepine and carbenoxolone in the treatment of chronic gastric ulcer. A double-blind endoscopic trial. Hepatogastroenterology 32:293, 1985.

292. Carmine, A. A., and Brogden, R. N. Pirenzepine: A review of its pharmacodynamic and pharmacokinetic properties and therapeutic efficacy in peptic ulcer disease and other allied diseases. Drugs 30:85, 1985.

293. Morelli, A., Pelli, A., Narducci, F., and Spadacini, A. Pirenzepine in the treatment of gastric ulcer. A double-blind short-term clinical trial. Scand. J. Gastroenterol. 14(Suppl. 57):51, 1979.

294. Richardson, C. T., and Walsh, J. H. The value of a histamine H_2-receptor antagonist in the management of patients with the Zollinger-Ellison syndrome. N. Engl. J. Med. 294:133, 1976.

295. McCarthy, D. M., and Hyman, P. E. Effect of isopropramide on response to oral cimetidine in patients with Zollinger-Ellison syndrome. Dig. Dis. Sci. 27:353, 1982.

296. Myren, J., and Berstad, A. The early effect of trimipramine (Surmontil) on gastric secretion in man. Scand. J. Gastroenterol. 10:817, 1975.

297. Valnes, K., Myren, J., and Ovigstad, T. Trimipramine in the treatment of gastric ulcer. Scand. J. Gastroenterol. 13:497, 1978.

298. Caldara, R., Romussi, M., and Ferrari, C. Inhibition of gastrin secretion by sulpiride treatment in duodenal ulcer patients. Gastroenterology 74:221, 1978.

299. Schiller, L. R., and Feldman, M. Medical therapy of peptic ulcer. In Baron, J. H., and Moody, F. G. (eds.). Foregut: Butterworth's International Medical Reviews. London, Butterworth, 1981, pp. 192–240.

300. Fellenius, E., Berglindh, T., Brandstrom, A., et al. The inhibitory action of substituted benzimidazoles on isolated oxyntic glands and H^+/K^+-ATPase. In Hydrogen Ion Transport in Epithelia. Schulz, I., Sachs, G., Forte, J. G., and Ullrich, K. J. (eds.). Amsterdam, Elsevier North/Holland Biomedical Press, 1980, pp. 193–202.

301. Fellenius, E., Elander, B., Wallmark, B., Haglund, U., Olbe, L., and Helander, H. Studies on acid secretory mechanism and drug action in isolated gastric glands from man. In Rosselin, G., Fromageot, P., and Bonfils, S. (eds.). Hormone Receptors in Digestion and Nutrition. Amsterdam, Elsevier North/Holland Biomedical Press, 1979, pp. 335–360.

302. Clissold, S. P., and Campoli-Richards, D. M. Omeprazole. A preliminary review of its pharmacodynamic and pharmacokinetic properties, and therapeutic potential in peptic ulcer disease and Zollinger-Ellison syndrome. Drugs 32:15, 1986.

303. Larsson, H., Carlsson, E., Mattsson, H., et al. Plasma gastrin and gastric enterochromaffin-like cell activation and proliferation. Studies with omeprazole and ranitidine in intact and antrectomized rats. Gastroenterology 90:391, 1986.

304. Hollander, D., and Harlan, J. Antacids vs. placebos in peptic ulcer therapy. A controlled double-blind investigation. JAMA 226:1181, 1973.

305. Butler, M. L., and Gersh, H. Antacid vs placebo in hospitalized gastric ulcer patients. A controlled therapeutic study. Am. J. Dig. Dis. 20:803, 1975.

306. Rydning, A., Weberg, R., Lange, O., and Berstad, A. Healing of benign gastric ulcer with low-dose antacids and fiber diet. Gastroenterology 91:56, 1986.

307. Berstad, A., and Weberg, R. Review. Antacids in the treatment of gastroduodenal ulcer. Scand. J. Gastroenterol. 21:385, 1986.

308. Hollander, D., Tarnawski, A., Krause, W. J., and Gergely, H. Protective effect of sucralfate against alcohol-induced gastric mucosal injury in the rat. Macroscopic, histologic, ultrastructural, and functional time sequence analysis. Gastroenterology 88:366, 1985.

309. Mayberry, J. F., Williams, R. A., Rhodes, J., and Lawrie, B. W. A controlled clinical trial of sucralfate in the treatment of gastric ulcer. Br. J. Clin. Pract. 32:291, 1978.

310. Marks, I. N., Wright, J. P., Denyer, M., Garisch, J. A. M., and Lucke, W. Comparison of sucralfate with cimetidine in the short-term treatment of chronic peptic ulcers. S. Afr. Med. J. 57:567, 1980.

311. Hallerback, B., Anker-Hansen, O., Carling, L., et al. Short term treatment of gastric ulcer: a comparison of sucralfate and cimetidine. Gut 27:778, 1986.

312. Lam, S.K., Lau, W. Y., Lai, C. L., et al. Efficacy of sucralfate in corpus, prepyloric, and duodenal ulcer–associated gastric ulcers. A double-blind, placebo-controlled study. Am. J. Med. 79(Suppl. 2C):24, 1985.

313. Weiss, G., and Serfontein, W. J. The efficacy of a bismuth-protein-complex compound in treatment of gastric and duodenal ulcers. S. Afr. Med. J. 45:467, 1971.

314. Boyes, B. E., Woolf, I. L., Wilson, R. Y., Cowley, D. J., and Dymock, I. W. Effective treatment of gastric ulceration with a bismuth preparation (De Nol). (Abstract.) Gut 15:833, 1974.

315. Tytgat, G. N., Rauws, E., and Langenberg, W. The role of colloidal bismuth subcitrate in gastric ulcer and gastritis. Scand. J. Gastroenterol. 122(Suppl.):22, 1986.

316. Parente, F., Lazzaroni, M., Petrillo, M., and Bianchi-Porro, G. Colloidal bismuth subcitrate and ranitidine in the short-term treatment of benign gastric ulcer. An endoscopically controlled trial. Scand. J. Gastroenterol. 122(Suppl.):42, 1986.

317. Fung, W., Karim, S. M. M., and Tye, C. Y. Effect of 15(R)15 methyl-prostaglandin E_2 methyl ester on the healing of gastric ulcers. Controlled endoscopic study. Lancet 2:10, 1974.

318. Fung, W., and Karim, S. M. Effect of prostaglandin E_2 on the healing of gastric ulcers: a double-blind endoscopic trial. Aust. N.Z. J. Med. 6:121, 1976.

319. Gibinski, K., Rybicka, J., Mikos, E., and Nowak, A. Double-blind clinical trial on gastroduodenal ulcer healing with prostaglandin E_2 analogues. Gut 18:636, 1977.

320. Rybicka, J., and Gibinski, K. Methyl-prostaglandin E_2 analogues for healing of gastro-duodenal ulcers. Scand. J. Gastroent. 13:155, 1978.

321. Fich, A., Goldin, E., Zimmerman, J., Ligumsky, M., and Rachmilewitz, D. Comparison of misoprostol and cimetidine in the treatment of gastric ulcer. Isr. J. Med. Sci. 21:968, 1985.

322. Rachmilewitz, D., Chapman, J. W., and Nicholson, P. A. A multicenter international controlled comparison of two dosage regimens of misoprostol with cimetidine in treatment of gastric ulcer in outpatients. Dig. Dis. Sci. 31(Suppl.):75S, 1986.

323. Shield, M. J. Interim results of a multicenter international comparison of misoprostol and cimetidine in the treatment of out-patients with benign gastric ulcers. Dig. Dis. Sci. 30(Suppl.):178S, 1985.

324. Agrawal, N. M., Saffouri, B., Kruss, D. M., Callison, D. A., and Dajani, E. Z. Healing of benign gastric ulcer. A placebo-controlled comparison of two dosage regimens of misoprostol, a synthetic analog of prostaglandin E_1. Dig. Dis. Sci. 30(Suppl.):164S, 1985.

325. Navert, H. Treatment of gastric ulcer with enprostil. Am. J. Med. 81(Suppl.):75, 1986.

326. Dammann, H. G., Huttemann, W., Kalek, H. D., Rohner, H. G., Simon, B. A comparative clinical trial of enprostil and ranitidine in the treatment of gastric ulcer. Am. J. Med. 81(Suppl.):80, 1986.

327. Sontag, S. J. Prostaglandins in peptic ulcer disease: an overview of current status and future directions. Drugs 32:445, 1986.

328. Banks, S., and Marks, I. N. Maintenance carbenoxolone sodium in the prevention of gastric ulcer recurrence. In Baron, J. H., and Sullivan, F. M. (eds.). Carbenoxolone Sodium. London, Butterworth, 1970, pp. 103–112.

329. Domschke, W., Domschke, S., Classen, H., and Demlins, L. N-acetylneuraminic acid in gastric mucosa: a possible mediator of carbenoxolone action in gastric ulcer patients. Acta Hepatogastroenterol. 19:204, 1972.

330. Cross, S., Rhodes, J., and Calcraft, B. Carbenoxolone: its protective action on gastric mucosa. In Biologie et Gastroenterologie, 9th International Congress of Gastroenterology, Paris 5:568C, 1972.

331. Lipkin, M. In "defense" of the gastric mucosa. Gut 12:599, 1971.

332. Meeroff, J. C., Rubinstein, M., Luis, A., Waciarz, M., Eguia, O., and Meeroff, M. Randomized double-masked trial of sodium oxyferriscorbone for the treatment of gastric ulcers. Dig. Dis. Sci. 24:680, 1979.

333. Frommer, D. J. The healing of gastric ulcers by zinc sulphate. Med. J. Aust. 2:793, 1975.

334. Doll, R., and Pygott, F. Factors influencing the rate of healing of gastric ulcers: admission to hospital, phenobarbitone, and ascorbic acid. Lancet 1:171, 1952.

335. Hermann, R. P., and Piper, D. W. Factors influencing the healing rate of chronic gastric ulcer. Am. J. Dig. Dis. 18:1, 1973.

336. Evans, P. R. C. Value of strict dieting, drugs and Robaden in peptic ulceration. Br. Med. J. *1*:612, 1954.

337. Doll, R., Friedlander, P., and Pygott, F. Dietetic treatment of peptic ulcer. Lancet *1*:5, 1956.

338. McArthur, K. E., Hogan, D. L., and Isenberg, J. I. Relative stimulatory effects of commonly ingested beverages on gastric acid secretion in humans. Gastroenterology *83*:199, 1982.

339. Rydning, A., and Berstad, A. Dietary aspects of peptic ulcer disease. Scand. J. Gastroenterol. *20*(Suppl. 110):29, 1985.

340. Lanza, F. L., Royer, G. L., and Nelson, R. S. Endoscopic evaluation of the effects of aspirin, buffered aspirin and enteric-coated aspirin on gastric and duodenal mucosa. N. Engl. J. Med. *303*:136, 1980.

341. Piper, D. W. The treatment of chronic peptic ulcer. Front. Gastrointest. Res. *6*:109, 1980.

342. Agrawal, N., Roth, S., Mahowald, M., et al. Misoprostol coadministration heals aspirin-induced gastric lesions in rheumatoid arthritis patients. (Abstract.) Gastroenterology *92*:1290, 1987.

343. Croker, J. R., Cotton, P. B., Boyle, A. C., and Kinsella, P. Cimetidine for peptic ulcer in patients with arthritis. Ann. Rheum. Dis. *39*:275, 1980.

344. Tragardh, B., and Haglund, U. Endoscopic diagnosis of gastric ulcer. Evaluation of the benefits of endoscopic follow-up observation for malignancy. Acta Chir. Scand. *151*:37, 1985.

345. Steigmann, F., and Shulman, B. The time of healing of gastric ulcers: implications as to therapy. Gastroenterology *20*:20, 1952.

346. Brown, J. J., and Blank, L. Carcinoma of the stomach disguised as a benign gastric ulcer. South. Med. J. *79*:1312, 1986.

347. Sakita, T., Oguro, Y., Takasu, S., Fukutomi, H., Miwa, T., and Yoshimori, M. Observations on the healing of ulcerations in early gastric cancer. The life cycle of the malignant ulcer. Gastroenterology *60*:835, 1971.

348. LaBrooy, S. J., Taylor, R. H., Ayrton, C., et al. Cimetidine in the maintenance treatment of gastric ulceration (GU). Hepatogastroenterology (Suppl.). XI Int. Cong. Gastroenterol., Hamburg, June 8–13, 1980, p. 205, Abstract E26.5.

349. Kang, J. Y., Canalese, J., and Piper, D. W. The use of long-term cimetidine in the prevention of gastric ulcer relapse—double blind trial. Ann. Sci. Mtg., Gastroenterology Society Australia, Bardon Professional Centre, Brisbane, May 14–15, 1979, Abstract A9.

350. Kinloch, J. D., Pearson, A. J. G., Woolf, I. L., and Young, P. H. The effect of cimetidine on the maintenance of healing of gastric ulceration. Postgrad. Med. J. *60*:665, 1984.

351. Miyake, T., Ariyoshi, J., Suzaki, T., Oishi, M., Sakai, M., and Ueda, S. Endoscopic evaluation of the effect of sucralfate therapy and other clinical parameters on the recurrence rate of gastric ulcers. Dig. Dis. Sci. *25*:1, 1980.

352. Marks, I. N., Wright, J. P., Girdwood, A. H., Gilinsky, N. H., and Lucke, W. Maintenance therapy with sucralfate reduces rate of gastric ulcer recurrence. Am. J. Med. *79*(Suppl. 2C):32, 1985.

353. Wormsley, K. G. Occasional report. Assessing the safety of drugs for the long-term treatment of peptic ulcers. Gut *25*:1416, 1984.

49

The Zollinger-Ellison Syndrome

JAMES E. McGUIGAN

In 1955, Zollinger and Ellison described the syndrome which now bears their names in two patients with the clinical triad characteristic of this syndrome, that is, gastric acid hypersecretion, severe ulcer disease of the upper gastrointestinal tract, and non-beta islet cell tumors of the pancreas.[1] They suggested that this syndrome was produced by tumor release of a humoral substance (a secretagogue) into the circulation that stimulated gastric acid secretion resulting in severe ulcer disease. Their hypothesis has been shown to be correct.[2]

The Zollinger-Ellison syndrome, although uncommon, is not rare. Its true incidence is not known. It has been estimated to occur in 0.1 to 1 per cent of all patients with duodenal ulcer. The Zollinger-Ellison syndrome appears to be slightly more frequent in males than in females.[3] Although it has been detected from early childhood through the tenth decade of life, initial clinical manifestations of the Zollinger-Ellison syndrome appear most commonly in patients from 30 to 50 years of age.[3, 4]

ETIOLOGY AND PATHOGENESIS

Five years after Zollinger and Ellison proposed that a substance that stimulated gastric acid was released from these tumors, Gregory and colleagues confirmed their prediction by demonstrating a potent acid secretagogue in extracts from these tumors.[2] The biologic behavior of this substance strongly suggested that it may be gastrin, a known powerful stimulant of gastric acid secretion. Subsequent investigations confirmed this suspicion and demonstrated large amounts of gastrin in Zollinger-Ellison tumors and in sera from patients with the Zollinger-Ellison syndrome.[5-7] These gastrin-containing and -releasing tumors have been designated as gastrinomas. Gastrin has been shown by use of immunocytochemistry to reside in numerous prominent granules in the cytoplasm of gastrinoma cells.[8]

The predominant form of gastrin in gastrinomas is heptadecapeptide gastrin (G17), whereas the major form of circulating gastrin in patients with gastrinoma is a larger form of gastrin which contains 34 amino acid residues (G34).[7, 9, 10] Most circulating gastrin in normal subjects is also G34, whereas antral gastrin in both normal subjects and patients with the Zollinger-Ellison syndrome is predominantly G17 (approximately 90 to 95 per cent). There is more variability in the proportion of G17 to G34 in gastrinoma tissue than in antral mucosa, and, on the average, 60 to 90 per cent of gastrin in gastrinomas is G17. Both sulfated (gastrin II) and non-sulfated (gastrin I) gastrin forms are present in the circulation of patients with gastrinoma as well as in normal subjects. The proportion of sulfated gastrin in the serum of patients with the Zollinger-Ellison syndrome (mean 57 per cent) has been reported to be higher than in patients with common duodenal or gastric ulcer or in healthy subjects without ulcers (mean 37 per cent).[11] Evidence has been provided, using peptide region–specific gastrin antibodies, that the ratio of amino-terminal to carboxyl-terminal G17 gastrin immunoreactivity is increased in the serum of patients with metastatic gastrinoma when compared with normal subjects and patients with nonmetastatic gastrinoma.[12] In addition to G17 and G34, smaller and larger forms of gastrin have been found in sera and gastrinomas from Zollinger-Ellison patients.[10, 13] These have included a form of gastrin slightly larger than G34, not yet characterized, which is referred to as component I gastrin; as well as small amounts of gastrin fragments, including the amino-terminal 1–13 fragment of G17 (which has no biologic activity) and the carboxyl-terminal tetradecapeptide amide ("minigastrin"), which has immunoreactivity and biologic activity similar to that of G17.

Gastrinomas in patients with the Zollinger-Ellison syndrome are usually located in the pancreas.[3, 14-16] Pancreatic gastrinomas are most frequent in the head of the pancreas (Figs. 49–1 to 49–3). Gastrinomas have been found in the wall of the duodenum, the most common site of extrapancreatic gastrinomas, in approximately 13 per cent of patients in whom the tumors have been localized.[17] Duodenal gastrinomas are usually located in the second portion of the duodenum and are solitary in approximately 50 per cent of instances. Gastrinomas vary enormously in size, ranging from approximately 0.2 to 20 cm or more in diameter.[3] At least half of gastrinomas are multiple and approximately two thirds are malignant. Sites of metastasis include regional lymph nodes, liver, spleen, bone, mediastinum, peritoneal surfaces, and skin.[3, 14] A disparity may exist between the histologic appearance and biologic behavior of these tumors, which when malig-

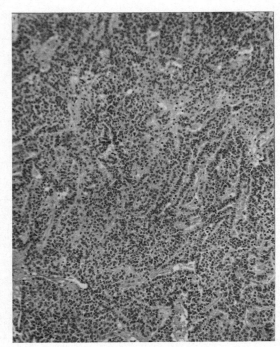

Figure 49–1. Pancreatic gastrinoma from patient with the Zollinger-Ellison syndrome. Hematoxylin and eosin stain, × 125. (Courtesy of Dr. Marie Greider.)

nant usually behave in a progressive, slow-growing, indolent fashion. In contrast, in a small proportion of patients with gastrinomas the tumor may grow rapidly and metastasize early and widely. Gastrinomas, which are apparently primary, have also been identified in the hilus of the spleen, rarely in the stomach or liver, and not infrequently in regional peripancreatic and mesenteric lymph nodes, or lymph node–like lymphoid tissue, in which they were originally considered to be metastatic.[18, 19] Characteristic histologic features that have been suggested to be of assistance in distinguishing these primary entrapancreatic gastrinomas in lymphoid tissue from metastatic gastrinoma have included a centrifugal expansive growth pattern with a thick fibrous capsule, hyalinized fibrous septa, and frequently cystic degenerative changes.[20] At surgery gastrinomas may be identified readily, almost as frequently may be relatively occult and difficult to localize, or may not be identified at all.[21-24] When carefully sought for and finally located, such occult gastrinomas have been reported to be most often within an anatomic triangle defined by the junction of the cystic and common bile ducts superiorly, the junction of the second and third portions of the duodenum inferiorly and the junction of the neck and body of the pancreas medially.[25] A small number of ovarian and parathyroid tumors have been shown to be gastrinomas and may produce the Zollinger-Ellison syndrome.[26-28]

The cells from which gastrinomas arise appear structurally distinct from antral mucosal gastrin cells (G cells). Although gastrin-containing cells are present in pancreatic islets of prenatal and newborn animals, there is very little if any immunoreactive gastrin in the

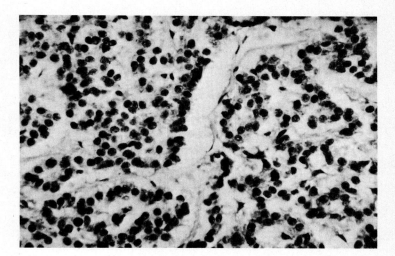

Figure 49–2. Same tumor as in Figure 49–1, at higher magnification (× 400). Cells are malignant. Hematoxylin and eosin stain. (Courtesy of Dr. Marie Greider.)

normal adult pancreas; for this reason pancreatic gastrinomas have been generally viewed as ectopic tumors. Hyperplasia of the pancreatic islets is found in approximately 10 per cent of patients with the Zollinger-Ellison syndrome.[18] In patients with the Zollinger-Ellison syndrome, in the presence or absence of detectable tumor, hyperplastic pancreatic islet tissue has not been shown to contain gastrin. Increased serum gastrin levels do not decrease following excision of this hyperplastic tissue. For these reasons islet hyperplasia is believed to be associated with, or result from, gastrinoma in circumstances in which the tumor may or may not be recognized; islet hyperplasia is not directly responsible for increased serum gastrin levels and gastric acid hypersecretion in patients with the Zollinger-Ellison syndrome.

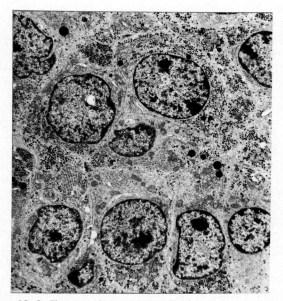

Figure 49–3. Electron photomicrograph of pancreatic gastrinoma from a patient with the Zollinger-Ellison syndrome. The well-differentiated cells contain small secretory granules. The large black granules are lipid bodies. × 4000. (Courtesy of Dr. Marie Greider.)

Approximately 25 per cent of patients with gastrinomas are found to have the multiple endocrine neoplasia syndrome, type I (MEN I), which is composed of tumors or hyperplasia of parathyroid, pancreatic islet, and pituitary glands.[29, 30] Tumors in these patients are frequently multiple or multifocal in the pancreas or in other locations. Microadenomatosis, with numerous islet cell tumors less than 5 mm in diameter, within the pancreas is much more common in gastrinoma patients with MEN I than in those with sporadic gastrinomas. Distant metastasis and biologic invasiveness of gastrinoma occurs less frequently in association with MEN I than with sporadic gastrinomas.

The gastric parietal cell mass is expanded enormously in patients with Zollinger-Ellison syndrome.[15] It has been estimated to be, on the average, at least three to six times as large as in normal individuals and two to three times that of patients with common duodenal ulcer. Expansion of the parietal cell mass, resulting in enhanced capacity to secrete gastric acid, is caused by direct trophic effects of excess circulating gastrin on the parietal cell. Multicentric, small, noninvasive gastric carcinoid tumors have been identified in the gastric mucosa of patients with the Zollinger-Ellison syndrome.[31] These carcinoid tumors may represent consequences of substantial and sustained hypergastrinemia.

In addition to ulcer disease, there are also frequently functional and morphologic abnormalities of the small intestine in patients with gastrinoma. The mucosa of the duodenum and proximal jejunum is often abnormal, with areas of denuded villi and infiltration of the lamina propria with polymorphonuclear leukocytes and eosinophils, often with accompanying edema, hemorrhage, and multiple superficial mucosal erosions.[32, 33] Remaining small intestinal mucosal villi are often stunted and broader than normal. These small intestinal mucosal abnormalities are nonspecific in appearance. Brunner's glands, normally restricted to the proximal duodenum, may be found as distal as the ligament of Treitz in patients with the Zollinger-Ellison syndrome.

CLINICAL FEATURES

The most common clinical manifestations, by far, in patients with the Zollinger-Ellison syndrome are those related to peptic ulcer.[3, 14–18] Ninety to 95 per cent of patients with gastrinomas develop ulceration of the upper gastrointestinal tract at some time during the course of their disease. Ulcer symptoms in patients with gastrinoma are often similar to those of patients with common peptic ulcer; alternatively, symptoms may be more persistent, progressive, and less responsive to therapy. The distribution of ulcers in the upper gastrointestinal tract in patients with gastrinoma is similar, but not identical, to that of patients with common peptic ulcer. Approximately 75 per cent of ulcers in patients with the Zollinger-Ellison syndrome are located in the first portion of the duodenum or (much less commonly) in the stomach. Ulcers are usually solitary, but may be multiple. In contrast to common peptic ulcer, ulcer associated with gastrinoma may involve the second, third, or fourth portions of the duodenum or even the jejunum.[3, 14, 34] In a review of patients with the Zollinger-Ellison syndrome, 14 per cent of ulcers were found in the duodenum beyond its first portion, and 11 per cent were found in the jejunum.[3]

The ulcers are usually moderate or small in size (less than 1 cm in diameter). However, uncommonly, ulcers in patients with gastrinoma may be large, exceeding 2 cm in diameter. Some patients with the Zollinger-Ellison syndrome have responded, but usually only transiently, to peptic ulcer management with antacids and anticholinergic agents.[35, 36] Recurrent ulcer, either at or distal to the anastomosis, is extremely frequent when gastric surgery for peptic ulcer is performed in Zollinger-Ellison patients harboring gastrinoma and the syndrome is not recognized in the patient.[3, 4] This is commonly accompanied by severe complications, including hemorrhage or perforation or both. Patients with gastrinomas may also develop reflux esophagitis, esophageal ulcerations, and esophageal strictures. Acid peptic reflux disease is probably more common in patients with the Zollinger-Ellison syndrome than had been appreciated initially.

Patients with gastrinoma may have symptoms other than, or in addition to, those associated with ulcer disease. Diarrhea is frequent and occurs in more than one third of patients with gastrinoma. Diarrhea may precede ulcer symptoms by as much as eight years. In approximately 7 per cent of symptomatic patients with gastrinoma, diarrhea occurs in the absence of clinical ulcer disease.[3] Diarrhea appears to be due principally to the effects of large amounts of hydrochloric acid secreted into the upper gastrointestinal tract by parietal cells in response to stimulation by circulating gastrin. In patients with diarrhea due to gastrinoma, the diarrhea may be reduced or eliminated by aspiration of gastric juice from the stomach. Although the major cause of diarrhea in patients with the Zollinger-Ellison syndrome is the large quantity of concentrated gastric acid passing into and through the small intestine, direct

effects of circulating gastrin on the secretory and absorptive properties of the small intestinal mucosa may play a role in producing diarrhea. Intravenous infusion of large amounts of gastrin has been shown to increase intestinal secretion of potassium and to reduce jejunal absorption of sodium and water, direct effects of gastrin that are not consequences of reduction of pH of the intestinal contents.[37] It has been proposed that, although gastric acid hypersecretion is necessary to produce diarrhea in these patients, gastrin may contribute by its direct effects on absorption and secretion by the small intestine. This hypothesis is supported by the observation that diarrhea is absent in those duodenal ulcer patients (without gastrinoma) with normal serum gastrin levels, who have gastric acid secretory rates comparable to those of gastrinoma patients with diarrhea. Gastric acid hypersecretion is also associated with increased pepsin secretion by gastric zymogen cells. Gastric acid hypersecretion produces pH values as low as 1 and 3.6 in the proximal and distal jejunum, respectively, converting pepsinogens to proteolytically active pepsin, which is believed to contribute to mucosal injury of the small intestine.

Patients with the Zollinger-Ellison syndrome may have reduced absorption of a variety of substances, including fat.[32] Steatorrhea, which is much less common in gastrinoma patients than diarrhea, is produced by several mechanisms. Pancreatic lipase is inactivated by enormous amounts of intraluminal acid in the upper small intestine of these patients. Pancreatic lipase is exquisitely susceptible to irreversible denaturation by acidification, rendering the lipase molecule inactive. Lipase inactivation results in failure to hydrolyze intraluminal triglycerides to their respective diglycerides, monoglycerides, and fatty acids in preparation for absorption. Hypersecretion of gastric acid may also produce steatorrhea by direct effects of low pH on bile acids. The acid environment of the small intestine renders some primary bile acids insoluble, reducing formation of micelles which are necessary for facilitation of fatty acid and monoglyceride absorption, therefore resulting in steatorrhea. Patients with the Zollinger-Ellison syndrome may develop vitamin B_{12} malabsorption which is not correctable by oral administration of intrinsic factor.[32] Although gastric secretion of intrinsic factor is normal in these patients, the low intraluminal pH in the intestine interferes with intrinsic factor facilitation of active absorption of vitamin B_{12} by the distal ileum. The precise mechanism by which low pH within the small intestinal lumen reduces intrinsic factor activity is not known. However, when the intraluminal pH is adjusted upward to 7, inhibition of intrinsic factor–mediated vitamin B_{12} absorption is abolished.

The possibility of gastrinoma should be considered in a variety of clinical circumstances, including those in patients with (1) multiple ulcers in the upper gastrointestinal tract, (2) ulcers distal to the first portion of the duodenum, (3) persistent peptic ulcer disease despite medical treatment with the usual doses and schedules, (4) rapid recurrence of ulcer following surgery for ulcer disease, (5) unexplained secretory diarrhea, (6) a strong familial history of peptic ulcer, (7) a personal or a family history suggesting parathyroid or pituitary tumors, and (8) as will be described, striking gastric acid hypersecretion and/or hypergastrinemia.

DIAGNOSIS

The Zollinger-Ellison syndrome should be suspected in patients with compatible clinical presentations, especially when rates of gastric acid secretion have been found to be substantially increased.

Gastric Acid Secretion

Hypersecretion of gastric acid, a direct effect of hypergastrinemia, is extremely frequent, but is not a universal phenomenon among Zollinger-Ellison patients, nor is gastric acid hypersecretion restricted to patients with gastrinoma, since a small proportion of patients with common duodenal ulcer have gastric acid secretory rates comparable to those of patients with the Zollinger-Ellison syndrome.[38] However, gastric acid hypersecretion with gastrinoma is sufficiently common and is sufficiently impressive in magnitude that it does provide valuable evidence in support of consideration of the Zollinger-Ellison syndrome. Most patients with the Zollinger-Ellison syndrome have unstimulated gastric acid secretory rates that exceed 15 mEq per hour, and may have rates of gastric acid secretion as high as 100 mEq per hour. It must be emphasized that there may be overlap among acid secretory rates of Zollinger-Ellison patients, with patients with common duodenal ulcers, and even with normal subjects.

It has been proposed that it may be of value in efforts to identify patients with gastrinoma to compare basal gastric acid output with that obtained following maximal stimulation with histamine, betazole (Histalog), or pentagastrin.[38, 39] In patients with the Zollinger-Ellison syndrome, stimulation by any of these agents often does not increase gastric acid output proportionately to the extent that it does in normal individuals and in patients with common peptic ulcer. In the latter groups, basal gastric acid output is usually less than 60 per cent of acid secreted after stimulation. Since the gastric parietal cell mass is already stimulated by endogenous hypergastrinemia prior to administration of the exogenous secretagogue, patients with the Zollinger-Ellison syndrome often increase their gastric acid output proportionately less than do normal subjects or patients with common duodenal ulcer; in Zollinger-Ellison patients basal acid output is often more than 60 per cent of maximal acid output in response to exogenous stimulation. However, it is usually not possible to distinguish gastrinoma patients from those with common peptic ulcer by comparing basal and stimulated gastric acid outputs. From one half to two thirds of patients with the Zollinger-Ellison syndrome have ratios of basal to maximum acid output

that are less than 60 per cent. Although detection of basal gastric acid hypersecretion may be of value in raising the suspicion of the diagnosis, neither its recognition or absence, nor the ratio of basal to maximal stimulated acid secretion can serve to establish or exclude the diagnosis of the Zollinger-Ellison syndrome.

Barium Contrast Radiographic Examination

Radiographic abnormalities may be of value in suggesting or supporting the diagnosis in patients with the Zollinger-Ellison syndrome (Fig. 49–4). The gastric rugal folds are often extremely prominent, and the stomach may contain large amounts of fluid. Large gastric folds in patients with the Zollinger-Ellison syndrome may be similar to those in patients with Menetrier's disease, gastric lymphoma, or other infiltrative processes. Prominent gastric mucosal folds, especially those on the greater curvature, also may occur occasionally in normal individuals and in patients with common peptic ulcer. In patients with the Zollinger-Ellison syndrome, mucosal folds also may be prominent throughout the duodenum and, in some instances, in the jejunum. The duodenum may be dilated. The normally fine small intestinal mucosal folds may be thickened and widened, and loops of small intestine may be abnormally separated from one another. Large amounts of fluid may be present in the lumen of the small intestine and may be associated with irregular flocculation of barium.

Although in patients with the Zollinger-Ellison syndrome barium examination of the upper gastrointes-

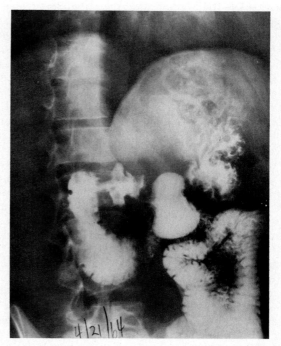

Figure 49–4. Large greater curvature and duodenal ulcers associated with the Zollinger-Ellison syndrome. Note also the edematous gastric and small bowel folds. (Courtesy of M. H. Sleisenger, M.D.)

tinal tract may be of value in identifying the consequences of excess gastrin release—ulcer disease or hypersecretion of fluid, or both—it seldom identifies the location of the gastrinoma. Gastrinomas in the pancreas are almost never identified by upper gastrointestinal barium examination. However, tumors arising within the wall of the duodenum or, more rarely, in the stomach or in other portions of the intestinal tract may occasionally be identified by barium studies.

Serum Gastrin

The most sensitive and specific method for identifying patients with the Zollinger-Ellison syndrome is demonstration of increased serum gastrin concentrations by radioimmunoassay.[6, 40] In normal subjects and in patients with common duodenal ulcer, fasting serum gastrin concentrations average approximately 50 to 60 pg/ml (or less), with an upper limit of normal, in most laboratories, approximating 150 mg/ml.[41] Patients with gastrinoma almost always have fasting serum gastrin levels greater than 150 mg/ml and may have serum gastrin concentrations as high as 450,000 pg/ml. Markedly increased fasting serum gastrin concentrations (greater than 1000 pg/ml) in patients with compatible clinical features and gastric acid hypersecretion establish the diagnosis of the Zollinger-Ellison syndrome.

It must be emphasized that marked hypergastrinemia is not specific for patients with gastrinoma. Strikingly elevated serum gastrin concentrations are found in many patients with pernicious anemia.[42] Approximately three fourths of patients with pernicious anemia have increased serum gastrin levels. Mean serum gastrin concentrations in patients with pernicious anemia approximate 1000 pg/ml and are in the same range as in patients with gastrinomas. Hypergastrinemia in patients with pernicious anemia appears to be produced by at least two mechanisms. First, there is an increase in the number of gastrin-containing cells (G cells) in the gastric mucosa of patients with pernicious anemia. (In general, in pernicious anemia the atrophic inflammatory process involves principally the mucosa of the body and fundus of the stomach with relative sparing of the antral mucosa, the normal residence of gastrin.) Second, in pernicious anemia there is failure of the normal acid-gastrin feedback control mechanism, which is important in regulation of antral gastrin release. The principal mechanism for inhibition of gastrin release in normal subjects is acidification of the antral contents; when the pH of antral contents is reduced to 3 (or lower), gastrin release is inhibited, and when the pH is reduced to 1.5, gastrin release is eliminated.[45] In pernicious anemia the pH of the gastric contents, even in response to maximal stimulation, is not reduced below 6. Instillation of 0.1 M hydrochloric acid into the stomachs of patients with pernicious anemia reduces increased serum gastrin toward normal levels.[40]

Patients with other varieties of gastric atrophy with chronic gastritis and substantially reduced or absent gastric acid secretion also frequently exhibit increased serum gastrin levels. These include patients with chronic gastritis and hypochlorhydria or achlorhydria in the absence of pernicious anemia, as well as those with gastric carcinoma with reduced or absent gastric acid secretion.[44–46] These groups of patients tend to have serum gastrin concentrations that are lower than those found in patients with pernicious anemia, but commonly higher than in normal subjects.

Elevated serum gastrin concentrations also have been reported in an assortment of other clinical states, including rheumatoid arthritis, vitiligo, and diabetes mellitus in the presence or absence of gastroparesis. Increased fasting serum gastrin levels have also been described in patients and experimental animals with renal insufficiency, in patients with the retained and excluded antrum syndrome, and in some patients with massive resection of the small intestine.[47–50] Hypergastrinemia in patients with renal insufficiency, in general, correlates directly with the severity of renal impairment. Hypergastrinemia was believed originally to be secondary to reduced renal cortical degradation of gastrin. However, it is unlikely that this explanation is complete or correct, since anephric patients exhibit normal rates of gastrin clearance. The mechanism for hypergastrinemia, which is usually transient, reported in some patients with massive intestinal resection has not been defined, but appears not to be due exclusively to reduced intestinal degradation of gastrin.[50] Small intestinal resection may remove the site of release of intestinal hormone(s) which normally inhibit gastrin release. Increased serum gastrin concentrations also have been described in patients with pheochromocytoma, with hypergastrinemia believed to be secondary to catecholamine-stimulated gastrin release.[51] Increased serum gastrin levels may be found in a very small proportion of patients with duodenal ulcer disease due to antral gastrin cell (G cell) hyperplasia and hyperfunction.[52]

Several *provocative tests* have been applied to identify patients with the Zollinger-Ellison syndrome.[53–59] These tests are of greatest value in those patients without striking hypergastrinemia, because, as indicated previously, in patients with compatible clinical presentation, marked gastric acid hypersecretion, and fasting serum gastrin concentrations that exceed 1000 pg/ml, the diagnosis of the Zollinger-Ellison syndrome is established. However, in patients with a clinical course consistent with, or suggestive of, the Zollinger-Ellison syndrome and marginal or slightly increased serum gastrin concentrations (150 to less than 1000 pg/ml), performance of provocative tests may be necessary to identify or exclude gastrinoma. Three major provocative tests have been used: (1) intravenous secretin injection, (2) intravenous calcium infusion, and (3) ingestion of a standard test meal, each performed with multiple measurements of serum gastrin concentrations.

In normal individuals and in patients with common duodenal ulcer, *intravenous secretin* slightly decreases, has no significant effect, or slightly increases serum gastrin levels.[60] In contrast, in patients with the Zollinger-Ellison syndrome, intravenous secretin evokes an often dramatic increase in serum gastrin concentration.[56, 57] The secretin injection test is the provocative test of greatest value in identifying patients with gastrinomas. Confident and consistent interpretations of the test have been difficult because performance of the test has not been well standardized; that is, different investigators have used different methods of administration (intravenous injection or infusion), different types of secretin (pure or impure), different doses of secretin, and different interpretation of positive responses, and radioimmunoassay has been performed in different laboratories with variable precision and antibody specificity.

The following is recommended as a method for performance and interpretation of the intravenous secretion injection test in patients suspected to have the Zollinger-Ellison syndrome.[61] Pure porcine GIH secretin (Kabi Group, Inc., Greenwich, CT), 2 units/kg, is given by intravenous injection over a 30-second interval. Serum samples are obtained for radioimmunoassay measurement of gastrin five minutes before administration of secretin, immediately before secretin administration, at two and five minutes, and then at five-minute intervals for a total of 30 minutes after secretin injection. In patients with gastrinoma serum gastrin concentrations increase promptly by at least 200 pg/ml (usually at two minutes and virtually always by ten minutes) after intravenous secretin injection (Fig. 49–5). The serum gastrin concentration then returns gradually to or toward the pre-injection level. An alternative and commonly used method for performance of the test employs GIH secretin, 1 unit/kg given by intravenous injection, with increases in serum gastrin levels greater than 110 pg/ml being characteristic of patients with gastrinoma.[62] Boot's secretin should not be used in the secretin injection test for gastrinoma, in part because it is much less potent than GIH secretin, but, more important, because it contains materials immunoreactive with many gastrin antibodies, which may produce spuriously elevated serum gastrin levels and erroneous false-positive results.[63]

In the *calcium infusion* test, calcium, as calcium gluconate, has been given by constant intravenous infusion at a rate of 5 mg of calcium per kilogram body weight per hour for a three-hour period. Serum samples are obtained for gastrin radioimmunoassay 30 minutes before initiation of calcium infusion, at the time when calcium infusion is begun, and at 30 minute intervals thereafter for four hours. In most patients with the Zollinger-Ellison syndrome, intravenous calcium infusion evokes substantial increases in serum gastrin concentrations, usually more than a 400 pg/ml increase, with smaller increases in patients with common duodenal ulcer. Maximum serum gastrin concentrations are usually achieved during the final hour of intravenous calcium infusion.

The third provocative test is that of *feeding a standard meal*; one meal proposed for this purpose includes one slice of bread, 200 ml of milk, one boiled egg, and 50 gm of cheese. This meal contains 20 gm of fat, 30 gm of protein, and 25 gm of carbohydrate. Serum samples for gastrin radioimmunoassay are obtained 15 minutes before and immediately before initiation of the meal, and then at 15-minute intervals for 90 minutes. In patients with gastrinomas the serum gastrin level does not increase or increases only slightly; the highest serum gastrin concentration after feeding is less than 50 per cent greater than the fasting serum gastrin level. In contrast, in patients with gastrin cell hyperplasia and hyperfunction serum gastrin levels usually increase strikingly (by more than 200 per cent) after ingestion of the standard meal.

Interpretation of Serum Gastrin. The characteristic serum gastrin profile in patients with gastrinoma includes fasting hypergastrinemia (greater than 150 pg/ml), prompt and substantial increase in serum gastrin in response to intravenous secretin (increase by more than 200 pg/ml), marked increase in serum gastrin concentration with calcium infusion (increase by more than 400 pg/ml), and a failure to increase the serum gastrin level by more than 50 per cent after a standard meal. The most frequent error in interpretation of

Figure 49–5. Serum gastrin responses to intravenous secretin injection (left) and to intravenous calcium infusion (right) in a patient with gastrinoma.

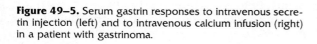
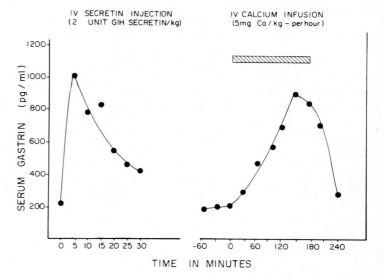

Table 49–1. COMPARISON OF SERUM GASTRIN RESPONSE*

Disorder	Calcium Infusion	Secretin Injection	Test Meal
Zollinger-Ellison syndrome (gastrinoma)	Exaggerated release of gastrin (usually serum gastrin increases by more than 400 pg/ml)	Substantial increase in serum gastrin (increase is usually greater than 200 pg/ml)	Little or no increase in serum gastrin (increase is less than 50%)
Antral G cell hyperfunction	May or may not have increase in serum gastrin greater than 400 pg/ml	Decrease, no change, or slight increase in serum gastrin (no increase greater than 200 pg/ml)	Exaggerated release of gastrin in response to feeding (increase by greater than 200%)
Common duodenal ulcer	Small increase in serum gastrin (less than 400 pg/ml)	Decrease, no change, or slight increase in serum gastrin (no increase greater than 200 pg/ml)	Moderate increase in serum gastrin (often slightly more than normal, but less than in G-cell hyperfunction)

*The responses indicated are based on currently available experience and must be viewed as tentative and subject to change as further information becomes available.

fasting serum gastrin levels is the presumption of a diagnosis of gastrinoma upon detection of hypergastrinemia. Achlorhydria or hypochlorhydria is a much more common cause of hypergastrinemia than is gastrinoma. When hypergastrinemia is identified, studies should be performed to determine the presence of gastric acid hypersecretion or, alternatively, achlorhydria (or acid hyposecretion).[64] This determination should be performed before initiating any provocative tests, such as secretin stimulation. Achlorhydria or profound hypochlorhydria can readily account for strikingly increased serum gastrin levels and, in such circumstances, no further search for gastrinoma is justified.

The provocative tests in the Zollinger-Ellison syndrome are summarized in Table 49–1. With intravenous injection of secretin, a positive response (increase greater than 200 pg/ml) occurs in over 95 per cent of patients with proven gastrinoma.[61] It is difficult to be certain of the true incidence of false-negative tests in patients with gastrinomas, because of variability in testing procedures, radioimmunoassay methods, and interpretation and difficulties in identifying occult gastrinoma even at surgery. False-positive tests with intravenous secretin, performed as suggested above and in Table 49–1, have been reported rarely.

The calcium infusion test is less sensitive and less specific than the secretin injection test in identifying patients with gastrinomas. Exaggerated gastrin release in response to calcium infusion is rarely, if ever, observed in patients with gastrinoma in the absence of a positive gastrin release response to secretin. Exaggerated gastrin release in response to calcium infusion occurs in more than 80 per cent of patients with gastrinoma. This exaggerated response to calcium infusion is not usually observed in normal subjects nor in patients with common duodenal ulcer. However, it may be obtained in some patients (approximately 50 per cent) with hypergastrinemia of antral origin, e.g., achlorhydria, in the presence or absence of pernicious anemia. For the reasons cited above, the calcium infusion test does not appear to have a role in the clinical diagnosis of the Zollinger-Ellison syndrome and related entities.

In a very small proportion of patients with duodenal ulcer, gastric acid hypersecretion is accompanied by elevated serum gastrin concentrations, which appear to be secondary to antral gastrin-cell (G-cell) hyperplasia and hyperfunction.[52, 59] Elevated serum gastrin levels in these patients are usually less than 1000 pg/ml. These subjects may be distinguished from those with gastrinomas by measurements of serum gastrin after secretin infusion and after the test meal. In contrast to patients with gastrinomas, patients with antral gastrin-cell hyperfunction show decreases, no change, or only slight increases in serum gastrin levels after intravenous secretin injection. Following the test meal these patients exhibit marked increases in serum gastrin concentrations (greater than 200 per cent increase); these increases greatly exceed those of normal subjects and patients with common duodenal ulcer or gastrinoma. Antral G-cell hyperplasia and hyperfunction, therefore, is characterized by gastric acid hypersecretion, elevated fasting serum gastrin concentrations, exaggerated gastrin release in response to feeding, and serum gastrin levels that do not increase dramatically after intravenous injection of secretin. The meal-stimulation test is not necessary in the evaluation of most patients in whom the Zollinger-Ellison syndrome is considered and usually provides less useful information than the secretin injection test.

Aspiration of gastric juice has been reported to reduce serum gastrin concentrations in some patients with gastrinoma.[65] Reduction of hypergastrinemia in Zollinger-Ellison patients by aspiration of gastric contents may be due to elimination of acid-induced stimulation of secretin release from the mucosa of the proximal small intestine.

In summation, in identifying patients with gastrinomas, the most valuable diagnostic information is detection of striking hypergastrinemia accompanied by acid hypersecretion and clinical features consistent with the Zollinger-Ellison syndrome. In patients with less prominent hypergastrinemia (less than 1000 pg/ml), performance of the intravenous secretin provocative test usually serves to identify or exclude gastrinoma. The secretin injection test is recommended in preference to the calcium infusion test because of its safety and its greater specificity and sensitivity. In patients with hypergastrinemia and gastric acid hypersecretion in whom gastrinoma has been excluded by the intravenous secretin test, a meal-stimulated test is recommended to determine whether excess gastrin release, characteristic of gastrin cell hyperplasia and hyperfunction, is present or absent in the patient.

Tumor Localization

Localization of gastrinomas is often difficult and frequently impossible even at surgery. In approximately 40 to 45 per cent of patients with clinical and laboratory evidence of gastrinomas, the tumor cannot be identified at surgery.[21–25] Imaging studies that have been utilized in efforts to localize tumors have included computerized axial tomography (CT scan), ultrasonography, and selective arteriography. Initial studies with selective arteriography in efforts to localize gastrinomas were disappointing, with only approximately 13 to 25 per cent of gastrinomas identified at surgery being detected, with a high frequency of false-positive arteriographic studies (70 per cent).[66–68] More recently, selective arteriography and computerized tomography have been reported to each detect about one third of patients with clinical and biochemical evidence of gastrinoma (approximately 60 per cent of those found at surgery). Performance of both selective arteriography and computerized tomography has been reported to detect 44 per cent of gastrinomas in Zollinger-Ellison patients and 80 per cent of those which could be located at surgery.[24] Ultrasound was found to be less sensitive, being positive in only about 15 per cent of patients with evidence of gastrinoma. Transhepatic portal venous sampling with identification of localized serum gastrin gradients, a technically demanding procedure, has also been utilized in efforts to localize gastrinoma, yielding results comparable to or slightly superior to the best results with computerized tomography.[24, 68–70] There is some evidence that this procedure may identify small gastrinomas not located by selective arteriography, computerized tomography, or surgical exploration. Selective venous sampling should not be used in efforts to distinguish patients with gastrinoma from those with other causes of hypergastrinemia, nor to select patients with the Zollinger-Ellison syndrome with MEN I for exploratory laparotomy, since attempts at gastrinoma resection are not justified in those patients.

TREATMENT

A variety of factors must be considered in the selection of treatment from the various therapeutic alternatives that are available for patients with the Zollinger-Ellison syndrome. Considerations regarding treatment selection in patients with the Zollinger-Ellison syndrome include those related to their ulcer disease and/or diarrhea secondary to gastric acid hy-

persecretion produced by gastrin released from the gastrinoma, and to those related to the potentially malignant biologic behavior of the tumor.[3] Selection of appropriate therapy for individual patients with the Zollinger-Ellison syndrome must be individualized. Choice of the best treatment may be difficult and, in some instances, may be controversial. Both medical and surgical treatment alternatives must be considered carefully on behalf of each patient with Zollinger-Ellison syndrome.

Medical Treatment

Until the availability of H_2-receptor antagonists there had been no generally effective medical therapy for patients with the Zollinger-Ellison syndrome. The development of H_2-receptor antagonists has provided therapeutic agents that are effective in reducing gastric acid secretion, producing symptom relief, and inducing ulcer healing in these patients.[71, 72] Cimetidine, the first and most widely used H_2-receptor antagonist, was shown to decrease gastric acid secretion, improve clinical symptoms, and induce ulcer healing in approximately 80 to 85 per cent of patients with the Zollinger-Ellison syndrome. The doses of H_2-receptor antagonists required in treatment of patients with the Zollinger-Ellison syndrome exceed substantially those used in treatment of common duodenal ulcer. Cimetidine dosage is necessary at four- to six-hour intervals, usually requiring 5 to 9 gm per day. More recently, H_2-receptor antagonists of greater potency, ranitidine and famotidine, have been shown to be as effective as or more effective than cimetidine in the treatment of ulcer disease in patients with the Zollinger-Ellison syndrome.[73] Average total daily doses of H_2-receptor antagonist reported to be required to reduce gastric acid secretion to satisfactory levels in patients with the Zollinger-Ellison syndrome have been 7.8 gm (range 1.2 to 13.2 gm) for cimetidine, 2.1 gm (range 0.6 to 3.6 gm) for ranitidine, and 0.24 gm (range 0.08 to 0.48 gm) for famotidine.[73] The duration of action of famotidine has been estimated to be approximately 30 per cent longer than that of cimetidine and ranitidine.

Assessment of symptoms has been found not to correlate closely with ulcer healing response or ulcer recurrence in Zollinger-Ellison patients treated with H_2-receptor antagonists.[74] Ulcer disease may continue or recur in patients with the Zollinger-Ellison syndrome treated with H_2-receptor antagonists in the absence of clinical symptoms. For this reason, it has been proposed that the dosage of H_2-receptor antagonist be selected that reduces gastric acid output to less than 10 mEq/hr for a one- or two-hour period immediately preceding the next scheduled dose of H_2-receptor antagonist.[74] There is no evidence that treatment with H_2-receptor antagonist influences, either adversely or favorably, serum gastrin levels or the biologic behavior of the gastrinoma. Anticholinergic agents, including selective M_1 antagonists such as pirenzepine, have been utilized to enhance the effectiveness of concurrent administration of H_2-receptor antagonists in reducing gastric acid secretion in patients with the Zollinger-Ellison syndrome.

Treatment with H_2-receptor antagonists is indicated as initial treatment of patients with the Zollinger-Ellison syndrome as well as for prolonged treatment of those patients who are poor candidates for resection of the gastrinoma, for whom attempted resection of tumor has been unsuccessful and in whom total gastrectomy is not performed. When instituted for long-term management of patients with the Zollinger-Ellison syndrome H_2-receptor antagonist treatment should not lapse or be interrupted, since discontinuance is often followed by ulcer recurrence, frequently with complications including hemorrhage or perforation, or both.

It is not unusual for Zollinger-Ellison patients who were initially responsive to become resistant to treatment with H_2-receptor antagonists. With long-term treatment and extended observation as many as 50 per cent of patients with the Zollinger-Ellison syndrome have been reported to fail with H_2-receptor antagonist treatment.[75] The development of omeprazole has provided a potent antisecretory agent that is effective in inducing striking reductions in gastric acid secretion associated with ulcer healing and symptom relief in patients with the Zollinger-Ellison syndrome.[76-78] Omeprazole, a substituted benzimidazole, is an inhibitor of hydrogen potassium ATPase, the proton pump that is considered to constitute the terminal step in parietal cell secretion of hydrogen ions. Omeprazole, which reduces acid secretion by 77 to 100 per cent, has been found to be effective in Zollinger-Ellison patients whose symptoms were not adequately controlled by high doses of H_2-receptor antagonists with or without pirenzepine. Treatment of patients with the Zollinger-Ellison syndrome with omeprazole, including those considered to be resistant to treatment with H_2-receptor antagonists, has resulted in ulcer healing in more than 60 per cent at two weeks and in 90 to 100 per cent at four weeks. The daily dose required in most patients is from 60 to 80 mg per day in a single dose.

Somatostatin is known to inhibit gastric acid secretion and to inhibit release of a variety of hormones, including gastrin. Somatostatin reduces gastric acid secretion both by direct inhibitory effects of somatostatin on the parietal cell and by its effects in inhibiting gastrin release. Use of somatostatin as a therapeutic agent has been limited by its brief half-life. A synthetic analog of somatostatin (SMS201-995, Sandoz), with a much longer duration of biologic action, has been administered to patients with the Zollinger-Ellison syndrome.[79] This somatostatin analog reduced serum gastrin levels substantially for 16 hours and decreased gastric acid secretion for as long as 18 hours.

Patients with metastatic gastrinoma have been treated with a variety of chemotherapeutic programs, including streptozotocin, streptozotocin with 5-fluorouracil, or both agents with doxorubicin.[80-82] Decreases in both metastatic tumor mass and serum gastrin levels have been reported in more than half of patients treated by intra-arterial administration of streptozotocin. Because of reduced nephrotoxicity, the arterial route may be preferable to intravenous administration.[81] Chemotherapy in patients with metastatic gastrinoma may serve a useful role in reducing tumor size and improving symptoms due to invasive or mass effects of the tumor. Chemotherapy has no primary therapeutic role in attempts to reduce gastric acid hypersecretion and consequent ulcer disease associated with gastrinoma.

Surgical Treatment

Since shortly after general clinical recognition of the Zollinger-Ellison syndrome, total gastrectomy has been considered to be the surgical procedure of choice in treatment of patients with this syndrome. This conclusion has been based on recognition that mortality was lowest among those patients with the Zollinger-Ellison syndrome in whom total gastrectomy was performed as the initial surgical procedure, and not as a final procedure following earlier surgical attempts to treat the ulcer disease (Fig. 49–6). Total gastrectomy does remove the major target organ for gastrin and is therefore effective in curing the ulcer disease.

Earlier studies suggested that only a very small proportion of gastrinomas, probably less than 10 per cent, could be resected completely in Zollinger-Ellison patients. With enhanced methods for tumor detection

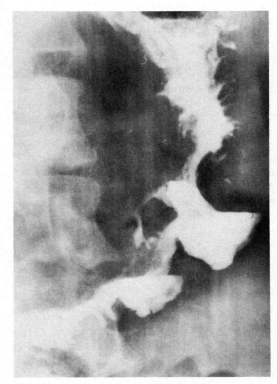

Figure 49–6. Huge jejunal ulcer in Zollinger-Ellison syndrome after subtotal gastrectomy. (Courtesy of M. H. Sleisenger, M.D.)

and localization it now appears that approximately 20 to 25 per cent of gastrinomas can be completely removed surgically with resultant cure.[22, 23, 83–85] Complete tumor removal is more often possible with extrapancreatic, extraintestinal gastrinomas, or gastrinomas located in the duodenal wall.[17, 19, 23] Approximately half of extrapancreatic gastrinomas that are identified can be completely resected.

Surgical resection, when possible, is the optimum treatment for patients with the Zollinger-Ellison syndrome. Patients with the Zollinger-Ellison syndrome should have a careful preoperative evaluation in an attempt to localize the gastrinoma. Surgical exploration should be performed, with the intention to resect the gastrinoma, in all patients with the Zollinger-Ellison syndrome except for those in whom surgery is contraindicated, in those with extensive metastatic disease, and in patients with MEN I. The invariably multifocal nature of gastrinomas in patients with MEN I makes it inadvisable to recommend attempts at surgical removal of gastrinoma in these patients. If gastrinoma is identified at surgery and is resectable, complete surgical removal is recommended. When this is performed successfully, it is not necessary to include gastrectomy. If at the time of abdominal exploration there is no evidence of metastasis or if metastasis is limited to regional lymph nodes, it is unlikely that these patients will succumb to metastatic disease.[85] The presence of demonstrable hepatic metastasis is an ominous finding in patients with gastrinoma.[82, 85] These patients usually continue with invasive tumor extension and death. When surgical removal of metastatic gastrinoma in the liver is possible, aggressive resection of metastatic gastrinoma with favorable clinical responses has been reported.[82] When surgical removal of hepatic metastases to the liver cannot be accomplished, therapeutic alternatives include chemotherapy and/or occlusion of the hepatic artery supplying the tumor by embolization of autologous clot. Reduction of metastatic hepatic tumor mass and associated symptoms can usually be achieved as palliative treatment with chemotherapy or tumor infarction produced by hepatic arterial embolization.[80–82, 86] These two modalities should be considered for treatment of patients with symptoms associated with substantial metastases of gastrinoma to the liver. It is important to attempt to distinguish hepatic metastatic disease from relatively rare primary hepatic gastrinomas, which may be readily cured by complete removal of the hepatic tumor.[19]

It has been estimated that using currently available diagnostic and surgical methods, it should be possible to resect gastrinomas successfully and thereby effect cure in approximately 25 per cent of Zollinger-Ellison patients with sporadic gastrinomas (non–MEN I) and in over 70 per cent of those who appear to have a solitary tumor. Total pancreatectomy is rarely, if ever, justified. Surgical options in those patients in whom gastrinomas cannot be localized and/or resected include total gastrectomy and proximal gastric vagotomy. Performance of proximal gastric vagotomy in patients with gastrinoma substantially reduces gastric acid secretion and reduces the doses of H_2-receptor antagonist required to treat the ulcer disease in these patients.[23] In a small portion of patients with gastrinoma, antisecretory drugs may not be required following proximal gastric vagotomy.

Decisions for Treatment

Appropriate decisions regarding selection of therapy for patients with gastrinoma are influenced by recognition that these tumors are often multifocal, usually malignant and slowly progressive, and frequently metastatic at the time of diagnosis, and that the tumors, even after careful preoperative evaluation and examination at surgery, often cannot be located.

The following is proposed as general guidelines for selection of therapy in patients with the Zollinger-Ellison syndrome. H_2-receptor antagonists (and omeprazole) are generally effective treatment and should be used for preoperative control in Zollinger-Ellison patients and during evaluation, as well as in treatment of those gastrinoma patients in whom surgery is not possible and when tumor cannot be found or resected. Following careful evaluation in an attempt to localize the gastrinoma, surgical exploration directed to resection of the tumor should be performed in all patients with the Zollinger-Ellison syndrome except those with MEN I. When a solitary tumor is found and is apparently completely resected, there is no need for total gastrectomy. Aggressive surgical removal of metastatic gastrinoma may benefit selected patients with invasive metastatic disease. When the diagnosis of gastrinoma appears certain, but despite maximum efforts it is not possible to localize the tumor, the physician and patient are faced with a difficult therapeutic decision. The options that should be considered by the physician and patient include lifelong treatment with an H_2-receptor antagonist, total gastrectomy, or a lesser surgical procedure such as proximal gastric vagotomy. In those patients in whom at surgical exploration gastrinoma cannot be found or resected, proximal gastric vagotomy is recommended; proximal vagotomy will reduce gastric acid secretion and will reduce and, in a minority of patients, will eliminate the dose of H_2-receptor antagonist required to control ulcer disease. In those patients in whom lifelong treatment with an H_2-treatment antagonist is not possible or accepted and in whom complete gastrinoma resection is not possible, total gastrectomy should be performed.

PROGNOSIS

Treatment with H_2-receptor antagonists usually induces substantial reductions in gastric acid secretion, improvement or disappearance of ulcer symptoms, and ulcer healing in patients with the Zollinger-Ellison syndrome. The H_2-receptor antagonist should be continued indefinitely, because of frequent, prompt, and often aggressive ulcer recurrence after discontinuance of the drug. H_2-receptor antagonist treatment has negligible effects on serum gastrin levels in patients with gastrinomas.

The optimum treatment for patients with the Zollinger-Ellison syndrome is complete surgical removal of the gastrinoma. With currently available diagnostic and therapeutic methods, this can be achieved in approximately 25 per cent of patients with gastrinoma who do not have MEN I. Complete tumor removal is followed promptly by reductions in serum gastrin levels and rates of gastric acid secretion and by disappearance of ulcer disease and/or diarrhea. Patients in whom gastrinoma cannot be resected and who are treated by proximal gastric vagotomy are able to reduce their dose of antisecretory medication with good ulcer response to such treatment and, less commonly, may discontinue antisecretory medications.

As a result of removal of the target organ, symptoms in patients with gastrinoma improve dramatically and ulcers disappear following total gastrectomy. Patients with the Zollinger-Ellison syndrome treated by total gastrectomy are subject to the same complications as other patients after total gastrectomy. However, they live longer and exhibit less severe metabolic consequences than do patients in whom total gastrectomy is performed for carcinoma of the stomach. After total gastrectomy, these patients require intramuscular administration of vitamin B_{12} (100 µg per month). Oral administration of calcium and vitamin D is recommended in an effort to reduce the development of osteoporosis and osteomalacia, which occur commonly after total gastrectomy.

In most patients, serum gastrin concentrations remain unchanged after total gastric resection. In approximately one-third of Zollinger-Ellison patients there may be modest decreases in serum gastrin levels after total gastric resection.[87] This may reflect the absence of secretin-stimulated release of tumor gastrin due to elimination of contact of secreted gastric acid with secretin-secreting duodenal mucosa. In a very small number of patients with metastatic gastrinoma, regression of primary tumor and/or metastases has been reported after total gastrectomy.[87, 88] The explanation of this distinctly unusual event after total gastrectomy is not understood, although ablation of trophic influences on the gastrinoma exerted by the stomach has been suggested. Substantial progressive increases in serum gastrin concentrations have been reported to parallel invasive and metastatic tumor progression.

Because of earlier diagnosis and more effective therapeutic alternatives, malignant invasion by tumor has replaced ulcer complication as the major factor responsible for mortality in patients with gastrinoma. Poorest survival is among patients with sporadic gastrinoma unassociated with MEN I, especially in those with hepatic metastases.[22, 85] Life expectancy in these patients, without resective surgery, has been estimated to average approximately two years.[86] Complete resection of gastrinomas, which should be performed whenever possible, appears to be associated with an otherwise normal life expectancy and complete resolution of ulcer disease.

RELATIONSHIP BETWEEN THE ZOLLINGER-ELLISON SYNDROME AND MULTIPLE ENDOCRINE NEOPLASIA (TYPE I)

Multiple endocrine neoplasia type I (MEN I) is an autosomal dominant disorder associated with a high degree of penetrance and substantial variability in expressivity.[29, 30] The endocrine glands most frequently involved with hyperplasia, adenoma, or carcinoma include the parathyroids, pancreatic islets, and pituitary, in that order. In addition, thyroid nodules, carcinoid tumors, and hyperplasia of the adrenal cortices have been noted in family members. Hyperparathyroidism has been detected in 87 per cent of patients with the MEN I syndrome, and gastrinoma has been found in 40 to 60 per cent of these patients. Approximately 25 per cent of patients with gastrinomas have been found to have MEN I or are members of families with MEN I. It has been noted that, with increasing age, those patients with hyperparathyroidism initially, who are members of families with this syndrome, frequently progress later to development of the Zollinger-Ellison syndrome. The development of hyperparathyroidism, with associated hypercalcemia, in patients with MEN I may unmask a latent gastrinoma.[89] This results from the effects of calcium in inducing gastrin release from the gastrinoma, which may then produce clinical manifestations of the Zollinger-Ellison syndrome.

The possibility of gastrinoma should be considered in all first-degree relatives of patients with MEN I. Fasting serum gastrin levels should be measured and intravenous secretin provocative tests should be performed on first-degree members of these families. Determination of serum gastrin concentrations in MEN I family members in this manner provides a satisfactory method for identifying both latent and overt Zollinger-Ellison syndrome due to gastrinoma in this high-risk population of patients (see pp. 914 to 917). In the absence of gastrinoma or other reasons for hypergastrinemia, for example, achlorhydria, almost all patients with hyperparathyroidism have normal fasting serum gastrin levels.

ISLET CELL TUMORS CONTAINING MULTIPLE PEPTIDES

When sought for using immunocytochemical techniques, islet cell tumors have been shown almost invariably to contain multiple polypeptide hormones.[90–92] These peptides may or may not be released into the circulation with their resultant individual and diverse physiologic effects. In general, although these islet cell tumors contain multiple polypeptide hormones and may release more than one peptide hormone, there is usually one dominant hormone released by the tumor into the circulation that is responsible for the clinical manifestations in symptomatic patients, for example, gastric acid hypersecretion and ulcer disease secondary to hypergastrinemia in patients with gastrinomas.

Etiology and Pathogenesis. The mechanism responsible for development of tumors containing multiple peptides and the factors resulting in selective release of the dominant circulating peptide with its associated pathophysiologic consequences have not been elucidated. An islet cell carcinoma of the pancreas has been described that contained large amounts of ACTH, melanocyte-stimulating hormone, gastrin, and glucagon.[90] Islet tumors have also been described containing parathyroid hormone, antidiuretic hormone, growth hormone releasing factor (GRF), vasoactive intestinal peptide, and pancreatic polypeptide, among others.[90–92]

ACTH is particularly frequent in endocrine tumors containing multiple polypeptide hormones. Approximately 30 per cent of gastrinomas display ACTH-like immunoreactivity. In most instances biologically significant amounts are not released into the circulation. However, increased serum ACTH levels with associated Cushing's syndrome have been noted in 8 per cent of 75 patients with the Zollinger-Ellison syndrome.[93] Three of the 59 patients (5 per cent) with sporadic gastrinoma had Cushing's syndrome, with severe symptoms produced by ACTH secretion by the islet cell tumor. Each of those patients had metastatic gastrinoma, which responded poorly to chemotherapy, and each died within three years of diagnosis. Three of 16 MEN I patients (19 per cent) with the Zollinger-Ellison syndrome had Cushing's syndrome consequent to pituitary release of ACTH and, in general, their symptoms are mild. Gastrinomas in those patients were not metastatic and prognosis was excellent.

Careful evaluation has indicated that 30 to 40 per cent of patients with the Zollinger-Ellison syndrome as a manifestation of gastrinoma have laboratory and/or clinical evidence of excess release of additional peptide hormones either from tumors in other locations, such as parathyroid or pituitary, or from the gastrinoma-containing islet cell tumor.[94] Patients with pancreatic islet cell tumors containing and releasing gastrin and glucagon may exhibit clinical manifestations of both Zollinger-Ellison and glucagonoma syndromes.[95]

Increases in serum pancreatic polypeptide concentration may be due to rare pancreatic polypeptide–secreting tumors, or be caused by release from pancreatic polypeptide cells from mixed endocrine cell tumors of the pancreas, or, most commonly, be associated with hyperplasia of pancreatic polypeptide cells, often accompanying islet tumors of the pancreas, including gastrinomas.[91, 95–97] Increased serum pancreatic polypeptide levels have not, as yet, been associated with production of a recognized characteristic clinical syndrome. Serum concentrations of pancreatic polypeptide are increased in 10 to 20 per cent of patients with gastrinoma. Although the increase in gastrinoma

patients as a group is significant, the frequency of this increase is insufficient to make this determination a marker of value in identifying patients with gastrinoma.[98] In general, in normal subjects serum levels of pancreatic polypeptide increase with age. This variation of pancreatic polypeptide level with age must be taken into consideration in assessing the significance of potentially increased serum pancreatic polypeptide levels.

Peptide-containing and -secreting islet tumors of the pancreas, including gastrinomas, when examined by immunocytochemical techniques, have been found to stain positively for neuron-specific enolase, a marker of their neurocrine origin.[91, 92] Neuron-specific enolase has been localized by immunohistochemistry as diffuse cytoplasmic staining in neuroendocrine cells in these tumors. Twenty per cent of patients with malignant gastrinomas have been reported with increased serum concentrations of alpha–human chorionic gonadotropin (α-hCG).[99] Patients with extensive metastatic gastrinoma are more likely to have strikingly increased α-hCG serum levels. Increased serum α-HcG levels have not been found in patients with benign gastrinoma.

Clinical Features and Diagnosis. The clinical features and necessary diagnostic measures are dictated by the single or multiple peptides released by these islet cell tumors. The physician should be aware of the potential of islet cell tumors, such as gastrinomas, to secrete additional peptides with resulting endocrine disorders. The frequency of ACTH-secreting gastrinomas deserves special attention in patients with the Zollinger-Ellison syndrome.

Treatment. When possible, the preferred teatment of these tumors is resection, which, when complete, results in relief of symptoms caused by release of the physiologically active hormonal agents.

Prognosis. Total removal of the tumor produces disappearance of the pathophysiologic manifestations of excess hormone release. Solitary gastrinomas that release multiple biologically active hormones tend to be more often malignant and to behave in an aggressive fashion. Tumors that are widely metastatic at the time of diagnosis may be benefited by attempts at surgical reduction of tumor mass and/or by treatment with chemotherapeutic agents, such as streptozotocin and/or 5-fluorouracil.

ISLET CELL HYPERPLASIA

In some patients with clinical features of the Zollinger-Ellison syndrome, marked hyperplasia of the islets of Langerhans may be found in the pancreas.[100]

Etiology and Pathogenesis. Islet cell hyperplasia is characterized by an increase in both the number and size of the islets of Langerhans in the pancreas; frequently the islets are also densely cellular. Islet cell hyperplasia in patients with the clinical symptom complex of the Zollinger-Ellison syndrome has been observed both in the presence and in the absence of demonstrated gastrinoma. The Zollinger-Ellison syndrome does not appear to be caused by islet hyperplasia, since removal of hyperplastic islet tissue does not result in resolution of the syndrome nor does it decrease serum gastrin concentrations. Gastrin has not been shown to be present in the hyperplastic islet cells, which frequently contain pancreatic polypeptide. It is believed, therefore, that islet cell hyperplasia in patients with Zollinger-Ellison syndrome is most commonly the result of or is associated with gastrinoma, which may or may not be able to be located. Islet cell hyperplasia appears to be associated with sporadic gastrinoma but not with MEN I, in which multiple microadenomas (less than 5 mm diameter) are characteristically present.[101]

Clinical Features and Diagnosis. The symptoms and complications in patients with the Zollinger-Ellison syndrome with hyperplasia of the islet cells are not distinguishable from those in other patients with demonstrable gastrinoma. Islet cell hyperplasia in the absence of identified gastrinoma may be found at surgery early in the course of the Zollinger-Ellison syndrome. Later, gastrinomas of the pancreas or other locations that escaped prior recognition may be found.

Treatment. Treatment of patients with symptoms and complications characteristic of the Zollinger-Ellison syndrome with islet cell hyperplasia is similar to that of other patients in whom gastrinoma is identified. Blind resection of the pancreas is not recommended in these patients.

Prognosis. In general, patients with hyperplasia of the islets of Langerhans with the Zollinger-Ellison syndrome have the same potential complications as those with recognized gastrinomas.

HYPERPARATHYROIDISM AND PEPTIC ULCER DISEASE

An assortment of questions remain to be answered concerning possible relationships between hyperparathyroidism and peptic ulcer disease. Some investigators have suggested that there is an increased incidence of peptic ulcer disease in patients with hyperparathyroidism; however, at present such an increased association of common peptic ulcer disease with hyperparathyroidism has not been proved. The frequency of peptic ulcer disease in the general population in the United States has been estimated to be approximately 10 to 15 per cent; however, the varying expressions of peptic ulcer disease make it difficult to make this estimate with satisfactory confidence.[102] Some retrospective studies of patients with hyperparathyroidism have suggested an incidence of peptic ulcer disease ranging from 20 to 30 per cent.[103, 104] Conversely, there have been reports of the incidence of ulcer disease with hyperthyroidism as low as 9.1 per cent, thus failing to affirm a clear-cut statistical association between hyperparathyroidism and peptic ulcer disease[105] (see pp. 490–491).

Clinical Features and Diagnosis. When peptic ulcer disease occurs in association with hyperparathyroidism and is not due to simultaneously occurring gastrinoma,

the clinical features are those of common peptic ulcer. The ulcer disease is more prevalent in males; 80 per cent of the ulcers are in the duodenum, and, just as with usual duodenal ulcer, almost always in its first portion. In contrast to the Zollinger-Ellison syndrome, marked gastric hypersecretion is not present. Following parathyroidectomy, there have been instances in which the rate of gastric acid secretion has decreased substantially. More commonly, there is no significant change in the status of the ulcer disease.[106–109] In many patients, the peptic ulcer responds to conventional therapy without parathyroidectomy. In other instances, symptoms have been reported to improve remarkably after parathyroidectomy.

Because of potential relationships between peptic ulcer and hyperparathyroidism, a variety of studies have been conducted in attempts to define factors that may relate serum calcium levels and gastric acid secretion. Patients with hypoparathyroidism, whose serum calcium levels are less than 7.0 mg/dl, are usually achlorhydric. Following treatment with calcium, vitamin D, or parathyroid hormone, with resultant elevation of plasma calcium to eucalcemic levels, gastric acid secretory rates usually return to normal.[110] In normal human subjects, calcium infusion, with consequent increases in plasma calcium concentrations, produces increases in gastric acid secretion and minimal increases in serum gastrin levels.[111] These related, and perhaps relevant, observations, however, do not substantiate a direct relationship between hyperparathyroidsm and peptic ulcer disease; nor do they prove that peptic ulcer disease, if resulting from hyperparathyroidism, is necessarily produced by excessive gastrin release.

A substantial portion of patient with hyperparathyroidism who develop peptic ulcer disease may harbor gastrinomas. This must be suspected particularly in individuals with elevated fasting serum gastrin concentrations. In order to enhance detection of such individuals, it is recommended that the secretin stimulation test be performed in patients with documented hyperparathyroidism and peptic ulcer. In general, in the absence of associated gastrinoma or other causes for hypergastrinemia, patients with hyperparathyroidism do not have increased serum gastrin levels.

Treatment. Treatment of peptic ulcer disease associated with hyperparathyroidism is that indicated for treatment of the two individual diseases. The approach to the hyperparathyroidism usually would be surgical, and the treatment of the peptic ulcer would be that indicated by the clinical features in the patient.

The presence of gastrinoma in these patients requires appropriate treatment for this disorder. In patients with gastrinoma and hyperparathyroidism, in addition to treatment with an H_2-receptor antagonist, it is recommended, when possible, that parathyroidectomy be performed.

Prognosis. The bulk of currently available information indicates that the prognosis of peptic ulcer disease in association with hyperparathyroidism is similar to that in usual peptic ulcer disease. When the ulcer disease is a manifestation of the Zollinger-Ellison syndrome, treatment and prognosis are the same as for MEN I patients with gastrinoma.

References

1. Zollinger, R. M., and Ellison, E. H. Primary peptic ulcerations of the jejunum associated with islet cell tumors of the pancreas. Ann. Surg. *142*:709, 1955.
2. Gregory, R. A., Tracy, H. J., French, J. M., and Sircus, W. Extraction of gastrin-like substance from pancreatic tumour in case of Zollinger-Ellison syndrome. Lancet *1*:1045, 1960.
3. Ellison, E. H., and Wilson, S. D. The Zollinger-Ellison syndrome: reappraisal and evaluation of 260 registered cases. Ann. Surg. *160*:512, 1964.
4. Wilson, S. D., and Ellison, E. H. Total gastric resection in children with the Zollinger-Ellison syndrome. Arch. Surg. *91*:165, 1965.
5. Gregory, R. A., Grossman, M. I., Tracy, H. J., and Bentley, P. H. Nature of gastric secretagogue in Zollinger-Ellison tumors. Lancet *2*:543, 1967.
6. McGuigan, J. E., and Trudeau, W. L. Immunochemical measurement of elevated levels of gastrin in the serum of patients with pancreatic tumors of the Zollinger-Ellison variety. N. Engl. J. Med. *278*:1308, 1968.
7. Gregory, R. A., Tracy, H. J., and Agarwal, K. L. Amino acid constitution of two gastrins isolated from Zollinger-Ellison tumor tissue. Gut *10*:603, 1969.
8. Greider, M. H., Rosai, J., and McGuigan, J. E. The human pancreatic islet cells and their tumors. II. Ulcerogenic and diarrheogenic tumors. Cancer *33*:1423, 1974.
9. Yalow, R. S., and Berson, S. A. Size and charge distinctions between endogenous human plasma gastrin in peripheral blood and heptadecapeptide gastrins. Gastroenterology *58*:609, 1970.
10. Rehfeld, J. F., Stadil, F., and Vikelsoe, J. Immunoreactive gastric components in human serum. Gut *15*:102, 1974.
11. Andersen, B. N., Petersen, B., Borch, K., and Rehfeld, J. F. Variations in the sulfation of circulating gastrins in gastrointestinal disease. Scand. J. Gastroenterol. *18*:565, 1983.
12. Kothary, P. C., Fabri, P. J., Gower, W., O'Dorisio, T. M., and Ellis, J. Evaluation of NH2-terminus gastrins in gastrinoma syndrome. J. Clin. Endocrinol. Metab. *62*:970, 1986.
13. Dockray, G. J., and Walsh, J. H. Amino terminal gastrin fragment in serum of Zollinger-Ellison syndrome patients. Gastroenterology *68*:222, 1975.
14. Way, L., Goldman, L., and Dunphy, J. E. Zollinger-Ellison syndrome: an analysis of twenty-five cases. Am. J. Surg. *116*:293, 1968.
15. Zollinger, R. M., and Moore, F. T. Zollinger-Ellison syndrome comes of age. JAMA *204*:361, 1968.
16. Thompson, J. C., Reeder, D. D., Villar, H. V. Natural history and experience with diagnosis and treatment of the Zollinger-Ellison syndrome. Surg. Gynecol. Obstet. *140*:5, 1975.
17. Hofmann, J. W., Fox, P. S., and Wilson, S. D. Duodenal wall tumors and the Zollinger-Ellison syndrome. Surgical management. Arch. Surg. *107*:334, 1973.
18. Fox, P. S., Hofmann, J. W., Wilson, S. D., and Decosse, J. J. Surgical management of the Zollinger-Ellison syndrome. Surg. Clin. North Am. *54*:395, 1974.
19. Wolfe, M. M., Alexander, R. W., and McGuigan, J. E. Extrapancreatic, extraintestinal gastrinoma: effective treatment by surgery. N. Engl J. Med. *306*:1533, 1982.
20. Bhagavan, B. S., Salvin, R. E., Goldberg, J., and Rao, R. N. Ectopic gastrinoma and Zollinger-Ellison syndrome. Hum. Pathol. *17*:584, 1986.
21. Thompson, J. C., Lewis, B. G., Weiner, I., and Townsend, C. M., Jr. The role of surgery in the Zollinger-Ellison syndrome. Ann. Surg. *197*:594, 1983.
22. Malagelada, J. R., Edis, A. J., Adson, M. A., van Heerden, J. A., and Go, V. L. Medical and surgical options in the management of patients with gastrinoma. Gastroenterology *84*:1524, 1983.
23. Richardson, C. T., Peters, M. N., Feldman, M., et al. Treatment of Zollinger-Ellison syndrome with exploratory laparotomy, proximal gastric vagotomy, and H$_2$-receptor antagonists. A prospective study. Gastroenterology *89*:357, 1985.
24. Cherner, J. A., Doppman, J. L., Norton, J. A., et al. Selective venous sampling for gastrin to localize gastrinomas. Ann. Intern. Med. *105*:841, 1986.
25. Stabile, B. E., Morrow, D. J., and Passaro, E., Jr. The gastrinoma triangle: operative implications. Am. J. Surg. *147*:25, 1984.
26. Stremple, J. F., and Watson, C. Serum calcium, serum gastrin, and gastric acid secretion before and after parathyroidectomy for hyperparathyroidism. Surgery *75*:841, 1974.
27. Cocco, A. E., and Conway, S. J. Zollinger-Ellison syndrome with ovarian mucinous cystadenocarcinoma. N. Engl. J. Med. *293*:485, 1975.
28. Long, T. T., Barton, T. K., Draffin, R., Reeves, W. J., and McCarty, K. S. Conservative management of the Zollinger-Ellison syndrome. JAMA *243*:1837, 1980.
29. Ballard, H. S., Frame, B., and Hartsock, R. J. Familial multiple endocrine adenoma–peptic ulcer complex. Medicine *43*:481, 1964.
30. Wermer, P. Multiple endocrine adenomatosis: multiple hormone producing tumors, a familial syndrome. *In* Bonfile S. (ed.) Endocrine-Secreting Tumors of the Gastrointestinal Tract. London, W. B. Saunders Company, 1974, p. 671.
31. Morgan, J. E., Kaiser, C. W., Johnson, W., et al. Gastric carcinoid (gastrinoma) associated with achlorhydria (pernicious anemia). Cancer *51*:2332, 1983.
32. Shimoda, S. S., Saunders, D. R., and Rubin, C. E. The Zollinger-Ellison syndrome with steatorrhea. Mechanisms of fat and vitamin B$_{12}$ malabsorption. Gastroenterology *55*:705, 1968.
33. Mansbach, C. M., Wilkins, R. M., Dobbins, W. O., and Taylor, M. P. Intestinal mucosal function and structure in the steatorrhea of Zollinger-Ellison syndrome. Arch. Intern. Med. *121*:487, 1968.
34. Guida, P. M., Todd, J. E., Moore, S. W., and Beal, J. M. Zollinger-Ellison syndrome with interesting variations. Am. J. Surg. *112*:807, 1966.
35. Shimoda, S. S., and Rubin, C. E. The Zollinger-Ellison syndrome with steatorrhea. Anticholinergic treatment followed by total gastrectomy and colon interposition. Gastroenterology *55*:695, 1968.
36. Shuster, F., and Alexander, H. C. Antacid relief of diarrhea in Zollinger-Ellison syndrome. JAMA *208*:2162, 1969.
37. Wright, H. K., Hersh, T., Floch, M. H., and Weinstein, L. D. Impaired intestinal absorption in the Zollinger-Ellison syndrome independent of gastric hypersecretion. Am. J. Surg. *119*:250, 1970.
38. Ayogi, T., and Summerskill, W. H. J. Gastric secretion with ulcerogenic islet cell tumor: importance of basal acid output. Arch. Intern. Med. *117*:667, 1966.
39. Marks, I. N., Selzer, G., Louw, J. H., and Bank, S. Zollinger-Ellison syndrome in Bantu woman, with isolation of gastrin-like substance from primary and secondary tumors. I. Case report. Gastroenterology *41*:77, 1961.
40. Yalow, R. S., and Berson, S. A. Radioimmunoassay of gastrin. Gastroenterology *58*:1, 1970.
41. Trudeau, W. L., and McGuigan, J. E. Serum gastrin levels in patients with peptic ulcer disease. Gastroenterology *59*:6, 1970.
42. McGuigan, J. E., and Trudeau, W. L. Serum gastrin concentrations in pernicious anemia. N. Engl. J. Med. *282*:358, 1970.
43. Unvas, B. Discussion of Schofield B. Inhibition by acid of gastrin release. *In* Grossman, M. I. (ed.). Gastrin (UCLA Forum in Medical Sciences No. 5). Berkeley, University of California Press, 1966, p. 186.
44. Korman, M. G., Strickland, R. G., and Hansky, J. Serum gastrin in chronic gastritis. Br. Med. J. *2*:16, 1971.
45. Ganguli, P. C., Cullen, D. R., and Irvine, W. J. Radioimmunoassay of plasma-gastrin in pernicious anemia, achlorhydria without pernicious anemia, hypochlorhydria, and in controls. Lancet *1*:155, 1971.
46. McGuigan, J. E., and Trudeau, W. L. Serum and tissue gastrin concentrations in patients with carcinoma of the stomach. Gastroenterology *64*:22, 1973.

47. Korman, M. G., Scott, D. H., Hansky, J., et al. Hypergastrinanemia due to an excluded gastric antrum: a proposed method of differentiation from the Zollinger-Ellison syndrome. Aust. N.Z. J. Med. 3:266, 1972.
48. Korman, M. G., Laver, M. C., and Hansky, J. Hypergastrinanemia in chronic renal failure. Br. Med. J. 1:209, 1972.
49. Davidson, W. D., Springberg, P. D., and Falkinburg, N. R. Renal extraction and excretion of endogenous gastrin in the dog. Gastroenterology 64:955, 1973.
50. Straus, E., Gerson, C. D., and Yalow, R. S. Hypersecretion of gastrin associated with the short bowel syndrome. Gastroenterology 66:175, 1974.
51. Hayes, J. R., Ardill, J., Kennedy, T. L., et al. Stimulation of gastrin release by catecholamines. Lancet 1:819, 1972.
52. Walsh, J. H., Nair, P. K., Kleibeuker, J., et al. Pathological acid secretion not due to gastrinoma. Scand. J. Gastroenterol. 82:45, 1983.
53. Trudeau, W. L., and McGuigan, J. E. Effects of calcium on serum gastrin in the Zollinger-Ellison syndrome. N. Engl. J. Med. 281:862, 1969.
54. Basso, N., and Passaro, E., Jr. Calcium-stimulated gastric secretion in the Zollinger-Ellison syndrome. Arch. Surg. 101:3399, 1970.
55. Passaro, E., Jr., Basso, N., Sanchez, R. E., and Gordon, H. E. Newer studies in the Zollinger-Ellison syndrome. Am. J. Surg. 120:138, 1970.
56. Isenberg, J. I., Walsh, J. H., Passaro, E., Jr., et al. Unusual effect of secretin on serum gastrin, serum calcium, and gastric acid secretion in a patient with suspected Zollinger-Ellison syndrome. Gastroenterology 62:626, 1972.
57. Kolts, B. E., Herbest, C. A., and McGuigan, J. E. Calcium- and secretin-stimulated gastrin release in the Zollinger-Ellison syndrome. Ann. Intern. Med. 81:758, 1974.
58. Straus, E., and Yalow, R. S. Differential diagnosis in hyperchlorhydric hypergastrinemia. Gastroenterology 66:867, 1974.
59. Ganguli, P. C., Elder, J. B., Polak, J. M., et al. Antral–gastrin cell hyperplasia in peptic-ulcer disease. Lancet 1:1288, 1974.
60. Hansky, J., Soveny, C., and Korman, M. G. Effect of secretin on serum gastrin as measured by immunoassay. Gastroenterology 61:62, 1971.
61. McGuigan, J. E., and Wolfe, M. M. Secretin injection test in the diagnosis of gastrinoma. Gastroenterology 79:1324, 1980.
62. DeVeney, C. W., DeVeney, K. S., Jaffe, B. M., Jones, R. S., and Way, L. W. Use of calcium and secretin in the diagnosis of gastrinoma (Zollinger-Ellison syndrome). Ann. Intern. Med. 87:680, 1977.
63. Brady, C. E., Johnson, R. C., Williams, J. R., and Boran, K. False positive serum gastrin stimulation due to impure secretin. Gastroenterology 76:1106, 1979.
64. Spindel, E., Harty, R. F., Leibach, J. R., and McGuigan, J. E. Decision analysis in evaluation of hypergastrinemia. Am. J. Med. 80:11, 1986.
65. Stadil, F., Rehfeld, J. F., and Hess Thaysen, E. Gastric juice as gastrin-releasing factor in the Zollinger-Ellison syndrome. Lancet 2:102, 1971.
66. Mills, S. R., Doppman, J. L., Dunnick, N. R., and McCarthy, D. M. Evaluation of angiography in Zollinger-Ellison syndrome. Radiology 131:317, 1979.
67. Damgaard-Petersen, K., and Stage, J. G. CT scanning in patients with Zollinger-Ellison syndrome and carcinoid syndrome. Scand. J. Gastroenterol. 53:117, 1979.
68. Roche, A., Raisonnier, A., and Gillon-Savouret, M. C. Pancreatic venous sampling and arteriography in localizing insulinomas and gastrinomas: procedure and results in 55 cases. Radiology 198:621, 1982.
69. Burcharth, F., Stage, J. G., Stadil, F., Jensen, L. I., and Fischermann, K. Localization of gastrinomas by transhepatic portal catheterization and gastrin assay. Gastroenterology 77:444, 1979.
70. Glowniak, J. V., Shapiro, B., Vinik, A. I., Glaser, B., Thompson, N. W., and Cho, K. J. Percutaneous transhepatic venous sampling of gastrin: value in sporadic and familial islet-cell tumors and G-cell hyperfunction. N. Engl. J. Med. 307:293, 1982.
71. McCarthy, D. M. Report on the United States experience with cimetidine in Zollinger-Ellison syndrome and other hypersecretory states. Gastroenterology 74:453, 1978.
72. Bonfils, S., Nignon, M., and Gratton, J. Cimetidine treatment of acute and chronic Zollinger-Ellison syndrome. World J. Surg. 3:597, 1979.
73. Howard, J. M., Chermos, A. N., Collen, M. J., et al. Famotidine, a new, potent, long-acting histamine H$_2$-receptor antagonist: comparison with cimetidine and ranitidine in the treatment of Zollinger-Ellison syndrome. Gastroenterology 88:1026, 1985.
74. Raufman, J. P., Collins, S. M., Pandol, S. J., et al. Uncertainties in the management of the Zollinger-Ellison syndrome. Gastroenterology 84:108, 1983.
75. Stabile, B. E., Ippoliti, A. F., Walsh, J. H., and Passaro, E., Jr. Failure of histamine H$_2$-receptor antagonist therapy in Zollinger-Ellison syndrome. Am. J. Surg. 145:17, 1983.
76. Lambers, C. B., Lind, T., Moberg, S., Jansen, J. B., and Olbe, L. Omeprazole in Zollinger-Ellison syndrome. Effects of a single dose and of long-term treatment in patients resistant to histamine H$_2$-receptor antagonists. N. Engl. J. Med. 310:758, 1984.
77. McArthur, K. E., Collen, M. J., Maton, P. N., et al. Omeprazole: effective convenient therapy for Zollinger-Ellison syndrome. Gastroenterology 88:939, 1985.
78. McArthur, K. E., Jensen, R. T., and Gardner, J. D. Treatment of acid-peptic diseases by inhibition of gastric H+, K+-ATPase. Annu. Rev. Med. 37:97, 1986.
79. Ellison, E. C., O'Dorisio, T. M., Sparks, J., et al. Observations on the effect of a somatostatin analog in the Zollinger-Ellison syndrome: implications for the treatment of apudomas. Surgery 100:437, 1986.
80. Stadil, F., Stage, G., Rehfeld, J. F., Efsen, F., and Fischermann, K. Treatment of Zollinger-Ellison patients with streptozotocin. N. Engl. J. Med. 294:1440, 1976.
81. Huard, G. S., II, Stephens, R. L., and Friesen, S. R. Zollinger-Ellison syndrome. Streptozotocin therapy for metastatic gastrinomas. J. Kansas Med. Soc. 82:216, 1981.
82. Norton, J. A., Sugarbaker, P. H., Doppman, J. L., et al. Aggressive resection of metastatic disease in selected patients with malignant gastrinomas. Ann. Surg. 149:144, 1985.
83. Deveney, C. W., Deveney, K. E., Stark, D., Moss, A., Stein, S., and Way, L. W. Resection of gastrinomas. Ann. Surg. 198:546, 1983.
84. Jensen, R. T., Maton, P. N., and Gardner, J. D. Current management of Zollinger-Ellison syndrome. Drugs 32:188, 1986.
85. Stabile, B. E., and Passaro, E., Jr. Benign and malignant gastrinoma. Am. J. Surg. 149:144, 1985.
86. Clouse, M. E., Lee, R. G., Duszlak, E. J., Lokich, J. J., and Alday, M. T. Hepatic artery embolization for metastatic endocrine-secreting tumors of the pancreas. Gastroenterology 85:1183, 1983.
87. Friesen, S. R., Bolinger, R. E., Pearse, A. G. E., and McGuigan, J. E. Serum gastrin levels in malignant Zollinger-Ellison syndrome after gastrectomy and hypophysectomy. Ann. Surg. 172:504, 1970.
88. Fox, P. S., Hofmann, J. W., Decosse, J. J., and Wilson, S. D. The influence of total gastrectomy on survival in malignant Zollinger-Ellison tumors. Ann. Surg. 180:558, 1974.
89. Gogel, H. K., Buckman, M. T., Cadieux, D., and McCarthy, D. M. Gastric secretion and hormonal interactions in multiple endocrine neoplasia type I. Arch. Intern. Med. 145:855, 1985.
90. O'Neal, L. W., Kipnis, D. M., Luse, S. A., Lacy, P. E., and Jarret, L. Secretion of various endocrine substances by ACTH-secreting tumors—gastrin, melanotropin, norepinephrine, serotonin, parathormone, vasopressin, glucagon. Cancer 21:1219, 1968.
91. Tomita, T., Kimmbel, J. R., Friesen, S. R., Doull, V., and Pollock, H. G. Pancreatic polypeptide in islet cell tumors. Morphologic and functional correlations. Cancer 56:1649, 1985.
92. Simpson, S., Vinik, A. I., Marangos, P. J., and Lloyd, R. V. Immunohistochemical localization of neuron-specific enolase in gastroenteropancreatic neuroendocrine tumors. Correlation

with tissue and serum levels of neuron-specific enolase. Cancer *54*:1364, 1984.

93. Maton, P. N., Gardner, J. D., and Jensen, R. T. Cushing's syndrome in patients with the Zollinger-Ellison syndrome. N. Engl. J. Med. *315*:1, 1986.

94. Bardram, L., and Stage, J. G. Frequency of endocrine disorders in patients with the Zollinger-Ellison syndrome. Scand. J. Gastroenterol. *20*:233, 1985.

95. Dawson, J., Bloom, S. R., and Cockel, R. A unique apudoma producing the glucagonoma and gastrinoma syndromes. Postgrad. Med. J. *59*:315, 1983.

96. Lamers, C. B. H., Diemel, J., and Roeffen, W. Serum levels of pancreatic polypeptide in Zollinger-Ellison syndrome, and hyperparathyroidism from families with multiple endocrine adenomatosis type I. Digestion *18*:297, 1978.

97. Schwartz, T. W. Pancreatic-polypeptide (PP) and endocrine tumours of the pancreas. Scand. J. Gastroenterol. *14*:93, 1979.

98. Byrnes, D. J., Marjason, J., Henderson, L., Gallagher, N., and Fabricatorian, D. Is pancreatic polypeptide estimation of value in diagnosing gastrinomas (Zollinger-Ellison syndrome). Aust. N.Z. J. Med. *9*:364, 1979.

99. Stabile, B. E., Braunstein, G. D., and Passaro, E., Jr. Serum gastrin and human chorionic gonadotropin in the Zollinger-Ellison syndrome. Arch. Surg. *115*:1090, 1980.

100. Bloodworth, J. M. B., Jr., and Elliott, D. W. The histochemistry of pancreatic islet cell lesions. JAMA *183*:1011, 1968.

101. Kloppel, G., Willemer, S., Stamm, B., Hacki, W. H., and Heitz, P. U. Pancreatic lesions and hormonal profile of pancreatic tumors in multiple endocrine neoplasia type I. An immunocytochemical study of nine patients. Cancer *57*:1824, 1986.

102. Kirsner, J. B. The parathyroids and peptic ulcer. Gastroenterology *34*:145, 1958.

103. Black, B. H. Hyperparathyroidism. Springfield, IL, Charles C Thomas, 1953.

104. Ellis, C., and Nicoloff, D. M. Hyperparathyroidism and peptic ulcer disease. Arch. Surg. *96*:114, 1968.

105. Ostrow, J. D., Blandshard, G., and Gray, S. J. Peptic ulcer in primary hyperparathyroidism. Am. J. Med. *29*:769, 1960.

106. Ward, J. T., Adesola, A. O., and Welbourne, R. B. The parathyroids, calcium and gastric secretion in man and the dog. Gut *5*:173, 1964.

107. Barrearas, R. F., and Donaldson, R. M. Role of calcium in gastric hypersecretion, parathyroid adenoma and peptic ulcer. N. Engl. J. Med. *276*:1122, 1967.

108. Barrearas, R. F., and Donaldson, R. M. Effects of induced hypercalcemia on human gastric secretion. Gastroenterology *52*:670, 1967.

109. Patterson, M., Wolma, F., Drake, A., and Ong, H. Gastric secretion and chronic hyperparathyroidism. Arch. Surg. *99*:9, 1969.

110. Donegan, W. L., and Spiro, H. M. Parathyroids and gastric secretion. Gastroenterology *38*:750, 1960.

111. Smallwood, R. A. Effect of intravenous calcium administration on gastric secretion of acid and pepsin in man. Gut *8*:592, 1967.

Complications of Peptic Ulcer Disease and Indications for Surgery

50

DAVID Y. GRAHAM

INDICATIONS FOR SURGERY

The major complications of peptic ulcer disease are intractability, hemorrhage, perforation, penetration, and obstruction. The presence of any of these complications suggests that the peptic ulcer disease is no longer a trivial matter in that particular patient and that a permanent solution should be considered.

A variety of therapies for peptic ulcer are available, including drugs, recommendations for alterations in lifestyle or habits, and changes in gastric anatomy and physiology. Goals of therapy may be (1) to cure the disease, (2) to alter the natural history of the disease in a beneficial direction, (3) to treat any existing complications, or (4) to prevent future complications. Any of the above-described complications constitutes an indication for surgery unless there are extenuating circumstances.

The internist/gastroenterologist usually makes the decision to refer an ulcer patient for surgery and then, too often, views that referral as some sort of personal defeat. This attitude is probably related to the high frequency of complications associated with the types of ulcer surgery most commonly employed in the past. The relative reluctance to recommend a patient for ulcer surgery will reflect the anticipated results. Surgeons usually score the success of ulcer operations in terms of recurrence rates; a better measure of success would be to consider what the operation has done to the natural history of the disease and at what cost to the patient. Many surgeons would declare an operation a failure if it transformed almost daily symptoms to infrequent and easily treated ulcer recurrences, whereas an operation that was followed by no recurrence but resulted in an anemic, underweight patient with diarrhea would be scored as a success. In contrast, from a gastroenterologist's point of view, a "good" operation is one in which (1) the patient survives, (2) there is little or no acute or chronic morbidity, and (3) the natural history of the disease is influenced in a beneficial direction. The availability of a particular operation in a given locale will strongly influence the decision as to whether surgical therapy is best for an individual patient. The development of a less mutilating operation with very low mortality or morbidity (the highly selective vagotomy) has made surgical therapy more attractive for ulcer patients. Access to surgeons experienced in highly selective vagotomy should soften the reticence of responsible gastroenterologists to refer patients for ulcer surgery.

INTRACTABILITY

Definition

Intractability was once equated with failure of peptic ulcer to respond to good medical therapy delivered in a hospital. However, medical therapies have improved to the point that even the most virulent hypersecretory states can be medically managed, making the diagnosis of intractability more difficult. It is still appropriate to base the diagnosis of intractability on the history and clinical severity of the peptic ulcer disease. A modern definition of intractability would be sufficient severity of symptoms of peptic ulcer disease to recommend surgery as a preferred method of treatment. Intractability relates to symptoms and not to delayed ulcer healing. The diagnosis of intractability requires clinical confirmation that an ulcer is responsible for the patient's symptoms. Intractability remains the most common reason for surgery in peptic ulcer disease.

Clinical Severity of Peptic Ulcer

The clinical severity of peptic ulcer disease can be divided into three general groups: mild, average, and severe. When ranked on such a scale, patients with ulcer disease can be thought as exhibiting a normal or bell-shaped distribution (Fig. 50–1). The group "Clinical Severity: Average" encompasses the mean clinical severity plus and minus one standard deviation. This group will contain 67 per cent of patients. The remaining one third of patients will be divided equally into the "Mild" and "Severe" categories (approximately 16 per cent each). This concept fits the reported data. For example, Fry[1] followed 265 patients prospectively and 16 per cent required surgical therapy because of "such severe symptoms that their lives were completely disorganized" and 15 per cent of the ulcer patients followed long term by Elashoff and colleagues[2] were classified as having severe symptoms (Table 50–1). Patients with combined duodenal and gastric ulcer may more often fall toward the "Clinical Severity: Severe" end of the scale (Fig. 50–1).

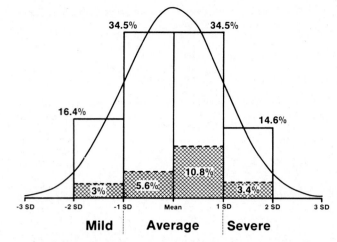

Figure 50–1. Clinical severity of peptic ulcer disease. Clinical severity is depicted as occurring in a normal distribution. Data from population of ulcer patients[2] of whom 15 per cent were classified as having severe symptoms. Data from patients with combined duodenal and gastric ulcer are shown in the hatched area, in which there is a more skewed distribution toward severe symptoms.

Relation Between Frequency of Ulcer Recurrence and Intractability

Recent clinical trials of ulcer healing have shown that about half the population of patients with duodenal ulcer will experience a symptomatic recurrence within one year.[3] Those with severe disease will average three or more recurrences per year. Symptomatic ulcer recurrences are so much more common in smokers than in nonsmokers[4] that a recommendation to stop smoking should be given to all ulcer patients and especially to those with disease in the "Clinical Severity: Severe" category. This recommendation is made despite the current lack of proof that stopping smoking will result in a reduction in clinical severity classification.

Table 50–1. SEVERITY CLASSIFICATION OF PEPTIC ULCERS

Severity	Definition
Mild	Mean pain score ≤34 and those not meeting criteria for moderate or severe
Moderate	Mean pain score ≥35 but <80, and night pain <80% of the time, or mean H_2-receptor antagonist use ≥0.5 with no complications
Severe	Mean pain score ≥80, or night pain reported 80% of time or more or at least one complication (bleeding requiring transfusion, obstruction, or perforation).

Pain score = pain intensity times days of pain in last 2 months, where days of pain may range from 0 to 60 and pain intensity scores are: 0 = no pain, 1 = mild pain, 2 = moderate pain that interfered with daily activities, 3 = severe pain (bedridden). Pain scores can vary from 0 to 180.
H_2-receptor antagonist code average of 1 = prn usage; 2 = less than full dose per day, 3 = full dose per day.
Modified from Elashoff JD, Van Deventer G, Reedy TJ, et al. J Clin Gastroenterol 5:509, 1983.

Relationship Between Intractability and Duration of Ulcer Disease

The natural history of peptic ulcer disease is still ill-defined. Fry suggested that the natural history of ulcer disease is to "burn out."[1] In a long-term study, he found that symptoms occurred in repeated attacks over many years, reached a peak, and then decreased in both frequency and severity. "Burn-out" tended to occur within 10 years of the onset of disease. This tendency has been confirmed.[5] More recent studies have evaluated patient populations largely consisting of those who already had ulcer disease for more than 10 years.[2] Therefore it seems prudent to consider that a patient with ulcer disease of less than 10 years' duration might experience burn-out of the disease, so that referral of that patient to surgical therapy might be delayed, even if clinically severe ulcer disease is present. In contrast, a patient with a 20-year history of clinically severe disease would not be expected to have spontaneous remission, so there would be little to be gained from deferring surgical therapy.

Diagnosis

The diagnosis of intractability rests upon an assessment of the symptoms and the course of ulcer disease in a particular patient. Once the physician decides that a patient has intractable ulcer disease, possible responsible factors should be reviewed (Table 50–2).[6–11] It is especially important to distinguish those complaints that have a neuropsychiatric basis from symptoms of ulcer disease. Surgical therapy in the former group of patients will not often result in improvement. Successful surgical therapy may not lead to the patient returning to work, as those patients may simply change their symptoms (e.g., back pain) and continue their pattern of sick leave.[12]

HEMORRHAGE

Peptic ulcer disease is responsible for approximately half of all admissions for major upper gastrointestinal hemorrhage. The proportion of all bleeding patients

Table 50–2. FACTORS RESPONSIBLE FOR INTRACTABILITY

Intrinsic
    Penetration of ulcer
    Pyloric obstruction
    Postbulbar ulcer
    Channel ulcer
    Hypersecretory drive
       states
Extrinsic
    Smoking
Neuropsychiatric
    Psychic stress
    Inadequate personality
Improper treatment

with duodenal ulcer or gastric ulcer has remained relatively constant over the last 20 years, averaging 26 and 20 per cent, respectively.[13] Between 15 and 20 per cent of ulcer patients will experience hemorrhage during the course of their disease, with a larger proportion of duodenal ulcer patients than of those with gastric ulcer experiencing bleeding.[1, 14, 15]

Clinical Manifestations

Bleeding is most common in the sixth decade. The average age of the bleeding patient has gradually increased coincident with the aging of the population and with the increased use of nonsteroidal anti-inflammatory drugs, especially in elderly women.[16–18] Approximately 80 per cent of patients will relate a history of symptomatic ulcer disease prior to the onset of bleeding.[14, 19–21] About one third will have suffered a previous hemorrhage, and about 10 per cent of patients will have bled more than once.[19, 21, 22] Hematemesis, melena, or a combination of both, will be evident in more than 95 per cent by the time the hospital is reached.[19] About 15 per cent of patients will present in shock, and about one quarter will have a hemoglobin concentration less than 8 gm/dl.[23–25] Physical examination will reflect the degree to which the circulatory status is compromised. The physical findings and treatment of upper gastrointestinal bleeding are detailed in pages 400 to 411.

There are several clinical features that help stratify patients at the time of entry as to their ability to survive a bleeding episode. Factors that suggest a poor outcome include age greater than 60, hematemesis, the presence of shock, severe bleeding requiring multiple transfusions, and the presence of clinically active co-morbid disease (particularly of cardiovascular, respiratory, hepatic, or malignant origin).[26–33] Physical examination should include a search for evidence suggesting causes other than ulcer for the upper gastrointestinal hemorrhage, such as features of chronic liver disease or cutaneous telangiectasias.

Mortality of Bleeding

The majority of deaths that occur following bleeding from a peptic ulcer do not result from exsanguination but, rather, as a result of either co-morbid disease or complications related to a surgical procedure performed to stop bleeding. Most deaths happen more than three days after the bleeding episode; cancer, stroke, hepatic failure, respiratory failure, chronic renal failure, and sepsis are frequently cited as causes of death.[19, 27, 28, 32, 34–38] Emergency surgery is associated with greater mortality than elective surgery, but the usual indication for emergency surgery is to prevent exsanguination in patients who either continue to bleed or who suffer rebleeding. Such patients are at higher risk of dying, even when treated with emergency surgery. The mortality associated with gastric ulcers is twice that of duodenal ulcers, possibly a reflection of the fact that gastric ulcers are more common in elderly people with co-morbid diseases.[16]

Diagnosis

A history of symptomatic ulcer or a previous documentation of ulcer disease strongly suggests a peptic ulcer as the bleeding site, but it does not exclude the presence of some other etiologic lesion, such as Mallory-Weiss tear.[39] Peptic ulcer will prove to be the bleeding site in 75 per cent of patients reporting a positive ulcer history.[20]

Initial Therapy

Bleeding from a peptic ulcer is usually self-limited. Rebleeding occurs in about one third of patients, and 80 to 90 per cent of rebleeding episodes occur within 8 hours of entry into the hospital.[24, 29] Rebleeding is more frequent in patients with gastric ulcer (32 to 48 per cent) than in those with duodenal ulcer (12 to 32 per cent).[22, 24, 26, 29, 33, 40]

The goal of initial therapy is to prevent patient death and includes an assessment of the severity of the bleeding along with restoration of both the blood volume and the oxygen-carrying capacity of the blood (Table 50–3). After the patient is stabilized, the site of bleeding should be diagnosed so that specific therapy, if available, might be employed. Endoscopy plays a major role in the diagnosis of the bleeding site and should be employed early, within 12 to 24 hours of hospitalization.[13] No diagnostic or therapeutic intervention can improve the outcome of those destined to stop bleeding and leave the hospital alive and well, making it important to restrict those procedures and therapies that carry inherent risks.

An intravenous line should be inserted in all patients; a central venous catheter is useful for those with known cardiovascular disease or those presenting in shock. A nasogastric tube should be inserted to ascertain whether there is fresh blood or clots within the stomach. Transfusions should generally be given in order to maintain the hemoglobin around 10 gm/dl. Overtransfusion should be avoided, as there are data suggesting transfusion to a normal or near-normal hemoglobin level may be associated with a worse prognosis.[32]

Most patients with major upper gastrointestinal bleeding should receive initial management in an intensive care unit. The patient most likely to do well is one taken care of by a group of health care professionals who are experienced in all phases of management of the bleeding patient. Studies designed to evaluate the role of early endoscopy and aggressive surgery in patients with bleeding ulcers suggested that early surgery would significantly reduce patient mortality, especially for those over age 60,[21] but further assessment revealed that improved survival was the result of treatment being provided by a well-trained and experienced team that included a gastroenterologist, a surgeon, and experienced nursing personnel.[16, 41]

One component of modern management is early

Table 50–3. IMPORTANT CONSIDERATIONS IN PEPTIC ULCER PATIENTS WITH MAJOR HEMORRHAGE

1. Factors associated with an increase in mortality
    Age greater than 60 years
    Clinically active co-morbid disease, especially cardiac, respiratory, hepatic, or malignancy
    Continued bleeding or rebleeding
    Onset of bleeding in hospital
    No history of aspirin or ethanol use
    Gastric ulcer
2. Presence of shock at entry predicts a high frequency of rebleeding
3. The presence of a visible vessel or fresh clot adherent to the ulcer at endoscopy predicts increased probability of rebleeding
4. The mortality rate associated with emergency surgery is three to four times that of elective surgery
5. There is no contraindication to emergency surgery in the face of exsanguinating hemorrhage

endoscopy, that is, endoscopy performed within 24 hours of entry. Endoscopy will provide a precise diagnosis, either by identifying the bleeding site or by localizing it to a particular portion of the stomach or duodenum. An accurate diagnosis can improve outcome only if a specific therapy is available or if it results in avoidance of a therapy that would be associated with complications. Endoscopy offers direct access to the bleeding site so that specific treatment, such as injection or coagulative therapy, can be applied.[42, 43] Endoscopy also provides prognostic information as to the probability of rebleeding. Examination of the ulcer crater may reveal an adherent fresh clot or a visible vessel, signs that correlate with increased risk of bleeding.[33, 40, 44–46] In contrast, the presence of a flat spot or a clean ulcer base correlates with a low risk of rebleeding. Importantly, the presence of shock correlates with endoscopic findings suggesting rebleeding, and thus endoscopy probably has little additional predictive power and should not be done simply to search for predictive stigmata.[25] Rather, endoscopy should be used to identify the bleeding site to assist the surgeons or to attempt endoscopically applied hemostasis. A method using an endoscopically applied Doppler device has shown promise in categorizing patients as to risk of rebleeding, as the Doppler device can identify the presence of an arterial vessel under the ulcer base.[47] The coexistence of a positive Doppler test and a fresh clot adherent to the ulcer was associated with a 67 per cent chance of rebleeding, versus only a 14 per cent chance with the combination of a clot and a negative Doppler study.

Emergency Surgery

The goal of surgery, in the emergency situation, is to prevent exsanguination. Coincidentally, the peptic ulcer disease should be treated to prevent recurrent ulcer and bleeding. Emergency surgery carries a higher mortality rate than does elective operation. Surgery that involves gastric resection has a higher mortality than vagotomy and pyloroplasty or highly selective vagotomy and oversewing of the ulcer.

Most patients can be resuscitated and evaluated to determine the site of bleeding and the nature of any co-morbid conditions. If bleeding is of such severity that it cannot be controlled, immediate surgery is indicated. Diagnostic studies, such as endoscopy, can be performed in the operating room if the information is deemed necessary. The most common reason for emergency surgery is rebleeding that occurs within hours of entry into the hospital. Many "rules" have been proposed to help decide when surgery should be performed, but application of any set of guidelines must be tempered by the clinical situation. For example, those under age 60 almost never die from bleeding ulcers, whereas an elderly person with advanced carcinoma will probably die regardless of the therapy employed. The difficulty in applying rules is well illustrated by the results of a recent prospective study in which patients were randomly assigned to early or delayed surgery.[48] Criteria for early surgery included a requirement for 4 units of blood or plasma expander to correct blood loss in the first 24 hours, one rebleed, endoscopic evidence of stigmata (active bleeding, visible vessel, adherent clot, spots), or previous upper gastrointestinal hemorrhage plus a two-year history of dyspepsia. Criteria for delayed surgery included a requirement for 8 units of blood or plasma expander to correct blood volume in 24 hours, two rebleeds in hospital, or persistent bleeding requiring transfusions (12 units in 48 hours or 16 units in 72 hours). Fewer operations were performed in the delayed group compared to the early group, 21 versus 59 per cent. The operation rate was low (6 per cent) in those under age 60 and no patient younger than 60 died in either group. The overall mortality was 7 per cent, with the highest mortality occurring in gastric ulcer patients over age 60 who received delayed surgery. Mortality was generally related to postoperative complications or co-morbid conditions.

Mortality rates among patients with hemorrhage would be lower if emergency surgery could be avoided. Endoscopically applied therapy offers the yet unfulfilled promise of an alternative to surgery. Noncontact therapy such as laser therapy appears to offer limited benefit, as it relies on obliterative coagulation (shrinkage and constriction of the open vessel by application of heat to the vessel and surrounding tissues), it is not portable, and the frequency of rebleeding has been high.[43] Following a long history of successful application in surgery, endoscopists have developed methods to coaptively coagulate bleeding vessels (coaptive closure is the physical apposition of tissue during heating, such as by grasping a blood vessel with a hemostat and then passing an electric current through it).[49] Prospective studies are still needed to establish the general applicability of these therapies. Candidates for endoscopic therapy include those who continue bleeding or rebleed. Because the presence of shock at entry is the best predictor of rebleeding or continued bleeding, if endoscopic therapy is to be employed, such patients should undergo endoscopy soon after resuscitation.

The goals of endoscopic therapy are to change an emergency situation into a less dangerous elective one, and to obviate the need for surgery in those ill suited to withstand any operation.

Patients who have nonremediable near-terminal illnesses are often not candidates for either endoscopic evaluation or surgical therapy.

Management after Resuscitation

A nasogastric tube is useful during the period of resuscitation to monitor the bleeding and, in confused or semicomatose patients, to prevent aspiration. H_2-receptor antagonists are often unnecessarily administered intravenously as part of the initial resuscitative efforts (as if they would somehow stop arterial hemorrhage). Antacids and agents that inhibit acid secretion are part of the therapy of the underlying ulcer and can be delayed until the patient is stabilized, the diagnosis of peptic ulcer confirmed, and oral feeding begun (usually within 12 to 24 hours of entry into the hospital).

Course after Bleeding

Patients who have bled from peptic ulcer are at an increased risk of having additional episodes of hemorrhage in the future. This increased risk does not decrease with time; more than half of the patients treated medically will suffer another bleeding episode during the ensuing 10 to 15 years.[23, 50–56] The risk of another episode remains equally high after each subsequent bleed. This phenomenon is also reflected by the finding that the increased risk of bleeding following surgery for hemorrhage exceeds that pursuant to ulcer surgery for intractability, penetration, or perforation.

The surgical literature has documented that rebleeding is frequent following surgical therapy for bleeding ulcer and that such rebleeding is almost always a reflection of recurrent ulcer disease. Operations such as hemigastrectomy without vagotomy have been associated with relatively high rates of ulcer recurrence and with high rates of recurrent gastrointestinal bleeding. Modern operations that include vagotomy are associated with low rates of both ulcer recurrence and recurrent bleeding.

The frequency with which recurrent episodes of hemorrhage complicate the course of the medically treated patient suggests that elective surgery should be seriously considered after any major bleeding episode. The low mortality rate associated with hemorrhage in patients less than 50 years old suggests that, unless there has been a long history of ulcer disease, operation can be deferred until after two or three bleeding episodes have occurred. An elective, highly selective vagotomy is an operation with very low mortality in a good-risk patient. However, the risk:benefit calculation for an elderly patient with several clinically active co-morbid diseases usually favors long-term therapy with an H_2-receptor antagonist.

PERFORATION

Incidence

The incidence of ulcer perforation is 7 to 10 per 100,000 population per year.[57, 58] Perforation is less common than hemorrhage but more common than obstruction. Pyloroduodenal perforations are 6 to 8 times more common than gastric perforations.[57, 59, 60] The site of pyloroduodenal perforation is usually the anterior wall, whereas the majority of perforated gastric ulcers are located on the lesser curvature.

Manifestations

Perforation is four to eight times more common in men than in women, although that ratio may be changing as the frequency of gastric perforation appears to be increasing in association with nonsteroidal anti-inflammatory drug use in elderly women.[57, 58, 61] The peak incidence for perforation is between ages 40 and 49.

The most common presentation is an abrupt onset of severe abdominal pain, followed rapidly by signs of peritoneal inflammation.[60-63] The pain typically begins in the epigastrium and rapidly spreads throughout the abdomen. The abruptness, severity, and rapid progression of symptoms convinces the patient that something bad has happened and there is usually little delay in seeking medical attention.

The typical patient will appear to be acutely and seriously ill, lying immobile in bed with grunting and shallow respirations. The physical findings will depend upon the duration of the perforation and the amount of spillage into the peritoneal cavity. At entry, the patient may have a normal pulse and blood pressure, but unless spillage is minimal and the perforation seals rapidly, the patient will develop progressive hypotension and fever. Spillage of gastric and intestinal contents into the peritoneum causes a chemical peritonitis and the outpouring of fluid soon results in hypovolemia.

Signs of acute peritonitis develop rapidly, with abdominal tenderness being particularly pronounced in the epigastrium and with spasm of the abdominal musculature usually approaching board-like rigidity. Loss of hepatic dullness may be present and, if elicited, is a valuable clue to the correct diagnosis.[64] Bowel sounds are absent in two thirds of cases,[60] but the presence of bowel sounds does not exclude the diagnosis.

Leukocytosis appears rapidly. The blood chemistries are usually normal with the exception of the serum amylase, which may be slightly increased (in 19 per cent of patients).[65] The increase in serum amylase will be approximately twice normal in about 8 per cent of cases and will seldom be greater than three times normal.

The diagnosis of perforation is usually suggested by the history and physical examination. The suspected diagnosis can be confirmed by the identification of the presence of free intraperitoneal air, a finding that is demonstrable in about 80 per cent of cases.[66-69] An erect chest X-ray or a left decubitus film of the abdomen is better than a plain abdominal film for detecting the presence of free air.[70] When the diagnosis is suspected and the X-rays are negative, it is worthwhile to repeat the radiographic evaluation after an interval of several hours. Alternatively, the diagnosis may be confirmed by an upper gastrointestinal series using Gastrografin.[68] This approach will often demonstrate the duodenal ulcer, as well as confirm perforation by the intraperitoneal spillage of contrast media.

The diagnosis may be difficult if the disease presents in one of the possible variant forms.[68] For example, the ulcer may seal soon after perforation such that the physical findings are less intense. Alternatively, perforation localized to the right upper quadrant may simulate biliary tract disease. The picture may resemble acute appendicitis when leakage is shunted to the right lower quadrant by the falciform ligament, the liver, and the hepatic flexure of the colon. Finally, in patients with markedly elevated serum amylase, there may be confusion between a perforated ulcer and pancreatitis.[65] Elevation of the serum amylase is thought to be secondary to absorption of salivary and pancreatic amylase after spillage of gastric and intestinal contents into the peritoneal cavity. The increased serum amylase is usually a late finding and is correlated with a large perforation, a large amount of peritoneal soilage, and increased patient mortality. These diagnostic difficulties are usually resolved by the identification of free intraperitoneal air or by a positive Gastrografin upper GI series. Peritoneal aspiration may be helpful in selected cases, as the peritoneal fluid obtained from perforated ulcer disease is usually cloudy and bile-stained, contains organisms, and has a low glucose concentration.

The diagnosis of perforation is most commonly missed in elderly female patients with gastric perforation who have been admitted to nonsurgical wards and for whom surgical consultations have not been requested.[57, 64, 71] Perforation is also frequently misdiagnosed in elderly patients who are already hospitalized with neuropsychiatric disease. Unexplained hypotension is a common clinical finding in patients in whom perforation was missed. One aid to increased diagnostic accuracy may be to include perforated viscus in the differential diagnosis of patients with unexplained shock.

The Role of Acute versus Chronic Ulcers in Perforation

Attempts have been made to classify perforations on the basis of whether the responsible ulcer was acute or chronic. Presumably, an acute ulcer is not an expression of chronic ulcer disease and additional ulcer symptoms or complications would not be expected to occur in the future. All recognize the difficulty in obtaining an accurate history prior to surgery in severely ill patients. When the history has been carefully obtained after surgery, more than 80 per cent of patients have related symptoms consistent with peptic ulcer disease for more than one year.[59] Therefore, probably less than 20 per cent of patients presenting with perforation will not have underlying chronic peptic ulcer disease. Possible exceptions to this conclusion are those individuals taking nonsteroidal anti-inflammatory drugs.[61]

Management

The goal of initial management of perforation is to prepare the patient for surgery. The steps include resuscitation by correction of fluid and electrolyte abnormalities, treatment of complications, continuous nasogastric suction, parenteral administration of broad-spectrum antibiotics and, if a tension pneumoperitoneum is present, needle aspiration of the peritoneal cavity.[68] Nasogastric suction is one of the mainstays of therapy, and it is important to confirm that the aspirating ports of the nasogastric tube are positioned in the most dependent portion of the stomach. A decision not to operate should be based upon the clinical condition of the patient.[68, 72] A nonoperative approach is suitable in patients that satisfy two criteria: a very poor surgical risk and a Gastrografin upper GI series that shows no free leakage into the peritoneal cavity. A nonoperative approach may also be chosen for a patient presenting in shock who has significant co-morbid disease (e.g., carcinoma of the lung). The response to nonoperative therapy employing nasogastric suction and antibiotics is usually rapid unless the perforation continues to leak. If there is evidence of increasing peritoneal irritation after six hours of treatment, it is best to declare nonoperative therapy a failure and to proceed to surgery.

Prognosis and Surgery

Perforation is a complication of the underlying chronic peptic ulcer disease. Both problems, the chronic ulcer disease and the perforation, must be considered in designing long-term treatment. The primary issue is not whether to operate but to decide which operation is optimal for the particular patient. Follow-up of patients treated by simple suture of the perforated ulcer has revealed that the percentage of those individuals who develop complications will increase over time.[73–76] It is not surprising that simply closing a hole will not alter the natural history of peptic ulcer disease, that is, it will not move a patient already categorized in the group with severe clinical disease into a ranking of average or mild clinical severity. Prior to the introduction of the highly selective vagotomy, surgeons were faced with the dilemma of whether to offer the patient an operation that provided no protection against recurrent ulceration or a more destructive procedure associated with a high morbidity rate, a particularly undesirable outcome for those patients

destined to remain free of ulcer symptoms. Closure of the perforation and proximal selective gastric vagotomy is now the preferred operation.[77–79] It is associated with little morbidity and drastically lowers the rate of ulcer recurrence, thereby obviating the need for subsequent medical or surgical therapy in most patients.

Not only are patients who experience one perforation more likely to experience further complications, but ulcers that recur following gastric resection (anastomotic ulcers) are more likely to perforate than when the indication for original operation was intractability, obstruction, or hemorrhage.[80]

Mortality

The age and the condition of the patient at the time of admission or operation are the primary determinants of survival.[57, 81, 82] Prospective studies have shown that concurrent medical disease, presence of shock, and a perforation present for more than 48 hours are independent risk factors, all predicting poor outcome. Old age, extensive peritoneal contamination, and a short history of ulcer prior to surgery are also important, but are not independent factors. An elevated serum creatinine in patients without chronic renal failure is also a sign of poor prognosis.[62] The mortality rate for good-risk patients undergoing surgery is less than 3 per cent. Following the simple closure of a perforated ulcer, at least half the individuals will eventually develop hemorrhage, perforation, or obstruction.

The overall mortality from perforated pyloroduodenal ulcers is approximately 10 per cent (including nonoperative cases). Perforated gastric ulcers have a higher mortality (10 to 40 per cent), reflecting the greater age and larger perforations typical of gastric ulcer patients. Perforations that occur at night in elderly women tend to have an even higher mortality rate, possibly owing to a delay in seeking medical attention. Patients who go to surgery moribund, who have had the correct diagnosis missed, and who suffer perforations while hospitalized represent the groups that contain most of the reported fatalities.

PENETRATION

Penetration signifies erosion of an ulcer through the entire thickness of the wall of the stomach or intestine without leakage of digestive contents into the peritoneal cavity. The ulcerative process is limited by dense fibrous adhesions or adjacent structures. The incidence of penetration is unknown because penetration can be diagnosed reliably only at surgery, by autopsy, when a biopsy of an ulcer reveals liver or pancreatic tissue, or when there is a fistulous communication evident between the stomach or intestine and adjacent structures such as the biliary tree or colon. Data from surgical series reveal that penetration is identified in approximately 20 per cent of patients who require surgery for peptic ulcer disease.

Sites of Penetration

In order of decreasing frequency, penetration occurs into the pancreas, gastrohepatic omentum, biliary tract, liver, greater omentum, mesocolon, and colon.[83] The pancreas is the most common site for penetration by either gastric or duodenal ulcers.

Manifestations

The average patient with penetration has had characteristic ulcer symptoms for many years.[83–86] Penetration is suggested by an alteration in the typical spectrum of symptoms experienced by that patient. Typically, the alteration in pattern is gradual and changes may occur in the frequency, intensity, radiation, or duration of pain. The most common symptom is a new onset of pain referred to the back, usually to the level of the lower thoracic and upper lumbar vertebrae and often slightly to the left. Initially, the back pain is coincident with the anterior abdominal distress, but later it may become unrelenting and predominant. The patient may relate the new occurrence of night pain. Typically, the rhythmic pain-food-relief pattern is distorted and the pain becomes refractory to the simple measures that had previously given relief (i.e., the patient develops intractable ulcer pain).

The diagnosis of posterior penetration is made by taking a careful history. In a small percentage of patients, hyperamylasemia may be demonstrated or radiographic evidence of penetration or abscess may be obtained.[87] A nondeformed duodenal bulb does not exclude the presence of a posterior penetrating duodenal ulcer, but weighs against its existence.

Management of Simple Penetration

Patients with penetrating ulcer have peptic ulcer disease that is clinically severe. In our experience, penetrating ulcers respond well to therapy with H_2-receptor antagonists.

Complicated Penetration

The two most frequently recognized special types of penetration involve fistulous communications between the stomach and colon, the gastrocolic fistula, or between the duodenum and biliary tree, the choledochoduodenal fistula. A gastrocolic fistula occurs most frequently as a complication of a marginal ulcer but can occur secondary to a deeply penetrating gastric ulcer located on the greater curvature or on the posterior wall of the stomach.[88, 89] Typical features are the combination of pain, weight loss, and diarrhea. Fecal vomiting is an especially helpful sign diagnostically, but is rarely present. Barium enema remains the most reliable method of diagnosing the presence of the fistula, although on occasion the diagnosis can be confirmed by barium upper gastrointestinal series or endoscopy. Treatment is surgical.

A choledochoduodenal fistula may complicate the course of duodenal ulcer disease.[90, 91] In most cases the diagnosis is made incidentally by the demonstration of the fistula by upper gastrointestinal series, although cases presenting with cholangitis, jaundice, or hemorrhage have been described. Most patients have typical complaints of ulcer disease of long duration, and the fistula resolves with therapy directed at the ulcer disease. Surgery is not required unless biliary complications are present or the ulcer disease is of such severity as to otherwise require surgical therapy.

GASTRIC OUTLET OBSTRUCTION (PYLORIC STENOSIS)

Severe gastric emptying disorders are clinically evident, whereas minor degrees of gastric motor abnormalities are difficult to identify and to quantify.[92, 93] The stomach readily discriminates between liquids and solids, with liquids normally leaving the stomach rapidly. The rate of gastric emptying is governed by duodenal receptors (e.g., for fat or for acid) that regulate the rate at which the duodenum will accept gastric contents. The tonic activity of the gastric fundus provides the energy necessary for transfer of liquids into the duodenum.[94] Saline does not stimulate duodenal receptors and is emptied more rapidly than even water. The emptying of solids from the stomach is a relatively slow process, as particles greater than 2 mm in diameter are retained. When particles are adequately ground to small size, they leave the stomach suspended in fluid. Large, nondigestible solids do not exit the stomach until the individual fasts and then leave as a result of the "interdigestive migrating motor complex." It is possible for the stomach to display a normal emptying of liquids but an abnormal emptying of solids, or vice versa. Clinical features that suggest gastric retention are shown in Table 50–4.[95]

Table 50–4. CRITERIA FOR GASTRIC RETENTION

History
    Vomiting of stale food (food ingested over 4 hours previously)
    Repetitive vomiting, often projectile or nocturnal
Physical examination
    Visible gastric peristalsis
    Succussion splash more than four hours after eating
Gastric aspirate
    Gastric residue greater than 300 ml four hours after eating
    Overnight fasting gastric residue greater than 200 ml
Radiology
    Retention of barium—50 per cent at four hours
    Large atonic stomach
Special studies
    Saline load: positive for retention when more than 400 ml of 750 ml of normal saline is retained after 30 minutes
    Barium-burger: barium residue after six hours in intact stomach and three hours in resected stomach
    External scanning techniques—technetium label
        Liquid: fractional emptying rate of less than 10%/min
        Solid: fractional emptying rate of less than 0.5%/min

Frequency

Approximately 2 per cent of all ulcer patients will develop gastric outlet obstruction.[96] Pyloric obstruction is a less frequent complication of ulcers than either perforation or bleeding; the ratio among obstruction, perforation, and bleeding is approximately 1:2.1:2.3.[97] The clinical severity of ulcer disease in patients with gastric outlet obstruction is severe. Eighty per cent of patients with gastric outlet obstruction admit a history of previous ulcer disease, 20 per cent relate previous gastrointestinal hemorrhage, 18 per cent have had previous ulcer perforation, and 11 per cent have suffered a previous gastric outlet obstruction.[96–103] The magnitude of the problem is reflected by the fact that 30 per cent of ulcer patients who undergo surgery do so because of gastric outlet obstruction.

Gastric retention may develop due to different mechanisms: cicatricial narrowing, inflammatory swelling surrounding an active ulcer, muscular spasm, impaired motility in the pyloric region associated with nearby peptic ulceration, gastric muscular atony, or a combination of factors. Ninety per cent of cases of obstruction are caused by previous or coexistent duodenal or channel ulcers, whereas gastric ulcers are associated with only 4 to 5 per cent of cases.[96] Active ulcer is present in more than 75 per cent, and the ulcer is penetrating in about 40 per cent of these.[96–98, 100] A miscellaneous group of causes is responsible for the remainder of the cases (Table 50–5).

Symptoms of Obstruction

The average patient is middle-aged or older and has a history of symptomatic peptic ulcer disease that exceeds ten years. The symptoms of underlying peptic ulcer disease exhibited by obstructed patients are usually indistinguishable from those of nonobstructed patients with peptic ulcer disease. Vomiting is the most frequent symptom of obstruction and is absent in only 10 per cent of cases. Other features of the disorder include abdominal pain (in 87 per cent of patients), weight loss (65 per cent), early satiety (60 per cent), and nausea (40 per cent). Constipation is reported by about 45 per cent of affected individuals and, depending upon completeness of obstruction, sometimes progresses to obstipation (approximately 7 per cent). Diarrhea occurs in approximately 5 per cent of obstructed patients. Physical examination will often reveal evidence of weight loss or malnutrition, and weight loss in excess of 5 pounds is common. Dehydration occurs in 20 per cent of cases. Abdominal tenderness is common, but nonspecific. Abdominal distention may be present (in 20 per cent), and a succussion splash can be elicited in at least 25 per cent of patients with outlet obstruction.

Character of the Vomiting. Vomiting is often the presenting symptom for obstructed patients (about 80 per cent of cases). Vomiting may occur daily (34 per cent), more frequently than daily (41 per cent), or only occasionally (25 per cent).[96] Although the vomiting of recognizable food particles is relatively infrequent, when vomitus contains recognizable food eaten 12 or more hours previously it is highly suggesitve of gastric retention. The difficulties in diagnosis that are encountered in approximately one third of cases of obstruction usually occur because physicians fail to appreciate the significance of any reported vomiting.

Pain. Pain associated with obstruction is localized to the epigastrium in more than 80 per cent of patients. It can best be described as typical ulcer pain. It may be characterized as a "fullness" or may radiate. Nocturnal pain is reported by about one third of the patients.

Duration of Symptoms of Obstruction. Obstructive symptoms are present for less than one month in about one third of patients, for one to three months in another third of patients, and for longer than three months in the final third. Only 10 per cent of patients reported suffering obstructive symptoms for more than one year. The most common interval is one month.[103]

Laboratory Features of Pyloric Obstruction

The frequency of abnormal laboratory findings is proportional to the severity and the duration of the obstruction suffered by a given patient. Malnutrition, anemia, and low serum albumin commonly occur. Electrolyte and acid-base abnormalities, often associated with prerenal azotemia, are exhibited by about 20 per cent of patients. These disturbances result from vomiting and decreased fluid intake. Vomiting causes loss of hydrogen and chloride from the stomach, which results in contraction of the extracellular volume and metabolic alkalosis.[104] The renal response to these volume and electrolyte derangements is to conserve sodium at the expense of potassium; this may ultimately lead to a severely dehydrated patient with hyponatremia and a hypokalemic metabolic alkalosis.

Evaluation of Gastric Emptying. The saline load test is a simple means of evaluating the stomach's ability to empty a fluid load efficiently and rapidly.[105] The test

Table 50–5. CAUSES OF OUTLET OBSTRUCTION

Peptic ulcer disease
Tumors
  Benign
    Adenomatous polyp
    Ectopic pancreas
  Malignant
    Gastric carcinoma
    Carcinoma of pancreatic head
    Lymphomas
Inflammatory
  Cholecystitis
  Acute pancreatitis
  Crohn's disease
Miscellaneous
  Adult hypertrophic pyloric stenosis
  Postsurgical stenosis
  Pyloric diaphragm
  Duodenal diaphragm
  Caustic stricture
  Annular pancreas

is performed by passing a 16 French nasogastric tube (a sump type tube is best) into the stomach until the tip is 65 cm from the nares. The patient should be positioned right-side down so as to enhance gastric emptying. Within three to five minutes, 750 ml of 0.9 per cent sodium chloride is infused into the stomach. Thirty minutes after the infusion is begun, the gastric contents are aspirated with a syringe and the recovery volume measured. The test is scored as positive (diagnostic) when there is retention of more than 400 ml; volumes of 300 to 400 ml are highly suggestive of gastric retention.

The saline load test provides semiquantitative information about the degree of outlet obstruction. Serial saline load tests allow the physician to assess a patient's response to medical therapy (see below).

The barium-burger test is a useful assay that provides information about the gastric emptying of solids.[106, 107] The barium-burger test may be positive when the saline load test is negative, and vice versa. Disadvantages of the barium-burger test are the amount of time required, the radiation exposure, and the fact that some patients dislike hamburger. The positive aspect of the test is that it does not require intubation. Newer radionuclide tests of gastric emptying are still primarily research tools; they provide semiquantitative measurements of gastric emptying of both liquids and solids.[108, 109] Although a number of problems complicate the performance and interpretation of radionuclide tests, they promise to provide objective data that physicians will be able to use to compare with clinical outcome. In general the barium-burger and radionuclide tests are not needed to manage patients with outlet obstruction.

Endoscopy is the best method for evaluating the stomach, pylorus, and duodenum for the presence of obstruction and for determining the cause of any obstruction. Although endoscopy will provide valuable anatomic information, it is unable to yield useful data concerning gastric motility or gastric emptying.

Initial Management

After a diagnosis of gastric retention is confirmed, it is important to determine whether the retention is secondary to mechanical obstruction, to gastric atony, or to both. The presence of gastric atony is suggested by the history and physical examination; for example, the concomitant presence of diabetes mellitus or the use of anticholinergic drugs are possible contributing factors.

Recent studies have failed to confirm early optimism that many obstructed patients would respond to medical therapy and not require surgery. It appears that only 25 to 35 per cent of patients with gastric outlet obstruction due to chronic ulcer disease will respond to medical management and, unfortunately, more than 90 per cent of those responders will subsequently require surgery for either recurrent obstruction or recurrent ulcer disease.[101, 110] When a patient does respond to medical therapy, it may take up to 12 months for gastric size to return completely to normal, although the patient will be asymptomatic.

The stomach responds to outlet obstruction by vigorous peristalsis such that, following chronic obstruction, the gastric musculature is described by surgeons as thickened or hypertrophic. By the time a patient contacts a physician, decompensation of the gastric musculature (reflected by gastric dilatation) is often evident; the distended stomach may occupy a significant proportion of the abdominal cavity.

Once gastric retention is suspected, the problem should be documented by passage of a nasogastric tube. Retention is confirmed by a gastric residue in excess of 300 ml four hours after eating. The pH of the recovered fluid should be measured. In cases of mechanical outlet obstruction, a pH greater than 3 suggests the presence of gastric carcinoma, whereas a more acidic pH suggests ulcer disease.

If gastric retention is documented, the nasogastric tube should be replaced with a large-bore tube, such as a Ewald tube. The large tube is passed through the mouth and is particularly useful for removing any large food particles present. The stomach should be thoroughly lavaged with water or saline to move all debris. Once the stomach is cleansed, the large-bore tube is removed and a nasogastric tube reinserted. Constant suction should be applied to the nasogastric tube for about 72 hours.

Diagnostic and therapeutic measures occur concurrently during the early management of gastric retention. The first 12 to 24 hours of therapy should focus on the correction of fluid, electrolyte, and acid-base abnormalities and on the decompression of the obstructed stomach. The typical patient is in no acute distress, and there is no need to be overly vigorous in treatment. However, aggressive resuscitative measures involving fluids and electrolytes are required for severely dehydrated patients with marked acid-base abnormalities. The initial treatment is to begin an infusion of isotonic saline to correct the extracellular fluid deficit. Once a urine output is confirmed, potassium replacement is begun at the rate of about 10 mEq/hr until hypokalemia is corrected. Occasionally, the alkalosis is of such severe magnitude that the intravenous infusion of isotonic hydrochloric acid (150 ml of 1.0 normal HCl in 1 liter of distilled water), given over several hours, is indicated.[111]

It is useful to perform a baseline saline load test after the stomach has been emptied and thoroughly cleansed. The test is repeated at 24-hour intervals for the first 72 hours. An excellent response to therapy would be evidenced by a saline residual of less than 200 ml.

Ancillary therapy should be directed toward the correction of any severe protein-calorie malnutrition. If the nutritional deficits are large, total parenteral nutrition should be considered and, if the patient is unable to take oral feedings within 48 to 72 hours, parenteral therapy should be instituted. Finally, an attempt should be made to reduce gastric acid secretion, not only to begin treatment of the presumed

Table 50–6. CAUSES OF CHRONIC GASTRIC RETENTION WITHOUT OUTLET OBSTRUCTION

Atropine-like drugs
Diabetic neuropathy
Prior gastric surgery
Severe pain or trauma, especially involving the peritoneum
Contiguous inflammation
Neuromuscular disorders
Central nervous system disease
Pseudo-obstruction
Collagen vascular disease
Idiopathic

active peptic ulcer disease but to reduce the volume of gastric secretions to facilitate recovery of normal tone by the stomach musculature.

Following the resuscitative period, the etiology of the gastric retention should be addressed. The history and physical examination and the screening laboratory tests will have provided additional data that might suggest diagnoses other than mechanical outlet obstruction, such as diabetic neuropathy, uremia, pancreatitis, or hepatitis (Table 50–6).

Surgical Therapy

Preoperative preparation consists primarily of an adequate medical decompression of the stomach and of appropriate fluid and electrolyte replacement. Recently, pylorus-conserving operations (highly selective vagotomy and stricture dilatation or duodenoplasty) have been attempted with patients suffering from gastric outlet obstruction.[112–121] The ulcer recurrence rate may be greater after highly selective vagotomy performed for obstruction than when used for intractability, but this procedure may prove to be the initial operation of choice.

Endoscopy in Pyloric Stenosis

Endoscopy is best delayed until after resuscitation and after nasogastric suction has been applied for 12 to 24 hours. This will allow the stomach to regain its normal shape and make the landmarks more evident. Sometimes the stomach will greatly dilate when air is insufflated, completely effacing the antrum and making it difficult to identify the location of the pylorus. Removal of most of the air by suction, however, will reveal familiar landmarks and identify the direction that one should proceed. Once the pylorus is identified, the pyloric canal, ring, and duodenum should be thoroughly inspected. When gastric or pyloric ulcer or malignancy is the cause of the obstruction, the diagnosis is usually obvious. In contrast, duodenal ulcer may be difficult to diagnose unless one obtains a peek through the pylorus.

Endoscopic Therapy of Gastric Outlet Obstruction. An ulcerated stenotic pyloric canal with a luminal diameter ≤5 mm is readily identifiable as an abnormal situation. The normal pyloric canal is 15 to 20 mm in diameter and dilates to 25 mm without difficulty.[125] The inability to pass a standard endoscope (approxi-

mate diameter, 11 to 12 mm) is highly suggestive of pyloric stenosis; failure to enter the duodenum with a slim endoscope is even more indicative. The problem with this evaluation is deciding whether failure to pass an endoscope is a problem with the endoscopist, the instrument, or the pyloric ring. There has been no systematic study comparing the diameter of the pyloric ring and disease symptomatology, but a pyloric ring ≤6 mm in diameter is generally associated with symptoms of gastric outlet obstruction.

Previous studies have demonstrated that although patients with gastric outlet obstruction may respond to medical management, the majority will subsequently require surgical intervention. Of note, however, those studies did not direct therapy toward the stenotic segment. Dilatation of the stenotic segment combined with highly selective vagotomy is usually successful in the long-term management of patients with pyloric stenosis. One would presume that the combination of H_2-receptor antagonist therapy and endoscopic dilatation of the pyloric ring should be equally effective. Reports in the literature tend to support this hypothesis, although the available data have not been collected in a systematic fashion.

Technique of Pyloric Dilatation. Balloon dilatation of the stenotic segment can resolve the acute problem of outlet obstruction in most patients and, thereby, greatly increase the options available to the physician. Balloon dilatation can be performed with either over-the-guide-wire or through-the-scope techniques. Most experience has been with over-the-guide-wire balloons, and they are probably superior as they will withstand higher pressures and are, consequently, more likely to accomplish dilatation.[126–129] However, the ease of use of the through-the-scope balloons makes them a practical first choice.

Through-the-Scope Balloon Dilatation. A 10- or 15-mm outside diameter balloon is used as the initial dilator. The well-lubricated balloon is passed through the biopsy channel of an endoscope with a large channel. The balloon is passed into the stricture. Balloons 6 to 8 cm in length are preferred because shorter balloons are difficult to maintain in position (they either advance or back out of the stricture during inflation). The balloon is inflated to maximum pressure with water or dilute contrast media, using a pressure gauge to ensure that the low-compliance (and expensive) balloon does not rupture. Dilatation is repeated three or four times, and it is probably best to maintain the balloon at maximum inflation for at least one minute during each dilatation. An attempt is made to pull the inflated balloon back through the pylorus, although failure to accomplish this does not signify failure of dilatation.

When the balloon is first distended, one should take the opportunity to look through the transparent balloon and inspect the walls of the duodenum and pyloric ring for presence of ulcers. After dilatation is complete, the balloon is withdrawn and the endoscope is passed through the pyloric ring for inspection of the duodenal bulb and beyond.

Over-the-Wire Balloon Dilatation. Dilatation over a wire requires fluoroscopy and may be safer than the through-the-scope approach. The guide wire is passed through the stricture using direct vision at endoscopy or with fluoroscopic guidance. The wire is advanced far enough to serve as an anchor. A heavy-gauge piano wire is preferred to a flexible wire because flexible wires are frequently dislodged during the dilatation procedure or when a small balloon is being exchanged for a larger one. Some investigators have used a Dormia basket, which can be passed beyond the ligament of Treitz and then opened to serve as an anchor.[128] We prefer spring-tip guide wires made of a heavy-gauge piano wire and with a long, flexible spring.

Dilatation is done under fluoroscopic guidance using dilute radiographic contrast material, such as diatrizoate meglumine. A waist form is initially seen in the balloon, and the subsequent effacement of that waist signifies dilatation. Following fluoroscopically directed balloon dilatation, endoscopy is employed to evaluate the pyloric ring and duodenal bulb. Endoscopy can either be performed immediately or be delayed for 24 hours.

Follow-up after Balloon Dilatation. The optimum diameter achieved during dilatation is unknown. Most surgeons use a 14-mm Hager dilator along with highly selective vagotomy. A 15-mm balloon is good for the first endoscopic attempt, whereas 18 to 20 mm may be the best final diameter. This question will be resolved only by prospective studies. Patients with active ulcer disease are begun on therapy with an H_2-receptor antagonist. For those patients with greatly dilated stomachs, nasogastric suction is continued for 24 to 48 hours to allow the stomach musculature to regain its normal strength. Alternatively, the gastric residual volume can be checked or a saline load test repeated each morning for several days following dilatation to ensure that the problem has been resolved. The results of therapy should be reviewed after a week to ten days (by either a saline load test or endoscopy), and the patient should be examined at three-month intervals for the next year. The liabilities, the long-term benefits, and comparisons with traditional therapy all remain unknown for balloon dilatation; prospective studies using objective criteria will be required in order to position this technique correctly within our armamentarium of therapies.

References

1. Fry, J. Peptic ulcer: A profile. Br. Med. J. *2*:809, 1964.
2. Elashoff, J. D., Van Deventer, G., Reedy, T. J., Ippoliti, A., Samloff, I. M., Kurata, J., Billings, M., and Isenberg, M. Long-term follow-up of duodenal ulcer patients. J. Clin. Gastroenterol. *5*:509, 1983.
3. Strum, W. B. Prevention of duodenal ulcer recurrence. Ann. Intern. Med. *105*:757, 1986.
4. Sontag, S., Graham, D. Y., Belsito, A., Weiss, J., et al. Cimetidine, cigarette smoking, and recurrence of duodenal ulcer. N. Engl. J. Med. *311*:689, 1984.
5. Greibe, J., Bugge, P., Gjorup, T., Lauritzen, T., Bonnevie, O., and Wulff, H. R. Long-term prognosis of duodenal ulcer: follow-up study and survey of doctors' estimates. Br. Med. J. *2*:1572, 1977.
6. Haubrich, W. S. The clinical recognition and pathological anatomy of intractability in peptic ulcer disease. Ann. NY Acad. Sci. *99*:114, 1962.
7. Ruffin, J. M., Johnston, D. H., Carter, D. D., and Baylin, G. J. Clinical picture of pyloric channel ulcer. Analysis of one hundred consecutive cases. JAMA *159*:668, 1955.
8. Foulk, W. T., Comfort, M. W., Butt, H. R., Dockerty, M. B., and Weber, H. M. Peptic ulcer near the pylorus. Gastroenterology *32*:395, 1957.
9. Lumsden, K., MacLarnon, J. C., and Dawson, J. Giant duodenal ulcer. Gut *11*:592, 1970.
10. Bullock, W. K., and Snyder, E. N., Jr. Benign giant duodenal ulcer. Gastroenterology *20*:330, 1952.
11. Mistilis, S. P., Wiot, J. F., and Nedelman, S. H. Giant duodenal ulcer. Ann. Intern. Med. *59*:155, 1963.
12. Graffner, H., Gulich, T., and Oscarson, J. The effect of highly selective vagotomy on sick-listing in peptic ulcer patients. Scand. J. Gastroenterol. *18*:439, 1983.
13. Graham, D. Y. Should emergency endoscopy be utilized in the management of upper gastrointestinal bleeding of unknown cause? Negative. *In* Gitnick, G. (ed.). Controversies in Gastroenterology. New York, Churchill Livingstone, 1984, pp. 153–169.
14. Chinn, A. B., and Weckesser, E. C. Acute hemorrhage from peptic ulceration: an analysis of 322 cases. Ann. Intern. Med. *34*:339, 1951.
15. Norbye, E. Ulcer statistics from Drammen Hospital, 1936–1945. Acta Med. Scand. *143*:50, 1952.
16. Hunt, P. S. Surgical management of bleeding chronic peptic ulcer. A 10-year prospective study. Ann. Surg. *199*:44, 1984.
17. Smart, H. L., and Langman, M. J. S. Late outcome of bleeding gastric ulcers. Gut *27*:926, 1986.
18. Bartle, W. R., Gupta, A. K., and Lazor, J. Nonsteroidal anti-inflammatory drugs and gastrointestinal bleeding: a case-control study. Arch. Intern. Med. *146*:2365, 1986.
19. Schiller, K. F. R., Truelove, S. C., and Williams, D. G. Haematemesis and melaena, with special reference to factors influencing the outcome. Br. Med. J. *2*:7, 1970.
20. Cotton, P. B., Rosenberg, M. T., Waldram, R. P. L., and Axon, A. T. R. Early endoscopy of oesophagus, stomach, and duodenal bulb in patients with haematemesis and melaena. Br. Med. J. *2*:505, 1973.
21. Donaldson, R. M., Jr., Handy, J., and Papper, S. Five-year follow-up study of patients with bleeding duodenal ulcer with and without surgery. N. Engl. J. Med. *259*:201, 1958.
22. Jones, P. F., Johnston, S. J., McEwan, A. B., Kyle, J., and Needham, C. D. Further haemorrhage after admission to hospital for gastrointestinal haemorrhage. Br. Med. J. *3*:660, 1973.
23. Macleod, I. A., and Mills, P. R. Factors identifying the probability of further haemorrhage after acute upper gastrointestinal haemorrhage. Br. J. Surg. *69*:256, 1982.
24. Crook, J. N., Gray, L. W., Jr., Nance, F. C., and Cohn, I., Jr. Upper gastrointestinal bleeding. Ann. Surg. *175*:771, 1972.
25. Bornman, P. C., Theodorou, N. A., Shuttleworth, R. D., Essel, H. P., and Marks, I. N. Importance of hypovolaemic shock and endoscopic signs in predicting recurrent haemorrhage from peptic ulceration: a prospective evaluation. Br. Med. J. (Clin. Res.) *291*:245, 1985.
26. Jones, F. A. Hematemesis and melena with special reference to causation and to the factors influencing the mortality from bleeding peptic ulcers. Gastroenterology *30*:166, 1956.
27. Read, R. C., Huebl, H. C., and Thal, A. P. Randomized study of massive bleeding from peptic ulceration. Ann. Surg. *162*:561, 1965.
28. Enquist, I. F., Karlson, K. E., Dennis, C., Fierst, S. M., and Shaftan, G. W. Statistically valid ten-year comparative evaluation of three methods of management of massive gastroduodenal hemorrhage. Ann. Surg. *162*:550, 1965.
29. Northfield, T. C. Factors predisposing to recurrent haemorrhage after acute gastrointestinal bleeding Br. Med. J. *1*:26, 1971.
30. Logan, R. F. A., and Finlayson, N. D. C. Death in acute upper gastrointestinal bleeding. Can endoscopy reduce mortality? Lancet *1*:1173, 1976.

31. Morgan, A. G., McAdam, W. A. F., Walmsley, G. L., Jessop, A., Horrocks, J. C., and deDombal, F. T. Clinical findings, early endoscopy, and multivariate analysis in patients bleeding from the upper gastrointestinal tract. Br. Med. J. 2:237, 1977.

32. Wara, P., Berg, V., and Amdrup, E. Factors influencing mortality in patients with bleeding ulcer. Review of 7 years' experience preceding therapeutic endoscopy. Acta Chir. Scand. 149:775, 1983.

33. Bordley, D. R., Mushlin, A. I., Dolan, J. G., Richardson, W. S., Barry, M., Polio, J., and Griner, P. F. Early clinical signs identify low-risk patients with acute upper gastrointestinal hemorrhage. JAMA 253:3282, 1985.

34. Vellacott, K. D., Dronfield, M. W., Atkinson, M., and Langman, M. J. S. Comparison of surgical and medical management of bleeding peptic ulcers. Br. Med. J. (Clin. Res.) 284:548, 1982.

35. Jensen, H. E., Amdrup, E., Christiansen, P., Fenger, C., Lindskov, J., Nielsen, J., and Nielsen, S. A. Bleeding gastric ulcer. Surgical and non-surgical treatment of 225 patients. Scand. J. Gastroenterol. 7:535, 1972.

36. Allan, R., and Dykes, P. A study of the factors influencing mortality rates from gastrointestinal hemorrhage. Q. J. Med. 45:533, 1976.

37. Graham, D. Y. Limited value of early endoscopy in the management of acute upper gastrointestinal bleeding. Prospective controlled trial. Am. J. Surg. 140:284, 1980.

38. Guth, P. H. Bleeding peptic ulcer in the elderly. Am. J. Gastroenterol. 39:43, 1963.

39. Graham, D. Y., and Schwartz, J. T. The spectrum of the Mallory-Weiss tear. Medicine (Baltimore) 57:307, 1977.

40. Foster, D. N., Miloszewski, K. J. A., and Losowsky, M. S. Stigmata of recent haemorrhage in diagnosis and prognosis of upper gastrointestinal bleeding. Br. Med. J. 1:1173, 1978.

41. Rofe, S. B., Duggan, J. M., Smith, E. R., and Thursby, C. J. Conservative treatment of gastrointestinal haemorrhage. Gut 26:481, 1985.

42. Sanowski, R. A. Thermal application for gastrointestinal bleeding. J. Clin. Gastroenterol. 8:239, 1986.

43. Fleischer D. Endoscopic therapy of upper gastrointestinal bleeding in humans. Gastroenterology 90:217, 1986.

44. Griffiths, W. J., Neumann, D. A., and Welsh, J. D. The visible vessel as an indicator of uncontrolled or recurrent gastrointestinal hemorrhage. N. Engl. J. Med. 300:1411, 1979.

45. Storey, D. W., Bown, S. G., Swain, C. P., Salmon, P. R., Kirkham, J. S., and Northfield, T. C. Endoscopic prediction of recurrent bleeding in peptic ulcers. N. Engl. J. Med. 305:915, 1981.

46. Wara, P. Endoscopic prediction of major rebleeding—a prospective study of stigmata of hemorrhage in bleeding ulcer. Gastroenterology 88:1209, 1985.

47. Beckly, D. E., and Casebow, M. P. Prediction of rebleeding from peptic ulcer experience with an endoscopic Doppler device. Gut 27:96, 1986.

48. Morris, D. L., Hawker, P. C., Brearley, S., Simms, M., Dykes, P. W., and Keighley, M. R. B. Optimal timing of operation for bleeding peptic ulcer: prospective randomised trial. Br. Med. J. (Clin. Res.) 288:1277, 1984.

49. Sigel, B., and Hatke, F. L. Physical factors in electrocoaptation of blood vessels. Arch. Surg. 95:54, 1967.

50. Serebro, H. A., and Mendeloff, A. I. Late results of medical and surgical treatment of bleeding peptic ulcer. Lancet 2:505, 1966.

51. Arias, I. M., Zamcheck, N., and Thrower, W. B. Recurrence of hemorrhage from medically treated gastric ulcers: 4-year to 8-year follow-up of 47 patients. Arch. Intern. Med. 101:369, 1958.

52. Harvey, R. F., and Langman, M. J. S. The late results of medical and surgical treatment for bleeding duodenal ulcer. Q. J. Med. 39:539, 1970.

53. Johansson, C., and Barany, F. A retrospective study on the outcome of massive bleeding from peptic ulceration. Scand. J. Gastroenterol. 8:113, 1973.

54. Hallenbeck, G. A. Elective surgery for treatment of hemorrhage from duodenal ulcer. Gastroenterology 59:784, 1970.

55. Borland, J. L., Sr., Hancock, W. R., and Borland, J. L., Jr. Recurrent upper gastrointestinal hemorrhage in peptic ulcer. Gastroenterology 52:631, 1967.

56. Boles, R. S., Jr., Cassidy, W. J., and Jordan, S. M. Medical versus surgical management for the complication of hemorrhage in duodenal ulcer. Gastroenterology 32:52, 1957.

57. Cohen, M. M. Treatment and mortality of perforated peptic ulcer: a survey of 852 cases. Can. Med. Assoc. J. 105:263, 1971.

58. Watkins, R. M., Dennison, A. R., and Collin, J. What has happened to perforated peptic ulcer? Br. J. Surg. 71:774, 1984.

59. Jordan, P. H., Jr. Proximal gastric vagotomy without drainage for treatment of perforated duodenal ulcer. Gastroenterology 83:179, 1982.

60. Kozoll, D. D., and Meyer, K. A. Symptoms and signs in the prognosis of gastroduodenal ulcers: an analysis of 1,904 cases of acute perforated gastroduodenal ulcer. Arch. Surg. 82:528, 1961.

61. Collier, D. S. T. J., and Pain, J. A. Non-steroidal anti-inflammatory drugs and peptic ulcer perforation. Gut 26:359, 1985.

62. Ferrara, J. J., Wanamaker, S., and Carey, L. C. Preoperative serum creatinine as a predictor of survival in perforated gastroduodenal ulcer. Am. Surg. 51:551, 1985.

63. Botsford, T. W., Wilson, R. E. The Acute Abdomen. Philadephia, W. B. Saunders Co., 1969, p. 79.

64. Felix, W. R., Jr., and Stahlgren, L. H. Death by undiagnosed perforated peptic ulcer: analysis of 31 cases. Ann. Surg. 177:344, 1973.

65. Rogers, F. A. Elevated serum amylase: a review and an analysis of findings in 1,000 cases of perforated peptic ulcer. Ann. Surg. 153:228, 1961.

66. Kristensen, E. S. Conservative treatment of 155 cases of perforated peptic ulcer. Acta Chir. Scand. 146:189, 1980.

67. Kirkpatrick, J. R., and Bouwman, D. L. A logical solution to the perforated ulcer controversy. Surg. Gynecol. Obstet. 150:683, 1980.

68. Donovan, A. J., Vinson, T. L., Maulsby, G. O., and Gewin, J. R. Selective treatment of duodenal ulcer with perforation. Ann. Surg. 189:627, 1979.

69. Greco, R. S., Cahow, C. E. Alternatives in the management of acute perforated duodenal ulcer. Am. J. Surg. 127:109, 1974.

70. Paster, S. B., Brogdon, B. G. Roentgenographic diagnosis of pneumoperitoneum. JAMA 235:1264, 1976.

71. Coleman, J. A., Denham, M. J. Perforation of the peptic ulceration in the elderly. Age Ageing 9:257, 1980.

72. Seeley, S. F., and Campbell, D. Nonoperative treatment of perforated peptic ulcer: a further report. Surg. Gynecol. Obstet. 102:435, 1956.

73. Hofkin, G. A. Course of patients with perforated duodenal ulcers. Am. J. Surg. 111:193, 1966.

74. Boey, J., Lee, N. W., Wong, J., and Ong, G. B. Perforations in acute duodenal ulcers. Surg. Gynecol. Obstet. 155:193, 1982.

75. Jarrett, F., and Donaldson, G. A. The ulcer diathesis in perforated duodenal ulcer disease. Experience with 252 patients during a twenty-five year period. Am. J. Surg. 123:406, 1972.

76. Jordan, G. L., Jr., DeBakey, M. E., and Duncan, J. M., Jr. Surgical management of perforated peptic ulcer. Ann. Surg. 179:628, 1974.

77. Boey, J., Lee, N. W., Koo, J., Lam, P. H. M., Wong, J., and Ong, G. B. Immediate definitive surgery for perforated duodenal ulcers: a prospective controlled trial. Ann. Surg. 196:338, 1982.

78. Sawyers, J. L., and Herrington, J. L., Jr. Perforated duodenal ulcer managed by proximal gastric vagotomy and suture plication. Ann. Surg. 185:656, 1977.

79. Wara, P., Kristensen, E. S., Sorensen, F. H., Bone, J., Skovgaard, S., and Amdrup, E. The value of parietal cell vagotomy compared to simple closure in a selective approach to perforated duodenal ulcer. Operative morbidity and recurrence rate. Acta Chir. Scand. 149:585, 1983.

80. Cleator, I. G. M., Holubitsky, I. B., and Harrison, R. C. Perforated anastomotic ulcers. Ann. Surg. 177:436, 1973.

81. Mattingly, S. S., Ram, M. D., and Griffen, W. O., Jr. Factors influencing morbidity and mortality in perforated duodenal ulcer. Am. J. Surg. 46:61, 1980.

82. Boey, J., Wong, J., and Ong, G. B. A prospective study of operative risk factors in perforated duodenal ulcers. Ann. Surg. 195:265, 1982.

83. Norris, J. R., and Haubrich, W. S. The incidence and clinical features of penetration in peptic ulceration. JAMA 178:386, 1961.

84. Caruolo, J. E., Hallenbeck, G. A., and Dockerty, M. B. A clinicopathologic study of posterior penetrating gastric ulcers. Surg. Gynecol. Obstet. 101:759, 1955.

85. Ross, J. R., and Reaves, L. E., III. Syndrome of posterior penetrating ulcer. Med. Clin. North Am. 50:461, 1966.

86. Cassel, C., Ruffin, J. M., and Bone, F. C. The clinical features of walled off perforated peptic ulcer: an analysis of 100 cases. South. Med. J. 44:1021, 1951.

87. Hashmonal, M., Abrahamson, J., Erlik, D., and Schramek, A. Retroperitoneal perforation of duodenal ulcers with abscess formation: report of four cases and survey of the literature. Ann. Surg. 173:409, 1971.

88. Cody, J. H., DiVincenti, F. C., Cowick, D. R., and Mahanes, J. R. Gastrocolic and gastrojejunocolic fistulae: report of twelve cases and review of the literature. Ann. Surg. 181:376, 1975.

89. Laufer, I., Thornley, G. D., and Stolberg, H. Gastrocolic fistula as a complication of benign gastric ulcer. Radiology 119:7, 1976.

90. Feller, E. R., Warshaw, A. L., and Schapiro, R. H. Observations on management of choledochoduodenal fistula due to penetrating peptic ulcer. Gastroenterology 78:126, 1980.

91. Sarr, M. G., Shepard, A. J., and Zuidema, G. D. Choledochoduodenal fistula: an unusual complication of duodenal ulcer disease. Am. J. Surg. 141:736, 1981.

92. Dubois, A. Pathophysiology of gastric emptying: methods of measurement and clinical significance. J. Clin. Gastroenterol. 1:259, 1979.

93. Malagelada, J. R. Physiologic basis and clinical significance of gastric emptying disorders. Dig. Dis. Sci. 24:657, 1979.

94. Kelly, K. A. Gastric emptying of liquids and solids: roles of proximal and distal stomach. Am. J. Physiol. 239:G671, 1980

95. Balint, J. A., and Spence, M. P. Pyloric stenosis. Br. Med. J. 1:890, 1959.

96. Rimer, D. G. Gastric retention without mechanical obstruction. A review. Arch. Intern. Med. 117:287, 1966.

97. Kozoll, D. D., and Meyer, K. A. Obstructing gastroduodenal ulcers: general factors influencing incidence and mortality. Arch. Surg. 88:793, 1964.

98. Dworken, H. J., and Roth, H. P. Pyloric obstruction associated with peptic ulcer: a clinicopathological analysis of 158 surgically treated cases. JAMA 180:1007, 1962.

99. Kreel, L., and Ellis, H. Pyloric stenosis in adults: a clinical and radiological study of 100 consecutive patients. Gut 6:253, 1965.

100. Moody, F. G., Cornell, G. N., and Beal, J. M. Pyloric obstruction complicating peptic ulcer. Arch. Surg. 84:462, 1962.

101. Weiland, D., Dunn, D. H., Humphrey, E. W., and Schwartz, M. L. Gastric outlet obstruction in peptic ulcer disease: an indication for surgery. Am. J. Surg. 143:90, 1982.

102. Kozoll, D. D., and Meyer, K. A. Obstructing gastroduodenal ulcer, symptoms and signs. Arch. Surg. 89:491, 1964.

103. Goldstein, H., Janin, M., Schapiro, M., and Boyle, J. D. Gastric retention associated with gastroduodenal disease: a study of 217 cases. Am. J. Dig. Dis. 11:887, 1966.

104. Kassirer, J. P., and Schwartz, W. B. The response of normal man to selective depletion of hydrochloric acid. Factors in the genesis of persistent gastric alkalosis. Am. J. Med. 40:10, 1966.

105. Goldstein, H., and Boyle, J. D. The saline load test—a bedside evaluation of gastric retention. Gastroenterology 49:375, 1965.

106. Raskin, H. F. Barium-burger roentgen study for unrecognized, clinically significant, gastric retention. South. Med. J. 64:1227, 1971.

107. Pelot, D., Dana, E. R., Berk, J. E., and Dixon, G. Comparative assessment of gastric emptying by the "barium-burger" and saline load tests. Am. J. Gastroenterol. 58:411, 1972.

108. Tothill, P., McLoughlin, G. P., and Heading, R. C. Techniques and errors in scintigraphic measurements of gastric emptying. J. Nucl. Med. 19:256, 1978.

109. Dubois, A., Price, S. F., and Castell, D. O. Gastric retention in peptic ulcer disease: a reappraisal. Am. J. Dig. Dis. 23:993, 1978.

110. Jaffin, B. W., and Kaye, M. D. The prognosis of gastric outlet obstruction. Ann. Surg. 201:176, 1985.

111. Abouna, G. M., Veazey, P. R., and Terry, D. B., Jr. Intravenous infusion of hydrochloric acid for treatment of severe metabolic alkalosis. Surgery 75:194, 1974.

112. Hai, A. A., Singh, A., and Mittal, V. K. Closed pyloroduodenal digital dilatation as a complementary drainage procedure to truncal vagotomy. Int. Surg. 71:87, 1986.

113. Rossi, R. L., Braasch, J. W., Cady, B., and Sedgwick, C. E. Parietal cell vagotomy for intractable and obstructing duodenal ulcer. Am. J. Surg. 141:482, 1981.

114. Ferraz, E. M., Ferreira Filho, H. A., Bacelar, T. S., Lacerda, C. M., Ponce de Souza, A., and Kelner, S. Proximal gastric vagotomy in stenosed or perforated duodenal ulcer. Br. J. Surg. 68:452, 1981.

115. Pringle, R., Irving, A. D., Longrigg, J. N., and Wisbey, M. Randomized trial of truncal vagotomy with either pyloroplasty or pyloric dilatation in the surgical management of chronic duodenal ulcer. Br. J. Surg. 70:482, 1983.

116. Johnston, D., Lyndon, P. J., Smith, R. B., and Humphrey, C. S. Highly selective vagotomy without a drainage procedure in the treatment of haemorrhage, perforation, and pyloric stenosis due to peptic ulcer. Br. J. Surg. 60:790, 1973.

117. Hooks, V. H., III, Bowden, T. A., Jr., Sisley, J. F., and Mansberger, A. R., Jr. Highly selective vagotomy with dilatation or duodenoplasty. A surgical alternative for obstructing duodenal ulcer. Ann. Surg. 203:545, 1986.

118. Barroso, F. L., Ornellas-Filho, A., Saboya, C. J., Frota-Pessoa, R., Oliveira, A., Vaz, O. P., and Galvao, J. B. Duodenoplasty and proximal gastric vagotomy in peptic stenosis. Experience with 43 cases. Arch. Surg. 121:1021, 1986.

119. Delaney, P. Preoperative grading of pyloric stenosis: a long-term clinical and radiological follow-up of patients with severe pyloric stenosis treated by highly selective vagotomy and dilatation of the stricture. Br. J. Surg. 65:157, 1978.

120. Dunn, D. C., Thomas, W. E. G., and Hunter, J. O. Highly selective vagotomy and pyloric dilatation for duodenal ulcer with stenosis. Br. J. Surg. 68:194, 1981.

121. Verhaeghe, P. J., Stoppa, R. E., Henry, X. F., and Myon, Y. L. Pyloric stenosis: organic or functional? The need for an intraoperative test in peptic ulcer surgery. Int. Surg. 65:301, 1980.

122. Kirk, R. M. The size of the pyloroduodenal canal: its relation to the cause and treatment of peptic ulcer. Proc. R. Soc. Med. 63:944, 1970.

123. Solt, J., Rauth, J., Papp, Z., and Bohenszky, G. Balloon catheter dilation of postoperative gastric outlet stenosis. Gastrointest. Endosc. 30:359, 1984.

124. Byrnes, D. J., and Blackie, J. D. Successful endoscopic treatment of pyloric and intestinal stenoses. Med. J. Aust. 2:516, 1982.

125. Benjamin, S. B., Glass, R. L., Cattau, E. L., Jr., and Miller, W. B. Preliminary experience with balloon dilation of the pylorus. Gastrointest. Endosc. 30:93, 1984.

126. Hogan, R. B., Hamilton, J. K., and Polter, D. E. Preliminary experience with hydrostatic balloon dilation of gastric outlet obstruction. Gastrointest. Endosc. 32:71, 1986.

127. Lindor, K. D., Ott, B. J., and Hughes, R. W., Jr. Balloon dilatation of upper digestive tract strictures. Gastroenterology 89:545, 1985.

128. Hogstrom, H., and Haglund, U. A technique for endoscopic balloon dilatation of pyloric stenoses. Endoscopy 17:224, 1985.

129. Gotberg, S., Afzelius, L. E., Hambraeus, J., Lunderquist, A., Owman, T., and Svensson, G. Balloon-catheter dilatation of strictures in the upper digestive tract. Radiologe 22:479, 1982.

Operations for Peptic Ulcer Disease and Early Postoperative Complications

51

PAUL H. JORDAN, JR.

Improved medical therapy for peptic ulcer disease has coincided with improved operative management. The indications for operating on patients electively for intractable peptic ulcer disease cannot be rigidly defined; however, severity and duration of symptoms, response to medication, patient compliance, and frequency of recurrences are factors that contribute to making this decision. Gastric surgeons have long recognized that the number of patients requiring elective gastric surgery for intractable peptic ulcers represents a small percentage of the total population with this disease. There comes a time, however, when patients with severe or recurrent ulcer distress should be informed that surgical treatment as well as continued, prolonged, cyclical medical therapy is an option.

Various operative procedures have been devised for the treatment of peptic ulcer disease. The intent of each new operation has been to improve the clinical results of surgical treatment, but the findings of controlled clinical trials of the more commonly used procedures suggest that, with the exception of the persistence or recurrence of ulcers, there is little to recommend one operation over another. The newest operation, parietal cell vagotomy without drainage, has been extensively studied for 17 years. These studies show that the undesirable side effects accompanying other gastric procedures are greatly reduced with parietal cell vagotomy while maintaining an acceptable recurrent ulcer rate. This operation has become the procedure of choice in many parts of the world, including England and Continental Europe. The operation has not yet gained the same acceptance in the United States, although it has become increasingly popular. Full assessment of its place in gastric surgery and its limitations in the treatment of peptic ulcer await the outcome of long-term, prospective randomized studies.

Sometimes technical factors—for example, the amount of inflammation in the area of the duodenum or the location of an ulcer—dictate the advisability of one type of operation over another. With these exceptions, it can be said that most surgeons perform a particular operation in preference to the others because in their opinion it is the best operation. In fact, a given operation may be best for a given surgeon because he is more experienced and more skilled with a particular operation which he therefore performs with greater safety.

It would be ideal if it could be determined that one operation was more suitable for a given patient than any other procedure. Although there are claims[1–7] that such discrimination can be made, the evidence for this is not convincing.

SELECTION OF OPERATIONS FOR ELECTIVE TREATMENT OF DUODENAL ULCER

Distal Subtotal (Two-Thirds to Three-Quarters) Gastrectomy without a Vagotomy

This operation was formerly used extensively for the treatment of duodenal ulcer. After resection, gastrointestinal continuity can be restored by gastroduodenostomy (Billroth I) or gastrojejunostomy (Billroth II) (Fig. 51–1). The number of recurrent ulcers after gastroduodenostomy has led to the abandonment of this procedure in favor of gastrojejunostomy unless the resection is accompanied by vagotomy.[8] The higher recurrence rate after Billroth I anastomosis was attributed to a lesser resection in order to approximate the stomach and duodenum without tension on the suture line. Another possible explanation for the unsatisfactory results after Billroth I anastomosis is that innervated parietal cells are more sensitive to gastrin, which,

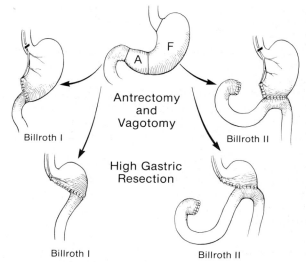

Figure 51–1. Diagram of antrectomy (A) and vagotomy and high subtotal gastric resection, which includes the antrum and a major portion of the fundus (F). Gastrointestinal continuity can be achieved by either gastroduodenostomy (Billroth I) or gastrojejunostomy (Billroth II).

Table 51–1. PERCENTAGE OF PATIENTS WITH SYMPTOMS REFERABLE TO THE ALIMENTARY TRACT AFTER OPERATION

Symptoms	Vagotomy and Gastroenterostomy n = 122	Vagotomy and Antrectomy n = 126	Subtotal Gastrectomy n = 112
Epigastric fullness	37	36	39
Early dumping	12	14	20
Late dumping	3	4	1
Nausea	18	18	21
Food vomiting	5	7	9
Bile vomiting	11	13	15
Heartburn	17	12	6
Flatulence	18	22	18
Dysphagia	1	2	0
Diarrhea	27	21	11

Modified from Goligher, J. C., Pulvertaft, C. N., and Watkinson, G. Br. Med. J. *1*:455, 1967. Used by permission.

in response to feeding, is released in greater amounts from the duodenum after gastroduodenostomy than from the jejunum after gastrojejunostomy.[9]

Undesirable postoperative sequelae increase as greater amounts of the stomach are removed to prevent recurrence of ulcers.[10] For this reason many surgeons no longer advocate high subtotal partial gastrectomy. Although the acceptance of this operation has greatly diminished, its only controlled evaluation demonstrated that the clinical results were as good as those obtained with the other operations tested.[11]

In the prospective, randomized study by Goligher and associates,[11] distal partial gastrectomy and Billroth II, vagotomy and antrectomy, and vagotomy and gastrojejunostomy were evaluated. Table 51–1 lists the common gastrointestinal symptoms encountered by patients after gastric surgery.[11] Except for a slightly higher rate of early dumping after distal partial gastrectomy, the patients seemed as well off after this operation as after the other two, and the overall results scored according to the Visick scale (an arbitrary scale for excellent, good, fair, and poor) showed no difference in the outcome achieved after the three operations. After four years, the results slightly favored vagotomy and antrectomy and distal partial gastrectomy, because they offered better protection against recurrent ulcer and marginally better Visick gradings than vagotomy and gastrojejunostomy. The operative mortality and the recurrent ulcer rates were the same after distal partial gastrectomy as they were after vagotomy and antrectomy. In other reports, both were lower after vagotomy and antrectomy than they were after distal partial gastrectomy. The wide variation in the recurrent ulcer rate after distal partial gastrectomy, which ranged from 1.2 to 12.7 per cent in the review by Rhea and associates,[12] was probably related to the varying and unknown amounts of stomach removed by different surgeons. As indicated, the use of high subtotal gastrectomy without vagotomy is diminishing, and this is due to the persuasive logic that (1) it is desirable to preserve as much gastric reservoir as possible, and

(2) there is little to recommend the operation over vagotomy and antrectomy, which appears to be a safer operation for most surgeons.

Some of the complications of distal partial gastrectomy and gastrojejunostomy are seen in Figure 51–2. The most frequent and significant complications include mechanical obstruction of the efferent and/or afferent limbs of the anastomosis, caused by angulation, twists, or inflammation secondary to an anastomotic leak or idiopathic fat necrosis. An afferent limb obstruction with resulting increased pressure within the duodenum enhances the chance for disruption of a duodenal stump closure. Leakage from an insecurely closed duodenal stump is a potential complication even when there is no distal obstruction. If, at the time of operation, this is considered as a possible complication, the duodenum can be drained with a tube to establish a controlled fistula that will close spontaneously after a fistulous tract is established and the tube is removed. These complications do not develop if a gastroduodenostomy is performed; but the high recurrent ulcer rate that occurs with this method of restoring gastrointestinal continuity precludes its use unless vagotomy is also done. The gastroduodenostomy method of reconstruction has its own complications, which include obstruction or leakage at the anastomosis.

Another potential complication associated with any operation that includes resection of the distal stomach is pancreatitis. Pancreatitis is associated with trauma at the time of dissection of the duodenal bulb. It may be mild or sufficiently acute and fulminating to result in death. Related to this complication is the possibility of injury to the common bile duct when the duodenum is foreshortened and the common bile duct is drawn into the inflammatory mass in which one must operate if a resection is being carried out.

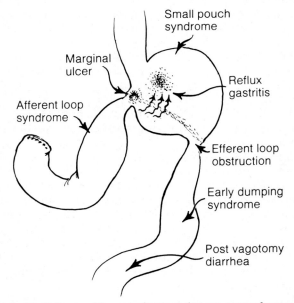

Figure 51–2. Some of the complications that can occur after gastric surgery.

Truncal Vagotomy and Drainage

Vagotomy removes the direct effect of vagal stimulation on the parietal cells, and it reduces the sensitivity of parietal cells to gastrin. For these reasons, vagotomy has exerted a profound influence on the treatment of duodenal ulcer.

Dragstedt and Owens[13] reintroduced vagotomy in 1943 in hope of finding a cure for duodenal ulcer that was associated with fewer undesirable sequelae and with a lower mortality rate than was generally obtained at that time with distal partial gastrectomy. Their initial operation was a transthoracic vagotomy, which was soon abandoned because of the number of patients who postoperatively developed gastric retention that led to the formation of a gastric ulcer in some. The procedure was changed to a transabdominal vagotomy accompanied by a gastroenterostomy to facilitate gastric emptying. Transthoracic vagotomy is now performed only in certain circumstances for the treatment of recurrent ulcer.

Because gastroenterostomy was considered a less than ideal drainage procedure, the Heineke-Mukulicz pyloroplasty (Fig. 51–3) was widely substituted and became the most popular drainage procedure. Nevertheless, many surgeons think that stasis is not prevented satisfactorily by this type of pyloroplasty even when it is performed using the single layer closure technique.

Lynch and colleagues[14] emphasized the importance of poor gastric emptying as a cause for the development of gastric ulcer after Heineke-Mikulicz pyloroplasty. Rather than risk resection or resort to gastroenteros-tomy, a Finney pyloroplasty or Jaboulay gastroduo-denostomy (Fig. 51–3) to promote satisfactory gastric drainage after vagotomy has been recommended.

Hayden and Read[15] concluded from their studies that for the average patient there was insufficient advantage to justify the more extensive Finney instead of the Heineke-Mikulicz pyloroplasty. Sometimes when one needs desperately to avoid gastric resection but the duodenum is opened and cannot be closed with a Heineke-Mikulicz pyloroplasty, a Finney type of closure will be a valuable procedure to use. Gastroen-terostomy as a drainage procedure has been down-graded in America but is still held in esteem by many in the British Isles. Kennedy and associates[16] consider gastroenterostomy the drainage procedure of choice, because, in patients with significant dumping, it may be dismantled after the stomach has regained its tone lost by vagotomy without fear of gastric retention. Goligher and colleagues[17] consider it preferable to pyloroplasty, because it is associated with a lower recurrent ulcer rate.

There is no disagreement that the number of recurrent ulcers is greater after vagotomy and drainage (4 to 27 per cent) than after high subtotal gastrectomy (4 per cent) or vagotomy and antrectomy (1 per cent). The causes for recurrent ulcer after vagotomy and drainage are (1) gastric stasis due to an unsatisfactory drainage procedure, (2) failure to cut a major vagal branch to the stomach and (3) the unrecognized presence of a Zollinger-Ellison tumor. But there must be other factors. Eisenberg and associates,[18] representing the Dragstedt school, reported an overall recurrence rate of 3.6 per cent among 443 patients followed 1 to

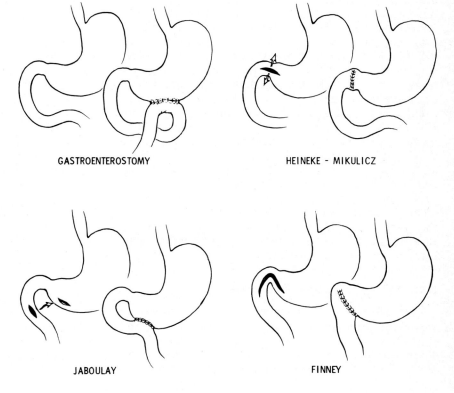

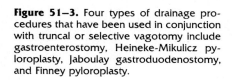

GASTROENTEROSTOMY

HEINEKE - MIKULICZ

JABOULAY

FINNEY

Figure 51–3. Four types of drainage procedures that have been used in conjunction with truncal or selective vagotomy include gastroenterostomy, Heineke-Mikulicz pyloroplasty, Jaboulay gastroduodenostomy, and Finney pyloroplasty.

10 years after vagotomy and drainage. By contrast, Stempien and coworkers[19] studied 161 patients 10 to 18 years after vagotomy and pyloroplasty was performed by Weinberg's group; the recurrent ulcer rate was 27 per cent. Why there should be such a wide divergence in the results observed by these two groups is unknown. Jordan and Condon,[20] in a prospective, randomized study, noted that the Hollander insulin test was positive in 50 per cent of patients after vagotomy and pyloroplasty and in 13 per cent of those patients undergoing vagotomy and antrectomy. Since the same surgeons performed the vagotomies in both groups of patients, one cannot conclude that vagotomy was anatomically less complete in one group than the other, but rather that insulin in some way exerted an effect on the secretory response through the retained antrum in patients undergoing vagotomy and pyloroplasty. By inference one can postulate that the recurrent ulcer rate is higher after vagotomy and pyloroplasty than after vagotomy and antrectomy because of the continued influence of the retained antrum on acid secretion.

For many surgeons, the higher recurrent ulcer rate associated with vagotomy and drainage is an acceptable trade for the perceived higher mortality rate associated with operations that include resection. On the other hand, if surgeons who prefer resection reserve vagotomy and drainage for patients in whom resection is contraindicated because of difficulty dissecting the duodenum or for the poor-risk medical patient, the mortality rate for patients undergoing resection should be equally low as for those in whom vagotomy and drainage is performed routinely.

The immediate complications of vagotomy and drainage procedures include obstruction of the pyloroplasty or gastroenterostomy leading to gastric stasis and gastric ulcer. Loss of gastric motility after vagotomy may cause delayed gastric emptying and can be differentiated from stomal obstruction by gastroscopic examination. A leaking pyloroplasty or gastroenterostomy is a major complication that can lead to stomal obstruction and fistulas. If the disruption of the anastomosis is of greater magnitude, peritonitis and death may result. Placement of a gastroenterostomy too high on the greater curvature of the stomach may cause the duodenal contents to re-enter the stomach through the gastroenterostomy stoma. This recirculation of gastric and duodenal contents will stimulate antral function, acid hypersecretion, and possibly recurrent marginal ulcer. Obstruction of the efferent or afferent limbs of the gastroenterostomy will create the same complications that are associated with gastrojejunostomy performed after gastric resection.

Truncal Vagotomy and Antrectomy

Currently vagotomy and antrectomy with gastrojejunostomy reconstruction (Fig. 51–1) is one of the most frequent operations used for the treatment of duodenal ulcer. Surgeons utilizing this operation remove 20 per cent (antrectomy) to 50 per cent (hemi-

gastrectomy) of the stomach. The procedure was introduced by Smithwick in 1946, because he thought it would be the most effective operation to produce achlorhydria while at the same time preserving a larger gastric reservoir than occurs with high subtotal gastric resection.[21]

A similar operation was performed independently by Edwards.[22] Later the operation was modified by Harkins and colleagues[23] so that reconstruction was by means of gastroduodenostomy (Billroth I), because it was expected that the number of patients with the dumping symptoms and weight loss would be fewer with this technique than after gastrojejunostomy (Billroth II). The combined procedure of antrectomy and vagotomy proposed by Smithwick and Edwards and modified by Harkins continued to be the preferred procedure of Herrington's group,[24] who in 1976 reported 95 per cent excellent to good results following the operation performed on 3771 patients who were followed for 10 to 22 years. The overall recurrence rate was 0.5 per cent, and the mortality rate was 1.5 per cent. If those patients who were operated upon for emergency bleeding were excluded, the mortality was 1 per cent. The mortality for massive hemorrhage in patients over age 60 was 6 per cent. The low mortality was attributed to the use of gastrojejunostomy (Billroth II) for reconstruction rather than gastroduodenostomy (Billroth I) in patients in whom the inflammation involving the duodenum created unusual technical difficulties.

The consensus of others who also favor vagotomy and antrectomy[25–27] is that nutritional deficits, anemia, and excessive weight loss occur less frequently than after distal partial gastrectomy. A higher mortality is the major criticism of vagotomy and antrectomy advanced by those who favor vagotomy and drainage. In a prospective study by Jordan[20] (Table 51–2), there was no mortality after vagotomy and antrectomy and a 2 per cent mortality after vagotomy and drainage. After a five-year follow-up period, the principal difference in the clinical results obtained in the two groups of patients was a recurrent ulcer rate of 8.3 per cent after vagotomy and pyloroplasty and 1.1 per cent after vagotomy and antrectomy. This study suggested that vagotomy and antrectomy for treatment of duodenal ulcer can be performed under elective conditions in patients who are reasonably good risk surgical candidates and who do not have severe inflammation sur-

Table 51–2. COMPARISON OF TRUNCAL VAGOTOMY–ANTRECTOMY AND TRUNCAL VAGOTOMY–DRAINAGE

	TV-A n = 92	TV-D n = 108
Operative mortality	0	2%
Ulcer recurrence	1.1%	8.3%
Diarrhea at 3 years	12%	13%
Dumping at 3 years	20%	18%

Data from Jordan, P. H., Jr., and Condon, R. E. Ann. Surg. *172*:547, 1970.

rounding the duodenum, with an operative mortality rate and clinical results equivalent to or better than those obtained with vagotomy and drainage. Therefore in choosing between the standard operative procedures already discussed, there is little justification for subjecting all healthy persons to the high risk of recurrent ulcer and the possible need for reoperation by performing vagotomy and pyloroplasty when there are no clinical advantages over vagotomy and antrectomy.

The early complications related to vagotomy and antrectomy are the same as for high subtotal partial gastrectomy but are fewer after gastroduodenostomy (Billroth I) than after gastrojejunostomy (Billroth II) reconstruction. Loss of gastric motility following vagotomy may cause gastric stasis and may simulate or potentiate stomal dysfunction.

Results of experiments on the intact stomach, after resection of the stomach, and after various types of gastric denervation are consistent with the hypothesis that proximal stomach contractions exert a major role on gastric emptying of liquids while contractions of the distal stomach exert a major role on gastric emptying of solids.[28] However, the reasons for delayed gastric emptying that occasionally occurs after operations on the stomach are not thoroughly understood. Fortunately, in most instances a stomach that has been slow to empty will regain its ability to do so if given adequate time.

In addition to operations that interfere with normal gastric motility, such as vagotomy, gastric paresis may also result from diabetes and gastric decompensation caused by gastric outlet obstruction. Edema of the gastric stoma has been implicated as the cause of delayed gastric emptying more frequently than seems justified.

A stoma poorly constructed or obstructed by an inflammatory process is not an uncommon cause for a stomach not to empty properly after operation. A less than perfect stoma and a degree of gastric paresis, neither of which by itself would cause delayed gastric emptying, may when combined cause such delay. By using contrast studies and endoscopy, the adequacy of a gastric stoma should be determined early and reoperation performed to correct mechanical problems that may exist rather than waiting long periods "for the stoma to open."

Other Types of Vagotomy

Selective Vagotomy. Since vagal denervation of viscera other than the stomach seemed neither necessary nor desirable in the treatment of duodenal ulcer, selective vagotomy which denervates only the stomach was introduced independently by Jackson[29] and Franksson[30] (Fig. 51–4). There is evidence that sacrifice of the extragastric vagi at the time of truncal vagotomy adversely affects small bowel function and causes the bile to become lithogenic. Retention of the extragastric vagi has been credited with preventing postvagotomy diarrhea. Clearly, an enteropancreatic reflex important

for pancreatic exocrine[31] and endocrine function is dependent on the extragastric vagi.[32] Several lines of evidence in dogs suggest that the extragastric branches of the vagi that are not sacrificed during selective vagotomy exert an inhibitory effect on gastric secretion by an unknown mechanism. Whether this is also true in human beings is unknown.[33, 34]

Selective vagotomy has been used[35–38] in combination with antrectomy or pyloroplasty in the belief that the clinical results achieved were superior, particularly in reducing the frequency of diarrhea, to those obtained with truncal vagotomy. Selective vagotomy permitted a degree of gastric denervation that was as good as that achieved with truncal vagotomy. In fact, there are reports suggesting that incomplete gastric vagotomy occurs less frequently after selective vagotomy than after truncal vagotomy.[39, 40] Some prospective, randomized studies of selective and truncal vagotomy[39–44] failed to show that the early or late results were better after one type of vagotomy than after the other. The effect of selective vagotomy on lowering acid secretion is controversial; however, several investigators are of the opinion that there are no clear differences between selective vagotomy and truncal vagotomy on basal,[43] maximal acid output,[43, 45] and insulin-stimulated acid output.[42–45] Yet there is some evidence that a clinical difference exists between the two types of vagotomy. In a randomized study, Sawyers and Scott[46] reported a recurrent ulcer rate after selective vagotomy and pyloroplasty that was as low as that observed after selective vagotomy and antrectomy. This is in contrast to the high recurrence rate they reported after truncal vagotomy and pyloroplasty.

Whether selective vagotomy is superior to truncal vagotomy in the treatment of duodenal ulcer is still controversial, but my personal bias supports selective vagotomy over truncal vagotomy. There appear to be no complications unique to selective vagotomy. The use of selective vagotomy does not obviate the necessity to perform a complementary resection or drainage procedure. Although vagotomy not accompanied by either resection or drainage has been attempted, it has been condemned by those who have tried it.

Parietal Cell Vagotomy without Drainage. This operation is the newest of the definitive operations for treatment of peptic ulcer disease. It is also called proximal gastric vagotomy or superselective vagotomy, as well as several other names. Parietal cell vagotomy, conceived by Griffith and Harkins,[47] was first performed in human beings by Holle,[48] but he combined it with pyloromyotomy and continues to do so. Parietal cell vagotomy without drainage was performed independently in human beings at about the same time by Amdrup and Jensen[49] and by Johnston and Wilkinson.[50]

The principle of the operation is to section all branches of the anterior and posterior vagus nerves that supply the fundic gland area of the stomach while preserving the hepatic, celiac, and antral branches. It is the preservation of the motor nerve branches to the

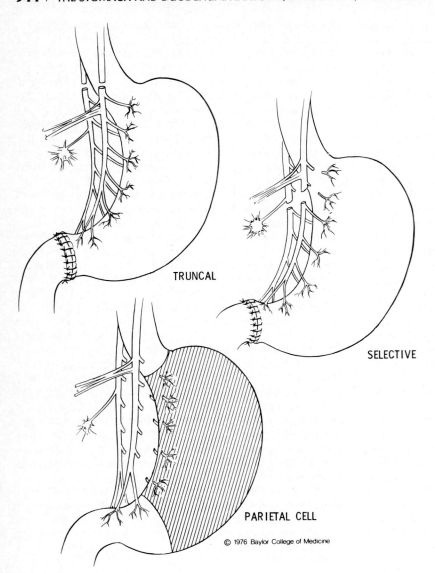

TRUNCAL

SELECTIVE

PARIETAL CELL

© 1976 Baylor College of Medicine

Figure 51—4. The three types of vagotomy in use are truncal or total intra-abdominal vagotomy, selective or total gastric vagotomy, and parietal cell vagotomy or vagotomy of the acid-secreting portion of the stomach.

antrum that makes it unnecessary to resect, destroy, or bypass the pylorus in order to ensure satisfactory gastric emptying.

The dumping syndrome is probably related only indirectly to total vagotomy. It is more likely the result of gastric incontinence that follows destruction or bypass of the pyloroantral pump mechanism by pyloroplasty, antrectomy, or gastroenterostomy. Diarrhea following gastric surgery is attributed to truncal vagotomy and/or loss of pyloric function. The cause for vagotomy diarrhea is unknown, but has been considered by some to be intestinal hurry. The diarrhea resulting from the loss of the pylorus is associated with unregulated gastric emptying. It was expected therefore that preservation of the intact pylorus and antral innervation would reduce dumping and diarrhea by permitting near-normal gastric emptying, whereas preservation of the extragastric vagi would reduce the incidence of vagotomy diarrhea. In one study,[51] the incidence of dumping and of diarrhea after parietal

cell vagotomy was 5 and 5.6 per cent, respectively, which was significantly less than that observed after truncal vagotomy and drainage or truncal vagotomy and antrectomy. Most investigations support these findings. In a recent study we showed no significant difference in the frequency of diarrhea between parietal cell vagotomy and selective vagotomy and antrectomy.[52] This may have been due to the use of selective rather than truncal vagotomy. The major differences between parietal cell vagotomy, which in the opinion of the author is the best, and selective vagotomy-antrectomy and Billroth I anastomosis, which is the operation with the widest range of application, are seen in Table 51–3.[52]

Parietal cell vagotomy is a less traumatic operation than the conventional gastric procedures. Because it does not require opening of the stomach or the creation of a suture line, the mortality and the immediate postoperative morbidity have been less than with other forms of gastric surgery. The absence of an anastomosis

Table 51–3. COMPARISON OF PARIETAL CELL VAGOTOMY AND SELECTIVE VAGOTOMY-ANTRECTOMY

	PCV	SV-A
Operative mortality	0	0
Ulcerative recurrence for 10 years	10.1%	2.2%
Diarrhea at 3 years	6%	12%
Dumping at 3 years	5%	38%
Weight loss at 3 years	27%	51%
Visick I (excellent results at 3 years)	89%	59%

From Jordan, P. H., Jr., and Thornby, J. Ann. Surg., *205*:572, 1986.

eliminates such complications as afferent and efferent loop syndromes. The mortality in several series of patients has been zero, and in a survey of 4557 patients operated upon by 40 different surgeons the mortality was 0.26 per cent.[53]

Unlike truncal vagotomy without a drainage procedure, gastric stasis after parietal cell vagotomy has not been a problem. The size of the pyloric lumen can be tested by having the anesthetist pass a mercury-weighted bougie into the stomach, where it can than be guided by the surgeon into the duodenum. If a No. 40 French bougie passes easily, the pyloric lumen is of adequate size. On the other hand, if the size of the pyloric lumen is inadequate and/or excessive denervation of the antrum is performed, gastric stasis and the development of a gastric ulcer may occur. This chain of events is suggested by the observation that in the experience of different investigators, about half of the recurrent ulcers after parietal cell vagotomy for duodenal ulcer occur in the stomach.

Another potential disadvantage of parietal cell vagotomy, which delayed its trial in the United States, was the possibility that retention of an innervated antrum would be a potent stimulus for acid secretion. Johnston and associates[54] demonstrated that acid production in response to a test meal was no greater in patients with a vagally innervated antrum than in those with a vagally denervated antrum. It has also been shown that the serum gastrin levels after parietal cell vagotomy are not significantly different from those observed after truncal vagotomy. From these studies as well as others, it can be reasonably concluded that the retained gastric antrum need not be vagally denervated in the duodenal ulcer patient provided it is well drained and is in continuity with the acid-secreting portion of the stomach. However, antral preservation, either innervated or denervated, is undesirable in some patients and recurrent ulcer can be successfully treated by antrectomy.[20, 55] Why antrectomy is required to control ulcerogenesis in some patients and not in the majority is unknown. It may be due to high adrenergic release of gastrin,[56] alteration in the number and responsiveness of "functional" parietal cells,[57] or some other mechanism. Parietal cell vagotomy failures could be reduced if it were possible to recognize preoperatively which patients required antrectomy.

Currently, parietal cell vagotomy without drainage has been used clinically for 17 years. It can be said

that the mortality, the immediate postoperative complications, and the late complications of dumping, diarrhea, and bilious vomiting are less than with almost any other operation used for the treatment of duodenal ulcer. The ultimate recurrent ulcer rate that will be associated with this operation is the remaining unanswered question that contributes to its slow acceptance in some parts of the world, including the United States. In several reports in which patients were studied five to ten years after parietal cell vagotomy, the recurrence rate has been 4 to 11 per cent.[52, 58–60] In other studies the recurrence rate was reported as high as 26 per cent.[61] The discrepancy in the recurrence rates reported by different investigators is the result of several factors. The first relates to the actual variation in the operative procedure that is performed by different surgeons. The second factor is the experience, training, and skill of the surgeon. This is not an easy operation to perform. The recurrence rate is highest for the first patients operated on by any surgeon and is related to a very steep learning curve for this procedure.[62–64] Further, a surgeon must perform parietal cell vagotomy at regular intervals to maintain competency. The operation requires dedication to learning its proper execution and every surgeon must not feel compelled to perform parietal cell vagotomy. Finally, it is important to note that the recurrence rate following parietal cell vagotomy in one study was 33 per cent for pyloric and prepyloric ulcers and only 15 per cent for duodenal ulcers.[60] This has been the experience of numerous authors but has been denied by others.[65] It seems reasonable until this question is finally settled that parietal cell vagotomy be used only under special circumstances for pyloric and prepyloric ulcers.

Although the ultimate recurrence rate is unknown, the evidence now at hand suggests that the eventual recurrence rate should be the same as or better than after vagotomy and pyloroplasty. Accepting this assumption, the benefits derived from the operation so outweigh the possibility and consequences of a recurrence that it is my operation of choice for all patients treated electively in whom the pylorus is adequately patent. I agree with Johnston and associates[66] that there is no evidence based on gastric acid secretory studies to suggest that the operation is more or less suitable for one group of patients than another.

Efforts on the part of surgeons to improve the operative treatment of duodenal ulcers have led to evaluating the possibility of removing the antral mucosa in conjunction with parietal cell vagotomy without destroying the motility of the antrum.[67] This operation has not yet been evaluated in man.

SELECTION OF OPERATION FOR BENIGN GASTRIC ULCER

Conservative data reveal that 42 per cent of patients with healed gastric ulcers develop recurrent ulcers and 8 per cent develop hemorrhage, obstruction, or perforation within two years once treatment is discontinued.[68] Because of the improvements in surgery and the excellent results that can be obtained, patients with a gastric ulcer that do not heal in a maximum of 12 to 15 weeks, a recurrent ulcer that does not heal in the same period, recurrence of an ulcer while under treatment, or large chronic gastric ulcers should be given the option of having an operation as well as continued medical treatment. Patients with ulcers suspected of cancer and those with obstruction, perforation, or uncontrolled hemorrhage should be operated upon emergently.

Gastric ulcers can occur in any portion of the stomach, but most benign ulcers occur in the prepyloric area or along the lesser curvature. A distinction should be made between gastric ulcers based on their location and the acid secretory potential of the stomach, because treatment will vary accordingly. Prepyloric ulcers occurring in younger people with high secretory rates (type III) or lesser curvature ulcers occurring in conjunction with duodenal ulcer (type II) should be treated as one would treat duodenal ulcers. The cause of lesser curvature ulcers that occur near the incisura (type I) in older patients may be different; they respond satisfactorily to antrectomy and Billroth I anastomosis without vagotomy, treatment that would be considered inadequate for a duodenal ulcer.

The recurrence rate reported by Pheils and colleagues[69] was 6 per cent after resection and gastroduodenostomy and less than 3 per cent after resection and gastrojejunostomy. When the ulcers were considered according to their location, the recurrence rates following both types of reconstruction were similar for ulcers located along the lesser curvature (type I). For prepyloric ulcers (type III), however, the recurrent ulcer rate was 11 per cent after resection and gastroduodenostomy and 0.7 per cent after resection and gastrojejunostomy. These recurrent ulcer rates are similar to those observed following Billroth I and Billroth II anastomoses in patients with duodenal ulcer treated by resection without vagotomy. These figures suggest that lesser curvature ulcers are satisfactorily treated by distal partial gastrectomy without vagotomy and either gastroduodenostomy or gastrojejunostomy reconstruction. Prepyloric gastric ulcers, on the other hand, since they behave like duodenal ulcers, should be treated surgically like duodenal ulcers. As has already been discussed, however, pyloric channel and prepyloric ulcers do not respond as favorably to parietal cell vagotomy as do duodenal ulcers. This operation is, therefore, to be avoided for treatment of gastric ulcers of these types.

Although distal partial gastrectomy without vagotomy has gained wide acceptance for treatment of benign gastric ulcer, vagotomy in conjunction with resection is performed by many surgeons because of the frequent (10 to 30 per cent) association of type I ulcer with duodenal ulcer and the similarity in the clinical behavior between prepyloric gastric ulcers (type III) and duodenal ulcers.

The theory that gastric stasis and antral hyperfunction cause gastric ulcer led to the proposal that a drainage operation alone would be adequate therapy. Based on this reasoning, pyloroplasty without vagotomy has been tried, with the result being an unacceptably high recurrence rate. The theory that gastric stasis is the cause of gastric ulcer remains unproved, except when there is an element of obstruction in a patient with duodenal ulcer and acid hypersecretion.

Nevertheless, the theory of gastric stasis and antral hyperfunction as the cause for gastric ulcer led to its treatment by combining vagotomy, to reduce acid secretion, and pyloroplasty, to prevent the hormonal effect of antral stasis. The reported recurrent ulcer rate for this operation, recommended as a safer procedure than gastric resection, ranges from zero[70] to 36 per cent.[71] In a randomized prospective study, Duthie and colleagues[72] came to the conclusion that partial gastrectomy should not be abandoned in favor of vagotomy and pyloroplasty, which has a higher morbidity, a higher recurrent ulcer rate, and a greater risk of overlooking cancer without the advantage of a lower mortality rate. When the ulcer is left behind, it is essential that adequate biopsy specimens be taken for frozen section analysis.

Gastric ulcers, particularly those along the lesser curvature, may be removed by a full-thickness wedge excision of the gastric wall, and the entire ulcer may be submitted for frozen section. The partial vagotomy that accompanies wedge resection is formally completed and a drainage procedure added. The recurrent ulcer rate reported for this type of operation ranges from 7[73] to 30[74] per cent and is no different from that following vagotomy and pyloroplasty without wedge resection. The operation may be indicated occasionally for juxtaesophageal ulcers, but otherwise the operation has little to recommend it.

An important theory for production of lesser curvature gastric ulcers is that gastric mucosa damaged by the detergent effect of bile is particularly sensitive to ulceration by acid. Davenport[75] suggests that the apparent hyposecretion of acid by patients with gastric ulcer is a consequence of a broken mucosal barrier permitting diffusion of hydrogen ions into the gastric mucosa. If one accepts these assumptions when contemplating surgical treatment of gastric ulcer, it is reasonable to perform vagotomy to reduce acid secretion, and it is unreasonable to perform a drainage procedure or resection that initiates duodenal reflux and mucosal damage.

Two new operations have been proposed that accommodate the aforementioned theoretic considerations. The first is the pylorus-preserving gastrectomy proposed by Maki and associates.[76] In this operation the distal 1.5 cm of the antrum and pylorus is preserved. A gastric resection without vagotomy and an end-to-end anastomosis are performed. A one- to nine-year follow-up of this operation by Sekine and coworkers[77] demonstrated excellent results. The other operation designed to preserve the pylorus is parietal cell vagotomy without drainage. We have combined the operation with resection of the ulcer from within the lumen of the stomach through a small gastrostomy. This operation reduces acid secretion, maintains good gastric emptying, provides the entire ulcer for pathologic examination, and does not facilitate duodenal reflux. This operation has had clinical trial but requires further study before conclusions can be drawn regarding its merit.[78]

Finally, gastric ulcer located near the esophagogastric junction presents special technical problems. The method of surgical treatment depends on the size, location, and degree of inflammation present. Among the different possibilities are high subtotal gastric resection including the ulcer and the Kelling-Madlender[79] operation, which consists of biopsy of the ulcer and distal gastric resection, leaving the ulcer in place.

Another approach is vagotomy combined with antrectomy or drainage, with either biopsy or complete excision of the ulcer. Proximal gastric resection and esophagogastrostomy might seem reasonable, but it is to be discouraged because of its high operative mortality and the complication of reflux resulting from loss of the lower esophageal sphincter.

Although numerous operations are in vogue for the treatment of gastric ulcer (Table 51–4), gastric resection, including the ulcer, with or without vagotomy is the most common procedure being utilized. Complications following gastric resection for gastric ulcer are fewer than those following resection for duodenal ulcer. It is easier to effect a closure or an anastomosis

Table 51–4. TYPES OF GASTRIC ULCER AND THEIR TREATMENT

Type and Location	Operations Available
Type I At incisura	1. Antrectomy-B_1, or B_2. 2. Antrectomy and vagotomy. 3. Pyloroplasty and vagotomy. 4. Submucosal resection of ulcer and PCV. 5. Sleeve resection.
Type II At incisura with evidence of present or previous duodenal ulcer	1. Antrectomy-B_1, or B_2 and vagotomy. 2. Pyloroplasty or gastroenterostomy and vagotomy.
Type III Prepyloric with or without evidence of duodenal ulcer	1. Antrectomy-B_1, or B_2 and vagotomy. 2. Pyloroplasty or gastroenterostomy and vagotomy.
Juxtaesophageal near esophago-gastric junction	1. High gastric resection including the ulcer-B_1, or B_2 or Roux-en-Y and vagotomy. 2. Subtotal gastric resection not including the ulcer-B_1, or B_2 and vagotomy; biopsy of ulcer. 3. Pyloroplasty or gastroenterostomy, vagotomy and biopsy of ulcer.
Drug Related Anywhere, most likely at greater curvature	Avoid operation except for emergencies.

with the duodenum. It is usually unnecessary to remove a large amount of stomach, and recurrent ulcer is uncommon.

SELECTION OF EMERGENCY OPERATION FOR BLEEDING PEPTIC ULCERS OF THE DUODENUM AND STOMACH

The majority of patients bleeding from the stomach and duodenum stop bleeding without operative intervention. Those patients who must be operated upon as an emergency measure to control bleeding represent an increased operative risk because of the adverse effect blood loss has upon vital organs. Foster and associates[80] reported a mortality rate of 28.5 per cent in 130 patients and attributed death in 31 of the 37 patients to delayed surgical intervention in the presence of continuous hemorrhage. It is therefore important in the management of these patients that replacement of blood loss be adequately maintained and that a clinical judgment be made to operate prior to the development of irreversible deterioration of vital organs. For the individual patient the decision of when to operate cannot be made solely on the basis of an alogorithm.

It was reported that early diagnosis by endoscopy has had no beneficial effect on the morbidity and mortality in patients with upper gastrointestinal bleeding.[81, 82] This may be so because in the natural course of bleeding such a large number of patients cease bleeding spontaneously and do not require emergency operation. Nevertheless, for the surgeon who must operate on patients emergently an accurate diagnosis of the bleeding source is important. Since we cannot predict which patient will fail to stop bleeding or which will rebleed, it is desirable to establish the diagnosis by endoscopy at a convenient time after the patient has been stabilized. Therapeutic endoscopy until now has been of questionable and limited value in treatment of bleeding, especially bleeding from a visible gastroduodenal artery.

In the selection of an operation for a patient with a bleeding duodenal ulcer, the basic choice is between (1) vagotomy and antrectomy, and (2) vagotomy, oversew of the bleeding ulcer, and pyloroplasty. The major factors to be considerd in making this selection are the mortality rates and the incidence of recurrent bleeding that follow the two procedures. In the opinion of most authors, vagotomy and antrectomy is the procedure of choice from the standpoint of ulcer cure and the prevention of rebleeding. The mortality rate is lower with vagotomy, oversew, and pyloroplasty; however, there is a difference of opinion regarding the effectiveness of the procedure to prevent rebleeding, particularly if the ulcer has a large calloused base.

Vagotomy, oversew, and pyloroplasty of a bleeding duodenal ulcer was first reported by Dorton and associates.[83] Using this method, Weinberg[84] reported a mortality rate of 2 per cent and an incidence of early and late rebleeding of 15 per cent. In 1957, Smith and Farris reported using vagotomy and pyloroplasty for bleeding with a mortality rate of 7 per cent. In their follow-up study, the rate of rebleeding was 1 per cent.[85]

Foster and colleagues[86] who had previously reported a mortality rate of 28.5 per cent following resection, later reported a mortality rate of 9 per cent and a rebleeding rate of 8 per cent after vagotomy, oversew of the ulcer, and pyloroplasty. This was less than for any other type of procedure, irrespective of the patient's age, and was their procedure of choice for gastric as well as duodenal ulcers, unless for technical reasons resection was necessary to control bleeding. Vagotomy, oversew, and pyloroplasty has been strongly supported by others,[18] but not all reports have been so favorable. The incidence of rebleeding was reported as 36 per cent by Kelley and associates[87] and 20 per cent by Herrington.[88]

Scott and colleagues[89] reported a mortality rate of 15 per cent following emergency vagotomy and antrectomy for bleeding. Rebleeding was not a problem, and the deaths occurred mainly in elderly patients. In view of the reported good results with vagotomy, oversew, and pyloroplasty, they used the procedure in 69 patients and incurred a 12 per cent mortality rate and a 22 per cent rate of rebleeding. On the basis of this experience, they concluded that vagotomy and antrectomy should be used in the younger, good-risk patient, and that vagotomy, oversew, and pyloroplasty should be reserved for the older, poorer-risk patients. This may be as close to the correct answer to this problem as can be obtained until a prospective, randomized study is performed.

As already mentioned, a major complication of any gastric surgery for bleeding peptic ulcer is the recurrence of bleeding. Also common to all gastric procedures for bleeding peptic ulcer is the high incidence of wound infections, the reason being that old blood, an ideal culture medium, may contaminate the wound when the stomach is opened. The patients operated on for bleeding gastric and duodenal ulcers are subject to all the early complications that occur after elective operations. The technical problems incurred as a result of dissecting the posterior penetrating duodenal ulcer from the pancreas during elective resection are magnified during emergency procedures, causing an increased number of complications, including leakage from the duodenal stump or gastroduodenostomy, pancreatic trauma and pancreatitis, and injury of the bile duct and obstructive jaundice. Ulcers located in the second portion of the duodenum are unusual because of their occurrence in an area of high concentration of alkaline secretions from the pancreas. Control of bleeding from a postbulbar ulcer creates a particularly difficult problem because of the close proximity of the bleeding point to the biliary and pancreatic ducts. In my opinion, an ulcer located in the postbulbar area is an indication for an elective operation when the diagnosis is made so that the surgeon will not subsequently be required to control hemorrhage in this critical area.

SELECTION OF OPERATION FOR PERFORATED PEPTIC ULCERS OF THE DUODENUM AND STOMACH

Few physicians continue to treat perforated duodenal ulcers by nasogastric suction except in very special circumstances in which surgery is contraindicated or in selected patients in whom it is perceived that the ulcer has sealed spontaneously. Simple closure of an ulcer with an omental patch continues to be widely practiced and it is considered by many as the method of choice whenever it can be used. It is also the preferred treatment of perforated acute ulcers by some surgeons who would otherwise advocate definitive treatment for perforated chronic ulcers.

Definitive treatment refers to operative procedures that not only deal with the emergency aspects of perforation but also attempt to prevent persistent or recurrent ulcer. When truncal vagotomy was introduced, its adoption for treatment of perforated ulcer was slow because of the fear of causing mediastinitis. This complication did not materialize, and truncal vagotomy combined with antrectomy[90] became an accepted method for treating perforated duodenal ulcers. Jordan and associates,[90] as well as others, support the performance of a curative type of operation for perforated ulcers in patients who have had a previous history of ulcer disease, who have no purulent peritonitis or abscess at the time of operation, and who have not been in shock.

According to Norberg,[91] patients presenting with a prior history consistent with duodenal ulcer and who demonstrate chronic inflammation surrounding the ulcer at operation can be predicted to have further difficulty after simple closure. Nemanich and Nicoloff,[92] summarizing the reports of nine different investigators, stated that the number of patients requiring subsequent reoperation following simple closure ranged from 35 to 50 per cent and increased to 66 per cent at ten years. We share the opinion of Greco and Cahow[93] that one cannot predict with accuracy at the time of perforation the patients who will require a subsequent operation if definitive surgery is not performed at the time of perforation.

It was the opinion of some surgeons that vagotomy and drainage was safer and was associated with fewer undesirable gastric symptoms than vagotomy and hemigastrectomy. For these reasons, vagotomy and drainage was potentially more acceptable than vagotomy and hemigastrectomy as definitive therapy. Failure of these potential advantages of vagotomy and pyloroplasty to materialize[20] makes it as unacceptable as vagotomy and hemigastrectomy for the universal treatment of perforated duodenal ulcer. In my opinion, before a definitive operation can be recommended to all patients who might be expected to tolerate operation, the procedure should be attended with virtually no mortality, it should produce no undesirable gastric complaints, and it should provide protection against recurrent ulcer.

Absence of debilitating symptoms and a low recurrent ulcer rate (6.0 per cent) following vagotomy of the fundic gland area of the stomach without a drainage procedure (parietal cell vagotomy) in the elective treatment of duodenal ulcer suggested that this highly effective method of treatment, when combined with closure of the ulcer, might fulfill the requirements of the ideal operation for the definitive treatment of perforated duodenal ulcer. We have now performed this procedure in 80 patients with perforated duodenal ulcer without mortality. The results obtained by us over 13 years,[94] as well as those of others,[95] make this operation the procedure of choice when it is appropriate that it be done.

The postoperative complications peculiar to simple closure consist of pyloric obstruction and the possibility that the perforated ulcer was a prepyloric perforated gastric cancer. The latter complication should not occur following any of the methods of treatment if the lesion is adequately biopsied. The occurrence of an intra-abdominal abscess, which one would think might occur rather commonly, is rare. In the event a patient manifests gastrointestinal bleeding at the time of perforation, care must be taken at the time of simple closure to avoid leaving unrecognized a second, posterior ulcer that is responsible for the bleeding.

In cases of perforated benign gastric ulcer, definitive therapy consists of distal partial gastrectomy with or without vagotomy. If the ulcer is prepyloric, a pyloroplasty through the ulcer or an antrectomy may be performed but always combined with vagotomy. When the patient is an unsuitable risk or when the ulcer is unsuitably located for definitive therapy, biopsy should be performed and the ulcer should be closed with an omental patch. If the lesion is malignant, resection should be attempted at the time of perforation if at all possible.

SELECTION OF OPERATION FOR OBSTRUCTING DUODENAL, PYLORIC, OR PREPYLORIC GASTRIC ULCER

Patients who appear to have gastric outlet obstruction may not have cicatricial obstruction but may instead have functional obstruction due to pylorospasm. The distinction between obstruction and spasm can be determined preoperatively by endoscopic examination, and can be verified at operation by guiding through the pylorus a tapered No. 40 French dilator that has been passed into the stomach by the anesthesiologist. If this cannot be done easily without force, parietal cell vagotomy should not be utilized because of the high complication rate associated with the operation performed in patients with obstruction. Gastric outlet obstruction caused by peptic ulcer disease must also be differentiated from obstruction caused by carcinoma in the gastric antrum. This is best done preoperatively by endoscopic biopsy.

Patients with gastric outlet obstruction should be operated on after several days of preparation. This time is used to correct electrolyte and metabolic imbalances and to give the stomach, decompensated by distention, an opportunity to regain its muscular tone by the use of gastric decompression. After this period of preoperative preparation, vagotomy combined with gastric resection or one of the previously described drainage procedures is a suitable form of therapy. Balloon dilatation has recently become popular in the treatment of pyloric obstruction by gastrointestinal endoscopists. There are no long-term follow-up reports evaluating this form of therapy. It is a form of therapy that appears to the author to be dangerous, time-consuming, and of extremely limited value, if any, in the management of cicatricial pyloric obstruction.

The results of operation in patients with gastric outlet obstruction are usually excellent; however, gastric ileus is a complication related to operations on the obstructed and grossly dilated stomach. It was previously thought that the loss of gastric motor activity that follows vagotomy would further aggravate gastric ileus, but this complication is no greater after vagotomy in the obstructed than in the nonobstructed stomach if the stomach has been adequately prepared by preoperative decompression.

References

1. Orr, I. M. Selective surgery for peptic ulcer. J. Roy. Coll. Surg. Edinburgh 8:270, 1963.
2. Small, W. P., Bruce, J., Falconer, C. W. A., Sircus, W., and Smith, A. N. N. The results of a policy of selective surgical treatment of duodenal ulcer. Br. J. Surg. 54:838, 1967.
3. Johnson, H. D. Duodenal ulcer in Britain. A sample of practice and results. Am. J. Surg. 105:320, 1963.
4. Frankel, A., Finkelstein, J., and Kark, A. E. The selection of operation for peptic ulcer. The use of the gastric secretory response to the augmented histamine test as a guide. Am. J. Gastroenterol. 46:206, 1966.
5. Kronborg, O. Gastric acid secretion and risk of recurrence of duodenal ulcer within six to eight years after truncal vagotomy and drainage. Gut 15:714, 1974.
6. Robbs, J. V., Bank, S., Marks, I. N., and Louw, J. H. Selection of operation for duodenal ulcer based on acid secretory studies. A reappraisal. Br. J. Surg. 60:601, 1973.
7. Coutsoftides, T., and Himal, H. S. The effect of vagotomy antrectomy or vagotomy pyloroplasty on the response of the antrum to meat extract in duodenal ulcer patients. Ann. Surg. 184:212, 1976.
8. Newton, S. E., III, and Judd, E. S. Long-term follow-up proves Billroth I gastric resection inadequate for permanent control of duodenal ulcer. Surg. Gynecol. Obstet. 116:170, 1963.
9. Stern, D. H., and Walsh, J. H. Gastrin release in postoperative ulcer patients: evidence for release of duodenal gastrin. Gastroenterology 64:363, 1973.
10. Price, W. E., Grizzle, J. E., Postlethwait, R. W., Johnson, W. D., and Grabicki, P. Results of operation for duodenal ulcer. Surg. Gynecol. Obstet. 131:233, 1970.
11. Goligher, J. C., Pulvertaft, C. N., and Watkinson, G. Controlled trial of vagotomy and gastroenterostomy, vagotomy and antrectomy and subtotal gastrectomy in elective treatment of duodenal ulcer: interim report. Br. Med. J. 1:455, 1964.
12. Rhea, W. G., Jr., Killen, D. A., and Scott, H. W., Jr. Long-term results of partial gastric resection without vagotomy in duodenal ulcer disease. Surg. Gynecol. Obstet. 120:970, 1965.
13. Dragstedt, L.R., and Owens, F. M., Jr. Supradiaphragmatic section of the vagus nerves in treatment of duodenal ulcer. Proc. Soc. Exp. Biol. Med. 53:125, 1943.
14. Lynch, J. D., Jernigan, S. K., Trotta, P. H., and Clemens, B. Incidence and analysis of failure with vagotomy and Heineke-Mikulicz pyloroplasty. Surgery 58:483, 1965.
15. Hayden, W. F., and Read, R. C. A comparative study of Heineke-Mikulicz and Finney pyloroplasty. Am. J. Surg. 116:755, 1968.
16. Kennedy, T., Johnston, G. W., Macrae, K. D., and Spencer, E. F. A. Proximal gastric vagotomy: interim results of a randomized controlled trial. Br. Med. J. 2:301, 1975.
17. Goligher, J. C., Pulvertaft, C. N., Irvin, T. T., Johnston, D., Walker, B., Hall, R. A., Willson-Pepper, J., and Matheson, T. S. Five to eight year results of truncal vagotomy and pyloroplasty for duodenal ulcer. Br. Med. J. 1:7, 1972.
18. Eisenberg, M. M., Woodward, E. R., Carson, T. J., and Dragstedt, L. R. Vagotomy and drainage procedure for duodenal ulcer: the result of ten years' experience. Ann. Surg. 170:317, 1969.
19. Stempien, S. J., Dagradi, A. E., Lee, E. R., and Simonton, J. H. Status of duodenal ulcer patients ten years or more after vagotomypyloroplasty (V-P). Gastroenterology 58:997, 1970.
20. Jordan, P. H., Jr., and Condon, R. E. A prospective evaluation of vagotomy-pyloroplasty and vagotomy-antrectomy for treatment of duodenal ulcer. Ann. Surg. 172:547, 1970.
21. Farmer, D. A., and Smithwick, R. H. Hemigastrectomy combined with resection of the vagus nerves. N. Engl. J. Med. 247:1017, 1952.
22. Edwards, L. W., and Herrington, J. L., Jr. Efficacy of 40 per cent gastrectomy combined with vagotomy for duodenal ulcer. Surgery 41:346, 1957.
23. Harkins, H. N., Schmitz, E. J., Nyhus, L. M., Kanar, E. A., Zech, R. K., and Griffith, C. A. The Billroth I gastric resection: experimental studies and clinical observations on 291 cases. Ann. Surg. 140:405, 1954.
24. Herrington, J. L., Jr. Truncal vagotomy with antrectomy—1976. Surg. Clin. North Am. 56:1335, 1976.
25. Barber, K. W., Jr., Judd, E. S., and Stauffer, M. H. Hemigastrectomy and vagotomy in the treatment of complications of duodenal ulcer. Arch. Surg. 86:710, 1963.
26. Thoroughman, J. C., Walker, L. G., Jr., and Raft, D. A review of 504 patients with peptic ulcer treated by hemigastrectomy and vagotomy. Surg. Gynecol. Obstet. 119:257, 1964.
27. Palumbo, L. T., and Sharpe, W. S. Distal antrectomy with vagotomy: over five-year follow-up in 158 cases. Arch. Surg. 91:684, 1965.
28. Kelly, K. Gastric emptying of liquids and solids: roles of proximal and distal stomach. Am. J. Physiol. 239:G71, 1980.
29. Jackson, R. G. Anatomic study of the vagus nerves; with a technic of transabdominal selective gastric vagus resection. Arch. Surg. 57:333, 1948.
30. Franksson, C. Selective abdominal vagotomy. Acta Chir. Scand. 96:409, 1948.
31. Singer, M. V., Solomon, T. E., Wood, J., and Grossman, M. I. Latency of pancreatic enzyme response to intraduodenal stimulants. Am. J. Phys. 238:G23, 1980.
32. Humphrey, C. S., Dykes, J. R. W., and Johnson, D. Effects of truncal, selective and highly selective vagotomy on glucose tolerance and insulin secretion in patients with duodenal ulcer. Br. Med. J. 2:112, 1975.
33. Everett, M. T., and Griffith, C. A. Selective and total vagotomy plus pyloroplasty: a comparative study of gastric secretion and motility in dogs. Ann. Surg. 171:31, 1970.
34. Stening, G. F., and Grossman, M. I. Gastric acid response to pentagastrin and histamine after extragastric vagotomy in dogs. Gastroenterology 59:364, 1970.
35. Harkins, H. N., Stavney, L. S., Griffith, C. A., Savage, L. E., Kato, T., and Nyhus, L. M. Selective gastric vagotomy. Ann. Surg. 158:448, 1963.
36. Burg, H. Vagotomy. Baltimore, Williams & Wilkins Company, 1964.
37. Hedenstedt, S., and Lundquist, G. Selective gastric vagotomy versus total abdominal vagotomy. Acta Chir. Scand. 131:448, 1966.
38. Amdrup, E., Clemmesen, T., and Andreassen, J. Selective gastric vagotomy technic and primary results. Am. J. Dig. Dis. 12:351, 1967.

39. Sawyers, J. L., Scott, H. W., Jr., Edwards, W. H., Shull, H. J., and Law, H., IV. Comparative studies of the clinical effects of truncal and selective gastric vagotomy. Am. J. Surg *115*:165, 1968.

40. Kennedy, T., and Connell, A. M. A double-blind controlled trial of the value of selective and total vagotomy in the surgical treatment of duodenal ulcer. Br. J. Surg. *56*:385, 1969.

41. Kraft, R. O., Fry, W. J., Wilhelm, K. G., and Ransom, H. K. Selective gastric vagotomy: a critical reappraisal. Arch. Surg. *95*:625, 1967.

42. Mason, M. C., Giles, G. R., Graham, N. G., Clark, C. G., and Goligher, J. C. An early assessment of selective and total vagotomy. Br. J. Surg. *55*:677, 1968.

43. Dignan, A. P. A laboratory appraisal of the effects of truncal and selective vagotomy. Br. J. Surg. *57*:249, 1970.

44. Kronborg, O., Malmstrom, J., and Christiansen, P. M. A comparison between the results of truncal and selective vagotomy in patients with duodenal ulcer. Scand. J. Gastroenterol. *5*:519, 1970.

45. Bank, S., Marks, I. N., and Louw, J. H. Histamine and insulin stimulated gastric acid secretion after selective and truncal vagotomy. Gut *8*:36, 1967.

46. Sawyers, J. L., and Scott, H. W., Jr. Selective gastric vagotomy with antrectomy or pyloroplasty. Ann. Surg. *174*:541, 1971.

47. Griffith, C. A., and Harkins, H. N. Partial gastric vagotomy. An experimental study. Gastroenterology *32*:96, 1957.

48. Holle, F. New method for surgical treatment of gastroduodenal ulceration. *In* Harkins, H. N., and Nyhus, L. M. (eds.). Surgery of the Stomach and Duodenum. 2nd ed. Boston, Little, Brown & Company, 1969, p. 629.

49. Amdrup, E., and Jensen, H.-E. Selective vagotomy of the parietal cell mass preserving innervation of the undrained antrum. Gastroenterology *59*:522, 1970.

50. Johnston, D., and Wilkinson, A. R. Highly selective vagotomy without a drainage procedure in the treatment of duodenal ulcer. Br. J. Surg. *57*:289, 1970.

51. Andrup, E., Jensen, H.-E., Johnston, D., Walker, B. E., and Goligher, J. C. Clinical results of parietal cell vagotomy (highly selective vagotomy) two to four years after operation. Ann. Surg. *180*:279, 1974.

52. Jordan, P. H., Jr., and Thornby, J. Should it be parietal cell vagotomy or selective vagotomy-antrectomy for treatment of duodenal ulcer? Ann. Surg. *205*:572, 1986.

53. Johnston, D. Operative mortality and postoperative morbidity of highly selective vagotomy. Br. J. Surg. *62*:160, 1975.

54. Johnston, D., Humphrey, C. S., Smith, R. B., and Wilkinson, A. R. Should the gastric antrum be vagally denervated if it is well drained and in the acid stream? Br. J. Surg. *58*:725, 1971.

55. Ingvar, C., Adami, H.-O., Enander, E. K., Enskog, L., and Rydberg, B. Clinical results of reoperation after failed highly selective vagotomy. Am. J. Surg. *152*:308, 1986.

56. Aaki, T., Kushida, M., and Nagao, F. Insulin and adrenalin infusion tests in the pathophysiologic analysis of hyperacidity in duodenal ulcer patients. *In* Drugs and Peptic Ulcer. Boca Raton, FL, CRC Press Inc., 1982.

57. Blair, A. J., Richardson, C. T., Walsh, J. H., Chew, P., and Feldman, M. Effect of parietal cell vagotomy on acid secretory responsiveness to circulating gastrin in humans. Relationship to postprandial serum gastrin concentration. Gastroenterology *90*:1001, 1986.

58. De Miguel, J. Late results of proximal gastric vagotomy without drainage for duodenal ulcer. Br. J. Surg. *69*:7, 1982.

59. Blackett, R. L., and Johnston, D. Recurrent ulceration after highly selective vagotomy for duodenal ulcer. Br. J. Surg. *68*:705, 1981.

60. Andersen, D., Amdrup, E., Høstrup, H., and Sorensen, F. H. The Aarhus County vagotomy trial: trends in the problem of recurrent ulcer after parietal cell vagotomy and selective gastric vagotomy with drainage. World J. Surg. *6*:86, 1982.

61. Madsen, P., and Kronborg, O. Recurrent ulcer 5½–8 years after highly selective vagotomy without drainage and selective vagotomy with pyloroplasty. Scand. J. Gastroenterol. *15*:193, 1980.

62. Donahue, P. E., Bombeck, C. T., Condon, R. E., and Nyhus,

L. M. Proximal gastric vagotomy versus selective vagotomy and antrectomy: results of a prospective, randomized clinical trial after four to twelve years. Surgery *96*:585, 1984.

63. Poppen, B., and Delin, A. Parietal cell vagotomy for duodenal and pyloric ulcers. I. Clinical factors leading to failure of the operation. Am. J. Surg. *141*:323, 1981.

64. Gorey, T. F., Lennon, F., and Heffernan, S. J. Highly selective vagotomy in duodenal ulceration and its complications. A 12 year review. Ann. Surg. *200*:181, 1984.

65. Jensen, H.-E, Kjaergaard, J., and Meisner, S. Ulcer recurrence two to twelve years after parietal cell vagotomy for duodenal ulcer. Surgery *94*:802, 1982.

66. Johnston, D., Pickford, I. R., Walker, B. E., and Goligher, J. C. Highly selective vagotomy for duodenal ulcer: do hypersecretors need antrectomy? Br. Med. J. *1*:716, 1975.

67. Becker, J. M., Kelly, K. A., Haddad, A. C., and Zinsmeister, A. R. Proximal gastric vagotomy and mucosal antrectomy: a possible operative approach to duodenal ulcer. Surgery *94*:58, 1983.

68. Sun, D. C. H., and Stempien, S. J. Site and size of the ulcer as determinants of outcome. The Veterans Administration cooperative study of gastric ulcer. Gastroenterology *61*:576, 1971.

69. Pheils, M. T., Mayday, G. B., Gillett, D. J., and Dunn, R. M. Surgery for benign gastric ulcer. Med. J. Aust. *1*:56, 1970.

70. Farris, J. M., and Smith, G. K. Some other operations for gastric ulcer. Surg. Clin. North Am. *46*:329, 1966.

71. Stemmer, E. A., Zahn, R. L., Hom, L. W., and Connolly, J. E. Vagotomy and drainage procedure for gastric ulcer. Arch. Surg. *96*:586, 1968.

72. Duthie, H. L., Moore, K. T. H., Bardsley, D., and Clark, R. G. Surgical treatment of gastric ulcers. Controlled comparison of Billroth I gastrectomy and vagotomy and pyloroplasty. Br. J. Surg. *57*:784, 1970.

73. Nyhus, L. M. Gastric ulcer. *In* Harkins, H. N., and Nyhus, L. M. (eds.). Surgery of the Stomach and Duodenum. 2nd ed. Boston, Little, Brown & Company, 1969, p. 203.

74. Herrington, J. L., Jr. Discussion of paper by Woodward, E. R., Eisenberg, M. M., and Dragstedt, L. R. Recurrence of gastric ulcer after pyloroplasty. A note of warning. Am. J. Surg.*113*:11, 1967.

75. Davenport, H.W. Is the apparent hyposecretion of acid by patients with gastric ulcer a consequence of a broken barrier to diffusion of hydrogen ions into the gastric mucosa? Gut *6*:513, 1965.

76. Maki, T., Shiratori, T., Hatafuku, T., and Sugawara, K. Pylorus-preserving gastrectomy as an improved operation for gastric ulcer. Surgery *61*:838, 1967.

77. Sekine, T., Sato, T., Maki, T., and Shiratori, T. Pylorus-preserving gastrectomy for gastric ulcer—one- to nine-year follow-up study. Surgery *77*:92, 1975.

78. Jordan, P. H., Jr. Treatment of gastric ulcers by parietal cell vagotomy and excision of the ulcer—rationale and results. Arch. Surg. *116*:1320, 1981.

79. Kelling, G. Ueber die operative Behandlung des chronischen Ulcus ventriculi. Arch. Klin. Chir. *109*:775, 1918.

80. Foster, J. H., Hickok, D. F., and Dunphy, F. E. Factors influencing mortality following emergency operation for massive upper gastrointestinal hemorrhage. Surg. Gynecol. Obstet. *117*:257, 1963.

81. Eastwood, E. L. Does early endoscopy benefit the patient with active upper gastrointestinal bleeding? Gastroenterology *72*:737, 1977.

82. Peterson, W. L. Evaluation and initial management of patients with upper gastrointestinal bleeding. J. Clin. Gastroenterol. *3*(Suppl. 2):79, 1981.

83. Dorton, H. E., Webb, J. G., and Royalty, D. M. Vagotomy and pyloroplasty. A simple safe solution to the bleeding ulcer problem. J. Kentucky Med. Assoc. *50*:16, 1952.

84. Weinberg, J. A. Treatment of the massively bleeding duodenal ulcer by ligation, pyloroplasty and vagotomy. Am. J. Surg. *102*:158, 1961.

85. Farris, J. M., and Smith, G. K. Vagotomy and pyloroplasty: a solution to the management of bleeding duodenal ulcer. Ann. Surg. *152*:416, 1960.

86. Foster, J. H., Hall, A. D., and Dunphy, J. E. Surgical management of bleeding ulcers. Surg. Clin. North Am. 46:387, 1966.

87. Kelley, H. G., Grant, G. N., and Elliott, D. W. Massive gastroduodenal hemorrhage. Changing concepts of management. Arch. Surg. 87:6, 1963.

88. Herrington, J. L., Jr. Vagotomy-pyloroplasty for duodenal ulcer: a critical appraisal of early results. Surgery 61:698, 1967.

89. Scott, H. W., Sawyers, J. L., Gobbel, W. G., Jr., and Herrington, J. L., Jr. Definitive surgical treatment in duodenal ulcer disease. Curr. Probl. Surg. 10:3, 1968.

90. Jordan, G. L., Jr., DeBakey, M. E., and Duncan, J. M., Jr. Surgical management of perforated peptic ulcer. Ann. Surg. 179:628, 1974.

91. Norberg, P. B. Results of the surgical treatment of perforated peptic ulcer; a clinical and roentgenological study. Acta Chir. Scand. (Suppl.) 249:74, 1959.

92. Nemanich, G. J., and Nicoloff, D. M. Perforated duodenal ulcer; long-term followup. Surgery 67:727, 1970.

93. Greco, R. S., and Cahow, C. E. Alternatives in the management of acute perforated duodenal ulcer. Am. J. Surg. 127:109, 1974.

94. Jordan, P. H., Jr. Proximal gastric vagotomy without drainage for treatment of perforated duodenal ulcer. Gastroenterology 83:179, 1982.

95. Boey, J., Lee, N. W., Koo, J., Lam, P. H. M., Wong, J., and Ong, G. B. Immediate definitive surgery for perforated duodenal ulcers. A prospective controlled trial. Ann. Surg. 196:338, 1982.

52

Postoperative Recurrent Ulcer

RICHARD C. THIRLBY
MARK FELDMAN

This chapter deals with the evaluation and management of the patients with postoperative recurrent ulcer. Although only a relatively small percentage of patients develop ulcer recurrences after surgery, this topic is important because of the large number of ulcer operations still being performed. Ulcers may recur in the duodenum, jejunum (adjacent to a gastrojejunal anastomosis), or stomach.

INCIDENCE

The incidence of ulcer recurrence after gastric surgery may depend upon several factors.

1. *Indication for original operation.* Ulcers recur more commonly when the original operative procedure had been for duodenal ulcer (3 to 10 per cent recurrence) and less commonly when the original procedure had been for gastric ulcer (2 per cent recurrence). Ulcers may also develop *de novo* when the original gastric operation had not been for peptic ulcer disease. For example, gastrojejunal (stomal) ulcers occur in approximately 3 per cent of patients treated for morbid obesity with gastric bypass plus gastrojejunostomy.[1] Peptic ulcers following gastric resection for gastric cancer are unusual. On the other hand, marginal ulcers may occur in up to 20 per cent of patients treated by distal gastrectomy and gastrojejunostomy (without vagotomy) for pancreatic cancer or duodenal trauma.[2, 3]

2. *Type of operation performed.* As shown in Table 52–1, the recurrence rate after different operations for duodenal ulcer varies depending on the operation performed. There is a relatively high recurrence rate after gastrojejunostomy, an intermediate recurrence rate after proximal gastric vagotomy or truncal vagotomy and drainage, a somewhat lower recurrence rate after subtotal gastrectomy alone, and a very low recurrence rate after truncal vagotomy plus antrectomy.[4]

3. *Experience of the surgeon.* The recurrence rate after a given operation varies with different surgeons and usually decreases as the surgeon gains experience.[5, 6] This is especially true for proximal gastric vagotomy, with reported recurrence rates in duodenal ulcer patients ranging from 2 to 28 per cent for individual surgeons at the same hospital.[7] In our opinion, sham

Table 52–1. INCIDENCE OF POSTOPERATIVE RECURRENT ULCER BASED UPON ORIGINAL OPERATION FOR DUODENAL ULCER

Original Operation	Incidence of Recurrence (%)
Gastrojejunostomy	30–35
Proximal gastric vagotomy	7–10
Truncal vagotomy and drainage	7–10
Subtotal gastrectomy	2–6
Truncal vagotomy and antrectomy	1

Modified from Stabile, B. E., and Passaro, E., Jr. Gastroenterology 70:124, 1976.

feeding testing (see below) should be performed after proximal gastric vagotomy to document complete vagotomy and thereby validate the individual surgeon's technique. Postoperative sham feeding testing may identify patients with incomplete vagotomy; such individuals are more likely to develop recurrent ulcer.

Surgical experience and awareness have markedly reduced the frequency of retained antrum syndrome as a cause of recurrent ulcer.

4. *Presence of hypersecretory state.* An operation that would be satisfactory for most ulcer patients may fail to prevent ulcer recurrences in patients with an acid hypersecretory state (e.g., Zollinger-Ellison syndrome with or without primary hyperparathyroidism).[8–10] Therefore, fasting serum gastrin and calcium concentrations should be determined to exclude Zollinger-Ellison syndrome and primary hyperparathyroidism, respectively, in all patients about to undergo operation for peptic ulcer. The value of preoperative acid secretion studies in all patients before the initial operation is controversial. If preoperative fasting and/or secretin-stimulated serum gastrin concentrations suggest the diagnosis of Zollinger-Ellison syndrome, then acid secretion studies are imperative (see pp. 000–000). On the other hand, preoperative acid secretion rates play little role in choosing which operation to perform. For example, the recurrence rate after proximal gastric vagotomy is unrelated to preoperative basal and peak acid output.[11–15] Thus, normogastrinemic patients about to undergo elective operation for peptic ulcer generally do not require preoperative acid secretion studies.

5. *Behavioral risk factors for ulcer.* There is epidemiologic[16] and endoscopic[17] evidence suggesting a relationship between chronic gastric ulceration and ingestion of aspirin or other nonsteroidal anti-inflammatory drugs. If a patient resumes aspirin use postoperatively, gastric ulcer may recur. Cigarette smoking is thought to play a pathogenic role in duodenal and gastric ulcer;[18–20] continued smoking after surgery might predispose to ulcer recurrence.

It must be emphasized that incidences of ulcer recurrence mentioned above and in Table 52–1 are clinically recognized. Postoperative ulcer recurrence is probably more common, but some patients are asymptomatic.

CLINICAL PRESENTATIONS[21]

Abdominal Pain. Pain is present in over 90 per cent of patients with peptic ulcer who have not had ulcer surgery. On the other hand, the incidence of pain in patients with *postoperative* recurrent ulcers is only about 40 per cent[23] and possibly even lower in patients with marginal ulcers after gastrojejunostomy.[24] Even when present, the pain may be vague or atypical for ulcer. It can be difficult to distinguish symptoms of recurrent ulcer from other postoperative symptoms, especially when surgery has included partial gastrectomy. Pain is usually in the epigastrium but may occur in, or radiate to, other abdominal regions, the back, or the chest.

Hemorrhage. The 40 to 60 per cent incidence of hemorrhage as a presenting symptom of postoperative recurrent peptic ulcer[23–25] is more than twice that seen in unoperated patients initially presenting with peptic ulcer.[22] In many cases no history of ulcer-like pain prior to onset of hemorrhage can be elicited. Bleeding is usually slow and chronic, but may be voluminous and life-threatening.[26] Those who have chronic bleeding may develop iron-deficiency anemia, with or without occult blood in the stool. It is important to document the presence of recurrent ulcer in these patients because iron deficiency can be due to other causes (e.g., iron malabsorption, bleeding gastritis, or bleeding from carcinoma of the stomach or colon). Likewise, acute upper gastrointestinal hemorrhage presenting as melena, with or without hematemesis, can be due to causes other than recurrent ulcer (e.g., acute gastritis, Mallory-Weiss laceration, varices).

Obstruction. A recurrent ulcer in the pyloric channel, in the duodenum, or near a gastroenterostomy may lead to gastric outlet obstruction. The patient will have nausea, early satiety, vomiting of old food, and weight loss. Abdominal pain and signs of chronic blood loss also may be present. Differential diagnosis includes other causes of obstruction, (e.g., anastomotic stricture, gastric carcinoma, jejunal-gastric intussusception), postoperative atony without obstruction (gastroparesis), and alkaline ("bile") gastritis.

Perforation. Free perforation will lead to a clinical picture of peritonitis. Fortunately, this is an uncommon presentation of recurrent ulcer, although the rare patient with recurrent ulcer due to Zollinger-Ellison syndrome may be more likely to present with perforation.

Gastrojejunocolic Fistula. In some cases, a marginal ulcer at a gastrojejunostomy can penetrate into the adjacent transverse colon and result in a gastrojejunocolic fistula.[27, 28] Many patients with this complication will have diarrhea and weight loss due to bacterial overgrowth of the small bowel and stomach with colonic organisms and resultant malabsorption. This complication is now uncommon because (1) gastrojejunostomy without vagotomy is rarely used to treat peptic ulcer disease, and (2) most gastrojejunostomies are retrocolic instead of antecolic. Diarrhea that develops after ulcer surgery also can be a consequence of vagotomy and drainage procedure, malabsorption, or Zollinger-Ellison syndrome.

EVALUATION OF THE PATIENT

In evaluating the patient with complaints following ulcer surgery, it is important to have a high index of suspicion for the presence of recurrent ulcer. Careful history, physical examination, and testing of the stool for blood may give useful information. For example, the history may indicate a strong family history of ulcer and kidney stones (suggesting the possibility of gastrinoma), or physical examination may disclose a succussion splash several hours after a meal (suggesting the possibility of gastric outlet obstruction). Diagnostic procedures are usually necessary to establish the *presence* of recurrent ulcer before therapy is initiated. Additional tests will be necessary to help establish the *cause* of the recurrent ulcer.

Procedures to Demonstrate the Presence of Recurrent Peptic Ulcer

Barium Studies. Upper gastrointestinal series sometimes will be able to demonstrate the presence of recurrent ulcer (Fig. 52–1). However, accurate radiologic evaluation of the postoperative stomach is difficult and ulcers may be missed, or conversely, a collection of barium may be called an ulcer when in fact no ulcer is present.[29] Although the greatest difficulty occurs after gastrojejunostomy, there also can be uncertainty in assessing the presence of an ulcer after gastroduodenostomy or after pyloroplasty (Fig. 52–2). Barium studies are less expensive but are also less sensitive and specific than endoscopy in determining the presence of recurrent ulcer.[30] Many physicians now choose to omit barium studies and proceed directly to endoscopy in evaluating patients with signs or symptoms of recurrent ulcer after gastric surgery. When gastrojejunocolic fistula is suspected, barium enema is the diagnostic procedure of choice.[27]

Endoscopy. Because recurrent ulcers mostly occur within the first 1 or 2 cm of the jejunum or duodenum or in the stomach or gastric remnant, the ulcer usually can be demonstrated by endoscopy.[30] In some cases, however, because of edema, inflammation, or scarring, an ulcer cannot be located at endoscopy.[31] If the ulcer is in the duodenum or jejunum, there is usually no reason to obtain cytologic or biopsy specimens. On the other hand, if the ulcer appears to be in the stomach or gastric remnant, it is wise to obtain endoscopic biopsy specimens to exclude malignancy.

Procedures to Demonstrate Cause of Recurrent Peptic Ulcer

Clinically, it is important to try to demonstrate the cause of a postoperative recurrent peptic ulcer only if knowledge of the cause will affect the manner in which the patient will be treated. However, since some causes of ulcer recurrence may not respond well to standard medical treatment and should be treated specifically, it is desirable to try to exclude certain causes of ulcer recurrence. Table 52–2 lists the most common causes of recurrent ulcer, as well as several factors that may contribute to ulcer recurrence. Procedures that can be carried out to elucidate the specific cause in a given patient are listed below.

Review of Previous Operative Report and Pathology Slides. Review of previous records should disclose (1) the type of operation that was performed; (2) whether the entire distal margin of a gastrectomy specimen

Table 52–2. PRIMARY CAUSES AND POSSIBLE CONTRIBUTING FACTORS FOR POSTOPERATIVE RECURRENT ULCER

Primary causes
　Incomplete vagotomy
　Adjacent nonabsorbable suture
　Retained antrum syndrome
　Antral G cell hyperplasia
　Zollinger-Ellison syndrome (gastrinoma)
　Gastric cancer
Possible contributing factors
　Ulcerogenic drugs/smoking
　Gastric outlet obstruction/delayed gastric emptying
　Enterogastric reflux
　Primary hyperparathyroidism
　Gastric bezoar

included a portion of duodenum with Brunner's glands (if not, retained antrum is possible); and (3) whether or not at least two nerve trunks assumed to be vagal were confirmed histologically (if not, incomplete vagotomy is likely). It should be pointed out, however, that incomplete vagotomy can still be present despite division of two or more nerve trunks at a previous operation.

Endoscopy. In a few patients, endoscopy will determine not only presence of ulcer, but also its cause (Table 52–2). First, if the ulcer is related to a recently placed surgical suture, this can be visualized, the suture material can be removed through the endoscope, and ulcer healing may occur.[32, 33] Second, it may be possible to pass the endoscope to the proximal end of the afferent duodenal loop and obtain biopsy specimens in order to demonstrate retained antral mucosa.[34] Third, it is sometimes possible to identify a gastrinoma in the duodenum or stomach. Endoscopic biopsy of such a tumor can reveal an endocrine tumor resembling a carcinoid or islet cell tumor.[35] Fourth, if the ulcer is in the stomach, endoscopic biopsy of the gastric ulcer or an ulcerated gastric polyp[36] may reveal that the ulcer is malignant.[37–41] Fifth, endoscopy may raise the suspicion of gastric outlet obstruction or delayed gastric emptying as a contributing factor in ulcer recurrence.[42] Sixth, enterogastric reflux of bile-stained secretions with resultant gastritis may be identified. It has been proposed that postoperative recurrent gastric ulceration can be caused by excessive enterogastric reflux.[30] Lastly, endoscopy may identify a gastric bezoar, which may contribute to gastric ulcer formation (see pp. 741–744).

Measurement of Serum Gastrin Concentration. Table 52–3 lists causes of hypergastrinemia in patients with postoperative ulcers. With rare exceptions, a normal serum gastrin concentration ($\leq$100 or 200 pg/ml) excludes the possibility of Zollinger-Ellison syndrome,[43, 44] while a serum gastrin concentration greater than 1000 pg/ml in a patient with documented gastric acid hypersecretion is virtually diagnostic. Patients with retained antrum syndrome typically have fasting serum gastrin concentrations two to four times above the normal range,[45–47] although a recent study suggested that patients with clinically significant retained antrum

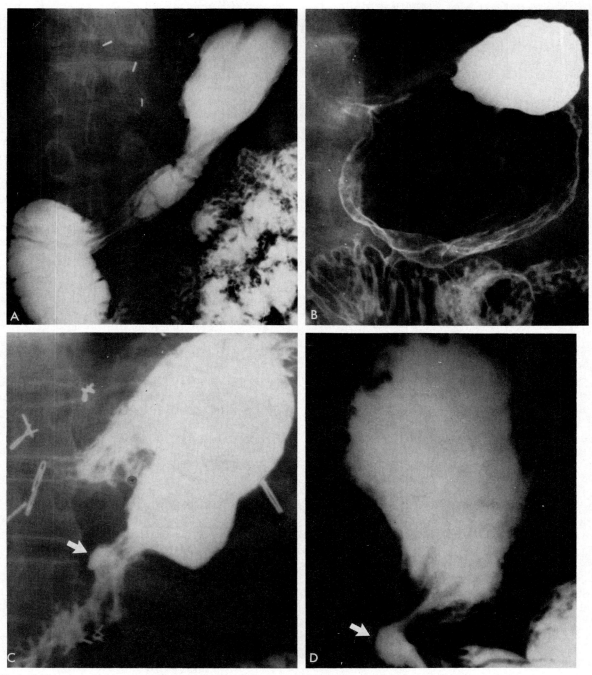

Figure 52–1. *A,* The normal appearance of the stomach after vagotomy and antrectomy with Billroth I gastroduodenostomy. *B,* The normal appearance of the stomach after antrectomy with Billroth II gastrojejunostomy. *C,* A postoperative recurrent ulcer in the duodenum *(arrow)* after vagotomy, antrectomy, and Billroth I gastroduodenostomy. *D,* A postoperative recurrent ulcer in the jejunum after antrectomy and Billroth II gastrojejunostomy.

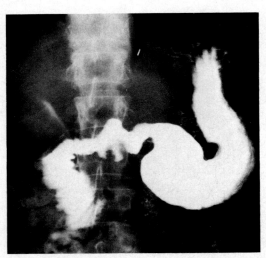

Figure 52–2. Upper gastrointestinal series following vagotomy and pyloroplasty. There are outpouchings at the pyloroplasty, which are easily confused wtih a recurrent ulcer.

may have only minimal elevations in fasting serum gastrin concentration.[25]

The differential diagnosis of a moderate elevation of serum gastrin concentration (200 to 900 pg/ml) in a patient with recurrent ulcer includes Zollinger-Ellison syndrome, postvagotomy hypergastrinemia,*[48] antral G cell hyperplasia,[52, 53] achlorhydria/hypochlorhydria, renal failure, gastric outlet obstruction, and retained antrum syndrome. Hypergastrinemia associated with gastric outlet obstruction should resolve after gastric evacuation and decompression with nasogastric suction. Zollinger-Ellison syndrome usually can be distinguished from the other causes of hypergastrinemia such as postvagotomy hypergastrinemia by the serum gastrin response to intravenous secretin. There is only a small increase (<100 pg/ml) above basal gastrin levels in patients with postvagotomy hypergastrinemia and a much larger (>100 pg/ml) increase in most (85 to 90 per cent) gastrinoma patients with or without previous vagotomy.[49] Similarly, the increase in serum gastrin concentration after secretin injection in patients with antral G cell hyperplasia or retained antrum syndrome is nearly always less than 100 pg/ml,[45–47, 52, 53] although rare exceptions have been reported.[54] Bombesin is a potent stimulant of antral gastrin release but has little effect on gastrin release from gastrinoma cells;[55] hence, bombesin increases serum gastrin concentration in patients with antral G cell hyperplasia, achlorhydria/hypochlorhydria, and retained antrum syndrome but not in patients with Zollinger-Ellison syndrome.†[34, 56]

Stimulation of gastrin release by a meal may be indicated in patients with peptic ulcer and an intact

---

*After vagotomy, fasting serum gastrin concentration increases so that about 40 per cent of patients have an abnormally high level,[49] in some patients as high as two to three times the upper limit of normal. After antrectomy, with or without vagotomy, fasting serum gastrin concentration should be normal or low normal.[50, 51]

†Bombesin is not commercially available at present in the United States.

antrum in whom fasting hypergastrinemia (200 to 900 pg/ml) and a negative secretin test suggest the possibility of antral G cell hyperplasia.[53] In patients with this syndrome, a standard high-protein meal results in a marked increase in serum gastrin concentration (mean maximal increase 300 per cent). In vagotomized patients or those with Zollinger-Ellison syndrome, the serum gastrin increase after a meal is usually less pronounced. In patients with retained antrum syndrome, a high-protein meal may also produce a large increase in the serum gastrin concentration.[45]

Measurement of Serum Calcium Concentration. In addition to serum gastrin, serum calcium concentration should be measured in a recurrent ulcer patient to screen for primary hyperparathyroidism that may or may not be associated with multiple endocrine neoplasia, type I.

Technetium Radionuclide Scan. Technetium pertechnetate ($Tc99mO_4$) is selectively concentrated in the thyroid gland, the salivary glands, and the entire gastric mucosa.[57] After concentration in the stomach, technetium is then secreted by the fundic and antral gastric mucosa. Thus, radioisotope scanning with $Tc99mO_4$ may play a role in diagnosing retained gastric antrum in patients with postoperative recurrent peptic ulcer and hypergastrinemia. Studies in animals indicate that an antral cuff as small as 1 cm may be detected by scanning the abdomen after intravenous bolus injection of $Tc99mO_4$.[57] Tests in humans have confirmed that retained gastric antrum can be diagnosed by radioisotope scanning (Fig. 52–3).[25, 58, 59] Positive tests are probably reliable; however, a negative scan does not rule out retained antrum since the false negative rate may be as high as 27 per cent.[60]

Measurement of Gastric Acid Secretion. Studies of gastric acid secretion are not necessary in the evaluation of all patients presenting with postoperative recurrent ulcer. The initial evaluation (history, endoscopy, serum gastrin, and calcium) should exclude causes of postoperative recurrent ulcer that require specific treatment (Table 52–4). The majority of the remaining patients can be successfully treated medically regardless of the results of the acid secretion tests (see below), and thus measurement of acid secretion

---

Table 52–3. CAUSES OF BASAL HYPERGASTRINEMIA IN PATIENTS WITH POSTOPERATIVE ULCER*

If antrum is present:
  Zollinger-Ellison syndrome (gastrinoma)
  Vagotomy
  Antral G cell hyperplasia
  Achlorhydria/hypochlorhydria
  Renal failure
  Gastric outlet obstruction (retained food)
If antrum has been resected:
  Zollinger-Ellison syndrome (gastrinoma)
  Retained antrum

---

*Occasionally an elevated basal serum gastrin concentration is due to a laboratory error. Therefore, the test should be repeated to confirm that basal hypergastrinemia is present.

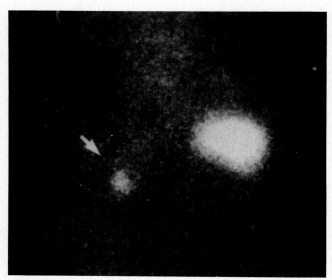

Figure 52–3. Positive sodium pertechnetate (Tc99mO₄) scan of retained gastric antrum *(arrow)* in a patient after gastrectomy with Billroth II gastrojejunostomy. The radionuclide is also secreted by the normal gastric remnant. (From Lee, C.-H., Peng, F.-K., and Lui, W.-Y. Arch. Surg. *121:*1181, 1986. Copyright 1986, American Medical Association. Used by permission.)

is probably necessary only when medical treatment has failed and when surgery is anticipated. Measurement of acid secretion can be difficult after ulcer surgery because of reflux of alkaline, bile-stained intestinal juice into the stomach after a drainage procedure and because of difficulty in positioning the nasogastric tube in the gastric remnant after partial gastrectomy. Nevertheless, if carefully performed, acid secretory studies can be useful in evaluating patients with postoperative recurrent ulcers.

Basal Acid Output (BAO) and Peak Acid Output (PAO). Methods for measuring BAO and PAO are described on pages 000 to 000. After vagotomy, a subcutaneous dose of 12 μg/kg pentagastrin, rather than the usual 6 μg/kg dose, is used to elicit PAO.[61] Values for BAO and PAO are difficult to interpret in postoperative patients for the following reasons: (1) in many patients, BAO and PAO had not been determined preoperatively, so that it is not usually possible to compare preoperative and postoperative values; (2) there is no absolute value for BAO and PAO that indicates with confidence an adequate vagotomy and/or antrectomy; and (3) the characteristic findings in Zollinger-Ellison syndrome patients who have not had surgery—very high BAO (>15 mM per hour) and BAO/PAO of 60 per cent or greater—often are not present in such patients who have already undergone surgery.[62] Thus, other than documenting that the patient with a recurrent ulcer still secretes acid, BAO and PAO do not usually aid in determining the specific cause of recurrent ulcer. The same statement can be made regarding the use of basal and betazole-stimulated serum pepsinogen concentrations.[63]

Insulin (Hollander) Test. Acid secretion during insulin-induced hypoglycemia has been widely used to

diagnose incomplete vagotomy.[64] In this test, 0.1 or 0.2 units of regular insulin per kilogram of body weight is injected intravenously as a bolus. Hypoglycemia results within about 30 minutes, and this stimulates vagal efferent pathways to the stomach and secretion of acid. Little or no increase in gastric acidity above basal acidity during hypoglycemia is said to indicate complete vagotomy, whereas a large increase suggests incomplete vagotomy.

Unfortunately, there are two major problems with the insulin test. First, insulin-induced hypoglycemia stimulates acid secretion by nonvagal as well as by vagal mechanisms.[65] Thus, an increase in acid secretion following administration of insulin may not necessarily indicate inadequate vagotomy (false-positive test). Second, hypoglycemia is dangerous, as evidenced by the occurrence of seizures, myocardial infarctions, and even deaths during performance of this test.[66, 67] Thus, the insulin test cannot be recommended.

Sham Feeding Test.[68, 69] The rationale for this test is that sham feeding (i.e., seeing, chewing, tasting, and smelling appetizing food without actually swallowing it) is thought to stimulate gastric acid secretion solely via vagal pathways.[70] Studies have shown that sham feeding stimulates as much acid secretion as 0.1 unit per kilogram of intravenous regular insulin.[71] After an adequate vagotomy, sham feeding does not stimulate acid secretion.[68, 69]

The sham feeding test as performed in our laboratory is a three-hour test during which BAO is measured in the first hour, sham feeding–stimulated acid output (SAO) in the second hour, and PAO in the third hour.[68] A meal of sirloin steak and French fried potatoes plus water is used for sham feeding. Feldman and associates studied a large number of non-vagotomized controls and found that SAO averaged approximately 40 per cent of the PAO and that the lower limit of normal for SAO was 10 per cent of PAO (95 per cent

Table 52–4. INITIAL EVALUATION AND TREATMENT OF PATIENTS WITH POSTOPERATIVE RECURRENT ULCER

Evaluation/Procedure	Cause Diagnosed or Excluded	Treatment
History	Ulcerogenic drugs/smoking	Discontinue drug/cigarettes
Endoscopy	Adjacent suture	Remove suture
	Zollinger-Ellison syndrome (gastrinoma)	See pages 917 to 919
	Gastric cancer	Surgery
	Gastric outlet obstruction	Surgery or dilatation
	Bezoar	Remove bezoar
Serum gastrin	Retained antrum syndrome	Resect duodenal stump/retained antrum
	Antral G cell hyperplasia	Antrectomy
	Zollinger-Ellison syndrome	See pages 914 to 917
Serum calcium	Primary hyperparathyroidism	Parathyroidectomy

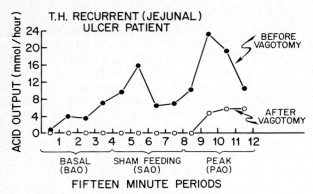

Figure 52–4. Example of a three-hour sham feeding test in a patient with a recurrent jejunal ulcer after truncal vagotomy, antrectomy, and Billroth II gastrojejunostomy. For four 15-minute periods, basal acid output (BAO) was measured by aspiration. Then sham feeding was performed, and sham feeding acid output (SAO) was measured for four 15-minute periods. A steak and potato meal was smelled, chewed, and tasted by the patient for 30 minutes, but the meal was expectorated into a basin rather than swallowed. After eight 15-minute periods (i.e., at the end of the second hour) a maximal dose of pentagastrin (12 μg/kg subcutaneously) was injected and peak acid output (PAO) measured. As shown by solid circles, BAO was 3.8, SAO 9.6, and PAO 21.2 mM/hour. Thus, the SAO was 45 per cent of PAO, compatible with incomplete vagotomy.[68] Basal serum gastrin concentration was 60 pg/ml. The patient then underwent transthoracic truncal re-vagotomy. Eight days later, BAO was zero, SAO was zero, and PAO was 5.7 mM/hour. If the original vagotomy had been complete, acid secretion would not have been expected to decrease after re-vagotomy. Complete ulcer healing occurred within six weeks of re-vagotomy.

confidence limits).[68, 72] They then studied vagotomized patients with no clinical evidence of ulcer recurrence and found that the majority (approximately 70 per cent) had an SAO less than 10 per cent of PAO, suggesting an adequate vagotomy (in most, SAO/PAO was zero). An example of the acid outputs during this three-hour test before and after complete vagotomy is shown in Figure 52–4. Note that after vagotomy, PAO was reduced and SAO was abolished. Approximately 70 per cent of patients with a history of vagotomy but with a postoperative recurrent ulcer had SAOs greater than 10 per cent of PAO, indicating normal vagally mediated acid secretion, which suggests incomplete vagotomy. In 15 of these latter patients with postoperative recurrent ulcer and incomplete vagotomy as diagnosed by sham feeding, transthoracic revagotomy was performed and acid secretion decreased in each patient, SAO and PAO decreasing by 91 and 68 per cent, respectively[73] (Table 52–5). This decrease in acid secretion after re-vagotomy would not have been expected if the original vagotomy had been complete, and thus confirmed that an SAO more than 10 per cent of PAO had indicated incomplete vagotomy.

The sham feeding test is safe and easy to perform. However, certain precautions must be taken. First, it is important to ensure that the patient does not accidentally swallow food during the test, since swallowed food may stimulate acid secretion and/or buffer acid.[74] However, it has been claimed that swallowing small amounts of food does not alter acid secretion results significantly.[75] If food is present in gastric aspi-

Table 52–5. MEAN ACID SECRETION (mM/H) BEFORE AND AFTER TRANSTHORACIC RE-VAGOTOMY IN 15 PATIENTS WITH POSTOPERATIVE RECURRENT ULCER AND INCOMPLETE VAGOTOMY SHOWN BY SHAM FEEDING TESTING

	BAO	SAO	PAO
Before transthoracic re-vagotomy	6.2	12.9	28.2
After transthoracic re-vagotomy	0.5*	1.1*	9.0*

*p <0.02 vs. before transthoracic re-vagotomy.
BAO, basal acid output; SAO, sham feeding stimulated acid output; PAO, peak acid output.

rates, the test ideally should be repeated. Second, if the PAO is very low, virtually any SAO will then produce a ratio of SAO to PAO greater than 0.10. Therefore, in patients with a PAO less than 4 or 5 mM per hour, the results must be interpreted with caution. Third, it must be remembered that in a patient with a high BAO (that is, greater than 10 per cent of PAO), the SAO also will be more than 10 per cent of PAO even if sham feeding does not increase acid secretion above BAO. Thus, in a postoperative patient with a recurrent ulcer and a BAO more than 10 per cent of PAO, it may be unnecessary to carry out a sham feeding test.

THERAPY

Not very long ago it was believed that postoperative recurrent ulcer almost always should be managed surgically.[4] This attitude has changed in the past few years with the advent of histamine H_2-receptor antagonists. Thus, current indications for reoperation for recurrent ulcer are less clear-cut.

Medical Therapy. Table 52–6 summarizes studies that evaluated the effect of cimetidine or ranitidine on healing of postoperative recurrent ulcer.[76–84] It is apparent that about 80 per cent of ulcers healed during

Table 52–6. EFFECT OF H_2-RECEPTOR ANTAGONISTS ON HEALING OF POSTOPERATIVE RECURRENT ULCER

	Healing (%)*		
Medication	*Medication*	*Placebo*	**Reference**
Cimetidine†	58	42	76
Cimetidine†	85		77
Cimetidine†	67	11	78
Cimetidine†	81		79
Cimetidine†	80	13	80
Cimetidine†	79		81
Cimetidine†	95		82
Cimetidine‡	80		83
Ranitidine§	96		84

*In most studies, healing was assessed endoscopically after four or six weeks of therapy. The number of patients per study ranged from 10 to 24.
†Cimetidine dosage: 200 mg T.I.D. and 400 mg at bedtime.
‡Cimetidine dosage: 400 mg B.I.D.
§Ranitidine dosage: 150 mg B.I.D.

a four- to six-week course of H_2-receptor antagonist therapy, and in placebo-controlled studies, healing rates were higher during H_2 blocker therapy than during placebo therapy.* In most studies, it was not specified whether an attempt was made to determine the etiology of the ulcer recurrence.

Endoscopic evaluation of whether or not healing has occurred is usually indicated in patients with postoperative peptic ulcer, especially in patients who present with an ulcer complication. After the ulcer has healed, maintenance H_2 blocker therapy will often prevent healed postoperative ulcers from recurring. In one study in which cimetidine was continued for one year, the recurrence rate was only 16 per cent,[78] whereas the recurrence rate after discontinuing cimetidine is at least 50 per cent within 18 weeks.[78, 79, 81, 82] Therefore, about 70 per cent of medically treated patients with postoperative recurrent ulcer can be treated successfully for at least one year. Medical treatment of recurrent ulcer in patients after proximal gastric vagotomy may be more successful than in patients with recurrent ulcer after other operations for peptic ulcer.[82] Lifetime maintenance treatment is probably indicated since relapse is very likely when medication is stopped, and the relapse frequently presents as painless gastrointestinal hemorrhage. Patients with Zollinger-Ellison syndrome and postoperative ulcer have also been treated successfully with H_2-receptor antagonists, although high doses may be required.[85]

In addition to pharmacologic therapy, patients with postoperative recurrent ulcer should be advised to stop smoking and discontinue ingestion of aspirin or other nonsteroidal anti-inflammatory agents.

Surgical Therapy. In our opinion, surgery is usually indicated for recurrent ulcer if (1) the postoperative recurrent ulcer fails to heal after 3 months of medical therapy; (2) the ulcer recurs while the patient is on maintenance medical therapy; (3) the recurrent ulcer presents as a complication such as perforation, obstruction, or serious hemorrhage; or (4) the patient cannot or will not comply with a medical regimen that includes close follow-up and lifetime medication. It is also preferable that the patient be an adequate surgical candidate from a general medical standpoint, although it is sometimes necessary to operate on high-risk patients under emergency conditions (e.g., bleeding, perforation).

The choice of surgical procedure for recurrent ulcer is made by some physicians solely on the basis of the previous operation.[32, 86] For example, if the patient has previously had a subtotal gastrectomy without vagotomy, the ulcer recurrence is treated by truncal vagotomy, performed through a thoracic or abdominal approach. If the patient has had previous vagotomy but no resection, antrectomy is performed. Other physicians recommend both resection (or re-resection) and vagotomy (or re-vagotomy) for all patients with recur-

rent ulcer.[87, 88] While another ulcer recurrence is prevented in most patients after revagotomy and resection or re-resection, long-term morbidity is frequent, and up to 45 per cent of patients will have an unsatisfactory long-term outcome.[4, 23, 89, 90]

Another approach is to try to tailor the surgical therapy to the probable cause of recurrent ulcer. If the patient has an incomplete truncal vagotomy with a satisfactory drainage procedure (pyloroplasty, gastrojejunostomy), re-vagotomy can be performed with good results.[73, 91, 92] Contraindications to re-vagotomy alone in patients with postoperative recurrent ulcer and incomplete vagotomy by sham feeding testing include gastric outlet obstruction, another indication for abdominal exploration (e.g., ongoing hemorrhage, retained antrum), and no previous drainage procedure. If the patient has had an incomplete proximal gastric vagotomy without a prior drainage procedure, it is most logical to perform an antrectomy plus truncal vagotomy, although truncal vagotomy and drainage might suffice in some patients.[93–95] Most surgeons recommend gastric resection for any patient with ulcer recurrence after an operation that did not include a resection (e.g., truncal vagotomy and drainage).[96] However, if excessive morbidity with abdominal exploration is anticipated and if preoperative sham feeding testing suggests incomplete vagotomy, transthoracic vagotomy can be performed safely with good results.[73]

If serum gastrin and acid secretory studies points to a diagnosis of Zollinger-Ellison syndrome as a cause for recurrent ulcer, most surgeons would perform total gastrectomy because lesser degrees of gastric resection may be associated with a high recurrence rate and increased morbidity.[8, 97] At the time of laparotomy, a search for a potentially resectable gastrinoma in or near the pancreas should be made prior to total gastrectomy. If such a lesion is located and removed, the surgeon should probably not remove the stomach, since resection of the tumor could possibly cure the patient (see pp. 918–919).

Retained antrum syndrome is curable by resecting the cuff of antral tissue at the end of the afferent limb.[25, 46, 98] In some cases, it also may be necessary to resect the stomal ulcer and revise the gastrojejunal anastomosis.

If the patient has had an adequate vagotomy, as judged by sham feeding testing, but nevertheless has a recurrent peptic ulcer not due to gastrinoma, retained antrum, or surgical suture, the surgical approach is either antrectomy (if it has not already been done) or gastric re-resection (if the patient has previously had antrectomy). In rare cases, total gastrectomy may be necessary. Simple revision of an obstructed gastroenteric anastomosis without vagotomy and/or resection is usually unsuccessful in patients with postoperative recurrent ulcer.

The role of Roux-en-Y gastrojejunostomy in the management of patients with postoperative recurrent peptic ulcer is unclear.[99, 100] Alkaline reflux and bilious vomiting are eliminated by this operation and the rate of ulcer recurrence is low.[100] However, at least 5 per

---

*No reported studies have evaluated the effect of sucralfate, omeprazole, or newer H_2-blockers such as famotidine on healing of postoperative recurrent ulcers.

cent of patients will require reoperation for delayed gastric emptying,[100] and a greater percentage will develop a syndrome of nausea, vomiting, and abdominal pain.[101, 102] It is possible that those patients with poor results after Roux-en-Y gastrojejunostomy had delayed gastric emptying prior to reoperation.[102, 103] Roux-en-Y gastrojejunostomy may be warranted in patients about to undergo reoperation for recurrent ulcer in whom severe alkaline reflux is thought to be contributing to the symptoms and/or causing the ulcer[30] and in whom gastric emptying is normal. Complete vagotomy should always be added to any Roux-en-Y reconstruction.

References

1. Printen, K. J., Scott, D., and Mason, E. E. Stomal ulcers after gastric bypass. Arch. Surg. *115:*525, 1980.
2. Scott, H. W., Jr., Dean, R. H., Parker, T., and Avant, G. The role of vagotomy in pancreaticoduodenectomy. Ann. Surg. *191:*688, 1980.
3. Martin, T. D., Feliciano, D. V., Mattox, K. L., and Jordan, G. L., Jr. Severe duodenal injuries: treatment with pyloric exclusion and gastrojejunostomy. Arch. Surg. *118:*631, 1983.
4. Stabile, B. E., and Passaro, E., Jr. Recurrent peptic ulcer. Gastroenterology *70:*124, 1976.
5. Kronborg, O., Holst-Christensen, J., and Joergensen, P. M. Influence of different techniques of proximal gastric vagotomy upon risk of recurrent duodenal ulcer and gastric acid secretion. Acta Chir. Scand. *143:*53, 1977.
6. Kronborg, O., Joergensen, P. M., Hansen, O. H., and Pedersen, T. Assessment of completeness of vagotomy and surgical experience 10 days and 3 months after proximal gastric vagotomy. Acta Chir. Scand. *144:*495, 1978.
7. Blackett, R. L., and Johnston, D. Recurrent ulceration after highly selective vagotomy for duodenal ulcer. Br. J. Surg. *68:*705, 1981.
8. Thompson, J. C., Reeder, D. D., Villar, H. V., and Fender, H. R. Natural history and experience with diagnosis and treatment of the Zollinger-Ellison syndrome. Surg. Gynecol. Obstet. *140:*721, 1975.
9. Primrose, J. N., Joffe, S. N., Ratcliff, J. G., and Buchanan, K. D. The prevalence of gastrinomas in recurrent peptic ulceration. Scott. Med. J. *28:*328, 1983.
10. Christiansen, J. Primary hyperparathyroidism and peptic ulcer disease. Scand. J. Gastroenterol. *9:*111, 1974.
11. Holst-Christensen, J., Hansen, O., Pedersen, T., and Kronborg, O. Recurrent ulcer after proximal gastric vagotomy for duodenal and pre-pyloric ulcer. Br. J. Surg. *64:*42, 1977.
12. Hauer-Jensen, M., Carlsen, E., and Semb, L. Prognostic value of the pentagastrin and insulin tests after proximal gastric vagotomy. Scand. J. Gastroenterol. *15:*721, 1980.
13. Johnston, D., Pickford, I., Walker, B., and Goligher, J. Highly selective vagotomy for duodenal ulcer: do hypersecretors need antrectomy? Br. Med. J. *1:*716, 1975.
14. Ornsholt, J., Amdrup, E., Andersen, D., and Hostrup, H. Arhus County vagotomy trial; ulcer recurrence rate related to alterations in gastric acid secretion after selective gastric and parietal cell vagotomy. Scand. J. Gastroenterol. *18:*465, 1983.
15. Adami, H., Enander, L., Enskog, L., Ingvar, C., and Rydberg, B. Recurrences 1 to 10 years after highly selective vagotomy in prepyloric and duodenal ulcer disease. Frequency, pattern, and predictors. Ann. Surg. *199:*393, 1984.
16. Levy, M. Aspirin use in patients with major upper gastrointestinal bleeding and peptic-ulcer disease. A report from the Boston collaborative drug surveillance program, Boston University Medical Center. N. Engl. J. Med. *290:*1158, 1974.
17. Lanza, F. L., Royer, G. L., and Nelson, R. S. Endoscopic evaluation of the effects of aspirin, buffered aspirin, and enteric-coated aspirin on gastric and duodenal mucosa. N. Engl. J. Med. *303:*136, 1980.
18. Korman, M. G., Shaw, R. G., Hansky, J., Schmidt, G. T., and Stern, A. Influence of smoking on healing rate of duodenal ulcer in response to cimetidine or high-dose antacid. Gastroenterology *80:*1451, 1981.
19. Korman, M. G., Hansky, J., Merrett, A. C., and Schmidt, G. T. Ranitidine in duodenal ulcer. Incidence of healing and effect of smoking. Dig. Dis. Sci. *27:*712, 1982.
20. Chuong, J. J. H., Fisher, R. L., Chuong, R. L. B., and Spiro, H. M. Duodenal ulcer. Incidence, risks factors, and predictive value of plasma pepsinogen. Dig. Dis. Sci. *31:*1178, 1986.
21. Wychulis, A. R., Priestley, J. T., and Foulk, W. T. A study of 360 patients with gastrojejunal ulceration. Surg. Gynecol. Obstet. *122:*89, 1966.
22. Crean, G. P., and Spiegelhalter, D. J. Symptoms of peptic ulcer. *In* Cohen, S., and Soloway, R. D. (eds.). Peptic Ulcer Disease. New York, Churchill-Livingstone, 1985, p. 1.
23. Schirmer, B. D., Meyers, W. C., Hanks, J. B., Kortz, W. J., Jones, R. S., and Postlethwait, R. W. Marginal ulcer—a difficult surgical problem. Ann. Surg. *195:*653, 1982.
24. Sharaiha, Z. K., Smith, J. L., Cain, G. D., Schwartz, J. T., and Graham, D. Y. Recurrent ulcers after gastric surgery: endoscopic localization to the gastric mucosa. Am. J. Gastroenterol. *78:*269, 1983.
25. Lee, C-H., P'eng, F-K., and Lui, W-Y. The clinical aspect of retained gastric antrum. Arch. Surg. *121:*1181, 1986.
26. Hunt, P. S., Dowling, J., Korman, M., and Hansky, J. Bleeding stomal ulceration. Aust. N. Z. J. Surg. *49:*15, 1979.
27. Amlicke, J. A., and Ponka, J. L. Gastrocolic and gastrojejunocolic fistulas. Am. J. Surg. *107:*744, 1964.
28. Cody, J. H., DiVincenti, F. C., Cowick, D. R., and Mahanes, J. R. Gastrocolic and gastrojejunocolic fistulae: report of twelve cases and review of the literature. Ann. Surg. *181:*376, 1975.
29. Ott, D. J., Munitz, H. A., Gelfand, D. W., Lane, T. G., and Wu, W. C. The sensitivity of radiography of the postoperative stomach. Radiology *144:*741, 1982.
30. Mosiman, F., Donovan, I. A., and Alexander-Williams, J. Pitfalls in the diagnosis of recurrent ulceration after surgery for peptic ulcer disease. J. Clin. Gastroenterol. *7:*133, 1985.
31. Neustein, C. L., Bushkin, F. L., Weinshelbaum, E. I., and Woodward, E. R. Reoperation for postsurgical peptic ulcer recurrence. Appraisal of ten years' experience. Ann. Surg. *185:*169, 1977.
32. Cohen, M. M. Practical management of recurrent peptic ulcer. Can. J. Surg. *21:*21, 1978.
33. Halvorsen, J. F., Solhaug, J. H., and Semb, B. K. H. Suture line ulcers after gastric surgery. Acta Chir. Scand. *141:*149, 1975.
34. Basso, N., Lezoche, E., Giri, S., Percoco, M., and Speranza, V. Acid and gastrin levels after bombesin and calcium infusion in patients with incomplete antrectomy. Dig. Dis. Sci. *22:*125, 1977.
35. Donovan, D. C., Dureza, R., and Jain, U. Gastrinoma of duodenum. Diagnosis by endoscopy. N. Y. State J. Med. *79:*1766, 1979.
36. Janunger, K.-G., and Domellof, L. Gastric polyps and precancerous mucosal changes after partial gastrectomy. Acta Chir. Scand. *144:*293, 1978.
37. Caygill, C. P. J., Kirkham, J. S., Hill, M. J., and Northfield, T. C. Mortality from gastric cancer following gastric surgery for peptic ulcer. Lancet *1:*929, 1986.
38. Sandler, R. S., Johnson, M. D., and Holland, K. L. Risk of stomach cancer after gastric surgery for benign conditions: a case-control study. Dig. Dis. Sci. *29:*703, 1984.
39. Schafer, L. W., Larson, D. E., Melton, J., Higgins, J. A., and Ilstrup, D. M. The risk of gastric carcinoma after surgical treatment for benign ulcer disease. N. Engl. J. Med. *309:*1210, 1983.
40. Schnapka, G., Hofstaedter, F., Schwamberger, K., and Reissigl, H. Gastric stump carcinoma following Billroth II resection for peptic ulcer disease. Endoscopy *16:*171, 1984.
41. Domellof, L., Eriksson, S., and Janunger, K. G. Carcinoma and possible precancerous changes of the gastric stump after Billroth II resection. Gastroenterology *73:*462, 1977.
42. Amdrup, E., Brandsborg, M., Brandsborg, O., and Lovgreen, N. A. Interrelationship between serum gastrin concentration, gastric acid secretion, and gastric emptying rate in recurrent peptic ulcer. World J. Surg. *3:*235, 1979.
43. Wolfe, M. M., Jain, D. K., and Edgerton, J. R. Zollinger-

Ellison syndrome associated with persistently normal fasting serum gastrin concentrations. Ann. Intern. Med. *103:*215, 1985.

44. McGuigan, J. E., and Wolfe, M. M. Secretin injection test in the diagnosis of gastrinoma. Gastroenterology *79:*1324, 1980.

45. Stremple, J. F., and Elliott, D. W. Gastrin determinations in symptomatic patients before and after standard ulcer operations. Arch. Surg. *110:*875, 1975.

46. Korman, M. G., Scott, D. F., Hansky, J., and Wilson, H. Hypergastrinaemia due to an excluded gastric antrum: a proposed method of differentiation from the Zollinger-Ellison syndrome. Aust. N. Z. J. Med. *3:*266, 1972.

47. Webster, M. W., Barnes, E. L., and Stremple, J. F. Serum gastrin levels in the differential diagnosis of recurrent peptic ulceration due to retained gastric antrum. Am. J. Surg. *135:*248, 1978.

48. Thompson, J. C., Lowder, W. S., Peurifoy, J. T., Swierczek, J. S., and Rayford, P. L. Effect of selective proximal vagotomy and truncal vagotomy on gastric acid and serum gastrin responses to a meal in duodenal ulcer patients. Ann. Surg. *188:*431, 1978.

49. Feldman, M., Walsh, J. H., and Richardson, C. T. Serum gastrin response to secretin after vagotomy. Dig. Dis. Sci. *25:*921, 1980.

50. Becker, H. D., Reeder, D. D., and Thompson, J. C. Effect of truncal vagotomy with pyloroplasty or with antrectomy on food-stimulated gastrin values in patients with duodenal ulcer. Surgery *74:*580, 1973.

51. Lam, S. K., Chan, P. K. W., Wong, J., and Ong, G. B. Fasting and postprandial serum gastrin levels before and after highly selective gastric vagotomy, truncal vagotomy with pyloroplasty and truncal vagotomy with antrectomy: is there a cholinergic antral gastrin inhibitory and releasing mechanism? Br. J. Surg. *65:*797, 1978.

52. Keuppens, F., Willems, G., De Graef, J., and Woussen-Colle, M. C. Antral gastrin cell hyperplasia in patients with peptic ulcer. Ann. Surg. *191:*276, 1980.

53. Friesen, S. R., and Tomita, T. Pseudo-Zollinger-Ellison syndrome: Hypergastrinemia, hyperchlorhydria without tumor. Ann. Surg. *194:*481, 1981.

54. Primrose, J., Ratcliffe, J., and Joffe, S. Assessment of the secretin provocation test in the diagnosis of gastrinoma. Br. J. Surg. *67:*744, 1980.

55. Basso, N., Lezoche, E., Materia, A., Giri, S., and Speranza, V. Effect of bombesin on extragastric gastrin in man. Dig. Dis. Sci. *20:*923, 1975.

56. Speranza, V., Basso, N., Lezoche, E., Materia, A., Bagarani, M., and Paduos, A. Management and long-term results in patients with two-thirds gastrectomy and stomal ulcer. Am. J. Surg. *141:*105, 1981.

57. Safaie-Shirazi, S., Chaudhuri, T. K., Chaudhuri, M. D. and Condon, R. E. Visualization of isolated retained antrum by using technetium-99m. Surgery 73:278, 1973.

58. Cortot, A., Fleming, C. R., Brown, M. L., Go, V. L. W., and Malagelada, J.-R. Isolated retained antrum: diagnosis by gastrin challenge tests and radioscintillation scanning. Dig. Dis. Sci. *26:*748, 1981.

59. Dunlap, J., McLane, R., and Roper, T. The retained gastric antrum, a case report. Radiology *117:*371, 1975.

60. Lee, C., P'eng, F., and Yeh, P. H. Sodium pertechnetate Tc99m antral scan in the diagnosis of retained gastric antrum. Arch. Surg. *119:*309, 1984.

61. Multicenter Study. Intramuscular pentagastrin compared with other stimuli as tests of gastric secretion. Lancet *1:*341, 1969.

62. Richardson, C. T., Peters, M. N., Feldman, M., McClelland, R. N., Walsh, J. H., Cooper, K. A., Willeford, G., Dickerman, R. M., and Fordtran, J. S. Treatment of Zollinger-Ellison syndrome with exploratory laparotomy, proximal gastric vagotomy, and H2-receptor antagonists. Gastroenterology *89:*357, 1985.

63. Samloff, I. M., Secrist, D. M., and Passaro, E., Jr. The effect of betazole on serum group I pepsinogen levels: studies in symptomatic patients with and without recurrent ulcer after vagotomy and gastric resection or drainage. Gastroenterology *70:*1007, 1976.

64. Hollander, F. The insulin test for the presence of intact nerve fibers after vagal operations for peptic ulcer. Gastroenterology 7:607, 1946.

65. Read, R. C., Thompson, B. W., and Hall, W. H. Conversion of Hollander tests in man from positive to negative. Arch. Surg. *104:*573, 1972.

66. Read, R. C., and Doherty, J. E. Cardiovascular effects of induced insulin hypoglycemia in man during the Hollander test. Am. J. Surg. *119:*155, 1970.

67. Decker, G. A. G., and Myburgh, J. A. A fatality during the Hollander insulin test. S. Afr. Med. J. *43:*869, 1969.

68. Feldman, M., Richardson, C. T., and Fordtran, J. S. Experience with sham feeding as a test for vagotomy. Gastroenterology *79:*792, 1980.

69. Kronborg, O., and Anderson, D. Acid response to sham feeding as a test for completeness of vagotomy. Scand. J. Gastroenterol. *15:*119, 1980.

70. Farrell, J. I. Contributions to the physiology of gastric secretion. The vagi as the sole efferent pathway for the cephalic phase of gastric secretion. Am. J. Physiol. *85:*685, 1928.

71. Stenquist, B., Knutson, U., and Olbe, L. Gastric acid responses to adequate and modified sham feeding and to insulin hypoglycemia in duodenal ulcer patients. Scand. J. Gastroenterol. *13:*357, 1978.

72. Feldman, M., Richardson, C. T., and Fordtran, J. S. Effect of sham feeding on gastric acid secretion in healthy subjects and duodenal ulcer patients: evidence for increased basal vagal tone in some ulcer patients. Gastroenterology *79:*796, 1980.

73. Thirlby, R. C., and Feldman, M. Transthoracic vagotomy for postoperative peptic ulcer: effects on basal, sham feeding- and pentagastrin-stimulated acid secretion and on clinical outcome. Ann. Surg. *201:*648, 1985.

74. Moore, E. The terminology and measurement of gastric acidity. Ann. N. Y. Acad. Sci. *140:*866, 1967.

75. Knutson, U., and Olbe, L. Gastric acid response to sham feeding in the duodenal ulcer subject. Scand. J. Gastroenterol. *8:*513, 1974.

76. Kennedy, T., and Spencer, A. Cimetidine for recurrent ulcer after vagotomy or gastrectomy: a randomised controlled trial. Br. Med. J. *1:*1242, 1978.

77. Hoare, A. M., Jones, E. L., and Hawkins, C. F. Cimetidine for ulcers recurring after gastric surgery. Br. Med. J. *1:*1325, 1978.

78. Festen, H. P. M., Lamers, C. B. H., Driessen, W. M. M., and Von Tongeren, J. H. M. Cimetidine in anastomotic ulceration after partial gastrectomy. Gastroenterology *77:*83, 1979.

79. Stage, J. G., Henriksen, F. W., and Kehlet, H. Cimetidine treatment of recurrent ulcer. Scand. J. Gastroenterol. *14:*977, 1979.

80. Gugler, R., Lindstaedt, H., Miederer, S., Mockel, W., Rohner, H. G., Schmitz, H., and Szekessy, T. Cimetidine for anastomotic ulcers after partial gastrectomy. A randomized controlled trial. N. Engl. J. Med. *301:*1077, 1979.

81. Koo, J., Lam, S. K., and Ong, G. B. Cimetidine versus surgery for recurrent ulcer after gastric surgery. Ann. Surg. *195:*406, 1982.

82. Berstad, A., Aadland, E., and Bjerke, K. Cimetidine treatment of recurrent ulcer after proximal gastric vagotomy. Scand. J. Gastroent. *16:*891, 1981.

83. Eaves, R., and Korman, M. G. Twice-a-day dosage of cimetidine in the short-term treatment of peptic ulcer. Med. J. Aust. *2:*518, 1982.

84. Stage, J. G., Friis, J., and Nielsen, O. V. Ranitidine treatment of patients with postoperative recurrent ulcers. Scand. J. Gastroenterol. *18*(Suppl. 86):80, 1983.

85. McCarthy, D. M. Report on the United States experience with cimetidine in Zollinger-Ellison syndrome and other hypersecretory states. Gastroenterology *74:*453, 1978.

86. Taylor, T. V., Pearson, K. W., and Torrance, B. Revagotomy for recurrent peptic ulceration. Br. J. Surg. *64:*477, 1977.

87. Green, W. E. R., Kennedy, T., Hassard, K. T., and Spencer, E. F. A. Management of recurrent peptic ulceration. Br. J. Surg. *65:*422, 1978.

88. Kennedy, T., and Green, W. E. R. Stomal and recurrent ulceration: medical or surgical management? Am. J. Surg. *139:*18, 1980.

89. Hoffmann, J., Shokouh-Amiri, M. H., Klarskov, P., Madsen, O. G., and Jensen, H. E. Gastrectomy for recurrent ulcer after vagotomy: five- to nineteen-year follow-up. Surgery 99:517, 1986.
90. Pietri, P., Gabrielli, F., and Pellis, G. Reoperation for recurrent peptic ulcer. Int. Surg. 68:301, 1983.
91. Hede, J. E., Temple, J. G., and McFarland, J. The place of transthoracic vagotomy in the management of recurrent peptic ulceration. Br. J. Surg. 64:332, 1977.
92. Lehr, L., and Pichlmayr, R. Low-risk thoracic vagotomy for anastomotic ulceration. World J. Surg. 6:93, 1982.
93. Lunde, O. C., Liavag, I., and Roland, M. Recurrent ulceration after proximal gastric vagotomy for duodenal ulcer. World J. Surg. 7:751, 1983.
94. Hoffmann, J., Meisner, S., and Jensen, H. E. Antrectomy for recurrent ulcer after parietal cell vagotomy. Br. J. Surg. 70:120, 1983.
95. Ingvar, C., Adami, H. O., Enander, L., Enskog, L., and Rydberg, B. Clinical results of reoperation after failed highly selective vagotomy. Am. J. Surg. 152:308, 1986.
96. Heppell, J., Bess, M. A., McIlrath, D. C., and Dozois, R. R. Surgical treatment of recurrent peptic ulcer disease. Ann. Surg. 198:1, 1983.
97. Lusby, R. J., Byrnes, D. J., and Hugh, T. B. Postoperative recurrent peptic ulcer. The significance of the Zollinger-Ellison syndrome. Med. J. Aust. 2:389, 1977.
98. Scobie, B. A., and Rovelstad, R. A. Anastomotic ulcer: significance of the augmented histamine test. Gastroenterology 48:318, 1965.
99. Cooper, G., and Bell, G. Combined antrectomy and Roux-en-Y anastomosis in the surgical treatment of recurrent peptic ulceration. Br. J. Surg. 69:646, 1982.
100. Herrington, J. L., Jr., Scott, H. W., and Sawyers, J. L. Experience with vagotomy-antrectomy and Roux-en-Y gastro-jejunostomy in surgical treatment of duodenal, gastric, and stomal ulcers. Ann. Surg. 199:590, 1984.
101. Mathias, J. R., Fernandez, A., Sninsky, C. A., Clench, M. H., and Davis, R. H. Nausea, vomiting, and abdominal pain after Roux-en-Y anastomosis: motility of the jejunal limb. Gastroenterology 88:101, 1985.
102. Davidson, E. D., and Hersh, T. The surgical treatment of bile reflux gastritis. Ann. Surg. 192:175, 1980.
103. Mackie, C., Hulks, G., and Cuschieri, A. Enterogastric reflux and gastric clearance of refluxate in normal subjects and in patients with and without bile vomiting following peptic ulcer surgery. Ann. Surg. 204:537, 1986.

53

Chronic Morbidity after Ulcer Surgery

JAMES H. MEYER

Chronic morbidity after ulcer surgery takes many forms. Nearly half the patients operated upon for ulcer disease experience some kind of chronic debility as the result of surgery. Physicians, surgeons, and many patients may dismiss symptoms as trivial and thus minimize these discomforts as an acceptable price for surgical cure of ulcer disease. Nevertheless, *postgastrectomy dysfunction* (the term is commonly used after any type of ulcer surgery whether or not a gastric resection was performed) is of considerable importance to patients and the medical community.

About one patient in ten operated upon for ulcer disease is unable to accommodate to the chronic effects of the surgery and is impaired to the point of losing time from work, at least temporarily. Such a patient seeks relief sequentially from a variety of physicians. Large sums are expended by way of time and diagnostic tests in search of unusual complicating conditions more amenable to treatment than commonplace postgastrectomy dysfunction. Although the number of ulcer operations annually in the United States has dropped to 25 per cent of the peak rates of the late 1960s, 80,000 to 100,000

Americans still undergo surgery each year.[1, 2] Thus, even a 10 per cent incidence of more severe postoperative debility results in a significant social and economic burden to the community.

PATHOPHYSIOLOGY OF OPERATIONS FOR ULCER DISEASE

Theoretical Possibilities

Gastric Secretion

Since all types of ulcer surgery reduce gastric secretion, it is possible that some postoperative problems might result from chronically suppressed secretion by the stomach. Principal components of gastric juice are *acid, pepsin,* and *intrinsic factor.* In addition to facilitating peptic hydrolysis, the secretion of acid serves to reduce the numbers of bacteria in the stomach and proximal bowel. Spontaneously achlorhydric subjects, as well as postoperative subjects, have an increased incidence of *gastric carcinoma*[3] associated with increased numbers of intragastric bacteria. One possibility for this is that bacterial degradation products in the stomach may be carcinogenic.[4] While both spontaneously and postoperatively hypochlorhydric subjects also have somewhat increased numbers of bacteria in the small bowel, spontaneously achlorhydric subjects do not commonly exhibit diarrhea or malabsorption as a consequence of bacterial proliferation; likewise, suppression of small bowel bacteria with antibiotics does not correct mild malabsorption or diarrhea seen in postoperative subjects. Apparently, the mild increase in populations of small intestinal bacteria in hypochlorhydric subjects without intestinal stasis is insufficient to cause digestive problems. Nevertheless, spontaneously hypochlorhydric patients or patients who have had ulcer surgery are more susceptible to *salmonellosis* and *cholera*,[5] probably because smaller per orum inocula are more infective.

Gastric acidification also may promote solubilization of salts of iron and calcium and thus facilitate absorption of these highly required nutrients. Deficiencies of *iron* and *calcium* are common after ulcer surgery, but, since it is unclear to what extent these same deficiencies are encountered in spontaneously hypochlorhydric subjects, the importance of gastric acid in mineral nutrition is unsettled. Recent studies indicate gastric acidity may be more important for the absorption of iron salts than for the absorption of calcium.[6, 7] Acid-peptic proteolysis facilitates the breakdown of meat into fine particles and the solubilization of dietary proteins, but, in the absence of peptic activity, the motor actions of the normal (canine) stomach are sufficient to grind food into fine particles.[8] Likewise, proteolysis by pancreatic enzymes appears to be sufficient for normal digestion in the absence of gastric secretion of pepsins or lipase. The adequate general nutrition of the achlorhydric subjects supports the idea that the digestive functions of gastric juice are dispensable.

The loss of gastric intrinsic factor leads to malabsorption of vitamin B_{12} and vitamin B_{12} deficiency. However, the stomach normally secretes 100 times the amount of intrinsic factor required for maintenance of normal B_{12} stores.[9, 10] Thus, *pernicious anemia* is *uncommon* in hypochlorhydria associated with Type B atrophic gastritis (antrum involved; absent parietal cell antibody), and it follows that the 50 to 90 per cent reduction in postcibal gastric secretion after ulcer surgery in itself should not regularly produce malabsorption of B_{12}.

Motility

See also pages 675 to 713.

In addition to reducing gastric secretion, surgical resection or surgical denervation of the stomach alters normal gastric motor function. Normal gastric motility is probably important in two respects: (1) the normal stomach functions as a reservoir, retaining food and allowing it to pass into the small intestine at a controlled rate; and (2) as food is retained, the normal stomach disperses the food into small particles, which are much more easily attacked in the small intestine by digestive enzymes.

Normal Gastric Motility and Emptying. In regard to its motility, the stomach really acts as two organs. The proximal half is a reservoir whose volume is governed by the tone of the muscular wall. Contractions in this portion of the stomach are sustained and result in increases in pressure over minutes. The distal half of the stomach, by contrast, undergoes "phasic contractions"; that is, circumferential bands of muscle contract forcefully over a few seconds to increase intraluminal pressure transiently. The phasic contractions in the distal stomach are usually peristaltic—that is, rings of muscular contraction sweep in an aboral direction along the antrum. The two parts of the stomach are in series with each other, and in turn with the pylorus, duodenum, and small bowel. Emptying of digesta from the stomach is controlled by a balance of forces between proximal and distal stomach and resistance to outflow at the pylorus and in the duodenum and small intestine.[11]

The proximal stomach serves as a reservoir for both solid and liquid nutrients. This function depends on how its tone can be modified. A variety of vagal reflexes modulate proximal gastric tone. Distention of the throat or esophagus inhibits proximal gastric tone in anticipation of incoming material. This reflex, called *receptive relaxation,* is abolished by truncal vagotomy. When the stomach is filled with a volume, its wall progressively relaxes, so that pressures do not rise much. This *gastric accommodation reflex* is also carried by the vagus nerves. After truncal vagotomy, the proximal stomach is still capable of relaxing its tone in response to distention, but the process takes longer; and as food enters the stomach, intraluminal pressures rise more than in the same animals before vagotomy. Tone of the proximal stomach is relaxed in response to duodenal distention, a reflex also carried in the vagal nerves.[12] Nutrients in the intestine relax the tone of the proximal stomach. This relaxation by intraintestinal nutrients may be in part hormonally mediated (gastrin, secretin, cholecystokinin, and GIP relax the proximal stomach) and may be in part neurally mediated. When dogs are fed, the proximal stomach relaxes and its volume expands for several minutes after a meal; but then increasing tone returns so that the luminal volume of the fundus decreases.[13]

Contractions in the distal stomach are also modulated by neural and hormonal stimuli. Distention of the proximal stomach increases the strength and frequencies of antral contractions, an *antral reflex* that is abolished by vagotomy. Distention of the small bowel inhibits antral contractions, a reflex carried in both vagal and splanchnic nerves. Acid or nutrients (especially fat) in the proximal intestinal lumen inhibit antral contractions and contract the pylorus. While these actions of intestinal nutrients are reduced after truncal vagotomy, indicating a vagal reflex, intestinal hormones (especially secretin and/or cholecystokinin) may also play a role. Nutrients in the small intestine decrease the tonic diameter of the pylorus and duodenum, decrease the peristaltic spread of contractions along the duodenum, and increase the number of segmenting contractions in the proximal small intestine.[14]

An interplay of these various regional motilities governs the normal gastric emptying of food in ways that are not, as yet, entirely understood. Scintigraphic studies of gastric emptying in humans indicate that both liquids and solid nutrients are stored initially in the proximal stomach and that emptying from the stomach does not begin until digesta are pressed into the antrum, which then propels food into the duodenum. Some believe this initial distribution of food depends on a balance between the accommodation reflex, which relaxes the proximal stomach, and the antral reflex, which increases contractility of the antrum. Collins and associates[15] observed that the distribution of food between the proximal and distal parts of the stomach is actively controlled and may be modified by infusion of fat into the proximal bowel: the fat infusion shifted food from the antrum into the fundus, and this change in distribution was accompanied by a marked slowing of gastric emptying. Because of their fluidity, liquid nutrients tend more than solid foods to flow by gravity into the dependent antrum; and correspondingly, liquid nutrients tend to empty from the stomach promptly—sooner than solids, which often begin to empty only many minutes after eating.

The size of particles of solid food or of plastic spheres that leave the food-filled stomach is tightly regulated. In both the dog and the human, meat particles passing into the duodenum are distributed in sizes almost entirely below 1 mm.[16, 17] In both species, plastic spheres 1 mm or less in diameter leave the stomach rapidly, but spheres larger than 1 mm empty more and more slowly, as sphere diameter increases. While the pyloric orifice may play some role in the selection or sieving of particles, recent evidence indicates much of this selective, sieving process is determined by hydrodynamic forces. For example, the speed at which spheres of a given size leave the stomach may be modified by changing the density of the spheres or the viscosity of the gastric contents.[18] Apparently, as they are propelled from the stomach by either antral contractions or tonic pressures of the proximal stomach, liquids will carry solid food particles with them; but how fast the particles are swept along in the liquid stream depends on their inertia and/or their tendency to sink or float out of the central, fast-moving stream of liquid. The process is analogous to the way stones of various sizes and silt are carried along by a fast-moving river. However sieving is accomplished, the gastric retention of particles larger than 1 mm may influence how fast food is emptied because of the time required to reduce food to small particles. Thus, when meat is fed as 0.25-mm and 10-mm particles, the smaller particles leave the stomach much more quickly.[16, 19]

Ulcer operations may significantly alter motor patterns. Truncal or selective vagotomies reduce tonic relaxation of the proximal stomach and increase postcibal pressures within the stomach cavity.[20] As a result, pressure gradients between proximal stomach and duodenum are increased so that liquids are propelled more quickly out of the stomach. Liquid emptying might be further sped if pyloric resistance to outflow is ablated by pyloroplasty or distal gastrectomy. By eliminating the narrow pyloric orifice or by changing the flow patterns, antrectomy may alter the size of particles that the stomach allows to empty. To the extent that the phasic contractions of the antrum may physically grind food into small particles, antrectomy may also slow the rate at which food is fragmented. If fragmentation is slowed but sieving is preserved, antrectomy might slow gastric emptying of solid food, as the time required to reduce food to the proper size would be increased. Similarly, if the antrum were not removed but its contractility and thus its grinding functions were decreased by vagal denervation, solid emptying would be slowed if selective sieving prevailed. Thus, the outcome of various operations on gastric emptying of solid food may depend on how the balance between grinding and sieving functions of the stomach is affected.

Observed Effects on Emptying

Subtotal Gastrectomy

This operation accelerates emptying of liquid meals whether the meals contain fat, carbohydrate, or protein,[21] which normally slow gastric emptying. Likewise, solid food[22, 23] leaves the stomach remnant more rapidly after this operation. Gastric emptying is disturbed after both subtotal gastrectomy with gastroduodenostomy (Billroth I) and subtotal gastrectomy with gastrojejunostomy (Billroth II). Data are too limited to detect possible differences between these two operations, but current indications are that both affect gastric emptying similarly. The effect of subtotal gastrectomy on gastric sieving has not been observed in human subjects. After distal gastric resection in dogs, 30 to 40 per cent of meat particles that emptied from the stomach were larger than 2 mm, a marked upward shift from the spectrum of particles emptied from intact canine stomachs.[16, 24] Resection of both the pylorus and the distal 6 cm of antrum was required to affect this change, as neither pyloroplasty or pylorectomy alone nor antral resection with preservation of the pylorus altered the normal sieving process.

The simplest interpretation of these findings is that the terminal antrum, together with the pylorus, forms an orifice that is small enough to limit the passage of particles larger than 1 mm. Such an orifice would have to be a functional opening, as there is no anatomic orifice that corresponds to the pylorus and distal antrum. Hydrodynamic sieving is an alternative explanation: as the food-filled stomach dilates, the proximal antrum extends downward so that the distal antrum and pylorus form a U-shaped trap. This shape forces fluid and particles upward before they can be ejected from the stomach. Particles with more inertia (that is, those with larger diameter or higher densities) are caught in this "trap" and retropelled backward as the pylorus and terminal antrum pylorus close. Resecting the distal stomach would destroy or distort the "trap."

Effects of Various Vagotomies

In dogs, truncal, selective (complete gastric), or proximal gastric vagotomies alter fundic tone, increase postcibal pressures, and speed the gastric emptying of liquids.[20] In man, proximal gastric and truncal vagotomies impair gastric accommodation reflexes.[25, 26] Proximal gastric vagotomy moderately speeds human gastric emptying of liquid nutrients;[27] this acceleration is increased further if a pyloroplasty is added to the proximal vagotomy.[28-30] Because of gastric obstruction in 20 per cent of patients with truncal[31] or selective[28] vagotomy alone, neither vagotomy is performed anymore in man without "drainage" (i.e., pyloroplasty, gastroenterostomy, or antrectomy). All reports indicate that truncal vagotomy with a "drainage" procedure accelerates the emptying of liquid nutrients.[21, 32, 33] Selective vagotomy with pyloroplasty speeds the emptying of liquids about as much as truncal vagotomy with pyloroplasty.[28] Proximal gastric vagotomy preserves antral innervation and antropyloric function. The rate of gastric emptying of solid food is unaffected by this procedure,[17, 27] and the size of food particles leaving the stomach is normal (Fig. 53–1).

Truncal vagotomy denervates the entire stomach so that this operation decreases antral contractility[26] and alters the tone of the proximal stomach. With either pyloroplasty or antrectomy, truncal vagotomy has a highly varied effect on gastric emptying of solid food. An occasional patient with truncal vagotomy plus pyloroplasty will empty solid food very rapidly.[22, 34] In most patients, however, emptying of solids is initially accelerated, but this initially rapid emptying is followed by a very slow emptying phase (Fig. 53–1). In about 40 per cent of subjects, the slow emptying phase predominates so that the overall emptying of solid food is slowed. Emptying patterns are similar for truncal vagotomy plus pyloroplasty and truncal vagotomy with antrectomy.

In patients with truncal vagotomy plus pyloroplasty, the size of liver particles emptied from the stomach was normal. A sieving defect was observed after truncal vagotomy plus antrectomy, however, so that on the average, about 30 per cent of meat particles emptied in sizes greater than 1 mm (Fig. 53–1). Despite the absence of an antrum, these patients were able to reduce 70 per cent of radiolabeled liver to small particles (just as in dogs with antrectomies). Thus, the grinding action of the stomach is not confined to the antrum.

In summary, all ulcer operations accelerate the gastric emptying of liquid nutrients. Proximal gastric vagotomy, without pyloroplasty, is the least disruptive in this regard. Proximal gastric vagotomy does not alter the speed of solid emptying or the character of solid food particles emptied. Distal gastric resections, with

Figure 53–1. Gastric emptying of radiolabeled liver (solid food) in normal subjects six patients with highly selective (i.e., proximal gastric) vagotomy (HSV), nine patients with truncal vagotomy and antrectomy (TVA), and seven patients with truncal vagotomy and pyloroplasty (TVP). Curves designated as "gamma camera" (solid circles, solid lines) indicate gastric emptying of all sizes of liver particles, while curves labeled "bubble trap" (hollow circles, dashed lines) indicate gastric emptying of particles ≤ 1 mm in diameter. Gastric empyting was similar in both normal subjects and patients with proximal gastric vagotomy: emptying began after a 30 min lag and then was linear until almost all of the radiolabeled liver had left the stomach. In both groups virtually all radiolabeled liver left the stomach as particles ≤ 1 mm (i.e., no difference between camera and bubble trap curves). By contrast, both groups with truncal vagotomy emptied 40 to 50 per cent of the radiolabeled liver in the first 40 minutes and little thereafter. Patients with TVA emptied about one third of the radiolabeled liver as particles > 1 mm (camera and bubble trap curves significantly differed), while those with TVP emptied the liver as particles ≤ 1 mm.[17]

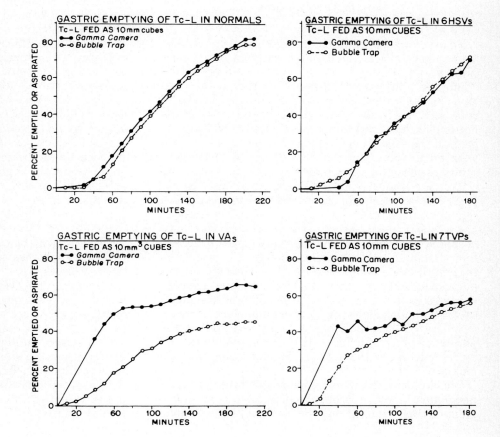

or without vagotomy, tend to accelerate emptying of solids and to disrupt normal gastric sieving. Truncal vagotomy with either antrectomy or pyloroplasty has a highly variable effect on rates of emptying of solid foods.[17] Though emptying patterns are similar after the two operations, sieving is normal after truncal vagotomy plus pyloroplasty but is disrupted when truncal vagotomy is combined with antrectomy.

Up to this point, we have been discussing effects of ulcer surgery on postcibal motility and gastric emptying. However, gastrointestinal motility has a different pattern in man during fasting. When the gastrointestinal tract is empty, the stomach does not contract most of the time. About every 100 to 120 minutes, contractions reappear in the antrum, building over about 15 minutes to a crescendo of frequent and very vigorous contractions. Over the next 100 to 120 minutes, this crescendo of contractile activity slowly migrates from the antrum down the entire small bowel, while the antrum is again quiet, until the next cycle begins. These cycles of migrating contractility are called migrating myoelectric complexes (MMCs). Another name for the MMC is the "housekeeper" because the complex sweeps the gastrointestinal tract free of debris, emptying in its path even very large materials (7-mm spheres, tablets, foreign bodies) from the stomach. In some patients who have had truncal vagotomy, the cycle is either absent or much weakened.[35] These individuals may develop gastric bezoars.

Rapid Gastric Emptying in the Genesis of Postcibal Symptoms

Many postcibal symptoms can be easily understood in the light of accelerated gastric emptying after ulcer surgery. For example, in his classic studies on the "dumping syndrome," Machella[36] observed that balloon distention in the proximal jejunum produced cramping, upper abdominal pain, nausea, or vomiting not unlike those symptoms experienced postcibally by patients who have been operated upon for ulcers. He went on to show that rapid instillation of hypertonic solutions (glucose, salt solutions, or solutions of amino acids) into the jejunum reproduced almost exactly postcibal symptoms in such patients and evoked a similar complex of symptoms even in volunteers who had not had ulcer surgery. He concluded that most postcibal symptoms arose from rapid egress of hypertonic liquids into the proximal bowel. He postulated that extracellular fluid entering the lumen during osmotic equilibration added to large volumes entering the intestine from the stomach, resulting in distention of the jejunum and symptoms related thereto. Similarly, in rats, satiety could be induced by filling the jejunum with nutrients; satiety appeared more and more quickly as the rate of jejunal filling was increased.[37]

We have since come to recognize that other postcibal phenomena can be reasonably ascribed to rapid movement of meal contents into the intestine. For example,

the appearance of milk (lactose) intolerance in adults following ulcer surgery[38] is easily understood; adults have limited capacity to hydrolyze lactose; rapid gastric emptying of ingested milk results in the entry of lactose into the jejunum at rates exceeding hydrolytic capacity. Likewise, postcibal hyperglycemia[34, 39] found postoperatively arises from prompt absorption of carbohydrates rapidly emptying from the stomach.

Despite such intuitively reasonable relationships between disturbed gastric motility and postoperative dysfunction, many problems remain unexplained. Since ulcer surgery destroys major motor mechanisms in the stomach, why are not all patients, instead of the minority, severely afflicted with symptomatic postsurgical dysfunction? What does rapid gastric evacuation have to do with general or specific types of malnutrition or with diarrhea continuing during periods of fasting? What other processes produce postgastrectomy dysfunction? Although these riddles have not been solved, hints can be found amid epidemiologic data, clinical observations, and reported experimental studies.

COMMON FORMS OF CHRONIC MORBIDITY AFTER ULCER SURGERY

Postcibal Alimentary Symptoms

Early Postcibal Symptoms

Some pattern of early satiety with or without postcibal vomiting (usually within 30 to 60 minutes of eating) is the most commonly encountered "postgastrectomy syndrome." A variety of other symptoms may be associated with the vomiting, most often pain.

Depending on the pattern of vomiting and the type of associated discomforts, this postsurgical dysfunction has been given a variety of names that frequently imply some perceptible pathophysiologic mechanism: *(early) dumping syndrome, small stomach syndrome, afferent loop syndrome, (alkaline, bile) reflux gastritis,* and *bilious vomiting syndrome.* The semantics are confusing and sometimes illogical. For example, the small stomach syndrome (early satiety sometimes culminating in vomiting) appears with equal frequency among those who have a small stomach as a result of gastric resection and those who have undergone nonresective ulcer surgery (vagotomy plus "drainage"). Similarly, some use the term "afferent loop syndrome" to describe postcibal bilious vomiting whether or not the patient actually has an afferent loop (subtotal gastrectomy, Billroth II).

Circumstantial evidence indicates that *early satiety* or *postcibal vomiting* or both are related to rapid gastric emptying after ulcer surgery with consequent distention of the proximal small intestine. First, the syndrome usually occurs during the period of most rapid transit of food from the stomach through the intestine—that is, in the first postcibal 30 minutes (Fig. 53–2). Second, the syndrome may be aggravated by consumption of meals with large volumes of liquids, which enhance the rate of transfer of material from the stomach. Third,

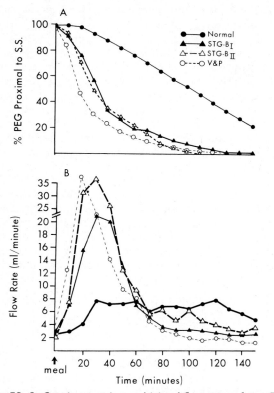

Figure 53–2. Gastric emptying and jejunal flow rates after a 500-ml liquid meal of fat, protein, and hypertonic glucose in normal subjects and in those who have had various ulcer operations. *A* expresses the percentage of ingested meal marker (PEG) remaining proximal to the jejunum (SS) as time elapses after ingesting the meal. The six normal subjects passed the meal into the intestine at a steady, slow rate, in contrast to the five or six subjects with each operation who passed 80 per cent of the meal precipitously into the intestine in the first postcibal hour. *B* illustrates the very high jejunal flow rates that followed the 500-ml meal in the subjects who had undergone surgery for ulcers versus the normal subjects. Jejunal flow rates in the postoperative subjects are increased by rapid gastric emptying of the meal as well as osmotic equilibration with meal contents in the jejunum.

many patients note that recumbency alleviates the syndrome; it is known that after ulcer surgery, recumbency slows gastric emptying.[33, 34] Fourth, the consumption of hypertonic liquids (for example, coffee laden with sugar or sweetened fruit juices) aggravates the syndrome in some patients, presumably as the result of adding an osmotic load to a volume load entering the small bowel.

On the other hand, patients who have had ulcer surgery usually ingest meals of solid food and small amounts of water. These meals are hypotonic, so that water is quickly absorbed after chyme enters the duodenum. Also, the secretion of gastric acid after ulcer operations is reduced, and, correspondingly, so is the secretion of pancreatic volume and bicarbonate in response to duodenal acidification. Consequently, rates of volume flow in the proximal jejunum of postoperative patients are low after more usual meals (Fig. 53–3), so that the concept of jejunal distention may apply only to meals of high liquid volume and osmolality.

Although the symptoms may vary from episode to episode in patients and among patients, the central characteristic of this syndrome is its temporal relationship to eating. If *early satiety* is experienced with sufficient intensity to prevent further intake of food, vomiting may not occur. Alternatively, the patient may *vomit* small amounts of food or, more often, bile-stained liquid (bilious vomiting). That the amount of food vomited is usually small or, more commonly, that the bile-stained vomitus does not contain food at all[40] attests to the association of this early postcibal syndrome with rapid gastric emptying. Abdominal *discomfort,* either steady upper abdominal pain or cramps, may be associated; since patterns of pain may resemble those experimentally produced by distention of segments of proximal jejunum,[36, 41] it is presumed that these symptoms are similarly caused by jejunal distention with rapidly emptied gastric contents. In addition, diarrhea is another common postcibal alimentary symptom (discussed separately later).

Patients also may experience postcibal *vasomotor* phenomena (flushing, palpitations, diaphoresis, lightheadedness, tachycardia, and postural hypotension) or peculiar affective symptoms (lassitude, intense desire to lie down, diminished attention span). Combinations of alimentary symptoms with these constitutional complaints are usually referred to as the "dumping syn-

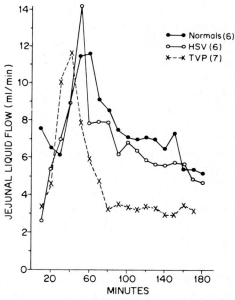

Figure 53–3. Flow patterns in the proximal jejunum of normal subjects, patients with highly selective (i.e., proximal gastric) vagotomies (HSV), and patients with truncal vagotomy and pyloroplasty (TVP) after a meal of 100 ml of water and 90 gm of meat. Flow patterns were similar in normals and patients with HSV. Although proximal jejunal flows peaked earlier after the meal in patients with TVP (probably because of very rapid gastric emptying), the magnitude of fluid flows was not much different from that in the normal subjects and contrasted greatly with large jejunal flows (see V & P, Fig. 53–2) after a hypertonic, sugar-laden liquid meal in patients with TVP. In other studies in patients with vagotomy and antrectomy, jejunal flows after this test meal were about half the flows in the normal subjects.

drome." Nevertheless, patients commonly experience alimentary symptoms (satiety, nausea, vomiting, cramps, pain, and/or diarrhea) without associated vasomotor phenomena[42-44] or, conversely, may experience postcibal constitutional symptoms without alimentary complaints.

The genesis of postcibal vasomotor abnormalities remains obscure. Like alimentary symptoms, these abnormalities can be evoked by rapid filling of the proximal small intestine with hypertonic material. In addition to distending the bowel, rapid osmotic equilibration of hypertonic luminal contents results in contraction of blood volume, usually by a few hundred milliliters.[45, 46] Using a liquid test of 50 per cent glucose in water, Ralphs and coworkers have shown that the degree of postprandial hemoconcentration or hypovolemia and the intensity of symptoms vary with the speed of gastric emptying,[47] but it is unclear to what extent these findings with meals of 50 per cent glucose may pertain to postcibal symptoms commonly encountered after less osmolar, ordinary meals. The role of hypovolemia in the production of vasomotor phenomena is uncertain: (1) there is only a poor correlation between the magnitude of hypovolemia and the appearance of symptoms,[48] and thus a modest contraction of a few hundred milliliters may be associated with marked postural hypotension and tachycardia; and (2) prevention of postcibal hypovolemia by intravenous infusion of saline or dextran does not invariably abort the development of symptoms.[46, 48] Rapid influx of (hypertonic) material into the small intestine may be associated with rapid and copious release of a variety of intestinal hormones into the bloodstream.

Serotonin, bradykinin, substance P, enteroglucagon, gastric inhibitory peptide, neurotensin[49] or vasoactive intestinal peptide[50] have been shown to be elevated to abnormally high postcibal blood concentrations, usually after meals of hypertonic glucose in symptomatic, postoperative patients. Such elevations may be epiphenomena and not necessarily the cause of symptoms, since intravenous infusion of one or another of these agents at rates producing comparable blood levels has not been shown to produce the pattern of postcibal symptoms.[49]

In summary, there are three likely mechanisms: (1) autonomic reflexes triggered by intestinal distention, (2) contraction of blood volume, and (3) excessive release of vasoactive hormones from the small intestine. Individually, none of these mechanisms has been conclusively implicated; all three could operate together to produce postcibal vasomotor symptoms.

The combination of postcibal vasomotor symptoms and alimentary symptoms (dumping syndrome) is so characteristic of uncomplicated postoperative dysfunction that it is seldom mimicked by other conditions. However, alimentary symptoms unaccompanied by vasomotor phenomena may be confused with other syndromes characterized by postcibal vomiting.

Probably the most easily confused situation is that of chronic *partial afferent loop obstruction* in patients with subtotal gastrectomy with a gastrojejunostomy. Partial afferent loop obstruction results in dilatation of the afferent loop with pancreatic and biliary secretion. Since these secretions are voluminous only in response to feeding, symptoms (upper abdominal pain sometimes radiating to the infrascapular region) from partial afferent loop obstruction characteristically arise postcibally. As the loop distends, pain mounts; the episode may terminate in the vomiting of moderate amounts of bile-stained secretions. From this description it is apparent that the suggested pathogenesis of symptoms (afferent loop distention relieved by vomiting) in partial afferent loop obstruction is very similar to the presumed pathogenesis of common postcibal vomiting (distention of the proximal jejunum); correspondingly, the two syndromes may be confused, as they may differ only by the intensity of the symptom (pain more severe and more consistently present in partial afferent loop obstruction). Such confusion is rare, because partial obstruction of the afferent loop is very uncommon. Diagnosis may be established by radiographic demonstration of the point of partial obstruction or a dilated afferent loop, or by endoscopic demonstration of a stenosis in the afferent loop.

Bile vomiting, either after eating or during fasting, and abdominal pain are major symptoms of a syndrome called *alkaline* or *bile reflux gastritis*.[51] As implied by the name of the syndrome, these patients have extensive gastritis (erythema, friability, or bleeding at endoscopy; histologic gastritis on biopsy); some patients may exhibit anemia, presumably the result of blood loss from the gastritis. Despite the name, the role of duodenogastric reflux and gastritis in the genesis of symptoms in this syndrome is unclear, since some degree of gastritis (erythema in the distal stomach at endoscopy; superficial and atrophic gastritis histologically) and reflux of duodenal contents is common to most patients with any of the traditional ulcer operations. Instillation of autologous duodenal contents into the stomachs of these fasting patients may trigger abnormal gastrointestinal motor activity and vomiting.[52, 53] Some postulate that abnormal concentrations of bile salts or abnormal bacterial degradation products in duodenal contents incite this response, while others believe that the stomach, owing to extensive gastritis or to a primary motor disorder, is abnormally sensitive to duodenal contents. Whatever the exact mechanisms, patients in whom bilious vomiting is induced by duodenogastric reflux should, and often do, benefit from an operation that prevents reflux of duodenal contents into the stomach. The difficult problem for the clinician is to distinguish the patients with bile vomiting incited by duodenogastric reflux from those with postcibal bile vomiting associated with the dumping syndrome, who are not so likely to be benefitted by corrective surgery.

Gastric obstruction (by the stomach cicatrix or recurrent ulcer) is usually less easily confused. Satiety and vomiting occur, but here more protracted sitophobia or vomiting is the rule; vomitus is copious and usually contains undigested food, sometimes from a preceding meal. Diagnosis can be established radiographically or endoscopically.

Recurrent ulcer (see pp. 952–962) may present with pain and/or vomiting. However, here pain usually persists during interdigestive periods and may in fact be temporarily relieved by eating. The diagnosis can be established by endoscopy.

Late Postcibal Symptoms

A few patients operated on for ulcer may experience diaphoresis, palpitations, lassitude, mental confusion, or even loss of consciousness between 90 and 180 minutes following a meal. The syndrome is usually called "late dumping" to distinguish it from the vasomotor symptoms associated with rapid gastric emptying earlier in the postcibal period.

Many authorities attribute these late symptoms to *reactive hypoglycemia.* Indeed, when a standard oral glucose tolerance test is performed in such patients with concentrated solutions of 50 to 100 grams of glucose, symptoms are frequently provoked both early after the glucose meal and 90 to 180 minutes later.[54] Characteristically, the early postcibal symptoms coincide with a hyperglycemic phase and the later postcibal symptoms arise when the blood glucose concentration has fallen to 60 mg/dl or below. At one time, clinical investigators ascribed early postcibal symptoms to "hyperglycemic shock," but this notion was abandoned when it was realized that (1) hyperglycemia *per se* usually does not cause symptoms, and (2) similar symptoms could be precipitated by carbohydrate-free meals, which were not associated with hyperglycemia. Late dumping has not been looked upon with equal circumspection. For example, very little information substantiates that late dumping arising spontaneously after ordinary meals is frequently coincident with, or caused by, hypoglycemia. Only a minority of patients who undergo surgery ever experience these late postcibal symptoms, and even these few susceptible individuals do not experience symptoms regularly or predictably after ordinary meals, so the chances are few for observing blood glucose concentrations during spontaneous attacks. In my limited experience, such spontaneous attacks are rarely associated with blood glucose concentrations so low as to be clearly the cause of symptoms.

Nevertheless, all current theories of pathogenesis assume hypoglycemia is the cause of late postcibal symptoms, and all hypotheses revolve around rapid gastric emptying of carbohydrate in the genesis of hypoglycemic symptoms. The simplest idea is that such rapidly emptied carbohydrate is absorbed at supranormal rates, releasing a large output of insulin early in the postprandial period, and that the persisting effect of this large bolus of endogenous insulin produces hypoglycemia at a later time. Other theories on pathogenesis invoke supranormal release of gut hormones, such as gastric inhibitory peptide (GIP), by rapidly emptied carbohydrate and postulate that abundantly released intestinal hormone in turn triggers a supranormal insulin release. For example, Radziuk and associates[55] observed increased breath hydrogen after meals of 100 grams of glucose in water and suggested significant malabsorption of glucose, as the bowel was overwhelmed by glucose entering the intestine very rapidly. These workers believe the rapid entry of glucose releases a correspondingly large bolus of GIP from the intestine, which is appropriate for the amount of glucose entering the intestine, but not for the lesser amount absorbed. Others have suggested that hormones released from the gut (such as enteroglucagon) may inhibit the hyperglycemic action of glucagon, blunting the ability of endogenous glucagon to prevent a hypoglycemic phase. Circumstantial but inconclusive evidence supports each of these theories.

It is probably not appropriate to study the pathogenesis of this syndrome with markedly atypical meals of concentrated glucose solutions. For example, meals of solid starch are emptied much more slowly from the stomachs of patients with truncal vagotomy plus pyloroplasty than are isocaloric meals of starch or glucose in solution; correspondingly, the time courses of blood glucose and insulin were normal after the former but abnormal after the latter meals. In the few symptomatic subjects, postcibal symptoms prevailed even when glucose tolerance was normal after the solid starch meals.[34] Since meals of solid carbohydrate are far more commonly consumed than liquid meals of sugar, the extremely rapid emptying and the hypertonicity of the latter create conditions that probably are uncommon after usual meals. Phenomena such as unstable glucose tolerance or shifts of body water may pertain only to these very atypical meals.

Diarrhea

Chronic *diarrhea* may follow any of the traditional ulcer operations. Most commonly, diarrhea appears within an hour or two of eating. Usually the patient recognizes that certain foods seem predictably to evoke loose, watery stools (common offenders are milk, sweetened fruit juices, or soft drinks). Most observations are thus consistent with the notion that rapid entry of hypertonic liquids into the small intestine overwhelms small intestinal absorptive capacity, with consequent passage of large volumes of unabsorbed water into the colon.

For many years, physicians and surgeons had been impressed by a seemingly higher prevalence of diarrhea among patients who had a truncal vagotomy than among those who had a subtotal gastrectomy for ulcers; this impression was conveyed by the commonly used term "postvagotomy diarrhea." Indeed, the first randomized, prospective trial of various ulcer operations confirmed that diarrhea was nearly four times as frequent after truncal vagotomy as after subtotal gastrectomy.[42] More recent prospective trials,[56-58] however, have failed to demonstrate striking differences. Although most observers still adhere to the belief that postvagotomy diarrhea is a unique postoperative syndrome, this notion has not yet been conclusively substantiated.

The idea that diarrhea is more common after truncal vagotomy has prompted many investigations of patients with postvagotomy diarrhea. Several workers believe that the patient who has diarrhea after truncal vagotomy suffers from excessively rapid gastric emptying as the basis of diarrhea—that is, the resulting excessive fluid loads entering the small intestine overwhelm small intestinal absorptive capacity, as just mentioned. In support of this thesis are the several observations that those with diarrhea after vagotomy have more rapid gastric emptying than those with vagotomy who do not have diarrhea.[32, 33] Likewise, the possibly higher prevalence of diarrhea after vagotomy versus subtotal gastrectomy may reflect a greater acceleration of gastric emptying of liquids[21, 32] produced by vagotomy.

Ladas and associates[59] found that patients with diarrhea after truncal vagotomy plus "drainage" had faster transit of a liquid meal (marker) from stomach to proximal jejunum or stomach to terminal ileum than control patients or postvagotomy patients who did not have diarrhea. In the same study, the authors measured fluid flow through the terminal ileum and ileal input of osmolytes into the colon. Flows and solute delivery to the colon were excessive after the liquid meal in patients with diarrhea, but were also increased even during fasting. We (Allison, J., Stern, D., and Meyer, J., unpublished) also observed abnormally high ileal flows and delivery of electrolytes to the colon over a 24-hour period in patients with postvagotomy diarrhea when they were compared with postvagotomy patients without diarrhea or to normal subjects. Like Ladas, we found ileal flows were especially high after meals; but some of the patients with diarrhea also had high ileal flows during nocturnal (fasting) hours. In the main, these observations support the idea that postvagotomy diarrhea arises from rapid gastric emptying of meals, which accelerates intestinal transit and augments ileal flow into the colon; but the high, fasting, ileal flows remain unexplained and are at variance with earlier observations[60] of normal jejunal water and electrolyte fluxes in postvagotomy patients (without diarrhea). Radiologic studies[32] and lactulose breath tests[61] have also documented that patients with (postvagotomy) diarrhea have rapid rates of gastrocolonic transit.

Others have looked for extragastric effects of truncal vagotomy that could produce diarrhea, comparing patients who have had truncal vagotomy with diarrhea versus those without diarrhea. Such searches have failed to uncover differences in (1) small intestinal morphology, (2) small intestinal bacteria,[62] (3) fasting small intestinal fluxes of fluid and electrolytes,[60] or (4) fecal output of fat.[62] However, some patients with postvagotomy diarrhea have been found to have increased fecal outputs of bile acids.[63, 64] Fecal bile acid output is frequently increased in patients with postvagotomy diarrhea, probably as the result of rapid intestinal transit of postcibal contents. However, the concentrations of bile salts in stool water are usually not elevated because low fecal pH limits bile salt solubility. Choleraic diarrhea is driven by the effects of high bile salt concentrations on colonic mucosa. Aqueous concentrations of bile salts in most patients with postvagotomy diarrhea are too low to cause diarrhea; and correspondingly, treatment with cholestyramine does not always ameliorate postvagotomy diarrhea.[65] In effect, high fecal outputs of bile salts are the result,

rather than the cause, of postvagotomy diarrhea in most patients.

Whatever the effects of truncal vagotomy on extragastric structures, limiting the vagotomy to the stomach (selective vagotomy) somewhat reduces the incidence of postoperative diarrhea,[66–68] whereas restricting the vagotomy to the proximal stomach (proximal gastric vagotomy) appears to reduce postoperative diarrhea[69, 70] even further.

Like selective vagotomy, proximal gastric vagotomy limits vagal denervation to the stomach, but proximal gastric vagotomy disturbs gastric emptying much less than selective vagotomy. Thus a much lower prevalence of diarrhea among patients who have had a proximal gastric vagotomy, as opposed to selective gastric vagotomy, would support the hypothesis that rapid gastric emptying of liquids is an important pathogenetic component of postvagotomy diarrhea. However, not enough data have been collected on the prevalence of diarrhea after proximal versus selective gastric vagotomy to make this judgment.

Occasionally, a patient will experience almost continuous diarrhea after truncal vagotomy or will have episodes of diarrhea that continue through the night or into periods of fasting.[71] Obviously, this pattern of diarrhea cannot be readily explained on the basis of rapid gastric emptying of meal contents and supports arguments in favor of extragastric mechanisms.

Weight Loss

Thirty to 40 per cent of patients *lose weight* after ulcer surgery, and many of those remain at postoperative weights significantly less than ideal body weight. In addition to general malnutrition, as evidenced by weight loss, many patients develop specific nutritional deficiencies, to be discussed later.

Much of medical literature is focused on maldigestion and malabsorption as the cause of postoperative malnutrition. Mild steatorrhea and milder azotorrhea are common after all traditional ulcer operations but do not follow proximal gastric vagotomy.[72] Occasionally, an emaciated patient is encountered with profound malabsorption. Moreover, defects in absorption of iron and vitamin B_{12} (see below) are prevalent among patients operated on for ulcer. Such clinical experiences reinforce the notion that malnutrition arises from postoperative malabsorption. However, a broader collective experience indicates that decreased consumption of food is the most common cause of postoperative weight loss.

Daily fecal fat output seldom exceeds 15 per cent of fat intake in patients with truncal vagotomy plus pyloroplasty or gastroenterostomy,[72, 73] subtotal gastric resection,[74, 75] or even total gastrectomy.[76, 77] The coefficient of fat absorption remains constant over a wide range of fat intake in subjects with gastrectomies. Fecal nitrogen loss likewise is small, rarely exceeding 20 per cent of nitrogen intake, and remains a fairly constant fraction of intake over a wide range of protein consumption. Nevertheless, such small fecal wastage alone cannot reasonably account for postoperative weight loss in most subjects. Thus, on a 100 gram fat, 100 gram protein intake, fecal wastage of fat and protein would not usually account for more than a loss of 200 kcal daily in a patient operated on for ulcer, and such a small loss could easily be compensated for by a 10 per cent increase in consumption of food. It is therefore not surprising that there is no correlation between postoperative weight loss and fecal wastage among patients with gastric resections.[76, 78] Such data indicate that it is *decreased intake* of *food*, not malabsorption, that accounts for most postoperative weight loss, a fact readily documented by a carefully taken dietary history or observation of daily intake in most patients with postoperative weight loss.[76, 78]

In the author's experience[17, 22, 79] direct observation of how postoperative patients eat is required to understand how profoundly early satiety may limit intake. Historical dietary surveys are known to be inaccurate in normal subjects. Patients with ulcer operations frequently develop distorted perspectives about food, for they commonly overestimate, by large amounts, the quantity of food they can or do eat. The inaccuracies of dietary surveys in such patients must be kept in mind when discussing the effects of limited intake on specific nutritional deficiencies (see below).

Direct observations confirm that patients with gastrectomies or vagotomies restrict their *ad libitum* intake of total calories, mostly by reducing consumption of carbohydrates, especially of sugar-laden foods and beverages.[78, 80] Some observers attribute such self-restrictions to early satiety or to the conscious or unconscious desire of the patient to avoid or mollify one or another food-related symptoms complex[80–83] (e.g., pain, vomiting, diarrhea, hypoglycemia).

There seems to be a consensus in the literature that nutrition is worse after subtotal gastrectomy with a gastrojejunostomy (STG-BII) than after subtotal gastrectomy with duodenostomy (STG-BI),[74, 75] although such comparisons have not been well controlled.[75, 83–85] Likewise, some believe that nutrition is worse after vagotomy plus gastrojejunostomy (V + GE) than after vagotomy plus pyloroplasty (V + P).[71] Significantly more weight loss after subtotal gastrectomy than after vagotomy plus drainage was noted in one prospective trial,[42] but not in another.[56] Explanations of these poorly codified differences have focused on (1) by-pass of the duodenum with the gastrojejunal anastomosis (differences between STG-BI and STG-BII or between V + P and V + GE), and (2) the smaller size of the stomach after resection than after vagotomy plus drainage. Nevertheless, because vagotomy impairs receptive relaxation and accommodation, it is moot whether the vagally denervated stomach in fact will accommodate more food than the resected stomach without producing satiety or fullness.

The above discussion indicates that satiety, by limiting intake, is perhaps the most important factor in undernutrition after ulcer surgery. Our understanding of satiety is primitive, even in normal subjects. Gastric distention and nutrients in the proximal small intestine appear to work together to induce satiety.[37, 86] Thus,

larger gastric resections might result in more distention from a given amount of food; and this effect, together with rapid entry of nutrients into the proximal bowel, might greatly increase satiation. But additional mechanisms are suggested by recent observations. Food reaching the distal small intestine and/or colon in normal subjects induces early satiety and slows gastrointestinal transit.[87, 88] After truncal vagotomy plus antrectomy in dogs, a large proportion of solid food escaped digestion and absorption in the proximal intestine[89] and thus reached distal bowel. Similar malabsorption in patients may allow food to reach distal intestine, where it may trigger satiety mechanisms. Since this malabsorptive process resulted from defective sieving of solid food after gastric resection (only large particles of food were maldigested), any satiating effects of unabsorbed food in the distal intestines would be worse after resective surgery.

Maldigestion

Many factors may contribute to maldigestion in patients who have had ulcer surgery:

1. Distal gastric resection accelerates gastric emptying of liquid and solid food, whereas truncal vagotomy (plus pyloroplasty) speeds the emptying of liquids but has a variable effect on the emptying of solid food. After gastric resection, pancreatic and biliary secretory responses are generally unimpaired, but, as a result of rapid gastric emptying, the ratio between entry of pancreatic and biliary secretions and the entry of food into the small intestine is lowered.

2. The effect is accentuated in patients with subtotal gastrectomy plus gastrojejunostomy (Billroth II), because some of the food has passed from the stomach down the efferent loop before food-stimulated biliary and pancreatic secretory outputs reach the efferent loop.[21] Consistent with this idea is the observation that longer afferent loops after Billroth II subtotal gastrectomy are associated with greater amounts of steatorrhea.[74]

3. After truncal vagotomy, pancreatic response to eating is about half of normal;[17, 21] this diminished response further reduces the ratio of pancreatic enzyme to food entering the small intestine postcibally. It is not clear to what extent these lowered ratios might contribute to maldigestion or malabsorption. For example, pancreatic output must drop to about 15 per cent of normal in patients with chronic pancreatitis or pancreatic resection (see p. 1847) before malabsorption is detected; presumably, therefore, ratios between entry of pancreatic enzymes and food can drop to 15 per cent of normal before digestive disturbance is detected. Nevertheless, the situation after ulcer surgery is more complex and thus not comparable to simple pancreatic insufficiency.

4. For example, transit of chyme through the entire small intestine is accelerated, paralleling accelerated emptying from the stomach. Time available for digestion in the small intestinal lumen is therefore shortened. Under such circumstances, considerable quantities of undigested protein and fat were observed to

pass from the ileum to the colon after liquid test meals.[90]

5. After distal gastrectomy, pieces of food larger than 2 mm empty into the small intestine.[17] Since these large pieces are much more slowly digested than food particles in the normal size range of 0.5 mm or less, they often reach midintestine after little digestion and absorption of their contents, even though they travel slowly along the intestine.[91] In dogs with truncal vagotomy plus Billroth I antrectomy, liquid fat in a test meal was normally absorbed, so that less than 10 per cent remained unabsorbed by the time digesta reached mid–small intestine; but fat within solid food remained mostly undigested and unabsorbed within large pieces of meat reaching the midintestine.[89] These observations indicate that postoperative gastric emptying of abnormally large, poorly digestible pieces of solid food accounts for significant malabsorption of fat and other nutrients within the solid food matrix (see discussion on anemia, below).

Luminal concentrations of pancreatic enzymes and bile salts were markedly reduced in the duodenum or proximal jejunum for the first 40 minutes after liquid test meals were fed to patients with subtotal gastrectomies[21, 90] (Fig. 53–4) or with truncal vagotomy plus pyloroplasty.[21] This marked reduction was the result of dilution of normal or near normal pancreatic and biliary secretions by test meals rapidly emptying from the stomach.[21] Under these circumstances bile salt concentrations dipped below the critical micellar concentrations so that solubilization of fat and lipolysis were impaired.[92] Likewise, impaired proteolysis was found when pancreatic proteases were similarly diluted.[90] As striking as these findings were, they seem to be peculiar to the use of liquid test meals. More recent experiments that utilized a predominantly solid test meal of beefsteak and liver have shown that flow rates and luminal concentrations of bile salts and pancreatic enzymes are normal or nearly normal in the proximal jejunum after this meal in patients with

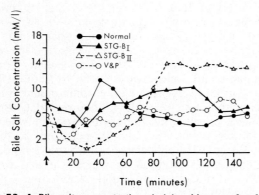

Figure 53—4. Bile salt concentrations in jejunal lumen after feeding a hypertonic liquid meal of fat, protein, and sugar to normal subjects and to patients who have had ulcer surgery. Note that in the first 40 minutes after the meal was taken *(arrow)*, the luminal concentration of bile salt was less than 2 mM in subjects who had undergone ulcer surgery. These low concentrations were noted despite normal postcibal outputs of bile from the biliary tract and resulted from dilution by contents rapidly leaving the stomach.

vagotomy plus antrectomy[17] (Fig. 53–3). Thus, the situation with liquid test meals was probably peculiar and not pertinent to general pathogenetic mechanisms, in much the same way that only very limited conclusions can be drawn from the study of the dumping syndrome after liquid meals of concentrated glucose.

Fecal bacterial flora colonize the small intestinal lumen in increased numbers (10^1 to 10^8 organisms per ml) after ulcer surgery. Colony counts are generally higher after resection than after vagotomy plus drainage, probably as the result of a more marked reduction of gastric acid secretion after gastric resection. Most authorities discount the role of small intestinal bacteria in the pathogenesis of the mild malabsorption commonly encountered after ulcer surgery.[93] For example, treatment with antibiotics does not usually correct the mild steatorrhea. Also, the combination of mild postoperative steatorrhea together with malabsorption of iron and creatorrhea does not typify the pattern of malabsorption arising from bacterial overgrowth. Only in an occasional patient does bacterial overgrowth play a major role in malabsorption, usually in association with other uncommon problems contributing to marked bacterial colonization, such as stasis associated with *partial intestinal obstruction,* or *gastrojejunocolic fistula.*

Anemia

Mild anemia (hemoglobin of 10 to 12 gm/dl) may appear after any of the traditional ulcer operations. In the absence of complicating disease, however, anemia develops gradually over a period of years after gastric resection (Fig. 53–5) and even more slowly after truncal vagotomy with a drainage procedure.[71, 81, 94–96] Because anemia evolves so slowly, it is too early to tell how often anemia will develop in patients who have had the newest operation, proximal gastric vagotomy. Most information on postoperative anemia has been derived from the study of patients who underwent subtotal gastrectomy for ulcer disease.

Anemia develops after partial gastrectomy as the result of deficiencies in iron, vitamin B_{12}, and/or folate. Often, multiple deficiencies are documented in anemic patients. Nevertheless, iron deficiency is the most common and appears to play the dominant role in the genesis of anemia. Thus, most postoperative anemias are microcytic and hypochromic. Mixed anemias with some macrocytosis are the next most common, whereas a purely macrocytic anemia is infrequent after ulcer surgery.[97–99] The fall in hemoglobin concentration parallels a decline in serum iron, and both are accelerated when blood (iron) loss complicates the postoperative situation, whether from normal causes (viz., menstruation) or intercurrent disease (Fig. 53–5). The serum concentration of vitamin B_{12} also declines over years after ulcer surgery but may reach a plateau at the lower limits of normal after five to eight years from surgery.[100, 101] Likewise, serum folate concentrations tend to drift downward with time after subtotal gastrectomy,[102] but findings are quite variable among

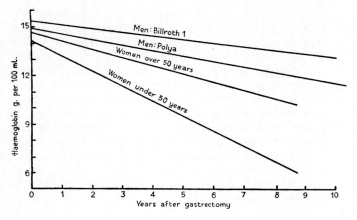

Figure 53–5. The fall of blood hemoglobin concentrations with time after subtotal gastrectomy in various groups of patients retrospectively surveyed by Baird and coworkers (Q. J. Med. *28*: 21, 1959). Note the significantly more rapid appearance of anemia in patients losing blood—viz., menstruating women (see text).

patients. Only a minority of anemic patients with subtotal gastrectomy have distinctly subnormal serum concentrations of iron, vitamin B_{12}, or folate. Therefore in any individual patient multiple mild deficiencies may account for the anemia; determining which deficiency predominates may be difficult and depends upon the morphology of blood or bone marrow and response to empiric treatment.

The causes of these deficiencies after ulcer surgery are multiple. Since food consumption is reduced in many patients, inadequate intake of iron, vitamin B_{12}, or folate might account for mild deficiencies. Nevertheless, several workers have observed that many patients deficient in iron or vitamin B_{12} consume adequate amounts of these nutrients despite other dietary restrictions.[94, 100] In general, there is no obvious correlation between the development of anemia and nutritional status, the degree of steatorrhea, or symptoms after surgery.[44, 82, 103] While chronic blood loss from a symptomatic or asymptomatic postoperative chronic gastritis might aggravate iron deficiency in some patients, it is clear that many individuals develop iron deficiency in the absence of gastrointestinal bleeding.[94, 104] These various observations suggest that some degree of specific malabsorption of iron, vitamin B_{12}, of folate complicates ulcer operations.

Normally, the intestine adapts to low body stores of iron by increasing its avidity for iron uptake. Most postoperative patients have an increased intestinal avidity for either iron salts or heme iron,[79, 94, 105–107] indicating this form of compensation is intact.

About two thirds of iron in the diet is food-bound, as iron salts; about one third is derived from heme iron in meat as muscle myoglobin or blood hemoglobin. Gastric acid dissociates iron salts from food and dissolves them. As a result, dissolved Fe^{+3} ions can be reduced in the stomach by glutathione and other organic matter to Fe^{+2} ions, which are about 100 times more soluble at intestinal pH (5.5 to 6.5) than ferric ions.[108] After they are dissolved by gastric acid, ferric ions may also be complexed by ascorbic acid or sugars, which keep them soluble at the more neutral pH levels of the proximal intestinal lumen. Thus, gastric acidity plays an important role in reducing and solubilizing inorganic, dietary iron so that it can be absorbed by the proximal intestine. This role can be illustrated by showing that normal subjects absorb significantly less iron from iron salts added to their food when their acid secretion is suppressed by cimetidine.[6] Likewise, the hypochlorhydria after ulcer surgery results in a diminished capacity to absorb iron salts from food. Postoperative patients have a high capacity to absorb iron when ferrous salts are ingested in acidified, aqueous solutions; but the same patients have a much reduced ability to absorb iron salts mixed with food at more neutral pH levels.[105–107]

Iron in heme is chelated by the heme porphyrin. Thus, gastric acidity is not important in the absorption of heme iron; all that is required is that heme proteins be digested by pancreatic proteases in the proximal bowel to liberate soluble heme-iron complexes, which are absorbed directly by a carrier for heme on the intestinal absorptive cell.[109] While subjects with spontaneous hypo- or achlorhydria have a modestly higher prevalence of iron deficiency than the normal population,[6] the fact that iron deficiency is not more widespread in this group is perhaps the result of this second pathway for absorption of heme iron. In contrast to subjects who have not had ulcer surgery, patients who have had gastric resections empty pieces of meat from their stomachs as large, poorly digestible fragments. Thus, they may not be able to digest and absorb iron from heme protein efficiently. Although postoperative patients share with spontaneously hypochlorhydric subjects a similar defect in solubilizing iron salts, an additionally defective digestion of heme protein would make the postoperative patient even more subject to iron deficiency.

Patients who had had a truncal vagotomy with antrectomy absorbed iron from myoglobin in pieces of lamb about half as well, on the average, as they absorbed iron from hemoglobin that was dissolved in a gravy in the same meal; whereas normal subjects were able to absorb both forms of heme iron equally well from this meal.[79] These findings confirm that the patients had difficulty digesting the heme iron in the meat. The patients with antrectomy absorbed the iron from the dissolved hemoglobin even better than the normal subjects, confirming that the heme pathway is intact after ulcer surgery. In the operated patients, the twice-normal capacity to absorb soluble heme from the gravy compensated for half-normal ability to absorb heme iron from the lamb. Since normally, most dietary heme is not in solution but is either myoglobin or cooked and denatured hemoglobin in pieces of meat, the above study suggests that dietary heme iron is less available for absorption to patients with gastric resections than to normal subjects. Additionally, some studies[105, 110, 111] indicate that a few postoperative patients with severe iron deficiency did not increase their capacity to absorb soluble heme iron. Those few patients appeared unable to offset defective digestion by increasing their avidity for heme iron.

Thus, three factors account for a high prevalence of iron deficiency among postoperative patients: (1) a mildly diminished dietary intake of iron; (2) a decreased availability of iron salts for absorption, because of postoperative hypochlorhydria; and (3) defective digestion of meat, a major source of heme iron. Excessive iron losses, for example, from gastritis, will aggravate these problems. In most patients who have undergone operation, low availability of iron can be compensated by an increased intestinal avidity for any soluble iron that enters the proximal intestinal lumen; but iron deficiency will follow in those who cannot increase intestinal avidity enough to offset the decreased availability of dietary iron. Patients with truncal vagotomy plus pyloroplasty have both decreased intake (because of early satiety and other postcibal symptoms) and hypochlorhydria but normal grinding and sieving of meat particles. Thus, they should not have as much difficulty absorbing heme iron as patients with antrectomy. Perhaps this difference accounts for the fact that it takes longer to develop iron deficiency after vagotomy plus pyloroplasty than after gastric resection.

Ingested vitamin B_{12} may be malabsorbed after ulcer surgery; several types of malabsorptive problems exist.[101] For example, some patients have an abnormal Schilling test, which corrects to normal with the addition of human intrinsic factor; these patients thus seem to suffer from a deficiency in intrinsic factor after ulcer surgery. Others have an abnormal Schilling test even after the addition of intrinsic factor; some may have bacterial overgrowth in the small bowel.[112] Still others have a normal Schilling test but food-bound $^{57}Co\text{-}B_{12}$ is malabsorbed,[113, 114] indicating impaired digestion. Likewise, causes of folate deficiency after gastrectomy appear to be multiple.[102]

Bone Disease

Since the 1960s, bone disease has been recognized as a consequence of ulcer surgery. Though it is often difficult to distinguish osteomalacia from osteoporosis and both conditions often coexist, bone disease after ulcer surgery most resembles osteomalacia. Thus, following ulcer surgery, various patients exhibit low serum calcium, low urinary calcium, elevated serum alkaline phosphatase, elevated immunoreactive parathyroid hormone, positive calcium infusion tests (i.e., abnor-

mally high retention of intravenously infused calcium), bone pain, loss of bone mineral content, occasional pseudofractures on X-ray, and widened osteoid seams and/or low phosphorus:hydroxyproline ratios in bone as shown by biopsy.[105, 115–122] The importance of bone disease after ulcer surgery is underscored by three studies from different parts of the world that have documented a fracture rate in postoperative patients that is two to three times that of age- and sex-matched controls from the normal population.[119, 122, 123]

Early studies depended on visual assessment of radiodensities of bones on X-ray films to document loss of bone mineral. This is an insensitive technique, because as much as 30 per cent of skeletal calcium must be lost before a loss of radiodensity can be appreciated. Despite their insensitivity, radiographic surveys indicated up to a 20 per cent higher prevalence of bone disease in patients who had been operated upon versus matched controls; a higher prevalence after gastric resections than after nonresective ulcer surgery; and a sharply increasing prevalence of bone loss with age and time after surgery.[124]

Gamma photon absorptiometry and/or computed X-ray tomography of the vertebral column are much more quantitative than conventional radiography for measuring loss of bone mineral content. Over the last decade, studies with these new techniques have confirmed and extended the earlier observations. Loss of bone mineral normally occurs with aging, and this process is more rapid in women. The newer studies have demonstrated that the rate of bone mineral loss is increased over the normal by ulcer operations.[122] Differences between subjects who have had ulcer surgery and age- and sex-matched controls widen with time after surgery.[84, 85, 125] Total gastrectomy accelerates bone loss more than partial gastric resection (Fig. 53–6), and some studies suggest that bone loss is more rapid after resection with Billroth II anastomosis than with Billroth I.

Because bone demineralization is a continuum with age in the normal population and because ulcer surgery accelerates this loss, one cannot define, in conventional terms, a postoperative prevalence of bone disease. Rather, one can only predict how much additional bone mineral would be lost as the result of surgery done a number of years before. One absorptiometry study[121] suggests the additional rate of bone mineral loss after antrectomy is 2 per cent per year; thus, at ten years after surgery patients will have 20 per cent less bone mineral than normal subjects of the same age and sex. Considering that radiographic bone demineralization is not detected until 20 to 30 per cent of calcium is lost, this projection with photon absorptiometry corresponds to the maxim based on the older, radiologic surveys that bone disease does not become evident until at least six years or more after ulcer surgery.[102, 124]

Surgical practice has changed repeatedly over the last 30 years. Thus, most of the newer studies with photon absorptiometry have focused on truncal vagotomy plus antrectomy, an operation favored in many centers since 1970. The older, radiographic surveys

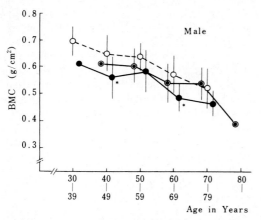
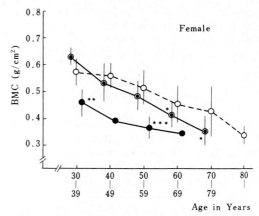

Figure 53–6. Average bone mineral content (BMC) measured in the distal radius (trabecular bone) by gamma photon absorptiometry in patients after gastric resection, compared with age- and sex-matched controls from the normal population (○ - - - -○). The figure shows that age-related bone loss was accelerated by subtotal (⊙——⊙) and especially by total (●——●) gastrectomy and that this acceleration was worse in women. *p<0.05; **p<0.01 and ***p<0.001 versus matched controls (○- - - -○). The time since surgery varied widely (5 to 34 years) among the subjects, and the separate influence of postoperative interval was not expressed in this figure; but more than 10 years after gastric surgery patients were more than three times as likely to have abnormally low BMCs than patients who had undergone gastric surgery less than 10 years previously. (From Nishimura, O., Furumoto, T., Nosaka, K., et al. Jpn. J. Surg. *16*:98, 1986. Used by permission.)

focused on subtotal gastrectomy, the standard procedure for ulcer treatment throughout this century until the early 1960s. Vagotomy plus pyloroplasty was extensively used only for about 15 years; and proximal gastric vagotomy, though very widely used in Europe, has been a recent innovation. Consequently, it is difficult to compare the effects of the various operations on bone loss. What data there are suggest that truncal vagotomy plus pyloroplasty produced less demineralization than resective surgery;[81, 116, 119] and because of this observation, the expectation would be that proximal gastric vagotomy will produce little bone loss.

Why patients lose bone mineral after ulcer surgery is not at all clear. Favored theories have invoked (1) decreased intake of calcium and/or vitamin D; (2) malabsorption of calcium; and (3) malabsorption of vitamin D. Since rapid gastric emptying of liquids may aggravate milk intolerance after ulcer surgery, the idea that calcium intake is reduced after such surgery[126] is quite plausible; but evaluations of calcium intake by historical, dietary survey have failed to establish a low calcium intake in some patients who have bone demineralization.[127] One might assume that gastric acidity would be important for the absorption of insoluble calcium salts (carbonates, phytates, phosphates) in the diet, so that hypochlorhydric, postoperative patients would have less of their dietary calcium available for absorption. However, at ambient intestinal pH (5.5 to 6.5) which is maintained by the proximal intestinal mucosa, calcium carbonates and phosphates are soluble in significant quantities.[7] Therefore, it is not surprising that patients with spontaneous achlorhydria may absorb calcium from calcium carbonate or that suppressing gastric secretion of acid with cimetidine in normal subjects did not affect calcium absorption.[7] Similarly, studies on the absorption of radiocalcium in small numbers of patients with gastric resections have not consistently delineated an absorptive defect.[128–130]

Many studies have revealed either low serum levels of 25-hydroxyvitamin D or an abnormal distribution of D metabolites in sera of patients with postoperative bone disease despite an adequate dietary intake of vitamin D.[117] Though vitamin D may be acquired from both endogenous and dietary sources, it is logical to assume that low levels of serum vitamin D arise from an impaired intestinal absorption of vitamin D after gastric surgery, which often gives rise to malabsorption of fat. However, steatorrhea after ulcer surgery is very mild and may be absent in patients who, nevertheless, exhibit postoperative bone loss.[117, 131] Thus, it is not likely that postoperative steatorrhea *per se* accounts for vitamin D malabsorption. Indeed, studies of absorption vitamin D after ulcer surgery have not consistently revealed malabsorption of the vitamin.[132–134]

Our understanding of vitamin D metabolism is incomplete. The various forms of vitamin D are stored in the blood on a specific, cholecalciferol binding protein; and vitamin D_3 is stored mainly in adipose tissue.[135] Pulvertaft[127] pointed out that postoperative patients with bone demineralization frequently had very low amounts of body fat, as measured by triceps skinfold. For unexplained reasons, patients with total and subtotal (Billroth II) resections may also develop low levels of vitamin D binding protein.[136] It is possible, therefore, that the osteomalacia-like bone disease that follows ulcer operations may arise from low fat and blood stores of vitamin D as a result of undernutrition in these patients, rather than from some specific defect in intestinal absorption of vitamin D.

Metabolic Neuropathy

A few reports[137, 138] indicate that clinical or subclinical *neuropathy* may afflict patients with ulcer operations, presumably as the result of vitamin B_{12} deficiency. Data suggest that patients with subtotal gastrectomy are more at risk than those with vagotomy plus drainage. Nevertheless, reporters failed to study appropriate control populations, so it is unclear just how often neuropathy arises as a complication of ulcer surgery.

Mechanical Problems

A variety of mechanical problems can befall the patient with an ulcer operation. *Bezoars*[139] in the stomach or stomach remnant may come and go without symptoms or may present as partial gastric obstruction with fullness, satiety, and vomiting. They befall patients with resective or nonresective surgery alike (see pp. 741–744). They are thought to form when indigestible residue is not normally swept from the stomach during phase III of the migrating myoelectric complex (MMC). Removal of the antrum, the main portion of the stomach generating the peristaltic phase III complex, or interruption of antral phase III peristalsis after vagal denervation[35] could quite easily account for postoperative bezoar formation.

Other mechanical problems affect patients who have had resective surgery. *Stomal stenosis, intussusception, herniation,* or *volvulus* involving a gastroenterostomy, *gastrojejunocolic fistulization*, and inadvertent *gastroileal* (rather than gastrojejunal) *anastomoses* are all problems that may affect ulcer surgery patients. They are discussed primarily on pages 939 to 962, as they frequently present acutely after surgery or are complications of recurrent ulceration.

Gastric Neoplasia

Both surveys of patients with gastric cancer and follow-up surveys of patients who underwent ulcer surgery have indicated a higher than expected association between ulcer surgery and *gastric cancer*. The most commonly reported association is between subtotal gastrectomy (Billroth I or II) and gastric cancer after either gastric or duodenal ulcer. The risk of cancer increases sharply about 15 to 20 years after subtotal gastrectomy, when it is about twice that of an age- and sex-matched population.[3] Susceptibility also seems to increase with the age of the postoperative patient. As a result of both trends, operated patients develop stomach cancer at about the same age as unoperated patients. Most investigators assume the association between gastric "stump carcinoma" and subtotal gastrectomy is somehow related to the aftereffects of the surgery, but two reports suggest gastric cancer may be more prevalent among patients with ulcer disease than in the general population, whether or not the patients have had surgery.[140]

There have been many reports of gastric cancer in patients who have had simple gastrojejunostomy for duodenal ulcer[140, 141] (an operation abandoned since the 1930s). Also, gastric cancer has been reported to follow truncal vagotomy plus pyloroplasty.[140] The predomi-

nant association of cancer with subtotal gastrectomy may simply reflect the almost exclusive use of that operation for ulcer disease many years ago, before the long latency for the development of cancer.

While reports from around the world[142–145] continue to indicate a two- to threefold increased risk for gastric carcinoma in patients who had ulcer surgery more than 20 years previously, other studies have failed to confirm such a risk.[146, 147] Thus, the very existence of "stump carcinoma" after ulcer surgery is somewhat controversial. An additional controversy is whether patients who had ulcer surgery more than 20 years ago should undergo frequent endoscopic surveillance to detect early cancer or dysplasia in the gastric mucosa. Aside from the controversy over whether postoperative patients are really at increased risk of carcinoma, proposals for endoscopic surveillance[148] raise issues about the natural history of dysplasia, cure rates for detected carcinomas, and cost-effectiveness of surveillance programs. The natural history of dysplasia in the gastric remnant is poorly defined. Mortensen and Savage[149] followed 13 postoperative patients with annual biopsies over 5 years; in none did the severity of dysplasia consistently increase over the period of surveillance. One patient with severe dysplasia underwent a prophylactic total gastrectomy, but no invasive carcinoma was found on histologic examination of the resected gastric remnant. On the other hand, most authors have reported that endoscopically detected carcinomas can rarely be cured by radical gastric resection.[144] Another aspect of the potential for cancer cure is the age of the patients: "stump carcinoma" afflicts the elderly, who have a high prevalence of other diseases that may affect their operability or their life expectancy regardless of their risk for gastric cancer. With all of these uncertainties, it would seem that endoscopic surveillance is not cost-effective.[150]

Benign gastric polyps are commonly found (in about 10 per cent of patients) after gastric resection, along the gastrointestinal anastomosis. These may be inflammatory pseudopolyps of granulation tissue or hyperplastic, adenomatous polyps.[143, 144, 151] Some believe the latter are premalignant.

Most clinical investigators believe that postoperative (reflux) gastritis predisposes the operated stomach to neoplasia. Gastritis is commonly found adjacent to the gastrointestinal anastomosis, where it is usually more intense than in the proximal stomach remnant. Both polyps and gastric carcinoma arise much more frequently near the stoma, in this intensely inflamed area.[151] Another idea is that the stomach, rendered hypochlorhydric by surgery, is abnormally colonized with bacteria that produce carcinogens.[4] Since cancer seems to follow simple gastrojejunostomy, an operation that does not reduce acid secretion but is associated with gastritis, epidemiologic information favors the first hypothesis. A third possibility is that postoperative cancer simply reflects the predisposition of ulcer patients to gastric cancer, whether or not they have undergone surgery. For example, excessive smoking peculiar to patients with ulcers could lead to increased rates of cancer.[152]

TIME COURSE OF POSTOPERATIVE MORBIDITY

Many surgeons and gastroenterologists are impressed that symptoms after ulcer surgery generally lessen with the passage of time, with psychologic and physiologic adaptation to surgical alterations. Few data bear on this question.

In the randomized, prospective trial of Jordan and Condon,[153] the prevalence of abdominal pain, vomiting, and postcibal vasomotor symptoms (sweating, weakness, palpitations) did not decline over five years of follow-up, while early satiety was about half as common after the first postoperative year. In the prospective Veterans Administration study, the frequency of diarrhea was about the same when operated patients were evaluated two[43] or more than five years[56] after surgery: other symptoms were not tabulated in such a way in the Veterans Administration study to allow assessment of the time course. Although both these studies provide an overview of what happens with time to the frequency of complaints among large numbers of patients, neither provides any clues about what happens to the nature or severity of complaints in an individual patient.

A few studies provide information about individual patients followed for many years. Although these reports are sometimes conflicting, they indicate a trend toward complete relief or partial amelioration of symptoms with the passage of time. Thus, one survey of 44 patients showed that about half who had had severe postcibal vasomotor symptoms or diarrhea were symptom-free 9 to 14 years postoperatively;[154] an additional 25 per cent were improved in this interval. Likewise, a follow-up of 13 patients with postcibal symptoms indicated complete relief or marked improvement in symptoms over an eight-year period in 60 per cent.[155] Bilious vomiting disappeared entirely over a seven-year period in about 25 per cent of those afflicted and lessened in frequency in a considerable number of the others.[40] Wastell found complete cessation of diarrhea over a nine-year period in about a quarter of patients suffering from postvagotomy diarrhea,[71] a finding that has been corroborated by Fromm and coworkers.[65] On the other hand, one report indicated that patients with mild symptoms improved but that those with moderate or severe symptoms did not show improvement over a 12-year period after ulcer surgery.[156]

Malabsorption or nutritional disturbances seem to persist unabated with time. Thus, outputs of fecal fat after subtotal gastrectomy remained equally abnormal among a group of patients studied at three months to three years postoperatively.[74] As detailed earlier, hemoglobin, serum iron, vitamin B_{12}, and perhaps folate levels seem to decline with time following surgery, suggesting cumulative effects of persistent maldigestion and malabsorption; bone rarefaction becomes more obvious with the passage of time from surgery.

PREVALENCE OF POSTOPERATIVE PROBLEMS

Reported prevalence rates vary widely among studies. The reasons for such variation are threefold: (1) sampling techniques vary, (2) methods of data collection differ, and (3) the various studies have involved different groups of patients. Since the perception of symptoms is subjective, sociocultural factors may influence reporting by patients; likewise, examiners may discount complaints.[157] Because of these cultural biases from both patients and examiners, absolute prevalence rates cannot be meaningfully established.

The only infallible method of establishing prevalence rates of various forms of postoperative morbidity would be to evaluate every patient operated on over a standard postoperative interaval. This approach has been prospective in some studies and retrospective in others; generally 20 to 40 per cent of patients (usually more in retrospective analyses) are lost to follow-up in such studies. The most fallible approach has been the evaluation of a small fraction of patients consecutively operated upon. There is no way to assure that such incomplete samples of populations of patients are unbiased—that is, that patients did not volunteer for evaluation because they were uniquely well or peculiarly sick. Variations in analysis and reporting have compounded problems with sampling. Terms have not been well defined, and often reports have not indicated the severity of a complaint.

Table 53–1, a compilation of available data, presents many of the problems connected with defining prevalence of postgastrectomy syndromes:

1. Alimentary symptoms are not reported under

Table 53–1. RANGE OF REPORTED PREVALENCE (PER CENT) OF VARIOUS PROBLEMS AFTER ULCER SURGERY*

	V + D	V + A	STG-BII	STG-BI†
GI symptoms (excluding diarrhea)	25–65	34–63	3–51	40
Hypoglycemic symptoms	6–12	4–16	1–12	—
Diarrhea	16–30	1–43	2–17	18
Weight loss	5–39	10–42	25–44	36
Anemia	3†–18§	7	9‡–44§	17§
Bone disease	—	—	1–13	—

*Data collected from selected reports (references 42, 44, 56, 66–68, 99, and 192–195) in which more than 70 per cent of patients who underwent ulcer surgery consecutively were followed for more than three years, either prospectively or retrospectively.

†In some instances only one pertinent report could be found; hence there is no reported range of prevalence.

‡Prevalence at five years after surgery.

§Prevalence in patients followed more than six years from surgery.

V, vagotomy; D, duodenostomy; A, antrectomy; STG, subtotal gastrectomy; BII, Billroth II operation; BI, Billroth I operation.

uniform headings. Hence the only possible comparison between studies is the prevalence of patients having any gastrointestinal complaints, however trivial. The range reported in Table 53–1 is wide.

2. Hypoglycemia symptoms were recorded on the basis of clinical history without laboratory confirmation.

3. Available information indicates that anemia and bone disease are late complications, arising more than five years after surgery (see above). Nevertheless, most reports represent follow-up data over intervals of five years or less; wide variations in reported prevalence of these late sequelae probably reflect non-uniformity in periods of follow-up.

4. Finally, patients usually undergo a Billroth I gastrectomy for gastric ulcer disease, whereas the other operations are employed for duodenal or (less commonly) gastric ulcer disease; thus results are being compared in two different populations of patients. Also, postoperative results have been infrequently reported for the Billroth I gastrectomy compared with the other operations.

Despite problems inherent in assessing available literature, Table 53–1 illustrates that *abdominal complaints, weight loss, diarrhea,* and *anemia* are common among patients who have had ulcer surgery. Some would argue that these higher reported prevalences are meaningless because they include some with only trivial complaints. Nevertheless, it is noteworthy that in the Veterans Administration cooperative study,[56] 35 to 44 per cent of patients who had undergone ulcer surgery were adhering to a restricted diet; such a finding indicates that gastrointestinal symptoms reported were sufficiently troublesome to the patients to require dietary restriction.

The reported prevalence of alimentary symptoms, diarrhea, or weight loss is consistently lower among the more affluent, private patients than among institutional patients such as those at Veterans Administration hospitals. On the other hand, other sequelae, such as ulcer recurrence or anemia, have strikingly uniform prevalence among institutional or private patients. This observation suggests that sociocultural factors affect the perception or development of some symptoms among groups of patients.

Self-Selection for Surgery and Postoperative Outcome

Most patients are operated upon electively for intractable ulcer disease. The definition of intractability is so vague and so subjective that many extraneous factors could influence both the selection for surgery and the postoperative outcome. Several reports suggest depression and smoking are two such factors.

Depression, social deprivation (i.e., bereavement, separation, divorce, loss of job), and disruptive changes in the lives of patients preoperatively are highly associated with a poor postoperative outcome—some form of chronic incapacitation.[158–162] One retrospective analysis[162] suggests these same adverse psychologic factors might have contributed to an intolerance to ulcer disease that prompted the original selection for surgery. In the pre-endoscopic era, several surgeons[163, 164] called attention to an unusually high prevalence of postoperative incapacitation among those patients who were operated upon for a presumed ulcer that could not be demonstrated at the time of ulcer surgery. The implication of these reports was that the intractable pain preoperatively was psychologically determined and that the same psychologic factors led to continuing postoperative morbidity. Nowadays, patients are seldom sent to surgery without prior endoscopic demonstration of an ulcer. Nevertheless, tolerance to pain from a demonstrable ulcer undoubtedly is influenced by what is going on in the patient's life. Since the selection for surgery most often depends on suffering reported by the patient, psychologic factors probably continue to influence the selection for surgery and the postoperative outcome. A higher prevalence of postoperative morbidity among institutional versus private patients could reflect a higher prevalence of depression among the economically disadvantaged and/or an insensitivity to psychologic factors on the part of institutional physicians who sent the patients to surgery.

Many controlled trials of ulcer therapy have shown that smoking delays healing of duodenal or gastric ulcers. It is therefore likely that a significant number of patients are referred for surgery because of refractoriness associated with smoking. One report[152] suggested that premature death after ulcer surgery stems largely from diseases associated with smoking. Thus, patients who had undergone ulcer surgery died of emphysema or carcinoma of the lung, pancreas, and colon (assumed to be smoking-related) nearly a decade before their contemporaries with ulcers who did not have surgery. Nevertheless, a large Danish series of 1000 operated patients has failed to confirm an excessive death rate from cancer or other smoking-related diseases.[165] Interestingly, the Danish report, like its American counterpart,[152] documented a high risk of suicide among patients with ulcer operations as compared with suicide rates in the normal population. In the Danish study, suicide was associated with antecedent histories of alcoholism or psychiatric illness. Of course, it is unclear whether patients with alcoholism or psychiatric illness were self-selected for ulcer surgery or whether somehow the surgery predisposed to later mental illness.

TREATMENT OF POSTGASTRECTOMY SYNDROMES

My approach to the problem of postgastrectomy syndromes is threefold. First, I try to identify promptly those small numbers of patients having intercurrent disease or unusual complications for which specific treatment is highly effective. Second, I undertake supportive medical treatment for a prolonged period of assessment for the majority of afflicted patients. This general support suffices in a large number of patients to reduce symptoms to an acceptable level, while at the same time it allows a period of evaluation of the patient and his or her psychologic adjustment to life and health problems. Third, for the minority who remain severely impaired with some objective evidence of physical, rather than solely psychologic, disability, I recommend remedial surgery. Usually, the last is in a situation in which the chance of permanent improvement by reoperation is about 50 per cent.

Evaluation

The tendency of many clinicians is to evaluate extensively every patient who complains of persistent problems after ulcer surgery. Such a practice is very expensive. It also reflects the conscious or unconscious bias of the physician that surgery itself rarely causes difficulty. On the contrary, ulcer surgery commonly produces patterns of symptoms (Table 53–1) that only infrequently result either from a recognizable complication of ulcer surgery (or ulcer disease) or from an unrelated, intercurrent illness.

Symptoms are very common after ulcer surgery and are usually characteristic. Thus combinations of postcibal alimentary symptoms with vasomotor symptoms ("dumping syndrome") are so characteristic of uncomplicated postsurgical dysfunction that they do not require extensive evaluation. On the other hand, sometimes one complaint is dissociated from the typical constellation of symptoms—it appears alone or, because of its unusual severity, dominates the history. It is with this less characteristic situation that physicians may worry that they are dealing with a complication or an intercurrent disease. Most often, an evaluation of this complaint is nonproductive; since no complication or intercurrent illness is recognized after extensive evaluation, the physician finally concludes that the less typical history is a variant of a more common "postgastrectomy syndrome."

Needless evaluation can be greatly reduced if only the physician is aware in advance that a spectrum of complaints typifies postgastrectomy dysfunction and senses when the presenting situation is sufficiently common that it most likely does not represent a complication or an intercurrent illness (guidelines follow). An alternate approach to limit the scope of evaluation is to recognize that there are only a few remediable conditions that might mimic the symptoms of postgastrectomy dysfunction and to direct evaluation specifically toward diagnosing these few conditions. These approaches can be combined.

The Presenting Problem

The most common presenting problems are *abdominal complaints, weight loss, diarrhea,* and *anemia.* Since the severity of abdominal complaints is almost always a subjective assessment, features other than severity (time of onset, frequency, associated signs) are required to formulate a differential diagnosis. Such historical distinctions are usually imperfect. Consequently, some form of diagnostic testing has to be targeted at uncovering the few treatable conditions that might give rise to abdominal complaints similar to those of uncomplicated postgastrectomy dysfunction. On the other hand, weight loss, diarrhea, and anemia can be objectively quantified. The problem with these complaints is to decide whether their magnitude is sufficiently unusual in the postsurgical patient to warrant further investigation.

Abdominal Complaints. In the absence of associated vasomotor phenomena (features of the dumping syndrome), *postcibal abdominal pain* or *vomiting* (Table 53–2) after ulcer surgery may suggest complications or intercurrent illness. The differential diagnosis has been outlined earlier in this chapter. Complications producing these complaints are *recurrent ulcer, gastric obstruction,* and *partial obstruction of the afferent loop* (in patients with gastrojejunostomy). Since more than three quarters of patients with any of these three complicating conditions are responsive to specific surgical correction,[166–168] diagnosis is important. A combination of gastrointestinal radiography and endoscopy will strongly supplement a detailed history in establishing the diagnosis of these three complicating conditions. Since patients may not be able to give a discerning history, we routinely employ radiography and endoscopy to exclude these conditions in which poorly described or atypical vomiting and pain dominate the clinical picture.

Thus *gastric obstruction* (from stomal stenosis) and

Table 53–2. PAIN AND VOMITING SYNDROMES AFTER ULCER SURGERY

Presenting Syndrome	Frequency	Objective Findings	Treatment	Efficacy
Vomiting satiety, pain ("dumping" variant)	Common	Mild gastritis	Medical	Partially effective
Pain, bilious vomiting ("reflux gastritis")	Poorly defined	Intense gastritis	Surgical	Unpredictably effective
Food vomiting, intense satiety (postvagotomy stasis)	Uncommon	Slow gastric emptying	Medical	Partially effective
Food vomiting, intense satiety (stomal stenosis)	Very uncommon	Stomach stenosis	Surgical	Effective
Pain, bilious vomiting ("afferent loop syndrome")	Rare	Obstructed afferent loop	Surgical	Probably effective
Epigastric pain, vomiting	Uncommon	Recurrent ulcer	Surgical H₂-blockers	Effective Probably effective

recurrent ulcer usually can be demonstrated with a combination of radiographic and endoscopic examinations. *Partial obstruction of the afferent loop,* a rather rare condition, may be difficult to demonstrate radiographically because of failure to fill the afferent loop on examination with a barium meal. Cholangiography may provide such visualization, and stenosis at the exit of the afferent loop or dilation of the loop proximally may be demonstrated at endoscopy.[168] Even so, the diagnosis of partial obstruction of an afferent loop sometimes is entirely clinical; however, failure of surgical correction in a significant number of cases may reflect an inappropriate clinical diagnosis preoperatively in some patients.[168, 169] *Cholelithiasis* causing bile duct obstruction is the common intercurrent disease that may be associated with postcibal pain and vomiting. Usually biliary colic is not historically confused with postgastrectomy dysfunction, because episodes of biliary colic do not occur with the same postcibal regularity and each episode tends to persist longer; or biliary colic may be complicated by fever, acholia, or icterus—signs not associated with postgastrectomy dysfunction. Cholecystography or abdominal ultrasonography may confirm cholelithiasis when symptoms are thought to stem from biliary colic.

Reflux gastritis and *postvagotomy gastric stasis* are syndromes that also show vomiting and abdominal pain. Their response to treatment is less predictable (Table 53–2).

Many believe that *bile* or *alkaline reflux gastritis* is an unusual and distinct clinical syndrome caused by excessive reflux of bile or duodenal contents into the stomach. The refluxed duodenal contents are postulated to produce severe gastritis or to excite abnormal gastrointestinal motility manifested by pain and vomiting.[51] While this syndrome is not responsive to medical therapy designed to reduce intragastric concentrations of bile salts,[170, 171] patients are sometimes dramatically relieved by surgery designed to prevent reflux of duodenal contents into the stomach (discussed further later). Reported cure rates with this kind of surgery range from 45 to 95 per cent.[172] The skeptic considers the 45 per cent response as a placebo effect of surgical treatment of an undefineable condition, while the enthusiastic surgeon focuses on the 95 per cent figure as a realizable goal, if only patients could be better diagnosed. Consequently, a large surgical literature has evolved around strengthening diagnosis.

Patients with reflux gastritis experience bile vomiting. The vomiting is most common shortly after eating, but, in addition, some patients also vomit bilious material while fasting, at night or in the early morning. Epigastric pain may be constant or made worse by eating. Some patients also experience heartburn, often in association with vomiting or regurgitation of bile-stained material. A few exhibit iron deficiency, presumed to be the result of blood loss from gastritis. All patients have severe gastritis and marked reflux of bile into the stomach at endoscopy in the absence of recurrent ulcers, but these findings are so common, even in asymptomatic individuals after ulcer surgery, that their relation to symptoms is questionable. Like-

wise, the pain, the vomiting, and the anemia are so common after ulcer surgery that, except by their intensity, they do not distinguish the patient who may be having excessive duodenogastric reflux.

Since endoscopic hyperemia/friabilty and histologic gastritis do not distinguish symptomatic from asymptomatic patients, two other approaches have been taken to develop objective criteria for reflux gastritis: (1) to quantitate the amount of reflux, with the idea that more than a certain minimum reflux will reliably predict those who will respond to surgery because they excessively reflux bile and/or (2) to provoke symptoms in a specific way that will predict benefit from surgery. The amount of bile reflux can be quantitated by aspiration of the stomach from an intragastric tube[173] or by radioscintigraphy.[174] Because many asymptomatic patients have large amounts of bile reflux, neither method has defined a minimum amount of reflux that is associated with symptoms; and thus far, neither has been used to identify prospectively patients who will benefit from surgery. Meshkinpour and associates[53] reported that autologous bile will evoke typical symptoms when placed into the stomach of a patient suffering from reflux gastritis, but there have been no formal attempts to use this provocation as a means for selecting patients for surgery. In a series of 20 patients referred for bile gastritis, Warshaw[175] found that among patients who developed typical pain after gastric instillation of 0.1 molar NaOH, surgery for reflux gastritis was 90 per cent successful, whereas the same operation did not help any patient who had a negative alkali infusion test preoperatively.

After truncal vagotomy, some patients develop *gastric stasis.* They often have a long history of recurrent bezoars but otherwise are similar to patients with anatomic outlet obstruction (marked early satiety, epigastric fullness and discomfort, weight loss, vomiting of food). The syndrome is thought to be the result of diminished antral motility after vagal denervation,[35] although it is not clear why only a few individuals with vagotomy are so affected. At endoscopy to ascertain gastric obstruction, no anatomic obstruction is found, yet on further testing with radiolabeled test meals or with barium-coated foods, gastric emptying of solid foods is markedly delayed. The syndrome may respond to treatment with metoclopramide[35, 176] or bethanechol;[35, 177] both are agents that increase antral peristalsis. While controlled trials have demonstrated the efficacy of metoclopramide, individual patients may not benefit.

Weight Loss. The differential diagnosis of this frequent complaint is outlined in Table 53–3. Although several conditions may complicate common weight loss after ulcer surgery, most of these are rare.[74] An extensive evaluation for *malabsorption,* therefore, is not practical in most patients with weight loss. Special situations may indicate more extensive investigation. These include a fecal fat output of greater than 15 gm per day, hypoproteinemia or hypoprothrombinemia in the absence of liver disease or proteinuria, and symptomatic vitamin deficiencies. These three situations are all manifestations of more severe malabsorptive disease

Table 53–3. OVERVIEW OF WEIGHT LOSS AS A CLINICAL PROBLEM AFTER ULCER SURGERY

Cause	Frequency	Method of Diagnosis	Treatment	Frequency of Successful Treatment*
Reduced intake	Most common	Dietary history Hospital observation Stool fat <15 gm/day	Dietary advice[196] Nonspecific support[196]	90% 20–30%
Chronic gastric obstruction (bezoar, stenosis, postvagotomy stasis)	Uncommon	Copious vomiting of food Endoscopy Emptying tests Upper GI X-ray studies	Lysis of bezoar[139] Surgical[168] Medical[176, 179]	75%† 80%† Unknown
Excessive fecal wastage of undefined cause	Uncommon	Diarrhea Stool fat >15 gm/day Diagnosis of exclusion	Medical[197] Surgical[167]	80% 100%‡
Blind loop syndrome (long or obstructed afferent loop, gastrojejunocolic fistula)	Rare	Multiple deficiencies Hypoproteinemia, diarrhea GI radiography Stool fat >15 gm/day Jejunal culture >4 × 10⁵/ml Therapeutic trial (antibiotics)	Antibiotics[198] Surgical[198]	77% 77%
Pancreatic insufficiency	Rare	Stool fat >15 gm/day RATO test Secretin test Therapeutic trial	Pancreatin[112]	Effective
Celiac sprue	Rare	Multiple deficiencies Stool fat >15 gm/day Positive biopsy	Gluten exclusion	Successful
Inadvertent gastroileostomy	Very rare	Profound diarrhea Stool fat >15 gm/day Radiography	Surgical	Successful

*Reported cases are too few to project generalization from quoted success rates.
†Success refers to relief of obstruction without comment on weight gain.
‡Other surgical series report that about 70 per cent of patients gain weight after surgery to correct postcibal symptoms. Fecal fat data are not available from these series.

than is usually encountered in uncomplicated postgastrectomy dysfunction and therefore indicate that an evaluation is needed to uncover a complicating illness. Since less than 1 per cent of ulcer surgery patients have such unusually severe malabsorption,[74, 178] the practice of extensively evaluating all patients with weight loss for complicated or intercurrent malabsorptive disease *is* a wasteful and futile exercise.

When weight loss (usually more than 10 to 15 pounds) is the clinical problem, our practice is to hospitalize the patient for three to four days. This period allows (1) time to take a careful dietary history, (2) direct observation of food consumption and postcibal symptoms, and (3) an adequate fecal fat collection. Such observation is usually sufficient to determine whether the patient suffers from common postgastrectomy weight loss caused by poor diet or, conversely, whether further work-up is indicated.

Those few patients requiring further evaluation for complicated postgastrectomy malabsorption may have to undergo evaluation at tertiary care centers where special diagnostic services are available. For example, the diagnosis of *bacterial overgrowth* in the proximal small intestine may be established by quantitative culture of small bowel contents, a technique not available in all hospitals. Likewise, the documentation of *exocrine pancreatic insufficiency* may be very difficult in those patients having had a gastric resection with a gastrojejunal anastomosis, which precludes direct aspiration of pancreatic juice from the duodenum during

a secretin test. In such patients a Lundh test is unreliable because of dilution of luminal trypsin by rapidly emptying gastric contents;[21] diagnosis may be established via special tests measuring output of pancreatic enzymes into the jejunum after liquid test meals. In lieu of these special diagnostic tests, a tentative diagnosis may be established by therapeutic trial, with antibiotics for suspected blind loop syndrome or oral pancreatic enzyme therapy for suspected pancreatic insufficiency.

Diarrhea. Mild (<400 ml per day of stool water) postcibal diarrhea is typical of uncomplicated postgastrectomy dysfunction and rarely presents the physician with a diagnostic problem requiring extensive evaluation. Protracted or more severe diarrhea or diarrhea coincident with severe malabsorption after ulcer surgery is atypical although occasionally seen after truncal vagotomy without demonstrable complication.[71] The evaluation of this problem is the same as that outlined in the appraisal of any protracted diarrheal illness. Such routine evaluation will usually uncover remediable conditions that complicate postgastrectomy dysfunction. For example, a barium enema examination will demonstrate the infrequent *gastrojejunocolic fistula* or *intercurrent colonic disease* underlying the protracted diarrhea. In the course of evaluation of diarrhea associated with malabsorption, small bowel films may demonstrate problems such as the very rare inadvertent gastroileostomy or a blind loop.

Anemia. This problem is usually uncovered in the

evaluation of some other presenting complaint. Mild anemia is such a common late complication of ulcer surgery that its discovery *per se* does not dictate an exhaustive search for a cause. Treatable causes include (1) *colonic neoplasia,* (2) *silent recurrent ulcer,* and (3) *blind loop syndrome.* As a general rule, more marked anemia (hemoglobin less than 10 gm/dl) or anemia appearing within the first five years of ulcer surgery indicates a complicating illness. An exception to this rule is the situation in which iron stores were not replenished at the time of ulcer surgery for hemorrhage, producing an earlier postoperative appearance of significant iron deficiency anemia.

Medical Measures

The medical treatment of uncomplicated postgastrectomy dysfunction consists almost entirely of dietary manipulations and nonspecific psychologic support.

Over the years, many remedies have been suggested for specific problems. Only a few have undergone clinical trials against placebos. These trials include cholestyramine for reflux gastritis,[170] which proved to be of no benefit; metoclopramide for postvagotomy gastric stasis,[176, 179] which reduced symptoms of nausea and vomiting among patients in a large, heterogeneous group; and cholestyramine for postvagotomy diarrhea,[62, 180] which reduced frequency of bowel motions. However, neither metoclopramide nor cholestyramine is universally successful in ameliorating, respectively, postvagotomy gastric stasis or diarrhea. Many patients with postvagotomy diarrhea do not have high fecal concentrations of bile salts, so they may not respond to cholestyramine.[65]

Other remedies have been proposed simply because their advocates believed they might remedy one or another perceived dysfunction. For example, some have suggested adding pectin to the diet because this agent (1) slows gastric emptying of liquids and (2) ameliorates dumping symptoms in ulcer surgery patients after liquid meals of concentrated glucose.[181] Whether this agent would be useful when added to ordinary meals remains to be determined. Others have suggested orally administered pancreatic enzymes or bile salts to improve malabsorption, but these agents generally have been unsuccessful in abolishing steatorrhea.[182]

More general measures consist of dietary restrictions. Thus, limiting the size of meals with more frequent feedings of smaller amounts per feeding, restricting carbohydrate intake in favor of protein, avoiding milk (lactose), and prescribing the intake of fluids between, rather than with, meals usually ameliorates postcibal symptoms. These dietary manipulations are designed to reduce loads of volume, sugar, and osmotic material entering the proximal small bowel postprandially and thus to reduce distention of the proximal bowel and delayed hypoglycemia. Likewise, deficiencies in iron, vitamin B_{12}, and folate may be established by appropriate diagnostic tests; their treatment with oral iron salts or parenteral vitamin B_{12} probably adds to the general well-being of the patient.

Although these measures serve only to reduce rather than to eliminate morbidity, the setting in which the medical treatment is undertaken allows the therapist to provide psychologic support for the patient as the latter learns to adapt to the aftermath of gastric surgery. Although the benefits of such support are difficult to quantify, most physicians and surgeons who have had experience with these patients attest to the positive effects. Also, whether as the result of therapy or as an outcome of an unrelated process, symptoms tend to lessen with time after surgery (as noted earlier). In fact, with the passage of time under medical supervision, only about 10 per cent of patients who have had ulcer surgery continue to experience symptoms of such severity as to be incapacitated. Even in some of those who do not improve, it is apparent that incapacitation may have actually preceded the ulcer surgery, that is, the new disability introduced by the surgical alteration is merely symptomatic of a chronically maladjusted personality.[163, 164] For this and other reasons (to be discussed), reoperation in patients who do not improve under medical supervision is fraught with ill success.

Remedy by Reoperation

Empiric observation has indicated that reoperation is predictably (70 per cent or more) successful in certain situations; as earlier outlined, these are *recurrent ulcer,*[166] *stomal stenosis,*[167, 168] and demonstrated *obstruction* of an *afferent loop* with[168] or without[183] an associated *malabsorption* from *bacterial overgrowth.* Likewise, surgical correction of an inadvertent gastroileostomy or a gastrojejunocolic fistula is predictably successful. All these situations are associated with a definable problem. They are, however, uncommon.

The more common types of morbidity after ulcer surgery arise from functional derangements that are poorly delineated. Circumstantial evidence suggests that many symptoms are the result of accelerated gastric emptying, but proof is tenuous. Moreover, even a rudimentary understanding of processes that regulate the movement of food in the upper gastrointestinal tract has escaped present scientific definition. In this situation of unverified hypotheses, surgical correction of postulated defects is, at best, presumptuous. Even so, if such operations were predictably successful (regardless of theoretical merit or demerit), remedial surgery would be a practical solution for the patient with refractory postgastrectomy dysfunction. Unfortunately, there is no uniform agreement on the outcome of various operations other than as listed in the preceding paragraph.

The problems are threefold. First, selection of patients for one or another of these operations has not been standardized. Second, the outcome of surgical treatment is not observed under controlled conditions that would negate placebo effects of the surgery, the supportive effects of surgical follow-up, or even the tendency for symptoms to regress spontaneously with time.[40, 155] Third, a successful outcome may be the fortuitous result of a surgical manipulation rather than the intended effect. For example, surgery for "dumping" has been judged successful in half the cases[167, 168] without a clue as to why it succeeds in some and not others.

A good example of the complexities involved is the currently popular operations for reflux gastritis that divert duodenal secretions away from the stomach, either by interposing a piece of jejunum between the stomach and duodenum or by draining the duodenum via a Roux-en-Y into the jejunum 30 centimeters below a gastrojejunostomy. Such surgery markedly reduces or eliminates detectable bile reflux, yet relief of symptoms is variable, with successes reported in 45 to 96 per cent of patients in various series.[169, 184, 185] The surgery prevents the reflux of bile and pancreatic enzymes and decreases gastric mucosal hyperemia/friability but does not reverse histologic gastritis and may reduce but frequently does not eliminate abdominal pain or vomiting.[186]

Because abdominal pain and vomiting may persist after Roux-en-Y diversion, some have postulated a motility disorder as the outcome of a *Roux syndrome*.[187, 188] In dogs[188, 189] as well as in patients,[187] motility may be reduced in the jejunal loop that was interposed in the Roux procedure. Furthermore, gastric emptying of solid food may be slow. The combination of continued abdominal pain and vomiting, slow gastric emptying, and diminished jejunal motility has prompted some to postulate that the interposed Roux-en-Y diversion is the cause of the clinical problems. Nevertheless, the abnormal gastric emptying of liquid nutrients[190] or solid food[188] observed in dogs with jejunal Roux-en-Y diversions after truncal vagotomy and/or antrectomy is no different than that usually found after truncal vagotomy and/or antrectomy without jejunal interposition; and jejunal interpositions in a large number of human subjects had no predictably deleterious outcome on gastrointestinal transit.[191] It seems more likely to this reviewer that the persistence of symptoms after Roux-en-Y interposition for bile gastritis is simply a failure in understanding and treating the original problem rather than the emergence of a new "syndrome."

Clearly, more fundamental understanding of normal alimentary processes is needed to gain insight into the adverse effects of ulcer surgery. Also, designed and controlled, rather than anecdotal, clinical trials of remedial surgery are needed to provide an empiric basis on which to judge the effectiveness of these operations. Until these goals are accomplished, the patient who continues to suffer from an ill-defined postgastrectomy dysfunction can expect only about a 50 per cent chance of benefit from one of these operations.

EPILOGUE

While much has been learned about the effects of gastric surgery, we are just beginning to understand the interplay between diverse alimentary processes, such as motility, secretion, and digestion, and the interactions between neighboring regions of the gastrointestinal tract. Given this state of ignorance and the insight that we are almost powerless to treat most forms of postoperative morbidity, we should avoid ulcer surgery whenever possible. This is particularly true because peptic ulcer diseases are rarely fatal, so operations are not often life-saving but are usually undertaken to relieve symptoms. All too often, they create other problems that are as bad or worse. Nevertheless, surgery will continue to be needed for a minority of patients, especially those with complications. Of all ulcer operations, proximal gastric vagotomy results in the fewest physiologic derangements and the mildest postoperative symptoms; but many surgeons are skeptical because of high recurrence rates after this procedure and limited long-term experience with it. Thus, there is little room for complacency; and together, physicians and surgeons must struggle for better operations and more wisdom.

References

1. Sonnenberg, A. Changes in physician visits for gastric and duodenal ulcer in the United States during 1958–1984 as shown by national disease and therapeutic index. Dig Dis Sci. *32*:1, 1987.
2. Larson, G. M., and Davidson, P. R. The decline in surgery for peptic ulcer disease. J. Kentucky Med. Assoc. *84*:233, 1986.
3. Domellof, L., and Janunger, K. G. The risk of gastric carcinoma after partial gastrectomy. Am. J. Surg. *134*:581, 1977.
4. Schlag, P., Bockler, R., Ulrich, H., et al. Are nitrite and N-nitroso compounds in gastric juice risk factors for carcinoma in the operated stomach? Lancet *1*:727, 1980.
5. Gianella, R. A., Broitman, S. A., and Zamcheck, N. Influence of gastric pH on bacterial and parasitic infections. A perspective. Ann. Intern. Med. *78*:271, 1973.
6. Skikne, B. S., Lynch, S. R., and Cook, J. D. Role of gastric acid in food iron absorption. Gastroenterology *81*:1068, 1981.
7. Bo-Linn, G. W., Davis, G. R., Buddrus, D. J., et al. An evaluation of the importance of gastric secretion in the absorption of dietary calcium. J. Clin. Invest. *73*:640, 1984.
8. Ohashi, H., and Meyer, J. H. Effect of peptic digestion on emptying of cooked liver in dogs. Gastroenterology *79*:305, 1980.
9. Ardeman, S., Chaarin, I., and Doyle, J. C. Studies on secretion of gastric intrinsic factor. Br. Med. J. *2*:600, 1964.
10. Heyssel, R. M., Bozian, R. C., Darby, W. J., et al. Vitamin B_{12} turnover in man. The assimilation of vitamin B_{12} from natural foodstuff by man and estimates of minimal daily dietary requirements. Am. J. Clin. Nutr. *18*:176, 1966.
11. Meyer, J. H. Motility of the stomach and gastroduodenal junction. *In* Johnson, L. R. (ed.). Physiology of the Gastrointestinal Tract. 2nd ed. New York, Raven Press, 1987.
12. DePonti, F., Azpiroz, F., and Malagelada, J. R. Neural control of gastric tone via long vagal reflexes. (Abstract.) Gastroenterology *90*:1392, 1986.
13. Azpiroz, F., and Malagelada, J. R. Physiological variations in canine gastric tone measured by electronic barostat. Am. J. Physiol. *248*:G249, 1985.
14. Keinke, O., and Ehrlein, H. J. Effect of oleic acid on canine gastroduodenal motility, pyloric diameter, and gastric emptying. Q. J. Exp. Physiol. *68*:675, 1983.
15. Collins, P. J., Heddle, R., Horowitz, M., et al. The effect of intraduodenal lipid on gastric emptying and intragastric distribution of a solid meal. (Abstract.) Gastroenterology *90*:1377, 1986.
16. Meyer, J. H., Thomson, J. B., Cohen, M. B., et al. Sieving of solid food by the normal and ulcer-operated canine stomach. Gastroenterology *76*:804, 1979.

17. Mayer, E. A., Thomson, J. B., Jehn, D., Reedy, T., Elashoff, J., Deveney, C., and Meyer, J. H. Gastric emptying and sieving of solid food and pancreatic and biliary secretions after solid meals in patients with nonresective ulcer surgery. Gastroenterology 87:1264, 1984.

18. Meyer, J. H., Gu, Y. G., Dressman, J., and Amidon, G. Effect of viscosity and flow rate on gastric emptying of solids. Am. J. Physiol. 250:G161, 1986.

19. Wiener, K., Grahn, L. S., Reedy, T., Elashoff, J., and Meyer, J. H. Simultaneous gastric emptying of two solid foods. Gastroenterology 81:257, 1981.

20. Wilbur, B. G., and Kelly, K. A. Effect of proximal gastric, complete gastric and truncal vagotomy on canine gastric electric activity, motility, and emptying. Ann. Surg. 178:295, 1973.

21. MacGregor, I. L., Parent, J. A., and Meyer, J. H. Gastric emptying of liquid meals and pancreatic and biliary secretion after subtotal gastrectomy or truncal vagotomy with pyloroplasty in man. Gastroenterology 72:195, 1977.

22. MacGregor, I. L., Martin, P., and Meyer, J. H. Gastric emptying of solid food in normal man and after subtotal gastrectomy and truncal vagotomy with pyloroplasty. Gastroenterology 72:206, 1977.

23. Buckler, K. G. Effects of gastric surgery upon gastric emptying in cases of peptic ulceration. Gut 8:137, 1967.

24. Hinder, R. A., and San-Garde, B. A. Individual and combined roles of the pylorus and antrum in the canine gastric emptying of a liquid and a digestible solid. Gastroenterology 84:281, 1983.

25. Aune, S. Intragastric pressure after vagotomy in man. Scand. J. Gastroenterol. 4:447, 1969.

26. Stadaas, J. O. Intragastric pressure/volume relationship before and after proximal gastric vagotomy. Scand. J. Gastroenterol. 10:129, 1975.

27. Lavigne, M. E., Wiley, Z. D., Martin, P., et al. Gastric, pancreatic, and biliary secretion and the rate of gastric emptying after parietal cell vagotomy. Am. J. Surg. 138:644, 1979.

28. Clarke, R. J., and Alexander-Williams, J. The effect of preserving antral innervation and of a pyloroplasty on gastric emptying after vagotomy in man. Gut 14:300, 1973.

29. Binswanger, R. O., Aeberhard, P., Walther, M., et al. Effect of pyloroplasty on gastric emptying: long-term results obtained with a labeled test meal 14–43 months after operation. Br. J. Surg. 65:27, 1978.

30. Faxen, A., Dotevall, N., Kock, G., et al. The influence of pyloroplasty on gastric emptying after parietal cell vagotomy. (Abstract.) Scand. J. Gastroenterol. (Suppl.) 20:14, 1973.

31. Dragstadt, L. R., and Schafter, P. W. Removal of the vagus innervation of the stomach in gastroduodenal ulcer surgery. Surgery 17:727, 1945.

32. Madsen, P., and Peterson, G. Postvagotomy diarrhea examined by means of a nutritional contrast medium. Scand. J. Gastroenterol. 3:545, 1968.

33. McKelvey, S. T. D. Gastric incontinence and postvagotomy diarrhea. Br. J. Surg. 57:741, 1970.

34. Gulsrud, P. O., Taylor, I. L., Watts, H. D., et al. How gastric emptying of carbohydrate affects glucose tolerance and symptoms after truncal vagotomy with pyloroplasty. Gastroenterology 79:305, 1980.

35. Malagelada, J. R., Rees, W. D., Mazzotta, L. J., and Go, V. L. W. Gastric motor abnormalities in diabetic and postvagotomy gastroparesis: effect of metoclopramide and bethanecol. Gastroenterology 78:286, 1980.

36. Machella, T. E. Mechanism of post-gastrectomy dumping syndrome. Gastroenterology 14:237, 1950.

37. Reidelberger, R. D., Kalogeris, T. J., and Leung, M. B. Postgastric satiety in the sham feeding rat. Am. J. Physiol. 244:R872, 1983.

38. Condon, J. E., Westerholm, P., and Tanner, N. C. Lactose malabsorption and postgastrectomy milk intolerance, dumping, and diarrhea. Gut 10:311, 1969.

39. Hall, W. H., Sanders, L. I., and Read, N. C. Effect of vagotomy and pyloroplasty: the oral glucose tolerance test. Gastroenterology 64:217, 1973.

40. Griffiths, J. M. T. The features and course of bile vomiting following gastric surgery. Br. J. Surg. 61:617, 1974.

41. Buckwald, H. The dumping syndrome and its treatment. A review and presentation of cases. Am. J. Surg. 116:81, 1968.

42. Goligher, J. C., Pulvertaft, C. N., deDombal, F. T., et al. Five to eight year results of Leeds-York controlled trial of elective surgery for duodenal ulcer. Br. Med. J. 2:781, 1968.

43. Price, W. E., Grizzle, J. E., Postlethwait, R. W., et al. Results of operation for duodenal ulcer. Surg. Gynecol. Obstet. 131:233, 1970.

44. McKeown, K. C. A prospective study of the immediate and long-term results of Polya gastrectomy for duodenal ulcer. Br. J. Surg. 59:849, 1972.

45. Roberts, K. E., Randall, H. T., Farr, H. W., et al. Cardiovascular and blood volume alterations resulting from intrajejunal administration of hypotonic glucose to gastrectomized patients: the relationship of these changes to the dumping syndrome. Ann. Surg. 140:631, 1954.

46. Butz, R. Dumping syndrome studied during maintenance of blood volume. Ann. Surg. 154:225, 1961.

47. Ralphs, D. N. L., Thomson, J. P. S., Haynes, S., et al. The relationship between the rate of gastric emptying and the dumping syndrome. Br. J. Surg. 65:637, 1978.

48. LeQuesne, L. P., Hobsley, M., and Hand, B. H. The dumping syndrome—I. Factors responsible for symptoms. Br. Med. J. 1:141, 1960.

49. Editorial. Dumping syndrome and gut peptides. Lancet 2:1173, 1980.

50. Sagar, G. R., Bryant, M. G., Ghatel, M. A., et al. Release of vasoactive intestinal peptide and the dumping syndrome. Br. Med. J. 282:507, 1981.

51. Meyer, J. H. Reflections on reflux gastritis. (Editorial.) Gastroenterology 77:1143, 1979.

52. Toye, D. K. M., and Williams, J. A. Postgastrectomy bile vomiting. Lancet 1:469, 1964.

53. Meshkinpour, H., Marks, J. W., Schoenfield, L. S., and Bonnoris, G. G. Reflux gastritis syndrome: mechanism of symptoms. Gastroenterology 79:1283, 1980.

54. Zollinger, R. M., and Hoerr, S. O. Gastric operations. Troublesome postoperative symptoms with special reference to carbohydrate ingestion. JAMA 134:574, 1947.

55. Radziuk, J., Bondy, D. C., Track, N., et al. Abnormal glucose tolerance and glucose malabsorption after vagotomy and pyloroplasty. A tracer method for measuring glucose absorption rates. Gastroenterology 83:1017, 1983.

56. Postlethwait, R. W. Five year follow-up results of operations for duodenal ulcer. Surg. Gynecol. Obstet. 137:387, 1973.

57. Howard, R. J., Murphy, W. R., and Humphrey, E. W. A prospective randomized study of elective surgical treatment for duodenal ulcer. Two to ten year follow-up study. Surgery 73:256, 1973.

58. Cox, A. G. Comparison of symptoms after vagotomy with gastrojejunostomy and partial gastrectomy. Br. Med. J. 1:288, 1968.

59. Ladas, S. D., Isaacs, P. E. T., Quereshi, Y., et al. Role of the small intestine in postvagotomy diarrhea. Gastroenterology 85:1088, 1983.

60. Bunch, G. A., and Shields, R. The effects of vagotomy on the intestinal handling of water and electrolytes. Gut 14:116, 1973.

61. Bond, J. H., and Levitt, M. D. Use of breath hydrogen (H_2) to quantitate small bowel transit time following partial gastrectomy. J. Lab. Clin. Med. 90:30, 1977.

62. Browning, G. C., Buchan, K. A., and MacKay, C. Clinical and laboratory study of postvagotomy diarrhea. Gut 15:644, 1974.

63. Allan, J. G., Gerskowitch, V. P., and Russell, R. I. The role of bile acids in the pathogenesis of postvagotomy diarrhea. Br. J. Surg. 61:516, 1974.

64. Duncombe, V. M., Bolin, T. D., and Davis, A. E. Double-blind trial of cholestyramine in post-vagotomy diarrhea. Gut 18:531, 1977.

65. Fromm, H., Tunuguntla, A. K., Malavolti, M., et al. Absence of significant role of bile acids in diarrhea of a heterogeneous group of postcholecystectomy patients. Dig. Dis. Sci. 32:33, 1987.

66. Kronborg, O., Malstrom, J., and Christiansen, P. M. A comparison between the results of truncal and selective vagotomy

in patients with duodenal ulcer. Scand. J. Gastroenterol. 5:519, 1970.

67. Kennedy, T., Connell, A. M., Love, A. H. G., et al. Selective or truncal vagotomy? Five-year results of a double-blind, randomized, controlled trial. Br. J. Surg. 60:944, 1973.

68. Sawyers, J. L., Scott, H. W., Edwards, W. H., et al. Comparative studies of the clinical effects of truncal and selective vagotomy. Am. J. Surg. 115:165, 1968.

69. Jordan, P. H. Current status of parietal cell vagotomy. Ann. Surg. 184:659, 1976.

70. Amdrup, E., Andersen, D., and Hostrup, H. The Aarhus County vagotomy trial. I. An interim report on primary results and incidence of sequelae following parietal cell vagotomy and selective vagotomy in 748 patients. World J. Surg. 2:85, 1978.

71. Wastell, C. Long-term clinical and metabolic effects of vagotomy with either gastrojejunostomy or pyloroplasty. Ann. R. Coll. Surg. Engl. 45:193, 1969.

72. Edwards, J. P., Lyndon, P. J., Smith, T. B., and Johnston, D. Fecal fat excretion after truncal, selective, and highly selective vagotomy for duodenal ulcer. Gut 15:521, 1974.

73. Enquist, I. F. Effects of vagotomy on digestion and absorption. In Williams, J. D., and Cox, A. G. (eds.). After Vagotomy. London, Butterworth, 1969, pp. 137–149.

74. Butler, T. J. The effect of gastrectomy on pancreatic secretion in man. Part II. The pattern of steatorrhea following gastrectomy. Ann. R. Coll. Surg. Engl. 29:311, 1961.

75. Wall, A. J., Ungar, B., Baird, C. W., et al. Malnutrition after partial gastrectomy. Influence of site of ulcer and type of anastomosis. Am. J. Dig. Dis. 12:1077, 1967.

76. Lawrence, W., Vanamee, P. L., Peterson, A. S., et al. Alterations in fat and nitrogen metabolism after total and subtotal gastrectomy. Surg. Gynecol. Obstet. 110:601, 1960.

77. Schwartz, M. K., Bodansky, O., and Randall, H. E. Metabolism in surgical patients. II. Fat and mineral metabolism in totally gastrectomized patients. Am. J. Clin. Nutr. 4:51, 1956.

78. Bradley, E. L., Isaacs, J., Hersh, T., et al. Nutritional consequences of total gastrectomy. Ann. Surg. 182:415, 1975.

79. Meyer, J. H., Porter-Fink, V., Crott, R., and Figueroa, W. Absorption of heme iron after truncal vagotomy with antrectomy. Abstract. Gastroenterology 92:1534, 1987.

80. Faxen, A., Rosander, R., and Kewenter, J. The effect of parietal cell vagotomy and selective vagotomy with pyloroplasty on body weight and dietary habits. Scand. J. Gastroenterol. 14:7, 1979.

81. Wheldon, E. J., Venable, C. W., and Johnson, I. D. S. Late metabolic sequelae of vagotomy and gastroenterostomy. Lancet 1:437, 1970.

82. Johnston, I. D. A. The management of side-effects of surgery for peptic ulceration. Br. J. Surg. 57:787, 1970.

83. Johnson, H. D., and Hoffbrand, A. V. The influence of extent of resection, type of anastomosis, and ulcer site on the haematological side effects of gastrectomy. Br. J. Surg. 57:33, 1970.

84. Paakonen, M., Alhava, E. M., Karajalainen, P., et al. Long-term follow-up after Billroth I and II partial gastrectomy. Acta Chir. Scand. 150:485, 1984.

85. Nishimura, O., Furumoto, T., Nosaka, K., et al. Bone disorder following partial and total gastrectomy with reference to bone mineral content. Jpn. J. Surg. 16:98, 1986.

86. Moran, T. H., and McHugh, P. R. Cholecystokinin suppresses food intake by inhibiting gastric emptying. Am. J. Physiol. 242:R491, 1982.

87. Koopmans, H. S. Satiety: signals from the gastrointestinal tract. Am. J. Clin. Nutr. 42:1044, 1985.

88. Welch, I., Saunders, K., and Read, N. W. Effect of ileal and intravenous infusions of fat emulsions on feeding and satiety in human volunteers. Gastroenterology 89:1293, 1985.

89. Doty, J. E., and Meyer, J. H. Vagotomy and antrectomy impairs absorption of fat from solid but not liquid dietary sources. Gastroenterology 94:50, 1988.

90. Lundh, G. Intestinal digestion and absorption after gastrectomy. Acta Chir. Scand. (Suppl.) 231:1, 1958.

91. Williams, N. S., Meyer, J. H., Jehn, D., et al. Canine intestinal transit and digestion of radiolabeled liver particles. Gastroenterology 86:1451, 1984.

92. Fields, M., and Duthie, H. L. Effect of vagotomy on intraluminal digestion of fat in man. Gut 6:301, 1965.

93. Tabaqchali, S. The pathophysiological role of small intestinal flora. Scand. J. Gastroenterol. 5(Suppl 6):139, 1970.

94. Baird, I. M., Blackburn, E. K., and Wilson, G. M. The pathogenesis of anemia after partial gastrectomy. Q. J. Med. 28:21, 1959.

95. Johnson, H. D., Kahn, T. A., Srivata, R., et al. The late nutritional and hematological effects of vagal section. Br. J. Surg. 56:4, 1969.

96. Tovey, F. I., and Clark, C. G. Anemia after partial gastrectomy: a neglected, curable condition. Lancet 1:956, 1980.

97. Ames, J. D., Hoffbrand, D. M., and Mollin, D. L. The hematologic complications following partial gastrectomy. Am. J. Med. 43:555, 1967.

98. Mahmud, K., Ripley, D., Swaim, W. R., and Doscherholmen, A. Hematologic complications of partial gastrectomy. Ann. Surg. 177:432, 1972.

99. Pryor, J. P., O'Shea, M. J., Brooks, P. L., and Datar, G. K. The long-term metabolic consequences of partial gastrectomy. Am. J. Med. 51:5, 1971.

100. Deller, D. H., and Witts, L. J. Changes in blood after partial gastrectomy with special reference to vitamin B_{12}. Q. J. Med. 31:71, 1952.

101. Rygvold, O. Hypovitaminosis B_{12} following partial gastrectomy by Billroth II method. Scand. J. Gastroenterol. (Suppl.) 29:57, 1974.

102. Deller, D. J., Ibboston, R. N., and Crompton, B. Metabolic effects of partial gastrectomy with special reference to calcium and folic acid. II. The contribution of folic acid deficiency to anemia. Gut 5:225, 1964.

103. Blake, J., and Rechnitzor, P. A. The hematological and nutritional effects of gastric operations. Q. J. Med. 22:419, 1953.

104. Stevens, A. R., Prizio-Biroli, G., Harkins, H. N., et al. Iron metabolism in patients after partial gastrectomy. Ann. Surg. 149:534, 1959.

105. Turnberg, L. A. The absorption of iron after partial gastrectomy. Q. J. Med. 35:107, 1966.

106. Magnasson, B. E. D. Iron absorption after antrectomy with gastroduodenostomy. Scand. J. Haematol. (Suppl.) 26:1, 1976.

107. Chaudhary, M. R., and Williams, J. Iron absorption after gastric operation. Clin. Sci. 18:527, 1959.

108. Conrad, M. E. Factors affecting iron absorption. In Halberg, L., Harworth, H. G., Vannotti, A. (eds.). Iron Deficiency. Pathogenesis, Clinical Aspects, Therapy. New York, Academic Press, 1970, pp. 87–115.

109. Conrad, M. E., Weintraub, L. R., Sears, D. A., and Crosby, W. H. Absorption of hemoglobin iron. Am. J. Physiol. 211:1123, 1966.

110. Baird, I. M., and Wilson, G. M. The pathogenesis of anemia after partial gastrectomy. Iron absorption after partial gastrectomy. Q. J. Med. 28:35, 1959.

111. Hallberg, L., Solvell, L., and Zederfeldt, B. Iron absorption after partial gastrectomy. A comparative study on the absorption from ferrous sulphate and hemoglobin. Acta Med. Scand. Suppl. 445:269, 1966.

112. Neale, G., Antcliff, A. C., Welbourn, R. B., et al. Protein malnutrition after partial gastrectomy. Q. J. Med. 36:369, 1967.

113. Doscherholmen, A., and Swaim, W. R. Impaired assimilation of egg ^{57}Co vitamin B_{12} in patients with hypochlorhydria and achlorhydria after gastric resection. Gastroenterology 64:913, 1973.

114. Streeter, A. M., Duraiappah, B., Boyle, R., et al. Malabsorption of vitamin B_{12} after vagotomy. Am. J. Surg. 128:340, 1974.

115. Clark, C. G., Crooks, J., Dawson, A. A., and Mitchell, P. E. G. Disordered calcium metabolism after Polya gastrectomy. Lancet 1:734, 1964.

116. Patterson, C. R., Pulvertaft, C. N., Wood, C. G., and Fourman, P. Search for osteomalacia in 1228 patients after gastrectomy and other operations on the stomach. Lancet 2:1085, 1965.

117. Morgan, D. B., Hunt, G., and Paterson, C. R. The osteomalacia syndrome after stomach operations. Q. J. Med. 155:395, 1970.

118. Garrick, R., Ireland, A. W., and Posen, S. Bone abnormalities after gastric surgery. A prospective histological study. Ann. Intern. Med. 75:221, 1971.

119. Eddy, R. L. Metabolic bone disease after gastrectomy. Am. J. Med. 50:442, 1971.

120. Tougaard, L., Rickers, H., Rodbro, P., et al. Bone composition and vitamin D after Polya gastrectomy. Acta Med. Scand. 202:47, 1977.

121. Alhava, E. M., Aukee, S., and Karjalainen, P. Bone mineral after partial gastrectomy. I. Scand. J. Gastroenterol. 9:463, 1974.

122. Klein, K. B., Orwoll, E. S., Lieberman, D. A., et al. Metabolic bone disease in asymptomatic men after partial gastrectomy with Billroth II anastomoses. Gastroenterology 92:608, 1987.

123. Nilsson, B. E., and Westin, N. E. The fracture incidence after gastrectomy. Acta Chir. Scand. 137:533, 1971.

124. Morgan, D. B., Pulvertaft, C. N., and Fourman, P. Effects of age on the loss of bone after ulcer surgery. Lancet 2:772, 1966.

125. Alhava, E. M., Aukee, S., and Karjalainen, P. Bone mineral after partial gastrectomy II. Scand. J. Gastroenterol. 10:165, 1975.

126. Koclan, J., Vuterinova, M., Bejblova, O., and Skala, I. Influence of lactose intolerance on the bones of patients after partial gastrectomy. Digestion 8:324, 1973.

127. Pulvertaft, C. N. Gastric resection and metabolic bone disease. Postgrad. Med. 44:618, 1968.

128. Paakonen, M., Alhava, E. M., and Karalainen, P. Bone mineral and intestinal calcium absorption after partial gastrectomy. Scand. J. Gastroenterol. 17:369, 1982.

129. Deller, D. J. Radiocalcium absorption after partial gastrectomy. Am. J. Dig. Dis. 11:10, 1966.

130. Canniga, A., Gennari, C., and Caesari, L. Intestinal absorption of ^{45}Ca and dynamics of ^{45}Ca in gastrectomy osteoporosis. Acta Med. Scand. 176:599, 1964.

131. Williams, J. A. Effects of upper gastrointestinal surgery on blood formation and bone metabolism. Br. J. Surg. 51:125, 1964.

132. Thompson, G. R. Studies in the absorption and metabolism of vitamin D after gastric surgery. Postgrad. Med. J. 44:626, 1958.

133. Gertner, J. M., Lilburn, M., and Domenech, M. 25-Hydroxy-cholecalciferol absorption in steatorrhea and postgastrectomy osteomalacia. Br. Med. J. 1:1310, 1977.

134. Lilienfeld-Toal, H., Mackes, K. G., Kodrat, G., et al. Plasma 25-hydroxyvitamin D and urinary cyclic AMP in German patients with subtotal gastrectomy (Billroth II). Am. J. Dig. Dis. 22:633, 1977.

135. Norman, A. W., and Miller, B. E. Vitamin D. In Maachlin, L. J. (ed.) Handbook of Vitamins. Nutritional, Biochemical and Clinical Aspects. New York, Marcel Dekker, 1984, pp. 45–98.

136. Imawari, M., Kozawa, K., Akanuma, Y., et al. Serum 25-hydroxyvitamin D and vitamin D binding protein levels and mineral metabolism after partial and total gastrectomy. Gastroenterology 79:255, 1980.

137. Roos, D. Neurological complications in an unselected group of patients partially gastrectomized for gastric ulcer. Acta Neurol. Scand. 50:753, 1974.

138. Koch, M. J., Hoffman, P., Brody, J. A., and Edgar, A. H. Neurologic disorders following surgery for peptic ulcer disease. Arch. Neurol. 32:206, 1975.

139. Ammjjad, H., Kumar, C. K., and McLaughey, R. Postgastrectomy bezoars. Am. J. Gastroenterol. 66:327, 1976.

140. Ellis, J., Kingston, R. D., Brookes, V. S., and Waterhouse, J. A. H. Gastric carcinoma and previous peptic ulceration. Br. J. Surg. 66:117, 1979.

141. Morgenstern, L., Yamakawa, T., and Seltzer, D. Carcinoma of the gastric stump. Am. J. Surg. 125:29, 1973.

142. Pickford, I. R., Craven, J. L., Hall, R., et al. Endoscopic examination of the gastric remnant 31–39 years after subtotal gastrectomy for peptic ulcer. Gut 25:393, 1984.

143. Schuman, B. M., Walbaum, J. R., and Hiltz, S. W. Carcinoma of the gastric remnant in a U.S. population. Gastrointest. Endosc. 30:71, 1984.

144. Loscos, J. M., Gutierrez del Olmo, A., Nisa, E., et al. Cancer of the gastric stump. Gastrointest. Endosc. 32:75, 1986.

145. Caygill, C. P. J., Hill, M. J., Kirkham, J. S., and Northfield, T. C. Mortality from gastric cancer following gastric surgery for peptic ulcer. Lancet 1:930, 1986.

146. Schafer, L. W., Larson, D. E., Melton, J., et al. The risk of gastric carcinoma after surgical treatment for benign ulcer disease. A population-based study in Olmsted County, Minnesota. N. Engl. J. Med. 309:1210, 1983.

147. Fischer, A. B., Graem, N., and Jensen, O. M. Risk of gastric cancer after Billroth II resection for duodenal ulcer. Br. J. Surg. 70:552, 1983.

148. Schuman, B. M. Endoscopic surveillance for cancer of the gastric stump. Gastrointest. Endosc. 32:117, 1986.

149. Mortensen, N. J. M., Savage, A. Endoscopic screening for premalignant changes 25 years after gastrectomy: results of a five-year prospective study. Br. J. Surg. 71:363, 1984.

150. Sonnenberg, A. Endoscopic screening for gastric stump cancer—would it be beneficial? Gastroenterology 87:489, 1984.

151. Domellof, L., Erickson, S., and Janunger, K. G. Carcinoma and possible precancerous changes of the gastric stump after Billroth II resection. Gastroenterology 73:462, 1977.

152. Ross, A. H. M., Smith, M. A., Anderson, J. R., and Small, W. P. Late mortality after surgery for peptic ulcer. N. Engl. J. Med. 307:519, 1982.

153. Jordan, P. H., Condon, R. E. A prospective evaluation of vagotomy-pyloroplasty and vagotomy-antrectomy for treatment of duodenal ulcer. Ann. Surg. 172:547, 1970.

154. Chaimoff, C., Dintsman, M., and Tiqua, P. The long-term fate of patients with the dumping syndrome. Arch. Surg. 105:554, 1972.

155. Eldh, J., Kewenter, J., Koch, N. G., and Olson, P. Long-term results of surgical treatment for dumping after partial gastrectomy. Br. J. Surg. 61:90, 1974.

156. Visick, A. H. A study of failures after gastrectomy. Ann. R. Coll. Surg. Engl. 3:266, 1948.

157. DeDombol, F. T., Horrocks, J. C., and Clamps, S. E. Observer variation in the assessment of results of surgery for peptic ulcer. (Abstract.) Gut 15:824, 1974.

158. Small, W. P., Cay, E. L., Dugard, P., et al. Peptic ulcer surgery: selection for operation by "earning." Gut 10:996, 1969.

159. Thoroughman, J. C., Pascal, G. R., Jenkins, W., et al. Psychological factors predictive of surgical success in patients with intractable ulcer disease. Psychosom. Med. 26:618, 1964.

160. McColl, I., Drinkwater, J. E., Hulme-Moir, I., and Donnan, S. P. B. Prediction of success and failure of gastric surgery. Br. J. Surg. 58:768, 1971.

161. Hulme-Moir, I. Psychological, social, and surgical factors which influence success of failure after gastric operations. Scand. J. Gastroenterol. 14:457, 1979.

162. Stevenson, D. K., Nabseth, D. C., Masuda, M., and Holmes, T. H. Life change and the postoperative course of duodenal ulcer patients. J. Human Stress 5:19, 1979.

163. Johnstone, F. R., Holbitsky, I. B., and Debas, J. T. Postgastrectomy problems in patients with personality defects. The "albatross" syndrome. Can. Med. Assoc. J. 96:1559, 1967.

164. Amdrup, E. Variations in food tolerance after partial gastrectomy. The relationship between pathological findings at operation and type and intensity of postgastrectomy symptoms. Acta Chir. Scand. 120:410, 1960.

165. Fischer, A. B., Knop, J., and Graem, N. Late mortality following Billroth II resection for duodenal ulcer. Acta Chir. Scand. 151:43, 1985.

166. Stabile, B. E., and Passaro, E. Recurrent peptic ulcer. Gastroenterology 70:124, 1976.

167. Reber, H. A., and Way, L. W. Surgical treatment of late postgastrectomy syndromes. Am. J. Surg. 129:71, 1975.

168. Brooke-Cowden, G. L., Braasch, J. W., Gibb, S. O., et al. Postgastrectomy syndromes. Am. J. Surg. 131:464, 1976.

169. Halpern, N. B., Hirshowitz, B. L., and Moody, F. G. Failure to achieve success with remedial gastric surgery. Am. J. Surg. 125:108, 1973.

170. Meshkinpour, H., Elashoff, J., Stewart, H., and Sturdevant, R. A. L. Effect of cholestyramine on the symptoms of reflux gastritis. Gastroenterology 73:441, 1977.

171. Malagelada, J. R., Phillips, S. F., and Higgins, J. A. A

prospective evaluation of alkaline reflux gastritis. Bile acid binding agents and Roux-en-Y diversion. Gastroenterology *76*:1192, 1979.

172. Ritchie, W. P. Alkaline reflux gastritis: a critical reappraisal. Gut *25*:975, 1984.

173. Ritchie, W. P. Alkaline reflux gastritis. An objective assessment of its diagnosis and treatment. Ann. Surg. *192*:288, 1982.

174. Mosimann, F., Sorgi, M., Wolverson, R. L., et al. Bile reflux after duodenal ulcer surgery. A study of 114 asymptomatic and symptomatic patients. Scand. J. Gastroenterol. *19*(Suppl. 92):224, 1984.

175. Warshaw, A. L. Intragastric alkali infusion. Simple, accurate provocative test for diagnosis of symptomatic alkaline reflux gastritis. Ann. Surg. *194*:297, 1983.

176. Perkel, M. S., Moore, C., Hersh, T., and Davidson, E. D. Metoclopramide therapy in patients with delayed gastric emptying. A randomized, double-blind study. Dig. Dis. Sci. *24*:662, 1979.

177. Sheiner, H. J., and Catchpole, B. N. Drug therapy for postvagotomy stasis. Br. J. Surg. *63*:608, 1976.

178. French, J. M., and Crain, C. W. Undernutrition, malnutrition, and malabsorption after gastrectomy. *In* Stammers, F. A. R., and Williams, J. A. (eds.). Partial Gastrectomy. Complications and Metabolic Consequences. London, Butterworth, 1963, pp. 227–262.

179. Saltzman, M., Meyer, C., Callachan, C., and McCallum, R. W. Effect of metoclopramide on chronic gastric stasis in diabetic and postgastrectomy surgery patients. (Abstract.) Gastroenterology *80*:1268, 1981.

180. Allan, J. G., and Russell, R. I. Cholestyramine in treatment of postvagotomy diarrhea—double-blind controlled trial. Br. Med. J. *1*:674, 1977.

181. Leeds, A. R., Ebeid, F., Ralphs, D. N. L., et al. Pectin in the dumping syndrome. Lancet *1*:1075, 1981.

182. Polack, M., and Pontes, J. F. The cause of postvagotomy diarrhea. Gastroenterology *30*:489, 1956.

183. Jordan, G. L. Surgical management of postgastrectomy problems. Arch. Surg. *102*:251, 1971.

184. Herrington, J. L., Sawyers, J. L., and Whitehead, W. A. Surgical management of reflux gastritis. Ann. Surg. *180*:526, 1974.

185. Boren, C. H., and Way, L. W. Alkaline reflux gastritis: a reevaluation. Am. J. Surg. *140*:40, 1980.

186. Malagelada, J. R., Phillips, S. F., Shorter, R. G., et al. Postoperative reflux gastritis: pathophysiology and long-term outcome after Roux-en-Y diversion. Ann. Intern. Med. *103*:178, 1985.

187. Mathias, J. R., Fernandez, A., Sninsky, C. A., et al. Nausea, vomiting, and abdominal pain after Roux-en-Y anastomosis: motility of the jejunal limb. Gastroenterology *88*:101, 1985.

188. Vogel, S. B., Vair, D. B., and Woodward, E. R. Alterations in gastrointestinal emptying of ^{99m}technetium-labeled solids following sequential antrectomy, truncal vagotomy, and Roux-en-Y gastroenterostomy. Ann. Surg. *198*:506, 1983.

189. Ehrlein, H. J., Thoma, G., Kernke O., et al. Effects of nutrients on gastrointestinal motility and gastric emptying after distal gastrectomy with Roux-Y gastrojejunostomy in dogs. Dig Dis Sci *32*:538, 1987.

190. Williams, N. S., Miller, J., Elashoff, J., and Meyer, J. H. Canine resistances to gastric emptying of liquids after ulcer surgery. Dig. Dis. Sci. *31*:273, 1986.

191. Pellegrini, C. A., Patti, M. G., Lewis, M., and Way, L. W. Alkaline reflux gastritis and the effect of biliary diversion on gastric emptying of solid food. Am. J. Surg. *150*:166, 1985.

192. Keefer, E. D. Life with subtotal gastrectomy. A follow-up study ten or more years after operation. Gastroenterology *37*:434, 1959.

193. Harvey, H. D. Twenty-four years of experience with elective gastric resection for duodenal ulcer. Surg. Gynecol. Obstet. *112*:203, 1961.

194. Feggetter, G. Y., and Pringle, R. The long-term results of bilateral vagotomy and gastrojejunostomy for chronic duodenal ulcer. Surg. Gynecol. Obstet. *116*:175, 1963.

195. Duthie, H. L., Moore, K. R. H., Bardsley, M. D., and Clark, R. G. Surgical treatment of gastric ulcers. Controlled comparison of Billroth I gastrectomy and vagotomy and pyloroplasty. Br. J. Surg. *57*:784, 1970.

196. Johnston, I. D., Welbourn, R., and Acheson, K. Gastrectomy and loss of weight. Lancet *1*:1242, 1958.

197. Hillman, H. S. Postgastrectomy malnutrition. Gut *9*:576, 1968.

198. Wirts, C. W., Templeton, J. V., Fineberg, C., and Goldstein, F. The correction of postgastrectomy malabsorption following a jejunal interposition operation. Gastroenterology *49*:141, 1965.

Note: Page numbers in *italics* refer to illustrations;
Roman numerals refer to illustrations in color section;
page numbers followed by (t) refer to tables.